Antibiotic and Chemotherapy

Anti-infective agents and their use in therapy

Commissioning Editor: **Jill Day**
Project Development Manager: **Tim Kimber**
Project Manager: **Alan Nicholson**
Design Manager: **Jayne Jones**
Illustration Manager: **Mick Ruddy**

EIGHTH EDITION

Antibiotic and Chemotherapy

Anti-infective agents and their use in therapy

Edited by

Roger G. Finch
MB BS FRCP FRCPath FRCPEd FFPM
Professor of Infectious Diseases, Division of Microbiology and Infectious Diseases,
Clinical Laboratory Sciences, The City Hospital, Nottingham, UK

David Greenwood
BSc PhD DSc FRCPath
Emeritus Professor of Antimicrobial Science, Division of Microbiology and
Infectious Diseases, Department of Clinical Laboratory Sciences, University
Hospital, Queen's Medical Centre, Nottingham, UK

S. Ragnar Norrby
MD PhD FRCP (Edin)
Professor and Director General
The Swedish Institute for Infectious Disease Control, Solna, Sweden

Richard J. Whitley
MD
Loeb Scholar in Pediatrics
Professor of Pediatrics, Microbiology, Medicine and Neurosurgery
Department of Pediatrics,
The University of Alabama at Birmingham,
Birmingham, Alabama, USA

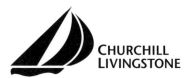

CHURCHILL LIVINGSTONE

Edinburgh London New York Philadelphia St Louis Sydney Toronto 2003

CHURCHILL LIVINGSTONE
An imprint of Elsevier Science Limited

First edition 1963
Second edition 1968
Third edition 1971
Fourth edition 1973
Fifth edition 1981
Sixth edition 1992
Seventh edition 1997
Eighth edition 2003

ISBN 0443071292

British Library Cataloguing in Publication Data
A catalogue record for this book is available from the British Library

Library of Congress Cataloging in Publication Data
A catalog record for this book is available from the Library of Congress

Notice
Medical knowledge is constantly changing. Standard safety precautions must be followed,
but as new research and clinical experience broaden our knowledge, changes in treatment
and drug therapy may become necessary or appropriate. Readers are advised to check the
most current product information provided by the manufacturer of each drug to be
administered to verify the recommended dose, the method and duration of administration,
and contraindications. It is the responsibility of the practitioner, relying on experience and
knowledge of the patient, to determine dosages and the best treatment for each individual
patient. Neither the Publisher nor the editors assumes any liability for any injury and/or
damage to persons or property arising from this publication.
The Publisher

Typeset by Phoenix Photosetting, Chatham, Kent
Printed in UK by MPG Books Ltd

The
Publisher's
policy is to use
**paper manufactured
from sustainable forests**

Preface

When the first edition of this book appeared in 1963, around 50 antibacterial agents, including 19 sulphonamides, and a handful of antifungal compounds were discussed. The demand for such a text was amply demonstrated by its popularity, and it rapidly became an indispensable guide to the properties and use of these drugs. Presently, there are over 250 different antibacterial agents available for the treatment of systemic infection on the world market. Add in the smaller, but increasingly substantial numbers of antiviral, antifungal, antiprotozoal and anthelmintic agents — to say nothing of the diverse formulations and names under which all these drugs are traded — and the formidable problems now facing prescribers become clear. The need for a comprehensive, globally relevant account of the agents available for the treatment of human infection, as well as the principles and practice of their use, is greater now than ever.

Much is at stake: multi-drug resistant organisms, notably (but certainly not exclusively) in high-dependency areas of modern high-technology hospitals cause frequent problems. In many countries, resistance severely constrains therapeutic choice in common infections like malaria, tuberculosis and typhoid fever. Such developments threaten to undermine much of the progress that was achieved in the treatment of infectious diseases during the second half of the 20th century. There is a general consensus that reversing this trend requires concerted action on several different fronts, but it is the selective pressure of the use of antimicrobial drugs that drives resistance. Encouragement of rational use in man and animals is plainly essential to the success of any strategy.

The aim of this book is to provide a reliable reference source to the properties of antimicrobial agents of all kinds and an authoritative 'user's guide' to antimicrobial chemotherapy relevant to clinical practice throughout the world. To achieve this end, we have been fortunate to be able to call on a distinguished panel of international experts, each bringing a wealth of experience to their topic. The book is again divided into three parts: Section 1 deals with general aspects of antimicrobial chemotherapy; Section 2 provides a systematic account of the properties of the various families of compounds and individual agents within those families; Section 3 surveys the specific clinical settings in which the drugs are used and explains their rational use. Several new chapters have been commissioned and many others have been completely rewritten; all have been fully revised. In order to make the book truly international, recommended International Non-proprietary Names (rINN) are used throughout. Readers' attention is also drawn to other conventions described in the Introduction to Section 2 (p. 154), many of which are applicable to the whole text.

Sincere thanks are due to our authors, who have patiently accepted our editorial demands and, sometimes, our extensive amendments to their contributions. We also gratefully acknowledge the expert assistance of Ian Hutchison in compiling the information in the *Preparations and Dosage* boxes in Section 2. The editorial team at Elsevier Science have seen the book through to production with their customary efficiency. Finally, we thank those who have contributed to previous editions of this book and may still find echoes of their labours in the text. In particular, we are most grateful to the former Editors, Francis O'Grady and Harold Lambert, who have done so much to encourage sensible use of antimicrobial agents throughout their long careers and who now leave the book after many years. We trust that this new edition will live up to the high standards that they have set.

Roger Finch, David Greenwood, Ragnar Norrby, Richard Whitley
Nottingham, UK; Solna, Sweden; Birmingham, USA
June 2002

Contributors

Vincent Andriole MD
Professor of Medicine
Department of Internal Medicine
Yale University School of Medicine
New Haven
Connecticut
USA

Anneli Bjöersdorff DVM, PhD
Consultant in Medical Microbiology
Department of Clinical Microbiology
Research Center for Zoonotic Ecology and
Epidemiology
Kalmar
Sweden

David Boehr BSc
Health Sciences Centre
Hamilton
Ontario
Canada

Anthony Bron BSc FRCS FRCOphth
Professor of Ophthalmology and Head of Department
Nuffield Laboratory of Ophthalmology
University of Oxford
Oxford
UK

André Bryskier MD
Director, Head of Clinical Pharmacology of
Anti-infectives
Infectious Disease Group
Aventis Pharma
Romainville
France

Karen Bush PhD
Senior Research Fellow
Drug Discovery
Johnson & Johnson Pharmaceutical Research and
Development
Raritan
New Jersey
USA

Jean-Paul Butzler MD PhD
Service de Microbiologie
Université Libre de Bruxelles
CHU Saint-Pierre
Brussels
Belgium

Claude J Carbon MD
Professor of Internal Medicine
Hôpital Bichat
Paris
France

Daniel Carrasco MD
Mount Sinai School of Medicine
Department of Dermatology
New York
New York
USA

Mark Casewell BSc MD FRCPath FRCP
Emeritus Professor of Medical Microbiology
King's College School of Medicine and Dentistry
London
UK

Kevin A. Cassady MD
Assistant Professor of Pediatrics
Division of Infectious Diseases
Department of Pediatrics
University of Alabama at Birmingham
Children's Harbor Research Center
Birmingham
Alabama
USA

Peter L Chiodini BSc MB BS PhD FRCP
Consultant Parasitologist
Department of Clinical Parasitology
The Hospital for Tropical Diseases
London
UK

Ian Chopra BA MA PhD DSc
Professor of Microbiology
Division of Microbiology, School of Biochemistry
and Molecular Biology
University of Leeds
Leeds
UK

George A. Conder PhD
Director, Clinical Development
Animal Health Group
Pfizer Inc
Groton
Connecticut
USA

David A. Cooper MD DSc
Professor of Medicine
National Centre in HIV Epidemiology and Clinicial Research
University of New South Wales
Darlinghurst
Sydney
NSW
Australia

Christopher J. Crnich MD
Infectious Disease Fellow
Section of Infectious Diseases, Department of Medicine
University of Wisconsin Hospital and Clinics
Madison
WI
USA

Simon L. Croft PhD
Reader in Parasitology
Dept. of Infectious and Tropical Diseases
London School of Hygiene and Tropical Medicine
London
UK

Peter Davey MD FRCP
Professor in Pharmacoeconomics
MEMO
Department of Clinical Pharmacology
Ninewells Hospital
Dundee
UK

Robert Davidson MD FRCP DTM&H
Consultant in Infectious Diseases
Department of Infection and Tropical Medicine
Northwick Park Hospital
Harrow
Middlesex
UK

David W. Denning MB BS FRCP FRCPath DCH
Senior Lecturer and Honorary Consultant in Medicine and Medical Mycology
ATR4, Education and Research Centre
Wythenshawe Hospital
Manchester
UK

Kari-ann Draker HBSc
Health Sciences Centre
Hamilton
Ontario
Canada

George Drusano MD
Professor of Medicine and Clinical Pharmacology
Department of Infectious Diseases
Albany Medical School
Albany
USA

David T. Durack MB DPhil
Medical Director Worldwide
Microbiology & Infectious Diseases
Becton Dickinson Technologies
Durham
NC
USA

David I. Edwards PhD FRCPath
Emeritus Professor
School of Bioscience
University of East London
London UK
and Senior Scientific Adviser (Academic)
Department of Health
Essex
UK

Sean Emery BSc (Hons) PhD
Head, Therapeutic Research Unit
National Centre in HIV Epidemiology and Clinical Research
Sydney
NSW
Australia

Robert Fass MD
Samuel Saslaw Professor of Infectious Diseases
Professor of Internal Medicine and Microbiology and Immunology, Director Division of Infectious Diseases
The Ohio State University College of Medicine
Columbus
Ohio
USA

Roger Finch MB BS FRCP FRCPath FRCPEd FFPM
Professor of Infectious Diseases
Department of Microbiology and Infectious Diseases
Nottingham City Hospital
Nottingham
UK

Arne Forsgren MD PhD
Professor
Department of Medical Microbiology
Malmö University Hospital
Malmö
Sweden

John M. Grange MSc MD
Visiting Professor
Centre for Infectious Diseases and International Health
Royal Free and University College Medical School
Windeyer Institute for Medical Science
London
UK

David Greenwood BSc PhD DSc FRCPath
Emeritus Professor of Antimicrobial Science
Division of Microbiology and Infectious Diseases, Department of Clinical Laboratory Sciences University Hospital
Queen's Medical Centre Nottingham
UK

Jeremy M. T. Hamilton-Miller MA PhD DSc FRCPath
Professor of Medical Microbiology
Dept of Medical Microbiology
Royal Free Hospital and University College Medical school
Royal Free Campus
London
UK

Phillip Hay MB BS FRCP
Senior Lecturer in Genitourinary Medicine
Courtyard Clinic
St George's Hospital
London
UK

Ian S Hutchison BPharm MRPharmS
Practice Pharmacist
Sheffield West Primary Care Trust
Sheffield
UK

Victoria Johnston MA MB MRCP
Research Registrar
Sexually Transmitted Infections Research Center
Westmead Hospital
Westmead
Australia

Gunnar Kahlmeter MD PhD
Associate Professor
Clinical Microbiology
Department of Clinical Microbiology
Central Hospital
Växjö
Sweden

Christopher Kibbler MA FRCP FRCPath
Consultant in Medical Microbiology
Royal Free Hospital
London
UK

Giancarlo Lancini PhD
Professor of Pharmacy
Biosearch Italia S.p.A.
Gerenzano (Varese)
Italy

Diana N J Lockwood BSc MD FRCP
Consultant Physician and Leprologist
Hospital for Tropical Diseases
London
UK

Donald Low MD FRCP
Microbiologist-in-chief
Dept of Microbiology
Mount Sinai Hospital
Toronto
Ontario
Canada

Alasdair MacGowan BMedBiol MD FRCP(Ed)
FRCPath
Professor of Clinical Microbiology and
Antimicrobial Therapeutics
Department of Medical Microbiology
North Bristol NHS Trust
Southmead Hospital
Bristol
UK

Janice Main FRCP (Edin and Lond)
Senior Lecturer in Infectious Diseases and
Medicine
Imperial College School of Medicine
St Mary's Hospital (QEQM Wing)
London
UK

Dennis Maki MD
Professor
Department of Infectious Diseases / Medicine
University of Wisconsin Hospital/Clinics
Madison
WI
USA

Lionel Mandell MD FRCPC
Professor of Medicine and Chief
Division of Infectious Diseases
McMaster University
Henderson General Hospital
Hamilton
Ontario
Canada

Sharon Marlowe MB ChB MRCP DTM&H
Clinical Research Fellow
Clinical Research Unit, Infectious and Tropical
Diseases Department
London School of Hygiene & Tropical Medicine
London
UK

Adrian Mindel MD FRCP FRACP
Director
Sexually Transmitted Infections Research Center
Westmead Hospital
Westmead
NSW
Australia

Peter Moss MD MRCP DTMH
Consultant in Infectious Diseases
Castle Hill Hospital
Cottingham
Yorkshire
UK

Dilip Nathwani MB FRCP(Ed & Glas) DTM & H
Consultant Physician
Infection Ward
Ninewells Hospital and Medical School
Dundee
UK

Una Ni Riain
Southmead Hospital
Bristol
UK

Ragnar Norrby MD PhD FRCP (Edin)
Professor and Director General
The Swedish Institute for Infectious Disease
Control
Solna
Sweden

Anna Norrby-Teglund PhD
Associate Professor
Center for Infectious Medicine
Karolinska Institutet
Stockholm
Sweden

Tim O'Dempsey DTM&H DTCH FRCP
Senior Lecturer in Clinical Tropical Medicine
Liverpool School of Tropical Medicine
Liverpool
UK

L. Peter Ormerod BSc MB ChB (Hons) MD DSc
(Med) FRCP
Professor of Medicine
Chest Clinic
Blackburn Royal Infirmary
Blackburn
Lancs
UK

Francesco Parenti PhD
Chief Scientific Officer
Biosearch Italia S.p.A.
Lainate
Italy

Jean-Claude Pechère MD
Professor of Genetics and Microbiology
Centre Médical Universitaire (CMU)
Université de Genève
Geneva
Switzerland

Rudi Pittrof MRCOG
Specialist Registrar
St Georges Hospital
London
UK

Ron Polk PharmD
Professor, Medical College of Virginia
Virginia Commonwealth University
Richmond
VA
USA

Anton L. Pozniak MD FRCP
Consultant Physician
Department of HIV and Genito-urinary Medicine
Chelsea and Westminster Hospital
London
UK

Steven J. Projan PhD
Director, Antibacterial Research
Wyeth Research
Pearl River
New York
USA

Roula B. Qaqish PharmD
Assistant Professor of Pharmacy
St. Louis College of Pharmacy
St. Louis
MO
USA

Beth Rasmussen PhD
Director, Pre-Development Project
Management
Wyeth Research
Pearl River
New York
USA

Kristian Riesbeck MD PhD
Associate Professor
Department of Medical Microbiology
Malmö University Hospital
Malmö
Sweden

Ethan Rubinstein MD LLB
Professor of Medicine
Infectious Diseases Unit
Chaim Sheba Medical Centre
Tel-Hashomer
Israel

John Ryan PhD MD
Senior Vice President, Clinical R&D
Infectious Diseases
Wyeth-Ayerst Research
Pearl River
NY
USA

Nasia Safdar MD
Fellow, Section of Infectious Diseases,
Department of Medicine
University of Wisconsin Hospital and Clinics
Madison
WI
USA

Helmut Schuster MRCP MSc DipRCPath
Specialist Registrar in Microbiology
Department of Clinical Microbiology
University College London Hospital
London
UK

David Seal MD FRCPath FRCOphth MIBiol DipBact
Visiting Professor
Applied Vision Research Centre
City University
London
UK

David Shlaes MD PhD
Executive Vice President of Research and
Development
Idenix Pharmaceuticals, Inc.
Cambridge
MA
USA

Stephen Streat FRACP
Specialist Intensivist
Department of Critical Care Medicine
Auckland Hospital
Auckland
New Zealand

Marc J Struelens MD PhD
Professor of Medical Microbiology
Laboratory of Microbiology
Erasme University Hospital
Bruxelles
Belgium

Eric Taylor MBBS FRCS
Consultant Surgeon
Vale of Leven District General Hospital
Alexandria
Dunbartonshire
UK

Rudolf Then PhD
Consultant Anti-infectives
Morphochem AG
Basel
Switzerland

Howard C. Thomas BSc PhD FRCP FRCPath
FMedSci
Professor of Medicine and Dean (Clinical)
Faculty of Medicine
Imperial College London
Department of Medicine
St Mary's Hospital
London
UK

Mark Thomas MB ChB MD DipObst FRACP
Associate Professor in Infectious Diseases
Division of Molecular Medicine, Faculty of
Medical
and Health Sciences
University of Auckland
Auckland
New Zealand

Professor Stephen K. Tyring MD PhD
Professor of Dermatology,
Microbiology/Immunology and Internal
Medicine
University of Texas Medical Branch
Houston
Texas
USA

David W Warnock MD PhD FRCPath
Chief Mycotic Diseases Branch
National Center for Infectious Diseases
Centers for Disease Control and Prevention
Atlanta
Georgia
USA

Nicholas White OBE DSc MD FRCP FMedSci
Professor of Tropical Medicine, Mahidol
University
and Oxford University
Faculty of Tropical Medicine
Mahidol University
Bangkok
Thailand

Richard J. Whitley MD
Professor of Pediatrics, Microbiology and
Medicine
Department of Microbiology and Medicine
The University of Alabama at Birmingham
Birmingham
AL
USA

Mark Wilcox MD MRCPath
Reader, Consultant in Medical Microbiology
Department of Microbiology
Old Medical School
Leeds General Infirmary
Leeds
UK

David Wininger MD
Associate Professor
Department of Clinical Internal Medicine
Ohio State University
Columbus
OH
USA

Gerard Wright PhD
Associate Professor
Department of Biochemistry
McMaster University
Hamilton
Ontario
Canada

Hisham Ziglam MB Bch MSc DIC MRCP
Specialist Registrar in Infectious Diseases
Department of Infectious Diseases
Nottingham City Hospital
Nottingham
UK

Contents

General aspects

1

Historical introduction

D. Greenwood

The first part of this chapter was written by Professor Lawrence Paul Garrod (1895–1979) co-author of the first five editions of *Antibiotic and Chemotherapy*. Garrod, after serving as a surgeon probationer in the Navy during the 1914–18 war, then qualified and practised clinical medicine before specializing in bacteriology, later achieving world recognition as the foremost authority on antimicrobial chemotherapy. He witnessed, and studied profoundly, the whole development of modern chemotherapy. A selection of over 300 leading articles written by him (but published anonymously) for the *British Medical Journal* between 1933 and 1979, was reprinted in a supplement to the *Journal of Antimicrobial Chemotherapy* in 1985*. These articles themselves provide a remarkable insight into the history of antimicrobial chemotherapy as it happened.

Garrod's original historical introduction was written in 1968 for the second edition of *Antibiotic and Chemotherapy* and updated for the fifth edition just before his death in 1979. It is reproduced here as a tribute to his memory. The development of antimicrobial chemotherapy is summarized so well, and with such characteristic lucidity, that to add anything seems superfluous, but a brief summary of events that have occurred since about 1975 has been added to complete the historical perspective.

THE EVOLUTION OF ANTIMICROBIC DRUGS

No one recently qualified even with the liveliest imagination, can picture the ravages of bacterial infection which continued until rather less than 40 years ago. To take only two examples, lobar pneumonia was a common cause of death even in young and vigorous patients, and puerperal septicaemia and other forms of acute streptococcal sepsis had a high mortality, little affected by any treatment then available. One purpose of this introduction is therefore to place the subject of this book in historical perspective.

This subject is chemotherapy, which may be defined as the administration of a substance with a systemic antimicrobic action. Some would confine the term to synthetic drugs, and the distinction is recognized in the title of this book, but since some all-embracing term is needed, this one might with advantage be understood also to include substances of natural origin. Several antibiotics can now be synthesized, and it would be ludicrous if their use should qualify for description as chemotherapy only because they happened to be prepared in this way. The essence of the term is that the effect must be systemic, the substance being absorbed, whether from the alimentary tract or a site of injection, and reaching the infected area by way of the blood stream. 'Local chemotherapy' is in this sense a contradiction in terms: any application to a surface, even of something capable of exerting a systemic effect, is better described as antisepsis.

THE THREE ERAS OF CHEMOTHERAPY

There are three distinct periods in the history of this subject. In the first, which is of great antiquity, the only substances capable of curing an infection by systemic action were natural plant products. The second was the era of synthesis, and in the third we return to natural plant products, although from plants of a much lower order, the moulds and bacteria forming antibiotics.

1. Alkaloids. This era may be dated from 1619, since it is from this year that the first record is derived of the successful treatment of malaria with an extract of cinchona bark, the patient being the wife of the Spanish governor of Peru.† Another South American discovery was the efficacy of ipecacuanha root in amoebic dysentery. Until the early years of this century these extracts, and in more recent times the alkaloids, quinine and emetine, derived from them, provided the only curative chemotherapy known.

---

* Waterworth PM (ed.) L.P. Garrod on antibiotics. *Journal of Antimicrobial Chemotherapy* 1985; 15 (Suppl. B)

† Garrod was mistaken in perpetuating this legend, which is now discounted by medical historians.

2. Synthetic compounds. Therapeutic progress in this field, which initially and for many years after was due almost entirely to research in Germany, dates from the discovery of salvarsan by Ehrlich in 1909. His successors produced germanin for trypanosomiasis and other drugs effective in protozoal infections. A common view at that time was that protozoa were susceptible to chemotherapeutic attack, but that bacteria were not: the treponemata, which had been shown to be susceptible to organic arsenicals, are no ordinary bacteria, and were regarded as a class apart.

The belief that bacteria are by nature insusceptible to any drug which is not also prohibitively toxic to the human body was finally destroyed by the discovery of Prontosil. This, the forerunner of the sulphonamides, was again a product of German research, and its discovery was publicly announced in 1935. All the work with which this book is concerned is subsequent to this year: it saw the beginning of the effective treatment of bacterial infections.

Progress in the synthesis of antimicrobic drugs has continued to the present day. Apart from many new sulphonamides, perhaps the most notable additions have been the synthetic compounds used in the treatment of tuberculosis.

3. Antibiotics. The therapeutic revolution produced by the sulphonamides, which included the conquest of haemolytic streptococcal and pneumococcal infections and of gonorrhoea and cerebrospinal fever, was still in progress and even causing some bewilderment when the first report appeared of a study which was to have even wider consequences. This was not the discovery of penicillin – that had been made by Fleming in 1929 – but the demonstration by Florey and his colleagues that it was a chemotherapeutic agent of unexampled potency. The first announcement of this, made in 1940, was the beginning of the antibiotic era, and the unimagined developments from it are still in progress. We little knew at the time that penicillin, besides providing a remedy for infections insusceptible to sulphonamide treatment, was also a necessary second line of defence against those fully susceptible to it. During the early 1940s, resistance to sulphonamides appeared successively in gonococci, haemolytic streptococci and pneumococci: nearly 20 years later it has appeared also in meningococci. But for the advent of the antibiotics, all the benefits stemming from Domagk's discovery might by now have been lost, and bacterial infections have regained their pre-1935 prevalence and mortality.

The earlier history of two of these discoveries calls for further description.

Sulphonamides

Prontosil, or sulphonamido-chrysoidin, was first synthesized by Klarer and Mietzsch in 1932, and was one of a series of azo dyes examined by Domagk for possible effects on haemolytic streptococcal infection. When a curative effect in mice had been demonstrated, cautious trials in erysipelas and other human infections were undertaken, and not until the evidence afforded by these was conclusive did the discoverers make their announcement. Domagk (1935) published the original claims, and the same information was communicated by Hörlein (1935) to a notable meeting in London.*

These claims, which initially concerned only the treatment of haemolytic streptococcal infections, were soon confirmed in other countries, and one of the most notable early studies was that of Colebrook and Kenny (1936) in England, who demonstrated the efficacy of the drug in puerperal fever. This infection had until then been taking a steady toll of about 1000 young lives per annum in England and Wales, despite every effort to prevent it by hygiene measures and futile efforts to overcome it by serotherapy. The immediate effect of the adoption of this treatment can be seen in Figure 1.1: a steep fall in mortality began in 1935, and continued as the treatment became universal and better understood, and as more potent sulphonamides were introduced, until the present-day low level had almost been reached *before penicillin became generally available.* The effect of penicillin between 1945 and 1950 is perhaps more evident on incidence: its widespread use tends completely to banish haemolytic streptococci from the environment. The apparent rise in incidence after 1950 is due to the redefinition of puerperal pyrexia as any rise of temperature to 38°C, whereas previously the term was only applied when the temperature was maintained for 24 h or recurred. Needless to say, fever so defined is frequently not of uterine origin.

---

* A meeting at which Garrod was present.

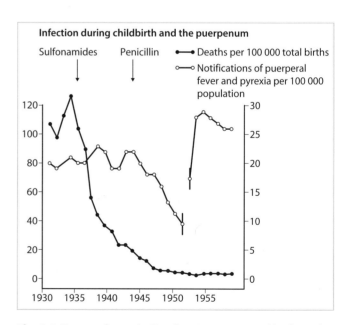

Fig. 1.1 Puerperal pyrexia. Deaths per 100 000 total births and incidence per 100 000 population in England and Wales, 1930–1957. N.B. The apparent rise in incidence in 1950 is due to the fact that the definition of puerperal pyrexia was changed in this year (*see text*). (Reproduced with permission from Barber 1960 Journal of Obstetrics and Gynaecology 67:727 by kind permission of the editor).

Prontosil had no antibacterial action in vitro, and it was soon suggested by workers in Paris (Tréfouel et al 1935) that it owed its activity to the liberation from it in the body of *p*-aminobenzene sulphonamide (sulphanilamide); that this compound is so formed was subsequently proved by Fuller (1937). Sulphanilamide had a demonstrable inhibitory action on streptococci in vitro, much dependent on the medium and particularly on the size of the inoculum, facts which are readily understandable in the light of modern knowledge. This explanation of the therapeutic action of Prontosil was hotly contested by Domagk. It must be remembered that it relegated the chrysoidin component to an inert role, whereas the affinity of dyes for bacteria had been a basis of German research since the time of Ehrlich, and was the doctrine underlying the choice of this series of compounds for examination. German workers also took the attitude that there must be something mysterious about the action of a true chemotherapeutic agent: an effect easily demonstrable in a test tube by any tyro was too banal altogether to explain it. Finally, they felt justifiable resentment that sulphanilamide, as a compound which had been described many years earlier, could be freely manufactured by anyone.

Every enterprising pharmaceutical house in the world was soon making this drug, and at one time it was on the market under at least 70 different proprietary names. What was more important, chemists were soon busy modifying the molecule to improve its performance. Early advances so secured were of two kinds, the first being higher activity against a wider range of bacteria: sulphapyridine (M and B 693), discovered in 1938, was the greatest single advance, since it was the first drug to be effective in pneumococcal pneumonia. The next stage, the introduction of sulphathiazole and sulphadiazine, while retaining and enhancing antibacterial activity, eliminated the frequent nausea and cyanosis caused by earlier drugs. Further developments, mainly in the direction of altered pharmacokinetic properties, have continued to the present day and are described in Chapter 1 (*now Ch. 32*).

ANTIBIOTICS

'Out of the earth shall come thy salvation.' – S.A. Waksman

Definition

Of many definitions of the term antibiotic which have been proposed, the narrower seem preferable. It is true that the word 'antibiosis' was coined by Vuillemin in 1889 to denote antagonism between living creatures in general, but the noun 'antibiotic' was first used by Waksman in 1942 (Waksman & Lechevalier 1962), which gives him a right to re-define it, and definition confines it to substances produced by micro-organisms antagonistic to the growth or life of others in high dilution (the last clause being necessary to exclude such metabolic products as organic acids, hydrogen peroxide and alcohol). To define an antibiotic simply as an antibacterial substance from a living source would embrace gastric juice, antibodies and lysozyme from man, essential oils and alkaloids from plants, and such oddities as the substance in the faeces of blowfly larvae which exerts an antiseptic effect in wounds. All substances known as antibiotics which are in clinical use and capable of exerting systemic effect are in fact products of micro-organisms.

Early history

The study of intermicrobic antagonism is almost as old as microbiology itself: several instances of it were described, one by Pasteur himself, in the seventies of the last century.* Therapeutic applications followed, some employing actual living cultures, others extracts of bacteria or moulds which had been found active. One of the best known products was an extract of *Pseudomonas aeruginosa*, first used as a local application by Czech workers, Honl and Bukovsky, in 1899: this was commercially available as 'pyocyanase' on the continent for many years. Other investigators used extracts of species of *Penicillium* and *Aspergillus* which probably or certainly contained antibiotics, but in too low a concentration to exert more than a local and transient effect. Florey (1945) gave a revealing account of these early developments in a lecture with the intriguing title 'The Use of Micro-organisms as Therapeutic Agents': this was amplified in a later publication (Florey 1949).

The systemic search, by an ingenious method, for an organism which could attack pyogenic cocci, conducted by Dubos (1939) in New York, led to the discovery of tyrothricin (gramicidin + tyrocidine), formed by *Bacillus brevis*, a substance which, although too toxic for systemic use in man, had in fact a systemic curative effect in mice. This work exerted a strong influence in inducing Florey and his colleagues to embark on a study of naturally formed antibacterial substances, and penicillin was the second on their list.

Penicillin

The present antibiotic era may be said to date from 1940, when the first account of the properties of an extract of cultures of *Penicillium notatum* appeared from Oxford (Chain et al 1940): a fuller account followed, with impressive clinical evidence (Abraham et al 1941). It had been necessary to find means of extracting a very labile substance from culture fluids, to examine its action on a wide range of bacteria, to examine its toxicity by a variety of methods, to establish a unit of its activity, to study its distribution and excretion when administered to animals, and finally to prove its systemic efficacy in mouse infections. There then remained the gigantic task, seemingly impossible except on a factory scale, of producing in the School of Pathology at Oxford enough of a substance, which was known to be excreted with unexampled rapidity, for the treatment of human disease. One means of maintaining

---

* i.e. the nineteenth century.

supplies was extraction from the patients' urine and re-administration.

It was several years before penicillin was fully purified, its structure ascertained, and its large-scale commercial production achieved. That this was of necessity first entrusted to manufacturers in the USA gave them a lead in a highly profitable industry which was not to be overtaken for many years.

Later antibiotics

The dates of discovery and sources of the principal antibiotics are given chronologically in Table 1.1. This is far from being a complete list, but subsequently discovered antibiotics have been closely related to others already known, such as aminoglycosides and macrolides. A few, including penicillin, were

Table 1.1 Date of discovery and source of natural antibiotics

Name	Date of discovery	Microbe
Penicillin	1929–40	*Penicillium notatum*
Tyrothricin {Gramicidin / Tyrocidine}	1939	*Bacillus brevis*
Griseofulvin	1939	*Penicillium griseofulvum Dierckx*
	1945	*Penicillium janczewski*
Streptomycin	1944	*Streptomyces griseus*
Bacitracin	1945	*Bacillus licheniformis*
Chloramphenicol	1947	*Streptomyces venezuelae*
Polymyxin	1947	*Bacillus polymyxa*
Framycetin	1947–53	*Streptomyces lavendulae*
Chlortetracycline	1948	*Streptomyces aureofaciens*
Cephalosporin C, N and P	1948	*Cephalosporium* sp.
Neomycin	1949	*Streptomyces fradiae*
Oxytetracycline	1950	*Streptomyces rimosus*
Nystatin	1950	*Streptomyces noursei*
Erythromycin	1952	*Streptomyces erythreus*
Oleandomycin	1954	*Streptomyces antibioticus*
Spiramycin	1954	*Streptomyces ambofaciens*
Novobiocin	1955	*Streptomyces spheroides*
		Streptomyces niveus
Cycloserine	1955	*Streptomyces orchidaceus*
		Streptomyces gaeryphalus
Vancomycin	1956	*Streptomyces orientalis*
Rifamycin	1957	*Streptomyces mediterranei*
Kanamycin	1957	*Streptomyces kanamyceticus*
Nebramycins	1958	*Streptomyces tenebraeus*
Paromomycin	1959	*Streptomyces rimosus*
Fusidic acid	1960	*Fusidium coccineum*
Spectinomycin	1961–62	*Streptomyces flavopersicus*
Lincomycin	1962	*Streptomyces lincolnensis*
Gentamicin	1963	*Micromonospora purpurea*
Josamycin	1964	*Streptomyces narvonensis* var. *josamyceticus*
Tobramycin	1968	*Streptomyces tenebraeus*
Ribostamycin	1970	*Streptomyces ribosidificus*
Butirosin	1970	*Bacillus circulans*
Sissomicin	1970	*Micromonospora myosensis*
Rosaramicin	1972	*Micromonospora rosaria*

chance discoveries, but 'stretching out suppliant Petri dishes' (Florey 1945) in the hope of catching a new antibiotic-producing organism was not to lead anywhere. Most further discoveries resulted from soil surveys, a process from which a large annual outlay might or might not be repaid a hundred-fold, a gamble against much longer odds than most oil prospecting. Soil contains a profuse and very mixed flora varying with climate, vegetation, mineral content and other factors, and is a medium in which antibiotic formation may well play a part in the competition for nutriment. A soil survey consists of obtaining samples from as many and as varied sources as possible, cultivating them on plates, subculturing all colonies of promising organisms such as actinomycetes and examining each for antibacterial activity. Alternatively the primary plate culture may be inoculated by spraying or by agar layering with suitable bacteria, the growth of which may then be seen to be inhibited in a zone surrounding some of the original colonies. This is only a beginning: many thousands of successive colonies so examined are found to form an antibiotic already known or useless by reason of toxicity.

Antibiotics have been derived from some odd sources other than soil. Although the original strain of *P. notatum* apparently floated into Fleming's laboratory at St. Mary's from one on another floor of the building in which moulds were being studied, that of *Penicillium chrysogenum* now used for penicillin production was derived from a mouldy Canteloupe melon in the market at Peoria, Illinois. Perhaps the strangest derivation was that of helenine, an antibiotic with some antiviral activity, isolated by Shope (1953) from *Penicillium funiculosum* growing on 'the isinglass cover of a photograph of my wife, Helen, on Guam, near the end of the war in 1945'. He proceeds to explain that he chose the name because it was non-descriptive, non-committal and not pre-empted, 'but largely out of recognition of the good taste shown by the mould... in locating on the picture of my wife'.

Those antibiotics out of thousands now discovered which have qualified for therapeutic use are described in chapters which follow.

FUTURE PROSPECTS

All successful chemotherapeutic agents have certain properties in common. They must exert an antimicrobic action, whether inhibitory or lethal, in high dilution, and in the complex chemical environment which they encounter in the body. Secondly, since they are brought into contact with every tissue in the body, they must so far as possible be without harmful effect on the function of any organ. To these two essential qualities may be added others which are highly desirable, although sometimes lacking in useful drugs: stability, free solubility, a slow rate of excretion, and diffusibility into remote areas.

If a drug is toxic to bacteria but not to mammalian cells the probability is that it interferes with some structure or function peculiar to bacteria. When the mode of action of sulphanilamide was elucidated by Woods and Fildes, and the theory was put forward of bacterial inhibition by metabolite analogues, the way seemed open for devising further antibacterial drugs on a rational basis. Immense subsequent advances in knowledge of the anatomy, chemical composition and metabolism of the bacterial cell should have encouraged such hopes still further. This new knowledge has been helpful in explaining what drugs do to bacteria, but not in devising new ones. Discoveries have continued to result only from random trials, purely empirical in the antibiotic field, although sometimes based on reasonable theoretical expectation in the synthetic.

Not only is the action of any new drug on individual bacteria still unpredictable on a theoretical basis, but so are its effects on the body itself. Most of the toxic effects of antibiotics have come to light only after extensive use, and even now no one can explain their affinity for some of the organs attacked. Some new observations in this field have contributed something to the present climate of suspicion about new drugs generally, which is insisting on far more searching tests of toxicity, and delaying the release of drugs for therapeutic use, particularly in the USA.

The present scope of chemotherapy

Successive discoveries have added to the list of infections amenable to chemotherapy until nothing remains altogether untouched except the viruses. On the other hand, however, some of the drugs which it is necessary to use are far from ideal, whether because of toxicity or of unsatisfactory pharmacokinetic properties, and some forms of treatment are consequently less often successful than others. Moreover, microbic resistance is a constant threat to the future usefulness of almost any drug. It seems unlikely that any totally new antibiotic remains to be discovered, since those of recent origin have similar properties to others already known. It therefore will be wise to husband our resources, and employ them in such a way as to preserve them. The problems of drug resistance and policies for preventing it are discussed in Chapters 13 and 14 (*now Chs* 3 and 11).

Adaptation of existing drugs

A line of advance other than the discovery of new drugs is the adaptation of old ones. An outstanding example of what can be achieved in this way is presented by the sulphonamides. Similar attention has naturally been directed to the antibiotics, with fruitful results of two different kinds. One is simply an alteration for the better in pharmacokinetic properties. Thus procaine penicillin, because less soluble, is longer acting than potassium penicillin; the esterification of macrolides improves absorption; chloramphenicol palmitate is palatable, and other variants so produced are more stable, more soluble and less irritant. Secondly, synthetic modification may also enhance antimicrobic properties. Sometimes both types of change can be achieved together; thus rifampicin is not only well absorbed after oral administration, whereas rifamycin, from which it is

derived, is not, but antibacterially much more active. The most varied achievements of these kinds have been among the penicillins, overcoming to varying degrees three defects in benzylpenicillin: its susceptibility to destruction by gastric acid and by staphylococcal penicillinase, and the relative insusceptibility to it of many species of Gram-negative bacilli. Similar developments have provided many new derivatives of cephalosporin C, although the majority differ from their prototypes much less than the penicillins.

One effect of these developments, of which it may seem captious to complain, is that a quite bewildering variety of products is now available for the same purposes. There are still many sulphonamides, about 10 tetracyclines, more than 20 semi-synthetic penicillins, and a rapidly extending list of cephalosporins, and a confident choice between them for any given purpose is one which few prescribers are qualified to make – indeed no one may be, since there is often no significant difference between the effects to be expected. Manufacturers whose costly research laboratories have produced some new derivative with a marginal advantage over others are entitled to make the most of their discovery. But if an antibiotic in a new form has a substantial advantage over that from which it was derived and no countervailing disadvantages, could not its predecessor sometimes simply be dropped? This rarely seems to happen, and there are doubtless good reasons for it, but the only foreseeable opportunity for simplifying the prescriber's choice has thus been missed.

References

Abraham EP, Chain E, Fletcher CM et al 1941 *Lancet* ii: 177–189.
Chain E, Florey HW, Gardner AD et al 1940 *Lancet* ii: 226–228.
Colebrook L, Kenny M 1936 *Lancet* i: 1279–1286.
Domagk G 1935 *Deutsche Medizinische Wochenschrift* 61: 250–253.
Dubos RJ 1939 *Journal of Experimental Medicine* 70: 1–10.
Florey HW 1945 *British Medical Journal* 2: 635–642.
Florey HW 1949 Antibiotics. Oxford University Press, London, ch. 1.
Fuller AT 1937 *Lancet* i: 194–198.
Honl J, Bukovsky J 1899 *Zentralblatt für Bakteriologie, Parasitenkunde, Infektionskrankheiten und Hygiene*, Abteilung 126: 305 (*see* Florey 1949).
Hörlein H 1935 *Proceedings of the Royal Society of Medicine* 29: 313–324.
Shope RE 1953 *Journal of Experimental Medicine* 97: 601–626.
Tréfouël J, Tréfouël J, Nitti F, Bovet D 1935 *Comptes Rendus des Séances de la Société de Biologie et de ses Filiales (Paris)* 120: 756–758.
Waksman SA, Lechevalier HA 1962 The Actinomycetes. Baillière, London, vol 3

LATER DEVELOPMENTS IN ANTIMICROBIAL CHEMOTHERAPY

ANTIBACTERIAL AGENTS

At the time of Garrod's death, penicillins and cephalosporins were still in the ascendancy: apart from the aminoglycoside, amikacin, the latest advances in antimicrobial therapy to reach the formulary in the late 1970s were the antipseudomonal penicillins, azlocillin, mezlocillin and piperacillin, the amidinopenicillin mecillinam (amdinocillin), and the β-lacta-mase-stable cephalosporins cefuroxime and cefoxitin. The latter compounds emerged in response to the growing importance of enterobacterial β-lactamases, which were the subject of intense scrutiny around this time. Discovery of other novel, enzyme-resistant, β-lactam molecules elaborated by microorganisms, including clavams, carbapenems and monobactams (*see* Ch. 17) were to follow, reminding us that Mother Nature still has some antimicrobial surprises up her copious sleeves.

The appearance of cefuroxime (first described in 1976) was soon followed by the synthesis of cefotaxime, a methoximino-cephalosporin that was not only β-lactamase stable but also exhibited a vast improvement in intrinsic activity. This compound stimulated a wave of commercial interest in cephalosporins with similar properties and the early 1980s were dominated by the appearance of several variations on the cefotaxime theme (ceftizoxime, ceftriaxone, cefmenoxime, ceftazidime and the oxa-cephem, latamoxef). Although they have not been equally successful, these compounds arguably represent the high point in a continuing development of cephalosporins from 1964, when cephaloridine and cephalothin were first introduced.

Among the aminoglycosides the search for new derivatives petered out in most countries after the development of netilmicin in 1976. However, in Japan, where amikacin was first synthesized in 1972 in response to concerns about aminoglycoside resistance (and where there is still an undiminished appetite for new antibacterial compounds) several novel aminoglycosides that are not exploited elsewhere appeared on the market.

Interest in most other antimicrobial drug families languished during this period, although a number of macrolides with rather undistinguished properties appeared during the 1980s and found use in Japan and some other countries, but not in the UK or the USA. More general interest in new macrolides had to await the appearance of compounds that claimed pharmacological advantages over erythromycin (*see* Ch. 24); two, azithromycin and clarithromycin, reached the UK market in 1991 (Table 1.2) and others became available elsewhere.

Quinolone antibacterial agents enjoyed a renaissance when it was realized that fluorinated, piperazine-substituted derivatives exhibited much enhanced potency and a broader spectrum of activity than earlier congeners (*see* Ch. 29). Norfloxacin, first described in 1980 and marketed in Japan in 1984, was the forerunner of this revival and other fluoroquinolones quickly followed. Soon manufacturers of the new fluoroquinolones such as ciprofloxacin, enoxacin and ofloxacin began to struggle for market dominance in Europe, the USA and elsewhere and competing claims of activity and toxicity began to circulate.

The domination of the cephalosporins among β-lactam agents began to decline in the late 1980s as novel derivatives such as the monobactam aztreonam and the carbapenem imipenem came on stream. The contrasting properties of these two compounds reflected a still unresolved debate about the relative merits of narrow-spectrum targeted therapy and ultra-

Table 1.2 Antibacterial agents introduced on the UK market 1987–2001

Agent	Type
1987–1989	
Aztreonam	Monobactam
Cefuroxime axetil	Oral cephalosporin
Ciprofloxacin	Fluoroquinolone
Enoxacin*	Fluoroquinolone
Imipenem	Carbapenem
Mupirocin	Monic acid (topical)
Temocillin*	Penicillin
Ticarcillin + clavulanate†	Penicillin/β-lactamase inhibitor combination
1990–1992	
Azithromycin	Macrolide (azalide)
Cefixime	Oral cephalosporin
Cefodizime*	Parenteral cephalosporin
Clarithromycin	Macrolide
Norfloxacin	Fluoroquinolone
Ofloxacin	Fluoroquinolone
Sulbactam (+ ampicillin)*	β-Lactamase inhibitor
Tazobactam (+ piperacillin)	β-Lactamase inhibitor
Teicoplanin	Glycopeptide
Temafloxacin*	Fluoroquinolone
1993–1995	
Cefpodoxime	Oral cephalosporin
Ceftibuten*	Oral cephalosporin
Ceftriaxone	Parenteral cephalosporin
Fosfomycin trometamol*	Phosphonic acid
Rifabutin	Rifamycin (antimycobacterial)
1996–1998	
Cefprozil	Oral cephalosporin
Grepafloxacin*	Fluoroquinolone
Levofloxacin	Fluoroquinolone
1999–2001	
Dalfopristin/quinupristin	Streptogramin
Linezolid	Oxazolidinone

*Later withdrawn from the UK market.
† A new combination of older compounds.

broad spectrum cover. Meanwhile, research emphasis among β-lactam antibiotics turned to the development of orally absorbed cephalosporins that exhibited the favorable properties of the expanded-spectrum parenteral compounds, and formulations that sought to improve on the successful combination of amoxicillin with clavulanic acid (Table 1.2).

As the 20th century drew to a close the spotlight of drug development turned from antibacterial to antiviral and antifungal compounds, stimulated by the increased importance of viral and fungal pathogens in immunocompromised patients, including those with AIDS. However, concerns about the development and spread of resistance to traditional agents among Gram-positive cocci kept some interest in antibacterial agents alive. This has so far borne fruit in three new agents:

the quinupristin-dalfopristin combination (Ch. 31), the oxazolidinone linezolid (Ch. 28) and the ketolide telithromycin (Ch. 24). A similar concern – and the commercial appeal of the respiratory tract infection market – has also ensured a sustained interest in new quinolones that reliably include the pneumococcus in their spectrum of activity. Several quinolones of this type are beginning to appear on the market, though enthusiasm has been muted to some extent by unexpected problems of serious toxicity: temafloxacin and grepafloxacin had to be withdrawn soon after they were launched because of unacceptable adverse reactions; trovafloxacin has had its licence severely curtailed for similar reasons.

The plea with which Garrod concluded his historical introduction, that prescribers' choice should be simplified by removing old agents from the formulary, was heeded with great alacrity during the latter part of the 20th century – though for commercial rather than the therapeutic reasons that Garrod envisaged. Many sulphonamides and other drugs have fallen by the wayside, and old agents are judged redundant as fast as new ones appear. At least 12 β-lactam antibiotics (azlocillin, carfecillin, cefodizime, ceftibuten, cephaloridine, cephalothin, ciclacillin, latamoxef, methicillin, mezlocillin, penamecillin and phenethicillin) were deleted from the *British National Formulary* between 1990 and 1999.

ANTIVIRAL AGENTS

The massive intellectual and financial investment that was brought to bear in the wake of the HIV pandemic began to pay off in the last decade of the century. In the late 1980s only a handful of antiviral agents was available to the prescriber, whereas nearly 30 are available today. Twenty new antiviral drugs were approved by the US Food and Drug Administration in the period 1992–2000 alone (Table 1.3);

Table 1.3 Antiviral agents newly approved by the US Food and Drug Administration 1992–2000

Year	Antiretroviral agents	Other antiviral agents
1992	Zalcitabine	
1993		Rimantadine
1994	Stavudine	Famciclovir
1995	Lamivudine	Valaciclovir
	Saquinavir	
1996	Ritonavir	Cidofovir
	Indinavir	
	Nevirapine	
1997	Nelfinavir	
	Delavirdine	
1998	Efavirenz	Fomivirsen
1999	Amprenavir	Zanamivir
		Oseltamivir
2000	Lopinavir	Docosanol*

* For topical use.

they included important new approaches to the attack on HIV, opening the way to effective combination therapy (*see* Ch. 39). In addition, new compounds for the prevention and treatment of influenza (zanamivir, oseltamivir; Ch. 40) and cytomegalovirus infection (cidofovir, fomivirsen; Ch. 40) have emerged in the last few years.

ANTIFUNGAL AGENTS

Many of the new antifungal drugs that appeared in the late 20th century were variations on older themes: antifungal azoles and safer (but expensive) formulations of amphotericin B. However, they included useful new triazoles (fluconazole and itraconazole) that are effective when given systemically and a novel allylamine compound, terbinafine, which offers a welcome alternative to griseofulvin in recalcitrant dermatophyte infections (Ch. 35). Investigation of antibiotics of the echinocandin class has borne fruit in the development of caspofungin (p. 421), which is licensed for use in serious *Aspergillus* infections. The emergence of *Pneumocystis carinii* (long a taxonomic orphan, but now accepted as a fungus) as an important pathogen in HIV-infected persons stimulated the investigation of new therapies, leading to the introduction of trimetrexate and atovaquone for cases unresponsive to older drugs.

ANTIPARASITIC AGENTS

The most serious effects of parasitic infections are borne by the economically poor countries of the world, and research into agents for the treatment of human parasitic disease has always received low priority. Nevertheless, some useful new antimalarial compounds have found their way into therapeutic use. These include mefloquine and halofantrine, which originally emerged in the early 1980s from the extensive antimalarial research program undertaken by the Walter Reed Army Institute of Research in Washington.

Another useful development, by the Wellcome Foundation in the UK, was the hydroxynaphthoquinone, atovaquone. Although this drug was first approved in the USA (in 1993) and the UK (in 1996) for the treatment of *P. carinii* pneumonia (*see above*), it was originally developed as an antimalarial agent. Early trials in malaria were disappointing, but interest has been revived by the demonstration of synergy with proguanil. Derivatives of artemisinin, the active principle of the Chinese herbal remedy qinghaosu, are also now in use in parts of the Far East and Africa. These developments have been slow, but are nonetheless welcome in view of the inexorable spread of chloroquine resistance in *Plasmodium falciparum*, which continues unabated (*see* Ch. 64).

There have been few noteworthy developments in the treatment of other protozoan diseases, but one, eflornithine (difluoromethylornithine), provides a long-awaited alternative to arsenicals in trypanosomiasis. Eflornithine has been dubbed the 'resurrection drug' in West Africa because of its effect in the late stages of sleeping sickness. Unfortunately, it appears ineffective in the East African form of the disease. Even more lamentably, its availability and, indeed, that of other antitrypanosomal drugs, is threatened because production (unless other uses can be found) is unprofitable (Pécoul & Gastellu 1999; Van Nieuwenhove 2000).

On the helminth front the late 20th century witnessed a revolution in the reliability of treatment. Amazingly, three agents – albendazole, praziquantel and ivermectin – emerged, which between them cover nearly all the important causes of human intestinal and systemic worm infections (*see* Chs 37 and 66). Most anthelminthic compounds enter the human anti-infective formulary by the veterinary route (praziquantel is an honorable exception), underlying the melancholy fact that animal husbandry is of relatively greater economic importance than the well-being of the approximately 1.5 billion people who harbor parasitic worms.

THE SCOPE OF ANTIMICROBIAL CHEMOTHERAPY AT THE BEGINNING OF THE 21ST CENTURY

Thousands of new antibacterial agents have been described in the world literature during the last 50 years. There have been many false dawns, but relatively few compounds have survived the stages of development and licensing to reach the pharmacist's shelf. The commercial reality behind this is plain: it has been estimated that the process of bringing a new drug to market takes about 12 years; the cost of development exceeds $350 million (about £250 million) and only about a third of the drugs that are launched yield a profit (Billstein 1994). Given this, and the already crowded market for antibacterial drugs, it is not surprising that anti-infective research in the pharmaceutical houses has been scaled down or turned to the potentially more lucrative fields of antifungal and antiviral drugs. Meanwhile, resistance continues to increase inexorably (Kunin 1993, Greenwood 1998). Although most bacterial infection remains amenable to therapy with common, well established drugs, the prospect of untreatable infection is already becoming an occasional reality among seriously ill patients in high-dependency units where there is intense selective pressure created by widespread use of potent, broad-spectrum agents. On a global scale, multiple drug resistance in a number of different organisms, including those that cause typhoid fever, tuberculosis and malaria, is an unsolved problem. These are life-threatening infections for which treatment options are limited, even when fully sensitive organisms are involved.

Science, with a little help from Lady Luck, has provided us with formidable resources for the treatment of infectious disease during the last 65 years. Garrod, surveying the scope of chemotherapy in 1968 (in the second edition of this book), warned of the threat of microbial resistance and the need to husband our resources. That threat and that need have not diminished. The challenge for the future is to preserve the precious assets that we have acquired by sensible regulation of the availability of antimicrobial drugs in countries in which controls are presently inadequate and by informed and cautious prescribing everywhere.

 References

Billstein SA 1994 How the pharmaceutical industry brings an antibiotic drug to market in the United States. *Antimicrobial Agents and Chemotherapy* 38: 2679–2682.

Greenwood D 1998 Resistance to antimicrobial agents: a personal view. *Journal of Medical Microbiology* 47: 751–755.

Kunin CM 1993 Resistance to antimicrobial agents – a worldwide calamity. *Annals of Internal Medicine* 118: 557–561.

Pécoul B, Gastellu M 1999 Production of sleeping-sickness treatment. *Lancet* 354: 955–996.

Van Nieuwenhove S 2000 Gambiense sleeping sickness: re-emerging and soon untreatable? *Bulletin of the World Health Organization* 78: 1283.

2 Modes of action

D. Greenwood and R. Whitley

At the basis of all antimicrobial chemotherapy lies the concept of selective toxicity. The necessary selectivity can be achieved in several ways: vulnerable targets within the microbe may be absent from the cells of the host or, alternatively, the analogous targets within the host cells may be sufficiently different, or at least sufficiently inaccessible, for selective attack to be possible. With agents like the polymyxins, the organic arsenicals used in trypanosomiasis, the antifungal polyenes and many antiviral compounds, the gap between toxicity to the microbe and to the host is small, but in most cases antimicrobial agents are able to exploit fundamental differences in structure and function within the microbial cell, and host toxicity generally results from unexpected secondary effects.

ANTIBACTERIAL AGENTS

The minute size and capacity for very rapid multiplication of bacteria ensures that they are structurally and metabolically very different from mammalian cells and, in theory, there are numerous ways in which bacteria can be selectively killed or disabled. In the event, it turns out that only the bacterial cell wall is structurally unique; other subcellular structures, including the cytoplasmic membrane, ribosomes and DNA, are built on the same pattern as those of mammalian cells, although sufficient differences in construction and organization do exist at these sites to make exploitation of the selective toxicity principle feasible.

Antibacterial agents have been discovered – rarely designed – that attack each of these vulnerable sites; the most successful compounds seem to be those that interfere with the construction of the bacterial cell wall, the synthesis of protein, or the replication and transcription of DNA. Relatively few clinically useful agents act at the level of the cell membrane or by interfering with specific metabolic processes of the bacterial cell (Table 2.1).

Unless the target is located on the outside of the bacterial cell, antimicrobial agents must be able to penetrate to the site of action. Access through the cytoplasmic membrane is usually achieved by passive or facilitated diffusion, or (as, for example,

Table 2.1 Sites of action of antibacterial agents

Site	Agent	Principal target
Cell wall	Penicillins	Transpeptidase
	Cephalosporins	Transpeptidase
	Bacitracin	Isoprenylphosphate
	Glycopeptides	Acyl-D-alanyl-D-alanine
	Cycloserine	Alanine racemase/synthetase
	Fosfomycin	Pyruvyl transferase
	Isoniazid	Desaturation of fatty acids
	Ethambutol	Arabinosyl transferases
Ribosome	Chloramphenicol	Peptidyl transferase
	Tetracyclines	Ribosomal A site
	Aminoglycosides	Initiation complex/translation
	Macrolides	Translocation
	Lincosamides	?Peptidyl transferase
	Fusidic acid	Elongation factor G
	Oxazolidinones	70S initiation complex formation
	Mupirocin	Isoleucyl-tRNA synthetase
Nucleic acid	Quinolones	DNA gyrase (α subunit)/ topoisomerase IV
	Novobiocin	DNA gyrase (β subunit)
	Rifampicin	RNA polymerase
	5-Nitroimidazoles	DNA strands
	Nitrofurans	DNA strands
Cell membrane	Polymyxins	Phospholipids
	Ionophores	Ion transport
Folate synthesis	Sulfonamides	Pteroate synthetase
	Diaminopyrimidines	Dihydrofolate reductase

with aminoglycosides and tetracyclines) by active transport processes. In the case of Gram-negative organisms the antibiotic must also negotiate an outer membrane, consisting of a characteristic lipopolysaccharide–lipoprotein complex, which is responsible for preventing many antibiotics from reaching an otherwise sensitive intracellular target. This lipophilic outer membrane contains aqueous transmembrane channels (porins), which selectively allow passage of hydrophilic molecules depending on their molecular size and ionic charge (Figure 2.1). Many antibacterial agents use porins to gain

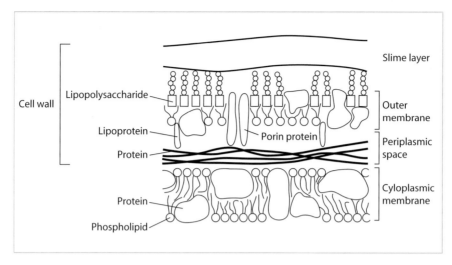

Fig. 2.1 Diagrammatic representation of the Gram-negative cell envelope. The periplasmic space contains the peptidoglycan and some enzymes. (Reproduced with permission from Russell AD, Quesnel LB, eds, *Antibiotics: assessment of antimicrobial activity and resistance. The Society for Applied Bacteriology Technical Series no. 18*, London: Academic Press, p. 62.)

access to Gram-negative organisms, although other pathways are also used.[1]

INHIBITORS OF BACTERIAL CELL WALL SYNTHESIS

Peptidoglycan forms the rigid, shape-maintaining layer of all medically important bacteria except mycoplasmas. Its structure is basically similar in Gram-positive and Gram-negative organisms, although there are important differences. In both types of organism the basic macromolecular chain consists of *N*-acetylglucosamine alternating with its lactyl ether, *N*-acetyl-muramic acid. Each muramic acid unit carries a pentapeptide, the third amino acid of which is L-lysine in most Gram-positive cocci and *meso*-diaminopimelic acid in Gram-negative bacilli. The cell wall is given its rigidity by cross-links between this amino acid and the penultimate amino acid (which is always D-alanine) of adjacent chains, with loss of the terminal amino acid (also D-alanine) (Figure 2.2). Gram-negative bacilli have a very thin peptidoglycan layer, which is loosely cross-linked; Gram-positive cocci, in contrast, possess a very thick peptido-glycan coat, which is tightly cross-linked through interpeptide bridges. The walls of Gram-positive bacteria also differ in containing considerable amounts of polymeric sugar alcohol phosphates (teichoic and teichuronic acids), while Gram-negative bacteria possess an external membrane-like envelope as described above.

Penicillins, cephalosporins and other β-lactam agents, as well as fosfomycin, cycloserine, bacitracin and the glycopep-tides vancomycin and teicoplanin, selectively inhibit different stages in the construction of the peptidoglycan (Figure 2.3).

In addition, the unusual structure of the mycobacterial cell wall is exploited by a number of antituberculosis agents.

Fosfomycin

The *N*-acetylmuramic acid component of the bacterial cell wall is derived from *N*-acetylglucosamine by the addition of a lactic acid substituent derived from phosphoenolpyruvate. Fosfomycin blocks this reaction by inhibiting the pyruvyl trans-ferase enzyme involved. The antibiotic enters bacterial cells by active transport mechanisms for α-glycerophosphate and glucose-6-phosphate. Glucose-6-phosphate induces the hexose phosphate transport pathway in some organisms (notably *Escherichia coli*) and potentiates the activity of fosfomycin against those bacteria.

The related phosphonic acid, fosmidomycin, uses the same transport pathways and is also potentiated by glucose-6-phos-phate. However, fosmidomycin acts differently by interfering with the formation of isopentyl diphosphate during isoprenoid biosynthesis.[2] The vulnerable enzyme is part of an alternative mevalonate-independent pathway of isoprenoid biosynthesis present in *E. coli*, malaria parasites and the chloroplasts of higher plants, but *Staphylococcus aureus* uses the normal meval-onate pathway, which probably explains the intrinsic resistance to fosmidomycin of Gram-positive bacteria.[3]

Cycloserine

The first three amino acids of the pentapeptide chain of muramic acid are added sequentially, but the terminal D-alanyl-D-alanine is added as a unit (Figure 2.3). To form this unit the natural form of the amino acid, L-alanine, must first

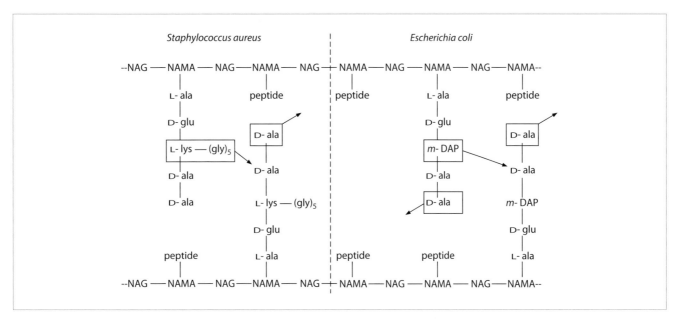

Fig. 2.2 Schematic representations of the terminal stages of cell wall synthesis in Gram-positive (*Staphylococcus aureus*) and Gram-negative (*Escherichia coli*) bacteria. See text for explanation. Arrows indicate formation of cross-links, with loss of terminal D-alanine; in Gram-negative bacilli many D-alanine residues are not involved in cross-linking and are removed by D-alanine carboxypeptidase. NAG, *N*-acetylglucosamine; NAMA, *N*-acetylmuramic acid; ala, alanine; glu, glutamic acid; lys, lysine; gly, glycine; *m*-DAP, *meso*-diaminopimelic acid.

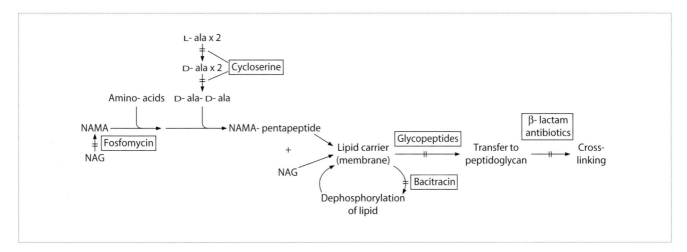

Fig. 2.3 Simplified scheme of bacterial cell wall synthesis, showing the sites of action of cell wall active antibiotics. NAG, *N*-acetylglucosamine; NAMA, *N*-acetylmuramic acid. (Reproduced from Greenwood D, Ogilvie MM, Antimicrobial Agents in: Greenwood D, Slack RCB, Peutherer JF, eds, 2002 *Medical Microbiology* 16th edn. Edinburgh: Churchill Livingstone.)

be racemized to D-alanine and two molecules are then joined together by D-alanine synthetase. Both of these reactions are blocked by the antibiotic cycloserine, which is a structural analog of D-alanine.

Glycopeptides

Once the muramylpentapeptide is formed in the cell cytoplasm, an *N*-acetylglucosamine unit is added, together with any amino acids needed for the interpeptide bridge of Gram-positive organisms. It is then passed to a lipid carrier molecule, which transfers the whole unit across the cell membrane to be added to the growing end of the peptidoglycan macromolecule (Figure 2.3). Addition of the new building block is prevented by the glycopeptides vancomycin and teicoplanin, which bind to the acyl-D-alanyl-D-alanine tail of the muramylpentapeptide. Strains of enterococci that are able to replace the terminal D-alanine with D-lactate exhibit resistance to glycopeptides.[4] Because these glycopeptides are large polar molecules they cannot penetrate the outer membrane of Gram-negative organisms, which explains their restricted spectrum of activity.

Bacitracin

The lipid carrier involved in transporting the cell wall building block across the membrane has been characterized as a C_{55} isoprenyl phosphate. The lipid acquires an additional phosphate group in the transport process and must be dephosphorylated in order to regenerate the native compound for another round of transfer. The cyclic peptide antibiotic bacitracin binds to the isoprenyl pyrophosphate and prevents this dephosphorylation. Unfortunately, analogous reactions in eukaryotic cells are also inhibited by bacitracin, and this may be the basis of the toxicity of the compound.

β-Lactam antibiotics

The final cross-linking reaction that gives the bacterial cell wall its characteristic rigidity was pinpointed many years ago as the primary target of penicillin and other β-lactam agents. These compounds were postulated to inhibit formation of the transpeptide bond by virtue of their structural resemblance to the terminal D-alanyl-D-alanine unit that participates in the transpeptidation reaction. This knowledge had to be reconciled with various concentration-dependent morphological responses that Gram-negative bacilli undergo on exposure to penicillin and other β-lactam compounds: filamentation (caused by inhibition of division rather than growth of the bacteria) at low concentrations, and the formation of osmotically fragile spheroplasts (peptidoglycan-deficient forms that have lost their bacillary shape) at high concentrations.

Three observations suggested that these morphological events could be dissociated:

- The oral cephalosporin cefalexin (and some other β-lactam agents, including cefradine, temocillin and the monobactam, aztreonam) causes the filamentation response alone over an extremely wide range of concentrations.
- Mecillinam (amdinocillin) does not inhibit division (and hence does not cause filamentation in Gram-negative bacilli), but has a generalized effect on the bacterial cell wall.
- Combining cefalexin and mecillinam evokes the 'typical' spheroplast response in *E. coli* that neither agent induces when acting alone.[5]

It was subsequently shown that isolated membranes of bacteria contain a number of proteins that are able to bind penicillin and other β-lactam antibiotics. These penicillin-binding proteins (PBPs) are numbered in descending order of their molecular weight according to their separation by polyacrylamide gel electrophoresis. The number found in bacterial cells varies from species to species: *E. coli* has at least seven and *Staph. aureus* four. β-Lactam agents that induce filamentation in Gram-negative bacilli bind to PBP3; similarly, mecillinam binds exclusively to PBP2. Most β-lactam antibiotics, when present in sufficient concentration, bind to both these sites and to others (PBP1a and PBP1b) that participate in the rapidly lytic response of Gram-negative bacilli to many penicillins and cephalosporins.

The low-molecular-weight PBPs (4, 5 and 6) of *E. coli* are carboxypeptidases, which may operate to control the extent of cross-linking in the cell wall. Mutants lacking these enzymes grow normally and have thus been ruled out as targets for the inhibitory or lethal actions of β-lactam antibiotics. The PBPs with higher molecular weights (PBPs 1a, 1b, 2 and 3) possess transpeptidase activity, and it seems that these PBPs represent different forms of the transpeptidase enzyme necessary to arrange the complicated architecture of the cylindrical or spherical bacterial cell during growth, septation and division.

The nature of the lethal event

In Gram-negative bacilli, the bactericidal effect of β-lactam antibiotics can be quantitatively prevented by providing sufficient osmotic protection. In these circumstances the bacteria survive as spheroplasts, which readily revert to the bacillary shape on removal of the antibiotic. It thus seems clear that cell death in Gram-negative bacilli is a direct consequence of osmotic lysis of cells deprived of the protective peptidoglycan coat.

The nature of the lethal event in Gram-positive cocci is more complex. Since these bacteria possess a much thicker, tougher peptidoglycan layer than that present in the Gram-negative cell wall, much greater damage has to be inflicted before death of the cell ensues. However, one of the first events that occurs on exposure of Gram-positive cocci to β-lactam antibiotics is a release of lipoteichoic acid, an event which appears to trigger autolysis of the peptidoglycan.

Optimal dosage effect

For many strains of Gram-positive cocci, an optimal bactericidal concentration of β-lactam antibiotics can be identified above which the killing effect is reduced, sometimes very strikingly. The basis of this effect, often called the 'Eagle phenomenon' after its discoverer, has never been satisfactorily explained. A plausible hypothesis is that the lethal event is triggered by low concentrations of the antibiotic as a consequence of binding to one particular target protein; binding at higher concentrations to other targets (PBPs) stops the bacterial cell from growing and this antagonizes the lethal effect, which requires continued cell growth.

Persisters

About 1 in 10^5 bacteria in a culture exposed to β-lactam antibiotics survive, even on prolonged exposure to an optimal bactericidal concentration. These 'persisters' have not acquired resistance, since, if the antibiotic is removed and they are allowed to grow, most of their immediate progeny are killed on re-exposure, just as the parent culture is. These bacteria may be cells in which the peptidoglycan exists transiently as a complete covalently linked macromolecule. Inhibition by the antibiotic of autolytic enzymes needed to create growth points in the peptidoglycan would effectively trap the cells in a state in which they could not grow (and therefore could not be killed) until the antibiotic is removed.

Tolerance

In some Gram-positive cocci there may be a marked dissociation between the concentrations of β-lactam agents (and glycopeptides) required to achieve a bacteristatic and a bactericidal effect. The organisms are not 'resistant' since they remain fully susceptible to the inhibitory activity of the antibiotic, although the bactericidal effect is reduced. Defective autolysins remain the most likely explanation of the effect, which has some similarities to the persister phenomenon.[6]

Antimycobacterial agents

Agents acting specifically against *Mycobacterium tuberculosis* and other mycobacteria have been less well characterized than other antimicrobial drugs. However, it is thought that several of them owe their activity to selective effects on the unique structure of the mycobacterial envelope.[7] Thus, although isoniazid has been found to interfere with various cellular functions of bacteria, it is likely that it owes its specific bactericidal activity against *M. tuberculosis* to interference with mycolic acid synthesis. The effect is achieved by inhibition of a fatty acid desaturase after intracellular oxidation of isoniazid to an active product.[8] Ethionamide, prothionamide and pyrazinamide, which are related nicotinic acid derivatives, are also thought to undergo intracellular modification and to act in a similar fashion.

Ethambutol, a slow acting and primarily bacteristatic antimycobacterial agent, inhibits arabinosyl transferases. These enzymes bring about the polymerization of arabinose to form arabinan, a polysaccharide component of the core polymers of the mycobacterial cell wall.[8]

INHIBITORS OF BACTERIAL PROTEIN SYNTHESIS

The amazing process by which the genetic message in DNA is translated into large and unique protein molecules is universal; in prokaryotic, as in eukaryotic cells, the workbench is the ribosome, composed of two distinct subunits, each a complex of ribosomal RNA (rRNA) and numerous proteins. However, bacterial ribosomes are open to selective attack because they differ from their mammalian counterparts in both protein and RNA content; indeed they can be readily distinguished in the ultracentrifuge: bacterial ribosomes exhibit a sedimentation coefficient of 70S (composed of 30S and 50S subunits), whereas mammalian ribosomes display a coefficient of 80S (composed of 40S and 60S subunits).

In the first stage of bacterial protein synthesis, messenger RNA (mRNA), transcribed from the appropriate region of DNA, binds to the smaller ribosomal subunit and attracts *N*-formylmethionyl transfer RNA (fMet-tRNA) to the initiator codon AUG. The larger subunit is then added to form a complete initiation complex. fMet-tRNA occupies the P (peptidyl donor) site; adjacent to it is the A (aminoacyl acceptor) site aligned with the next trinucleotide codon of the mRNA. Transfer RNA (tRNA) bearing the appropriate anticodon, and its specific amino acid, enters the A site, and a peptidyl transferase joins *N*-formylmethionine to the new amino acid with loss (via an exit site) of the tRNA in the P site; the first peptide bond of the protein has been formed. A translocation event then moves the remaining tRNA with its dipeptide to the P site and concomitantly aligns the next triplet codon of mRNA with the now vacant A site. The appropriate aminoacyl-tRNA enters the A site and the transfer process and subsequent translocation are repeated. In this way, the peptide chain is built up in precise fashion, faithful to the original DNA blueprint, until a so-called 'nonsense' codon is encountered on the mRNA that signals chain termination and release of the peptide chain. The mRNA is disengaged from the ribosome, which dissociates into its two subunits ready to form a new initiation complex. Within bacterial cells, many ribosomes are engaged in protein synthesis during active growth, and a single strand of mRNA may interact with many ribosomes along its length to form a polysome.

Many antibiotics interfere with the process of protein synthesis (Figure 2.4). Some, like puromycin, which is an analog of the aminoacyl tail of charged tRNA and causes premature chain termination, act on bacterial and mammalian ribosomes alike and are therefore unsuitable for systemic use in humans. Therapeutically useful inhibitors of protein synthesis include many of the naturally occurring antibiotics, such as chloramphenicol, tetracyclines, aminoglycosides, fusidic acid, macrolides, lincosamides and streptogramins. Some newer agents, including mupirocin and the oxazolidinones, also act at this stage.

Chloramphenicol

The molecular target for chloramphenicol is the peptidyl transferase enzyme that links amino acids in the growing peptide chain. The effect of the antibiotic is thus to freeze the process of chain elongation, bringing bacterial growth to an abrupt halt. The process is completely reversible, and chloramphenicol is fundamentally a bacteristatic agent. The binding of chloramphenicol to the 50S subunit of 70S ribosomes is highly specific. The basis for the rare, but fatal, marrow aplasia associated with this compound is not therefore a generalized effect on mammalian protein synthesis, although mitochondrial ribosomes, which are similar to those of bacteria, may be involved.

Tetracyclines

Antibiotics of the tetracycline group are actively transported into bacterial cells and attach to 30S ribosomal subunits in such a manner as to prevent binding of incoming aminoacyl-

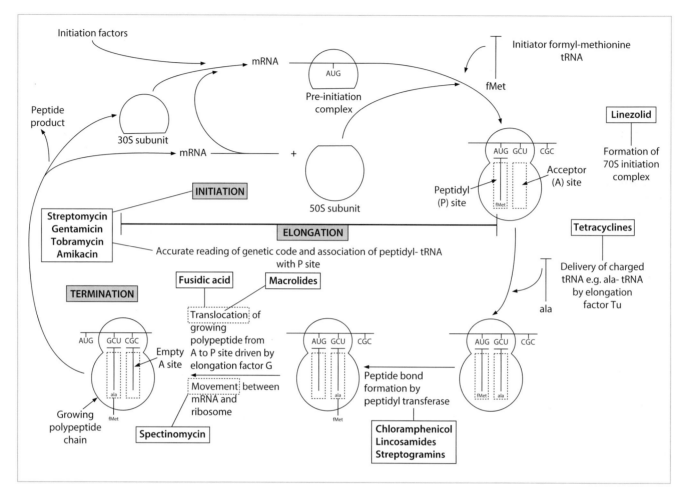

Fig. 2.4 The process of protein synthesis and the steps inhibited by various antibacterial agents. (Adapted from Chopra I, Greenwood D, Antibacterial agents: basis of action, in: *Encyclopedia of Life Sciences*, Nature Publishing Group, London: www.els.net).

tRNA to the A site.[9] The effect is to halt chain elongation and, like chloramphenicol, these antibiotics are predominantly bacteristatic.

Tetracyclines also penetrate into mammalian cells (indeed, the effect on chlamydiae depends on this) and can interfere with protein synthesis on eukaryotic ribosomes. Fortunately, cytoplasmic ribosomes are not affected at the concentrations achieved during therapy, although mitochondrial ribosomes are. The selective toxicity of tetracyclines thus presents something of a puzzle, the solution to which is presumably that these antibiotics are not actively concentrated by mitochondria as they are by bacteria and concentrations reached are insufficient to deplete respiratory chain enzymes.[9]

Aminoglycosides

Much of the literature on the mode of action of aminoglycosides has concentrated on streptomycin. However, the action of gentamicin and other deoxystreptamine-containing aminoglycosides is clearly not identical, since they bind at more than

one site on the ribosome, whereas streptomycin binds in a 1:1 ratio at a unique site. One consequence of this is that single-step, high-level resistance to streptomycin, which is due to a change in a specific protein of the 30S ribosomal subunit, does not extend to other aminoglycosides.

Elucidation of the mode of action of aminoglycosides has been complicated by the need to reconcile a variety of enigmatic observations:

- Streptomycin and other aminoglycosides cause misreading of mRNA on the ribosome while paradoxically halting protein synthesis completely by interfering with the formation of functional initiation complexes.
- Inhibition of protein synthesis by aminoglycosides leads not just to bacteristasis as with, for example, tetracycline or chloramphenicol, but also to rapid cell death.
- Susceptible bacteria (but not those with resistant ribosomes) quickly become leaky to small molecules on exposure to the drug, apparently because of an effect on the cell membrane.

- Mutations can occur that render the bacterial cell dependent on streptomycin for growth.
- Susceptibility is dominant over resistance in merozygotes that are diploid for the two allelic forms.

A well-lit path through this maze has not yet been definitively charted, but the situation is slowly becoming clearer. The two effects of aminoglycosides on initiation and misreading may be explained by a concentration-dependent effect on ribosomes engaged in the formation of the initiation complex and those in the process of chain elongation:[10] in the presence of a sufficiently high concentration of drug, protein synthesis is completely halted once the mRNA is run off because re-initiation is blocked; under these circumstances there is little or no opportunity for misreading to occur. However, at concentrations at which only a proportion of the ribosomes can be blocked at initiation, some protein synthesis will take place and the opportunity for misreading will be provided.

The dominance of susceptibility over resistance has been tentatively explained by the fact that the non-functional initiation complexes formed in the presence of aminoglycosides are unstable, so that the ribosomes continuously dissociate from mRNA and recycle in an inoperative form. These crippled ribosomes (of which there are twice as many as there are resistant ones in merozygotes) are hence continuously made re-available to sequester newly formed mRNA and prevent the resistant ribosomes from maintaining a supply of the polypeptides that the cell needs.[10]

The effects of aminoglycosides on membrane permeability, and the potent bactericidal activity of these compounds, remain enigmatic. However, the two phenomena may be related.[11] In bacteria, as in mammalian cells, some of the ribosomes (presumably those engaged in transmembrane protein transfer) may be membrane bound. Moreover, aminoglycosides enter bacteria by an active transport process (absent in anaerobes and streptococci, hence their inherent resistance) that is dependent on protein synthesis. It is possible that site-specific uptake of the drug at ribosomal attachment sites and subsequent binding to the ribosome–membrane complex may lead to membrane leakiness and cell death.[12]

Spectinomycin

The aminocyclitol antibiotic spectinomycin, often considered alongside the aminoglycosides, binds in reversible fashion (hence the bacteristatic activity) to ribosomal RNA of the 30S subunit. There it interrupts the translocation event that occurs as the next codon of mRNA is aligned with the A site in readiness for the incoming aminoacyl-tRNA.

Macrolides, lincosamides, streptogramins

These antibiotic groups are structurally very different, but bind to closely related sites on the 50S ribosome of bacteria. One consequence of this is that staphylococci exhibiting inducible resistance to erythromycin, which is caused by methylation of certain adenine residues in the rRNA, also become resistant to other macrolides, lincosamides and streptogramin B in the presence of erythromycin (p. 33 and 314).

The detailed mode of action of these antibiotics has not yet been definitively worked out. Erythromycin (like type A streptogramins; *see below*) binds almost exclusively to free ribosomes and brings protein synthesis to a halt after formation of the initiation complex, probably by interfering with the translocation reaction. The precise mechanism of action of lincosamides is less clear, but they appear to interfere indirectly with the peptidyl transferase reaction, possibly by blocking the P site.

The streptogramins are composed of two interacting components designated A and B (p. 382). The type A molecules bind to 50S ribosomal subunits and affect both donor and acceptor functions of peptidyl transferase by blocking attachment of aminoacyl-tRNA to the catalytic site of the enzyme and subsequent transfer of the growing peptide chain. Type B streptogramins occupy an adjacent site on the ribosome and prevent formation of the peptide bond, leading to the premature release of incomplete polypeptides.[13] Type A molecules bind to free ribosomes, but not to polysomes engaged in protein synthesis, whereas type B can prevent further synthesis during active synthesis. The bactericidal synergy between the two components arises mainly from conformational changes induced by Type A molecules that improve the binding affinity of Type B compounds.[14]

Fusidic acid

Fusidic acid forms a stable complex with an elongation factor (EF-G) involved in translocation and with guanosine triphosphate (GTP), which provides energy for the translocation process. One round of translocation occurs, with hydrolysis of GTP, but the fusidic acid–EF–G–GDP–ribosome complex blocks further chain elongation, leaving peptidyl-tRNA in the P site.

Although protein synthesis in Gram-negative bacilli – and, indeed, mammalian cells – is susceptible to fusidic acid, the antibiotic penetrates poorly into these cells and the spectrum of action is virtually restricted to Gram-positive bacteria, notably staphylococci.

Oxazolidinones

Linezolid and other oxazolidinones are bacteriostatic agents that act at an earlier stage than other inhibitors of protein synthesis. They prevent the process by which the 50S ribosomal subunit and the 30S unit (charged with mRNA and fMet-tRNA) come together to form the 70S initiation complex.[15,16] This is achieved by binding to the 50S subunit, at a site close to that of chloramphenicol and lincosamides.[17]

Mupirocin

Mupirocin also has a unique mode of action. The epoxide-containing monic acid tail of the molecule (*see* p. 326) is an analog of isoleucine and, as such, is a competitive inhibitor of isoleucyl-tRNA synthetase in bacterial cells.[18] It may be a bifunctional inhibitor of the synthetase, since it also binds to the ATP-binding site of the enzyme.[19] The corresponding mammalian enzyme is unaffected.

INHIBITORS OF NUCLEIC ACID SYNTHESIS

Compounds that bind directly to the double helix are generally highly toxic to mammalian cells and only a few – those that interfere with DNA-associated enzymic processes – exhibit sufficient selectivity for systemic use as antibacterial agents. These compounds include antibacterial quinolones, novobiocin and rifampicin (rifampin). Diaminopyrimidines, sulfonamides, 5-nitroimidazoles and (probably) nitrofurans also affect DNA synthesis and will be considered under this heading.

Quinolones

The problem of packaging the enormous circular chromosome of bacteria (>1 mm long) into a microscopic cell, while making adequate arrangements for transcription and replication, has necessitated some considerable ingenuity on the part of the microbe. The solution has been to condense the DNA down and to twist it into a 'supercoiled' state – a process aided by the natural strain imposed on a covalently closed double helix. The twists are introduced in the opposite sense to those of the double helix itself and the molecule is said to be negatively supercoiled. Relaxation and re-establishment of the supercoiled state involves precisely regulated nicking and resealing of the DNA strands, accomplished by enzymes called topoisomerases. One topoisomerase, DNA gyrase, is a tetramer composed of two pairs of α and β subunits, and the primary target of the action of nalidixic acid and other quinolones is the α subunit of DNA gyrase, although another enzyme, topoisomerase IV, is also affected.[20] Indeed, in Gram-positive bacteria, topoisomerase IV seems to be the main target.[21] This enzyme does not have supercoiling activity; it appears to be involved in relaxation of the DNA chain and chromosomal segregation. Fortunately, the corresponding mammalian topoisomerases are less susceptible to quinolone attack.

Curiously, the coumarin antibiotic novobiocin, which acts in a complementary fashion by binding specifically to the β-subunit of DNA gyrase, displays an exactly opposite spectrum of activity to that of nalidixic acid.

Rifampicin

Rifampicin and other compounds of the ansamycin group specifically inhibit DNA-dependent RNA polymerase; that is, they prevent the transcription of RNA species from the DNA template. Rifampicin is an extremely efficient inhibitor of the bacterial enzyme, but fortunately eukaryotic RNA polymerase is not affected. RNA polymerase consists of a core enzyme made up of four polypeptide subunits, and rifampicin specifically binds to the β subunit. However, since isolated β subunit does not bind rifampicin, the precise configuration in which it is locked into the core enzyme is important.

Sulfonamides and diaminopyrimidines

These agents act at separate stages in the pathway of folic acid synthesis and thus act indirectly on DNA synthesis, since the active form of the co-enzyme, tetrahydrofolic acid, serves as intermediate in the transfer of methyl, formyl and other single-carbon fragments in the biosynthesis of purine nucleotides and thymidylic acid, as well as of some amino acids.

Sulfonamides are analogs of p-aminobenzoic acid. They competitively inhibit dihydropteroate synthetase, the enzyme which condenses p-aminobenzoic acid with dihydropteroic acid in the early stages of folic acid synthesis. Most bacteria need to synthesize folic acid and cannot use exogenous sources of the vitamin. Mammalian cells, in contrast, require preformed folate and this is the basis of the selective action of sulfonamides. The antileprotic sulfone dapsone, and the antituberculosis drug p-aminosalicylic acid, act in a similar way; the basis for their restricted spectrum may reside in differences of affinity for variant forms of dihydropteroate synthetase in the bacteria against which they act.

Diaminopyrimidines act later in the pathway of folate synthesis. These compounds inhibit dihydrofolate reductase, the enzyme that generates the active form of the co-enzyme tetrahydrofolic acid. In most of the reactions in which tetrahydrofolate takes part it remains unchanged, but in the biosynthesis of thymidylic acid tetrahydrofolate acts as hydrogen donor as well as a methyl group carrier and is thus oxidized to dihydrofolic acid in the process. Dihydrofolate reductase is therefore crucial in recycling tetrahydrofolate, and diaminopyrimidines act relatively quickly to halt bacterial growth. Sulfonamides, in contrast, cut off the supply of folic acid at source and act slowly, since the existing folate pool can satisfy the needs of the cell for several generations.

The selective toxicity of diaminopyrimidines comes about because of differential affinity of these compounds for dihydrofolate reductase from various sources. Thus trimethoprim has a vastly greater affinity for the bacterial enzyme than for its mammalian counterpart, pyrimethamine exhibits a particularly high affinity for the plasmodial version of the enzyme and, in keeping with its anticancer activity, methotrexate has high affinity for the enzyme found in mammalian cells.

5-Nitroimidazoles

The most intensively investigated compound in this group is metronidazole, but other 5-nitroimidazoles are thought to act in a similar manner. Metronidazole siphons off electrons from ferredoxin (or other electron transfer proteins with low redox potential) causing the nitro group of the drug to be reduced. It is this reduced and highly reactive intermediate that is responsible for the antimicrobial effect, probably by binding to DNA, which undergoes strand breakage.[22] The requirement for interaction with low redox systems restricts the activity largely to anaerobic bacteria and certain protozoa that exhibit anaerobic metabolism. The basis for activity against micro-aerophilic species such as *Helicobacter pylori* and *Gardnerella vaginalis* remains speculative, though a novel nitroreductase, which is altered in metronidazole-resistant strains, is implicated in *H. pylori*.[23]

Nitrofurans

As with nitroimidazoles, the reduction of the nitro group of nitrofurantoin and other nitrofurans is a prerequisite for antibacterial activity. Micro-organisms with appropriate nitroreductases act on nitrofurans to produce a highly reactive electrophilic intermediate and this is postulated to affect DNA as the reduced intermediates of nitroimidazoles do. Other evidence suggests that the reduced nitrofurans bind to bacterial ribosomes and prevent protein synthesis;[24] inducible enzyme synthesis seems to be particularly susceptible. An effect on DNA has the virtue of explaining the known mutagenicity of these compounds in vitro and any revised mechanism relating to inhibition of protein synthesis needs to be reconciled with this property.

AGENTS AFFECTING MEMBRANE PERMEABILITY

Agents acting on cell membranes do not normally discriminate between microbial and mammalian membranes, although the fungal cell membrane has proved more amenable to selective attack (*see below*). The only membrane-active antibacterial agents to be administered systemically in human medicine, polymyxin B (now rarely used systemically) and the closely related compound colistin (polymyxin E), act like cationic detergents; they disrupt the cytoplasmic membrane of the cell, probably by attacking the exposed phosphate groups of the membrane phospholipid. They also have an effect on the external membrane of Gram-negative bacilli, which might explain their preferential action on these organisms. The end result is leakage of cytoplasmic contents and death of the cell. Various factors, including growth phase and incubation temperature, alter the balance of fatty acids within the bacterial cell membrane, and this can concomitantly affect the response to polymyxins.[25]

Several antibiotics, known collectively as ionophores, interfere with cation transport in cell membranes. These include the topical antibiotic gramicidin A, and some agents used in veterinary medicine, such as the macrotetralide monensin and the depsipeptide valinomycin. Naturally occurring antimicrobial peptides, such as the cecropins, magainins and defensins, as well as the lanthionine-containing lantibiotics, disrupt cell membranes, sometimes in a selective manner; some of these peptides appear to form aggregates with ionophoric properties.[26,27]

In view of the scarcity of antibacterial agents acting on the cytoplasmic membrane, it is surprising to find that the most successful groups of antifungal agents – the polyenes, azoles, and allylamines – all achieve their effects in this way.[28,29] However, the echinocandins, the latest addition to the antifungal armamentarium, differ in affecting the fungal cell wall.

POLYENES

The polyenes bind only to membranes containing sterols; ergosterol, the predominant sterol of fungal membranes, appears to be particularly susceptible. The effect is to make the membrane leaky, probably by the formation of transmembrane pores. Since bacterial cell membranes (except those of mycoplasmas) do not contain sterols, they are unaffected by polyenes, even in high concentration; unfortunately, this immunity does not extend to sterol-containing mammalian cells, and polyenes consequently exhibit a low therapeutic index.

AZOLES

The activity of the antifungal azoles is also dependent on the presence of ergosterol in the fungal cell membrane. These compounds block ergosterol synthesis by interfering with the demethylation of its precursor, lanosterol.[30] Lanosterol demethylase is a cytochrome P_{450} enzyme and, although azole antifungals have much less influence on analogous mammalian systems, some of the side effects are attributable to such action.

Antifungal azole derivatives are predominantly fungistatic but some compounds, notably miconazole and clotrimazole, kill fungi at concentrations higher than those which merely inhibit growth, apparently by causing direct membrane damage. Other, less well characterized, effects of azoles on fungal respiration have also been described.[31]

ALLYLAMINES

The antifungal allylamine derivatives terbinafine and naftifine inhibit squalene epoxidase, another enzyme involved in the biosynthesis of ergosterol.[32] The fungicidal effect may be due to accumulation of squalene rather than a deficiency of ergosterol. In *Candida albicans* the effect is fungistatic and the yeast form is less susceptible than is mycelial growth. In this species there is less accumulation of squalene than in dermatophytes, and ergosterol deficiency may be the limiting factor.[33]

ECHINOCANDINS

Caspofungin and related compounds inhibit the formation of glucan, an essential polysaccharide of the cell wall of many fungi, including *Pneumocystis carinii*. The vulnerable enzyme is β-1,3-glucan synthase, which is located in the cell membrane.[34]

FLUCYTOSINE

The spectrum of activity of flucytosine (5-fluorocytosine) is virtually restricted to yeasts. In these fungi flucytosine is transported into the cell by a cytosine permease; a cytosine deaminase then converts flucytosine to 5-fluorouracil, which is incorporated into RNA in place of uracil, leading to the formation of abnormal proteins. There is also an effect on DNA synthesis through inhibition of thymidylate synthetase.[35]

GRISEOFULVIN

The antidermatophyte antibiotic griseofulvin binds to the microtubules of the mitotic spindle, interfering with their assembly and function. However, the precise mechanism of action and the basis of the selectivity remain to be elucidated.

ANTIPROTOZOAL AGENTS

The actions of some antiprotozoal drugs overlap with, or are analogous to, those seen with the antibacterial and antifungal agents already discussed. Thus, the activity of 5-nitroimidazoles such as metronidazole extends to those protozoa that exhibit an essentially anaerobic metabolism; the antimalarial agents pyrimethamine and cycloguanil (the metabolic product of proguanil), like trimethoprim, inhibit dihydrofolate reductase; some polyenes and antifungal imidazoles display sufficient activity against *Leishmania* and certain other protozoa for them to have received attention as potential therapeutic agents.

There seems to be deep uncertainty about how other antiprotozoal agents actually work. Various sites of action have been ascribed to many of them and, with a few notable exceptions, the literature reveals only desultory attempts to pin down the primary target.

ANTIMALARIAL AGENTS

Quinoline antimalarials

Quinine and the various quinoline antimalarials were once thought to achieve their effect by intercalation with plasmodial DNA after concentration in parasitized erythrocytes. However, these effects occur only at concentrations in excess of those achieved in vivo; moreover, a non-specific effect on DNA does not explain the selective action of these compounds at precise points in the plasmodial life cycle, or the differential activity of antimalarial quinolines.

Clarification of the mode of action of these compounds has proved elusive, but it now seems likely that chloroquine and related compounds act primarily by inhibiting heme polymerase, thus preventing detoxification of ferriprotoporphyrin IX (heme), which is produced from the red cell hemoglobin in the food vacuole of the parasites.[36] Ferriprotoporphyrin IX is a toxic metabolite which is normally rendered innocuous by polymerization; malarial pigment consists of granules of this polymer.

Chloroquine achieves a very high concentration within the food vacuole of the parasite and this greatly aids its activity. However, quinine and mefloquine are not concentrated to the same extent, and have much less effect on heme polymerization, raising the possibility that other (possibly multiple) targets are involved in the action of these compounds.[37,38]

8-Aminoquinolines like primaquine, which, at therapeutically useful concentrations exhibit selective activity against liver-stage parasites and gametocytes, possibly inhibit mitochondrial enzyme systems after undergoing hepatic metabolism. However, the precise mechanism of action is unknown.

Artemisinin

Artemisinin, the active principle of the Chinese herbal remedy qinghaosu, has several effects on malaria parasites, but the activity appears to be due chiefly to the reactivity of the endoperoxide bridge. This is cleaved in the presence of heme or free iron within the parasitized red cell to form a short-lived, but highly reactive, free radical that irreversibly alkylates malaria proteins.[39]

Atovaquone

The hydroxynaphthoquinone atovaquone, which exhibits antimalarial and antipneumocystis activity, is an electron transport inhibitor that causes depletion of the ATP pool. The primary effect is on the iron flavoprotein dihydro-orotate dehydrogenase, an essential enzyme in the production of pyrimidines. Mammalian cells are able to avoid undue toxicity by use of preformed pyrimidines.[40] Dihydro-orotate dehydrogenase from *Plasmodium falciparum* is inhibited by concentrations of atovaquone that are very much lower than those needed to inhibit the pneumocystis enzyme, raising the possibility that the antimicrobial consequences might differ in the two organisms.[41]

OTHER ANTIPROTOZOAL AGENTS

Arsenical compounds, which are still the mainstay of treatment of African sleeping sickness, poison the cell by an effect on glucose catabolism and are consequently very toxic to the host. The mechanism by which this is achieved and the basis for any selective action are not well understood, though they are known to bind to essential thiol groups. The primary target may be trypanothione, which substitutes for glutathione in trypanosomes, and this may aid the selective toxicity.[42]

The actions of other agents with antitrypanosomal activity, including suramin and pentamidine, are also poorly characterized.[43] Various cell processes, mainly those involved in glycolysis within the specialized glycosomes of protozoa of the trypanosome family, have been implicated in the action of suramin.[44] Pentamidine and other diamidines disrupt the trypanosomal kinetoplast, a specialized DNA-containing organelle, probably by binding to DNA, though they also interfere with polyamine synthesis.[45]

Laboratory studies of leishmania are hampered by the fact that in-vitro culture yields promastigotes that are morphologically and metabolically different from the amastigotes involved in disease. Such evidence as is available suggests that the pentavalent antimonials commonly used for treatment inhibit glycolysis in leishmanial glycosomes. Antifungal azoles take advantage of similarities in sterol biosynthesis among fungi and leishmanial amastigotes.[46]

Eflornithine (difluoromethylornithine) is a selective inhibitor of ornithine decarboxylase and achieves its effect by depleting the biosynthesis of polyamines such as spermidine, a precursor of trypanothione.[47] The corresponding mammalian enzyme has a much shorter half-life than its trypanosomal counterpart, and this may account for the apparent selectivity of action. The preferential activity against *Trypanosoma brucei gambiense* rather than the related *rhodesiense* form may be due to reduced drug uptake or differences in polyamine metabolism in the latter subspecies.[48]

Several of the drugs used in amebiasis, including the plant alkaloid emetine and diloxanide furoate appear to interfere with protein synthesis within amebic trophozoites or cysts.[49]

ANTHELMINTIC AGENTS

Just as the cell wall of bacteria is a prime target for selective agents and the cell membrane is peculiarly vulnerable in fungi, so the neuromuscular system appears to be the Achilles' heel of parasitic worms. Despite the fact that present understanding of the neurobiology of helminths is extremely meagre, a considerable number of anthelmintic agents have been shown to work by paralysing the neuromusculature in various ways. Such compounds include piperazine, praziquantel, levamisole, pyrantel pamoate, ivermectin, metrifonate (trichlorfon) and dichlorovos.[50–52] Praziquantel induces schistosomes to disengage from their intravascular attachment site and migrate to the liver, but there is also a profound effect on schistosome metabolism and disruption of the tegument, causing exposure of parasite antigens. All these effects appear to be referable to alterations in calcium homeostasis.[53]

A notable exception to the general rule that anthelmintic agents act on the neuromuscular systems of worms is provided by the benzimidazole derivatives, including mebendazole and albendazole. These broad-spectrum anthelmintic drugs seem to have at least two effects on adult worms and larvae: inhibition of the uptake of the chief energy source, glucose;

and binding to tubulin, the structural protein of microtubules.[54]

The basis of the activity of the antifilarial drug diethylcarbamazine has long been a puzzle, since the drug has no effect on microfilaria in vitro. Consequently it seems likely that the effect of drug observed in vivo is due to alterations in the surface coat, making them responsive to immunological processes from which they are normally protected.[55] The source of its effect on adult filarial worms is unknown.

ANTIVIRAL AGENTS

The prospects for the development of selectively toxic antiviral agents were long thought to be poor, since the life cycle of the virus is so closely bound to normal cellular processes. However, closer scrutiny of the relationship of the virus to the cell reveals several points at which the viral cycle might be interrupted.[56] These include:

- Adsorption to and penetration of the cell.
- Uncoating of the viral nucleic acid.
- The various stages of nucleic acid replication.
- Assembly of the new viral particles.
- Release of infectious virions (if the cell is not destroyed).

NUCLEOSIDE ANALOGS

In the event, it is the process of viral replication (which is extremely rapid relative to most mammalian cells) that has proved to be the most vulnerable point of attack, and most clinically useful antiviral agents are nucleoside analogs. Among these, only aciclovir (acycloguanosine) and penciclovir (the active product of the oral agent famciclovir) exhibit a genuine selectivity. In order to achieve their antiviral effect, nucleoside analogs have to be converted within the cell to the triphosphate derivative. In the case of aciclovir and penciclovir the initial phosphorylation, yielding aciclovir or penciclovir monophosphate, is accomplished by a thymidine kinase coded for by the virus itself. The corresponding cellular thymidine kinase phosphorylates these compounds very inefficiently and consequently only cells harboring the virus are affected. Moreover, the triphosphates of aciclovir and penciclovir inhibit viral DNA polymerase more efficiently than the cellular enzyme; this is another feature of their selective activity. As well as inhibiting viral DNA polymerase, aciclovir and penciclovir triphosphates are incorporated into the growing DNA chain and cause premature termination of DNA synthesis.

Other nucleoside analogs, including the anti-HIV agents zidovudine, didanosine, zalcitabine, stavudine, lamivudine and abacavir, and the anti-cytomegalovirus agents ganciclovir and valganciclovir, act in a non-specific manner because they are phosphorylated by cellular enzymes and/or are less selective for viral versus host cell enzymes. Ribavirin is also a nucleoside analog that acts through the inosine monophosphate pathway. The anti-HIV compounds are thought to act primarily to inhibit reverse transcriptase activity by causing premature chain termination during the transcription of DNA from the single-stranded RNA template. Similarly, ganciclovir acts as a chain terminator and DNA polymerase inhibitor during the transcription of cytomegalovirus DNA. Since these compounds lack a hydroxyl group on the deoxyribose ring, they are unable to form phosphodiester linkages in the DNA chain.[57] Ribavirin, in contrast, allows DNA synthesis to occur, but prevents the formation of viral proteins, probably by interfering with capping of viral mRNA.[58] In vitro, ribavirin antagonizes the action of zidovudine, probably by feedback inhibition of thymidine kinase so that the zidovudine is not phosphorylated.[59]

NON-NUCLEOSIDE REVERSE TRANSCRIPTASE INHIBITORS

Although they are structurally unrelated, the non-nucleoside reverse transcriptase inhibitors nevirapine, delavirdine, and efavirenz (p. 480) all bind to HIV-1 reverse transcriptase in a non-competitive fashion.

PROTEASE INHIBITORS

An alternative tactic to disable HIV is to inhibit the enzyme that cleaves the polypeptide precursor of several essential viral proteins.[60] Such protease inhibitors in therapeutic use include saquinavir, ritonavir, indinavir, nelfinavir, amprenavir and lopinavir/ritonavir (see Chapter 39).

NUCLEOTIDE ANALOGS

One nucleotide analog is licensed for the treatment of cytomegalovirus disease in AIDS patients: hydroxy-propoxymethyl cytosine (cidofovir). It is phosphorylated by cellular kinases to the triphosphate derivative, which then becomes a competitive inhibitor of DNA polymerase.

PHOSPHONIC ACID DERIVATIVES

The simple phosphonoformate salt foscarnet and its close analog phosphonoacetic acid inhibit DNA polymerase activity of herpes viruses by preventing pyrophosphate exchange.[61] The action is selective in that the corresponding mammalian polymerase is much less susceptible to inhibition. Activity of foscarnet against HIV seems to be due to a different mechanism. Like the nucleoside analogs, it inhibits reverse transcriptase activity of retroviruses, but it binds to the enzyme at a site distinct from that of the nucleoside triphosphates. The effect is non-competitive and reversible.

AMANTADINE AND RIMANTIDINE

The anti-influenza A compound amantadine and its close relative rimantadine appear to act at the stage of viral uptake by preventing membrane fusion; these compounds also interfere with virus disassembly. Both effects may be due to specific interaction of the drugs with a membrane-associated protein of the virus.[62,63]

NEURAMINIDASE INHIBITORS

Two drugs target the neuraminidase of influenza A and B viruses: zanamivir and oseltamivir. Both directly bind to the neuraminidase enzyme and prevent the formation of infectious progeny virions.[64–66]

ANTISENSE DRUGS

Fomivirsen is the only licensed antisense oligonucleotide for the treatment of cytomegalovirus retinitis.[67] The nucleotide sequence of fomivirsen is complementary to a sequence in the messenger RNA transcript of the major immediate early region 2 of cytomegalovirus, which is essential for production of infectious virus. The binding is reversible.

 Further information

Detailed information on the mode of action of anti-infective agents can be found in the following sources:

Campbell WC, Few RS (eds) 1986 *Chemotherapy of parasitic disease*. Plenum, New York.

Dax SL 1997 *Antibacterial chemotherapeutic agents*. Blackie Academic, London.

Franklin TJ, Snow GA 1998 Biochemistry and molecular biology of antimicrobial action, 5th edn. Kluwer Academic Publishers, Dordrecht.

Frayha GJ, Smyth JD, Gobert JG, Savel J 1997 The mechanism of action of antiprotozoal and anthelmintic drugs in man. *General Pharmacology* 28: 273–299.

Gale EF, Cundliffe E, Reynolds PE, Richmond MH, Waring MJ 1981 *The molecular basis of antibiotic action*, 2nd edn. Wiley, Chichester.

Greenwood D, O'Grady F (eds) 1985 *The scientific basis of antimicrobial chemotherapy*. Cambridge University Press, Cambridge.

James DH, Gilles HM 1985 *Human antiparasitic drugs: Pharmacology and usage*. Wiley, Chichester.

Rosenthal PJ (ed) 2001 *Antimalarial Chemotherapy: mechanisms of action, resistance, and new directions*. Humana Press, Totowa, New Jersey.

Lancini G, Parenti F, Gallo G-C 1995 *Antibiotics: a multidisciplinary approach*. Plenum, New York.

Russell AD, Chopra I 1996 *Understanding antibacterial action and resistance*, 2nd edn. Ellis Horwood, London.

Scholar EM, Pratt WB 2000 *The antimicrobial drugs* 2nd edn. Oxford University Press, Oxford.

Williams RAD, Lambert PA, Singleton P 1996 *Antimicrobial drug action*. βios Scientific Publishers, Oxford.

References

1. Hancock REW, Bellido F 1992 Antibiotic uptake: unusual results for unusual molecules. *Journal of Antimicrobial Chemotherapy* 29: 235–239.

2. Lichtenthaler H 2000 Non-mevalonate isoprenoid biosynthesis: enzymes, genes and inhibitors. *Biochemical Society Transactions* 28: 785–789.

3. Kuzuyama T, Shimizu T, Takahashi S, Seto H 1998 Fosmidomycin, a specific inhibitor of 1-deoxy-D-xylose 5-phosphate reductoisomerase in the non-mevalonate pathway for terienoid biosynthesis. *Tetrahedron Letters* 39: 7913–7916.

4. Arthur M, Reynolds PE, Depardieu F et al 1993 Mechanisms of glycopeptide resistance in enterococci. *Journal of Infection* 32: 11–16.

5. Greenwood D, O'Grady F 1973 The two sites of penicillin action in *Escherichia coli. Journal of Infectious Diseases* 128: 791–794.

6. Handwerger S, Tomasz A 1985 Antibiotic tolerance among clinical isolates of bacteria. *Reviews of Infectious Diseases* 7: 368–386.

7. Brennan PJ, Nikaido H 1995 The envelope of mycobacteria. *Annual Review of Biochemistry* 64: 29–63.

8. Chopra I, Brennan P 1998 Molecular action of antimycobacterial agents. *Tubercle and Lung Disease* 78: 89–98.

9. Chopra I, Hawkey PM, Hinton M 1992 Tetracyclines, molecular and clinical aspects. *Journal of Antimicrobial Chemotherapy* 29: 245–277.

10. Tai PC, Davis BD 1985 The actions of antibiotics on the ribosome. In: Greenwood D, O'Grady F (eds) *The scientific basis of antimicrobial chemotherapy.* Cambridge University Press, Cambridge, p. 41–68.

11. Davis BD 1988 The lethal action of aminoglycosides. *Journal of Antimicrobial Chemotherapy* 22: 1–3.

12. Davis BD 1987 Mechanism of bactericidal action of aminoglycosides. *Microbiological Reviews* 51: 341–350.

13. Cocito C, Di Giambattista M, Nyssen E, Vannuffel P 1997 Inhibition of protein synthesis by streptogramins and related antibiotics. *Journal of Antimicrobial Chemotherapy* 39 (Suppl. A): 7–13.

14. Vannuffel P, Cocito C 1996 Mechanism of action of streptogramins and macrolides. *Drugs* 51 (Suppl. 1): 20–30.

15. Shinabarger DL, Marotti KR, Murray RW et al 1997 Mechanism of action of oxazolidinones: effect of linezolid and eperezolid on translation reactions. *Antimicrobial Agents and Chemotherapy* 41: 2132–2136.

16. Swaney SM, Aoki H, Ganoza MC, Shinabarger DL 1998 The oxazolidinone linezolid inhibits initiation of protein synthesis in bacteria. *Antimicrobial Agents and Chemotherapy* 42: 3251–3255.

17. Lin AH, Murray RW, Vidmar TJ, Marotti KR 1997 The oxazolidinone eperezolid binds to the 50S ribosomal subunit and competes with binding of chloramphenicol and lincomycin. *Antimicrobial Agents and Chemotherapy* 41: 2127–2131.

18. Parenti MA, Hatfield SM, Leyden JJ 1987 Mupirocin: a topical antibiotic with a unique structure and mode of action. *Clinical Pharmacology* 6: 761–770.

19. Yanagisawa T, Lee JT, Wu HC, Kawakami M 1994 Relationship of protein structure of isoleucyl-tRNA synthetase with pseudomonic acid resistance of *Escherichia coli.* A proposed mode of action of pseudomonic acid as an inhibitor of isoleucyl-tRNA synthetase. *Journal of Biological Chemistry* 269: 24304–24309.

20. Hooper DC 1995 Quinolone mode of action. *Drugs* 49 (Suppl. 2): 10–15.

21. Ng EYW, Trucksis M, Hooper DC 1996 Quinolone resistance mutations in topoisomerase IV: relationship to the *flqA* locus and genetic evidence that topoisomerase IV is the primary target and DNA gyrase is the secondary target of fluoroquinolones in *Staphylococcus aureus. Antimicrobial Agents and Chemotherapy* 40: 1881–1888.

22. Edwards DI 1993 Nitroimidazole drugs – action and resistance mechanisms. I. Mechanisms of action. *Journal of Antimicrobial Chemotherapy* 31: 9–20.

23. Goodwin A, Kersulyte D, Sisson G et al 1998 Metronidazole resistance in *Helicobacter pylori* is due to null mutations in a gene (*rdxA*) that encodes the oxygen-insensitive NADPH nitroreductase. *Molecular Microbiology* 28: 383–393.

24. McOsker CC, Fitzpatrick PM 1994 Nitrofurantoin: mechanism of action and implications for resistance development in common uropathogens. *Journal of Antimicrobial Chemotherapy* 33 (Suppl. A): 23–30.

25. Gilleland HE, Champlin FR, Conrad RS 1984 Chemical alterations in cell envelopes of *Pseudomonas aeruginosa* upon exposure to polymyxin: a possible mechanism to explain adaptive resistance to polymyxin. *Canadian Journal of Microbiology* 20: 869–873.

26. Boman HG, Marsh J, Goode JA (eds) 1994 *Antimicrobial peptides.* Ciba Foundation Symposium 186. Wiley, Chichester.

27. Boman HG 2000 Innate immunity and the normal microflora. *Immunological Reviews* 173: 5–16.

28. Elewski BE 1993 Mechanisms of action of systemic antifungal agents. *Journal of the American Academy of Dermatology* 28: S28–S34.

29. Ghannoum MA, Rice LB 1999 Antifungal agents: mode of action, mechanisms of resistance, and correlation of these mechanisms with bacterial resistance. *Clinical Microbiology Reviews* 12: 501–517.

30. Borgers M 1985 Antifungal azole derivatives. In: Greenwood D, O'Grady F (eds) *The scientific basis of antimicrobial chemotherapy.* Cambridge University Press, Cambridge, p. 133–153.

31. Fromtling RA 1988 Overview of medically important antifungal azole derivatives. *Clinical Microbiology Reviews* 1: 187–217.

32. Stütz A 1990 Allylamine derivatives – inhibitors of fungal squalene epoxidase. In: Borowski E, Shugar D (eds) *Molecular aspects of chemotherapy.* Pergamon, New York, p. 205–213.

33. Ryder NS 1989 The mode of action of terbinafine. *Clinical and Experimental Dermatology* 14: 98–100.

34. Georgopapadakou NH 2001 Update on antifungals targeted to the cell wall: focus on beta-1,3-glucan synthase inhibitors. *Expert Opinion in Investigational Drugs* 10: 269–280.

35. Odds FC 1988 *Candida and candidosis.* Baillière Tindall, London, p. 305–306.

36. Slater AFG, Cerami A 1992 Inhibition by chloroquine of a novel haem polymerase enzyme activity in malaria trophozoites. *Nature* 355: 167–169.

37. Foote SJ, Cowman AF 1994 The mode of action and the mechanism of resistance to antimalarial drugs. *Acta Tropica* 56: 157–171.

38. Foley M, Tilley L 1998 Quinoline antimalarials: mechanisms of action and resistance and prospects for new agents. *Pharmacology and Therapeutics* 79: 55–87.

39. Meshnick SR, Taylor TE, Kamchonwongpaison S 1996 Artemisinin and the antimalarial endoperoxides: from herbal remedy to targeted chemotherapy. *Microbiological Reviews* 60: 301–315.

40. Artymowicz RJ, James VE 1993 Atovaquone: a new antipneumocystis agent. *Clinical Pharmacy* 12: 563–569.

41. Ittarat I, Asawamahasakada W, Bartlett MS, Smith JW, Meshnick SR 1995 Effects of atovaquone and other inhibitors on *Pneumocystis carinii* dihydroorotate dehydrogenase. *Antimicrobial Agents and Chemotherapy* 39: 325–328.

42. Fairlamb AH, Henderson GB, Cerami A 1989 Trypanothione is the primary target for arsenical drugs against African trypanosomes. *Proceedings of the National Academy of Sciences, USA* 86: 2607–2611.

43. Denise H, Barrett MP 2001 Uptake and mode of action of drugs used against sleeping sickness. *Biochemical Pharmacology* 61: 1–5.

44. Voogd TE, Vansterkenburg ELM, Wilting J, Janssen LHM 1993 Recent research on the biological activity of suramin. *Pharmacological Reviews* 45: 177–203.

45. Sands M, Kron MA, Brown RB 1985 Pentamidine: a review. *Reviews of Infectious Diseases* 7: 625–635.

46. Berman JD 1988 Chemotherapy for leishmaniasis: biochemical mechanisms, clinical efficacy and future strategies. *Clinical Infectious Diseases* 10: 560–586.

47. McCann PP, Bacchi CJ, Clarkson AB et al 1986 Inhibition of polyamine biosynthesis by α-difluoromethylornithine in African trypanosomes and *Pneumocystis carinii* as a basis for chemotherapy: biochemical and clinical aspects. *American Journal of Tropical Medicine and Hygiene* 35: 1153–1156.

48. Bacchi CJ 1993 Resistance to clinical drugs in African trypanosomes *Parasitology Today* 9: 190–193.

49. Khaw M, Panosian CB 1995 Human antiprotozoal therapy: past, present and future. *Clinical Microbiology Reviews* 8: 427–439.

50. Fisher MH, Mrozik H 1992 The chemistry and pharmacology of avermectins. *Annual Review of Pharmacology and Toxicology* 32: 537–553.

51. Geary TG, Klein RD, Vanover L, Bowman JW, Thompson DP 1992 The nervous systems of helminths as targets for drugs. *Journal of Parasitology* 78: 215–230.

52. Rosenblatt JE 1992 Antiparasitic agents. *Mayo Clinic Proceedings* 67: 276–287.

53. Day TA, Bennett JL, Pax RA 1992 Praziquantel: the enigmatic antiparasitic. *Parasitology Today* 8: 342–344.

54. Lacey E 1990 The mode of action of benzimidazoles. *Parasitology Today* 6: 112–115.

55. Hawking F 1981 Chemotherapy for filariasis. *Antibiotics and Chemotherapy* 30: 135–162.

56. Crumpacker CS 1989 Molecular targets of antiviral therapy. *New England Journal of Medicine* 321: 163–172.

57. Lipsky JJ 1993 Zalcitabine and didanosine. *Lancet* 341: 30–32.

58. Hall CB 1987 Ribavirin. In: Peterson PK, Verhoef J (eds) *The antimicrobial agents annual – 2.* Elsevier, Amsterdam, p. 351–362.

59. Vogt MW, Hartshom KL, Furman PA et al 1987 Ribavirin antagonizes the effect of azidothymidine on HIV replication. *Science* 235: 1376–1379.

60. Debouck C 1992 The HIV-1 protease as a therapeutic target for AIDS. *AIDS Research and Human Retroviruses* 8: 153–164.

61. Crumpacker CS 1992 Mechanism of action of foscarnet against viral polymerases. *American Journal of Medicine* 92 (Suppl. 2A): 2A-35–2A-75.

62. Hay AJ, Wolstenholme AJ, Skehel JJ, Smith MH 1985 The molecular basis of the specific anti-influenza action of amantadine. *EMBO Journal* 4: 3021–3024.

63. Skehel JJ 1992 Amantadine blocks the channel. *Nature* 358: 110–111.

64. Waghorn SL, Goa KL 1998 Zanamivir. *Drugs* 55: 721–725.

65. Bardsley-Elliot A, Noble S 1999 Oseltamivir *Drugs* 58: 851–860.

66. Shitara E, Nishimura Y, Nerome K et al 2000 Synthesis of 6-acetamido-5-amino- and 5-guanidino-3, 4-dehydro-N-(2-ethylbutyrul)-3-piperideinecarboxylic acids related to zanamivir and oseltamivir, inhibitors of influenza virus neuraminidases. *Organic Letters* 2: 3837–3840.

67. Perry CM, Balfour JA 1999 Fomivirsen. *Drugs* 57: 375–380.

3 The problem of resistance

Marc J. Struelens

Antibiotic resistance is widespread and increasing worldwide at an accelerating pace, reducing the efficacy of therapy for many infections, fuelling transmission of epidemic pathogens and majoring health costs, morbidity and mortality related to infectious diseases.[1] This public health threat has been recognized as a priority for intervention by health agencies at national and international level.[2,3] In this chapter we will address the definition of resistance, its biochemical mechanisms, genetic basis, prevalence in major human pathogens, epidemiology and strategies for control.

DEFINITION OF RESISTANCE

There is no consensus definition of bacterial resistance to antibiotics. This is related to two issues: first, the resistance may be defined either from a biological or from a clinical standpoint; secondly, different 'critical breakpoint' values are often selected by national reference committees for categorization of bacteria as resistant or susceptible in various countries. In spite of these differences of opinion, resistance definitions are based on in-vitro quantitative testing of bacterial susceptibility to antibacterial agents. This is typically achieved by determination of the minimal inhibitory concentration (MIC) of a drug; that is, the lowest concentration that inhibits visible growth of a standard inoculum of bacteria in a defined medium within a defined period of incubation (usually 18–24 hours) in a suitable atmosphere (Ch. 9).

According to the US National Committee for Clinical and Laboratory Standards (NCCLS), infecting bacteria are considered *susceptible* when they can be inhibited by achievable serum or tissue concentration using a dose of the antimicrobial agent recommended for that type of infection and pathogen.[4] This 'target concentration' will not only depend on pharmacokinetic and pharmacodynamic properties of the drug (Ch. 4) but also on recommended dose, which may vary from one country of registration to another. According to the European Society of Clinical Microbiology and Infectious Diseases Committee for Antimicrobial Susceptibility Testing (EUCAST)[5] the *microbiological definition* of susceptible or sensitive bacteria includes those that belong to the most susceptible subpopulations and lack (acquired) mechanisms of resistance, whereas the *clinical definition* of susceptible bacteria is those that have been shown to respond to a standard therapeutic regimen based on in-vitro susceptibility level. In the absence of this clinical information, the definition is based on a consensus interpretation of the antibiotic's in-vitro properties and pharmacokinetics. The clinically susceptible category may include fully susceptible bacteria and borderline susceptible, or moderately susceptible, bacteria which have acquired low-level resistance mechanism(s) (Figure 3.1).

Resistance as defined by the NCCLS includes bacteria that are not inhibited by the usually achievable systemic concentrations of the agent with normal dosage schedule *and/or* fall in the minimal inhibitory concentration ranges where specific resistance mechanisms are likely and clinical efficacy has not been reliable in treatment studies. *Clinical resistance* is defined by EUCAST as when infection is highly unlikely to respond even to maximum doses of a given antibiotic. EUCAST defines as *microbiologically resistant* bacteria that possess any resistance mechanism demonstrated either phenotypically or genotypically. Some experts[6] have suggested that any statistically significant, inheritable increase of MIC observed in bacterial strains above those of the fully susceptible population is a biologically important antibiotic resistance phenomenon.

The *intermediate susceptible* category is used for bacteria with an MIC that lies between the breakpoints for clinically susceptible and clinically resistant (EUCAST), and are inhibited by concentrations of the antimicrobial that is close to either the usually or the maximally achievable blood or tissue level and for which therapeutic response rate may be less predictable than for infection with susceptible strains (NCCLS). It also provides a technical buffer zone that should limit the probability of misclassification of bacteria in susceptible or resistant categories, taking into account the precision limits of the reference quantitative susceptibility test method, the MIC determination, or alternative test methods that correlate with it, including the disk diffusion test.

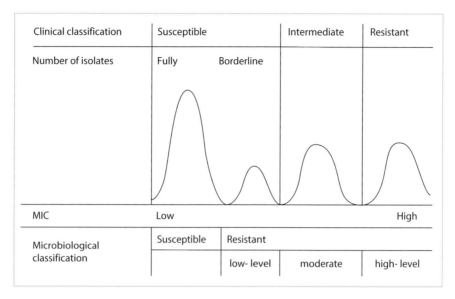

Fig. 3.1 Hypothetical distribution of MICs among clinical isolates of bacteria, classified clinically and microbiologically as susceptible or resistant. Adapted from EUCAST (2000).

Some strains of species that are normally inherently sensitive to an antibiotic may later *acquire* resistance to the drug. This phenomenon commonly arises when populations of bacteria have grown in the presence of the antibiotic which selects mutant strains that have increased their MIC by various adaptive mechanisms (*see below*). It may also result from horizontal gene transmission and acquisition of a resistance determinant, for example a β-lactamase, from a bacterial donor (see below). The range of MIC distribution of 'sensitive' and 'resistant' isolates of a given species may overlap and 'microbiologically resistant' strains may be classified as sensitive based on standard breakpoints. In such cases it will be necessary to demonstrate that some isolates have a resistance mechanism (see below) not present in others. This is particularly crucial if clinical studies demonstrate that such 'low-level resistant' strains are associated with an increased probability of treatment failure, as demonstrated for bacteremia caused by *Escherichia coli* and *Klebsiella pneumoniae* strains producing plasmid-mediated extended-spectrum β-lactamase treated with cephalosporins.[7]

Unfortunately, definitions that relate clinical response and microbiological susceptibility are less useful than might be expected because of the many confounding factors that may be present in patients. These range from relative differences of drug susceptibility dependent on the inoculum size and physiological state of bacteria grown in logarithmic phase in vitro versus those of biofilm-associated, stationary phase bacteria at the infecting site, limited distribution or reduced activity of the antibiotic in the infected site due to low pH or high protein binding, competence of phagocytic and immune response to the pathogen, presence of foreign body or undrained collections, to misidentification of the infective agent and straightforward sampling or testing error. In some infections there is a clear relationship between clinical success and in-vitro susceptibility, such as endocarditis, gonorrhea, meningitis, typhoid fever and even urinary tract infection, but clinical trials that would distinguish sensitive from resistant strains are unethical. In practice, much of the evidence on efficacy that is useful to refine breakpoints is gained post-marketing from observations of failures in patients treated empirically, from whom organisms are subsequently tested for antimicrobial susceptibility and demonstrate acquired resistance mechanisms. Recently, more systematic assessment of in-vitro activity on epidemiologically representative bacterial isolates and correlation of MIC value with treatment success in clinical trials has been required for antibiotic registration by regulatory agencies. Likewise, a process to periodically reassess the indications for registered antibiotics based on regional trends in resistance to the drug is being explored by these regulatory agencies.

From an early stage in the development of antibacterial agents it became clear that a knowledge of antibiotic pharmacokinetics and pharmacodynamics could be used to bolster the inadequate information gained from clinical use (Ch. 4). It is assumed that if an antibiotic reaches a concentration at the site of infection higher than the MIC for the infecting agent, the infection is likely to respond – at least to the extent possible in the presence of the other confounding factors discussed above. Depending on the antibiotic class, maximal antibacterial activity, defined not only by bacteristasis but including the killing rate, may be related either to the peak drug concentration over MIC ratio (as with the aminoglycosides) or to the proportion of the time interval between two doses when concentration is above the MIC (as with the β-lactams). Clearly, the antibiotic must be free to act at the site and not, for example, bound to protein and thus neutralized. Assays of antibiotics in sites of infection are complex both theoretically and practically: serum assays have been widely used as a proxy, even though there may be substantial intra- and interindividual variation depending on the patient pathophysiological conditions. For most antibiotics, this proxy has reasonable validity, but for some agents such as quinolones (Ch. 29) and newer macrolides such as azithromycin (Ch. 24) serum concentrations are considerably lower than those at the presumed site of infection and intracellular concentration may be an important predictor of efficacy against intracellular pathogens.

Different national committees have used different pharmacokinetic parameters in their correlations with pharmacodynamic characteristics. For example, the relevant serum concentration has variously been taken as the 'peak' concentration, the concentration midway between dosage, or various summations of concentrations under the concentration–time curve. The approach of the NCCLS has been based on wide consultation, and includes strong input from the antibiotic manufacturers. Their discussions usually lead to higher breakpoints, particularly for β-lactam antibiotics, than those used in Europe. Clearly, an international consensus on reference testing methods (EUCAST) and on susceptibility breakpoints is highly desirable, since it is confusing for a given strain to be labelled sensitive (or susceptible) in some countries and resistant in others.

MECHANISMS OF RESISTANCE

For an antimicrobial agent to be effective against a given micro-organism, two conditions must be met: a vital target susceptible to a low concentration of the antibiotic must exist in the micro-organism; the antibiotic must penetrate the bacterial envelope and reach the target in sufficient quantity.

There are five main mechanisms by which bacteria may circumvent the actions of antimicrobial agents:

- Specific enzymes may inactivate the drug before or after it enters the bacterial cell.
- The bacterial cell envelope may be modified so that it becomes less permeable to the antibiotic.
- The drug may be actively expelled from the cell by transmembrane efflux systems.
- The target may be modified so that it binds less avidly with the antibiotic.
- The target may be bypassed by acquisition of a novel metabolic pathway.

However, these resistance mechanisms do not exist in isolation, and two or more distinct mechanisms may interact to determine the actual level of resistance of a micro-organism to an antibiotic. Likewise, *multiple-drug resistance* is increasingly common in bacterial pathogens. It may be defined as resistance to two or more drugs or drug classes that are of therapeutic relevance, although more specific definitions apply to certain pathogens such as *Mycobacterium tuberculosis* (*see below*). Classically, *cross-resistance* is the term used for resistance to multiple drugs based on the same mechanism whereas *co-*resistance describes resistance to multiple antibiotics associated with multiple mechanisms in the same strain.

DRUG-MODIFYING ENZYMES

β-Lactamases

The most important mechanism of resistance to β-lactam antibiotics is the production of specific enzymes (β-lactamases). Over 340 β-lactamases with unique amino acid sequences or phenotype have been described from clinical isolates.[8] These enzymes bind to β-lactam antibiotics, usually via active serine sites, and the cyclic amide bonds of the β-lactam rings are hydrolyzed by the serine hydroxyl group. The open ring forms of β-lactams cannot bind to their target sites and thus have no antimicrobial activity. The ester linkage of the residual β-lactamase acylenzyme complex is usually readily hydrolyzed by water, regenerating the active enzyme. These enzymes have been classified based on functional and structural characteristics (*see* Table 17.1, p. 264).[9]

Among Gram-positive cocci, the only β-lactamase of major clinical significance is staphylococcal β-lactamase, which hydrolyses benzylpenicillin, ampicillin and related compounds, but is much less active against the antistaphylococcal penicillins and most cephalosporins. Among Gram-negative bacilli the situation is more complex, as these organisms produce many different β-lactamases with different spectra of activity (Table 3.1). All β-lactam drugs, including the latest cephems and carbapenems, are degraded by some of these enzymes, many of which have recently evolved through stepwise mutations selected in patients treated with cephalosporins.[10] Several groups of these β-lactamases are increasing in prevalence among Gram-negative pathogens in many parts of the world. The most widely dispersed are the group 2be extended-spectrum β-lactamases (ESBL) derived by mutational modifications from TEM and SHV enzymes. These ESBLs can hydrolyse most penicillins and all cephalosporins except the cephamycins. These enzymes are plasmid-mediated and can be produced by various Enterobacteriaceae, notably by *Klebsiella pneumoniae* strains that have caused hospital epidemics in all continents.[11] Another group of problematic β-lactamases is the group 1, which includes both the AmpC type, chromosomal, inducible cephalosporinases in *Enterobacter*, *Serratia*, *Citrobacter* and *Pseudomonas aeruginosa* and similar plasmid-mediated enzymes that are now spreading among Enterobacteriaceae such as *E. coli* and *K. pneumoniae*. Both hyperproduction of the chromosomal enzyme, often selected by cephalosporin therapy, and high-copy number plasmid-encoded enzymes are causing an increasing prevalence of resistance to all β-lactam drugs except some group 6 cephalosporins and carbapenems (*see* Chs 15 and 17). A third group of β-lactamases of emerging importance is the group 3 metalloenzymes that can hydrolyse all β-lactam drugs except monobactams. These β-lactamases, also called carbapenemases, include both diverse chromosomal enzymes found in aquatic bacteria such as *Stenotrophomonas maltophilia* and *Aeromonas hydrophila* and recently reported plasmid-mediated enzymes sporadically found in clinical isolates of *Pseudomonas aeruginosa*, *Acinetobacter* and Enterobacteriaceae in Asia and Europe.[12] Many anaerobic bacteria also produce β-lactamases, and this is the major mechanism of β-lactam antibiotic resistance in this group. The classification and properties of β-lactamases are described more fully in Chapter 17.

Aminoglycoside-modifying enzymes

Much of the resistance to aminoglycoside antibiotics observed in clinical isolates of Gram-negative bacilli and Gram-positive cocci is due to transferable plasmid-mediated enzymes that modify the amino groups or hydroxyl groups of the aminoglycoside molecule (*see* Ch. 14). The modified antibiotic molecules are unable to bind to the target protein in the ribosome. The genes encoding these enzymes are often transposable and in some cases have now transferred to the chromosome. These enzymes include many different types of acetyltransferases, phosphotransferases and nucleotidyl transferases, which vary greatly in their spectrum of activity and in the degree to which they inactivate different aminoglycosides (*see* Ch. 14).[13] Based on phylogenetic analysis, the origin of aminoglycoside modifying enzymes is believed to be aminoglycoside-producing streptomyces species. Certain aminoglycosides (such as amikacin and isepamicin) have been designed so that their three-dimensional structures prevent them from binding with many of these modifying enzymes, and organisms resistant to one of the earlier aminoglycosides by an enzymatic mechanism initially remained susceptible to amikacin. However, in recent years there has been a tendency for the amikacin-modifying 6′-acetyl-transferase to predominate and for multiply drug-resistant pathogens to acquire multiple modifying enzymes, often combined with additional mechanisms of resistance such as decreased uptake and active efflux (*see below*), rendering them resistant to all or most of the available aminoglycosides.

Chloramphenicol acetyltransferase

The major mechanism of acquired resistance to chloramphenicol in both Gram-positive and Gram-negative species is the production of a chloramphenicol acetyltransferase which converts the drug to either the monoacetate or diacetate. These derivatives are unable to bind to the bacterial 50S ribosomal subunit and thus cannot inhibit peptidyl transferase activity. There are several different types of chloramphenicol acetyltransferases produced by different bacterial species, and the enzymes are usually inducible in Gram-positive cocci and constitutive in Gram-negative bacilli. The gene is usually encoded on a plasmid or transposon and may transpose to the chromosome. Surprisingly, in view of the very limited use of chloramphenicol, resistance is not uncommon, even in *E. coli*, although it is most frequently seen in organisms that are also multiply resistant to other agents. In such species, resistance to chloramphenicol can be expressed as part of the MAR phenotype conferred by upregulation of AcrB multi-drug efflux system (*see below*).

Location and regulation of expression of drug-inactivating enzymes

In Gram-positive bacteria β-lactam antibiotics enter the cell easily because of the permeable cell wall, and β-lactamase is released freely from the cell. In *Staphylococcus aureus*, resistance to benzylpenicillin is caused by the release of β-lactamase into the extracellular environment, where it reduces the concentration of drug in the vicinity of the organism. This is a population phenomenon: a large inoculum of organisms is much more resistant than a small one. Furthermore, staphylococcal penicillinase is an inducible enzyme: up to 300 times more penicillinase is produced in the presence of penicillin than in its absence unless deletions or mutations in the regulatory genes lead to its constitutive expression.

In Gram-negative bacteria the outer membrane retards entry of penicillins and cephalosporins into the cell. The β-lactamase needs only to inactivate molecules of drug that penetrate within the periplasmic space between the cytoplasmic membrane and the cell wall. Each cell is thus responsible for its own protection – a more efficient mechanism than the external excretion of β-lactamase seen in Gram-positive bacteria. Enzymes are often produced constitutively (i.e. even when the antibiotic is not present) and a small inoculum of bacteria may be almost as resistant as a large one. A similar functional organization is exhibited by the aminoglycoside-modifying enzymes. These enzymes are located at the surface of the cytoplasmic membrane and only those molecules of aminoglycoside that are in the process of being transported across the membrane are modified.

ALTERATIONS TO THE PERMEABILITY OF THE BACTERIAL CELL ENVELOPE

The bacterial cell envelope consists of a capsule, a cell wall and a cytoplasmic membrane. This structure allows the passage of bacterial nutrients and excreted products, while acting as a barrier to harmful substances such as antibiotics. The capsule, composed mainly of polysaccharides, is not a major barrier to the passage of antibiotics. The Gram-positive cell wall is relatively thick but simple in structure, being made up of a network of cross-linked peptidoglycan complexed with teichoic and lipoteichoic acids. It is readily permeable to most antibiotics. The cell wall of Gram-negative bacteria is more complex, comprising an outer membrane of lipopolysaccharide, protein and phospholipid, attached to a thin layer of peptidoglycan (*see* p. 12). The lipopolysaccharide molecules cover the surface of the cell, with their hydrophilic portions pointing outwards. Their inner lipophilic regions interact with the fatty acid chains of the phospholipid monolayer of the inner surface of the outer membrane and are stabilized by divalent cation bridges. The phospholipid and lipopolysaccharide of the outer membrane form a classic lipid bilayer, which acts as a barrier to both hydrophobic and hydrophilic drug molecules. Natural permeability varies among different Gram-negative species and generally correlates with innate resistance. For example, the cell walls of *Neisseria* species and *Haemophilus influenzae* are more permeable than those of *E. coli*, while the walls of *Ps. aeruginosa* and *S. maltophilia* are markedly less permeable.

Hydrophobic antibiotics can enter the Gram-negative cell by direct solubilization through the lipid layer of the outer membrane, but the dense lipopolysaccharide cover may physically block this pathway. Changes in surface lipopolysaccharides may increase or decrease permeability resistance. However, most antibiotics are hydrophilic and cross through the outer membrane of Gram-negative cells via water-filled channels created by membrane proteins called porins. The rate of diffusion across these channels depends on size and physicochemical structure, small hydrophilic molecules with a zwitterionic charge showing the faster penetration. Some antimicrobial resistance in Gram-negative bacteria is due to reduced drug entry caused by decreased amounts of specific porin proteins, usually in combination with either overexpression of efflux pumps or β-lactamase production. This phenomenon is associated with significant β-lactam resistance, such as low-level resistance to imipenem in strains of *P. aeruginosa* and *Enterobacter* spp. that are hyperproducing chromosomal group 1 cephalosporinase and deficient in porins such as OprD in *Ps. aeruginosa* and OmpF and OmpC in *Enterobacter*.[14,15] Porin-deficient mutant strains emerge sporadically during therapy but appear less fit than their porin-proficient congeners, making these strains unstable and apparently unable to spread and cause epidemics.

The target molecules of antibiotics that inhibit cell wall synthesis, such as the β-lactam antibiotics and the glycopeptides, are located outside the cytoplasmic membrane, and it is not necessary for these drugs to pass through this membrane to exert their effect. Most other antibiotics must cross the membrane to reach their intracellular sites of action. The cytoplasmic membrane is freely permeable to lipophilic agents such as minocycline, chloramphenicol, trimethoprim, fluoroquinolones and rifampicin, but poses a significant barrier to hydrophilic agents such as aminoglycosides, erythromycin, clindamycin and the sulfonamides. These drugs are actively transported across the membrane by carrier proteins, and some resistances have been associated with various changes in these transporters. Resistance to aminoglycosides in both Gram-positive and Gram-negative bacteria may be mediated by defective uptake due to the mutational inactivation of proton motive force-driven cytoplamic pump systems, a defect which is associated with slow growth rate and production of 'small colony variants'.

RESISTANCE DUE TO DRUG EFFLUX

Single drug and multi-drug efflux pumps have been recognized recently to be ubiquitous systems in micro-organisms, and have been found in all bacterial genomes sequenced to date.[16] These systems are involved in the natural or innate resistance phenotype of many bacteria. Furthermore, they may produce clinically significant acquired resistance by mutational modification of the structural gene, overexpression due to mutation in regulatory genes or horizontal transfer of genetic elements. Most of the bacterial efflux pumps belong to the class of secondary transporters that mediate the extrusion of toxic compounds from the cytoplasm in a coupled exchange with protons.[17] Multidrug pumps can be subdivided into several superfamilies, including the major facilitator superfamily (MFS), small multidrug resistance family (SMR), resistance-nodulation-cell division family (RND) and multidrug and toxic compound extrusion family (MATE) (Table 3.1). RND and MATE

Table 3.1 Selected multidrug efflux systems determining multiple antibiotic resistance in pathogenic and commensal bacteria (adapted from Nikaido[16])

Transporter		Associated proteins		Regulator(s)	Organism	Antibiotic resistance profile
Class	Pump	Periplasmic	OM Channel			
MFS	NorA	–	–	–	*Staph. aureus*	Fluoroquinolones, chloramphenicol
MATE	NorM	–	–	–	*V. parahaemolyticus*	Fluoroquinolones, aminoglycosides
RND	AcrB	AcrA	TolC	AcrR, MarA	*E. coli*	β-lactams, tetracyclines, macrolides, fluoroquinolones, chloramphenicol
RND	MexB	MexA	OprM	MexR	*Ps. aeruginosa*	β-Lactams, tetracyclines, macrolides, fluoroquinolones, chloramphenicol
RND	MexD	MexC	OprJ	MexS	*Ps. aeruginosa*	Group 6 cephalosporins, tetracyclines, fluoroquinolones, chloramphenicol
RND	MexF	MexE	OprN	MexT	*Ps. aeruginosa*	Fluoroquinolones, chloramphenicol
RND	MexY	MexX	OprM	MexZ	*Ps. aeruginosa*	Macrolides, tetracyclines, aminoglycosides
RND	MtrD	MtrC	MtrE	MtrR	*N. gonorrhoeae*	β-Lactams, macrolides, tetracyclines, chloramphenicol

OM, outer membrane; MFS, major facilitator superfamily; MATE, multiple drug and toxic compound extrusion; RND, resistance-nodulation-division.

systems appear to function as detoxifying systems and transport heavy metals, solvents, detergents and bile salts whereas MFS pumps are closely related to specific efflux pumps and appear to function as major Na^+/H^+ transporters. MFS and SMR pumps are mostly found in Gram-positive bacteria whereas RND pumps are mostly found in Gram-negative bacteria, in which they function in association with special outer membrane channel proteins and periplasmic membrane fusion proteins, forming a tripartite transport system spanning both the inner and outer membranes (Table 3.1 and Figure 3.2). This allows the pumps to expel their substrates directly from the inner membrane or cytoplasm into the extracellular space. Although these pumps confer resistance mostly to a range of lipophilic and amphiphilic drugs (including β-lactams, fluoroquinolones, tetracyclines, macrolides and chloramphenicol) some pumps, such as MexY of *Ps. aeruginosa*, also transport aminoglycosides.

Among the best studied systems are the AcrB system of *E. coli* and the MexB system of *Ps. aeruginosa*. The AcrB pump is controlled by the Mar regulon, which is widespread among enteric bacteria. The MarA global activator, which can be derepressed by tetracycline or chloramphenicol, simultaneously upregulates the AcrAB–TolC transport complex and downregulates the synthesis of the larger porin OmpF, thereby acting in a synergistic manner to block the drug penetration into the cell. Constitutive overexpression of AcrAB is present in most ciprofloxacin-resistant *E. coli* clinical isolates.[18] In *Ps. aeruginosa*, overexpression of the

MexAB–OprM transport complex occurs commonly during β-lactam therapy by selection of mutants with altered specific repressor gene *mexR*. This increased efflux determines resistance to fluoroquinolones, penicillins, cephalosporins and meropenem. Paradoxically, it appears that these broad-spectrum resistance profiles mediated by efflux systems are more efficiently selected by newer antibiotics such as fluoroquinolones, meropenem or cefepime, presumably because other resistance mechanisms are not readily available. Another cause for concern is the selection of multidrug pumps by disinfectants such as triclosan, which is increasingly used in housekeeping products.

Active efflux of the drug from the bacterial cell is one of the major resistance mechanisms to tetracyclines, the second being 30S ribosome protection by elongation factor G-like proteins.[19] Efflux can be mediated either by tetracycline-specific efflux pumps or by multidrug transporter systems. Specific pumps of the TetA-E and TetG-H families are widespread in Gram-negative bacteria whereas the specific pumps TetK and TetL are common in Gram-positive bacteria (*see* p. 396). These determinants are often encoded by genes located on plasmids or transposons. Minocycline is not extruded by these proteins and remains active. These specific pumps are single proteins located on the inner membrane that export the drug into the periplasm, in contrast with multidrug transporter systems that extrude tetracyclines from the cytoplasm directly outside the cell.

More recently, specific efflux proteins have been shown to

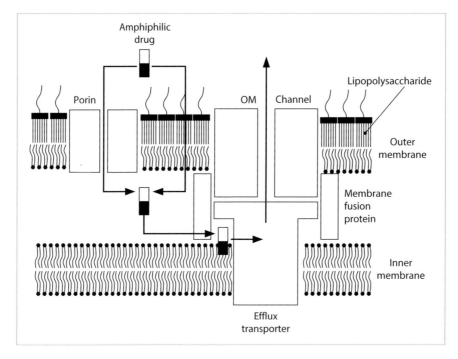

Fig. 3.2 Hypothetical structure of tricomponent efflux systems in Gram-negative bacteria. Amphiphilic drugs traversing the outer membrane (either directly or via porin channels) are partitioned into the outer leaflet of the inner membrane, where they are captured by the transporter protein and extruded directly outside the cell via the periplasmic-outer membrane protein channel. From Nikaido H, Zgurska HI. Antibiotic mechanisms. *Current Opinion in Infectious Diseases* 1999; 12: 529.

play a major role in macrolide resistance, including the Mef(A) transporters of the MFS superfamily that determine resistance to 14-C macrolides in pneumococci, β-hemolytic and oral streptococci, enterococci and corynebacteria and the Msr(A) ATP-binding transporters that confer resistance to erythromycin and streptogramin B in staphylococci.[20] The *mef* genes are located on conjugative elements that readily transfer across Gram-positive genera and species.

RESISTANCE DUE TO ALTERATIONS IN TARGET MOLECULES

β-Lactam resistance due to alterations to penicillin-binding proteins (PBPs)

These are proteins associated with the bacterial cell envelope that are the target sites for β-lactam antibiotics. Each bacterial cell has several PBPs, which vary with the species. PBPs are transpeptidases, carboxypeptidases and endopeptidases that are required for cell wall synthesis and remodelling during growth and septation. Some, but not all, PBPs are essential for cell survival (*see* p. 14). PBPs are related to β-lactamases, which also bind β-lactam antibiotics. However, unlike β-lactamases, PBPs form stable complexes with β-lactams and are themselves inactivated. β-Lactam antibiotics thus inactivate PBPs, preventing proper cell growth and division, and producing cell wall defects that lead to death by osmolysis. Alterations in PBPs, leading to decreased binding affinity with β-lactam antibiotics, are important causes of β-lactam resistance in a number of species, most commonly Gram-positive bacteria.

Penicillin-resistant strains of *Streptococcus pneumoniae* produce one or more altered PBPs that have reduced ability to bind penicillin. Stepwise acquisition of multiple changes in the genes encoding these PBPs produce various levels of penicillin resistance.[21] The genetic sequences encoding normal PBPs in sensitive strains of *Str. pneumoniae* are highly conserved; the genes in resistant strains are said to be 'mosaics' since they consist of blocks of conserved sequences interspersed with blocks of variant sequences. As more variant blocks are introduced into the mosaic, the more penicillin resistant the recipient strain tends to become. These gene sequences have probably been derived by transformation from oral streptococcal species such as *Streptococcus mitis* and *Streptococcus oralis*, although the donors may themselves be phenotypically penicillin sensitive and do not produce low-affinity PBPs.[22] Whereas high level resistance to penicillin involves changes in at least PBP 1a, PBP 2x and PBP 2a that require multiple transformation events, resistance to group 4 cephalosporins (*see* Ch. 15) can result from a single transformation event though cotransformation of the closely linked genes encoding PBP 1a and PBP 2x.

The relative penicillin resistance of enterococci is due to the normal production of PBPs with low binding affinity. The higher levels of penicillin and ampicillin resistance often seen in *Enterococcus faecium* are the result of overexpression of PBP 5 (which exhibits a lower affinity for penicillin than other PBPs), which can be further decreased by nucleotide point mutations in the very high level resistant strains. Other species showing β-lactam resistance due to altered PBPs include β-lactamase-negative strains of penicillin-resistant *Neisseria gonorrhoeae*, penicillin-resistant *Neisseria meningitidis* and ampicillin-resistant *H. influenzae*. The genes encoding altered PBPs in both *Neisseria* species appear to be mosaics, and the variant blocks may have been derived from *Neisseria flavescens* and other commensal *Neisseria*.

Methicillin resistance in *Staph. aureus* and in coagulase-negative staphylococci is caused by an acquired chromosomal gene (*mecA*) which results in the synthesis of a fifth penicillin-binding protein (PBP 2a), with decreased affinity for methicillin and other β-lactam agents, in addition to the intrinsic PBP 1 to 4.[23] Many MRSA strains exhibit heterogeneity in the expression of resistance, with only a small proportion of the total cell population expressing high-level resistance. The proportion of resistant cells is dependent on environmental conditions such as temperature and osmolality. This phenomenon is related to the presence of regulatory loci *mecI* and *mecR*1 upstream of *mecA*, which exhibit significant sequence and functional homology with the β-lactamase regulators *blaI-blaR*1. Deletion of these elements produce homogeneous expression of methicillin resistance. The *mecA* gene is located on a 20–60 kb-long antibiotic resistance island, called the staphylococcal cassette chromosome *mec* (SCC*mec*), a novel mobile element driven by two site-specific recombinases.[24]

Glycopeptide resistance due to metabolic bypass

Glycopeptides are large hexapeptides that inhibit bacterial peptidoglycan synthesis by binding the carboxy-terminal D-alanyl-D-alanine dipeptide residue of the muramyl pentapeptide precursor, thereby blocking access to three key steps in the peptidoglycan polymerization: transglycosylation, transpeptidation and carboxypeptidation (*see* Ch. 2). Most clinically important Gram-positive bacteria build their peptidoglycan from this conserved pentapeptide precursor and are naturally sensitive to the glycopeptides vancomycin and teicoplanin. After nearly 30 years of increasing vancomycin usage, acquired glycopeptide resistance was described in enterococci in 1986 and in coagulase-negative staphylococci in 1987, and decreased susceptibility to vancomycin was reported in *Staph. aureus* in 1997. The mechanisms of glycopeptide resistance are distinct in enterococci and staphylococci.

In enterococci, five different glycopeptide resistance phenotypes are now recognized:[25]

1. VanA, inducible high-level transferable resistance to both vancomycin and teicoplanin; this is usually seen in *E. faecium*, sometimes in *Enterococcus faecalis* and rarely in *Enterococcus avium*, *Enterococcus hirae*, *Enterococcus casseliflavus*, *Enterococcus mundtii*, and *Enterococcus durans*.

2. VanB, inducible low-level transferable resistance, usually to vancomycin alone; found in *E. faecium*, sometimes in *E. faecalis*.
3. VanC, constitutive low-level vancomycin resistance, seen in *Enterococcus gallinarum*, *E. casseliflavus* and *Enterococcus flavescens*.
4. VanD, constitutive or inducible moderate-level resistance, usually to vancomycin alone; rarely acquired in *E. faecium*.
5. VanE, low-level resistance to vancomycin alone; rarely acquired in *E. faecalis*.

Enterococcal resistance to glycopeptides is due to multi-enzymatic metabolic bypass, mediated by replacement of the normal D-alanyl-D-alanine termini of peptidoglycan precursors by abnormal precursors with D-alanyl-D-lactate, or D-alanyl-D-serine termini, none of which can bind glycopeptides. The *vanA* gene cluster is carried by a 10.8 kb transposon (Tn*1546*) that contains nine functionally related genes encoding mobilization of the element (resolvase and transposase) and co-ordinated replacement of muramyl pentapeptides. The *vanA* gene encodes an abnormal D-alanine-D-alanine ligase that synthesizes the D-alanine-D-lactate dipeptide. The *vanH* gene codes for a dehydrogenase that generates D-lactate. The *vanX* and *vanY* genes encode two enzymes that hydrolyse normal precursors: VanX, a D, D-dipeptidase that hydrolyzes D-alanyl-D-alanine dipeptides and VanY, a D,D-carboxypeptidase that cleaves terminal alanine from normal precursors. The *vanR* and *vanS* genes regulate the expression of the *vanHAX* operon through a two-component sensor system for glycopeptides. The *vanB* gene cluster has a similar organization, albeit with more heterogeneity, and is located on a large conjugative transposon (Tn*1547*) that is usually integrated in the chromosome and occasionally plasmid borne.

Over the past decade, the prevalence of glycopeptide resistance has increased markedly in clinical isolates of enterococci, particularly *E. faecium*, as a result of spread of transposons, plasmids and nosocomial outbreaks with multi-resistant clones. In Europe, the *vanA* genotype is predominant and polyclonal. It has a large reservoir in the community, with frequent fecal carriage in the healthy population and in farm animals fed avoparcin (a cross-selecting glycopeptide related to vancomycin) that was used for growth promotion between 1970 and 1998. In the USA, the *vanA* and *vanB* genotypes are widespread in many hospitals and frequently cause nosocomial infection but are rarely found in the community. This is presumably related to the lack of avoparcin use in animal husbandry in the USA. The *vanA* gene cluster has been transferred experimentally to other Gram-positive bacteria where it is expressed, including *Staph. aureus*.[26] It has not been reported in clinical isolates of *Staph. aureus* but has been found in *Bacillus circulans*, *Oerskovia turbata*, and *Arcanobacterium haemolyticum*.

Since 1997, clinical isolates of *Staph. aureus* with reduced susceptibility to vancomycin have been reported in patients failing glycopeptide therapy.[27,28] Interpretive criteria for vancomycin and teicoplanin susceptibility testing differ according to national guidelines. Therefore, strains with an MIC of 8 mg/l are considered vancomycin intermediate susceptible, or VISA, by the National Committee for Laboratory Standards and Comité de l'Antibiogramme- Société Française de Microbiologie standards but vancomycin resistant (VRSA) according to the British Society for Antimicrobial Therapy. Hiramatsu et al also described hetero-VISA or hetero-VRSA strains for which the MIC of vancomycin is ≤ 4 mg/l, but exhibit subpopulations at about 1 in 10^6 cells able to grow at 8 mg/l. Although laboratory detection methods are not well standardized, hetero-VISA strains appear to occur frequently as variants of endemic MRSA strains in various continents and are commonly found in patients not treated with glycopeptide. In contrast, infection with homogeneous VISA strains has been reported in a dozen cases. These infections developed in chronically ill patients failing prolonged glycopeptide therapy of infections associated with an indwelling device or undrained collections of pus.[28]

The mechanisms of decreased glycopeptide susceptibility in *Staph. aureus* are poorly understood. A number of abnormalities has been reported in clinical isolates and laboratory derived VISA strains: increased cell wall thickness, abnormal peptidoglycan with increased proportion of glutamine non-amidated muropeptides and decreased cross-linking, increased quantities of cell-wall precursors and overexpression of PBPs 2 and 2a. These abnormalities suggest that a mechanism of reduced susceptibility may be trapping of vancomycin by non-vital dipeptide termini outside the actively polymerising peptidoglycan adjacent to the cell membrane. In addition, VISA strains show other abnormalities, including slower growth and reduced autolytic activity. In some VISA strains, these abnormalities associated with increased vancomycin MIC levels are unstable in vitro in the absence of antibiotic.

Aminoglycoside resistance due to altered ribosomal proteins

Aminoglycoside resistance may be produced by alterations in specific ribosomal binding proteins, although this is uncommon in clinical isolates. Clinically important examples of this mechanism include high-level resistance to streptomycin in *Mycobacterium tuberculosis* and high-level resistance to streptomycin or gentamicin in some strains of enterococci, in which the combination of penicillin plus streptomycin or gentamicin fails to produce the usual synergistic bactericidal effect.

Quinolone resistance due to altered topoisomerases

The main targets for quinolones are the type 2 topoisomerases DNA gyrase and type IV topoisomerase, both of which are essential enzymes involved in chromosomal DNA replication and segregation (*see* Ch. 2). Fluoroquinolones exert their bactericidal action by trapping topoisomerase-DNA complexes, thereby blocking the replication fork. Both of these structurally related target enzymes are tetrameric. DNA gyrase is composed of two pairs of GyrA and GyrB subunits while topoisomerase type IV is composed of two pairs of the homologous ParC and ParE subunits. Bacterial resistance to fluoroquinolones is generally mediated by chromosomal mutations leading either to reduced affinity of DNA gyrase and/or topoisomerase IV, or to overexpression of endogenous MDR efflux systems (see above).[29] Plasmid mediated resistance was reported in *K. pneumoniae* and is of undetermined prevalence.[30] The commonest target resistance modifications arise from spontaneous mutations, occurring at a frequency of 1 in 10^6 to 1 in 10^9 cells, that substitute amino acids in specific domains of GyrA and ParC subunits and less frequently in GyrB and ParE. These regions of the enzymes, called the quinolone resistance determining regions, either contain the active site, a tyrosine that covalently binds to DNA, or constitute parts of quinolone binding sites. Fluoroquinolones have different potencies of antibacterial activity against different bacteria, a variance which is to a large part related to the different potency against their enzyme targets. The more sensitive of the two enzymes is the primary target. In general, DNA gyrase is the primary target in Gram-negative bacteria and topoisomerase IV is the primary target in Gram-positive bacteria. Resistance develops progressively by stepwise mutations. The first step in increasing resistance level results from amino acid change in the primary target and is followed by second-step mutational modifications of amino acid in the secondary target. The higher the difference in drug potency against the two enzymes, the higher the MIC increase provided by first-step mutation. Fluroquinolones with a low therapeutic index (defined as the drug concentration at the infected site divided by the MIC of that drug) are more likely to select first-step mutants. This explains why resistance to quinolones has emerged rapidly after the introduction of ciprofloxacin and ofloxacin for human therapeutics in two species, *Ps. aeruginosa* and *Staph. aureus*, which develop significant resistance after only a single mutation in *gyrA*. In *Staph. aureus*, fluoroquinolone resistance quickly became associated with methicillin resistance. This was the consequence of two factors: increased likelihood of exposure of multi-resistant strains to therapy with these drugs, leading to multiple mutations and high level resistance; and the further selective advantage for nosocomial spread conferred by this resistance.[31] In organisms in which multiple mutational changes are required to reach clinical resistance to these drugs, such as *E. coli*, *Campylobacter jejuni* and *N. gonorrhoeae*, it appeared later and was accelerated by other epidemiologic factors. For *C. jejuni*, this was related to the massive use of the cross-selecting fluoroquinolone enrofloxacin in the poultry industry followed by food-borne transmission to humans.[32] For *N. gonorrhoeae*, the emergence of fluoroquinolone resistance was soon followed with outbreaks of person-to-person transmission.

MLS resistance due to ribosomal modification

Macrolides inhibit protein synthesis by dissociation of the peptidyl-tRNA molecule from the 50S ribosomal subunit.

Macrolides bind to a ribosomal site that is overlapping with the binding site of the structurally unrelated lincosamides and streptogramins B antibiotics. The most common type of acquired resistance to erythromycin and clindamycin (and other macrolides and lincosamides) is seen in streptococci, enterococci and staphylococci and is called macrolide-lincosamide-streptogramin B (MLS_B) resistance. This is due to the production of enzymes that methylate a specific adenine residue in 23S rRNA, resulting in reduced ribosomal binding of the three antibiotic classes.[20] Low concentrations of erythromycin induce resistance to all the macrolides and lincosamides (so-called 'dissociated' resistance), but some strains may produce the methylase constitutively following mutations or deletions in the regulatory genes. More than 20 *erm* genes encode the MLS_B resistance. Most are located on conjugative and non-conjugative transposons that predominantly insert in the chromosome and are occasionally plasmid borne. They are frequently associated with other resistance genes, particularly those encoding tetracycline resistance by ribosomal protection. Over the past decade, increased use of macrolides has been related to spread of MLS resistance in group A β-hemolytic streptococci and pneumococci.[33]

In bacteria with a low copy number of ribosomal operons, such as the mycobacteria, *C. jejuni* and *Helicobacter pylori*, macrolide resistance is commonly caused by mutational modification of the 23S rRNA peptidyl-transferase region at the same adenine that is modified by *erm* methylases or adjacent nucleotides (A2057 to A2059). In most other bacteria, such mutations are recessive due to multi-copy rRNA genes.

Rifampicin resistance due to modification of RNA polymerase

Rifampicin resistance is commonly the result of a mutation that alters the β-subunit of RNA polymerase, reducing its binding affinity for rifampicin. Mutation usually produces high-level resistance in a single step, but intermediate resistance is sometimes seen. Mutational resistance occurs relatively frequently, and for this reason rifampicin is combined with other agents for the treatment of tuberculosis and staphylococcal infection. Meningococcal carriers have been treated with rifampicin alone, and this has resulted in the emergence of rifampicin resistance in strains of *N. meningitidis*.

Mupirocin resistance due to metabolic bypass

Mupirocin (pseudomonic acid), is widely used for topical treatment of Gram-positive skin infections and the clearance of nasal carriers of methicillin-sensitive and methicillin-resistant *Staph. aureus*. It acts by inhibiting bacterial isoleucyl-tRNA synthetase, and resistance is mediated by the production of modified enzymes. Isolates showing low-level resistance have a single chromosomally encoded synthetase modified by point mutation, while those with high-level resistance have a second enzyme that cannot bind the drug encoded on a transferable plasmid.[34]

Sulfonamide and trimethoprim resistance due to metabolic bypass

Acquired sulfonamide resistance is usually due to the production of an altered dihydropteroate synthetase that has reduced affinity for sulfonamides. Resistance is encoded on transferable plasmids and associated with transposons. Trimethoprim resistance occurs much less commonly. It is usually due to plasmid-mediated synthesis of new dihydrofolate reductases, which are much less susceptible to trimethoprim than the natural ones. The resistance genes are again associated with transposons.

Fusidic acid resistance due to modification of elongation factor G

Fusidic acid acts by inhibiting protein synthesis by interfering with ribosome translation. Resistance to fusidic acid results from mutational alteration of the target molecule, elongation factor G, causing reduced affinity for fusidic acid. This occurs at high frequency in *Staph. aureus* in vitro, and therefore it is recommended that fusidic acid should not be used alone to treat staphylococcal infections.

Failure to metabolize the drug to the active form

Both metronidazole and nitrofurantoin must be converted to an active form within the bacterium before they can have any effect. Resistance to them arises if the pathogen cannot effect this conversion. Aerobic organisms cannot reduce metronidazole to its active form and are therefore inherently resistant, but resistance in anaerobic organisms is very uncommon. Resistant strains of *Bacteroides fragilis* that have been investigated have reduced levels of pyruvate dehydrogenase, the enzyme necessary for the reduction of metronidazole to the active intermediate. Nitrofurantoin must be reduced to an active intermediate by NADH or NADPH reductases. One of these enzymes acts aerobically and another anaerobically. Resistance to nitrofurans is uncommon, since such strains must lose more than one reductase to become resistant.

GENETIC BASIS OF RESISTANCE

INTRINSIC RESISTANCE

Resistance of bacteria to antimicrobial agents may be intinsic or acquired. Intrinsic (or innate) resistance to some antibiotics is the natural resistance possessed by most strains of a bacterial species and is part of their genetic make-up, encoded on the chromosome. Intrinsic multiple resistance is characteristic of free-living organisms, which may have evolved because of metabolic polyvalence and exposure to natural antibiotics and other toxic compounds in the environment. Multiresistance is due mostly to decreased antibiotic uptake by highly selective outer membrane porins and multiple efflux systems. These organisms have low virulence, but their multiple resistance allows them to persist in hospital environments and cause nosocomial infections. An example of a free-living opportunistic pathogen with a high degree of intrinsic resistance is *P. aeruginosa*. From before the beginning of the antibiotic era, virtually all strains of this organism were already resistant to many antibiotics that subsequently became available.

MUTATIONAL RESISTANCE

Acquired resistance may be due to mutations affecting genes on the bacterial chromosome, to acquisition of mobile foreign genes, or to mutation in acquired mobile genes. Mutations usually involve deletion, substitution, or addition of one or a few base pairs, causing substitution of one or a few amino acids in a crucial peptide. Mutational resistance can affect the structural gene coding for the antibiotic target. This usually results in a gene product with reduced affinity for the antibiotic. Examples are the high-level resistance to streptomycin seen in *M. tuberculosis* and *E. faecalis*, caused by a mutation affecting the specific streptomycin-binding protein of the 30S subunit of the ribosome and the fluoroquinolone resistance from alterations in DNA topoisomerases found in many bacteria. Mutational resistance can also involve regulatory loci, leading to overproduction of detoxifying systems. Examples discussed above are resistance to group 4 cephalosporins seen in de-repressed AmpC β-lactamase hyper-producing mutants of *Enterobacter cloacae* and the multiple resistance expressed by MexAB-OprD efflux pump overproducing mutants of *Ps. aeruginosa*.

Although the basal rate of mutation is low in bacterial genomes, it is not constant but varies by a factor of 10 000 according to a number of intrinsic and external factors.[5] Among these factors are the sequence of the gene, with some hypermutable loci associated with short tandem repeats that are prone to deletions and duplications by slippped-strand mispairing; the mutator phenotype associated with defective mismatch repair system; stress-induced mutagenesis, including exposure to antibiotics and host defenses. Once a resistant mutant has been selected during exposure to the antibiotic, it usually shows a decreased fitness for competing with the wild-type ancestor, defined as the competitive efficiency of multiplication in the absence of the antibiotic. This deficiency is called the biological cost of resistance. It has been observed, however, that this reduction in fitness may be compensated by secondary mutations in other chromosomal loci, thereby ensuring the persistence of the mutant. The probability that antibiotic treatment will select a resistant mutant depends on a complex network of factors including the drug, its concentration, the organism, its resistance mutation rate, inoculum size, physiological state and structure of the bacterial population.[35]

TRANSFERABLE RESISTANCE

Horizontal spread of resistance gene from organism to organism occurs by conjugation (intercellular passage of plasmid or transposon), transduction (DNA transfer via bacteriophage), or transformation (uptake of naked DNA). The acquisition of resistance by transduction is rare in nature (the most important example in pathogenic bacteria is the transfer of penicillinase plasmid from strain to strain of *Staph. aureus*). Transformation of resistance factors is an important mechanism in the few bacterial species that are readily transformable during part of their life cycle and are said to be naturally competent. These organisms, which include, *Str. pneumoniae*, *H. influenzae*, *Helicobacter*, *Acinetobacter*, *Neisseria* and *Moraxella* spp., show extensive genetic variation resulting from natural transformation. They may also acquire chromosomally encoded antimicrobial resistance. Examples, as discussed above, include penicillin- or ampicillin-resistant *Str. pneumoniae* and *N. meningitidis* that acquired mosaic genes for the production of altered PBPs by transformation and site-specific recombination from phylogenetically related, co-resident commensal bacteria.

Plasmids

These are molecules of DNA that replicate independently from the bacterial chromosome. 'R-plasmids' carry one or more genetic determinants for drug resistance. This type of resistance is due to a dominant gene, usually one resulting in production of a drug-inactivating or drug-modifying enzyme. Conjugation is the most common method of resistance transfer in clinically important bacteria.[36] Conjugative plasmids, which are capable of self-transmission to other bacterial hosts, are common in Gram-negative enteric bacilli and are relatively large; non-conjugative plasmids, common in Gram-positive cocci, *H. influenzae*, *N. gonorrhoeae* and *Bacillus fragilis*, are usually small. Non-conjugative plasmids can transfer to other bacteria if they are mobilized by conjugative plasmids present in the same cell, or by transduction or transformation. Large plasmids are usually present at one or two copies per cell, and their replication is closely linked to replication of the bacterial chromosome. Small plasmids may be present at more than 30 copies per cell, and their distribution to progeny during cell division is ensured by the large number present. Plasmids tend to have a restricted host range: for example, those from Gram-negative bacteria cannot generally transfer to or maintain themselves in Gram-positive organisms, and vice versa. Conjugative transfer of plasmids has been observed, however, between these distant bacterial groups and even between bacteria and eukaryotic cells such as yeasts.

Transposons

These are discrete sequences of DNA, capable of translocation from one replicon (plasmid or chromosome) to another – hence the epithet 'jumping gene'. They may encode genes for resistance to a wide variety of antibiotics, as well as many other metabolic properties. They are circular segments of double-stranded DNA, 4–25 kb in length, and usually consist of a functional central region flanked by long terminal repeats, usually inverted repeats. Complex transposons also carry genes for the transposition enzymes transposase and resolvase and their repressors. They need not share extensive regions of homology with the replicon into which they insert, as is required in classical genetic recombination. Depending upon the transposon involved, they may transpose into a replicon randomly or into favored sites, and they may insert at only a few or at many different places.

A special type of element, called conjugative transposons, can transfer directly between the chromosome of one strain to the chromosome of another without plasmid intermediate. Antibiotics can function as pheromones that are capable of inducing conjugation of conjugative transposons that in turn mobilize the transfer of co-resident R-plasmids. These transposons are less restrictive than plasmids in host range. A well studied example is Tn*416*, which has spread the *tetM* gene from Gram-positive cocci to diverse bacteria such as *Neisseria*, *Mycoplasma*, and *Clostridium*.[37] Another example is the efficient spread by other conjugative transposons of resistance to tetracycline, clindamycin and cefoxitin between species and strains of *Bacteroides* in the human gut.

Other important genetic elements by which transposons and plasmids acquire multiple antibiotic resistance determinants by site-specific recombination are called integrons. These are site-specific recombination systems that recognize and capture antibiotic resistance gene cassettes in a high-efficiency expression site.[36,38] The structure of class 1 integrons (Figure 3.3) includes an integrase gene (*int*), an adjacent integration site (*attI*) that can contain one or more gene cassette, and one or more promotor. Class I integrons, the most frequently observed type, also contain a 3′-conserved segment that includes the genes encoding resistance to quaternary ammonium compounds (*qacEΔ*) and sulfonamides (*sul1*). The integrase is capable of excision and integration of up to five gene cassettes, each of which is associated with a related 59 bp palindromic element that acts as recombination hotspot. More than 60 different gene cassettes are known. They include determinants of β-lactamases, aminoglycoside-modifying enzymes, chloramphenicol acetyltransferases, and trimethoprim-resistant DFR enzymes. Integrons are widespread among antibiotic-resistant clinical isolates of diverse Gram-negative species and have also been reported in Gram-positive bacteria. They are involved in gene mobilization and plasmid fusion and are usually found associated with transposons and conjugative plasmids. The genetic linkage of resistance to sulfonamides and to newer antibiotics in these integrons may explain the persistence of sulfonamide resistance in *E. coli* in spite of a huge decrease in sulfonamide use.[39] Likewise, mercury released from dental amalgams has been suggest to select for antibiotic resistance in the oral and intestinal flora of humans because of the physical linkage between integron and mercury resistance in the ubiquitous Tn21-like transposons.[40] Clearly, transposons and inte-

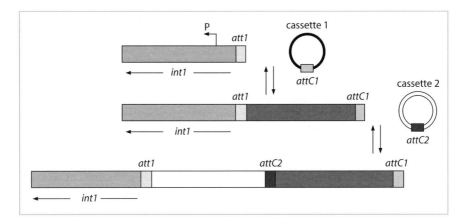

Fig. 3.3 Integron structure and gene cassette movement. The *intI* gene encodes the integrase that mediates site-specific integration of circular gene cassettes between the *attI* and *attC* sites. P denotes the common promoter. Adapted from Ploy (2000).

grons are responsible for much of the diversity observed among plasmids, and play a major role in the evolution and dissemination of antibiotic resistance among bacteria.[37,40]

CURRENT THERAPEUTIC PROBLEMS WITH RESISTANCE

STAPHYLOCOCCUS AUREUS

Approximately 85% of *Staph. aureus* are resistant to penicillin by plasmid-mediated β-lactamase. This is often associated with resistance to erythromycin and other agents. During the 1950s, large epidemics of hospital infection were caused by 'the hospital staphylococcus', a virulent strain of *Staph. aureus* resistant to penicillin, tetracycline, erythromycin, chloramphenicol and other drugs. After the introduction of the penicillinase-stable methicillin (followed later by cloxacillin and flucloxacillin), the incidence of hospital infection with multiresistant staphylococci gradually declined during the 1960s and 1970s. Although strains of methicillin-resistant *Staph. aureus* (MRSA) were seen as early as 1961, gentamicin-resistant MRSA emerged later as a major pathogen of hospital infection throughout the world in the 1980s. Since then, MRSA has continued to increase in prevalence in several countries, including the USA, UK, and countries in Southern and Eastern Europe, but was well contained in others such as Scandinavian countries and the Netherlands (Figure 3.4). Epidemic strains of MRSA have been associated with large nosocomial outbreaks spreading to whole regions by inter-hospital transfer of colonized patients or staff.[41,42] Deep-seated MRSA infections have been associated with increased mortality compared with oxacillin-susceptible *Staph. aureus* infection in some settings.[43] In recent years, community-acquired MRSA infections have emerged in several parts of the world, including USA, Western Australia and Europe.[44]

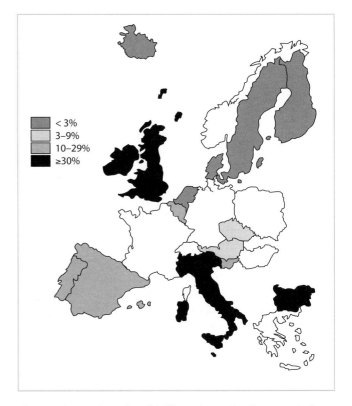

< 3%
3–9%
10–29%
≥30%

Fig. 3.4 Proportion of methicillin-resistant *Staph. aureus* isolates from bloodstream infections, EARSS participating countries. 2000. Available at http://www.earss.rivm.nl

MRSA strains have become multiresistant by a number of mechanisms. The chromosomal DNA region harboring the *mecA* gene, the staphylococcal cassette chromosome *mec*, contains a number of insertion sites. These permit the accumulation of multiple mobile genetic elements encoding resistances to other classes of antibiotics such as macrolides, lincosamides, streptogramins, sulfonamides and tetracyclines. In addition,

MRSA may acquire other resistances encoded on plasmids and transposons, including β-lactamase production and resistance to trimethoprim and the aminoglycosides. Aminoglycoside resistance is mediated by at least six aminoglycoside-modifying enzymes, of which a bifunctional protein with both aminoglycoside acetyltransferase and phosphotransferase activities determines gentamicin resistance. This transposon-encoded enzyme decreased in prevalence in MRSA strains in Europe in recent years.

Following the rapid emergence of mutational resistance to quinolones and to other drugs such as rifampicin and mupirocin, fuelled by clonal spread,[45] many strains of MRSA remain sensitive only to the glycopeptides vancomycin and teicoplanin. The recent recognition of MRSA strains with reduced susceptibility to glycopeptides (GISA, *see above*) is likely to further complicate therapy of serious staphylococcal infection. Infections caused by these strains leave very few therapeutic options and therefore their emergence adds to the rationale for containing both MRSA transmission and vancomycin use in hospitals. Among the recently available anti-staphylococcal antibiotics, such as linezolid and quinupristin-dalfopristin, partial or full resistance to the latter has already been reported due to cross-resistance by constitutive ErmA methylase or plasmid-mediated streptogramin-modifying enzymes and efflux pumps.

COAGULASE-NEGATIVE STAPHYLOCOCCI

These organisms are important causes of nosocomial infections associated with prosthetic and indwelling devices. In the community, people are normally colonized by relatively sensitive strains of *Staphylococcus epidermidis*; after admission to hospital and treatment with antibiotics, patients often become colonized with more resistant strains of *Staph. epidermidis* or *Staphyloccocus haemolyticus*. A majority of coagulase-negative staphylococci isolated in hospitals show multiple antibiotic resistance, including resistance to methicillin (and other β-lactams), gentamicin and, to a lesser extent, quinolone. *Staph. haemolyticus* frequently shows low-level, inducible, teicoplanin resistance.[46] Resistance in coagulase-negative staphylococci appears to be increasing, and multiresistant strains may act as a reservoir of resistance genes that can be transferred to *Staph. aureus* and enterococci.

ENTEROCOCCI

The enterococci are naturally sensitive to ampicillin, but are intrinsically relatively resistant to other β-lactams such as cloxacillin, the cephalosporins and the carbapenems. They are also usually resistant to trimethoprim and the sulfonamides, the quinolones, low levels of aminoglycosides and low levels of clindamycin. These organisms have a remarkable ability to acquire new resistances to ampicillin, vancomycin and teicoplanin, chloramphenicol, erythromycin, tetracyclines, high levels of aminoglycosides and clindamycin.[47]

E. faecalis is the most common enterococcal species to be isolated from clinical specimens, but *E. faecium* is increasing in frequency as a human pathogen. *E. faecium* is inherently more resistant to penicillin and ampicillin than *E. faecalis*, and hospital isolates tend to show increasing high-level resistance due to altered PBPs (*see above*). Transferable β-lactamase-mediated ampicillin resistance has been reported in *E. faecalis* but, although such strains have caused several large hospital outbreaks in the USA, they remain rare.

In the USA, acquired vancomycin resistance increased more than 40-fold among nosocomial isolates of enterococci, from 0.3% in 1989 to over 20% in 1999. This rise followed an increase by more than 100-fold in the use of vancomycin in American hospitals in the last 20 years. Initially, clonal epidemics of vancomycin-resistant enterococci broke out in intensive care units and later in whole hospitals. This was followed by spread of resistance plasmids and transposons among multiple strains of *E. faecium* and *E. faecalis*.[47] Transmission is enhanced by cross-contamination via the hands of healthcare personnel, by contaminated environment and is favored by exposure to antimicrobial therapy, particularly with glycopeptides, cephalosporins and drugs with anti-anaerobic activity.[48] In the USA, most of the vancomycin-resistant strains are resistant to all other available antimicrobials, making therapy extremely difficult and requiring multiple combinations of drugs based on specific mechanisms of resistance of infecting strains, or the use of new drugs such as quinupristin-dalfopristin and linezolid.[47] In some studies of patients with sepsis and bacteremia due to these strains, the mortality attributable to the infection was significant, although the specific impact of antibiotic therapy is difficult to ascertain because of the severity of the underlying disease.[49] In Europe, the incidence of nosocomial infection caused by multiple-resistant enterococci remains lower, with rates of <5% glycopeptide resistance and about 20% high-level gentamicin resistance in clinical isolates.[50] Outbreaks have also been reported in European hospitals, however, especially in transplant and intensive care units.[41]

STREPTOCOCCUS PNEUMONIAE

Acquired multidrug resistance in *Str. pneumoniae* has become a worldwide health problem, with increasing incidence of resistance to β-lactams, macrolides, lincosamides and tetracyclines in most parts of the world in the last two decades.[51,52] The MIC of penicillin for sensitive strains of pneumococci is <0.01 mg/l; the first penicillin-resistant isolates, reported in 1967 from Papua New Guinea, showed 'low-level' resistance with MICs of up to 1 mg/l, but in 1977 pneumococci were isolated in South Africa showing 'high-level' resistance with penicillin MICs of >1 mg/l. High-level penicillin resistance has so far been confined to a small number of serotypes, whereas low-level resistance is now found in nearly all the common serotypes. There is a wide geographical variation in the prevalence of penicillin-resistant pneumococci, even between regions of a particular country. There is conclusive evidence of international spread of multiresistant clones, such as the Spanish serotype 23F clone that was apparently 'exported' from Spain to the USA.[53] According to two recent worldwide surveys and Europe-wide surveillance data (www.earss.rivm.nl), in some countries, such as in Northern Europe, only a few per cent of pneumococcal isolates show low-level penicillin resistance and high-level resistance is rare; however, in other countries such as France, Hungary, Spain, Israel, and the USA, 30% or more of isolates are resistant (Figure 3.5), of which more than 15% of isolates are high-level resistant.[52,54] Resistance to cefotaxime varied between 2 and 4%. A high prevalence of macrolide resistance among *Str. pneumoniae* was reported from all continents (11–39%). In the USA it is mostly caused by MefA efflux and does not affect lincosamides, whereas in Europe and the Asia-Pacific regions the predominant mechanism of resistance is ribosomal methylation conferring the MLS_B phenotype. There is a strong association of co-resistance to penicillin, macrolides, lincosamides, chloramphenicol, tetracycline and co-trimoxazole. It is likely that the worldwide prevalence of penicillin and multiple-antibiotic resistant pneumococci will continue to increase.

Respiratory and bloodstream infections with strains of pneumococci showing low- to moderate-level penicillin resistance

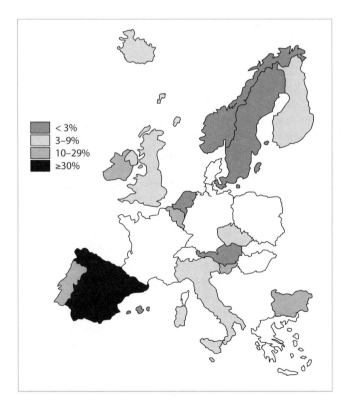

Fig. 3.5 Proportion of penicillin non-susceptible *Str. pneumoniae* isolates from meningitis and bloodstream infections, EARSS participating countries, 2000. Available at http://www.earss.rivm.nl

(MIC < 4.0 mg/l) can be treated with high doses of penicillin, amoxicillin or cephalosporins as there is no firm evidence that this level of penicillin resistance is associated with increased risk of treatment failure. On the other hand, meningitis treatment failures have been documented in infections with even low-level penicillin-resistant strains. Therefore, initial treatment of meningitis in areas with high levels of penicillin and cephalosporin resistance includes high-dose cefotaxime or ceftriaxone in association with vancomycin. Both drugs should be continued in case of infection with cefotaxime-intermediate resistant pneumococci (MIC of 1.0 mg/l), and rifampicin should be added if the cefotaxime MIC is ≥2 mg/l (*see* Ch. 53). Emerging resistance to fluoroquinolones has been reported in respiratory isolates of pneumococci from Canada, Spain and Hong Kong. This is a cause for concern, given the potential usefulness of newer generation fluoroquinolones for treatment of respiratory infections.[29]

HAEMOPHILUS INFLUENZAE

Ampicillin resistance due to plasmid-mediated TEM-1 β-lactamase production was first noted in 1972, and is now widespread. Repeated worldwide surveys from 1992 to 1999 of clinical isolates of *H. influenzae* recovered from lower respiratory and blood specimens have shown a rise in the prevalence of β-lactamase-producing strains, from 26% to 33% of isolates in the USA and from 14% to 19% in Europe. In 1999, these rates were about 17% in the Asia-Pacific and 16% in Latin America.[52,54] Non β-lactamase-mediated ampicillin resistance has been identified, associated with changes in penicillin-binding proteins, but this form of ampicillin resistance remains rare (<0.5%). Cephalosporins and amoxicillin-clavulanate remain very active (>99% sensitivity), as are fluoroquinolones, tetracyclines, rifampicin and chloramphenicol. Rates of chloramphenicol resistance in excess of 10% were occasionally found in some Latin American and Asian countries. Co-trimoxazole resistance rates vary markedly by region, with the highest rates reported from Latin America, the Middle East and Spain (about 30%), followed by Eastern Europe and North America (10–20%). *H. influenzae* is intrinsically resistant to erythromycin.

NEISSERIA MENINGITIDIS

The emergence of sulfonamide resistance in *N. meningitidis*, due to mutational or recombinational modification of the target dihydropterate synthase, emerged in the early 1960s and is now widespread.[55] Of greater concern today is the emergence of penicillin resistance. The MIC of penicillin for meningococci is usually <0.08 mg/l, but this may be increased in moderately susceptible isolates up to 0.5 mg/l. These strains were first reported in the 1960s but have increased in frequency in the past 15 years in some countries, especially in Spain. This low-level penicillin resistance is due to alterations in PBP 2, with mosaic gene structure arising as a result of transformation from commensal *Neisseria* species. In the 1990s, Spain has suffered a clonal epidemic associated with a penicillin moderately susceptible C:2b:P1.2,5 strain that accounted for more than 60% of invasive serogroup C isolates. There are only scant clinical data (two case reports) indicating that meningitis with the moderately susceptible meningococcal strains may be associated with penicillin treatment failures. Third-generation cephalosporins remain very active on these strains. In addition, β-lactamase production by meningococci has been reported in four cases and appears to be encoded on a gonococcal plasmid. Chloramphenicol resistance has been reported recently from Vietnam and was determined by a *catP* gene located on a defective transposon from *Clostridium perfringens*. Although up to 10% of carriers treated with rifampicin are subsequently found to harbor rifampicin-resistant meningococci, caused by a point mutation in the *rpoB* gene, such strains remain extremely rare in invasive disease. Ciprofloxacin is widely used for the eradication of throat carriage in adults but no resistant meningococci have yet been reported.

NEISSERIA GONORRHOEAE

Low-level resistance to benzylpenicillin (MIC 0.1–2 mg/l) has been increasing in strains of *N. gonorrhoeae* for several decades, and is now very common. This type of resistance is due to mutational alterations in the penicillin-binding proteins PBP 1 and PBP 2 and to impermeability associated with alteration of PI porin. Since 1976, a high-level plasmid-mediated type of resistance to penicillin, caused by production of TEM-1 β-lactamase, appeared in South-East Asia and West Africa and spread to Western countries.[56] These penicillinase-producing strains of *N. gonorrhoeae* remain common (30–65%) in many developing countries, but account for only 5–10% of gonococcal isolates in the West. Low-level resistance to tetracyclines is often associated with multiple resistance to penicillin, erythromycin and fusidic acid. It is caused by mutational derepression of the MtrRCDE efflux system.[16] Plasmid-mediated high-level resistance to all tetracyclines, including doxycycline, determined by the ribosomal protection protein TetM carried on a transposon, emerged in 1985. It has reached a high prevalence, which unfortunately reduces the clinical utility of this group of drugs for the treatment of dual infection with gonococci and chlamydia. Spectinomycin resistance, due to mutational alteration of the 30S ribosomal subunit, remains rare. Resistance to fluoroquinolones, due to GyrA and/or ParC mutational alteration, emerged in several countries during the 1990s and increased by clonal spread to reach prevalence rates up to 20% in South-East Asia and Africa.[29]

ESCHERICHIA COLI

Acquired resistance to ampicillin is conferred to *E. coli* by a plasmid-encoded, Tn3-associated TEM-1 β-lactamase. First described in 1965, this mobile gene has spread so extensively throughout the world that 40–60% of both hospital and community strains are now resistant by this mechanism. Up to 50% of these ampicillin-resistant organisms are also resistant to the combination of amoxicillin with the β-lactamase inhibitor clavulanic acid, either because of hyperproduction of TEM-1 β-lactamase or by production of mutant, inhibitor-resistant TEM enzyme. Other plasmid-encoded β-lactamases are seen in *E. coli* with increasing frequency, including extended-spectrum β-lactamases of the TEM, SHV and AmpC families. In a recent worldwide survey, the rates of decreased susceptibility to oxyiminocephalosporins among clinical isolates ranged from 3% in the USA, 5% in Europe, to 8% in the Western Pacific and 9% in Latin America.[57] This resistance was frequently associated with co-resistance to gentamicin (15–75%), tetracycline (45–77%), co-trimoxazole (6–26%) and ciprofloxacin (14–66%). Fluoroquinolone resistance in *E. coli* is an increasingly common problem in Europe, reaching prevalence rates of 5–10% in several surveys. It is particularly common in patients with complicated urinary tract infections and in neutropenic patients developing bacteremia during fluoroquinolone prophylaxis.[29] Furthermore, sequence determination of the gyrase genes in fluoroquinolone susceptible isolates has shown frequent first step mutations. This indicates that these organisms may rapidly evolve into the resistant category by acquisition of a second mutation.

KLEBSIELLA, ENTEROBACTER AND SERRATIA SPP.

These organisms are intrinsically resistant to ampicillin, and *Enterobacter* and *Serratia* spp. are resistant to older cephalosporins. They all have the ability to cause hospital outbreaks of opportunistic infection, and they often exchange plasmid-borne resistances. *K. pneumoniae* is the most common nosocomial pathogen of the three, and appears to have the greatest ability to receive and disseminate multiresistance plasmids. The ampicillin resistance of *K. pneumoniae* is mediated by chromosomal SHV-1 β-lactamase. In the 1970s, organisms carrying plasmid-borne aminoglycoside resistance often caused large outbreaks of hospital infection and sometimes disseminated their resistances to *Enterobacter*, *Serratia* and other enterobacterial species. These outbreaks diminished when the newer cephalosporins and aminoglycosides became available. Starting in the mid-1980s in Europe and Latin America and in the 1990s in the USA, hospital outbreaks due to *K. pneumoniae* with resistance to third-generation cephalosporins by plasmid-borne production of extended-spectrum β-lactamases (ESBL) were reported, particularly in ICUs.[10] ESBL-encoding plasmids were also transferred to *Klebsiella oxytoca*, *Citrobacter* spp., *E. coli*, *Proteus mirabilis*, and *Enterobacter* spp. Recent pan-European surveys in ICUs showed that the proportion of ESBL-producing klebsiellae varies markedly by hospital and by country, from 3% in Sweden to 60% in Turkey.[58,59] The proportion of *K. pneumoniae* clinical isolates with potential

ESBL expression found in a 1997–99 survey ranged from 8% in the USA, to 25% in the Western Pacific, to 45% in Latin America.[57] Co-resistance to aminoglycosides, co-trimoxazole, tetracyclines and fluoroquinolones is common. About 30% of hospital isolates of *Enterobacter* spp. show cephalosporinase hyperproduction.[59] More recently, ESBL-producing (mostly TEM-24), multiresistant *Enterobacter aerogenes* strains have emerged in France and Belgium as a common cause of noso-comial infection. Epidemic strains were first reported in ICUs and have since disseminated hospital-wide to cause large regional epidemics.[60] Many of these ESBL-producing strains remain susceptible only to carbapenems, which are the drugs of choice for treatment of serious infection with these organisms.[11] In *Enterobacter* strains with high-level cephalosporinase combined with ESBL production, however, emergence of porin-resistant mutants during imipenem therapy may lead to treatment failure, requiring the use of polymyxin B or doxy-cycline for infections with strains resistant to all β-lactams and fluoroquinolones.[15,61]

SHIGELLA

Shigellae were among the first organisms to be shown in the 1950s to harbor transferable antibiotic resistance determinants on conjugative plasmids. In developing countries, rates of multiple resistance are high, with 30–70% of isolates resistant to ampicillin, chloramphenicol, tetracycline, co-trimoxazole or nalidixic acid,[62] but most isolates remain susceptible to fluoroquinolones. Multiresistance is most common in *Shigella dysenteriae*, followed by *Shigella flexneri* and *Shigella sonnei*. In developed countries rates of resistance are higher in patients with a history of travel abroad.

SALMONELLA

Salmonella enterica serotype Typhi has developed multiple resistance to first-line antibiotics in many developing countries. In the 1970s, strains with plasmid-mediated resistance to ampicillin and chloramphenicol caused epidemics in Latin America. In the 1980s, strains with plasmid-mediated resistance to ampicillin, chloramphenicol and co-trimoxazole emerged in South-East Asia and have since become widespread in Asia and Latin America, where rates of 30–70% multiresistant *Salmonella* Typhi were reported in the 1990s. Fluoroquinolone resistance is now emerging in MDR strains and has been associated with recent outbreaks of typhoid fever in Tajikistan, Vietnam and the Indian subcontinent. The proportion of *Salmonella* Typhi with low level resistance to ciprofloxacin showed a rapid increase to more than 20% in 1999 in the UK, and was mostly seen in travelers returning from the Indian subcontinent.[63]

In the 1990s, multiple resistance also rose rapidly in non-typhoidal salmonellae in Europe and in the USA. Although the subject has stimulated considerable debate, there is conclusive evidence that antibiotics used in animal husbandry have contributed to antibiotic resistance in human isolates. In the UK and other European countries, the incidence of human infections with multiresistant *Salmonella* ser. Typhimurium DT104 resistant to ampicillin, chloramphenicol, streptomycin, co-trimoxazole and tetracycline increased markedly during the period 1990–1996, at a time when penicillin and tetracycline were commonly used in cattle feed. In Denmark, an outbreak of food-borne salmonellosis caused by a multidrug and low-level fluoroquinolone-resistant *Salmonella* ser. Typhimurium was traced to an infected swine herd. This strain was nalidixic acid resistant and showed increased ciprofloxacin MIC (0.06–0.12 mg/l). Although this level of susceptibility is categorized as sensitive by current breakpoints, patients treated with fluoroquinolones showed poor clinical response.[64] Soon after the introduction of enrofloxacin for veterinary use in the UK in 1993, human *Salmonella* isolates with decreased susceptibility to ciprofloxacin increased tenfold from 1994 to 1997. In 1999, soon after the introduction of codes of good practice for the prophylactic use of fluoroquinolones in animal husbandry in the UK, there was a 75% decline in isolations of multiresistant *Salmonella* ser Typhimurium DT104 from clinical specimens, which may indicate a favorable impact of more prudent antibiotic use.[65] The extended-spectrum β-lactamases have appeared in some *Salmonella* strains, possibly as a result of plasmid transfer from commensal enterobacteria in the human gut. ESBL-producing salmonellae caused epidemics in Greece and spread to other European countries in the 1990s.[66] The first case of infection by ceftriaxone-resistant *Salmonella* reported in the USA was linked to contact with infected cattle treated with cephalosporins on a Nebraska farm.[67] A recent worldwide survey of clinical isolates from hospital patients has found 2–3% ESBL-producing strains in salmonellae from Latin America and the Western Pacific but less than 1% in isolates from Europe and the USA.[57]

CAMPYLOBACTER

Campylobacter spp. have also shown increasing antimicrobial resistance in the past decade, and again much of this resistance appears related to the veterinary use of antibiotics. Although there is considerable geographic variation, macrolide resistance in *C. jejuni*, which is due to mutational alteration of 23S rRNA, has remained stable in recent years in Europe but is increasing in South-East Asia.[68] *Campylobacter coli* shows higher erythromycin resistance rates (0–68%) than *C. jejuni* (0–10%). In contrast, the proportion of isolates resistant to fluoroquinolones, which is caused by stepwise mutations in *gyrA* and/or *parC* genes, has increased dramatically around the world over the last 10 years (from 0% to over 80% in some areas). There is consistent evidence that this is a result of the addition of quinolones to chicken feed.[32,68] In every country where this has been investigated, quinolone resistance in human *Campylobacter* isolates increased in frequency soon after the introduction of these drugs in animal husbandry, but long after their licensing in human medicine. In the USA, domestic chickens were determined by epidemiologic and molecular investigations as the predominant source of quinolone-resistant *C. jejuni* infection in the years after these drugs were licensed for use in poultry in 1995.[69] In Thailand and Taiwan, very high rates of multiple resistance to quinolones, macrolides, tetracyclines and ampicillin leave often no effective antimicrobial treatment for *Campylobacter* enteritis.[68]

HELICOBACTER PYLORI

Peptic ulcer disease caused by *Helicobacter pylori* infection is treated by associations of antibiotics, which may include amoxicillin, tetracyclines, clarithromycin and metronidazole. Eradication fails, however, in 10–30% of cases. This is in part due to primary or secondary resistance to one or more of these drugs, most commonly to metronidazole or clarithromycin.[70] Development of secondary resistance may occur in over 50% of cases with suboptimal regimens. Nitroimidazole resistance is mostly related to mutational inactivation of the *rdxA* gene encoding an oxygen-sensitive NADPH nitroreductase.[71] The cure rate with most combination regimens drops by about 50% in case of nitroimidazole resistance. The prevalence of this resistance is rising and ranges currently from 10% to 50% of isolates in the West and 80% to 90% in developing countries. Resistance to clarithromycin is caused by mutation at position 2142 or 2143 in 23S rRNA. Its impact on cure rate appears similar to that of nitroimidazole resistance for most treatment regimens. The prevalence of primary macrolide resistance varies by region between 3% and 15% and is increasing. Standardization of resistance detection methods for this pathogen is much needed to assess the efficacy of treatment regimens based on primary resistance patterns and to guide local recommendations based on surveillance data.[70]

PSEUDOMONAS AERUGINOSA

Ps. aeruginosa is a leading cause of nosocomial infection in critically ill patients[59] and is associated with the highest attributable mortality among opportunistic Gram-negative bacteria. It is intrinsically resistant to most β-lactam antibiotics, tetracyclines, chloramphenicol, sulfonamides and nalidixic acid, due to the interplay of impermeability with multidrug efflux, principally mediated by MexAB-OprM.[72] Acquired resistance to anti-pseudomonal antibiotics develops rapidly and can emerge in more than 10% of patients during treatment. This occurs most commonly with imipenem and ciprofloxacin.[73] Multiple types of acquired β-lactam resistance are expressed by this adaptable organism, often in combination: hyperproduction of AmpC cephalosporinase, acquisition of transposon and plasmid-mediated ESBLs, oxacillinases, or carbapenemases; mutational loss of porins or upregulation of efflux pumps.[14] Three types of aminoglycoside resistance are seen: high-level, plasmid-mediated resistance to one or two aminoglycosides, due to the production of aminoglycoside-modifying enzymes, and broad-spectrum resistance to all the aminoglycosides, due to a reduction in the permeability of the cell envelope and/or overexpression of an efflux pump. Fluoroquinolone resistance is mediated by topoisomerase gene mutations, decreased permeability and efflux overexpression. Recent surveys of clinical isolates of *Ps. aeruginosa* from ICUs have indicated resistance rates >10% to all drugs in most European countries.[59] A global survey showed increasing resistance to most drugs between 1997 and 1999 and indicated that no antipseudomonal agent was still active on >80% of strains sampled hospital wide in 1999 from Europe and Latin America.[74] Resistance rates varied by region, with Latin America showing the highest prevalence, followed by Europe with high β-lactam resistance (>25% to ceftazidime) and fluoroquinolone resistance rates (>30% to ciprofloxacin), particularly in Southern Europe. Multidrug resistant strains were found in 1% of isolates from the USA, 5% from Europe and 8% from Latin America, and their distribution by participating center suggested local outbreaks. Multiresistant *Ps. aeruginosa* is becoming one of the most problematic nosocomial pathogens,[75] particularly in view of the lack of new antimicrobial classes active on this organism in clinical development.

ACINETOBACTER SPP.

Acinetobacters are free-living non-fermenting organisms that often colonize human skin and cause opportunistic infections. Furthermore, these organisms resist desiccation and are able to survive for prolonged periods in inanimate environments. The most frequently isolated species, and one most likely to acquire multiple antibiotic resistance, is *Acinetobacter baumannii*.[76] In the early 1970s, acinetobacters were usually sensitive to many common antimicrobial agents but many hospital strains are now resistant to most available agents, including co-trimoxazole, aminoglycosides, cephalosporins, quinolones and, to a lesser extent, carbapenems. The mechanisms and genetics of resistance in this species are complex, but they involve several plasmid-borne β-lactamases and aminoglycoside-modifying enzymes, as well as alterations in membrane permeability and penicillin-binding proteins. The acquisition of these multiple mechanisms may be due to the fact that this group of organisms is physiologically competent and can acquire DNA by transformation in vivo. Multiresistant *A. baumannii* strains have caused epidemics in several countries and nosocomial infections with these strains have been associated with excess mortality.[49] Polymyxins and sulbactam may be the only active drugs available to treat infections caused by multiresistant strains. Some epidemic strains have spread across Europe by transfer of colonized patients.[76]

OTHER NON-FERMENTING ORGANISMS

S. maltophilia and *Burkholderia cepacia* have recently emerged as significant nosocomial pathogens. These organisms are intrinsically resistant to many of the antimicrobial agents used for infection with Gram-negative organisms, including the aminoglycosides and cephalosporins, and often acquire further resistance to co-trimoxazole and fluoroquinolones. Because of this, and despite their relatively low virulence, they are seen with increasing frequency in areas of high antibiotic usage such as intensive care units. *S. maltophilia* is intrinsically resistant to all the aminoglycosides, to imipenem and most β-lactams, and up to 10% of isolates have acquired resistance to co-trimoxazole and tetracyclines. It has considerable ability to develop further multiple resistance by several mechanisms, including decrease in outer membrane permeability, active efflux and the production of inducible broad-spectrum β-lactamases. Bacteria of the *B. cepacia* complex are also generally resistant to the aminoglycosides and most β-lactam antibiotics, but sensitive to ciprofloxacin, temocillin and meropenem. However, additional acquired multiple resistance was found in epidemic strains that are associated with rapid deterioration in infected cystic fibrosis patients with advanced lung disease.

MYCOBACTERIUM TUBERCULOSIS

M. tuberculosis has limited susceptibility to standard antimicrobial agents, but can be treated by combinations of antituberculosis drugs, of which the common first-line agents are rifampicin, isoniazid, ethambutol and pyrazinamide (*see* Ch. 36 and 61). Resistance is the result of spontaneous chromosomal mutations at various loci. Mutational resistance occurs at the rate of about 1 in 10^8 for rifampicin, 1 in 10^8 to 1 in 10^9 for isoniazid, 1 in 10^6 for ethambutol and 1 in 10^5 for streptomycin. Since a cavitating lung lesion contains up to 10^9 organisms, mutational resistance appears quite frequently when these drugs are used singly for treatment, but is uncommon if three or more are used simultaneously. The action of isoniazid against *M. tuberculosis* may involve multiple mechanisms, including transport and activation of the drug by mechanisms involving catalase-peroxidase, pigment precursors, NAD and peroxide; generation of reactive oxygen radicals; and inhibition of mycolic acid biosynthesis. Mutations at several loci might be involved in decreased susceptibility to isoniazid, including the *katG* gene that encodes catalase-peroxidase activity, the *inhA* gene which is involved in mycolic acid synthesis, and the *aphC* gene which encodes alkylhydroxyperoxide reductase.[77] Likewise, resistance to ethambutol may result from diverse mutations in the *embCAB* operon, which is involved in the biosynthesis of cell wall arabinan, or in other genes. Resistance to rifampicin, fluoroquinolones and streptomycin appears to be caused in *M. tuberculosis* by mechanisms similar to those seen in other species, as the result of mutations in the *rpoB* gene that encodes the β-subunit of RNA polymerase, the *gyrA* gene encoding the A subunit of bacterial DNA polymerase and either the *rrs* gene encoding 16S rRNA or the *rpsL* gene encoding the S12 ribosomal protein, respectively. Resistance to pyrazinamide, however, does not appear to be due to altered target but to inactivation of the *pncA* gene encoding pyrazinamidase, an enzyme which is necessary for transformation of the pro-drug into active pyrazinic acid.[78]

Drug-resistant tuberculosis emerged in the 1990s as a major health problem in several parts of the world, occurring in up to 14% of new cases in some countries (e.g. Estonia).[79] Multidrug-resistant tuberculosis (MDR-TB) implies resistance to at least two of the first-line antituberculosis drugs: rifampicin and isoniazid. These two drugs are essential for most initial or short-course treatment regimens, and strains of *M. tuberculosis* resistant to them soon develop resistance to other drugs. Patients with MDR-TB thus fail to respond to standard therapy and disseminate resistant strains to their contacts (including healthcare workers), both before and after the resistance is discovered. MDR-TB is more difficult and expensive to treat and is associated with high mortality rates in all patients, but especially so in people infected with HIV, which is a common association in hospital outbreaks. Large nosocomial and community outbreaks of MDR-TB were seen in some American cities in the early 1990s, and later reported in Western Europe and Brazil.[80] The main factor for the appearance of MDR-TB is probably failure of patients to comply with their treatment regimens, resulting in inadequate therapy and the emergence of resistant mutants. Factors that contribute to this situation include deterioration of public-health services directed towards control of tuberculosis; inadequate training of healthcare workers in the diagnosis, treatment and control of tuberculosis; laboratory delays in the detection and sensitivity testing of *M. tuberculosis*; admission to hospitals unprepared and ill-equipped for control of airborne transmission of pathogens; addition of single drugs to failing treatment regimens; an increase in the number and promiscuity of individuals at high-risk of acquiring and disseminating tuberculosis, including those infected with HIV, the poor and the homeless; and increasing migration of people from areas where tuberculosis is common.[80] The single most important factor in the prevention and successful control of further emergence of MDR-TB is probably the reintroduction of supervised observed therapy. In addition, substantial commitment of resources, healthcare planning and the use of appropriate hospital isolation facilities has brought nosocomial MDR-TB under control. Although the median worldwide prevalence of MDR-TB among new cases of tuberculosis is 1%, these rates can reach 5–14% in some areas of Eastern Europe, Russia, Iran and China.[79] A higher prevalence of drug resistance is also seen in immigrants to Western countries.

EPIDEMIOLOGY OF ANTIBIOTIC RESISTANCE

Epidemiologic and biologic studies have shown that the rise of antibiotic resistance among human pathogenic bacteria is a global phenomenon which is related to the interplay of several factors that interact in various fashions in different ecosystems

(Figure 3.6).[1] These factors include the development of environmental and human reservoirs of antibiotic resistance genes and resistant bacteria, patterns of antibiotic use in medicine and agriculture that select for and amplify these reservoirs, and socio-economic changes that influence the transmission of pathogens. The genetic mechanisms that confer antibiotic resistance on bacteria must have existed long before the antibiotic era. Conjugative plasmids devoid of resistant genes were detected in clinical isolates of bacteria collected before the 1940s. Many resistance genes have presumably evolved from detoxifying mechanisms in antibiotic-producing fungi and streptomycetes living in soil and water and were later mobilized by genetic transfer to commensal and pathogenic bacteria.[10,36] Whatever the origins of resistance genes, there has clearly been a major increase in their prevalence during the past 60 years. This can be closely correlated with the use of antibiotics in humans and animals, and it is clear that resistance has eventually emerged to each new agent.

Antibiotic use is the driving force that promotes the selection, persistence and spread of resistant organisms. The phenomenon is common to hospitals, which have seen the emergence of a range of multidrug resistant pathogens,[81] to the community at large, where respiratory and gut pathogens have become resistant to often freely available antibiotics,[82] and to animal husbandry, where the use of antibiotics for growth promotion and for mass therapy has promoted resistance in *Salmonella* and *Campylobacter*[68] and created a reservoir of glycopeptide-resistant enterococci that can be transmitted to humans.[83]

In the community, where about 80% of human antibiotic consumption takes place, a large proportion of antibiotics is inappropriately prescribed for upper respiratory infections. Patients' misperceptions about the utility of antibiotics in self-resolving viral infections, commercial promotion, poor compliance with prescriptions and over-the-counter sales of antibiotics in some countries are contributing to this misuse of antimicrobials.[82] The factors relating prescription patterns to increasing resistance are only incompletely understood.[84] Low dosage and prolonged administration has been associated with increased risk of development of β-lactam resistance in pneumococci.[85] Finnish surveillance data show that macrolide resistance in *Streptococcus pyogenes* has increased as the national use has increased – and, conversely, has declined as a result of the much diminished use of erythromycin.[33] There are wide variations in per capita antibiotic consumption in Europe, with lowest levels of consumption in the Nordic countries correlating with a much lower prevalence of resistance in most bacterial pathogens than in the other parts of Europe (Figure 3.4). Socio-economic changes are also powerful drivers of the resurgence of infectious diseases and drug resistance.[1,3] The impoverishment of large sections of the population and disruption of the healthcare system in the former Soviet Union has had a clear impact on the spread of MDR-TB.[79] Globalization is stimulating international circulation of goods and people, and plays a role in accelerating the dissemination of pathogens, including resistant strains.

The hospital, particularly the intensive care unit, is a major breeding ground for antibiotic-resistant bacteria. Here, a high density population of patients with compromised host defences is exposed to a usage of antibiotics that is about 100 times more concentrated than in the community, and frequent contact with healthcare personnel creates ceaseless opportunities for cross-infection.[81] Most new drugs and injectable agents are first administered to hospital patients. Topical antibiotics are particularly likely to select for resistance, as illustrated by the emergence of gentamicin-resistant *P. aeruginosa* and fusidic-acid or mupirocin-resistant *S. aureus* that has often followed heavy topical use of gentamicin in burns and fusidic acid or mupirocin in dermatological patients. Multiple drug resistance can be encouraged even by the use of a single agent, since this may select for plasmids conferring resistance to multiple antibiotics.

Selection of resistance during antibiotic therapy in infecting or colonizing bacteria is enhanced by factors related to the patient: immune suppression, presence of a large bacterial inoculum, and biofilm-associated infection of foreign bodies which impede local host defences.[35] Other resistance-predisposing factors relate to the modalities of treatment: use of monotherapy as opposed to combination therapy may favor selection of resistance in certain infections, as will drug underdosing or inappropriate route of administration which causes failure to achieve bactericidal drug levels at the site of infection.[86] Alteration of the endogenous microflora during antibiotic therapy also enhances replacement of susceptible organisms by resistant strains from the hospital microflora.[48]

Nosocomial transmission of MDR bacteria occurs most commonly by indirect contact between patients (via the contaminated hands of healthcare personnel) and, less commonly, by contaminated fomites. Patient factors predisposing to this

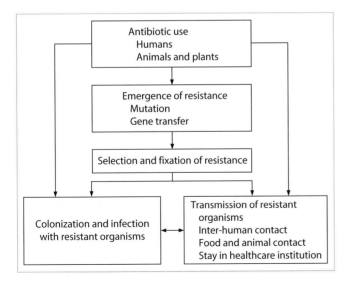

Fig. 3.6 Factors contributing to the emergence and spread of antibiotic resistance in interconnected ecosystems.

transmission include the severity of underlying illness, length of stay in hospital, intensity and duration of exposure to broad-spectrum antibiotics, and use of invasive devices (such as intravenous catheters) or procedures.[48,61,87] Hospital patients and staff colonized with resistant bacteria, especially in the feces or on the skin, further disseminate these organisms both within the hospital and into the community. Cost containment in hospital management has resulted in chronic understaffing, increased patient turnover and inter-institutional transfer, both factors which have been well documented to enhance nosocomial transmission of MDR bacteria such as MRSA and ESBL-producing Gram-negative bacteria.[11]

About 30% of the patients in acute care hospitals receive antibiotics for therapy or prophylaxis. Although antibiotics are essential for modern hospital care, many studies have shown that up to 50% of these prescriptions may be unnecessary or inappropriate. Insufficient training in antibiotic therapy, difficulty of selecting the appropriate anti-infective drugs empirically, underuse of microbiologic testing, drug promotion by pharmaceutical companies and fear of litigation are some of the factors that are stimulating the use of broad spectrum drugs.

PUBLIC HEALTH AND ECONOMIC IMPACT

Antibiotic resistance places an increasing burden on society in terms of increased morbidity, mortality and costs. In spite of methodologic complexities of the study of impact of antibiotic resistance on clinical outcomes, it is recognized that, for many diseases, individuals infected with resistant pathogens are more likely to receive ineffective therapy, to more frequently require hospital care, to stay in for longer, to develop complications and to die of the disease.[2,49] The cost of care is also increased for such patients, due to the need for more costly second-line drugs, longer duration of hospital stay, increased need for intensive care and diagnostic testing, higher incidence of complications, and expenses incurred by use of isolation precautions. There are also longer term costs for the society such as increased disease incidence and loss of profit for the pharmaceutical industry.[49]

CONTROL AND PREVENTION

Several societies and expert panels have published guidelines for optimizing antibiotic use and curtailing antibiotic resistance in hospitals.[88–91] Key components of these guidelines include:

- better undergraduate and postgraduate training;
- multidisciplinary cooperation between hospital administrators, clinicians, infectious disease specialists, infection control team, microbiologists and hospital pharmacists;
- formulary-based local guidelines on anti-infective therapy and prophylaxis, education and regulation of prescriptions

by consultant specialists, monitoring and auditing drug use, surveillance and reporting of resistance patterns of the hospital flora;
- surveillance and early detection of outbreaks by molecular typing, detection and notification of patients colonized with communicable resistant bacteria to infection control team when useful for patient isolation and/or decolonization;
- promotion and monitoring of basic hospital infection control practices such as hand hygiene.

These guidelines are mostly based on local experience and on the results of before–after and analytic studies.[92–94] Few strategies have been formally tested for cost-effectiveness in controlled intervention studies.[95] Mathematical modelling provides interesting insights into the prediction of epidemiologic factors that are the most vulnerable to effective interventions.[41,48] Antibiotic policies can slow down the development of resistance in hospitals by antibiotic cycling or rotation, whereby different classes of antibiotics are preferentially used in successive periods of time. Although this strategy has contributed to control MDR bacteria in outbreaks, its general efficacy as a preventive strategy requires further study.[96] The applicability of guidelines may be limited by heterogeneity in human and microbial populations and in healthcare organizations. Because each hospital has its own ecosystem and micro-society where determinants of antibiotic resistance are quite specific and evolve rapidly, effective solutions should be tailored to local circumstances and resources. On the other hand, early coordination of policies at regional or national level has been successful to control the transmission of emerging MDR nosocomial pathogens.[97]

In the past few years, antibiotic resistance has been universally identified as a public health priority and action plans to combat resistance have been developed by several national health agencies and international organizations such as the European Commission and WHO.[2,3,98] These strategic plans call for:

- public and professional education toward rational use of antimicrobials;
- coordination of surveillance of antibiotic resistance and antibiotic use in human and animal health sectors;
- refined regulation of antibiotic registration for use in both sectors;
- development and evaluation of improved diagnostic methods;
- promotion and evaluation of medical and veterinary practice guidelines;
- restriction of antibiotic use as growth promoters in food animals;
- promotion of infection control practice in healthcare institutions;
- development of novel antimicrobial drugs and vaccines;
- closer international cooperation.

A number of international surveillance systems and action programs are in development to provide early warning of the emergence of threatening antibiotic resistant bacteria in the hope of more timely interventions.[90,99]

Physicians can no longer avoid their responsibilities as antibiotic prescribers and their impact on the global ecosystem of microbial pathogens. They should contribute to the design and application of sound policies of antibiotic use and infection control. If we want to prove wrong the prediction of an impending post-antibiotic era, the time has come to drastically improve our antibiotic prescribing practices and to strengthen research to identify cost-effective strategies for controlling resistance.

References

1. Cohen ML 1992 Epidemiology of drug resistance: implications for a post-antimicrobial era. *Science* 257: 1050–1055.
2. US Interagency Task Force on antimicrobial drug resistance 2001 Public health action plan to combat antimicrobial drug resistance. Online. Available at *http://www.cdc.gov/drugresistance/actionplan/index.html*
3. WHO 2001 Global strategy for containment of antimicrobial resistance Geneva. Online. Available at: *http://who.int/emc/amr.html*
4. NCCLS 2000 Methods for dilution antimicrobial susceptibility testing for bacteria that grow aerobically; NCCLS document M7-A5. Approved standard 5th edition 20: 16–17. Pennsylvania, NCCLS.
5. European Committee for Antimicrobial Susceptibility Testing of the ESCMID (EUCAST), 2000 Terminology relating to methods for the determination of susceptibility of bacteria to antimicrobial agents. *Clinical Microbiological Infections* 6: 503–508.
6. Martinez JL, Baquero F 2000 Mutation frequencies and antibiotic resistance. *Antimicrobial Agents and Chemotherapy* 44: 1771–1777.
7. Paterson DL, Ko WC, Von Gottberg A et al 2001 Outcome of cephalosporin treatment for serious infections due to apparently susceptible organisms producing extended-spectrum beta-lactamases: Implications for the clinical microbiology laboratory. *Journal of Clinical Microbiology* 39: 2206–2212.
8. Bush K 2001 New beta-lactamases in Gram-negative bacteria: Diversity and impact on the selection of antimicrobial therapy. *Clinical Infectious Diseases* 32: 1085–1089.
9. Bush K, Jacoby GA, Medeiros AA 1995 A functional classification scheme for beta-lactamases and its correlation with molecular structure. *Antimicrobial Agents and Chemotherapy* 39: 1211–1233.
10. Medeiros AA 1997 Evolution and dissemination of beta-lactamases accelerated by generations of beta-lactam antibiotics. *Clinical Infectious Diseases* 24(Suppl 1): S19–S45.
11. Paterson DL, Yu VL 1999 Extended-spectrum beta-lactamases: a call for improved detection and control. *Clinical Infectious Diseases* 29: 1419–1422.
12. Livermore DM, Woodford N 2000 Carbapenemases: a problem in waiting? *Current Opinion in Microbiology* 3: 489–495.
13. Mingeot-Leclercq MP, Glupczynski Y, Tulkens PM 1999 Aminoglycosides: activity and resistance. *Antimicrobial Agents and Chemotherapy* 43: 727–737.
14. Livermore DM 2001 Of *Pseudomonas*, porins, pumps and carbapenems. *Journal of Antimicrobial Chemotherapy* 47: 247–250.
15. Charrel RN, Pages JM, De Micco P et al 1996 Prevalence of outer membrane porin alteration in beta-lactam-antibiotic-resistant *Enterobacter aerogenes*. *Antimicrobial Agents and Chemotherapy* 40: 2854–2858.
16. Nikaido H, Zgwiskaya HI 1999 Antibiotic efflux mechanisms. *Current Opinion in Infectious Diseases* 12: 529–536.
17. Nikaido H 1998 Antibiotic resistance caused by gram-negative multidrug efflux pumps. *Clinical Infectious Diseases* 27(Suppl. 1): S32–S41.
18. Mazzariol A, Tokue Y, Kanegawa TM et al 2000 High-level fluoroquinolone-resistant clinical isolates of *Escherichia coli* overproduce multidrug efflux protein AcrA. *Antimicrobial Agents and Chemotherapy* 44: 3441–3443.
19. Chopra I, Roberts M 2001 Tetracycline antibiotics: Mode of action, applications, molecular biology, and epidemiology of bacterial resistance. *Microbiology and Molecular Biology Reviews* 65: 232–260.
20. Roberts MC, Sutcliffe J, Courvalin P et al 1999 Nomenclature for macrolide and macrolide-lincosamide-streptogramin B resistance determinants. *Antimicrobial Agents and Chemotherapy* 43: 2823–2830.
21. Hakenbeck R, Kaminski K, Konig A et al 1999 Penicillin-binding proteins in beta-lactam-resistant *Streptococcus pneumoniae*. *Microbial Drug Resistance* 5: 91–99.
22. Dowson CG, Coffey TJ, Kell C et al 1993 Evolution of penicillin resistance in *Streptococcus pneumoniae*, the role of *Streptococcus mitis* in the formation of a low affinity PBP2B in *S. pneumoniae*. *Molecular Microbiology* 9: 635–643.
23. Chambers HF 1997 Methicillin resistance in staphylococci: molecular and biochemical basis and clinical implications. *Clinical Microbiology Reviews* 10: 781–791.
24. Katayama Y, Ito T, Hiramatsu K 2000 A new class of genetic element, *Staphylococcus* cassette Chromosome *mec*, encodes methicillin resistance in *Staphylococcus aureus*, *Antimicrobial Agents and Chemotherapy* 44: 1549–1555.
25. Gholizadeh Y, Courvalin P 2000 Acquired and intrinsic glycopeptide resistance in enterococci. *International Journal of Antimicrobial Agents* 16(Suppl. 1): S11–S17.
26. Noble WC, Virani Z, Cree RGA 1992 Co-transfer of vancomycin and other resistance genes from *Enterococcus faecalis* NCTC12201 to *Staphylococcus aureus*. *FEMS Microbiological Letters*, 93: 195–198.
27. Hiramatsu K, Aritaka N, Hanaki H et al 1997 Dissemination in Japanese hospitals of strains of *Staphylococcus aureus* heterogeneously resistant to vancomycin [see comments]. *Lancet* 350: 1670–1673.
28. Tenover FC 1999 Implications of vancomycin-resistant *Staphylococcus aureus*. *Journal of Hospital Infection* 43(Suppl): S3–S7.
29. Hooper DC 2001 Emerging mechanisms of fluoroquinolone resistance. *Emergency and Infectious Diseases* 7: 337–341.
30. Martinez-Martinez L, Pascual A, Jacoby GA 1998 Quinolone resistance from a transferable plasmid. *Lancet* 351: 797–799.
31. Deplano A, Zekhnini A, Allali N et al 1997 Association of mutations in *grlA* and *gyrA* topoisomerase genes with resistance to ciprofloxacin in epidemic and sporadic isolates of methicillin-resistant *Staphylococcus aureus*. *Antimicrobial Agents and Chemotherapy* 41: 2023–2025.
32. Endtz HP, Ruijs GJ, van Klingeren B et al 1991 Quinolone resistance in campylobacter isolated from man and poultry following the introduction of fluoroquinolones in veterinary medicine. *Antimicrobial Agents and Chemotherapy* 27: 199–208.
33. Seppala H, Klaukka T, Vuopio-Varkila J et al 1997 The effect of changes in the consumption of macrolide antibiotics on erythromycin resistance in group A streptococci in Finland. Finnish Study Group for Antimicrobial Resistance. *New England Journal of Medicine* 337: 441–446.
34. Gilbart J, Perry CR, Slocombe B 1993 High-level mupirocin resistance in *Staphylococcus aureus*: evidence for two distinct isoleucyl-tRNA synthetases. *Antimicrobial Agents and Chemotherapy* 37: 32–38.
35. Lewis K 2001 Riddle of biofilm resistance. *Antimicrobial Agents and Chemotherapy* 45: 999–1007.
36. Davies J 1994 Inactivation of antibiotics and the dissemination of resistance genes. *Science* 264: 375–382.
37. Salyers AA, Amabilc-Cuevas CF 1997 Why are antibiotic resistance genes so resistant to elimination? *Antimicrobial Agents and Chemotherapy* 41: 2321–2325.
38. Ploy MC, Lambert T, Couty JP et al 2000 Integrons: an antibiotic resistance gene capture and expression system. *Clinical Chemistry and Laboratory Medicine* 38: 483–487.
39. Enne VI, Livermore DM, Stephens P et al 2001 Persistence of sulphonamide resistance in *Escherichia coli* in the UK despite national prescribing restriction. *Lancet* 357: 1325–1328.
40. Liebert CA, Hall RM, Summers AO 1999 Transposon Tn*21*, flagship of the floating genome. *Microbiology and Molecular Biology Reviews* 63: 507–522.
41. Austin DJ, Anderson RM 1999 Transmission dynamics of epidemic methicillin-resistant *Staphylococcus aureus* and vancomycin-resistant enterococci in England and Wales. *Journal of Infectious Diseases* 179: 883–891.
42. Deplano A, Witte W, van Leeuwen WJ et al 2000 Clonal dissemination of epidemic methicillin-resistant *Staphylococcus aureus* in Belgium and neighboring countries. *Clinical Microbiology Infection* 6: 239–245.
43. Mekontso-Dessap A, Kirsch M, Brun-Buisson C et al 2001 Poststernotomy mediastinitis due to *Staphylococcus aureus*: Comparison of methicillin-resistant and methicillin-susceptible cases. *Clinical Infectious Diseases* 32: 877–883.
44. Chambers HF 2001 The changing epidemiology of *Staphylococcus aureus*? *Emergency and Infectious Diseases* 7: 178–182.

45. Schmitz FJ, Fluit AC, Hafner D et al 2000 Development of resistance to ciprofloxacin, rifampin, and mupirocin in methicillin-susceptible and -resistant *Staphylococcus aureus* isolates. *Antimicrobial Agents and Chemotherapy* 44: 3229–3231.

46. Sieradzki K, Villari P, Tomasz A 1998 Decreased susceptibilities to teicoplanin and vancomycin among coagulase-negative methicillin-resistant clinical isolates of staphylococci. *Antimicrobial Agents and Chemotherapy* 42: 100–107.

47. Murray BE 2000 Vancomycin-resistant enterococcal infections. *New England Journal of Medicine* 342: 710–721.

48. Austin DJ, Bonten MJ, Weinstein RA et al 1999 Vancomycin-resistant enterococci in intensive-care hospital settings: transmission dynamics, persistence, and the impact of infection control programs. *Proceedings of the National Academy of Sciences of the USA* 96: 6908–6913.

49. Niederman MS 2001 Impact of antibiotic resistance on clinical outcomes and the cost of care. *Critical Care Medicine* 29 (Suppl. 4): N114–120.

50. Schouten MA, Voss A, Hoogkamp-Korstanje JA 1999 Antimicrobial susceptibility patterns of enterococci causing infections in Europe. The European VRE Study Group. *Antimicrobial Agents and Chemotherapy* 43: 2542–2546.

51. Klugman KP 1990 Pneumococcal resistance to antibiotics. *Clinical Microbiology Reviews* 3: 171–196.

52. Hoban DJ, Doern GV, Fluit AC et al 2001 Worldwide prevalence of antimicrobial resistance in *Streptococcus pneumoniae*, *Haemophilus influenzae*, and *Moraxella catarrhalis* in the SENTRY Antimicrobial Surveillance Program, 1997–1999. *Clinical Infectious Diseases* 32 (Suppl. 2): S81–S93.

53. Munoz R, Coffey TJ, Daniels M, et al 1991 Intercontinental spread of a multiresistant clone of serotype 23F *Streptococcus pneumoniae*. *Journal of Infectious Diseases* 164: 302–306.

54. Felmingham D, Brown DF, Soussy CJ 1998 European Glycopeptide Susceptibility Survey of gram-positive bacteria for 1995. European Glycopeptide Resistance Survey Study Group. *Diagnostic Microbiology and Infectious Disease* 31: 563–571.

55. Vazquez JA 2001 The resistance of *Neisseria meningitidis* to the antimicrobial agents: an issue still in evolution. *Reviews in Medical Microbiology* 12: 39–45.

56. Phillips I 1976 Beta-lactamase-producing, penicillin-resistant gonococcus. *Lancet* ii,: 656–657.

57. Winokur PL, Canton R, Casellas JM et al 2001 Variations in the prevalence of strains expressing an extended-spectrum beta-lactamase phenotype and characterization of isolates from Europe, the Americas, and the Western Pacific Region. *Clinical Infectious Diseases* 32 (Suppl. 2): S94–S103.

58. Livermore DM, Yuan M 1996 Antibiotic resistance and production of extended-spectrum beta-lactamases amongst *Klebsiella* spp. from intensive care units in Europe. *Journal of Antimicrobial Chemotherapy* 38: 409–424.

59. Hanberger H, Gareia-Rodriguez JA, Gobernado M et al 1999 Antibiotic susceptibility among aerobic gram-negative bacilli in intensive care units in 5 European countries. French and Portuguese ICU Study Groups. *Journal of the American Medical Association* 281: 67–71.

60. De Gheldre Y, Struelens MJ, Glupczynski Y et al 2001 National Epidemiologic Surveys of *Enterobacter aerogenes* in Belgian Hospitals from 1996 to 1998. *Journal of Clinical Microbiology* 39: 889–896.

61. De Gheldre Y, Maes N, Rost F et al 1997 Molecular epidemiology of an outbreak of multidrug-resistant *Enterobacter aerogenes* infections and in vivo emergence of imipenem resistance. *Journal of Clinical Microbiology* 35: 152–160.

62. Bennish ML, Salam MA, Hossain MA et al 1992 Antimicrobial resistance of *Shigella* isolates in Bangladesh, 1983–1990: increasing frequency of strains multiply resistant to ampicillin, trimethoprim-sulfamethoxazole, and nalidixic acid. *Clinical Infectious Diseases* 14: 1055–1060.

63. Threlfall EJ, Ward LR 2001 Decreased susceptibility to ciprofloxacin in *Salmonella enterica* serotype Typhi, United Kingdom. *Emergency and Infectious Diseases* 7: 448–450.

64. Molbak K, Baggesen DL, Aarestrup FM et al 1999 An outbreak of multidrug-resistant, quinolone-resistant. *Salmonella enterica* serotype typhimurium DT104. *New England Journal of Medicine* 341: 1420–1425.

65. Threlfall EJ, Ward LR, Skinner JA, Graham A 2000 Antimicrobial drug resistance in non-typhoidal salmonellas from humans in England and Wales in 1999: decrease in multiple resistance in *Salmonella enterica* serotypes Typhimurium, Virchow, and Hadar. *Microbial Drug Resistance* 6: 319–325.

66. Tassios PT, Gazouli M, Tzelepi E et al 1999 Spread of a *Salmonella typhimurium* clone resistant to expanded-spectrum cephalosporins in three European countries. *Journal of Clinical Microbiology* 37: 3774–3777.

67. Fey PD, Safranek TJ, Rupp ME et al 2000 Ceftriaxone-resistant salmonella infection acquired by a child from cattle. *New England Journal of Medicine* 342: 1242–1249.

68. Engberg J, Aarestrup FM, Taylor DE et al 2001 Quinolone and macrolide resistance in *Campylobacter jejuni* and *C. coli*: resistance mechanisms and trends in human isolates. *Emergency and Infectious Diseases* 7: 24–34.

69. Smith KE, Besser JM, Hedberg CW et al 1999 Quinolone-resistant *Campylobacter jejuni* infections in Minnesota, 1992–1998. Investigation Team. *New England Journal of Medicine* 340: 1525–1532.

70. Houben MH, Van Der BD, Hensen EF et al 1999 A systematic review of *Helicobacter pylori* eradication therapy – the impact of antimicrobial resistance on eradication rates. *Alimentary Pharmacology and Therapeatics* 13: 1047–1055.

71. Megraud F 1998 Epidemiology and mechanism of antibiotic resistance in *Helicobacter pylori*. *Gastroenterology* 115: 1278–1282.

72. Li XZ, Nikaido H, Poole K 1995 Role of mexA-mexB-oprM in antibiotic efflux in *Pseudomonas aeruginosa*. *Antimicrobial Agents and Chemotherapy* 39: 1948–1953.

73. Carmeli Y, Troillet N, Eliopoulos GM et al 1999 Emergence of antibiotic-resistant *Pseudomonas aeruginosa*: comparison of risks associated with different antipseudomonal agents. *Antimicrobial Agents and Chemotherapy* 43: 1379–1382.

74. Gales AC, Jones RN, Turnidge J et al 2001 Characterization of *Pseudomonas aeruginosa* isolates: Occurrence rates, antimicrobial susceptibility patterns, and molecular typing in the global SENTRY antimicrobial surveillance program, 1997–1999. *Clinical Infectious Diseases* 32 (Suppl. 2): S146–S155.

75. Carmeli Y, Troillet N, Karchmer AW et al 1999 Health and economic outcomes of antibiotic resistance in *Pseudomonas aeruginosa*. *Archives of Internal Medicine* 159: 1127–1132.

76. Towner KJ 1997 Clinical importance and antibiotic resistance of *Acinetobacter* spp. Proceedings of a symposium held on 4–5 November 1996 at Eilat, Israel. *Journal of Medical Microbiology* 46: 721–746.

77. Telenti A 1997 Genetics of drug resistance in tuberculosis. *Clinics in Chest Medicine* 18: 55–64.

78. Lemaitre N, Sougakoff W, Truffot-Pernot C et al 1999 Characterization of new mutations in pyrazinamide-resistant strains of *Mycobacterium tuberculosis* and identification of conserved regions important for the catalytic activity of the pyrazinamidase PncA. *Antimicrobial Agents and Chemotherapy* 43: 1761–1763.

79. Espinal MA, Laszlo A, Simonsen L et al 2001 Global trends in resistance to antituberculosis drugs. World Health Organization-International Union against Tuberculosis and Lung Disease Working Group on Anti-Tuberculosis Drug Resistance Surveillance. *New England Journal of Medicine* 344: 1294–1303.

80. Nolan CM 1997 Nosocomial multidrug-resistant tuberculosis – global spread of the third epidemic. *Journal of Infectious Diseases* 176: 748–751.

81. Struelens MJ 1998 The epidemiology of antimicrobial resistance in hospital acquired infections: problems and possible solutions. *British Medical Journal* 317: 652–654.

82. Okeke IN, Lamikanra A, Edelman R 1999 Socioeconomic and behavioral factors leading to acquired bacterial resistance to antibiotics in developing countries. *Emergency and Infectious Diseases* 5: 18–27.

83. Wegener HC, Aarestrup FM, Jensen LB et al 1999 Use of antimicrobial growth promoters in food animals and *Enterococcus faecium* resistance to therapeutic antimicrobial drugs in Europe. *Emergency and Infectious Diseases* 5: 329–335.

84. Magee JT 2001 Antibiotic resistance and prescribing in the community. *Reviews in Medical Microbiology* 12: 87–96.

85. Guillemot D, Carbon C, Balkau B et al 1998 Low dosage and long treatment duration of beta-lactam: risk factors for carriage of penicillin-resistant *Streptococcus pneumoniae*. *Journal of the American Medical Association* 279: 365–370.

86. Richard P, Le Floch R, Chamoux C et al 1994 *Pseudomonas aeruginosa* outbreak in a burn unit: role of antimicrobials in the emergence of multiply resistant strains. *Journal of Infectious Diseases* 170: 377–383.

87. Asensio A, Oliver A, Gonzalez-Diego P et al 2000 Outbreak of a multiresistant *Klebsiella pneumoniae* strain in an intensive care unit: antibiotic use as risk factor for colonization and infection. *Clinical Infectious Diseases* 30: 55–60.

88. Working Party of the British Society for Antimicrobial Chemotherapy 1994 Hospital antibiotic control measures in the UK. *Journal of Antimicrobial Chemotherapy* 34: 21–42.

89. Goldmann DA, Weinstein RA, Wenzel RP et al 1996 Strategies to prevent and control the emergence and spread of antimicrobial-resistant microorganisms

in hospitals. A challenge to hospital leadership. *Journal of the American Medical Association* 275: 234–240.

90. Gould IM, MacKenzie FM, Struelens MJ et al 2000 Towards a European strategy for controlling antibiotic resistance, Nijmegen, Holland August 29–31, 1999. *Clinical Microbiology Infection* 6: 670–674.

91. Struelens MJ, Peetermans WE 1999 The antimicrobial resistance crisis in hospitals calls for multidisciplinary mobilization. *Acta Clinica Belgica* 54: 2–6.

92. Peterson LR, Noskin GA 2001 New technology for detecting multidrug-resistant pathogens in the clinical microbiology laboratory. *Emergency and Infectious Diseases* 7: 306–311.

93. Lucet JC, Decre D, Fichelle A et al 1999 Control of a prolonged outbreak of extended-spectrum beta-lactamase-producing enterobacteriaceae in a university hospital. *Clinical Infectious Diseases* 29: 1411–1418.

94. Souweine B, Traore O, Aublet-Cuvelier B et al 2000 Role of infection control measures in limiting morbidity associated with multi-resistant organisms in critically ill patients. *Journal of Hospital Infection* 45: 107–116.

95. Chaix C, Durand-Zaleski I, Alberti C et al 1999 Control of endemic methicillin-resistant *Staphylococcus aureus*: a cost-benefit analysis in an intensive care unit. *Journal of the American Medical Association* 282: 1745–1751.

96. McGowan JE, Jr 2000 Strategies for study of the role of cycling on antimicrobial use and resistance. *Infection Control and Hospital Epidemiology* 21 (Suppl 1): S36–S43.

97. Ostrowsky BE, Trick WE, Sohn AH et al 2001 Control of vancomycin-resistant enterococcus in health care facilities in a region. *New England Journal of Medicine* 344: 1427–1433.

98. Department of Health, UK 1998 Standing Medical Advisory Committee. The path of least resistance. Available at: http://www.doh.gov.uk/smacsyn.htm

99. Richet HM, Mohammed J, McDonald LC et al 2001 Building communication networks: international network for the study and prevention of emerging antimicrobial resistance. *Emergency and Infectious Diseases* 7: 319–322.

Pharmacodynamics of anti-infectives: target delineation and target attainment

G. L. Drusano

The goal of anti-infective chemotherapy is to administer a dose of drug that will generate the highest probability of a good outcome while also having the lowest probability of a drug-related toxicity event that is concentration-related.

While this is the stated goal of most drug therapy, anti-infective therapy differs in kind. This is because we are trying to dock the therapeutic agent into a receptor for which it is almost always possible to obtain information about how much of the agent is required to inhibit the pathway that receptor serves. There are certainly exceptions, such as with the hepatitis C virus. However, whether one talks about bacteria, fungi or viruses, there is virtually always an in-vitro test (MIC, EC_{50}, etc.) that provides information about the potency of the drug for the pathogen in question. This allows more straightforward development of exposure–response relationships. This does not, however, affect the development of exposure–toxicity relationships.

CHOICE OF ENDPOINTS AND ANALYSIS METHODS

The endpoint chosen is an important first step in developing an exposure–response relationship. It should be immediately clear that there are a number of different endpoints that may be examined, each of which will drive the analysis in a different direction and for which different analytical tools should be employed.

The typical endpoints examined for clinical trials data include clinical and microbiological outcomes. These endpoints are good, but have specific weaknesses. Their strong points are that they are the outcomes that we most care about. Their weaknesses are that they are usually dichotomous in nature. Further, the positive microbiologic endpoint (eradication) is most often inferred (no specimen available, eradication presumed).

These endpoints and other important dichotomous endpoints (e.g. emergence of resistance) are often modeled with logistic regression analysis or classification and regression tree (CART) analysis. These allow delineation of continuous (logistic regression) and breakpoint relationships to be determined.

They also have their limitations. As pointed out by Forrest (A. Forrest, personal communication), logistic regression explicitly assumes that the probability of the response assumes a value of 1.0 at some infinitely large value of the continuous exposure variable being examined. This assumption may not be true in the clinical arena. For physiologic reasons (e.g. clinical failure, even with microbiological success for a patient with nosocomial pneumonia, due to inadequate gas exchange), clinical outcome may not approach a probability of 1.0, even with very large drug exposures. For CART analysis, the breakpoint determined is a direct function of the data, as this approach relies upon a recursive partitioning algorithm.

More recently, other endpoints have been examined. For endpoints that may be determined serially, the time to attainment of that endpoint can be examined. An example is the time to clearance of the primary pathogen from lower respiratory tract infections. This endpoint has been examined[1,2] on several different occasions. These analyses have pointed out the pitfalls attendant on such endpoints. In the first analysis, an improper analytic tool was employed (linear regression analysis), which does not allow for right censoring of data. Both the first and the second of these analyses also suffer from a much more serious flaw: the endpoint itself was never validated. Many (if not all) of the patients studied had endotracheal tubes inserted as part of their support therapy. Many nosocomial pathogens are able to adhere to the surface of such endotracheal devices. Since neither quantitative culture techniques nor protected brush techniques were employed, the endpoint measured (time to organism eradication) is clearly open to question, as the presence or absence of the pathogen may have been influenced simply by contamination from a suction device inserted down an endotracheal tube.

There are, however, other well validated endpoints where the time to the end point and how this is altered by drug exposure is the appropriate analysis to perform. This was seen with the time to change of retinal lesions in the therapy in HIV-positive patients with cytomegalovirus (CMV) retinitis. The time to the next exacerbation of chronic bronchitis was used as an endpoint in a trial where a fluoroquinolone was compared to a non-quinolone therapy of acute exacerbations of chronic bronchitis. In Phase I/II challenge trials for respiratory virus (e.g. Influenza A or B virus), the measurement of the time to cessation of viral shedding has been examined.[3] This is important, because this endpoint has a direct effect not only on the individual patient but also on how infectious that patient is and with what probability they will spread their infectious virus. In these analyses, Cox Proportional Hazards modeling (or a fully parametric variant) or Kaplan–Meier analysis would be the appropriate analytical tool.

There are times when an endpoint is a continuous variable, for example in the area of HIV chemotherapy, where the endpoint is measured as the number of circulating viral copies as measured by reverse transcriptase polymerase chain reaction, or an equivalent methodology. In this circumstance, one can relate the change in the circulating viral copy number to some measure of drug exposure (e.g. time $> EC_{95}$ for protease inhibitors) for a population of patients.[4] This situation is often dealt with through use of a sigmoid–E_{max} effect model.

In Table 4.1, common endpoints and analytical approaches that are reasonable to employ are listed. It should be noted that this list is certainly not exhaustive and other equally appropriate statistical methodologies are available.

Table 4.1 Analytical tools useful for certain clinical trial endpoints

Endpoint	Analysis Tools
Clinical success/failure	Logistic regression, CART analysis
Eradication/persistence	Logistic regression, CART analysis
Time to pathogen clearance	Kaplan–Meier analysis, Cox regression
Time to disease exacerbation	Kaplan–Meier analysis, Cox regression
Change in a continuous variable	Sigmoid–E_{max} effect model

Once an endpoint has been determined for study, there are other issues that must be examined. The ultimate outcome of the analysis is directly dependent on having a validated endpoint to be examined and on collecting the data as carefully as possible. In the same vein, it is important to carefully collect data on drug exposure and on some measure of the potency of the drug for the pathogen in question (MIC, $EC_{50/95}$, etc.). While MIC and EC_{50} determinations are well standardized, less attention is paid to the care with which the drug exposure is estimated in an individual patient.

ESTIMATION OF DRUG EXPOSURE FOR DEVELOPMENT OF PHARMACODYNAMIC RELATIONSHIPS

Part of the recent success in delineating pharmacodynamic relationships in the clinical arena is related to developments in the area of mathematical pharmacology over the past two decades. Sheiner and colleagues pioneered the development of population pharmacokinetic modeling;[5] D'Argenio, and

DiStefano et al, published seminal papers in the areas of optimal sampling strategy for patients[6–9] and populations of patients.

Sheiner's breakthrough allows robust estimation of drug handling by a population of interest (e.g. in patients with nosocomial pneumonia) and how different demographic variables (age, sex, weight, creatinine clearance, APACHE II score, etc.) have an impact upon important pharmacokinetic variables such as clearance or volume of distribution.

Optimal sampling allows informative sampling times to be identified, so that robust pharmacokinetic information can be obtained with minimal invasion for sick patients. The optimal sampling approach has been extensively validated clinically,[10–12] but has been employed only sparingly in prospective pharmacodynamic trials. It is particularly important that this methodology is employed more widely.

The use of population modeling without optimal sampling is frequently seen. This means that patient data is collected randomly. Certainly, if the n of the sample is large enough, the error will have a mean of zero and an identifiable dispersion if good clinical practice is employed in collecting the data. This will, indeed, provide adequate estimates of the population pharmacokinetic parameters and the associated covariance matrix. This is certainly important (*see* p. 53). However, it is suboptimal for use in the development of pharmacodynamic relationships.

The estimation of the drug exposure achieved in a specific patient is achieved through the use of maximum a-posteriori probability (MAP) Bayesian estimation. If well-timed but random sampling is employed, there may be few samples obtained in a specific patient (sometimes only a single sample). Arguably worse, the sample(s) obtained may be from a portion of the dosing interval that is non-informative with respect to parameter estimation. Therefore, the Bayesian estimates may be poor and the actual drug exposure calculated can be biased. It is important, therefore, to attempt to obtain sufficient samples from every patient and to obtain them from portions of the dosing interval that are informative. Optimal sampling strategies calculated for populations of patients is a straightforward way of guarding against the twin sins of inadequate sample number and informativeness in pharmacodynamic relationship development.

An example of population modeling with population-based optimal sampling was shown by Preston's examination of the pharmacokinetics of levofloxacin in 272 patients with community-acquired pneumonia (Figure 4.1).[13]

Clearly, the combination of population modeling and population optimal sampling has provided robust estimates of the way in which all the patients handled the drug.

The question arises as to why it is only in the last 5–10 years that pharmacodynamic relationships have been generated with any frequency. As stated above, the lack of the mathematical tools is one explanation. However, this misses the important point that the earlier use of dose as a surrogate measure of drug failed. The reason for failure is straightforward and is illustrated in Figure 4.2. In the study of Preston et al,[13] over 250 of the

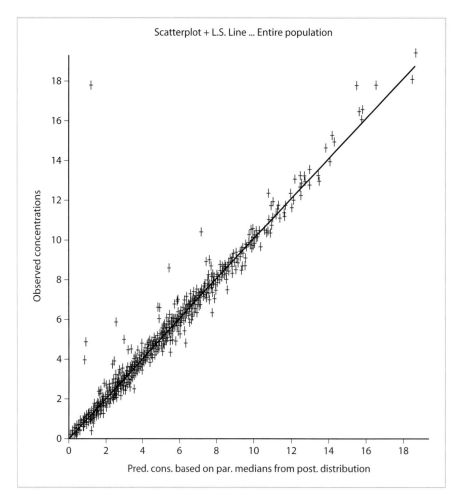

Fig. 4.1 Predicted-observed plot from the study of Preston et al,[13] examining the pharmacokinetics of levofloxacin in 272 patients. The best fit line was: observed = 1.001 × predicted +0.0054; $r^2 = 0.966$; $p \ll 0.001$

272 patients were administered 500 mg of levofloxacin. In none of the patients did the serum creatinine exceed 1.5, so renal functional impairment could not be the explanation for high exposures; rather, true between-patient variance in clearance would be responsible for high areas under the curve (AUCs) (low clearances). Such between-patient variance would prevent dose functioning as an adequate exposure surrogate. The dose exposure range was 2-fold. The clearance range (Figure 4.2) is greater than 10-fold. It is no surprise, then, that attempts at using dose as an exposure surrogate often fail.

Once we have Bayesian estimates of the pharmacokinetic parameter values for an individual patient, we must make a decision regarding the measure of exposure to employ. As stated above, for exposure–response relationships (effect relationships), we must employ the measure of drug potency for the pathogen in question (MIC, EC_{50}, etc.). For the example used here, MIC will be employed. In general, the most common choices for exposure variables for effect outcomes are peak/MIC ratio, AUC/MIC ratio and time > MIC. If sufficient doses and schedules are studied (normally at least three doses and two or more schedules), the appropriate dynamically linked variable can be chosen statistically. Unfortunately, such a wealth of doses and schedules is almost never available. These data are much easier to obtain in in-vitro or animal model pharmacodynamic systems but in the absence of the ability to obtain them in the clinical arena, it is best to choose the exposure variable for analysis directly from the animal model or in-vitro systems.

EXAMPLES OF DEVELOPMENT OF CLINICAL PHARMACODYNAMIC RELATIONSHIPS

The first prospective multicenter study for the development of a pharmacodynamic relationship was undertaken for a fluoroquinolone, levofloxacin[14] (earlier clinical analyses were retrospective in nature). In this analysis population optimal sampling design, population pharmacokinetic modeling, MAP-Bayesian estimation and CART analysis were all employed.

For both clinical and microbiological outcomes, it was possible to generate relationships between exposure and response.

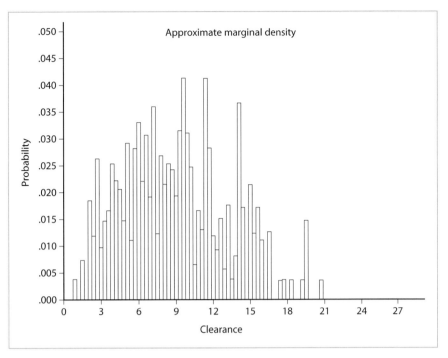

Fig. 4.2 Bayesian clearance estimates for levofloxacin for 272 patients.[13]

These are presented in Figure 4.3. Clearly, it is possible to study large numbers of patients and generate relationships between measures of exposure and response. The ability to have a breakpoint generated is particularly important.

It is also possible to examine both therapeutic and toxic endpoints for a drug or drug class. For example, it is possible to link aminoglycoside exposure to the probability of temper-

ature resolution by day 7 of therapy. Kashuba et al[15] examined this issue for patients with nosocomial pneumonia. In Figure 4.4, the probability curve is demonstrated with AUC/MIC ratio as the independent variable. While this is important for optimization of effect, aminoglycosides have traditionally been molecules associated with considerable toxicity, particularly nephrotoxicity. This issue was addressed in a randomized,

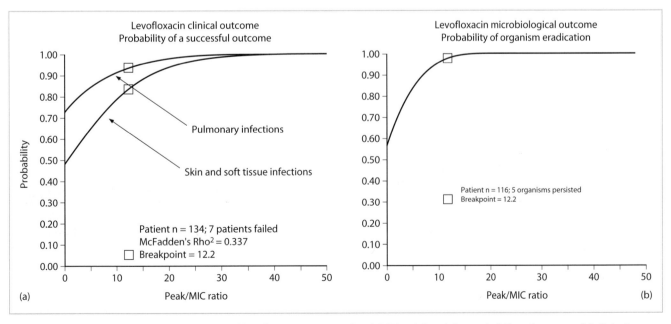

Fig. 4.3 (a) Relationship between a measure of levofloxacin exposure (peak/MIC ratio) and the probability of a successful clinical outcome, as determined by logistic regression analysis. The probabilities differ by infection site. CART analysis demonstrated a breakpoint at a peak/MIC ratio of 12.2/1. (b) The probability of organism eradication is displayed as a function of peak/MIC ratio. The CART-determined breakpoint is unchanged.

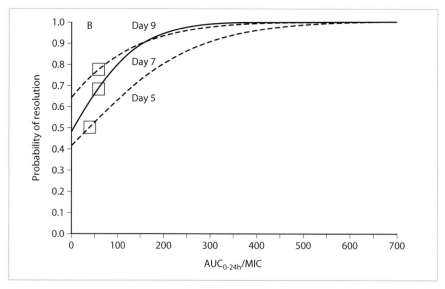

Fig. 4.4 The probability of temperature resolution as a function of AUC/MIC ratio for therapy days 5, 7 and 9. The boxes are breakpoint values determined by CART analysis.[15]

prospective double-blind trial,[16] testing the hypothesis that once-daily aminoglycoside dosing would be less nephrotoxic and examining other factors that would influence the probability of occurrence of aminoglycoside nephrotoxicity in a multivariate analysis (Table 4.2, Figure 4.5). These display the model-building approach, where the factors that affect the probability univariately are included in a model-building analysis to generate the final model.

It is important to recognize that pharmacodynamic relationships can be developed for both efficacy and toxicity. This allows attainment of the goal of chemotherapy. We can, by employing these relationships, define a dose of drug that will produce the highest probability of the desired clinical outcome while encumbering the patient with the lowest probability of having a drug exposure-related toxic event. To formally calculate this dose, approaches such as open loop with feedback stochastic control can be employed.

Other examples of pharmacokinetic/pharmacodynamic relationship development have employed a time-to event endpoint and Cox proportional hazards modeling. Before more potent agents came into our armamentarium, HIV-infected patients often had fewer than 50 CD4 cells and very high viral loads, frequently complicated by CMV retinitis. As therapy for this disease was (and remains) suboptimal, the endpoint for trials of new therapy was the time to observed progression of the retinitis. In an analysis of foscarnet therapy for CMV retinitis, Drusano et al found that only the daily AUC of foscarnet and whether or not the patient had a positive blood culture for CMV at baseline affected the time to progression of CMV retinitis (Figure 4.6).[17] Consequently, it is straightforward to use Cox proportional hazards modeling to link measures of exposure to the time to occurrence of the endpoint event. As above, these endpoints can also include time to clearance of the pathogen from an infection site that can be re-sampled (e.g. pneumonia).

Table 4.2 Risk factors tested univariately for affecting the probability of aminoglycoside toxicity. The second part of the table provides the final model

Covariate	Constant	Estimate	Standard error	p value
Site	−2.639	0.732		>0.1
Skin or soft tissue		0.0		
Respiratory tract		−0.069	1.266	
Urosepsis or pyelonephritis		−0.357	1.259	
Bacteremia or sepsis		1.723	1.112	
AUC	−4.751	1.309		0.04
		0.031	0.015	
DOT	−2.614		0.595	>0.1
		0.017	0.035	
Schedule[a]	−30.202		0.444	0.004
Once daily		0.0		
Twice daily		1.822	28.497	
Cumulative AUC[b]	−2.911		0.597	>0.1
		0.001	0.0004	
Vanco	−3.418	0.719		0.002
Non-use		0.0		
Use		2.858	0.954	
AmphoB	−2.595	0.464		>0.1
Non-use		0.0		
Use		2.595	1.488	
Final model				
Vanco	−37.239		2.482	0.000065
Non-use		0.0		
Use		3.531	1.411	
Schedule				
Once daily		0.0		
Twice daily		30.757	<0.001	
AUC		0.049	0.026	

[a] Schedule: once-daily versus twice-daily aminoglycoside administration.
[b] Calculated as AUC × DOT.
Vanco, use of systemic vancomycin; AmphoB, use of systemic amphotericin B; AUC, area under concentration – time curve; DOT, days of therapy.

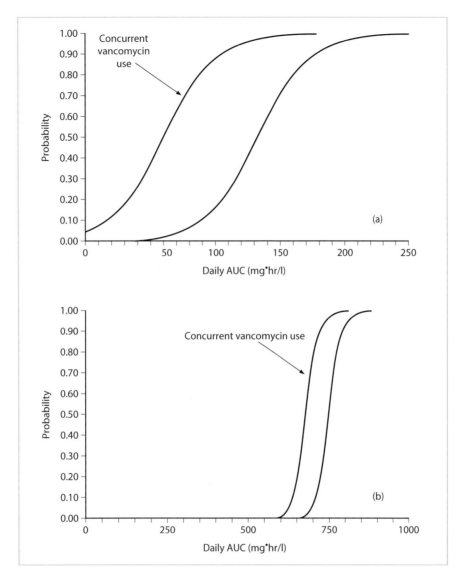

Fig. 4.5 (a) The probability of aminoglycoside toxicity for drug administration every 12 h. Increasing aminoglycoside exposure, as indexed to AUC, increases the probability of nephrotoxicity, as does concurrent vancomycin administration. (b) The data for once-daily administration.

Whether one employs logistic regression, Cox modeling or some other analytic tool, it is possible to link some measure of drug exposure to the outcome measure desired. Because of this, it is possible to choose a target of exposure. This target can be some probability of response that is empiric (e.g. 10% probability of aminoglycoside nephrotoxicity at a particular AUC), or is identified by CART analysis (e.g. 12/1 peak/MIC ratio for pathogen eradication). This then poses the next important question: What drug dose will achieve the stated target with a high probability?

TARGET ATTAINMENT ANALYSES

The optimal outcome of anti-infective chemotherapy is to achieve the highest probability of a positive outcome (clinical cure, pathogen eradication, etc.) while having no greater than a targeted maximal probability of having an exposure-driven toxicity. Stochastic control processes can play a central role in achieving such an optimal exposure.[18] However, in many cases of anti-infective therapy the duration of therapy is too short to attain the desired impact because the cycle time of sampling drug concentrations, making the appropriate calculation and feeding back to the patient with a changed dose is difficult to achieve in the appropriate time frame.

In this circumstance, it is still possible to choose a dose to achieve the desired therapeutic endpoint, particularly when the drug in question has a relatively broad therapeutic-toxic window.

There are a limited number of factors influencing the ability of a fixed drug dose to achieve a specific exposure target, such as an AUC/MIC ratio or a time > MIC (EC_{95}). These are:

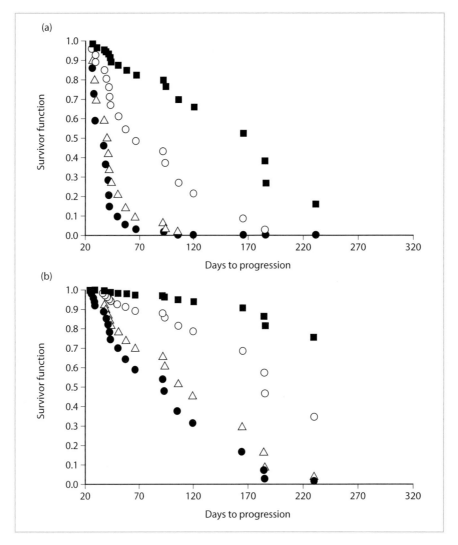

Fig. 4.6 (a) Time to CMV retinitis progression in patients with positive blood cultures for cytomegalovirus. ●, Lowest AUC in the population; △, 20th; ○, 50th; ■, 80th percentile of AUC in the population. (b) The same times to progression in patients whose baseline CMV blood cultures were negative.

- The variability of the drug's pharmacokinetics in the target population.
- The variability of the measure of drug potency for the pathogen (MIC, EC_{95}, etc.).
- The exposure target desired.
- The protein binding of the drug.

Using Monte Carlo simulation to create enough simulated subjects (multiple thousands) allows the full range of drug exposure that will be achieved in the clinic to be observed (*see* Figure 4.2). The protein binding allows free drug exposure to be estimated (it is only the free drug that is microbiologically active[19]). An exposure target must be chosen that produces a desired effect (e.g. achieving a free drug AUC/MIC ratio of 35–40 for therapy of pneumococcal pneumonia with fluoroquinolones, which will achieve a high likelihood of organism eradication[20]). Each of the simulated subject AUCs may then be divided by a specific MIC (e.g. 0.25 mg/l) and the fraction

of simulated subjects whose AUC/MIC ratio will achieve the target at that specific MIC determined. This process is then repeated for higher MICs. Such a process allows creation of a figure that will allow rational decisions regarding choosing an MIC breakpoint for a drug that is specific to an endpoint. That is, at the MIC breakpoint, the desired goal has a high (and explicitly defined) probability of attainment with a specific drug dose.

Further, the MIC distribution can be used to determine the overall probability of attaining the desired endpoint in the clinic. The frequency with which a specific drug MIC occurs in a population of organisms can be multiplied by the target attainment rate at that MIC. This is repeated for all the MICs in the distribution and all the results summed up (this is referred to as taking an expectation over the MIC distribution and serves to weight the target attainment rates by their own probability). This technique was first described by Drusano using everninomicin at an FDA Anti-Infectives Drug Product

Advisory Panel (FDA Website, October 15, 1998) and subsequently published.[21]

An example is given below for levofloxacin. The AUC/MIC exposure target was defined in the mouse thigh infection model of Craig et al (personal communication). The population model employed for the simulation was that of Preston et al for this drug in 272 patients with community-acquired infections.[13] This was used to generate a 10 000 subject Monte Carlo simulation (Figure 4.7). The MIC distribution was taken from the TRUST3 study. It was not necessary to factor in protein binding, as the protein binding in mice and humans is virtually identical. The AUC/MIC target of 27.5 is a stasis exposure, while that of 34.5 is for a 1 $\log_{10}$ CFU/ml drop in the number of pneumococci recovered in the Craig animal model. The MIC distribution represents 4296 pneumococcal isolates from the TRUST3 (1998–1999) study. When an expectation is taken over the MIC distribution, the overall probability of attaining the stasis target is 0.978, while the 1 $\log_{10}$ CFU/ml drop target has a probability of attainment of 0.947. These numbers are quite reasonable when the results of the study of File et al[23] are taken into account. Further, Preston and colleagues had 20 patients with documented pneumococcal pneumonia in their study.[14] In these patients, a 500 mg dose of levofloxacin had a 95% positive clinical outcome rate (19/20) and a 100% eradication rate, concordant with the Monte Carlo simulation results.

Perhaps the best examples with attendant validation are seen in the HIV arena. For the HIV-1 protease inhibitor atazanavir (previously known as BMS 232632), the in-vitro hollow fiber pharmacodynamic model demonstrated that time > EC_{90} is the pharmacodynamically linked variable and that the effect maximizes at free drug concentrations above the

EC_{90} for 80% of a 24-h dosing interval.[24] Monte Carlo simulation was then performed for two drug doses, oral 400 mg or 600 mg daily. The plasma concentrations were corrected for protein binding and the target attainment rate calculated. These data are presented in Figure 4.8. As can be seen in Figure 4.8(a) (the in-vitro experiment), once-daily drug administration requires four times as much drug to suppress viral replication as a continuous infusion. This is not surprising, as time > threshold rises as the logarithm of the dose (because the drug concentration falls exponentially). Figure 4.8(b) demonstrates target attainment rates for the two doses as a function of HIV EC_{50}. A total of 43 HIV other isolates were tested for EC_{50} for atazanavir from patients who were treatment naïve. It is immediately clear that, as long as the viral EC_{50} is less than 2 nmol (i.e. in the wild-type range), it would be difficult to differentiate these two doses by their antiviral effect. This was demonstrated in the Phase I/II environment for this agent.

Yet another study employing Monte Carlo simulation for rational dose selection examined a non-nucleoside reverse transcriptase inhibitor.[25] Three doses were evaluated (50 mg, 100 mg and 200 mg). The target chosen for this agent was free drug concentration in excess of the EC_{90} for the entire 24-h dosing interval. Monte Carlo simulation was performed and the target attainment calculated (Figure 4.9).

Wild-type isolates all had an EC_{50} value for GW420867X below 10 nmol/l. Again, it is straightforward to posit that all three doses of drug would demonstrate near-maximal activity in the clinic. A phase I/II trial was performed with these doses: monotherapy for one week followed by combination therapy beginning on the morning of study day 8, continuing to study day 28 (Figure 4.10).

Clearly, the Monte Carlo simulation and target attainment

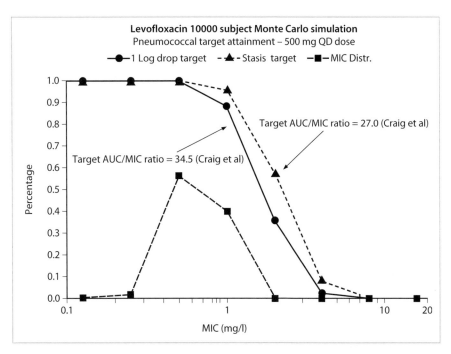

Fig. 4.7 Levofloxacin Monte Carlo simulation for *Streptococcus pneumoniae*[22]

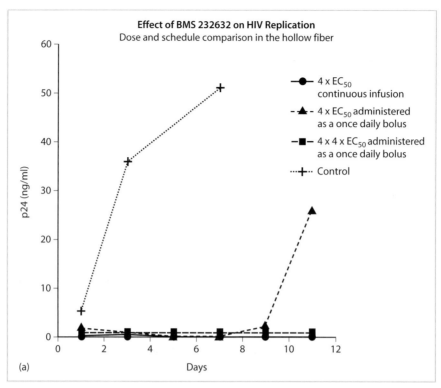

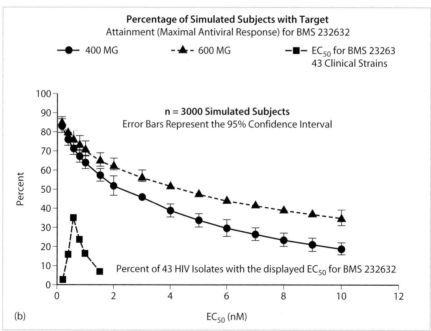

Fig. 4.8 (a) Pharmacodynamic target delineation for atazanavir by in-vitro hollow fiber system experimentation. (b) Monte Carlo simulation and target attainment for atazanavir by EC_{50}.

analyses demonstrated allowed the rational selection of dose to achieve the desired exposure targets. Were exposure–toxicity relationships also to be developed (*see* Figure 4.5, for aminoglycosides), it would be possible to ascertain the probability of developing an exposure-related toxicity for a fixed dose. Again, this would allow the rational choice of a dose for a population

of patients that would have the highest probability of achieving the desired effect while having the lowest probability of encountering a dose-related toxicity.

For all of the Monte Carlo simulation data displayed above, the validity of the approach rests upon a few, critically important, assumptions. First, it is critical that the target chosen is

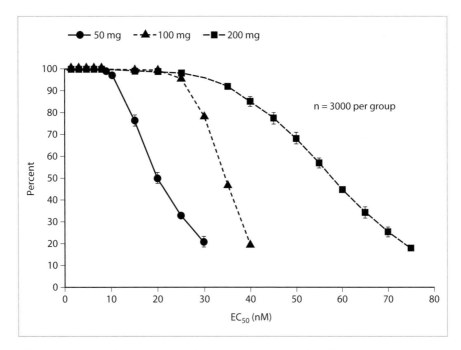

Fig. 4.9 Monte Carlo simulation and target attainment analysis for GW420867X (see text for details).

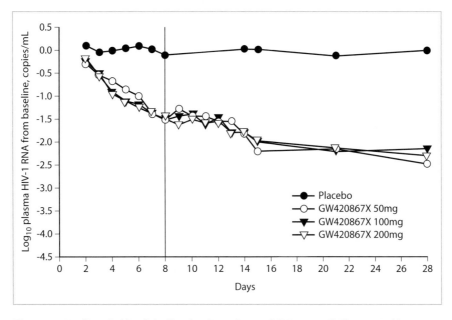

Fig. 4.10 Median viral load decline for three doses of GW420867X. The vertical bar indicates the viral load at the end of monotherapy. Neither study day 8 viral load (monotherapy) nor the viral load at study day 28 (combination therapy) differ by dose of GW420867X.

appropriate. Second, it is also important that the pharmacokinetic data employed is appropriate for the population for which the dose is intended. For effect modeling (but not toxicity modeling), the distribution of potency measures (MIC, $EC_{50/95}$, etc.) should be representative of that seen in the population for which the drug dose is intended.

This last issue is particularly crucial. For instance, looking at the data for either atazanavir or GW420867X, the wild-type EC_{50} makes it clear that it would be difficult to differentiate the doses in a trial. However, if viral isolates from drug class-experienced patients were studied, where the EC_{50} values exceeded 2 nmol for atazanavir and exceeded 10 nmol for

GW420867X, then higher doses of these agents would perform significantly better than the lower doses. Specifically, for GW420867X, while 50 mg would perform well for isolates with an EC_{50} as high as 10 nmol, 100 mg would perform well for isolates with EC_{50} values as high as 30 nmol.

SUMMARY

The advent and broad availability of sophisticated mathematical and statistical techniques has started a revolution in our ability to delineate exposure–response and exposure–toxicity relationships for anti-infective agents. This group of drugs is particularly straightforward to model (at least for effect) because we frequently have measures of potency of the drug for the pathogen in question. Such techniques as stochastic design, population pharmacokinetic modeling, MAP-Bayesian estimation, along with statistical techniques such as CART analysis, logistic regression analysis and Cox proportional hazards analysis, allow delineation of effect relationships for a variety of different endpoints.

Once these relationships are in place, exposure targets can be chosen to meet specific needs, such as 90% of maximal bactericidal effect or time to viral clearance of a specific value (e.g. clearance of influenza virus from secretions by 5 days). Once a target is chosen, Monte Carlo simulation is a useful mathematical tool for predicting the utility of different drug doses and which has been prospectively validated in the clinic.

Clearly, for diseases with long time lines of therapy (HIV disease, hepatitis C, etc.) stochastic control techniques will allow achievement of goals of therapy with a high probability. However, when therapy timelines are short or it is impractical to obtain drug concentrations from patients in a timely manner, Monte Carlo simulation and subsequent target attainment analysis still allow rational dose choice for populations of patients.

References

1. Schentag JJ, Smith IL, Swanson DJ et al 1984 Role for dual individualization with cefmenoxime. *American Journal of Medicine* 77 (6A): 43–50.
2. Forrest A, Ballow CH, Nix DE, Birmingham MC, Schentag JJ 1993 Development of a population pharmacokinetic model and optimal sampling strategies for intravenous ciprofloxacin. *Antimicrobial Agents and Chemotherapy* 37: 1065–1072.
3. Drusano GL, Treanor J, Fowler C et al 2000 Time to viral clearance after experimental infection with influenza B is related to the cumulative area under the curve of RWJ 270201. Abstracts of the 38th Annual Meeting of the Infectious Diseases Society of America, New Orleans.
4. Stein DS, Fish DG, Bilello LA et al 1996 A 24 week open label phase I evaluation of the HIV protease inhibitor MK-639. *AIDS* 10: 485–92.
5. Sheiner LB, Rosenberg B, Marathe VV 1977 Estimation of population characteristics of pharmacokinetic parameters from routine clinical data. *Journal of Pharmacokinetics and Biopharmaceutics* 5: 445–479.
6. D'Argenio DZ 1990 Incorporating prior parameter uncertainty in the design of sampling schedules for pharmacokinetic parameter estimation experiments. *Mathematics and Bioscience* 99: 105–118.
7. D'Argenio DZ 1981 Optimal sampling times for pharmacokinetic experiments. *Journal of Pharmacokinetics and Biopharmaceutics* 9: 739–756.
8. DiStefano JJ III 1981 Optimized blood sampling protocols and sequential design of kinetic experiments. *American Journal of Physiology* 9: R259–265.
9. DiStefano JJ III 1983 Algorithms, software and sequential optimal sampling schedule designs for pharmacokinetic and physiologic experiments. *Mathematics and Computer Simulations* 24: 531–534.
10. Drusano GL, Forrest A, Snyder MJ, Reed MD, Blumer JL 1988 An evaluation of optimal sampling strategy and adaptive study design. *Clinical Pharmacology and Therapeutics* 44: 232–238.
11. Drusano GL, Forrest A, Plaisance KI, Wade JC 1989 A prospective evaluation of optimal sampling theory in the determination of the steady state pharmacokinetics of piperacillin in febrile neutropenic cancer patients. *Clinical Pharmacology and Therapeutics* 45: 635–641.
12. Drusano GL, Forrest A, Yuen JG, Plaisance KI 1994 Optimal Sampling Theory: Effect of error in a nominal parameter value on bias and precision of parameter estimation. *Journal of Clinical Pharmacology* 34: 967–974.
13. Preston SL, Drusano GL, Berman AL et al 1998 Levofloxacin population pharmacokinetics in hospitalized patients with serious community-acquired infection and creation of a demographics model for prediction of individual drug clearance. *Antimicrobial Agents and Chemotherapy* 42: 1098–1104.
14. Preston SL, Drusano GL, Berman AL et al 1998 Prospective development of pharmacodynamic relationships between measures of levofloxacin exposure and measures of patient outcome: a new paradigm for early clinical trials. *Journal of the American Medical Association* 279: 125–129.
15. Kashuba AD, Nafziger AN, Drusand GL, Bertino JS Jr 1999 Optimizing aminoglycoside therapy for nosocomial pneumonia caused by Gram-negativ bacteria. *Antimicrobial Agents and Chemotherapy* 43: 623–629.
16. Rybak MJ, Abate BJ, Kang SL, Ruffing MJ, Lerner SA, Drusano GL 1999 Prospective evaluation of the effect of an aminoglycoside dosing regimen on rates of observed nephrotoxicity and ototoxicity. *Antimicrobial Agents and Chemotherapy* 43: 1549–1555.
17. Drusano GL, Aweeka F, Gambertoglio J et al 1996 Relationship between foscarnet exposure, baseline Cytomegalovirus blood culture and the time to progression of Cytomegalovirus retinitis in HIV-positive patients. *AIDS* 10: 1113–1119.
18. Schumitzky A 1991 Applications of stochastic control theory to optimal design of dosage regimens. In: D'Argenio D-Z (ed.) *Advanced Methods of Pharmacokinetic and Pharmacodynamic Systems Analysis* New York, Plenum Press 137–152.
19. Merriken DJ, Briant J, Rolinson GN 1983 Effect of protein binding on antibiotic activity *in vivo*. *Antimicrobial Agents and Chemotherapy* 11: 233–238.
20. Ambrose PG, Grasela DM, Grasela TH, Passarell J, Mayer HB, Pierce PF 2001 Pharmacodynamics of fluoroquinolones against *Streptococcus pneumonia* in patients with community-acquired respiratory tract infections. *Antimicrobial Agents and Chemotherapy* 45: 2793–2797.
21. Drusano GL, Preston SL, Hardalo C et al 2001 Use of pre-clinical data for the choice of a Phase II/III dose for SCH27899 with application to identification of a pre-clinical MIC breakpoint. *Antimicrobial Agents and Chemotherapy* 45: 13–22.
22. Drusano GL 2001 Human pharmacodynamics of anti-infectives: determination from clinical trial data. In: Nightengale CH, Murakawa T, Ambrose PG (eds). *Antimicrobial pharmacodynamics in theory and clinical practice*. New York and Basel Marcel Dekker, pp. 303–325.
23. File TM Jr, Segreti J, Dunbar L et al 1997 A multicenter, randomized study comparing the efficacy and safety of intravenous and/or oral levofloxacin versus ceftriaxone and/or cefuroxim axetil in treatment of adults with community-acquired pneumonia. *Antimicrobial Agents and Chemotherapy* 41: 1965–1972.
24. Drusano GL, Bilello JA, Preston SL et al 2001 Hollow fiber unit evaluation of a new Human Immunodeficiency Virus (HIV)-1 protease inhibitor, BMS 232632, for determination of the linked pharmacodynamic variable. *Journal of Infectious Diseases* 183: 1126–1129.
25. Drusano GL, Moore KHP, Kleim JP, Prince W, Bye A 2002 Rational dose selection for a nonnucleoside reverse transcriptase inhibitor through the use of population pharmacokinetic modeling and Monte Carlo simulation. *Antimicrobial Agents and Chemotherapy* 46: 913–916.

5 Antimicrobial agents and the kidneys

S. Ragnar Norrby

Antimicrobial drugs may interact with the kidneys in several ways. Decreased renal function often results in slower excretion of drugs or their metabolites. In the extreme situation the patient lacks renal function and is treated with hemodialysis, peritoneal dialysis or hemofiltration; since most antimicrobial drugs are low-molecular-weight compounds they are often readily eliminated from blood by such treatments. However, more and more drugs (e.g. the fluoroquinolones and many of the macrolides) are so widely distributed in tissue compartments and/or so highly protein bound that only a small fraction is available for elimination from the blood.

Another type of interaction between drugs and the kidneys is nephrotoxity. Some of the most commonly used antimicrobial drugs (e.g. the aminoglycosides and amphotericin B) are also nephrotoxic when used in normal doses relative to the patient's renal function.

This chapter deals with general aspects on interactions between antimicrobial drugs and the kidneys. The readers are referred to section 2 for details about dosing in patients with reduced renal function.

RENAL FUNCTION AND AGE

The prematurely born child has reduced renal function. Thereafter the glomerular filtration rate (GFR) is higher than in the adult. The young, healthy adult has a GFR of about 120 ml/min. Creatinine clearance overestimates GFR by 8–10%. With increasing age GFR becomes markedly reduced and in the very old (>85 years) is often lower than 30 ml/min even if there are no signs of renal disease. For drugs that are excreted only by glomerular filtration, which are not metabolized, and which have low protein binding (e.g. the aminoglycosides and many of the cephalosporins) the renal clearances are normally directly proportional to GFR. As shown in Figure 5.1,[1] the elimination time (the plasma half-life) of the drug increases slowly in the range from normal GFR to markedly reduced GFR but then increases drastically. Clinically this means that the drug will not accumulate markedly until renal function is profoundly decreased. However, when that is the case, only very slight further reductions of renal function will result in a marked increase in the elimination time and an obvious risk of accumulation to toxic levels.

Measurement of GFR is difficult because it requires precise collection and volume measurement of urine over time for determination of creatinine clearance or repeated plasma samples when ^{51}Cr clearance or inulin clearance are studied. For ^{51}Cr clearance there is also a need to administer and handle an isotope, and none of these methods is suitable for routine clinical use. The most frequently used way to measure renal function is by serum creatinine assay, which in the last decades has replaced blood urea nitrogen. However, serum creatinine depends on renal function and muscle mass. Therefore, in a very old person with reduced muscle mass, serum creatinine may be within normal values despite the fact that GFR is <25 ml/min. As a consequence, serum creatinine must be related to age, sex and weight (or preferably lean body mass). Two widely used routine methods are available; the Cockroft and Gault formula (Figure 5.2[2]) and a nomogram (Figure 5.3[3]).

ELIMINATION OF ANTIMICROBIAL DRUGS IN RENAL FAILURE

GENERAL ASPECTS

Only water-soluble drugs are eliminated via the kidneys: liver metabolism normally aims at producing water-soluble metabolites that can be excreted renally. In the kidneys water-soluble compounds that are not bound to protein are eliminated by glomerular filtration, tubular secretion or both of these mechanisms. For protein-bound drugs, only the free fraction is available for glomerular filtration. Following glomerular filtration some drugs (e.g. the aminoglycosides) are reabsorbed into, and sometimes accumulate in, proximal tubular cells.

In renal failure glomerular filtration is reduced while tubular secretion is often maintained. The effect of renal failure depends to a large degree on whether the drug is also metab-

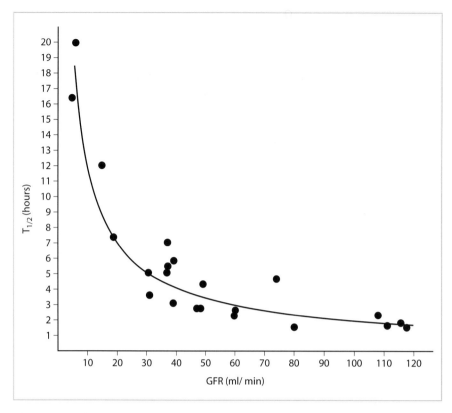

Fig. 5.1 Correlation between glomerular filtration rate (GFR) and serum half-life ($T_{1/2}$ of ceftazidime. After Alestig et al. Ceftazidime and renal function. *Journal of Antimicrobial Chemotherapy* 1989; 13: 177–181 with permission of Oxford University Press.

$$\text{Creatinine clearance (ml/min)} = \frac{f \times (140 - \text{age (years)}) \times \text{body weight (kg)}}{\text{Serum creatinine (\mu mol/l)}}$$

f = 1.23 for men and 1.04 for women

Fig. 5.2 Cockroft and Gault[2] formula for estimation of creatinine clearance.

olized or eliminated through the bile. For example, among the cephalosporins cefuroxime has low protein binding and is not metabolized; its plasma clearance will be virtually identical to creatinine clearance. Ceftriaxone, on the other hand, has a relatively high protein binding and is eliminated via the bile; in patients with renal failure the elimination half-life of ceftriaxone will not increase markedly because the proportion of drug eliminated by biliary excretion will increase. Another example is imipenem, which is excreted by glomerular filtration but which also has a (non-hepatic) metabolism that is constant over time. In renal failure the plasma half-life of imipenem will increase, but only to about 3 h in the anuric patient (compared with 1 h in an individual with normal renal function). In contrast, cilastatin, the enzyme inhibitor administered with imipenem, has relatively little metabolism and low protein binding

and its half-life will increase from about 1 h to > 10 h in severe renal failure.

It is essential to know the mode of elimination of all antimicrobial drugs used as well as the effects on elimination time of renal failure. Many compounds are toxic if given in overdose, and failure to correct dosages in patients with markedly reduced renal function may result in serious adverse effects.

ANTIMICROBIAL DRUGS THAT ARE INDEPENDENT OF RENAL FUNCTION FOR THEIR ELIMINATION

Some antimicrobial drugs can be given at full doses even to patients with severe renal failure (Table 5.1). However, also in

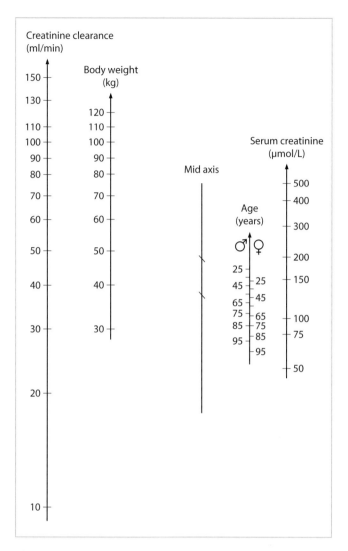

Fig. 5.3 Nomogram for calculation of creatinine clearance. Connect body weight and age with a ruler and mark the crossing on the mid axis. Connect the crossing with the serum creatinine value and read the estimated creatinine clearance. After Siersback-Nielsen et al.[3] © by The Lancet Ltd, 1971.

Table 5.1 Antimicrobial drugs that can be given at full doses to patients with severe renal failure

Drug	Comments
Azithromycin	
Ceftriaxone	The manufacturer recommends a maximum daily dose of 2 g if GFR <10 ml/min
Chloramphenicol	
Clarithromycin	
Clindamycin	
Doxycycline	Other tetracyclines should not be used in renal failure
Erythromycin	It has been proposed that the risk of toxicity should increase in patients with renal failure
Ethambutol	
Indinavir	No data but minimal renal excretion
Itraconazole	
Ketoconazole	
Mebendazole	
Mefloquine	
Metronidazole	
Mezlocillin	Liver metabolism
Praziquantel	
Primaquine	
Pyrazinamide	
Quinine	
Rifampicin	
Ritonavir	No data but minimal renal excretion
Saquinavir	No data but minimal renal excretion
Sulfonamides	
Tinidazole	

such patients elimination by hemodialysis or hemofiltration should be considered. A relatively simple rule of thumb is that drugs that are highly protein bound (≥90%) and drugs that have a large volume of distribution tend not to be eliminated. Alternatively, for most drugs with low protein binding and/or low volume of distribution a further dose should be considered after peritoneal dialysis, hemodialysis or hemofiltration.

ANTIMICROBIAL DRUGS THAT SHOULD BE AVOIDED IN SEVERE RENAL FAILURE

Nephrotoxic drugs should not be used in patients with renal failure unless they are anephric. When using formulations that are combinations of two drugs, it should be noted that the pharmacokinetics of the two components in renal failure may differ from those in patients with normal kidney function. Examples are imipenem/cilastatin and piperacillin/tazobactam: the elimination times of cilastatin and tazobactam increase far more drastically than those of imipenem and piperacillin, which both undergo substantial metabolism.

PERITONEAL DIALYSIS

Modern medicine offers several replacement treatments of severe renal failure: hemodialysis, continuous peritoneal dialysis (CAPD), continuous arteriovenous hemofiltration (CAVHF), venovenous hemofiltration (CVVHF), and continuous venovenous hemodiafiltration (CVVHDF). The degrees of elimination of individual antimicrobial drugs by these methods vary and are sometimes incompletely studied.

In terms of reproducibility of the elimination rate, CAPD is likely to be the least reproducible both with the same patient and between patients. The main reason for this is that, with time, a person undergoing CAPD is likely to develop fibrin adherence, which limits the peritoneal surface area available for dialysis. The efficacy of the dialysis may also vary with the position of the patient and the amount of dialysis fluid

Table 5.2 Antimicrobial drugs which are removed during hemodialysis. Data are partly taken from Livornese et al[4]. Doses, when specified, are for adults.

Drug	Dose recommendation
Aciclovir	Maximal oral dose 800 mg twice daily. New parenteral dose after dialysis and then half normal dose every day
Amikacin	Two-thirds of normal dose after dialysis. Monitor serum concentrations
Amoxicillin	New dose after dialysis
Ampicillin	New dose after dialysis
Amoxicillin/clavulanic acid	New dose after dialysis
Aztreonam	Half normal dose after dialysis and one-quarter of normal dose between dialyses
Cefaclor	New dose after dialysis
Cefadroxil	New dose after dialysis
Cefamandole	New dose after dialysis
Cefazolin	New dose (maximum 1 g) after dialysis
Cefdinir	New dose after dialysis
Cefepime	New dose (maximum 1 g) after dialysis
Cefixime	New dose after dialysis
Cefoperazone	New dose after dialysis
Cefotaxime	New dose (maximum 1 g) after dialysis
Cefotetan	New dose (maximum 1 g) after dialysis
Cefpodoxime	New dose after dialysis
Cefprozil	250 mg after dialysis
Ceftazidime	New dose (maximum 1 g) after dialysis
Cefuroxime	New dose after dialysis
Cefalexin	New dose after dialysis
Cefapirin	New dose after dialysis
Cefradine	New dose after dialysis
Clarithromycin	New dose after dialysis
Didanosine	New dose after dialysis and then once daily
Famciclovir	New dose after dialysis and then every 48 h
Fluconazole	New dose after dialysis
Flucytosine	New dose after dialysis. Monitor serum concentrations
Ganciclovir	Half dose after dialysis and then 0.625 mg/kg 3 times/week
Gentamicin	Two-thirds normal dose after dialysis. Monitor serum concentrations
Imipenem/cilastatin	New dose after dialysis and then 0.5 g every 12 h
Lamivudine	25 mg once daily
Levofloxacin	125 mg daily
Mecillinam	New dose after dialysis
Meropenem	New dose after dialysis
Metronidazole	New dose after dialysis
Netilmicin	Two-thirds normal dose after dialysis. Monitor serum concentrations
Ofloxacin	100 mg twice daily
Penicillin V and G	New dose after dialysis
Piperacillin	1 g after dialysis and then 2 g every 8 h
Piperacillin/tazobactam	2 g (of piperacillin) after dialysis and then 4 g (of piperacillin) every 12 h
Stavudine	New dose after dialysis and then once daily
Sulfamethoxazole	New dose after dialysis
Sulfisoxazole	New dose after dialysis
Teicoplanin	Dose for GFR <10 ml/min. Monitor serum concentrations
Ticarcillin	New dose after dialysis
Trimethoprim	New dose after dialysis
Tobramycin	Two-thirds normal dose after dialysis. Monitor serum concentrations
Valaciclovir	Maximal dose 1 g once daily
Vancomycin	Dose for GFR <10 ml/min. Monitor serum concentrations

administered during a specified time. Other factors limiting elimination of drugs with CAPD are protein binding and molecular size. There is often limited information about rate of elimination of an antimicrobial agent in patients using CAPD. For renally eliminated antibiotics, the most common recommendation is to give the dose normally administered to a patient with a GFR <10 ml/min. When aminoglycosides are given to patients on CAPD, about 50% of the dose given is found in the dialysate fluid but regular serum concentration assays are recommended (*see below*).

In patients undergoing CAPD antibiotics are also frequently used as additives to peritoneal dialysate fluid to treat peritonitis, a common complication in these patients. Since the most common agent causing these infections is coagulase-negative staphylococci that are often methicillin resistant, vancomycin is most frequently used. In such treatment varying but generally quite high plasma concentrations are achieved as a result of passage of the antibiotic from the dialysate fluid to plasma. This is especially important to note if the patient is also on systemic antibiotic treatment.

HEMODIALYSIS

In hemodialysis toxic substances are cleared from blood through passive diffusion across a membrane. Drug elimination via hemodialysis depends on molecular size of the drug, protein binding and volume of distribution (drugs with a molecular weight <500 Da normally pass through the dialysis filter easily if they are not protein bound). Factors of the dialysis technique that influence drug elimination are dialysis time, blood and dialysate flow rates, and dialysis membrane permeability, pore size and surface area. Elimination of molecules of 500–5000 Da will depend largely on the type of filter used; some of the modern filters also allow passage of relatively large molecules.

For most antibiotics, the effect of hemodialysis on the elimination is known, although information is more limited on antifungal, antiparasitic and antiviral drugs (Tables 5.2 and 5.3). With drugs that are readily eliminated during hemodialysis it is necessary to give a new dose directly after hemodialysis; no dose corrections are needed for those that are not significantly eliminated.

No information has been found on elimination of the following in patients on hemodialysis: foscarnet, indinavir, itraconazole, ketoconazole, moxifloxacin, ritonavir, saquinavir, sparfloxacin, trovafloxacin, zalcitabine, and zidovudine. The manufacturer of isoniazid states that it is eliminated during hemodialysis but gives no dosage recommendations.

HEMOFILTRATION AND HEMODIAFILTRATION

There is far less information on elimination of drugs in patients on hemofiltration than there is for those on hemodialysis. The

Table 5.3 Antimicrobial drugs that are not removed by hemodialysis

Drug	Comments
Amphotericin B	Large molecular weight
Azithromycin	Large molecule; very large volume of distribution
Ceftriaxone	High protein binding; alternative biliary excretion
Chloramphenicol	Large volume of distribution
Chloroquine	Large volume of distribution
Ciprofloxacin	Large volume of distribution
Clindamycin	Large volume of distribution, High protein binding
Cloxacillin	High protein binding
Dicloxacillin	High protein binding
Doxycycline	High protein binding; large volume of distribution
Erythromycin	Large molecule; large volume of distribution
Fusidic acid	High protein binding
Mefloquine	High protein binding
Minocycline	High protein binding; large volume of distribution
Nafcillin	High protein binding
Quinine	Large volume of distribution
Quinupristin/ dalfopristin	Large volumes of distribution, large molecules
Rifabutin	Large volume of distribution, high protein binding
Rifampicin	Large volume of distribution
Spectinomycin	Always single dose
Tetracycline	High protein binding; large volume of distribution

principle of removal of compounds by hemofiltration is convection of the compound in solution in plasma water over a filter, while hemodialysis involves diffusion against a dialysis fluid. In hemofiltration the drug is removed by drag of plasma water. Only free drug can be removed by this process and protein binding is a major factor restricting elimination. Large molecular size is also a restrictive factor. The efficiency with which a drug is removed is measured as the *sieving coefficient*; a drug with sieving coefficient of 1 will cross the filter freely; one with a coefficient of 0 is unable to cross. Amikacin has a sieving coefficient of 0.9, amphotericin B (which has a high molecular weight) 0.3 and oxacillin (which has a very high protein binding) 0.02.

Hemofiltration is generally less efficient than hemodialysis in eliminating drugs from plasma. The most common recommendation for drugs which are normally given in a full dose after each intermittent hemodialysis is to give the dose used in patients with moderate renal failure (GFR 10–50 ml/min) during CVVH or CAVH. In patients treated with aminoglycosides or glycopeptides, serum concentrations should be monitored to avoid toxic reactions.

Another way of treating patients with acute renal failure is to use continuous venovenous hemodiafiltration (CVVDHF), which combines hemofiltration and hemodialysis. This technique is more efficient in eliminating filterable and dialysable

Table 5.4 Comparison of meropenem pharmacokinetics in patients treated with continuous venovenous hemofiltration (CVVHF) or hemodiafiltration (CVVHDF). Data from Valtonen et al[5].

Parameter (mean ± SD)	CVVHF	CVVHDF (1 l/h)	CVVHDF (2 l/h)
Meropenem half-life (h)	7.5±2.0	5.6±1.4[a]	4.8±1.2[a,b]
Meropenem clearance (l/h)	3.3±2.3	4.7±2.7[a]	5.7±3.6[a]

[a] Significantly ($p<0.05$) different from the CVVHF
[b] Significantly ($p<0.05$) different from the CVVHDF (1 l/h) phase

drugs. Table 5.4 gives a comparison of CVVHF and CVVHDF when used in patients treated with meropenem.

NEPHROTOXICITY OF ANTIMICROBIAL DRUGS

Some antimicrobial drugs – such as the aminoglycosides, vancomycin, and amphotericin B – are also nephrotoxic when dosed correctly in relation to the renal function of the patients. Others (e.g. cefaloridine; no longer available) are nephrotoxic if overdosed while a large number of drugs, especially the penicillins and rifampicin, have been reported to cause interstitial nephritis in a very low frequency of patients treated. Some antimicrobial agents (e.g. older sulfonamides, quinolones, and indinavir) may cause urolithiasis as a consequence of precipitation in the renal pelvis.

AMINOGLYCOSIDE NEPHROTOXICITY

This subject has been excellently reviewed by Mingeot-Leclerq and Tulkens.[6] Following glomerular filtration, approximately 5% of an aminoglycoside dose is reabsorbed in the proximal tubular cells of the kidneys. This process is assumed to be, at least partially, the result of adsorptive endocytosis and most of the reabsorbed aminoglycoside is found in endosomal and lyso-somal vacuoles. However, part of the reabsorbed drug is found in the Golgi complex. The tubular reabsorption of aminoglycosides results in accumulation of drug in the proximal tubular cells since the release from the cells is far slower than the rate of uptake. Important for the discussion below of optimal dosing of aminoglycosides is the fact that the uptake into the tubular cells seems to be saturable.

At normal aminoglycoside doses, signs of nephrotoxicity can be observed after a few days, manifest as release of brush border and lysosomal enzymes and increased excretion of potassium, magnesium, calcium, glucose, and phospholipids. After prolonged treatment (>7 days) serum creatinine increases as a consequence of reduced GFR. At the subcellular level, accumulation of polar lipids into so-called 'myeloid bodies' is seen. There is some evidence that generation of toxic oxygen metabolites (hydrogen peroxide) plays an important role in this pathological process.[7] If these early changes are overlooked and if the patient is overdosed, the end result will be tubular necrosis and renal failure.

The best way to reduce the effects of aminoglycoside nephrotoxicity is to adjust doses in order to avoid overdosing and subsequent risks for serious nephrotoxicity and for ototoxicity. This can be achieved by regular monitoring of serum concentrations of the aminoglycoside used (*see later*).

The pharmacodynamics of aminoglycosides are characterized by a direct correlation between antibacterial efficacy and the area under the serum concentration curve, i.e. the higher the individual dose the more bactericidal the aminoglycoside. This speaks in favor of using few doses per time unit. Fortunately several studies show there to be no increase in toxicity of aminoglycosides when once-a-day regimens have been used rather than regimens with two or three daily doses. Table 5.5 shows the results of a meta-analysis of studies comparing single and multiple daily dosing of aminoglycosides. From the results of that study (and others) it seems clear that aminoglycosides should be administered once daily. This has been questioned for neutropenic patients in whom there may be a reduced post-antibiotic effect of the aminoglycoside. However, studies have indicated no reduction in efficacy or safety of aminoglycosides when single and multiple daily dosing have been compared in neutropenic patients.

Table 5.5 Results of a meta-analysis of single versus multiple daily dosing of aminoglycosides. Data modified from Ali & Goetz.[8]

Parameter	Mean difference[a]	95% confidence interval
Overall clinical response	3.06% ($p = 0.04$)	0.17–5.95%
Overall microbiological response	1.25% (not significant)	−0.40–2.89%
Nephrotoxicity	−0.18% (not significant)	−2.17–1.81%
Ototoxicity	1.38% (not significant)	−0.99–3.75%
Vestibular toxicity	−3.05% (not significant)	−10.7–4.59%

[a] A positive result for response or a negative result for toxicity favors single daily dose regimens

GLYCOPEPTIDE NEPHROTOXICITY

Both vancomycin and teicoplanin are nephrotoxic but the latter appears to be less so.[9] The mechanism by which these antibiotics are nephrotoxic is not completely known. It has been postulated that glycopeptides accumulate in proximal tubular cells as a result of passage from the blood rather than by tubular reabsorption.

The risk of developing nephrotoxicity seems to vary with certain risk factors. In one study cisplatin administration, high Apache scores and administration of carboplatin, cyclophosphamide or non-steroidal anti-inflammatory drugs correlated to increased nephrotoxicity of vancomycin in cancer patients.[10] High individual doses (high area under the serum concentration curve) and prolonged treatment seem to increase the risk of nephrotoxicity.

Nephrotoxicity of glycopeptides seems to be reversible in most cases. However, vancomycin therapy should be monitored with serum concentration assays (*see below*). Teicoplanin concentrations should also be monitored but this is more to achieve therapeutic levels, e.g. in a patient with endocarditis, than to prevent nephrotoxicity.

NEPHROTOXICITY OF β-LACTAM ANTIBIOTICS

Cefaloridine (no longer available for therapeutic use) was the first cephalosporin with marked dose-related nephrotoxicity. Cefaloridine accumulates in proximal renal tubular cells probably by active anionic transport. Thus, probenecid, which blocks such transport, eliminates the nephrotoxicity of cephaloridine.

Nephrotoxicity of the cefaloridine type has been seen with imipenem given intravenously to rabbits. That toxicity is completely blocked if imipenem is administered as a 1:1 combination with cilastatin, an inhibitor of the brush border renal enzyme (dehydropeptidase-I) which metabolizes imipenem and which also has a probenecid-like effect.

Ceftazidime, which has a mode of elimination and renal handling very similar to that of cefaloridine, has shown slight nephrotoxicity in overdose.

Dicloxacillin, when used as prophylaxis in orthopedic surgery, increases serum creatinine. So far no explanation has been offered as to why single doses of dicloxacillin (with or without single dose of gentamicin) should result in increased serum creatinine.

AMPHOTERICIN B NEPHROTOXICITY

Amphotericin B acts by binding to ergosterol in the cytoplasmic membrane of the fungal cell. It is fungicidal and, for systemic treatment of several clinically important mycoses, is often the only therapeutic choice. Unfortunately, amphotericin B also binds to ergosterol in the human cell and in particular the proximal tubular cells of the kidney. Thus, treatment of mycoses such as aspergillosis and disseminated candidiasis with normal doses of amphotericin B results in reduced renal function manifested by loss of potassium, loss of magnesium, signs of tubular necrosis, and decreased GFR. Factors of importance for how long treatment can continue are total dose given and renal function at the start of treatment.

The nephrotoxicity of amphotericin B can be reduced considerably, but not eliminated, by administration of the drug as a lipid formulation. Several variants of such formulations (e.g. incorporation of amphotericin B in liposomes and complex binding to phospholipids) have been developed (*see* Ch. 35).

ACUTE INTERSTITIAL NEPHRITIS AND ANTIMICROBIAL DRUGS

The following antimicrobial drugs have been reported to cause acute nephritis: aciclovir, cephalosporins, chloramphenicol, erythromycin, ethambutol, fluoroquinolones (ciprofloxacin and norfloxacin), gentamicin, minocycline, penicillins, rifampicin, sulfonamides, trimethoprim, and vancomycin.[11] Typically, the patient develops hematuria and proteinuria after more than 10 days of treatment. Other common symptoms are fever and rash, often with eosinophilia. These conditions are normally rapidly reversible if treatment is stopped.

UROLITHIASIS CAUSED BY ANTIMICROBIAL DRUGS

Sometimes a drug may precipitate in the kidney as a result of poor solubility in urine. Important factors in the risk of formation of precipitates are urine volume, urine pH, and drug solubility. Drugs with a high tendency to precipitate and cause symptoms of urolithiasis include the older sulfonamides and indinavir, an HIV protease inhibitor. For ciprofloxacin and some other fluoroquinolones, the solubility is very poor at alkaline pH. Thus, a patient with a renal infection caused by *Proteus* spp., may be at risk of clinically significant precipitation of the quinolone.

MONITORING OF SERUM CONCENTRATIONS OF ANTIMICROBIAL DRUGS

Serum concentration assays have two purposes: to avoid exceeding drug levels known to increase the risk of toxicity and to ensure that the dose given is sufficient to achieve therapeutic activity (*see* p. 118). For most antimicrobial drugs, serum concentration assays are not meaningful because there are no defined limits for toxicity or therapeutic efficacy. With some antibiotics (e.g. imipenem) concentration assays should be avoided because the drug is very unstable and transportation of the sample may lead to degradation of imipenem and falsely low concentrations in the assay. However, for some antimicrobial agents serum concentration assays are clinically indicated (Table 5.6).

Table 5.6 Antimicrobial drugs for which serum concentration monitoring is indicated

Drug	Comments
Aminoglycosides	High trough levels clearly related to nephrotoxicity and ototoxicity; low peak levels related to increased risk of therapeutic failure
Flucytosine	Concentrations <25 mg/l increase risk of emergence of resistance; concentrations >100 mg/l may result in toxicity
Glycopeptides	High trough levels related to nephrotoxicity and ototoxicity; low peak levels related to increased risk of therapeutic failure
Isoniazid	Concentration assay helps in identifying fast and slow acetylators; concentrations may be too low in the former and toxic in the latter

References

1. Alestig K, Trollfors B, Andersson R, Olaison L, Suurküla M, Norrby SR 1984 Ceftazidime and renal function. *Journal of Antimicrobial Chemotherapy* 13: 177–181.
2. Cockroft DW, Gault MH 1976 Prediction of creatinine clearance from serum creatinine. *Nephron* 16: 31–41.
3. Siersbaeck-Nielsen K, Mølholm Hansen J, Kampmann J, Kristensen M 1971 Rapid evaluation of creatinine clearance. *Lancet* i: 1333–1334.
4. Livornese LL, Slavin D, Benz RL, Ingerman MJ, Santoro J 2000 Use of antibacterial agents in renal failure. *Infectious Disease Clinics of North America* 14: 371–390.
5. Valtonen M, Tiula E, Backman JT, Neuvonen PJ 2000 Elimination of meropenem during continuous veno-venous haemofiltration and haemodiafiltration in patients with acute renal failure. *Journal of Antimicrobial Chemotherapy* 45: 701–704.
6. Mingeot-Leclecq MP, Tulkens PM 1999 Aminoglycosides: Nephrotoxicity. *Antimicrobial Agents and Chemotherapy* 43: 1003–1012.
7. Walker PD, Barry Y, Shah SV 1999 Oxidant mechanisms in gentamicin nephrotoxicity. *Renal Failure* 21: 433–442.
8. Ali MZ, Goetz B 1997 Meta-analysis of the relative efficacy and toxicity of single daily dosing versus multiple daily dosing of aminoglycosides. *Clinical Infectious Diseases* 24: 796–809.
9. Wood MJ 1996 The comparative efficacy and safety of teicoplanin and vancomycin. *Journal of Antimicrobial Chemotherapy* 37: 209–222.
10. Elting LS, Rubenstein EB, Kurtin D et al 1998 Mississippi mud in the 1990s. Risks and outcomes of vancomycin-associated toxicity in general oncology praxis. *Cancer* 15: 2597–2607.
11. Alexopoulos E 1998 Drug-induced acute intertstitial nephritis. *Renal Failure* 20: 809–819.

 Further Information

Alestig K, Trollfors B, Andersson R, Olaison L, Suurkula M, Norrby SR 1984 Ceftazidime and renal function. *Journal of Antimicrobial Chemotherapy* 13: 177–181.

Bailey TC, Little JR, Littenberg B, Reichley RM, Dunagan WC 1995 A meta-analysis of extended-interval dosing versus multiple daily dosing of aminoglycosides. *Clinical Infectious Diseases* 24: 786–195.

Baliga R, Ueda N, Walker PD, Shah SV 1999 Oxidant mechanisms in toxic acute renal failure. *Drug Metabolism Reviews* 31: 971–997.

Beauchamps D, Laurent G, Grenier L et al 1997 Attenuation of gentamicin-induced nephrotoxicity in rats by fleroxacin. *Antimicrobial Agents and Chemotherapy* 41: 1237–1245.

Brown NM, Reeves DS, McMullin CM 1997 The pharmacokinetics and protein-binding of fusidic acid in patients with severe renal failure requiring either haemodialysis or continuous ambulatory peritoneal dialysis. *Journal of Antimicrobial Chemotherapy* 39: 803–809.

Chow AW, Azar RW 1994 Glycopeptides and nephrotoxicity. *Intensive Care Medicine* 20: 523–529.

De Vriese AS, Robbrecht DL, Vanholder RC, Vogelaers DP, Lamiere NH 1998 Rifampicin-associated acute renal failure: pathophysiologic, immunologic, and clinical features. *American Journal of Kidney Diseases* 31: 108–115.

Fanos V, Cataldo L 1999 Antibacterial-induced nephrotoxicity in the newborn. *Drug Safety* 20: 245–267.

Gilbert DN, Lee BL, Dworkin RJ et al 1998 A randomized comparison of the safety of once-daily or thrice-daily gentamicin combination with ticarcillin-clavulanate. *American Journal of Medicine* 105: 182–191.

Hatal R, Dinh TT, Cook DJ 1997 Single daily dosing of aminoglycosides in immunocompromised adults: a systematic review. *Clinical Infectious Diseases* 24: 810–815.

Krueger WA, Schroeder TH, Hutchison M et al 1998 Pharmacokinetics of meropenem in critically ill patients with acute renal failure treated with continuous hemodiafiltration. *Antimicrobial Agents and Chemotherapy* 42: 2421–2424.

Murray KR, McKinnon PS, Mitrzyk B, Rybak MJ 1999 Pharmacodynamic characterization of nephrotoxicity associated with once-daily aminoglycoside. *Pharmacotherapy* 19: 1252–1260.

Norrby SR 1998 Carbapenems: Imipenem/cilastatin and meropenem. *Antibiotics for Clinicians* 2: 25–33.

Nucci M, Loureiro M, Silveira F et al 1999 Comparison of the toxicity of amphotericin B in 5% dextrose with that of amphotericin B in fat emulsion in a randomized trial with cancer patients. *Antimicrobial Agents and Chemotherapy* 43: 1445–1448.

Rohde B, Werner U, Hickstein H, Ehmcke H, Drewelow B 1997 Pharmacokinetics of mezlocillin and sulbactam under continuous veno-venous hemodialysis (CVVHD) in intensive care patients with acute renal failure. *European Journal of Clinical Pharmacology* 53: 111–115.

Ryback MJ, Abate BJ, Kang SL, Ruffing MJ, Lerner SA, Drusano GL 1999 Prospective evaluation of the effect of an aminoglyoside dosing regimen on rates of observed nephrotoxicity and ototoxicity. *Antimicrobial Agents and Chemotherapy* 43: 1549–1555.

Sánches Alcaraz A, Vargas A, Quintana MB et al 1998 Therapeutic drug monitoring of tobramycin: once-daily versus twice-daily dosage schedules. *Journal of Clinical Pharmacy and Therapeutics* 23: 367–373.

Solgaard T, Tuxoe JI, Mafi M, Due Olofsen S, Toftgaard Jensen T 2000 Nephrotoxicity by dicloxacillin and gentamicin in 163 patients with trochanteric hip fractures. *Orthopedics International* 24: 155–157.

Swan SK 1997 Aminoglycoside nephrotoxicity. *Seminars in Nephrology* 17: 27–33.

Takeda M, Tojo A, Sekine T, Hosoyamada M, Kanai Y, Endou H 1999 Role of organic anion transporter 1 in cephaloridine (CER)-induced nephrotoxicity. *Kidney International* 56: 2128–2136.

Tegeder FI, Neumann F, Bremer F, Brune K, Lötsch J, Geisslinger G 1999 Pharmacokinetics of meropenem in critically ill patients with acute renal failure undergoing continuous venovenous hemofiltration. *Clinical Pharmacology and Therapeutics* 65: 50–57.

Van der Verf TS, Mulder POM, Zijlstra JG, Uges DRA, Stegeman CA 1997 Pharmacokinetics of piperacillin and tazobactam in critically ill patients with renal failure, treated with continuous veno-venous hemofiltration (CVVH). *Intensive Care Medicine* 23: 873–877.

Van der Verf TS, Fijen JW, Van de Merbel NC et al 1999 Pharmacokinetics of cefpirome in critically ill patients with renal failure treated by continuous venovenous hemofiltration. *Intensive Care Medicine* 25: 1427–1431.

Warkentin D, Ippoliti C, Bruton J, Van Besien K, Champlin R 1999 Toxicity of single daily dose of gentamicin in stem cell transplantation. *Bone Marrow Transplantation* 24: 57–61.

Wingard JR, Kabilkis P, Lee L et al 1999 Clinical significance of nephrotoxicity in patients treated with amphotericin B for suspected or proven aspergillosis. *Clinical Infectious Diseases* 29: 1402–1407.

Wingard JR, White HM, Anaisse E, Raffalli J, Goodman J, Arrieta A 2000 A randomized, double-blind comparative trial evaluating the safety of liposomal amphotericin B versus an amphotericin B lipid complex in the empirical treatment of febrile neutropenia. L Amph/ABLC Collaborative Study Group. *Clinical Infectious Diseases* 31: 1155–1163.

6 Drug interactions involving antimicrobial agents

Ronald Polk and Roula B. Qaqish

The adverse clinical consequences of drug–drug interactions have been the focus of much attention,[1] and anti-infective drugs contribute disproportionately to this problem.[2] For example, between July 1993 and May 1999, 270 cases of cardiac arrhythmias in patients receiving cisapride (Propulsid™) were reported to the FDA.[3] There were 70 fatalities. In most cases, patients had known risk factors for arrhythmias, including concomitant drug therapy that often included antimicrobial drugs. The morbidity and mortality associated with cisapride occurred despite considerable attention previously given to terfenadine for causing similar problems.[4] On January 24, 2000, a boxed warning was added to the cisapride prescribing information (Figure 6.1). In July 2000 cisapride was removed from general distribution in the USA. A retrospective survey of over 141 119 prescriptions for cisapride dispensed between 1993 and 1998 revealed that 4414 patients (3.4%) received concomitant treatment with a contraindicated drug. Three antimicrobial drugs – clarithromycin, erythromycin and fluconazole – accounted for 91% of the contraindications.[3]

Increasingly, drug–drug interactions are also recognized between antimicrobials and herbal products. For example, St. John's Wort reduces serum concentrations of HIV-1 protease inhibitors, leading to the recommendation that this combination be avoided in all patients with HIV.[5,6] Our understanding of the mechanisms of these interactions has evolved to the point were we can predict with near certainty other interactions with St. John's Wort, and a list of contraindicated drugs in patients receiving St. John's Wort can be proposed, despite the lack of prospective clinical investigations (see below).

This chapter will discuss the mechanisms of drug–drug interaction, followed by a review of some of the more important and recently described drug–drug interactions for each antimicrobial class (antiviral, antibacterial, antifungal and antiprotozoal drugs). Extensive tables summarize drug–drug interactions for each class. Because of space limitations, secondary literature sources are cited where available. An excellent textbook of antimicrobial drug–drug interactions has been published,[2] as well as a number of reviews.[7–15] The literature is expanding rapidly, especially among the antiretroviral drugs. Some of the information in this chapter will become quickly dated and the most recent prescribing information and online references should be consulted.

CLASSIFICATION AND MECHANISMS OF DRUG–DRUG INTERACTIONS

Drug interactions are frequently classified as pharmacokinetic, pharmacodynamic, or physiochemical.[16]

PHARMACOKINETIC INTERACTIONS

A pharmacokinetic drug–drug interaction occurs when one drug changes the absorption, distribution, metabolism or excretion of another. These interactions may or may not cause a measurable change in clinical symptoms or in response to therapy, depending upon a number of variables (see below). For antimicrobial compounds, pharmacokinetic interactions involving absorption and metabolism are numerous and are most likely to be clinically significant. A brief review of these mechanisms as they apply to antimicrobial drugs follows.

Fig. 6.1 Warning statement in the cisapride prescribing information (Propulsid® Revised Prescribing Information, Janssen Pharmaceutica, Titusville, NJ, January 2000). As is evident, antimicrobials are a common cause of serious drug–drug interactions

PROPULSID is contraindicated in patients taking certain macrolide antibiotics (such as clarithromycin, erythromycin, and troleandomycin), certain antifungals (such as fluconazole, itraconazole, and ketoconazole), protease inhibitors (such as indinavir and ritonavir), phenothiazines (such as prochlorperazine and promethazine). Class IA and Class III antiarrhythmics (such as quinidine, procainamide, and sotalol): tricylic antidepressants (such as amitriptyline); certain antidepressants (such as nefazodone and maprotiline); certain antipsycotic medications (such as sertindole) as well as other agents (such as bepridil, sparfloxacin, and grapefruit juice).

Absorption interactions

Absorption interactions can occur by many mechanisms. For instance, one drug can alter the physiology of the gastrointestinal tract, such as pH or motility, changing the absorption of another drug. Itraconazole capsules require an acidic environment for dissolution and subsequent absorption, and drugs that increase gastric pH (including antacids, histamine-2 (H-2) blockers and proton-pump inhibitors) dramatically impair itraconazole absorption (*see below*). A second mechanism is chelation of an antibiotic when it is given with metal cations found in many antacids and mineral supplements. The best examples include chelation of fluoroquinolones and tetracyclines by di- and trivalent cations (*see below*). A final mechanism involves a change in gastrointestinal absorption at the level of the enterocyte. Metabolic enzymes including cytochrome P_{450} 3A4 (*see below*) are present in enterocytes and metabolize many drugs before they reach the systemic circulation ('first pass' metabolism). In addition, transporter proteins including P-glycoprotein (P-gp) reduce absorption of many drugs by pumping them back into the gastrointestinal lumen.[17] Both inhibition and induction of gastrointestinal enzymes and transporter proteins are major causes of drug interactions. There is currently great effort to develop inhibitors of these proteins to increase absorption of poorly bioavailable drugs. The use of ritonavir to increase the absorption of saquinavir and lopinavir is an example of an interaction that exploits inhibition of P-gp and CYP3A4 to increase systemic exposure of otherwise poorly absorbed drugs.[9,11,13,14,18]

Distribution interactions

One drug can alter the distribution of another drug, most commonly by changing receptor binding or plasma protein binding. Displacement of warfarin from albumin by certain sulfonamides is an example of a pharmacokinetic interaction involving altered distribution (*see below*). These interactions have generally not been of major importance for antimicrobial drugs. Recently however, ketoconazole has been used to increase the concentration of protease inhibitors in the central nervous system, raising the possibility that the distribution of antimicrobial drugs in the body may be altered for patient benefit by exploiting distribution drug interactions.[19]

Metabolism interactions

Most clinically relevant antimicrobial drug–drug interactions result from altered metabolism. Because of their importance, a brief review of drug metabolism is appropriate. There are numerous and more extensive reviews.[17,20–22]

Steps in drug metabolism are commonly divided into two phases. Phase I metabolism most commonly occurs in the gastrointestinal tract and liver, and includes oxidation, reduction and hydrolysis reactions. Different cytochrome P_{450} enzymes most commonly mediate these metabolic reactions. The prefix CYP is used to designate cytochrome P_{450} enzymes. Depending on the degree of homology for the amino acids making up each enzyme, an Arabic number distinguishes three major families (i.e. CYP1, CYP2, CYP3). These families are further divided into subfamilies, such as CYP3A, and further to the specific enzyme, such as CYP3A4.

It is now common for a new chemical entity to be investigated in vitro using preparations of human enzymes to determine if it is a substrate, inhibitor or inducer of the common CYP enzymes. This has resulted in more rational drug development and it allows for early investigations of potential interactions with a new antimicrobial.[21] Table 6.1 includes the most common enzymes in each of the three families and the more important known substrates, inhibitors and inducers. Anti-infective drugs commonly alter the activity of these enzymes, and the clinical consequences of combining drugs that are metabolized by similar pathways are often predictable.

Many antimicrobials are inhibitors of drug metabolizing enzymes, including certain fluoroquinolones, macrolides, azole antifungals and HIV-1 protease inhibitors.[12] Enzyme inhibition usually occurs immediately following the first dose of an inhibitor antibiotic. The subsequent rise in serum concentration of the interactant drug will happen rapidly and will reach a new steady-state serum concentration in 3–5 half-lives. An adverse clinical consequence can occur before steady-state is achieved, or after the new steady-state concentration is achieved, depending on a number of variables (*see below*). In contrast, antimicrobials such as rifampicin, pleconaril and nevirapine induce metabolic enzymes. The maximal induction effect is not observed for at least a few days, as synthesis of new protein is required.[15] The resulting reduction in serum concentration of the interacted drug may not result in clinical consequences for a few more days, depending on the specific drug and its new half-life.

Many antimicrobials alter the activity of CYP3A4 (Table 6.1).[12] This enzyme is present in hepatic tissue and gastrointestinal tissue and consequently an interaction can result from increased absorption, decreased hepatic metabolism, or by both mechanisms. Grapefruit juice is known to inhibit the gastrointestinal form of CYP3A4, and can increase the absorption of many drugs that are metabolized in the gut.[16,17] Many CYP3A4 inhibitors, such as the HIV-1 protease inhibitors and itraconazole, nearly always cause an increase in the area under the curve (AUC) of a CYP3A4 substrate, such as cyclosporine, sildenafil and simvastatin. However, it is difficult to determine if serum concentrations have increased because of inhibition of hepatic or gastrointestinal CYP3A4, or inhibition of gastrointestinal P-glycoprotein, or a combination of these mechanisms (or some yet undiscovered mechanism).[17] Drug interactions involving substrates of CYP3A4 will be discussed below as if hepatic CYP3A4 is the major or only mechanism for a metabolic interaction, unless other mechanisms are known to be involved. In part, this is because many of the cited investigations were published before the role of gastrointestinal CYP3A4 and P-glycoprotein was appreciated. However, as newer transport proteins are discovered, and as investigational techniques are developed to sort

Table 6.1 Substrates, inducers and inhibitors of the CYP$_{450}$ isoenzymes[16,20,22]

	CYP1A2	CYP2C9	CYP2C19	CYP2D6	CYP3A4	CYP2E1
Substrates	Caffeine	Amitriptyline	Imipramine	Amitriptyline	Alprazolam	Dapsone
	Clozapine	Celecoxib	Diazepam	Amphetamine	Amiodarone	Chloroxazone
	Estradiol	Diclofenac	Omeprazole	Captopril	Amitriptyline	
	Grepafloxacin	Glyburide	Propranolol	Codeine	Astemizole	
	Haloperidol	Glipizide	(S)-Mephenytoin	Debrisquine	Atorvastatin	
	Mirtazapine	Naproxen	Voriconazole	Desipramine	Buspirone	
	Mexiletine	Nelfinavir		Ecanide	Cisapride	
	(R)-Warfarin	Phenytoin		Flecanide	Clarithromycin	
	Tacrine	Piroxicam		Fluoxetine	Cyclosporine	
	Theophylline	Pravastatin		Haloperidol	Dapsone	
	Zileuton	Rosiglitazone		Imipramine	Docetaxel	
		(S)-Warfarin		Mirtazapine	Efavirenz	
		Tolbutamide		Methoxyamphetamine	Erythromycin	
				Nortriptyline	Estrogens	
				Paroxetine	Etoposide	
				Risperidone	Fentanyl	
				Venlafaxine	Granisetron	
					Glyburide	
					Itraconazole	
					Lidocaine	
					Loratadine	
					Lovastatin	
					Midazolam	
					Mirtazapine	
					Nefazadone	
					NNRTIs	
					Paclitaxel	
					Pioglitazone	
					Posaconazole	
					Prednisone	
					Protease inhibitors	
					Quinidine	
					Repaglinide	
					Sertraline	
					Sildenafil	
					Sirolimus	
					Simvastatin	
					Tacrolimus	
					Telithromycin	
					Testosterone	
					Triazolam	
					Verapamil	
					Vinblastine	
					Ziprazidone	
					Zolpidem	
Inhibitor	Cimetidine	Fluconazole	Fluoxetine	Cimetidine	Amprenavir	Disulfiram
	Ciprofloxacin	Fluoxetine	Fluvoxamine	Fluoxetine	Clarithromycin	Isoniazid
	Clarithromycin	Fluvoxamine		Omeprazole	Delavirdine	
	Erythromycin	Isoniazid		Paroxetine	Diltiazem	
	Fluvoxamine	Sertraline		Quinidine	Efavirenz	
	Paroxetine	Omeprazole			Erythromycin	
					Fluconazole	
					Fluoxetine	
					Fluvoxamine	
					Grapefruit juice (GI only)	
					Indinavir	

Table 6.1 *Continued*

	CYP1A2	CYP2C9	CYP2C19	CYP2D6	CYP3A4	CYP2E1
Inhibitor *contd*					Itraconazole	
					Ketoconazole	
					Mibefradil	
					Nefazodone	
					Nelfinavir	
					Lopinavir/ritonavir	
					Posaconazole	
					Quinupristin/dalfopristin	
					Ritonavir	
					Saquinavir	
					Telithromycin	
Inducer	Carbamazepine	Rifampicin		Carbamazepine	Carbamazepine	Isoniazid
	Cigarette smoke			Phenytoin	Dexamethasone	
	Phenytoin			Phenobarbital	Efavirenz	
	Phenobarbital			Rifampicin	Nevirapine	
	Rifampicin				Phenytoin	
	Ritonavir				Phenobarbital	
					Pleconaril	
					Rifampicin	
					Rifabutin	
					Ritonavir	
					St. John's Wort	
					Troglitazone	

CYP = Cytochrome P$_{450}$ enzyme; NNRTI = non-nucleoside reverse transcriptase inhibitor; GI = gastrointestinal

out competing mechanisms, this overly simplistic view will undoubtedly change.

Since inhibition of CYP3A4 is such a common cause of drug–drug interactions between antimicrobials, a brief summary of some of the important interactions mediated by CYP3A4 is appropriate.

Cisapride, terfenadine, astemizole and pimozide
All of these drugs are substrates for CYP3A4 and if there is a reduced rate of metabolism when given with CYP3A4 inhibitors, the resulting prolongation of the QTc interval can cause torsade de pointes, syncope and sudden death (Figure 6.1).[1,3,4,20,23] The US Food and Drug Administration removed terfenadine from the US market in February 1998,[4] and the manufacturer of astemizole removed it from the US market in June 1999.[24] Restrictions on use of cisapride are so severe (Figure 6.1) that it is little used. A warning letter was mailed to all US healthcare practitioners in September 1999, alerting them to potentially fatal cardiac arrhythmias in patients taking pimozide for whom a CYP3A4 inhibitor is prescribed.[25]

Ergot alkaloids
Ergot alkaloids, including ergotamine and dihydroergotamine, are metabolized by CYP3A4 and can lead to serious peripheral ischemia when given with potent inhibitors of CYP3A4 such as protease inhibitors, certain non-nucleoside reverse transcriptase inhibitors (NNRTIs), azoles and macrolides (*see below*).[7,20]

Sildenafil
Sildenafil is especially susceptible to increases in serum concentrations when combined with inhibitors of CYP3A4. For example, the HIV-1 protease inhibitor ritonavir increases the AUC of sildenafil by 2–11-fold and this may lead to syncope, hypotension, visual disturbances, and prolonged erection.[11,26,27]

HMG-CoA reductase inhibitors ('Statins')
Lovastatin and simvastatin and, to a lesser extent, atorvastatin are metabolized by CYP3A4 and serum concentrations increase dramatically when coadministered with CYP3A4 inhibitors.[20] CYP3A4 inhibitors should be avoided with lovastatin and simvastatin due to the increased risk of rhabdomyolysis, although the pathology of this effect is not well understood. Fluvastatin and pravastatin are less dependent on CYP3A4 for metabolism and are preferred for patients who will be treated with CYP3A4 inhibitors. Cerivastatin was removed from the US market in August 2001 because it caused a higher incidence of rhabdomyolysis than the other statins.

Rifabutin
Rifabutin is dependent on CYP3A4 for its metabolism, and the main metabolite is further metabolized by CYP3A4. When coadministered with CYP3A4 inhibitors, rifabutin and metabolite concentrations increase dramatically and can cause a high incidence of severe flu-like symptoms, including fever and myalgia, uveitis and neutropenia.[15] When rifabutin is indi-

cated in patients receiving inhibitors of CYP3A4, it is often recommended that half of the normal dose be given.[11,15,26] However, this dose reduction does not always compensate for the large interaction effects, and patients should be monitored closely.

HIV-1 protease inhibitors and NNRTIs

All HIV-1 protease inhibitor drugs are substrates of CYP3A4 and they are some of the most potent inhibitors of CYP3A4 in clinical use.[11,13,14,26,28,29] Their coadministration may have profound effects on the pharmacokinetics of other drugs (see below). When they are administered with other CYP3A4 inhibitors, there is frequently a decrease in clearance of the protease inhibitor. However, the magnitude of the effect is generally small, and is unlikely to be clinically important.

As a result of the central role for CYP3A4 in drug metabolism, there is a predictable list of concomitantly administered drugs for which caution should be exercised when CYP3A4 inhibitory drugs, including many antimicrobials, are prescribed (Table 6.2). Many of these Phase I metabolic interactions should be known to every practitioner because of their common mechanism, and the high potential for adverse clinical consequences.

Phase II metabolism occurs in the cytosol of hepatocytes and includes conjugation reactions such as glucuronidation and sulfation.[16,30] Fluconazole inhibits zidovudine metabolism, presumably by reducing Phase II acetylation of zidovudine, since zidovudine is not known to be a substrate of P_{450} enzymes.[11] In general, drug–drug interactions involving Phase II metabolism have not been as thoroughly investigated as those involving Phase I metabolism.

Excretion interactions

Excretion drug–drug interactions include an alteration in renal elimination of one drug as a result of changes in glomerular filtration, tubular secretion, and tubular reabsorption caused by another.[16] For example, administration of probenecid is recommended before each dose of cidofovir to decrease tubular secretion and nephrotoxicity.[31] Similarly, cilastatin is added to the commercial formulation of imipenem to increase renal clearance of imipenem (this interaction can also be thought of as having a metabolic basis). Excretion interactions are not common causes of important antimicrobial drug interactions.

PHARMACODYNAMIC DRUG–DRUG INTERACTIONS

Pharmacodynamic interactions result when one drug alters the pharmacological response of another, but without a change in the pharmacokinetics of either. The increase in QTc interval when cisapride is combined with sparfloxacin (Figure 6.1) is an example: sparfloxacin does not change the pharmacokinetics of cisapride, but instead both drugs increase QTc interval independently.[23] Pharmacodynamic interactions are more difficult to predict a priori than pharmacokinetic interactions, and the literature is less extensive.

PHYSIOCHEMICAL INTERACTIONS

Physiochemical interactions represent those that take place ex-vivo between drugs in packaging or with administrative device

Table 6.2 Substrates of CYP3A4 with a narrow therapeutic index and pharmacologic effects when administered with CYP3A4 inhibitors (*see text for references*)

CYP 3A4[a] substrate	Pharmacologic effect	Comments
Ergot alkaloids	Ergotism and peripheral ischemia	Contraindicated
Cisapride, terfenadine, astemizole, pimozide	Increase QTc interval, arrhythmias, sudden death	Contraindicated
Cyclosporine, tacrolimus, sirolimus	Nephrotoxicity	Avoid use or monitor serum concentrations
HMG Co-A[b] reductase inhibitors ('Statins')	Rhabdomyolysis may be most likely with simvastatin and lovastatin	Pravastatin or fluvastatin are preferred when CYP3A4 inhibitors are used
Rifabutin	Neutropenia, flu-like syndrome	Reduce dose of rifabutin
Oncology drugs (vincristine, vinblastine etoposide, irinotecan, taxol, tamoxifen)	Decreased metabolism, increased drug toxicity	Avoid concomitant therapy (although erythromycin has been used to reverse antitumor drug resistance)
Sildenafil	Hypotension, priapism	Reduce dose of sildenafil or avoid use entirely
Triazolam, midazolam	Excessive sedation	Avoid or reduce dose
HIV-1 Protease inhibitors and NNRTIs[c]	Enhanced efficacy and possibly greater toxicity	Usually not a contraindication

[a] Cytochrome P_{450}, 3A4
[b] 3 hydroxy-3 methylglutaryl coenzyme A
[c] Non-nucleoside reverse transcriptase inhibitors

systems. The inadvertent mixing of most aminoglycosides in the same intravenous bag containing high concentrations of β-lactams such as ticarcillin, resulting in inactivation of the aminoglycoside, is an example of a physiochemical interaction. These are relatively uncommon problems with antimicrobial drugs and will not be discussed.

EFFECTS OF INFECTION ON DRUG METABOLISM

Infection can alter the pharmacokinetics of drugs.[32] It is increasingly appreciated that interleukin-1 (IL-1 alpha and IL-1 beta), IL-6 and tumor necrosis factor (TNF-α), and free oxygen radicals released during infection can disrupt drug disposition and metabolism. These cytokines reduce CYP gene expression and the activity of drug metabolizing enzymes. Consequently it is possible to see an exaggerated response to a drug that the patient has previously tolerated during an infection episode. Another practical consequence is that many case reports of 'antibiotic drug–drug interactions' are probably caused by infection and not the antimicrobial used to treat the infection. For example, case reports of cyclosporine and warfarin interactions with some fluoroquinolones probably reflect the inhibition of cyclosporine and warfarin metabolism as a consequence of infection (see below). The fluoroquinolones are probably innocent bystanders in these 'interactions' and are inappropriately blamed for an effect that is cytokine induced.

MANAGEMENT OF CLINICALLY SIGNIFICANT DRUG INTERACTIONS

Antibiotic drug–drug interactions most commonly result from administration of an antimicrobial to a patient already receiving multiple drugs. The most important step to avoid the adverse consequences of a drug–drug interaction is to recognize the potential before the antibiotic is given. The tragic consequences of terfenadine and cisapride interactions occurred despite multiple warnings in the medical literature, warnings in the official prescribing information, and warnings to the lay public. Despite this effort to educate, physicians continued to write prescriptions for potentially lethal combinations and pharmacists continued to fill these prescriptions. Computer technology is widely available to warn the prescriber and the dispenser of the adverse consequences of drug combinations,[33,34] however, it will still take a human being to assess the potential clinical consequences when an antibiotic is prescribed to a patient receiving other drugs and to make a rational decision.

Potential drug–drug interactions are usually categorized as either an absolute or a relative contraindication, depending on the probability of occurrence and the clinical significance of the consequences:

● *Absolute contraindication*: A well documented interaction with serious consequences, or the potential for serious con-

sequences. For example, rifampicin cannot be coadministered with most HIV-1 protease inhibitors.[11] Likewise, itraconazole cannot be given to a patient receiving pimozide, dofetilide or cisapride.[25,35] The drugs listed in Table 6.2 are generally considered to represent absolute contraindications, although there may be little firm data to document serious consequences.

● *Relative contraindication*: These represent well documented interaction for which adverse clinical consequences are unlikely if appropriate steps are taken. For example, antacids can be administered with fluroquinolones if administration times are staggered by 2 hours. Most drug–drug interactions with antimicrobials are relative contraindications.

The clinical consequences of a pharmacokinetic drug–drug interaction depend on many variables, including the magnitude of the effect, the therapeutic index of the interactant drug, and the patient's 'sensitivity' to the pharmacological effect of the interactant drug. The terfenadine and cisapride interactions were critically important because the changes in serum concentrations were relatively large, these drugs have a relatively narrow therapeutic index, and the clinical consequences (arrhythmia and death) were obvious. In contrast, the clinical importance of many other antibiotic drug–drug interactions is often unclear. Drug interaction trials are typically performed in healthy (uninfected) young volunteer subjects. The effects of an antibiotic on the pharmacokinetics of another drug (or vice versa) are typically determined by measuring changes in serum concentrations, but usually without measuring changes in pharmacological response. These studies can reliably detect relatively small changes in the AUC if an interaction exists.

A typical finding from a drug interaction trial is illustrated by a statement found in the quinupristin-dalfopristin (Synercid™) package insert:

> 'Concomitant administration of Synercid™ ... and midazolam (intravenous bolus dose) in healthy volunteers lead to elevated plasma concentrations. The C_{max} increased by 14% (median value) and the AUC increased by 33% ...'.[36]

Often the clinical consequences of an increase in AUC for the interactant drug, midazolam in this example, is unknown. Furthermore, it is easy to forget that some subjects in this study had a much larger increase in AUC than the mean increase of 33%. Finally, the subjects studied in these investigations are not the target population. To bring this example to the bedside, if Synercid™ is administered to an elderly patient who is receiving midazolam (and possibly multiple other drugs), and if midazolam clearance is already decreased by the presence of 'infection' or concomitant drug therapy, then a real (but relatively small) interaction following administration of Synercid™ to this individual may result a clinically important effect. This can occur even though the interaction is judged to be 'of no clinical significance' on the basis of a trial in normal volunteers. This caution against assuming that an interaction is not likely to be clinically important, based on normal volunteer investigations, can be applied to most antimicrobial drug interactions.

The clinician who is faced with a patient who needs an antibiotic, yet is also receiving a drug that may interact adversely, has a number of choices:

- Administer the antibiotic if the interaction is not likely to be clinically important. For example, fluconazole will increase the AUC of zidovudine, but the combination has been extensively used and is not known to result in adverse clinical effects.
- Administer the antibiotic, but change the dosage of the interactant drug to reflect the mean magnitude of the interaction. This is the current recommendation for patients who are receiving a HIV-1 protease inhibitor and for whom rifabutin is to be used. It is common to reduce the rifabutin dose by 50% in such patients.[11,37]
- Administer the antibiotic but monitor the serum concentration of the interactant drug. This may be possible for a few drugs when assays are readily available, such as for digoxin and cyclosporine.
- Administer an alternative antibiotic that does not have an interaction potential. This is the most appropriate decision in most cases, since it avoids the problem entirely. For example, azithromycin does not result in metabolic interactions and may be a safe alternative to the subject receiving a 'statin', who must be treated with a macrolide compound. However, use of an alternative antimicrobial is not always possible.

ANTIVIRAL DRUG INTERACTIONS

NUCLEOSIDE/NUCLEOTIDE REVERSE TRANSCRIPTASE INHIBITORS (NRTIs)

There are few pharmacokinetic interactions with this class because the NRTIs are eliminated via the kidneys as parent compound (tenofovir, lamivudine) or as metabolites that do not require CYP_{450} pathways (zidovudine, didanosine, zalcitabine, stavudine, abacavir). The most significant types of interactions caused by the NRTIs are pharmacodynamic and are due to overlapping toxicities.

Pharmacodynamic interactions[11,13,14]

Overlapping toxicities

These pharmacodynamic interactions occur at the intracellular level, resulting in increased toxicity that may be of clinical significance (Table 6.3).

The combination of zalcitabine with stavudine or didanosine causes severe cases of peripheral neuropathy. Neurotoxicity may also occur when isoniazid is given with didanosine, stavudine or zalcitabine, and patients should be monitored for signs and symptoms of peripheral neuropathy.

The combination of zidovudine with ganciclovir results in additive bone marrow toxicity, especially neutropenia. This combination should be avoided, especially during ganciclovir induction therapy, and a different NRTI such as stavudine should be considered as a substitute for zidovudine. If this combination is necessary, it is recommended that a complete blood count with a differential be initially monitored three times weekly, then once weekly.

When didanosine is combined with agents that can cause pancreatitis (e.g. stavudine, pentamidine, zalcitabine, alcohol) there is a potential for an increased risk. Concomitant use of these agents should be avoided, or monitored closely.

Pharmacokinetic interactions[11,13,14]

Absorption

Didanosine tablets contain an antacid buffer to improve bioavailability. The antacid can interfere with the absorption of agents that require acidic media, such as indinavir or delavirdine (Table 6.3). Didanosine should be administered at least 30 minutes before indinavir or delavirdine (Table 6.3). The buffer can also decrease absorption of ketoconazole and itraconazole, and didanosine tablets must be administered at least 2 hours before these antifungal drugs (Table 6.3). Similarly, didanosine cannot be administered with fluoroquinolones or tetracyclines because metal cations chelate these antibiotics and reduce absorption. The enteric coated formulation of didanosine does not cause these absorption interactions.

Metabolism

NRTI activity requires intracellular phosphorylation for conversion to the active form. Both zidovudine and stavudine are phosphorylated via thymidine kinase. Combining thymidine analogs results in antagonism and a compromise in the anti-HIV effects (Table 6.3). This is also true for the combination of lamivudine and zalcitabine, where both cytosine analogs use the same pathway for activation (Table 6.3). Currently the Department of Health and Human Services (DHHS) in the US recommends against such combinations.[26]

Beneficial interactions are occasionally observed with NRTIs. In vitro, hydroxyurea improves didanosine's antiviral activity by increasing phosphorylation of didanosine to dideoxyadenosine phosphate.[38] However, long-term use of hydroxyurea with didanosine has been associated with reports of hepatitis and pancreatitis.

Zidovudine is glucuronidated and metabolite formation can be reduced by probenecid, fluconazole or valproic acid resulting in an increase in the area under the concentration curve (AUC) of zidovudine (Table 6.3). Conversely, the AUC of zidovudine is decreased 35% and 25%, respectively, by the protease inhibitors nelfinavir and ritonavir, presumably via induction of glucuronyl transferases. Similarly, rifampicin decreases the AUC of zidovudine by 47% by inducing more rapid glucuronidation. These interactions are believed to be of little clinical significance since it is the intracellular concentrations of zidovudine that are important for the pharmacologic effect.

Table 6.3 Nucleoside/Nucleotide reverse transcriptase inhibitor drug interactions (*see text for references*)

NRTI	Drug altered by or altering NRTI	Pharmacokinetic interactions	Pharmacodynamic interactions	Clinical management
Abacavir	Alcohol	↑ ABC AUC by 40%	N/A	Use with caution
Didanosine	Delavirdine	Antacid in DDI reduces absorption of DLV	N/A	Separate DDI from DLV by at least 30 min
	Ganciclovir (p.o.)	↑ DDI AUC by >100%; ↓ ganciclovir AUC by 20%	N/A	Separate DDI from ganciclovir by 2 h; monitor for toxicity of DDI and progression of CMV
	Ganciclovir (i.v.)	↑ DDI AUC by >70%		
	Hydroxyurea	N/A	Hydroxyurea potentiates the antiretroviral effect of DDI	Combined use is controversial
	Indinavir	Antacid in DDI decreases absorption of IDV	N/A	Separate DDI from IDV by at least 30 min
	Itraconazole	Antacid in DDI reduces absorption of itraconazole (capsule only)	N/A	Separate DDI from itraconazole capsules by 2 h
	Isoniazid	N/A	Additive PN	Monitor for PN
	Ketoconazole	Antacid in DDI reduces absorption of ketoconazole	N/A	Separate DDI from ketoconazole by 2 h
	Methadone	↓ DDI AUC by 40%		Uncertain clinical significance
	Quinolones	Antacid in DDI reduces absorption of quinolones	N/A	Separate DDI from quinolone by 2 h
	Stavudine	N/A	Additive PN	Monitor for PN
	Zalcitabine		Additive PN	Avoid concomitant use
Lamivudine	Zalcitabine	N/A	Antagonistic anti-HIV effect	Avoid concomitant use
Stavudine	Didanosine	N/A	Additive PN	Monitor for PN
	Isoniazid	N/A	Additive PN	Monitor for PN
	Methadone	↓ stavudine AUC by 27%	N/A	Minimal clinical significance
	Zalcitabine		Additive PN	Monitor for PN
	Zidovudine	N/A	Antagonistic anti-HIV effect	Avoid concomitant use
Tenofovir	didanosine	↑ DDL AUC by 44%	Increased virologic response?	Uncertain importance. Separate doses by 2 hours
Zalcitabine	Lamivudine	N/A	Antagonistic anti-HIV effect	Avoid concomitant use
	Probenecid	↑ zalcitabine AUC by 50%	N/A	Monitor for zalcitabine toxicity
	Stavudine		Additive PN	Avoid concomitant use

Table 6.3 *Continued*

NRTI	Drug altered by or altering NRTI	Pharmacokinetic interactions	Pharmacodynamic interactions	Clinical management
Zidovudine	Fluconazole	↑ AZT AUC by 60% (depends on fluconazole dose)	N/A	Monitor AZT toxicities
	Ganciclovir	N/A	Additive bone marrow toxicity	Monitor CBC, or switch to alternative NRTI
	Methadone	↑ AZT glucuronidation, ↓ AZT AUC by 1.4 fold	N/A	Monitor for suboptimal virologic response
	Nelfinavir	↑ AZT glucuronidation, ↓ AZT AUC by 35%	N/A	Monitor for suboptimal virologic response to AZT
	Probenacid	↑ AZT glucuronidation, ↓ AZT AUC by 80% (RQ:AUC goes *up*!)	N/A	Monitor excessive AZT toxicities
	Ribavirin	N/A	Antagonistic anti-HIV effect	Avoid concomitant use
	Ritonavir	↑ AZT glucuronidation, ↓ AZT AUC by 25%	N/A	Monitor for suboptimal virologic response to AZT
	Stavudine		Antagonistic anti-HIV effect	Avoid concomitant use
	Valproic acid	↓ AZT glucuronidation, ↑ AZT AUC by 80%	N/A	Monitor AZT toxicities

ABC = Abacavir; AUC = area under the concentration curve; AZT = zidovudine; CBC = complete blood count; DDI = didanosine; DLV = delavirdine; IDV = indinavir; N/A = not anticipated; NRTI = nucleoside reverse transcriptase inhibitor; PN = peripheral neuropathy; ↑ = increase; ↓ decrease.

Methadone causes a decrease in the AUC of didanosine and stavudine by 40% and 27% respectively, although the clinical significance of this interaction is unknown.[39]

Abacavir is metabolized via alcohol dehydrogenase. Concomitant use of alcohol with abacavir can increase the AUC of abacavir by 40% and the combination should be used with caution.

Elimination
In HIV-infected patients, probenecid is combined with cidofovir to improve its renal safety profile. However, probenecid increases the AUC of zalcitabine by 50% and of zidovudine by 75–115%, probably by inhibiting renal tubular secretion. The clinical significance of these changes is unknown.

NON-NUCLEOSIDE REVERSE TRANSCRIPTASE INHIBITORS (NNRTIs)

NNRTIs have pronounced effects on CYP3A4 and are common causes of drug–drug interactions (Table 6.4).[11,13,14,26,29]

Pharmacokinetic interactions

Absorption
Didanosine must be administered 2 hours before administering delavirdine (above), but absorption of nevirapine and efavirenz is not affected by gastric pH (Table 6.3).

Metabolism
NNRTIs are primarily metabolized by CYP3A4 and the potential for metabolic interactions is very high. Delavirdine is a potent inhibitor of CYP3A4, whereas efavirenz and nevirap-

Table 6.4 Non-nucleoside reverse transcriptase inhibitor – drug pharmacokinetic interactions (*see text for references*)

NNRTI	Interacting Drug (ID)	Anticipated effect of NNRTI on ID	Anticipated effect of ID on NNRTI	Clinical management
Delavirdine	*Anticonvulsant:*			
	Carbamazepine	No data*	May ↓ DLV levels	Use with caution, monitor anticonvulsant levels
	Phenobarbital			
	Phenytoin			
	Antihistamines:			
	Astemizole	↑ astemizole levels	No data*	Combination contraindicated, may cause QTc prolongation
	Terfenadine	↑ terfenadine levels	No data*	Combination contraindicated, may cause QTc prolongation
	Antifungals:			
	Fluconazole	↔ on fluconazole levels	↔ in DLV levels	Standard dosing used
	Ketoconazole	No data*	No data*	
	Itraconazole	No data*	No data*	
	Antimycobacterials:	↑ clarithromycin AUC by 100%	↑ DLV AUC by 44%	Reduce clarithromycin dose in renal failure
	Clarithromycin			
	Rifabutin	↑ rifabutin AUC by 100%	↓ DLV AUC by 80%	Not recommended
	Rifampicin	No data*	↓ DLV AUC by 96%	Contraindicated combination
	Lipid lowering agents:			
	Lovastatin	↑ in statin levels, rhabdomyolysis	No data*	Avoid concomitant use
	Simvastatin			
	Miscellaneous:			
	Cisapride	↑ Cisapride levels	No data*	Combination contraindicated, may cause QTc prolongation
	Methadone	↑ methadone levels	No data*	Monitor patients mental and respiratory status
	Sildenafil	↑ Sildenafil levels	No data*	Maximum sildenafil dose may not exceed 25 mg in 48 h
	Oral contraceptives:	Potential ↑ in estrogen and progesterone levels	No data*	
	Protease inhibitors:			
	Amprenavir	↑ AUC APV by 4-fold	No data*	↓ IDV dose to 600 mg per 8 h
	Indinavir	↑ IDV AUC by >40%	No effect on DLV	Consider dosing IDV 600 mg per 8 h with DLV 400 mg t.i.d.
	Lopinavir/ritonavir	No data*	No data*	
	Nelfinavir	↑ NFV AUC by 2-fold	↓ DLV AUC by 50%	No data*, monitor for neutropenic complications
	Ritonavir	↑ RTV AUC by 70%	No effect on DLV	Limited data, may consider dosing RTV 400 mg b.i.d. with standard DLV dose
	Saquinavir	↑ SQV AUC by 5-fold	No effect on DLV	↓ SQV-HGC dose to 800 mg t.i.d. with standard DLV dose
Efavirenz	*Anticonvulsant:*			
	Carbamazepine	No data*	No data*	Use with caution, monitor anticonvulsant levels
	Phenobarbitol			
	Phenytoin			
	Antifungals:			
	Fluconazole	↔ in fluconazole levels	↔ in EFV levels	Standard dosing used of both drugs
	Ketoconazole	No data*	No data*	
	Itraconazole	No data*	No data*	
	Antimycobacterials:	↓ clarithromycin AUC by 39%	↑ EFV AUC by 11%	Alternative therapy recommended
	Clarithromycin			
	Rifabutin	↓ rifabutin AUC by 35%	↔ in EFV AUC	↑ rifabutin dose to 450–600 mg q.d. or 600 q. 2–3 weeks with standard EFV dose
	Rifampicin	No data*	↓ EFV AUC by 25%	Not likely to require dosing adjustment

Table 6.4 *Continued*

NNRTI	Interacting Drug (ID)	Anticipated effect of NNRTI on ID	Anticipated effect of ID on NNRTI	Clinical management
Efavirenz (*contd*)	*Lipidlowering agents:*			
	Lovastatin	No data*	No data*	Use with caution, monitor anticonvulsant levels
	Simvastatin			
	Miscellaneous:			
	Methadone	↓ methadone AUC by 25–50%	No data*	Consider ↑ methadone dose
	Warfarin	No data*	No data*	Monitor warfarin levels with standard NVP dose
	Oral contraceptives:			
	Ethinylestradiol	↑ Ethinylestradiol AUC by 37%	No data*	Clinical significance unknown
	Protease inhibitors:			
	Amprenavir	↓ APV AUC by 39%	No data*	↑ APV dose to 1200 mg t.i.d., or 1200 mg b.i.d. + RTV 200 mg b.i.d. with standard EFV dose
	Indinavir	↓ IDV AUC by 31%	No data*	↑ IDV dosing to 1000 mg q. 8 h with standard EFV dose
	Lopinavir/ritonavir	↓ LPV AUC by 40%	↔ EFV in AUC	↑ LPV/RTV dosing to 533/133 mg b.i.d. with standard EFV dose
	Nelfinavir	↑ NLV AUC by 20%	No data*	Standard NFV dose
	Ritonavir	↑ RTV AUC by 18%	↑ EFV AUC by 21%	Consider dose reduction of RTV with standard EFV dose
	Saquinavir-SGC	↓ SQV-HGC AUC by 62%	↓ EFV AUC by 12%	Avoid concomitant use
Nevirapine	*Anticonvulsant:*			
	Carbamazepine	No data*	No data*	Use with caution, monitor anticonvulsant levels
	Phenobarbitol			
	Phenytoin			
	Antifungals:			
	Ketoconazole	↓ Ketoconazole AUC by 63%	↑ NVP AUC by 15–30%	Not recommended
	Antimycobacterials:			
	Clarithromycin	↓ clarithromycin AUC by 30%	↑ NVP AUC by 26%	Standard dosing of both drugs
	Rifabutin	No data*	↓ NVP AUC by 16%	May administer with caution, no dose adjustment needed
	Rifampicin	↔ rifampin	↓ NVP AUC by 37%	Not recommended
	Fluconazole	No data*	No data*	
	Itraconazole	No data*	No data*	
	Lipidlowering agents:	No data*	No data*	
	Lovastatin			
	Simvastatin			
	Miscellaneous:			
	Methadone	↓ 46–60% methadone levels	NVP unchanged	Titrate methadone dose to effect with standard NVP dose
	Oral contraceptives:			
	Ethinylestradiol	No data*	No data*	
	Protease inhibitors:			
	Amprenavir	No data*	No data*	
	Indinavir	↓ IDV AUC by 28%	NVP unchanged	↑ IDV dose to 1000 mg q. 8 h with standard NVP dose
	Lopinavir	↓ AUC LPV by 20–25%	1.08-fold ↑ in NVP AUC	↑ LPV/RTV dosing to 533/133 mg b.i.d. with standard NVP dose
	Nelfinavir	↑ NFV AUC by 10%	NVP unchanged	Standard dosing of both drugs
	Ritonavir	↓ RTV AUC by 11%	NVP unchanged	Standard dosing of both drugs
	Saquinavir	↓ SQV-HGC AUC by 27%	NVP unchanged	No data* on SQV-SGC, avoid combining NVP with SQV-HGC when used as sole protease inhibitor

APV = amprenavir; AUC = area under the concentration curve; DLV= delavirdine; EFV = efavirenz; IDV = indinavir; LPV = lopinavir; NFV = nelfinavir; NNRTI = non-nucleoside reverse transcriptase inhibitor; NRTI = nucleoside reverse transcriptase inhibitor; NVP = nevirapine; RTV = ritonavir; SQV = saquinavir; SQV-HGC = saquinavir hard-gel capsule; SGC = soft gel capsule; ↑ = increase; ↓ = decrease; ↔ = no change. * No data = Current recommendations should be consulted for updated effect and clinical management.

ine are modest inducers of CYP3A4.[11,13,14,26,29] Efavirenz may also inhibit CYP3A4 and there are extensive drug–drug interaction warnings in the prescribing information for these drugs. Most of the drugs listed as substrates of CYP3A4 in Table 6.1 are known to interact with the NNRTIs, or are expected to do so.

NNRTI INTERACTIONS WITH PROTEASE INHIBITORS

Delavirdine increases the AUC of saquinavir by 5-fold, nelfinavir by 2-fold; indinavir by 40%, and ritonavir by 70%. The protease inhibitors have little effect on the AUC of delavirdine, however. Nelfinavir decreased the AUC of delavirdine by 50%, presumably because nelfinavir induces various microsomal pathways including CYP3A4 (Table 6.4).[28,29]

Efavirenz is a substrate and an inducer of CYP3A4 and CYP2B6. Therefore, efavirenz can enhance its own metabolism and the metabolism of protease inhibitors (Table 6.4). Efavirenz can inhibit CYP3A4 and CYP2C19 isoenzymes and increase the AUC of nelfinavir and ritonavir by 20% and 18%, respectively (Table 6.4).[28]

Nevirapine is also a substrate and an inducer of CYP3A4 and CYP2B6 isoenzymes. Nevirapine metabolism is minimally affected by protease inhibitors and standard dosing of nevirapine is used with a protease inhibitor (Table 6.4). However, nevirapine induces its own metabolism and the metabolism of several protease inhibitors (Table 6.4).[29]

HIV-1 PROTEASE INHIBITORS

Protease inhibitors are all substrates and potent inhibitors of CYP3A4, and metabolic interactions are common.[11,13,14] Ritonavir is the most potent inhibitor of CYP3A4 and it alters activity of various other cytochrome P450 isoenzymes, including CYP2D6, CY2C9, and CYP2C19. Indinavir, nelfinavir and amprenavir are somewhat less potent inhibitors of CYP3A4, while lopinavir and saquinavir appear least inhibiting. Nelfinavir and ritonavir induce glycuronyl transferase and appear to induce both CYP2C9 and CYP2C19. Further, HIV protease inhibitors are substrates and inhibitors of P-glycoprotein.[11] Consequently, before a patient is placed on a protease inhibitor, concomitant drug therapy – including 'herbal' therapies – must be reviewed for contraindications.

PHARMACOKINETIC INTERACTIONS

Protease inhibitor interactions with other protease inhibitors

Current recommendations for first-line treatment of HIV-1 often include dual protease inhibitors.[26] One protease inhibitor may increase serum concentrations – and clinical response – to another protease inhibitor by inhibiting presystemic clearance, first-pass metabolism, and/or hepatic CYP3A4 mediated systemic clearance. In general, a more potent inhibitor of CYP3A4 or P-glycoprotein such as riton-

avir is combined with a second protease inhibitor that is less potent. For example, low-dose ritonavir (100 mg) will increase the AUC of the poorly absorbed drug, saquinavir, by up to 50-fold.[11,26] The combination product, Kaletra™, exploits the inhibitory activity of ritonavir toward CYP3A4 and P-glycoprotein to increase the AUC of lopinavir by up to 20-fold. Other protease inhibitor combinations and their effects are summarized in Table 6.5.

Clarithromycin

Clarithromycin is metabolized via CYP3A4 to its hydroxy metabolite. Protease inhibitors generally increase the AUC of clarithromycin, presumably via an increase in absorption and/or decrease in systemic metabolism. Hydroxy-clarithromycin serum concentrations are substantially decreased, presumably due to inhibition of CYP3A4 by the protease inhibitor. However, these effects are believed to be of little clinical significance. Clarithromycin may slightly increase the AUC of the protease inhibitor, but the effects are modest and no dosage adjustment is recommended (Table 6.5).

Itraconazole

Itraconazole is a potent inhibitor of CYP3A4 and significantly increases the AUC of protease inhibitors. The combination of itraconazole with ritonavir increased the half-life of itraconazole by greater than 5-fold and is associated with an increased incidence of pruritic dry skin, and eczematous eruptions. Caution is advised when protease inhibitors and itraconazole are coadministered.[35] Other protease inhibitor and azole interactions are listed in Table 6.5.

Sildenafil

Sildenafil is a substrate of CYP3A4 and the AUC of sildenafil is increased in the presence of potent inhibitors of CYP3A4, including all of the protease inhibitors and some of the NNRTIs.[11,26,27] The maximum dose of sildenafil should not exceed 25 mg in 48 hours in patients receiving any of the protease inhibitors (Table 6.5).

Miscellaneous

Efficacy of hormonal oral contraceptives may be compromised in the presence of nelfinavir, lopinavir/ritonavir and ritonavir, reflected by a decrease in the AUC of ethinylestradiol.[11,40,41] Hormone metabolism is complex and not completely understood, and the effects of these antimicrobials are often perplexing (see below). Changes in hormone concentrations, usually ethinylestradiol, norethindrone or levonorgestrol, presumably reflect induction of glucuronyl transferase by the protease inhibitor and/or induction of CYP isoenzymes. Patients are advised to use an alternative or additional contraceptive method when hormonal contraceptives are combined with nelfinavir, lopinavir/ritonavir, ritonavir or amprenavir. Indinavir increases the AUC of ethinylestradiol, but the clinical significance of this interaction is unclear (Table 6.5).

Most antiepileptic drugs, including carbamazepine, pheno-

Table 6.5 Protease inhibitor–drug pharmacokinetic interactions (*see text for references*)

Protease inhibitor	Interacting drug (ID)	Anticipated effect of PI on ID	Anticipated effect of ID on PI	Clinical management
Amprenavir	*Anticonvulsants:*			
	Carbamazepine Phenobarbital Phenytoin	No data*	Unknown, may ↓ APV levels	Use with caution. Monitor anticonvulsant levels
	Antifungals:			
	Fluconazole	No data*	No data*	
	Itraconazole	No data*	No data*	
	Ketoconazole	↑ ketoconazole AUC by 44%	↑ APV AUC by 31%	Clinical significance unclear. Monitor for ketoconazole and APV toxicity
	Antihistamines:			
	Astemizole	↑ astemizole levels by inhibiting CYP3A4	No data*	Contraindicated combination. May result in QTc prolongation
	Terfenadine	↑ terfenadine levels by inhibiting CYP3A4	No data*	Contraindicated combination. May result in QTc prolongation
	Antimycobacterials:			
	Clarithromycin	↔ in clarithromycin AUC	↑ APV AUC by 18%	Standard dosing of both drugs
	Rifabutin	↑ rifabutin AUC by 193%	↓ APV AUC by 15%	↓ rifabutin dosing to 150 mg q.d. or 300 mg 2–3×/week with standard APV dose
	Rifampicin	↔ in rifampicin AUC	↓ APV AUC by 82%	Avoid concomitant use
	HMG-CoA reductase inhibitors:			
	Atorvastatin Lovastatin Simvastatin }	A potential interaction exists	A potential interaction exists	Avoid concomitant use
	Miscellaneous:			
	Cisapride	↑ Cisapride levels	No data*	Combination contraindicated, may cause QTc prolongation
	Ergot alkaloids	DHE levels may ↑	No data*	Combination contraindicated, may cause increased risk of ergotism (nausea, vomiting, vasospastic ischemia)
	Methadone	Unknown, a potential for ↓ methadone levels	No data*	Monitor response to methadone
	Sildenafil	May ↑ sildenafil level	No data*	Maximum sildenafil dose may not exceed 25 mg in 48 h
	NNRTIs	*See* Table 6.4	*See* Table 6.4	
	NRTIs:			
	Abacavir	No data*	↑ APV AUC by 29%	Not established
	Lamivudine	↔ in 3TC AUC	↔ in APV AUC	Standard dosing of both drugs
	Zidovudine	↑ AZT AUC by 35%	↑ APV AUC by 13%	Not established
	Oral contraceptives:	A potential interaction exists	A potential interaction exists	Use alternative or additional method of contraception
	Protease inhibitors:			
	Indinavir	↓ IDV AUC by 38%	↑ APV AUC by 32%	Standard dosing of both drugs
	Lopinavir/ Ritonavir	0.85-fold ↓ in LPV AUC	↑ APV AUC. Dose reduction of APV recommended	Dose APV at 750 mg b.i.d. with standard LPV/RTV dosing
	Nelfinavir	↔ in NFV AUC	↑ APV AUC by 46%	Standard dosing of both drugs
	Ritonavir	No data*	2.5-fold ↑ in APV AUC	Not established, may consider ↓ APV to 600 mg b.i.d. with RTV 100 mg b.i.d. or APV to 1200 mg q.d. with 200 mg RTV q.d.
	Saquinavir	↓ SQV AUC by 19%	↓ APV AUC by 32%	Not established

Table 6.5 *Continued*

Protease inhibitor	Interacting drug (ID)	Anticipated effect of PI on ID	Anticipated effect of ID on PI	Clinical management
Indinavir	*Anticonvulsants:*			
	Carbamazepine	A potential interaction exists	Carbamazipine ↓ IDV AUC	Use with caution
	Phenobarbital			Monitor anticonvulsants levels
	Phenytoin			
	Antifungals:			
	Fluconazole	↔ in fluconazole levels	↔ in IDV levels	Standard dosing of both drugs
	Itraconazole	No data*	↑IDV AUC at IDV 600 mg q. 8 h with itraconazole 200 mg b.i.d.	↓IDV dosing to 600 mg q. 8 h with itraconazole 200 mg b.i.d.
	Ketoconazole	No data*	↑IDV AUC by 68% at IDV 400 mg q. 8 h with ketoconazole 400 mg q.d.	↓IDV dosing to 600 mg q. 8 h with ketoconazole 400 mg q.d.
	Antihistamines:			
	Astemizole	↑astemizole levels by inhibiting CYP3A4	No data*	Contraindicated combination. May result in QTc prolongation
	Terfenadine	↑terfenadine levels by inhibiting CYP3A4	No data*	Contraindicated combination. May result in QTc prolongation
	Antimycobacterials:			
	Clarithromycin	↑clarithromycin AUC by 53%	No data*	Standard clarithromycin dosing
	Rifabutin	2-fold ↑ in rifabutin AUC	↓IDV AUC by 32%	↓rifabutin dose to 150 mg q.d. or 300 mg 2–3×/week with ↑IDV dosing to 1000 mg q. 8 h
	Rifampicin	No data*	↓IDV AUC by 89%	Contraindicated
	Miscellaneous:			
	Cisapride	↑cisapride levels	No data*	Combination contraindicated. May cause QTc prolongation
	Ergot alkaloids	DHE levels may ↑	No data*	Combination contraindicated, may cause increased risk of ergotism (nausea, vomiting, vasospastic ischemia)
	Grapefruit juice		↓IDV by 26%	Clinical significance unknown
	Sildenafil	4.4 X ↑ in sildenafil AUC	No data*	Maximum dose may not exceed 25 mg in 48 h
	NNRTIs	*See* Table 6.4	*See* Table 6.4	
	NRTIs	*See* Table 6.3	*See* Table 6.3	
	HMG-CoA reductase inhibitors:			
	Lovastatin	A potential interaction exists	No data*	Avoid concomitant use
	Simvastatin			
	Oral contraceptives:			
	Norethindrone	↑norethindrone by 26%	No data*	Standard dosing of both drugs
	Ethinylestradiol	↑ethinylestradiol by 24%		
	Protease inhibitors:			
	Amprenavir	↑APV AUC by 32%	↓IDV AUC by 38%	Standard dosing of both drugs
	Lopinavir/ ritonavir	No data* of IDV effect on LPV	IDV 600 mg b.i.d. dosing, may produce ↔ in IDV AUC	↓IDV dosing to 600 mg b.i.d. with standard LPV/RTV dosing
	Nelfinavir	↔ NFV AUC	↑IDV AUC by 51%	IDV 1200 mg b.i.d. with NFV 1250 mg b.i.d.
	Ritonavir	No data*	2–5 fold ↑ in IDV AUC	Consult recent guidelines for combination therapy
	Saquinavir	4–7 fold ↑ in SQV AUC	↔ IDV AUC	Not established
Lopinavir/ Ritonavir	*Anticonvulsants:*			
	Carbamazepine	Unknown	May ↓ LPV levels	Use with caution. Monitor anticonvulsants levels
	Phenobarbital			
	Phenytoin			
	Antifungals:			
	Fluconazole	No data*	No data*	
	Itraconazole	No data*	No data*	
	Ketoconazole	3-fold ↑ in ketoconazole AUC	↓ in LPV AUC by 13%	High dose ketoconazole (>200 mg/day) not recommended with standard LPV/RTV dose

Table 6.5 *Continued*

Protease inhibitor	Interacting drug (ID)	Anticipated effect of PI on ID	Anticipated effect of ID on PI	Clinical management
Lopinavir/ Ritonavir (*contd*)	*Antihistamines:*			
	Astemizole	↑ astemizole levels by inhibiting CYP3A4	No data*	Contraindicated combination. May result in QTc prolongation
	Terfenadine	↑ terfenadine levels by inhibiting CYP3A4	No data*	Contraindicated combination. May result in QTc prolongation
	Antimycobacterials:			
	Clarithromycin	No data*	1.17-fold ↑ in LPV AUC	Adjust clarithromycin dose in patients with renal insufficiency with standard LPV/RTV dose
	Rifabutin	3-fold ↑ rifabutin AUC	0.25-fold ↓ in LPV AUC	↓ rifabutin dosing to 150 mg q.o.d. with standard LPV/RTV dose
	Rifampicin	No data*	↓ in LPV AUC by 75%	Contraindicated
	HMG-CoA reductase inhibitors:			
	Atorvastatin	5.88-fold ↑ in atorvastatin AUC	10% ↓ in LPV AUC	Use lowest dose possible of atorvastatin with standard LPV dose
	Pravastatin	33% ↑ pravastatin AUC	5% ↓ in LPV AUC	Monitor for HMG-Co reductase inhibitors side effects with standard LPV dose
	Miscellaneous:			
	Cisapride	↑ cisapride levels	No data*	Combination contraindicated. May cause QTc prolongation
	Ergot alkaloids	DHE levels may ↑	No data*	Combination contraindicated, may cause increased risk of ergotism (nausea, vomiting, vasospastic ischemia)
	Methadone	53% ↓ methadone AUC	No data*	Use with caution. May need to ↑ methadone dosing
	Sildenafil	May ↑ sildenafil levels	No data*	Maximum dose may not exceed 25 mg in 48 h
	NNRTIs	*See* Table 6.4	*See* Table 6.4	
	Oral contraceptives:			
	Ethinylestradiol	42% ↓ in ethinylestradiol AUC	No data*	Alternative or additional contraceptive method should be used if OC contains estrogen
	Norethindrone	17% ↓ in norethindrone AUC	No data*	Alternative or additional contraceptive method should be used if OC contains norethindrone
	Protease inhibitors:			
	Amprenavir	Increase APV AUC	0.85-fold ↓ in LPV AUC	↓ APV to 750 mg b.i.d. with standard LPV/RTV dosing
	Indinavir	Increase IDV AUC may produce ↔ in IDV AUC	No data* of IDV effect on LPV	↓ IDV to 600 mg b.i.d. dosing with standard LPV/RTV dose
	Nelfinavir	No data*	No data*	
	Ritonavir	Minimal change to RTV	1.46-fold ↑ in LPV AUC	Standard dose of LPV 400 mg/RTV 100 mg b.i.d.
	Saquinavir	SQV 800 mg b.i.d. dosing may produce ↔ in LPV/RTV AUC	No data*	↓ SQV to 800 mg b.i.d. dosing with standard LPV/RTV
Nelfinavir	*Anticonvulsants:*			
	Carbamazepine Phenobarbital Phenytoin	Unknown	May ↓ NFV	Use with caution. Monitor anticonvulsants levels
	Antifungals:			
	Fluconazole	↔ in fluconazole levels	↑ NFV levels by 35%	Standard dosing of both drugs
	Itraconazole	No data*	No data*	
	Ketoconazole	↔ in ketoconazole levels	↔ in NFV levels	Standard dosing of both drugs
	Antihistamines:			
	Astemizole	↑ astemizole levels by inhibiting CYP3A4	No data*	Contraindicated combination. May result in QTc prolongation
	Terfenadine	↑ terfenadine levels by inhibiting CYP3A4	No data*	Contraindicated combination. May result in QTc prolongation

Table 6.5 *Continued*

Protease inhibitor	Interacting drug (ID)	Anticipated effect of PI on ID	Anticipated effect of ID on PI	Clinical management
Nelfinavir (contd)	*Antimycobacterials*:			
	Clarithromycin	No data*	No data*	
	Rifabutin	2-fold ↑ in rifabutin AUC	↓ NFV AUC by 32%	↓ rifabutin dosing to 150 mg q.d. or 300 mg 2–3 × week with ↑ NFV dose to 1000 mg t.i.d.
	Rifampicin	No data*	↓ NFV AUC by 82%	Contraindicated
	HMG-CoA reductase inhibitors:			
	Atorvastatin, lovastatin, simvastatin	A potential interaction	Little effect anticipated	Pravastatin, fluvastatin preferred
	Miscellaneous:			
	Cisapride	↑ Cisapride levels	No data*	Combination contraindicated, may cause QTc prolongation
	Ergot alkaloids	DHE levels may ↑	No data*	Combination contraindicated, may cause increased risk of ergotism (nausea, vomiting, vasopastic ischemia)
	Methadone	↓ methadone by 34–47%	No data*	Titrate for response to methadone
	Sildenafil	May ↑ sildenafil levels	No data*	Maximum dose may not exceed 25 mg in 48 h
	NNRTIs	*See* Table 6.4	*See* Table 6.4	
	Oral contraceptives:			
	Ethinylestradiol	↓ ethinylestradiol by 47%	No data*	Use alternative or additional contraceptive method
	Norethindrone	↓ norethindrone by 18%	No data*	Use alternative or additional contraceptive method
	Protease inhibitors:			
	Amprenavir	↑ APV AUC by 46%	↔ in NFV AUC	Not established
	Indinavir	↑ IDV AUC by 51%	↔ in NFV AUC	IDV 1200 mg b.i.d. with NFV 1250 mg b.i.d.
	Lopinavir/ ritonavir	No data*	No data*	Not established
	Ritonavir	↔ in RTV AUC	1.5-fold ↑ in NFV AUC	Limited data.
	Saquinavir	3–5 fold in ↑ SQV-SGC AUC	↑ NFV AUC by 20%	↓ SQV-SGC dosing to 800 mg t.i.d. or 1200 mg b.i.d. with standard NFV dose
Ritonavir	*Anticonvulsants*:			
	Carbamazepine		Unknown	Use with caution.
	Phenobarbital			Monitor anticonvulsants levels
	Phenytoin			
	Antifungals:			
	Fluconazole	↔ in fluconazole levels	↔ in RTV levels	Standard dosing of both drugs
	Itraconazole	↑ itraconazole $t_{1/2}$ by 5-fold	No data*	Caution when combined
	Ketoconazole	3-fold ↑ in ketoconazole levels	No data*	Use with caution
	Antihistamines:			
	Astemizole	↑ astemizole levels by inhibiting CYP3A4	No data*	Contraindicated combination. May result in QTc prolongation
	Terfenadine	↑ terfenadine levels by inhibiting CYP3A4	No data*	Contraindicated combination. May result in QTc prolongation
	Antimycobacterials:			
	Clarithromycin	↑ clarithromycin by 77%	No data*	Adjust clarithromycin dose in patients with renal insufficiency
	Rifabutin	4-fold ↑ in rifabutin levels	No data*	↓ rifabutin dosing to 150 mg q.o.d., or dose rifabutin 300 mg 3×/week with standard RTV dose
	Rifampicin	No data*	↓ RTV levels by 35%	Contraindicated, possibly increased liver toxicity

Table 6.5 *Continued*

Protease inhibitor	Interacting drug (ID)	Anticipated effect of PI on ID	Anticipated effect of ID on PI	Clinical management
Ritonavir (contd)	*HMG-CoA reductase inhibitors:*			
	Atorvastatin Lovastatin Simvastatin	A potential interaction exists	A potential interaction exists	Avoid concomitant use
	Miscellaneous:			
	Cisapride	↑ cisapride levels	No data*	Combination contraindicated, may cause QTc prolongation
	Desipramine	↑ desipramine levels by 145%	No data*	Reduce desipramine dosing
	Ergot alkaloids	DHE levels may ↑	No data*	Combination contraindicated, may cause increased risk of ergotism (nausea, vomiting, vasospastic ischemia)
	Methadone	↓ methadone levels by 37%	No data*	May require dose increase
	Sildenafil	11-fold ↑ in sildenafil AUC	No data*	Maximum dose may not exceed 25 mg in 48 hrs
	Theophylline	↓ theophylline levels by 47%	No data*	Monitor theophylline levels
	NNRTIs	*See* Table 6.4	*See* Table 6.4	
	Oral contraceptives:			
	Ethinylestradiol	↓ ethinylestradiol levels by 40%	No data*	Use alternative or additional method of contraception
	Protease inhibitors:			
	Amprenavir	2.5-fold ↑ in APV AUC	No data*	Not established, may ↓ APV to 600 mg b.i.d. with RTV 100 mg b.i.d. or APV to 1200 mg q.d. with 200 mg RTV q.d.
	Indinavir	2–5-fold ↑ in IDV AUC	No data*	Not established. Limited data for b.i.d. dosing of: IDV 400 mg/RTV 400 mg or IDV 800 mg/RTV 100 mg or 200 mg
	Lopinavir/ritonavir	1.46-fold ↑ in LPV AUC	Minimal change to RTV	Standard dose of LPV 400 mg/RTV 100 mg b.i.d.
	Nelfinavir	1.5-fold ↑ in NFV AUC	↔ in RTV AUC	Limited data on RTV 400 mg with NFV 500–750 mg b.i.d.
	Saquinavir	20-fold ↑ in SQV AUC	↔ in RTV AUC	Frequently used in combination therapy
Saquinavir	*Anticonvulsants:*			
	Carbamazepine Phenobarbital Phenytoin	Unknown	May ↓ SQV levels	Use with caution. Monitor anticonvulsant levels
	Antifungals:			
	Fluconazole	↔ in fluconazole levels	↔ in SQV levels	Standard dosing of both drugs
	Itraconazole	↑ itraconazole t$_{1/2}$ by 5-fold	No data*	Caution when combined
	Ketoconazole	No data*	1.5-fold ↑ in SQV-HGC	Standard dosing of both drugs
	Antihistamines:			
	Astemizole	↑ astemizole levels by inhibiting CYP3A4	No data*	Contraindicated combination. May result in QTc prolongation
	Terfenadine	↑ terfenadine levels by inhibiting CYP3A4	No data*	Contraindicated combination. May result in QTc prolongation
	Antimycobacterials:			
	Clarithromycin	↑ clarithromycin levels by 45%	↑ SQV levels by 177%	Standard dosing of both drugs
	Rifabutin	No data*	↓ SQV levels by 40%	Concomitant use not recommended, unless using RTV/SQV, then ↓ rifabutin to 150 mg 2–3 ×/week
	Rifampicin	No data*	↓ SQV levels by 84%	Contraindicated

Table 6.5 *Continued*

Protease inhibitor	Interacting drug (ID)	Anticipated effect of PI on ID	Anticipated effect of ID on PI	Clinical management
Saquinavir (*contd*)	*HMG-CoA reductase inhibitors:*			
	Lovastatin Simvastatin	A potential interaction exists	A potential interaction exists	Avoid concomitant use
	Miscellaneous:			
	Cisapride	↑ Cisapride levels	No data*	Combination contraindicated, may cause QTc prolongation
	Ergot alkaloids	DHE levels may ↑	No data*	Combination contraindicated, may cause increased risk of ergotism (nausea, vomiting, vasospastic ischemia)
	Grapefruit juice		May ↑ SQV levels	Not established
	Methadone	Conflicting data on SQV/RTV combined with methadone	No data*	Monitor patients for response to methadone
	Sildenafil	3.1-fold ↑ in sildenafil AUC	No data*	Maximum dose may not exceed 25 mg in 24 h
	NNRTIs	*See* Table 6.4	*See* Table 6.4	
	Oral contraceptives	No data*	No data*	
	Protease inhibitors:			
	Amprenavir	↓ APV AUC by 32%	↓ SQV AUC by 19%	Not established
	Indinavir	↔ in IDV AUC	4–7-fold ↑ in SQV AUC	Not established
	Lopinavir/ ritonavir	No data*	Increased saquinavir AUC	↓ SQV dosing to 800 mg b.i.d. with standard LPV/RTV
	Nelfinavir	↑ NFV AUC by 20%	3–5-fold in ↑ SQV-SGC AUC	↓ SQV-SGC dosing to 800 mg t.i.d. or 1200 mg b.i.d. with standard NFV dose
	Ritonavir	↔ in RTV AUC	20-fold ↑ in SQV AUC	Frequently used in combination therapy

APV = amprenavir; AUC = area under the concentration curve; AZT = zidovudine; DHE = dihydroergotamine; HGC = hard-gel capsule; IDV = indinavir; LPV = lopinavir; NFV = nelfinavir; NNRTI = non-nucleoside reverse transcriptase inhibitor; OC = oral contraceptive; PI = protease inhibitor; RTV = ritonavir; SQV = saquinavir; SGC = soft-gel capsule; $t_{1/2}$ = half-life; 3TC = lamivudine; ↑ = increase; ↓ = decrease; ↔ = no change.
* No data = Current recommendations should be consulted for updated effect and clinical management

barbital and phenytoin, induce CYP3A4 and are expected to decrease the AUC of protease inhibitors, although this is an area in need of additional investigations.[11,42] Carbamazepine is a partial substrate of CYP3A4 and concentrations of carbamazepine may increase when given with protease inhibitors. Phenytoin doses may have to be increased when given with ritonavir or nelfinavir, both of which are inducers of CYP2C9, the isoenzyme that metabolizes phenytoin (Table 6.5). In general, anticonvulsants known to induce CYP enzymes should be used with caution in the patient receiving a protease inhibitor.[11]

ANTIFUNGAL DRUG INTERACTIONS

Pharmacokinetic and pharmacodynamic interactions are common with many systemically active antifungals.[8,39] In particular the azoles are potent inhibitors of P_{450} isoenzymes and are the cause of many metabolic interactions. Even the small quantities of miconazole that reach the systemic circulation after intravaginal administration can impair systemic metabo-

lism of other drugs, such as warfarin.[43] Drug interactions may be especially common in immunocompromised patients, who are likely to require antifungal therapy while taking many other drugs.

AMPHOTERICIN B

Pharmacodynamic interactions

Amphotericin B is often combined with flucytosine for treatment of meningitis caused by *Cryptococcus neoformans*. However, nephrotoxicity from amphotericin B can decrease renal elimination of flucytosine and result in excessive serum concentrations, leading to bone marrow suppression.[39] This interaction requires that renal function, flucytosine concentrations (if available), and blood counts be monitored periodically (Table 6.6).

Overlapping pharmacodynamic toxicities are anticipated when amphotericin B is combined with other nephrotoxic agents such as aminoglycosides, cyclosporine, cisplatin, fos-

Table 6.6 Antifungal drug interactions (*see text for references*)

Drug	Amphotericin	Fluconazole	Itraconazole	Ketoconazole
Flucytosine	May ↓ flucytosine renal elimination. Monitor flucytosine levels, serum creatinine, and clinical response			
Nephrotoxins	Overlapping nephrotoxicity. Monitor serum creatinine and BUN			
Zidovudine	Overlapping toxicity. Monitor CBC	*See* Table 6.3		
Anticonvulsants:				
Carbamazepine	↑ Carbamazepine levels.	Marked ↓ itraconazole levels. Monitor carbamazepine levels	↑ Carbamazepine levels. Avoid concomitant use.	Monitor carbamazepine levels
Phenobarbital		Potential interaction exists Monitor phenobarbital levels while on fluconazole	↓ itraconazole levels. Avoid concomitant use.	Potential interaction exists. Monitor phenobarbital levels while on ketoconazole
Phenytoin		↑ phenytoin AUC by 75% Monitor phenytoin levels while on fluconazole	↓ itraconazole AUC by >90% Avoid concomitant use	May ↓ ketoconazole. Monitor phenytoin levels and response to ketoconazole
Non-sedating antihistamines:				
Astemizole		Potential interaction exists Avoid combination	≈ 3-fold ↑ in astemizole AUC. Contraindicated combination	Potential interaction exists Contraindicated combination
Terfenadine		↑ in terfenadine AUC by 34% Contraindicated combination	↓ terfenadine metabolism, ↑ QTc on ECG. Contraindicated combination	↓ terfenadine metabolism, ↑ QTc on ECG. Contraindicated combination
Antimycobacterials:				
Rifabutin		↑ in rifabutin AUC by 80%; ↔ fluconazole Maximum rifabutin dose of 300 mg q.d., monitor for s/sx of uveitis	↑ in rifabutin levels, uveitis has been reported. ↓ itraconazole AUC by 74%. Avoid concomitant use	Potential interaction exists Monitor rifabutin toxicity
Rifampicin		↓ fluconazole AUC by 23%. Monitor clinical response to fluconazole therapy	Undetectable levels of itraconazole Avoid concomitant use	↓ ketoconazole AUC by 50%, may ↓ rifampicin C_{max} by 40%. Dose adjustment of both is required
Antiretrovirals		*See* Tables 6.4, 6.5 and 6.6	*See* Tables 6.3, 6.4 and 6.5	*See* Tables 6.2, 6.3 and 6.4
Benzodiazepines:				
Midazolam		≈ 2-fold ↑ in midazolam AUC. Monitor for excessive sedation	≈ 2-fold ↑ in midazolam bioavailability and AUC. Monitor for excessive sedation	↑ in midazolam AUC by 1490%. Significant interaction. Avoid combination
Triazolam		≈ 1.25–2.5-fold ↑ in triazolam AUC. Use with caution	≈ 3–27-fold ↑ in triazolam bioavailability and AUC. Use with caution	≈ 22-fold ↑ in triazolam AUC (Liver and intestine CYP3A4). Significant interaction. Avoid
HMG-CoA reductase inhibitors:				
Atorvastatin		Potential interaction	≈ 3-fold ↑ in atorvastatin AUC	Fluvastatin, pravastatin preferred
Lovastatin		Potential interaction	≈ 20-fold ↑ in lovastatin AUC Avoid concomitant use	Fluvastatin, pravastatin preferred
Simvastatin		Potential interaction	≈ 10-fold ↑ in simvastatin AUC Avoid concomitant use	Fluvastatin, pravastatin preferred

Table 6.6 *Continued*

Drug	Amphotericin	Fluconazole	Itraconazole	Ketoconazole
Immuno-suppressants:				
Cyclosporine		↑ CyA AUC by ≈ 50%	↑ CyA C_{min} by ≈ 50%	↑ CyA levels. If ketoconazole needed, consider 50% ↓ in CyA dose. Monitor CyA levels
		Monitor CyA levels. Dose dependent inhibition	Monitor CyA levels.	
Sirolimus		Potential interaction exists	Potential interaction exists	Potential interaction exists
Tacrolimus		↔ in tacrolimus levels	↑ tacrolimus C_{min} by ≈ 5-fold Monitor tacrolimus levels	↑ tacrolimus levels Monitor tacrolimus levels
Gastric pH modifiers:				
Antacids		↔ in fluconazole levels	↓ itraconazole levels (capsules), separate dosing of itraconazole by 2 h	↓ ketoconazole tablets levels, separate dosing of ketoconazole by 2 h
Famotidine		↔ in fluconazole levels	↓ itraconazole AUC by 30%, consider itraconazole solution	↓ ketoconazole levels. Avoid
Lansaprozole		↔ in fluconazole levels	Expected interaction exists, consider itraconazole solution	↓ ketoconazole levels. Avoid
Omeprazole		↔ in fluconazole levels	↓ itraconazole AUC by 64%, consider itraconazole solution	↓ ketoconazole levels. Avoid
Miscellaneous:				
Celecoxib		2-fold ↑ in celecoxib levels	No data*	No data*
Cisapride		↑ in cisapride AUC by 102–192%, and QTc prolonged. Contraindicated combination	≈ 8-fold ↑ in cisapride, and QTc prolonged. Contraindicated combination	≈ 8-fold ↑ in cisapride, and QTc prolonged. Contraindicated combination
Felodipine		↑ in felodipine levels Consider alternate therapy or ↓ felodipine dose	≈ 5–7-fold ↑ in felodipine AUC Consider alternate therapy or ↓ felodipine dose	↑ in felodipine levels Consider alternate therapy or ↓ felodipine dose
Haloperidol		No data*	↑ haloperidol concentration by 30%. Monitor haloperidol neurologic side effects	No data*
Warfarin		↑ (S)-warfarin enantiomer by 284%. ↑ PT by 2-fold. Monitor PT and INR	Expected increase in (S)-warfarin levels. Monitor INR and PT	Reported increase in (S)-warfarin levels. Monitor INR and PT

AUC = area under the concentration curve; BUN = blood urea nitrogen; CBC = complete blood count; CYP = cytochrome P_{450}; C_{min} = minimum serum concentration; CyA = cyclosporine; ECG = electrocardiogram; INR = international normalization ratio; P-gp = P-glycoprotein; PT = Prothrombin time; QTc = Corrected QT interval; ↑ = increase; ↓ = decrease; ↔ = no change; ?questionable; s/sx = signs/symptoms;
* No data = current recommendations should be consulted for updated effect and clinical management

carnet, and tacrolimus. Amphotericin-associated electrolyte disturbances can be additive to those of other drugs such as diuretics, or it may augment the pharmacologic effects of drugs such as nondepolarizing skeletal muscle relaxants and digoxin. For example, amphotericin B-induced hypokalemia can increase cardiac automaticity and facilitate inhibition of the Na^+–K^+ ATPase pump by digoxin.

AZOLE ANTIFUNGALS

Azole antifungals cause dose-dependent inhibition of P_{450} enzymes, especially CYP3A4, and some Phase II enzymes.[8,39] In addition, itraconazole and ketoconazole absorption is impaired by concomitant administrations of agents that increase gastric pH such as antacids and H_2 blockers. Finally, induction of azole metabolism, especially itraconazole voriconazole and posaconazole.

PHARMACOKINETIC INTERACTIONS

Absorption

The dissolution of ketoconazole tablets and itraconazole capsules is optimal under acidic conditions. In the presence of drugs that increase gastric pH (e.g. antacids and H_2 antagonists, and proton pump inhibitors), absorption of ketoconazole and itraconazole capsules is dramatically decreased (Table 6.6) and the risk of clinical failure is high. The administration of antacids should precede ketoconazole and itraconazole administration by at least 1 hour. Itraconazole has been administered with an acidic cola beverage in patients taking H_2 antagonists or a proton pump inhibitor to facilitate dissolution. Itraconazole oral solution does not require dissolution in the stomach, thus its absorption is unaffected by gastric acid modifiers. The absorption of oral fluconazole is unaffected by gastric acid modifiers and can be safely administered with antacids or H_2 blockers (Table 6.6).

Distribution

Ketoconazole inhibits P-glycoprotein, both in the gastrointestinal tract and in the central nervous system and may be useful to enhance penetration of drugs into the cerebrospinal fluid. Pharmacological manipulation of drug distribution may eventually become an important mechanism to improve penetration of drugs to the site of action.

Metabolism

INHIBITION OF CYP3A4

Itraconazole posaconazole, voriconazole and ketoconazole are potent inhibitors of CYP3A4, and interactions are similar as those described for the HIV-1 protease inhibitors and delavirdine (above).[8,39] In addition, other CYPs are inhibited, depending on the specific azole, and additional interactions involving drugs other than those metabolized by CYP3A4 are well described (see below). Fluconazole also causes dose-dependent inhibition of CYP3A4, but is less potent at usual doses (100–200 mg/day) than the other azoles. Ketoconazole is used less often and this discussion will focus on the other azoles. Itraconazole increases the AUC of atorvastatin, simvastatin, and lovastatin by 3-, 10- and 20-fold, reflecting the degree to which each of these statins is dependent on CYP3A4 for metabolism. Itraconazole increases the AUC of midazolam by 2-fold and triazolam by 3- to 27-fold, which results in prolongation of the benzodiazepine effects. The combination of itraconazole and triazolam is generally contraindicated, and patients receiving midazolam should be monitored carefully for prolonged or excessive sedation (Table 6.6). These interactions are dose dependent and are more significant as the dose of the azole increases. Ketoconazole and itraconazole increase the AUC of cyclosporine, serolimus and tacrolimus and serum concentrations should be monitored upon initiation of azole therapy (Table 6.6). Itraconazole can interact with protease inhibitors and NNRTIs (Tables 6.4 and 6.5). Like all inhibitors of CY3A4, azoles increase the risk of uveitis when given to the patient receiving rifabutin (Table 6.6).

Other isoenzymes

Fluconazole is a 'broad-spectrum' inhibitor of cytochrome P_{450} enzymes. In addition to inhibiting CYP3A4, it is an inhibitor of CYP2C9, CYP2C19 and is an inducer of phase II enzymes such as glucuronyl transferase. Fluconazole increases the AUC of phenytoin by 75%, probably by inhibition of CYP2C9, which is the main metabolizing enzyme for phenytoin (Table 6.1). Warfarin exists in a racemic mixture of the pharmacologically active (S)-enantiomer and the less active (R)-enan-

tiomer. The (S)-enantiomer is metabolized by CYP2C9 isoenzyme and fluconazole increases the international normalization ratio (INR) in patients previously stable on warfarin by about 38% (Table 6.6). Bleeding has been precipitated in women who were receiving warfarin when miconazole vaginal cream was used.[43] Fluconazole was found to slightly increase the AUC of theophylline but this is unlikely to be clinically important.

Fluconazole inhibits the phase II enzyme uridine diphosphate glucuronosyl transferase, resulting in a decrease in the metabolism of drugs requiring glucuronidation. This is presumed to be the mechanism by which fluconazole increases zidovudine concentrations, though this is not considered a clinically important interaction.

Voriconazole is extensively metabolized by CYP2C19. Omeprazole is a potent inhibitor of CYP2C19 and significantly increases voriconazole serum concentrations. Both rifampicin and rifabutin significantly reduce the AUC for voriconazole. Phenytoin induces the metabolism of voriconazole, and voriconazole inhibits the metabolism of phenytoin. In contrast, voriconazole did not change indinavir concentrations, nor did indinavir alter voriconazole concentrations.

Induction of CYP3A4

CYP3A4 inducers, such as most anticonvulsants and the rifamycins, will decrease the AUC of itraconazole voriconazole and posaconazole substantially and clinical failures to itraconazole are well described. Phenytoin decreases the AUC of itraconazole by 90%, and itraconazole serum levels are virtually undetectable when rifampicin is given. Gabapentin does not induce microsomal enzymes and may be an option in patients requiring anticonvulsive therapy. Although rifabutin is a less potent inducer of metabolic enzymes than rifampicin, it will nevertheless decrease itraconazole and posaconazole levels significantly (~50–90%). Therefore, patients receiving these combinations must be closely monitored for poor clinical response to itraconazole therapy or adverse effects of the rifabutin.[33]

Phenytoin does not change the pharmacokinetics of fluconazole, presumably because fluconazole is mostly eliminated unchanged. Rifampicin can decrease the AUC of fluconazole by 23%, perhaps because rifampicin is inducing a minor metabolic pathway for fluconazole.

P-glycoprotein interactions

Case reports of patients who developed digoxin toxicity when itraconazole was prescribed were initially confusing. Digoxin is eliminated mostly by the kidneys as the parent compound, so it is unclear why itraconazole was having an effect (the same is true for reports of clarithromycin-induced increases in digoxin concentrations – see below). Itraconazole increases digoxin concentration by inhibiting P-glycoprotein mediated efflux of digoxin in the gastrointestinal tract and renal tubules. Patients should be monitored carefully when itraconazole is taken while receiving digoxin.

The itraconazole prescribing information (Figure 6.2) illustrates the numerous interactions likely from these multiple mechanisms.[35] This prescribing information is very similar to that found for other potent inhibitors of P_{450} enzymes, including the HIV-1 protease inhibitors and the NNRTIs. The prescribing information for posaconazole and voriconazole have similar lengthy warnings.

Fig. 6.2 Selected drugs that are predicted to alter the plasma concentration of itraconazole or have their plasma concentration altered by SPORANOX

Drug plasma concentration increased by itraconazole
Antiarrhythmics: digoxin, quinidine
Anticonvulsants: carbamazepine
Antihistamines: astemizole
Antineoplastics: busulfan, docetaxel, vinca alkaloids
Antipsychotics: pimozide
Benzodiazepines: alprazolam, diazepam, midazolam, triazolam
Calcium channel blockers: dihydropyridines, verapamil
Gastrointestinal motility agents: cisapride
HMG CoA-reductase inhibitors: atorvastatin, cerivastatin, lovastatin, simvastatin
Immunosuppressants: cyclosporine, tacrolimus, sirolimus
Oral hypoglycemics: glipizide,
Protease inhibitors: indinavir, ritonavir, saquinavir
Other: alfentanil, buspirone, methylprednisolone, trimetrexate, warfarin
Decrease plasma concentration of itraconazole
Anticonvulsants: carbamazepine, phenobarbital, phenytoin
Antimycobacterials: isoniazid, rifabutin, rifampicin
Gastric acid suppressors/neutralizers: antacids, H2-receptor antagonists, proton pump inhibitors
Non-nucleoside reverse transcriptase inhibitors: nevirapine
Increase plasma concentration of itraconazole
Macrolide antibiotics: clarithromycin
Protease inhibitors: indinavir, ritonavir
This list is not all-inclusive.

ANTIBACTERIAL DRUG INTERACTIONS

FLUOROQUINOLONES

Fluoroquinolones can cause both pharmacodynamic and pharmacokinetic interactions.[45] Quinolones are usually administered orally, and absorption interactions are common. In addition, some quinolones are potent inhibitors of CYP1A2 and can cause metabolic interactions. Table 6.7 lists the most significant quinolone–drug interactions.

Pharmacodynamic interactions

QTc prolongation and quinolones

Certain fluoroquinolone antibiotics, along with many other drugs, can increase QTc interval and precipitate fatal arrhythmias in the susceptible individual.[23,45] Grepafloxacin was removed from the world market in November 1999 after seven deaths were reported, presumably from arrhythmias associated with a prolonged QTc interval.[46] In addition, when quinolones are given with other drugs with similar cardiovascular effects, such as antiarrhythmics class I, II, and III, cisapride, macrolides (clarithromycin and erythromycin), and tricyclic antidepressants, a pharmacodynamic interaction (increased QTc interval) may occur. Caution should be used when fluoroquinolones are combined with such agents.

NSAIDs and quinolones

Central nervous system (CNS) toxicities, including tremulousness and seizure, can occur in patients receiving quinolones. There is believed to be additional potential for a pharmacodynamic interaction between some non-steroidal anti-inflammatory drugs (NSAIDs) in conjunction with select quinolones.[47] When patients received both enoxacin and the NSAID fenbufen, tremulousness and seizure were reported. However, quinolones and NSAIDS are commonly prescribed together and CNS effects appear to be very uncommon, suggesting that this interaction is unlikely to be clinically important.

Pharmacokinetic interactions

Absorption

Divalent and trivalent cations chelate all fluoroquinolones and reduce bioavailability when these drugs are given together. The magnitude of effect depends on the specific cation and quinolone, the dose and dosage form of the cation, and the timing of administration. Magnesium or aluminum-containing antacids, and sucralfate, have the greatest effects and decrease the AUC for quinolones by about 90%. Absorption remains decreased when the cation is given 2 h before the quinolone, though the effect is less pronounced than with simultaneous administration. Coadministration with calcium can also decrease absorption, though the magnitude of effect is less than that seen with magnesium and aluminum. Similarly, quinolone absorption is reduced when concomitantly administered with iron preparations or multiple vitamins with minerals such as zinc, magnesium, copper, and manganese. The clinical importance of the interaction will depend on the location of the infection, the in-vitro susceptibility of the pathogen, and the magnitude of the effect. Therefore, concomitant use of quinolones with magnesium-, aluminum-, or calcium-containing antacids, sucralfate, or iron/vitamin-mineral preparations should be avoided, unless the quinolone is administered at least 2 h before the cation. Ciprofloxacin and norfloxacin bioavailability are decreased when concomitantly administered with milk or yogurt. In contrast, absorption of other quinolones appears unaffected.

Table 6.7 Quinolone drug interactions (*see text for references*)

Drug name	Anticipated pharmacokinetic interactions		Anticipated pharmacodynamic interactions	Clinical management
	Absorption interaction	Metabolic interaction		
Antacids containing di- and trivalent cations	↓ absorption of all quinolones			Separate doses by 2 h, give quinolone first
Antiarrhythmics Class I, II, III			Theoretical potential for QTc prolongation	Uncertain significance. Use cautiously with quinolones that increase QTc interval
Caffeine		↑ caffeine levels with certain quinolones (*see text*)		Unclear clinical significance
Cisapride			Theoretical potential for QTc prolongation and quinolones with similar effect	Unclear clinical significance; Use cautiously with quinolones that increase QTc interval
Cyclosporine		Care reports that CyA levels may ↑ with ciprofloxacin and norfloxacin	Possible ↑ nephrotoxicity effect	Unlikely to be clinically important (*see text*)
Didanosine standard tablet formulation	↓ absorption of all quinolones			Separate doses by 2 h, give quinolone first, or use enteric-coated didanosine
Iron	↓ absorption of all quinolones			Separate doses by 2 h, give quinolone first
Macrolides (clarithromycin/ erythromycin)			Theoretical potential for QTc prolongation if used with quinolones with similar effects	Caution if used with quinolones that increase QTc interval
Multivitamins	Multivitamins with zinc cause a small ↓ absorption of ciprofloxacin			Best to separate doses by 2 h, give quinolone first
NSAIDs			Early reports of seizures with fenbufen and enoxacin	Interaction appears to be of little clinical relevance with current quinolones and NSAIDS
Sucralfate	↓ absorption of all quinolones			Avoid combination, or give quinolone 2 h before sucralfate
Theophylline		↑ theophylline levels with certain quinolones (*see text*)		Ciprofloxacin is most likely to result in an interaction; most other quinolones safe (*see text*)
Tricyclic antidepressants			Theoretical potential for QTc prolongation	Caution if used with quinolones that increase QTC interval. Uncertain clinical significance
Warfarin		Conflicting data, (*see text*)		Monitor INR and PT when a quinolone is administered to patients receiving warfarin

CyA = cyclosporine; INR = International normalization ratio; PT = Prothrombin time; QTc = corrected QT interval; ↑ = increase; ↓ = decrease.

The concomitant administration of quinolones and enteral feedings can result in decreased absorption of quinolones. Osmolite™, Pulmocare™, continuous dosing of Jevity™ enteral feeding through gastrostomy and jejunostomy tubes, and Sustacal™ enteral feedings decrease the AUC and C_{max} of ciprofloxacin. However, one study reported no significant interactions between single-dose ciprofloxacin and Osmolite™.

Metabolism

METHYLXANTHINES

Some quinolone antibiotics inhibit CYP1A2 and can impair the metabolism of a limited number of drugs, including methylxanthines (Table 6.1). This interaction was initially reported for enoxacin, when a number of patients receiving theophylline had seizures. Gemifloxacin is similar in inhibitory potency to enoxacin. Ciprofloxacin is less potent an inhibitor of theophylline metabolism compared with enoxacin and gemifloxacin, but at high doses (>500 mg) it can also precipitate seizures in the susceptible patient. Most other fluoroquinolones, including ofloxacin, levofloxacin, sparfloxacin, gatifloxacin, and moxifloxacin, do not result in important inhibition of methylxanthine metabolism.

WARFARIN AND CYCLOSPORINE A

Many case reports describe increased anticoagulant effect to warfarin in patients who also received ciprofloxacin, norfloxacin, and ofloxacin. Other reports suggest that quinolones may decrease the clearance of cyclosporine A, resulting in nephrotoxicity. However, multiple studies in healthy volunteers and anticoagulated patients have shown no significant effect on either warfarin pharmacokinetics or measures of anticoagulation (prothrombin time and INR) when various quinolones are given. Similarly, prospective investigations have found that quinolones do not alter cyclosporine pharmacokinetics or increase its adverse effects. In retrospect, the lack of a warfarin and cyclosporine interaction in prospective investigations is consistent with the known effects of the quinolones on drug metabolizing enzymes. The most potent sterioisomer of warfarin is S-warfarin, which is metabolized by CYP2C9 (Table 6.1). Cyclosporine is metabolized by CYP3A4. Neither of these enzymes is inhibited by the available quinolones, consistent with the lack of a pharmacokinetic interaction in prospective investigations. The case reports of clinically important interactions when quinolones are administered to patients receiving warfarin and cyclosporine may be secondary to inhibitory effects of 'infection' on hepatic metabolizing enzymes, resulting in elevations in cyclosporine and warfarin concentrations (*see introduction*). One prospective investigation did report statistically significant increases in INR in healthy volunteers receiving warfarin who received a 2-week course of clinafloxacin. There was no significant effect on warfarin pharmacokinetics, and the increase in INR was attributed to a reduction in vitamin K-producing bacteria in the gut by clinafloxacin. Although 'antibiotics' have commonly been said to result in enhancement of the warfarin response because of this local effect on gastrointestinal micro-organisms, it remains a poorly investigated phenomenon. Consequently, it remains prudent to monitor prothrombin time/international normalized ratio (PT/INR) in patients who are receiving warfarin when any antimicrobial, including quinolones, is prescribed to an infected patient.

Elimination

Quinolones are generally excreted in the urine, with tubular secretion being a prominent excretory pathway. Administration of probenecid, a blocker of the anionic renal tubular secretory pathway, significantly decreases the renal elimination of norfloxacin, levofloxacin, and ciprofloxacin, but not moxifloxacin. These are not likely to be clinically important effects.

MACROLIDES/KETOLIDES/AZALIDES

Many macrolide antibiotics are well known inhibitors of CYP3A4 and pharmacokinetic interactions are common and mostly predictable[7] (Table 6.1). The 14-membered ring macrolides, including erythromycin, clarithromycin and troleandomycin, are substrates and inhibitors of CYP3A4 (Table 6.1). The ketolide antimicrobial telithromycin is also an inhibitor of CYP3A, similar to erythromycin in potency. In the discussion below, these macrolides and ketolides will be collectively referred to as 'inhibitory macrolides'. In contrast, dirithromycin, the azalide antibiotic azithromycin, and 16-membered ring macrolides (josamycin, flurithromycin, midecamycin, miokamycin, roxithromycin rokitamycin, and spiramycin) do not significantly inhibit metabolic enzymes. Inhibitory macrolides are also substrates and inhibitors of P-glycoprotein and significant drug–drug interactions may result from effects on this transporter protein.

Pharmacokinetic interactions

Metabolism

THEOPHYLLINE

Theophylline is a substrate of CYP1A2, a pathway which macrolides are not known to inhibit (Table 6.1). Nevertheless, there is an abundant literature demonstrating that certain macrolides can inhibit theophylline metabolism in some patients. Inhibitory macrolides increase the AUC of theophylline by 20–25%, although there appears to be a subset of patients who are more likely to experience an interaction. Azithromycin and the other macrolides do not appear to interact with theophylline.

CARBAMAZEPINE

Carbamazepine is a partial substrate of CYP3A4 and inhibitory macrolides increase the AUC of carbamazepine by a clinically significant amount. The combination of inhibitory macrolides and carbamazepine should be avoided or the carbamazepine dose should be decreased. This interaction has also been reported between carbamazepine and flurithromycin, josamycin and miocamycin. Azithromycin and roxithromycin have no affect on serum levels of carbamazepine.

CYCLOSPORINE

Cyclosporine is a prototype CYP3A4 substrate and administration of CYP3A4 inhibitors predictably decrease cyclosporine clearance and can result in nephrotoxicity. Clarithromycin and erythromycin increase cyclosporine serum levels by approximately 50% and the combination of cyclosporine and inhibitory macrolides should be avoided, or cyclosporine levels must be monitored closely (Table 6.8).

BENZODIAZEPINES

Aside from its clinical use as a short-acting sedative, midazolam is frequently used in pharmacokinetic drug–drug interaction studies as a marker for the activity of hepatic CYP3A4.

Table 6.8 Macrolide/azalide and ketolide drug interactions (*see text for references*)

Macrolide	Interacting drug	Mechanism of interaction	Anticipated effect	Clinical management
Azithromycin	Rifabutin	Unknown	No significant ↑ in rifabutin AUC	Use with caution. Monitor CBC, patients appear at greater risk of developing neutropenia, rash, and GI disturbances
Clarithromycin and erythromycin	Astemizole	Inhibition of CYP3A4	↑ astemizole levels	Contraindicated combination. May result in QTc prolongation
	Benzodiazepines: Midazolam Triazolam	Inhibition of CYP3A4 (intestinal and liver)	3–4 × ↑ in AUC, excessive sedation	Avoid combination or decrease benzodiazepine dose by 50–75%. Result in increased CNS depression, lethargy and ataxia
	Carbamazepine	Inhibition of CYP3A4	2 × ↑ CBZ C_{min}, excess sedation	Consider ↓ CBZ dose by 25–50%, monitor CBZ serum levels closely
	Cisapride	Inhibition of CYP3A4	3-fold ↑ in cisapride AUC	Contraindicated combination. Prolonged QTc interval observed
	Cyclosporine	Inhibition of CYP3A4	↑ CyA C_{min} levels	Monitor CyA levels, and toxicities
	Digitalis	Decreased gastrointestinal metabolism or increased absorption from P-gp inhibition	↑ digoxin levels	Avoid if possible, or monitor digoxin levels
	Ergotamine	Decreased metabolism	Ergotism; peripheral ischemia	Avoid
	NNRTIs	*See* Table 6.3		
	Protease inhibitors	*See* Table 6.4		
	Rifabutin	Inhibition of CYP3A4; *see* Table 6.8 for effect of rifabutin on clarithromycin	↑ rifabutin AUC and ↑ 25-O-desacetyl-rifabutin AUC by 37%. Some patients develop fever, myalgia, neutropenia and thrombocytopenia	Use with caution and monitor closely. Consider ↓ rifabutin dose to 300 mg q.d.
	Rifampicin	Induction of clarithromycin and erythromycin metabolism	Possible subtherapeutic macrolide concentrations	Not established. Monitor patients for clinical response to clarithromycin
	Simvastatin and lovastatin	Inhibition of CYP3A4	↑ concentrations and possible rhabdomyolysis	Monitor s/sx of myopathy and creatine kinase
	Terfenadine	Inhibition of CYP3A4	Doubling of active terfenadine AUC and C_{max}	Contraindicated combination. Prolonged QTc interval observed
	Sildenafil	Inhibition of CYP3A4 metabolism	Cardiotoxicity, priapism	Reduce sildenafil dose
	Theophylline	Inhibition of CYP1A2	20% ↑ in theophylline AUC (highly variable)	Monitor theophylline levels
	Verapamil	Inhibition of CYP3A4	↑ verapamil	↑ verapamil toxicty, monitor blood pressure and heart rate
	Vincristine/vinblastine	Inhibition of metabolism	Increased toxicity	Avoid
	Warfarin	Inhibition of warfarin metabolism	↑ INR and PT	Monitor INR and PT when a macrolide is used
	Zidovudine	Unknown	12% ↓ in zidovadine AUC	Not likely to be important

Table 6.8 *Continued*

Macrolide	Interacting drug	Mechanism of interaction	Anticipated effect	Clinical management
Josamycin	Caffeine	No hepatic CYP inhibition	Caffeine $t_{1/2}$ $\uparrow$ ≈15% 26% $\downarrow$ in clearance	May be important in neonates who receive caffeine therapy
	Carbamazepine	No hepatic CYP inhibition	17–20% $\uparrow$ in CBZ AUC	No patients experienced CBZ toxicity, clinical significance unknown
	Cyclosporine	No hepatic CYP inhibition P-gp is most likely mechanism	5 × $\downarrow$ in CyA clearance	Clinical ramifications unknown, may chose to $\downarrow$ CyA dose, monitor CyA levels or use another antibiotic
	Theophylline	No hepatic CYP inhibition	No change in adults. $\downarrow$ theophylline clearance by 39% in children	This may be of clinical significance in children Monitor theophylline levels when given with josamycin
Miokamycin	Carbamazepine	Unknown	13% $\uparrow$ in CBZ AUC, 26% $\downarrow$ in CBZ-10, 11-epoxide	Monitor CBZ serum levels
	Cyclosporine	Unknown	Doubling of CyA plasma levels	Monitor CyA serum levels
	Theophylline	Unknown	$\leftrightarrow$ theophylline	Standard dosing of theophylline
Telithromycin	Preliminary data strongly suggests telithromycin inhibits CYP3A4 similar to erythromycin. All precautions applied to erythromycin and clarithromycin are appropriate.	CYP3A4 inhibitor		

AUC = area under the concentration curve; CBC = complete blood count; CBZ = carbamazepine; C_{max} = maximum serum concentration; C_{min} = minimum serum concentration; CYP = cytochrome P450; CyA = cyclosporine; ECG = Electrocardiogram; GI = gastrointestinal; INR = international normalization ratio; P-gp = P-glycoprotein; PT = Prothrombin time; QTc = corrected QT interval; s/sx = signs and symptoms; $\uparrow$ = increase; $\downarrow$ = decrease; $\leftrightarrow$ = no change; ? questionable. *No data = current recommendations should be consulted for updated effect and clinical management

Consequently, inhibitors of CYP3A4 have predictable consequences when midazolam is coadministered (Table 6.8). Erythromycin and clarithromycin decrease the clearance of midazolam and triazolam by up to 50%, and can result in prolonged sedation and amnesia. These combinations should be avoided or the doses of the benzodiazepines should be decreased by 50–75%.

PROTEASE INHIBITORS

Inhibitory macrolides and protease inhibitors both compete for CYP3A4 and P-glycoprotein in the liver and gastrointestinal tissues. The pharmacokinetic drug interactions that result tend to be bidirectional; there is inhibition of clearance of both drugs. However, because both drugs have a reasonably wide therapeutic index, macrolides are thought to be safe in patients receiving protease inhibitors and normal doses of both drugs are generally recommended.

NNRTIs

The CYP3A4 inhibitor delavirdine increases the AUC of clarithromycin by 100%, whereas, delavirdine AUC is increased by 44%.[29] In contrast, efavirenz and nevirapine induce CYP3A4 and decrease the AUC of clarithromycin while clarithromycin increases the AUC of efavirenz and nevirapine (Table 6.4). Associated with an increase in the AUC of efavirenz is an increase in the incidence of rash and this combination should be avoided.

RIFAMPICIN AND RIFABUTIN

The interactions between macrolides and the rifamycins are bidirectional. Clarithromycin increases the AUC of rifabutin and the bioactive metabolite 25-O-desacetyl rifabutin by 57% and 375%, respectively. Conversely, rifabutin decreased the AUC of clarithromycin by 50% and increased the AUC of its active metabolite, 14-hydroxyclarithromycin, by 40% as a result of inducing CYP3A4 (Table 6.8).[11,20] For reasons that are unclear, azithromycin given with rifabutin is poorly tolerated, although there is no pharmacokinetic interaction.

DIGOXIN

Digoxin is a substrate of renal and intestinal P-glycoprotein. Digoxin is normally absorbed and transported through duodenal epithelial cells. P-glycoprotein partially pumps digoxin back into the gut lumen, lowering overall bioavailability. Inhibitors of intestinal P-glycoprotein, such as erythromycin, clarithromycin and azoles, can increase the bioavailability of digoxin and result in toxicity. A second reported mechanism involves the anaerobic gut bacterium *Eubacterium lentum*. This organism metabolizes digoxin in about 10% of the population. Macrolides and other antibiotics are proposed to increase digoxin serum concentrations in these patients by reducing the numbers of these organisms.[7]

WARFARIN

There are many reports of exaggerated response to anticoagulation in patients receiving warfarin who are treated with macrolides, and prospective pharmacokinetic investigations have shown that macrolides can increase warfarin concentrations (for example, erythromycin decreased warfarin clearance by 14%). The mechanism of this interaction is not clear since erythromycin is not known to inhibit the enzymes responsible for S-warfarin metabolism. Inhibition of vitamin K-producing gut bacteria by macrolides is also a possible mechanism for some patients who experience bleeding. Patients receiving warfarin should be closely monitored if a macrolide is required.

HMG-CoA REDUCTASE INHIBITORS

CYP3A4 inhibitors are believed to be a risk factor for rhabdomyolysis in patients receiving certain 'statins'. (Table 6.8). Like other CYP3A4 inhibitors, macrolides can dramatically increase the AUC of statins that are dependent on CYP3A4 for metabolism. Inhibitory macrolides should be avoided in patients receiving statins that are dependent on CYP3A4 for metabolism.

SILDENAFIL

The warning statement in the sildenafil package insert (Figure 6.3) illustrates the degree of interaction with clarithromycin and contrasts the effect to other CYP3A4 inhibitors.[27]

Fig. 6.3 Warning statement in the sildenafil prescribing information

When a single 100 mg dose of VIAGRA was administered with erythromycin, a specific CYP3A4 inhibitor, at steady state (500 mg b.i.d. for 5 days), there was a 182% increase in sildenafil systemic exposure (AUC). Stronger CYP3A4 inhibitors such as ketoconazole, itraconazole or mibefradil would be expected to have still greater effects, and population data from patients in clinical trials did indicate a reduction in sildenafil clearance when it was co-administered with CYP3A4 inhibitors (such as ketoconazole, erythromycin, or cimetidine). It can be expected that concomitant administration of CYP3A4 inducers, such as rifampin, will decrease plasma levels of sildenafil.

QUINUPRISTIN-DALFOPRISTIN (SYNERCID™)

Synercid™ is an inhibitor of CYP3A4 and clinical studies have confirmed that the metabolism of cyclosporine and other CYP3A4 substrates is impaired (Table 6.1, Figure 6.4). As with any other inhibitor, concomitant drug therapy must be reviewed before Synercid™ is prescribed.[36]

LINEZOLID

Linezolid is extensively metabolized but it is not a substrate of P_{450} enzymes, and it does not alter their activity.[47] However, linezolid is a monoamine oxidase enzyme inhibitor, and the product labeling warns patients to avoid consumption of high-

Fig. 6.4 Warning statement in the Synercid™ prescribing information

> **WARNINGS**
>
> **Drug interactions**: In vitro drug interaction studies have demonstrated that **Synercid** significantly inhibits cytochrome P_{450} 3A4 metabolism of cyclosporine A, midazolam, nifedipine and terfenadine. In addition, 24 subjects given Synercid 7.5 mg/kg q8h for 2 days and 300 mg of cyclosporine on day 3 showed an increase of 63% in the AUC of cyclosporine, an increase of 30% in the C_{max} of cyclosporine, a 77% increase in the $t_{1/2}$ of cyclosporine, and a decrease of 34% in the clearance of cyclosporine. **Therapeutic level monitoring of cyclosporine should be performed when cyclosporine must be used concomitantly with Synercid.**
>
> It is reasonable to expect that the concomitant administration of Synercid and other drugs primarily metabolized by the cytochrome P_{450} 3A4 enzyme system is likely to result in increased plasma concentrations of these drugs that could increase or prolong their therapeutic effect and/or increase adverse reactions (see table below). Therefore, coadministration of Synercid with drugs that are cytochrome P_{450} 3A4 substrates and possess a narrow therapeutic window requires caution and monitoring of these drugs (e.g. cyclosporine), whenever possible. Concomitant medications metabolized by the cytochrome P_{450} 3A4 enzyme system that may prolong the QTc interval should be avoided.
>
> Concomitant administration of **Synercid** and nifedipine (repeated oral doses) and midazolam (intravenous bolus dose) in healthy volunteers led to elevated plasma concentrations of these drugs. The C_{max} increased by 18% and 14% (median values) and the AUC increased by 44% and 33% for nifedipine and midazolam, respectively.

tyramine content foods, or concomitant administration of adrenergic or serotonergic foods. In a few case reports linezolid potentiated the effects of phenylpropalonalmine. Serotonin syndrome in patients taking linezolid and selective serotonin re-uptake inhibitors has been reported.

METRONIDAZOLE

Metronidazole has been reported to be an inhibitor of hepatic metabolism.[48] The most significant interaction involves the combination of metronidazole with warfarin, resulting in accumulation of warfarin and an enhanced anticoagulant effect. Avoidance of this combination is recommended. If use of metronidazole therapy for >1 week is necessary, patients should be monitored closely for increased anticoagulant effects.

A disulfiram-like reaction (flushing, increased respiratory rate, increased pulse rate) between alcohol and metronidazole intravenous, oral, and vaginal tablet dosage forms has been described in some patients. Therefore, patients should avoid ingesting alcohol while receiving metronidazole.

β-LACTAM ANTIBIOTICS

The β-lactam group of agents cause few drug interactions. The most common types are elimination interactions. For example, large doses of penicillin can inhibit the renal elimination of methotrexate, resulting in accumulation and toxicity. Probenecid is a well known inhibitor of renal secretion of many types of penicillin, though this has little current clinical utility.

Nafcillin and dicloxacillin have been reported to increase the anticoagulant effects of warfarin. The mechanism of these interactions remain unknown, and monitoring patients' INR/PT while receiving such combinations is recommended.

Cephalosporins rarely cause drug–drug interactions. Absorption of two oral drugs, cefpodoxime proxetil and cefuroxime axetil, is pH-dependent and they should not be administered with gastric acid modifiers such as antacids, H_2 blockers, and proton pump inhibitors. The absorption of cefdinir is significantly reduced by iron. The effect of iron on the absorption of other cephalosporins is unknown.

TETRACYCLINES

Similar to the penicillins, tetracyclines have been associated with menstrual cycle interruptions and unplanned pregnancies. Therefore patients using oral contraceptives who require the use of tetracycline should be advised to use an additional contraceptive method. Tetracyclines are mainly associated with pharmacokinetic absorption types of interactions and the same precautions for fluoroquinolones are appropriate for tetracyclines.[48] Tetracyclines are minimally metabolized by the liver, except for doxycycline. Rifampicin and the antiepileptics carbamazepine, phenobarbital, and phenytoin can reduce the AUC of doxycycline when administered concomitantly. These interactions may be of clinical importance.

CHLORAMPHENICOL

Chloramphenicol can inhibit phenytoin metabolism, resulting in phenytoin toxicity, and anticonvulsants can increase chloramphenicol concentrations.[48] Because so little chloramphenicol is used presently, the full spectrum of interactions and their mechanisms are unclear.

ANTIMYCOBACTERIALS

Many drugs from this class cause multiple pharmacokinetic interactions and a few pharmacodynamic interactions.[49]

Pharmacodynamic interactions

Overlapping toxicities

Prolonged isoniazid therapy can cause peripheral neuropathy. When it is given with other neurotoxic agents such as the NRTIs stavudine, didanosine, and zalcitabine, peripheral neuropathy may result. Administration of pyridoxine can minimize neuropathy associated with isoniazid but has no effect on NRTI neuropathy.

Pharmacokinetic Interactions

Rifampicin (rifampin), rifapentine and rifabutin

Rifampicin is one of the most potent inducers of multiple Phase 1 and Phase 2 enzymes, as well as being a potent inducer of P-glycoprotein.[15,37,49,50,51] Rifapentine is also a potent inducer of cytochrome P_{450} 3A4, 2C8, and 2C9 enzymes. Rifabutin is least likely to result in clinically important induction. However, rifabutin is a substrate for CYP3A4 and when its metabolism is impaired, accumulation of rifabutin and its metabolite can cause severe side effects, including uveitis, a flu-like syndrome and neutropenia (*see above*). Every patient who receives any of these three drugs should be evaluated closely for potential interactions. Many of the interactions with rifampicin and rifabutin have been discussed, and only a brief review follows. The drug interactions with rifampicin, rifapentine and rifabutin are summarized in Table 6.9.

PROTEASE INHIBITORS

Interactions between rifampicin, rifapentine, and rifabutin are particularly problematic in patients infected with HIV-1. Because the AUC of most protease inhibitors is reduced by about 80% when taken with rifampicin, rifampicin is contraindicated with most protease inhibitors and NNRTIs.[11,15,20,28,37,50] Since rifampicin is not a substrate of CYP3A4, protease inhibitors have no effect on rifampicin kinetics. Similarly, rifapentine decreases indinavir AUC by 70% (Table 6.9), and its use with protease inhibitors should be avoided. In contrast, rifabutin is a substrate of CYP3A4 but is believed to be a poor inducer of this enzyme. Consequently, rifabutin can be given to patients receiving protease inhibitors and is one of the recommended treatments for infection with *Mycobacterium tuberculosis* in patients receiving protease inhibitors. However, rifabutin has a low therapeutic index and serum concentrations of parent drug and metabolite are markedly increased in the presence of protease inhibitors, and severe adverse events including neutropenia and flu-like syndrome are common. The dosage of rifabutin must be reduced by at least one-half to avoid excessive accumulation in the patient receiving protease inhibitors (Table 6.9).

Other clinically significant interactions involving rifampicin, rifapentine and rifabutin include the interactions with other CYP3A4, CYP2C9 and CYP1A2 substrates. Examples of these substrates include antiarrhythmic agents (Classes I–IV) (Table 6.9), antifungals (Table 6.6), oral contraceptives, corticosteroids, cyclosporine, dapsone, digoxin, methadone, theophylline, and warfarin (Table 6.9). All patients receiving such combinations should thus be monitored appropriately for clinical response and dosing adjustments should be considered as needed.

Other antimycobacterial drug interactions[49]

Absorption interactions

Ethambutol absorption is reduced when given with antacids. The data describing the interactions between isoniazid and antacids are conflicting. Several studies have found a reduction in isoniazid AUC from zero to 19% when combined with aluminum salts, and it has been suggested that the drug be given at least 2 h before aluminum-containing antacids. A

Table 6.9 Antimycobacterial drug interactions (*see text for references*)

Anti-mycobacterial	Interacting drug	Anticipated mechanism interaction	Anticipated effect	Clinical management
Azithromycin	*See* Table 6.8			
Clarithromycin	*See* Table 6.8			
Ethambutol	Aluminum salts	↓ ethambutol absorption	↓ ethambutol AUC by 10%	Separate dosing from ethambutol by at least 2 hrs
Ethionamide	Azole antifungals Delavirdine Protease inhibitors	All listed drugs may inhibit metabolism of ethionamide	↑ ethionamide levels	Clinical significance unclear. Monitor for ethionamide toxicity
Isoniazid	Acetaminophen	Pharmacodynamic interaction	↑ hepatotoxicity risk when combined	Limit acetaminophen use, although a causal relationship has not been established
	Aluminum salts	↓ INH absorption	↓ INH AUC by ≈ 19%	Separate dosing from aluminum salts by at least 2 h
	Carbamazepine	Hepatic enzyme inhibition	INH may ↑ CBZ levels	Monitor for signs and symptoms of CBZ toxicity
	Cycloserine	Pharmacodynamic interaction and hepatic enzyme inhibition	Overlapping toxicity due to ↓ vitamin B_6 metabolism	Monitor for central nervous system toxicities
	Disulfiram	Dopamine metabolic pathway alterations	Behavioral changes when both are given concomitantly	A true relationship has not been fully established Monitor for changes in behavior and coordination
	Phenytoin	Metabolic inhibition	↑ phenytoin levels	Monitor for phenytoin toxicity and levels
	Theophylline	Metabolic inhibition	↓ theophylline clearance by 16–23%	Monitor for theophylline toxicity
	Zalcitabine	↓ INH absorption	↓ INH levels	Separate dosing from INH by at least 1 h Monitor for increased peripheral neuropathy

Table 6.9 *Continued*

Anti-mycobacterial	Interacting drug	Anticipated mechanism interaction	Anticipated effect	Clinical management
Quinolones	*See* Table 6.7			
Rifabutin	Antifungals	See Table 6.6		
	Clarithromycin	CYP3A4 induction	↓ clarithromycin AUC by 44%, *see also* Table 6.8	Not established. Monitor for clinical response to clarithromycin
	Oral contraceptives	Hepatic enzyme induction	↓ ethinylestradiol AUC ↓ norethindrone AUC Increase the risk of unintended pregnancies, and irregular menstrual cycle	Use additional (barrier) contraceptive methods
	Cyclosporine	CYP3A4 induction	↑ in CyA clearance	Monitor CyA levels, may require increase in CyA dose
	Methadone	Induction	Because rifabutin is similar to rifampicin, increased methadone clearance may occur	Monitor for clinical response to methadone, may require methadone dose increase
	NNRTIs	*See* Table 6.4		
	Protease inhibitors	*See* Table 6.5		
	Warfarin	Induction	Possible increase in warfarin clearance	Monitor for clinical response to warfarin, may require warfarin dose increase
Rifampicin and rifapentine	Beta blockers	Hepatic enzyme induction	↓ levels of propranolol, metoprolol, bisoprolol	Increase in beta blocker dose
	Calcium channel blockers	Hepatic enzyme induction	↓ levels of verapamil, diltiazem and nifedipine	Increase in calcium channel blocker dose
	Clarithromycin	CYP3A4 induction	Significant ↓ in clarithromycin levels	Not established. Monitor for clinical response to clarithromycin
	Oral contraceptives	Hepatic enzyme induction	↓ ethinylestradiol AUC ↓ norethindrone AUC Increase the risk of unintended pregnancies, and irregular menstrual cycle	Use additional (barrier) contraceptive methods
	Corticosteroids	CYP3A4 induction	↓ prednisolone AUC by 66%, ↑ clearance by 45%	↑ prednisolone dose, monitor for clinical response to corticosteroids
	Cyclosporine, tacrolimus, sirolimus	CYP3A4 induction	↑ clearance	Avoid combination
	Dapsone	Hepatic enzyme induction	7–10 × ↓ in dapsone levels	Monitor for clinical response to dapsone, may require dapsone dose increase
	Digoxin	P-gp induction	↑ digoxin clearance	Monitor digoxin levels. May require ↑ digoxin dose
	Methadone	Hepatic enzyme induction	Methadone levels ↓ by 30–65%	Monitor for clinical response to methadone, may require methadone dose increase
	NNRTIs	*See* Table 6.4		
	Phenytoin	Hepatic enzyme induction	Doubling in phenytoin clearance, and 53% ↓ in phenytoin $t_{1/2}$	Monitor phenytoin levels, may require phenytoin dose increase
	Protease inhibitors	*See* Table 6.5		
	Sulfonylurea	Hepatic enzyme induction	Rifampicin increases sulfonylurea clearance	Monitor glucose and clinical response to sulfonylurea, may require sulfonylurea dose increase
	Theophylline	Hepatic enzyme induction	↑ theophylline clearance	↑ theophylline dose as needed, monitor theophylline levels and clinical response
	Warfarin	Hepatic enzyme induction	2–3 × ↑ (S) and (R)-warfarin clearance, ↓ warfarin levels	Avoid combination if possible. If concomitant use is necessary, monitor INR and PT

AUC = area under the concentration curve; CBZ = carbamazepine; CYP = cytochrome P_{450}; CyA = cyclosporine; INH = isoniazid; INR = International normalization ratio; PT = Prothrombin time; ↑ = increase; ↓ = decrease.

more recent investigation found no significant change in the AUC of isoniazid when a magnesium-aluminum hydroxide antacid (Mylanta™) was coadministered. Similarly, didanosine did not change the AUC of isoniazid and standard doses of both drugs may be used, although patients should be monitored for increased risk of peripheral neuropathy.

Metabolism

Isoniazid is reported to inhibit the activity of CYP2E1, CYP1A2, CYP2C9, and 3A4.[49] It can increase levels of carbamazepine (a CYP3A4, 2C8, and 2C9 substrate), and phenytoin (a CYP2C9 substrate). These are well studied interactions and antiepileptic serum levels should be monitored closely.

ANTIPARASITIC AGENTS

Interactions in this class of drugs may be pharmacodynamic or pharmacokinetic in nature (Table 6.10).

PHARMACODYNAMIC INTERACTIONS

Dapsone causes multiple overlapping neurotoxicities when concomitantly administered with didanosine, primaquine and stavudine.[26,50] Therefore, patients receiving such combinations should be closely monitored for signs and symptoms of peripheral neuropathies. In addition, the combination of dapsone with zidovudine has resulted in increased risk of bone marrow toxicity (Table 6.9). A complete blood count with differential should be obtained to monitor for overlapping toxicities.

The nephrotoxicity from pentamidine is additive when combined with other nephrotoxic agents such as amphotericin B, foscarnet, ganciclovir, cyclosporine and aminoglycosides (Table 6.9).[26] Other pharmacodynamic interactions involving pentamidine include its concomitant use with pancreotoxins such as didanosine and stavudine, and other antibiotics that cause QTc prolongation (Table 6.9).

PHARMACOKINETIC INTERACTIONS

Absorption

Atovaquone decreases the absorption and AUC of didanosine but this interaction is not considered clinically significant. However, didanosine is usually administered on an empty stomach, whereas atovaquone should be administered with meals. The coadministration of these agents should thus be avoided.

Metabolism

Sulfadiazine/pyrimethamine and trimethoprim/sulfamethoxazole decrease the clearance of phenytoin by 80% and 27%, respectively (Table 6.9) presumably via inhibition of phenytoin hepatic metabolism. Similarly, some sulfonamides can inhibit the hepatic metabolism of warfarin or displace it from binding sites. Therefore patients should be monitored for an increase in PT/INR when sulfonamide containing products are administered with warfarin.

Atovaquone AUC is decreased by 50% when coadministered with rifampicin, whereas it increases the AUC of rifampicin by 35%. This combination should be avoided, and an alternative should be considered. Atovaquone can inhibit glucuronidation; thus it can increase the AUC of zidovudine. The AUC of dapsone is increased by up to 50% when coadministered with probenecid and by 40% with trimethoprim.[26]

Hypoglycemia has been reported when sulfonylureas were coadministered with trimethoprim/sulfamethoxazole and sulfadiazine/pyrimethamine. Therefore patients receiving such combinations must be monitored closely.

Elimination

Trimethoprim decreases renal tubular secretion of the NRTIs, lamivudine, zidovudine and zalcitabine, leading to an increase in the AUC of 43%, 23% and 37%, respectively (Table 6.10). The clinical significance of these interactions is unclear, because therapeutic efficacy of NRTIs depends on the intracellular concentration of these agents, and not their plasma levels.

References

1. Woosley RL 2000 Drug labeling revisions – Guaranteed to fail? *Journal of the American Medical Association* 284: 3047–3049.
2. Piscitelli JH, Rodvold K (eds) 2000 *Drug Interaction in Infectious Diseases.* Humana Press, Totowa.
3. Jones JK, Fife D, Curkendall S, Goehring E, Guo JJ, Shannon M 2001 Coprescribing and codispensing of cisapride and contraindicated drugs. *Journal of the American Medical Association* 286: 1607–1609.
4. Seldane and generic terfenadine withdrawn from market. Online. Available: *http://www.fda.gov/bbs/topics/ANSWARS/ANS00853.html* 27 February 1998.
5. Piscitelli SC, Burstein AH, Chaitt D, Alfaro RM, Falloon J 2000 Indinavir concentrations and St John's wort. *Lancet* 355: 547–548.
6. Henney JH 2000 Drug interactions with St John's Wort. *Journal of the American Medical Association* 283: 679.
7. Westphal, J-F 2000 Macrolide-induced clinically relevant drug interactions with cytochrome P-450A (CYP) 3A4: an update focused on clarithromycin, azithromycin and dirithromycin. *British Journal of Clinical Pharmacology* 50: 285–295.
8. Venkatakrishnan K, von Moltke LL, Greenblatt DJ 2000 Effects of the antifungal agents on oxidative drug metabolism: Clinical relevance. *Clinical Pharmacokinetics* 38: 111–180.
9. Flexner C 2000 Dual protease inhibitor therapy in HIV-infected patients: Pharmacologic rationale and clinical benefit. *Annual Review of Pharmacology and Toxicology* 40: 649–674.
10. Giao P, de Vries P 2001 Pharmacokinetic interactions of antimalarial agents. *Clinical Pharmacokinetics* 40: 343–373.
11. Piscitelli S, Gallicano KD 2001 Interactions among drugs for HIV and opportunistic infections. *New England Journal of Medicine* 344: 984–996.
12. Polk RE. 2000 Antimicrobials and antiparasitics. In Levy RH, Thummel KE, Trager WF et al. (eds). *Metabolic drug interactions*, pp. 615–622 Lippincott Williams and Wilkins, Philadelphia.
13. Kosel BW, Aweeka F 2000 Drug interactions of antiretroviral agents. *AIDS Clinical Reviews* 193–227.

Table 6.10 Antiparasitic drug interactions[2,10,12,15,26,28,42,49,50]

Drug	Interacting drug	Pharmacokinetic interactions		Pharmacodynamic interactions	Clinical management
		Absorption interactions	Metabolic interactions		
Atovaquone	Didanosine	↓ didanosine AUC by 24%			Not clinically significant, however didanosine should be administered without food, while atovaquone is given with food
	Phenytoin		↔ atovaquone AUC ↔ phenytoin AUC		Not clinically significant
	Rifabutin		May ↓ atovaquone AUC May ↑ rifabutin AUC		Because rifabutin is similar to rifampicin, interactions may occur
	Rifampicin		↓ atovaquone AUC by 50% ↑ rifampicin AUC by 35%		Avoid concomitant use. Potential failure of response to atovaquone
	Ritonavir		↓ atovaquone AUC		Monitor for failure to response to atovaquone, may need to ↑ atovaquone doses
	Sulfamethoxazole/ trimethoprim		↓ SMX/TMP plasma levels ↔ atovaquone AUC		Not clinically significant
	Zidovudine		↑ zidovudine plasma levels due to inhibition of zidovudine glucuronidation		Not clinically significant. Monitor for zidovudine toxicity
Dapsone	Didanosine			Overlapping toxicity, may ↑ risk of neurotoxicity	Monitor for s/sx of peripheral neuropathy
	Probenecid		↑ dapsone levels by 25–50%		Monitor for dapsone toxicity, CBC
	Pyrimethamine		Inhibition of dapsone metabolism		Monitor for dapsone toxicity, CBC
	Primaquine			Overlapping toxicity, may ↑ risk of neurotoxicity	Monitor for s/sx of peripheral neuropathy
	Rifabutin		See Table 6.8		
	Rifampicin		See Table 6.8		
	Stavudine			Overlapping toxicity, may ↑ risk of neurotoxicity	Monitor for s/sx of peripheral neuropathy
	Trimethoprim		40% ↑ in both trimethoprim and dapsone levels		Consider trimethoprim dose ↓ in patients with baseline anemia. Monitor CBC
	Zalcitabine		↔ dapsone AUC, but ↓ dapsone oral clearance		Monitor for additive peripheral neuropathy
	Zidovudine			Overlapping toxicity, may ↑ risk of bone marrow toxicity	Monitor toxicities and CBC
Pentamidine	Amphotericin B			Overlapping toxicity, may ↑ risk of nephrotoxicity	Caution when used together. Monitor toxicities
	Foscarnet			Overlapping toxicity, may ↑ risk of nephrotoxicity	Consider avoiding this combination Monitor toxicities
	Nephrotoxins			Overlapping toxicity, may ↑ risk of nephrotoxicity	Consider avoiding this combination Monitor toxicities
	Sparfloxacin			Overlapping toxicity, may cause QTc prolongation	Contraindicated, unless appropriate cardiac monitoring can be assured

Table 6.10 *Continued*

Drug	Interacting drug	Pharmacokinetic interactions		Pharmacodynamic interactions	Clinical management
		Absorption interactions	**Metabolic interactions**		
Sulfadiazine/ pyrimethamine	Phenytoin		Sulfadiazine ↑ pheyntoin's $t_{1/2}$ by 80% and ↓ phenytoin clearance by 45%		Monitor patient for signs and symptoms of phenytoin toxicity
	Sulfonylureas		Hypoglycemia has been reported		Avoid combining sulfonamide antibiotics with sulfonylureas
	Zidovudine			Antagonistic antibacterial effects	Clinical significance unclear
Sulfamethoxazole/ trimethoprim	Atovaquone		*See above*		
	Cyclosporine		↑ CyA levels	Overlapping toxicity, ↑ risk of nephrotoxicity	Monitor CyA levels and renal function
	Lamivudine		TMP inhibits renal tubular secretion of lamivudine (lamivudine AUC ↑ by 43%)		Standard dosing use. Monitor for lamivudine toxicities
	Phenytoin		Sulfadiazine ↑ pheyntoin's $t_{1/2}$ by 39%		Monitor patient for signs and symptoms of phenytoin toxicity
	Pyrimethamine			Additive toxicity due to additive inhibition of dihydrofolate reductase	Monitor CBC with differential. Give in low doses if possible
	Sulfonylureas		Hypoglycemia has been reported		Avoid combining sulfonamide antibiotics with sulfonylureas
	Warfarin		↑ warfarin levels and risk of bleeding		Monitor PT and INR
	Zalcitabine		Trimethoprim inhibits renal tubular secretion of zalcitabine, ↓ zalcitabine AUC by 37%		Clinical significance unclear. Monitor for zalcitabine toxicities
	Zidovudine		Trimethoprim inhibits renal tubular secretion of zidovudine, ↓ zidovudine AUC by 23%		Clinical significance unclear. Monitor for zidovudine toxicities

AUC = area under the concentration curve; CBC = complete blood count; CyA = cyclosporine; INR = international normalization ratio; PT = prothrombin time; QTc = corrected QT interval; s/sx = signs and symptoms; ↑ = increase; ↓ = decrease; ↔ = no change.

14. Gerber JG 2000 Using pharmacokinetics to optimize antiretroviral drug–drug interactions in the treatment of human immunodeficiency virus infection. *Clinical Infectious Diseases* 30(Suppl. 2): S123–129.

15. Burman WJ, Gallicano K, Peloquin C 2001 Comparative pharmacokinetics and pharmacodynamics of the rifamycin antibacterials. *Clinical Pharmacokinetics* 40: 327–341.

16. Kashuba ADM, Bertino, JS 2000. Mechanisms of drug interactions. In Piscitelli JH, Rodvold KA, Masur H, (eds). *Drug Interaction in Infectious Diseases*, pp. 13–38. Humana Press, Totowa.

17. Zhang Y, Benet LZ 2001 The gut as a barrier to drug absorption: Combined role of cytochrome P_{450} 3A and P-Glycoprotein. *Clinical Pharmacokinetics* 40: 159–168.

18. Kaletra™ Prescribing Information, Abbott Laboratories, Abbott Park, IL. September 2000.

19. Khaliq Y, Gallicano K, Venance S, Kravcik S, Cameron DW 2000 Effect of ketoconazole on ritonavir and saquinavir concentrations in plasma and cerebrospinal fluid from patients infected with human immunodeficiency virus. *Clinical Pharmacology and Therapeutics* 68: 637–646.

20. Dresser GK, Spence JD, Bailey DG 2000 Pharmacokinetic-pharmacodynamic consequences and clinical relevance of cytochrome P_{450} 3A4 inhibition. *Clinical Pharmacokinetics* 38: 41–57.

21. Tucke GT, Houston JB, Huang S-M 2001 Optimizing drug development: Strategies to assess drug metabolism/transporter interaction potential – toward a consensus. *Clinical Pharmacology and Therapeutics* 70: 103–114.

22. Levy RH, Thummel KE, Trager WF, et al (eds) 2000 *Metabolic drug interactions*. Lippincott Williams and Wilkins, Philadelphia.

23. Owens RC Jr 2001 Risk assessment for antimicrobial agent-induced QTc interval prolongation and torsades de pointes. *Pharmacotherapy* 21(3): 301–319.

24. Withdrawal of astemizole (Hismanal®) from the U.S. market. Online. Available: *http://www.pharminfo.com/pubs/medbrief/mb7 7.html* 28 June 1999.

25. Orap™ (Pimizide) Revised Prescribing Information, Gate Pharmaceuticals, Montgomeryville, PA. September 1999.

26. Panel on Clinical Practices for Treatment of HIV Infection 2002 Guidelines for the use of antiretroviral agents in HIV-infected adults and adolescents. Department of Health and Human Services and Henry J. Kaiser Family Foundation. Online. Available: www.hivatis.org.

27. Sildenafil (Viagra™) Prescribing information, Pfizer US Pharmaeuticals Group, New York, NY. March 1998 (update).

28. Piscitelli SC, Struble KA 2000 Drug interactions with antiretrovirals for HIV Infection. In Piscitelli JH, Rodvold KA (eds) *Drug Interaction in Infectious Diseases*, pp. 39–60. Humana Press, Totowa.

29. Tran JQ, Gerber JG, Kerr BM 2001 Delavirdine: clinical pharmacokinetics and drug interactions. *Clinical Pharmacokinetics* 40(3): 207–226.

30. Tephly TR, Breen MD 2000 UDP-Glucuronosyltransferases. In Levy RH, Thummel KE, Trager EF et al. (eds). *Metabolic drug interactions*, pp. 161–173. Lippincott Williams and Wilkins, Philadelphia.

31. Vistide® (Cidofovir injection), (Vistide) Prescribing information, Gilead Sciences, Inc. Foster City, CA September 2000.

32. Hass C 2000 Drug–cytokine interactions. In Piscitelli JH, Rodvold KA (eds). *Drug Interaction in Infectious Diseases*, pp. 287–310. Humana Press, Totowa.

33. Halkin H, Katzir I, Kurman I, Jan J, Malkin B 2001 Preventing drug interactions by online prescription screening in community pharmacies and medical practices. *Clinical Pharmacology and Therapeutics* 69: 260–265.

34. Bailey TC, McMullin ST 2001 Using information systems technology to improve antibiotic prescribing. *Critical Care Medicine* 29(4) (Suppl.): N87–N91.

35. Itraconazole (Sporonax®) Prescribing Information, Janssen Pharmaceutical Products, Titusville, NJ. April 2001.

36. Quinupristine-dalfopristine (Syercid™) Prescribing Information, Aventis Pharmaceutical, Collegeville, PA. July 1999.

37. Centers for Disease Control and Prevention 2000 Updated guidelines for the use of rifabutin or rifampin for the treatment and prevention of tuberculosis among HIV-infected patient taking protease inhibitors or nonnucleoside reverse transcriptase inhibitors. *Morbidity and Mortality Weekly Report* 49: 185–189.

38. Lori F, Lisziewicz J 2000 Rationale for the use of hydroxyurea as an antihuman immunodeficiency virus drug. *Clinical Infectious Diseases* 30 (Suppl 2): S193–197.

39. Gubbins PO, McConnell SA, Penzak SR 2000 Drug interactions associated with antifungal agents. In Piscitelli JH, Rodvold KA. *Drug Interaction in Infectious Diseases*, pp. 185–217. Humana Press, Totowa.

40. Weisberg E 1999 Interactions between oral contraceptives and antifungals/antibacterials. Is contraceptive failure the result? *Clinical Pharmacokinetics* 36: 309–313.

41. Dickinson BD, Altman RD, Nielsen NH, Sterling ML 2001 Drug Interactions between oral contraceptives and antibiotics. *Obstetrics and Gynecology* 98: 853–860.

42. Romanelli F, Jennings HR, Nath A, Ryan M, Berger J 2000 Therapeutic dilemma: the use of anticonvulsants in HIV-positive individuals. *Neurology* 54: 1404–1407.

43. FDA Talk paper. FDA updates safety information for miconazole vaginal cream and suppositories. Online. Available: *http://www.fda.gov/cder/drug/infopage/miconazole/default.htm* 5 March 2001.

44. Sabo JA, Abdel-Rahman SM 2000 Voriconazole: a new triazole antifungal. *Annals of Pharmacotherapy* 34: 1032–1043.

45. Guay DP 2000 Quinolones. In Piscitelli JH, Rodvold KA (eds). *Drug interaction in infectious diseases*, pp. 121–150. Humana Press, Totowa.

46. Withdrawal of Product: RAXAR (grepafloxacin HCl) 600 mg Tablets, 400 mg Tablets, and 200 mg Tablets. Online. Available: *http://www.fda.gov/medwatch/safety/1999/raxhcp.html* 1 November 1999.

47. Zyvox™ (linezolid) prescribing information, Pharmacea and Upjohn, Kalamazoo. MI. January 2002.

48. Susla GM 2000 Miscellaneous antibiotics. In Piscitelli JH, Rodvold KA (eds). *Drug interaction in infectious diseases*, pp. 219–248. Humana Press Totowa.

49. Kuper JI, D'Aprile M 2000 Drug–drug interactions of clinical significance in the treatment of patients with *Mycobacterium avium complex* disease. *Clinical Pharmacokinetics* 39: 203–214.

50. Tseng A 2000 AIDS/HIV Drugs for opportunistic infections. In Piscitelli JH, Rodvold KA (eds). *Drug interaction in infectious diseases* pp. 61–107. Humana Press, Totowa.

51. Finch CK, Crisman CR, Baciewicz AM, Self TH. Rifampin and Rifabutin drug interactions: an update. *Arch Int Med* 2002; 162: 985–992.

7 Antibiotics and the immune system

Arne Forsgren and Kristian Riesbeck

Numerous reports on the effect of antibacterial agents on the immune system have accumulated in recent years. However, immune capacity is difficult to examine, and different results, sometimes conflicting, will be obtained depending on the derivative, incubation time, cell type, analysis method, or experimental animal used. In this chapter, selected current literature is reviewed.

Comprehensive reviews on effects of antibiotics on the immune reponse have been published over the last two decades. Hauser and Remington in 1983 concluded that a potential for immunosuppression exists for several antibiotics,[1] although the clinical relevance of the experimental observations remained to be elucidated. Milatovic characterized the published results on phagocytosis to a large extent as controversial, thus rendering the evaluation rather difficult.[2] More recently, Van Vlem et al, searched the Medline database for negative and positive statements on effects of antibiotics on the immune system,[3] thereby enabling calculation of an immune index for different phagocyte and lymphocyte functions. Since publications in high-quality journals were, however, given the same value as non-peer-reviewed preliminary reports the pattern obtained can be questioned. Finally, Labro concluded that her review of the therapeutic relevance of the observed effects and future research prospects will certainly raise more questions than answers.[4]

During an infection antibiotics interfere with both the infecting bacterium and the host in a complicated fashion (Figure 7.1). In addition to the conventional effects of an antibiotic, i.e. bacteriostasis and bactericidial activity (A), some antibiotics act directly on important components in the host defense such as granulocytes and lymphocytes (B). Antibiotics can alter the susceptibility of bacteria to host defenses and alter release of toxins and inflammatory products, with secondary effects on the host (C). Phagocytic or other host cells can also protect bacteria against antibiotics (D).

CHEMOTAXIS

Most studies on the direct effect of antibiotics on phagocytic cells concern chemotaxis. The in-vitro effect of 20 different antibiotics on chemotaxis towards an *Escherichia coli* filtrate

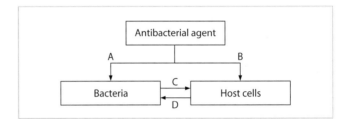

Fig. 7.1 Schematic drawing demonstrating host–cell interactions and different levels of intervention by antibacterial agents. See text for details.

was studied using an agarose technique.[5] Human leukocytes pre-incubated with clinically obtainable concentrations of rifampicin and sodium fusidate showed markedly depressed directional migration, and at concentrations slightly above those clinically achievable doxycycline also inhibited chemotaxis. The clinical implications of these results must, however, be questioned as the experiments were performed in a low-protein tissue culture suspension, and fusidic acid particularly is heavily protein bound. In patients and healthy volunteers given doxycycline, leukocyte migration was studied ex vivo with an agarose technique and in vivo with a skin window technique (Figure 7.2). The very high dose 600 mg doxycycline administered intravenously had only an insignificant effect, while controls given non-steroidal anti-inflammatory drugs (NSAIDs) had significantly reduced values both ex vivo and in vivo (Scheja A., Forsgren A., unpublished results). Aminoglycosides, β-lactams, macrolides, clindamycin, sulfamethoxazole, trimethoprim and fluoroquinolones have shown no interactions with agarose chemotaxis. In contrast to those results, it has been reported that macrolides potentiate human neutrophil locomotion in vitro by inhibition of leukoattractant-activated superoxide generation and auto-oxidation. In addition, aminoglycosides have been reported to inhibit chemotaxis. The effects of macrolides and aminoglycosides have not been confirmed in in-vivo studies.

PHAGOCYTOSIS AND KILLING

Studies of the direct influence of antibiotics on other phagocytic cell functions such as engulfment, killing and metabolic responses are more scarce. Tetracyclines at clinical concentrations slightly above the levels obtained in vivo have been shown to inhibit the uptake of different bacteria, yeasts and particles in vitro. Furthermore, leukocytes harvested from healthy volunteers after ingestion of tetracycline also demonstrated decreased phagocytic capacity for yeasts, although results are conflicting. In various studies aminoglycosides have decreased, increased or had no effect on uptake. Other antibiotics have not been studied or have no apparent effect on phagocyte engulfment or killing functions. At clinically achievable concentrations, for example, fluoroquinolones in general do not affect phagocyte functions.

INTRACELLULAR EFFECTS

The penetration of antibiotics into human cells has been addressed by different methods, often including the use of radiolabeled drugs. Again results vary with experimental conditions: for example, using different media with (or without) albumin considerably affects the outcome.[6] Penicillins, cephalosporins and aminoglycosides have in general limited access to the intracellular space with cellular/extracellular ratio (C/E) less than 1, whereas quinolones, tetracyclines, ethambutol and rifampicin are enriched intracellularly: azithromycin, clarithromycin, clindamycin, erythromycin, roxithromycin, telithromycin and teicoplanin demonstrate C/Es of 10:1 to 100:1, or higher. Host cells also differ greatly in their capacity to accumulate antibiotics. Most authors have reported a lack of intracellular accumulation of β-lactams in phagocytic cells. However, during longer incubation, β-lactam antibiotics diffuse through membranes into the cell cytosol. Macrophages and fibroblasts incubated with aminoglycosides for several days accumulate these drugs to an apparent C/E of 2–4. Macrophages take up penicillins and aminoglycosides by pinocytosis; granulocytes lack this uptake mechanism. In macrophages actively ingesting bacteria, and in resting macrophages obtained from smokers, the rate of penetration of the drugs is increased. The intracellular distribution of antibiotics will influence their ultimate biological activity. A prerequisite for a beneficial intracellular antibacterial effect is the localization of the antibiotic and the pathogen in the same intracellular compartment. Thus, intracellular bioactivity is not a common property among antibacterial agents even though they are accumulated intracellularly.

Bacteria are internalized by both professional and non-professional phagocytic cells, in which they not only survive but also multiply.[7] The ability of bacteria to enter non-phagocytic host cells such as epithelial cells, endothelial cells and fibroblasts requires specific uptake mechanisms including invasins, which interact with specific host cell receptors or bacterial proteins, triggering membrane ruffling and concomitant bacterial uptake. Although the molecular details in the uptake mechanism differ, the first event following the specific interaction between the bacterial cell and the host cell is always the formation of a primary phagosome. After being taken up most bacteria are inactivated by the generation of reactive oxygen intermediates, nitrous oxide and lytic enzymes. However, it is widely recognized that intracellular survival or even multiplication of many bacteria traditionally referred to as extracellular parasites play a significant role in the pathogenesis of the diseases these organisms cause. This is evident in infections caused by *Staphylococcus aureus* but is also seen in *Haemophilus influenzae*, pneumococcal and streptococcal infections. In order to escape the hostile conditions in the phagosome, intracellular bacteria have invented strategies either to modify the phagosomal compartment in a variety of ways to prevent the bactericidal attack or to escape from the primary phagosome into the cytosol of the host cell. The first strategy is used by *Salmonella* spp., *Mycobacterium tuberculosis*, *Legionella pneumophila* and *Chlamydia* spp. In contrast, *Listeria*, *Shigella* and *Rickettsia* spp. escape from the primary phagosome into the host cytosol, where they continue replicating.

The activity of antibiotics against intracellular bacteria was reviewed by van den Broek, who commented on the difficulties in comparing data generated by different laboratories.[8] Most antibiotics have not been tested in vitro for intracellular effect against microbes with different locations. Intracellular *Staph. aureus* have been shown to present a problem in antibiotic therapy and staphylococci phagocytosed by granulocytes have often been used as a model. Although there are discrepancies in the literature on the ability of antibiotics to kill intracellular *Staph. aureus* most studies have shown a good intraphagocytic activity for rifampicin and ciprofloxacin. In contrast, macrolides, clindamycin, vancomycin, and teicoplanin, although giving high intracellular levels, have shown inability to kill intracellular *Staph. aureus*. This may be due to the fact that clindamycin (and also erythromycin) is associated more with the cytosol fraction and less with the lysosomal fraction, where the staphylococci are found. Macrolides and clindamycin are also negatively affected by acidic pH in the lysosomal fraction. β-Lactam antibiotics and aminoglycosides have in most studies not shown reduction of *Staph. aureus* within neutrophils, although phenoxymethylpenicillin, cloxacillin, flucloxacillin, and aminoglycosides exert some activity against staphylococci within macrophages. It is widely believed that aminoglycosides only affect extracellular bacteria. However, as pointed out above, aminoglycosides enter macrophages and accumulate slowly. The activity of aminoglycosides against intracellular *M. tuberculosis* has been confirmed in classic macrophage studies. The activity of rifampicin against intracellular *L. pneumophila* and *M. tuberculosis* is well accepted, and the intraphagocytic bactericidal effects of erythromycin on *Legionella* and *Chlamydia* spp. seem well established. This may, however, vary due to the cell type in question, as infection with *Chlamydophila* (*Chlamydia*) *pneumoniae* in circulating human monocytes is refractory to antibiotic treatment with azithromycin and rifampicin.[9]

Extracellular respiratory tract pathogens such as *H. influenzae*, pneumococci and streptococci can enter epithelial cells and macrophages and survive intracellularly. In studies of the activity of azithromycin, gentamicin, levofloxacin, moxifloxacin, penicillin G, rifampicin, telithromycin and trovafloxacin against intracellular pneumococci moxifloxacin, trovafloxacin and telithromycin were most active. Telithromycin killed all intracellular organisms.[10]

STRUCTURAL CHANGES IN BACTERIA EXPOSED TO ANTIBIOTICS

Altered uptake and killing of bacteria exposed to antibiotics has been clearly documented.[11] Bacteria exposed to various antibiotics (including β-lactam antibiotics, vancomycin, macrolides, and quinolones) have been reported as more easily phagocytosed and killed. In contrast, tetracycline and gentamicin have been reported to decrease phagocytosis. The reason for the improvement in killing varies, but some bacteria exposed to low concentrations of antibiotics (i.e. sub MIC), often show increased killing. Structural changes in the pathogen can be one reason for changed uptake and killing, and β-lactam antibiotics produce the most dramatic alteration of the bacterial morphology. The functional role of penicillin binding proteins (PBPs) in bacterial growth and morphologic integrity provides the biochemical base for most of the alterations occurring in the presence of β-lactam antibiotics. Each β-lactam antibiotic has a characteristic binding activity for each PBP and at sub-MIC concentrations the antibiotic binds to that PBP for which it has the highest affinity, resulting in antibiotic-dependent specific changes – for example, filaments or oval cells. All β-lactam antibiotics have similar morphologic effects on staphylococci and other Gram-positive cocci because there is little variation in PBP affinity in these bacteria. Fosfomycin and vancomycin, which inhibit earlier stages of cell wall synthesis (*see* Fig. 2.3, p. 13), produce similar morphologic alterations in Gram-positive cocci. Sub-MIC concentrations of antibiotics with targets other than cell wall synthesis induce different morphologic changes: exposure of staphylococci to chloramphenicol, tetracycline, rifampicin, and quinupristin/dalfopristin results in bacteria with multiple layers of cell wall; in Gram-negative bacteria, ciprofloxacin and trimethoprim leads to production of filaments.

Antibiotics may also inhibit the synthesis of key surface molecules. The enhanced phagocytosis and killing of clindamycin-exposed group A streptococci and *Bacteroides* spp. appear to be due to the disappearance of M protein and capsule, respectively, from the bacterial surface. Similarly, clindamycin reduces the amount of protein A on the surface of *Staph. aureus*; consequently the bacteria become more susceptible to phagocytic uptake and killing. Ceftriaxone and monobactams reduce antiphagocytic antigen of *E. coli*. In parallel, ampicillin and chloramphenicol alter the antiphagocytic capsule of *H. influenzae* type b, resulting in increased uptake.

ENDOTOXIN AND EXOTOXIN RELEASE

An effect of great importance of antibacterial agents is their potential ability to limit release of exotoxin and endotoxin (lipopolysaccharide; LPS), the major constituent of the outer membrane of Gram-negative bacteria, in the critically ill patient. As early as 1960 Hinton and Orr, for example, observed that α-hemolysin production by *Staph. aureus* is inhibited by streptomycin or bacitracin at concentrations below those interferring with bacterial growth.[11] These findings were confirmed using other antibiotics (tetracyclines, clindamycin, chloramphenicol, and erythromycin). Specific inhibition of, for example, toxic shock syndrome toxin is possible with sub-MIC levels of clindamycin. Treatment of several other species, such as *Clostridium difficile*, *Pseudomonas aeruginosa*, group A streptococci, and *E. coli*, with mainly protein synthesis inhibitors reduces both toxin synthesis and the production of other virulence factors. Clindamycin has recently been used as a supplement to benzylpenicillin to lower exotoxin levels in patients suffering from infections with β-hemolytic group A streptococci.[12]

In recent years, interest has focused on developing antibiotics that kill bacteria with minimal endotoxin release. Initial investigations favored imipenem over ceftazidime and meropenem; however, in a recent randomized, multicenter, double-blind study, no differences in the levels of proinflammatory cytokines were detected in patients with Gram-negative urosepsis treated with either imipenem or ceftazidime.[13] Thus, well controlled clinical investigations are required to shed light on complicated biological phenomena. Another example of reduced endotoxin shedding (production) is that pretreatment of *E. coli* with clindamycin suppresses endotoxin release in bacteria subsequently killed by ceftazidime.[4]

CELL PROLIFERATION AND CYTOKINE PRODUCTION

The effects of antibiotics on lymphoid cells or cells of other origins have been described for most antibiotics that accumulate intracellularly. Fluoroquinolones reach concentrations within human leukocytes 3–20 times the extracellular concentration. Importantly, these drugs are not associated with any specific cellular organelle and do not require cell viability for accumulation. At concentrations slightly above those clinically achievable, the effects of fluoroquinolones on the immune system have been thoroughly investigated. Using ciprofloxacin as a model drug for this large group of derivatives, ciprofloxacin (5–80 mg/l), and to a lower degree other fluoroquinolones, superinduces IL-2 synthesis by mitogen-activated peripheral blood lymphocytes.[14–16] Experiments with T-cell lines and primary T lymphocytes transiently transfected with a plasmid containing the IL-2 promoter region, show ciprofloxacin to enhance IL-2 gene activation. In parallel with these observations, under certain in-vitro conditions, ciprofloxacin (20–80 mg/l) counteracts the effect of the immunosuppressive agent cyclosporin A that normally inhibits the phosphatase activity of calcineurin inhibiting NF-AT-1 activity. Ciprofloxacin thus interferes with a regulative pathway common to several cytokines. Indeed, analysis of cytokine mRNAs in ciprofloxacin-treated peripheral blood lymphocytes revealed that not only IL-2 mRNA but also an array of other cytokine mRNAs, including IFN-γ and IL-4, are enhanced (Figure 7.2A). An earlier and stronger ciprofloxacin-dependent activation of the transcriptional regulation factors, nuclear factor of activated T cells-1 (NF-AT-1) and activator protein-1 (AP-1), has been observed in T-cell lines, whereas ciprofloxacin in primary T cells increases the levels of immediate early transcripts and upregulates AP-1 only (Figure 7.2B). These data suggest a program commonly observed in mammalian stress responses. Ciprofloxacin and trovafloxacin at experimental concentrations potentiate IL-8 and E-selectin (CD62E) synthesis in stimulated endothelial cells.[17]

Several reports exist on ciprofloxacin-dependent immunomodulation in vivo, strongly indicating that the observed cytokine upregulation is not an in-vitro artefact.[4] It is thus clear that the fluoroquinolone ciprofloxacin stimulates bone marrow regeneration in both transplanted and sublethally irradiated mice by interferring with IL-3 and GM-CSF syn-

thesis. The treated mice demonstrated a higher number of white blood cells and myeloid progenitor cells in bone marrow and spleen on days 4 and 8 post-irradiation than in saline-treated animals. Despite promising results in mouse models, there has been only one successful study on this phenomenon in human subjects. Irrespective of the antibacterial effect, fluoroquinolones (75% and 50% for trovafloxacin and tosufloxacin, respectively) protect mice from LPS-dependent mortality when animals were injected with lethal doses.[18] IL-6 and TNF-α serum concentrations were significantly lower in fluoroquinolone-treated animals than in drug-free controls. Several studies have shown that fluoroquinolones inhibit monokine production by LPS-activated monocytic cells albeit at drug concentrations higher than the ones achieved in serum.

Macrolides, including erythromycin, clarithromycin and roxithromycin, have been analysed in several cell systems using various stimulatory compounds such as cytokines and endotoxins. Since macrolides are strongly accumulated intracellularly (>10- to 200-fold) this group of antibiotics has the prerequisite to interfere with eukaryotic cell activities. The molecular target for macrolides (as tested with erythromycin) seems to be the nuclear transcription factor NF-kB or a target upstream.[19] A common feature of the macrolides in in-vitro

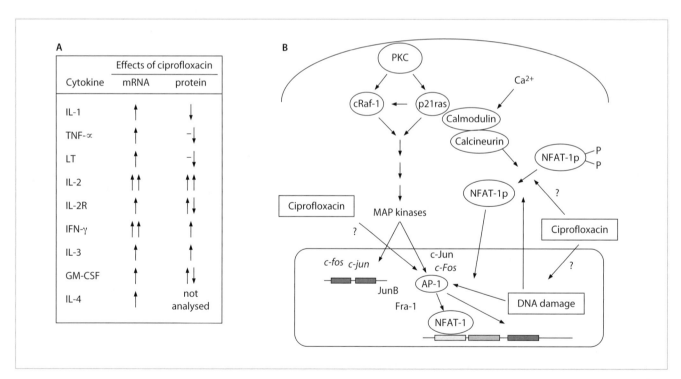

Fig. 7.2 Immunomodulatory effects of the representative fluoroquinolone ciprofloxacin and its putative site(s) of action. Ciprofloxacin upregulates virtually all examined mRNA transcripts in mitogen-activated peripheral blood lymphocytes, whereas only T helper 1 and 2 cytokines are paralleled by an increased protein synthesis[14,15] (A). B delineates the signaling events in a T lymphocyte stimulated through the T-cell receptor/CD3 complex resulting in protein kinase C (PKC) activation followed by triggering of the MAP kinase cascade on one hand and the increased Ca²⁺ mobilization on the other, causing dephosphorylation of the pre-existing nuclear factor of activated T cells-1 (NFAT-1p). It is not completely clear, however, whether ciprofloxacin directly interferes with the transcriptional regulation factors activator protein-1 (AP-1) or NFAT-1, or inhibits the DNA topoisomerase II resulting in DNA damage and genotoxic stress and leading to a secondary activation of the transcription factors (as indicated by the question marks).

experimental systems is inhibition of production of pro-inflammatory cytokines, such as IL-6, TNF-α and IL-8. The effects of the macrolides are similar on epithelial and monocytic cells. Macrolides also interfere directly with eosinophils (inhibited IL-8 synthesis) and neutrophils (decreased superoxide anion production), suggesting that, together with available data on inhibitory effects on proinflammatory cytokines, macrolides may inhibit the inflammatory response on different levels. In fact, clarithromycin postoperatively administered to women undergoing mastectomy effectively suppressed several inflammatory parameters exemplified by reduced febrile response and postoperative pain.[20]

Tetracycline derivatives, and in particular doxycycline, have repeatedly been reported to interfere with the components of the immune system. For example, doxycycline inhibits proliferation of mitogen-activated peripheral blood lymphocytes,[5] minocycline has been shown to decrease T-helper cell cytokines such as IL-2 and IFN-γ. The primary target for tetracyclines may be mitochondria as tetracyclines inhibit mitochondrial protein synthesis, leading to a reduced mitochondrial mass and consequently a decreased oxidative phosphorylation and energy supply.[21] However, a recent study demonstrated that immunoglobulin secretion was suppressed by doxycycline and that the most likely targets were metalloproteinases.[22]

Fusidic acid at clinically achievable concentrations in low protein tissue culture suspension significantly inhibits mitogen-activated peripheral blood lymphocytes.[5] Nitrofurantoin also interferes with lymphocyte proliferation, whereas penicillins, cephalosporins, aminoglycosides, and trimethoprim do not appear to exert any specific effects on lymphocyte immune functions.

Rifampicin modifies several aspects of the immune response:[1] it interferes with lymphocyte proliferation as demonstrated by decreased thymidine incorporation,[5] and significantly prolongs graft survival up to 40% when examined in a split-heart allograft transplantation model. The mechanism responsible for this has not yet been thoroughly elucidated, but it is most likely that the drug inhibits the cellular immune response to the transplanted tissue. Interestingly, cytokine-activated monocytes incubated with rifampicin show an increased CD1b expression,[4] a phenomenon that might be beneficial in tuberculosis patients on rifampicin therapy since CD1b plays a role in presentation of non-peptide antigens.

Cephalosporins do not in general potentiate or modify the immune system. The results obtained in several studies on cefodizime are contradictory and the precise mechanisms have not yet been defined, although the effects of cefodizime have been summarized by Bergeron et al.[23] The drug has been reported to exert negative, neutral or positive effects on neutrophil chemotaxis; to have no effect or positive effects on phagocytosis; to downregulate TNF-α, IL-1, and IL-6 released by stimulated human monocytes; to have no effect on IL-1 release; and to upregulate IL-8 release and GM-CSF from monocytes and bronchial epithelial cells, respectively. Ex vivo, cefodizime shows either neutral or positive effects on chemotaxis and phagocytosis. In vivo, cefodizime restores IL-1 and interferon production in immunocompromised hosts, and enhances phagocytosis and survival of mice infected with cefodizime-resistant pathogens. The drug decreases TNF-α synthesis and inflammation in mice infected by *Streptococcus pneumoniae*, whereas TNF-α production is increased in cefodizime-treated mice administered heat-killed *Klebsiella pneumoniae*.

CONCLUDING REMARKS

Since the field of immunology expanded in the early 1980s, many studies have been performed in order to elucidate the effects of clinically useful antibiotics on different immune functions. Several antibiotics (e.g. certain fluoroquinolones, macrolides, tetracyclines, and rifampicin) significantly interfere with the immune response although despite much effort, only a few of the precise mechanisms behind the immunomodulatory capacities have been elucidated. The term *biological response modifiers* has been coined for some drugs, but an antibiotic that is solely chosen for its immunomodulatory activity in lieu of others is not yet available. We are still awaiting drug derivatives with defined antibacterial activities in addition to well clarified chemical structures that superinduce or inhibit specific immune functions. The field is still in its infancy; structural chemistry followed by high-throughput screening and modern molecular immunology should point us towards new drugs.

References

1. Hauser WE, Remington JS 1982 Effect of antibiotics on the immune response. *American Journal of Medicine* 72: 711–716.
2. Milatovic D 1983 Antibiotics and phagocytosis. *European Journal of Clinical Microbiology* 2: 414–425.
3. Van Vlem B, Vanholder R, De Paepe P, Vogelaers D, Ringoir S 1996 Immunomodulating effects of antibiotics: literature review. *Infection;* 24: 275–291.
4. Labro MT 2000 Interference of antibacterial agents with phagocyte functions: immunomodulation or 'immuno-fairy tales'? *Clinical Microbiological Reviews* 13: 615–650.
5. Forsgren A, Banck G, Beckman H, Bellahsène A 1980 Antibiotic-host defence interactions *in vitro* and *in vivo*. *Scandinavian Journal of Infectious Diseases* (Suppl 24) 195–203.
6. Tulkens PM 1991 Intracellular distribution and activity of antibiotics. *European Journal of Clinical Microbiology and Infectious Diseases* 10: 100–106.
7. Goebel W, Kuhn M 2000 Bacterial replication in the host cytosol. *Current Opinion in Microbiology* 3: 49–53.
8. van den Broeck PJ 1989 Antimicrobial drugs, microorganisms and phagocytes. *Reviews of Infectious Diseases* 11: 213–245.
9. Gieffers J, Fullgraf H, Jahn J et al 2001 *Chlamydia pneumoniae* infection in circulating human monocytes is refractory to antibiotic treatment. *Circulation* 103: 351–356.
10. Mandell GL, Coleman EJ 2000 Activities of antimicrobial agents against intracellular pneumococci. *Antimicrobial Agents and Chemotherapy* 44: 351–356.
11. Gemmell CG, Lorian V 1996 Effects of low concentrations of antibiotics on ultrastructure, virulence, and susceptibility to immunodefenses: Clinical significance. In Lorian V (ed.) *Antibiotics in laboratory medicine.* Williams and Wilkins, Maryland; pp. 397–452.
12. Norrby SR, Norrby-Teglund A 1997 Infections due to group A streptococcus: new concepts and potential treatment strategies. *Annals of the Academy of Medicine Singapore* 26: 691–693.

13. Luchi M, Morrison DC, Opal S et al 2000 A comparative trial of imipenem versus ceftazidime in the release of endotoxin and cytokine generation in patients with gram-negative urosepsis. Urosepsis Study Group. *Journal of Endotoxin Research* 6: 25–31.

14. Riesbeck K, Andersson J, Gullberg M, Forsgren A 1989 Fluorinated 4-quinolones induce hyper-production of interleukin-2. *Proceedings of the National Academy of Sciences of the USA* 86: 2809–2813.

15. Riesbeck K, Forsgren A, Henriksson A, Bredberg A 1998 Ciprofloxacin induces an immunomodulatory stress response in human T lymphocytes. *Antimicrobial Agents and Chemotherapy* 42: 1923–1930.

16. Shalit I 1991 Immunological aspects of new quinolones. *European Journal of Clinical Microbiology and Infectious Diseases* 10: 262–266.

17. Galley HF, Nelson SJ, Dubbles AM, Webster NR 1997 Effect of ciprofloxacin on the accumulation of interleukin-6, interleukin-8, and nitrite from a human endothelial cell model of sepsis. *Critical Care Medicine* 25: 1392–1395.

18. Khan AA, Slifer TR, Araujo FG, Suzuki Y, Remington JS 2000 Protection against lipopolysaccharide-induced death by fluoroquinolones. *Antimicrobial Agents and Chemotherapy* 44: 3169–3173.

19. Aoki Y, Kao PN 1999 Erythromycin inhibits transcriptional activation of NF-kappaB, but not NFAT, through calcineurin-independent signaling in T cells. *Antimicrobial Agents and Chemotherapy* 43: 2678–2684.

20. Chow LW, Yuen KY, Woo PC, Wei WI 2000 Clarithromycin attenuates mastectomy-induced acute inflammatory response. *Clinical Diagnosis and Laboratory Immunology* 7: 925–931.

21. Riesbeck K, Bredberg A, Forsgren A 1990 Ciprofloxacin does not inhibit mitochondrial functions but other antibiotics do. *Antimicrobial Agents and Chemotherapy* 34: 167–169.

22. Bottaro A, Kuzin II, Snyder JE et al 2001 Tetracyclins inhibit activated B cell function. Keystone Symposia, B cell immunobiology and Disease, Snowbird, Utah, April 2001, poster abstract 310, p. 98.

23. Bergeron Y, Deslauriers AM, Ouellet N, Gauthier MC, Bergeron MG 1999 Influence of cefodizime on pulmonary inflammatory response to heat-killed *Klebsiella pneumoniae* in mice. *Antimicrobial Agents and Chemotherapy* 43: 2291–2294.

8 General principles of antimicrobial chemotherapy

R.G. Finch

Antimicrobial drugs active in the laboratory against a large number of infectious agents are available, many of them of established value in the treatment of the diseases caused by these agents. But, as with most other drugs, their administration may be accompanied by unwanted effects. These naturally differ in their nature and severity from agent to agent, varying in their effects from trivial to life-threatening. However, in addition to the familiar problem of deciding the balance between benefit and risk (the therapeutic ratio) in the individual for whom any drug is prescribed, the administration of antimicrobial agents carries another problem, that of the selection and dissemination of resistant organisms. Drug resistance is discussed in detail in Chapter 3, but it is important here to note the cycle in which increasing use of a drug begets drug resistance and thus the requirement for new agents, only to be followed by resistance to the new agent in its turn. The problem of antibiotic resistance is far from theoretical, having led to the loss of many once-valuable agents: sulfonamides for meningococcal disease, low-dose penicillin for gonorrhea, ampicillin for *Haemophilus influenzae* meningitis or enteric fever, can no longer be employed; many other examples are described in these pages. The constraints imposed by increasing drug resistance on antibiotic choice are most severe in the hospital environment, in which selection of resistant and virulent organisms takes place most easily. However, the past decade has seen the global problem of reduced susceptibility of *Streptococcus pneumoniae* to penicillin with an increasing incidence of therapeutic failures among community infections such as otitis media and, more seriously, pneumococcal meningitis.

Drug resistance is by no means exclusive to bacteria. In the few years in which effective chemotherapy has become available to treat HIV infection, drug resistance (phenotypic as well as genotypic) is the major reason for disease progression in developed countries. Among fungi, primary and acquired resistance to azole antifungals is increasingly recognized among *Candida* spp. Worldwide resistance of *Plasmodium falciparum* to chloroquine and other drugs is a major cause of failure of therapeutic and prophylactic control of this disease.

The optimal use of antimicrobial agents can best be considered first in the context of choice for the individual patient, and second in the context of policies for the control of antibiotic usage in general. These may be devised for a particular clinical problem or unit, or may form part of a control program used in a hospital, in community practice or even nationally or internationally (see Ch. 11).

ANTIBIOTIC PRESCRIBING FOR THE INDIVIDUAL PATIENT

L.P. Garrod, the senior co-author of earlier editions of this book, wrote that:

> successful chemotherapy must be rational, and rational treatment demands a diagnosis. This may only be provisional, and it may later be proved wrong, but the treatment chosen should be based on some explicit assumption as to the nature of the disease process. This may or may not carry with it an implication that the cause is a particular micro-organism.

Many failures of therapy, sometimes with tragic consequences, result from neglecting to observe this basic precept. Thus, a patient may be treated for presumed postoperative septicemia with agents appropriate only for Gram-negative aerobic bacteria when such a syndrome can as well be caused by Gram-positive cocci. The treatment must in fact be aimed at the micro-organism and not at the disease as such. For a few diseases, the clinical diagnosis implies a specific microbial diagnosis with a known, or at least highly probable, drug susceptibility pattern. Thus, diagnoses of erysipelas or scarlet fever imply causation by *Streptococcus pyogenes* and susceptibility to penicillin, meningococcal septicemia with its almost pathognomonic rash implies causation by *Neisseria meningitidis* and, with occasional exceptions, susceptibility to penicillin, and severe chicken pox with primary pneumonia indicates causation by varicella-zoster virus and susceptibility to aciclovir.

In another group of infections, the causal organism is implicit in the clinical diagnosis but its antibiotic susceptibility cannot be inferred from the diagnosis. Examples, such as typhoid fever caused by *Salmonella enterica* serotype Typhi or a carbuncle caused by *Staphylococcus aureus* can be cited. In these cases, when antibiotics need to be used before or without laboratory help, factors in drug choice must include previous local laboratory or epidemiological information which may indicate the likely susceptibility pattern.

Unfortunately, a large number of infections fit into neither of these categories. Syndromes such as pneumonia, meningitis or pyelonephritis can each be caused by diverse organisms, and clinical information is of limited value in deciding between them. Initial management, if early microbiological information is unavailable or has not contributed – indeed, management throughout if laboratory facilities do not exist – must therefore be based on an explicit analysis of the likely or possible causal organisms and of their relative importance as pathogens. Clearly the decision pathway pursued by the clinician must vary considerably depending on the availability of laboratory services and on their degree of sophistication and skill, and on the time taken to produce a clinically meaningful result. The role of microbiological diagnosis is crucial in the optimal management of infectious diseases and is discussed in Chapter 9.

Decision-making about antibiotic choice in the individual patient can be facilitated by the use of a simple checklist, which may also be found of value in teaching students and junior staff good habits of antimicrobial drug use.

Beginning with the premise that the patient has a microbial infection requiring treatment, the following aspects can be systematically considered:

- Which organism(s) is (are) the likely cause(s) of the syndrome and what is their relative importance?
- In the light of the presumed diagnosis what other steps should be taken to further diagnostic precision? Which specimens should be taken and how should they be handled? The answers obviously depend on the facilities available. Even when full laboratory facilities are available, many diagnostic failures are caused by poor handling of specimens, an aspect of diagnosis deserving more attention than it often receives.
- Which agents are available and active against the presumed cause or causes of the illness? Is their range of antimicrobial activity appropriate and what information is available about the likelihood of drug resistance?
- What is the mode of action of a particular drug? Is it bactericidal or bacteristatic against particular pathogens? This has relevance when treating infective endocarditis and febrile neutropenic patients in whom phagocytic function is either absent (as it is within an infected vegetation) or grossly impaired (as is the case in persons treated with cytotoxic drug regimens for malignant disease).
- What are the unwanted effects of the agents under consideration, and how may they be balanced against the likely benefits of therapy with each agent? Special attention should be paid to the patient's renal function and possible deleterious effects on it, and any known contraindication such as a previous hypersensitivity reaction; pre-existing disease such as epilepsy precludes the use of imipenem. Marrow suppressive agents such as ganciclovir should be avoided or used with utmost caution in granulocytopenic patients such as recent recipients of bone marrow transplants. Likewise,

the potential for toxicity resulting from drug interactions should be considered. For example, ciprofloxacin can result in toxic concentrations of theophylline if coadministered.

These preliminary considerations are used to determine initial choice of therapy and should lead to a proper balance between appropriate and unnecessary use.

- Having decided the most appropriate agent, what is the correct dose and dose interval and what is the correct route of administration?

The object of systemic treatment is to attain a drug concentration in blood and tissue at least several times the minimal concentration necessary to inhibit or kill the infecting organism. Standard dose regimens, based as they are on antimicrobial susceptibility of the relevant organisms and on the pharmacological properties of the drugs concerned, are usually satisfactory. More recently, pharmacodynamic principles in which the in-vitro susceptibility of a target pathogen is modeled against the usual dose–response curve of a drug has emerged as a useful predictor of clinical performance and is discussed in Chapter 4. Dosage often has to be reduced if the patient's renal function is impaired and the drug has a mainly renal route of excretion. On the other hand, the dose may have to be increased when the site of infection is relatively inaccessible to the agent chosen, for example, in the treatment of meningitis by penicillins or cephalosporins (*see* Ch. 53). Thus it is essential to consider dose in the individual patient.

Oral administration should be used if possible, but parenteral therapy is often necessary when speed of action is essential, when high serum concentrations need to be attained and when vomiting, bowel dysfunction or impaired consciousness make oral treatment potentially unreliable or impossible.

Topical treatment at the site of infection is appropriate in the management of a number of localized infections. For example, candidiasis of the vagina responds to topically applied antifungal agents such as azoles. Likewise, superficial infections of the eye and middle ear can be effectively treated with topically administered agents such as chloramphenicol and fluoroquinolones. However, for most deep-seated infections, local treatment at the site of infection is seldom necessary. Adequate antimicrobial drug concentrations can usually be achieved by high systemic dosage, even at relatively inaccessible sites such as cerebrospinal fluid (CSF) or joint cavities, and against the apparent advantage of local administration must be set the possibility of local tissue damage by the antibiotic solution used. If local treatment is thought necessary, careful attention to the correct preparation and dose is essential. The potential dangers of intrathecal or intraventricular administration are especially to be borne in mind, and many tragedies have resulted from miscalculation of the dose of penicillin appropriate for intrathecal use. Intrathecal agents, which are in any case rarely needed, should never be given except after careful discussion with informed authorities of the necessity of doing so, and most rigorous checking of preparation and dose.

- What is the correct duration of treatment? Antimicrobial drugs are often continued for an unnecessarily prolonged time or are discontinued too soon. It is regrettable that the correct duration of therapy has been established for relatively few infectious diseases. Good clinical trials data support the current regimens for treating pulmonary tuberculosis and infective endocarditis resulting from penicillin-susceptible or insusceptible viridans streptococci and enterococci. Support for single-dose therapy of uncomplicated bacteriuria exists but this has to be balanced against slower resolution of the inflammatory response to infection. Hence many authorities recommend a 3-day regimen. However, for the vast majority of common infectious diseases treatment duration relies on resolution of the host response to infection rather than a microbiological eradication. Duration of therapy is discussed in relation to individual indications throughout this book, but in hospital patients frequent, at least daily, review of drug charts is a sound rule.

- Is the treatment working? Antimicrobial drug therapy cannot of course be considered in isolation and other aspects of therapy, many of them crucially important, must be taken into account in judging the effect of treatment. Even an 'appropriate' antibiotic may be ineffective if pus is not drained, bacterial shock treated and hypoxia and anemia corrected. The main criteria of success are the normal clinical ones: well-being, resolution of fever, tachycardia and abnormal signs. In some infections, however, therapeutic drug monitoring employs antibiotic assays in order to ensure that concentrations have reached effective but not toxic levels. The most common example in frequent use is the need for aminoglycoside assays (*see* pp. 118 and 161).

- What is the cost of the drug? In publicly funded hospitals, this aspect is considered mainly in the formulation of hospital antibiotic policies rather than in individual treatment. In many countries and in private facilities, antibiotic cost is a major constraint on choice of agent. Regrettably, acquisition costs frequently dominate thinking rather than cost-effectiveness, cost-benefit and cost-utility, which assess the impact of an intervention in relation to total disease management. These issues are discussed further in Chapter 11.

ANTIBIOTIC COMBINATIONS

Treatment with more than one agent is sometimes necessary but all too often is not. It should be noted that unnecessary polypharmacy not only adds to the cost of therapy but potentially exposes the recipient to a greater risk of drug toxicity. The rationale for combination therapy can be classified under five headings:

1. To achieve adequate 'cover' of the range of possible pathogens before full diagnosis is reached.
2. Mixed infections.
3. Prevention of drug resistance.
4. Reducing dosage of toxic agents.
5. Antibacterial synergy.

1. The most frequent indication is found on the many occasions when treatment of a seriously ill patient has to be initiated before the microbial diagnosis is established, and when the organisms to be considered as possible pathogens cannot all be 'covered' by the use of one agent. It is rarely required when treating patients in the community. The use is diminishing with the increasing variety of broad-spectrum agents. It is often then possible to switch to monotherapy when the responsible organism and its antimicrobial susceptibility are established.

2. In mixed infections, two agents are sometimes necessary to ensure activity against the pathogens concerned.

3. Combined treatment as a means of preventing the development of drug resistance is especially relevant to chronic infections and is of course firmly established as a cardinal feature in the treatment of tuberculosis and of leprosy (Chs. 60 and 61).

4. Occasionally, combined treatment can be used as a method of reducing dosage of a potentially toxic drug while achieving the same therapeutic end by its use in combination. The best authenticated example is the use of reduced dosage of amphotericin B in combination with flucytosine (itself unfortunately possessing substantial toxicity) in the treatment of cryptococcal meningitis (p. 849), although now less commonly adopted with the availability of fluconazole for this disease.

5. When antibiotics are combined in laboratory conditions, the combinations may prove additive, indifferent, synergistic or antagonistic. Where the effect is additive, the agents together behave as though the concentration of either had been increased; where indifferent, the combined effect is no different from that of either alone; and where antagonistic, the effect of the combination is less than that of either agent alone. The word 'synergy' is used with slightly different connotations in the contexts of bacteristatic and bactericidal tests. In the former, synergy denotes a combined effect significantly greater than that of either drug acting alone. The best known example is that of sulfonamides and trimethoprim, acting as they do on different stages of bacterial folate synthesis. The clinical significance of this type of combined action is uncertain.

   Bactericidal synergy is used to describe the phenomenon in which two drugs are individually incompletely bactericidal but which acting together are able to kill the inoculum completely. An inhibitory concentration of one drug will be required, but complete killing may be produced by the addition of a subinhibitory concentration of the second.

   This type of combined action is clinically important and is needed to achieve cure in certain cases of infective endocarditis, especially when the responsible organism is shown to be drug tolerant (p. 15), and in the treatment of septicemia in the immune suppressed, notably by combining an antipseudomonal β-lactam antibiotic such as ceftazidime and gentamicin to treat *Pseudomonas aeruginosa* infection.

These laboratory interactions and their clinical significance are discussed further in Section 3.

THE ROLE OF THE LABORATORY IN DIAGNOSIS AND TREATMENT

Since it is often impossible to determine by clinical analysis the identity, let alone the drug susceptibility, of the causal agent, the importance of sound microbiological practice and of good liaison between ward or clinic and laboratory cannot be overemphasized. Nevertheless, even when laboratory service is not available, it is often possible, by employing the foregoing principles of antibiotic use, to make a logical and successful choice of agent. In many parts of the world sophisticated laboratory facilities and trained staff are absent, but simple laboratory methods are often available to the clinician, and the scope for diagnosis can be much enlarged by the ability to reliably perform a Gram stain and a Ziehl–Neelsen stain on CSF or pus, to examine urine microscopically and to do blood, CSF and urine cultures.

When full laboratory facilities are available, it is essential that all appropriate specimens are taken before treatment is started (an occasional exception is the need sometimes to begin treatment in acute meningitis before lumbar puncture is done), and for the specimens to be handled properly and expeditiously. The responsibility for this stage in diagnosis, falling as it does between clinician and laboratory, is often badly executed and the cause of many missed opportunities for diagnosis. The proper collection, handling and examination of specimens in the diagnosis and management of infection is most important.

In most regimens of antibiotic treatment it is assumed from data acquired before marketing that concentrations achieved at the site of infection are adequate and not excessive. The low toxicity of many antibiotic groups, notably of the β-lactam compounds, makes this a reasonable assumption in most circumstances. For compounds with a low therapeutic ratio, notably the aminoglycosides, assay of concentrations in blood and occasionally in other body fluids is essential, to establish both that adequate concentrations have been achieved and that concentrations are not excessive. This is especially important in patients with impaired renal function.

The stages of laboratory control of antibiotic therapy may thus be summarized:

- Collection of appropriate specimens at the earliest possible moment and whenever possible before therapy has been started.
- Efficient and rapid transport of specimens to the laboratory.
- Microscopy, culture and identification.
- Susceptibility testing of significant isolates.

- When indicated, antibiotic assay in body fluids.
- When indicated, tests of combined antibiotic action.

ANTIBIOTIC CONTROL POLICIES (*SEE* CH. 11)

The search for rational and effective policies of antibiotic usage arises from increasing concern about the spread of resistant strains, the burden of unwanted effects from antimicrobial drugs and the mounting cost of the agents. Earlier studies on the use of antimicrobial drugs, mainly in hospitals, painted an alarming picture of widespread misuse, with a large proportion of prescriptions thought to be inappropriate, either because no antibiotic was indicated or because the agent and/or the dose chosen was incorrect. Later studies painted a less lurid picture, but it remains clear that, whether used wisely or not, antibiotic prescription is extremely common. Whilst most therapeutic use appears reasonably judicious, some is undoubtedly inappropriate, with particular difficulty in prophylactic use (this is considered further here and in Chapter 10), which in a number of surveys has accounted for about one-third of antibiotic prescriptions.

Antibiotic prescribing has also been studied in general practice. As might be supposed, variations in social and psychological history significantly affected the doctor's response and, despite a reasonably conservative prescribing pattern, there has been a trend towards an increase in antibiotic prescribing and a tendency to use a wider range of compounds. General practice formularies are doing much to improve and standardize antibiotic prescribing practice.

In any type of practice, whether in hospital or in the community, the use of drugs is affected by a number of pressures: uncertainties of diagnosis, the wish to treat the patient successfully, the desire for treatment on the part of the patient and the cultural framework affecting expectations of drug treatment in the particular community. It is perhaps simpler for a research team to define the criteria for proper antimicrobial drug usage than for the practising clinician to follow them. Moreover, even when social and psychological pressures are excluded, there is often substantial disagreement about what constitutes rational or irrational use of antimicrobial drugs, and in some of the studies the criteria might have been unreasonably rigorous. Nonetheless, for all these caveats, there is no doubt that antibiotic prescribing habits leave much room for improvement and much effort has been put into attempts to improve them.

There seems to be a strong case in favor of a positive policy for antibiotic prescribing which includes a prominent audit component enabling judgments to be made about the effect of the program. While it is not unduly difficult to measure unwanted clinical effects of antibiotics and to monitor the consumption and cost of drugs, measurement of the spread of drug resistance, the third major disadvantage of antibiotic use, presents much greater difficulties. Many individual studies show that drug-resistant organisms can be controlled by restrictive antibiotic policies, but the overall effects of even the most judicious prescribing policies are difficult to predict and require extensive study. These issues, and the measures which can be taken to develop antibiotic policies, are discussed fully in Chapter 11.

Three further general comments should be borne in mind in formulating antibiotic policies.

1. Many rational methods proposed for antibiotic control rely heavily on feedback from laboratory information (on isolation rates, antibiotic susceptibility patterns, etc.) and are thus inapplicable to antibiotic prescribing as it is practised in most parts of the world, including most general practice usage.
2. An important component of the problem is that of the initial clinical assessment (does the patient have an infection? What might be the cause?). Thus, standards of undergraduate and postgraduate teaching in medicine and especially infectious diseases are likely to be as important as, or more important than, administrative policies in determining patterns of antibiotic usage.
3. Efforts to control antibiotic usage in order to limit the spread of resistant strains are likely to be unsuccessful unless they are combined with vigorous cross-infection control policies. Their success depends, too, on a combination of sound administrative policies with adequate staffing levels and high standards of professional practice.

WORLD HEALTH ORGANIZATION ESSENTIAL DRUG LIST

Control of antibiotic usage on a much larger canvas than that so far discussed is being attempted through the medium of the WHO Essential Drug List, a series of recommendations proposed by an international group of experts which, together with advice on other aspects of drug usage such as quality control, is published to act as a model for national policies.[1] The list is updated from time to time and Table 8.1 gives the antibacterial agents included in current recommendations. It is important to note that some of the agents (as indicated in the table) are given as examples of a therapeutic group and that in these cases alternative agents may be preferred, depending on national factors such as cost and availability. The full list includes routes of administration, dosage forms and strengths, together with other information such as the need for dose adjustment in renal failure.

Table 8.1 Antibacterial agents included in the WHO Essential Drug List[1]

Penicillins
Amoxicillin
Ampicillin
Benzathine penicillin
Benzylpenicillin
Cloxacillin
Phenoxymethylpenicillin
Piperacillin
Procaine benzylpenicillin
Restricted indications
Amoxicillin-clavulanic acid
Ceftazidime
Ceftriaxone
Imipenem-cilastatin
Other antibacterial drugs
Chloramphenicol
Ciprofloxacin
Doxycycline
Erythromycin
Gentamicin
Metronidazole
Spectinomycin
Sulfadiazine
Sulfamethoxazole + trimethoprim
Trimethoprim
Antileprosy drugs
Clofazimine
Dapsone
Rifampicin
Antituberculous drugs
Ethambutol
Isoniazid
Isoniazid + ethambutol
Pyrazinamide
Rifampicin
Rifampicin + isoniazid
Rifampicin + isoniazid + pyrazinamide + ethambutol
Streptomycin
Thiacetazone + isoniazid

Reference

1. World Health Organization Model List of Essential Drugs; definition, selection process, essential drug lists, 11th edition 1999: http://www.who.int/medicines/edl.html.

9 Laboratory control of antimicrobial therapy

Gunnar Kahlmeter

Most antimicrobial therapy is empirical. However, empirical therapy is based on the scientific evaluation of the outcome of clinical trials in which the result of drug therapy has been related to laboratory tests of the antimicrobial susceptibility of the causative micro-organisms and on clinical experience built up during the years following registration of a new antibiotic. The scientific proof of the effectiveness of a drug against certain micro-organisms in specific clinical situations is usually based on results with micro-organisms that lack resistance mechanisms because acquired resistance (i.e. resistance caused by a genetic alteration) is rare when the drug is new or because organisms with resistance to the drug are excluded by the clinical trials protocol. If factors determining therapeutic success (indications for therapy, drug formulation and dosing, target micro-organisms and antimicrobial susceptibility of target micro-organisms) were constant over time antimicrobial susceptibility testing in the routine microbiological laboratory would be unnecessary. However, due to the worldwide rapid increase of acquired antimicrobial resistance, empirical therapy becomes more and more uncertain and the foundation for empirical therapy needs constant re-evaluation. Due to sometimes major local differences in the occurrence of resistance, this re-evaluation has to be based on local resistance frequencies.

WHY SUSCEPTIBILITY TESTING?

Susceptibility testing is performed:

- To predict the outcome of antimicrobial chemotherapy in individual patients, i.e. as an instrument for directing antimicrobial chemotherapy.
- To predict the outcome of antimicrobial chemotherapy in future patients, i.e. for continuous evaluation of the basis for empirical therapy.
- To permit epidemiological intervention through:
  - the early detection of bacteria with certain resistance mechanisms in the hospital (methicillin-resistant *Staphylococcus aureus* (MRSA), glycopeptide non-susceptible enterococci or staphylococci, extended spectrum β-lactamase (ESBL) producing Gram-negative bacteria) and in the community (multiresistant *Mycobacterium tuberculosis*, multiresistant *Salmonella enterica* serotype Typhimurium, penicillin and/or multiresistant *Streptococcus pneumoniae*);
  - the early detection of trends in resistance frequencies and the identification of factors affecting the dynamics of such trends: consumption of antibiotics, infection control, associated resistance towards other antibiotics or other substances, crowding, etc. Knowledge obtained in this way forms the basis for national and local antibiotic policies and interventions and affects national and international legislation (i.e. the inhibition of the use of some antimicrobials as growth promoters in animal husbandry).

DEFINITION OF RESISTANCE AND THE CLASSIFICATION OF ANTIMICROBIAL SUSCEPTIBILITY

The antimicrobial susceptibility of bacteria and fungi is traditionally classified with the letters S, I and R for *Susceptible* or *Sensitive*, *Intermediate* or *Indeterminate* and *Resistant*. A bacterium classified susceptible is considered therapeutically available at standard doses of the antibiotic, provided the antibiotic is documented for use in that type of infection; 'resistance' implies the opposite. 'Intermediate' confers the message that, if the drug can be used at a higher dose or the antibiotic for pharmacokinetic reasons is concentrated at the site of infection, the micro-organism could be treated despite the presence of inferred low-level resistance. 'Indeterminate', as used by the Swedish Reference Group of Antibiotics, is a signal from the microbiologist to the clinician that the bacterium is now compromised (i.e. has acquired some degree of resistance) and that the interpretation is difficult in the individual patient.

A major problem with the classical definitions of susceptibility and resistance is that they confer different messages in different situations. We use the same classification system for predicting outcome of therapy in the individual patient (irrespective of patient age, type of infection, immune status, etc.) as we do for measuring resistance development as a function of the spread of resistance genes and the use and misuse of antimicrobials in human medicine, veterinary medicine, for growth promotion in animal husbandry and in food production. Clinicians often cry 'resistance must mean something to the clinician!' Their skepticism of susceptibility testing is expressed in Alan Percival's now classical 'Resistance is much more common in microbiologists than in microbes!' – a statement which was, but unfortunately is no longer, true. Consider the fact that NCCLS (the National Committee for Clinical Laboratory Standards of United States of America) breakpoints for erythromycin in *Haemophilus influenzae* for years have divided perfectly normal *Haemophilus* (without biological variation among the individual bacteria and without resistance mechanisms to macrolide antibiotics) into three almost 'equal' parts classified as S, I and R, respectively. It not only makes poor clinical sense to divide bacteria lacking in biological variation, it prevents reproducibility of susceptibility testing results and makes the measurement of resistance development and its correlation to macrolide consumption meaningless. The same population of *Haemophilus* was classified resistant by the BSAC (British Society for Antimicrobial Chemotherapy) breakpoints and indeterminate by the breakpoints of the SRGA (Swedish Reference Group of Antibiotics). So the R for resistance may on one hand convey the decision that an antibiotic is generally unsuitable in the treatment of a given bacterium and on the other hand announce the rather frightening acquisition of genes not normally present. The latter implies a dynamic situation, a 'development', an unwanted surprise to the clinician trusting empirical experience. Thus, our classical definitions of susceptibility and resistance need to be reconsidered. We should consider the use of two sets of breakpoints: 'clinical' breakpoints reflecting the clinical limits for antimicrobial chemotherapy and 'epidemiological' (or 'microbiological') breakpoints designed for early detection and quantitative description of the emergence of resistance. The former should be based on the correlation between minimum inhibitory concentrations (MICs) and clinical outcome of therapy where doses and duration of therapy were selected on the basis of pharmacologic and pharmacodynamic data. The latter should be based on the correlation between MICs and the presence and absence of resistance mechanisms. Epidemiological breakpoints should be used for epidemiological surveillance, for determining factors important for resistance development and for planning and measuring the effects of intervention.

DETECTION OF ANTIMICROBIAL RESISTANCE

The detection of resistance can be phenotypic or genotypic. Phenotypic methods are always in some way related to the MIC of the bacterium. Genotypic methods detect either a defined gene, such as *mecA* coding for methicillin resistance in staphylococci or the *van*-genes coding for glycopeptide resistance in enterococci, or the product of one or more related genes, such as the detection of β-lactamases with nitrocefin or of PBP2a with antibody kits. Genotypic tests tend to be either/or, i.e. if 'positive' the bacterium is considered resistant to the drug or to a complete class of drugs. Thus, with genotypic tests the clinical and epidemiological breakpoints are allowed to converge or expressed differently: the microbiological breakpoint is allowed to define the clinical breakpoint.

Phenotypic tests, such as MIC determination or agar disk diffusion, require interpretation and thus standardization of interpretative criteria as well as methodology to become meaningful. However, so far international agreement on interpretative criteria is lacking and there is no international standardization of methodology. While the international community is adressing these shortcomings, it is of utmost importance that phenotypic susceptibility testing is performed with quantitative methods and that the results of the tests (the MIC value or the inhibition zone diameter) are saved in databases for geographical and temporal comparisons.

THE MINIMUM INHIBITORY CONCENTRATION (MIC)

Antimicrobial susceptibility testing is traditionally based on the minimum inhibitory concentration (MIC; mg/l) for the antibiotic in question. All other methods relate to the MIC in one way or another. MIC values are at best determined in defined and highly standardized in-vitro systems. These give relative results – i.e. when the systems are at all manipulated (medium, additives, pH, ion content, incubation time, temperature, etc.) the results are very different.

The MIC determination is performed by subjecting the micro-organism to a series of two-fold concentrations, most often between 256 and 0.008 mg/l, in solid or liquid medium, in a defined atmosphere and for a defined period of time. The macroscopic inhibition of further cell division is measured as the lack or near lack of growth on a solid medium or as the lack of clouding in a liquid medium.

Most models for susceptibility testing use two MIC breakpoints to divide bacteria into the three susceptibility categories S, I and R defined above. In some techniques the breakpoint concentrations are incorporated in solid or liquid media, in which case two plates or two vials are needed. Growth at neither concentration equals susceptible, growth at the lower but not the higher concentration equals intermediate susceptibility and growth at neither concentration is interpreted as resistance, provided failure of the system can be ruled out (a control must be included). A number of automated or semi-automated systems on the market utilize this principle. Either the MIC value of the isolate and the corresponding S-, I- and R-interpretation is obtained, or the one- or two-concentration breakpoint system just described is utilized, whereby only the interpretation is given. Using one or two plates or vials with breakpoint concentrations is more difficult to control than using a purely quantitative technique such as MIC determination or agar disk diffusion with the measurement of zone diameters.

Etest®

The Etest® is a variation on MIC determination, which the manufacturer (AB Biodisk, Stockholm, Sweden) has calibrated against MIC determination. It is a diffusion method that enables MIC values to be estimated directly. A series of two-fold dilutions of an antibiotic are distributed along a special carrier strip from which the antibiotic can diffuse freely into the agar, creating a series of diffusion gradients. After incubation overnight, the MIC is read as being where the growth inhibition ellipse intersects the scale. Recommendations are provided by the manufacturers about standardization of the inoculum, type of medium to be used for different organisms and reading of the plates.

The Etest® has brought MIC determination to those clinical laboratories that did not previously do the rather elaborate work needed to set up a standard MIC test in solid or liquid medium. In the hands of someone with reasonable expertise the reproducibility is +/- 1 dilution step. When 25 Swedish laboratories were asked to Etest three type strains (*Staphylococcus aureus*, *Streptococcus pneumoniae* and *Enterococcus faecalis*) and a random fresh clinical isolate of respective species there was no difference in the distributions of MIC-values of the type strains and the clinical isolates, in both instances covering MICs of 2–3 dilution steps. This demonstrates the achievable interlaboratory variation of the Etest and the lack of biological variation among organisms within a species lacking resistance mechanisms.

Agar disk diffusion

The growth inhibition zone diameter obtained around a paper disk impregnated with a calibrated amount of antibiotic, which, during the incubation of the agar plate, creates a concentration gradient around the disk, constitutes a measure of the sensitivity of the bacterium to the antibiotic. The zone diameter is traditionally correlated to MIC determination through a regression analysis performed on the parallel MIC and disk results obtained with collections of clinical and type culture isolates. The MIC breakpoints are then transformed into corresponding zone diameter breakpoints through the regression analysis curve. In the classic Kirby–Bauer[2] and Ericsson & Sherris[3] regression analyses of parallel MIC values and zone diameters, a collection of bacteria are analyzed in a regression analysis involving many different species and all species receive common MIC and zone diameter breakpoints. To be able to characterize the slope of the regression line, it is often necessary to include species inherently insensitive to the drug, which are poorly representative of bacteria with acquired resistance. Thus, multi-species regression lines often do not reflect the relationship between MIC and zone diameter for future isolates with acquired resistance. A further complication is that although many species share a regression line, the compromise is not valid for some species. This means that despite the fact that the consensus breakpoints are common for all species, they may not be valid for all species.

The Kirby–Bauer method, described by Bauer and co-workers[2], is still the basis of the recommendations of the NCCLS in the USA The NCCLS-approved version of Kirby–Bauer emphasizes strict adherence to the NCCLS documents and standardization. The use of Mueller–Hinton agar as the only approved medium and an inoculum of confluent growth (rather than a semiconfluent growth) sets it apart from the recommendations of the Ericsson & Sherris[3] ICS report and most disk diffusion methods recommended by European groups. A reason for the European groups to adhere to the semiconfluent inoculum is that it is easier to control by eye and the results obtained (zone diameters) are less sensitive to variations in the inoculum.

Agar disk diffusion as a screening test

In situations where resistance is rare but clinically or epidemiologically important, and provided the zone diameter breakpoints are specific to the species and set very close to the native population, a routine standard disk diffusion test can be used as a screen test to single out suspicious isolates for further testing (i.e. methicillin resistance in *Staph. aureus*, penicillin resistance in *Str. pneumoniae*, glycopeptide resistance in enterococci, erythromycin resistance in streptococci, non-β-lactamase penicillin resistance in *H. influenzae*). In some cases the next step is a confirmatory test such as a polymerase chain reaction for the detection of the specific gene responsible for a known resistance mechanism (*mecA*-gene coding for methicillin resistance in staphylococci, the *van*-genes coding for glycopeptide resistance in enterococcal species). In other cases a follow-up MIC test in broth or agar, or an Etest®, provides a means for laboratories to more closely define the degree of reduced susceptibility. This is certainly true of *Str. pneumoniae* and of β-lactamase-negative *H. influenzae* with decreased sensitivity to β-lactam drugs.

MIC and zone diameter breakpoints

To decide on national MIC and zone diameter breakpoints, and in some instances to describe national methods and standards for susceptibility testing, many countries have formed breakpoint committees or antibiotic reference groups (*see below*) consisting of clinical microbiologists and infectious disease specialists and sometimes pediatricians, general practitioners, clinical pharmacologists and occasionally representatives of the pharmaceutical industries.

The MIC and zone diameter breakpoints published during the 1960s and 1970s were, with a few exceptions (*Neisseria gonorrhoeae*, *M. tuberculosis*), common for all bacterial species and for all clinical situations.

The Swedish Reference Group of Antibiotics (SRGA) was first to systematically collect large species-defined parallel databases of MIC values and zone diameter distributions of bacteria lacking resistance mechanisms. Their database of MIC and disk diffusion zone diameter distributions is in the public domain on the internet: http://www.srga.org. As the species-defined database grew two things became obvious:

- Unimodal distributions of MIC or zone diameters were identical irrespective of where in the world the isolates were collected, and in bimodal distributions only that part of the distribution consisting of non-native strains was affected (Figure 9.1).
- Breakpoints common for all species often failed in one of two principal ways. Either the breakpoint would divide biologically homogenous populations of a species in such a way that organisms without biological difference in their relationship to the drug in question would be classified as being

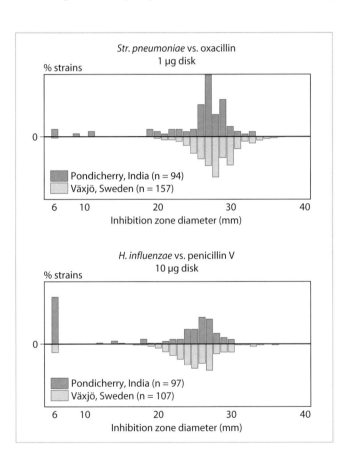

Fig. 9.1 Distributions of *Streptococcus pneumoniae* (top) tested against a disk of oxacillin 1 µg (as a screen test for penicillin resistance) and *Haemophilus influenzae* (bottom) tested against a disc of penicillin V 10 µg (as a screen test for both β-lactamase and resistance due to changes in penicillin-binding proteins in *H. influenzae*). In both graphs consecutive clinical isolates from India and Sweden were investigated simultaneously in one laboratory.[1] The graphs show that the distributions of pneumococci and *Haemophilus* in Sweden and India are very similar although there are more β-lactamase-producing *Haemophilus* in India.

different (this was detrimental to the reproducibility of susceptibility results) or, because the drug would be very active against a certain species (fluoroquinolones and *Neisseria* or *Haemophilus*), the common breakpoint would be so generous that resistance development would go undetected.

Figure 9.2 clearly suggests that the S/I breakpoint of 1 mg/l, as decided by most breakpoint committees, was originally set to ensure that *Pseudomonas aeruginosa* was classified as susceptible to ciprofloxacin. This was inevitable as the fluoroquinolones were welcomed as the first oral therapy against *Pseudomonas* infections. This breakpoint is thus well suited to ensure (1) that *Ps. aeruginosa* lacking quinolone resistance mechanisms are classified as susceptible to ciprofloxacin, (2) that *Ps. aeruginosa* that have acquired resistance mechanisms are immediately detected as having acquired new properties and as not fully susceptible. Furthermore, for *Ps. aeruginosa* it permits methodological reproducibility of susceptibility testing because the breakpoint is in a concentration interval where there are few or no native isolates. However, it should be obvious that a breakpoint of 1 mg/l is less suited for other species. The breakpoint divides biologically homogenous populations of wild-type staphylococci, streptococci and enterococci, which reduces the credibility of testing and obviates reproducibility. For *Neisseria*, *Haemophilus* spp. and Enterobacteriaceae reproducibility of susceptibility classification will not be a problem since even major resistance development will go undetected because the breakpoints are wide of the native population.

The only solution to this problem is to make species-related adjustments of breakpoints. This need is now recognized by most of the breakpoint committees. For more detailed discussions on species related breakpoints, see the web-site of the SRGA.

TESTS FOR β-LACTAMASE

Various methods are available for detection of β-lactamase activity. The most specific and also the most commonly used is the nitrocefin test. Alternative methods are the so-called 'cloverleaf' test, the acidometric method and the iodometric method.

The nitrocefin test is based on the use of a chromogenic cephalosporin, which is yellow when intact but changes color to red when its β-lactam bond is hydrolyzed by β-lactamase. Nitrocefin can be used in solution, as paper disks or strips. The color change is often rapid and can be read within 30 minutes. The nitrocefin test works well with *Staph. aureus* (preferably after induction with penicillin), *H. influenzae*, *Moraxella catarrhalis*, *N. gonorrhoeae*, *Neisseria meningitidis* and *E. faecalis* – β-lactamase production in the last two being very rare. Because of false-positive reactions, the nitrocefin test should not be used in *Staphylococcus saprophyticus*.

Enterobacteriaceae exhibit a multitude of enzymes, some of which hydrolyze nitrocefin and some of which do not. For this reason the detection of relevant β-lactamases in the clini-

Organism	MIC (mg/l)														
	≤0.004	0.008	0.016	0.032	0.064	0.125	0.25	0.5	1	2	4	8	16	32	≥64
Staphylococcus aureus						●	●	●							
Coagulase-negative staphylococci						●	●	●							
Staphylococcus saprophyticus								●	●	●					
Streptococcus pyogenes (GAS)							●	●	●						
Streptococcus agalactiae (GBS)								●	●	●					
Streptococcus pneumoniae								●	●	●					
Streptococcus miscellaneous							●	●	●	●					
Enterococcus spp.								●	●	●					
Listeria monocytogenes								●	●	●	●				
Pasteurella multocida			●	●	●										
Haemophilus influenzae		●	●	●	●										
Moraxella catarrhalis			●	●	●										
Neisseria meningitidis	●	●	●												
Neisseria gonorrhoeae	●	●													
Escherichia coli	●	●	●	●											
Klebsiella spp.	●	●	●	●											
Enterobacter spp.		●	●	●	●										
Proteus mirabilis		●	●	●	●										
Providencia spp.		●	●	●	●										
Pseudomonas aeruginosa						●	●	●	●						
Stenotrophomonas maltophilia									●	●	●	●			
Pseudomonas fluorescens		●	●	●	●										
Pseudomonas stutzeri		●	●	●	●										
Burkholderia cepacia						●	●	●	●	●					
Acinetobacter spp.				●	●	●	●	●							

Fig. 9.2 Ciprofloxacin MIC values of native bacteria lacking quinolone resistance mechanisms (from the website of the SRGA, URL www.srga.org/mictab/mic/miccip.html).

cal laboratory must be based on the outcome of phenotypic susceptibility testing of combinations of penicillins (with and without β-lactamase inhibitors) and cephalosporins. It is especially important to include an antibiotic which will make the laboratory suspect the presence of an extended-spectrum β-lactamase. Provided disk diffusion breakpoints are set close to the wild type populations of relevant species of Enterobacteriaceae the inclusion of cefotaxime and ceftazidime in the susceptibility test will disclose most producers of 'difficult β-lactamases', including the ESBLs.

DETECTION OF RESISTANCE GENES WITH MOLECULAR TECHNIQUES

The polymerase chain reaction (PCR) can be used for the detection of many resistance mechanisms. Examples are methicillin resistance in staphylococci (MRSA, MRSE) where the detection of the *mecA* gene coding for the rogue penicillin binding protein 2, PBP2a, classifies the staphylococcus as resistant to all marketed β-lactam antibiotics; and glycopeptide resistance in enterococci mediated by the *vanA*, *vanB* and *vanC* genes. PCR techniques for the detection of genes coding for β-lactamases, aminoglycoside-inactivating enzymes, macrolide resistance and others have also been described. However, in most of these instances the phenotypic susceptibility testing, utilizing disk diffusion or MIC determination, easily discriminates between resistant and susceptible isolates. This is not the case with MRSA (where there is considerable overlap in MIC values of *mecA*-positive and *mecA*-negative staphylococci) and glycopeptide-resistant enterococci (where MIC or disk diffusion techniques quite often fail to separate *vanB*-positive from native enterococci). In these cases, the polymerase chain reaction (PCR) is a very useful tool, especially in low-prevalence areas where epidemiological intervention in the form of sometimes cumbersome activities to prevent dissemination requires confirmation of the results of phenotypic methods.

QUALITY CONTROL

INTERNAL QUALITY CONTROL

All susceptibility testing needs tight quality control. Collaboration is vital between the clinical laboratory and the manufacturers of media, antibiotic disks, Etest®s, microtiter plates with ready-made antibiotic concentrations, producers of automated or semiautomated systems, etc. Disk diffusion testing can be performed with the same accuracy and precision as MIC determination.

Quality control must also be part of the daily routine in the laboratory to be of any real value. A choice of well-defined strains representing Gram-negative and Gram-positive bacteria and fastidious bacteria can be obtained from national reference groups of antibiotics and from type culture collections (e.g. ATCC, NCTC, CCUG). Choose 4–6 type strains (usually *E. coli, Ps. aeruginosa, Staph. aureus, Str. pneumoniae, Streptococcus pyogenes, N. gonorrhoeae*) and test them daily against the panels of antibiotics used in the daily routine. Control strains should be handled exactly as patient isolates. Record the MICs or the zone diameters and plot them graphically in a Shewart diagram for visual inspection. Define target values and action levels and decide on which actions should be taken if results fall outside these limits. Boards of accreditation require that laboratories can demonstrate valid internal and external quality control programs. Irrespective of method there is a need for saving and analysing consecutive clinical data and for repeatedly calibrating one's antimicrobial susceptibility testing.

EXTERNAL QUALITY ASSESSMENT

Most external quality assessment programs distribute microorganisms with defined resistance mechanisms. The international external quality assessment scheme for clinical microbiology organized from the UK (the NEQAS program: www.pcug.co.uk/~ukneqasm) has a wide coverage, with laboratories from all over Europe and many other parts of the world as subscribers. Evaluations of the proficiency of European laboratories have been published on several occasions, showing that in many laboratories there is still a lack of know-how and quality control.[4]

The Swedish Reference Group of Antibiotics has devised a model for combined external quality assessment and national surveillance of antimicrobial resistance.[5] It is based on the fact that MIC and zone diameter distributions of consecutive wild-type clinical isolates are invariably unimodal. For most bacteria the wild-type population (the remnant of the unimodal distribution) can be easily identified, and compared between laboratories. Laboratories subscribing to a standardized AST methodology (NCCLS, BSAC, SRGA) should exhibit closely similar wild-type distributions. The median value (reflecting accuracy and basic methodology) and the width and shape (reflecting reproducibility of inoculum, temperature, etc. within the laboratory) of the distributions form the basis for discussions on standardization of methodology and proficiency within and between laboratories. The percentage of isolates deviating from the identifiable wild-type population constitute the frequency of true resistance (isolates harboring resistance mechanisms) of bacteria, and when many laboratories partake in the program it becomes a useful tool for combined external quality control and resistance surveillance. The Swedish program has run for 8 years and today forms a successful part of national methodological standardization and national surveillance of antimicrobial resistance development. See ResNet on http://www.smittskyddsinstitutet.se.

External quality assessment programs are sometimes criticized for distributing strains with too obvious results and without challenge. However, with ambiguous strains the discussion will focus on what the correct result should be rather than on the proficiency of the laboratory. A proportion of the laboratories fail even though the chosen strains harbor obvious resistance mechanisms. One should also consider that laboratories subscribing to quality assurance programs are probably more proficient than those that do not. National efforts to encourage laboratories to take part in such programs are needed. Regulatory or otherwise 'encouraged' accreditation is now a reality in many countries. Hopefully the bodies responsible for accreditation will work closely together with the profession to further the cause of reliable and meaningful susceptibility testing and thus create a foundation for useful antimicrobial resistance surveillance.

ANTIBIOTIC BREAKPOINT COMMITTEES AND/OR REFERENCE GROUPS FOR ANTIBIOTICS

Many countries have their own antibiotic breakpoint committees and/or reference groups for antibiotics. Some of these, are listed here.

- **BSAC** (British Society for Antimicrobial Chemotherapy, http://www.bsac.org.uk, UK).
- **CA-SFM** (Comité de l'ántibiogramme de la Société Française de Microbiologie, http://www.sfm.asso.fr).
- **CRG** (Commissie Richtlijnen Gevoeligheids-bepalingen, The Netherlands).
- **DIN** (Deutsches Institut für Normung, http://www.din.de, Germany).
- **MENSURA** (Spain).
- **FIRe** (Finland).
- **NCCLS** (National Committee for Clinical Laboratory Standards, http://www.nccls.org).
- **NWGA** (Norwegian Working Group on Antibiotics, Norway).
- **SRGA** and **SRGA-M** (Swedish Reference Group of Antibiotics and its subcommittee on methodology, http://www.srga.org).

Many of the reference groups are more than just breakpoint committees. Several publish guidelines on methodology, on internal and external quality assurance, on the characterization and use of reference strains; some take on education of laboratory personnel, surveillance of antimicrobial resistance and liaison with authorities, regulatory bodies, the medical profession and pharmaceutical industry.

Apart from the national groups, ESCMID (European Society of Clinical Microbiology and Infectious Diseases, www.escmid.org) has formed a joint committee, the EUCAST (The European Committee on Antimicrobial Susceptibility Testing), with the purpose of bringing together the national efforts of the European countries.

ANTIBIOTIC ASSAY

Assays of antibiotic concentrations in serum and other body fluids were developed with the introduction of the modern aminoglycosides during the 1960s and 1970s. A vast number of articles described various assay methods and nomograms for ensuring therapeutic and non-toxic concentrations of gentamicin, tobramycin, amikacin and netilmicin. At the same time the first serious attempts were made to measure and describe antimicrobial tissue concentrations and their relation to therapeutic effect. Pharmacokinetic and eventually pharmacodynamic modeling also depended on the development of assays for measuring the concentration of antimicrobial drugs.

The monitoring of antimicrobial drug therapy is performed for four main reasons.

- To ensure therapeutic concentrations – especially where the therapeutic margin is narrow (aminoglycosides) or where there are wide individual variations in the pharmacokinetics of the drug (e.g. rifampicin, isoniazid).
- To avoid potentially toxic concentrations (e.g. aminoglycosides, vancomycin).
- To prevent accumulation of drug (aminoglycosides, fluoroquinolones in the elderly) – most often caused by deteriorating renal function.
- To ensure compliance and bioavailability in long-term oral therapy.

Apart from the listed reasons, it is preferable to optimize drug therapy in the very sick patients on multidrug therapy in whom drug interactions, failing renal function, dialysis and other factors affecting pharmacokinetics may make dosing difficult even at the best of times. Assaying and reporting drug concentrations in mg/l may be a job well done, provided it has been performed with relevant and well maintained equipment, well educated staff, and appropriate internal and external quality control programs. However, anyone who takes on antimicrobial assaying should also be prepared to interpret the results and give advice as to actions needed to bring drug concentrations to within the appropriate range.

A routine clinical laboratory should be able to measure and advise on the serum concentrations of at least one, possibly two, aminoglycosides and vancomycin.

The measurement of aminoglycoside concentrations is important for three reasons:

1 Aminoglycosides are potentially oto- and nephrotoxic. Ototoxicity is to some degree directly related to high drug serum levels, whereas nephrotoxicity causes increasing serum levels of drugs cleared by glomerular filtration, among which are the aminoglycosides.
2 In trying to avoid potentially toxic serum levels the clinician runs the risk of under-dosing the patient.
3 Aminoglycoside therapy administered as part of intensive care or over longer periods is always accompanied by some degree of renal function deterioration (i.e. the drug negatively affects its own major pathway of elimination). Accumulation of drug, common when therapy goes beyond 3–5 days, and should be prevented by monitoring pre-dose levels.

Vancomycin serum levels are measured mainly to ensure that therapeutic levels are attained but high levels of vancomycin should be avoided.

ENZYME IMMUNOASSAYS

Many clinical laboratories measure aminoglycoside and vancomycin concentrations with the Abbott fluorescence polarization immunoassay (which can be used with the Abbott TDx, FLx or AxSYM analyzers depending on the equipment of the laboratory). Teicoplanin can be measured with the same equipment but in that case the reagents for the teicoplanin assay must be obtained from Innofluor FPIA (Oxis, Portland, Oregon, USA).

PLATE DIFFUSION METHODS

Assaying modern antibiotics in modern multidrug medicine using plate assays is a juggling act with many pitfalls. To validate a battery of test organisms with the appropriate susceptibilities and resistancies and a proper stability to additive and synergistic activities between modern antimicrobial and anticancer chemotherapeutics is a challenge best avoided. However, in skilful hands and when the pitfalls can be avoided, plate assays can be performed with a high degree of reproducibility.

HIGH-PERFORMANCE LIQUID CHROMATOGRAPHY (HPLC)

This technique depends on the test drugs, in a mobile phase, having differential retention times when passed under pressure down a particle column. Metabolites of antimicrobial agents usually exhibit different retention times and the method has the advantage of being able to quantify metabolites as well as parent substance. Aminoglycosides, vancomycin, teicoplanin and several cephalosporins can be measured with HPLC.

RADIOIMMUNOASSAY

Radioimmunoassays for the detection of antibiotics in clinical samples are no longer used.

The reader is referred to the excellent and recently updated *Clinical Antimicrobial Assays*[6] for more detailed information on assaying antimicrobial drugs.

References

1. Larsson C et al 1999 *Clinical Microbiology and Infection* 5: 740–747.
2. Bauer AW, Kirby W, Sherris J, Turck M 1966 Antibiotic susceptibility testing by a standardized single disk method. *American Journal of Clinical Pathology* 45: 493–496.
3. Ericsson HM, Sherris JC 1971 Antibiotic sensitivity testing. Report of an international collaborative study. *Acta Pathologica et Microbiologica Scandinavica, Section B* (Suppl. 217): 1–90.
4. Snell JJ, Brown DF 2001 External quality assessment of antimicrobial susceptibility testing in Europe. *Journal of Antimicrobial Chemotherapy* 47: 801–810.
5. Kahlmeter G, Olsson-Liljequist B, Ringertz S 1997 Antimicrobial susceptibility testing in Sweden. Quality assurance. *Scandinavian Journal of Infectious Diseases, Supplement* 105: 24–31.
6. Reeves DS, Wise R, Andrews JM, White LO 1999 *Clinical Antimicrobial Assays*. Oxford University Press, Oxford.

10 Principles of chemoprophylaxis

S. Ragnar Norrby

Chemoprophylaxis aims at preventing clinical infections and should be separated from early treatment. Prophylactic use of antimicrobial drugs has been established in several types of surgery to prevent post-operative infections. In patients with certain heart disorders antibiotic treatment is recommended to prevent endocarditis following invasive procedures that may lead to bacteremia (e.g. dental treatment and urogenital surgery). Patients who are neutropenic or otherwise immunocompromised often receive prophylactic antibiotics and/or antifungal or antiviral agents to prevent infections.

These are all examples of primary prophylaxis; the aim is to prevent infections occurring. Other examples include prophylactic use of antimalarial drugs in travelers (see Ch. 64) and prophylaxis against *Pneumocystis carinii* pneumonia in HIV-infected patients with low CD4-lymphocyte counts. Following certain infections in immunocompromised patients (e.g. those with AIDS who have had *P. carinii* pneumonia or *Cryptococcus neoformans* meningitis) secondary chemoprophylaxis is used to prevent recurrences of the infections for as long as the patient remains immunodeficient.

SURGICAL PROPHYLAXIS

Several surgical procedures (such as abdominal surgery with enterotomies, transvaginal surgery and lung surgery) will result in spillage of material, that contains the normal bacterial flora. In other types of surgery the risk of postoperative infection is increased by the use of foreign material, such as hip and knee prostheses. Prophylactic use of antibiotics has been found to reduce the incidence of postoperative bacterial infections in these procedures. In other types of surgery in which spillage is not a major problem and where foreign bodies are not implanted, advantages of prophylaxis cannot be proven and its use is often doubtful. Table 10.1 gives examples of types of surgery where antibiotic prophylaxis has been proven to be beneficial, where it is routinely used but with no solid documentation of efficacy and where it has been proven not to reduce the incidence of postoperative infections.[1]

Correct timing of antibiotic prophylaxis in surgery is essential. Treatment should aim at obtaining high antibiotic con-

Table 10.1 Need for antibiotic prophylaxis in various surgical procedures.[1]

Procedures for which antibiotic prophylaxis is documented and indicated
- Esophageal, gastric and duodenal surgery
- Intestinal surgery
- Acute laparotomy
- Transurethral or tranvesical prostatectomy
- Total hysterectomy
- Cesarean section
- Surgical legal abortion
- Amputations
- Reconstructive vascular surgery (not surgery on the carotid arteries) with or without the use of grafts
- Cardiac surgery
- Pulmonary surgery

Procedures for which antibiotic prophylaxis is often used but with incompletely documented efficacy
- Pancreatic surgery
- Liver surgery (resection)
- Urological surgery with enteric substitutes
- Implanted urological prostheses
- Transrectal prostate biopsy
- Hemiplastic surgery in patients with cervical hip fractures
- Back surgery with metal implantation
- Aortic graft-stents
- Neck surgery

Procedures for which antibiotic prophylaxis is not documented or indicated
- Biliary tract surgery in patients with normal bile ducts and no stents
- Endoscopic examination of the urinary tract
- Reconstructive urethral surgery
- Arthroscopic procedures

centration in tissue and tissue fluids during the surgical procedure, and in particular when there is a high risk of contamination (e.g. when an enterotomy is performed). One study demonstrated that if antibiotics with short plasma half-lives were used, administration more than 2 h before or 3 h after surgery resulted in poor prophylactic effect.[2] Today it is agreed that surgical prophylaxis should be perioperative, i.e. it should be administered during surgery and terminated when the wound is closed.[3–6] Prolonged antibiotic prophylaxis is costly, gives no further benefits and increases the risk of selection of antibiotic-resistant bacteria.

ENDOCARDITIS PROPHYLAXIS

It is generally recommended that patients who have had endocarditis or known cardiac valvular defects and/or prostheses should be considered for antibiotic prophylaxis when subjected to certain procedures, including extensive dental surgery and treatment and genitourinary, gastrointestinal and respiratory tract surgery (i.e. medical interventions which increase the risk of bacteremia and the number of bacteria in bacteremia).[7] However, the scientific background for using antibiotic prophylaxis has recently been questioned.[8]

The choice of antibiotics in endocarditis prophylaxis has been modified in the latest recommendations from the American Heart Association.[7] For example, the standard regimen before dental and respiratory procedures is today 2 g amoxicillin 1 h before dental treatment or surgery; in patients hypersensitive to penicillin, erythromycin has been replaced by clindamycin or azithromycin.

PREVENTION OF TRAVELERS' DIARRHEA

Up to 50% of travelers to tropical and subtropical countries will develop travelers' diarrhea. The most common pathogens causing this condition are strains of *Escherichia coli* producing enterotoxin (ETEC), *Campylobacter* spp., *Vibrio parahaemolyticus*, *Vibrio cholerae*, *Salmonella enterica* serotypes, and *Shigella* spp. In addition diarrhea may be the result of food poisoning with bacterial toxins produced by *Staphylococcus aureus*, *Bacillus cereus* or *Clostridium perfringens*. Vaccines are available only against *V. cholerae* (one of the cholera vaccines may also give short-term protection against ETEC) and *Salmonella* Typhi.

Chemoprophylaxis using trimethoprim/sulfamethoxazole, doxycycline, fluoroquinolones or other antibiotics effectively decreases the incidence of travelers' diarrhea. Arguments against such use of antibiotics are the risks of adverse effects and of emergence of resistance. However, prophylaxis should be considered in individuals with underlying diseases that may be complicated by acute diarrhea, e.g. people with diabetes mellitus, reactive arthritis or inflammatory bowel disease. Patients treated with drugs that reduce the gastric acidity should also be considered for prophylaxis because they are at increased risk of developing diarrhea due to a defective acidic barrier.

PROPHYLAXIS AGAINST MENINGOCOCCAL DISEASE

It is well known that individuals who have had close contact with a patient with meningococcal disease are at increased risk of developing the disease. Two types of prophylaxis have been used. The most common one is to use ciprofloxacin or rifampicin in order to eradicate carriage of *Neisseria meningitidis*. Another approach, commonly used in Norway, is to treat contacts of a patient with meningococcal disease with penicillin V for 7 days. Such a regimen will prevent disease but will not eradicate carriage. For further details, see Chapter 53.

CHEMOPROPHYLAXIS IN PATIENTS WITH IMMUNE DEFICIENCIES

Prophylactic antibiotics and antiviral drugs are commonly used in patients with various types of immune deficiencies and are summarized in Table 10.2. The use of primary and secondary

Table 10.2 Primary chemoprophylaxis in immunodeficient patients

Type of immune deficiency	Prophylaxis against	Drugs used
Organ transplantation (Chapter 43)	*Pneumocystis carinii*	Trimethoprim/sulfamethoxazole
	Herpes simplex	Aciclovir
	Cytomegalovirus	Ganciclovir, aciclovir
	Candida infections	Azole antifungals
Neutropenia (Chapter 43)	Bacterial infections	Various
	Candida infections	Azole antifungals
Asplenia	Pneumococcal infections	Penicillin V
HIV-infection (Chapter 46)	*Pneumocystis carinii*	Trimethoprim/sulfamethoxazole
	Toxoplasma gondii	Trimethoprim/sulfamethoxazole
	Atypical mycobacteria	Various
	Neonatal transmission	Antiretroviral drugs

prophylaxis against *P. carinii* pneumonia with trimethoprim/sulfamethoxazole (which also seems to prevent *Toxoplasma gondii* encephalitis) and secondary prophylaxis against *C. neoformans* meningitis have been proven to be effective. Primary prophylaxis against fungal infections, especially those caused by *Candida* spp. in HIV-positive patients, seems more doubtful since the time during which prophylaxis is used by necessity must be long and might result in selection of resistant strains, especially when oral treatment with an azole antifungal agent such as fluconazole or itraconazole is used. Importantly, it has been demonstrated that during effective, so-called 'highly active' antiretroviral treatment (HAART), pneumocystis prophylaxis can be discontinued without negative effects.[9]

Another type of prophylaxis in HIV-infected patients that has been proven to be effective is the administration of zidovudine or other antiretroviral drugs to pregnant women and to their newborn children in order to prevent intrauterine and neonatal transmission of HIV.

References

1. Swedish-Norwegian Consensus Group 1998 Antibiotic prophylaxis in Surgery: summary of a Swedish-Norwegian consensus conference. *Scandinavian Journal of Infectious Diseases* 30: 547–557.
2. Classen DC, Evans RS, Pestotnik SL, Horn SD, Menlove RL, Burke JP 1992 The timing of prophylactic administration of antibiotics and the risk of surgical wound infections. *New England Journal of Medicine* 326: 161–169.
3. Waddell TK, Rotstein OD 1994 Antimicrobial prophylaxis in Surgery. *Canadian Medical Association Journal* 151: 925–931.
4. Page CP, Bohnen JMA, Fletcher JR, McManus AT, Solomkin JS, Wittman DH 1993. Antimicrobial prophylaxis for surgical wounds. *Archives of Surgery* 128: 79–88.
5. Norrby SR 1996 Cost-effective prophylaxis in surgical infections. *Pharmaco-Economics* 10: 129–140.
6. Bucknell SJ, Mohajeri M, Low J, McDonald M, Hill DG 2000 Single-versus multiple-dose antibiotic prophylaxis for cardiac surgery. *Australian and New Zealand Journal of Surgery* 70: 409–411.
7. Dajani AS, Taubert KA, Wilson W et al 1997 Prevention of bacterial endocarditis: recommendations by the American heart Association. *Clinical Infectious Diseases* 25: 1448–1458.
8. Strom BL, Abrutyn E, Berlin JA et al 1998 Dental and cardiac risk factors for infective endocarditis. A population-based, case-control study. *Annals of Internal Medicine* 129: 761–769.
9. Furrer H, Egger M, Opravil M et al 1999 Discontinuation of primary prophylaxis against *Pneumocystis carinii* pneumonia in HIV-1-infected adults treated with combination antiretroviral therapy. Swiss HIV Cohort Study. *New England Journal of Medicine* 340: 1301–1306.

 ## Further Information

Benson CA, Williams PL, Cohn DL et al 2000 Clarithromycin or rifabutin alone or in combination for primary prophylaxis of *Mycobacterium avium* complex disease in patients with AIDS: A randomized, double-blind, placebo-controlled trial. The AIDS Clinical Trials Group 196/Terry Beirn Community Programs for Clinical Research on AIDS 009 Protocol Team. *Journal of Infectious Diseases* 181: 1289–1297.

Dobay KJ, Freier DT, Albear P 1999 The absent role of prophylactic antibiotics in low-risk patients undergoing laparoscopic cholecystectomy. *American Surgeon* 65: 226–228.

Fleschner SM, Avery RK, Fisher R et al 1998 A randomized prospective controlled trial of oral acyclovir versus oral ganciclovir for cytomegalovirus prophylaxis in high-risk kidney transplant recipients. *Transplantation* 66: 1682–1688.

Kreter B, Woods M 1992 Antibiotic prophylaxis for cardiothoracic operations. Meta-analysis of thirty years of clinical trials. *Journal of Thoracic and Cardiovascular Surgery* 13: 606–608.

Lallemant M, Jourdian G, Le Coeur S et al 2000 A trial of shortened zidovudine regimens to prevent mother-to-child transmission of human immunodeficiency virus type 1. Perinatal HIV Prevention Trial (Thailand) Investigators. *New England Journal of Medicine* 343: 1036–1037.

Mittendorf R, Aronson MP, Berry RE et al 1993 Avoiding serious infections associated with abdominal hysterectomy; a meta-analysis of antibiotic prophylaxis. *American Journal of Obstetrics and Gynecology* 142: 1119–1124.

Nucci M. Biasoli I, Aiti T et al 2000 A double-blind, randomized, placebo-controlled trial of itraconazole capsules as antifungal prophylaxis for neutropenic patients. *Clinical Infectious Diseases* 30: 300–305.

Salminen US, Viljanen TU, Valtonen VV, Ikonen TE, Sahlman AE, Harjula AL 1999 Ceftriaxone versus vancomycin prophylaxis in cardiovascular surgery. *Journal of Antimicrobial Chemotherapy* 44: 287–290.

Sawaya GF, Grady D, Kerlikowske K, Grimes DA 1996 Antibiotics at the time of induced abortions: the case for universal antibiotic prophylaxis based on a meta-analysis. *Obstetrics and Gynecology* 87: 884–890.

Wiström J, Norrby SR 1995 Fluoroquinolones and bacterial enteritis. *Journal of Antimicrobial Chemotherapy* 36: 23–40.

11 Antibiotic policies

P. Davey, D. Nathwani and E. Rubinstein

Increasing antibiotic resistance is a global public health problem and control of antibiotic prescribing is a crucial part of any strategy to limit the development of resistance.[1-3] In 1990 the *Drug and Therapeutics Bulletin* concluded that local prescribing formularies are worth the time and money they take to produce, improve the quality of prescribing and reduce the overall costs in hospitals and in general practice.[4] Nonetheless, in 1994 only 62% of 427 UK hospitals had a policy for antibiotic therapy and only 75% an antibiotic formulary.[5] In 2001 the House of Lords Select Committee on Science and Technology again had to urge the Department of Health to pursue any hospitals which do not yet have a formal prescribing policy.[2] In the USA all of the 47 hospitals surveyed in 2000 had an antibiotic formulary[6] but only 47% had written policies for surgical prophylaxis, a key area of antibiotic misuse.[7] The problems of antibiotic resistance linked to widespread prescribing of antibiotics are even more pressing in developing countries: in India and Sri Lanka 66% of community prescriptions include an antimicrobial; in Bangladesh and Egypt antibiotic use accounts for 54% and 61% respectively of all hospital prescribing.[8]

In this chapter we review the aims of antibiotic policies, the methods for policy implementation or evaluation and the evidence that policies achieve their aims.

STIMULI FOR THE INTRODUCTION OF ANTIBIOTIC POLICIES

Many of the stimuli for antibiotic policies are common to policies for other drug groups, but some are unique to antibiotics (Table 11.1). The general advantages of defining a core list of drugs that are used regularly have been recognized for many years by the World Health Organization.[9] The aim is to encourage rational prescribing, which is based on knowledge of pharmacology, efficacy, safety and cost. Drug resistance among microbes is a unique stimulus to control of antibiotic prescribing.

PRACTICAL ADVANTAGES OF LIMITING THE RANGE OF ANTIMICROBIALS PRESCRIBED

In the hospital, the prescription of an antimicrobial by a clinician has implications for nurses, pharmacists and microbiologists, who will all be involved in preparation, administration and monitoring of the prescribed drug. Limiting the range of drugs used allows the team to become familiar with the necessary processes.[10] Many of the staff who take responsibility for these processes will rotate through several departments in the hospital or will provide cross-cover outside working hours. Having common policies within and between clinical directorates reduces the need for time-consuming retraining of staff as they move between clinical units. The need for antibiotic policies in primary care has also been recognized.[11] In the microbiology laboratory sensitivity testing of bacteria will clearly be facilitated by restricting the range of drugs prescribed both in primary and secondary care. This has implications for the range of reagents the laboratory must stock, the number of separate tests that must be carried out on each microbe and the range of procedures for which staff must be trained.

Providers of healthcare are increasingly being asked for evidence about quality assurance. Auditing practice is possible only if standards of care have been defined. The narrower the range of drugs, the easier it is to write and audit detailed standards of care. It is also likely that staff will find it easier to comply with policies that cover a limited range of drugs.

COST

Antibiotics account for 3–25% of all prescriptions, 2–21% of the total market value of drugs in a single country,[12] and up to 50% of the drug budget in a hospital.[13] New drugs are inevitably more expensive than old drugs and new drugs will

Table 11.1 General and specific advantages of an antibiotic policy

Category	Benefits
Knowledge	*General*
	Promotes awareness of benefits, risks and cost of prescribing
	Facilitates educational and training programs within the healthcare setting
	Reduces the impact of aggressive marketing by the pharmaceutical industry
	Encourages rational choice between drugs based on analysis of pharmacology, clinical effectiveness, safety and cost
	Specific to antimicrobials
	Provides education about local epidemiology of pathogens and their susceptibility to antimicrobials
	Promotes awareness of the importance of infection control
Attitudes	*General*
	Acceptance by clinicians of the importance of setting standards of care and prescribing
	Acceptance of peer review and audit of prescribing
	Specific to antimicrobials
	Recognition of the complex issues underlying antimicrobial chemotherapy
	Recognition of the importance of the special expertise required for full evaluation of antimicrobial chemotherapy:
	Diagnostic microbiology
	Epidemiology and infection control
	Clinical diagnosis and recognition of other diseases mimicking infection
	Pharmacokinetics and pharmacodynamics
Behavior	*General*
	Increased compliance with guidelines and treatment policies
	Reduction of medical practice variation
	Specific to antimicrobials
	Improved liaison between clinicians, pharmacists, microbiologists and the infection control team
Outcome	*General*
	Improved efficiency of prescribing by increasing sensitivity (patients who can benefit receive treatment) and specificity (treatment is not prescribed to patients who will not benefit)
	Improved clinical outcome
	Reduces medicolegal liability
	Specific to antimicrobials
	Limit emergence and spread of drug-resistant strains

be heavily promoted by pharmaceutical companies. One of the aims of antibiotic policies is to encourage prescribers to continue to use older, more familiar drugs unless there are good reasons not to. Intravenous antibiotics are usually about 10 times more expensive than equivalent oral formulations and their administration requires additional consumables and staff time.[14] Policies that include specific recommendations about route of administration may reduce costs considerably.[15] Finally, limiting the range of drugs stocked allows the pharmacy to negotiate better prices for larger quantities of individual drugs and reduces the range of stock that is sitting on the pharmacy shelves.

QUALITY AND SAFETY OF PRESCRIBING

The importance of iatrogenic disease has been recognized and most countries now have national and local systems for monitoring drug safety. Iatrogenic disease caused by avoidable prescribing errors is relatively difficult to study but published data suggests that it is disturbingly common. For example, 47% of patients leaving a hospital emergency room in the USA received a prescription for a new drug, and 10% of these prescriptions introduced a potentially harmful drug interaction.[16] Errors in prescribing, monitoring, or administering drugs account for a quarter of successful claims for damages against general practitioners in the UK.[17] The risk of adverse drug reactions is non-linearly related to the number of drugs prescribed: in other words, if the number of drugs a patient is prescribed is increased from three to six, the risk of adverse effects is more than doubled.[18] Prescribing drugs that do not benefit the patient exposes them to unnecessary risk, and one study found that 26% of all adverse drug reactions in a hospital were caused by drugs that were prescribed unnecessarily.[19] Given that 36% of in patients will show some evidence of adverse drug reaction,[16] this means that 1 in 10 inpatients have an adverse reaction to a drug that they did not need to receive. Unnecessary prescribing of antimicrobials carries additional risks for the patient (increased risk of superinfection with *Clostridium difficile*) and the environment (selection of drug resistant bacteria, e.g. *Enterococcus faecalis*). Therefore, assessment of the quality of prescribing must consider several elements, including the risks and benefits of introducing another drug and of parenteral versus oral administration.

In practice it is very difficult to assess the appropriateness of an entire course of treatment, particularly in hospital: what is appropriate on one day may be inappropriate the next. This problem has been recognized in a practical system for reviewing each day of an antibiotic prescription and then computing the proportion of inappropriate days.[20] The term 'inappropriate' covers a multitude of sins, and encompasses both undertreatment and unnecessary overtreatment (Figure 11.1). Inappropriate prescribing is associated with increased costs of care, although prescribing errors may just be a marker for a generally poor quality of care.[20]

Monitoring of community prescribing is more difficult, especially where drugs are freely available over the counter. Self-medication rates reported include 51% in Ecuador, 70% in Thailand, 75% in Brazil, 82% in Ethiopia and 92% in the Philippines.[8] There are undoubtedly some potential advantages to increasing the availability of antibacterials without prescription, such as convenience for the patient, faster initiation of treatment and reduction in primary care workload;[21] however, in the European Union[1,3] and in North America[22] the risks of increasing access to antibacterials are thought to outweigh these benefits. The degree of control of supply of antibiotics is highly variable between countries (Table 11.2).

Until recently there was an inexorable increase in the number of prescriptions for antibiotics in the community in developed countries.[23] This trend has recently reversed and several countries have reported significant reduction of antibiotic prescribing in primary care.[2,24–26] Nonetheless there is still plenty of room for improvement. For example, in the Netherlands 75% of prescriptions for otitis media in primary care were judged to be unnecessary.[27]

RESISTANCE

Other chapters in this book describe the mechanisms and epidemiology of drug resistance. Control of antibiotic resistance has always been a primary stimulus to the development of antibiotic policies.[28] The global escalation of antibiotic resistance might be seen as evidence that policies have failed, but that

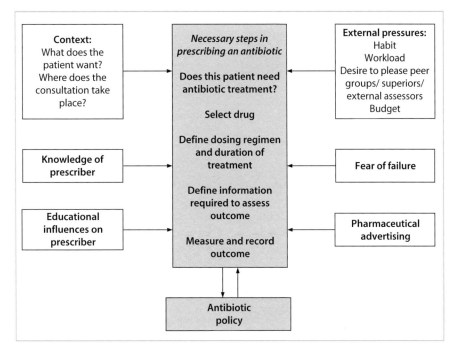

Fig. 11.1 Factors involved in antibiotic prescribing.

Table 11.2 Definition of categories for policies, laws and regulations pertaining to antibiotics (adapted from the report of a NIH taskforce)[86]

Category and designation	Basis for assignment
A. Comprehensive	1. *No* free sale allowed 2. Professional limits placed on prescription practices by law 3. Statutory control of advertising; *no* advertising allowed to lay public 4. Content of advertising limited by law
B. Partial	1. *No* free sale allowed 2. *And* at least one of controls 2–4 above
C. Minimal	1. *No* free sale allowed 2. *But* none of controls 2–4 above
D. None	1. Free sale allowed without any restrictions
Application in practice and enforcement of compliance with regulation	
A. Complete	Tightly controlled availability; regulations rigorously enforced
B. Partial	Incomplete enforcement of controls, associated with limited availability of antibiotics to the public for other reasons, such as economics and/or logistic factors
C. Minimal	Incomplete enforcement of controls, associated with widespread availability of antibiotics as a result of failure to apply regulations in practice and absence of other constraining factors
D. None	No restrictive legislation; widespread availability

Grouping of 35 countries by laws/regulations and enforcement/compliance assessed by questionnaire in 1986. Countries were selected from Eastern and Western Europe, North, Central and South America, Africa, Asia and Oceania. Data were reported anonymously (locality within each category not reported).
For explanation of categories of laws/regulations and Enforcement/compliance see the table above.

Laws/regulations	Enforcement/compliance			
	1. Complete	2. Partial	3. Minimal	4. None
A. Comprehensive	11 (31.4%)	2 (0.6%)	5 (14.3%)	1 (0.3%)
B. Partial	2 (0.6%)	1 (0.3%)	3 (0.9%)	1 (0.3%)
C. Minimal		2 (0.3%)	1 (0.3%)	
D. None				6 (1.7%)

question is addressed in more detail at the end of this chapter. At this stage we can conclude that the existence and increase in antibiotic resistance are both powerful stimuli to antibiotic policies.

IMPLEMENTATION OF ANTIBIOTIC POLICIES

It is very easy to be too ambitious in setting aims for guidelines or policies. The first aim should be to change medical practice,[29] which may have a variety of secondary aims (e.g. reducing drug costs, improving quality of prescribing, limiting drug resistance). The success of a policy at achieving these secondary aims cannot be assessed unless it has achieved or maintained a specified standard of practice. Ideally, antibiotic policies should recognize the complex process of prescribing an antibiotic (Figure 11.1). Nevertheless, a great deal of information can be captured within a simple flow chart, providing an easily accessible reminder to prescribers either on the wall of a treatment room or in a pocket-sized antibiotic policy.[30] However comprehensive or limited the policy, it is essential that information flows both ways. The policy will only truly succeed if the results of implementation are audited and the policy adapted in response to the information col-

Table 11.3 Core indicators for audit from the Scottish Intercollegiate Guidelines Network (SIGN) guidelines on surgical prophylaxis

Process measures
- Was prophylaxis given for an operation included in local guidelines?
- If prophylaxis was given for an operation not included in local guidelines, was a clinical justification for prophylaxis recorded in the case notes?
- Was the first dose of prophylaxis given within 30 minutes of the start of surgery?
- Was the prescription written in the 'once-only' section of the drug prescription chart?
- Was the duration of prophylaxis greater than 24 hours?

Outcome measures
- Surgical Site Infection (SSI) rate = number of SSIs occurring postoperatively/total number of operative procedures
- Rate of SSIs occurring postoperatively in patients who receive inappropriate prophylaxis (as defined in guideline) compared with rate of this infection in patients who receive appropriate prophylaxis, expressed as a ratio
- Rate of *C. difficile* infections occurring postoperatively in patients who receive inappropriate prophylaxis (as defined in guideline) compared with rate of this infection in patients who receive appropriate prophylaxis, expressed as a ratio

Minimum data set (MDS) for surgical antibiotic prophylaxis
- Date
- Operation performed
- Justification for prophylaxis (e.g. evidence of high risk of SSI) if prophylaxis is given for an operation that is not one of the indications for routine prophylaxis
- Time of antibiotic administration
- Elective or emergency
- Name, dose, route of antibiotic
- Time of surgical incision
- Number of doses given
- Classification of operation (clean/clean-contaminated/contaminated)
- Previous adverse reactions to antibiotics?
- Duration of operation
- Name of anesthesiologist
- Name of surgeon
- Designation of surgeon

lected.[31] It follows that it is necessary to develop indicators of whether or not the policy is being followed. These can be indicators of process or outcome and ideally should be agreed during the development phase of the policy and integrated into the overall quality assurance system for the organization.[32] Inclusion of targets for audit of implementation is a key component of the assessment of evidence-based guidelines.[33] Examples of core indicators for audit of a surgical antibiotic prophylaxis policy are given in Table 11.3. In the UK infection control has become a key target for clinical governance and risk management and will be incorporated into external review of quality and accreditation of institutions.

vide concurrent feedback of information about implementation (Table 11.4). However, this approach requires considerable investment of time by both the professionals carrying out the intervention and those who are its targets, plus information systems that are capable of providing concurrent, patient-specific feedback. Simply providing prescribers with educational information may be relatively unsuccessful (Table 11.4), but it also requires much less resource and so it could be a more cost-effective method for achieving change. As in most areas of medicine, the most complex and effective intervention available is not necessarily the most appropriate.[35]

METHODS FOR IMPLEMENTATION OF ANTIBIOTIC POLICIES

There is now a considerable literature of interventions to improve professional practice: a systematic review published in 1995 identified 102 trials in this area.[34] The title of this review states that there are 'No magic bullets', meaning that it is not possible to provide general guidance about the most appropriate method for improving professional practice in any context. There are three phases to any intervention that aims to change practice: development, dissemination and implementation (Table 11.4). There is undoubtedly evidence that the most successful interventions are those which involve the professionals who are the targets for change in both the development and dissemination phases, and pro-

PUBLISHED EVIDENCE ABOUT INTERVENTIONS TO IMPROVE PROFESSIONAL PRACTICE

The Cochrane database contains seven systematic reviews of evidence about the effectiveness of six different methods for changing practice: audit and feedback of information; computerized advice on drug dosage; educational outreach visits; local opinion leaders; mass media interventions; and printed educational materials (Table 11.5). There are two reviews about audit and feedback: one deals with this intervention alone[36] and the second with complementary interventions to enhance its effectiveness.[37] Each of the seven reviews includes studies that are directly relevant to antibiotic policies or to improvement in professional practice in infection (Table 11.5).

Table 11.4 Probability that antibiotic policies will change practice related to a classification of strategies for development, dissemination and implementation. Based on a table in Grimshaw and Russell.[87] Note that while there is good evidence to support the ranking of probability of success within each column, it is less clear how the columns link together. For example, how will an intervention that ranks 4 under development but 1 under dissemination and implementation compare with an intervention that ranks third for all three strategies?

Probability	Development strategy: Who develops the policy and sets the standards against which practice will be measured?	Dissemination strategy: How will the target professionals be made aware of the policy or standards?	Implementation strategy: How will the target professionals be told about whether or not they are following the policy or standards?
High	Internal: the professionals who are the targets for behavior change	Educational intervention targeted at specific professionals or clinical teams (primary care or hospital)	Concurrent (e.g. patient-specific reminders at the time of consultation, or feedback of information while the patient is still being treated)
	Intermediate: opinion leaders are identified from within each clinical unit (primary care practice or hospital team)	Educational intervention targeted at groupings (e.g. all primary care practitioners or all junior hospital doctors)	Retrospective, patient-specific feedback (e.g. the percentage of patients in whom targets were met) with peer comparison (averages compared with those of all local professionals or teams)
	External, local: a local group without any input from the target professionals	Mailed or web-based information targeted at groupings (e.g. all primary care practitioners or all junior hospital doctors)	Retrospective general feedback (e.g. Defined Daily Doses per 1000 population or bed days)
Low	External, national: a national group without any local input	Publication of guidelines/standard (in a journal or newsletter or on the web)	General reminder

Table 11.5 Summary of seven systematic reviews in the Cochrane database about evidence to support methods for achieving behavior change, with examples of evidence from the reviews that is relevant to antibiotic policies

Review topic and reference(s)	General conclusions	Example of evidence relevant to antibiotic policies or the management of infection
Audit and feedback[36,37]	Audit and feedback can sometimes be effective in improving the practice of healthcare professionals, in particular prescribing and diagnostic test ordering. When it is effective, the effects appear to be small to moderate but potentially worthwhile. Those attempting to enhance professional behavior should not rely solely on this approach.[88] It is not possible to recommend a complementary intervention to enhance the effectiveness of audit and feedback. Few trials have investigated the effect of varying different characteristics of the audit and feedback process. Consideration should be given to testing the effects of modifying important characteristics such as the content, source, timing, recipient and format[89]	Increasing generic prescribing in primary care[88] Reducing the cost of prescribing in primary care[59] Improving the management of cystitis and vaginitis in primary care[90] Improving outpatient management of acute bronchitis and cystitis[91] Improving inpatient management of acute bacterial pneumonia and urinary tract infection[92]
Computerized advice on drug dosage[93]	This systematic review provides evidence to support the use of computer assistance in determining drug dosage. Further clinical trials are necessary to determine whether the benefits seen in specialist applications can be realized in general use	Reduction in the incidence of toxicity and length of stay of patients receiving aminoglycosides in a controlled trial of the cost benefit of computerized support for dose adjustment[94] Reduction in duration of fever and hospital stay in a controlled trial of a clinical pharmacokinetic service[95]
Educational outreach visits[96]	Educational outreach visits, particularly when combined with social marketing, appear to be a promising approach to modifying health professional behavior, especially prescribing. Further research is needed to assess the effects of outreach visits for other aspects of practice and to identify key characteristics of outreach visits that are important to its success. The cost-effectiveness of outreach visits is not well evaluated	Improving use of cefalexin in primary care[97] Reducing use of tetracycline for upper respiratory tract infections in primary care[42] Reducing over the counter sale of antibiotics for diarrhea by community pharmacies[98] Reducing prescribing of antibiotics for diarrhea in primary care[99]
Local opinion leaders[100]	Using local opinion leaders results in mixed effects on professional practice. However, it is not always clear what local opinion leaders do and replicable descriptions are needed. Further research is required to determine if opinion leaders can be identified and in which circumstances they are likely to influence the practice of their peers	Reducing inappropriate care of urinary catheters in hospitals by using local opinion leaders on wards to give tutorials compared with in-service lectures to all nurses[101]
Mass media interventions[102]	Despite the limited information about key aspects of mass media interventions and the poor quality of the available primary research, there is evidence that these channels of communication may have an important role in influencing the use of healthcare interventions. Those engaged in promoting better uptake of research information in clinical practice should consider mass media as one of the tools that may encourage the use of effective services and discourage those of unproven effectiveness	None about antibiotic prescribing. Two about improved uptake of HIV testing and two about improved uptake of immunization
Printed educational materials[103]	The effects of printed educational materials compared with no active intervention appear small and of uncertain clinical significance. These conclusions should be viewed as tentative due to the poor reporting of results and inappropriate primary analyses. The additional impact of more active interventions produced mixed results. Audit and feedback and conferences/workshops did not appear to produce substantial changes in practice; the effects in the evaluations of educational outreach visits and opinion leaders were larger and likely to be of practical importance. None of the studies included full economic analyses, and thus it is unclear to what extent the effects of any of the interventions may be worth the costs involved	Improving knowledge of pediatricians about compliance enhancing strategies for mothers of children prescribed antibiotics for otitis media. Significant increase in the use of these strategies by pediatricians and in the mothers' compliance with antibiotic regimens[104]

However, while each of the reviews shows that all six of these interventions can be effective, overall they provide little evidence about the relative effectiveness of the different methods in specific contexts or about the importance of other potential effect modifiers, such as content, source, timing, recipient and format. The potential importance of these effect modifiers is illustrated by the few studies that do address these issues. For example, in a randomized controlled trial that included 186 family physicians the impact of a drug bulletin was evaluated on changes in knowledge, perceived drug utility, and prescribing. Information in the bulletin on the treatment of renal colic changed physicians' knowledge, their perceived utility of drugs used for renal colic and their prescribing ($p < 0.05$). On the other hand, advice in the same bulletin on the treatment of the irritable bowel syndrome (IBS) had no impact at all: it did not even improve the knowledge of the physicians about the drugs used for IBS. Apparently, the message about the treatment of IBS failed to gain the attention of the physicians. The authors suggested that some messages are sufficiently transmitted through written information, and others that are seen as less relevant or too difficult to implement need more intensive strategies.[38] In another randomized trial the effect of an educational and feedback intervention on H_2-blocker prescribing patterns was compared on network versus group-model health maintenance organization (HMO) physicians and in academic versus non-academic settings. Physicians were randomized to receive an educational memorandum alone or the memorandum combined with feedback regarding their individual prescribing behavior. Thirty group-model (at two academic and four non-academic sites) and 33 network-model (all in full-time private practice) primary care physicians participated in the study. A significant response to the intervention was noted among academic and non-academic group-model HMO physicians, but not among network physicians (adjusted mean absolute prescribing changes of +9.9% and +8.9% versus –2.8%, $p = 0.02$). There was no difference in prescribing change based on type of intervention (education versus feedback). The authors concluded that a simple passive educational intervention can be effective at changing group-model HMO physician behavior but that even the more complex strategy of providing feedback had no impact on the network physicians.[39]

METHODS FOR EVALUATION OF INTERVENTIONS TO IMPROVE PROFESSIONAL PRACTICE

The Cochrane Collaboration group on Effective Practice and Organization of Care (EPOC) was responsible for the reviews summarized in Table 11.5. The group has a website (http://www.abdn.ac.uk/public_health/hsru/epoc/) where they have posted a checklist for evaluating interventions with detailed criteria for the assessment of the quality of intervention studies. Three basic study designs are considered for review by the Cochrane EPOC groups (Table 11.6). In addition to clinical trials the group includes two forms of quasi-experimental study design: controlled before and after or interrupted time series (Table 11.6). Studies with single measures of prescribing before and after an intervention are not accepted because there is a large literature showing that this design is subject to unacceptable levels of bias and confounding.[40, 41] Controlled before and after studies are relatively simple to understand and to analyze (Table 11.6). The two minimum criteria that are required for this design are that data are collected at the same time at the intervention and control sites and that the sites are truly comparable (Table 11.6). The analysis of data is similar to a standard controlled trial that compares changes in the primary endpoint in the intervention and control arms. The interrupted time series design is likely to be less familiar to a clinical audience, although it has been used widely in other fields such as education and psychology. This design does not require a control group but does require multiple data points to be collected before and after the intervention (Figure 11.2). The advantage of an interrupted time series is that it quantifies background fluctuations in prescribing, and any trends in prescribing or other outcomes that were occurring before the intervention. In both examples in Figure 11.2 there is considerable fluctuation of the primary outcome measure (cefazolin dosing in Figure 11.2a and cases of *Clostridium difficile*-associated diarrhea in Figure 11.2b). In Figure 11.2a there is a downward trend in the percentage of incorrect dosing of cefazolin before the intervention, but the intervention clearly accelerated the elimination of incorrect dosing. In contrast, Figure 11.2b shows an upward trend in the number of cases of *C. difficile*-associated diarrhea before the intervention to restrict prescribing of clindamycin. Methods for evaluation and analysis of interrupted time series analyses are available from the Cochrane EPOC website.

The Cochrane EPOC methods paper *Issues Related to Baseline Measures of Performance* is essential to critical review of either randomized trials or controlled before and after studies. In a very large randomized trial there should be little or no difference at baseline between the study arms but this is often not true when the unit of randomization is a cluster such as a practice or a hospital. The following example is used in the paper to illustrate the problem. It comes from a trial in which hospitals were randomly assigned to one of three groups (Table 11.7). The relevant comparisons are between or among groups, not comparisons within groups before and after an intervention. However, comparison of the three groups after the intervention would be quite misleading, suggesting that the education intervention had a negative effect (49% receiving prophylaxis versus 51% in the control group) and the education plus audit intervention had only a small positive effect (55% versus 51%). There are two reasons for this: the three groups were not balanced at baseline and there was significant improvement in the control hospital. The solution is to present the changes in the intervention groups adjusted for the change in the control group. When the primary outcome measure is continuous variable, such as the number of prescriptions, then analysis of covariance can be used to compare changes in the

Table 11.6 Rigorous designs for the evaluation of antibiotic policies or other interventions designed to achieve changes in practice. The criteria for assessment of quality are taken from the checklist used by the Cochrane Effective Practice and Organization of Care (EPOC) group

Design	Description	Criteria for assessment of quality	Examples relevant to antibiotic policies
Controlled trial	A trial in which the participants (patients, doctors, healthcare teams etc.) were assigned prospectively to alternative forms of interventions. *Randomized controlled trial:* assignment by random allocation (e.g. random number generation, coin flips) *Controlled clinical trial:* quasi-random allocation method (e.g. alternation, date of birth, patient identifier)	Minimum criteria for any design (controlled trial, before and after or interrupted time series): Objective measurement of performance, behavior or health outcomes in a clinical not test situation. Relevant and interpretable data presented or obtainable. Additional desirable criteria for any design: Concealment of allocation to intervention or control groups Follow-up of 80–100% of subjects Blinded assessment of outcome(s) Outcomes were measured before the intervention, with no substantial differences across study groups. Reliable primary outcome measures Protection against contamination: allocation was by community, institution or practice and it is unlikely that the control received the intervention	Randomized controlled parallel group trial of educational mailing supplemented with visits by a project pharmacist to improve prescribing of recommended antibiotics (erythromycin and penicillin V) for tonsillitis in primary care. There was a significant increase in use of recommended antibiotics in the control group (19% absolute increase), but a greater (27%) increase in the intervention group[105] Randomized controlled trial of the impact of suggestions from a multidisciplinary infection consultation team on clinical and microbiological outcomes of inpatients receiving three or more days of parenteral antibiotics. There was a $400 per patient reduction in antibiotic charges with a trend towards shorter hospital stay (20 vs 25 days) but no difference in clinical or microbiological response, in-hospital mortality or readmission[61]
Controlled before and after study	Involvement of intervention and control groups other than by random process, and inclusion of baseline period of assessment of main outcomes	Two minimum criteria in addition to those for controlled trials: *Contemporaneous data collection:* pre and post intervention periods for study and control sites are the same *Appropriate choice of control site:* study and control sites are comparable with respect to dominant reimbursement system, level of care, setting of care and academic status	Controlled before and after study of an educational program designed to increase use of recommended drugs (erythromycin and penicillin V) for tonsillitis in one community health centre in comparison with two control community centres from the same county. Significantly greater change in the intervention group (Table 11.7)[106] Follow up 5 years later showed sustained differences between the intervention and control health centres[107] Crossover study on two intensive care units of the impact on antibiotic resistance in surveillance cultures of an antibiotic policy eliminating use of broad-spectrum β-lactams. The relative risk for colonization with resistant strains per 1000 patient days at risk was 18 times higher without antibiotic restriction[66]
Interrupted time series	A change in trend attributable to the intervention, with repeated measures of the main outcomes before and after the intervention	Two minimum criteria in addition to those for controlled trials: Clearly defined point in time when the intervention occurred At least three data points before and three after the intervention	Time series analysis of the effect of a structured antibiotic order form designed to improve dosing of clindamycin and cefazolin. The intervention virtually eliminated incorrect prescribing (Fig 11.2)[108] Switchback study of the impact on carriage of glycopeptide-resistant *Enterococcus* spp. of antibiotic policy on a hematology unit. Switching from ceftazidime to piperacillin/tazobactam was associated with a significant reduction in risk, with return to baseline levels when the policy was switched back to ceftazidime[67]

intervention and control groups.[42] In this example the aim was to reduce prescribing of tetracycline for upper respiratory tract infection. In the intervention group the mean number of prescriptions over 6 months reduced from 12.6 to 1.8. However, the mean number of prescriptions also reduced in the control group, from 7.5 to 3.2. Analysis of covariance showed that the reduction in mean number of prescriptions in the intervention group was significantly greater than in the control group.

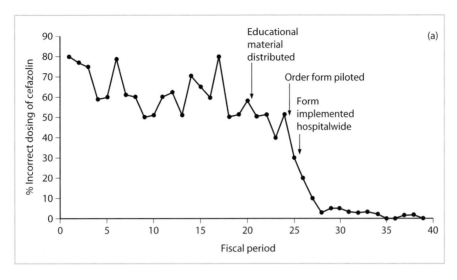

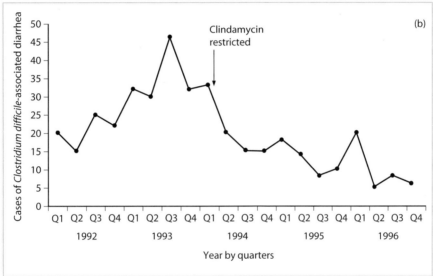

Fig. 11.2 Examples of interrupted time series study design (see text for explanation)

Table 11.7 Example of a randomized trial with potentially misleading results (see text for explanation).

Percentage of patients receiving prophylaxis	Baseline	Post	Difference	Adjusted change*
Control	40%	51%	11%	NA
Education alone	21%	49%	28%	155%
Education + quality assurance	27%	55%	28%	155%

* Adjusted change = (intervention baseline – post score) ÷ (control baseline – post score)

HOW SHOULD COMPLIANCE WITH ANTIBIOTIC POLICIES BE MONITORED?

Hospitals fortunate enough to have sophisticated information systems may be able to use these to monitor compliance with policies.[43,44] However, this is the exception rather than the rule.

Less sophisticated information systems can still provide valuable information but there is often no substitute for collection of data by hand.[45] This is not necessarily as daunting as it may seem; a one-day prevalence survey of an entire hospital can be achieved in a few hours and may be a useful tool to detect deviations from guidelines and provide physicians with educational feedback.[45–47] In Tayside, Scotland we have involved a variety of staff in auditing policies, including trainee nurses, pharmacists, doctors and medical students.[30]

In primary care routine data about antibiotic prescribing can be used to measure the impact of prescribing interventions.[48] More sophisticated data systems that include diagnosis may be required to monitor the impact of targeted interventions, for example to reduce prescribing for bronchitis.[49] However, as in hospitals, hand collection of data may be the only practical method available. Community pharmacists have an important potential role in the audit of antibiotic prescribing in primary care.

Audit is an educational activity; the process of data collection and analysis provides a valuable learning opportunity.[9] As with implementation, there are few studies comparing more than one method for monitoring compliance with policies and the published data do not allow for conclusions to be drawn about the relative merits of different methods.

WHAT SHOULD BE INCLUDED IN AN ANTIBIOTIC POLICY?

Most antibiotic policies focus on which drug to prescribe but there are several other important considerations (route of administration, dose, and duration of treatment). Perhaps the most important step in prescribing is the assessment of need for any antibiotic at all (Figure 11.1). In hospital, the decision to prescribe is often made by junior staff faced with a seriously ill patient and little or no results of investigation. It is unrealistic, and may well be undesirable, to try to prevent antibiotic prescribing under these circumstances. An alternative method for limiting unnecessary antimicrobial prescribing is to recommend that senior staff review the need for prescription at 48–72 h after initiation. At this time laboratory information will be available, a non-infectious cause for the patient's symptoms may have been identified and the antibiotic can be stopped. This approach led to a sustained reduction in antibiotic prescribing on one neonatal intensive care unit.[50] In a recent randomized trial, early cessation of antibiotics in patients with suspected ventilator-associated pneumonia but culture-negative bronchoalveolar lavage was associated with improved clinical outcome.[51] Outside intensive care units patients with suspected infection will be less severely ill and the clinical evidence supporting prescription may be minimal.[47,52–54] Audit of antibiotic prescribing would be greatly enhanced by the development of evidence-based minimum datasets, which should be recorded in every patient who receives an antibiotic.[55]

In the community, regular review of the patient's need for antibiotic is unrealistic. In this situation development of decision rules may help to define the probability of bacterial infection and hence the risks and benefits of antibiotic prescription.[55–58] At the national level campaigns directed at professionals and the public have resulted in sustained decreases in antibiotic prescribing in the community.[2,24,26] This is

encouraging but will be sustained only if antibiotic policies deal with the need for prescribing any antibiotic at all in addition to providing guidance about which antibiotic to prescribe.

In hospitals bacteremia provides a manageable focus for attention. Our own experience[59] is very similar to previously published audits.[43] Review of patients with bacteremia identifies patients who are being overtreated, including those with contaminated blood cultures. However, we regularly identify patients with significant bacteremia who are receiving no antibiotic treatment at all.

TO WHAT EXTENT DO ANTIBIOTIC POLICIES ACHIEVE THEIR SECONDARY AIMS?

A definitive answer to this question requires systematic review of the literature with rigorous methods for assessment of the quality of studies, extraction and analysis of data. No such reviews are currently available but two reviews on measures to control antibiotic prescribing have recently been registered with the Cochrane EPOC group, one dealing with interventions in hospitals and the other in primary care. The EPOC website will provide information about progress with these reviews and contact details for the reviewers. Until these reviews are completed it is only possible to provide examples of evidence to show that antibiotic policies can achieve their secondary aims.

CAN ANTIBIOTIC POLICIES REDUCE HEALTHCARE COSTS?

Many published examples claim to show that implementation of policies reduces antibiotic costs, in hospital or in the community. However, these studies suffer from two limitations. First, they do not always quantify the cost of designing, implementing and monitoring the policy, which may be considerable. The Cochrane EPOC checklist includes the cost of any intervention as an essential component of evaluation. Secondly, monitoring of the effects of the policy is generally restricted to antibiotic costs alone. When treatment failure results in hospitalization, prescription of cheaper but less effective drugs may dramatically increase healthcare costs.[60] In several examples the costs of drug utilization reviews or other prescribing interventions are offset by the savings achieved.[35] There are fewer comprehensive analyses that include adequate measurement of the clinical impact of prescribing interventions but there is growing evidence to show that reduction in antibiotic prescribing and costs can be achieved without compromising clinical outcome.[61] In summary, before embarking on a drug utilization review it is important to estimate the costs of the program and to compare these with the estimated benefits. Potential adverse effects of restricting antibiotic prescribing should also be considered, together with the availability of routine data such as length of hospital stay, which may be used as an indicator of clinical outcome.[61]

CAN ANTIBIOTIC POLICIES IMPROVE THE QUALITY OF PRESCRIBING?

Published Cochrane reviews about methods for achieving behavior change contain several examples of high-quality studies that have shown that interventions can improve the quality of antibiotic prescribing (Table 11.5). In addition we have recently reviewed evidence about the impact of guidelines for the management of community-acquired pneumonia and identified several studies which show that increase in the proportion of patients who receive prompt, appropriate antibiotic therapy is associated with improvements in outcome measures such as mortality and length of hospital stay.[62] In all of these examples the keys to success have been identification of a problem that prescribers agree to be important followed by identification of a practical method for improving practice.

CAN ANTIBIOTIC POLICIES CONTROL RESISTANCE?

There is clearly a crude relationship between the overall use of antibiotics and the development of bacterial resistance;[1,3] the question is whether or not antibiotic policies can limit the development of resistance. The literature contains many examples of control of outbreaks of infection with drug-resistant bacteria that may be attributed to antibiotic control measures (Table 11.8). However, it has been very difficult to eliminate confounding variables, such as other infection control measures or change in patient case mix (Table 11.8). The methodology of earlier studies was crude, both in terms of microbiology and epidemiology. More recent studies have used molecular techniques for precise definition of cross-infection and more rigorous case control to minimize the impact of confounding variables.[63,64] Association between prescribing and resistance is strengthened if the relationship can be demonstrated across a range of institutions. A study conducted in 18 centres in the USA identified a significant correlation between ceftazidime prescribing in intensive care units and the prevalence of ceftazidime-resistant *Enterobacter cloacae*.[65] However, the best evidence comes from studies that relate changes in antibiotic prescribing to changes in resistance.[66] These examples provide evidence that either reducing overall prescribing or modifying the choice of empirical antibiotics can reduce the prevalence of antibiotic-resistant bacteria.[26,67]

The previous examples dealt with the difficulty of proving that antibiotic policies help to resolve a problem of resistance that has already developed. It is even more difficult to prove that policies prevent the development of resistance. It *is* clear that prescribing antibiotics does increase the prevalence of drug-resistant bacteria in the normal human flora and that this acts as a reservoir of resistant bacteria.[25] As we have already noted, most antibiotic policies are concerned with which antibiotic is prescribed and it is more likely that development of resistance will be contained by policies which also try to limit unnecessary prescribing of antibiotics. Although it is encouraging when hos-

Table 11.8 Evidence in support of a link between antimicrobial prescribing and the prevalence of drug-resistant strains of bacteria, with some of the potential confounding variables which could mean that it is wrong to interpret the association as simple cause and effect. For more detailed analysis see McGowan[109] and Richard et al[63,64]

Supporting evidence	Potential confounding variables
1. In the pre-antibiotic era pneumococci and other streptococci were common causes of nosocomial infection. In the antibiotic era they have been replaced by organisms such as *Pseudomonas aeruginosa*. In general, antimicrobial resistance is more prevalent in bacterial strains causing nosocomial infection than in organisms from community-acquired cases	1. There have been many other changes which may account for these observations (case mix, new medical technology)
2. Patients with resistant organisms are more likely to have received prior antibiotic therapy than are controls	2. Antibiotic use may just be a marker for patients who are more ill
3. Concurrent variation between antimicrobial utilization and resistance has been noted for both increases and decreases in these two factors	3a. Other reports document decreased prevalence of antimicrobial resistance without a corresponding decrease in antimicrobial use
	3b. It is difficult to separate control of antimicrobial prescribing from other infection control measures which are used in the context of an outbreak of nosocomial infection with drug resistant strains
4. There is a dose–response relationship between antimicrobial prescribing and the probability of infection with drug-resistant strains which operates at several different levels (individual patient, ward unit, hospital and country)	4. The association may be because of differences in underlying disease and/or aspects of management other than antimicrobial therapy
5. Interruption of transmission of resistant organisms (e.g. barrier isolation techniques) and control of antimicrobial prescribing are the only two measures that have been shown to be successful in limiting the prevalence of drug-resistant bacteria	5. It is virtually impossible to separate the effects of these two measures, which are almost always implemented concurrently

pitals that enforce policies also report low resistance rates it is impossible to prove cause and effect. It is unrealistic to expect policies to completely prevent the development of drug resistance because policies have a limited sphere of influence and reservoirs of resistant bacteria will inevitably arise elsewhere. For example, there is ample evidence of community reservoirs of resistance arising from prescribing of antibiotics in general medical or veterinary practice[68] or from travel to countries with high rates of resistance;[69] consequently tight control of antibiotic prescribing in hospitals cannot eliminate the risk of introduction of drug-resistant bacteria. Finally it is important to note that resistance to a drug may persist even when use of the drug has been virtually eliminated. Examples include streptomycin resistance in hospitals[70] and sulfamethoxazole resistance in the community.[71]

In summary, demonstration of the impact of antibiotic policies on the spread of bacterial resistance is challenging because of the virtual impossibility of controlling for all of the other factors that influence development of resistance. Advocates of antibiotic policies should not be discouraged by this situation and should certainly not allow it to be used as an argument against implementation of policies. We hope that the evidence that we have reviewed shows that antibiotic policies can definitely improve the quality of prescribing and may be used to limit prescribing costs. Limiting superinfection and antibiotic resistance should be viewed as additional potential benefits but they are probably not realistic primary aims for most policies.

LEGAL IMPLICATIONS OF ANTIBIOTIC POLICIES

It is important to be aware of the legal implications of antibiotic policies. It is not unusual for audits to show that only a minority of professionals' practice is fully consistent with antibiotic policies. In that case are most professionals guilty of negligence? Moreover, is the organization in which the professionals practice also guilty of negligence unless it takes action and achieves 100% adherence to policies? Although interventions can improve adherence to policies, the changes are often small (Table 11.5) and, even when the best methods for development, dissemination and implementation (Table 11.4) are used a majority of professionals may still not adhere to the policy.[72] Reasons include lack of knowledge, awareness, familiarity, agreement, outcome expectancy and ability to overcome the inertia of previous practice.[73] Guidelines by their very nature consider common problems in typical patients and may fail to adequately address the needs of individual patients, particularly the elderly and the patient with a complicated course.[72] Guidelines frequently lack objective parameters, lack graded recommendations and do not favor a multidisciplinary approach.[74] As has already been noted, a major flaw of much of the literature on the implementation of guidelines is the failure to include measures of clinical outcome in studies of interventions designed to reduce the cost of care. A systematic review of the effects of clinical practice guidelines on patient outcomes in primary care found that only 13 of 91 studies included patient outcome as an end result.[75] Guidelines have frequently been instituted by hospitals, payers (insurance agencies or sick funds) or large providers (health maintenance organizations or the military) in order to reduce treatment expenditures, with the justification that cutting costs benefits the patient in the long run but without adequate measurement of the impact on clinical outcome. For all of these reasons 100% concordance between clinical practice and guidelines is neither desirable nor achievable.

Written policies and practice guidelines have a major impact on courts of law, particularly if they are endorsed by national societies or other professional bodies. As a legal standard, their testimonial relevance, or 'weight' in that respect, is just below regulations issued by the primary or secondary lawmaker. The legal implication of this position is that presentation of a policy or guideline in court may overcome expert opinion, results of well conducted studies and even meta-analysis (particularly if published after the guideline was written). Most courts will assign a written policy/guideline a burden of evidence far beyond the importance assigned to the policy/guideline by those who wrote it or use it. Writers of guidelines, such as the Scottish Intercollegiate Guidelines Network, often clearly state that the intention is to provide guidance rather than to impose stiff regulations. Nonetheless, courts of law may still interpret guidelines as minimum standards of care.

Conversely, a court can even declare a policy or guideline as insufficient or unacceptable; the court is sovereign to decide upon the standard according to its own legal policies – which are usually aimed at improving the health of the public. Thus, if the court finds a certain policy, even if approved by official bodies, to be insufficient it can declare it as a non-standard and set its own standard. The following quote is from the book *International Medical Malpractice Law*.[76] 'A common practice (regardless if founded on guidelines) simply may not be good enough to fulfill the standard required by the law.' In 1993 the supreme court of Canada expressed the view that 'conformity with standard practice (based on policy or guidelines) in a profession does not necessarily insulate a doctor from negligence where the standard of practice itself is negligent.'[77] In the UK, the House of Lords has stated the view that the court can, in rare cases, reach a conclusion that a professional standard is not based on a rational analysis, and that the experts express views that are not logical or responsible.[78] These judgments have important implications for antibiotic policy makers. Concerns about antibiotic resistance may be used to justify restriction of antibiotics even when there is compelling evidence to suggest that this is not in the interests of the individual patient.[79] However, a court may not agree with this decision; indeed the court is likely to decide that a doctor's primary duty is care of the individual patient. The problem of antibiotic resistance confronts prescribers and the healthcare organizations in which they work with two conflicting ethical duties: one is their duty of fidelity to the individual patient, the other is their duty of stewardship for the resources that have been entrusted to them.[80] Rigid enforcement of the duty of fidelity would result in prescription of antibiotics to any patient who might conceivably have infection and selection of an empirical regimen that covers all possible pathogens. Such a policy is clearly not in the long-term interests of the public. However, would a court of law support a healthcare organization that put the long-term interests of the public before the interests of the individual patient?[81]

Legislation should also be considered as an instrument for helping to achieve the aims of antibiotic policies. Once antimicrobial drug resistance has been recognized as a concern by public health authorities they will ask for legal as well as scientific analysis of the problem and international organizations such as the European Union and the World Health Organization will also seek legal solutions.[82] However, cooperative initiatives may be more practical and speedy than legislation, at least in the first instance.[82] Similarly, at the national level it has been recognized that development of local solutions may be more productive than imposing national legislation.[82] Nonetheless, Fidler[82] provides several practical proposals for introducing legislation to help to control antimicrobial prescribing:

1. International legal harmonization of principles for prudent antimicrobial drug use will have to include monitoring and enforcement, as well as financial, technical, and legal assistance by industrialized countries to developing countries.
2. In the USA, Congress could regulate use of antimicrobial drugs by monitoring interstate commerce in these products. Congress probably does not have the authority to regulate antimicrobial prescription practices directly; such authority rests with the states.
3. Perhaps the most powerful US federal strategy would be to make implementation of state policies to curb the misuse of antimicrobial drugs mandatory before states receive federal funds earmarked for public health. In countries where governments subsidize the purchase of antimicrobial drugs, legislative or regulatory changes in these subsidies could lead to a decline in the use of the drugs.
4. Fulfilment of legal duties often hinges on sufficient resources. In many developing countries public health systems may be inadequate. Thus, financial and technical leadership is needed from national governments towards local authorities and from international organizations towards developing countries. A precedent can be found in the proposed Convention on the Provision of Telecommunication Resources for Disaster Mitigation and Relief Operations, which obligates the parties, where possible, to lower or remove regulatory barriers for using telecommunication resources during disasters.
5. Lessons from international environmental efforts suggest that international law must play a major role in setting international standards for implementation domestically and creating the political, technical, and financial conditions necessary to integrate international and national law.

IMPORTANT UNANSWERED QUESTIONS ABOUT ANTIBIOTIC POLICIES

WHAT IS THE MOST COST-EFFECTIVE METHOD FOR IMPLEMENTING POLICIES?

It is probably unrealistic to expect a definitive answer to this question because of the influence of context as well as the knowledge, attitudes and beliefs of both the professionals who are the targets for change and of the patients that they serve. Healthcare professionals should acknowledge the expertise of other disciplines such as psychology, which can certainly help to identify appropriate interventions for specific contexts.[73] Currently there are far too few studies that have compared the cost effectiveness of different methods within a single context, or a single method within different contexts. Furthermore, standardized reporting of trials of interventions would improve comparison between studies.[34]

WHEN SHOULD RESTRICTIVE STRATEGIES BE USED TO IMPLEMENT ANTIBIOTIC POLICIES?

Restrictive methods for controlling antibiotic prescribing include restricting access to the formulary, not allowing prescription outside the formulary list, therapeutic substitution of non-formulary drugs and automatic stop orders that limit the duration of antibiotic prescriptions. These strategies are perceived as dictatorial or punitive and are likely to be less appealing to clinicians.[83] It is generally acknowledged that practice guidelines achieve their greatest good by expanding medical knowledge, which may not be achieved by punitive measures.[84] Arguments can certainly be made for enforcing guidelines that define optimal care and are founded on high-quality evidence.[84] Nonetheless, the best evidence always leaves some element of uncertainty and even the best-supported guidelines do not necessarily define all options. Enforcement of policies may be justified when persuasive strategies have failed but there is still a dearth of good quality evidence to support the use of restrictive strategies and the few published examples deal with relatively simple issues such as different dosing regimens for the same antibiotic.[85] Restrictive strategies for antibiotic control are not covered by any of the published Cochrane reviews (Table 11.5) but will be addressed by the ongoing reviews of strategies to control antibiotic prescribing.

WHAT KIND OF DIFFERENCE (IN PRESCRIBING) MAKES A DIFFERENCE (TO RESISTANCE)?

The key to answering this question is to develop models that relate current antibiotic use to the future development of resistance.[79] Models have been developed but there is an urgent need for data that can be used to test their predictions.[25] We are not aware of any examples of explicit use of this type of information in decision making about antibiotic policies. However, policy makers must be prepared to support their decisions with more than just concerns about the future development of resistance.[79] It is ethical to make trade offs between the needs of future and current patients provided that the final decision is supported by evidence.[80]

References

1. House of Lords Select Committee on Science and Technology 1998 *Resistance to Antibiotics and Other Antimicrobial Agents.* Session 1997–98 /th Report, 1–108. The Stationery Office, London.

2. House of Lords Select Committee on Science and Technology 2001 *Resistance to Antibiotics.* Session 2000–01 3rd Report, 1–34. The Stationery Office, London.

3. Anonymous 1998 The Copenhagen Recommendations. Report from the Invitational EU Conference on The Microbial Threat, Copenhagen, Denmark, 9–10 September 1998. Rosdahl, V. K. and Pedersen, K. B. 1–52. Copenhagen, Denmark, Ministry of Health, Ministry of Food, Agriculture and Fisheries; http://www.sum.dk/publika/micro98/.

4. Anonymous 1990 Implementing a local prescribing policy 3409. *Drug and Therapeutics Bulletin* 28: 93–95.

5. Working party of the British Society of Antimicrobial Chemotherapy 1994 Working Party Report – Hospital antibiotic control measures in the UK. *Journal of Antimicrobial Chemotherapy* 34: 21–42.

6. Lawton RM, Fridkin SK, Gaynes RP, McGowan JE 2000 Practices to improve antimicrobial use at 47 US hospital: the status of the 1997 SHEA/IDSA position paper recommendations. *Infection Control and Hospital Epidemiology* 21: 256–259.

7. Scottish Intercollegiate Guidelines Network 2000 Antibiotic Prophylaxis in Surgery. SIGN Guideline 45. Royal College of Physicians of Edinburgh, Edinburgh.

8. Bapna JS, Tripathi CD, Tekur U 1996 Drug utilisation patterns in the third world. *PharmacoEconomics* 9: 286–294.

9. Hogerzeil HV 1995 Promoting rational prescribing: an international perspective. *British Journal of Clinical Pharmacology* 39: 1–6.

10. Barber N 1993 Improving quality of drug use through hospital directorates. *Quality Health Care* 2: 3–4.

11. Wyatt TD, Passmore CM, Morrow NC, Reilly PM 1990 Antibiotic prescribing: the need for a policy in general practice. *British Medical Journal* 300: 441–444.

12. Simon HJ, Folb PI, Rocha H 1987 Policies, laws and regulations pertaining to antibiotics: Report of Task Force 3. *Reviews of Infectious Disease* 9(Suppl. 3) S261–S269.

13. Barriere SL 1985 Cost containment of antimicrobial therapy. *Drug Intelligence and Clinical Pharmacology* 19: 278–281.

14. Parker SE, Davey PG 1992 Pharmacoeconomics of intravenous drug administration. *Pharmaco Economics* 1: 103–115.

15. Davey P, Nathwani D 1998 Sequential antibiotic therapy: the right patient, the right time and the right outcome. *Journal of Infection* 37: 37–44.

16. Beers MH, Storrie M, Lee G 1990 Potential adverse drug interactions in the emergency room. *Annals of Internal Medicine* 112: 61–64.

17. Goldbeck-Wood S 1996 MDU exposes drug errors. *British Medical Journal* 312: 1439.

18. Smith JW, Seidl LG, Cluff LE 1996 Studies on the epidemiology of adverse drug reactions V. Clinical factors influencing susceptibility. *Annals of Internal Medicine* 65: 629–640.

19. Ponge T, Cottin S, Fruneau P, Ponge A, Van Wassenhove L, Larousse C 1989 Iatrogenic disease. Prospective study, relation to drug consumption. *Therapie* 44: 63–66.

20. Dunagan WC, Woodward RS, Medoff G et al 1991 Antibiotic misuse in two clinical situations: Positive blood culture and administration of aminoglycosides. *Reviews of Infectious Disease* 13: 405–412.

21. Reeves DS, Finch RG, Bax RP et al 1999 Self-medication of antibacterials without prescription (also called 'over-the-counter' use). A report of a Working Party of the British Society for Antimicrobial Chemotherapy. *Journal of Antimicrobial Chemotherapy* 44: 163–177.

22. Wenzel RP, Kunin CM 1994 Should oral antimicrobial drugs be available over the counter? *Journal of Infectious Diseases* 170: 1256–1259.

23. Davey PG, Bax RP, Newey J et al 1996 Growth in the use of antibiotics in the community in England and Scotland in 1980–1993. *British Medical Journal* 312: 613– 11/36 .

24. Molstad S, Cars O 1999 Major change in the use of antibiotics following a national programme: Swedish Strategic Programme for the Rational Use of Antimicrobial Agents and Surveillance of Resistance (STRAMA). *Scandinavian Journal of Infectious Diseases* 31: 191–195.

25. Austin DJ, Kristinsson KG, Anderson RM 1999 The relationship between the volume of antimicrobial consumption in human communities and the frequency of resistance. *Proceedings of the National Academy of Sciences of the USA* 96: 1152–1156.

26. Seppala H, Klaukka T, Vuopio-Varkila J et al 1997 The effect of changes in the consumption of macrolide antibiotics on erythromycin resistance in group A streptococci in Finland. *New England Journal of Medicine* 337: 441–446.

27. Damoiseaux RA, de Melker RA, Ausems MJ, van Balen FA 1999 Reasons for non-guideline-based antibiotic prescriptions for acute otitis media in The Netherlands. *Family Practice* 16: 50–53.

28. Kunin CM, Tupasi T, Craig WA 1973 Use of Antibiotics. A brief exposition of the problem and some tentative solutions. *Annals of Internal Medicine* 79: 555–560.

29. Mant D 1992 Facilitating prevention in primary care. *British Medical Journal* 304: 652–653.

30. Nathwani D, Davey PG 1998 Strategies to rationalize sepsis management – a review of 4 years' experience in Dundee. *Journal of Infection* 37: 10–17.

31. Grimshaw JM, Russell IT 1993 Effect of clinical guidelines on medical practice: a systematic review of rigorous evaluations. *Lancet* 342: 1317–1321.

32. Donabedian A 1966 Evaluating the quality of medical care. *Millbank Memorial fund Quarterly* 4: 155.

33. Scottish Intercollegiate Guidelines Network. SIGN Guidelines: An introduction to SIGN methodology for the development of evidence-based clinical guidelines. SIGN Guideline 39, 1–34. 1999. Royal College of Physicians of Edinburgh, Edinburgh.

34. Oxman AD, Thomson MA, Davis DA, Haynes RB 1995 No magic bullets: a systematic review of 102 trials of interventions to improve professional practice. *Canadian Medical Association Journal* 153: 1423–1431.

35. Kreling DH, Mott DA 1993 The cost effectiveness of drug utilisation review in an outpatient setting. *PharmacoEconomics* 4: 414–436.

36. Thomson O'Brien MA, Oxman AD, Davis DA, Haynes RB, Freemantle N, Harvey EL 2001 Audit and feedback: effects on professional practice and health care outcomes (Cochrane Review). Update Software, Oxford.

37. Thomson O'Brien MA, Oxman AD, Davis DA, Haynes RB, Freemantle N, Harvey EL 2001 Audit and feedback versus alternative strategies: effects on professional practice and health care outcomes (Cochrane Review). Update Software, Oxford.

38. Denig P, Haaijer-Ruskamp FM, Zijlsing DH 1990 Impact of a drug bulletin on the knowledge, perception of drug utility, and prescribing behavior of physicians. *Drug Intelligence and Clinical Pharmacology* 24: 87–93.

39. Schectman JM, Kanwal NK, Schroth WS, Elinsky EG 1995 The effect of an education and feedback intervention on group-model and network-model health maintenance organization physician prescribing behavior. *Medical Care* 33: 139–144.

40. Soumerai SB, McLaughlin TJ, Avorn J 1989 Improving drug prescribing in primary care: A critical analysis of the experimental literature. *Millbank Quarterly* 67: 268–317.

41. Cook TD, Campbell DT 1979 *Quasi Experimentation. Design & Analysis Issues for Field Settings.* Houghton Mifflin Company, Boston.

42. McConnell TS, Cushing AH, Bankhurst AD, Healy JL, McIlvenna PA, Skipper BJ 1982 Physician behavior modification using claims data: tetracycline for upper respiratory infection. *Western Journal of Medicine* 137: 448–450.

43. Horn DL, Opal SM 1992 Computerized clinical practice guidelines for review of antibiotic therapy for bacteremia. *Infectious Disease in Clinical Practice* 1: 169–173.

44. Pestotnik SL, Classen DC, Evans RS, Burke JP 1996 Implementing antibiotic practice guidelines through computer-assisted decision support: clinical and financial outcomes. *Annals of Internal Medicine* 124: 884–890.

45. Cooke DM, Salter AJ, Phillips I 1983 The impact of antibiotic policy on prescribing in a London Teaching Hospital. A one-day prevalence survey as an indicator of antibiotic use. *Journal of Antimicrobial Chemotherapy* 11: 447–453.

46. Berild D, Ringertz SH, Lelek M, Fosse B 2001 Antibiotic guidelines lead to reductions in the use and cost of antibiotics in a university hospital. *Scandinavian Journal of Infectious Diseases* 33: 63–67.

47. Seaton RA, Nathwani D, Phillips G, Millar R, Davey P 1999 Clinical record keeping in patients receiving antibiotics in hospital. *Health Bulletin* 57: 128–133.

48. Cates C 1999 An evidence based approach to reducing antibiotic use in children with acute otitis media: controlled before and after study. *British Medical Journal* 318: 715–716.

49. Gonzales R, Steiner JF, Lum A, Barrett PH, Jr 1999 Decreasing antibiotic use in ambulatory practice: impact of a multidimensional intervention on the treatment of uncomplicated acute bronchitis in adults. *Journal of the American Medical Associations* 281: 1512–1519.

50. Isaacs D, Wilkinson AR, Moxon ER 1987 Duration of antibiotic courses for neonates. *Archives of Disease in Childhood* 62: 727–728.

51. Fagon JY, Chastre J, Wolff M 2000 Invasive and noninvasive strategies for management of suspected ventilator-associated pneumonia. A randomized trial. *Annals of Internal Medicine* 132: 621–630.

52. Moss F, McNicol MW, McSwiggan DA, Miller DL 1981 Survey of antibiotic prescribing in a district general hospital 1. pattern of use. *Lancet* ii: 349–352.

53. Moss F, McNicol MW, McSwiggan DA, Miller DL 1981 Survey of antibiotic prescribing in a district general hospital II. lower respiratory tract infection. *Lancet* ii: 407–409.

54. Moss F, McNicol MW, McSwiggan DA, Miller DL 1981 Survey of antibiotic prescribing in a district general hospital III. urinary tract infection. *Lancet* ii: 461–462.

55. Loeb M, Bentley DW, Bradley S 2001 Development of minimum criteria for the initiation of antibiotics in residents of long-term-care facilities: results of a consensus conference. *Infection Control and Hospital Epidemiology* 22: 120–124.

56. Del Mar C 1992 Managing sore throat: a literature review – 1: Making the diagnosis. *Medical Journal of Australia* 156: 572–575.

57. Gorelick MH, Shaw KN 2000 Clinical decision rule to identify febrile young girls at risk for urinary tract infection. *Archives of Pediatric and Adolescent Medicine* 154: 386–390.

58. Jaskiewicz JA, McCarthy CA, Richardson AC et al 1994 Febrile infants at low risk for serious bacterial infection – an appraisal of the Rochester criteria and implications for management. Febrile Infant Collaborative Study Group. *Pediatrics* 94: 390–396.

59. Nathwani D, Davey P, France AJ, Phillips G, Orange G, Parratt D 1996 Impact of an infection consultation service for bacteraemia on clinical management and use of resources. *Quarterly Journal of Medicine* 89: 789–797.

60. Roach AC, Kernodle DS, Kaiser AB 1990 Selecting cost-effective antimicrobial prophylaxis in surgery: are we getting what we pay for? *Drug Intelligence and Clinical Pharmacology* 24: 183–185.

61. Fraser GL, Stogsdill P, Dickens JD, Wennberg DE, Smith RP, Prato S 1997 Antibiotic opitimization: an evaluation of patient safety and economic outcomes. *Archives of Internal Medicine* 157: 1689–1694.

62. Nathwani D, Rubinstein E, Barlow G, Davey P 2000 Do Guidelines for Community Acquired Pneumonia Improve the Cost-Effectiveness of Hospital Care? *Clinical Infectious Diseases* 32: 728–741.

63. Richard P, Delangle M-H, Merrien D et al 1994 Fluoroquinolone Use and Fluoroquinolone Resistance: Is there an Association? *Clinical Infectious Diseases* 19: 54–59.

64. Richard P, Le Floch R, Chamoux C, Pannier M, Espaze E, Richet H 1994 *Pseudomonas aeruginosa* outbreak in a Burn Unit: Role of Antimicrobials in the Emergence of Multiply Resistant Strains. *Journal of Infectious Disease* 170: 377–383.

65. Ballow CH, Schentag JJ 1992 Trends in antibiotic utilization and bacterial resistance: report of the National Nosocomial Resistance Surveillance Group. *Diagnostic Microbiology and Infectious Disease* 15: 37S–42S.

66. de Man P, Verhoeven BAN, Verbrugh HA, Vos MC, van den Anker JN 2000 An antibiotic policy to prevent emergence of resistant bacilli. *Lancet* 355: 973–978.

67. Bradley SJ, Wilson ALT, Allen MC, Sher HA, Goldstone AH, Scott GM 1999 The control of hyperendemic glycopeptide-resistant *Enterococcus* spp. on a haematology unit by changing antibiotic usage. *Journal of Antimicrobial Chemotherapy* 43: 261–266.

68. Shanahan PMA, Thomson CJ, Amyes SGB 1994 The global impact of antibiotic-resistant bacteria: their sources and resevoirs. *Reviews of Medical Microbiology* 5: 174–182.

69. Murray BE, Mathewson JJ, DuPont HL, Ericsson CD, Reves RR 1990 Emergence of resistant fecal *Escherichia coli* in travelers not taking prophylactic antimicrobial agents. *Antimicrobial Agents and Chemotherapy* 34: 515–518.

70. Chiew Y-F, Yeo S-F, Hall LMC, Livermore DM 1998 Can susceptibility to an antimicrobial be restored by halting its use? The case of streptomycin versus Enterobacteriaceae. *Journal of Antimicrobial Chemotherapy* 41: 247–251.

71. Enne VI, Livermore DM, Stephens P, Hall LM 2001 Persistence of sulphonamide resistance in *Escherichia coli* in the UK despite national prescribing restriction. *Lancet* 357: 1325–1328.

72. Halm EA, Atlas SJ, Borowsky LH et al 2000 Understanding physician adherence with a pneumonia practice guideline: effects of patient, system, and physician factors. *Archives of Internal Medicine* 160: 98–104.

73. Cabana MD, Rand CS, Powe NR et al 1999 Why don't physicians follow clinical practice guidelines? A framework for improvement. *Journal of the American Medical Association* 282: 1458–1465.

74. Grilli R, Magrini N, Penna A, Mura G, Liberati A 2000 Practice guidelines developed by specialty societies: the need for a critical appraisal. *Lancet* 355: 103–106.

75. Worrall G, Chaulk P, Freake D 1997 The effects of clinical practice guidelines on patient outcomes in primary care: a systematic review. *Canadian Medical Association Journal* 156: 1705–1712.

76. Giesen D 1988 *International Medical Malpractice Law*. Kluwer Academic Publishers, Dordrecht.

77. Dominion Law Reports. ter Neuzen v. Korn. 103, 473–520, 2001. Ontario Canada, Canada Law Book, 4th Series.

78. House of Lords 1997 Judgments – Bolitho v. City and Hackney Health Authority. 13–11–1997. Judicial Office, House of Lords, London.

79. Pauker SG, Rothberg M 1999 Commentary: resist jumping to conclusions. *British Medical Journal* 318: 1616–1617.

80. Sabin JE 1998 Fairness as a problem of love and the heart: a clinician's perspective on priority setting. *British Medical Journal* 317: 1002–1004.

81. Leibovici L, Shraga I, Andreassen S 1999 How do you choose antibiotic treatment? *British Medical Journal* 318: 1614–1618.

82. Fidler DP 1998 Legal issues associated with antimicrobial drug resistance. *Emergency Infectious Diseases* 4: 169–177.

83. Murray MD, Kohler RB, McCarthy MC, Main JW 1988 Attitudes of house physicians concerning various antibiotic use control programs. *American Journal of Hospital Pharmacology* 45: 584–588.

84. Woolf SH 1993 Practice guidelines: A new reality in medicine. *Archives of Internal Medicine* 153: 2646–2655.

85. Bunz D, Gupta S, Jewesson P 1990 Metronidazole cost containment: a two-stage intervention. *Hospital Formulary* 25: 1167–1169, 1177.

86. NIH Task Forces on Antibiotic Use and Antibiotic Resistance Worldwide 1987 Reports of the NIH Task Forces on Antibiotic Use and Antibiotic Resistance Worldwide. Infectious Diseases Society of America, Washington.

87. Grimshaw JM, Russell IT 1993 Effect of clinical guidelines on medical practice: a systematic review of rigorous evaluations. *Lancet* 342: 1317–1321.

88. Gehlbach SH, Wilkinson WE, Hammond WE et al 1984 Improving drug prescribing in a primary care practice. *Medical Care* 22: 193–201.

89. Hershey CO, Porter DK, Breslau D, Cohen DI 1986 Influence of simple computerized feedback on prescription charges in an ambulatory clinic: a randomized clinical trial. *Medical Care* 24: 472–481.

90. Norton PG, Dempsey LJ 1985 Self-audit: its effect on quality of care. *Journal of Family Practice* 21: 289–291.

91. Putnam RW, Curry L 1985 Impact of patient care appraisal on physician behaviour in the office setting. *Canadian Medical Association Journal* 132: 1025–1029.

92. Sanazaro PJ, Worth RM 1978 Concurrent quality assurance in hospital care. Report of a study by Private Initiative in PSRO. *New England Journal of Medicine* 298: 1171–1177.

93. Walton RT, Harvey E, Dovey S, Freemantle N 2001 Computerised advice on drug dosage to improve prescribing practice (Cochrane Review). Update Software; Oxford.

94. Burton ME, Ash CL, Hill DP, Handy T, Shepherd MD, Vasko MR 1991 A controlled trial of the cost benefit of computerized bayesian aminoglycoside administration. *Clinical Pharmacology and Therapeutics* 49: 685–694.

95. Destache CJ, Meyer SK, Bittner MJ, Hermann KG 1990 Impact of a clinical pharmacokinetic service on patients treated with aminoglycosides: a cost-benefit analysis. *Therapeutic Drug Monitoring* 12: 419–426.

96. Thomson O'Brien MA, Oxman AD, Davis DA, Haynes RB, Freemantle N, Harvey EL 2001 Educational outreach visits: effects on professional practice and health care outcomes (Cochrane Review). Update Software, Oxford.

97. Avorn J, Soumerai SB 1983 Improving drug-therapy decisions through educational outreach. A randomized controlled trial of academically based detailing. *New England Journal of Medicine* 308: 1457–1463.

98. Ross-Degnan D, Soumerai SB, Goel PK et al 1996 The impact of face-to-face educational outreach on diarrhoea treatment in pharmacies. *Health Policy Planning* 11: 308–318.

99. Santoso B, Suryawati S, Prawaitasari JE 1996 Small group intervention vs formal seminar for improving appropriate drug use. *Social Science and Medicine* 42: 1163–1168.

100. Thomson O'Brien MA, Oxman AD, Haynes RB, Davis DA, Freemantle N, Harvey EL 2001 Local opinion leaders: effects on professional practice and health care outcomes (Cochrane Review). Update Software, Oxford.

101. Hong SW, Ching TY, Fung JP, Seto WL 1990 The employment of ward opinion leaders for continuing education in the hospital. *Medical Teacher* 12: 209–217.

102. Grilli R, Freemantle N, Minozzi S et al 2001 Mass media interventions: effects on health services utilisation (Cochrane Review). Update Software, Oxford.

103. Freemantle N, Harvey EL, Wolf F et al 2001 Printed educational materials: effects on professional practice and health care outcomes (Cochrane Review). Update Software, Oxford.

104. Maiman LA, Becker MH, Liptak GS, Nazarian LF, Rounds KA 1988 Improving pediatricians' compliance-enhancing practices. A randomized trial. *American Journal of Diseases in Childhood* 142: 773–779.

105. De Santis G, Harvey KJ, Howard D, Mashford ML, Moulds RFW 1994 Improving the quality of antibiotic prescription patterns in general practice. The role of educational intervention 1820. *Medical Journal of Australia* 160: 502–505.

106. Molstad S, Hovelius B 1989 Reduction in antibiotic usage following an educational programme. *Family Practice* 6: 33–37.

107. Molstad S, Ekedahl A, Hovelius B, Thimansson H 1994 Antibiotics prescription in primary care: a 5-year follow-up of an educational programme. *Family Practice* 11: 282–286.

108. Avorn J, Soumerai SB, Taylor W, Wessels MR, Janousek J, Weiner M 1988 Reduction of incorrect antibiotic dosing through a structured educational order form. *Archives of Internal Medicine* 148: 1720–1724.

109. McGowan JE 1983 Antimicrobial resistance in hospital organisms and its relation to antibiotic use. *Reviews of Infectious Disease* 5: 1033–1048.

110. Climo MW, Israel DS, Wong ES, Williams D, Coudron P, Markowitz SM 1998 Hospital-wide restriction of clindamycin: effect on the incidence of *Clostridium difficile*-associated diarrhea and cost. *Annals of Internal Medicine* 128: 989–995.

Useful websites

Relevant guidelines about antibiotic prescribing and infection control

Antibiotic Prescribing Guidance for primary care, issued by Public Health Laboratory Service, London:
http://www.phls.co.uk/advice/Antibiotic%20guidance.htm

Antibiotic Prophylaxis in Surgery, SIGN Guideline 45: http://www.sign.ac.uk/

The SIGN website also has a Guideline Developers Handbook (SIGN 50), a guideline (Number 34) on the management of sore throat, which includes a section on antibiotics and will publish new guidelines on Lower Respiratory Tract and on Otitis Media in 2001/2002 epic – National Evidence-based Guidelines for Preventing Healthcare-associated Infections: http://www.epic.tvu.ac.uk/

Community acquired pneumonia: a new guideline will be published in *Thorax* in mid 2001 and will be available on the British Thoracic Society website: http://www.brit-thoracic.org.uk

Guidelines on the management of infection issued by the Infectious Diseases Society of America: http://www.idsociety.org/

Swedish Strategic Programme for the Rational Use of Antimicrobial Agents and Surveillance of Resistance (STRAMA): http://www.strama.org/English/english.html

Websites with relevant background information and links

Alliance for the Prudent Use of Antibiotics: www.apua.org

American Medical Association: www.ama-assn.org/insight/gen hlth/Antibiot/antibi01.htm

American Society for Microbiology: http://www.asmusa.org/

British Society for Antimicrobial Chemotherapy: http://www.bsac.org.uk

Centers for Disease Control and Prevention: www.cdc.org

Cochrane Effective Practice and Organisation of Care (EPOC): http://www.abdn.ac.uk/public health/hsru/epoc/

National Institute of Allergy and Infectious Diseases: www.niaid.nih.gov/factsheets/antimicro/htm

NIPA: Canada's National Information Program on Antibiotics. http://www.antibiotics-info. org/anti01.html

Nosocomial Infection Control in Europe: http://nice.univ-lyon1.fr/nice/index.htm

Project Icare: Intensive Care Antimicrobial Resistance Epidemiology: http://www.sph.emory.edu/ICARE/

The Copenhagen Recommendations. Report of the EU conference 'The Microbial Threat': http://www.sum.dk/publika/micro98/.

The Hot Zone: Emerging Infectious Diseases Reports and Web Sites: http://www/qis.net/~edwardmc/eid.htm

USA National Center for Infectious Diseases: http://www.cdc.gov/ncidod/eidtopics.htm

WHO Antimicrobial Resistance InfoBank: http://oms2.b3e.jussieu.fr/arinfobank/

WHO Communicable Diseases home page: http://www.who.int/health-topics/idindex.htm

World Health Organization: http://www.who.int/

12 Antibacterial drug discovery: what's in the pipeline?

Beth A. Rasmussen and Steven J. Projan

With the discovery of penicillin, followed by other antibacterial drugs such as tetracycline, came an air of false confidence that bacterial infections had been conquered and a thing of the past. However, bacteria are adapters and survivors. These characteristics have given them the ability to overcome the antibacterial drug assault. It is known all too well that with the use of any antibacterial agent eventually comes the development of resistance to that agent; with resistant bacteria come treatment failures and increased medical expenses. For the majority of clinically important bacterial species the percentage of resistant isolates is continually increasing. As an example, a recent survey of clinical *Streptococcus pneumoniae* isolates from the USA found, not unexpectedly, increasing resistance rates for many antibacterial drugs.[1] Between 1994–1995 and 1999–2000 resistance rates increased 10.6% for penicillin, 16.1% for erythromycin, 9.0% for tetracycline, 9.1% for trimethoprim/sulfamethoxazole and 4.0% for chloramphenicol. The number of multiresistant clinical isolates increased 13.3%. This trend is expected to continue not only for *Str. pneumoniae* but for all clinical species as long as the use of antibacterial drugs continues. The increasing prevalence of resistant and multiresistant isolates is the driving force for the need for new antibacterial drugs. Compounds with unique chemical structures and novel targets are often touted as being preferred since it is expected that such compounds will be effective against isolates harboring multiple resistance mechanisms. This chapter was designated to focus on new preclinical antibacterial drug candidates that are being developed to meet these needs. Unfortunately, most pharmaceutical companies do not disclose information on individual future drug candidates far in advance of their selection as a clinical lead, and for this reason it is difficult to pinpoint specific chemical entities that are destined for future clinical development. Despite this one can gather information from the literature about the approaches and directions that companies are taking to identify the next new antibacterial drug that they hope to take forward into clinical trials. This chapter will give an overview of the challenge in finding a new agent and some of the types of new agents that are being sought with a glimpse at what may be on the horizon in terms of new types of antibacterial drugs.

To begin, the concept of an antibacterial drug is very simple: find a compound that arrests bacterial growth, or kills the bac-

Table 12.1 Characteristics of a new antibacterial agent

Characteristic	Preferred	Acceptable
Spectrum of activity	Broad spectrum Gm+ and Gm–	Gm+ and fastidious Gm– or Gm+ only
Bioavailability	Orally active	Parenteral
Dosing	Once a day	More than once per day
Compound Class	Novel	'Next generation'
Antibacterial Activity	Bactericidal	Bacteristatic
Safety	Non-toxic	

Gm+ = Gram-positive; Gm– = Gram-negative

terium, but does not harm the infected individual. However, finding a compound that meets these criteria is not as simple as the statement may lead one to believe. There are boundaries that need to be placed on this statement. The first half of the statement appears straightforward: an antibacterial drug needs to be able to arrest bacterial growth or kill the bacterium. However, all bacterial species are not alike, each bacterial species has unique characteristics that make it susceptibile to an antibacterial agent in different ways from other species. When initiating treatment of an infection a physician often does not know the causative organism(s). To limit the number of drugs a patient receives, an antibacterial drug needs to be effective against a broad spectrum of bacterial species. With very few exceptions an antibacterial drug effective against a single bacterial species would be neither practical nor cost effective to develop. For this reason, the target of an antibacterial drug needs to be essential for many different pathogenic bacterial species. This in turn means that the drug must be active against a target that is conserved but unlikely to be identical among diverse pathogenic bacterial species. In addition to having this broad spectrum of activity, an antibacterial agent must be highly effective. The object of an antibacterial drug is to arrest growth or kill the infecting bacterial species, an agent that only slows bacterial growth would not be an effective antibacterial agent.

The highest hurdle for a new antibacterial drug is safety (as is the case for all pharmaceuticals). Antibacterial drugs currently on the market are not only active but also very safe, and the same level of activity and safety is expected of any new antibacterial drug that comes to market. One might argue that there is a need for new antibacterial agents in light of the increasing number of antibiotic resistant bacteria that are being identified; however, most bacterial isolates are still susceptible to one or more marketed antibacterial agents. A new antibacterial agent with even limited toxicity would have severely restricted (if any) use. The sales of such a drug would therefore be small, and the compound would probably not find wide use. Importantly, to gain enough use to warrant its development, a new antibacterial drug needs to be safe enough to be used to treat infections caused by susceptible as well as resistant bacterial isolates.

Besides safety, any new pharmaceutical agent needs to have a pharmacological profile that makes administration of the drug convenient and demonstrates that the drug will be distributed to the region of the body where it is needed. For an antibacterial drug it is preferred that the compound can be administered orally and as few times a day as possible.

A combination of a broad-spectrum, highly active agent with a good safety profile and a good pharmacological profile is very difficult to find. Despite these hurdles the challenge to find new, effective antibacterial drugs is being taken on by numerous large and small pharmaceutical and biotech companies. To achieve this goal a variety of different approaches are being applied.

Perhaps the most obvious approach, and one that has proven successful for decades, is the identification of 'next generation' agents, agents that are structurally related to an already marketed compound. These compounds belong to the same chemical class and work via the same mechanism of action as the existing drug, but have chemical modifications that give them improved attributes such as an increased spectrum of activity, effectivity against isolates that are resistant to the 'earlier generation(s)' of this drug class, or improved toxicity or pharmacology profiles. A second approach is to develop a compound that is able to inhibit a major resistance mechanism (for example a β-lactamase inhibitor). Such an inhibitor would be used in combination with the original antibacterial drug, shielding it from the resistance mechanism and restoring its activity. One very active area of research for new antibacterial agents is the identification of completely new chemical structures with antibacterial activity. To find these compounds researchers are looking for inhibitors of known, but underexploited, antibacterial targets as well as newly identified antibacterial targets that have come from the analysis of bacterial genomes. There are also novel approaches that are being considered as potential avenues to antibacterial chemotherapy. One such avenue is the targeting of bacterial virulence.

Table 12.2 Potential new antibacterial agents

Compound class	Target	Requirements of new compounds/Comments
'Next generation'		
β-Lactams	Cell wall synthesis	Overcome existing resistance
Ketolides	Protein synthesis	Overcome existing resistance
Quinolones	Gyrase, topoisomerase	Overcome existing resistance
		Improved Gram positive activity
Oxazolidinones	Protein synthesis	Improved spectrum of activity
		Improved potency
Resistance inhibitors		
β-Lactamase inhibitors	β-Lactamases	Improved spectrum of activity. Used in combination with a β-lactam
Efflux pump inhibitors	Tetracycline efflux pumps	Active against multiple efflux pumps. Ineffective against other mechanisms of resistance. Used in combination with a tetracycline
	Pseudomonas efflux pumps	Active against multiple efflux pumps. Used in combination with an antibacterial drug
New compound classes		
Actinoin, novel structures	Peptide deformylase	Rapid development of resistance
Cationic peptides	Bacterial cell membrane, others	High production costs. Topical utility demonstrated
New targets		
	Peptidoglycan synthesis (MurA-F)	Essential, MurB-F non-validated targets
	LxpC, lipid A synthesis	Essential, Gram negative only
	Era, RAS-like GTPase	Essential, non-validated target
	Acyl carrier protein synthase	Essential, non-validated target
New approaches		
	Virulence, sortase enzyme	Non-validated antibacterial target. May have prophylactic utility

'NEXT GENERATION' DRUGS

β-LACTAMS

When the term 'next generation' is used along with an anti-bacterial agent the first drug class that comes to mind is the β-lactam family. β-Lactam drugs are highly effective inhibitors of bacterial cell wall synthesis, inhibiting the formation of the peptide cross-bridges of peptidoglycan. β-Lactam drugs fall into four basic structure classes (penicillins, cephalosporins, carbapenems, and monobactams), determined by the core structure of the lactam ring-containing portion of the molecule. Several classes of β-lactam drugs already have three or more generations in their family tree.

Among the β-lactam antibiotics currently being studied are the next generation of cepahlosporins. Several companies are involved in the identification of cephalosporins that are active against methicillin-resistant *Staphylococcus aureus* (MRSA).[2–4] Any drug active against MRSA could be used in place of van-comycin to treat these infections. It is anticipated that this would decrease the use of vancomycin, thus decreasing the selection and spread of vancomycin-resistant *Enterococcus* (VRE) and glycopeptide-intermediate resistant *Staph. aureus* (GISA). In addition to including MRSA in the antibacterial spectrum, the increased anti-pseudomonal activity is also being sought.

Like the cephalosporins the carbapenem class of β-lactams is also being improved upon. Among the activities that are looking to be improved with this class are oral bioavailability[5] (all currently marketed carbapenems are parenteral[6,7]), activity of the compounds against MRSA;[8,9] and stability of the compounds to the human renal dehydropeptidase I enzyme,[10,11] a major metabolic enzyme for this class of β-lactams. Also of concern with the carbapenem antibiotics (and many other β-lactams) is serum albumin binding. Reduced albumin binding is another area where next generation β-lactams may show improvement. There is a considerable amount of research being performed to find improved cephalosporins and carbapenems. It is anticipated that newer versions of both types will eventually find their way to the marketplace.

KETOLIDES

The ketolides, telithromycin being the first member of this class, are another class of antibiotic that is experiencing a strong next generation surge. Ketolides themselves are a modi-fied version of the macrolides. The first improved versions of the macrolide class of antibacterial drugs were designed to improve their half-life and gastrointestinal toxicity. The next generation ketolides are now being developed to overcome resistance, which has been steadily increasing.[12–16] The chal-lenge here is that more than one mechanism of resistance is of clinical importance. Resistance can be achieved by expression of an efflux pump that is able to pump the drug out of the cell, reducing the intracellular concentration. For many inhibitors of protein synthesis decreasing the intracellular concentration is an effective resistance mechanism. The second major mech-anism of resistance is enzymatic ribosomal modification (MLS phenotype; *see* p. 33), leading to a reduced affinity of the inhibitor for its site of action on the ribosome. Several com-panies are developing compounds designed to overcome both mechanisms of resistance. Some of these compounds are already headed to clinical development. However, one problem with some of these new agents is that they do not truly over-come the ribosomal modification resistance mechanism. The compounds are effective against bacterial isolates harboring the MLS resistance mechanism, because they are not effective at inducing expression of this resistance mechanism. However, if the resistance is activated by other means, such as by muta-tion to constitutive expression, the strains *are* resistant to these new ketolides. Thus, resistance to these compounds will develop rapidly in isolates harboring the MLS resistance genes by mutation to constitutive expression.[13] This will limit the effective lifespan of these agents and may hinder their devel-opment.

QUINOLONES

The quinolones are also continuing to grow in number. Quinolones are unique in that they are actually inhibitors of two essential structurally related bacterial enzymes, gyrase and topoisomerase. The relative susceptibility of each target differs among bacterial species. High-level resistance to this class of drugs is associated with mutational changes in both target genes.

New fluoro- and non-fluorinated quinolones are under development to overcome one or more mechanisms of resis-tance. The 2-hydroxyisoquinolones are being developed as a new class of gyrase inhibitors said to be active against quinolone resistant gyrase mutants.[17] Acidic quinolones having an amino or alkylamino group at the 7 position have shown improved activity against Gram-positive bacteria including quinolone-resistant isolates.[18] Other positions of the molecule are also being looked at for substitutions that will improve the activity of the compounds against Gram-positive bacteria.[19,20] Several companies are developing new non-fluorinated quinolones in the hope of having activity against resistant iso-lates. These compounds show improved MIC against quinolone-resistant Gram-positive bacterial isolates.[20,21] However, the level of susceptibility of the resistant isolates is not equivalent to that of the susceptible isolates. Analysis of the MIC data indicates that these compounds are more potent than the earlier quinolones. However, there is still a large increase in the MIC values of quinolone-resistant versus sus-ceptible isolates. This suggests that the compounds are more potent, and that the MICs against both resistant and suscep-tible isolates are equally improved but that the resistance allele is still rendering the isolates less susceptible to the drug.

One very important issue that needs to be kept in mind with the quinolones is toxicity. Several quinolones have been removed from the market or restricted in their use due to toxicity issues:[22] liver toxicity, QTc interval prolongation, and other safety issues that will have to be addressed by the newer generation compounds. It is anticipated that at least some newer quinolone compounds will make it to clinical trials.

OXAZOLIDINONES

Another class of next generation compounds is the oxazolidinones. The first marketed oxazolidinone, linezolid, has just arrived on the market. Yet, before its approval newer versions of this drug class had been developed. The main features that are being sought in the next generation oxazolidinones are improved potency and an expansion of the spectrum of activity.[23] Linezolid is active against Gram-positive isolates including MRSA, VRE and penicillin-resistant *Streptococcus pneumoniae*. However, it lacks activity against Gram-negative bacteria, including the fastidious Gram-negative bacteria that contribute to respiratory infections. The minimal addition of the fastidious Gram-negative species, including *Haemophilus influenzae* and *Moraxella catarrhalis*, would greatly improve the utility of this drug class. Some newer compounds are showing improvements in the spectrum of activity.[24–28] There are also slight improvements in the antibacterial potency of some of these newer compounds. It is anticipated that additional oxazolidinones will become antibacterial drugs.

INHIBITORS OF RESISTANCE MECHANISMS

Another method of saving a good antibacterial drug, whose utility is threatened by increasing resistance, is to find an inhibitor of the resistance mechanism as described above. The inhibitor would be used in combination with the drug, inactivating the resistance mechanism and in so doing potentiating the activity of the antibacterial drug.

β-LACTAMASE INHIBITORS

This method has worked well with β-lactam antibacterials, for which the major resistance mechanism is inactivation by a β-lactamase. There are currently four β-lactam/β-lactamase inhibitor drug combinations on the market (*see* Ch. 17). Although these combinations are very effective they are limited in that enzymes from only one class (class A) of the four classes (classes A, B, C, and D) of β-lactamases are effectively inhibited. Class A enzymes were the predominant clinically important β-lactamases at the time these inhibitors were developed; however, the β-lactamase profile of clinical isolates is changing. Increasing numbers of isolates express β-lactamases that are not susceptible to inhibition by the currently marketed

inhibitors, and to continue the reign of the β-lactam researchers are looking to find new β-lactamase inhibitors, among them broad-spectrum inhibitors that work against the two most common classes of β-lactamase enzymes (the class A and class C active site serine enzymes; *see* p. 262).[29]

The challenge in finding a broad-spectrum inhibitor is multifold. First there are hundreds of β-lactamases. Although most of these enzymes fall into a few principal families and perform the same enzymatic function, there are differences in the details of the mechanism of hydrolysis that make finding one universal inhibitor difficult. Despite this, there have been reports of several inhibitors that are active against more than one class of active site serine β-lactamases.[29,30]

Perhaps the most diverse class of β-lactamases is the class B metallo-β-lactamases. Although still limited in their distribution, these enzymes are increasing in prominence. Many enzymes in this class have the unique ability to inactivate multiple classes of β-lactams, including the carbapenems, which are generally resistant to inactivation by the serine β-lactamases. For this reason the metalloenzymes have been identified as an inhibitor target. A series of mercaptoacetic compounds having metallo-β-lactamase inhibitory activity have been identified.[31] Although these compounds show good activity against the *Pseudomonas aeruginosa* IMP-1 metallo-β-lactamase as well as the *Aeromonas hydrophilia* CphA enzyme they lack effective inhibitor activity against the *Bacteriodes fragilis* metallo-β-lactamase.

Another potential β-lactamase inhibitor for future consideration is a series of 1β-methyl carbapenem-based inhibitors. One inhibitor of this structure was found to be active against IMP-1 and other metallo-β-lactamases, also active against class A and class C beta-lactamases.[30] Further development of multiclass β-lactamase inhibitors is expected.

EFFLUX PUMP INHIBITORS

Efflux pumps may be specific, as in the case of the tetracycline efflux pumps, or non-specific, as is the case for the multidrug resistance pumps capable of effluxing a host of drugs and other toxic agents.

Inhibitors of the efflux pumps are being developed along two avenues. One is the development of pump inhibitors designed to block the efflux of tetracycline by the tetracycline efflux pumps.[32] A tetracycline pump inhibitor would be used in combination with a tetracycline in the same way that a β-lactamase inhibitor is used in combination with a β-lactam. There are two major complications to this approach. The first is that there are multiple tetracycline efflux pumps. An effective inhibitor would need to be active against at least the most common subset of these pumps. The bigger problem is that efflux is not the only mechanism of tetracycline resistance. A second major mechanism, ribosomal protection, is also of clinical importance. Clinical isolates have been identified which harbor such genes and express both resistance mechanisms.

At the present time the ribosomal protection resistance

mechanism is not the major mechanism of resistance among the Gram-negative bacteria. It does, however, play a large role in Gram-positive tetracycline resistance. It is possible that a tetracycline efflux inhibitor could be developed specifically against the major Gram-negative bacterial efflux pumps for use against Gram-negative bacteria; however, it is anticipated that this would foster the spread of the ribosomal protection resistance mechanism.

Another more promising area, where pump inhibitors could make an impact on antibacterial therapy, is in inhibitors directed against the *Pseudomonas aeruginosa* endogenous efflux pumps. *Ps. aeruginosa* is one of only a few bacterial species for which a specific antibacterial agent would potentially be commercially viable. *Ps. aeruginosa* is known for being refractory to antibacterial chemotherapy; in general being less permeable to antibacterial agents than most other infectious bacterial species due to its restrictive outer membrane. It also harbors a collection of efflux pumps that are capable of effluxing a large number and variety of antibacterial agents. The organism is capable of upregulating expression of one or more efflux pumps to decrease its susceptibility to most any given antibiotic. An inhibitor of these efflux pumps could be used to enhance the activity of many antibacterial drugs.

Inhibitors of the major *Ps. aeruginosa* efflux pumps have been identified and have been shown to enhance the antibacterial activity of levofloxacin and some macrolides.[33–35] These peptidomimetic inhibitors are able to reduce the MIC of *Ps. aeruginosa* isolates overexpressing one of the major efflux pumps. The compounds have also been demonstrated to reduce the ED_{50} of levofloxacin in a mouse sepsis model using efflux pump overexpressing *Ps. aeruginosa* isolates.[36] The effectiveness of these compounds in enhancing the activity of levofloxacin is demonstrable even when the organism harbors a *gyrA* (one of the two cellular targets of the quinolones) resistance mutation.[36] These compounds have potential as enhancers of antibacterial activity of several classes of antibacterial drugs.[35] Improvements in the original series have been made to stabilize the compound to serum proteases as well as chemical instability. It remains to be seen if the current compounds have sufficient breadth of activity against multiple different efflux pumps to be effective antibacterial drug enhancers. However, the concept of using an efflux pump inhibitor in combination with an antibacterial drug has been validated with the current compounds.

NEW ANTIBACTERIAL DRUG CLASSES AND TARGETS

An example of a new antibacterial target is peptide deformylase (PDF), the enzyme that removes the formyl group from the *N*-terminal methionine of nascent polypeptides. The enzymatic activity is essential and highly conserved among bacteria, but is absent from eukaryotes, which do not use a formyl-methionine to initiate protein synthesis. A natural product inhibitor, actinoin, and several synthetic chemical structures, have been identified as inhibitors of this enzymatic activity.[37–41] These compounds have antibacterial activity against a variety of bacterial species and by all measures are acting through inhibition of PDF. However, the utility of these compounds as antibacterial drugs is questionable. Studies indicate that resistance among *Escherichia coli* to PDF inhibitors develops at a frequency of one in 10^{-7}.[38] Interestingly, the resistance is mediated by mutations in the formyltransferase gene.[38,42] The formyltransferase is responsible for attachment of the formyl group to the methionine-charged tRNA. These mutant strains do not produce formyl-methionine-charged tRNA and initiate protein synthesis with a met-tRNA. There is consequently no formyl group to be removed from the nascent polypeptides. Formyltransferase-negative bacteria grow more slowly than wild-type bacteria and have been demonstrated to be less virulent, but not avirulent.[42] Because of the rapid development of resistance to inhibitors of PDF it is unlikely that compounds active against this target will be developed into antibacterial drugs.

An area of research that has spawned the formation of several biotech companies is antibacterial cationic peptides. The progenitors of these peptides are part of the natural defense mechanism of plants and animals.[43] The first antibacterial peptides were identified in the early 1980s in the pupae of the silk moth, and have since been found in plants, insects, frogs, humans, and numerous other species. These peptides contain excess lysine and arginine and can be α-helical or β-sheet peptides with or without disulfide bridges. The site of action of many of these peptides is the cytoplasmic membrane, where the peptides assemble, forming pores or channels.[43,44] However, the exact mechanism by which this process kills the bacteria is still unclear. The selectivity of these peptides for bacterial cells is due to differences in the composition of bacterial and eukaryotic membranes. Synthetic peptides based on the natural versions are being designed as antibacterial agents,[45–47] with the goal of improving the metabolic stability and antibacterial activity and broadening the spectrum of activity to include both Gram-positive and Gram-negative bacteria. The advantages of using cationic peptides are that the compounds are usually bactericidal, the development of resistance is extremely low, and they are active against bacterial isolates harboring resistance mechanisms to other antibacterial drugs.[45] However, their breadth of utility is as yet unknown as the compounds of this class that have been developed to date have been developed for topical or wound applications,[46] and it is unclear whether they will be amenable to systemic application.

In the quest to identify antibacterial agents with a unique chemical structure new potential drug targets are being exploited. There are two hoped-for advantages to doing this: (a) identification of a new antibacterial drug class: (b) that the active compounds will not be limited in their efficacy by pre-existing resistance mechanisms. Within the past few years the complete DNA sequence of numerous bacterial genomes have been elucidated, which has facilitated the identification and validation of new essential targets. The development of polymerase chain reaction technology has expedited the cloning and manipulation of these targets for study and screen development. Together this knowledge and technology base has led to an explosion of new antibacterial targets for which inhibitors are being sought. These targets cross the spectrum of essential activities from inhibitors of the underexplored cell wall synthetic enzymes (MurB-F)[48,49] to LxpC,[50–52] an enzyme involved in Lipid A synthesis, to ACPS (acyl carrier protein synthase),[53] an enzyme essential in fatty acid synthesis, to Era,[54] a RAS-like GTPase that is essential in both Gram-positive and Gram-negative bacteria. For these the essential nature of the targets is known, but their ability to serve as good targets for antibacterial chemotherapy has yet to be documented. There is little doubt that inhibitors of each of these enzymes can be identified; the question is whether these inhibitors can be developed into safe and effective antibacterial drugs.

One last area of antibacterial drug discovery to be discussed is the area of virulence. If one can disarm a bacterium will this assist in the clearance or prevention of infection. Keeping in mind that disease-causing bacteria often express more then one virulence factor and that eliminating any one virulence factor reduces the virulence but rarely renders a strain avirulent, are virulence factors viable antibacterial targets? If so, how many of the factors need to be inhibited to see a positive effect? Is the inhibition of virulence factors going to have an antibacterial effect? One of the best chances of answering these questions is to target a broader mechanism such as the attachment of virulence factors to the bacterial cell surface. This would potentially have the effect of disabling several virulence factors at once. Inhibitors of the bacterial enzyme sortase are being sought,[55] (sortase is the enzyme that attaches Gram-positive bacterial virulence factors to the bacterial cell wall, tethering them to the cell surface[56]). Will these compounds function as antibacterial agents or can they be used prophylactically, sparing the use of 'true' antibacterial drugs? The answer to this question is unknown, and will only become known with the identification of an inhibitor.

The search for new antibacterial agents encompasses a plethora of approaches. The risk and reward for each approach is different. The 'next generation' compounds come from a family of compounds with a generally proven track record. However, the development of resistance may be more rapid and the market share may be smaller due to competition with other members of the same class. The identification of a completely new chemical structure with antibacterial drug-like properties is more challenging and has greater risk, but the returns in finding a new antibacterial drug class can be very high. A blend of both approaches is needed to provide compounds that will fill the needs of the community, which is to provide new antibacterial drugs that will effectively treat bacterial infections without further injury to the infected person.

References

1. Doem GV, Heilmann KP, Huynh HK, Rhomberg PR, Coffman SL, Brueggemann AB 2001 Antimicrobial resistance among clinical isolates of *Streptococcus pneumoniae* in the United States during 1999–2000, including a comparison of resistance rates since 1994–1995. *Antimicrobial Agents and Chemotherapy* 45: 1721–1729.
2. Chamberland S, Blais J, Hoang M et al 2001 In vitro activities of RWJ-54428 (MC-02,479) against multiresistant Gram-positive bacteria. *Antimicrobial Agents and Chemotherapy* 45: 1422–1430.
3. Ohki H, Kawabata K, Inamoto Y, Okuda S, Kamimura T, Sakane K 1997 Studies on 3'-quaternary ammonium cephalosporins-III. Synthesis and antibacterial activity of 3'-(3-aminopyrazolium)cephalosporins. *Bioorganic and Medicinal Chemistry* 5: 557–567.
4. Tsushima M, Iwamatsu K, Tamura A, Shibahara S 1998 Novel cephalosporin derivatives processing a bicyclic heterocycle at the 3-position. Part I: Synthesis and biological activities of 3-(benzothiazol-2-yl) thiocephalosporin derivatives, CP0467 and related compounds. *Bioorganic and Medicinal Chemistry* 6: 1009–1017.
5. Kanno O, Miyauchi M, Shibayama T, Ohya S, Kawamoto I 1999 Synthesis and biological evaluation of new oral carbapenems with 1-methyl-5-oxopyrrolidin-3-ylthio moiety. *Journal of Antibiotics* 52: 900–907.
6. Kato N, Tanaka K, Kato H, Watanabe K 2000 In vitro activity of R-95867, the active metabolite of a new oral carbapenem, CS-834, against anaerobic bacteria. *Journal of Antimicrobial Chemotherapy* 45: 357–361.
7. Hikida M, Itahashi K, Igarashi A, Shiba T, Kitamura M 1999 In vitro antibacterial activity of LJC 11,036, an active metabolite of L-084, a new oral carbapenem antibiotic with potent antipneumococcal activity. *Antimicrobial Agents and Chemotherapy* 43: 2010–2016.
8. Laub JB, Greenlee ML, DiNinno F, Huber JL, Sundelof JG 1999 The synthesis and anti-MRSA activity of amidinium-substituted 2-dibenzofuranylcarbapenems. *Bioorganic and Medicinal Chemistry Letters* 9: 2973–2976.
9. Ohtake N, Imamura H, Jona H et al 1998 Novel dithiocarbamate carbapenems with anti-MRSA activity. *Bioorganic and Medicinal Chemistry* 6: 1089–1101.
10. Shin KJ, Yoo KH, Kim DJ et al 1998 Synthesis and biological properities of new 1β-methylcarbapenems. *Bioorganic and Medicinal Chemistry Letters* 8: 1607–1612.
11. Kang YK, Shin KJ, Yoo KH et al 2000 Synthesis and antibacterial activity of new carbapenems containing isoxazole moiety. *Bioorganic and Medicinal Chemistry Letters* 10: 95–99.
12. Agouridas C, Denis A, Auger J-M et al 1998 Synthesis and antibacterial activity of Ketolides (6-O-Methyl-3-oxoerythromycin derivatives): A new class of antibacterials highly potent against macrolide-resistant and -susceptible respiratory pathogens. *Journal of Medicinal Chemistry* 41: 4080–4100.
13. Or YS, Clark RF, Wang S et al 2000 Design, synthesis, and antimicrobial activity of 6-O-substituted ketolides active against resistant respiratory tract pathogens. *Journal of Medicinal Chemistry* 43: 1045–1049.
14. Kaneko T, Mcmillen W, Sutcliffe J, Duignan J, Petitpas J 2000 Synthesis and in vitro activity of C2-substituted C9-oxime ketolides. Abstracts of 40th Interscience Conference on Antimicrobial Agents and Chemotherapy. American Society for Microbiology, Toronto, Ontario, Canada, p. 213.
15. Girard D, Mathieu HW, Fnegan SM, Cimochowski CR, Kaneko TK, Mcmillen W 2000 In vitro antibacterial activity of CP-654, 743, a new C2-fluoro ketolide, against macrolide resistant Pneumonocci and *Haemophilus influenzae*. Abstracts of 40th Interscience Conference on Antimicrobial Agents and Chemotherapy. American Society for Microbiology, Toronto, Ontario, Canada, p. 213.
16. Bush K, Abbanat D, Ashley G et al 2000 In vitro and in vivo SAR of ketolides derived from R13-modified erythromycin A and picromycin core structures. Abstracts of 40th Interscience Conference on Antimicrobial Agents and Chemotherapy. American Society for Microbiology, Toronto, Ontario, Canada, p. 214.
17. Stier Ma, Watson BM, Domagala JM et al 2000 The synthesis and SAR of a series of 2-hydroxyisoquinolones: New antibacterial gyrase inhibitors. Abstracts of 40th Interscience Conference on Antimicrobial Agents and Chemotherapy. American Society for Microbiology, Toronto, Ontario, Canada, p. 209.
18. Kuramoto Y, Ohshita Y, Amano H, Hirao Y, Hayashi N, Aoki S 2000 Structure-activity relationships of novel acidic, 7-amino or 7-alkylamino-1-(5-amino-2,4-difluorophenly)-8-methylquinolones. Abstracts of 40th Interscience Conference on Antimicrobial Agents and Chemotherapy. American Society for Microbiology, Toronto, Ontario, Canada, p. 209.
19. Takahashi H 2000 Synthesis and biological evaluation of D61-1113, a novel fluoroquinolone having potent activity against Gram-positive bacteria including MRSA, PRSP and VRE. Abstracts of 40th Interscience Conference on Antimicrobial Agents and Chemotherapy. American Society for Microbiology, Toronto, Ontario, Canada, p. 209.

20. Sahm DF, Staples A, Critchley I, Thornsberry C, Murfitt K, Mayfield D 2000 Activities of non-fluorinated quinolones against recent clinical isolates of Gram-positive cocci, including those resistant to currently available fluoroquinolones. Abstracts of 40th Interscience Conference on Antimicrobial Agents and Chemotherapy. American Society for Microbiology, Toronto, Ontario, Canada, p. 210.

21. Brown SD, Fuchs PC, Barry AL 2000 In vitro activities of 3 non-fluorinated quinolones and 3 fluoroquinolones against consecutive clinical isolates from eleven U. S. medical centers. Abstracts of 40th Interscience Conference on Antimicrobial Agents and Chemotherapy. American Society for Microbiology, Toronto, Ontario, Canada, p. 210.

22. Berito JJ, Fish D 2000 The safety profile of the fluoroquinolones. *Clinical Therapeutics* 22: 798–817.

23. Gleave DM, Brickner SJ, Manninen PR et al 1998 Synthesis and antibacterial activity of [6,5,5] and [6,6,5] tricyclic fused oxazolidinones. *Bioorganic and Medicinal Chemistry Letters* 8: 1231–1236.

24. Genin MJ, Hutchinson DK, Allwine DA et al 1998 Nitrogen-carbon-linked (Azolylphenyl) oxazolidinones with potent antibacterial activity against the fastidious Gram-negative organisms *Hemophilus influenzae* and *Moraxella catarrhalis*. *Journal of Medicinal Chemistry* 41: 5144–5147.

25. Cynamon MH, Klemens SP, Sharpe CA, Chase S 1999 Activities of several novel oxazolidinones against *Mycobacterium tuberculosis* in a murine model. *Antimicrobial Agents and Chemotherapy* 43: 1189–1191.

26. Genin MJ, Allwine DA, Anderson DJ et al 2000 Substituent effects on the antibacterial activity of nitrogen-carbon-linked (azolylphenyl)oxazolidinones with expanded activity against the fastidious Gram-negative organisms *Haemophilus influenzae* and *Moraxella catarrhalis*. *Journal of Medicinal Chemistry* 43: 953–970.

27. Rhee JK, Im WB, Lee TH et al 2000 In vitro and in vivo activities of 10 new pyridine-containing oxazolidinone derivatives including DA-7686. Abstracts of 40th Interscience Conference on Antimicrobial Agents and Chemotherapy. American Society for Microbiology, Toronto, Ontario, Canada, p. 214.

28. Endermann R, Bartel S, Guarnieri W et al 2000 Novel imidazo-benzoxazinlyoxazolidinones: In vitro and in vivo activities and pharmacokinetics in mice. Abstracts of 40th Interscience Conference on Antimicrobial Agents and Chemotherapy. American Society for Microbiology, Toronto, Ontario, Canada, p. 215.

29. Tondi D, Powers RA, Caselli E, Costi PM, Shoichet BK 2000 Structure-based design and in parallel synthesis of boronic acid inhibitors of AmpC β-lactamase. Abstracts of 40th Interscience Conference on Antimicrobial Agents and Chemotherapy. American Society for Microbiology, Toronto, Ontario, Canada, p. 204.

30. Nagano R, Adachi Y, Imamura H, Yamada K, Hashizume T, Morishima H 1999 Carbapentem derivatives as potential inhibitors of various β-lactamases, Including class B metallo-β-lactamases. *Antimicrobial Agents and Chemotherapy* 43: 2497–2503.

31. Payne DJ, Bateson JH, Gasson BC et al 1997 Inhibition of metallo-β-lactamases by a series of mercaptoacetic acid thiol ester derivatives. *Antimicrobial Agents and Chemotherapy* 41: 135–140.

32. Hirata T, Wakatabe R, Nielsen J, Satoh T, Nihira S, Yamaguchi A 1998 Screening of an inhibitor of the tetracycline efflux pump in a tetracycline-resistant clinical-isolate of *Staphylococcus aureus*. *Biological and Pharmaceutical Bulletin* 21: 678–681.

33. Renau TE, Leger R, Flamme EM et al 1999 Inhibitors of efflux pumps in *Pseudomonas aeruginosa* potentiate the activity of the fluoroquinolone antibacterial levofloxacin. *Journal of Medicinal Chemistry* 42: 4928–4931.

34. Leger R, Renau TE, Zhang JZ et al 2000 Peptidomimetics of dipeptide amide efflux pump inhibitors potentiate the activity of levofloxacin in Pseudomonas aeruginosa. Abstracts of 40th Interscience Conference on Antimicrobial Agents and Chemotherapy. American Society for Microbiology, Toronto, Ontario, Canada, p. 207.

35. Cho D, Lofland D, Blais J et al 2000 An efflux pump inhibitor (EPI), MC-04, 124, enhances the activity of macrolides against Gram-negative bacteria. Abstracts of 40th Interscience Conference on Antimicrobial Agents and Chemotherapy. American Society for Microbiology, Toronto, Ontario, Canada, p. 208.

36. Griffith D 2000 Potentiation of Levofloxicin (Levo) by MC-02, 595, a broad-spectrum efflux pump inhibitor (EPI) in mouse models of infection due to *Pseudomonas aeruginosa* (PA) with combinations of different Mex pump

expression and *gyrA*. Abstracts of 40th Interscience Conference on Antimicrobial Agents and Chemotherapy. American Society for Microbiology, Toronto, Ontario, Canada, p. 207.

37. Chen DZ, Patel DV, Hackbarth CJ et al 2000 Actinonin, a naturally occuring antibacterial agent, is a potent deformylase inhibitor. *Biochemistry* 39: 1256–1262.

38. Apfel CM, Locher H, Evers S et al 2001 Peptide deformylase as an antibacterial drug target: Target validation and resistance development. *Antimicrobial Agents and Chemotherapy* 45: 1058–1064.

39. Hu Y-J, Rajagopalan PTR, Pei D 1998 H-phosphonate derivatives as novel peptide deformylase inhibitors. *Bioorganic and Medicinal Chemistry Letters* 8: 2479–2482.

40. Apfel C, Banner DW, Bur D et al 2000 Hydroxamic acid derivatives as potent peptide derofmylase inhibitors and antibacterial agents. *Journal of Medicinal Chemistry* 43: 2324–2331.

41. Huntington KM, Yi T, Wei Y, Pei D 2000 Synthesis and antibacterial activity of peptide deformylase inhibitors. *Biochemistry* 39: 4543–4551.

42. Margolis PS, Hackbarth CJ, Young DC et al 2000 Peptide deformylase in *Staphylococcus aureus*: Resistance to inhibitors is mediated by mutations in the formyltransferase gene. *Antimicriobial Agents and Chemotherapy* 44: 1825–1831.

43. Hancock REW, Lehrer R 1998 Cationic peptides: a new source of antibiotics. *Trends in Biotechnology* 16: 82–88.

44. Friedrich CL, Moyles D, Beveridge TJ, Hancock REW 2000 Antibacterial action of structurally diverse cationic peptides on Gram-positive bacteria. *Antimicrobial Agents and Chemotherapy* 44: 2086–2092.

45. Ge Y, MacDonald DL, Holroyd KJ, Thomsberry C, Wexler H, Zasloff M 1999 In vitro antibacterial properities of Pexiganan, an analog of Magainin. *Antimicrobial Agents and Chemotherapy* 43: 782–788.

46. Oren Z, Shai Y 2000 Cyclization of a cytolytic amphipathic α-helical peptide and its diastereomer: Effect on structure, interaction with model membranes, and biological function. *Biochemistry* 39: 6103–6114.

47. Otvos LJ, Bokonyi K, Vara I et al 2000 Insect peptides with improved protease-resistance protect mice against bacterial infection. *Protein Science* 9: 742–749.

48. Sun D, Chhen S, Rothstein DM 2000 A sensitive and specific high-throughput screen that detects cell wall-active agents. Abstracts of 40th Interscience Conference on Antimicrobial Agents and Chemotherapy. American Society for Microbiology, Toronto, Ontario, Canada, p. 223.

49. Wu CYE, Cox K, Yao R et al 2000 The development of a high throughput screen to select inhibitors of MurD from *Streptococcus pneumoniae*. Abstracts of 40th Interscience Conference on Antimicrobial Agents and Chemotherapy. American Society for Microbiology, Toronto, Ontario, Canada, p. 224.

50. Young D, Rafanan N, Margolis P, Trias J 2000 Role of LpxC, a target for novel antibiotic discovery, in natural resistance to antibiotics. Abstracts of 40th Interscience Conference on Antimicrobial Agents and Chemotherapy. American Society for Microbiology, Toronto, Ontario, Canada, p. 224.

51. Rafanan N, Lopez S, Hackbarth C et al 2000 Resistance in *E. coli* to LpxC inhibitor L-161, 240 is due to mutations in the *lpxC* gene. Abstracts of 40th Interscience Conference on Antimicrobial Agents and Chemotherapy. American Society for Microbiology, Toronto, Ontario, Canada, p. 225.

52. Wang W, Maniar M, Jain R, Jacobs J, Trias J, Yuan Z 2001 A flourescence-based homogeneous assay for measuring activity of UDP-3-O-(R-3-hydroxymyristoyl)-N-acetylglucosamine deacetylase. *Analytical Biochemistry* 290: 338–346.

53. McAllister KA 2001 The use of a flourescein-labeled Co-enzyme A for the detection of acyl carrier protein synthase (AcpS) activity. Abstracts of 40th Interscience Conference on Antimicrobial Agents and Chemotherapy. American Society for Microbiology, Toronto, Ontario, Canada, p. 225.

54. Snyder NJ, Meier TI, Wu CE, Letourneau DL, Zhao G, Tebbe MJ 2000 Discovery of a series of compounds that demonstrate potent broad-spectrum antibacterial activity and inhibition of Era, an essential bacterial GTPase. Abstracts of 40th Interscience Conference on Antimicrobial Agents and Chemotherapy. American Society for Microbiology, Toronto, Ontario, Canada; p. 225.

55. Ton-That H, Schneewing O 1999 Anchor structure of staphylococcal surface proteins. IV. Inhibitors of the cell wall sorting reaction. *Journal of Biological Chemistry* 274: 24316–24320.

56. Mazmanian SK, Liu G, Ton-That H, Schneewind O 1999 *Staphylococcus aureus* sortase, an enzyme that anchors surface protein to the cell wall. *Science* 285: 760–763.

Strategic and regulatory considerations in the clinical development of anti-infectives

David M. Shlaes and John L. Ryan

The clinical development of new therapeutic and prophylactic entities for infectious diseases has come under increasing regulatory scrutiny in the last several years. During the early years of the HIV pandemic there was a strong community-based movement to pressure both industry and regulatory agencies (e.g. the Food and Drug Administration FDA) to expedite drug development and make new drugs available more quickly. Both industry and the FDA responded to this pressure and several antiviral drugs were approved based on surrogate endpoints. This was in contrast to the requirements for more traditional antibiotics that required both microbiological and clinical endpoints to be met to achieve approval.

The FDA Division of Antiviral Drug Products, in the Center for Drug Evaluation and Research[1] has published a guidance for industry which represents the FDA's current approach to antiretroviral drug development for accelerated and traditional approval. This guidance was published in August 1999, to assist sponsors in the clinical development of drugs for HIV infection. The guidance focused on the use of HIV RNA measurements to support approvals of antiretroviral drugs.[2] Accelerated approvals based on surrogate markers (e.g. CD4 counts and RNA levels), had been recognized officially since 1997 when an advisory panel convened by the FDA recommended the use of a virologic endpoint without extending trials to achieve a clinical endpoint by HIV infection. In fact, combination therapy had already demonstrated a decline in opportunistic infections associated with an increase in CD4 counts and a decrease in RNA levels; thus, longer studies requiring a clinical endpoint for new drugs was no longer feasible. Clearly, community pressure played a central role in motivating the FDA to take this action.

The FDA has published accelerated approval regulations for drugs that 'have been studied for their safety and efficacy in treating serious and/or life-threatening illnesses and that provide meaningful therapeutic benefit to patients over existing treatments (e.g. the ability to treat patients unresponsive to, or intolerant of, available therapy or improved patient response over available therapy).'[3] These regulations apply to *all* drugs and are not restricted to infectious diseases or HIV.

However, there are many areas of clinical development within the field of infectious diseases that fit the criteria specified in these regulations very well. New therapies for chronic viral diseases such as hepatitis B and hepatitis C are examples. While therapies for each of these exist, they are only partially effective and may be associated with significant adverse effects that prevent continuing therapy. The same is true in the HIV field. In spite of the availability of multiple drugs in multiple classes (e.g. nucleoside analogs, non-nucleoside reverse transcriptive inhibitors, protease inhibitors, immunodulators), many patients cannot or will not continue long-term therapy because of tolerability issues. Thus new antiviral agents are needed and the FDA has encouraged industry to study patients who have limited approved treatment options due to lack of therapeutic response or intolerance. The FDA has gone as far as to encourage the use of multiple investigational agents, with the strong caveat that the treatment effect of each drug can be isolated and the potential for drug–drug interactions considered. Isolating the treatment effect of each drug may be challenging, but innovative clinical trial design will often succeed in achieving this goal.

Ribavarin as a single agent has minimal, if any, demonstrable therapeutic benefit in hepatitis C as a single agent, but in combination with interferon has nearly doubled the clinical response rate compared to interferon alone.[4] While the mechanism of this increased activity is unknown, the striking increase in clinical response rate in patients who have few, if any, alternative options for therapy, facilitated regulatory approval of the combination. In hepatitis C, as in HIV, the sustained decrease in viral RNA levels has proven to be a reasonable surrogate marker for clinical activity. A sustained response for hepatitis C, however, necessitates a prolonged eradication of virus for at least 6 months after cessation of therapy. This has not been possible in HIV therapy and to the present continuous therapy is required to maintain viral suppression.

The Committee for Proprietary Medicinal Products has independently issued a 'points to consider' document in the assessment of anti-HIV medicinal products.[5] This document gives guidance similar to the FDA guidance discussed earlier for HIV. New products can be approved under exceptional circumstances. If comprehensive clinical data are not available at the time of submission 24-week data on biological markers (viral load and CD4 counts) along with an acceptable tolerability profile need to be filed.

Thus accelerated approval could be a reasonable approach for a new therapeutic entity in the antiviral area specifically, for either HIV or hepatitis C. These regulations do not diminish the need for an adequate safety database. Unfortunately, the definition of an adequate safety database differs widely in various infectious diseases. In HIV, a relatively small database (less than 1000 patients) is generally acceptable to the FDA. Of interest, the International Committee on Harmonization (ICH)[6,7] guidelines for drugs intended for long-term treatment for non-life-threatening infections is only 300–600 patients for 6 months and a total safety database of 1500 patients. More long-term safety data are also advised, on at least a cohort of patients. It is advisable to maintain close communications with regulatory agencies in the USA and abroad during the conduct of clinical trials if accelerated approval is contemplated. Controlled and comparative data are required to adequately demonstrate both safety and efficacy. Most Phase 2 trials are open and uncontrolled. While impressive efficacy may be observed, the size and duration of such trials is not adequate, in general, to fulfill the safety requirements for accelerated approvals. The FDA has clearly emphasized that casual relationships between a drug and an adverse event are more difficult to ascertain in uncontrolled trials. This is an issue when there is no approved therapy for the illness studied. For instance, what would be the appropriate control in a study of interferon/ribavirin failures for hepatitis C where there is no approved therapy? These challenges are constantly faced by industry in the quest to develop drugs that are able to meet the needs of specific underserved patient populations. As mentioned earlier, the best approach is to work closely and cooperatively with the agencies in designing the trials to be used to seek approval.

Clinical development of new antibacterial compounds has also been exposed to a dynamic regulatory environment and a new set of challenges for industry. Resistance to antibacterial compounds, especially among Gram-positive pathogens, has reawakened the public perception of antibiotics, and the approach of government and the pharmaceutical industry. In the 1980s, the antibacterial market was viewed by physicians and industry as saturated and satisfied, with many drugs becoming generic and with continued competition for sales of branded products, especially among the injectable antibiotics used in hospitals. This led to a significant decline in antibacterial research and development, which lasted throughout the decade.[8] In 1990, with the continuing epidemic of methicillin-resistant staphylococci, the emergence of vancomycin-resistant enterococci in US hospitals, and penicillin-resistant pneumococci in communities globally, interest in antibacterial research and development was revitalized, particularly for Gram-positive infections. In the USA, the groundbreaking publication of the National Academy of Sciences *Emerging Infectious Diseases, a Threat to Public Health*, appeared in 1992.[9] This was followed by increased awareness from the lay press, a number of books from journalists on the topic, and action by Congress to craft a government-wide response. The newly focused research effort by the pharmaceutical industry during the early 1990s led to the development and ultimate registration of a number of new compounds with activity against resistant Gram-positive pathogens. These included quinupristin–dalfopristin, linezolid, the first novel class antibacterial to be introduced since rifampin in 1965, and several fluoroquinolones with increased activity against Gram-positive pathogens. A number of new antibiotics are also in late-stage development including oritavancin, a vancomycin-like glycopeptide with improved activity against vancomycin-resistant Gram-positives, daptomycin, a lipopeptide, and tigilcycline, a glycylcycline with broad spectrum activity including Gram-negative pathogens, anaerobes, atypicals, and Gram-positives (including resistant strains).

Governments in general, the FDA, the European Agency for the Evaluation of Medicinal Products (EMEA), and the WHO in particular are aware of the emergence of life-threatening Gram-positive infections. They are also cognizant of the increasing threat of antimicrobial resistance. There is now pressure from both the public and a variety of scientific groups (including the American Society for Microbiology, the Infectious Diseases Society of America, and the Royal Society) to act to deal with this emerging threat.[10–13] Towards this end, in 2000 the WHO published a report dealing with antimicrobial resistance, antimicrobial use and the development of new antibacterials.[13] The US recently issued a multiagency task force report on the problem of antibiotic resistance.[11] In the section entitled 'product development' the top priority issue to be addressed was to 'better inform researchers and drug manufacturers of current and projected gaps in the arsenal of antimicrobial drugs, vaccines and diagnostics and of potential markets for these products.' The top priority action item under that heading was to create an interagency antimicrobial resistance product development working group coordinated by the FDA, US Department of Agriculture (USDA) and Centers for Disease Control and Prevention (CDC) with a timeline to begin within 1–2 years. A second top priority issue was that existing market incentives and regulatory processes might be insufficient to stimulate development of certain priority products related to antimicrobial resistance while fostering their appropriate use. The goal for this issue was 'to investigate and act upon potential approaches for stimulating and speeding the entire antimicrobial resistance product development process, from drug discovery through licensing.' The action items were to explore the economics of this situation, and explore incentives, with coordinators being the FDA and CDC within 1–5 years. These timelines, unfortunately, suggest that the reports will not really bear fruit until after 2010 given the pace of antibacterial discovery and clinical development.

Ongoing processes noted in the report include the expedited approval process, use of surrogate endpoints, development of more targeted approaches for life-threatening resistance problems and other initiatives. Such incentives and process-improvement possibilities have been explored both by the WHO and the US National Academy of Sciences.[13–15] Table 13.1 is a modification of proposals discussed at the Forum for Emerging Infections of the National Academy of Sciences.[14] Part of this effort would include the development and approval of rapid bedside diagnostic tests for bacterial pathogens, which would allow immediate implementation of focused therapy rather than the current empiric approach taken by most physicians in the absence of an immediate etiological diagnosis. However, such rapid, bedside testing of clinical specimens faces a number of substantial scientific challenges:

Table 13.1 Incentives for increasing pharmaceutical research and development for priority infectious diseases

What is needed	Demand side	Supply side: basic research	Supply side: clinical phases
More information	Market identification • epidemiologic/burden of disease data • ongoing, accessible, integrated, comprehensive surveillance data on disease trends and resistance patterns Priority setting • well articulated, consensus-based public health agendas • clear portrayals of specific disease priorities • product characterization	Disease-specific bioinformation system • research data from universities, research councils, biotechnology companies on product leads for possible development by industry	Development of surrogate endpoints • generic categories of endpoints for use with a range of infectious diseases • alternatives to correlates of protection for vaccines for which clinical trials difficult or impossible
More predictability	Market assessment • early forecasting of demand based on epidemiologic criteria from surveys, demographic analysis • segmentation by size, ability to pay, disease profile • cost-effectiveness analysis	International regulatory harmonization/reinforcement of intellectual property rights	Restricted distribution/product labeling • systematic exploration of tension between need to conserve usable life of antimicrobials while conserving market appeal for R&D investment
More cost- and risk-sharing	Market creation • procurement guarantees via: high-volume bulk orders, extended contracts, product bundling subsidies for poorest countries • revolving funds for national and/or regional purchasing • ODA for health infrastructure and education, drug logistics Multi-tiered pricing • careful articulation of rationales to re-start legislative dialog	Patent extension • exploration of extension of patents for expired compounds with potential utility in new antimicrobials; exploration of extension of non-antimicrobial drug patents • explicit inclusion of antibiotics under Patent Term Restoration Act Stabilization of funding • examination of R&D implications of ODA decreases, annual volatility Financial support to universities and biotechnology companies for taking promising leads to proof-of-principle Venture fund for early-stage development of product leads	Orphan drug legislation • exploration of applications of orphan drug law in developing products for emerging infections, especially niche products, with primary market outside the USA Accelerated regulatory approval • accelerated enrollment in trials • aggregation of efficacy data from multiple sources • continuing the progress in predictability and efficiency in regulatory oversight processes Building contact research organization capability in developing countries to reduce costs and enhance infrastructure for clinical trials Financial subsidy for phase II/III trials, with payback on success

ODA = Official Development Assistance; R&D = research and development.
We want to acknowledge the importance to this table of the list, presented at the workshop by the representative from the World Bank, of suggestions from a survey of pharmaceutical company executives on how to promote health product development for low-income countries. The tabular material presented here is a broader synthesis that draws on the whole range of workshop presentations, including discussions of public-sector needs and priorities; industry perspectives on needs: lessons learned from the Children's Vaccine Initiative and other models; and legal and regulatory issues involved in development of drugs and vaccines for emerging infections. That there is so much concordance about which areas merit attention, as well as the kind of attention they require, is impressive.

- Bedside detection of organisms in specimens where pathogen numbers might be low, like blood, is probably still years from realization.
- A multiplex testing to detect both species and resistance mechanism might be required to specifically guide therapy.

These technical issues make the development of such rapid testing devices unlikely in the next decade or so. Thus, empiric therapy will be with us for at least the next decade. Therefore, we must have a continued supply of broad-spectrum agents available to us until such time as targeted therapy becomes feasible.

Unfortunately, while government struggles to develop incentives for the pharmaceutical industry to continue their research and development activities in antibacterials, they simultaneously send signals that tend to discourage investment. The FDA recently issued draft guidelines[16] in which the in-vitro activity of antibacterials would be deleted from the product label. This proposed guideline, even though it would apply across the industry, represents a clear disincentive for antibacterial discovery and development as it limits the ability to appropriately educate physicians and promote products. At the same time, pharmaceutical companies are currently appropriately required to carry out post-market surveillance studies for resistance and to update their label on a regular basis. Thus, an entire global surveillance effort, with significant support provided by the pharmaceutical industry, has arisen. This surveillance serves the public by keeping health authorities abreast of new developments in resistance to licensed antibiotics. However, if in-vitro data are eliminated from the label, there would be significantly less incentive for industry to continue microbiological surveillance studies on resistance and valuable data may be lost.

In addition, the FDA approves automated antibacterial susceptibility testing devices. In the USA and the major European markets, most hospitals and private laboratories practice such automated testing. Susceptibility testing provides data for treatment of individual patients as well as a repository of surveillance data on resistance. However, without the in-vitro label, it is unclear how regulatory agencies would approve such testing devices.

The pressures on the pharmaceutical industry continue to make the development of antibacterials a high-risk venture. The cost of development has skyrocketed in the last 10–15 years, to the point where overall costs to bring a drug to market have risen to between $170 and $500 million.[17–20] The antibacterial market continues to be a crowded one, with downward price pressure from generics. Price pressures, especially outside the USA, continue to increase, with ever-higher standards being applied to achieve desired pricing. Further, there is continuing pressure to increase the stringency of trials. The FDA guidelines and recent ICH guidelines[6,7] are vaguely worded since trial design tends to be individualized to the compound under development and its comparators. For the last several decades, trials showing equivalence at the 20% level powered to an 80% confidence were acceptable both to the US and EMEA. Now, based on the experience of a number of companies in designing recent trials, there appears to be pressure to change this approach to one of 10–15% non-inferiority powered at the 90% level. This policy, if adopted, would have significant cost implications for running clinical trials because the number of patients required to meet these criteria would increase substantially.

Another issue that tends to increase costs of development include the rising healthcare costs, where the per patient charges for clinical studies are steadily increasing. Institutional review boards are, appropriately, scrutinizing trials of ever-increasing complexity with greater care. This causes delays in starting trials, which slows clinical development and, ultimately, increases costs by delaying entry to market. Although none of these issues is specifically addressed in the US Multi-Agency Task Force Report or by the WHO, they should be discussed as part of the agendas described.

Another key approach to the problem of antimicrobial resistance is pressure to decrease inappropriate use of antibiotics. This concept is supported by industry because it has the potential to prolong the utility of marketed products. The global surveillance for resistance now mandated by EMEA and the FDA (described above) is an important part of this effort. Changing the manner in which antibiotics are prescribed, however, is a long-term educational effort that will require cooperation between practitioners and patients in the interest of public welfare. Academic infectious disease specialists and the major professional associations need to emphasize the issue of appropriate usage of antibiotics to a greater extent. Industry will be a partner in these efforts. Nevertheless, prescribing habits will probably change only slowly, and changes will be dependent to a large extent on available diagnostic testing. The disincentive perceived to exist within managed care for diagnostic testing represents a negative influence on this process.[15]

Another approach, which is not discussed in any of the published guidelines, is to encourage the development of antiviral agents, especially for respiratory viral infections. It is clear that at least 25 million inappropriate antibiotic prescriptions are written every year in the USA for the treatment of viral respiratory infections.[21,22] A safe and effective antiviral that can be used by physicians for viral infections will decrease inappropriate use of antibiotic and specifically treat the etiologic agent causing such disease. Several such agents have recently been developed or are in development: in 1999 and 2000 zanamivir and oseltamivir were approved for the treatment and prevention of influenza; pleconaril for picornavirus (rhinovirus and enterovirus) infections just completed Phase III trials; several compounds are now in early stages of development for respiratory syncytial virus infections in adults and children. Clearly, the pharmaceutical industry sees important opportunities in these therapeutic arenas. There will probably be important public health benefits, both direct and indirect, from these efforts, including a lower risk of the emergence of antimicrobial resistance.

Most antibacterial use is empiric. That is, when physicians prescribe an antibiotic they usually have not yet identified a specific pathogen. There seems to be a growing disincentive for even obtaining a specific diagnosis,[15] so this percentage (now about 70%) may increase. In the clinical development of antibacterials, however, there is no specific indication of 'empiric' therapy. There is not even a specific indication for 'bacteremia.' The old FDA indication for 'septicemia' was abrogated a number of years ago under the hypothesis that most bacteremia was secondary to some primary source, and that the primary source should be the focus of drug development. Thus, indications now exist for skin and skin structure infections (complicated and uncomplicated), complicated intra-abdominal infections, community and hospital-acquired pneumonia, complicated and uncomplicated urinary tract infections, among others. However, the most common source of bacteremia in hospitals is probably so-called 'primary' bacteremia, for which a source is usually not identified.[23,24] It is thought that about 80–90% of these cases have an intravascular catheter as the source of infection. The FDA is currently struggling to provide guidelines for the development of antibiotics for this indication,[25] but no clear consensus has yet emerged. Thus, industry cannot yet develop or promote drugs for one of the most common uses in hospital practice.

There has been increasing regulatory pressure to include diverse patient populations in all infectious disease (as well as other) national drug authorities. The same is true under International Conference on Harmonization guidelines. Gender, age, and race are obvious patient populations that must be treated as well as advanced and early disease (for chronic diseases) and naïve and previously treated patients. Most recently attention has been focused on pediatric populations, and two sets of guidelines have become regulations.

1. One is the 'pediatric rule' which requires each New Drug Application (NDA) to contain data from pediatric populations. This rule (63 FR 66632), called *Regulations Requiring Manufacturers to Assess the Safety and Effectiveness of New Drugs and Biologic Products in Pediatric Patients* represents a change and a mandate to industry to include children before NDA approval. The rationale is obvious: most infectious diseases occur in children as well as adults, yet the safety and activity of new drugs has not been generally assessed before marketing new drugs. This new regulation mandates that pediatric studies be done before submission of a dossier. This should insure that pediatric populations have the benefit of new drugs and that pediatricians have guidance on doses and schedules that are proven safe and effective in children. There has, however, been a negative side to this regulation. Children are now exposed to new drugs earlier in development before the full risk/benefit profile has been defined. There have already been instances of severe adverse experiences, including death, as complications of early clinical testing in children. These events, although rare, have elicited criticism for including children in trials before the full toxicologic profile of a new drug is established. In order to minimize such events while following the 'pediatric rule' the timing and length of pediatric studies pre-NDA approval must be very carefully planned in close cooperation with the FDA and other agencies.

2. The second set of pediatric regulations recently implemented is known as 'pediatric exclusivity'. These regulations allow for a 6-month extension of marketing exclusivity (patent life) for submission of pediatric data by agreement with the FDA. This is permitted in Section 505A of the Federal, Food, Drug and Cosmetic Act (21 U.S.C.355a). This rule benefits both industry and the public in that pediatric data are generated at company expense to provide guidance on the utility of licensed drugs for pediatric use. The company gets a patent extension and the community receives data on risk/benefit for pediatric populations.

European regulations have been updated as the Committee for Proprietary Medicinal Products (CPMP) published its *Note for Guidance on Evaluation of New Anti-Bacterial Medicinal Products*.[26] Emphasis has been placed on microbiologic data for both urinary tract infections and sexually transmitted diseases where the microbiology represents the primary endpoint. Frequency of resistance of targeted pathogens at baseline must be described, as well as susceptibility data on targeted patients classified as failures or recurrences.

General indications such as upper respiratory tract infections or urinary tract infections are not acceptable for licensure. More specific indications such as pharyngitis, otitis media and prostatitis are now required, similar to the FDA mandate that Phase III trials must be randomized and controlled.[26] Open trials are not acceptable, particularly when clinical endpoints are primary endpoints. Double-blind trials should be carried out whenever possible. Emphasis is also placed on performing high-quality active comparator trials. Careful choice of the comparative agent to be used is necessary as it must be effective in the clinical setting under study. Active control studies rather than placebo-control studies are the norm for most infectious diseases. There are specific instances where a placebo control may be used (e.g. exacerbation of chronic bronchitis) but the recent revisions in the Declaration of Helsinki have essentially banned the use of placebo controls in most clinical investigation. In general, placebo controls are not relevant for antibacterial clinical studies.

One important issue within the European Union is that there are regional differences in resistance patterns based on regional uses of licensed drugs. It is the responsibility of the sponsor to take these differences into account in the selection of comparitor drugs within the protocol such that clinical trial data on efficacy are applicable throughout the European Union. An approved indication is applicable only to the population studied in the clinical trial. Extension to other populations will require new studies. Pharmacokinetic and pharmacodynamic data will often help bridge the data sets for different indications.

Specific attention must be paid to ensure the specificity of the microbiologic diagnosis. This is a particular issue where sputum cultures or nasopharyngeal cultures are used. Microbiologic data from these sources is notoriously non-specific and may not reflect the organism in the lung or the middle ear. Specific diagnoses must be made, if possible; if not, clinical diagnoses based on strict predetermined criteria need to be established and accepted by the Agency before the trial.

The analysis of data represents another area that is receiving detailed attention by regulatory agencies. Intent to treat (ITT) analyses are always required, but there must be consistent conclusions from the ITT, the modified ITT and the per protocol (PP) analyses. In the ITT, all randomized patients are included in the analysis and lost patients are regarded as failures. This analysis reflects most closely the manner in which the drug will be used in clinical practice, but is not the best manner of assessing true efficacy because patients with inaccurate diagnoses make the data less amenable to the detection of treatment differences. It is a critical issue in protocol design to try to assure that inclusion criteria are sufficiently unambiguous to allow a minimum of protocol violations. This will help keep the ITT analysis similar to the PP analysis. The modified ITT should fall within the ITT and PP analyses. In this situation, unqualified patients are excluded and patients with appropriately documented infections who have received at least one dose of the test drug, but who may not have completed the protocol, are included in the analysis. Excluded patients must be clearly discussed to assure lack of bias in this analysis.

The most critical aspect of protocol design is the definition of the endpoint for the primary analysis of efficacy. Response to therapy is based on both clinical and microbiological endpoints, with the clinical endpoint usually representing the primary endpoint. For certain infections (e.g. urinary tract infections) the microbiological endpoint may be the primary endpoint. To confirm eradication of pathogens long-term follow-up after cessation of therapy is generally required. The rationale for the timing of such cultures must be detailed in the protocol. Most post-therapy evaluations are done 72 hours after cessation of therapy and may be done 10 days after therapy. This culture will often be the primary endpoint and must be timed such that no drug remains in the system cultured (e.g. no drug in urine). CPMP guidance on endpoints for selected infections is shown in Table 13.2

CPMP guidance on safety analysis has also been specified.[26] Very thorough evaluation of adverse effects from controlled studies is often the best data available because placebo controls are not cured. Targeted monitoring is necessary for certain classes of antibiotics (e.g. phototoxicity for tetracyclines and quinolones). Whenever possible, control agents should be of the same class as the test drug to facilitate the analysis of the safety profile of the new drug. It is also useful to assess the safety data by indication in order to distinguish side effects more related to the underlying disease than to the new drug.

References

1. Center for Drug Evaluation and Research. Guidance for Industry. FDA published Good Guidance Practices in February 1997. Online. Available: http://www.fda.gov/cder/guidance/index.html.
2. Food and Drug Administration 1991 Department of Health and Human Service. Draft Guidance for Industry on Clinical Considerations for Accelerated and Traditional Approval of Antiretroviral Drugs Using Plasma HIV RNA Measurements; Availability. Federal Register, Vol. 64 No. 169, September 1, 1999.
3. Subpart H-Accelerated Approval of New Drugs for Serious or Life-Threatening Illnesses. 21 CFR 314,500 Scope, 57 FR 58958, Dec. 11, 1992, as amended at 64 FR 402, Jan 5, 1999.
4. McHutchison JG et al 1998 Interferon Alfa-2B alone or in combination with ribavirin as initial treatment for chronic hepatitis C. *New England Journal of Medicine* 339: 1485–1492.
5. CPMP 1997 Points to Consider in the Assessment of Anti-HIV Medicinal Products. CPMP/602/95, rev. 1, November 19, 1997.
6. International Conference on Harmonisation of Technical Requirements for Registration of Pharmaceuticals for Human Use. ICH Expert Working Group. ICH Harmonised Tripartite Guideline. Choice of Control Group and Related Issues in Clinical Trials.
7. International Conference on Harmonisation of Technical Requirements for Registration of Pharmaceuticals for Human Use. ICH Harmonised Tripartite Guideline. Statistical Principles for Clinical Trials.
8. Shlaes DM et al 1991 Antimicrobial resistance: New directions. *ASM News.* 57: 455–458.
9. Lederberg J, Shope RE, Oaks SC (eds) 1992 Institute of Medicine Emerging infections. Microbial threats to health in the United States. National Academy Press, Washington, DC.
10. Report of the ASM Taskforce on Antibiotic Resistance 1994 Antibiotic Resistance: Current Status and Future Directions Workshop. ASM. Washington, DC, July 6, 1994.
11. Centers for Disease Control and Prevention. A Public Health Action Plan To Combat Antimicrobial Resistance. Interagency Task Force on Antimicrobial Resistance.

Table 13.2 Committee for Proprietary Medicinal Products guidance on endpoints

Infection	Possible endpoints	Endpoint
Urinary tract infection	Clinical/Microbiological/Laboratory	Microbiological
Skin and soft tissue infection	Clinical/Microbiological	Clinical
Respiratory infection	Clinical/Microbiological/Laboratory	Clinical/Microbiological
Abdominal infection	Clinical/Microbiological/Laboratory	Clinical
Sexually transmitted disease	Clinical/Microbiological/Laboratory	Microbiological
Endocarditis	Clinical/Microbiological/Laboratory	Clinical/Microbiological

Clinical endpoints of cure, failure or indeterminate are acceptable but must be clearly defined within the protocol. Microbiological efficacy is defined as either elimination, persistence, or reinfection

12. Shlaes DM et al 1997 Society for Healthcare Epidemiology of America and Infectious Diseases Society of America Joint Committee on the Prevention of Antimicrobial Resistance: Guidelines for the Prevention of Antimicrobial Resistance in Hospitals. *Infection Control and Hospital Epidemiology* 18: 275–291.

13. World Health Organization 2000 Overcoming Antimicrobial Resistance. World Health Report on Infectious Diseases 2000. Online. Available: http://www.who.int/infectious-disease-report/2000/index-rpt2000 text.html.

14. Harrison PF, Lederberg J (eds) 1997 Institute Of Medicine Forum on Emerging Infections. Orphans and Incentives: Developing Technologies to Address Emerging Infections Workshop Report. National Academy Press, Washington, DC.

15. Harrison PF, Lederberg J (eds) 1998 Institute of Medicine. Forum on Emerging Infections. Antimicrobial Resistance: Issues and Options Workshop Report. National Academy Press, Washington, DC.

16. Food and Drug Administration 2000 Department of Health and Human Service, Part III. Requirements on Content and Format of Labeling for Human Prescription Drugs and Biologics; Requirements for Prescription Drug Product Labels; Proposed Rule. Federal Register. December 22, 2000.

17. Pharmaceutical Research and Manufacturers of America. The Pharmaceutical Industry's R&D Investment. Online. Available: http://www.phrma.org/publications/backgrounders/development/invest.phtml

18. DiMasi JA et al 1995 Research and development costs for new drugs by thera-peutic category, A study of the US pharmaceutical industry. *Pharmaco Economics* 7: 152–169.

19. DiMasi JA 1995 Success rates for new drugs entering clinical testing in the United States. *Clinical Pharmacology and Therapeutics* 58: 1–14.

20. DiMasi JA, Seibring MA, Lasagna L 1994 New drug development in the United States from 1963 to 1992. *Clinical Pharmacology and Therapeutics* 55: 609–622.

21. Gonzales R, Steiner JF, Sande MA 1997 Antibiotic prescribing for adults with colds, upper respiratory tract infections, and bronchitis by ambulatory care physicians. *Journal of the American Medical Association* 278: 901–904.

22. Nyquist AC et al 1998 Antibiotic prescribing for children with colds, upper respiratory tract infections, and bronchitis. *Journal of the American Medical Association* 279: 875–877.

23. Mermel LA 2000 Review – Prevention of intravascular catheter-related infections. *Annals of Internal Medicine* 132: 391–402.

24. National Nosocomial Infections Surveillance (NNIS) system report, data summary from October 1986-April 1998, issued June 1998. *American Journal of Infection Control* 26: 522–533.

25. Food and Drug Administration 1999 Center for Drug Evaluation and Research. Guidance for Industry. Catheter-Related Bloodstream Infections – Developing Antimicrobial Drugs for Treatment. Federal Register.

26. CPMP/EWP 1997 Note for Guidance on Evaluation of New Anti-Bacterial Medicinal Products. CPMP/EWP/558/95, October.

Agents

INTRODUCTION TO SECTION 2

The number and variety of antimicrobial agents has expanded inexorably since the appearance of the first edition of this book nearly forty years ago and successive editors have struggled to organize the information on individual compounds in a way that helps the reader to make sense of the profusion. The problem has not diminished for the present editorial team and we have again tried to restructure the information provided in a more uniform and accessible manner.

As always, the aim has been to be as inclusive and up to date as possible and we have sought to include all but the most obscure compounds that are available worldwide. Compounds used exclusively in veterinary medicine are mentioned by name if appropriate, but are not otherwise dealt with.

The amount of detail provided for older or less important drugs has been reduced to a short summary of their most important properties. For the rest we have tried to present the most important information in a standard and logical manner, tabulating such information as could be easily accommodated in this form. For large groups of agents, such as the penicillins, cephalosporins, macrolides, aminoglycosides and quinolones, the individual drug monographs are preceded by a general account of the group and its classification.

For the individual monographs, the following conventions have been adopted:

Drug names: The recommended International Non-proprietary Name (rINN) is used throughout, with the United States Adopted Name (USAN) and any other commonly used alternative name given at the beginning of each monograph. An exception has been made for methicillin (rINN: meticillin), since this antibiotic is no longer generally available and the original spelling is universally used in the context of 'methicillin-resistant *Staphylococcus aureus*'.

Structures: Simple two-dimensional structures of the most important compounds are given, together with the molecular weights and those of appropriate salts.

Antimicrobial activity: For antibacterial agents, minimum inhibitory concentration (MIC) values for the most common Gram-positive and Gram-negative pathogens are tabulated with members of the same drug group appearing in the same Table. Since published MIC values differ, sometimes quite widely, depending on the methodology used and the source of the micro-organisms tested, those given are representative ones, usually based on fully susceptible strains. Activity against other relevant pathogens is described in the text. Nomenclature of micro-organisms follows current recommendations (e.g. all clinically important salmonellae are described as *Salmonella enterica* serotypes rather than individual species).

Acquired resistance: Common mechanisms of acquired resistance and its general prevalence are described.

Pharmacokinetics: Basic pharmacokinetic parameters are tabulated: oral absorption (if relevant); maximum plasma concentration (C_{max}) for common dosage forms; plasma half-life; volume of distribution (usually in liters or, preferably, l/kg); and plasma protein binding. Values given normally refer to data from healthy adult volunteers and may be altered in disease or at the extremes of age. Unless otherwise stated, the plasma half-life is the β-phase value; when the terminal half-life differs substantially, this is described in the following text.

Wherever possible, a more extensive account of absorption, distribution, metabolism and excretion characteristics is added, at least for the more important compounds.

Interactions: Some important interactions are described, but a more extensive account is provided in Section 1 (Chapter 6).

Toxicity and side effects: The most important adverse reactions are given. For compounds for which class effects are prominent, this information is to be found in the section on general properties of the class earlier in the chapter.

Clinical use: The most common uses are listed. Information on the mode of use in different clinical settings is dealt with in appropriate chapters of Section 3.

Preparations and dosage: Common proprietary names are given, except for older compounds for which many generic preparations are available. Dosages are commonly accepted regimens for adults and children. Since recommended dosage regimens sometimes vary in different countries, the information may differ from that found in local formularies.

Further information: No in-text references are provided, but appropriate up-to-date sources of information are listed. Extensive monographs on many anti-infective drugs can be found in *Therapeutic Drugs* 2nd edn (Dollery, C. ed.) Churchill Livingstone, Edinburgh, 1999.

14 Aminoglycosides and aminocyclitols

David D. Boehr, Kari-ann Draker and Gerard D. Wright

The aminoglycoside antibiotics comprise a large group of naturally occurring or semi-synthetic polycationic compounds, several of which have therapeutic importance. Most are potent bactericidal agents and share the same general range of antibacterial activity, pharmacokinetic behavior, a tendency to damage one or other branch of the eighth nerve and some propensity to cause renal damage, or at least to impair further the function of an already damaged kidney. The degree of toxicity varies among compounds and for some it is so great as to preclude systemic use.

The therapeutically important members of the group have amino sugars glycosidically linked to aminocyclitols – cyclic alcohols that are also substituted with amino functions. Consequently, they should properly be described as 'aminoglycosidic aminocyclitols', but the name 'aminoglycosides', which was used before the detailed structures of the compounds was known, is now too well established to be easily displaced by a more cumbersome title. At the extremes of the group are kasugamycin, which contains an aminoglycoside but no aminocyclitol and is hence a 'pure aminoglycoside', and spectinomycin, which contains an aminocyclitol but no aminoglycoside and is hence a 'pure aminocyclitol'.

Streptomycin was the first aminoglycoside, identified in 1944 by Waksman's group as a natural product of a soil bacterium, *Streptomyces griseus*. This was followed by the discovery of neomycin by the same group in 1949 and by kanamycin by Umezawa and his colleagues in 1957. Gentamicin, the most important aminoglycoside in use today, was first reported in 1963; thereafter there followed an era in which research on new aminoglycosides concentrated on the chemical modification of known compounds, largely in response to developing resistance, rather than the discovery of new antibiotics from soil microbes.

CLASSIFICATION

In most aminoglycosides in regular clinical use, the aminocyclitol moiety is 2-deoxystreptamine; these compounds can be subdivided into the neomycin group, in which there are carbohydrate substitutions at positions 4 and 5 of deoxystreptamine, and the kanamycin and gentamicin groups, in which the aminocyclitol is 4,6-disubstituted. In streptomycin (and its close relatives dihydrostreptomycin and bluensomycin, neither of which is used clinically) the aminocyclitol ring is another derivative of streptamine, streptidine. Several less important compounds exhibit other structural variations on the aminoglycoside-aminocyclitol theme.

2-Deoxystreptamine-containing glycosides			
Neomycin group	Kanamycin group	Gentamicin group	Other aminoglycosides/ aminocyclitols
Neomycin	Amikacin	Gentamicin	Apramycin
Paromomycin	Arbekacin	Isepamicin	Astromicin
	Dibekacin	Netilmicin	Kasugamycin
	Kanamycin	Sisomicin	Spectinomycin
	Tobramycin	Verdamicin	Streptomycin

Several of the natural agents consist of mixtures of closely related compounds. For example, there are numerous gentamicins, three kanamycins and two neomycins. Moreover, there are close relationships between some of the differently named compounds. For example, tobramycin is 3'-deoxykanamycin B and the substitution of an amino for a hydroxyl group in paromomycin I gives neomycin B. The chemical differences are particularly important in determining sensitivity of the compounds to inactivation by bacterial aminoglycoside resistance enzymes (p. 157).

The nomenclature of the aminoglycoside structure is illustrated by that of kanamycin B:

The carbon atoms in the 2-deoxystreptamine ring are labelled 1 to 6; those in the amino sugar substituted at position 4 are labelled 1' to 6' and those in the 6-position amino sugar 1" to 6".

ANTIMICROBIAL ACTIVITY

The activity of the more important aminoglycosides against common pathogens is summarized in Table 14.1. They are active to different degrees against *Staphylococcus aureus*, coagulase-negative staphylococci and *Corynebacterium* spp., but the activity against many other Gram-positive bacteria, including streptococci, is generally limited. However, they interact synergistically with antibiotics such as penicillin against strepto-

cocci, enterococci and some other organisms and this combination is used as first-line therapy in enterococcal endocarditis (p. 663).

As a group, they are widely active against the Enterobacteriaceae and other aerobic Gram-negative bacilli including, for some compounds, *Pseudomonas aeruginosa*. Several, including streptomycin, are active against *Mycobacterium tuberculosis* and some other mycobacteria. Aminoglycosides require a threshold membrane potential to cross the bacterial cell membrane and are not active against anaerobic bacteria.

They are generally bactericidal in concentrations close to the minimum inhibitory concentration (MIC) and the rate of killing increases directly with the concentration.

AMINOGLYCOSIDE TRANSPORT

Diffusion of such highly polar cationic compounds across the cell membrane is very limited and intracellular accumulation of the drugs is brought about by active transport, which occurs in three phases:

- an initial energy-independent binding of the compounds to the exterior of the cell, which is inhibited by Ca^{2+} and Mg^{2+} ions
- energy-dependent phase I (so called because it is abolished by molecules that inhibit energy metabolism), in which the aminoglycosides are driven across the cytoplasmic membrane by the electrical potential difference, which is negative on the interior of the membrane

Table 14.1 Median MICs (mg/l) of aminoglycosides for common pathogenic bacteria

Bacterium	Gentamicin	Netilmicin	Tobramycin	Amikacin	Kanamycin	Neomycin	Streptomycin	Spectinomycin
Staph. aureus	0.25	0.25	0.25	1	1	0.5	4	64
Coagulase-negative staphylococci	0.03	0.03	0.03	0.25	0.5	0.06	2	32
Str. pyogenes	4	4	16	32	32	16	8	32
Str. pneumoniae	4	8	16	64	64	128	32	8
E. faecalis	16	8	16	128	64	32	128	64
N. meningitidis	16	16	16	32	32	4		8
N. gonorrhoeae	4	4	4	16	16	16	8	16
H. influenzae	0.5	0.5	1	1	1	2	2	4
Esch. coli	0.5	0.5	1	2	4	1	8	8
K. pneumoniae	0.5	0.5	0.5	2	2	1	4	16
B. fragilis	R	R	R	R	R	R	R	R
M. tuberculosis	R		R	1	8	0.5	0.5	
M. avium	4			8	4		2	

R, resistant (MIC >64 mg\l).

- a faster, energy-dependent phase II, which starts after aminoglycosides have bound to ribosomes and seems to be an effect, rather than a cause, of their action on the cell.

Uptake is adversely affected by low pH and reduced oxygen tension. Consequently, activity of the drugs in vitro is reduced in acid media or anaerobic conditions and by the presence of divalent cations; the susceptibility of *Ps. aeruginosa* is particularly sensitive to the cation concentration. Because of the effects of pH on activity, it is hard to be sure that the relatively high MICs seen for organisms that require carbon dioxide truly reflect their degree of resistance.

ACQUIRED RESISTANCE

Resistance in many organisms originally susceptible to the older compounds such as kanamycin is now widespread, and resistance to the more recently introduced agents has increased. The geographical distribution of resistant strains is diverse. Marked changes have also occurred over the years. For example, resistance to streptomycin or kanamycin was fairly common by the mid-1970s in the UK but resistance to gentamicin, tobramycin or amikacin was very rare. Not surprisingly, as a result of the increased use of gentamicin, resistance increased to upwards of 13% in the Enterobacteriaceae by the year 2000. A survey in 20 European university hospitals indicated that the incidence of gentamicin resistance had increased up to 5% in some Gram-negative bacteria and over 10% in *Staphylococcus aureus* between 1987 and 1998. Many strains with plasmid-encoded extended-spectrum β-lactamases (p. 263) are also aminoglycoside resistant, so outbreaks of infection with such strains may result in an increase in aminoglycoside resistance rates.

There are four general mechanisms of resistance to aminoglycosides:

- alteration in the ribosomal binding of the drug
- reduced uptake
- inactivation by specific aminoglycoside-modifying enzymes
- active efflux.

Single-step mutation to high-level resistance occurs only to streptomycin in clinical isolates. It results from alteration of a single ribosomal protein or rRNA, usually in the *rpsL* gene. The level of resistance conferred by reduced uptake is generally modest.

Resistance mediated by modifying enzymes usually confers a higher degree of resistance and is the most common mechanism. The enzymes are usually, though not always, plasmid encoded and the resistances conferred are frequently transferable. This mechanism of resistance shares many features with β-lactamase production by organisms resistant to penicillins or cephalosporins in that the cells owe their survival to the inactivation of the agent to which they remain intrinsically susceptible and in that a considerable, and growing, number of

enzymes have been identified from different bacterial species and strains.

AMINOGLYCOSIDE-MODIFYING ENZYMES

There are three classes of aminoglycoside-modifying enzyme, which differ in the nature of the sites modified:

- *N*-acetyltransferases (AAC) modify amino groups
- *O*-phosphotransferases (APH) modify hydroxyl groups
- *O*-nucleotidyltransferases (ANT) modify hydroxyl groups.

The sites of attack of these enzymes on gentamicin are shown below:

Gentamicin C1a

The position of the group attacked and the ring that carries it are indicated by the number of the enzyme: thus AAC(3) is the acetyltransferase that modifies the amino group in the 3-position on the central aminocyclitol ring; AAC(2′) is the acetyltransferase that modifies the amino group in the 2-position on the 4-substituent ring; AAC(6′) is the acetyltransferase that modifies the amino group in the 6-position on the 4-substituent ring; ANT(2″) and APH(2″) modify the hydroxyl group at the 2-position on the 6-substituent ring.

If two enzymes act at the same position on the molecule, but differ in the aminoglycosides modified (resistance phenotype), they are distinguished by roman numerals. For example, all types of AAC(3) modify gentamicin; AAC(3)-I modifies tobramycin so poorly that it does not confer resistance to it; AAC(3)-II confers resistance to tobramycin and netilmicin as well as to gentamicin; AAC(3)-III adds kanamycin and neomycin but loses netilmicin, and AAC(3)-IV is one of the few enzymes to modify apramycin. Other AAC(3) enzymes have also been described. The widespread AAC(3)-V has subsequently been recognized to be the same as AAC(3)-II. The resistance of important 2-deoxystreptamine-containing aminoglycosides to the principal enzymes so far characterized is shown in Table 14.2. Various phosphotransferases and nucleotidyltransferases modify streptomycin and its relatives (and sometimes also spectinomycin), but there is no crossover

Table 14.2 Range of activity of enzymes that modify 2-deoxystreptamine-containing aminoglycosides

Enzyme	Kanamycin A	Neomycin	Amikacin	Tobramycin	Gentamicin	Netilmicin	Sisomicin
APH(3′)-I & II	+	+	–	0	0	0	0
APH(3′)-III & VI	+	+	+	0	0	0	0
APH(2″)	+	0	–	+	+	–	0
ANT(4′,4″)	+	+	+	+	0	0	0
ANT(2″)	+	0	–	+	+	–	0
AAC(3)-I	–	–	–	–	+	–	–
AAC(3)-II	±	–	–	+	+	+	+
AAC(3)-III	+	+	–	+	+	–	–
AAC(3)-IV	±	+	–	+	+	+	+
AAC(2′)	0	+	0	+	+	+	0
AAC(6′)-I	+	+	+	+	Variable*	+	0
AAC(6′)-II	+	–	–	+	+	+	0

+, Modified; ±, poorly modified; –, not modified; 0, substituent necessary for modification absent.
* Gentamicin C_{1a}, C_2 and sisomicin +, gentamicin C_1 ±/–.

between the streptomycin and 2-deoxystreptamine groups in terms of sensitivity to aminoglycoside-modifying enzymes.

Many aminoglycoside-modifying enzymes that are apparently identical in terms of resistance profile have different amino acid sequences (genotype). Lower case letters are used to designate the different subgroups: thus, AAC(6′)-Ia and AAC(6′)-Ib are two unique proteins conferring identical resistance profiles. It is often found that one particular subgroup is responsible for most instances of the resistance profile. For example, in one study the *aac(3)-IIa* gene was found in 85% of isolates with the AAC(3)-II phenotype, while *aac(3)-IIb* was found in 6%. The *aac(3)-IIb* gene was 72% identical to *aac(3)-IIa*. A third gene, *aac(3)-IIc*, was 97% identical to *aac(3)-IIa* with changes in only 26 bases resulting in 12 amino acid changes; it is likely that strains possessing this gene would hybridize with a DNA probe for the *aac(3)-IIa* gene. Consequently, the subgroups of enzymes should perhaps be regarded as related families of enzymes, analogous to the TEM and SHV groups of plasmid-determined β-lactamases (p. 264), rather than as particular amino acid sequences. As with β-lactamases, single amino acid changes can have significant effects on substrate profiles; for example, changing the leucine at position 119 of AAC(6′)-Ib to serine results in an enzyme with the AAC(6′)-II phenotype.

Resistance to aminoglycosides results from the interplay between the rate of drug inactivation by the modifying enzyme and the rate of drug transport. Thus the resistance phenotype of a particular micro-organism depends on the concentration of enzyme, the ratio of V_{max} to K_m for a given substrate and the rate of drug uptake. Resistance caused by modifying enzymes is sometimes expressed not as a decrease in bacteristatic activity but rather as reduced bactericidal activity or abolition of bactericidal synergy with other antibiotics.

REDUCED PERMEABILITY

Another variety of resistance, which is not caused by antibiotic inactivation by specific modifying enzymes, may also be clinically significant. This resistance is manifested by impaired uptake of the drugs as a result of changes in energy metabolism or outer membrane structure, and is conveniently, though probably inaccurately, termed 'reduced permeability'. It often occurs by selection of mutants following exposure to the drug. Its clinical significance lies in the possibility that newer aminoglycosides that are active against strains resistant to older members of the group by virtue of their resistance to aminoglycoside-modifying enzymes may show no advantage against relatively impermeable strains – in fact the reverse may be true.

DISTRIBUTION OF MODIFYING ENZYMES

Most aminoglycoside-modifying enzymes are plasmid- or transposon-encoded; however, some are chromosomally determined with the presence of the gene, if not its expression in terms of resistance profile, characteristic of the species. The most notable examples are:

● *aac(2′)-Ia*; characteristic of *Providencia stuartii*
● *aac(6′)-Ic*; characteristic of *Serratia marcescens*
● *aac(6′)-Ii*; present in all *Enterococcus faecium* strains.

The expression of these genes appears to be tightly regulated. Although the chromosomal *aac(6′)-Ic* gene is found in all *Ser. marcescens* strains, most are aminoglycoside-susceptible with little or no *aac(6′)-Ic* mRNA detectable. Mutation to aminoglycoside resistance is accompanied by abundant mRNA production. AAC(6′)-Ic in *P. stuartii* is linked with peptido-glycan acetylation, which renders the organism more resistant against muramidases such as lysozyme. The actual biochemical role of ACC(6′)-Ii from *E. faecium* is not known, but it can acetylate proteins.

Genome sequences have identified several putative aminoglycoside resistance genes, even in organisms known to be sensitive to these drugs. Some have been characterized in vitro to be bona fide resistance enzymes, but most have not. However, this finding indicates a substantial reservoir of potential aminoglycoside resistance genes within bacterial genomes.

Expression of the plasmid- or transposon-encoded aminoglycoside-modifying enzymes does not appear to be regulated by the presence of the antibiotics. Transcription of these genes is constitutive, which, although costly in terms of cellular energy, provides constant protection against the presence of aminoglycosides.

Differences occur between organisms, both in location and with time, in the aminoglycoside-modifying enzymes detected.

- Enterobacteriaceae tend to produce AAC(3)-I, II or IV, AAC(6′)-I, ANT(2″) and APH(3′).
- *Ps. aeruginosa* tends to produce AAC(3)-I, AAC(3)-III, AAC(6′)-I or II, ANT(2″) and APH (3′).
- Staphylococci and *E. faecalis* tend to produce ANT (4′,4″) or a protein with bifunctional AAC(6′) + APH(2″) activity.

The use of specific aminoglycosides has a significant impact on the acquisition and expression of specific resistance genes and these vary among geographical areas over time, often reflecting policies of aminoglycoside use. Strains resistant to gentamicin or tobramycin often also produce a phosphotransferase or nucleotidyltransferase that confers resistance to streptomycin. An increasing number of strains appear to produce two or more enzymes active against gentamicin group aminoglycosides.

Formal demonstration of the presence of these enzymes is beyond the capability of most diagnostic microbiology laboratories. However, their presence can often be deduced with varying degrees of confidence from the resistance patterns of the organisms. The predominance of some enzymes such as the bifunctional AAC(6′)-APH(2′) in staphylococci lends itself well to the use of PCR-based diagnostics, and multiplex methods that include primers specific to a number of aminoglycoside and other antibiotic resistance genes have been developed.

Since the prevalence of these enzymes differs from place to place and time to time, as a result of local differences in the availability of organisms receptive to the plasmids that encode them, in antibiotic prescribing habits and in the opportunities for resistant organisms to spread, it is imperative that the local prevalence of resistance to individual agents be established when choosing between aminoglycosides. This is particularly important for the treatment of severe sepsis of undetermined origin. Sensitive PCR-based methods developed locally should be especially powerful in this regard.

PHARMACOKINETICS

Being highly polar polycations, the aminoglycosides are very poorly absorbed from the gut, less than 1% of the oral dose reaching the plasma. Some absorption may occur on prolonged administration or in the presence of inflammatory bowel disease. All are rapidly absorbed after intramuscular injection or instillation into serous cavities. Their binding to plasma protein is low and they are distributed in the extracellular water. There is little penetration into cells, tissues or secretions, including the aqueous humor and cerebrospinal fluid (CSF), although this may unpredictably increase in the presence of inflammation. It has been suggested that dosage would be more appropriately based on the lean body mass, of which the body water is consistently 70%. There is widespread binding to tissue sites, and saturation of these is responsible for incomplete excretion of the drugs over the first few days of administration and their relatively prolonged excretion after cessation of treatment. The normal serum half-life is roughly 2 h, but there is considerable variability among patients dependent on kidney function.

β-LACTAM DEGRADATION

β-Lactam antibiotics, particularly penicillins and cephalosporins, are commonly prescribed in combination with aminoglycosides to secure bactericidal synergy, or breadth of spectrum, and it is unfortunate that the agents frequently inactivate one another if mixed together in infusion fluids. For example, in the presence of carbenicillin and piperacillin, gentamicin and tobramycin show considerable loss of activity over 8 h at 25°C or 4°C. The process is due to the opening of the β-lactam ring with inactivation of the penicillin and reaction with the methylamino group of the aminoglycoside to form an inactive amine. This takes several hours and is seen in clinical practice only if the agents are mixed in a bottle for slow parenteral infusion and in severe renal failure where the agents persist for long periods in the plasma.

EXCRETION

Excretion of aminoglycosides is almost entirely by glomerular filtration. High concentrations of unchanged agent are found in the kidney substance and the urine. Consequently, they are retained in relation to the degree of reduction of renal function, and dosage must be appropriately monitored and adjusted in renal failure. Clearance depends in part on accumulation in the deep compartment, which can be saturated. It is the reabsorption by the proximal tubule and subsequent build up in the renal cortex, where very high concentrations may be found, that is associated with renal toxicity. Aminoglycosides are removed reasonably effectively by hemodialysis but not by peritoneal dialysis.

BLOOD CONCENTRATIONS AND DOSAGE ADJUSTMENT

Because aminoglycosides can produce concentration-related ototoxicity and nephrotoxicity, it is important to ensure that plasma concentrations do not exceed toxic concentrations. It is equally important to ensure that fear of toxicity does not result in therapeutically inadequate dosage. For gentamicin and related aminoglycosides target concentrations are 5–10 mg/l at peak and <2 mg/l at trough. Plasma concentrations in patients receiving aminoglycosides must be monitored, and dosage adjusted appropriately. Means of achieving this in patients with renal impairment are described in Chapter 5, but retention of the drugs because of relatively inefficient renal excretion must also be anticipated and the dosage appropriately adjusted in infants and elderly people. Repeated courses of aminoglycoside therapy, for example in patients with cystic fibrosis, may also lead to toxic effects, at least subclinically.

The need for individualized rather than standard dosage and the benefits of less frequent dosage have been repeatedly emphasized but – no doubt in part as a result of the heterogeneity of patient groups – unequivocal benefit in terms of efficacy or toxicity is difficult to establish. Nevertheless, once-daily aminoglycoside therapy, which tends to produce higher peak plasma concentrations but lower trough levels, is believed to be at least as efficacious and safe as conventional dosing regimens for non-neutropenic patients. This approach is attractive because of the dose-dependent bactericidal activity of aminoglycosides and their long postantibiotic effect. It may also dampen toxic effects on susceptible tissues. Once-daily dosing is not recommended in patients with enterococcal endocarditis, children, neutropenic individuals, pregnant women, or patients with marked renal problems.

Several special situations alter the pharmacokinetics of aminoglycosides. Since the compounds do not penetrate adipose tissue well, excessively high serum concentrations will be achieved in obese patients if the dose is based on total body weight; it has been suggested that addition of 40% of the adipose mass to the lean body mass be used to calculate the dose for patients who are less than 80% overweight with 60% added for patients more than 80% overweight. Higher doses and perhaps more frequent doses may be necessary in patients with cystic fibrosis. Higher and more frequent doses may also be necessary for burns patients.

Various methods have been developed to monitor aminoglycoside concentrations during therapy. Because of the need for rapidity and specificity, immunological methods (e.g. the commercial EMIT and TDx systems) that can give answers in a few minutes are now generally used.

Both manual and computerized nomograms have been used to select an appropriate loading dose and initial maintenance dosage, but no standard recommendations are yet available. A comparison of various guidelines found that a large percentage of patients would have achieved concentrations outside of the target ranges, no matter which nomogram was used. It was concluded that serum concentration monitoring is still recommended to confirm dose requirements.

Even if a nomogram is used, it is essential that the doses are administered and documented accurately and that blood samples are collected for assay at the correct times; assay results must be analyzed, and changes in dosage made promptly when necessary.

TOXICITY AND SIDE EFFECTS

Adverse effects include pain and irritation at the site of infection, hypersensitivity, eosinophilia with or without other allergic manifestations, circumoral paresthesias and other peripheral and central nervous effects, mild hematological disturbances and abnormal liver function tests. However, by far the most important toxic effects are those exerted on the eighth nerve and kidney.

There are considerable differences among the agents in their relative toxicities, which are summarized for some of the older compounds in Table 14.3. A comparison of clinical trials suggested that netilmicin is less ototoxic and nephrotoxic than gentamicin, tobramycin or amikacin when conventional two or three times daily doses were given. When once-daily gentamicin and netilmicin were compared, no significant differences were found between the regimens with regard to hearing loss, prodromal signs of ototoxicity or nephrotoxicity.

Table 14.3 Relative toxicity index* of aminoglycosides

	Vestibular	Auditory	Renal
Streptomycin	4	1	<1
Neomycin	1	4	4
Kanamycin	1	2	1
Gentamicin	3	2	2
Tobramycin	2	2	2

* 1–4: least to most toxic. Based on Price KE, Godfrey JC, Kawaguchi H 1974 *Advances in Applied Microbiology* 18: 191–307

OTOTOXICITY

The aminoglycosides are potentially toxic to varying degrees to the vestibular and cochlear branches of the eighth nerve. Ototoxicity results from accumulation of the drugs in the perilymph of the inner ear. Penetration is facilitated by high plasma concentrations and persistence by elevated trough concentrations, which impair back diffusion of the agents into the plasma. It follows that the danger of ototoxicity is likely to be markedly increased in the presence of impaired renal function. Toxicity is due to injury to the sensory cells of the inner ear, which may progress to destructive changes with consequent permanent functional impairment. Ataxia and oscillopsy may be less well recognized (and more distressing) manifestations of toxicity than vertigo.

Vestibular toxicity develops before the cochlear effects. Both may be prevented by stopping the drug when caloric irrigation indicates vestibular impairment, but formal testing of auditory or vestibular function commonly reveals evidence of subclinical injury.

Simultaneous or sequential administration of other potentially ototoxic agents, including repeated treatment with the same or other aminoglycosides, potent diuretics such as ethacrynic acid or furosemide (frusemide) or certain cephalosporins, may potentiate the adverse effects of aminoglycosides, which are likely to be greater in elderly people and those with pre-existing hearing impairment. The predictive value of such factors has been disputed and auditory toxicity has also been correlated with longer treatment, bacteremia, higher temperature, liver dysfunction, urea/serum creatinine ratio and low hematocrit.

NEPHROTOXICITY

Renal damage is produced to very different degrees by the various agents and is related to the accumulation of high concentrations of the drugs in the renal cortex. The frequency of nephrotoxicity from the systematically administered agents differs markedly, from around 2% to 60% depending on the patient population, dosage and criteria of renal damage. In volunteers, the percentage of drug excreted was highest for netilmicin (99%) and lowest for gentamicin (80%), which showed the highest degree of net reabsorption and is generally regarded as the more nephrotoxic. The abnormal persistence of aminoglycosides in the plasma between doses may be the earliest and most sensitive indication of the onset of renal impairment.

If acute tubular necrosis develops it usually does so towards the end of the first week of administration, during which time the drugs are accumulated at tissue binding sites. Regeneration of damaged tubular epithelium with the restoration of function usually occurs if the drug is discontinued. The precise value of measurements of renal enzymes or β_2 microglobulin excretion as early indicators of renal damage has been debated, but the appearance of brush border membrane fragments in the urine or new cylindruria are strongly correlated with decline of renal function.

Many putative risk factors including dosage and duration of therapy, plasma concentrations and renal function are related to age, which has emerged in some studies as the dominant or even sole independent determinant of toxicity risk.

Renal damage is probably more likely and more severe with simultaneous use of other agents that act on the kidney, including some diuretics, cisplatin and cephalosporins, especially cefaloridine (p. 193).

NEUROMUSCULAR BLOCKADE

Aminoglycosides can produce neuromuscular blockade, probably by functioning as membrane stabilizers in the same way as curare. Their effect is relatively feeble, and they rarely produce any effect in those with normal neuromuscular function. However, antibiotics are customarily given in much larger amounts than curare, and patients who are also receiving muscle relaxants or anesthetics or who are suffering from myasthenia gravis are at special risk. Analogous effects, which can be reversed by calcium, have been described on the gut and uterus.

CLINICAL USE

Aminoglycosides are the mainstay of the treatment of severe sepsis caused by enterobacteria and some other Gram-negative aerobic bacilli. For the treatment of severe sepsis of undetermined cause they are frequently administered in combination with agents active against Gram-positive or anaerobic bacteria as appropriate. Some are also used for a number of specialized infections described under the individual agents, including endocarditis, respiratory infections and tuberculosis.

For general clinical purposes, gentamicin, netilmicin, tobramycin or amikacin are commonly used. There is no clear choice on the grounds of toxicity because differences between the various members of the group are of no proven clinical relevance. Differences in in-vitro activity depend largely on the local prevalence of particular resistance mechanisms.

Gentamicin is a sensible choice for the treatment of suspected or confirmed infections caused by Gram-negative bacilli unless resistance is a major problem. It is often used as first-choice therapy for patients without renal functional deficit. Tobramycin may have some advantage for proven *Ps. aeruginosa* or *Acinetobacter* infections. Amikacin is preferred if there is resistance to other aminoglycosides, and netilmicin is preferred in patients with auditory or vestibular deficits or with established or impending renal insufficiency, including the elderly. These drugs can also be combined with amoxicillin and metronidazole as appropriate for microbiologically undiagnosed severe infection, unless microbiological or epidemiological evidence indicates a high probability of resistance in any individual case.

 Further information

Aminoglycoside Resistance Study Groups 1994 Resistance to aminoglycosides in *Pseudomonas*. *Trends in Microbiology* 2: 347–353.

Bryan LE 1988 General mechanisms of resistance to antibiotics. *Journal of Antimicrobial Chemotherapy* 22 (suppl A): 1–15.

D'Amico DJ, Caspers-Velu L, Libert J et al 1985 Comparative toxicity of intravitreal aminoglycoside antibiotics. *American Journal of Ophthalmology* 100: 264–275.

Davey PG, Finch RG, Wood MJ (eds) 1991 Once daily amikacin. *Journal of Antimicrobial Chemotherapy* 27 (suppl C): 1–152.

Edson RS, Terrell CL 1999 The aminoglycosides. *Mayo Clinic Proceedings* 74: 519–528.

Flournoy DJ 1985 Influence of aminoglycoside usage on susceptibilities. *Chemotherapy* 31: 178–180.

Franson TR, Quebbeman EJ, Whipple J et al 1988 Prospective comparison of traditional and pharmakokinetic aminoglycoside dosing methods. *Critical Care Medicine* 16: 840–843.

Gilbert DN 1991 Once-daily aminoglycoside therapy. *Antimicrobial Agents and Chemotherapy* 35: 399–405.

Jedeikin R, Dolgunski E, Kaplan R, Hoffman S 1987 Prolongation of neuromuscular blocking effect of vecuronium by antibiotics. *Anaesthesia* 42: 858–860.

Klastersky J, Phillips I (eds) 1986 Aminoglycosides in combination in severe infections. *Journal of Antimicrobial Chemotherapy* 17 (suppl A): 1–66.

Kumana CR, Yuen KY 1994 Parenteral aminoglycoside therapy: selection, administration and monitoring. *Drugs* 47: 902–913.

Mattie H, Craig WA, Pechère JC 1989 Determinants of efficacy and toxicity of aminoglycosides. *Journal of Antimicrobial Chemotherapy* 24: 281–293.

Mendelman PM, Smith AL, Levy J, Weber A, Ramsey B, Davis RL 1985 Aminoglycoside penetration, inactivation and efficacy in cystic fibrosis sputum. *American Review of Respiratory Diseases* 131: 761–765.

Miller GH, Sabatelli FJ, Hare RS et al 1997 The most frequent aminoglycoside resistance mechanisms – changes with time and geographic area: A reflection of aminoglycoside usage patterns? *Clinical Infectious Diseases* 24(Suppl 1): S46–S62.

Nordström L, Ringberg H, Cronberg S, Tjernström O, Walder M 1990 Does administration of an aminoglycoside in a single daily dose affect its efficacy and toxicity? *Journal of Antimicrobial Chemotherapy* 25: 159–173.

Palla R, Marchitiello M, Tuoni M 1985 Enzymuria in aminoglycoside-induced kidney damage. Comparative study of gentamicin, amikacin, sisomicin and netilmicin. *International Journal of Clinical Pharmacology Research (Geneva)* 5: 351–355.

Prins JM, Büller HR, Kuijper EJ, Tange RA, Speelman P 1994 Once daily gentamicin versus once-daily netilmicin in patients with serious infections: a randomized clinical trial. *Journal of Antimicrobial Chemotherapy* 33: 823–835.

Rybak ML, Abate BJ, Kang SL et al 1999 Prospective evaluation of the effect of an aminoglycoside dosing regimen on rates of observed nephrotoxicity and ototoxicity. *Antimicrobial Agents and Chemotherapy* 43: 1549–1555.

Schmitz F-J, Verhoef J, Fluit AC, SENTRY Participants Group 1999 Prevalence of aminoglycoside resistance in 20 European university hospitals participating in the European SENTRY antimicrobial surveillance programme. *European Journal of Microbiology and Infectious Diseases* 18: 414–421.

Shaw KJ, Rather PN, Hare RS, Miller GH 1993 Molecular genetics of aminoglycoside resistance genes and familial relationships of the aminoglycoside-modifying enzymes. *Microbiological Reviews* 57: 138–163.

Silva VL, Gil FZ, Nascimento G, Cavanal MF 1988 Aminoglycosides and nephrotoxicity. *Renal Physiology* 10: 327–337.

Thomson AH, Campbell KC, Kelman AW 1990 Evaluation of six gentamicin nomograms using a bayesian parameter estimation program. *Therapeutic Drug Monitoring* 12: 258–263.

Wright GD, Berghuis AM, Mobashery S 1998 Aminoglycoside antibiotics: Structures, functions, and resistance. *Advances in Experimental Medical Biology* 456: 27–69.

Young EJ, Sewell CM, Koza MA, Clarridge JE 1985 Antibiotic resistance patterns during aminoglycoside restriction. *American Journal of the Medical Sciences* 290: 223–227.

Zetany RG, El Saghir NS, Santosh-Kumar CR, Sigmon MA 1990 Increased aminoglycoside requirements in haematological malignancy. *Antimicrobial Agents and Chemotherapy* 34: 702–708.

GENTAMICIN GROUP

 ## GENTAMICIN

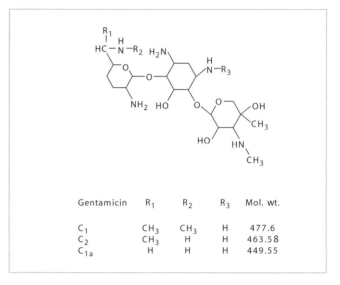

A mixture of fermentation products of *Micromonospora purpurea*. The commercial product is a mixture of gentamicin Cs in which C_1, C_{1a} and C_2 are required to be present in certain proportions. Minute amounts of gentamicin C_{2b} (micronomicin; sagamicin) are also present. The compound is supplied as the sulfate, and usually sterilized by filtration, but aqueous solutions to which sodium metabisulfate (80 mg/l) is added can be autoclaved without discoloration or loss of activity.

Antimicrobial activity

The activity against common pathogenic bacteria is shown in Table 14.1 (p. 156). It is active against staphylococci, but streptococci are at least moderately resistant. Gram-positive bacilli, including *Actinomyces* and *Listeria* spp. are moderately susceptible, but clostridia and other obligate anaerobes are resistant. There is no useful activity at clinically attainable concentrations against mycobacteria. Gentamicin is active against most enterobacteria, including *Citrobacter*, *Enterobacter*, *Proteus*, *Serratia* and *Yersinia* spp., and also against some other aerobic Gram-negative bacilli including *Acinetobacter*, *Brucella*, *Francisella* and *Legionella* spp., although its in-vitro activity against intracellular parasites such as *Brucella* spp. is of doubtful usefulness. It is active against *Ps. aeruginosa* and other members of the fluorescens group, but other pseudomonads are often resistant and *Flavobacterium* spp. are always resistant.

As with other aminoglycosides, activity is increased by low Mg^{2+} and Ca^{2+} concentrations and diminished under anaerobic or hypercapnic conditions. The MIC for susceptible strains of *Ps. aeruginosa* can vary more than 300-fold with the Mg^{2+} content of the medium. Activity against *Ps. aeruginosa* has also been found to be significantly lower in serum or sputum than in ion-depleted broth, as a result both of binding (more in sputum than in serum) and antagonism by ions.

The action is bactericidal and increases with pH, but to different degrees against different bacterial species. Marked bactericidal synergy is commonly demonstrable with β-lactam antibiotics, notably with ampicillin or benzylpenicillin against *E. faecalis*, and with vancomycin against streptococci and staphylococci. Bactericidal synergy with a wide variety of β-lactam antibiotics can also be demonstrated in vitro against many Gram-negative rods, including *Ps. aeruginosa*. Antagonism has been demonstrated in vitro with chloramphenicol, but the clinical significance of this is doubtful.

Acquired resistance

Gentamicin-resistant strains of staphylococci, enterobacteria, *Pseudomonas* and *Acinetobacter* spp. have been reported from many centers, often from burns and intensive care units where the agent has been used extensively. There are considerable geographical differences in the overall prevalence of resistance, with figures ranging from 3% to around 50% reported for Gram-negative organisms in various countries. Countries in which control of the prescription of antibiotics is lax often have very high rates.

Acquired resistance in Gram-negative organisms is usually, but not exclusively, caused by aminoglycoside-modifying enzymes. There is some geographical variation in the prevalence of the different enzymes. ANT(2″) is the most common in the USA, but in Europe various forms of AAC(3), particularly AAC(3)-II, are widely prevalent. ANT(2″) is also common in the Far East, usually accompanied by AAC(6′). Strains that owe their resistance not to the enzymatic degradation of the agent but to a non-specific decrease in uptake of aminoglycosides have been involved in outbreaks of hospital-acquired infection, and are cross-resistant to all aminoglycosides.

Gentamicin resistance in staphylococci and high-level resistance in enterococci is usually caused by the bifunctional APH(2″)-AAC(6′) enzyme. Other aminoglycoside-modifying enzymes, e.g. ANT(4′, 4″) and APH(3′), may also occur in these organisms, but do not contribute to gentamicin resistance. Gentamicin-resistant staphylococci began to emerge in the mid-1970s. By 1986 about 3% of *Staph. aureus* and 25% of coagulase-negative staphylococci in the UK were gentamicin resistant. A follow-up study in 1999 showed an increase in resistance to gentamicin, with 23% of *Staph. aureus* isolates resistant, and 33% of coagulase-negative staphylococci resistant. Gentamicin resistance was also found to be closely related to methicillin resistance: 75% of methicillin-resistant *Staph. aureus* (MRSA) were fully resistant to gentamicin compared with only 4% of methicillin-sensitive strains.

Since first being described in 1979, high-level resistance to gentamicin (MIC >2000 mg/l) in enterococci has spread worldwide, reaching levels of around one-third of blood culture isolates in some places. Penicillin–gentamicin combinations do not exert synergistic bactericidal activity against such strains. High-level gentamicin resistance is much less common in *E. faecium*, but has been reported in the UK, the USA and Asia.

Pharmacokinetics

C_{max} 1 mg/kg intramuscular	4–7.6 mg/l after 0.5–1 h
80 mg intramuscular	4–12 mg/l after 0.5–2 h
Plasma half-life (mean)	2 h
Volume of distribution	0.25 l/kg
Plasma protein binding	<10%

In normal subjects wide variations are observed between individuals in the peak plasma concentrations and half-lives of the drug after similar doses, but individual patients tend to behave consistently. Some patients with normal renal function develop unexpectedly high, and some develop unexpectedly low, peak values on conventional doses. Fever appears to be a significant factor in reducing the peak concentration, and anemia has been found to be a significant factor in raising it. The mechanisms involved in these effects have not been elucidated, but hemodynamic changes associated with fever and anemia might facilitate mobilization of the drug from intramuscular injection sites to raise the peak concentration or to modify drug distribution and renal handling in such a way as to lower it.

Intravenous infusion over 20–30 min achieves concentrations similar to those after intramuscular injection. The peak plasma concentration increases proportionally with dose. Mean initial serum peak concentrations were 10.2 mg/l in patients given 4 mg/kg once daily, compared with 5.2 mg/l in patients given 1.33 mg/kg three times daily. Despite the very high bronchial concentrations achieved, aerosol administration does not give rise to detectable plasma concentrations.

There is a marked effect of age: in children up to 5 years the peak plasma concentration is about half, and for children between 5 and 10 years about two-thirds, of the concentration produced by the same dose per kilogram in adults. This difference can be eliminated to a large extent by calculating dosage not on the basis of weight but on surface area, which is more closely related to the volume of the extracellular fluid in which gentamicin is distributed.

Some febrile neutropenic patients do not differ from normal subjects in their pharmacokinetics, but in others, as in patients with cystic fibrosis, gentamicin clearance is enhanced and dosage adjustment is necessary.

β-Lactam degradation

Like other aminoglycosides, gentamicin is degraded in the presence of high concentrations of some β-lactam agents. The serum concentration of gentamicin in patients given 80 mg of the drug plus 5 g ticarcillin by intravenous infusion over 30 min was consistently lowered, while that of ticarcillin was unaffected. The ureidopenicillins mezlocillin and piperacillin were without effect.

Absorption

Gentamicin is almost unabsorbed from the alimentary tract, but well absorbed after intramuscular injection. Absorption of half the dose was achieved when 100 mg was added to 2 l of dialysate in patients on continuous ambulatory peritoneal dialysis (CAPD). On a 6 h cycle, clearance by dialysis was 2.9 ml/min.

Distribution

Gentamicin does not enter cells so intracellular organisms are protected from its action. Fat contains less extracellular fluid than other tissues and pharmacokinetic comparisons indicate that the volume of distribution in obese patients approximates to the lean body mass plus 40% of the adipose mass.

SPUTUM

Access to the lower respiratory tract is limited, and it appears that rapid intravenous infusion produces the highest but shortest-lived intrabronchial concentrations, while intramuscular injection produces lower but more sustained concentrations.

CSF

Gentamicin does not reach the CSF in useful concentrations after systemic administration. In patients receiving 3.5 mg/kg per day plus 4 mg intrathecally, CSF concentrations of 20–25 mg/l have been found.

SEROUS FLUIDS AND EXUDATES

Concentrations in pleural, pericardial and synovial fluids are less than half the simultaneous plasma concentrations but may rise in the presence of inflammation. In cirrhotic patients with bacterial peritonitis treated with 3–5 mg/kg per day, concentrations of 4.2 mg/l were found in the peritoneal fluid with a fluid to serum ratio of 0.68. The maximum concentration in inflammatory exudate is less than that in the plasma, partly because it is reversibly bound (it is thought by chromatin released from lysed neutrophils) in purulent exudates, but it persists much longer.

SKIN AND MUSCLE

Concentrations in skin and muscle, as judged from assay of decubitus ulcers excised 150 min after patients had received 80 mg intramuscularly, were 5.8 and 6.5 mg/kg, respectively, the serum concentrations at that time being 5.1 and 5.4 mg/l.

FETUS

Concentrations in fetal blood are about one-third of that in the maternal blood.

Excretion

The initial plasma half-life is about 2 h, but a significant proportion is eliminated much more slowly, the terminal half-life being of the order of 12 days. There is much individual variation.

Gentamicin accumulates in the renal cortical cells, and over the first day or two of treatment only about 40% of the dose is recovered. The renal clearance is around 60 ml/min.

Subsequently it is excreted almost quantitatively unchanged in the urine, principally by glomerular filtration, but there is probably an element of tubular secretion. In severely oliguric patients some extrarenal elimination by unidentified routes evidently occurs. Urinary concentrations of 16–125 mg/l are found in patients with normal renal function receiving 1.5 mg/kg per day. In the presence of severe renal impairment with persistence of the drug in the circulation, urinary concentrations as high as 1000 mg/l may be found. The clearance of the drug is linearly related to that of creatinine, and this relationship is used as the basis of the modified dosage schedules that are required in patients with impaired renal function in order to avoid accumulation of the drug.

Hemodialysis can remove the drug at about 60% of the rate at which creatinine is cleared, but the efficiency of different dialysers varies markedly. Peritoneal dialysis removes only about 20% of the administered dose over 36 h – a rate that does not add materially to normal elimination.

Concentrations in bile are less than half the simultaneous plasma concentration.

Toxicity and side effects

Ototoxicity

Vestibular function is usually affected, but labyrinthine damage has been reported in about 2% of patients, usually in those with peak plasma concentrations in excess of 8 mg/l. Symptoms range from acute Ménière's disease to tinnitus and are usually permanent. Deafness is unusual but may occur in patients treated with other potentially ototoxic agents. Onset of ototoxicity after the cessation of treatment is very rare. In an extensive study, the overall incidence of ototoxicity was 2%. Vestibular damage accounted for two-thirds of this and impaired renal function was the main determinant.

Nephrotoxicity

Some degree of renal toxicity has been observed in 5–10% of patients. Among 97 patients receiving 102 courses of the drug in dosages adjusted in relation to renal function, nephrotoxicity was described as definite in 9.8% and possible in 7.8%. In patients treated for 39–48 days, serum creatinine has been reported to increase initially with retention of gentamicin, but renal function recovered after 3–4 weeks despite continuing treatment. However, many patients are treated for severe sepsis associated with shock or disseminated intravascular coagulopathy, or from other disorders that are themselves associated with renal failure. In critically ill patients with severe sepsis, treatment has been complicated by nephrotoxicity in 23–37%.

MECHANISM

Selective accumulation of the drug by the proximal renal tubules may lead to cloudy swelling and progress to tubular necrosis. Autoradiographic localization indicates that gentamicin is very selectively localized in the proximal convoluted tubules, and a specific effect on potassium excretion may both indicate the site of toxicity and provide an early indication of renal damage. There is accumulating evidence that redox-active aminoglycoside–iron complexes may be involved at the molecular level, and a variety of antioxidants have been shown to prevent toxic effects in rats and guinea pigs. Accumulation of the drug and excretion of proximal tubular enzymes may precede any rise in the serum creatinine.

DETECTION

Alanine aminopeptidase excretion is very variable in normal subjects and an unreliable predictor of renal damage. β_2-microglobulin excretion has been found by some observers to show decreased tubular function both before and during treatment of patients with urinary tract infection which improved with successful therapy. Excretion of the protein has also been shown to parallel increases in elimination half-life in patients on well controlled therapy in whom reduction of creatinine clearance occurred, although the serum creatinine concentration remained within normal limits. When more severe and less readily reversible nephrotoxicity occurs, it is almost invariably seen in patients with pre-existing renal disorders.

Other effects

Neuromuscular blockade is possible but unlikely in view of the small amounts of the drug administered. Intrathecal injection may result in radiculitis, fever and persistent pleocytosis. Significant hypomagnesemia may occur, particularly in patients also receiving cytotoxic agents.

Clinical use

- Suspected or documented Gram-negative septicemia, particularly when shock or hypotension are present.
- Enterococcal endocarditis (with a penicillin).
- Respiratory tract infection caused by Gram-negative bacilli.
- Urinary tract infection.
- Bone and soft-tissue infections, including peritonitis, burns complicated by sepsis and infected surgical and traumatic wounds.
- Serious staphylococcal infection when other conventional antimicrobial therapy is inappropriate.

In severe sepsis of unknown origin, it is usually combined with an agent active against Gram-positive organisms, and where they are thought likely to be implicated, an agent active against anaerobes. In systemic *Ps. aeruginosa* infections it is advisable to combine gentamicin with an antipseudomonal penicillin or cephalosporin.

Gentamicin eye drops are effective for the treatment of conjunctival infections with susceptible organisms. Gentamicin drops, often in combination with hydrocortisone, are also used for infections of the external ear.

Preparations and dosage

Proprietary names: Genticin, Cidomycin.

Preparations: Injection, various topical.

Dosages: Adult, i.m., i.v., i.v. infusion 2–5 mg/kg per day in divided doses every 8 hours.

Children aged up to 2 weeks, 3 mg/kg every 12 h; aged 2 weeks to 12 years, 2 mg/kg every 8 h. In the elderly and those with renal impairment the dose must be suitably modified.

Widely available.

Further information

Aran JM, Erre JP, Lima da Costa D, Debbarh I, Dulon D 1999 Acute and chronic effects of aminoglycosides on cochlear hair cells. *Annals of the New York Academy of Sciences* 884: 60–68.

Bianco TM, Dwyer PN, Bertino JS Jr 1989 Gentamicin pharmacokinetics, nephrotoxicity and prediction of mortality in febrile neutropenic patients. *Antimicrobial Agents and Chemotherapy* 33: 1890–1895.

Freeman CD, Nicolau DP, Belliveau PP, Nightingale CH 1997 Once-daily dosing of aminoglycosides: review and recommendations for clinical practice. *Journal of Antimicrobial Chemotherapy* 39: 677–686.

Glasser DB, Gardner S, Ellis JG, Pettit TH 1985 Loading doses and extended dosing intervals in topical gentamicin therapy. *American Journal of Ophthalmology* 99: 329–332.

Miller GH, Sabatelli FJ, Hare RS et al 1997 The most frequent aminoglycoside resistance mechanisms- changes with time and geographic area: a reflection of aminoglycoside usage patterns? Aminoglycoside Resistance Study Groups. *Clinical Infectious Diseases* 24 (Suppl 1): S46–62.

Pons G, d'this P, Rey E et al 1988 Gentamicin monitoring in neonates. *Therapeutic Drug Monitoring* 10: 421–427.

Meunier F, Van der Auwera P, Schmitt H, de Maertelaer V, Klastersky J 1987 Pharmacokinetics of gentamicin after i.v. infusion or i.v. bolus. *Journal of Antimicrobial Chemotherapy* 19: 225–231.

Triggs E, Charles B 1999 Pharmacokinetics and therapeutic drug monitoring of gentamicin in the elderly. *Clinical Pharmacokinetics* 37: 331–341.

Walker PD, Barri Y, Shah SV 1999 Oxidant mechanisms in gentamicin nephrotoxicity. *Renal Failure* 21: 433–442.

Winstanley TG, Hastings JGM 1990 Synergy between penicillin and gentamicin against enterococci. *Journal of Antimicrobial Chemotherapy* 25: 551–560.

ISEPAMICIN

Hydroxyamino propionyl gentamicin B. Molecular weight (free base): 569.6

A semi-synthetic derivative of gentamicin B, modified in such a way as to preserve its activity, but render it resistant to microbial inactivation.

Antimicrobial activity

In-vitro activity is comparable to or slightly greater than amikacin against *Staph. aureus* and most enterobacteria; it is much more active against *Ser. marcescens*, *Enterobacter* spp. and *K. pneumoniae*. It is also active in vitro against the *M. avium* complex and *Nocardia asteroides*. It is less susceptible than amikacin or gentamicin to inactivation by β-lactam antibiotics.

Acquired resistance

Because of its resistance to most aminoglycoside-modifying enzymes, isepamicin retains activity against some strains resistant to most other aminoglycosides. However, like amikacin, it is inactivated by AAC(3)-III and ANT(4′, 4″) (mostly from Gram-positive organisms) and AAC(3)-VI (mostly from *Acinetobacter*). Unlike amikacin it is resistant to AAC(6′).

Pharmacokinetics

The pharmacokinetics have been evaluated in neonatal, pediatric, adult, elderly and renally impaired patients, and do not appear different from those of other aminoglycosides, although there is some evidence that it has less tissue accumulation.

The clearance is reduced in both neonates and elderly people. A 7.5 mg/kg once-daily dosage is recommended for children less than 16 days old; no dosage adjustment is required for the elderly. Clearance is proportional to creatinine clearance ($CL_{(CR)}$) in patients with chronic renal impairment, where the recommended regimen is 8 mg/kg with an administration interval of 24 h in moderate impairment, 48 h in severe impairment, 72 h for $CL_{(CR)}$ of 0.6–1.14 l/h (10–19 ml/min) and 96 h for $CL_{(CR)}$ 0.36–0.54 l/h (6–9 ml/min). It is eliminated by hemodialysis.

Toxicity, side effects and clinical use

Isepamicin has been used in respiratory tract infections, urinary tract infections and intra-abdominal infections, in adults and children. It appears to be as effective and well tolerated as amikacin.

Preparations and dosage

Preparations: Injection.

Dosages: Adult, i.m., i.v. infusion 8–15 mg/kg per day in one to two divided doses.

Children aged up to 16 days, 7.5 mg/kg daily; over 16 days, 7.5 mg/kg twice daily. The dose should be reduced in renal impairment.

Available in Japan.

Further information

Barrett MS, Jones RN, Erwin ME, Koontz FP 1992 CI-960 (PD 127391 or AM-1091), sparfloxacin, WIN 57273, and isepamicin activity against clinical isolates of *Mycobacterium avium–intracellularae* complex, *M. chelonae*, and *M. fortuitum*. *Diagnostic Microbiology and Infectious Disease* 15: 169–171.

Barr WH, Colucci R, Radwanski E et al 1995 Pharmacokinetics of isepamicin. *Journal of Chemotherapy* 7 (Suppl 2): 53–61.

Blum D 1995 An overview of the safety of isepamicin in adults. *Journal of Chemotherapy* 7 (Suppl 2): 87–93.

Carbon C 1995 Overview of the efficacy of isepamicin in the adult core clinical trial programme. *Journal of Chemotherapy* 7 (Suppl 2): 79–85.

Mainardi JL, Zhou XY, Goldstein F et al 1994 Activity of isepamicin and selection of permeability mutants to beta-lactams during aminoglycoside therapy of experimental endocarditis due to *Klebsiella pneumoniae* CF 104 producing an aminoglycoside acetyltransferase 6′ modifying enzyme and a TEM-3 β-lactamase. *Journal of Infectious Diseases* 169: 1318–1324.

Petrikkos G, Giamarellou H, Tsagaraki C, Pefanis A 1995 Evaluation of the efficacy and safety of isepamicin in the treatment of various bacterial infections. *Journal of Chemotherapy* 7 (Suppl 2): 161–164.

Qadri SM, Ueno Y, Tullo D, Saldin H 1995 In vitro activity of isepamicin (Sch 21420), a new aminoglycoside. *Chemotherapy* 21: 14–17.

Tod M, Padoin C, Petitjean O 2000 Clinical pharmacokinetics and pharmacodynamics of isepamicin. *Clinical Pharmacokinetics* 38: 205–223.

Walterspiel JN, Feldman S, Van R, Ravis WR 1991 Comparative inactivation of isepamicin, amikacin, and gentamicin by nine β-lactams and two β-lactamase inhibitors, cilastatin and heparin. *Antimicrobial Agents and Chemotherapy* 35: 1875–1878.

NETILMICIN

Molecular weight (free base): 475.58

The semi-synthetic 1-*N*-ethyl derivative of sisomicin supplied as the sulfate salt.

Antimicrobial activity

The susceptibility of common pathogenic bacteria is shown in Table 14.1 (p. 156). Netilmicin is active against staphylococci, including methicillin-resistant and coagulase-negative strains. Nocardiae are inhibited by 0.04–1 mg/l. It is active against a wide range of enterobacteria, *Acinetobacter* and *Pseudomonas*, *Citrobacter*, some *Proteus* spp, and some *Serratia* spp. *Providencia* spp. and anaerobic bacteria are generally resistant.

It is active against some gentamicin-resistant strains, particularly those that synthesize ANT(2″) or AAC(3)-I. It exhibits typical aminoglycoside properties such as bactericidal activity at or close to the MIC, greater activity at alkaline pH, depression of activity against *Pseudomonas* by divalent cations and synergy with β-lactam antibiotics. Bactericidal synergy can be demonstrated regularly with benzylpenicillin against viridans streptococci and *E. faecalis*, including penicillin-tolerant strains, but seldom against *E. faecium*, which characteristically synthesizes AAC(6′), to which netilmicin is sensitive.

Acquired resistance

Netilmicin is resistant to ANT(2″), AAC(3)-I and AAC(3)-III, but sensitive to AAC(6′) (Table 14.2). AAC(3)-II confers resistance to netilmicin, but generally to a lesser degree than to gentamicin.

Resistance rates are generally about the same as, or a little lower than, those for gentamicin.

Pharmacokinetics

C_{max} 1 mg/kg intramuscular	3–5 mg/l after 30–40 min
2 mg/kg intravenous 30 min infusion	*c.* 12 mg/l end infusion
Plasma half-life	3 h
Volume of distribution	0.25 l/kg
Plasma protein binding	Low

Doubling the dose approximately doubles the peak plasma concentration. In patients receiving 200 mg (2.2–3.6 mg/kg) intramuscularly 8 hourly for 10 days a mean peak plasma concentration of around 14 mg/l was found. When once-daily doses of about 6 mg/kg were used in febrile neutropenic patients, the peak plasma concentrations were about 15 mg/l. Peak concentrations of about 10 mg/l were found in children with pyelonephritis treated with 5 mg/kg once daily, compared with peaks of about 5 mg/l in children given 2 mg/kg three times per day. The serum half-life is linearly inversely related to creatinine clearance.

In the newborn, intramuscular injection of 2.5 mg/kg produced peak plasma concentrations of 1–5 mg/l 1 h after the dose, with a plasma half-life of 4 h. In children with cystic fibrosis, a terminal half-life of 2.3 h (versus 1.4 h in unaffected children) has been found.

Distribution

Netilmicin is distributed in the extracellular water. In patients with cystic fibrosis the apparent volume of distribution is increased and the total body clearance prolonged.

Very little reaches the CSF even in the presence of inflammation. Concentrations of 0.13–0.45 mg/l were found in the CSF of patients without meningeal inflammation following an intravenous dose of 400 mg. In patients with meningitis, the drug was still undetectable in some, although concentrations of 0.2–5 mg/l could be found later in the course of treatment in others.

Excretion

Netilmicin is incompletely excreted unchanged in the urine over 24 h in the glomerular filtrate, with some tubular reabsorption. Over the first 6 h, about 50% and by 24 h about 80% of the dose appears. The remainder is metabolized or disposed of by unidentified mechanisms. Clearance on hemodialysis is similar to that reported for gentamicin.

Toxicity and side effects

Netilmicin appears to be distinctly less nephrotoxic than gentamicin, a difference not easily explained since the renal clearance and renal and medullary concentrations of the drugs appear to be similar. Both vestibular and cochlear toxicity appear to be low and vestibular toxicity without audiometric abnormality is rare. In some patients, plasma concentrations up to 30 mg/l over periods exceeding 1 week have not resulted in ototoxicity. Evidence of some renal toxicity in the excretion of granular casts has occurred fairly frequently in patients receiving 7.5 mg/kg per day, and is more likely to occur in the elderly and in those receiving higher doses or longer courses. In patients treated for an average of 35 days with 2.4–6.9 mg/kg per day, there was no effect on initially normal renal function, even in the elderly. Long-term treatment led to an increase in elimination half-life from 1.5 to 1.9 h. Nephrotoxicity has been observed in some diabetic patients. Overall estimates of the frequency of nephrotoxicity have ranged from 1–18%. Increases in serum transaminase and alkaline phosphatase concentrations have been seen in some patients without other evidence of hepatic impairment.

Once-daily dosing is thought to be safer than twice or three times daily dosing.

Clinical use

- Severe infections (including septicemia, lower respiratory tract infections, urinary tract infections, peritonitis, endometritis) caused by susceptible strains of Gram-negative bacilli and staphylococci.

Preparations and dosage

Proprietary name: Netillin, Netromycin

Preparation: Injection.

Dosage: Adults: i.m., i.v., i.v. infusion 4–6 mg/kg per day in a single dose or divided doses every 8–12 h. In severe infections up to 7.5 mg/kg per day in divided doses every 8 h, reduced as soon as is clinically indicated, usually within 48 h.

Children: 6–7.5 mg/kg per day, divided into three equal doses and administered every 8 hours. This should be reduced to 6 mg/kg per day as soon as clinically indicated.

Infants and neonates (more than 1 week of age): 7.5–9 mg/kg per day, divided into three equal doses and administered every 8 h. Premature and full-term neonates (less than 1 week of age): 6 mg/kg per day, divided into two equal doses and administered every 12 h.

Widely available.

Further information

Blaser J, Simmen HP, Thurnheer U, Konig C, Luthy R 1995 Nephrotoxicity, high frequency ototoxicity, efficacy and serum kinetics of once versus thrice daily dosing of netilmicin in patients with serious infections. *Journal of Antimicrobial Chemotherapy* 36: 803–814.

Craig WA, Gudmundsson S, Reich RM 1983 Netilmicin sulfate: a comparative evaluation of antimicrobial activity, pharmacokinetics, adverse reaction and clinical efficacy. *Pharmacotherapy* 3: 305–315.

Ettlinger JJ, Bedford KA, Lovering AM, Reeves DS, Speidel BD, MacGowan AP 1996 Pharmacokinetics of once-a-day netilmicin (6 mg/kg) in neonates. *Journal of Antimicrobial Chemotherapy* 38: 499–505.

Dahlager JI 1980 The effect of netilmicin and other aminoglycosides on renal function. A survey of the literature on the nephrotoxicity of netilmicin. *Scandinavian Journal of Infectious Diseases* 23 (suppl): 96–102.

Kahlmeter G 1980 Netilmicin: clinical pharmacokinetics and aspects of dosage schedules. An overview. *Scandinavian Journal of Infectious Diseases* 23 (suppl): 74–81.

Kuhn RJ, Nahata MC, Powell DA, Bickers RG 1986 Pharmacokinetics of netilmicin in premature infants. *European Journal of Clinical Pharmacology* 29: 635–637.

Manoharan A, Lalitha MK, Jesudason MV 1997 In vitro activity of netilmicin against clinical isolates of methicillin resistant and susceptible *Staphylococcus aureus*. *National Medical Journal of India* 10: 61–62.

Schwank S, Blaser J 1996 Once-versus thrice-daily netilmicin combined with amoxicillin, penicillin, or vancomycin against *Enterococcus faecalis* in a pharmacodynamic in vitro model. *Antimicrobial Agents and Chemotherapy* 40: 2258–2261.

Solberg CO, Reeves D, Phillips I (eds) 1984 Netilmicin. *Journal of Antimicrobial Chemotherapy* 13 (Suppl A): 1–81.

Treyluyer JM, Merle Y, Semlali A, Pons G 2000 Population pharmacokinetic analysis of netilmicin in neonates and infants with use of a nonparametric method. *Clinical Pharmacology and Therapeutics* 67: 600–609

 SISOMICIN

Sissomicin; rickamicin. Molecular weight (free base): 447.53.

A fermentation product of *Micromonospora inyoensis*. It is a dehydro derivative of gentamicin C_{1a}, supplied as the sulfate salt.

Antimicrobial activity

It is active against *Staph. aureus*, enterobacteria and *Ps. aeruginosa*. As with other aminoglycosides, its action against *Pseudomonas* is depressed in the presence of Mg^{2+} and Ca^{2+}. Streptococci and anaerobes are resistant. Its bactericidal activity, exerted at concentrations close to the MIC, increases with pH. Typical aminoglycoside synergy with appropriate β-lactam agents can be demonstrated against *Staph. aureus*, streptococci, enterobacteria and *Ps. aeruginosa*.

Acquired resistance

Cross-resistance with gentamicin is due to almost identical sensitivity of the two drugs to aminoglycoside-modifying enzymes (Table 14.2). Sisomicin, being a derivative of gentamicin C_{1a}, is sensitive to AAC(6′).

Pharmacokinetics

C_{max} 1–1.5 mg/kg intramuscular	1.5–9.0 mg/l after 0.5–1 h
Plasma half-life	2.5 h
Volume of distribution	0.25 l/kg
Plasma protein binding	Low

Sisomicin appears to be virtually identical to gentamicin in pharmacokinetic behavior. It is widely distributed in the body water, but concentrations in CSF are low, even in the presence of inflammation.

It is eliminated unchanged almost completely over 24 h in the glomerular filtrate. Excretion decreases proportionately with renal impairment and because of the virtual identity of the behavior of the two compounds, a gentamicin nomogram can be used to adjust dosage. About 40% of the dose is eliminated during a 6 h dialysis period, during which the elimination half-life falls to about 8 h.

Toxicity and side effects

Mild and reversible impairment of renal function, as evidenced by a 50% rise in serum creatinine concentration, occurs in about 5% of patients. Nephrotoxicity is more likely to be seen in those with pre-existing renal disease or treated concurrently with other potentially nephrotoxic drugs.

Ototoxicity mainly affecting vestibular function has been found in about 1% of patients. Neuromuscular blockade and other effects common to aminoglycosides including rashes, paresthesiae, eosinophilia and abnormal liver function tests have been described.

Clinical use

Its uses are identical with those of gentamicin, which it closely resembles.

Preparations and dosage

Proprietary names: Baymicine, Sissoline (France),

Extramycin (Germany), Mensiso, Sisobiotic, Sisomin (Italy), Sisomina (Spain).

Preparation: Injection.

Dosages: Adult i.m., i.v., i.v. infusion 3 mg/kg per day in two to three divided doses. The dose should be reduced in renal impairment.

Limited availability, not UK or USA.

Further information

Symposium 1979 New aspects in aminoglycoside therapy: sisomicin. *Infection 7* (Suppl 3): S240–S304.

Tamura K, Iwakiri R, Amamoto T, Seith M 1985 Serum concentration of sisomicin by intravenous infusion and its clinical response as a single agent. *Japanese Journal of Antibiotics* 38: 1552–1556

OTHER GENTAMICIN GROUP AMINOGLYCOSIDES

5-Epi-sisomicin

A semisynthetic derivative of sisomicin in which the hydroxyl group at position 5 of the deoxystreptamine ring is reorientated. It is more resistant than the parent compound to aminoglycoside-modifying enzymes including ANT(2″), APH(2″), AAC(3)-I, AAC(3)-II and AAC(2′).

Micronomicin (sagamicin; gentamicin C$_{2b}$)

A compound produced in substantial amounts, together with its precursor, gentamicin C$_{1a}$, by a mutant of *Micromonospora purpurea* and by *Micromonospora sagamiensis* var. *nonreducans*. It closely resembles gentamicin in antibiotic activity and spectrum, but is more resistant to AAC(6′).

Available in Japan.

Verdamicin

The dehydro derivative of gentamicin C$_2$. Its in-vitro activity resembles that of gentamicin and sisomicin.

KANAMYCIN

Kanamycin	R$_1$	Mol. wt.
A	OH	484.50
B	NH$_2$	483.51

A fermentation product of *Streptomyces kanamyceticus*, containing a mixture of kanamycins A, B and C. Commercial preparations consist predominantly of kanamycin A; the content of kanamycin B is required to be less than 3% (BP) or less than 5% (USP). Kanamycin A is very stable, losing less than 10% of its activity on autoclaving at 120°C for 1 h. Kanamycin B (available as bekanamycin in Japan) has twice the activity and twice the acute toxicity of kanamycin A. Kanamycin C is significantly less active and more toxic than kanamycin A.

Antimicrobial activity

The susceptibility of common pathogenic bacteria is shown in Table 14.1 (p. 156). Kanamycin is active against staphylococci, including methicillin-resistant strains. Other aerobic and anaerobic Gram-positive cocci and most Gram-positive rods are resistant. *M. tuberculosis* is susceptible. It is widely active against enterobacteria; *Acinetobacter*, *Alkaligenes*, *Campylobacter*, *Legionella* and *Pasteurella* spp. are also susceptible in vitro, but *Burkholderia cepacia* and *Stenotrophomonas maltophilia* are resistant. *Flavobacterium* spp. and *Bacteroides melaninogenicus* are moderately susceptible, but most other *Bacteroides* spp. are resistant. *Treponema pallidum*, *Leptospira* and *Mycoplasma* spp. are all resistant. It is more active at alkaline pH and exerts a rapid bactericidal effect at concentrations a little above the MIC. Bactericidal synergy is generally demonstrable with penicillins against *E. faecalis*.

Acquired resistance

Clinically significant resistance is usually multiple, plasmidborne and due to enzymatic inactivation of the drug. Kanamycin A is sensitive to many of the aminoglycoside-modifying enzymes that inactivate gentamicin or tobramycin and in addition is sensitive to APH(3′); however, it is resistant to AAC(2′) so *Prov. stuartii* is usually susceptible (*see* Table 14.2). Resistance due to reduced permeability is also encountered.

Pharmacokinetics

C_{max} 500 mg intramuscular	*c.* 15–20 mg/l after 1 h
Plasma half-life	2.5 h
Volume of distribution	0.3 l/kg
Plasma protein binding	Low

Absorption

Very little is absorbed from the intestinal tract. After an oral dose of 6 g, the concentration in feces was found to be 25 mg/g. The peak plasma concentration in the neonate is dose related: concentrations of 8–30 mg/l (mean 18 mg/l) have been found 1 h after a 10 mg/kg dose.

Distribution

The drug is confined to the extracellular fluid. The concentration in serous fluids is said to equal that in the plasma, but it does not enter the CSF in therapeutically useful concentrations even in the presence of meningeal inflammation.

Excretion

Kanamycin is excreted almost entirely by the kidneys and almost exclusively in the glomerular filtrate, so that probenecid has no effect on its plasma concentration. Renal clearance is about 80 ml/min, indicating some tubular reabsorption. Up to 80% of the dose appears unchanged in the urine over the first 24 h, producing concentrations around 100–500 mg/l. It is retained in proportion to reduction in renal function. Less than 1% of the dose appears in the bile. In patients receiving 500 mg intramuscularly preoperatively, concentrations of 2–23 mg/l have been found in bile and 8–14 mg/g in gallbladder wall, through which some entry evidently occurs since the drug can still be detected when the cystic duct is obstructed. The fate of the remaining 20% or so has not been established.

Toxicity and side effects

Intramuscular injections are moderately painful, and minor side effects similar to those encountered with streptomycin have been described. Eosinophilia in the absence of other manifestations of allergy occurs in up to 10% of patients. Other manifestations of hypersensitivity are rare. As with other aminoglycosides, the most important toxic effects are on the eighth nerve and much less frequently, but more importantly, on the kidney.

Nephrotoxicity

Renal damage is seen principally in patients with pre-existing renal disease or treated concurrently or sequentially with other potentially nephrotoxic agents. The drug accumulates in the renal cortex, producing cloudy swelling, which may progress to acute necrosis of proximal tubular cells with oliguric renal failure. The resulting renal impairment may take months to resolve. The appearance of protein, red cells and casts in the urine of treated patients is relatively common. Less dramatic deterioration of renal function, particularly exaggeration of the potential nephrotoxicity of other drugs or of existing renal disease, is principally important because it increases the likelihood of ototoxicity.

Ototoxicity

Vestibular damage is uncommon but may be severe and prolonged. Hearing damage is usually bilateral, and typically affects frequencies above the conversational range. Acute toxicity is most likely in patients in whom the plasma concentration exceeds 30 mg/l, but chronic toxicity may be seen in patients treated with the drug over long periods. Toxicity has been seen in up to 40% of patients treated for tuberculosis but in less than 2% of patients treated for acute conditions. Auditory toxicity may be potentiated by concurrent treatment with potent diuretics like ethacrynic acid. If tinnitus – which usually heralds the onset of auditory injury – develops, the drug should be withdrawn.

Neuromuscular blockade

This is seen particularly in patients receiving other muscle relaxants or suffering from myasthenia gravis and may be reversed by neostigmine. Prolonged oral use may be associated with malabsorption or, rarely, complicated by superinfection with resistant *Staph. aureus* leading to severe enteritis.

Clinical use

- Severe infection with susceptible organisms.

Kanamycin has largely been superseded by other aminoglycosides.

Preparations and dosage

Proprietary name: Kannasyn.

Preparations: Injection, ophthalmic, capsules.

Dosage: Adults, i.m. injection 250 mg every 6 h, or 500 mg every 12 h. Adults and children, i.v. infusion, 15–30 mg/kg per day in divided doses every 6–12 h. **The dose should be reduced in renal impairment.**

Widely available.

Further information

Davis RR, Brummett RE, Bendrick TW, Himes DL 1984. Dissociation of maximum concentration of kanamycin in plasma and perilymph from ototoxic effect. *Journal of Antimicrobial Chemotherapy* 14: 291–302.

Garrod LP, Lambert HP, O'Grady F 1981 Antibiotic and chemotherapy, 5th edn. Churchill Livingstone, Edinburgh

AMIKACIN

Molecular weight (free base): 585.62; (sulfate): 781.8.

A semisynthetic derivative of kanamycin A, in which the 1-amino group of the deoxystreptamine moiety is replaced by the hydroxyaminobutyric acid group also found in the natural aminoglycoside, butirosin. Supplied as the sulfate.

Antimicrobial activity

The activity of amikacin against common pathogenic bacteria is shown in Table 14.1 (p. 156). Among other organisms, *Acinetobacter, Alkaligenes, Campylobacter, Citrobacter, Hafnia, Legionella, Pasteurella, Providencia, Serratia* and *Yersinia* spp. are usually susceptible in vitro. *Sten. maltophilia*, many non-aeruginosa pseudomonads and *Flavobacterium* spp. are resistant. *M. tuberculosis* (including most streptomycin-resistant strains) and some other mycobacteria (including *M. fortuitum* and the *M. avium* complex) are susceptible; most other mycobacteria, including *M. kansasii* are resistant. *Nocardia asteroides* is susceptible.

Amikacin exhibits typical aminoglycoside characteristics, including an effect of divalent cations on its activity against *Ps. aeruginosa* analogous to that seen with gentamicin and synergy with β-lactam antibiotics. Synergy has been demonstrated with imipenem against about a third of *Staph. aureus* and gentamicin-resistant enterobacteria, but rarely against *Ps. aeruginosa*.

Acquired resistance

Amikacin is unaffected by most of the modifying enzymes that inactivate gentamicin and tobramycin (Table 14.2) and is consequently active against staphylococci, enterobacteria and pseudomonas that owe their resistance to the elaboration of those enzymes. However, AAC(6′), AAD(4′)(4″) and some forms of APH(3′) can confer amikacin resistance; because these enzymes generally do not confer gentamicin resistance, amikacin-resistant strains can be missed in routine susceptibility tests when gentamicin is used as the representative aminoglycoside.

There have been reports of amikacin resistance arising during treatment of infections due to *Serratia* spp. and *Ps. aeruginosa*. Outbreaks of infection due to multiresistant strains of enterobacteria and *Ps. aeruginosa* have occurred where amikacin has been used extensively, particularly in burns units. Strains of *Staph. aureus* and coagulase-negative staphylococci that owe their resistance to the expression of AAD(4′)(4″) have been described; this enzyme has also been found in *Esch. coli, Klebsiella* spp. and *Ps. aeruginosa*. In *E. faecalis*, resistance to penicillin-aminoglycoside synergy has been associated with plasmid-mediated APH(3′); a derivative of amikacin that lacks the 4′-OH group (BB-K311) is a very poor substrate for the enzyme and is active against strains that produce it.

Resistance in Gram-negative organisms is usually caused by reduced uptake of the drug or by the aminoglycoside-modifying enzymes AAC(6′) or AAC(3)-VI. The latter enzyme is usually found in *Acinetobacter* spp., but has also been found, encoded by a transposon, in *Prov. stuartii*. One type of AAC(6) is chromosomally encoded by *Ser. marcescens*, though not usually expressed.

The prevalence of resistance can change rapidly with increased usage of the drug, although no significant increase in amikacin resistance has been observed in the past decade. In New York, resistant strains rose from 2% to almost 8% in 18 months, during which there had been a threefold increase in usage; most resistance, associated with AAC(6′), was seen in *Klebsiella, Serratia* and *Pseudomonas* spp. The spread of extended spectrum β-lactamases belonging to the TEM and SHV families may result in an increase in amikacin resistance, since most strains that produce such enzymes also produce AAC(6′).

Pharmacokinetics

C_{max} 7.5 mg/kg intramuscular	*c.* 30 mg/l after 1 h
500 mg 30-min infusion	35–50 mg/l end infusion
Plasma half-life	2.2 h
Volume of distribution	0.25–0.3 l/kg
Plasma protein binding	3–11%

Amikacin is readily absorbed after intramuscular administration. Rapid intravenous injection of 7.5 mg/kg produced concentrations in excess of 60 mg/l shortly after injection. In volunteers, intravenous infusion of 3.33 mg/kg for 6 h followed by 1 mg/kg produced a steady state concentration around 12 mg/l.

Most pharmacokinetic parameters follow an almost linear correlation when the high once-daily doses (15 mg/kg) are compared with the traditional 7.5 mg/kg twice daily. In patients on CAPD, there was no difference in mean peak plasma concentration or volume of distribution whether the drug was given intravenously or intraperitoneally.

In infants receiving 7.5 mg/kg by intravenous injection, peak plasma concentrations were 17–20 mg/l. No accumulation occurred on 12 mg/kg per day for 5–7 days, but infusion over

20 min produced very low concentrations. There was little change in the plasma concentration or the half-life (1.7 and 1.9 h) on the third and seventh days of a period over which 150 mg/m² was infused over 30 min every 6 h. When the dose was raised to 200 mg/m² the concentration never fell below 8 mg/l. The plasma half-life was longer in babies of lower birth weight and was still 5–5.5 h in babies aged 1 week or older. The importance of dosage control in the neonate is emphasized by the findings that there is an inverse linear relationship between postconception age and plasma elimination half-life – leading to potential underdosing on standard regimens – with the complication that toxicity in the neonate is not clearly related to plasma concentration.

Distribution

The apparent volume of distribution indicates distribution throughout the extracellular water. Following an intravenous bolus of 0.5 g, peak concentrations in blister fluid were around 12 mg/l, with a mean elimination half-life of 2.3 h. In patients with impaired renal function, penetrance and peak concentration increased linearly with decrease in creatinine clearance.

In patients with purulent sputum, a loading dose of 4 mg/kg intravenously plus 8 h infusions of 7–12 mg/kg produced concentrations around 2 mg/l, with a mean sputum:serum ratio of 0.15. With brief infusions over 10 min for 7 days, sputum concentrations of around 9% of the simultaneous serum values have been found.

Concentrations of amikacin in the CSF of adult volunteers receiving 7.5 mg/kg intramuscularly were less than 0.5 mg/l and virtually the same in patients with meningitis. Rather higher, but variable, concentrations up to 3.8 mg/l have been found in neonatal meningitis.

Amikacin crosses the placenta, and concentrations of 0.5–6 mg/l have been found in the cord blood of women receiving 7.5 mg/kg in labor. Concentrations of 8 mg/l and 16.8 mg/l were reached in the fetal lung and kidney, respectively, after a standard dose of 7.5 mg/kg given to healthy women before therapeutic abortion.

Excretion

Only 1–2% of the administered dose is excreted in the bile, with the remainder excreted in the urine, producing urinary concentrations of 150–3000 mg/l. Renal clearance is 70–84 ml/min, and this, with the ratio of amikacin to creatinine clearance (around 0.7), indicates that it is filtered and tubular reabsorption is insignificant. Amikacin accumulates in proportion to reduction in renal function, although there may be some extrarenal elimination in anephric patients. The mean plasma half-life in patients on, or recently off, hemodialysis was around 4 h, while that on peritoneal dialysis was 28 h.

In patients receiving 500 mg/kg preoperatively, concentrations in gallbladder wall reached 34 mg/l and in bile 7.5 mg/l in some patients. In patients given 500 mg intravenously 12 h before surgery and 12 hourly for four doses thereafter, the mean bile:serum ratio 1 h after the dose was around 0.4.

Toxicity and side effects

Ototoxicity

Neurosensory hearing loss (mainly high-tone deafness) has been detected by audiometry and labyrinthine injury by caloric testing, but have seldom been severe. High-frequency hearing loss and vestibular impairment have been described in about 5% of patients and conversational loss in about 0.5%; more in patients monitored audiometrically (29%) and by caloric testing (19%). Toxicity is significantly more common in men. Cochlear damage has appeared after cessation of treatment.

Hearing loss appears to be reversible when the drug is discontinued. Patients with high-tone hearing loss have generally received more drug for longer than patients without. Over half the patients with peak serum concentrations exceeding 30 mg/l or trough concentrations exceeding 10 mg/l developed cochlear damage. The main contributory factor was previous treatment with other aminoglycosides.

Nephrotoxicity

Impairment of renal function, usually mild or transient, has been observed in 3–13% of patients, notably in the elderly or those with pre-existing renal disorders or treated concurrently or previously with other potentially nephrotoxic agents.

Other reactions

Adverse effects common to aminoglycosides occur, including hypersensitivity, gastrointestinal disturbances, headache, drug fever, peripheral nervous manifestations, eosinophilia, mild hematological abnormalities and disturbed liver function tests without other evidence of hepatic derangement.

Clinical uses

- Severe infection (including septicemia, neonatal sepsis, osteomyelitis, septic arthritis, respiratory tract, urinary tract, intra-abdominal, peritoneal and soft tissue infections) caused by susceptible micro-organisms.
- Sepsis of unknown origin (combined with a β-lactam or anti-anaerobe agent as appropriate).

Amikacin is principally used for the treatment of infections caused by organisms resistant to other aminoglycosides because of their ability to degrade them. Peak concentrations should not exceed 30 mg/l, and trough concentration of 10 mg/l should be maintained to achieve therapeutic effects. However, higher peak concentrations would be expected if the once-daily regimen with 15 mg/kg were used.

Preparations and dosage

Proprietary name: Amikin.

Preparation: Injection.

Dosage: Adults and children, i.m., i.v., i.v. infusion 15 mg/kg per day in two divided doses.

Neonates and premature infants, an initial loading dose of 10 mg/kg followed by 15 mg/kg per day in two equally divided doses.

The dose must be reduced if renal function is impaired, and in elderly patients.

Widely available.

Further information

Edson RS, Terrel CL 1999 The aminoglycosides. *Mayo Clinic Proceedings* 74: 519–528.

Fujimura S, Tokue Y, Takahashi H et al 2000 Novel arbekacin- and amikacin-modifying enzymes of methicillin-resistant *Staphylococcus aureus*. *FEMS Microbiology Letters* 190: 299–303.

Gerding DN, Larson TA, Hughes RA, Weiler M, Shanholtzer C, Peterson LR 1991 Aminoglycoside resistance and aminoglycoside usage: ten years of experience in one hospital. *Antimicrobial Agents and Chemotherapy* 35: 1284–1290.

Gonzalez LS, Spencer JP 1998 Aminoglycosides: A Practical Review. *American Family Physician* 58: 1811–1820.

Jacoby GA, Blaser MJ, Santanam P et al 1990 Appearance of amikacin and tobramycin resistance due to 4'-aminoglycoside nucleotidyltransferase [ANT(4')-II] in Gram-negative pathogens. *Antimicrobial Agents and Chemotherapy* 34: 2381–2386.

Kenyon CF, Knoppert DC, Lee SK, Vandenberghe HM, Chance GW 1990 Amikacin pharmacokinetics and suggested dosage modifications for the preterm infant. *Antimicrobial Agents and Chemotherapy* 34: 265–268.

Lambert T, Gerbaud G, Courvalin P 1994 Characterization of transposon Tn1528, which confers amikacin resistance by synthesis of aminoglycoside 3'-O-phosphotransferase type VI. *Antimicrobial Agents and Chemotherapy* 38: 702–706.

Lima Da Costa D, Erre JP, Pehourq F, Aran JM 1998 Aminoglycoside ototoxicity and the medial efferent system: II. comparison of acute effects of different antibiotics. *Audiology* 37: 162–173.

Tran Van Nhieu G, Bordon F, Collatz E 1992 Incidence of an aminoglycoside 6'-N-acetyltransferase, ACC(6')-Ib, in amikacin-resistant clinical isolates of Gram-negative bacilli, as determined by DNA-DNA hybridisation and immunoblotting. *Journal of Medical Microbiology* 36: 83–88

DIBEKACIN

Molecular weight (free base): 451.54.

A semisynthetic aminoglycoside also referred to as 3',4'-dideoxy kanamycin B. It is closely related to the natural compound tobramycin (3'-deoxy kanamycin B). Supplied as the sulfate.

Antimicrobial activity

Dibekacin is active against staphylococci including methicillin-resistant strains, a wide range of enterobacteria, *Acinetobacter* and *Pseudomonas* spp. It is also active against *M. tuberculosis* and the *M. avium* complex (MICs 4–16 mg/l). It exhibits the usual aminoglycoside properties of bactericidal activity at concentrations close to the MIC and bactericidal synergy with selected β-lactam antibiotics.

Acquired resistance

Absence of hydroxyl groups present in the parent kanamycin B renders dibekacin resistant to phosphorylation by APH(3'). It is also resistant to some forms of ANT(4'). However, the type of this enzyme, ANT(4')(4''), found in some Gram-positive organisms modifies dibekacin at the 2''-hydroxyl group; nevertheless dibekacin has much greater activity than tobramycin against organisms that produce the enzyme.

Pharmacokinetics

C_{max} 1 mg/kg intravenous bolus	*c.* 5 mg/l
Plasma half-life	2.3 h
Volume of distribution	0.25–0.38 l/kg
Plasma protein binding	3–12%

As with other aminoglycosides, dibekacin is inactivated in the presence of high concentrations of certain β-lactam antibiotics and at a dibekacin:β-lactam ratio of 1:100, the loss of activity over 48 h in the presence of different penicillins was: ticarcillin, 99%; carbenicillin, 90% and ampicillin 65%.

It is eliminated principally by the renal route, 75–80% of the dose appearing in the urine in the first 24 h. Elimination is inversely related to renal function, and in patients maintained on chronic hemodialysis, the half-life has been found to rise to 54 h between dialyses and fall to 6–7 h on dialysis.

Toxicity and side effects

Toxic effects are those typical of aminoglycosides with a frequency similar to or less than those of gentamicin. In a study in guinea pigs, dibekacin was found to have greater auditory toxicity than tobramycin but lower vestibular toxicity.

Clinical use

- Severe infections caused by susceptible micro-organisms, especially those resistant to established aminoglycosides.

Preparations and dosage

Proprietary name: Dibekacin

Preparation: Injection, ophthalmic.

Dosage: Adults and children, i.m., i.v., 1–3 mg/kg per day in divided doses.

Available in continental Europe and Japan, but not in the UK or USA.

Further information

Arancibia A, Chavez J, Ibarra R et al 1987 Disposition kinetics of dibekacin in normal subjects and in patients with renal failure. *International Journal of Clinical Pharmacology, Therapy and Toxicology* 25: 38–43.

Jacoby GA, Blaser MJ, Santanam P et al 1990 Appearance of amikacin and tobramycin resistance due to 4'-aminoglycoside nucleotidyltransferase [ANT(4')-II] in Gram-negative pathogens. *Antimicrobial Agents and Chemotherapy* 34: 2381–2386.

Kitsato I, Yokota M, Inouye S, Igarishi M 1990 Comparative ototoxicity of ribostamycin, dactimicin, dibekacin, kanamycin, amikacin, tobramycin, gentamicin, sisomicin and netilmicin in the inner ear of guinea pigs. *Chemotherapy* 36: 155–168.

Navarro AS, Lanao JM, Dominguez-Gil Huale A 1986 In vitro interaction between dibekacin and penicillin. *Journal of Antimicrobial Chemotherapy* 17: 83–89.

Noone P 1984 Sisiomicin, netilmicin and dibekacin. A review of their antibacterial activity and therapeutic use. *Drugs* 27: 548–578.

ARBEKACIN

Habekacin. Molecular weight (free base): 552.63.

The 1-*N*-(4-amino-2-hydroxybutyryl) derivative of dibekacin, to which it bears the same relation as amikacin bears to kanamycin A. Supplied as the sulfate.

Antimicrobial activity

Activity is comparable with that of amikacin against susceptible and a number of gentamicin- and tobramycin-resistant strains. It is also active against many strains of methicillin-resistant *Staph. aureus*, either alone or in combination with β-lactam or other agents. Synergy with ampicillin has been observed for high-level gentamicin- and vancomycin-resistant enterococci.

Acquired resistance

As with amikacin, several modifying enzymes that inactivate tobramycin and gentamicin do not modify arbekacin, making it active against some strains of enterococci, staphylococci and *Pseudomonas* spp. *N*-acetylation at the 4''' position of arbekacin and amikacin by an AAC(4''') modifying enzyme have been observed in arbekacin-resistant MRSA strains.

Pharmacokinetics

C_{max} 3 mg/kg intravenous	*c.* 8 mg/l after 1 h
Plasma half-life	2.1 h
Volume of distribution	0.25–0.38 l/kg
Plasma protein binding	3–12%

Urinary recovery rate was about 85% over a 48 h period. It is retained in renal failure, but moderately well removed by hemodialysis.

Toxicity and side effects

Typical of the aminoglycoside class.

Clinical use

- Severe infection cause by susceptible micro-organisms.

Preparations and dosage

Proprietary name: Habekacin

Preparation: Injection.

Dosage: Adults i.m., i.v., 4 mg/kg per day maximum in one to two divided doses.

Available in Japan.

Further information

Akins RL, Rybak MJ 2000 In vitro activities of daptomycin, arbekacin, vancomycin, and gentamicin alone and/or in combination against glycopeptide intermediate-resistant *Staphylococcus aureus* in an infection model. *Antimicrobial Agents and Chemotherapy* 44: 1925–1929.

Fujimura S, Tokue Y, Takahashi H et al 2000 Novel arbekacin- and amikacin-modifying enzymes of methicillin-resistant *Staphylococcus aureus*. *FEMS Microbiology Letters* 190: 299–303.

Hamilton-Miller JM, Shah S, 1995 Activity of the semi-synthetic kanamycin B derivative, arbekacin against methicillin-resistant *Staphylococcus aureus*. *Journal of Antimicrobial Chemotherapy* 35: 865–868.

Kak V, Donabedian SM, Zervos MJ, Kariyama R, Kumon H, Chow JW 2000 Efficacy of ampicillin plus arbekacin in experimental rabbit endocarditis caused by an *Enterococcus faecalis* strain with high-level gentamicin resistance. *Antimicrobial Agents and Chemotherapy* 44: 2545–2546.

Kak V, You, I, Zervos MJ, Kariyama R, Kumon H, Chow JW 2000 In vitro synergistic activity of the combination of ampicillin and arbekacin against vancomycin and high-level gentamicin-resistant *Enterococcus faecium* with the aph(2″)-Id gene. *Diagnostic Microbiology and Infectious Disease* 37: 297–299.

Matsuo H, Hayashi J, Ono K et al 1997 Administration of aminoglycosides to hemodialysis patients immediately before dialysis: a new dosing modality. *Antimicrobial Agents and Chemotherapy* 41: 2597–2601.

You I, Kariyama R, Zervos MJ, Kumon H, Chow JW 2000 In vitro activity of arbekacin alone and in combination with vancomycin against gentamicin- and methicillin-resistant *Staphylococcus aureus*. *Diagnostic Microbiology and Infectious Disease* 36: 37–41.

 ## TOBRAMYCIN

Nebramycin factor 6; 3′-deoxy kanamycin B. Molecular weight (free base): 467.52.

A natural fermentation product of *Streptomyces tenebraeus*, supplied as the sulfate in various preparations.

Antimicrobial activity

The susceptibility of common pathogenic organisms is shown in Table 14.1 (p. 156). In general it has somewhat greater in-vitro activity than gentamicin against *Ps. aeruginosa*, but against other organisms its activity is generally the same as, or a little lower than, that of gentamicin. Other *Pseudomonas* species are generally resistant, as are streptococci and most anaerobic bacteria. Other organisms usually susceptible in vitro include *Acinetobacter*, *Legionella*, and *Yersinia* spp. *Alkaligenes*, *Flavobacterium* spp. and *Mycobacterium* spp. are resistant. It exhibits bactericidal activity at concentrations close to the MIC and bactericidal synergy typical of aminoglycosides in combination with penicillins or cephalosporins.

Acquired resistance

Many aminoglycoside-modifying enzymes that attack gentamicin also attack tobramycin (Table 14.2). However, AAC(3′)-I does not confer tobramycin resistance and AAC(3′)-II confers a lower degree of tobramycin resistance than of gentamicin resistance. Conversely, ANT(4′)(4″) confers tobramycin but not gentamicin resistance, as do some types of AAC(6′). Overproduction of APH(3′) has been reported to confer a low degree of tobramycin resistance (MIC 8 mg/l), but not gentamicin resistance (MIC 2 mg/l); the resistance was ascribed to 'trapping' rather than phosphorylation.

Resistance rates are generally similar to those of gentamicin, although they may vary locally because of the prevalence of particular enzyme types.

Pharmacokinetics

C_{max} 80 mg intramuscular	3–4 mg/l after 30 min
1 mg/kg intravenous	6–7 mg/l after 30 min
Plasma half-life	1.5–3 h
Volume of distribution	c. 0.3 l/kg
Plasma protein binding	<30%

The pharmacokinetic behavior of tobramycin after systemic administration closely resembles that of gentamicin. In patients treated for prolonged periods with 2.5 mg/kg intravenously 12 hourly, average peak steady-state values were 6.5 mg/l after 30 weeks and 7.1 mg/l after 40 weeks. Continuous intravenous infusion of 6.6 mg/h and 30 mg/h produced steady-state concentrations of 1 and 3.5–4.5 mg/l, respectively. Higher concentrations (10–12 mg/l) have been obtained by bolus injection over about 3 min. Peak concentrations of around 50 mg/l have been reported in cystic fibrosis patients given 9 mg/kg once daily. Ten minutes after a 300 mg dose of tobramycin solution for inhalation mean concentration of drug in the sputum of cystic fibrosis patients was 1.2 mg/g and ranged from 0.04 to 1.4 mg/g. In general, the concentration found in the sputum of cystic fibrosis patients is high when administered by inhalation, but varies widely depending on individual airway pathology and nebulizer efficiency. Mean serum concentrations were 0.95 mg/l 1 h after administration by inhalation.

In patients dosed repeatedly or continuously for some weeks, the elimination half-life declined from 9.3–11.3 h initially to 5.6 h. Accumulation occurs over the first few days of treatment, due probably to tissue binding, and excretion continues for up to 3 weeks after cessation of treatment.

As with a number of other agents, clearance is more rapid in patients with cystic fibrosis. In the neonate, peak plasma concentrations of 4–6 mg/l have been found 0.5–1 h after doses of 2 mg/kg. Mean plasma elimination half-lives of 4.6–8.7 h were inversely proportional to the birth weight and creatinine clearance. The half-life was found to be initially extremely variable (3–17 h) in infants weighing 2.5 kg at birth, but considerably more stable (4–8 h) at the end of therapy 6–9 days later.

β-Lactam inactivation

In common with other aminoglycosides, tobramycin interacts with certain β-lactam agents, but is said to be stable in the presence of ceftazidime, imipenem and aztreonam. In mixtures containing tobramycin 80 mg/l and carbenicillin or ticarcillin 4–5 mg/l, 30–40% of tobramycin activity was lost over 1 h. Of the penicillins tested, piperacillin caused least inactivation in vitro.

Distribution

The volume of distribution slightly exceeds the extracellular water volume. In tracheostomized or intubated patients given a loading dose of 1 mg/kg and then 8-hourly intravenous infusions of 2–3.5 mg/kg, average concentrations in the bronchial secretions were 0.7 mg/l with a mean serum:secretion ratio of 0.18.

In patients with cystic fibrosis receiving 10 mg/kg of the drug per day, the bronchial secretions may contain 2 mg or more (2 mg or more/l). Concentrations are low in peritoneal fluid but can rise to 60% of the plasma concentration in peritonitis and in synovial fluid.

Tobramycin crosses the placenta, and concentrations of 0.5 mg/l have been found in the fetal serum when the mother was receiving a dose of 2 mg/kg.

Access to the CSF resembles that of gentamicin.

Excretion

Tobramycin is eliminated in the glomerular filtrate and is unaffected by probenecid. Renal clearance is 90 ml/min. About 60% of the administered dose is recovered from the urine over the first 10 h, producing urinary concentrations after a dose of 80 mg of 90–500 mg/l over the first 3 h. The nature of the extrarenal disposal of the remaining 40% of the drug has not been established. In the neonate, urinary concentrations after doses of 2 mg/kg ranged around 10–100 mg/l over the first 8 h, but the total urinary recovery has varied widely. In patients with impaired renal function, urinary concentrations of the drug are depressed and the plasma half-life prolonged in proportion to the rise in serum creatinine, reaching 6–8 h at a creatinine concentration of 350 μmol/l. In view of the virtually identical behavior of the two drugs, modification of tobramycin dosage in patients with impaired renal function may be based on the procedures used for gentamicin. About 70% of the drug is removed by hemodialysis over 12 h, but the efficiency of different dialysers varies markedly.

Toxicity and side effects

Ototoxicity

The effect is predominantly on the auditory branch of the eighth nerve; vestibular function is seldom affected. Experimental evidence suggests that comparable effects on cochlear electrophysiology and histology require doses about twice those of gentamicin. In patients, electrocochleography has shown an immediate dramatic reduction of cochlear activity when the serum tobramycin concentration exceeded 8–10 mg/l, but there were no associated symptoms and function recovered fully as the drug was eliminated. Clinical ototoxicity is rare and most likely to be seen in patients with renal impairment or treated concurrently or sequentially with other potentially ototoxic agents.

Nephrotoxicity

Renal impairment with proteinuria, excretion of granular casts, oliguria and rise of serum creatinine has been noted in 1–2% of patients. Some evidence of nephrotoxicity has been found in about 10% of patients, depending on the sensitivity of the tests employed. In patients treated for urinary tract infection, $β_2$-microglobulin excretion indicated reduced renal tubular function before and during treatment, which improved as infection was eliminated. In patients treated with a 120 mg loading dose and 80 mg 8-hourly, renal enzyme excretion increased and there was a small but significant reduction in chrome-EDTA clearance even when the clinical condition improved. It has been suggested that intermittent dosage with large but infrequent plasma peaks may be less toxic than, and as efficacious as, continuous dosing.

It is generally held that the likelihood of toxicity increases with pre-existing renal impairment and higher or more prolonged dosage, but in a comparison of patients treated with 8 mg/kg per day for *Pseudomonas* endocarditis with those treated with 3 mg/kg per day for Gram-negative sepsis there was no evidence of renal impairment in either group. Although there was audiological evidence of high-frequency loss in some patients receiving the high dosage, there was no sustained loss of conversational hearing. Nor does there seem to be a significant effect of age: in patients aged 20–39 years the mean elimination half-life of the drug at the end of treatment was 2.3 h while in those aged 60–79 years it was 2.4 h. Evidence of renal toxicity may be found in 20% of severely ill patients.

Other reactions

Other toxic manifestations are rare. Local reactions sometimes occur at the site of injection. Rashes and eosinophilia in the absence of other allergic manifestations are seen. Voice alterations and tinnitus were rare in cystic fibrosis patients receiving tobramycin by inhalation. Increased transaminase levels may occur in the absence of other evidence of hepatic derangement.

Clinical use

- Severe infections caused by susceptible micro-organisms.
- *Ps. aeruginosa* infections, including chronic pulmonary infections in cystic fibrosis (administration by injection or nebulizer).

For practical purposes use is identical to that of gentamicin, except possibly for *Pseudomonas* infection, where it has somewhat greater activity against gentamicin-susceptible and some gentamicin-resistant strains. Its use as a possible substitute for gentamicin in the speculative treatment of severe undiagnosed infection is offset by its lower activity against other possibly implicated organisms.

Preparations and dosage

Proprietary names: Nebcin, Tobradex, Tobrex, TOBI.

Preparations: Injections, topical and inhalation formulations.

Dosage: Adults i.m., i.v., 3 mg/kg per day in three equal doses every 8 h; 5 mg/kg per day in three to four equal doses may be used for life-threatening infections. The higher dose should be reduced as soon as clinically indicated.

Children, 6–7.5 mg/kg per day in three to four equally divided doses.

Premature or full-term term neonates up to 4 mg/kg per day in two equal doses every 12 h. The dose should be reduced in renal impairment.

Adults and children TOBI inhalation, 300 mg twice daily for management of cystic fibrosis.

Widely available.

Further information

Bonsignore CL 1998 Inhaled tobramycin (TOBI). *Pediatric Nursing* 24: 258–259.

Edson RS, Terrel CL 1999 The aminoglycosides. *Mayo Clinic Proceedings* 74: 519–528.

Gonzalez LS 3rd, Spencer, JP 1998 Aminoglycosides: a practical review. *American Family Physician* 58: 1811–1820.

Jacoby GA, Blaser MJ, Santanam P et al 1990 Appearance of amikacin and tobramycin resistance due to 4′-aminoglycoside nucleotidyltransferase [ANT(4′)-II] in Gram-negative pathogens. *Antimicrobial Agents and Chemotherapy* 34: 2381–2386.

Lima da Costa L, Erre JP, Pehourq F, Aran JM 1998 Aminoglycoside ototoxicity and the medial efferent system: II. Comparison of acute effects of different antibiotics. *Audiology* 37: 162–173.

Menard R, Molinas C, Arthur M, Duval J, Courvalin P, Leclercq R 1993 Overproduction of 3′-aminoglycoside phosphotransferase type I confers resistance to tobramycin in *Escherichia coli. Antimicrobial Agents and Chemotherapy* 37: 78–83.

Robinson P 2001 Cystic fibrosis. *Thorax* 56: 237–241.

Spruill WJ, McCall CY, Francisco GE 1985 In vitro inactivation of tobramycin by cephalosporins. *American Journal of Hospital Pharmacy* 42: 2506–2509.

Winslade NE, Adelman MH, Evans EJ, Schentag JJ 1987 Single-dose accumulation pharmacokinetics of tobramycin and netilmicin in normal volunteers. *Antimicrobial Agents and Chemotherapy* 31: 605–609.

NEOMYCIN GROUP

NEOMYCIN

Fradiomycin. Molecular weight (sulfate): 711.7; (free base): 614.7.

Neomycin	R_1	R_2	R_3
B	NH_2	H	CH_2NH_2
C	NH_2	CH_2NH_2	H

Neomycins A, B and C are fermentation products of *Streptomyces fradii*. The product marketed as 'neomycin' is an isomeric mixture of neomycins B and C supplied as the sulfates. Solutions are stable at room temperature.

Neomycin B, a fermentation product of *Streptomyces fradii* and *Streptomyces lavendulae*, is available alone under the name framycetin and is supplied as the sulfate for topical use. It is required to contain not more than 3% neomycin C and not more than 1% neomycin A. Buffered aqueous solutions (pH 7) are stable at room temperature.

Antimicrobial activity

The susceptibility of common pathogenic bacteria is shown in Table 14.1 (p. 156). Among other organisms susceptible in vitro (MIC 4–8 mg/l) are *Pasteurella*, *Vibrio*, *Borrelia* and *Leptospira* spp. It is active against *M. tuberculosis*, including streptomycin-resistant strains.

Neomycin exerts a rapid bactericidal effect that is enhanced at alkaline pH; when the pH is raised from 5.5 to 8.5, activity is increased 64-fold.

Acquired resistance

Resistance is acquired in a stepwise fashion and staphylococci may become resistant as a result of prolonged topical use. The use of neomycin–bacitracin–polymyxin mixtures may contribute to this, as many strains resistant to neomycin are also resistant to bacitracin. Resistant enterobacteria may appear in the feces of patients treated orally and in those treated for prolonged periods; most have been found to possess multiple transferable antibiotic resistance. Cross-resistance with kanamycin is often due to the synthesis of APH(3'), though AAC(6'), some forms of AAC(3) and ANT(4')(4") also modify both neomycin and kanamycin. Resistant strains of *Staph. aureus* are usually more resistant to kanamycin than to neomycin. The rare enzyme AAC(1) confers resistance to neomycin, paromomycin and apramycin, but not to other aminoglycosides.

Pharmacokinetics

C$_{max}$ 0.5 g intramuscular	20 mg/l after 1 h
Plasma half-life	2–3 h
Volume of distribution	0.25–0.35 l/kg
Plasma protein binding	Low

Very little is absorbed after oral administration and more than 95% is eliminated unchanged in the feces. Peak plasma concentrations of less than 4 mg/l have been found after an oral dose of 3 g. Distribution and excretion resemble that of streptomycin, but the toxicity of neomycin precludes systemic administration except in the most extreme cases.

Toxicity and side effects

Neomycin is the most likely of all the aminoglycosides to damage the kidneys and the auditory branch of the eighth nerve (Table 14.3; p. 160). This has almost entirely restricted it to topical and oral use.

Irreversible deafness may develop even if the drug is stopped at the first sign of damage. Loss of hearing may occur as a result of topical applications to wounds or other denuded areas, particularly if renal excretion is impaired. Instillation of ear drops containing neomycin can result in deafness. This generally develops in the second week of treatment and is usually reversible.

Rashes have been described in 6–8% of patients treated topically and these patients may be rendered allergic to other aminoglycosides. Nausea and protracted diarrhea may follow oral administration. Sufficient drug may be absorbed from the gut on prolonged oral administration to produce deafness but not renal damage. Intestinal malabsorption and superinfection have been seen in patients receiving 4–9 g/day and may develop in patients receiving as little as 3 g of the drug/day. Precipitation of bile salts by the drug may impair the hydrolysis of long-chain triglycerides. Large doses instilled into the peritoneal cavity at operation may be absorbed, with resultant systemic toxicity, and patients concurrently exposed to anesthetics and muscle relaxants are liable to suffer neuromuscular blockade, which is reversible by neostigmine.

Neomycin is a useful reagent in the investigation of phospholipase activity as, for example, in arachidonic acid release.

Clinical use

- Superficial infections with staphylococci and Gram-negative bacilli (topical; alone or in combination with bacitracin, chlorhexidine or polymyxin).
- Treatment of staphylococcal nasal carriers (topical, in combination with chlorhexidine or bacitracin).
- Eye infections (topical; alone or in combination).
- Otitis externa (alone or with a corticosteroid).
- Gut decontamination before abdominal surgery (oral).
- Prophylaxis after urinary tract instrumentation (instillation).

The use of neomycin is discouraged because of the possibility of promoting the appearance of aminoglycoside-resistant strains, and because of the risk of absorption with the consequent danger of systemic toxicity or neuromuscular blockade.

 ## Preparations and dosage

Neomycin
Proprietary names: Mycifradin, Nivemycin.
Preparations: Tablets, elixir, topical.
Dosage: Adults, oral, 1 g every 4 h for a maximum of 72 h.
Children 6–12 years, 250–500 mg every 4 h.
Widely available.

Framycetin (neomycin B)
Proprietary name: Soframycin.
Preparations: Tablets, topical ophthalmic, aural.
Dosage: Adult, oral, 2–4 g/day in divided doses.
Widely available in topical preparations.

 ## Further information

DiPitro JT 1985 Oral neomycin sulfate and erythromycin base before colon surgery: a comparison of serum and tissue concentrations. *Pharmacotherapy* 5: 91–94.

Dire DJ, Coppola M, Dwyer DA, Lorette JJ, Karr JL 1995 Prospective evaluation of topical antibiotics for preventing infections in uncomplicated soft-tissue wounds repaired in the ED. *Academic Emergency Medicine* 2: 4–10.

Langman AW 1994 Neomycin ototoxicity. *Otolaryngology and Head and Neck Surgery* 110: 441–444.

Lima da Costa L, Erre JP, Pehourq F, Aran JM 1998 Aminoglycoside ototoxicity and the medial efferent system: II. Comparison of acute effects of different antibiotics. *Audiology* 37: 162–173.

PAROMOMYCIN

Aminosidine, catenulin, crestomycin, hydroxymycin, estomycin, monomycin A, neomycin E, paucimycin. Molecular weight (free base): 615.65.

A fermentation product of *Streptomyces rimosus* var. *paromomycinus*, supplied as the sulfate. The commercial product is a mixture of the two isomeric paromomycins I and II, which are closely related to neomycin.

Antimicrobial activity

The antibacterial activity of paromomycin is almost identical to that of neomycin. Since it differs from neomycin in having a hydroxyl rather than an amino group at the 6′-position it is not sensitive to AAC(6′) modifying enzymes. It is active against *M. tuberculosis*, including multidrug-resistant strains, and the *M. avium* complex.

Unlike other aminoglycosides paromomycin is active against some protozoa, including *Entamoeba histolytica*, *Cryptosporidium parvum*, *Leishmania* spp., *Giardia lamblia* and *Trichomonas vaginalis*. It also exhibits activity against the tapeworms *Taenia saginata*, *Taenia solium*, *Diphyllobothrium latum* and *Hymenolepis nana*.

In its pharmacokinetic behavior and liability to produce deafness and intestinal malabsorption paromomycin closely resembles neomycin.

Clinical use

- Intestinal amebiasis (oral).
- Cutaneous leishmaniasis (topical).
- Nitroimidazole-resistant trichomoniasis (topical).

Its antiprotozoal activity has attracted some attention, but it has largely been superseded by more active and less toxic compounds. Success in treating nitroimidazole-resistant trichomoniasis with topical paromomycin has been reported.

 ## Preparations and dosage

Proprietary names: Gabbomycin, Humagel, Humatin.

Preparations: Capsules, syrup, topical.

Dosage: Adult oral dose 25–35 mg/kg per day in three divided doses for 5–10 days.

Limited availability. Available in the USA and continental Europe, but not in the UK.

Further information

Davidson RN 1998 Practical guide for the treatment of leishmaniasis. *Drugs* 56: 1009–1018.

Donald PR, Sirgel FA, Kanyok TP et al 2000 Early bactericidal activity of paromomycin (aminosidine) in patients with smear-positive pulmonary tuberculosis. *Antimicrobial Agents and Chemotherapy* 44: 3285–3287.

Kayok TP, Reddy MV, Chinnaswamy J, Danziger LH, Gangadharam PR 1994 Activity of aminosidine (paromomycin) for *Mycobacterium tuberculosis* and *Mycobacterium avium*. *Journal of Antimicrobial Chemotherapy* 33: 323–327.

Murray HW 2000 Treatment of visceral leismaniasis (kala-azar): a decade of progress and future approaches. *International Journal of Infectious Diseases* 4: 158–177.

Nyirjesy P, Sobel JD, Weitz MV, Leaman DJ, Gelone SP 1998 Difficult-to-treat trichomoniasis: results with paromomycin cream. *Clinical Infectious Diseases* 26: 986–988.

Coelho DD 1997 Metronidazole resistant trichomoniasis successfully treated with paromomycin. *Genitourinary Medicine* 73: 397–398.

Scott JA, Davidson RN, Moddy AH et al 1992 Aminosidine (paromomycin) in the treatment of leishmaniasis imported into the United Kingdom. *Transactions of the Royal Society of Tropical Medicine and Hygiene* 86: 617–619.

OTHER AMINOGLYCOSIDES AND AMINOCYCLITOLS

 ## STREPTOMYCIN

Molecular weight (free base): 581.58.

A fermentation product of *Streptomyces griseus*. It is available in some countries as the calcium chloride or as the hydrochloride, but usually supplied as the sulfate. Solutions are stable for long periods in the cold.

Antimicrobial activity

Activity against common bacterial pathogens is shown in Table 14.1 (p. 156). It is less active than gentamicin group compounds against most micro-organisms within the spectrum, but it is particularly active against mycobacteria, including *M. kansasii* and most strains of *M. ulcerans*. *Brucella* (MIC 0.5 mg/l), *Francisella*, *Pasteurella* spp. and *Yersinia pestis* are susceptible.

Streptomycin is actively bactericidal, the speed of killing increasing progressively with concentration. The antibacterial activity is greatest in a slightly alkaline medium (pH 7.8) and is considerably reduced in media with a pH of 6.0 or less. It is so sensitive to the effect of pH that the natural acidity of a solution of streptomycin sulfate may be sufficient to depress its antibacterial activity.

Acquired resistance

In contrast to most other aminoglycosides, high level resistance can result from a single-step mutation in the gene encoding ribosomal protein S12 (*rpsL*), which alters the protein so that binding of streptomycin is reduced. Resistance in some clinical isolates of *M. tuberculosis* is associated either with missense mutations in the *rpsL* gene, or with base substitutions at position 904 in the 16S rRNA.

Resistance can also be caused by aminoglycoside-modifying enzymes: phosphotransferases that modify the 3″-hydroxyl group have been found in both Gram-negative and Gram-positive organisms; a phosphotransferase that modifies the 6-hydroxyl group in *Pseudomonas* spp.; and a nucleotidyltransferase that modifies the 3″-hydroxyl group (plus the 9-hydroxyl of spectinomycin) in Gram-negative organisms.

Increase in resistance often occurs within a few days (for *M. tuberculosis* a few weeks) of the beginning of treatment, and resistance of many species is now common. Primary streptomycin resistance in *M. tuberculosis* had become uncommon in the UK and USA, though found in more than one-third of cases in the Far East. However, since 1990 several clusters of multidrug-resistant tuberculosis have been identified among hospital patients with AIDS in the USA. No streptomycin resistance was found in the isolates of *Yersinia pestis* from the 1991 outbreak of plague in Tanzania.

Strains of streptococci and enterococci showing moderate resistance (MIC 64–500 mg/l) exhibit synergy with penicillin, but strains showing high levels of resistance (MIC >500 mg/l) have ribosomes that are resistant to streptomycin and hence simultaneous treatment with penicillin is without effect.

It is not uncommon to find strains of bacteria, including *M. tuberculosis*, that are actually favored by the presence of the antibiotic or completely dependent on it. Isolated ribosomes from streptomycin-dependent *Esch. coli* show a change in the same single ribosomal protein that determines resistance and synthesize peptides only in the presence of the drug.

Streptomycin-resistant bacteria usually remain sensitive to other aminoglycosides. Enterococci with high-level resistance to gentamicin, and consequent resistance to gentamicin–β-lactam synergy, may show synergy between the β-lactam and streptomycin.

Pharmacokinetics

C_{max} 1 g intramuscular	26–58 mg/l after 0.5–1.5 h
Plasma half-life	2.4–2.7 h
Volume of distribution	0.3 l/kg
Plasma protein binding	35%

Absorption

Streptomycin is not absorbed in any quantity from the intestinal tract. In patients treated for tuberculosis, considerable variation has been encountered on repeat dosing, the peak concentrations following a dose of 0.75 g sometimes differing by as much as 50 mg/l. In premature infants, 10 mg/kg produced peak plasma concentrations of 17–42 mg/l at about 2 h with a half-life of 7 h. In patients over the age of 40 years, excretion is delayed and in older subjects commonly incomplete at 24 h. In such patients a dose of 0.75 g intramuscularly produces peak plasma concentrations around 25–60 mg/l with a half-life up to 9 h.

Distribution

Streptomycin diffuses fairly rapidly into most body tissues, but is distributed only in the extracellular fluid. It appears in the peritoneal fluid in concentrations of about one-quarter to one-half those present in the blood, and in pleural fluid the concentrations may equal those in the blood. It does not penetrate into the CSF or thick-walled abscesses, but significant amounts are usually present in tuberculous cavities. Concentrations in cord blood are similar to those in maternal blood.

Excretion

Streptomycin is rapidly excreted by glomerular filtration and is unaffected by agents that block tubular secretion. The renal clearance is 30–70 ml/min and 30–90% of the dose is usually excreted in the first 24 h. Concentrations in the urine often reach 400 mg/l after doses of 0.5 g and 1000 mg or more/l after doses of 1 g. In oliguria, the plasma half-life is prolonged and dosage must be reduced if toxic concentrations are to be avoided. Less than 1% appears in the bile, where concentrations of 3–12.5 mg/l have been recorded.

Toxicity and side effects

Pain and irritation at the site of injection are common, and sterile inflammatory reactions or peripheral neuritis from direct involvement of a nerve sometimes occur. Many patients experience paresthesia in and around the mouth, vertigo and ataxia, headaches, lassitude and 'muzziness in the head'.

Renal dysfunction is rare but has been described in patients receiving 3–4 g/day.

Ototoxicity

The most common serious toxic effect is vestibular disturbance, which is related to total dosage and excessive blood concentrations, and hence to the age of the patient and the state of renal function. In older patients the risk of damage is higher and compensation is less than in young patients. Active secretion into the endolymph or persistence of the drug in the perilymph after the plasma concentration has fallen may play an important part in such ototoxicity. There is no significant relation between incidence of dizziness and peak streptomycin concentration, but a highly significant relation to plasma concentrations exceeding 3 mg/l at 24 h. The risk to hearing is much less, but damage sometimes occurs after only a few doses. Congenital hearing loss or abnormalities in the caloric test or audiogram have several times been described in children born to women treated with streptomycin in pregnancy. There is considerable individual variation in susceptibility to its toxic effects, which may be partly genetically determined.

Allergy

In addition to eosinophilia unassociated with other allergic manifestations, rashes and drug fever occur in about 5% of treated patients. These are usually trivial and respond to antihistamine treatment, so that in most cases therapy can be continued, although this should be done with caution, since occasionally severe and even fatal exfoliative dermatitis may develop. Skin sensitization is also common in nurses and dispensers who handle streptomycin and may lead to severe dermatitis, sometimes associated with periorbital swelling and conjunctivitis. Reactions most frequently develop between 4 and 6 weeks, but may appear after the first dose or after 6 months' treatment. Patients who develop hypersensitivity during prolonged therapy can generally be desensitized by giving 20 mg prednisolone daily plus 10 daily increments from 0.1 to 1.0 g when normal dosage will usually be tolerated, or by giving increased doses of streptomycin every 6 h.

Neuromuscular blockade

It is rare for neuromuscular blockade to develop in those whose neuromuscular mechanisms are normal, but patients who are also receiving muscle relaxants or anesthetics or are suffering from myasthenia gravis are at special risk.

Other effects

Rare neurological manifestations include peripheral neuritis and optic neuritis with scotoma. Other rare effects have been aplastic anemia, agranulocytosis, hemolytic anemia, thrombocytopenia, hypocalcemia and severe bleeding associated with a circulating factor V antagonist.

Clinical use

- Tuberculosis (in combination with other antituberculosis drugs).
- Infections caused by *M. kansasii* (in combination with other antimycobacterial agents).
- Plague and tularemia, including tularemia pneumonia.
- Bacterial endocarditis (in combination with a penicillin).
- Brucellosis
- Whipple's disease (in combination with other antibiotics)

The most important use of streptomycin is in the treatment of tuberculosis (Ch. 61). Depression of vestibular function by streptomycin has been used in the treatment of patients suffering from Ménière's disease.

 ## Preparations and dosage

Proprietary names: Streptomycin sulfate, Strepto-Fatol (Germany), Streptocol (Italy), Novostrep, Solustrep (South Africa), Cidan Est (Spain).

Preparation: Injection.

Dosage: Tuberculosis: Adults, i.m., 1 g daily (750 mg daily for adults over 40 years of age or less than 50 kg body weight. Children, i.m., 15–20 mg/kg per day.

Widely available.

 ## Further information

Bagger-Sjoback D 1997 Effect of streptomycin and gentamicin on the inner ear. *Annals of the New York Academy of Science* 830: 120–129.

Edlin BR, Tokars JI, Grieco MH et al 1992 An outbreak of multidrug-resistant tuberculosis among hospitalized patients with the acquired immunodeficiency syndrome. *New England Journal of Medicine* 326: 1514–1521.

Gill V, Cunha BA, 1997 Tularemia pneumonia. *Seminars in Respiratory Infection* 12: 61–67.

Honore N, Cole ST 1994 Streptomycin resistance in mycobacteria. *Antimicrobial Agents and Chemotherapy* 38: 238–242.

Lyamuya EF, Nyanda P, Mohammedali H, Mhalu FS 1992 Laboratory studies on *Yersinia pestis* during the 1991 outbreak of plague in Lushoto, Tanzania. *Journal of Tropical Medicine and Hygiene* 95: 335–338.

Nachamkin I, Axelrod P, Talbot GH et al 1988 Multiply high-level-aminoglycoside-resistant enterococci isolated from patients in a University Hospital. *Journal of Clinical Microbiology* 26: 1287–1291.

Shea JJ Jr 1997 The role of dexamethasone or streptomycin perfusion in the treatment of Meniere's disease. *Otolaryngologic Clinics of North America* 30: 1051–1059.

SPECTINOMYCIN

Aminospectacin; actinospectacin. Molecular weight (free base): 332.35.

An aminocyclitol that lacks an aminoglycosidic function. A fermentation product of *Streptomyces spectabilis* and *Streptomyces flavopersicus*. It is supplied as the dihydrochloride and the sulfate. A propyl derivative, trospectinomycin, is more active than the parent compound, but is not available clinically.

Antimicrobial activity

Its activity is modest (Table 14.1; p. 156) and markedly affected by medium composition and pH. Spectinomycin exerts only moderate activity against Gram-positive organisms. It is widely active against enterobacteria but *Providencia* spp. are resistant. Anaerobic bacteria are also resistant.

Of particular interest is its activity against *N. gonorrhoeae*, including β-lactamase-producing strains. Among other sexually acquired organisms, *Ureaplasma urealyticum* is susceptible and *Chlamydia trachomatis* and *T. pallidum* are resistant.

For most organisms, the MBC is at least four times the MIC and it is regarded as essentially bacteristatic. In contrast, it is bactericidal for gonococci in concentrations close to the MIC, which is of the order of 2–16 mg/l for both penicillin-susceptible and resistant strains.

Acquired resistance

N. gonorrhoeae resistant to spectinomycin have emerged in South-East Asia, the USA and the UK; the resistance of UK isolates was not attributable to aminoglycoside-modifying enzymes. Spectinomycin was first used as the primary drug of choice against gonorrhea in the Philippines and Korea in 1981 and in Thailand in 1983; spectinomycin resistance reached 22% in the Philippines by 1988 and 9% in Thailand by 1990.

Acquired resistance in enterobacteria, enterococci and staphylococci can be caused by nucleotidyltransferases that modify the drug at position 9. The enzyme from Gram-negative organisms ANT(3″)(9) also modifies streptomycin at position 3″, thus conferring cross-resistance to the two drugs. There is no enzymatic cross-resistance with 2-deoxystreptamine-containing aminoglycosides.

Pharmacokinetics

C_{max} 25 mg/kg intramuscular	60–80 mg/l after 1 h
3 g intramuscular	40–160 mg/l after 1 h
Plasma half-life	2–3 h
Volume of distribution	10–13.4 l/kg
Plasma protein binding	<10%

Spectinomycin is poorly absorbed on oral administration. It is almost completely excreted unchanged in the urine over 24 h, concentrations on conventional dosage reaching 1 g/l. Excretion is unaffected by probenecid.

Toxicity and side effects

Transient headache, dizziness, pain at the site of injection and occasional fever have been described. No evidence of ototoxicity or renal toxicity has been found in volunteers receiving doses of 2 g 6-hourly for 3 weeks, amounts much in excess of those used therapeutically.

Clinical use

- Gonorrhea in penicillin-allergic patients or due to penicillin-resistant strains (single-dose treatment).

 Preparations and dosage

Proprietary name: Trobicin, Trobicine, Stanilo, Kempi (Sweden).

Preparation: Injection.

Dosage: Deep i.m. injection adults, 2 g as a single dose; or 4 g in two separate i.m. sites in those difficult to treat and in areas of resistance.

Children, i.m. 40 mg/kg as a single dose (maximum 2 g per day)

Widely available.

Further information

Clendennen TE, Echeverria P, Saengeur S, Kees ES, Boslego JW, Wignall FS 1992 Antibiotic susceptibility survey of *Neisseria gonorrhoeae* in Thailand. *Antimicrobial Agents and Chemotherapy* 36: 1682–1687.

Ison CA 1996 Antimicrobial agents and gonorrhoea: therapeutic choice, resistance and susceptibility testing. *Genitourinary Medicine* 72: 253–257.

Moran JS, Levine WC 1995 Drugs of choice for the treatment of uncomplicated gonococcal infections. *Clinical Infectious Diseases* 20 (Suppl 1): S47–65.

Suter TM, Viswanathan VK, Cianciotto NP 1997 Isolation of a gene encoding a novel spectinomycin phosphotransferase from *Legionella pneumophila*. *Antimicrobial Agents and Chemotherapy* 41: 1385–1388.

APRAMYCIN

Nebramycin factor 2. Molecular weight (free base): 539.6.

One of a group of antibiotics produced by a strain of *Streptomyces tenebrarius*. It is a 4-substituted deoxystreptamine with a unique octadiose in bicyclic form together with the rare 4-aminoglucose.

It has relatively low intrinsic activity and is used in veterinary medicine for the treatment of intestinal bacterial infections in animals. It is resistant to all known aminoglycoside-modifying enzymes apart from AAC(3)-IV and the rare AAC(1). AAC(3)-IV was initially found in bacteria from animals, but subsequently has appeared in human strains.

 Further information

Hunter JE, Hart CA, Shelley JC, Walton JR, Bennett M 1993 Human isolates of apramycin-resistant *Escherichia coli* which contain the genes for the AAC(3)IV enzyme. *Epidemiology and Infection* 110: 253–259.

Johnson AP, Burns L, Woodford N et al 1994 Gentamicin resistance in clinical isolates of *Escherichia coli* encoded by genes of veterinary origin. *Journal of Medical Microbiology* 40: 221–226.

Lovering AM, White LO, Reeves DS 1987 AAC(1): a new aminoglycoside-acetylating enzyme modifying the C1 aminogroup of apramycin. *Journal of Antimicrobial Chemotherapy* 20: 803–813.

van den Bogaard AE, Stobberingh EE 2000 Epidemiology of resistance to antibiotics. Links between animals and humans. *International Journal of Antimicrobial Agents* 14: 327–335.

 ASTROMICIN

Fortimicin A. Molecular weight: 405.65.

A pseudodisaccharide aminoglycoside produced by *Micromonospora olivoasterospora*. Two derivatives, 3-*O*-demethyl fortimicin A and dactimicin, originally isolated from *Dactylosporangium matsuzakienzae* and which chemically is the formimidoyl derivative of fortimicin A, have also been investigated.

Antimicrobial activity

Intrinsic activity is similar to that of amikacin for most groups of organisms, but activity against *Ps. aeruginosa* is relatively poor. 3-*O*-Demethyl fortimicin A tends to have slightly higher activity; its activity against *Ps. aeruginosa* is approximately threefold greater than that of astromicin. Dactimicin is similar to astromicin in activity.

Acquired resistance

Astromicin and its relatives are active against many strains that produce aminoglycoside-modifying enzymes. Astromicin and 3-*O*-demethyl fortimicin A are sensitive to AAC(3) and the APH(2″)/AAC(6′) bifunctional enzyme, but dactimicin is more resistant than astromicin to AAC(3)-I, probably owing to the protective action of the formimidoyl group.

Pharmacokinetics

Peak concentrations of 10–12 mg astromicin/l were found in the blood following 200 mg intravenous or intramuscular administration to volunteers; over 85% of the drug was recovered in urine during the 8 h following administration.

Toxicity and side effects

The fortimicins have toxicity and side effects similar to those observed for other aminoglycosides such as amikacin.

Clinical use

Astromicin may be used instead of amikacin in the treatment of infections caused by susceptible organisms where the drug is available.

Preparations and dosage

Proprietary names: Astromicin.

Preparation: Injection.

Dosage: Adults, i.m., i.v. 400 mg daily in 2 divided doses.

Available in Japan. Not available in the USA or UK.

Further information

Matsuhashi Y, Yoshida T, Hara T, Kazuno Y, Inouye S 1985 In vitro and in vivo antibacterial activities of dactimicin, a novel pseudodisaccharide aminoglycoside, compared with those of other aminoglycoside antibiotics. *Antimicrobial Agents and Chemotherapy* 27: 589–594.

Schwocho LR, Schaffner CP, Miller GH, Hare RS, Shaw KJ 1995 Cloning and characterization of a 3-*N*-aminoglycoside acetyltransferase gene, aac(3)-Ib, from *Pseudomonas aeruginosa*. *Antimicrobial Agents and Chemotherapy* 39: 1790–1796.

Uematsu T 1993 Population pharmacokinetic analysis of new aminoglycosides, astromicin and isepamicin, and evaluation of Bayesian prediction method for approximation of individual clearance of drug. *International Journal of Clinical Pharmacology, Therapy and Toxicology* 31: 606–610.

 KASUGAMYCIN

Molecular weight (free base): 379.36.

A fermentation product of *Streptomyces kasugaensis*. It is unusual among aminoglycosides in having a cyclitol ring that is not amino substituted. Its antibacterial activity is generally weak, but attention has been paid to its activity against mycobacteria, *Ps. aeruginosa* (MIC 16–32 mg/l) and *Leptospira*. The most striking contrast with major aminoglycosides is that up to 40% can be recovered from the urine after oral administration. After a dose of 1 g intravenously peak plasma concentrations are around 100 mg/l and after the same dose intramuscularly between 20 and 25 mg/l at 1–2 h. The plasma elimination half-life is around 3 h and peak concentrations in the urine exceed 1000 mg/l. The drug has been used in the treatment of pseudomonas urinary infection, but anorexia, which is often severe, is relatively common and this, combined with indications of nephrotoxicity, has deprived it of much therapeutic interest. It is used in crop protection and as an animal feed supplement where it is available.

Further information

Tamamura T, Sato K 1999 Comparative studies on in vitro activities of kasugamycin and clinically-used aminoglycosides antibiotics. *Japanese Journal of Antibiotics.* 52: 57–67.

15 β-Lactam antibiotics: cephalosporins

D. Greenwood

All cephalosporins are based on cephalosporin C, which was discovered by Edward Abraham and his colleagues in Oxford as a minor component of the antibiotic complex produced by *Cephalosporium acremonium*, a mould cultivated from a Sardinian sewage outfall by Giuseppe Brotzu in 1948. Interest in cephalosporin C was fuelled by its stability to staphylococcal β-lactamase (shared by all subsequent cephalosporins), which was causing concern at the time, and they probably owe their continued development to this property. Over 100 semisynthetic cephalosporins have since been marketed, although not all have survived into present-day use.

In all cephalosporins the β-lactam ring is fused to a 6-membered dihydrothiazine ring in place of the 5-membered thiazolidine ring of penicillins (*see* pp. 259–260). The basic 7-aminocephalosporanic acid skeleton can be modified at a number of positions.

- Alterations at the C-3 position tend to affect the pharmacokinetic and metabolic properties.
- Introduction of a methoxy group at C-7 yields a cephamycin with enhanced stability to β-lactamases, including the cephalosporinases of certain *Bacteroides* spp.
- Changes at the 7-amino position alter, in general, the antibacterial activity or β-lactamase stability or both.

Other compounds conveniently considered alongside the cephalosporins, since their properties are very similar, include:

- the oxacephems, in which the sulfur of the dihydrothiazine ring is replaced by oxygen
- the carbacephems, in which the sulfur is replaced by carbon.

CLASSIFICATION

As new cephalosporins have become available they have been loosely classified into 'generations', but these descriptions are too simplistic, and are to be discouraged. The following grouping is adopted here:

Group 1: parenteral compounds of moderate antimicrobial activity and susceptible to hydrolysis by a wide variety of enterobacterial β-lactamases.

Group 2: oral compounds of moderate antimicrobial activity and moderately resistant to some enterobacterial β-lactamases.

Group 3: parenteral compounds of moderate antimicrobial activity resistant to a wide range of β-lactamases. Some are available as esters for oral administration.

Group 4: parenteral compounds with potent antimicrobial activity and resistance to a wide range of β-lactamases.

Group 5: oral compounds (often achieved by esterification) resistant to a wide range of β-lactamases. Most exhibit potent activity against enterobacteria; activity against Gram-positive cocci is variable.

Group 6: parenteral compounds with activity against *Pseudomonas aeruginosa*. They vary widely in their spectrum of activity against other bacterial species.

Although the 'generation' categories often used are imprecise, 'first-generation' compounds roughly correspond to Groups 1 and 2; 'second-generation' to group 3; 'third-generation' to groups 4–6. Certain group 6 compounds are sometimes allocated to a so-called 'fourth generation'.

Some cephalosporins, including cefalonium and cefaloram (group 1) and cefquinone and ceftiofur (group 4) are used only in veterinary medicine and are not discussed further here.

ANTIMICROBIAL ACTIVITY

Cephalosporins are generally active against *Staphylococcus aureus* and coagulase-negative staphylococci, including β-lactamase-producing strains, although the degree of activity varies among different members of the group. Methicillin-resistant staphylococci are nearly always resistant. Streptococci, including pneumococci, are susceptible but *Enterococcus faecalis*, *Enterococcus faecium* and *Listeria monocytogenes*, despite their susceptibility to ampicillin and benzylpenicillin, are virtually completely resistant. *Streptococcus pneumoniae* strains with reduced susceptibility to penicillins are also less susceptible to the cephalosporins; cephalosporins of groups 4–6 are often more active than others against these strains, but susceptibility

Group 1	Group 2	Group 3	Group 4	Group 5	Group 6
Cefacetrile	Cefaclor	Cefbuperazone*	Cefmenoxime	Cefcapene	Cefepime
Cefaloridine	Cefadroxil	Cefmetazole*	Cefodizime	Cefdinir	Cefoperazone
Cefalotin	Cefalexin	Cefminox*	Cefotaxime	Cefditoren	Cefpimizole
Cefamandole	Cefatrizine	Cefotetan*	Ceftizoxime	Cefetamet	Cefpiramide
Cefapirin	Cefprozil	Cefotiam	Ceftriaxone	Cefixime	Cefpirome
Cefazolin	Cefradine	Cefoxitin*	Flomoxef†	Cefpodoxime	Cefsulodin
Cefonicid	Cefroxadine	Cefuroxime	Latamoxef†	Cefteram	Ceftazidime
Ceforanide	Loracarbef‡			Ceftibuten	

*7-Methoxycephalosporin (cephamycin).
†7-Methoxyoxacephem.
‡1-Carbacephem.

should be confirmed by titration in each case. Many Gram-negative species including neisseriae, *Haemophilus influenzae*, *Escherichia coli*, salmonellae, some klebsiellae and *Proteus mirabilis* are sensitive to varying degrees. Inoculum-related effects are common, particularly when compounds of groups 1 and 2 are tested against Gram-negative bacilli. *Ps. aeruginosa* is sensitive only to group 6 compounds. Except for cephamycins activity against many anaerobes is unreliable. Mycobacteria, mycoplasmas, chlamydiae and fungi are resistant.

Bactericidal synergy is commonly demonstrable with aminoglycosides and a number of other agents, and cephalosporins figure prominently in combinations intended to provide very broad-spectrum cover, particularly in immunocompromised patients.

Cephalosporins are usually bactericidal at concentrations above the MIC, but some, notably group 2 compounds such as cefalexin and cefradine, inhibit only penicillin-binding protein 3 at therapeutic concentrations (*see* p. 14), and are more slowly bactericidal.

ACQUIRED RESISTANCE

The most important form of resistance is that due to the elaboration of β-lactamases (p. 27). All cephalosporins are relatively stable to staphylococcal β-lactamase although some group 1 compounds, notably cefazolin and cefaloridine, are hydrolyzed more rapidly than others.

Resistance among Gram-negative genera is a good deal more complicated. The chromosomal β-lactamase of *Esch. coli*, which has virtually no hydrolytic activity against ampicillin, slowly degrades some of the earlier cephalosporins, including cefalotin, cefaloridine and cefazolin, and is responsible for the inoculum effect observed with *Esch. coli*. The *Bacteroides fragilis* group also possess chromosomal β-lactamases that are more active against cephalosporins than against penicillins, but

cephamycins and oxacephems are unusual in their stability to these enzymes. Genera, including *Citrobacter*, *Enterobacter* and *Serratia*, with an inducible, or derepressible chromosomal β-lactamase (p. 264) exhibit decreased susceptibility to a wide variety of β-lactam agents, including group 4 cephalosporins; some group 6 agents (cefepime and cefpirome) have a low affinity for these enzymes and retain activity. Cephalosporins vary in their efficiency as inducers. Cefoxitin and cefmetazole are more potent inducers than are cefazolin and cefotiam of the *Enterobacter cloacae* and *Citrobacter* enzymes and cefazolin and cefuroxime are more potent inducers of those of *Serratia* and *Morganella*. Cefmenoxime, cefotaxime, ceftizoxime, ceftriaxone and cefuroxime are poor inducers.

In addition to chromosomal β-lactamases, Gram-negative bacilli may possess plasmid-mediated enzymes (p. 264) against which different cephalosporins exhibit considerable variation in stability. Variants of the TEM-1, TEM-2 and SHV series of β-lactamases can hydrolyze all cephalosporins and may exhibit selectivity towards a particular compound. For example, the TEM-5 enzyme hydrolyzes ceftazidime more efficiently than cefotaxime, whereas TEM-9 has the reverse activity. Generally, group 5 oral agents are more resistant to plasmid-mediated β-lactamase hydrolysis than are the group 2 agents. The common TEM and PSE enzymes are predominantly responsible for the resistance of *Ps. aeruginosa* to cefoperazone and cefsulodin, but other mechanisms are involved in resistance to other antipseudomonal cephalosporins. The zinc-dependent metalloenzymes of *B. fragilis* and some other organisms (p. 264) rapidly hydrolyze cephamycins; other cephalosporins are inactivated somewhat more slowly.

The resistance of Gram-negative bacilli does not depend solely on β-lactamase formation. It varies also with the extent to which the antibiotic can penetrate the outer cell membrane and reach the site of enzyme formation. This property, known as crypticity, can be measured by comparing the enzyme activity of intact and disrupted cells. Resistance may also result from a change in the biochemical target of the antibiotic (i.e. the penicillin-binding proteins).

PHARMACOKINETICS

ABSORPTION

The oral agents in group 2 are generally well absorbed, with bioavailability often exceeding 85%. The bioavailability of some of the agents in other groups is enhanced by prodrug formulation; for example, cefuroxime axetil and cefpodoxime proxetil. These agents tend to have improved absorption following food, whereas food has little or a deleterious effect on the absorption of group 2 compounds.

DISTRIBUTION

Cephalosporins are usually well distributed, achieving high concentrations in the interstitial fluid of tissues and in serous cavities. Penetration into the eye and the cerebrospinal fluid (CSF) is poor, though some cephalosporins achieve adequate levels in the CSF in the presence of meningeal inflammation. They cross the placenta.

METABOLISM

Cephalosporins carrying an acetoxymethyl group at C-3, which include cefalotin, cefaloglycin, cefapirin, cefacetrile and cefotaxime, are susceptible to mammalian esterases that remove the acetyl group to form the corresponding hydroxymethyl compound. Such desacetyl-cephalosporins generally exhibit poorer antibacterial activity than the parent compounds, and spontaneous cyclization of the hydroxyl group with the carboxyl at C-4 may occur. The relevance (if any) of deacetylation to therapy has not been established.

EXCRETION

Cephalosporins are generally excreted in high concentrations in the urine by both glomerular filtration and tubular secretion and their elimination is depressed by probenecid and renal failure. Most cephalosporins are rapidly eliminated with plasma half-lives of 1–2 h but some are more persistent, with half-lives of 3.5 h (cefotetan), 4.5 h (cefonicid), 5 h (cefpiramide) and 8 h (ceftriaxone). The less active metabolites resulting from removal of acetoxymethyl groups at C-3 are also excreted in the urine. Some excretion is via the bile, and certain compounds, notably cefoperazone and cefpiramide, are preferentially excreted by this route. Substantial amounts of ceftriaxone are also excreted in bile and transient biliary 'sludge' of calcium ceftriaxone may occur.

Hepatic clearance tends to be lower in biliary obstruction than in cirrhosis, but the correlation with type of disease is poor, partly because compensatory changes in drug distribution and renal excretion may be extensive. Where compounds are deacetylated to inactive metabolites that are excreted predominantly by the kidney, hepatic failure has little effect on the plasma half-life, in part because deacetylating enzymes are widely distributed. The presence of ascites and edema in liver failure increases the volume of distribution, reducing the plasma concentration and increasing the elimination half-life; reduction of serum albumin and accumulation of inhibitors of protein binding such as bilirubin can increase the unbound fraction of highly bound compounds, facilitating their elimination in the glomerular filtrate. The compensatory role of the kidney is well exemplified, for example, by cefoperazone, of which the renal excretion rises from around 20% in normal subjects to around 90% in patients in hepatic failure.

TOXICITY AND SIDE EFFECTS

HYPERSENSITIVITY

Hypersensitivity occurs in 0.5–10% of patients, mostly in the form of rashes, eosinophilia, drug fever and serum sickness. In addition to immediate reactions, a maculopapular rash with or without fever, lymphadenopathy and eosinophilia may appear after several days' treatment. As with penicillins, allergy to cephalosporins is probably based on major and minor antigenic determinants, but they are less well characterized than with penicillins. Clinical reactions to cephalosporins in penicillin-allergic patients are uncommon and severe reactions are very rare. About 10% of such reactions are said to occur, generally in patients who react to a variety of drugs. Nonetheless, the generally accepted advice is that cephalosporins should not be given to patients who have previously suffered a well documented severe reaction to penicillins. The degree of cross-allergenicity with penicillin does not appear to differ among the various members of the group. Specific allergy to cephalosporins also occurs, but there is no evidence that the compounds differ markedly in allergenicity.

RENAL TOXICITY

The drug-related renal toxicity of cefaloridine is related to the special transport characteristics of the drug and is much less likely to occur with other agents. Cefazolin renal toxicity can be inhibited by probenecid and appears to depend on the same mechanism, but weight for weight cefazolin is 3 or 4 times less toxic than cefaloridine. Rare disturbances of renal function attributed to other agents in this group appear to have the direct toxic or allergic origins described for penicillins. Claims that the nephrotoxicity of cephalosporins is potentiated by aminoglycosides have been disputed.

HEMATOLOGIC TOXICITY

Rare reversible abnormalities of platelet function and coagulation resulting from several different mechanisms have been described. Thrombocytopenia and neutropenia are occasionally seen.

Abnormalities of coagulation have been associated with β-lactam agents since platelet dysfunction was first attributed to benzylpenicillin. Patients with severe renal impairment are most at risk from the combination of high plasma concentrations of β-lactam antibiotics and uremic platelet dysfunction. The effect results from interference with platelet–receptor interaction and is common to all β-lactam agents, but is particularly noted in patients receiving carbenicillin and ticarcillin in high dosage. It is much less frequently seen with cephalosporins, with the exception of latamoxef, which shares an α-carboxy substituent with the carboxypenicillins.

Although penicillins have long been associated with clotting abnormalities, it was cephalosporins that brought bleeding associated with β-lactam antibiotics into prominence when cefamandole, cefoperazone, latamoxef and other compounds with a methylthiotetrazole side-chain at the C-3 position were found to induce severe hypoprothrombinemia, especially in patients who were malnourished, had renal failure or were treated for prolonged periods. The deficiency is readily reversed by vitamin K_1.

DIARRHEA

Diarrhea occurs in about 5% of patients and pseudomembranous colitis has been described. Changes in bowel flora, accompanied by emergence of resistant organisms, including *Clostridium difficile*, are particularly likely with those potent agents which are extensively excreted in the bile and because of their non-absorption achieve substantial fecal concentrations. Cephalosporins of groups 4–6 are among the antibiotics most frequently associated with *Cl. difficile* diarrhea and pseudomembranous colitis.

OTHER ADVERSE REACTIONS

Pain at the site of intramuscular injection and phlebitis at the site of intravenous administration is fairly common. *Candida* overgrowth with vaginitis has been a feature of some studies.

As with other β-lactam antibiotics, if very high concentrations are achieved, there may be central nervous system (CNS) disturbances and, if they are given in excessive doses, particularly to patients with renal failure, there may be convulsions. Transient abnormalities of liver function tests without other evidence of hepatotoxicity and gastrointestinal disturbances have also occurred. The more recent agents do not appear to be significantly different in their renal, hepatic or CNS toxicity.

In addition to hypoprothrombinemia (*see above*) cephalosporins with a methylthiotetrazole side-chain may cause a disulfiram-like reaction, evidently due to inhibition of aldehyde dehydrogenase. Most problems have been associated with latamoxef and there is some evidence that the mechanism of ethanol metabolism inhibition by this compound is different, despite the presence of the offending side chain. Patients should be advised to avoid alcohol during and 3 days after treatment with these agents.

INTERFERENCE WITH LABORATORY TESTS

Many cephalosporins cause false-positive reactions in copper reduction tests for glucose, but not enzyme-based tests. Falsely elevated values may occur in the Porter-Silber reaction for 17-hydroxycorticosteroids and the Jaffé technique for creatinine determination.

CLINICAL USE

GROUP 1

Group 1 cephalosporins are no longer widely used. They are not reliable for the treatment of severe respiratory tract infection, severe undiagnosed sepsis or meningitis. They should be avoided in the treatment of diseases where *H. influenzae* or enterococci may be implicated. Cefazolin is used in surgical prophylaxis and, because of its higher biliary concentration, in the treatment of biliary infection.

GROUP 2

The older oral agents have had widespread use for the treatment of upper respiratory, urinary, soft tissue and various other infections. They are possible alternatives to benzylpenicillin in allergic patients for the treatment of streptococcal, pneumococcal and staphylococcal infections. With the exception of cefaclor, loracarbef and cefprozil they should not be used for the treatment of infections in which *H. influenzae* is known, or likely, to be implicated.

GROUPS 3 AND 4

The properties of the β-lactamase-stable cephalosporins strongly commend them for the treatment of severe sepsis of unknown or mixed bacterial origin. It is not established that the superior activity in vitro of group 4 over group 3 compounds is reflected in greater clinical efficacy. Despite the difference in potency, it is customary to give similar doses of compounds in both groups, partly because the very high activity seen against enterobacteria is not exhibited against staphylococci. They have been successfully used in hospital-acquired pneumonia, particularly that due to enterobacteria. They are inactive against *Legionella pneumophila*, *Mycoplasma pneumoniae* and *Coxiella burnetii*.

Where pseudomonas infection is unlikely and infection does not arise from sites in which enterococci or bacteroides are likely to be involved, cefuroxime and cefotaxime have been used successfully for the treatment of severe undiagnosed infection, either alone or in conjunction with other agents. Superinfection with enterococci may complicate treatment and relatively frequently resistance has developed during treatment of infections due to *Ps. aeruginosa* or *Enterobacter* spp.

Group 4 agents now have an established place in the treatment of meningitis due to many enterobacteria, β-lactamase-producing *H. influenzae* and penicillin-resistant pneumococci. They are not effective in the treatment of meningitis due to *Listeria monocytogenes*, *Enterobacter*, *Ps. aeruginosa* or *Serratia* spp. Despite their in-vitro potency, they do not appear to offer any advantage over established therapy in the treatment of meningitis due to *Neisseria meningitidis*. Their activity and resistance to β-lactamases has led to their successful use for the treatment of infection due to β-lactamase-producing gonococci.

GROUP 5

Those oral compounds may replace the group 2 agents if resistance to the earlier compounds becomes significant. The relatively lower activity of cefixime and ceftibuten against Gram-positive cocci suggests they should be used with caution in infections with these organisms. The incidence of side effects is generally low, but gastrointestinal problems may be higher with these more active compounds than with those in group 2.

GROUP 6

Ceftazidime has been widely used in infection due to *Ps. aeruginosa*, particularly in patients with cystic fibrosis, and as a single agent in the management of such problems as sepsis of unidentified origin in immunocompromised patients. Cefsulodin and cefoperazone are indicated only in proven or highly suspected pseudomonas infection and have often been given in combination with an appropriate aminoglycoside.

Other group 6 compounds are appropriate for use in patients with severe infections caused by bacteria with plasmid and chromosomally mediated β-lactamases. Their main use is in hospital-acquired infections or in serious problems in the neutropenic patient.

 Further information

Anonymous 1993 Antimicrobial prophylaxis in surgery. *Medical Letter* 35: 91–94.

Asbel LE, Levison ME 2000 Cephalosporins, carbapenems, and monobactams. *Infectious Disease Clinics of North America* 14: 435–437.

Baldo BA 1999 Penicillins and cephalosporins as allergens – structural aspects and cross-reactions. *Clinical and Experimental Allergy* 29: 744–749.

Cherubin CE, Eng RH, Norrby R, Modal J, Humbert G, Overturf G 1989 Penetration of newer cephalosporins into cerebrospinal fluid. *Reviews of Infectious Diseases* 11: 526–548.

Cojocel C, Gottsch U, Tolle KL, Baumann K 1988 Nephrotoxic potential of first-, second-, and third-generation cephalosporins. *Archives of Toxicology* 62: 458–464.

de Lalla F, Privitera G, Ortisi G et al 1989 Third generation cephalosporins as a risk factor for *Clostridium difficile* associated disease: a four year survey in a general hospital. *Journal of Antimicrobial Chemotherapy* 23: 623–631.

Eichenwald HF, Schmitt HJ 1986 The cephalosporin antibiotics in pediatric practice. *European Journal of Pediatrics* 144: 532–538.

Freeman J, Wilcox MH 1999 Antibiotics and *Clostridium difficile*. *Microbes and Infection/Institut Pasteur* 1: 377–384.

Harding SM 1985 Pharmacokinetics of the third-generation cephalosporins. *American Journal of Medicine* 79 (2A): 21–24.

Izhar M 1994 Cephalosporins: a guide to use in general practice. *Prescriber* 5: 55–74.

Kitson TM 1987 The effect of cephalosporin antibiotics on alcohol metabolism: a review. *Alcohol* 4: 143–148.

Klugman KP, Mahdi SA 1999 Emergence of drug resistance. Impact on bacterial meningitis. *Infectious Disease Clinics of North America* 13: 637–646.

Marshall WF, Blair JE 1999 The cephalosporins. *Mayo Clinic Proceedings* 74: 187–195.

Meyers BR 1985 Comparative toxicities of third generation cephalosporins. *American Journal of Medicine* 79: 96–103.

Moellering RC (ed.) 1995 *Oral Cephalosporins* (Antibiotics and Chemotherapy vol. 47). Karger, New York.

Murphy MF, Metcalf P, Grint PC et al 1985 Cephalosporin-induced immune neutropenia. *British Journal of Haematology* 59: 9–14.

Nathwani D 2000 Place of parenteral cephalosporins in the ambulatory setting: clinical evidence. *Drugs* 59 (Suppl. 3): 37–46.

Nichols RL, Wikler MA, McDevitt JT, Lentek AL, Hosutt JA 1987 Coagulopathy associated with extended-spectrum cephalosporins in patients with serious infections. *Antimicrobial Agents and Chemotherapy* 31: 281–285.

Norrby SR 1986 Adverse reactions and interactions with newer cephalosporin and cephamycin antibiotics. *Medical Toxicology* 1: 32–46.

Seminar-in-print 1987 The cephalosporin antibiotics. *Drugs* 34 (Suppl. 2): 1–258.

Shearer MJ, Bechtold H, Andrassy K et al 1988 Mechanism of cephalosporin-induced hypoprothrombinaemia: relation to cephalosporin side chain vitamin K metabolism and vitamin K status. *Journal of Clinical Pharmacology* 28: 88–95.

Tan JS, Salstrom SJ 1984 Diffusibility of the newer cephalosporins into human interstitial fluids. *American Journal of Medicine* 77 (4C): 33–36.

Thompson JW, Jacobs RF 1993 Adverse effects of newer cephalosporins – an update. *Drug Safety* 9: 132–142.

Thornberry C 1985 Review of the in vitro activity of third-generation cephalosporins and other newer beta-lactam antibiotics against clinically important bacteria. *American Journal of Medicine* 79 (2A): 14–20.

Williams JD 1987 The cephalosporin antibiotics. *Drugs* 34 (Suppl 2): 1–258.

Wise R 1990 The pharmacokinetics of the oral cephalosporins – a review. *Journal of Antimicrobial Chemotherapy* 26 (Suppl. E): 13–20.

Wise R 1994 Antibacterial agents: oral cephalosporins. *Prescribers Journal* 34: 110–115.

GROUP 1 CEPHALOSPORINS

 CEFALOTIN

Cephalothin. Molecular weight (sodium salt): 418.4.

An image of the chemical structure of cefalotin.

A semisynthetic cephalosporin supplied as the sodium salt.

Antimicrobial activity

Its activity against common pathogenic bacteria is shown in Table 15.1. Cefalotin is active against staphylococci, including β-lactamase-producing strains. Streptococci, including penicillin-sensitive pneumococci, but not enterococci, are highly susceptible. It is active against a range of enterobacteria, but is hydrolyzed by many enterobacterial β-lactamases. *Pasteurella* and *Vibrio* spp., *H. influenzae*, *Bordetella* and *Brucella* spp. are moderately resistant. *Campylobacter*, *Citrobacter*, *Enterobacter*, *Pseudomonas* and *Listeria* spp. are resistant. Most anaerobes, with the exception of *B. fragilis*, are susceptible: *Treponema pallidum* and *Leptospira* spp. are susceptible, but mycobacteria and mycoplasma are resistant.

PHARMACOKINETICS

C$_{max}$ 1 g intravenous	30 mg/l after 15 min
1 g intramuscular	15–20 mg/l after 0.5–1 h
Plasma half-life	c. 0.8 h
Volume of distribution	0.26 l
Plasma protein binding	60–70%

Distribution

Intramuscular adminstration is commonly painful and the normal route of administration is intravenous. Continuous infusion of 12 g/day produces steady-state plasma levels of 10–30 mg/l. An intravenous dose of 1 g has achieved concentrations of 70 mg/l in pleural fluid, but concentrations in ascitic fluid are much lower, around 3 mg/l. Penetration into the CSF is very poor, rising in the presence of inflammation to less than 2 mg/l after a 2 g intravenous dose. Concentrations in sputum are 10–25% of the corresponding serum levels. The sputum content has been said to improve markedly from a maximum of around 3 mg/l to around 13 mg/l when serum concentrations in excess of 20 mg/l are achieved. Concentrations in bone around 4 mg/kg have been described following an intravenous dose of 1 g. Concentrations of 2–6 mg/l in amniotic fluid and around 3 mg/l in cord blood have been found after a 1 g intramuscular dose. Concentrations about 25% of the simultaneous plasma levels have been found in prostatic fluid.

Metabolism

Cefalotin is metabolized by hepatic esterases to the microbiologically less active desacetyl compound. The metabolite has about 20% of the activity of the parent compound and accounts for 20–30% of the concentrations in serum and urine.

Excretion

Most of the dose is recovered in the urine, producing urinary concentrations of 500–2000 mg/l during the first 6 h after a 1 g dose. Urinary excretion is depressed by probenecid, indicating significant tubular secretion, and by renal failure although, because of metabolism, the plasma half-life of the drug is only moderately prolonged to about 3 h, while that of the principal metabolite rises to 12 h or more. Impaired tubular secretion is responsible for the elevated levels of the drug found in newborn and premature infants. Biliary excretion is trivial, producing levels of 1–17 mg/l after 1 g intravenously, and liver disease has little effect on its half-life or plasma protein binding.

Table 15.1 Activity of group 1 cephalosporins against common pathogenic bacteria: MIC (mg/l)

	Cefamandole	Ceforanide	Cefacetrile	Cefaloridine	Cefalotin	Cefapirin	Cefazolin	Cefonicid
Staph. aureus	0.5–1	1–4	0.5–1	0.1–0.25	0.25–0.5	0.25	0.25–0.5	1–4
Str. pyogenes	0.06–1	0.1–0.5	0.1–0.25	0.01–0.03	0.1	0.1	0.1–0.25	0.5–2
Str. pneumoniae	0.06–16	0.1–0.5	0.25	0.03–0.06	0.06–0.1	0.1	0.1	1–2
E. faecalis	32–R	R	16	16–32	32	32	R	R
N. gonorrhoeae	0.06	1–2	4	0.25–2	0.25–2	4	0.1–0.5	1
N. meningitidis	0.1–0.5	0.1		0.5	0.5			0.25
H. influenzae	0.25–2	4–8	2	4–8	4–8	2–4	2–8	0.5–1
Esch. coli	0.5–4	1–4	4–8	2–4	4–8	4	0.5–4	1
K. pneumoniae	0.5–2	1–8	4–8	4	4	4	1–4	4–8
Ps. aeruginosa	R	R	R	R	R	R	R	R
B. fragilis	R	R		32–64	32–64		16–32	R

R, resistant (MIC >64 mg/l)

Toxicity and side effects

Severe local pain, requiring the addition of lidocaine (lignocaine) and thrombophlebitis are common. In volunteers receiving very large doses (8 g daily for 2–4 weeks) a serum-sickness-like illness developed. Positive Coombs' reactions associated with red cell agglutination, but very seldom with hemolysis, are common. Thrombocytopenia and leukopenia, possibly mediated by analogous mechanisms, have been described. A coagulopathy with prolonged prothrombin time has been encountered in patients with renal failure or very high plasma levels resulting from excessive dosage. Evidence has been cited of exaggeration of pre-existing renal disease or renal damage, perhaps enhanced by simultaneous administration of aminoglycosides or furosemide (frusemide), in which direct tubular injury or allergic nephritis may have been involved.

Clinical use

Cefalotin has been used principally in staphylococcal and streptococcal infections in penicillin-allergic patients, but is no longer widely recommended.

Preparations and dosage

Proprietary name: Keflin.

Preparation: Injection.

Dosage: Adults, i.m., i.v., 0.5–1 g every 4–6 h; up to 12 g daily in severe infections.

Children, 50–150 mg/kg per day in divided doses.

Widely available, not UK.

Further information

Anonymous 1999 Cephalothin (sodium). In: Dollery C, (ed.) *Therapeutic Drugs* 2nd edn. Churchill Livingstone, Edinburgh, pp. C147–C149.

Klein JO, Eickhoff TC, Tilles JG, Finland M 1964 Cephalothin: activity, in vitro absorption and excretion in normal subjects and clinical observations in 40 patients. *American Journal of Medical Science* 248: 640–656.

Munch R, Steurer J, Luthy R, Seigenthaler W, Kuhlmann U 1983 Serum and dialysate concentrations of intraperitoneal cephalothin in patients undergoing continuous ambulatory peritoneal dialysis. *Clinical Nephrology* 20: 40–43.

Nilsson-Ehle I, Nilsson-Ehle P 1979 Pharmacokinetics of cephalothin: accumulation of its deacetylated metabolite in uremic patients. *Journal of Infectious Diseases* 139: 712–716.

 ## CEFAMANDOLE

Cephamandole. Molecular weight: (sodium salt) 512.5.

A semisynthetic cephalosporin supplied as the nafate, an antibacterially inactive ester hydrolyzed in the body to cefamandole.

Antimicrobial activity

The activity is shown in Table 15.1. It resembles cefalotin in its resistance to staphylococcal β-lactamase. It is more stable than other group 1 agents to enterobacterial β-lactamases, but the stability is inferior to that of cephalosporins of groups 3–6. It is generally active against both aerobic and anaerobic Grampositive rods and cocci. It is active against many enterobacteria, but there is considerable strain variation in susceptibility. *Citrobacter*, *Providencia* and *Yersinia* spp. are commonly susceptible, but *Pr. vulgaris*, *Morg. morganii* and *Providencia rettgeri* are often resistant, as are *Acinetobacter*, *Serratia* and *Pseudomonas* spp. Some anaerobic Gram-negative rods are susceptible but *B. fragilis* is resistant.

Pharmacokinetics

C_{max} 1 g intramuscular	20–35 mg/l after 1 h
1 g infusion (20–30 min)	90 mg/l end infusion
Plasma half-life	0.7–1 h
Volume of distribution	12.5–19 l
Plasma protein binding	65–80%

Distribution

Cefamandole is widely distributed in body tissues. It enters serous fluids, achieving levels in the synovial fluid of 30–50 mg/l after a 2 g intravenous dose. CSF levels are poor in the absence of meningeal inflammation. Therapeutically effective concentrations (*c.* 9 mg/kg) are found in bone after an intravenous dose of 2 g. In patients given 1 g intravenously at the time of induction of anesthesia, mean concentrations in the femoral head were 12.6 mg/l 20–70 min after the dose, giving a bone:serum ratio of 0.36.

Metabolism and excretion

The drug is not significantly metabolized. Excretion is mainly by both glomerular and tubular routes into urine, where about 75% of the unchanged drug is found within the first 6 h of administration. Concentrations of 200–400 mg/l are found in urine after an intramuscular dose of 500 mg and up to 2000 mg/l following a 1 g dose. Renal clearance is 230–260 ml/min per 1.72 m² and declines in renal failure. Only about 5% is removed by hemodialysis.

A small amount is excreted in the bile and concentrations around 150–250 mg/l are found in T-tube bile following a 1 g intravenous dose. In hepatobiliary disease, concentrations of 1.6–1400 mg/l have been found in gallbladder bile and between 9 and >2000 mg/l in common duct bile following 4–6-hourly intravenous infusions of 1 g over 15–20 min. It was absent only in complete aseptic common duct obstruction, following relief of which levels were still depressed 7 days later.

Toxicity and side effects

Most side effects common to cephalosporins have been described and cefamandole is one of the analogs containing the methylthiotetrazole side-chain associated with bleeding (p. 188). Rare renal damage or enhancement of exisiting renal damage has been described. Thrombophlebitis on intravenous administration is relatively common.

Clinical use

Cefamandole has been used as a general-purpose cephalosporin in the treatment of a variety of infections and for surgical prophylaxis, but experience with it has been mixed.

Preparations and dosage

Proprietary name: Kefadol.

Preparation: Injection.

Dosage: Adults, i.m., i.v., 500 mg to 2 g every 4–8 h, depending on severity of infection. Children over 1 month, 50–100 mg/kg per day in divided doses every 4–8 h; increase dose to 150 mg/kg per day in severe infections (do not exceed the maximum adult dose).

Widely available.

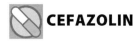

Further information

Anonymous 1999 Cefamandole (nafate). In Dollery C, (ed.) *Therapeutic Drugs* 2nd edn. Churchill Livingstone, Edinburgh, pp. C86–C88.

Colaizzi PA, Goodwin SD, Poynor WJ, Karnes HT, Polk RE 1987 Single dose pharmacokinetics of cefuroxime and cefamandole in healthy subjects. *Clinical Pharmacology* 6: 894–899.

Fraser DG 1979 Drug therapy reviews: antimicrobial spectrum, pharmacology and therapeutic use of cefamandole and cefoxitin. *American Journal of Hospital Pharmacy* 36: 1503–1508.

Lovering AM, Perez J, Bowker KE, Reeves DS, MacGowan AP, Bannister G 1997 A comparison of the penetration of cefuroxime and cefamandole into bone, fat and haematoma fluid in patients undergoing total hip replacement. *Journal of Antimicrobial Chemotherapy* 40: 99–104.

Ridley PD 1990 Comparative evaluation of cefotaxime and cephamandole in the prevention of post-operative infective complications of abdominal surgery. *British Journal of Clinical Pharmacology* 44: 17–21.

Townsend TR, Reitz BA, Bilker WB, Bartlett JG 1993 Clinical trial of cefamandole, cefazolin, and cefuroxime for antibiotic prophylaxis in cardiac operations. *Journal of Thoracic and Cardiovascular Surgery* 106: 664–670.

 CEFAZOLIN

Cephazolin. Molecular weight (sodium salt): 476.5.

A semisynthetic cephalosporin supplied as the sodium salt.

Antimicrobial activity

Its activity against common pathogenic bacteria is shown in Table 15.1. Its susceptibility to staphylococcal β-lactamase is intermediate between those of cefalotin and cefaloridine. *Enterobacter, Klebsiella, Providencia, Serratia* spp. and *Pr. vulgaris* are all resistant. *B. fragilis* is resistant, but other anaerobes are susceptible.

Pharmacokinetics

C_{max} 1 g intramuscular	65–70 mg/l at 1 h
1 g intravenous bolus	180–200 mg/l end infusion
Plasma half-life	1.5–2.0 h
Volume of distribution	c. 10 l
Plasma protein binding	75–85%

Distribution

The volume of distribution of cefazolin is the smallest of the cephalosporins in group 1 and can be an indication of relative confinement to the plasma space. It crosses inflamed synovial membranes, but the levels achieved are well below those of the simultaneous serum levels and entry to the CSF is poor. In patients receiving 10 mg/kg by intravenous bolus mean concentrations in cancellous bone were 3.0 mg/kg when the mean serum concentration was 33 mg/l, giving a bone:serum ratio of 0.09. Some crosses the placenta, but the concentrations found in the fetus and membranes are low.

Metabolism and excretion

Cefazolin is not metabolized. Around 60% of the dose is excreted in the urine within the first 6 h, producing concentrations in excess of 1 g/l. The involvement of tubular secretion is shown by the depression of excretion by probenecid. The renal clearance is around 65 ml/min and declines in renal failure, when the half-life may rise to 40 h, although levels in the urine sufficient to inhibit most urinary pathogens are still found. It is moderately well removed by hemodialysis and less well by peritoneal dialysis.

Levels sufficient to inhibit a number of enteric organisms likely to infect the biliary tract are found in T-tube bile (17–31 mg/l after a 1 g intravenous dose), but this is principally due to the high serum levels of the drug and the total amounts excreted via the bile are small.

Toxicity and side effects

Side effects are those common to other cephalosporins (pp. 187–188), including rare bleeding disorders and encephalopathy in patients in whom impaired excretion or direct instillation leads to very high CSF levels. Neutropenia has been described and hypoprothrombinemic bleeding has been attributed to the side-chain.

Clinical use

Cefazolin has been widely used in surgical prophylaxis, especially in biliary tract (because of the moderately high concentrations achieved in bile), orthopedic, cardiac and gynecological surgery.

Preparations and dosage

Proprietary name: Kefzol.

Preparation: Injection.

Dosage: Adults, i.m., i.v., i.v. infusion 0.5–1 g every 6–12 h, up to 12 g per day in severe infections Children, 25 mg/kg daily in divided doses, increasing to 100 mg/kg daily in severe infection.

Widely available.

Further information

Anonymous 1999 Cefazolin (sodium). In: Dollery C (ed.). *Therapeutic Drugs* 2nd edn. Churchill Livingstone, Edinburgh, pp. C89–C93.

Decroix MO, Zini R, Chaumeil JC, Tillementi P 1988 Cefazolin serum protein binding and its inhibition by bilirubin, fatty acids and other drugs. *Biochemical Pharmacology* 37: 2807–2814.

Jewesson PJ, Stiver G, Wai A et al 1996 Double-blind comparison of cefazolin and ceftizoxime for prophylaxis against infections following elective biliary tract surgery. *Antimicrobial Agents and Chemotherapy* 40: 70–74.

Ortiz A, Martin-Llonch N, Garron MP et al 1991 Cefazolin-induced encephalopathy in uremic patients. *Reviews of Infectious Diseases* 13: 772–774.

Periti P, Mazzei T, Orlandini F et al 1988 Comparison of the antimicrobial prophylactic efficacy of cefotaxime and cephazolin in obstetric and gynaecological surgery: a randomised multicentre study. *Drugs* 35: 133–138.

Thompson JR, Garber R, Ayers J, Oki J 1987 Cefazolin-associated neutropenia. *Clinical Pharmacy* 6: 811–814.

Townsend TR, Reitz BA, Bilker WB, Bartlett JG 1993 Clinical trial of cefamandole, cefazolin, and cefuroxime for antibiotic prophylaxis in cardiac operations. *Journal of Thoracic and Cardiovascular Surgery* 106: 664–670.

OTHER GROUP 1 CEPHALOSPORINS

Cefacetrile (cephacetrile)

Antimicrobial activity

Its spectrum resembles that of cefalotin (Table 15.1). Following an intramuscular dose of 1 g, a peak plasma concentration around 15 mg/l is achieved at 1 h. A few minutes after intravenous injection of 1 g the plasma level is around 100 mg/l. About 25% is bound to plasma protein and the apparent volume of distribution is 19–23 mg/l. Penetration into the CSF is limited. About 80% of the drug is excreted in the urine, producing concentrations in excess of 1 g/l, 25% of which is in the desacetylated form. Clearance is depressed by probenecid and in renal failure. Little is excreted in the bile.

Eosinophilia in the absence of other manifestations of hypersensitivity and in patients not known to be allergic to β-lactam antibiotics is common and fever occurs.

Preparations and dosage

Proprietary name: Celospor.

Preparation: Injection.

Dosage: Adults, i.m., i.v., 2–6 g daily in four divided doses, up to 12 g daily in severe infections.

Limited availability.

Further information

Gladtke E, Marget W, Muller AA (eds) 1977 Cephacetrile – a review of progress to date. CIBA, Basel.

Cefaloridine (cephaloridine)

Its activity and spectrum are similar to those of cefalotin (Table 15.1). It is much less resistant to staphylococcal β-lactamase than was at first believed and its activity against β-lactamase-producing *Staph. aureus* declines rapidly as the inoculum size is increased.

Intramuscular doses of 0.5 and 1 g produce peak plasma levels at 1 h of 18–20 and 20–40 mg/l, respectively. A 1 g dose given by rapid intravenous injection produces levels a few minutes after administration of 80–100 mg/l. The plasma half-life is 1.5 h. It is not significantly metabolized. It is about 20% bound to plasma protein. In the presence of inflammation, CSF concentrations are around 25% of simultaneous plasma levels.

Cefaloridine is excreted unchanged in the urine, mainly in the glomerular filtrate. Less than 0.1% of the total drug administered is excreted in bile. Moderate doses produce many hyaline casts in the urine and larger doses (6 g/day or more) have sometimes caused proximal tubular necrosis with increasing proteinuria and raised blood urea, occasionally leading to oliguria and renal failure. The renal toxicity is enhanced by furosemide (frusemide) and ethacrynic acid. Nephrotoxicity has led to its withdrawal in a number of countries.

Preparations and dosage

Preparation: Injection.

Dosage: Adults, i.m., i.v., 0.5–1 g 2–4 times daily. Children, 30–100 mg/kg per day in three divided doses.

Limited use and availability.

Further information

Mandell GL 1973 Cephaloridine. *Annals of Internal Medicine* 79: 561–565.
Tune BM 1975 Relationship between the transport and toxicity of cephalosporins in the kidney. *Journal of Infectious Diseases* 132: 189–194.

Cefapirin (cephapirin)

Its antibacterial spectrum is almost identical to that of cefalotin (Table 15.1), but it is more labile to staphylococcal β-lactamase. Intramuscular injections can be painful, but the inflammation resulting from intravenous infusion is said to be less than that produced by cefalotin. A peak plasma concentration of 15–25 mg/l is obtained 0.5 h after intramuscular injection of 1 g. A few minutes after intravenous administration of the same dose, the plasma concentration is 100–130 mg/l. The plasma half-life is 0.4–0.8 h. It is 45–55% bound to plasma protein and metabolized to the desacetyl form; only 5–10% of the metabolite appears in the plasma, but it accounts for almost half the drug in the urine. Less than 1% of the dose appears in the bile.

A serum-sickness-like illness analogous to that seen with cefalotin has been observed.

 Preparations and dosage

Proprietary name: Cefadyl.

Preparation: Injection.

Dosage: Adults, i.m., i.v., 0.5–1 g every 4–6 h; up to 12 g daily in severe infections.

Children > 3 months, 10–20 mg/kg every 6 h.

Limited availability, including USA; not UK.

 Further information

Axelrod J, Meyers BR, Hirschman SZ 1972 Cephapirin: pharmacology in normal human volunteers. *Journal of Clinical Pharmacology* 12: 84–88.
Creatsas G, Pavlatos M, Lolis D, Kaskarelis D 1980 A study of the kinetics of cephapirin and cephalexin in pregnancy. *Current Medical Research and Opinion* 7: 43–46.

Cefonicid

It is widely active against Gram-positive and Gram-negative organisms (Table 15.1) but its activity in vitro is depressed by the presence of 50% serum. It is highly bound to plasma protein (98%) and has an unusually extended plasma half life of 4.5–5 h. A 1 g intramuscular dose achieves a mean peak plasma concentration of around 83 mg/l. Following a 1 g intravenous bolus dose mean peak plasma concentrations of 130–300 mg/l have been reported. In patients treated for community-acquired pneumonia, concentrations of 2–4 mg/l have been found in sputum.

Cefonicid is predominantly excreted by renal secretion, 83–89% being recovered unchanged in the urine over 24 h. Plasma half-life is linearly related to creatinine clearance. As a result of its high protein binding it is not removed by hemodialysis.

It is generally well tolerated; pain on injection, rash and positive Coombs' test are reported in some patients. It has been used to treat respiratory, soft tissue and urinary infections.

 Preparations and dosage

Preparation: Injection.

Dosage: Adults, i.m., i.v., 500 mg to 2 g once daily, depending on severity of infection.

Available in Italy.

 Further information

Furlan G, Besa G, Broccali G, Gusmitta A 1989 Pharmacokinetics of cefonicid in serum and its penetration into lung tissue, bronchial mucosa and plasma. *International Journal of Clinical Pharmacology Research* 9: 49–53.
Furlanut M, D'Elia R, Riva E, Pasinelli F 1989 Pharmacokinetics of cefonicid in children. *European Journal of Clinical Pharmacology* 36: 79–82.
Saltier E, Brogden RN 1986 Cefonicid. A review of its antibacterial activity pharmacological properties and therapeutic use. *Drugs* 32: 222–259.
Trang JM, Monson TP, Ackermann BH, Underwood FL, Manning JT, Kearns GL 1989 Effect of age and renal function on cefonicid pharmacokinetics. *Antimicrobial Agents and Chemotherapy* 33: 142–146.

Ceforanide

A semisynthetic parenteral cephalosporin with activity broadly similar to that of cephalothin (Table 15.1). Its activity in vitro is significantly reduced in the presence of serum.

Pharmacokinetics

C_{max} 1 g intravenous	c. 135 mg/l end infusion
Plasma half-life	c. 2.5 h
Plasma protein binding	81–88%

The response is essentially linear, with mean end-infusion concentrations of around 40, 70 and 135 mg/l respectively after 0.25, 0.5 and 1 g intravenous doses. Similar intramuscular doses produced mean peak values of around 20, 40 and 70 mg/l. Administration of 2 g probenecid orally has no effect on the plasma, urinary or salivary levels.

Ceforanide is almost entirely eliminated in the urine, 80–95% being recovered in the first 12 h. The half-life is inversely related to renal function, rising to around 20 h when the creatinine clearance falls below 5 ml/min. About half the dose is removed by hemodialysis over 6 h, reducing the plasma half-life in renal failure to about 5 h.

It is generally well tolerated; phlebitis and pain at the site of injection are reported in some patients with occasional transient neutropenia and increased transaminase levels. Pseudomembranous colitis has been described.

Clinical use

It has been principally used for the treatment of infections due to Gram-positive cocci, including staphylococcal and streptococcal soft-tissue infections.

Preparations and dosage

Proprietary name: Precef.

Preparation: Injection

Dosage: Adults, i.m., i.v., i.v. infusion, 0.5–1 g every 12 h. Children, 10–20 mg/kg every 12 h.

Available in the USA. Not available in UK.

Further information

Campoli-Richards DM, Lackner TE, Monk JP 1987 Ceforanide. A review of its antibacterial activity, pharmacokinetic properties and clinical efficacy. *Drugs* 34: 411–437.

Lefrock JL, Holloway W, Carr BB, Schell RF 1984 In vitro and clinical evaluation of ceforanide. *American Journal of Medical Science* 287: 21–25.

Souney PF, Fisher S, Tuomala RE, Polk BF, Simpson C 1988 Plasma and tissue concentrations of ceforanide and cefazolin in women undergoing hysterectomy. *Chemotherapy* 34: 185–190.

GROUP 2 CEPHALOSPORINS

CEFACLOR

Molecular weight (monohydrate): 385.8.

A semisynthetic oral cephalosporin available as the monohydrate. Aqueous solutions are stable at room temperature and 4°C for 72 h at pH 2.5 but rapidly lose activity at pH 7. A delayed-release formulation is available.

Antimicrobial activity

Its activity against common pathogenic bacteria is shown in Table 15.2. It is less resistant than other group 2 cephalosporins to staphylococcal β-lactamase. It is active against *N. gonorrhoeae* and *H. influenzae* and against most enterobacteria, but it is susceptible to common enterobacterial β-lactamases. *Pr. vulgaris* and *Providencia*, *Acinetobacter* and *Serratia* spp. are resistant. *B. fragilis* and clostridia are resistant but other anaerobes are commonly susceptible.

Pharmacokinetics

Oral absorption	*c.* 90%
C_{max} 250 mg oral	*c.* 6–7 mg/l after 50 min
Plasma half-life	0.5–1 h
Volume of distribution	0.37 l
Plasma protein binding	25%

Absorption

Food intake increases the time taken to reach peak plasma levels and reduces the peak by 25–50%. The actual amount absorbed is unaffected. In children receiving 15 mg/kg per day (maximum daily dose 1 g) the mean peak serum level was 16.8 mg/l at 0.5–1 h. There is no accumulation of the drug during repeated administration.

Distribution

In patients receiving 500 mg 8-hourly for 10 days, concentrations were 0–1.7 (mean 0.5) mg/l in mucoid sputum and 0–2.8 (mean 1.0) mg/l in purulent sputum. In children with chronic serous otitis media receiving 15 mg/kg daily, the mean peak

Table 15.2 Activity of group 2 cephalosporins against common pathogenic bacteria: MIC (mg/l)

	Cefaclor	Cefadroxil	Cefatrizine	Cefroxadine	Cefalexin	Cefradine	Cefprozil	Loracarbef
Staph. aureus	2–4	2–4	0.5–1	2	2–4	2–4	0.25–4	1–8
Str. pyogenes	0.25	0.1–0.5	0.03–0.1	0.5	0.5–2	0.5–2	0.06–0.25	0.12–1
Str. pneumoniae	0.5–1	1	0.25–0.5	2	2	2–4	0.06–0.25	0.5–2
E. faecalis	R	R	R	R	R	R	16	R
N. gonorrhoeae	0.1–0.5	4	0.25–0.5	0.5	0.5–4	0.5–4	0.12–0.25	0.004–1
H. influenzae	1–2	16–32	2–8	8	8–32	8–32	0.006–8	0.5–2
Esch. coli	2–8	8–16	2–8	16	8	16	1–4	1–2
K. pneumoniae	4–8	8–16	8	16	8	16	1–64	1–8
Ps. aeruginosa	R	R	R	R	R	R	R	R
B. fragilis	R	R	R	32	R	R	R	R

R, resistant (MIC >64 mg/l)

concentration in middle ear secretion was 3.8 mg/l within 30 min of the dose when the mean simultaneous serum concentration was 12.8 mg/l.

Excretion

About half of the dose is recovered from the urine in the first 6 h and 70% in 24 h. Probenecid prolongs the plasma levels but in renal insufficiency the plasma half-life is only moderately increased, suggesting non-renal mechanisms of elimination, although no metabolites have been identified. The drug probably chemically degrades in serum. In patients with creatinine clearance values of 5–15 ml/min the mean plasma elimination half-life rose to 2.3 h and the 24 h urinary excretion fell to less than 10%. In patients requiring intermittent hemodialysis and receiving 500 mg 8-hourly for 10 days, the half-life rose to 2.9 h between and 1.5 h on dialysis. Dialysis was calculated to remove 34% of the dose. The corrected creatinine clearance proved to be the best indicator of plasma half-life.

Toxicity and side effects

Apart from mild gastrointestinal disturbance, the drug is well tolerated. Transiently increased transaminase levels and symptomatic vaginal candidosis have all been noted. Clusters of a serum sickness-like illness have been described in children.

Clinical use

Uses are similar to those of other group 2 cephalosporins. It is among the few suitable for use in respiratory infections because of its activity against *H. influenzae*.

 Preparations and dosage

Proprietary name: Distaclor.

Preparations: Tablets, suspension, capsules.

Dosage: Adults, oral, 250–500 mg every 8 h, depending on severity of infection (maximum dose 4 g per day). Children > 1 month, 20 mg/kg per day in divided doses every 8 h. In more severe infections, 40 mg/kg per day in divided doses, up to a daily maximum of 1 g.

Widely available.

 Further information

Anonymous 1999 Cefaclor. In: Dollery C, (ed.). *Therapeutic Drugs* 2nd edn. Churchill Livingstone, Edinburgh, pp. C83–C86.

Blumer JL, McLinn SE, DeAbate CA et al 1995 Multinational multicenter controlled trial comparing ceftibuten with cefaclor for the treatment of acute otitis media. *Pediatric Infectious Disease Journal* 14: S115–S120.

Brady MT, Barson WJ, Cannon HJ Jr, Grossman LK 1987 Onset of *Haemophilus influenzae* type-b meningitis during cefaclor therapy for preseptal cellulitis. *Clinical Pediatrics (Philadelphia)* 26: 132–134.

Brumfitt W, Hamilton-Miller JMT 1999 Cefaclor into the millennium. *Journal of Chemotherapy* 11: 163–178.

Hyslop DL 1988 Cefaclor safety profile: a ten-year review. *Clinical Therapeutics* 11 (Suppl. A): 83–94.

Meyers BR 2000 Cefaclor revisited. *Clinical Therapeutics* 22: 154–166.

Verhoef J 1988 Cefaclor in the treatment of skin, soft tissue and urinary tract infections: a review. *Clinical Therapeutics* 11 (Suppl. A): 71–82.

Vial T, Pont J, Pham E, Rabilloud M, Descotes J 1992 Cefaclor-associated serum sickness-like disease: eight cases and review of the literature. *Annals of Pharmacotherapy* 26: 910–914.

 CEFADROXIL

Molecular weight (monohydrate): 381.4.

p-Hydroxycephalexin, available as the mono- and trihydrate.

Antimicrobial activity

Resembles closely that of cefalexin (Table 15.2).

Pharmacokinetics

Oral absorption	>90%
C_{max} 250 mg oral	*c.* 9 mg/l after 1.2 h
500 mg oral	*c.* 18 mg/l after 1.2 h
Plasma half-life	1–1.5 h
Plasma protein binding	20%

Absorption and distribution

Absorption is little affected by administration with food. Distribution is similar to that of cefalexin.

Metabolism and elimination

Cefadroxil is eliminated unchanged by both glomerular filtration and tubular secretion, and 90% of the dose appears in the urine over 24 h, most in the first 6 h, producing concentrations exceeding 500 mg/l. Loss of linearity in the relation between peak plasma concentration and dose above 500 mg may be due to saturation of renal tubular clearance.

Toxicity and side effects

It is generally well tolerated. Such side effects as have been described are those common to oral cephalosporins.

Clinical use

Cefadroxil has been successfully used for the treatment of upper respiratory tract infection and community-acquired pneumonia.

Preparations and dosage

Proprietary name: Baxan.

Preparations: Capsules, suspension, tablets.

Dosage: Adults, oral, 40 kg and over, 0.5–1 g twice a day. Children under 1 year, 25 mg/kg daily in divided doses; children 1–6 years, 250 mg twice daily; children over 6 years, 500 mg twice daily.

Widely available.

Further information

Akimoto Y, Komiya M, Kaneko K, Fujii A, Peterson LJ 1994 Cefadroxil concentrations in human serum, gingiva, and mandibular bone following a single oral administration. *Journal of Oral and Maxillofacial Surgery* 52: 397–401.

Hampel B, Lode H, Wagner J, Koeppe P 1982 Pharmacokinetics of cefadroxil and cefaclor during an 8-day dosage period. *Antimicrobial Agents and Chemotherapy* 22: 1061–1063.

Hebert AA, Still JG, Reuman PD 1993 Comparative safety and efficacy of clarithromycin and cefadroxil suspensions in the treatment of mild to moderate skin and skin structure infections in children. *Pediatric Infectious Disease Journal* 12 (Suppl.): S112–S117.

Miller LM, Mooney CJ, Hansbrough JF 1989 Comparative evaluation of cefaclor versus cefadroxil in the treatment of skin and skin structure infections. *Current Therapeutic Research* 46: 405–410.

Stromberg A, Friberg U, Cars O 1987 Concentrations of phenoxymethylpenicillin and cefadroxil in tonsillar tissue and tonsillar surface fluid. *European Journal of Clinical Microbiology* 6: 525–529.

Tanrisever B, Santella PJ 1986 Cefadroxil. A review of its antibacterial, pharmacokinetic and therapeutic properties in comparison with cephalexin and cephradine. *Drugs* 32 (Suppl. 3): 1–16.

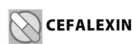

CEFALEXIN

Cephalexin. Molecular weight (monohydrate): 365.4.

Antimicrobial activity

Its antibacterial spectrum is similar to that of group 1 cephalosporins, but it is somewhat less active against most species, particularly Gram-positive cocci (Table 15.2). Cefalexin is relatively resistant to staphylococcal β-lactamase. Gram-positive rods and fastidious Gram-negative bacilli, such as *Bordetella* spp. and *H. influenzae* are relatively resistant. It is active against a range of enterobacteria, but it is degraded by many enterobacterial β-lactamases. *Citrobacter, Edwardsiella, Enterobacter, Hafnia, Providencia* and *Serratia* spp. are all resistant. Gram-negative anaerobes other than *B. fragilis* are susceptible. Because of its mode of action (p. 14) it is only slowly bactericidal to Gram-negative bacilli.

Pharmacokinetics

Oral absorption	> 90%
C~max~ 500 mg oral	*c.* 10–20 mg/l after 1 h
Plasma half-life	0.5–1 h
Volume of distribution	15 l
Plasma protein binding	10–15%

Absorption

It is stable to gastric acid and almost completely absorbed when given by mouth, the peak concentration being depressed or delayed by food. Intramuscular preparations are not available: injection is painful and produces delayed peak plasma concentrations considerably lower than those obtained by oral administration.

Distribution

In synovial fluid, levels of 6–38 mg/l have been described after a 4 g oral dose, but penetration into the CSF is poor: 1.3 mg/l 3–4 h after an oral dose of 0.75 g. Useful levels are achieved in bone (9–44 mg/kg after 1 g orally) and in purulent sputum. Concentrations of 10–20 mg/l have been found in breast milk. Concentrations in cord blood following a maternal oral dose of 0.25 g were minimal.

Metabolism and excretion

There is no biodegradation or transformation. Almost all the dose is recoverable from the urine within the first 6 h, producing urinary concentrations exceeding 1 g/l. The involvement of tubular secretion is indicated by the increased plasma peak concentration and reduced urinary excretion produced by probenecid. Renal clearance is around 200 ml/min and is depressed in renal failure, although a therapeutic concentration is still obtained in the urine. Cefalexin is removed by both peritoneal dialysis and hemodialysis. Some is excreted in the bile, in which therapeutic concentrations may be achieved.

Toxicity and side effects

Nausea, vomiting and abdominal discomfort are relatively common. Pseudomembranous colitis has been described and overgrowth of *Candida* with vaginitis may be troublesome. Otherwise, mild hypersensitivity reactions and biochemical changes common to cephalosporins occur. Very rare neurological disturbances have been described, particularly in patients in whom very high plasma levels have been achieved.

There are also rare reports of Stevens–Johnson syndrome and toxic epidermal necrolysis.

Clinical use

As for group 2 cephalosporins (p. 188). Cefalexin should not be used in infections in which *H. influenzae* is, or is likely to be, implicated. It should not be used as an alternative to penicillin in syphilis.

Preparations and dosage

Proprietary names: Keflex, Ceporex.

Preparations: Capsules, tablets, suspension.

Dosage: Adults, oral, 1–2 g/day in divided doses; for severe infections, increase dose to 1 g three times daily or 3 g twice daily. Children, 25–50 mg/kg per day; for severe infection increase dose to 100 mg/kg per day, with a maximum of 4 g/day.

Widely available.

Further information

Anonymous 1999 Cephalexin. In: Dollery C (ed.) *Therapeutic Drugs* 2nd edn. Churchill Livingstone, Edinburgh, pp. C144–C146.
Dave J, Heathcock R, Fenelon L, Bihari DJ, Simmons NA 1991 Cephalexin induced toxic epidermal necrolysis. *Journal of Antimicrobial Chemotherapy* 28: 477–488.
Martine FC, Kindrachuk RW, Thomas E, Stamey TA 1985 Effect of prophylactic, low dose cephalexin on fecal and vaginal flora. *Journal of Urology* 133: 994–996.
Speight TM, Brogden RN, Avery GS 1972 Cephalexin: a review of its antibacterial, pharmacological and therapeutic properties. *Drugs* 3: 9–76.

CEFPROZIL

Molecular weight (monohydrate): 407.5.

A semisynthetic oral cephalosporin formulated as the monohydrate. It exists as *cis-* and *trans-* isomers, 90% being in the *cis-* form.

Antimicrobial activity

Its activity against Gram-positive cocci and Gram-negative bacilli is better than that of cefadroxil (which it structurally resembles) but is not as good as that of group 5 agents (Table 15.2; *see also* Table 15.5). Cefprozil is moderately stable to hydrolysis by the common plasmid-mediated β-lactamases, but is hydrolyzed by the chromosomal enzymes of Gram-negative bacilli (pp. 263–264).

Pharmacokinetics

Oral absorption	>90%
C_{max} 250 mg oral	5–7 mg/l after 1 h
500 mg oral	10 mg/l after 1 h
Plasma half-life	1–1.4 h
Volume of distribution	15–20 l
Plasma protein binding	35–45%

Absorption and distribution

Cefprozil is almost completely absorbed and well distributed, penetrating well into tonsillar and other tissues and inflammatory exudate. Absorption is unaffected by food or antacids and there is no accumulation on multiple dosing regimens.

Metabolism and excretion

Most of the dose is excreted unchanged, mostly in urine, though about 20% is found in feces. Urinary concentrations after a 500 mg oral dose usually exceed 1000 mg/l. The elimination half-life is prolonged in patients with renal impairment, reaching 6 h in anuric patients. About half the drug is removed in 3 h by hemodialysis.

Toxicity and side effects

Cefprozil is well tolerated. Diarrhea and gastrointestinal discomfort are prominent among reported side effects. There have been a few reports of pseudomembranous colitis and serum sickness-like reactions.

Clinical use

Cefprozil has primarily been used to treat upper and lower respiratory tract infections, urinary tract infections and infections of skin and soft tissue.

Preparations and dosage

Proprietary name: Cefzil.

Preparation: Tablets, suspension.

Dosage: Adults, oral, 250–500 mg once or twice daily depending on infection being treated. Children, 7.5–15 mg/kg twice daily.

Available in the UK, USA, and continental Europe.

Further information

Anonymous 1999 Cefprozil (monohydrate). In: Dollery C (ed.) *Therapeutic Drugs* 2nd edn. Churchill Livingstone, Edinburgh, pp. C118–C120.
Barriere SL 1993 Review of in vitro activity, pharmacokinetic characteristics, safety, and clinical efficacy of cefprozil, a new oral cephalosporin. *Annals of Pharmacotherapy* 27: 1082–1089.
Lowery N, Kearns GL, Young RA, Wheeler JG 1994 Serum-sickness-like reactions associated with cefprozil therapy. *Journal of Pediatrics* 125: 325–328.

Nolen T 1994 Comparative studies of cefprozil in the management of skin and soft tissue infections. *European Journal of Clinical Microbiology and Infectious Diseases* 13: 866–871.

Saez-Llorens X, Shyu WC, Shelton S, Kumiesz H, Nelson J 1990 Pharmacokinetics of cefprozil in infants and children. *Antimicrobial Agents and Chemotherapy* 34: 2152–2155.

Shyu WC, Haddad J, Reilly J et al 1994 Penetration of cefprozil into middle ear fluid of patients with otitis media. *Antimicrobial Agents and Chemotherapy* 38: 2210–2212.

Wise R 1994 Comparative microbiological activity and pharmacokinetics of cefprozil. *European Journal of Clinical Microbiology and Infectious Diseases* 13: 839–845.

Wiseman LR, Benfield P 1993 Cefprozil. A review of its antibacterial activity, pharmacokinetic properties, and therapeutic potential. *Drugs* 45: 295–317.

 # CEFRADINE

Cephradine. Molecular weight 349.4.

A semisynthetic cephalosporin available in both oral and injectable forms.

Antimicrobial activity

Its antibacterial spectrum is almost identical to that of cefalexin (Table 15.2). It is active against aerobic and anaerobic Gram-positive cocci (with the exception of enterococci) and bacilli. *H. influenzae* is resistant. It is active against a variety of enterobacteria but susceptible to many enterobacterial β-lactamases.

Pharmacokinetics

Oral absorption	>90%
C_{max} 500 mg oral	*c.* 18–20 mg/l after 1 h
1 g intramuscular	10–12 mg/l after 1–2 h
1 g intravenous	50–90 mg/l
Plasma half-life	0.8–1 h
Volume of distribution	0.3 l
Plasma protein binding	*c.* 10%

Absorption

Cefradine is almost completely absorbed when given by mouth. The peak is delayed and reduced by food, but the half-life is not altered. Absorption is depressed by some intestinal disorders.

Distribution

Concentrations of up to 40% of those simultaneously found in the serum have been demonstrated in lung tissue. Penetration into the CSF is poor, concentrations of 1.4–4.5 mg/l being found after doses of 150–300 mg/kg in children. Levels in sputum were about 20% of those simultaneously present in the plasma following a 1 g oral dose and similar levels have been found in bone – around 10 mg/kg 20 min after 1 g intravenously. Breast milk concentrations approaching 1 mg/l have been found after 500 mg orally 6-hourly and similar concentrations have been found in amniotic fluid. Cord blood concentration is said to be similar to that in the maternal blood.

Metabolism and excretion

Cefradine is excreted unchanged in the urine, 90–100% being recovered in the first 6 h, achieving concentrations exceeding 1 g/l. The excretion is more rapid after oral than intramuscular administration. Probenecid produces a marked delay in the peak and a 40–70% increase in the plasma concentration. There is some biliary excretion, concentrations of 2–40 mg/l being found up to 8 h after an oral dose of 500 mg.

Toxicity and side effects

The parenteral forms may give rise to local pain or thrombophlebitis. Side effects common to cephalosporins have been described. In some patients *Candida* vaginitis has been troublesome. Increase of blood urea has been reported in some patients but there is no unequivocal evidence of renal toxicity. Joint pain is reported in some patients. Very rarely, diffuse interstitial infiltrates occur.

Clinical use

As for group 2 cephalosporins (p. 188). The intramuscular formulation is used for the prophylaxis and treatment of bone infection.

Preparations and dosage

Proprietary name: Velosef.

Preparations: Capsules, syrup, injection.

Dosage: Adults, oral, 250–500 mg every 6 h, or 0.5–1 g every 12 h (maximum dose 4 g per day). Children, 25–100 mg/kg per day in two or four equally divided doses.

Adults, i.m., i.v., 2–8 g/day in divided doses depending on severity of infection. Children, 50–100 mg/kg per day in four divided doses; more serious illnesses may require 200–300 mg/kg per day.

Widely available.

Further information

Adam D, Hofstetter AG, Jacoby W, Reichart B 1976 Studies on the diffusion of cephradine and cephalothin into human tissue. *Infection* 4 (Suppl. 2): S105–S107.

Anonymous 1999 Cephradine. In: Dollery C (ed.): *Therapeutic Drugs* 2nd edn. Churchill Livingstone, Edinburgh, pp. C150–C152.

Klastersky J, Daneau D, Weerts D 1973 Cephradine. Antibacterial activity and clinical effectiveness. *Chemotherapy* 18: 191–204.

Leigh DA 1989 Determination of serum and bone concentrations of cephradine and cefuroxime by HPLC in patients undergoing hip and knee replacement surgery. *Journal of Antimicrobial Chemotherapy* 23: 877–883.

Wicks MH, Rich GE, Ratcliffe RM, Hone MR 1981 The importance of cephradine in hip surgery. *Journal of Bone and Joint Surgery (B)* 63: 413–416.

LORACARBEF

Molecular weight (monohydrate): 367.8.

An oral carbacephem, with carbon replacing sulfur in the fused ring structure. Its structure and properties are otherwise closely related to those of cefaclor, but it has improved chemical stability.

Antimicrobial activity

Its activity corresponds closely to that of cefaclor, with moderate activity against staphylococci (but not methicillin-resistant strains), streptococci and some enterobacteria. Enterococci, *Ps. aeruginosa* and *B. fragilis* are resistant (Table 15.2). Like cefaclor, it is hydrolyzed by many enterobacterial β-lactamases, including the common TEM and OXA enzymes (p. 264).

Pharmacokinetics

Oral absorption	>90%
C_{max} 500 mg oral	16 mg/l after 1.3 h
Plasma half-life	*c.* 1 h
Volume of distribution	0.3 l
Plasma protein binding	25%

Absorption and distribution

Food delays absorption. In a study of children with upper respiratory tract infection, concentrations of 12.6 mg/l and 18.7 mg/l were achieved 45 min after doses of 7.5 and 15 mg/kg, respectively, given as an oral suspension. Similar doses administered to children with acute otitis media achieved concentrations of 2 and 4 mg/l (48% and 42% of the corresponding plasma level) in middle ear fluid after 2 h. Sputum concentrations have been found to be around 2% of the corresponding plasma level.

Metabolism and excretion

Loracarbef is very stable and most of the dose is excreted unchanged into urine, 60% within 12 h. The elimination half-life is increased in patients with impaired renal function. Probenecid delays excretion.

Toxicity and side effects

The drug is well tolerated. Diarrhea is the most prominent side effect, occurring in about 4% of patients. Other gastrointestinal upsets are also reported.

Clinical use

Loracarbef is used for the oral treatment of upper respiratory tract infection, particularly acute otitis media in children, in skin and soft-tissue infections, and in uncomplicated urinary tract infection caused by sensitive organisms.

 Preparations and dosage

Proprietary name: Lorabid.

Preparation: Capsules, suspension.

Dosage: Adults, oral, 200–400 mg twice daily. Children, 7.5–15 mg/kg twice daily.

Limited availability, not UK.

 Further information

Anonymous 1999 Loracarbef. In: (Dollery C (ed.) *Therapeutic Drugs* 2nd edn. Churchill Livingstone, Edinburgh, pp. L89–L95.

Brogden RN, McTavish D 1993 Loracarbef: a review of its antimicrobial activity, pharmacokinetic properties and therapeutic efficacy. *Drugs* 45: 716–736.

Force RW, Nahata MC, Perez A, Demers D 1993 Loracarbef: a new orally administered carbacephem antibiotic. *Annals of Pharmacotherapy* 27: 321–329.

Gan VN, Kusmiesz H, Shelton S, Nelson JD 1991 Comparative evaluation of loracarbef and amoxicillin-clavulanate for acute otitis media. *Antimicrobial Agents and Chemotherapy* 35: 967–971.

Hill SL, Bilton D, Johnson MM et al. 1994 Sputum and serum pharmacokinetics of loracarbef (LY 163892) in patients with chronic bronchial sepsis. *Journal of Antimicrobial Chemotherapy* 33: 129–136.

Jones RN, Barry AL 1988 Antimicrobial activity of LY163892, an orally administered 1-carbacephem. *Antimicrobial Agents and Chemotherapy* 22: 315–320.

Kusmiesz H, Shelton S, Brown O, Manning S, Nelson JD 1990 Loracarbef concentrations in middle ear fluid. *Antimicrobial Agents and Chemotherapy* 34: 2030–2031.

Nahata MC, Koranyi KI 1992 Pharmacokinetics of loracarbef in pediatric patients. *European Journal of Drug Metabolism and Pharmacokinetics* 17: 201–204.

Sitar DS, Hoban DJ, Aoki FY 1994 Pharmacokinetic disposition of loracarbef in healthy young men and women at steady state. *Journal of Clinical Pharmacology* 34: 924–929.

Therasse DG 1992 The safety profile of loracarbef: clinical trials in respiratory, skin and urinary tract infections. *American Journal of Medicine* 92 (Suppl. 6A): 20S–25S.

OTHER GROUP 2 CEPHALOSPORINS

Cefatrizine

The spectrum is similar to that of cefalexin but it is more active against *H. influenzae* (Table 15.2). Wide strain variations in susceptibility have been reported.

Pharmacokinetics

C_max 500 mg oral	c. 6 mg/l after 1–2 h
Plasma half-life	2.5 h
Plasma protein binding	40–60%

Cefatrizine is only partially absorbed when given by mouth. The half-life is extended to 5.5 h in end-stage renal failure. Distribution resembles that of cefalexin. It crosses the placenta readily.

Urinary recovery in 6 h is 35% of an oral dose, producing urinary levels of 50–1500 mg/l. It is presumed that the remainder is metabolized, but no metabolites have been identified.

Apart from some mild diarrhea, it appears to be well tolerated.

Preparations and dosage

Preparation: Capsules, suspension.

Dosage: Adults, oral, 500 mg twice daily.

Very limited availability. Available in Japan.

Further information

Carlone NA, Cuffini AM, Forno P, Izzoglio M, Cavallo G 1985 Susceptibility of clinical isolates of Gram-positive and Gram-negative organisms to cefatrizine. *Drugs Under Experimental and Clinical Research* 11: 447–451.

Pfeffer M, Gaver RC, Ximinez J 1983 Human intravenous pharmacokinetics and absolute oral bioavailability of cefatrizine. *Antimicrobial Agents and Chemotherapy* 24: 915–920.

Santella PJ, Tanrisever B 1985 Cefatrizine: a clinical overview. *Drugs Under Experimental and Clinical Research* 11: 441–445.

Cefroxadine

Cefroxadine is closely related to cefradine, the structure differing only by the presence of a methoxy group replacing methyl at the C-3 position. The antimicrobial spectrum is identical to that of cefradine and cefalexin (Table 15.2), but it is slightly more actively bactericidal. A dose of 1 g as film-coated tablets produced mean peak plasma levels of 25 mg/l at 1 h. Absorption is depressed and delayed by administration with food. The plasma elimination half-life is 0.8 h, rising to 40 h in end-stage renal failure and falling to 3.4 h during hemodialysis. Around 85% of an oral dose is excreted unchanged in urine.

Preparations and dosage

Proprietary name: Oraspor.

Dosage: Adults, oral, 0.5–2 g/day in divided doses.

Very limited availability. Available in Japan.

Further information

Gerardin A, Lecaillon JB, Schoeller JP, Humbert G, Guibert J 1982 Pharmacokinetics of cefroxadine (CGP 9000) in man. *Journal of Pharmacokinetics and Biopharmacy* 10: 15–26.

Lecaillon JB, Hirtz JL, Schoeller JP, Humbert G, Vischer W 1980 Pharmacokinetic comparison of cefroxadine (CGP 9000) and cephalexin by simultaneous administration to humans. *Antimicrobial Agents and Chemotherapy* 18: 656–660.

Nieto MJ, Lanao JM, Dominiguez-Gil A, Tabernero JM, Macias JF 1983 Elimination of cefroxadine from patients undergoing dialysis. *European Journal of Clinical Pharmacology* 24: 109–112.

Yasuda K, Kurashige S, Mitsuhashi S 1980 Cefroxadine (CGP 9000), an orally active cephalosporin. *Antimicrobial Agents and Chemotherapy* 18: 105–110.

GROUP 3 CEPHALOSPORINS

CEFOTETAN

Molecular weight (disodium salt): 603.

A semisynthetic cephamycin available as the disodium salt.

Antimicrobial activity

The activity is similar to that of cefoxitin, but cefotetan exhibits more potent activity against enterobacteria and more modest activity against *Staph. aureus* (Table 15.3).

Pharmacokinetics

C_max 500 mg intravenous	80–120 mg/l end injection
1 g intravenous	140–180 mg/l end injection
Plasma half-life	3–3.5 h
Volume of distribution	10.3 l
Plasma protein binding	88%

Distribution

There is no evidence of accumulation on a dosage of 1 g 12-hourly. Tissue fluid concentrations were about 30% of the

Table 15.3 Activity of group 3 cephalosporins against common pathogenic bacteria: MIC (mg/l)

	Cefbuperazone	Cefmetazole	Cefminox	Cefotetan	Cefotiam	Cefoxitin	Cefuroxime
Staph. aureus	8	1	8–16	8–16	1	2–8	1–4
Str. pyogenes	2–8	0.5	4–8	1	0.03	0.25–1	0.03–0.1
Str. pneumoniae	2–4	0.5	0.5–2	2	0.25	1–2	0.03–0.1
E. faecalis	R	R	R	R	R	R	R
N. gonorrhoeae		0.5	0.5–1	0.5–1	0.1	0.1–0.5	0.06–0.1
N. meningitidis		0.25		0.1	0.06	0.25	0.06
H. influenzae	1	4–8	0.25–2	1–4	0.5	2–4	0.5
Esch. coli	0.25	1–2	0.25–2	0.1–0.5	0.1	2–8	1–4
K. pneumoniae	0.5	1–2	0.5–1	0.1–0.5	0.5	2–8	2–4
Ps. aeruginosa	R	R	R	R	R	R	R
B. fragilis	2	4–R	0.5–4	4–32	R	4–32	4–64

R, resistant (MIC >64 mg/l)

simultaneous serum level. In patients given 1 g by intravenous bolus preoperatively, concentrations were detectable within minutes in the peritoneal fluid, reaching 44% of the simultaneous serum level at 0.5 h and 115% at 3 h.

Metabolism and excretion

Cefotetan is partially converted to a tautomer, which can occasionally be detected in the plasma. About 85% of the drug is eliminated in the urine over 24 h. Accumulation in renal failure is inversely linearly related to the creatinine clearance, the plasma half-life rising to 20 h in patients requiring hemodialysis. During hemodialysis the half-life falls to around 7.5 h and on continuous ambulatory peritoneal dialysis (CAPD) it falls to 15.5 h, 5–10% of the dose being recovered in the dialysate over 24 h. Excretion of the tautomer is not affected by the degree of renal failure.

Toxicity and side effects

Reactions are those typical of the group. Anaphylaxis has been described. Because of the methylthiotetrazole side-chain there is some risk of hypoprothrombinemia and disulfiram-like reactions can occur. Marked changes in the bowel flora, with appearance of *Cl. difficile*, have been reported.

Clinical uses

Similar to those of other cephamycins.

Preparations and dosage

Proprietary name: Cefotan.

Preparation: Injection.

Dosage: Adults, i.m., i.v., 1–3 g every 12 h, depending on severity of infection.

Available in Italy, France, USA.

Further information

Browning MJ, Holt HA, White LO et al 1986 Pharmacokinetics of cefotetan in patients with end-stage renal failure on maintenance dialysis. *Journal of Antimicrobial Chemotherapy* 18: 103–106.

Eckrich RJ, Fox S, Mallory D 1994 Cefotetan-induced immune hemolytic anemia due to the drug-adsorption mechanism. *Immunohematology* 10: 51–54.

Jones RN 1988 Cefotetan: a review of the microbiologic properties and antimicrobial spectrum. *American Journal of Surgery* 155: 16–23.

Kline SS, Mauro VF, Forney RB, Freimer EH, Somani P 1987 Cefotetan-induced disulfiram-type reactions and hypoprothrombinemia. *Antimicrobial Agents and Chemotherapy* 31: 1328–1331.

Martin C, Thomachet L, Albanese J 1994 Clinical pharmacokinetics of cefotetan. *Clinical Pharmacokinetics* 26: 248–258.

Shwed JA, Danziger LH, Wojtynek J, Rodvold KA 1991 A comparative evaluation of the safety and efficacy of cefotetan and cefoxitin in surgical prophylaxis. *Drug Intelligence and Clinical Pharmacy, Annals of Pharmacotherapy* 25: 10–13.

Wagner BKJ, Heaton AH, Flink JR 1992 Cefotetan disodium-induced hemolytic anemia. *Annals of Pharmacotherapy* 20: 199–200.

Ward A, Richards DM 1985 Cefotetan. A review of its antibacterial activity, pharmacokinetic properties and therapeutic use. *Drugs* 30: 382–426.

CEFOXITIN

Molecular weight (sodium salt): 449.4.

A semisynthetic cephamycin available as the sodium salt for intramuscular or intravenous injection.

Antimicrobial activity

Its activity against common pathogenic bacteria is shown in Table 15.3. Most Gram-positive bacilli are susceptible, but

L. monocytogenes is resistant. It is resistant to many Gram-negative β-lactamases and is active against organisms elaborating them, including some *Citrobacter, Providencia, Serratia* and *Acinetobacter* spp. *Enterobacter* spp. are resistant. It is moderately active against *Bacteroides* spp., but the MIC_{90} for *B. fragilis* is 16–32 mg/l and considerable strain variation in susceptibility occurs.

Acquired resistance

Resistant strains of *Bacteroides*, some of which produce β-lactamases that hydrolyze cefoxitin, have been described. Resistance may be transferable to other *Bacteroides* spp. It is a potent inducer of chromosomal cephalosporinases of certain Gram-negative bacilli (pp. 263–264) and can antagonize the effect of cefotaxime and other β-lactam agents.

Pharmacokinetics

C_{max} 500 mg intramuscular	11 mg/l after 20 min
1 g intravenous	c. 150 mg/l end injection
Plasma half-life	0.7–1 h
Volume of distribution	c. 10 l
Plasma protein binding	65–80%

Absorption

Cefoxitin is not absorbed by oral administration, but is very rapidly absorbed from intramuscular sites. Doubling the dose approximately doubles the plasma level. It is absorbed from suppositories to varying degrees depending on the adjuvants: peak serum levels around 9.8 mg/l have been obtained after a dose of 1 g, giving a bioavailability of around 20%. In infants and children treated with 150 mg/kg daily, mean serum concentrations 15 min after intravenous and intramuscular administration were 81.9 and 68.5 mg/l, with elimination half-lives of 0.70 and 0.67 h, respectively.

Distribution

About 20% of the corresponding serum levels are found in sputum. In patients given 1 g by intravenous bolus preoperatively concentrations in lung tissue at 1 h were around 13 mg/g. Penetration into normal CSF is very poor, in most patients with aseptic meningitis receiving 2 g intravenously none could be detected in the CSF. Even in patients with purulent meningitis CSF concentrations seldom exceed 6 mg/l. In children with meningitis receiving 75 mg/kg 6-hourly, peak concentrations of 5–6 mg/l were found around 1 h after the dose. In patients receiving 2 g intravenously before surgery, the mean penetrance into peritoneal fluid was 86%. In patients receiving 2 g intramuscularly before hysterectomy, mean concentrations in pelvic tissue were 7.8 mg/g. Breast milk has been found to contain 5–6 mg/l after 1 g intravenous dose. Concentrations up to 230 mg/l have been found in bile after 2 g intravenously.

Metabolism

Less than 5% of the drug is desacetylated and in a few subjects deacylation of 1 or 2% of the dose to the antibacterially inactive descarbamyl form also occurs.

Excretion

Cefoxitin is almost entirely excreted in the urine by both glomerular filtration and tubular secretion, 80–90% being found in the first 12 h following a parenteral dose, producing concentrations in excess of 1 g/l. Furosemide, in doses of 40–160 mg, had no effect on the elimination half-life of doses of 1 or 2 g. Probenecid delays the plasma peak and decreases the renal clearance and urine concentration. The renal clearance has been calculated variously to lie between 225 and 330 ml/min. The plasma half-life increases inversely with creatinine clearance to reach 24 h in oliguric patients, with corresponding reduction in total body clearance. In patients on CAPD, peritoneal clearance accounted for only 7.5% of mean plasma clearance and the mean plasma half-life during 6 h dialysis was 7.8 h.

Toxicity and side effects

Reactions have been those common to cephalosporins. Pain on intramuscular, and thrombophlebitis on intravenous, injection occur. Substantial changes can occur in the fecal flora, with virtual eradication of susceptible enterobacteria and non-*fragilis Bacteroides* and appearance of, or increase in, yeasts, enterococci and other resistant bacteria including *Cl. difficile*. Development of meningitis due to *H. influenzae* and *Str. pneumoniae* in patients treated for other infections has been observed.

Clinical use

As for other group 3 cephalosporins, with particular emphasis on mixed infections including anaerobes, notably abdominal and pelvic sepsis. In considering its use, its low activity against aerobic Gram-positive cocci should be noted.

Preparations and dosage

Proprietary name: Mefoxin.

Preparation: Injection.

Dosage: Adults, i.m., i.v., 1–2 g every 6–8 h with a maximum of 12 g/day. Children <1 week, 20–40 mg/kg every 12 h; children 1–4 weeks, 20–40 mg/kg every 8 h; children >1 month, 20–40 mg/kg every 6–8 h (maximum dose 200 mg/kg per day).

Widely available.

Further information

Anonymous 1999 Cefoxitin. In: Dollery C (ed.). *Therapeutic Drugs* 2nd edn. Churchill Livingstone, Edinburgh, pp. C106–C109.

Brogden RN, Heel RC, Speight TM, Avery GS 1979 Cefoxitin: a review of its antibacterial activity, pharmacological properties and therapeutic use. *Drugs* 17: 1–37.

Carver PL, Nightingale CH, Quintiliani R 1989 Pharmacokinetics and pharmacodynamics of total and unbound cefoxitin and cefotetan in healthy volunteers. *Journal of Antimicrobial Chemotherapy* 23: 99–106.

Feldman WE, Moffitt S, Manning NS 1982 Penetration of cefoxitin into cerebrospinal fluid of infants and children with bacterial meningitis. *Antimicrobial Agents and Chemotherapy* 21: 468–471.

Goodwin CS 1995 Cefoxitin 20 years on: is it still useful? *Reviews in Medical Microbiology* 6: 146–153.

Shwed JA, Danziger LH, Wojtynek J, Rodvold KA 1991 A comparative evaluation of the safety and efficacy of cefotetan and cefoxitin in surgical prophylaxis. *Drug Intelligence and Clinical Pharmacy, Annals of Pharmacotherapy* 25: 10–13.

Sieradzan RR, Bottner WA, Fasco MJ, Bertoni JS Jr 1988 Comparative effects of cefoxitin and cefotetan on vitamin K metabolism. *Antimicrobial Agents and Chemotherapy* 32: 1446–1449.

Van Hoogdalem EJ, Wackwitz AT, DeBoer AG, Cohen AF, Breimer DD 1989 Rate-controlled rectal absorption enhancement of cefoxitin by coadministration of sodium salicylate or sodium octanoate in healthy volunteers. *British Journal of Clinical Pharmacology* 27: 75–81.

CEFUROXIME

Molecular weight (sodium salt): 446.4.

A semisynthetic cephalosporin supplied as the sodium salt, or as the acetoxyethyl ester (cefuroxime axetil).

Antimicrobial activity

Its activity against common pathogenic bacteria is shown in Table 15.3. The methoximino side-chain provides stability to most Gram-negative β-lactamases and it is active against most enterobacteria, including many multiresistant strains. *Acinetobacter* spp., *Ser. marcescens* and *Ps. aeruginosa* are resistant, although some *Burkholderia cepacia* strains are susceptible. Some anaerobic Gram-negative rods are susceptible, but *B. fragilis* is resistant. The minimum immobilizing concentration for the Nichol's strain of *T. pallidum* is 0.01 mg/l.

Pharmacokinetics

Oral absorption (axetil)	40–50%
C_{max} 500 mg intramuscular	*c.* 18–25 mg/l after 0.5–1 h
0.75 g intravenous infusion	*c.* 50 mg/l end infusion
500 mg oral (axetil)	6–9 mg/l after 1.8–2.5 h
Plasma half-life	1.1–1.4 h
Volume of distribution	11–15 l
Plasma protein binding	30%

Absorption

The acetoxyethyl ester (cefuroxime axetil) is rapidly hydrolyzed on passage through the intestinal mucosa and in the portal circulation to liberate cefuroxime, acetaldehyde and acetic acid. No unchanged ester is detectable in the systemic circulation. Early problems of inconsistent absorption have been ameliorated by reformulation. Absorption is independent of dose in the range 0.25–1 g, and there is no accumulation on repeated dosing.

Bioavailability is improved after food to around 50%. In elderly subjects receiving doses of 500 mg two or three times daily peak plasma levels were 5.5 mg/l after 1.5–2 h in the fasting state, rising to 7.6 mg/l after 20 min when the dose was administered with food.

Distribution

In patients with severe meningeal inflammation, the mean CSF concentration after a 1.5 g intravenous dose was in the range 1.5–3.7 mg/l. In about a third of patients with normal CSF, no drug could be detected and in the remainder concentrations were 0.2–1 mg/l. In children treated for meningitis with 50 or 75 mg/kg, the CSF:serum ratios were 0.07 and 0.10, respectively. Concentrations in pleural drain fluid after thoracic surgery approximated to serum levels at 2 h after doses of 1 or 1.5 g and exceeded serum levels at 4 h, when they were still around 10 mg/l. Levels in pericardial fluid were similar, with fluid:serum ratios of 0.44 between 0.5 and 2 h. In patients receiving 1.5 g by intravenous bolus preoperatively, concentrations around 22 mg/g were found in subcutaneous tissue at about 5 h with an elimination half-life of about 1.5 h.

Mean bone:serum ratios in the femoral head after 750 mg intramuscular and 1.5 g intravenous bolus injections were 0.14 and 0.23, respectively. In patients with chronic otitis media treated with 0.75 g 8-hourly for 6–8 days, peak concentrations in middle ear of 0.7–1.7 mg/l were reached about 2 h after the dose. In patients given 750 mg intramuscularly on five consecutive days the mean sputum concentration rose from 0.57 mg/l on the first day to 1.15 mg/l on the third.

Excretion

The drug is excreted unchanged in the urine mostly within 6 h of administration, producing concentrations exceeding 1000 mg/l. About 45–55% of the drug is excreted by tubular secretion, so that the administration of probenecid increases the serum peak and prolongs the plasma half-life. Renal clearance is slightly affected by the route of administration but lies between 95 and 180 l/min. The plasma half-life is prolonged in the elderly up to 2.4 h.

Toxicity and side effects

Cefuroxime is well tolerated with little pain or phlebitis on injection. Reactions described are minor hypersensitivity manifestations and biochemical changes common to cephalosporins.

The axetil ester may cause diarrhea and, in some cases,

vomiting. Changes in the bowel flora, sometimes with the appearance of *Cl. difficile*, have been reported in about 15% of patients. Vaginitis is reported in about 2% of female patients.

Clinical use

Cefuroxime has been successfully used to treat urinary, soft-tissue, pulmonary infections, septicemia, and as a single-dose treatment (with probenecid) of gonorrhea due to β-lactamase-producing strains. It has been widely used for surgical prophylaxis.

Preparations and dosage

Cefuroxime

Proprietary name: Zinacef.

Preparation: Injection.

Dosage: Adults, i.m., i.v., 750 mg every 6–8 h; 1.5 g every 6–8 h in severe infections. Children, 30–100 mg/kg per day in 3–4 divided doses; 60 mg/kg per day in divided doses is appropriate for most infections. Neonates, 30–100 mg/kg per day in 2–3 divided doses.

Widely available.

Cefuroxime axetil

Proprietary name: Zinnat.

Preparation: Tablets, suspension, sachets.

Dosage: Adults, oral, 250–500 mg twice daily depending on severity of infection.

Children over 3 months, oral, 125 mg twice daily; if necessary, dose doubled in children over 2 years with otitis media.

Widely available.

Further information

Anonymous 1999 Cefuroxime (sodium and axetil). In: Dollery C (ed.) *Therapeutic Drugs* 2nd edn. Churchill Livingstone, Edinburgh, pp. C135–C140.

Baldwin DR, Andrews JM, Wise R, Honeybourne D 1992 Bronchoalveolar distribution of cefuroxime axetil and in-vitro efficacy of observed concentrations against respiratory pathogens. *Journal of Antimicrobial Chemotherapy* 30: 377–385.

Brogden RN, Heel RC, Speight TM, Avery GS 1979 Cefuroxime: a review of its antibacterial activity, pharmacological properties and therapeutic use. *Drugs* 17: 233–266.

Colaizzi PA, Goodwin SD, Poynor WJ, Karnes HT, Polk RE 1987 Single dose pharmacokinetics of cefuroxime and cefamandole in healthy subjects. *Clinical Pharmacy* 6: 894–899.

Dellamonica P 1994 Cefuroxime axetil. *International Journal of Antimicrobial Agents* 4: 23–36.

Donn KH, James NC, Powell JR 1994 Bioavailability of cefuroxime axetil formulations. *Journal of Pharmaceutical Sciences* 83: 842–844.

Finn A, Straughan A, Meyer M, Chubb J 1987 Effect of dose and food on the bioavailability of cefuroxime axetil. *Biopharmaceutics and Drug Disposition* 8: 519–526.

Ginsburg CM, McCracken GH, Petruska M, Olson K 1985 Pharmacokinetics and bactericidal activity of cefuroxime axetil. *Antimicrobial Agents and Chemotherapy* 28: 504–507.

Gold B, Rodriguez WJ 1983 Cefuroxime: mechanisms of action, antimicrobial activity, pharmacokinetics, clinical application, adverse reactions and therapeutic indications. *Pharmacotherapy* 3: 82–100.

Leigh DA, Walsh B, Leung A, Tait S, Peatey K, Hancock P 1990 The effect of cefuroxime axetil on the faecal flora of healthy volunteers. *Journal of Antimicrobial Chemotherapy* 26: 261–268.

Lovering AM, Perez J, Bowker KE, Reeves DS, MacGowan AP, Bannister G 1997 A comparison of the penetration of cefuroxime and cefamandole into bone, fat and haematoma fluid in patients undergoing total hip replacement. *Journal of Antimicrobial Chemotherapy* 40: 99–104.

Perry CM, Brogden RN 1996 Cefuroxime axetil. A review of its antibacterial activity, pharmacokinetic properties and therapeutic efficacy. *Drugs* 52: 125–158.

OTHER GROUP 3 CEPHALOSPORINS

Cefbuperazone

A semisynthetic cephamycin antibiotic with properties similar to those of cefoxitin, but somewhat more active against *B. fragilis* and enterobacteria. It is not hydrolyzed by common β-lactamases and as a result its activity is not affected by inoculum size. Its activity against common pathogenic bacteria is shown in Table 15.3. It is not active against cefoxitin-resistant strains.

Preparations

Proprietary names: Keiperazon, Tomiproan.

Available in Japan.

Further information

Del Bene VE, Carek PJ, Twitty JA, Burkey LJ 1985 In vitro activity of cefbuperazone compared with that of other new β-lactam agents against anaerobic Gram-negative bacilli and contribution of β-lactamase to resistance. *Antimicrobial Agents and Chemotherapy* 27: 817–820.

Karger L 1986 Impact of cefbuperazone on the colonic microflora in patients undergoing colorectal surgery. *Drugs under Experimental and Clinical Research* 12: 983–986.

Tanaka H, Nishino H, Sawada T et al 1987 Biliary penetration of cefbuperazone in the presence and absence of obstructive jaundice. *Journal of Antimicrobial Chemotherapy* 20: 417–420.

Cefmetazole

A semisynthetic cephamycin antibiotic. Its activity against common pathogenic bacteria is shown in Table 15.3. It is active against *Pr. mirabilis*, *Pr. vulgaris*, *Morganella morganii*, *Yersinia* spp. and most anaerobes. *Ser. marcescens* is moderately susceptible, but *Ps. aeruginosa* and *E. faecalis* are resistant. It is active against *Mycobacterium fortuitum* and some strains of *Mycobacterium chelonei*. It is resistant to a wide range of β-lactamases.

Pharmacokinetics

C_{max} 1 g intravenous (1 h infusion)	77 mg/l end infusion
Plasma half-life	*c.* 1.3 h
Volume of distribution	17.5 l
Plasma protein binding	68%

The principal route of excretion is the urine, where 70% is recovered over the first 6 h. In patients whose creatinine clearance is less than 10 ml/min, plasma levels are elevated and the plasma half-life is increased to around 15 h.

Side effects associated with the methylthiotetrazole group at position C-3 have been reported. Its uses are similar to those of cefoxitin.

Preparations and dosage

Preparation: Injection.

Dosage: Adults, i.m., i.v., 2 g every 6–12 h.

Available in Spain, Italy and Japan.

Further information

Borin MT, Peters GR, Smith TC 1990 Pharmacokinetics and dose proportionality of cemetazole in healthy young and elderly volunteers. *Antimicrobial Agents and Chemotherapy* 34: 1944–1948.

Cornick NA, Jacobus NV, Gorbach SL 1987 Activity of cefmetazole against anaerobic bacteria. *Antimicrobial Agents and Chemotherapy* 31: 2010–2012.

Halstenson CE, Guay DRP, Opsahl JA et al 1990 Disposition of cefmetazole in healthy volunteers and patients with impaired renal function. *Antimicrobial Agents and Chemotherapy* 34: 519–523.

Jones RN, Barry AL, Fuchs PC, Thornsberry C 1986 Antimicrobial activity of cefmetazole (CS-1170) and recommendations for susceptibility testing by disk diffusion, dilution and anaerobic methods. *Journal of Clinical Microbiology* 24: 1055–1059.

Schentag JJ 1991 Cefmetazole sodium: pharmacology, pharmacokinetics, and clinical trials. *Pharmacotherapy* 11: 2–19.

Cefminox

A semisynthetic cephamycin. Its activity is similar to that of cefoxitin and cefotetan, but the activity against enterobacteria and *B. fragilis* is somewhat better (Table 15.3). *Cl. difficile* is inhibited by 4–16 mg/l. It is stable to the common β-lactamases of enterobacteria and *Bacteroides* spp. The effect is bactericidal at concentrations close to the MIC and there is little inoculum effect. Some immunomodulatory activity has been claimed.

Pharmacokinetics

C$_{max}$ 1 g intravenous (15 min infusion)	30 mg/l after 1 h
Plasma half-life	c. 2 h
Plasma protein binding	68%

Its safety profile and uses are similar to those of other cephamycins.

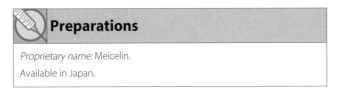

Preparations

Proprietary name: Meicelin.

Available in Japan.

Further information

Aguilar L, Esteban C, Frias J, Pérez-Balcabao I, Carcas AJ, Dal-Ré R 1994 Cefminox: correlation between in-vitro susceptibility and pharmacokinetics and serum bactericidal activity in healthy volunteers. *Journal of Antimicrobial Chemotherapy* 33: 91–101.

Corrales I, Aguilar L, Mato R, Frias J, Prieto J 1994 Immunomodulatory effect of cefminox. *Journal of Antimicrobial Chemotherapy* 33: 372–374.

Inouye S, Goi H, Watanabe T et al 1984 In vitro and in vivo antibacterial activities of a new semisynthetic cephalosporin compared with those of five cephalosporins. *Antimicrobial Agents and Chemotherapy* 26: 722–729.

Mayama T, Koyama Y, Sebata K, Tanaka Y, Shirai S, Sakai H 1995 Postmarketing surveillance on side-effects of cefminox sodium (Meicelin). *International Journal of Clinical Pharmacology and Therapeutics* 33: 149–155.

Soriano F, Edwards R, Greenwood D 1991 Comparative susceptibility of cefminox and cefoxitin to β-lactamases of *Bacteroides* spp. *Journal of Antimicrobial Chemotherapy* 28: 55–60.

Watanabe S, Omoto S 1990 Pharmacology of cefminox, a new bactericidal cephamycin. *Drugs under Experimental and Clinical Research* 16: 461–467.

Cefotiam

The activity is similar to that of cefuroxime, but it is somewhat more active against a range of enterobacteria (Table 15.3). Formulation as a prodrug ester, cefotiam hexetil, allows oral administration.

Pharmacokinetics

Absorption (hexetil ester)	*c.* 65%
C$_{max}$ 1 g intravenous (30 min infusion)	35 mg/l 15 min after end of infusion
1 g intramuscular	17 mg/l
Plasma half-life	0.6–1.1 h
Volume of distribution	35 l
Plasma protein binding	40%

Food delays absorption of the prodrug ester, cefotiam hexetil. In patients with chronic maxillary sinusitis given two 200 mg doses of the prodrug 12 h apart, plasma concentrations 1 h after the second dose were about 1 mg/l with similar concentrations in sinus fluid.

Urinary excretion is almost complete 4 h after the end of intravenous infusion, but only 50–67% is recovered unchanged; there is substantial non-renal elimination and some evidence of saturation of renal tubular excretion at doses above 2 g. In anuria the plasma elimination half-life rises to 13 h and plasma and renal clearances parallel creatinine clearance. A small amount is excreted in bile. In patients with cholelithiasis given 0.5 or 1 g intravenously mean concentrations in gall-bladder bile and gall-bladder wall 30 min after the dose were around 17 and 32 mg/l, respectively. In patients with normal liver function hepatic bile concentrations can exceed 1 g/l.

Cefotiam is generally well tolerated and has been successfully used to treat lower respiratory infections, skin and soft-tissue infection.

Preparations and dosage

Preparation: Injection

Dosage: Adults, i.m., i.v., up to 8 g per day in divided doses.

Limited availability in continental Europe.

Further information

Brogard JM, Jehl F, Willemin B, Lamalle AM, Blickle JF, Monteil H 1989 Clinical pharmacokinetics of cefotiam. *Clinical Pharmacokinetics* 17: 163–174.

Cherrier P, Tod M, Le-Gros V, Petitjean O, Brion N, Chatelin A 1992 Cefotiam concentrations in the sinus fluid of patients with chronic sinusitis after administration of cefotiam hexetil. *European Journal of Clinical Microbiology and Infectious Diseases* 12: 211–215.

Imada A, Hirai S 1995 Cefotiam hexetil. *International Journal of Antimicrobial Agents* 5: 85–99.

Maier H, Attalan M, Weidauer H 1992 Efficacy and safety of cefotiam hexetil in the treatment of ear, nose and throat infections. *Arzneimittelforschung* 42: 980–982.

Rouan MC, Binswanger U, Bammater F, Theobald W, Schoeller JP, Guibert J 1984 Pharmacokinetics and dosage adjustment of cefotiam in renal impaired patients. *Journal of Antimicrobial Chemotherapy* 13: 611–618.

GROUP 4 CEPHALOSPORINS

CEFOTAXIME

Molecular weight (sodium salt): 478.5.

A semisynthetic cephalosporin available as the sodium salt for parenteral administration.

Antimicrobial activity

The aminothiazoyl and methoximino groups at the 7-amino position confer, respectively, potent activity against many Gram-negative rods and cocci (Table 15.4) and stability to most β-lactamases. *Ps. aeruginosa*, *Sten. maltophilia* and other pseudomonads are often resistant. *Brucella melitensis* and some strains of *Nocardia asteroides* are susceptible. Cefotaxime exhibits poor activity against *L. monocytogenes* and *B. fragilis*. Desacetyl cefotaxime has about 10% of the activity of the parent against enterobacteria, less against *Staph. aureus*.

Acquired resistance

Many enterobacteria resistant to other β-lactam agents are susceptible, but selection of resistant strains with derepressed chromosomal molecular class C cephalosporinases (*see* pp. 263–264) may occur. Gram-negative bacilli producing variants of the TEM enzymes (p. 264) are resistant.

Pharmacokinetics

C$_{max}$ 500 mg intramuscular	10–15 mg/l after 0.5–1 h
1 g intravenous (15 min infusion)	90 mg/l end infusion
Plasma half-life	*c.* 1 h
Volume of distribution	32–37 l
Plasma protein binding	*c.* 40%

Distribution

It is widely distributed, achieving therapeutic concentrations in sputum, lung tissue, pleural fluid, peritoneal fluid, prostatic tissue and cortical bone. In patients receiving 2 g 8-hourly, mean CSF concentrations in aseptic meningitis were 0.8 mg/l. Levels of 2–15 mg/l can be found in the CSF in the presence

Table 15.4 Activity of group 4 cephalosporins against common pathogenic bacteria: MIC (mg/l)

	Cefmenoxime	Cefodizime	Cefotaxime	Ceftizoxime	Ceftriaxone	Latamoxef
Staph. aureus	2–4	2–8	2–4	2–4	4	8–16
Str. pyogenes	0.03	0.06–0.1	0.03–0.06	0.03	0.03	1
Str. pneumoniae*	0.06	0.03–0.25	0.1	0.1	0.25	1
E. faecalis	R	8–R	R	R	R	R
N. gonorrhoeae	<0.01–0.03	0.008	<0.01–0.03	<0.01–0.03	<0.01–0.06	0.03–0.1
N. meningitidis	<0.01	0.008	0.01	<0.01	<0.01	<0.01
H. influenzae	0.03	0.008	<0.01–0.03	0.03	<0.01–0.03	0.1
Esch. coli	0.06–0.1	0.1–1	0.03–0.1	0.03	0.06–0.1	0.1–0.25
K. pneumoniae	0.03	0.1–2	0.03–0.1	0.01	0.03–0.06	0.1–0.25
Ps. aeruginosa	16–32	R	8–32	32–64	16–32	4–16
B. fragilis	8–64	8-R	2–32	8–64	16–64	0.5–4

R, resistant (MIC >64 mg/l); *Penicillin-resistant strains are often less susceptible.

of inflammation after doses of 50 mg/kg by intravenous infusion over 30 min. A single dose of 40 mg/kg injected into the ventricle produced levels at 2, 4 and 6 h of 6.4, 5.7 and 4.5 mg/l.

Metabolism

About 15–25% of a dose is metabolized by hepatic esterases to the desacetyl form, which may have some clinical importance because of its concentration in bile and accumulation in renal failure. Its half-life in normal subjects is around 1.5 h.

Excretion

Elimination is predominantly by the renal route, more than half the dose being recovered in the urine over the first 24 h, about 25% as the desacetyl derivative. Excretion is depressed by probenecid and declines in renal failure with accumulation of the metabolite. In patients with creatinine clearances in the range 3–10 ml/min, the plasma half-life rose to 2.6 h while that of the metabolite rose to 10 h.

Toxicity and side effects

Minor hematological and dermatological side effects common to group 4 cephalosporins have been described. Superinfection with *Ps. aeruginosa* in the course of treatment has occurred. Occasional cases of pseudomembranous colitis have been reported.

Clinical uses

Cefotaxime is widely used in neutropenic patients, respiratory infection, meningitis, intra-abdominal sepsis, osteomyelitis, typhoid fever, urinary tract infection, neonatal sepsis and gonorrhea.

Preparations and dosage

Proprietary name: Claforan.

Preparation: Injection.

Dosage: Adults, i.m., i.v., 1–2 g every 8–12 h depending on severity of infection, with a maximum dose of 12 g/day. Neonates, 50 mg/kg per day in 2–4 divided doses, increased to 150–200 mg/kg per day in severe infections; children, 100–150 mg/kg per day in 2–4 divided doses, increased to 200 mg/kg per day in severe infections.

Widely available.

Further information

Aldridge KE 1995 Cefotaxime in the treatment of staphylococcal infections: comparison of in vitro and in vivo studies. *Diagnostic Microbiology and Infectious Disease* 22: 195–201.

Anonymous 1999 Cefotaxime (sodium). In: Dollery C (ed.) *Therapeutic Drugs* 2nd edn. Churchill Livingstone, Edinburgh, pp. C100–C106.

Beyssac E, Cardot JM, Colnel G, Sirot J, Aiache JM 1987 Pharmacokinetics of cefotaxime and its desacetyl metabolite in plasma and cerebrospinal fluid. *European Journal of Drug Metabolism and Pharmacokinetics* 12: 91–102.

Brogden RN, Spencer CM 1997 Cefotaxime. A reappraisal of its antibacterial activity and pharmacokinetic properties, and a review of its therapeutic efficacy when administered twice daily for the treatment of mild to moderate infections. *Drugs* 53: 483–510.

Davies A, Speller DCE (eds) 1990 Cefotaxime – recent clinical investigations. *Journal of Antimicrobial. Chemotherapy* 26 (suppl A): 1–83.

Fick RB Jr, Alexander MR, Prince RA, Kaslik JE 1987 Penetration of cefotaxime into respiration secretions. *Antimicrobial Agents and Chemotherapy* 11: 815–817.

Jacobs RF, Darville T, Parks JA, Enderlin G 1992 Safety profile and efficacy of cefotaxime for the treatment of hospitalized children. *Clinical Infectious Diseases* 14: 56–65.

Nau R, Prange HW, Muth P et al 1993 Passage of cefotaxime and ceftriaxone into cerebrospinal fluid of patients with uninflamed meninges. *Antimicrobial Agents and Chemotherapy* 37: 1518–1524.

Odio CM 1995 Cefotaxime for treatment of neonatal sepsis and meningitis. *Diagnostic Microbiology and Infectious Disease* 22: 111–117.

Plosker GL, Foster RH, Benfield P 1998 Cefotaxime. A pharmacoeconomic review of its use in the treatment of infections. *Pharmacoeconomics* 13: 91–106.

Todd PA, Brogden RN 1990 Cefotaxime: an update of its pharmacology and therapeutic use. *Drugs* 40: 608–651.

 CEFTRIAXONE

Molecular weight (disodium salt) 600.6.

A semisynthetic cephalosporin supplied as the disodium salt. Its main feature is a long plasma elimination half-life.

Antimicrobial activity

Its activity, which includes most β-lactamase-producing enterobacteria, is almost identical to that of cefotaxime (Table 15.4). Streptococci (but not enterococci) are highly susceptible, as are most fastidious Gram-negative bacilli, although Brucellae are less sensitive (MIC 0.25–2 mg/l). Treatment failure has been reported in tularemia. Mycoplasmas, mycobacteria and *Listeria monocytogenes* are resistant.

Acquired resistance

Ceftriaxone is hydrolyzed by some chromosomal enzymes, including those of *Enterobacter* spp. and *B. fragilis*. Derepression of chromosomal β-lactamase production (*see* p. 264) can result in the appearance of resistance in some species of Gram-negative bacilli in vitro and has been observed in patients.

Pharmacokinetics

C_{max} 500 mg/l intramuscular 1 g intravenous (15–30 min infusion)	c. 40 mg/l after 2 h c. 120–150 mg/l end infusion
Plasma half-life	6–9 h
Volume of distribution	0.15 l/kg
Plasma protein binding	95%

Distribution

Ceftriaxone penetrates well into normal body fluids and natural and experimental exudates. In children treated for meningitis with 50 or 75 mg/kg intravenously over 10–15 min, mean peak CSF concentrations ranged from 3.2 to 10.4 mg/l, with lower values later in the disease. In patients receiving 2 g before surgery, concentrations in cerebral tissue reached 0.3–12 mg/l. In patients with pleural effusions of variable etiology given a 1 g intravenous bolus, concentrations of 7–8.7 mg/l were found at 4–6 h. In patients with exacerbations of rheumatoid arthritis receiving the same dose, joint fluid contained concentrations close to those in the serum, but with wide individual variation. Tissue fluid:serum ratios have varied from around 0.05 in bone and muscle to 0.39 in cantharides blister fluid. The apparent volume of distribution is increased in patients with cirrhosis where the drug rapidly enters the ascitic fluid, but its elimination kinetics are unaffected.

It rapidly crosses the placenta, maternal doses of 2 g intravenously over 2–5 min producing mean concentrations in cord blood of 19.5 mg/l, a mean cord:maternal serum ratio of 0.18; and in amniotic fluid 3.8 mg/l, a fluid:maternal serum ratio of 0.04. The plasma elimination half-life appears to be somewhat shortened in pregnancy (5–6 h). Some appear in the breast milk, the milk:serum ratio being about 0.03–0.04, secretion persisting over a long period with a half-life of 12–17 h.

Metabolism and excretion

Ceftriaxone is not metabolized. Biliary excretion is unusually high, 10–20% of the drug appearing in the bile in unchanged form, with concentrations up to 130 mg/g in biopsied liver tissue from patients receiving 1 g intravenously over 30 min. The insoluble calcium salt may precipitate in the bile leading to pseudolithiasis. About half the dose appears in the urine over the first 48 h, somewhat more (c. 70%) in neonates. Excretion is almost entirely by glomerular filtration, since there is only a small effect of probenecid on the excretion of the drug. The half-life is not linearly correlated with creatinine clearance in renal failure and, in keeping with the low free plasma fraction, it is not significantly removed by hemodialysis. The volume of distribution is not affected by renal failure.

Toxicity and side effects

It is generally well tolerated, reactions being those common to other cephalosporins. Mention has been made of thrombocy-topenia, thrombocytosis, leukopenia, eosinophilia abdominal pain, phlebitis, rash, fever and increased values in liver function tests. Diarrhea is common and pronounced suppression of the aerobic and anaerobic fecal flora has been associated with the appearance of resistant bacteria and yeasts.

Biliary pseudolithiasis due to concretions of insoluble calcium salt has been described in adults but principally in children. The precipitates can be detected in a high proportion of patients by ultrasonography and can occasionally cause pain, but resolve on cessation of treatment. The drug is better avoided in patients with pre-existing biliary disease, but the principal hazard appears to be misdiagnosis of gallbladder disease and unnecessary surgery.

Clinical uses

Uses are similar to those of cefotaxime, the long half-life offering the advantage of once-daily administration. It is used in the treatment of acute bacterial meningitis and as an alternative to rifampicin in the prophylaxis of meningococcal disease (p. 716). Reference is made to its use in osteomyelitis, impetigo and spirochetoses.

 Preparations and dosage

Proprietary name: Rocephin.

Preparation: Injection.

Dosage: Adults, i.m., i.v., 1 g/day as a single dose, 2–4 g/day as a single dose in severe infections. Children over 6 weeks, 20–50 mg/kg per day as a single dose; in severe infections, 80 mg/kg per day as a single dose. Doses over 50 mg/kg must be given as an i.v. infusion. Neonates, i.v. infusion, 20–50 mg/kg per day.

Widely available.

 Further information

Anonymous 1999 Ceftriaxone (sodium). In: Dollery C (ed.) *Therapeutic Drugs* 2nd edn. Churchill Livingstone, Edinburgh pp. C130–C135.

Brogden RN, Ward A 1988 Ceftriaxone: a reappraisal of its antibacterial activity and pharmacokinetic properties, and an update on its therapeutic use with particular reference to once-daily administration. *Drugs* 35: 604–645.

Cometta A, Gallot-Lavallee-Villars S, Iten A et al 1990 incidence of gallbladder lithiasis after ceftriaxone treatment. *Journal of Antimicrobial Chemotherapy* 25: 689–695.

Cross JT, Jacobs RF 1993 Tularemia: failures with outpatient use of ceftriaxone. *Clinical Infectious Diseases* 17: 976–980.

Dansey RD, Jacka PJ, Strachan SA, Hay M 1992 Comparison of cefotaxime with ceftriaxone given intramuscularly 12-hourly for community-acquired pneumonia. *Diagnostic Microbiology and Infectious Disease* 15: 81–84.

Fraschini F, Braga PC, Scarpazza G et al 1986 Human pharmacokinetics and distribution in various tissues of ceftriaxone. *Chemotherapy* 32: 192–199.

Holazo AA, Patel IH, Weinfeld RE, Konikoff JJ, Parsonnet M 1986 Ceftriaxone pharmacokinetics following multiple intramuscular dosing. *European Journal of Clinical Pharmacology* 30: 109–112.

Lopez AJ, O'Keefe P, Morrissey M, Pickleman J 1991 Ceftriaxone-induced cholelithiasis. *Annals of Internal Medicine* 115: 712–714.

Lucht F, Dorche G, Aubert G, Boissier C, Bertrand AM, Brunon J 1990 The penetration of ceftriaxone into human brain tissue. *Journal of Antimicrobial Chemotherapy* 26: 81–86.

Nahata MC, Durrell DE, Barnes WJ 1986 Ceftriaxone kinetics and cerebrospinal fluid penetration in infants and children with meningitis. *Chemotherapy* 32: 89–94.

Schaad VB, Tshappeler H, Lentze MJ 1986 Transient formation of precipitations in the gallbladder associated with ceftriaxone therapy. *Pediatric Infectious Diseases* 5: 708–710.

Spector R 1987 Ceftriaxone transport through the bloodbrain barrier. *Journal of Infectious Diseases* 156: 209–211.

Stratton CW, Anthony LB, Johnston PE 1988 A review of ceftriaxone: A long-acting cephalosporin. *American Journal of Medical Science* 296: 221–222.

Yuk JH, Nightingale CH, Quintiliani R 1989 Clinical pharmacokinetics of ceftriaxone. *Clinical Pharmacokinetics* 17: 223–235.

 # LATAMOXEF

Moxalactam. Molecular weight (disodium salt): 564.4.

A semisynthetic 7-methoxyoxacephem, supplied as the disodium salt. There are two epimeric forms, (*R*) and (*S*) of which (*R*) has about twice the activity, but is slightly less stable at 37°C in serum, in which the mixture has a half-life in vitro of about 8 h.

Antimicrobial activity

Its activity against common pathogenic bacteria is shown in Table 15.4. Latamoxef is generally slightly less active than cefotaxime, especially against *Staph. aureus*, but unlike other group 4 cephalosporins it exhibits fairly good activity against *B. fragilis*. *B. thetaiotaomicron* (MIC 2 mg/l) and *B. ovatus* (MIC 4–8 mg/l) are less susceptible than *B. fragilis* and *B. vulgatus*. *Acinetobacter* is moderately resistant.

Acquired resistance

The 7-methoxy substitution, also found in cephamycins such as cefoxitin and cefotetan, confers resistance to hydrolysis by a wide range of β-lactamases including those of *Staph. aureus*, various enterobacteria and *B. fragilis*.

Resistance, predominantly in *Enterobacter* spp., *Ps. aeruginosa* and *Ser. marcescens* due to induction of chromosomal enzymes (p. 264), has been found in vitro and in some patients. Resistance also arises in some organisms through reduced entry into the cell due to modification of outer membrane proteins and to change in penicillin-binding proteins (p. 14). Resistant strains of bacteroides other than *B. fragilis* have been commonly found in some series and have emerged in occasional patients treated for anaerobic infections.

Pharmacokinetics

C_{max} 500 mg intramuscular	12–22 mg/l after 1.2 h
1 g intravenous (30 min infusion)	60 mg/l end infusion
Plasma half-life	c. 2 h
Volume of distribution	8.5 l
Plasma protein binding	40–50%

Distribution

There is reasonably good penetration into serous fluids, the concentration in ascitic fluid reaching 75% and in pleural fluid 50% of the concentration simultaneously present in the serum. After 1 g intravenously, the concentration in pleural fluid 4–6 h after the dose was 9–35 mg/l, with a half-life 2–5 times that of the serum. In volunteers given 1 g intravenously, mean peak concentrations in cantharides blister fluid around 16 mg/l were found at 3–4 h.

Levels of 5–35 mg/l or 10–20% of the corresponding plasma levels have been obtained in inflamed meninges. In adults with bacterial meningitis receiving 2 g intravenously over 30–60 min 4–8 hourly, mean concentrations around 14 mg/l were found in lumbar CSF and 12 mg/l in ventricular CSF. Sputum levels are of the order of 2 mg/l following 1 g of the drug intravenously.

Concentrations achieved in bone are insufficient for the reliable treatment of staphylococcal osteomyelitis. In patients receiving two doses of 500 mg 2 h preoperatively and at the time of surgery, mean concentrations in enucleated or transurethrally resected prostate tissue were 4.0 and 5.2 mg/l. Concentrations in T-tube bile in excess of 170 mg/l 2 h after a 2 g intravenous dose, and 30 mg/l 30 min after a 2 g intramuscular dose have been found.

It is well absorbed after instillation into the peritoneal cavity in patients on CAPD. When 1 g was instilled into the peritoneum, 60% of the dose was absorbed during the dwell time of 1 h, giving mean peak plasma concentrations around 25 mg/l, with a half-life around 13 h.

The volume of distribution is larger and the half-life longer in infants under 1 year.

Metabolism and excretion

No active metabolites have been detected. Renal elimination accounts for 90% of the clearance, but significant concentrations are found in the feces, presumably via biliary excretion. There is little tubular excretion because the effect of probenecid is negligible. Excretion is depressed in renal failure, the elimination half-life rising with falling creatinine clearance to around 50 h. Binding to plasma protein is reduced to 35% in uremic serum. Hemodialysis removes 48–51% of the drug in 4 h, a mean half-life of 18 h between dialyses falling to 2.7 h on dialysis. Peritoneal dialysis has little or no effect.

Toxicity and side effects

Latamoxef is generally well tolerated. Increased bleeding and decreases in platelet function associated with the methylthio-tetrazole side-chain are sufficiently common to have been cited as reasons for restricting use of the agent.

Mention has been made of reversible neutropenia, eosinophilia and increased values in liver function tests and prothrombin time. The agent is contraindicated in patients on anticoagulant therapy.

Overgrowth of resistant cocci, pseudomonads, yeasts and the occasional appearance of *Cl. difficile* may occur.

Clinical uses

Uses are similar to those of group 4 cephalosporins. It is generally less successful in the treatment of infections due to Gram-positive organisms.

Preparations and dosage

Preparation: Injection.

Dosage: Adults, i.m., i.v., 0.5–4 g/day in two divided doses. Children, 25–100 mg/kg per day in divided doses.

Available in continental Europe and Japan; not available in the UK or USA.

Further information

Anonymous. Moxalactam disodium. In: Dollery C (ed.) *Therapeutic Drugs* 2nd edn. Churchill Livingstone, Edinburgh, pp. M232–M235.

Benno Y, Shiragami N, Uchida K, Yoshida T, Mitsuoka T 1986 Effect of moxalactam on human fecal microflora. *Antimicrobial Agents and Chemotherapy* 29: 175–178.

Carmine AA, Brogden RN, Heel RC, Romankiewicz JA, Speight TM, Avery GS 1983 Moxalactam (latamoxef). A review of its antibacterial activity, pharmacokinetic properties and therapeutic use. *Drugs* 26: 279–333.

Drusand GL, Standiford HC, Fitzpatrick B et al 1984 Comparison of the pharmacokinetics of ceftazidime and moxalactam and their microbiological correlates in volunteers. *Antimicrobial Agents and Chemotherapy* 26: 388–393.

Morris DL, Frabricius PJ, Ambrose NS, Scammell B, Burdon DW, Keighley MR 1984 A high incidence of bleeding is observed in a trial to determine whether addition of metronidazole is needed with latamoxef for prophylaxis in colonic surgery. *Journal of Hospital Infection* 5: 398–408.

Oturai PS, Hollander NH, Hansen OP et al 1993 Ceftriaxone versus latamoxef in febrile neutropenic patients: empirical monotherapy in patients with solid tumours. *European Journal of Cancer Part A: General Topics* 29: 1274–1279.

Uchida K, Kakushi H, Shike T 1987 Effect of latamoxef (moxalactam) and its related compounds on platelet aggregation in vitro–structure activity relationships. *Thrombosis Research* 47: 215–222.

OTHER GROUP 4 CEPHALOSPORINS

Cefmenoxime

A semisynthetic cephalosporin supplied as the hydrochloride. The *syn* stereoisomer is about 30 times more active than the *anti* isomer, of which commercial preparations contain less than 0.8%. Its activity is very similar to that of cefotaxime (Table 15.4).

Pharmacokinetics

C_{max} 500 mg intramuscular	15 mg/l after 40 min
1 g intravenous	200 mg/l end injection
Plasma half-life	*c.* 1 h
Volume of distribution	9–14 l
Plasma protein binding	77%

Probenecid increases peak plasma levels and extends the plasma half-life to 1.8 h. Therapeutic concentrations are achieved in CSF. There is a degradation product with a long half-life (around 40 h), but 80–92% of the drug is recovered unchanged from the urine. In patients with renal insufficiency, no significant relation was found between creatinine clearance and peak serum concentrations but there was a linear relationship with plasma half-life and total body clearance. About 10% of the dose appears in the feces, mostly extensively degraded, possibly by the fecal flora.

Toxicity, side effects and clinical use are those common to group 4 cephalosporins.

Preparations and dosage

Preparation: Injection.

Dosage: Adults, i.m., i.v., 1–4 g/day in 2–4 divided doses (maximum dose 12 g per day).

Limited availability in France, Germany and Japan.

Further information

Campoli-Richards DM, Todd PA 1987 Cefmenoxime. A review of its antibacterial activity, pharmacokinetic properties and therapeutic use. *Drugs* 34: 188–221.

Humbert G, Veyssier P, Fourtillan JB et al 1986 Penetration of cefmenoxime into cerebrospinal fluid of patients with bacterial meningitis. *Journal of Antimicrobial Chemotherapy* 18: 503–506.

Konishi K 1986 Pharmacokinetics of cefmenoxime in patients with impaired renal function and in those undergoing haemodialysis. *Antimicrobial Agents and Chemotherapy* 30: 901–905.

Cefodizime

Its antimicrobial activity is typical of the group (Table 15.4) but its overall activity is somewhat less than that of cefotaxime against enterobacteria. There has been some interest in its immunomodulating properties, which affect a number of functions.

Pharmacokinetics

C_{max} 1 g intramuscular	55–60 mg/l after about 1.5 h
Plasma half-life	3.5–3.7 h
Volume of distribution	11–15 l
Plasma protein binding	c. 88%

Cefodizime penetrates into lung, sputum, serous fluids and prostate. Excretion is mainly renal with about 60% of the dose appearing in the urine over 12 h in adults and 80–90% in children. Elimination is inversely correlated with creatinine clearance.

It is well tolerated apart from some pain at the site of injection, mild gastrointestinal upset and rash in a few patients. It has been used mainly to treat respiratory and urinary tract infection.

Preparations and dosage

Proprietary name: Timecef.

Preparation: Injection.

Dosage: Adults, i.m., i.v., 1 g every 12 h (maximum dose 4 g per day). Children, 20–100 mg/kg per day in divided doses.

Not available in the UK. Limited availability in continental Europe.

Further information

Anonymous 1999 Cefodizime (sodium). In: Dollery C (ed.) *Therapeutic Drugs* 2nd edn. Churchill Livingstone, Edinburgh, pp. C96–C100.

Barradell LB, Brogden RN 1992 Cefodizime: a review of its antibacterial activity, pharmacokinetic properties and therapeutic use. *Drugs* 44: 800–834.

Conte JE 1994 Pharmacokinetics of cefodizime in volunteers with normal or impaired renal function. *Journal of Clinical Pharmacology* 34: 1066–1070.

Fietta A, Bersani C, Bertoletti R, Grassi FM, Grassi GG 1988 In vitro and in vivo enhancement of non-specific phagocytosis by cefodizime. *Chemotherapy* 34: 430–436.

Symposium 1990 Cefodizime: a third generation cephalosporin with immunomodulating properties. *Journal of Antimicrobial Chemotherapy* 26 (Suppl. C): 1–34.

Ceftizoxime

A semisynthetic cephalosporin supplied as the sodium salt. It is very similar to cefotaxime, but lacks the acetoxymethyl group at position C-4 and is therefore not subject to deacetylation. Its activity against common pathogenic bacteria (Table 15.4) is very similar to that of cefotaxime.

Pharmacokinetics

C_{max} 500 mg intramuscular	14 mg/l
1 g intravenous (30 min infusion)	85–90 mg/l end infusion
Plasma half-life	1.3–1.9 h
Volume of distribution	23–27 l
Plasma protein binding	30%

Like cefotaxime, ceftizoxime is widely distributed. In children with meningitis receiving 200–250 mg/kg daily as four daily doses for 14–21 days, mean CSF concentrations 2 h after a dose were 6.4 mg/l on day 2 and 3.6 mg/l on day 14.

It is excreted in the urine, from which 70–90% of the dose is recovered in the first 24 h. Excretion is principally by glomerular filtration, but there is some tubular secretion. A 1 g oral dose of probenecid increases the plasma half-life by about 50%. In patients receiving 1 g intravenously over 30 min, the plasma elimination half-life rose to 35 h when the corrected creatinine clearance was <10 ml/min. It is partly removed by peritoneal and hemodialysis.

Clinical use

Reported adverse reactions are few, reversible and typical of those of agents of its class. It has had wide use in the treatment of infections with otherwise resistant organisms, particularly in immunocompromised patients. Infections of the lower respiratory and urinary tracts and soft tissue, and intra-abdominal sepsis have all been successfully treated.

Preparations and dosage

Proprietary name: Cefizox.

Preparation: Injection.

Dosage: Adult, i.m., i.v., 1–2 g every 8–12 h, increased in severe infections up to 12 g/day in three divided doses. Children >3 months, 30–60 mg/kg per day in 2–4 divided doses, increased in severe infections to 100–150 mg/kg per day.

Widely available. Not available in the UK

Further information

Anonymous 1999 Ceftizoxime sodium. In: Dollery C (ed.) *Therapeutic Drugs* 2nd edn. Churchill Livingstone, Edinburgh, pp. C125–C130.

Richards DM, Heel RC 1985 Ceftizoxime. A review of its antibacterial activity, pharmacokinetic properties and therapeutic use. *Drugs* 29: 281–329.

Vallee F, LeBel M 1991 Comparative study of pharmacokinetics and serum bactericidal activity of ceftizoxime and cefotaxime. *Antimicrobial Agents and Chemotherapy* 35: 2057–2064.

Yangco BG, Baird I, Lorber B et al 1987 Comparative efficacy and safety of ceftizoxime, cefotaxime and latamoxef in the treatment of bacterial pneumonia in high risk patients. *Journal of Antimicrobial Chemotherapy* 19: 239–248.

Flomoxef

An oxa-cephem which differs from latamoxef in the side-chains carried at the 7-amino and C-3 positions, but which retains the 7-methoxy group that confers β-lactamase stability. The methyl group of the methylthiotetrazole side-chain of latamoxef has been modified to hydroxymethyl in an attempt to avoid the undesirable side effects, while the side chain at the 7-amino position is F_2-CH-S-CH$_2$-.

The antibacterial activity is similar to that of latamoxef, but activity against *Staph. aureus* is improved and it is claimed to be a poor inducer of penicillin-binding protein 2′, which is associated with resistance in methicillin-resistant strains.

Intravenous injection of 2 g achieves a peak plasma concentration of around 50 mg/l, falling to 2.6 mg/l after 6 h. The plasma half-life is about 50 min. It appears to be well distributed and penetrates moderately well into lung, mucosal tissue of the middle ear and bone.

Flomoxef does not seem to be prone to the effects on platelet function of latamoxef and it has a less marked effect on vitamin K metabolism. It does not cause a disulfiram-like reaction with alcohol.

Clinical experience is limited, but it seems safe and effective in a wide range of infections.

Preparations and dosage

Preparation: Injection.

Dosage: Adult, i.v., 1–2 g twice daily.

Available in Japan.

Further information

Andrassy K, Koderisch J, Gorges K, Sonntag H, Hirauchi K 1991 Pharmacokinetics and hemostasis following administration of a new, injectable oxacephem (6315-S, flomoxef) in volunteers and in patients with renal insufficiency. *Infection* 19 (Suppl. 5): S296–S302.

Cazzola M, Brancaccio V, De Giglio C, Paterno D, Matera MG, Rossi F 1993 Flomoxef, a new oxacephem antibiotic, does not cause hemostatic effect. *International Journal of Clinical Pharmacology, Therapeutics and Toxicology* 31: 148–152.

Ito M, Ishigami T 1991 The meaning of the development of flomoxef and clinical experience in Japan. *Infection* 19 (Suppl. 5): S253–S257.

Saito H, Kimura T, Takeda T, Kishimoto S, Oguma T, Shimamura K 1990 Pharmacokinetics of flomoxef in mucosal tissue of the middle ear and mastoid following intravenous administration in humans. *Chemotherapy* 36: 193–199.

Shimada M, Takenaka K, Sugimachi K 1994 A comprehensive multi-institutional study of empiric therapy with flomoxef in surgical infections of the digestive organs. The Kyushu research group for surgical infection. *Journal of Chemotherapy* 6: 251–256.

Uchida K, Matsubara T 1991 Effect of flomoxef on blood coagulation and alcohol metabolism. *Infection* 19 (Suppl. 5) S284–S295.

GROUP 5 CEPHALOSPORINS

CEFIXIME

Molecular weight (anhydrous): 453.4; (trihydrate): 507.5.

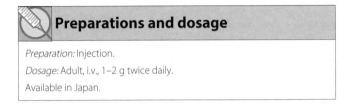

An oral cephalosporin formulated as the anhydrous compound or the trihydrate.

Antimicrobial activity

Its activity against common pathogenic bacteria is shown in Table 15.5. It is active against *N. gonorrhoeae*, *M. catarrhalis*, *H. influenzae* and a wide range of enterobacteria, including most strains of *Citrobacter*, *Enterobacter* and *Serratia* spp. Its antistaphylococcal activity is poor. It is not active against *Acinetobacter* spp., *Ps. aeruginosa* or *B. fragilis*. It is resistant to hydrolysis by common β-lactamases.

Pharmacokinetics

Oral absorption	*c.* 50%
C_{max} 400 mg oral	4–5.5 mg/l after 4 h
Plasma half-life	3–4 h
Volume of distribution	0.1 l/kg
Plasma protein binding	60–70%

Absorption and distribution

Oral absorption is slow and incomplete, but is unaffected by aluminum magnesium hydroxide. Penetration into cantharides blister fluid was very slow but exceeded the plasma level. CSF concentrations are poor even in the presence of meningeal inflammation, reaching an average of around 0.22 mg/l in children with meningitis.

Metabolism and excretion

Cefixime is not metabolized and is excreted unchanged into urine (mainly by glomerular filtration) and into bile, in which concentrations exceeding 100 mg/l have been found. Less than 20% of an oral dose is recovered from the urine over 24 h, falling to less than 5% in patients with severe renal impairment, with a corresponding increase in plasma concentration. It is not removed by peritoneal or hemodialysis.

Toxicity and side effects

It is well tolerated, but diarrhea is fairly common and pseudomembranous colitis has been reported. Other side effects common to cephalosporins are occasionally seen.

Clinical use

Cefixime has been successfully used in uncomplicated cystitis, upper and lower respiratory tract infections and various other infections. Its failure to provide adequate cover for staphylococci should be noted.

Preparations and dosage

Proprietary name: Suprax.

Preparation: Tablets, suspension.

Dosage: Adults, oral, 200–400 mg/day as a single dose or in two divided doses.

Children > 6 months, 8 mg/kg per day as a single dose or in two divided doses.

Widely available.

Further information

Anonymous 1999 Cefixime. In: Dollery C. (ed.) *Therapeutic Drugs* 2nd edn. Churchill Livingstone, Edinburgh, pp. C93–C96.

Brogden RN, Campoli-Richards DM 1989 Cefixime: a review of its antibacterial activity, pharmacokinetic properties and therapeutic potential. *Drugs* 38: 524–550.

Gremse DA, Dean PC, Farquhar DS 1994 Cefixime and antibiotic-associated colitis. *Pediatric Infectious Disease Journal* 13: 331–333.

Guay DR, Meatherall RC, Harding GK, Brown GR 1986 Pharmacokinetics of cefixime (CL 284, 635; FK 027) in healthy subjects and patients with renal insufficiency. *Antimicrobial Agents and Chemotherapy* 30: 485–490.

Leroy A, Oser B, Grise P, Humbert G 1995 Cefixime penetration in human renal parenchyma. *Antimicrobial Agents and Chemotherapy* 39: 1240–1242.

Markham A, Brogden RN 1995 Cefixime. A review of its therapeutic efficacy in lower respiratory tract infections. *Drugs* 49: 1007–1022.

Nahata MC, Kohlbrenner VM, Barson WJ 1993 Pharmacokinetics and cerebrospinal fluid concentrations of cefixime in infants and young children. *Chemotherapy* 39: 1–5.

Symposium 1987 Clinical pharmacology and efficacy of cefixime. *Pediatric Infectious Disease Journal* 6: 949–1009.

Wu DHA 1993 Review of the safety profile of cefixime. *Clinical Therapeutics* 15: 1108–1119.

CEFPODOXIME

Molecular weight (proxetil ester): 557.6.

A semisynthetic cephalosporin supplied as the prodrug ester, cefpodoxime proxetil.

Antimicrobial activity

The hydrolysis product is very similar to cefotaxime and it shares its potent, broad-spectrum activity (Table 15.5). It is stable to a wide range of plasmid-mediated β-lactamases. It induces the chromosomal β-lactamases of *Ps. aeruginosa*, *Enterobacter* spp., *Ser. marcescens* and *Citrobacter* spp., but is a less potent inducer than cefoxitin.

Pharmacokinetics

Oral absorption	*c.* 50%
C_{max} 200 mg oral	2.1 mg/l after 3 h
Plasma half-life	*c.* 2.2 h
Volume of distribution	*c.* 35 l
Plasma protein binding	20–30%

Absorption

The ester is rapidly hydrolyzed to the parent compound in the small intestine. Bioavailability increases to 65% if taken with food, but antacids and H_2-receptor antagonists reduce absorption. Unabsorbed drug is hydrolyzed and excreted in the feces.

Distribution

It is well distributed and penetrates well into tissues (including lung tissue) and inflammatory exudate to achieve concentrations inhibitory to common pathogens. There is no information on penetration into CSF, but oral cephalosporins are unlikely to be used for meningeal infections.

Metabolism and excretion

The hydrolyzed prodrug is not subject to further metabolism. About 80% of the absorbed compound (30–40% of the original dose) appears in the urine over 24 h. Excretion is by glomerular filtration and tubular secretion; probenecid delays secretion and increases the peak plasma concentration.

Toxicity and side effects

The drug is well tolerated, but gastrointestinal disturbance with diarrhea is common. Pseudomembranous colitis has been reported occasionally. Other side effects are those common to cephalosporins.

Clinical use

Cefpodoxime has been used principally for the treatment of upper and lower respiratory tract infections in children and adults.

Preparations and dosage

Proprietary name: Orelox.

Preparation: Tablets and suspension.

Dosage: Adults, oral, 100–200 mg twice daily depending on infection being treated.

Children, 8 mg/kg per day in two divided doses.

Widely available.

Table 15.5 Activity of group 5 cephalosporins against common pathogenic bacteria: MIC (mg/l)

	Cefdinir	Cefetamet	Cefixime	Cefpodoxime	Ceftibuten
Staph. aureus	0.002–1	16–R	4–16	0.5	32
Str. pyogenes	<0.06–0.25	0.015–0.25	0.01–0.25	0.06	8–16
Str. pneumoniae	0.03–0.5	0.06–0.25	0.01–0.25	0.06	0.5–32
E. faecalis	2–R	R	R	R	R
N. gonorrhoeae	0.002–0.06	<0.03–0.25	0.01–0.1	<0.06	0.008–0.06
H. influenzae	0.25–1	0.06–0.25	0.06–0.25	0.06–0.12	0.01–1
Esch. coli	0.008–1	0.125–8	0.25–8 0.25	0.25	0.01–16
K. pneumoniae	0.008–0.5	0.06–1	0.01–1	0.12	0.12
Ps. aeruginosa	R	R	2–32	R	R
B. fragilis	R	R	R	R	R

R, resistant (MIC >64 mg/l)

 Further information

Anonymous 1999 Cefpodoxime proxetil. In: Dollery C (ed.) *Therapeutic Drugs* 2nd edn. Churchill Livingstone, Edinburgh, pp. C113–C117.

Borin MT, Driver MR, Forbes KK 1995 Effect of timing of food on absorption of cefpodoxime proxetil. *Journal of Clinical Pharmacology* 35: 505–509.

Frampton JE, Brogden RN, Langtry HD, Buckley MM 1992 Cefprodoxime proxetil: a review of its antibacterial activity, pharmacokinetic properties and therapeutic potential. *Drugs* 44: 889–917.

Fulton B, Perry CM 2001 Cefpodoxime proxetil: a review of its use in the management of bacterial infections in paediatric patients. *Paediatric Drugs* 3: 137–158.

Moore EP, Speller DCE, White LO, Wilkinson PJ (eds) 1990 Cefpodoxime proxetil: a third-generation oral cephalosporin. *Journal of Antimicrobial Chemotherapy* 26 (Suppl. E): 1–100.

Todd WM 1994 Cefpodoxime proxetil: a comprehensive review. *International Journal of Antimicrobial Agents* 4: 37–62.

Wise R, Andrews JM, Ashby JP, Thornlier D 1990 The in vitro activity of cefpodoxime: a comparison with other oral cephalosporins. *Journal of Antimicrobial Chemotherapy* 25: 541–550.

OTHER GROUP 5 CEPHALOSPORINS

Cefcapene

A semisynthetic cephalosporin formulated for oral administration as the prodrug ester cefcapene pivoxil. Activity seems to be similar to that of cefpodoxime.

Available in Japan.

Cefdinir

An oral cephalosporin similar in structure to cefixime, but with a slightly modified side-chain at the 7-amino position.

Its activity is similar to that of cefixime, but it is somewhat more active, especially against staphylococci, (Table 15.5). It is not hydrolyzed by staphylococcal or the common plasmid-mediated enterobacterial β-lactamases. An enhancing effect on phagocytosis has been demonstrated in vitro.

Pharmacokinetics

Oral absorption	*c.* 35%
C_{max} 200 mg oral	1 mg/l after *c.* 3 h
400 mg oral	2.15 mg/l after *c.* 3 h
Plasma half-life	1.5 h
Plasma protein binding	60–70%

Absorption is reduced after a fatty meal. Maximum concentrations in suction-induced blister fluid were achieved later than in plasma, but were more prolonged. Concentrations equal to or higher than corresponding plasma levels were present in blister fluid 6–12 h after administration of an oral dose. A total of 12–20% of the dose was excreted into urine within 12 h, the renal elimination declining with increasing dose. The elimination half life and peak plasma concentration are increased in renal failure. About 60% of the drug is removed by hemodialysis.

Cefdinir appears to be well tolerated, although some volunteers receiving the drug experienced diarrhea. Its uses are similar to those of cefixime and other oral cephalosporins with improved β-lactamase stability.

 Preparations and dosage

Proprietary name: Omnicef.

Preparation: Capsules and suspension.

Dosage: Adults, oral, 600 mg per day in 1–2 divided doses. Children, 14 mg/kg per day.

Available in the USA and Japan. Not available in the UK.

 Further information

Cohen MA, Joannides ET, Roland GE et al 1994 In vitro evaluation of cefdinir (FK482), a new oral cephalosporin with enhanced antistaphylococcal activity and beta-lactamase stability. *Diagnostic Microbiology and Infectious Disease* 18: 31–39.

Gerlach EH, Jones RN, Allen SD et al 1992 Cefdinir (FK482), an orally administered cephalosporin in vitro activity comparison against recent clinical isolates from five medical centers and determination of MIC quality control guidelines. *Diagnostic Microbiology and Infectious Disease* 15: 537–543.

Guay DR 2000 Cefdinir: an expanded-spectrum oral cephalosporin. *Annals of Pharmacotherapy* 34: 1469–1477.

Hishida A, Ohishi K, Nagashima S, Kanamura M, Obara M, Kitada A 1998 Pharmacokinetic study of an oral cephalosporin, cefdinir, in haemodialysis patients. *Antimicrobial Agents and Chemotherapy* 42: 1718–1721.

Payne DJ, Amyes SGB 1993 Stability of cefdinir (CI-N983, FK482) to extended-spectrum plasmid-mediated β-lactamases. *Journal of Medical Microbiology* 38: 114–117.

Richer M, Allard S, Manseau L, Vallee F, Pak R, LeBel M 1995 Suction-induced blister fluid penetration of cefdinir in healthy volunteers following ascending oral doses. *Antimicrobial Agents and Chemotherapy* 39: 1082–1086.

Scriver SR, Willey BM, Low DE, Simor AE 1992 Comparative in vitro activity of cefdinir (CI-983; FK-482) against staphylococci, Gram-negative bacilli and respiratory tract pathogens. *European Journal of Clinical Microbiology and Infectious Diseases* 11: 646–652.

Wise R, Andrews JM, Thornber D 1991 The in-vitro activity of cefdinir (FK482), a new oral cephalosporin. *Journal of Antimicrobial Chemotherapy* 28: 239–248.

Cefditoren

A semisynthetic cephalosporin formulated for oral use as the pivaloyloxymethyl ester, cefditoren pivoxil.

It exhibits good activity against staphylococci, streptococci (but not enterococci) and most enterobacteria, including many *Enterobacter*, *Citrobacter*, *Serratia* and *Proteus* species. It is not active against *Ps. aeruginosa* or *Sten. maltophilia*. It is stable to staphylococcal and most enterobacterial β-lactamases.

An oral dose of 200 mg achieves a plasma concentration of around 2.5 mg/l after 1.5 h. It is excreted unchanged into urine.

Clinical experience is limited, but it appears to be well tolerated.

Available in USA and Japan.

 Further information

Felmingham D, Robbins MJ, Ghosh G, et al 1994 An in vitro characterization of cefditoren, a new oral cephalosporin. *Drugs Under Experimental and Clinical Research* 20: 127–147.

Jones RN, Biedenbach DJ, Johnson DM 2000 Cefditoren activity against nearly 1000 non-fastidious bacterial isolates and the development of in vitro susceptibility test methods. *Diagnostic Microbiology and Infectious Diseases* 37: 143–146.

Li JT, Hou F, Lu H, Li TY, Li H 1997 Phase I clinical trial of cefditoren pivoxil (ME 1207). Tolerance in healthy volunteers. *Drugs Under Experimental and Clinical Research* 23: 131–138.

Li JT, Hou F, Lu H, Li TY, Li H 1997 Phase I clinical trial of cefditoren pivoxil (ME 1207): pharmacokinetics in healthy volunteers. *Drugs Under Experimental and Clinical Research* 23: 145–150.

Cefetamet

A semisynthetic cephalosporin formulated for oral use as the prodrug ester, cefetamet pivoxyl.

It is less active than cefaclor and cefadroxil against *Staph. aureus*, but as active against streptococci and more active against enterobacteria, *H. influenzae* and *N. gonorrhoeae*, including β-lactamase-producing strains (Table 15.5). *L. mono-*cytogenes, *Cl. difficile*, *Sten. maltophilia* and *Burk. cepacia* are all resistant. It is resistant to hydrolysis by common plasmid-mediated enzymes.

The pivaloyl ester is orally absorbed and rapidly cleaved by esterases in the gut wall and hepatic circulation to liberate the active parent compound. The absolute bioavailability is about 50%. The plasma peak is delayed by food. Binding to plasma protein is about 20%. The volume of distribution approximates to the extracellular water.

Cefetamet is excreted by the renal route, predominantly in the glomerular filtrate. Elimination is linearly related to creatinine clearance. The normal elimination half-life is 2–2.5 h, but may reach 30 h in anuric subjects. The plasma peak concentration is elevated and delayed, but bioavailability and distribution at steady state are not altered. Cirrhosis has no effect on the bioavailability, and renal and non-renal clearance are not altered.

Its safety profile is similar to that of other oral cephalosporins. It uses are similar to those of cefixime and other oral cephalosporins that exhibit improved β-lactamase stability.

 Preparations and dosage

Preparation: Tablets and suspension.

Dosage: Adult, oral, 0.5–1 g twice daily. Children, 10–20 mg/kg twice daily.

Limited availability.

 Further information

Angehrn P, Hohl P, Then RL 1989 In vitro antibacterial properties of cefetamet and in vivo activity of its orally absorbable ester derivative, cefetamet pivoxil. *European Journal of Clinical Microbiology and Infectious Diseases* 8: 536–543.

Bernstein-Hahn L, Valdes E, Gehanno P et al 1989 Clinical experience with 1000 patients treated with cefetamet pivoxil. *Current Medical Research and Opinion* 11: 442–452.

Blouin R, Stoekel K 1993 Cefetamet pivoxil clinical pharmacokinetics. *Clinical Pharmacokinetics* 25: 172–188.

Bryson HM, Brogden RN 1993 Cefetamet pivoxil: a review of its antibacterial activity, pharmacokinetic properties and therapeutic use. *Drugs* 45: 589–621.

Stoekel K, Tam YK, Kneer J 1989 Pharmacokinetics of oral cefetamet pivoxil (Ro 15–8075) and intravenous cefetamet (Ro 15–8074) in humans: a review. *Current Medical Research and Opinion* 11: 432–441.

Tam YK, Kneer J, Dubach UC, Stoeckel K 1990 Effects of timing and food and fluid volume on cefetamet pivoxil absorption in healthy normal volunteers. *Antimicrobial Agents and Chemotherapy* 34: 1556–1559.

Cefteram

A semisynthetic cephalosporin formulated for oral administration as the prodrug ester cefteram pivoxil. Activity appears to be similar to that of cefixime, but with slightly better activity against staphylococci and some Gram-negative rods.

Available in Japan.

Further information

Jones RN, Fuchs PC, Barry AL, Ayers LW, Gerlach EH, Gavan TL 1987 Antimicrobial activity of Ro 19-5247 (T-2525), a new oral cephalosporin, tested against 7,745 recent clinical isolates. *Diagnostic Microbiology and Infectious Diseases* 6: 193–198.

Ceftibuten

A semisynthetic cephalosporin formulated as the dihydrate for oral administration.

The activity against common pathogens is shown in Table 15.5. It exhibits good activity against many Gram-negative bacilli, but its activity against Gram-positive cocci is very poor. It is stable to hydrolysis by the common plasmid-mediated β-lactamases, but not derepressed chromosomal enzymes (*see* p. 264).

It is rapidly and almost completely absorbed by mouth and is excreted into urine with a half-life of 1.5–3 h. An oral dose of 400 mg achieves a peak plasma concentration of around 15 mg/l. Binding to plasma proteins is 65–77%.

Side effects mostly consist of mild gastrointestinal symptoms and mild liver function test changes. Clinical trials have mainly been conducted in urinary tract and respiratory tract infections which, despite the poor in-vitro activity against *Str. pneumoniae*, have shown ceftibuten to be as efficacious as comparator agents.

Preparations and dosage

Proprietary name: Cedax.

Preparations: Capsules, suspension.

Dosage: Adults and children over 10 years (over 45 kg), oral, 400 mg daily as a single dose. Children over 6 months, 9 mg/kg daily as a single dose.

Available in USA and Japan. Not UK.

Further information

Andrews JM, Wise R, Baldwin DR, Honeybourne D 1995 Concentrations of ceftibuten in plasma and the respiratory tract following a single 400 mg oral dose. *International Journal of Antimicrobial Agents* 5: 141–144.

Guay DR 1997 Ceftibuten: a new expanded-spectrum oral cephalosporin. *Annals of Pharmacotherapy* 31: 1022–1033.

Kearns GL, Young RA 1994 Ceftibuten pharmacokinetics and pharmacodynamics: focus on paediatric use. *Clinical Pharmacokinetics* 26: 169–189.

Owens RC, Nightingale CH, Nicolau DP. 1997 Ceftibuten: an overview. *Pharmacotherapy* 17: 707–720.

Perrotta R, McCabe R, Rumans L, Nolen T 1994 Comparison of the efficacy and safety of ceftibuten and cefaclor in the treatment of acute bacterial bronchitis. *Infectious Diseases in Clinical Practice* 3: 270–276.

Wise R, Andrews JM, Ashby JP, Thornber D 1990 Ceftibuten-in vitro activity against respiratory pathogens, β-lactamase stability and mechanism of action. *Journal of Antimicrobial Chemotherapy* 26: 209–213.

Wiseman LR, Balfour JA 1994 Ceftibuten. A review of its antibacterial activity, pharmacokinetic properties and clinical efficacy. *Drugs* 47: 784–808.

GROUP 6 CEPHALOSPORINS

CEFTAZIDIME

Molecular weight (anhydrous): 546.6; (pentahydrate): 636.7.

A semisynthetic parenteral cephalosporin formulated as the pentahydrate.

Table 15.6 Activity of group 6 cephalosporins against common pathogenic bacteria: MIC (mg/l)

	Cefoperazone	Cefpimizole	Cefpiramide	Cefsulodin	Ceftazidime	Cefepime	Cefpirome
Staph. aureus	1–4	R	1	2–4	4–8	2–4	0.5–1
Str. pyogenes	0.1	1	0.1	2	0.1–0.25	0.1	0.03
*Str. pneumoniae**	0.1–0.25	1	0.1	4–8	0.25	<0.05	<0.05
E. faecalis	64–R	R	R	R	R	R	4–R
N. gonorrhoeae	0.06	0.08		4–8	0.06–0.1	0.1	0.03
N. meningitidis	0.06			4–8	<0.01		
H. influenzae	0.1	0.25	0.5	32	0.1		
Esch. coli	0.1–2	0.5	0.5	64–R	0.1	0.1–0.5	0.1–0.5
K. pneumoniae	0.5–8	4	2	64–R	0.1	0.1–0.5	0.1–0.5
Ps. aeruginosa	4–8	8	2	2	1–4	8–16	2–8
B. fragilis	16–32	R	R	R	16–64	R	R

R, resistant (MIC >64 mg/l) *Penicillin-resistant strains are often less susceptible.

Antimicrobial activity

Its activity against common pathogenic bacteria is shown in Table 15.6. Its activity is comparable to that of cefotaxime and ceftizoxime, but it is more active against *Ps. aeruginosa*, including almost all gentamicin-resistant strains, and *Burk. cepacia*. It is, however, less active against *Staph. aureus*. It is stable to a wide range of β-lactamases, but is hydrolyzed by some TEM variants (*see* p. 264).

Pharmacokinetics

C_{max} 500 mg intramuscular	18–20 mg/l
2 g intravenous (20 min infusion)	185 mg/l end infusion
Plasma half-life	1.5–2 h
Volume of distribution	16 l
Plasma protein binding	*c.* 10%

No accumulation was seen in subjects receiving 2 g 12-hourly over 8 days. In premature infants given 25 mg/kg twice daily, mean peak plasma concentrations were 77 mg/l after intravenous and 56 mg/l after intramuscular administration, with plasma elimination half-lives of 7.3 and 14.2 h, respectively. Postnatal age was the most important determinant of elimination rate, which was halved after 5 days. In newborn infants given 50 mg/kg intravenously over 20 min, mean peak plasma concentrations varied inversely with gestational age from 102 to 124 mg/l, with half-lives of 2.9–6.7 h.

Distribution

There is ready penetration into serous fluids, the concentration reaching 50% or more of those of the simultaneous serum level. In patients given 1 g intravenously during abdominal surgery, detectable concentrations appeared within a few minutes in the peritoneal fluid reaching a peak around 67 mg/l with a half-life of 0.9 h. Following a similar intravenous dose, a mean peak of 9.4 mg/l was reached at 2 h in ascitic fluid. Concentrations in middle ear fluid after 1 g intravenously were broadly comparable to those of the plasma.

In patients with meningitis, CSF concentrations of 2–30 mg/l have been found 2–3 h after doses of 2 g intravenously over 30 min given 8-hourly for four doses. Mean concentrations in patients receiving 2 or 3 g doses were substantially less (0.8 mg/l) in the absence of meningitis than in its presence (22.6 mg/l). Penetration occurred into intracranial abscesses with concentrations of 3–27 mg/g being found in patients treated with 0.5–2 g three times daily. Concentrations around 0.4 mg/g in skin, 0.6 mg/g in muscle and 0.2 mg/g in fatty tissue have been found in patients given 2 g intravenously over 5 min preoperatively. A similar dose has produced mean prostate tissue:serum ratios of around 0.14. Effective concentrations are achieved in bone: in patients given 1 g intravenously mean bone concentrations were 14.4 mg/kg 35–40 min after the dose.

Metabolism and excretion

No metabolites of the drug have been detected. There is secretion in breast milk, peak concentrations being around 5 mg/l at about 1 h in patients receiving 2 g intravenously 8-hourly. Elimination is almost exclusively renal, predominantly via the glomerular filtrate, with 80–90% of the dose appearing in the urine in the first 24 h. A slight but significant increase in the fraction filtered has been noted on repeated dosage. Renal clearance is between 90 and 115 ml/min. Elimination half-life is inversely correlated with creatinine clearance: as the values fall to 2–12 ml/min, the mean plasma half-life rises to 16 h. In patients maintained on hemodialysis the half-life fell to 2.8 h on dialysis. No accumulation occurred over 10 days in severe renal impairment on a daily dose of 0.5–1 g.

There is some excretion in bile, concentrations of 6.6–58 mg/l being found 25–160 min after the dose at times when the mean serum concentration was 77.4 mg/l. In T-tube bile there was considerable interpatient variation, with mean concentrations of 34 mg/l at 1–2 h after the dose. No accumulation occurs in patients with impaired hepatic function, but the presence of ascites, low plasma albumin and accumulation of protein-binding inhibitors may increase the volume of distribution.

Toxicity and side effects

Ceftazidime is generally well tolerated. Pain on intramuscular injection experienced with preparations containing sodium carbonate is now avoided by formulations containing arginine. Reactions common to cephalosporins have been observed in some patients, including positive antiglobulin tests without hemolysis, raised liver function test values, eosinophilia, rashes, leukopenia, thrombocytopenia and diarrhea, occasionally associated with the presence of toxigenic *Cl. difficile*.

Failure of therapy has been associated with superinfection with resistant organisms, including *Staph. aureus*, enterococci and *Candida*, or emergence of resistance principally in *Ps. aeruginosa*, *Ser. marcescens* or *Enterobacter* spp. associated with induction of chromosomal β-lactamases. Fecal enterobacterial counts may fall significantly on therapy, while anaerobes remain intact. An increase in ampicillin-resistant enterobacteria after treatment is common.

Clinical use

Ceftazidime has been successfully used, often combined with an aminoglycoside, to treat a wide range of severe urinary, respiratory and wound infections, mostly due to enterobacteria or *Ps. aeruginosa*. Reference is made to its use in pneumonia, septicemia, meningitis (especially if caused by *Ps. aeruginosa*), peritonitis, osteomyelitis, neonatal sepsis, burns and melioidosis. Concern has been expressed at the relative frequency with which failure is associated with superinfection or the emergence of resistance.

Preparations and dosage

Proprietary names: Fortum, Kefadim.

Preparation: Injection.

Dosage: Adults i.m., i.v., 1–6 g/day in divided doses, depending on severity of infection. Neonates and children up to 2 months, 25–60 mg/kg per day in two divided doses; children >2 months 30–100 mg/kg per day in 2–3 divided doses (maximum dose 150 mg/kg per day).

Widely available.

Further information

Anonymous 1999 Ceftazidime. In: Dollery C (ed.) *Therapeutic Drugs* 2nd edn. Churchill Livingstone, Edinburgh, pp. C120–C125.

Boogaerts MA, Demuynck H, Mestdagh N et al 1995 Equivalent efficacies of meropenem and ceftazidime as empirical monotherapy of febrile neutropenic patients. *Journal of Antimicrobial Chemotherapy* 36: 185–200.

Burwen DR, Banerjee SN, Gaynes RP 1994 Ceftazidime resistance among selected nosocomial Gram-negative bacilli in the United States. *Journal of Infectious Diseases* 170: 1622–1625.

Chaowagul W 2000 Recent advances in the treatment of severe melioidosis. *Acta Tropica* 74: 133–137.

Demotes-Mainard F, Vincon G, Ragnaud JM, Morlat P, Bannwarth B, Dangoumau J 1993 Pharmacokinetics of intravenous and intraperitoneal ceftazidime in chronic ambulatory peritoneal dialysis. *Journal of Clinical Pharmacology* 33: 475–479.

De Pauw BE, Deresinski SC, Feld R, Lane Allman EF, Donnelly JP, Elahi N 1994 Ceftazidime compared with piperacillin and tobramycin for the empiric treatment of fever in neutropenic patients with cancer: a multicenter randomized trial. *Annals of Internal Medicine* 120: 834–844.

Fong IN, Tomkins KB 1985 Review of *Pseudomonas aeruginosa* meningitis with special emphasis on treatment with ceftazidime. *Reviews of Infectious Diseases* 7: 604–612.

Green HT, O'Donoghue MAT, Shaw MDM, Dowling C 1989 Pentration of ceftazidime into intracranial abscess. *Journal of Antimicrobial Chemotherapy* 24: 431–436.

Jonsson M, Walder M 1992 Pharmacokinetics of ceftazidime in acutely ill hospitalised elderly patients. *European Journal of Clinical Microbiology and Infectious Diseases* 11: 15–21.

Lin MS, Wang LS, Huang JD 1989 Single- and multiple-dose pharmacokinetics of ceftazidime in infected patients with varying degrees of renal function. *Journal of Clinical Pharmacology* 29: 331–337.

Norrby SR, Finch RG, Glauser M et al 1993 Monotherapy in serious hospital-acquired infections: a clinical trial of ceftazidime versus imipenem/cilastatin. *Journal of Antimicrobial Chemotherapy* 31: 927–937.

O'Donoghue MA, Green HT, Mackenzie IJ, Durham L, Dowling CA 1989 Ceftazidime in middle ear fluid. *Journal of Antimicrobial Chemotherapy* 23: 664–666.

Rains CP, Bryson HM, Peters DH 1995 Ceftazidime: An update of its antibacterial activity, pharmacokinetic properties and therapeutic efficacy. *Drugs* 49: 577–617.

Tessin I, Trollfors B, Thiringer K, Thorn Z, Larsson P 1989 Concentrations of ceftazidime, tobramycin and ampicillin in the cerebrospinal fluid of newborn infants. *European Journal of Pediatrics* 148: 678–681.

Walstad RA, Aanerud L, Thurmann-Nielsen E 1988 Pharmacokinetics and tissue concentrations of ceftazidime in burn patients. *European Journal of Clinical Pharmacology* 35: 543–549.

Walstad RA, Dahl K, Hellum KB, Thurmann-Nielsen E 1988 The pharmacokinetics of ceftazidime in patients with impaired renal function and concurrent frusemide therapy. *European Journal of Clinical Pharmacology* 35: 272–279.

CEFPIROME

Molecular weight (sulfate): 612.7.

A semisynthetic aminothiazoyl cephalosporin formulated as the sulfate for parenteral administration.

Antimicrobial activity

Activity against common pathogens (Table 15.6) is similar to that of cefotaxime and ceftriaxone, but it is more active against *Ps. aeruginosa*. Unlike other cephalosporins cefpirome exhibits activity against some strains of enterococci (MIC 4–16 mg/l), but this is of doubtful clinical benefit. It is generally very stable to β-lactamases. There is very low affinity for the molecular class C (functional group 1) cephalosporinases of many enterobacteria (*see* p. 262) and is active against producer strains such as *Enterobacter* spp., *Citrobacter* spp., *Hafnia* spp. *Providencia* spp. *Ser. marcescens* and *Pr. vulgaris* (MIC 0.03–0.25 mg/l). *Sten. maltophilia* is resistant.

Pharmacokinetics

C_{max} 1 g intramuscular	25 mg/l after 1.6–2.3 h
1 g intravenous	97 mg/l end injection
Plasma half-life	1.4 2.3 h
Volume of distribution	*c.* 17 l
Plasma protein binding	10%

Absorption and distribution

Cefpirome is not absorbed by the oral route, but is rapidly absorbed after intramuscular injection. It is well distributed and achieves therapeutic concentrations in tissues and exudates. It penetrates poorly into CSF in the absence of meningeal inflammation, but concentrations around 2–4 mg/l have been found in patients with purulent meningitis.

Metabolism and excretion

Little, if any, of the drug is metabolized and most is excreted unchanged into urine within 12 h, mainly by glomerular filtration. Clearance declines in proportion to renal function. Around 60% of the drug is removed in 3 h by hemodialysis. Low concentrations are found in breast milk.

Toxicity and side effects

Side effects are those common to other cephalosporins. Diarrhea is common and occasional cases of pseudomembranous colitis have been reported.

Clinical use

It is mainly used in the treatment of serious sepsis, particularly nosocomial infections in which resistant Gram-negative pathogens are known or suspected to be involved.

Preparations and dosage

Proprietary name: Cefrom.

Preparation: Injection.

Dosage: i.v., 1–2 g every 12 h. Not recommended for children under 12. Available in the UK and continental Europe.

Further information

Anonymous 1999 Cefpirome. In Dollery C (ed.) *Therapeutic Drugs* 2nd edn. Churchill Livingstone, Edinburgh, pp. C109–C113.

Kavi J, Andrews JM, Ashby JP, Hillman G, Wise R 1988 Pharmacokinetics and tissue penetration of cefpirome, a new cephalosporin. *Journal of Antimicrobial Chemotherapy* 22: 911–916.

Kearns GL, Weber W, Harnisch L et al 1995 Single-dose pharmacokinetics of cefpirome in paediatric patients. *Clinical Drug Investigation* 10: 71–78.

Kobayashi S, Arai S, Hayashi S, Fujimoto K 1986 β-Lactamase stability of cefpirome (HR 810) a new cephalosporin with a broad antimicrobial spectrum. *Antimicrobial Agents and Chemotherapy* 30: 713–718.

Mitsukude M, Inoue M, Mitsuhashi S 1989 In vitro and in vivo antibacterial activity of the new semisynthetic cephalosporin cefpirome. *Arzneimittelforschung* 39: 26–30.

Neu HC, Chin NX, Labthavikul P 1985 The in vitro activity and beta-lactamase stability of cefpirome (HR 810), a pyridine cephalosporin agent active against staphylococci, enterobacteriaceae and *Pseudomonas aeruginosa*. *Infection* 13: 146–155.

Rubinstein E, Labs R, Reeves A 1993 A review of the adverse effects profile of cefpirome. *Drug Safety* 9: 340–345.

Strenkoski LC, Nix DE 1993 Cefpirome clinical pharmacokinetics. *Clinical Pharmacokinetics* 25: 263–273.

Wiseman LR, Lamb HM 1997 Cefpirome. A review of its antibacterial activity, pharmacokinetic properties and clinical efficacy in the treatment of severe nosocomial infections and febrile neutropenia. *Drugs* 54: 117–140.

OTHER GROUP 6 CEPHALOSPORINS

Cefepime

A semisynthetic parenteral cephalosporin formulated as the hydrochloride.

Its activity against common pathogens (Table 15.6) is comparable to that of group 4 cephalosporins, but it is somewhat more active against *Ps. aeruginosa*. Like cefpirome it has low affinity for the molecular class C cephalosporinases of many Gram-negative rods (p. 262) and is consequently active against most strains of *Citrobacter* spp., *Enterobacter* spp., *Serratia* spp. and *Ps. aeruginosa* that are resistant to cefotaxime and ceftazidime. It has poor activity against *L. monocytogenes* and against anaerobic organisms.

Pharmacokinetics

C_{max} 2 g intravenous (30 min infusion)	190 mg/l end infusion
Plasma half-life	*c.* 2 h
Volume of distribution	14–20 l
Plasma protein binding	10–19%

Its penetration into tissues, including lung, appears to be similar to that of other aminothiazoyl cephalosporins. Virtually the whole dose is excreted into urine over 8 h. It is used for the treatment of serious infection due to organisms resistant to group 4 compounds. It appears to be well tolerated.

Preparations and dosage

Proprietary name: Maxipime.

Preparation: Injection.

Dosage: Adult, i.m., i.v., 1–6 g per day in divided doses. Available in USA and Japan. Not available in UK.

Further information

Barbhaiya RH, Forgue ST, Gleason CR et al 1992 Pharmacokinetics of cefepime after single and multiple intravenous administrations in healthy subjects. *Antimicrobial Agents and Chemotherapy* 36: 552–557.

Barradell LB, Bryson HM 1994 Cefepime: a review of its antibacterial activity, pharmacokinetic properties and therapeutic use. *Drugs* 47: 471–505.

Brown EM, Finch RG, White LO (eds) 1993 Cefepime: a β-lactamase-stable extended-spectrum cephalosporin. *Journal of Antimicrobial Chemotherapy* 32 (Suppl. B): 1–214.

Fung-Tomc J, Dougherty TJ, DeOrio FJ, Simich-Jacobson V, Kessler RE 1989 Activity of cefepime against ceftazidime- and cefotaxime-resistant Gram-negative bacteria and its relationship to β-lactamase levels. *Antimicrobial Agents and Chemotherapy* 33: 498–502.

Kieft H, Hoepelman AIM, Rozenberg Arska M et al 1994 Cefepime compared with ceftazidime as initial therapy for serious bacterial infections and sepsis syndrome. *Antimicrobial Agents and Chemotherapy* 38: 415–42.

Liu YC, Huang WK, Cheng DL 1994 Antibacterial activity of cefepime in vitro. *Chemotherapy* 40: 384–390.

Rybak M 1996 The pharmacokinetic profile of a new generation of parenteral cephalosporin. *American Journal of Medicine* 100 (6A): 39S–44S.

Saez Llorens X, Castano E, Garcia R et al 1995 Prospective randomized comparison of cefepime and cefotaxime for treatment of bacterial meningitis in infants and children. *Antimicrobial Agents and Chemotherapy* 39: 937–940.

Wynd MA, Paladino JA 1996 Cefepime: a fourth-generation parenteral cephalosporin. *Annals of Pharmacotherapy* 30: 1414–1424.

Cefoperazone

A semisynthetic parenteral cephalosporin. It is unstable, losing activity on storage even at –20°C.

Its activity against common pathogenic bacteria is shown in Table 15.6. It exhibits moderate activity against carbenicillin-sensitive strains of *Ps. aeruginosa*. Activity against *Burk. cepacia* and *Sten. maltophilia* is unreliable. It is much less stable to enterobacterial β-lactamases than most other cephalosporins of groups 4–6 and consequently has unreliable activity against many species, including β-lactamase-producing strains of *H. influenzae* and *N. gonorrhoeae*. It is active against *Achromobacter*, *Flavobacterium*, *Aeromonas* and associated non-fermenters. *Past. multocida* is extremely susceptible (MIC <0.01–0.02 mg/l). It exhibits modest activity against most Gram-negative anaerobes, but not *B. fragilis*.

Combination with β-lactamase inhibitors renders many resistant strains susceptible and a formulation with sulbactam is available in some countries (*see* p. 275). Sulbactam increases activity against many, but not all, enterobacteria and non-fermenters, and almost all *B. fragilis*.

Pharmacokinetics

C_{max} 2 g intravenous (15–30 min infusion)	250 mg/l end infusion
Plasma half-life	1.5–2 h
Volume of distribution	10–17 l
Plasma protein binding	85–95%

It achieves therapeutic concentrations in tissue and inflammatory exudates. Variable low levels are found in the sputum up to 1.5% of simultaneous serum levels. Penetration into CSF is unreliable even in the presence of meningeal inflammation.

The bile is a major route of excretion, accounting for almost 20% of the dose. About 20–30% is eliminated in urine, almost entirely by glomerular filtration. The fate of the rest is unknown. Clearance is effectively unchanged by renal failure or dialysis.

It is generally well tolerated. Side effects associated with the methylthiotetrazole side-chain have been reported. Diarrhea has been notable in some studies. Marked suppression of fecal flora, with the appearance of *Cl. difficile*, has been found in some patients. There is a 5–10% incidence of mild transient increases in liver function tests.

It has been widely used, especially in circumstances in which the antipseudomonal activity has been felt to be an advantage. It potential toxicity and the availability of compounds with better β-lactamase stability and more reliable antipseudomonal activity have undermined its popularity.

Preparations and dosage

Preparation: Injection.

Dosage: Adults, i.m., i.v., 2–4 g/day in two divided doses; in severe infections up to 12 g/day in 2–4 divided doses. Children, 25–100 mg/kg twice daily.

Widely available, except UK.

Further information

Brogden RN, Carmine A, Heel RC, Morley PA, Speight TM, Avery GS 1981 Cefoperazone: a review of its in vitro antimicrobial activity, pharmacological properties and therapeutic efficacy. *Drugs* 22: 423–460.

Fass RJ, Gregory WW, D'Amato RF, Matsen JM, Wright DN, Young LS 1990 In vitro activities of cefoperazone and sulbactam singly and in combination against cefoperazone-resistant members of the family Enterobacteriaceae and non-fermenters. *Antimicrobial Agents and Chemotherapy* 34: 2256–2259.

Greenberg RN, Cayavec P, Danko LS et al 1994 Comparison of cefoperazone plus sulbactam with clindamycin plus gentamicin as treatment for intra-abdominal infections. *Journal of Antimicrobial Chemotherapy* 34: 391–401.

Reitberg DP, Whall TJ, Chung M, Blickens D, Swarz H, Arnold J 1988 Multiple-dose pharmacokinetics and toleration of intravenously administered cefoperazone and sulbactam when given as single agents and in combination. *Antimicrobial Agents and Chemotherapy* 32: 42–46.

Silva M, Cornick MA, Gorbach SL 1989 Suppression of colonic microflora by cefoperazone and evaluation of the drug as potential prophylaxis in bowel surgery. *Antimicrobial Agents and Chemotherapy* 33: 835–838.

Symposium 1983 Evaluation of cefoperazone. *Reviews of Infectious Diseases* 5 (Suppl. 1): S108–S209.

Welage IS, Borin MT, Wilton JH, Hejmanowski LG, Wels PB, Schentag JJ 1990 Comparative evaluation of the pharmacokinetics of *N*-methyl-thiotetrazole following administration of cefoperazone, cefotetan, and cefmetazole. *Antimicrobial Agents and Chemotherapy* 34: 2369–2374.

Cefpimizole

A semisynthetic parenteral cephalosporin.

It exhibits modest activity compared to other antipseudomonal cephalosporins (Table 15.6). Like cefoperazone, it is susceptible to many enterobacterial β-lactamases. In volunteers receiving 0.1–1 g intramuscularly mean peak plasma concentrations reached 15–20 and 35–40 mg/l respectively. There was no accumulation when the dose was repeated 8-hourly for 7 days. No metabolites have been detected. The plasma elimination half-life is 1.8–2.1 h. The principal route of elimination is renal, 70–80% being recovered unchanged in the urine.

Significant pain at the site of infection has been a prominent adverse event. A single dose of 1 g, but not less, has been successful in curing urethral but not rectal or pharyngeal gonorrhea.

Preparations

Available in Japan.

Further information

Jones RN, Ayers LW, Gavan TL, Gerlach EH, Sommers HM 1985 In vitro comparative antimicrobial activity of cefpimizole against clinical isolates from five medical centers. *Antimicrobial Agents and Chemotherapy* 27: 982–984.

Novak E, Lakings DB, Paxton LM 1987 Tolerance and disposition of cefpimizole in normal human volunteers after intramuscular administration. *Antimicrobial Agents and Chemotherapy* 31: 1706–1710.

Cefpiramide

A semisynthetic parenteral cephalosporin.

It exhibits a broad range of activity, which includes *Ps. aeruginosa*, though the overall activity is rather modest (Table 15.6). It is moderately stable to most β-lactamases but less so than ceftazidime or cefpirome.

In volunteers given 0.5 or 1 g by intravenous bolus, the mean plasma concentration shortly after injection was around 150 or 300 mg/l, respectively. There was no accumulation when the same doses were repeated 12-hourly for 11 doses. It is highly bound to plasma protein (*c.* 95%). The mean plasma half-life is around 5 h. Less than a quarter of the dose appears in the urine over 24 h. The rest is excreted in bile and high concentrations are found in feces.

Renal impairment has little effect on elimination in patients with normal liver function. Diarrhea may be associated with marked suppression of gut flora resulting from biliary excretion of the drug. The molecule includes a C-3 methylthio-tetrazole side-chain and side effects associated with that substituent are to be expected.

Preparations and dosage

Preparation: Injection.

Dosage: Adult, i.v., 1–2 g per day in two divided doses.

Available in Japan.

Further information

Barry AL, Jones RN, Thornsberry C et al 1985 Cefpiramide: comparative in-vitro activity and β-lactamase stability. *Journal of Antimicrobial Chemotherapy* 16: 315–325.

Brogard JM, Jeal F, Adloff M, Bickle JF, Montell H 1988 High hepatic excretion in humans of cefpiramide, a new cephalosporin. *Antimicrobial Agents and Chemotherapy* 32: 1360–1364.

Conte JE 1987 Pharmacokinetics of cefpiramide in volunteers with normal or impaired renal function. *Antimicrobial Agents and Chemotherapy* 31: 1585–1588.

Demontes-Mainard F, Vinccon G, Labat L et al 1994 Cefpiramide kinetics and plasma protein binding in cholestasis. *British Journal of Clinical Pharmacology* 37: 295–297.

Matsui H, Okada T 1988 Renal tubular mechanisms for excretion of cefpiramide (SM-1 652) in association with its longlasting pharmacokinetic properties. *Journal of Pharmacobiodynamics* 11: 67–73.

Nakagawa K, Koyama M, Matsui H et al 1984 Pharmacokinetics of cefpiramide (SM-1652) in humans. *Antimicrobial Agents and Chemotherapy* 25: 221–225.

Quentin C, Noury P, Titonel M 1989 Comparative in vitro activity of cefpiramide, a new parenteral cephalosporin. *European Journal of Clinical Microbiology and Infectious Diseases* 7: 544–549.

Cefsulodin

A semisynthetic parenteral cephalosporin supplied as the sodium salt.

Its activity against *Ps. aeruginosa* contrasts strikingly with poor activity against many other organisms (Table 15.6).

Anaerobic Gram-negative rods, Gram-positive rods and cocci are all resistant. It is stable to many β-lactamases, including the *Ps. aeruginosa* chromosomal enzyme, and is a poor substrate for the enzymes of *Enterobacter* spp. and *Morg. morganii*. It is slowly hydrolyzed by TEM β-lactamases and more rapidly by the enzymes of some carbenicillin-resistant strains of *Ps. aeruginosa*, with which distinct inoculum effects may be seen.

Pharmacokinetics

C$_{max}$ 500 mg intramuscular	15 mg/l
500 mg intravenous (bolus)	70 mg/l end injection
Plasma half-life	1.5 h
Volume of distribution	18 l
Plasma protein binding	15–30%

There is some metabolism of the drug, but the main route of excretion is via the kidneys, most appearing in the urine in the first 6 h. It accumulates in renal failure, but the volume of distribution is unaffected. The plasma half-life is linearly related to creatinine clearance, rising to a mean of 10–13 h in patients where clearance was <10 ml/min, falling to around 2 h on hemodialysis.

It is well tolerated, apart from nausea and vomiting in some subjects. It has been used in severe pseudomonas infections, usually in combination with an aminoglycoside, but treatment has been complicated on a number of occasions by the emergence of resistance or superinfection.

Preparations and dosage

Proprietary name: Monaspor.

Preparation: Injection.

Dosage: Adults, i.m., i.v., 1–4 g/day in 2–4 divided doses, increased in severe infections to 6 g/day. Children, 20–50 mg/kg per day (maximum dose 100 mg/kg per day).

Limited availability.

Further information

Granneman GR, Sennello LT, Sonders RC, Wynne B, Thomas EW 1982 Cefsulodin kinetics in healthy subjects after intramuscular and intravenous injection. *Clinical Pharmacology and Therapeutics* 31: 95–103.

King A, Shannon K, Phillips I 1980 In vitro antibacterial activity and susceptibility of cefsulodin, an antipseudomonal cephalosporin, to beta-lactamases. *Antimicrobial Agents and Chemotherapy* 17: 165–169.

Reed MD, Stern RC, Yamashita TS, Ackers I, Myers CM, Blumer JL 1984 Single-dose pharmacokinetics of cefsulodin in patients with cystic fibrosis. *Antimicrobial Agents and Chemotherapy* 25: 579–581.

Wright DB 1986 Cefsulodin. *Drug Intelligence and Clinical Pharmacy* 20: 845–849.

Young LS 1984 *Pseudomonas aeruginosa* – biology, immunology and therapy: a cefsulodin symposium. *Reviews of Infectious Diseases* 6 (Suppl. 3): S603–S776.

INVESTIGATIONAL CEPHALOSPORINS

The search (possibly futile) for the 'ideal' cephalosporin with favorable antimicrobial, pharmacological and toxicological properties continues unabated, mainly in Japan. The hunt continues for oral and parenteral compounds with further enhanced activity against *Ps. aeruginosa* and other refractory Gram-negative rods, as well as – most elusive of all – molecules with potent activity against enterococci and methicillin-resistant staphylococci. Among cephalosporins described in recent years that aspire to these properties are cefoselis, cefclidin, cefluprenam and cefozopran. Available literature on these compounds makes them difficult to assess at the time of writing and it remains to be seen whether any of them will emerge to challenge the agents that are presently favored in therapeutic practice.

16 β-Lactam antibiotics: penicillins

K. Bush

The penicillin class of antibiotics comprises a large group of bicyclic penam compounds (p. 259) differing in the nature of the acyl side chain attached to the fused β-lactam–thiazolidine ring system. Most are semisynthetic derivatives of the penicillin nucleus, 6-aminopenicillanic acid (6-APA), prepared synthetically by the addition of acyl side chains at the 6-amino group.

Fleming reported the discovery of penicillin as the compound responsible for the antibacterial activity displayed by the mold *Penicillium notatum* in 1929, but it was not until 1940 that Florey and his collaborators at Oxford isolated the active material. Later studies showed that the product derived from industrial fermentations of *Penicillium chrysogenum* was, in fact, a family of closely related compounds differing only in the nature of the acyl side chain. These natural penicillins consisted of penicillins F (pentenylpenicillin), G (benzylpenicillin), K (heptylpenicillin) and X (*p*-hydroxybenzylpenicillin). From this family, benzylpenicillin (penicillin G) was selected as the penicillin most suitable for clinical development based on biological properties and ease of commercial production.

The limitations of benzylpenicillin as an antibacterial agent soon led to efforts to produce novel penicillins with superior properties to the naturally occurring substance. In early work acidic side-chain precursors that could be assimilated by the mold during biosynthesis were added during the fermentation. However, only a limited number of different side chains could be introduced this way; the only penicillin produced by this process with any advantage over penicillin G was phenoxymethylpenicillin (penicillin V), the product of fermentations to which phenoxyacetic acid had been added as a precursor. The development of penicillin V as a clinically useful agent was based on its improved antibacterial activity and oral absorption, combined with acid stability, compared with penicillin G.

Another approach was the preparation of the first semisynthetic penicillins by chemical substitution of the *p*-hydroxy group of the naturally occurring penicillin X (*p*-hydroxybenzylpenicillin); however none of these derivatives was better than penicillin G. This approach was also unsuccessful in a later program to prepare novel penicillins by modification of the amino group of *p*-aminobenzylpenicillin. Although failing in its original objective to produce clinically useful semisynthetic penicillins, this research led to the important identification in 1957 of the penicillin nucleus in fermentations carried out in the absence of side-

chain precursors. This nucleus, 6-aminopenicillanic acid (6-APA), was first isolated and produced as a naturally occurring substance in fermentations of *P. chrysogenum*. It was later obtained more easily by removal of the benzylpenicillin side chain by microbial enzymes or by chemical modification, the process now used for commercial production.

The significance of the identification of 6-APA is that there is almost no limit to the number of semisynthetic penicillins that can be prepared by adding acyl side-chain structures to the 6-amino group of the molecule. Since 1959 thousands of novel structures have been reported in the literature. With the exceptions of penicillin G and penicillin V, the penicillins in clinical use are all derived from 6-APA, and display advantages over benzylpenicillin in antibacterial activity, stability to bacterial β-lactamases or pharmacokinetic properties. Attempts to further modify the penicillin nucleus have been disappointing. Only two clinically useful compounds have resulted: mecillinam (amdinocillin), in which the side chain is joined in an amidino linkage; and temocillin, in which a 6-methoxy group has been incorporated in the β-lactam ring. After the late 1970s, research emphasis in the β-lactam field switched from penicillins to other β-lactam agents, notably the cephalosporins, cephamycins, carbapenems, penems, monobactams and penicillanic acid sulfones (pp. 259–260), and the development of novel penams appears to have come to a halt.

CLASSIFICATION

Essentially, the objectives of research initiated following the isolation of 6-APA were:

- Synthesis of narrow-spectrum penicillins similar to benzylpenicillin in activity but with superior oral absorption characteristics.
- Preparation of penicillins stable to staphylococcal β-lactamase and active against penicillin-resistant staphylococci.
- Development of penicillins with broader spectra of antibacterial activity than benzylpenicillin and stability to plasmid-encoded class A β-lactamases (p. 262).

The first two objectives were achieved with some success but the third with less success, in that the extended-spectrum penicillins (with the exception of temocillin) are largely inactive against β-lactamase-producing bacteria. Some broad-spectrum penicillins, however, have achieved clinical success when combined with β-lactamase inhibitors (p. 272).

The large number of semisynthetic penicillins in clinical use may be divided into six major groups.

- *Group 1*: Benzylpenicillin and its long-acting parenteral forms.
- *Group 2*: Orally absorbed penicillins similar to benzylpenicillin.
- *Group 3*: Penicillins that are relatively stable to staphylococcal β-lactamase, but which have no useful activity against Gram-negative bacilli. Several are structurally related isoxazoylpenicillins.
- *Group 4*: Compounds with enhanced activity against certain Gram-negative bacilli, including many enterobacteria and *Haemophilus influenzae*, but which are inactivated by staphylococcal and many enterobacterial β-lactamases. They include several aminopenicillins, such as ampicillin and amoxicillin, and the amidinopenicillin mecillinam. Various esters and condensates of ampicillin and a mecillinam ester, pivmecillinam, have been developed to improve the poor oral absorption of the parent compounds to which they owe their antimicrobial activity.
- *Group 5*: Penicillins active against *Pseudomonas aeruginosa*. These include carboxypenicillins (and their orally absorbed esters) and acyl or acylureido derivatives of ampicillin.
- *Group 6*: Penicillins resistant to enterobacterial β-lactamases.

MODE OF ACTION

The target sites for penicillins and other β-lactam antibiotics are cell-wall synthesizing enzymes, 'penicillin-binding proteins' (PBPs), attached to the cytoplasmic membrane (p. 14). PBPs are not found in mammalian cells, which accounts for the low toxicity of penicillins and the consequent clinical popularity of this class of antibiotics.

Because of their mode of action, penicillins can facilitate the access of compounds acting on internal targets, potentiating inhibition or killing, as in classical synergy with aminoglycosides.

ACQUIRED RESISTANCE

Bacteria may exhibit resistance to penicillins and other β-lactam antibiotics by several mechanisms (*see also* Ch. 3).

- Acquisition of PBPs with reduced affinity for penicillin. This is a frequent cause of resistance in Gram-positive bacteria such as staphylococci, pneumococci and enterococci. This mechanism is also responsible for low-level penicillin resistance in *Haemophilus influenzae*, *Neisseria gonorrhoeae* and viridans streptococci.
- The production of a bacterial enzyme, β-lactamase, that opens the β-lactam ring, causing inactivation of the antibiotic.
- Modification of the outer membrane in Gram-negative bacteria creating a permeability barrier to the passage of penicillins into the bacterial cell. Recently, efflux mechanisms have been described in which bacteria pump out β-lactam antibiotics.

Frequently bacteria display more than one resistance mechanism. For example: methicillin-resistant staphylococci typically produce β-lactamase but have resistance primarily due to altered target sites; Gram-negative bacteria that produce β-lactamases in organisms with efflux mechanisms or altered outer membrane proteins.

Methicillin-resistant strains of *Staphylococcus aureus* (MRSA) are considered to be resistant to all β-lactam antibiotics and are frequently multiresistant, being susceptible only to glycopeptides (Ch. 22), or to newer agents such as linezolid (Ch. 28). The prevalence of MRSA is variable, with very low incidence in some countries of northern Europe, but high incidence in Japan and many other countries. In the USA the frequency increased from 2.4% in 1975 to 35% in 1996. Although largely confined to hospitals, where its appearance can cause the closure of wards and units and a halt to patient transfer, MRSA is increasingly being seen in community settings.

Group 1	Group 2	Group 3	Group 4	Group 5	Group 6
Benzylpenicillin	Azidocillin	Cloxacillin[a]	Ampicillin	Apalcillin	Temocillin
Benzathine penicillin	Phenethicillin	Dicloxacillin[a]	Amoxicillin	Aspoxicillin	
Clemizole penicillin	Phenoxymethyl	Flucloxacillin[a]	Ciclacillin	Azlocillin[b]	
Procaine penicillin	penicillin	Methicillin	Epicillin	Carbenicillin[c]	
	Propicillin	Nafcillin	Mecillinam	Mezlocillin[b]	
		Oxacillin[a]		Piperacillin[b]	
				Ticarcillin[c]	

[a] Isoxazolylpenicillins; [b]acyureidopencillins; [c]carboxypenicillins.

Methicillin resistance is even higher among *Staphylococcus epidermidis* and other coagulase-negative staphylococci, which, together with *Staph. aureus* and enterococci, represent the three most common causes of nosocomial bloodstream infections in the USA.

Until comparatively recently, clinical isolates of *Streptococcus pneumoniae* were uniformly susceptible to penicillin, but this has changed dramatically. The prevalence of pneumococci with reduced susceptibility to penicillins and other β-lactam agents is increasing worldwide. In 1990 the frequency of isolation of penicillin-resistant pneumococci was 51% in Hungary, 4% in the USA and 2% in the UK; in 1998 the incidence of insusceptible pneumococci was 24% in the USA and 9% in the UK. For most isolates the minimum inhibitory concentration (MIC) is in the intermediate category (penicillin MIC 0.1–1.0 mg/l), implying that high dosage will still provide effective concentrations, except in difficult-to-reach compartments such as cerebrospinal fluid (CSF); however, the frequency of isolation of pneumococci with full resistance (penicillin MIC ≥ 2 mg/l) is increasing.

As with pneumococci, enterococci were perceived always to be susceptible to ampicillin and benzylpenicillin, but resistant strains are being encountered with increasing frequency. Resistance is less prevalent among the most common species, *Enterococcus faecalis*, in which β-lactamase production is the major mechanism, than in *Enterococcus faecium*, the next most clinically important enterococcal species, in which high-level penicillin resistance is usual. Unlike *E. faecalis*, penicillin resistance of *E. faecium* is due to modified PBPs.

IMPERMEABILITY RESISTANCE

The PBPs of Gram-negative bacteria are protected by the outer membrane, which can function as a permeability barrier. The passage of β-lactam antibiotics across the outer membrane proceeds through porin proteins (pp. 11 and 29) and resistance can occur when alterations in porin production lead to decreased permeability. The isolation of porin-deficient mutants in clinical isolates of enterobacteria is being reported more frequently, especially when coupled with β-lactamase production in organisms such as *Escherichia coli*, *Klebsiella pneumoniae* and *Serratia marcescens*. Resistance due to decreased permeability is also important among *Pseudomonas aeruginosa* strains, which possess a less permeable membrane and contain significant efflux pump mechanisms for β-lactam antibiotics, coupled with production of chromosomally mediated β-lactamase activity. Because Gram-positive bacteria lack an outer membrane, this mechanism of resistance does not apply to them.

EFFLUX-MEDIATED RESISTANCE

Efflux mechanisms for β-lactam-containing antimicrobial agents were described in the 1990s. These multidrug, active efflux mechanisms have been best studied in *Ps. aeruginosa*, where an operon consisting of *mexA-mexB-oprM* has been shown to be involved in an energy-dependent pumping out of diverse agents such as tetracyclines, fluoroquinolones and chloramphenicol, as well as penicillins. Knockout mutations in MexA and OprM, the outer membrane components of this system, have resulted in increased accumulation of these agents. Related pumps are now being identified frequently in the pseudomonads, as well as in other Gram-negative bacteria.

TOXICITY AND SIDE EFFECTS

HYPERSENSITIVITY REACTIONS

Penicillins and other β-lactam agents are among the safest antibacterial agents used therapeutically. The most important untoward reactions are those resulting from hypersensitivity. Although serious or life-threatening reactions are rare, allergic reactions present a more serious problem with benzylpenicillin than with other antibiotics. There is cross-reaction among penicillins, and the agent to which the patient reacts is not necessarily the sensitizing agent.

The most dangerous form of drug allergy is acute anaphylactic shock, which may develop between a few minutes and 30 minutes after administration. It is characterized by profound circulatory collapse, nausea, vomiting, abdominal pain, severe bronchospasm and coma, and may be rapidly fatal. Anaphylaxis is said to occur in 0.005–0.05% of treated patients, with a mortality rate of approximately 10%.

The most common manifestation of hypersensitivity is a variety of skin eruptions, usually maculopapular with itching but sometimes urticarial or mixed, and occasionally purpuric. Penicillins should not be applied to the skin as topical preparations are likely to lead to contact dermatitis. Rashes are said to occur in 1–7% of patient courses of penicillin. Contact dermatitis or local swelling and edema can occur at sites of topical application. Although reactions can occur after any route of administration, the severe forms are much more common after injections than after oral administration. A serum sickness form of allergy can arise 7–10 days after first treatment (earlier in previously sensitized patients), in which fever, malaise, urticaria, joint pains, lymphadenopathy and possibly angioneurotic edema, sometimes erythema nodosum and, rarely, Stevens–Johnson syndrome occur.

Some patients develop allergic reactions only after repeated administration of penicillin but in others reactions develop on the first occasion penicillin is prescribed, often as a result of non-medicinal exposure to penicillin in the environment. Preparations for injection should always be freshly made.

Anaphylaxis is much less common with penicillins other than benzylpenicillin. Ampicillin, however, is much more likely to produce rashes (9.5%), which may be severe, especially in patients with coexisting viral infections caused by cytomegalovirus or Epstein–Barr virus, notably infectious mononucleosis. It has been claimed that this propensity is not exhibited to the same degree by amoxicillin, epicillin, ciclacillin or mecillinam.

Allergens

The principal antigen responsible for these reactions is generated by opening the β-lactam ring, allowing the carbonyl group to react with the amino groups of proteins. This benzylpenicilloyl hapten, accounting for 95% of tissue-bound penicillin, is the major determinant for hypersensitivity. A number of other reactions within and between the molecules can occur, leading to the 'minor determinants' – minor components of the complex mixtures, but potentially important determinants of penicillin allergy. Penicillins with different side chains have different sensitizing capacities and may lead to different populations of antibodies in treated patients.

Detection and control

Many patients without a history of penicillin allergy have circulating antibodies to the drug, and their presence is of no prognostic value. Skin testing for cutaneous reactivity to specific IgE is the most widely accepted test used to detect patients likely to suffer immediate hypersensitivity reactions to penicillins. Only about 10% of the patients who claim to have a history of penicillin hypersensitivity respond positively to the determinants used in skin testing. This testing, currently the most accepted and reliable testing method, uses all relevant antigens, including both major and minor determinants.

The use of benzylpenicillin itself is generally regarded as hazardous because it may lead to a severe reaction in the highly susceptible patient and may sensitize the previously non-allergic individual. For this reason, agents such as penicilloyl–polylysine, in which the amino groups of an artificial peptide are virtually saturated with penicilloyl residues, are used. As there are other antigens concerned, excellent predictive performance has been claimed for penicilloyl–polylysine plus a 'minor determinant' mixture. A positive penicillin skin test indicates that a patient is at risk for immediate hypersensitivity; a negative test cannot preclude a future hypersensitivity reaction upon subsequent therapy with penicillin. It is extremely rare, however, that life-threatening reactions occur in patients with a negative skin test.

The management of penicillin reactions relies on the use of antihistamines, corticosteroids and, in anaphylaxis or dangerous angioedema, adrenaline. Desensitization can sometimes be achieved by careful control of treatment in patients for whom penicillin is strongly indicated. This involves a gradual increase in exposure of the patient to the penicillin being used for treatment. It has sometimes been recommended that allergic patients may be successfully treated with the coadministration of corticosteroids or antihistamines, together with penicillin, where that is much the most appropriate agent. However, this has some major risks, as there is a possibility that any allergic reaction to the penicillin would be masked by the action of these agents.

Cross-reactions with cephalosporins

A major interest in early cephalosporins was the belief that they could be safely administered to patients allergic to penicillin. This appears to be mostly true, but about 3–9% of patients are cross-allergic to penicillins and cephalosporins; specific allergy to cephalosporins in the absence of reactions to penicillin also occurs, albeit rarely. It is generally recommended that cephalosporins should be avoided in patients with a clear history of severe reaction to penicillin. Cross-reactivity between penicillins and carbapenems is even less frequent, while the monobactam aztreonam (p. 270) is only very weakly immunogenic and does not show cross-reactivity with penicillin.

OTHER REACTIONS

Leukopenia has occurred in patients receiving various penicillins, including methicillin and piperacillin. Neutropenia in patients treated with benzylpenicillin for bacterial endocarditis is related both to high dosage (18 g/day) and to low neutrophil counts before treatment. Prolonged bleeding times due to platelet abnormalities have been noted, particularly with carboxypenicillins and, to a lesser extent, with acylureidopenicillins. Various nephrotoxic manifestations have been described with carbenicillin, dicloxacillin and methicillin, and reversible abnormalities of liver function tests with carboxypenicillins and less frequently acylureidopenicillins.

Because penicillins are given in large doses as sodium salts, sodium overload and hypokalemia may develop, particularly with the disodium salts of extended spectrum penicillins. Large doses of penicillins, especially in patients with impaired renal function, may result in convulsions. Access to the central nervous system of neurotoxic concentrations is related to lipophilicity and protein binding of the compounds.

 ## Further information

Anderson JA 1986 Cross-sensitivity to cephalosporins in patients allergic to penicillin. *Pediatric Infectious Diseases* 5: 557–561.

Brenner S, Wolf R, Ruocco V 1993 Drug induced pemphigus. I. A survey. *Clinical Dermatology* 11: 501–505.

Bush K 2001 New β-lactamases in gram-negative bacteria: diversity and impact on the selection of antimicrobial therapy. *Clinical Infectious Diseases* 32: 1085–1089.

de Haan P, Bruynzeel P, van Ketel WG 1986 Onset of penicillin rashes: relation between type of penicillin administered and type of immune reactivity. *Allergy* 41: 75–78.

Derendorf H 1989 Pharmacokinetic evaluation of β-lactam antibiotics. *Journal of Antimicrobial Chemotherapy* 24: 407–413.

Fass RJ, Copelan EA, Brandt JT, Moeschberger ML, Ashton JJ 1987 Platelet mediated bleeding caused by broad-spectrum penicillins. *Journal of Infectious Diseases* 155: 1242–1248.

Henwood CJ, Livermore DM, Johnson AP, James D, Warner M, Gardiner A 2000 Susceptibility of gram-positive cocci from 25 UK hospitals to antimicrobial agents including linezolid. The Linezolid Study Group. *Journal of Antimicrobial Chemotherapy* 46: 931–940.

Holgate ST 1988 Penicillin allergy: how to diagnose and when to treat. *British Medical Journal* 296: 1213–1214.

Karchmer AW 2000 Nosocomial bloodstream infections: organisms, risk factors, and implications. *Clinical Infectious Diseases* 31 (Suppl. 4): S139–143.

Kishiyama JL, Adelman DC 1994 The cross-reactivity and immunology of β-lactam antibiotics. *Drug Safety* 10: 318–327.

Klugman KP 1990 Pneumococcal resistance to antibiotics. *Clinical Microbiology Reviews* 3: 171–196.

Leitman PS 1988 Pharmacokinetics of antimicrobial drugs in cystic fibrosis. Beta-lactam antibiotics. *Chest* 94 (Suppl. 2): 115S–120S.

Li XZ, Nikaido H, Poole K 1995 Role of *mexA-mexB-oprM* in antibiotic efflux in *Pseudomonas aeruginosa*. *Antimicrobial Agents and Chemotherapy* 39: 1948–1953.

Lin RY 1992 A perspective on penicillin allergy. *Archives of Internal Medicine* 152: 930–937.

Livermore DM 1991 Mechanisms of resistance to β-lactam antibiotics. *Scandinavian Journal of Antibiotics* 78 (Suppl.): 7–16.

Markowitz M 1985 Long-acting penicillins: historical perspectives. *Pediatric Infectious Diseases* 4: 570–573.

Nathwani D, Wood MJ 1993 Penicillins. A current review of their clinical pharmacology and therapeutic use. *Drugs* 45: 866–894.

Olaison L, Alestig K 1990 A prospective study of neutropenia by high doses of β-lactam antibiotics. *Journal of Antimicrobial Chemotherapy* 25: 449–453.

Sogn DD, Evans R, Shepherd GM et al 1992 Results of the National Institute of Allergy and Infectious Diseases Collaborative Clinical Trial to test the predictive value of skin testing with major and minor penicillin derivatives in hospitalised patients. *Archives of Internal Medicine* 152: 1025–1032.

Stark BJ, Earl HS, Gross GN, Lumry WR, Goodman EL, Sullivan TJ 1987 Acute and chronic desensitization of penicillin-allergic patients using oral penicillin. *Journal of Allergy and Clinical Immunology* 79: 523–532.

Sutherland R 1993 Bacterial resistance to β-lactam antibiotics; problems and solutions. *Progress in Drug Research* 41: 95–149.

Symposium 1988 New developments in resistance to beta-lactam antibiotics among non-fastidious Gram-negative organisms. *Reviews of Infectious Diseases* 10: 677–914.

Weiss ME, Adkinson NF 1988 Immediate hypersensitivity reactions to penicillin and related antibiotics. *Clinical Allergy* 18: 515–540.

Whitney CG, Farley MM, Hadler J et al 2000 Active Bacterial Core Surveillance Program of the Emerging Infections Program Network. Increasing prevalence of multidrug-resistant *Streptococcus pneumoniae* in the United States. *New England Journal of Medicine* 343: 1917–1924.

Witte W 1999 Antibiotic resistance in gram-positive bacteria: epidemiological aspects. *Journal of Antimicrobial Chemotherapy* 44 (Suppl. A): 1–9.

GROUP 1: BENZYLPENICILLIN AND ITS LONG-ACTING PARENTERAL FORMS

Benzylpenicillin, the first naturally produced penicillin, is poorly absorbed orally and must be given by injection. The plasma half-life is short and in order to prolong its effect benzylpenicillin was first mixed with oils or waxes, so that the release of penicillin from intramuscular injection sites was delayed. Later, insoluble salts of penicillin were prepared that similarly act as intramuscular depots for the release of penicillin into the bloodstream. Several repository penicillins are in use: procaine penicillin, benzathine penicillin and clemizole penicillin, which was designed to combine slow release with antihistaminic properties of clemizole. Penethamate or penicillin diethylaminoethyl ester hydriodide (no longer commercially available) was of interest because of a particular capacity to penetrate into lung tissue.

 BENZYLPENICILLIN

Penicillin G. Molecular weight (free acid): 334.4.

Archetypal penicillin produced by *P. chrysogenum*; supplied as the highly soluble potassium or sodium salts for intramuscular or intravenous administration. Potency has traditionally been expressed in units (1 unit = 0.6 μg), but use of milligram or gram quantities is now preferred.

Antimicrobial activity

Activity against common pathogenic bacteria is shown in Table 16.1. It has intrinsic activity against almost all Gram-positive pathogens. Most species of streptococci are susceptible (typical MIC 0.03 mg/l), but group B streptococci, an important cause of neonatal infections, are about 10-fold less sensitive. Enterococci are more resistant than other Gram-positive cocci, but group D non-enterococcal streptococci are fully susceptible. Other susceptible Gram-positive organisms include non-β-lactamase-producing producing *Bacillus anthracis*, *Erysipelothrix rhusiopathiae* and *Listeria monocytogenes*. The spirochetes *Borrelia burgdorferi* and *Treponema pallidum* are also susceptible.

The aerobic Gram-negative cocci *Neisseria gonorrhoeae* and *Neisseria meningitidis* were initially highly susceptible to benzylpenicillin, but β-lactamase-producing strains of gonococci are now common. *Haemophilus influenzae* and *Moraxella* (*Branhamella*) *catarrhalis* are usually resistant due to β-lactamase production. *Pasteurella multocida* and *Streptobacillus moniliformis* are susceptible; *Legionella pneumophila* is inhibited by 0.5–2.0 mg/l in vitro but benzylpenicillin is inactive in tests against intracellular legionellae. The Enterobacteriaceae are almost all resistant, as a result of β-lactamase production or the impermeability of the bacterial cell wall to the antibiotic. However, some strains of *Esch. coli*, *Salmonella enterica* serotypes Typhi and Paratyphi, and many strains of *Proteus mirabilis* are inhibited by 8 mg/l. Most other aerobic Gram-negative bacilli, including *Brucella* spp., *Vibrio cholerae*, *Ps. aeruginosa* and *Stenotrophomonas maltophilia* are resistant. Other resistant organisms include mycobacteria, mycoplasmas, *Nocardia* spp, rickettsiae and chlamydiae.

Anaerobic Gram-positive cocci are very susceptible in the absence of β-lactamase production, and non-sporulating Gram-positive bacilli including *Actinomyces israelii* are also susceptible. Most strains of *Clostridium perfringens* and many strains of other clostridial species are susceptible, but resistance is observed. Anaerobic Gram-negative bacilli vary in their sensitivity: the *B. fragilis* group is resistant as the result of β-

Table 16.1 Activity of benzylpenicillin and group 2 penicillins against common non-β-lactamase-producing pathogenic bacteria: MIC (mg/l)

	Benzylpenicillin	Azidocillin	Phenethicillin	Phenoxymethylpenicillin
Staph. aureus	0.03	0.03	0.06	0.06
Str. pyogenes	0.01	0.01	0.06	0.03
Str. pneumoniae	0.01–0.03	0.06	0.06	0.03
E. faecalis	2	1	4–8	4–8
N. gonorrhoeae	0.01–0.03	0.01	0.1	0.03–0.1
N. meningitidis	0.03	ND	0.1	0.06
H. influenzae	1.0	0.25	4–8	4–8
Esch. coli	64	64	R	R
K. pneumoniae	R	R	R	R
Ps. aeruginosa	R	R	R	R
B. fragilis	32	ND	ND	ND

R, resistant (MIC ≥ 128 mg/l). ND, no data.

lactamase action, but most *Prevotella* and *Fusobacterium* spp. are susceptible.

Benzylpenicillin exhibits concentration-dependent bactericidal activity against growing organisms, the effect being maximum at about four times the MIC, above which no increase in killing occurs. Against many strains of *Staph. aureus* and *E. faecalis* further increase in the concentration actually reduces the death rate. Killing of highly susceptible Gram-positive cocci seldom proceeds to eradication, with measurable numbers of survivors (called 'persisters'), which on retesting are fully susceptible (p. 14). Combination with aminoglycosides results in pronounced bactericidal synergy. Some strains of staphylococci, streptococci (including group B) and pneumococci show very large numbers of survivors, resulting in a large difference between the MIC and MBC, the phenomenon known as 'tolerance' (p. 15).

Acquired resistance

Staph. aureus was originally highly susceptible to benzylpenicillin, but at least 85–90% of clinical isolates are now β-lactamase-producing strains. Most clinical isolates of *Staph. epidermidis* are also resistant. A few isolates of the urinary pathogen *Staphylococcus saprophyticus* display intermediate resistance, possibly as a result of β-lactamase production. β-Lactamase-producing strains of *E. faecalis* have been isolated worldwide since 1993, but are uncommon; the β-lactamase is identical to staphylococcal penicillinase. The frequency of β-lactamase production also appears to be increasing among clostridial species. The emergence of penicillin-resistant pneumococci, due to the acquisition of mosaic PBPs with decreased binding affinity for penicillin, has been described worldwide. Most strains of penicillin-resistant pneumococci also demonstrate reduced susceptibility to other β-lactam agents but, in rare cases, cross-resistance is not seen for all cephalosporins.

Penicillin-resistant strains of *E. faecium* and viridans group streptococci also result from production of modified PBPs that have reduced affinity for penicillin.

Strains of *N. gonorrhoeae* for which the MIC of benzylpenicillin increased from 0.06 mg/l to >2 mg/l appeared in the 1970s, as the result of the production of modified PBPs with reduced affinity for β-lactam antibiotics. Even after the emergence of these strains, gonorrhea could still be treated with high doses of penicillin; however, in 1976 TEM-1 β-lactamase-producing strains of *N. gonorrhoeae* fully resistant to benzylpenicillin were isolated in Africa and the Philippines. Currently more than 40% of *N. gonorrhoeae* isolates produce β-lactamase, and in most areas of the world, benzylpenicillin is no longer considered for empirical treatment of gonorrhea. *H. ducreyi* has also acquired TEM-1 β-lactamase, so that most isolates now display high level resistance.

Pharmacokinetics

Oral absorption	2–25%
C_{max} 0.6 g intramuscular	12 mg/l
3 g intravenous (3–5 min)	400 mg/l
Plasma half-life	0.5 h
Volume of distribution	0.2–0.7 l/kg
Plasma protein binding	60%

Absorption

Benzylpenicillin is unstable in acid and destroyed in the stomach. As a result, plasma concentrations obtained after oral administration are irregular and unreliable, and are further depressed by administration with food. Absorption may be better in the elderly due to the relative frequency of achlorhydria. It is absorbed from serous cavities, joints and the subarachnoid space. It is not absorbed following applications to the skin, which should in any case be avoided because of the likelihood of sensitization.

Distribution

The drug is widely distributed, penetrating into the pleural, pericardial, peritoneal and synovial fluids. Highest levels are found in the kidney, with lower levels in the liver, skin and intestines. Low concentrations appear in saliva and in maternal milk. It does not enter uninflamed bone or the cerebrospinal fluid (CSF). Its entry is limited by its low pK_a (2.6), which results in its almost complete ionization and very low lipid/water partition coefficient at pH 7.4. When the meninges are inflamed, the concentrations obtained in CSF are very variable, around 5% of the plasma level, active transport via the choroid plexus out of the CSF being depressed by meningitis. It is also reduced by probenecid, which inhibits the transport of weak acids from the CSF, giving rise to 2–3-fold increases in CSF concentrations – a potential cause of toxicity if large doses are given. In uremia, accumulated organic acids may enter the CSF and compete for transport of penicillin, causing the concentration to reach convulsive levels.

About 10% of the distributed drug enters erythrocytes, where the concentration may slightly exceed that of the plasma and the lower rate of release from the cells (elimination half-life 50–60 min) helps to maintain the tail of penicillin concentration. It diffuses into wound exudates and experimental transudates when the serum level is high and persists there longer than in the serum. Average sputum levels 2 h after 0.6 g are 0.3 mg/l. It enters glandular secretions and the fetal circulation, whence it is excreted in increased concentrations into the amniotic fluid.

Metabolism

About 40% is metabolized in the liver, mainly to penicilloic acid.

Excretion

After oral dosing, unabsorbed drug is largely degraded by colonic bacteria and very little activity remains in the feces. Concentrations 2–4 times those of the plasma are found in bile, but 60–90% is excreted in the urine, largely in the first hour, 90% by tubular secretion. This can be blocked by probenecid, with consequent doubling of the peak concentration and prolongation of the plasma half-life. Claims that this results partly from confining the drug to the vascular space have not been confirmed. Other drugs, especially organic acids, including aspirin, sulfonamides and some non-steroidal anti-inflammatory drugs and diuretics, may prolong the half-life, which naturally increases with decrease of renal function including that which occurs with advancing age.

Toxicity and side effects

Benzylpenicillin has low toxicity, except for the nervous system (to which it is normally denied access), where it is one of the most active convulsants among the β-lactam agents.

Concentrations in CSF above 10 mg/l are associated with drowsiness, occasional hallucinations, hyperreflexia, loss of consciousness, and myoclonic movements progressing to focal convulsions that may proceed to coma and death. Toxic levels may reach the CSF in three ways:

- By intrathecal injection (the dose should never exceed 12 mg (20 000 units) in the adult or 3 mg (5000 units) in the child as a single daily dose).
- In the presence of meningitis.
- Excessive dosage (60 g [100 megaunits] or more per day), or more modest dosage in the presence of unidentified predisposing factors or impaired renal function.

Inadvertant intravascular administration, especially direct injection into arteries, can cause severe neurovascular damage.

Massive intravenous doses of the sodium or potassium salts can lead to severe electrolyte disturbance. In patients treated with large doses of the potassium salt (60 g or more per day) hyponatremia, hyperkalemia and metabolic acidosis can develop.

Thrombocytopenia and platelet dysfunction resulting in coagulopathy and involving several different mechanisms has been described.

Large doses (24 g [40 megaunits]/day intravenously), or smaller doses given to patients with impaired renal function may interfere with platelet function in a manner analogous to that seen with carbenicillin, with resulting coagulation defects that persist for 3–4 days after cessation of therapy.

The most dramatic untoward response is anaphylactic shock due to allergy (p. 226). In addition to the generalized allergic reactions, particular organs may be damaged by a variety of immunological mechanisms. Hemolytic anemia occurs only in patients who have been treated previously with penicillin, and again receive a prolonged course of large doses (commonly 12 g/day). Reversible hemolysis is due to the action of anti-penicillin immunoglobulin G (IgG) on cells that have absorbed the antibiotic. Nephritis, resulting in dysuria, pyuria, proteinuria, azotemia and histological evidence of nephritis of allergic origin is only rarely seen, usually in patients receiving large doses (12–36 g [20–60 megaunits]/day).

A few cases of neutropenia associated with fever and allergic rash have been reported which appear to be related to total dose, usually in excess of 90 g. It can be very severe, but in most patients, recovery occurs within a few days of withdrawal of treatment.

Clinical use

- Streptococcal infections, including bacteremia, empyema, severe pneumonia, pericarditis, endocarditis and meningitis (other than meningitis caused by penicillin-resistant pneumococci).
- Staphylococcal infections caused by susceptible strains.
- Meningococcal septicemia and meningitis.
- Gonorrhea, gonorrheal endocarditis and arthritis caused by susceptible strains.

- Syphilis, including congenital syphilis, and other spirochetal infections.
- Anthrax.
- Actinomycosis.
- Clostridial infections (including tetanus).
- Diphtheria (to prevent carrier state).
- Infections with other susceptible organisms, including *Listeria monocytogenes*, *Pasteurella multocida*, *Erysipelothrix insidiosa*, *Spirillum minus* and *Streptobacillus moniliformis*, peptostreptococci and *Fusobacterium*.

Preparations and dosage

Proprietary name: Crystapen, Pfizerpen and numerous generic forms.

Preparation: Injection.

Dosage: Adults, i.m., i.v., 600 mg to 1.2 g daily in 2–4 divided doses; adult meningitis, up to 14.4 g/day may be given in divided doses; bacterial endocarditis, 4.8 g/day or more in divided doses. Children 1 month to 12 years, 10–20 mg/kg per day in four divided doses; newborn infants, 30 mg/kg per day in two divided doses in first few days of life, then in 3–4 divided doses. Meningitis in children and neonates; neonates ≤7 days old, 60–90 mg/kg per day in two divided doses; neonates >7 days old, 90–120 mg/kg per day as three divided doses; children 1 month to 12 years, 150–300 mg/kg per day in 4–6 divided doses. Intrathecal, see manufacturer's literature.

Widely available.

Further information

Anonymous 1999 Penicillin G (sodium or potassium). In: Dollery C (ed.) *Therapeutic Drugs* 2nd edn. Churchill Livingstone, Edinburgh, pp. P32–P36.

Ducas J, Robson HG 1981 Cerebrospinal fluid penicillin levels during therapy for latent syphilis. *Journal of the American Medical Association* 246: 2583–2584.

Kim KS 1988 Clinical perspectives on penicillin tolerance. *Journal of Pediatrics* 112: 509–514.

Neftel KA, Walti M, Spengler H, de Weck AL 1982 Effect of storage of penicillin-G solutions on sensitization to penicillin-G intravenous administration. *Lancet* i: 986–988.

Nicholls PJ 1980 Neurotoxicity of penicillin. *Journal of Antimicrobial Chemotherapy* 6: 161–164.

Overbosch D, van Gulpen C, Hermans, J, Mattie H 1988 The effect of probenecid on the renal tubular excretion of benzylpenicillin. *British Journal of Clinical Pharmacology* 25: 51–58.

Sáez-Nicto JA, Fontanals D, Garcia de Jalon J et al 1987 Isolation of *Neisseria meningitidis* strains with increase of penicillin minimal inhibitory concentrations. *Epidemiology and Infection* 99: 463–469.

Schoth PE, Wolters EC 1987 Penicillin concentration in serum and CSF during high-dose intravenous treatment for neurosyphilis. *Neurology* 37: 1214–1216.

Sullivan TJ 1982 Cardiac disorders in penicillin-induced anaphylaxis. Association with intravenous epinephrine therapy. *Journal of the American Medical Association* 248: 2116–2162.

COMPOUNDS LIBERATING BENZYLPENICILLIN

Antimicrobial activity and systemic effects of the long-acting forms are due to the liberation of benzylpenicillin.

Intramuscular injection, particularly of benzathine penicillin, may produce local pain or tenderness, and accidental intravascular injection of procaine penicillin may produce acute agitation, hallucinations and collapse.

Long-acting forms have their principal use in the treatment of gonorrhea, syphilis, in the follow-on treatment of patients requiring prolonged therapy after initial treatment with benzylpenicillin and in prophylaxis, particularly of rheumatic fever. Severe pneumonia, empyema, bacteremia, pericarditis, meningitis, peritonitis, and arthritis of pneumococcal etiology are better treated with benzylpenicillin during the acute stage of the illness.

Benzathine penicillin

N, *N*′-dibenzolylethylene diamine dipenicillin salt of benzylpenicillin. It is poorly soluble (1:6000) in water. Available as an intramuscular preparation and in various mixtures with benzyl- and procaine penicillins. It has a local anesthetic effect comparable with that of procaine penicillin.

It is very slowly absorbed after intramuscular injection, yielding very low plasma concentrations: a dose of 1.2 megaunits produces mean plasma concentrations of 0.1 mg/l 1 week after injection, 0.02 mg/l after 2 weeks and 0.002 mg/l after 4 weeks.

Preparations and dosage

Proprietary name: Permapen.

Preparation: Intramuscular injection.

Dosage: Varies according to infection being treated.

Limited availability; not available in the UK.

Further information

Kaplan EL, Berrios X, Speth J, Siefferman T, Guzman B, Quesny F 1989 Pharmacokinetics of benzathine penicillin G: serum levels during the 28 days after intramuscular injection of l 200 000 units. *Journal of Pediatrics* 115: 146–150.

Peter G, Dudley MN 1985 Clinical pharmacology of benzathine penicillin G. *Pediatric Infectious Diseases* 4: 586–591.

CLEMIZOLE PENICILLIN

A long-acting preparation of benzylpenicillin with the antihistamine, clemizole, given by deep intramuscular injection.

Preparations

Proprietary name: Clemipen, Antipen.

Preparation: Intramuscular Injection.

Limited availability in continental Europe.

Procaine penicillin

A poorly soluble (1:200 in water) equimolecular compound of penicillin and procaine, administered intramuscularly as a suspension of crystals which slowly dissolve at the site of the injection. It is also available in some countries as an oily suspension with aluminum monostearate.

It must not be given intravenously. Intramuscular administration produces a flat sustained plasma concentration of penicillin, which is much lower than that achieved by an equivalent dose of benzylpenicillin, with plasma levels still detectable 24 h later. An injection of 0.6 g yields a peak plasma concentration of 1–2 mg benzylpenicillin/l after 2–4 h. Free procaine is detectable in the plasma within 30 min.

Very severe and potentially fatal reactions resembling those of anaphylactic shock, but non-allergic in character, may occur, probably due to accidental entry into the vascular system at the site of injection and blockage of pulmonary and cerebral capillaries by crystals of the suspension. Some untoward reactions may be due to liberated procaine. There may be acute anxiety and angor animi without physical signs or fever, hypertension, tachycardia, vomiting, audiovisual hallucinations and acute psychotic disturbance. The most severe reactions lead to convulsions and cardiac arrest. Other reactions are those to liberated benzylpenicillin.

Preparations and dosage

Proprietary name: Bicillin and numerous generic forms.
Preparation: Injection.
Dosage: Adults, i.m., 300 mg (plus 60 mg benzylpenicillin) every 12–24 h. Widely available.

Further information

Shann F, Linnemann V, Gratten M 1987 Serum concentration of penicillin after intramuscular administration of procaine, benzyl and benethamine penicillin in children with pneumonia. *Journal of Pediatrics* 110: 299–302.
Silber TJ, D'Angelo L 1985 Psychosis and seizures following the injection of penicillin G procaine. *American Journal of Diseases of Children* 139: 335–337.

GROUP 2: ORALLY ABSORBED PENICILLINS RESEMBLING BENZYLPENICILLIN

Early efforts to improve the oral absorption characteristics of benzylpenicillin concentrated on esterification of the C-3 carboxyl group. Simple methyl or alkyl esters were ineffective, as humans do not produce the necessary esterase to release active penicillin. The acetoxymethyl ester, at one time available as penamecillin, is hydrolyzed by non-specific esterases to yield benzylpenicillin and formaldehyde. Benzathine penicillin, the sparingly soluble long-acting parenteral salt of benzylpenicillin (p. 231), produces low plasma concentrations after oral use but is rarely used.

The first natural penicillin to be identified as a useful oral agent on its own was phenoxymethylpenicillin (penicillin V), produced by addition of phenoxyacetic acid as a precursor to the fermentation. Penicillin V is more acid stable than benzylpenicillin and is absorbed after oral administration, producing therapeutically useful plasma penicillin concentrations. After the identification of the penicillin nucleus, 6-APA, a number of phenoxypenicillins, analogs of penicillin V, were developed with claims for superior oral absorption characteristics. The most important of these semisynthetic penicillins are phenethicillin (the immediate homolog of penicillin V) and propicillin, which were both successful in the clinic. Another phenoxypenicillin, phenbenicillin (phenoxybenzylpenicillin), which exhibits superior oral absorption, is no longer available due to its high protein binding and extensive metabolism.

The remaining oral narrow-spectrum penicillin that is still used therapeutically is azidopenicillin. Although it is not a phenoxypenicillin, its properties are similar.

ANTIMICROBIAL ACTIVITY

The phenoxypenicillins exhibit slightly lower activity than benzylpenicillin against Gram-positive cocci and are distinctly less active against Gram-negative bacteria. Azidocillin, an analog of benzylpenicillin, resembles benzylpenicillin in potency and range of activity. All group 2 penicillins lack stability to β-lactamase.

PHARMACOKINETICS

In general, the absorption efficiency of the phenoxypenicillins increases in parallel with molecular weight. The peak plasma levels obtained from the phenoxypenicillins and from azidocillin are well in excess of those required to inhibit the organisms for which benzylpenicillin is normally used.

CLINICAL USE

These drugs may be prescribed for many indications for which benzylpenicillin is suitable, including streptococcal pharyngitis and skin sepsis, but are not recommended for initial therapy of serious infections. They are useful for continuation therapy after initial control of the disease by parenteral benzylpenicillin when prolonged treatment is required, as in osteomyelitis due to penicillin-susceptible *Staph. aureus* or bacterial endocarditis due to fully penicillin-susceptible streptococci. In such potentially dangerous conditions, it must be established that the organisms are killed by the particular oral penicillin used, and that bactericidal levels for the infecting organisms are achieved in the patient's plasma; although they are much more reliably absorbed than benzylpenicillin, there are still some patients who absorb them poorly. They have been used prophylactically in recurrent pneumococcal meningitis after head injury and in rheumatic fever. They are not appropriate for respiratory infections where *H. influenzae* may be implicated, and are not recommended for the treatment of gonorrhea, syphilis or leptospirosis, or for infections caused by Gram-negative bacilli.

 ## PHENOXYMETHYLPENICILLIN

Penicillin V. Molecular weight (free acid): 350.4; (potassium salt): 388.5.

A naturally occurring penicillin produced by *P. chrysogenum* in media containing phenoxyacetic acid as a precursor. It is supplied as the potassium salt for oral administration.

Antimicrobial activity

The antibacterial spectrum and level of activity is similar to that of benzylpenicillin (Table 16.1). It is generally 2- to 8-fold less active than benzylpenicillin against streptococci, staphylococci, gonococci, meningococci and *H. influenzae*. Enteric Gram-negative bacilli are highly resistant.

Pharmacokinetics

Oral absorption	40–70%
C_{max} 250 mg oral	2 mg/l after 1 h
Plasma half-life	*c.* 0.5 h
Volume of distribution	0.2 l/kg
Plasma protein binding	80%

Absorption

Owing to acid stability, it is not destroyed in the stomach, but absorption is variable and incomplete, about 30% remaining in the feces. Absorption is better from a rapidly disintegrating tablet and after administration in the fasting state.

Metabolism and excretion

It is fairly extensively metabolized and degraded in the bowel. Some 60% of the dose is excreted in the urine, 25% in the unchanged form and the remainder as metabolites.

Toxicity and side effects

Those common to penicillins (p. 226). As with all penicillins, patients with a history of hypersensitivity to penicillins should be treated cautiously, as serious anaphylactic responses may occur.

Clinical uses

Those of group 2 penicillins (*see above*).

 ### Preparations and dosage

Proprietary name: Numerous generic forms.

Preparations: Tablets, oral solution.

Dosage: Adults, oral, 250–500 mg every 6 h. Doses can be doubled. Children <1 year, 62.5 mg every 6 h; children 1–5 years, 125 mg every 6 h; children 6–12 years, 250 mg every 6 h.

Widely available.

Further information

Anonymous 1999 Penicillin V (potassium). In: Dollery C (ed.) *Therapeutic Drugs* 2nd edn. Churchill Livingstone, Edinburgh, pp. P36–P38.

Josefsson K, Nord CE 1982 Effects of phenoxymethylpenicillin and erythromycin in high doses on the salivary microflora. *Journal of Antimicrobial Chemotherapy* 10: 325–333.

Overbosch D, Mattie H, vanFurth R 1985 Comparative pharmacodynamics and clinical pharmacokinetics of phenoxymethyl penicillin and pheneticillin. *British Journal of Clinical Pharmacology* 19: 657–668.

OTHER GROUP 2 PENICILLINS

Azidocillin

D-azidobenzylpenicillin. It is as active as benzylpenicillin and more active than the phenoxypenicillins against susceptible strains of *Staph. aureus*, *Str. pyogenes* and *Str. pneumoniae* (Table 16.1). Activity against susceptible *H. influenzae* is almost equal to that of ampicillin. Other Gram-negative bacteria are not notably susceptible. Protein binding (80%) is generally similar to phenoxymethylpenicillin and phenethicillin. It is well absorbed after oral administration and produces plasma concentrations higher than those of phenoxymethylpenicillin and comparable with phenethicillin. Urinary excretion is 68% of an oral dose and 80% of an intravenous dose, indicating about 75% absorption by the oral route. It has been used for the treatment of upper respiratory tract infection.

 ### Preparations and dosage

Dosage: Adult, oral, 750 mg twice daily.

Limited availability in continental Europe.

Further information

Bergan T, Sorensen G 1980 Pharmacokinetics of azidocillin in healthy adults. *Arzneimittelforschung* 30: 185–191.

Phenethicillin

Phenoxyethylpenicillin. The immediate homolog of penicillin V and the first semisynthetic penicillin to be used therapeutically after the discovery of 6-APA. Its antibacterial spectrum and activity is similar to that of penicillin V and differs slightly from that of benzylpenicillin (Table 16.1). Its slightly increased stability to staphylococcal β-lactamase compared to benzylpenicillin is not considered to be clinically significant.

A 250 mg oral dose achieves a peak plasma level of 3.5 mg/l after 1 h. The peak is depressed, but prolonged, on administration with food. Plasma protein binding is 75%. It is well distributed into serous and synovial fluid but does not reach the normal CSF. The bulk of the dose appears in the urine, about 25% as penicilloic acid and 50% as unchanged penicillin. Small amounts also appear as other metabolites, some of which are biologically active.

As with all penicillins, hypersensitivity occurs, but severe reactions are much less common than with benzylpenicillin. A serum-sickness-like illness has been noted relatively frequently. Hemolytic anemia has been reported, and overdosage may result in potassium intoxication. Its uses are those of group 2 penicillins (p. 232).

Preparations and dosage

Dosage: Adults, oral, 250–500 mg every 6 h.
Limited availability, not available in the UK.

Further information

Overbosch D, Mattie H, vanFurth R 1985 Comparative pharmacodynamics and clinical pharmacokinetics of phenoxymethylpenicillin and pheneticillin. *British Journal of Clinical Pharmacology* 19: 657–668.

Propicillin

Phenoxypropylpenicillin. A semisynthetic penicillin supplied as the potassium salt. Up to 30% is excreted in the urine as biologically active metabolites. Superior absorption is offset by its protein binding (90%) and inferior activity against some organisms. Clinical uses are those of group 2 penicillins (p. 232). It is no longer widely available.

GROUP 3: ANTISTAPHYLOCOCCAL β-LACTAMASE-STABLE PENICILLINS

The members of this group include methicillin, nafcillin and four isoxazolylpenicillins: oxacillin, cloxacillin, dicloxacillin and flucloxacillin. All have less intrinsic microbiological activity than benzylpenicillin, but they are stable to staphylococcal β-lactamase and, as a result, display improved activity against penicillinase-producing strains of *Staph. aureus*. Oxacillin is rather less stable to hydrolysis by staphylococcal β-lactamase than the other compounds, with the order of stability: methicillin >nafcillin >cloxacillin, dicloxacillin and flucloxacillin >oxacillin. Their resistance to β-lactamase hydrolysis is caused by poor binding, due to the C-6 side-chain substitutions.

Methicillin has been replaced in clinical practice because of low activity, poor oral absorption and a propensity to cause interstitial nephritis. Cloxacillin and flucloxacillin are used clinically in Europe and elsewhere, whereas nafcillin, oxacillin and dicloxacillin are preferred in North America.

ANTIMICROBIAL ACTIVITY

The compounds are active against staphylococci, streptococci, gonococci and meningococci but have no useful activity against enterococci, *H. influenzae* or enterobacteria (Table 16.2). Methicillin is approximately 10 times less active than the others against *Staph. aureus* and is 100-fold less active than benzylpenicillin against penicillin-susceptible *Staph. aureus*.

ACQUIRED RESISTANCE

Strains of *Staph. aureus* resistant to methicillin (MRSA; p. 31) were thought at first not to exist, but their prevalence has risen rapidly. MRSA and other methicillin-resistant staphylococci

Table 16.2 Antibacterial activity of group 3 penicillins against common pathogenic bacteria: MIC (mg/l)

	Cloxacillin*	Methicillin	Nafcillin
Staph. aureus	0.1	1	0.1
Staph. epidermidis	0.1	1	0.1
Str. pyogenes	0.1	0.25	0.06
Str. pneumoniae	0.25	0.25	0.1
E. faecalis	16–32	16–32	16
N. gonorrhoeae	0.1	0.1–0.5	2
N. meningitidis	0.25	0.25	8
H. influenzae	8–16	2	4
Esch. coli	R	R	R
K. pneumoniae	R	R	R
Ps. aeruginosa	R	R	R
B. fragilis	R	R	R

*Activities of dicloxacillin, flucloxacillin and oxacillin are similar.
R, resistant (MIC ≥ 128 mg/l).

produce large amounts of β-lactamase, but they do not inactivate methicillin. Resistance is due to the acquisition of the supplementary PBP 2a with low affinity for methicillin and other β-lactam antibiotics. The bacterial population is highly heterogeneous in its response to the agent and only a small minority of cells may appear to be resistant in conventional media. The resistance of individual cells can differ by more than two orders of magnitude, and the progeny of resistant colonies are similarly heterogeneous. The population can be rendered homogeneously resistant by growth either at 30°C or in a medium containing an excess of electrolytes, such as 5% NaCl; or by lowering the pH. For the above reasons, standard susceptibility testing may not detect MRSA and the use of large inocula plus media supplemented with NaCl and/or incubation at 30°C is recommended. Oxacillin is now the penicillin of choice for detection of these strains.

MRSA are resistant to almost all β-lactam agents, including imipenem and meropenem, and many isolates are also resistant to other antistaphylococcal antibiotics, with the exception of vancomycin and the related glycopeptide, teicoplanin. Some newer agents, including quinupristin-dalfopristin (p. 383) and linezolid (p. 345) include MRSA in their spectrum of activity.

PHARMACOKINETICS

Methicillin is the most metabolically stable and least protein bound of the group 3 penicillins. It is unstable in acid and not absorbed when given orally. Nafcillin is also relatively acid labile and poorly and irregularly absorbed when dosed orally. The isoxazolylpenicillins are considerably better absorbed from the gut than are methicillin or nafcillin, but differ among themselves. The mean peak plasma levels of cloxacillin are about twice those resulting from similar doses of oxacillin; those of dicloxacillin and flucloxacillin are about twice those of cloxacillin. Levels, especially those of oxacillin, are depressed when they are given with food.

Oxacillin is metabolized to a greater extent than dicloxacillin or flucloxacillin. All are highly protein bound. Levels obtained by intravenous bolus injection of isoxazolylpenicillins are higher than those produced by the extensively metabolized nafcillin, but this advantage is offset by their higher protein binding. Overall, dicloxacillin and flucloxacillin are superior to oxacillin and cloxacillin for oral administration. Flucloxacillin is better absorbed and provides more unbound drug than does dicloxacillin.

They are widely distributed in the extracellular fluid, and their plasma levels are correspondingly depressed when the extracellular volume is increased (as in pregnancy or in the newborn). They are well distributed into serous fluids, but as highly protein-bound agents their access to blister fluid is limited though their persistence there is prolonged. They do not enter normal CSF, but their entry is somewhat erratically increased by inflammation, nafcillin penetrating better than others.

Little of these drugs appears in the bile, and they are excreted principally unchanged in the urine by both glomerular filtration and tubular secretion to produce very high urinary levels. Plasma half-lives are consequently prolonged by probenecid and in the newborn and (with the exception of oxacillin, which is the most extensively metabolized) in renal failure. Patients with cystic fibrosis clear the drugs unusually rapidly, and allowance for this must be made in their dosage.

TOXICITY AND SIDE EFFECTS

As with all penicillins, serious anaphylactic responses may occur, but acute anaphylaxis is much less common than with benzylpenicillin. Most side effects are similar to those observed for other penicillins. Drug fever occurs most commonly with methicillin. Some patients develop diarrhea, and pseudomembranous colitis has been reported. Among rare hematological disorders are reversible dose-related leukopenia and platelet abnormalities. Reversible abnormalities of liver function tests can develop, particularly with oxacillin, and cholestatic jaundice has been described. Renal damage (generally reversible) has been described, usually in patients receiving large doses, and most frequently the interstitial nephritis associated with methicillin.

CLINICAL USE

The only, but important, therapeutic use for these agents is in the treatment of proven staphylococcal infection or (usually in combination therapy) where staphylococcal infection is suspected, and the causative organism is susceptible to the agent. The injectable forms are used in severe staphylococcal infections, including those of the bones, joints, heart valves and meninges, and in brain abscess and disseminated infection. The oral drugs are valuable in the treatment of staphylococcal infections of soft tissues and as continuation therapy in infections of bone and joints. The reservations concerning oral drugs in the treatment of severe infection must be considered if this form of therapy is contemplated.

CLOXACILLIN

Molecular weight (free acid): 435.9.

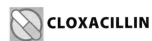

A semisynthetic isoxazolylpenicillin supplied as the sodium salt for oral or parenteral administration.

Antimicrobial activity

Cloxacillin is active against most Gram-positive cocci, but *E. faecalis* is relatively resistant (Table 16.2). It shows the same order of activity against β-lactamase-producing and β-lactamase-negative strains of staphylococci (MIC 0.1–0.25 mg/l), but is not active against MRSA. Other susceptible bacteria include *N. gonorrhoeae*, *N. meningitidis* and Gram-positive anaerobes (MIC 0.1–0.25 mg/l). *H. influenzae* is relatively resistant, Enterobacteriaceae and *Ps. aeruginosa* are highly resistant (MIC >512 mg/l) and Gram-negative anaerobes may be moderately or highly resistant. The compound is highly bound to serum protein and activity in vitro is substantially diminished in the presence of serum.

Acquired resistance

Cloxacillin exhibits complete cross-resistance with methicillin and other group 3 penicillins. Penicillin-tolerant strains are also tolerant to cloxacillin.

Pharmacokinetics

Oral absorption	40–60%
C_{max} 500 mg oral	8 mg/l (fasting) after 1 h
500 mg intramuscular	15 mg/l after 0.5–1 h
Plasma half-life	0.5 h
Plasma protein binding	93–95%

Absorption

Cloxacillin is moderately well absorbed by mouth but absorption is depressed by food.

Distribution

Being highly protein bound, it diffuses poorly into normal interstitial fluid, serous cavities and CSF, but enters pus and inflamed bones and joints. It crosses the placenta.

Metabolism

Some inactivation occurs in the liver and about 10% of the plasma content is in the form of metabolites.

Excretion

About 10% of an oral dose is excreted in the bile, but the main route of excretion is renal. Around 30% of an oral dose and 40–60% of an intramuscular dose appears in the urine as active antibiotic, with 10–20% in the form of metabolites. Excretion is by both glomerular filtration and tubular secretion and is depressed by probenecid, which elevates and prolongs the plasma concentration. Excretion is impaired in renal failure and there is some accumulation of metabolites. In patients with cystic fibrosis, tubular secretion is enhanced and elimination increased two- to three-fold.

Toxicity and side effects

In addition to hypersensitivity common to penicillins, nausea and diarrhea may occur on oral dosage, but are usually mild. Elevated transaminase levels have been described in some patients. As with other penicillins, large doses, especially in patients in renal failure, can be neurotoxic, and occasional neutropenia has been described.

Clinical uses

Those of Group 3 penicillins (p. 235).

Preparations and dosage

Proprietary name: Orbenin.

Preparations: Capsules, injection, oral solution.

Dosage: Adults, oral, 250–500 mg every 6 h; i.m., i.v., 250–500 mg every 4–6 h, the dose may be doubled in severe infections. Children <2 years, all routes, quarter adult dose; children 2–12 years, all routes, half adult dose.

Widely available; not UK.

Further information

Bergeron MG, Desaulnier SD, Lessard C et al 1985 Concentrations of fusidic acid, cloxacillin and cefamandole in sera and atrial appendages of patients undergoing cardiac surgery. *Antimicrobial Agents and Chemotherapy* 27: 928–932.

Grimm PC, Ogborn MR, Larson AJ, Crocker JF 1989 Interstitial nephritis induced by cloxacillin. *Nephron* 51: 285–286.

Spino M, Chai RP, Isles AF et al 1984 Cloxacillin absorption and disposition in cystic fibrosis. *Journal of Pediatrics* 105: 829–835.

DICLOXACILLIN

Molecular weight (free acid): 470.4.

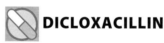

A semisynthetic isoxazolylpenicillin which differs from cloxacillin by an additional chlorine atom. It is supplied as the sodium monohydrate for oral administration.

Antimicrobial activity

Its activities are generally similar to those of other isoxazolylpenicillins (Table 16.2) but it is slightly more active than cloxacillin and oxacillin against streptococci and some strains of penicillin-susceptible and penicillin-resistant staphylococci. It is very highly bound to serum protein, and its activity in the presence of human serum in vitro is depressed to a greater extent than that of other isoxazolylpenicillins.

Pharmacokinetics

Oral absorption	c. 50%
C_{max} 250 mg oral	9 mg/l after 1 h
500 mg intramuscular	14–16 mg/l after 0.5–1 h
Plasma half-life	0.5 h
Plasma protein binding	95–97%

Absorption

Absorption in the very young is poor and unpredictable.

Metabolism

Dicloxacillin is partly metabolized in the liver and about 10% of the circulating drug is in the form of metabolites. Some 50–70% of a dose is excreted in the urine, about 20% as metabolites.

Excretion

Dicloxacillin is eliminated both in the glomerular filtrate and by tubular secretion, and plasma concentrations are raised by probenecid. Parent drug and increased proportions of metabolites accumulate in renal failure. Elimination is increased through enhanced tubular secretion in patients with cystic fibrosis.

Toxicity and clinical use

Phlebitis is common after intravenous injection. Its toxicity is otherwise similar to that of other penicillins (p. 226). Clinical uses are those of the group 3 penicillins (p. 235).

Preparations and dosage

Proprietary names: Dynapen, Dycill, Pathocil.

Preparations: Capsules, oral suspension.

Dosage: Adults, oral, 125–250 mg, four times daily. Children, oral, 12.5–25 mg/kg/day in divided doses. Doses can be doubled in severe infections.

Available in continental Europe and the USA.

Further information

Bergdahl S, Eriksson M, Finkel Y 1987 Plasma concentration following oral administration of di- and flucloxacillin in infants and children. *Pharmacology and Toxicology* 60: 233–234.

Lofgren S, Bucht G, Hermansson B, Holm SE, Winblad B, Norrby SR 1986 Single-dose pharmacokinetics of dicloxacillin in healthy subjects of young and old age. *Scandinavian Journal of Infectious Diseases* 18: 365–369.

Pacifici GM, Viani A, Taddeuchi-Brunelli G, Rizzo G, Carrai M 1987 Plasma protein binding of dicloxacillin: effects of age and disease. *International Journal of Clinical Pharmacology Therapy and Toxicology* 25: 622–626.

FLUCLOXACILLIN

Floxacillin. Molecular weight (free acid): 453.9; (sodium salt): 494.9.

A semisynthetic isoxazolylpenicillin that differs from dicloxacillin by the substitution of a fluorine atom for a chlorine atom. It is supplied as the sodium salt for oral or parenteral administration and as a suspension of the magnesium salt in a syrup formulation. It is also formulated as a combination product with ampicillin (co-fluampicil).

Antimicrobial activity

Its antibacterial activity is almost identical to that of cloxacillin (Table 16.2). It exhibits a uniform level of activity against β-lactamase-negative and β-lactamase-positive strains of *Staph. aureus*. There is complete cross-resistance with other penicillinase-stable penicillins.

Pharmacokinetics

Oral absorption	c. 80%
C_{max} 250 mg (oral)	11 mg/l after 0.5–1 h
Plasma half-life	2 h
Plasma protein binding	95%

Absorption and distribution

It is well absorbed after oral administration and penetrates rapidly into extravascular exudates. Its high protein binding limits its diffusion, notably into the normal CSF.

Metabolism and excretion

Flucloxacillin is partly metabolized in the liver and about 10% of the plasma concentration is made up of metabolites. It is more slowly eliminated than cloxacillin. Some appears in the bile but about 50–80% of an oral dose is recovered from the urine, about 20% as metabolites.

Toxicity and side effects

In patients treated by intravenous infusion, about 5% developed phlebitis by the first and 15% by the second day, after which the proportion rose dramatically. Side effects are otherwise those common to penicillins (p. 226).

Clinical use

Uses are those of group 3 penicillins (p. 235).

> ### Preparations and dosage
>
> *Proprietary name:* Floxapen.
>
> *Preparations:* Capsules, oral solution, injection.
>
> *Dosage:* Adults, oral, 250 mg every 6 h; i.m., i.v., 250 mg to 1 g every 6 h, the dose may be doubled in severe infections. Endocarditis, 12 g per day in six divided doses. Children <2 years, any route, quarter adult dose; children 2–10 years, any route, half adult dose.
>
> Widely available. Not available in the USA.

> ### Further information
>
> Anonymous 1999 Floxacillin (sodium). In Dollery C (ed.) *Therapeutic Drugs* 2nd edn. Churchill Livingstone, Edinburgh, pp. F57–F62.
>
> Basker MJ, Edmondson RA, Sutherland R 1980 Comparative stabilities of penicillins and cephalosporins to staphylococcal β-lactamase and activities against *Staph. aureus. Journal of Antimicrobial Chemotherapy* 6: 333–341.
>
> Bergan T, Engeset A, Olszewski W, Ostby N, Solberg R 1986 Extravascular penetration of highly protein-bound flucloxacillin. *Antimicrobial Agents and Chemotherapy* 30: 729–732.
>
> Frank U, Schmidt-Eisenlohr E, Schlosser V, Spillner G, Schindler M, Daschner FD 1988 Concentrations of flucloxacillin in heart valves and subcutaneous and muscle tissues of patients undergoing open-heart surgery. *Antimicrobial Agents and Chemotherapy* 32: 930–931.
>
> Herngren L, Ehrnebo M, Broberger U 1987 Pharmacokinetics of free and total flucloxacillin in newborn infants. *European Journal of Clinical Pharmacology* 32: 403–409.

METHICILLIN

2,6-Dimethoxyphenylpenicillin; meticillin (international non-proprietary name). Molecular weight (free acid): 380.4.

The first β-lactamase-resistant semisynthetic penicillin. It was initially used widely but has been superseded by other group 3 members. Supplied as the sodium salt for parenteral administration. Aqueous solutions are unstable, particularly at low pH.

Antimicrobial activity

Methicillin is active against most Gram-positive bacteria and against *Neisseria* spp., but it is much less active than benzylpenicillin (Table 16.2) or other group 3 penicillins. It is very stable to staphylococcal β-lactamase and is equally active against penicillin-susceptible and β-lactamase-producing strains of *Staph. aureus* that do not produce a functional PBP 2a (p. 235). It is bactericidal at concentrations close to the MIC; antibacterial activity in vitro is not affected by the presence of serum.

Acquired resistance

Resistance to methicillin is very common among strains of *Staph. epidermidis* and other coagulase-negative staphylococci, which are now responsible for many nosocomial bloodstream infections. As is the case with MRSA, most methicillin-resistant isolates of coagulase-negative staphylococci display multiresistance.

Pharmacokinetics

Oral absorption	Negligible
C_{max} 1 g intravenous (rapid infusion over 5 min)	60 mg/l
1 g intramuscular	17 mg/l after 0.5 h
Plasma half-life	0.5 h
Plasma protein binding	17–45%

Absorption and distribution

It is not acid resistant, and must therefore be administered parenterally. It is widely distributed, levels in serous fluids approximating to those in the serum, but it does not enter the CSF except, irregularly, in the presence of meningitis. Concentrations close to the simultaneous serum level have been found in infected bone.

Metabolism and excretion

About 10% is metabolized. This is enhanced in renal impairment and depressed in hepatic failure. A small amount (2–3%) appears in the bile but 60–80% is excreted in the urine by glomerular filtration and tubular secretion. Administration of probenecid significantly elevates and prolongs the plasma level. It is only slowly removed by hemodialysis.

Toxicity and side effects

Reversible leukopenia is fairly common and agranulocytosis and thrombocytopenia are described. Acute hemorrhagic cystitis is a rare reaction, and interstitial nephritis is common in patients receiving large doses, who may be slow to recover and subsequently relapse on administration of the same or another β-lactam antibiotic. Nephritis appears to be more common than with other penicillins, and therapy with nafcillin or an isoxazolylpenicillin is preferred. Concurrent appearance of neutropenia due to maturation arrest, hematuria and renal tubular atrophy associated with intense C_3 fixation, suggests all may be of immunological origin.

Maculopapular and urticarial rashes have been noted, particularly in children. Other reactions are those common to the group (p. 226).

Clinical use

Indications are those of group 3 penicillins (p. 235), but it is now seldom used.

Preparations and dosage

Preparation: Injection.

Dosage: Adults, i.m., i.v., 1 g every 4–6 h; in severe infections up to 12 g/day may be given. Children <2 years, quarter adult dose; children 2–10 years, half the adult dose.

Limited availability.

Further information

Blumberg HM 1991 Rapid development of ciprofloxacin resistance in methicillin-susceptible and -resistant *Staphylococcus aureus. Journal of Infectious Diseases* 163: 1279–1285.

Brown DF, Yates VS 1986 Methicillin susceptibility testing of *Staphylococcus aureus* on media containing five per cent sodium chloride. *European Journal of Clinical Microbiology* 5: 726–728.

Chambers HF 1988 Methicillin-resistant staphylococci. *Clinical Microbiology Reviews* 1: 173–186.

Coudron PE, Jones DL, Dalton HP, Archer GL 1986 Evaluation of laboratory tests for detection of methicillin-resistant *Staphylococcus aureus* and *Staphylococcus epidermidis. Journal of Clinical Microbiology* 24: 764–769.

Hackbarth CJ, Chambers HF 1989 Methicillin-resistant staphylococci. *Antimicrobial Agents and Chemotherapy* 33: 991–999.

Jarløv JO, Rosdahl VT, Mortensen I, Bentzon MW 1988 In vitro activity and beta-lactamase stability of methicillin, isoxazolyl penicillins and cephalothin against coagulase-negative staphylococci. *Journal of Antimicrobial Chemotherapy* 22: 119–125.

Livermore DM 2000 Antibiotic resistance in staphylococci. *International Journal of Antimicrobial Agents* 16 (Suppl. 1): S3–10.

Vigeral P, Kanfer A, Kenouch S, Blanchet F, Mougenot B, Méry JP 1987 Nephrogenic diabetes insipidus and distal tubular acidosis in methicillin-induced interstitial nephritis. *Advances in Experimental Biology and Medicine* 212: 129–134.

Wakefield DS, Pfaller M, Massanari RM, Hammons GT 1987 Variation in methicillin-resistant *Staphylococcus aureus* occurrence by geographic location and hospital characteristics. *Infection Control* 8: 151–157.

 NAFCILLIN

Molecular weight (free acid): 414.4.

A semisynthetic penicillin supplied as the sodium salt for oral or parenteral use.

Antimicrobial activity

The antibacterial spectrum is similar to that of the isoxazolylpenicillins but it is more active against streptococci and pneumococci (Table 16.2, p. 234). Activity in vitro is depressed in the presence of serum. It is as stable as methicillin, and more stable than the isoxazolylpenicillins, to staphylococcal β-lactamase. There is complete cross-resistance with other group 3 penicillins. Bactericidal synergy with rifampicin and aminoglycosides is demonstrable against *Staph. aureus.* Synergy is also seen with ampicillin against β-lactamase-negative ampicillin-resistant strains of *H. influenzae.*

Pharmacokinetics

Oral absorption	*c.* 35%
C_{max} 1 g intramuscular	8 mg/l after 1 h
Plasma half-life	0.5 h
Plasma protein binding	87%

Absorption

Nafcillin is poorly and irregularly absorbed after oral administration, even on an empty stomach, and absorption is further depressed if the drug is given with food.

Distribution

Penetration into tissues is similar to that of the isoxazolylpenicillins. Penetration into normal meninges is low. In patients with bacterial ventriculitis, CSF concentrations ranged from 1% to 20% of the simultaneous plasma value. Penetration was inversely related to ventricular fluid glucose, but poorly correlated with pleocytosis.

Metabolism

About 60–70% is inactivated in the liver.

Excretion

After oral administration only about 11% is recovered in the urine over 12 h. Following intramuscular administration, about 30% appears in the urine, producing concentrations up to 1000 mg/l. Administration of probenecid reduces the urinary excretion and raises and prolongs the plasma level. About 8% of the dose is excreted in the bile.

Toxicity and side effects

There is cross-allergenicity with other penicillins, and reappearance of methicillin-induced nephropathy on treatment with nafcillin has been described. In addition to side effects common to penicillins, reversible neutropenia may occur. Abnormal platelet aggregation responses with normal platelet counts and morphology have been associated with bleeding in some cases.

Clinical use

Uses are those of group 3 penicillins (p. 235). Nafcillin has been particularly recommended for the treatment of staphylococcal meningitis.

Preparations and dosage

Proprietary names: Unipen, Nafcil.

Preparations: Injection, tablets, capsules, oral solution.

Dosage: Adults, oral, 250 mg to 1 g every 4–6 h. Children, 6.25–12.5 mg/kg four times daily; neonates, 10 mg/kg 3–4 times daily. Adults, i.m., i.v., 0.5–1.5 g every 4–6 h. Children, 25 mg/kg twice a day; neonates, 10 mg/kg twice a day.

Available in USA.

Further information

Alexander DP, Russo ME, Fohrman DE, Rothstein G 1983 Nafcillin-induced platelet dysfunction and bleeding. *Antimicrobial Agents and Chemotherapy* 23: 59–62.

Banner W Jr, Gooch WM, Burckart G, Korones SB 1980 Pharmacokinetics of nafcillin in infants with low birth weights. *Antimicrobial Agents and Chemotherapy* 17: 691–694.

Tilden SJ, Craft JC, Cano R, Daum RS 1980 Cutaneous necrosis associated with intravenous nafcillin therapy. *American Journal of Disease of Children* 134: 1046–1048.

Zenk KE, Dungy CI, Greene GR 1981 Nafcillin extravasation injury. *American Journal of Diseases of Children* 135: 1113–1114.

OXACILLIN

Molecular weight (free acid): 401.5.

A semisynthetic penicillin supplied as the sodium salt for oral or intravenous administration. The first of the isoxazolyl series of β-lactamase-resistant penicillins.

Antimicrobial activity

Its spectrum and activity are those of isoxazolylpenicillins (Table 16.2, p. 234). Resistant and tolerant strains show complete cross-resistance and tolerance with other group 3 penicillins. Oxacillin has replaced methicillin for standardized susceptibility testing to detect resistant staphylococci due to its more reliable predictive value.

Acquired resistance

In addition to methicillin-resistant strains producing the low affinity PBP 2a, a small proportion of methicillin-susceptible isolates of *Staph. aureus* display reduced susceptibility to oxacillin, possibly due to hyperproduction of penicillinase.

Pharmacokinetics

Oral absorption	30–35%
C_{max} 500 mg oral	4 mg/l after 0.5 h
Plasma half-life	2 h
Plasma protein binding	92–96%

Absorption

It is the least well absorbed of the isoxazolylpenicillins. Approximately twice the oral fasting level is produced by the same dose administered intramuscularly.

Distribution

Oxacillin is widely distributed into interstitial fluid despite its high protein binding. Some appears in the bile.

Metabolism and excretion

Oxacillin is rapidly metabolized, but the main route of elimination is renal, about 25% of the dose being recovered from the urine as active material and another 25% as inactive metabolites. It is rapidly inactivated in the body and there is no accumulation in patients with end-stage kidney disease. It is still more rapidly eliminated in patients with cystic fibrosis.

Toxicity and side effects

There is cross-allergy with other penicillins and reactions are generally typical of the group. Abnormalities of liver function, especially elevation of transaminase levels, sometimes accompanied by fever, nausea, vomiting and eosinophilia, occur with biopsy evidence of non-specific hepatitis. There is rapid reversal on withdrawal of treatment and the response appears to be peculiar to oxacillin in that recrudescence was not observed on subsequent administration of benzylpenicillin or nafcillin. Neurotoxicity may develop on high dosage of patients with renal failure.

Clinical use

Uses are those of group 3 penicillins (p. 235).

Preparations and dosage

Proprietary names: Bactocill, Prostaphin.

Preparations: Capsules, oral solution, injection.

Dosage: Adults, oral, 500 mg to 1 g every 4–6 h; i.m., i.v., 250 mg to 1 g every 4–6 h. Children (under 40 kg), 12.5–25 mg/kg every 4–6 h. Newborn and premature infants, 25 mg/kg per day in divided doses may be given, but used with caution.

Available widely in continental Europe, North America, South America and Japan. Not available in the UK.

Further information

Hilty MD, Venglarcik JS, Best GK 1980 Oxacillin-tolerant staphylococcal bacteremia in children. *Journal of Pediatrics* 96: 1035–1037.

Massanari RM, Pfaller MA, Wakefield DS et al 1988 Implications of acquired oxacillin resistance in the management and control of *Staphylococcus aureus* infections. *Journal of Infectious Diseases* 158: 702–709.

McDougal LK, Thornsberry C 1986 The role of β-lactamase in staphylococcal resistance to penicillinase-resistant penicillins and cephalosporins. *Journal of Clinical Microbiology* 23: 832–839.

National Committee for Clinical Laboratory Standards 2000 Methods for dilution antimicrobial susceptibility tests for bacteria that grow aerobically. Approved standard – Fifth edition. Vol. M7-A5.

Pfaller MA, Wakefield DS, Stewart B, Bale M, Hammons GT, Massanari RM 1988 Evaluation of laboratory methods for the classification of oxacillin-resistant and oxacillin-susceptible *Staphylococcus aureus*. *American Journal of Clinical Pathology* 89: 120–125.

GROUP 4: EXTENDED-SPECTRUM PENICILLINS

The introduction of an amino group in the α-position of the side-chain of benzylpenicillin confers a high degree of acid stability together with enhanced activity against Gram-negative bacteria. Ampicillin, the first of the aminopenicillins to be developed, retains the activity of benzylpenicillin against Gram-positive cocci but exhibits increased activity against *H. influenzae* and certain Gram-negative bacilli, notably *Esch. coli*, *S. enterica* serotypes, *Shigella* spp. and *Pr. mirabilis*. The aminopenicillins lack stability to β-lactamases and are readily inactivated by β-lactamase-producing bacteria; but in combination with β-lactamase inhibitors (p. 272) they display enhanced activity against many β-lactamase-producing isolates.

The clinical success of ampicillin resulted in the development of a number of modified aminopenicillins with claims for superior properties. Compounds closely related structurally to ampicillin include amoxicillin, epicillin and ciclacillin.

Amoxicillin differs from ampicillin in possessing a *p*-hydroxy group in the benzene ring of the side chain and has a spectrum of activity essentially identical to that of ampicillin, but is bactericidal to susceptible Gram-negative bacilli at rather lower concentrations. Also, amoxicillin has superior oral absorption characteristics and the combination of improved antibacterial and pharmacokinetic properties has resulted in the newer compound largely displacing ampicillin as single-agent therapy.

The antibacterial activity of epicillin is virtually identical to that of ampicillin, while that of ciclacillin is substantially less. Neither of these agents is widely used.

Four esters of ampicillin (bacampicillin, lenampicillin, pivampicillin, talampicillin) have been developed as prodrugs with oral absorption characteristics superior to those of the parent penicillin. The esters are lipophilic compounds that are devoid of antibacterial activity in their own right but which are hydrolyzed by tissue esterases during absorption to liberate ampicillin. Two condensation products, hetacillin and metampicillin, formed by combination of ampicillin with acetone and formaldehyde respectively, hydrolyze spontaneously to release ampicillin. The antibacterial activity of all these compounds is due solely to the ampicillin liberated.

Two other group 4 penicillins, mecillinam (amdinocillin) and its prodrug pivmecillinam, are structurally different from the aminopenicillins. Like other semisynthetic penicillins they are derived from 6-APA but differ in being 6-α-amidinopenicillanates rather than 6-α-acylaminopenicillanates. This is reflected in the antibacterial spectrum of mecillinam, which is atypical of the penicillins in displaying high activity against Gram-negative bacteria but poor activity against Gram-positive cocci. The mechanism of action of mecillinam differs from that of other penicillins in binding almost exclusively to PBP 2 (p. 14) in Gram-negative bacteria.

PHARMACOKINETICS

The aminopenicillins are acid stable and can be given orally. Ampicillin is the least well absorbed, about one-third of the dose appearing in the urine as active drug, and absorption is further reduced by food. The esters and amoxicillin are substantially better absorbed and not significantly affected by food, peak plasma levels generally being at least twice those achieved by equivalent doses of ampicillin. The condensates and epicillin offer no material advantage over ampicillin in terms of absorption, whereas ciclacillin is more similar to amoxicillin in producing high plasma antibiotic concentrations. Plasma elimination half-lives are generally around 1 h and plasma protein binding is low (around 20%). Excretion is primarily renal, resulting in high concentrations of active antibiotic in urine; a proportion of an oral dose (10–20%) is metabolized in the liver and small amounts are found in the bile. With metampicillin, comparatively high biliary concentrations of ampicillin appear after parenteral administration. The aminopenicillins and the condensates may be administered by parenteral routes, but the esters are given only by mouth. Mecillinam is not absorbed by mouth but its pivaloyloxymethyl ester, pivmecillinam, is relatively well absorbed by the oral route.

TOXICITY AND SIDE EFFECTS

Patients with a history of hypersensitivity to penicillins should be treated cautiously, as serious anaphylactic responses may occur. Ampicillin appears to be less likely than benzylpenicillin to elicit true allergic reactions, but much more likely to give rise to rashes that appear not to be of allergic origin, especially in patients with infectious mononucleosis or other lymphoid disorders. It was originally thought that the prevalence of rashes was lower in patients treated with amoxicillin, but this appears not to be so. Ampicillin esters naturally have the same potential to give rise to rashes, but it has been claimed that they are less common after epicillin, ciclacillin and mecillinam.

Gastrointestinal side effects are relatively common in

patients treated with oral ampicillin. Ampicillin esters and the ester of mecillinam are more likely to cause upper abdominal discomfort, nausea and vomiting, but are less likely, being better absorbed (as are amoxicillin and ciclacillin), to cause diarrhea. Upper abdominal symptoms are substantially ameliorated if the esters are taken with food. Although questions have been raised about the potential toxicity of unhydrolyzed esters in circulation, it appears that these esters are very rapidly degraded and no toxic manifestation has been traced to the various degradation products. Liver function should be monitored in patients receiving prolonged courses, or in those in whom renal or hepatic function is impaired.

CLINICAL USE

Aminopenicillins are all recommended for the wide range of infections that made ampicillin one of the most commonly prescribed agents, notably for urinary and respiratory infections. However, the increasing frequency of isolation of β-lactamase-producing pathogens has resulted in a reduction of the usefulness of the aminopenicillins and often relegation to second-line treatment in these areas. This difficulty is overcome by combining ampicillin or amoxicillin with β-lactamase inhibitors (p. 272). Ampicillin and amoxicillin also have a role in the treatment of severe infections, including endocarditis, meningitis and septicemia, often in combination with other antibacterial agents, particularly aminoglycosides. Mecillinam is suitable only for infections involving Gram-negative bacteria and should not be used where Gram-positive organisms may be implicated.

 AMOXICILLIN

Amoxycillin. Molecular weight (free acid): 365.4; (trihydrate): 419.5.

p-Hydroxy ampicillin. Supplied as the trihydrate for oral administration and as the sodium salt for parenteral use. A formulation with clavulanic acid (co-amoxiclav) is also available (*see* p. 273).

Antimicrobial activity

The antibacterial spectrum is identical to that of ampicillin and there are few differences in antibacterial activity (Table 16.3). Like ampicillin, amoxicillin is unstable to most β-lactamases. It produces a more rapid bactericidal effect than ampicillin against Gram-negative bacilli at concentrations close to

Table 16.3 Activity of group 4 penicillins against common pathogenic bacteria: MIC (mg/l)

	Ampicillin	Amoxicillin	Epicillin	Mecillinam
Staph. aureus	0.06–1	0.1	0.1	128
Str. pyogenes	0.03	0.01	0.03	2
Str. pneumoniae	0.03–0.06	0.03	ND	2
E. faecalis	1	0.5	1	R
N. gonorrhoeae	0.03–0.06	0.1	0.06	0.1
N. meningitidis	0.03–0.06	0.06	ND	ND
H. influenzae	0.25	0.5	0.25	16
Esch. coli	4	4	4	0.25
K. pneumoniae	R	R	R	1
Ps. aeruginosa	R	R	R	R
B. fragilis	32	32	32	R

R, resistant (MIC ≥ 128 mg/l). ND, No data.

MIC values as a consequence of higher affinity for the lytic set of PBPs. It also has useful activity against *Helicobacter pylori*, although occasional isolates are resistant due to modified PBPs.

Acquired resistance

There is complete cross-resistance with ampicillin. Its action against many strains that owe their resistance to elaboration of β-lactamases can be restored by coadministration with β-lactamase inhibitors (p. 272).

Pharmacokinetics

Oral absorption	75–90%
C_{max} 500 mg oral	5.5–7.5 mg/l after 1–2 h
500 mg intramuscular	*c.* 14 mg/l after 1–2 h
Plasma half-life	1 h
Volume of distribution	0.3 l/kg
Plasma protein binding	17–20%

Absorption

Oral absorption is comparable with that of the ampicillin esters, producing around 2.5 times the peak concentration achieved by comparable doses of ampicillin. Absorption is unaffected by food.

Distribution

In patients receiving 500 mg 8-hourly for 10 days, concentrations in mucoid and purulent sputum were 0–1.2 (mean 0.2) mg/l and 0–3.0 (mean 1.0) mg/l, respectively. In patients receiving 750 mg, mean concentrations of 1.56 mg/l were achieved in pleural fluid. Levels of 84% of those in the serum were found in the peritoneal fluid of patients given 1 g by intravenous bolus. In children with chronic serous otitis media given 15 mg/kg, variable peak concentrations up to those in the serum were found in middle ear fluid at 2–3 h when the mean serum concentration was 5.8 mg/l

Metabolism
Some 10–25% is converted to the penicilloic acid.

Excretion
Between 50 and 70% of unchanged drug is recovered in the urine in the first 6 h after a dose of 250 mg. Plasma levels are elevated and prolonged by the administration of probenecid.

Toxicity and side effects

Amoxicillin is generally well tolerated, side effects (including non-allergic rashes in patients with glandular fever) being those common to penicillins. As the drug is well absorbed, diarrhea is generally infrequent and rarely sufficiently severe to require withdrawal of treatment.

Clinical use

- Upper respiratory tract infection (other than pharyngitis, which may mask glandular fever) due to streptococci, pneumococci, and *H. influenzae*.
- Lower respiratory tract infection.
- Urinary tract infection.
- Infections of skin and soft tissues due to streptococci and susceptible staphylococci.
- Gonorrhea.
- *Helicobacter pylori* infection (in combination with a proton pump inhibitor and a second antimicrobial agent such as clarithromycin).
- Dental prophylaxis in patients at risk of endocarditis (single high dose).

Isolates should be tested for susceptibility before use, especially for serious infections.

Preparations and dosage

Proprietary names: Amoxil (and many generic formulations).

Preparations: Capsules, suspension, injection, dispersible tablets, oral sachets.

Dosage: Adults, oral, 250–500 mg every 8 h high-dose therapy, 3 g twice daily; short course therapy, simple acute urinary tract infection, two 3 g doses with 10–12 h between doses, gonorrhea, single 3 g dose; i.m., i.v., 500 mg every 8 h, the dose may be increased to 1 g i.v. every 6 h in severe infections. Children up to 10 years, oral, 125–250 mg three times daily. In severe otitis media, 750 mg twice daily for 2 days may be used in children 3–10 years; i.m., i.v., 50–100 mg/kg per day in divided doses.

Widely available.

Further information

Anonymous 1999 Amoxicillin. In: Dollery C (ed.) *Therapeutic Drugs* 2nd edn. Churchill Livingstone, Edinburgh, pp. A162–A165.

Brogden RN, Speight TM, Avery GS 1975 Amoxycillin: a review of its antibacterial and pharmacokinetic properties and therapeutic use. *Drugs* 9: 88–140.

Cannon PD, Black HJ, Kitson K 1987 Serum concentrations of amoxycillin in children following an oral loading dose prior to general anesthesia: relevance for the prophylaxis of infective endocarditis. *Journal of Antimicrobial Chemotherapy* 19: 795–797.

Clumeck N, Thys JP, Vanhoof R, Vanderlinden MP, Butzler JP, Yourassowsky E 1978 Amoxicillin entry into human cerebro-spinal fluid: comparison with ampicillin. *Antimicrobial Agents and Chemotherapy* 14: 531–532.

Feder HM 1982 Comparative tolerability of ampicillin, amoxicillin and trimethoprim–sulfamethoxazole suspensions in children with otitis media. *Antimicrobial Agents and Chemotherapy* 21: 426–427.

MacGregor AJ, Hart P 1986 The effect of a single large dose of amoxycillin on oral streptococci. *Journal of Antimicrobial Chemotherapy* 18: 113–117.

Mattie H, Van der Voet GB 1981 The relative potency of amoxycillin and ampicillin in vitro and in vivo. *Scandinavian Journal of Infectious Diseases* 13: 291–296.

Peura D 1998 *Helicobacter pylori*: rational management options. *American Journal of Medicine*. 105: 424–430.

Shah PM 1981 Bactericidal activity of ampicillin and amoxicillin. *Journal of Antimicrobial Chemotherapy* 8 (Suppl. C): 93–99.

Sjovall J, Alvan G, Huitfeldt B 1986 Intra- and inter-individual variation in pharmacokinetics of intravenously infused amoxycillin and ampicillin to elderly volunteers. *British Journal of Clinical Pharmacology* 21: 171–181.

Todd PA, Benfield P 1990 Amoxicillin/clavulanic acid; an update of its antibacterial activity, pharmacokinetic properties and clinical use. *Drugs* 39: 264–307.

AMPICILLIN

Molecular weight (free acid): 349.4; (sodium salt): 471.4.

A semisynthetic penicillin administered orally as the trihydrate and parenterally as the soluble sodium salt. Formulations with sulbactam are also available (*see* p. 275).

Antimicrobial activity

Its activity against common pathogenic bacteria is shown in Table 16.3. Ampicillin is slightly less active than benzylpenicillin against most Gram-positive bacteria but is more active against *E. faecalis*. It is destroyed by staphylococcal β-lactamases and strains of *Str. pneumoniae* with reduced susceptibility to benzylpenicillin are usually resistant. Most group D streptococci, anaerobic Gram-positive cocci and bacilli, including *L. monocytogenes*, *Actinomyces* spp. and *Arachnia* spp., are susceptible. Mycobacteria and nocardia are resistant.

Ampicillin is slightly less active than benzylpenicillin against *N. gonorrhoeae* and *N. meningitidis*, slightly more active against

M. catarrhalis, and 2–4 times more active against *H. influenzae*. It is 4–8 times more active than benzylpenicillin against *Esch. coli*, *Pr. mirabilis*, *S. enterica* serotypes and *Shigella* spp., but β-lactamase-producing strains are resistant, as are *K. pneumoniae* and most other Enterobacteriaceae that produce at least one chromosomal β-lactamase. *Pseudomonas* spp. are resistant. *Bordetella*, *Brucella* and *Legionella* spp. are susceptible and *Campylobacter* spp. are frequently so. Certain Gram-negative anaerobes such as *Prevotella melaninogenica* and *Fusobacterium* spp. are susceptible, but *B. fragilis* is resistant, as are mycoplasmas and rickettsiae.

Activity against molecular class A β-lactamase-producing strains of staphylococci, gonococci, *H. influenzae*, *M. catarrhalis*, certain Enterobacteriaceae and *B. fragilis* is enhanced by the presence of β-lactamase inhibitors.

Its bactericidal activity resembles that of benzylpenicillin. Bactericidal synergy occurs with aminoglycosides against *E. faecalis* and many enterobacteria, and with mecillinam against a number of ampicillin-resistant enterobacteria. Bactericidal activity against group B streptococci, *H. influenzae* and *L. monocytogenes* is antagonized by chloramphenicol.

Acquired resistance

β-Lactamase-producing pathogens, including most clinical isolates of *Staph. aureus*, are resistant. All penicillin-resistant pneumococci and enterococci have reduced susceptibility to ampicillin. Strains of *N. gonorrhoeae* and *H. influenzae* with altered PBPs are less common than isolates with a TEM plasmid-mediated β-lactamase. The former may be moderately susceptible, but β-lactamase-producing strains of *H. influenzae* are fully resistant. β-Lactamase production is much higher among capsulate type B strains than in non-capsulate strains. Resistance among *H. influenzae* is often linked with resistance to chloramphenicol, erythromycin or tetracycline, due to plasmid-encoded resistance markers that are co-transferred with the gene for the TEM enzyme.

The widespread use of ampicillin and other aminopenicillins has led to resistance becoming common in formerly susceptible species of enteric pathogens as a result of the widespread dissemination of plasmid-mediated β-lactamases. Surveillance data from North America indicate only 52–54% susceptibility to ampicillin in *Esch. coli*. The identification of β-lactamase-producing isolates of *M. catarrhalis* has increased dramatically; such strains were unknown before 1977, whereas 90% of current isolates are β-lactamase-producing strains. Most strains of the sexually transmitted pathogen *H. ducreyi* have acquired TEM plasmid-mediated β-lactamases and are resistant.

β-Lactamase-producing strains of salmonellae, notably *S. enterica* serotypes Typhi and Typhimurium, are commonly isolated, and strains resistant to other antibiotics (including chloramphenicol, sulfonamides and tetracyclines) present a serious problem in Africa, Asia and South America. Multi resistant strains of shigellae also predominate in many parts of the world.

Pharmacokinetics

Oral absorption	30–40%
C_{max} 500 mg oral	2–6 mg/l after *c.* 2 h
500 mg intramuscular	5–15 mg/l after 1 h
500 mg intravenous infusion	12–29 mg/l
Plasma half life	1–1.5 h
Volume of distribution	0.38 l/kg
Plasma protein binding	20%

Absorption

Ampicillin is highly stable to acid: in 2 h at pH 2 and 37°C, only 5% of activity is lost. Absorption is impaired when it is given with meals, but is not affected by administration of antacids or cimetidine.

Distribution

Ampicillin is distributed in the extracellular fluid. Adequate concentrations are obtained in serous effusions. Effective CSF levels are obtained only in the presence of inflammation and then irregularly, peak concentrations around 3 mg/l being found in the first 3 days of treatment in patients receiving 150 mg/kg per day.

Ampicillin accumulates and persists in the amniotic fluid, evidently in consequence of renal excretion by the fetus, the levels generally exceeding 2.5 mg/l after three maternal doses of 500 mg, with corresponding cord blood levels of 0.2–2 mg/l.

Metabolism

A small proportion is converted to penicilloic acid.

Excretion

About 30% of an oral dose and 60–80% of parenteral doses are recoverable from the urine, where concentrations around 250–1000 mg/l appear. Excretion is partly in the glomerular filtrate and partly by tubular secretion, which can be blocked by probenecid. Impairment of renal function reduces the rate of excretion, the plasma half-life rising to 8–9 h in anuric patients.

Although excretion is mainly renal, fairly high concentrations are attained in the bile, up to 50 times the corresponding serum level. There are wide variations among patients with normal biliary tracts, and in those with obstructive lesions concentrations are very low or nil. There is a degree of enterohepatic recirculation and significant quantities appear in the feces. Bioavailability may be affected in severe liver disease.

Toxicity and side effects

Ampicillin appears generally free from severe toxicity and, apart from gastrointestinal intolerance, the only significant side effects seen have been rashes. In common with other semisynthetic penicillins, it appears to be less likely than benzylpenicillin to elicit true allergic reactions. However, it is more likely to give rise to rashes, which are found in approximately 9% of treated patients. These may be of toxic rather than allergic origin and there is some evidence of dose relation, since rashes occur more frequently in patients receiving large doses or in renal failure. Rashes occur with almost diagnostic frequency (95%) in patients with infectious mononucleosis or other lymphoid disorders. This unusual susceptibility disappears when the disease resolves. In keeping with a toxic rather than an allergic origin, skin tests to ampicillin and to mixed-allergen moieties of benzylpenicillin are negative. Since the typical maculopapular rash of ampicillin does not have an allergic origin, its development does not indicate penicillin allergy and is not a contraindication to the use of other penicillins.

Gastrointestinal side effects are relatively common (around 10%) in patients treated with oral ampicillin, and occur in 2–3% of patients given the drug parenterally, presumably as a result of drug entering the gut through the bile. The very young and the old are most likely to suffer. Diarrhea can be sufficiently severe to require withdrawal of treatment and pseudomembranous colitis occurs, rates of 0.3–0.7% being quoted. Interference with the bowel flora, which is presumably implicated in diarrhea, can also affect enterohepatic recirculation of steroids, and the derangement can be sufficient to impair the absorption of oral contraceptives and affect the interpretation of estriol levels.

Clinical use

- Urinary tract infections.
- Gonorrhea.
- Respiratory tract infections.
- Gastrointestinal infections, including typhoid fever and severe shigellosis.
- Enterococcal endocarditis (in combination with an aminoglycoside).
- Listeriosis (in combination with an aminoglycoside).

Isolates should be tested for susceptibility before use, especially for serious infections. For oral therapy, amoxicillin is preferable to ampicillin.

 Preparations and dosage

Proprietary name: Penbritin, Omnipen and many generic preparations.

Preparations: Capsules, syrup, injection.

Dosage: Adults, oral, 250 mg to 1 g every 6 h; i.m., i.v., 500 mg every 4–6 h. Meningitis, i.v., 2 g every 4 h. Children under 10 years, any route, half the adult dose. Meningitis, i.v., 150–200 mg/kg/day in divided doses.

Widely available.

 Further information

Anonymous 1999 Ampicillin. In: Dollery C (ed.) *Therapeutic Drugs* 2nd edn. Churchill Livingstone, Edinburgh, pp. A172–A176.

Feder HM Jr 1982 Comparative tolerability of ampicillin, amoxicillin and trimethoprim-sulfamethoxazole suspensions in children with otitis media. *Antimicrobial Agents and Chemotherapy* 21: 426–427.

Givner LB, Abramson JS, Wasilauskas B 1989 Meningitis due to *Haemophilus influenzae* type B resistant to ampicillin and chloramphenicol. *Reviews of Infectious Diseases* 11: 329–334.

Mendelman PM, Chaffin DO, Stull TL, Rubens CE, Mack KD, Smith AL 1984 Characterization of non-beta-lactamase-mediated ampicillin resistance in *Haemophilus influenzae*. *Antimicrobial Agents and Chemotherapy* 26: 235–244.

Mikhail IA, Sippel JF, Girgis NI, Yassin MW 1981 Cerebrospinal fluid and serum ampicillin levels in bacterial meningitis patients after intravenous and intramuscular administration. *Scandinavian Journal of Infectious Diseases* 13: 237–238.

Overturf GD, Cable D, Ward J 1987 Ampicillin-chloramphenicol-resistant *Haemophilus influenzae*: plasmid-mediated resistance in bacterial meningitis. *Pediatric Research* 22: 438–441.

Pfaller MA, Jones RN, Doern GV, Kugler K, The SENTRY Participants Group 1998 Bacterial pathogens isolated from patients with bloodstream infection: frequencies of occurrence and antimicrobial susceptibility patterns from the SENTRY antimicrobial surveillance program (United States and Canada, 1997) *Antimicrobial Agents and Chemotherapy* 42: 1762–1770.

Sapico FL, Canawat HN, Ginunas VJ et al 1989 Enterococci highly resistant to penicillin and ampicillin: an emerging clinical problem? *Journal of Clinical Microbiology* 27: 2091–2095.

AMPICILLIN ESTERS

Bacampicillin

The ethoxycarbonyloxyethyl ester of ampicillin. There is near-complete oral absorption and swift hydrolysis of the ester by tissue esterases with rapid release of ampicillin, resulting in identical microbiological and toxicological profiles. It is absorbed from the intestine more rapidly and more completely than ampicillin, with average peak plasma levels 2–3 times those produced by equivalent doses of ampicillin. Mean absorption differed considerably among hospital patients and was less than in healthy volunteers.

 Preparations and dosage

Proprietary name: Ambaxin; Spectrobid.

Preparations: Tablets, oral suspension.

Dosage: Adults, oral, 400 mg, 2–3 times daily; dose doubled in severe infections. Children over 5 years, 200 mg three times daily.

Widely available; not available in the UK.

 Further information

Ginsburg CM, McCracken GH, Clahsen JC, Zweighaft TC 1981 Comparative pharmacokinetics of bacampicillin and ampicillin suspensions in infants and children. *Reviews of Infectious Diseases* 3: 117–120.

Neu HC 1981 The pharmacokinetics of bacampicillin. *Reviews of Infectious Diseases* 3: 110–116.

Sjovall J 1981 Tissue levels after administration of bacampicillin, a prodrug of ampicillin and comparisons with other aminopenicillins: a review. *Journal of Antimicrobial Chemotherapy* 8 (Suppl. C): 41–58.

Lenampicillin

The daloxate ester of ampicillin. It is metabolized to acetoin and ampicillin, to which it owes its microbiological and toxicological profile. In volunteers receiving 400 mg orally, peak concentrations were around 6.0 mg/l at about 1 h – about twice those seen with an equimolar dose (250 mg) of ampicillin. Peak plasma concentration is slightly lower and delayed by food, but the area under the curve (AUC) is unaltered. Urinary excretion is blocked by probenecid.

Preparations

Available in Japan.

Further information

Saito A, Nakashima M 1986 Pharmacokinetic study of lenampicillin (KBT-1585) in healthy volunteers. *Antimicrobial Agents and Chemotherapy* 29: 948–950.

Sum ZM, Sefton AM, Jepson AP, Williams JD 1989 Comparative pharmacokinetic study between lenampicillin, bacampicillin and amoxycillin. *Journal of Antimicrobial Chemotherapy* 23: 861–868.

Pivampicillin

The pivaloyloxymethyl ester of ampicillin. Its antimicrobial activity is that of liberated ampicillin to which it owes its microbiological and toxicological profile.

Its absorption is considerably better than that of the parent ampicillin and is less affected by food. Plasma levels rise more rapidly to 2–3 times those produced by corresponding doses of ampicillin: mean peak concentrations around 10 mg/l being obtained 1–2 h after an oral dose of 700 mg (equivalent to 500 mg ampicillin).

In the intestine it is rapidly hydrolyzed to pivalic acid and an unstable hydroxymethyl ester, which decomposes to ampicillin. More than 99% conversion to ampicillin is achieved in less than 15 min and not more than 2% of the unchanged ester can be detected in the peripheral blood. Relative excretions in the urine as a measure of degree of absorption are: ampicillin 30–45%, pivampicillin 55–75%.

Preparations and dosage

Proprietary names: Pondocillin, Miraxid.

Preparations: Tablets, suspension.

Dosage: Adults, oral, 500 mg every 12 h. Children, 6–10 years, 525–700 mg/day in 2–3 divided doses; children 1–5 years, 350–525 mg/day in 2–3 divided doses; children up to 1 year, 40–60 mg/kg per day in 2–3 divided doses. Doses may be doubled in severe infections.

Widely available.

Further information

Roholt K, Nielsen B, Kristensen E 1974 Clinical pharmacology of pivampicillin. *Antimicrobial Agents and Chemotherapy* 6: 563–571.

Verbist L 1974 Triple crossover study on absorption and excretion of ampicillin, pivampicillin and amoxycillin. *Antimicrobial Agents and Chemotherapy* 6: 588–593.

Talampicillin

The phthalidyl thiazolidine carboxylic ester of ampicillin. Its antimicrobial activity and toxicity profile are those of liberated ampicillin.

It is well absorbed when administered by mouth, doses of 250 or 500 mg producing mean peak plasma levels of 4 or 11 mg/l, respectively, about 2 h after the dose. Administration with food delays and depresses the peak concentration but the AUC is unaffected.

Preparations and dosage

Dosage: Adults, oral, 250–500 mg three times daily.

Limited availability.

Further information

Jones KH, Langley PF, Lees LJ 1979 Bioavailability and metabolism of talampicillin. *Chemotherapy* 24: 217–226.

Symonds J, Georg RH 1978 The effect of talampicillin on faecal flora. *Journal of Antimicrobial Chemotherapy* 4: 92–94.

AMPICILLIN CONDENSATES

Hetacillin

A condensation product of ampicillin and acetone. It is disputed whether it has any antibacterial action distinct from that of ampicillin, but any such activity is of no therapeutic significance since hetacillin hydrolyzes rapidly in the body to liberate ampicillin, leaving only trace amounts of the parent compound detectable in the plasma for about 90 min. Although there is disagreement, in general it appears that absorption, peak levels and excretion are all rather lower than those for ampicillin. Its toxicity profile is comparable to that of ampicillin.

Preparations and dosage

Dosage: Adults, oral, 250–500 mg four times daily.
Very limited availability.

Further information

Kahrimanis R, Pierpaoli P 1971 Hetacillin vs ampicillin. *New England Journal of Medicine* 285: 236–237.

Metampicillin

A condensation product of ampicillin with formaldehyde. It hydrolyzes sufficiently rapidly to ampicillin for no unchanged drug to be detectable in the plasma after oral dosage. When high levels are produced by parenteral administration, the drug bound to protein is more slowly hydrolyzed at the neutral pH of the plasma and unchanged compound is detectable and is excreted, in part in the bile, where it may give elevated free ampicillin levels.

Preparations and dosage

Dosage: Adults, oral, 1–2 g/day in 2–4 divided doses.
Available in Spain.

Further information

Sutherland R, Elson S, Croydon EA 1972 Metampicillin: antibacterial activity and absorption and excretion in man. *Chemotherapy* 17: 145–160.

MECILLINAM

Amdinocillin. Molecular weight (free acid): 325.4.

6-β-Amidinopenicillin. Supplied as the hydrochloride dihydrate for parenteral administration and as the hydrochloride salt of the pivaloyloxymethyl ester (pivmecillinam; amdinocillin pivoxil) for oral use.

Antimicrobial activity

The antibacterial spectrum differs greatly from that of the aminopenicillins in that the compound displays high activity against many Gram-negative bacteria but only low activity against Gram-positive organisms (Table 16.3, p. 242). Mecillinam is active against many Enterobacteriaceae, including *Esch. coli*, *Enterobacter*, *Klebsiella*, *Salmonella*, and *Yersinia* spp. The susceptibility of *Proteus* and *Providencia* spp. is variable, *H. influenzae* is less susceptible than enteric bacilli, *Acinetobacter* spp., *B. fragilis* and *Ps. aeruginosa* are resistant. The activity is greatly reduced in media with high osmolality and in tests using high inocula.

Mecillinam is readily inactivated by many β-lactamases, although it is more stable than ampicillin, possibly because of poor affinity for the enzymes coupled with rapid penetration of the bacterial cell. Combination with β-lactamase inhibitors results in increased activity against many β-lactamase-producing strains of Enterobacteriaceae.

As a consequence of the mode of action (p. 14), cell division is not prevented; bactericidal activity is slow, inoculum dependent and varies inversely with salt and sucrose content of the medium. After exposure to the drug, the round forms generated can continue to grow and divide in spheroplast-like forms. These variants are phenotypically resistant in that they can grow in high mecillinam concentrations, but growth is relatively slow and their therapeutic importance is unclear.

Acquired resistance

Intrinsic resistance in susceptible species of enterobacteria is uncommon and many ampicillin-resistant enterobacteria are susceptible. Bacteria that are resistant to both ampicillin and mecillinam are usually those producing large amounts of β-lactamase, most commonly plasmid-mediated enzymes.

Pharmacokinetics

Oral absorption (pivmecillinam)	*c.* 75%
C_{max} 200 mg intravenous infusion	12 mg/l end infusion
200 mg intramuscular	*c.* 6 mg/l after 45 min
400 mg oral (pivmecillinam)	2–5 mg/l after *c.* 1 h
Plasma half-life	50 min
Volume of distribution	0.2–0.4 l/kg
Plasma protein binding	5–10%

Absorption

Oral absorption is very poor, with conventional doses producing plasma levels of <1 mg/l and recovery of only about 5% in the urine.

A 400 mg dose of the pivaloyl ester is equivalent to 273 mg mecillinam. It is relatively well absorbed and rapidly liberates the parent compound. Administration with food has little or no effect on its absorption.

Metabolism

Mecillinam is not metabolized, but the amidino side chain undergoes spontaneous aqueous hydrolysis to the *N*-formyl derivative, which retains some antibacterial activity. Hydrolysis of the β-lactam ring also occurs.

Excretion

Approximately 60% is excreted unchanged in the urine in the first 6 h, achieving concentrations exceeding 1 g/l. Plasma clearance and creatinine clearance are linearly related. The concentration in bile can reach 40 or 50 mg/l in patients with normally functioning gall-bladders treated with 800 mg intramuscularly.

Toxicity and side effects

Mecillinam is generally well tolerated, and serious anaphylactic responses are said to be very rare. Nausea and vomiting, which may be persistent, occur with diarrhea in some patients treated with pivmecillinam.

Clinical use

- Urinary tract infection (pivmecillinam).
- Other infections with susceptible Gram-negative bacilli (usually in combination with other agents.

Preparations and dosage

Proprietary names: Selexid, Selexidin

Preparation: Injection, suspension, tablets.

Dosage: Adults, mecillinam: 5–10 mg/kg every 6–8 h depending on the severity of the infection; pivmecillinam: 200–400 mg 3–4 times daily.

Limited availability; pivmecillinam available in UK.

Further information

Anonymous 1999 Amdinocillin. In: Dollery C (ed.) *Therapeutic Drugs* 2nd edn. Churchill Livingstone, Edinburgh, pp. A119–A122.

Geddes AM, Wise R 1977 Mecillinam. *Journal of Antimicrobial Chemotherapy* 3 (Suppl. B): 1–160.

Patel IH, Bornemann LD, Brocks VM, Fang LST, Tolkoff-Rubin NE, Rubin RH 1985 Pharmacokinetics of intravenous amdinocillin in healthy subjects and patients with renal insufficiency. *Antimicrobial Agents and Chemotherapy* 28: 46–50.

Roholt K 1977 Pharmacokinetic studies with mecillinam and pivmecillinam. *Journal of Antimicrobial Chemotherapy* 3 (Suppl. B): 71–81.

Symposium 1983 An international review of amdinocillin: a new beta-lactam antibiotic. *American Journal of Medicine* 75 (Suppl.): 1–138.

OTHER GROUP 4 PENICILLINS

Ciclacillin

Cyclacillin. The structure differs from other aminopenicillins in that the benzene ring is completely saturated and the amino substituent is attached directly to it instead of being linked to an adjacent carbon atom. It is some 10–20 times less active than ampicillin against staphylococci, streptococci and *H. influenzae*, but is better absorbed by mouth, peak plasma levels of 10–18 mg/l being reached 30–60 min after a 500 mg oral dose. Its pharmacokinetic properties, side effects and use resemble those of ampicillin.

Preparations and dosage

Preparations: Tablets, oral suspension.

Dosage: Adults, oral, 250–500 mg four times daily. Children, oral, 50–100 mg/kg/day in four divided doses.

Available in Japan.

Further information

Gonzaga AJ, Antonio-Velmonte M, Tupasi TE 1974 Cyclacillin: a clinical and in vitro profile. *Journal of Infectious Diseases* 129: 545–551.

Epicillin

An analog of ampicillin in which the benzene ring is partially saturated. It closely resembles ampicillin in its antibacterial properties. Although it is somewhat more active against *Ps. aeruginosa*, this is of no therapeutic significance (Table 16.3, p. 242). It is moderately well absorbed, a 500 mg oral dose producing mean peak plasma levels of 2–3 mg/l. Its behavior on intramuscular injection, distribution, excretion, toxicity and uses resemble those of ampicillin.

Preparations and dosage

Available fairly widely in continental Europe, and in Argentina and South Africa.

Further information

Gadebusch H, Miraglia G, Pansy F 1971 Epicillin: experimental chemotherapy, pharmacodynamics and susceptibility testing. *Infection and Immunity* 4: 50–53.

Table 16.4 Activity of group 5 and 6 penicillins against common pathogenic bacteria: MIC (mg/l)

	Apalcillin	Azlocillin	Mezlocillin	Piperacillin	Carbenicillin	Ticarcillin	Sulbenicillin	Temocillin
Staph. aureus	1	1	1	0.5	1	1	2	R
Str. pyogenes	0.03	0.03	0.06	0.03	0.5	0.25	0.5	R
Str. pneumoniae	0.03	0.03	0.03	0.03	1	0.5	1	R
E. faecalis	4	2	2	2	16–32	32	32	R
N. gonorrhoeae	<0.01	<0.01	<0.01	<0.01	0.06–0.1	0.06	0.1	0.01–1
N. meningitidis			0.03	0.06	0.06	0.06	ND	ND
H. influenzae	0.06	0.06	0.1	0.03	0.25–0.5	0.5	ND	0.1–2
Esch. coli	4	16	4	2	4–8	4	4	1–8
K. pneumoniae	16	64	32	16	R	R	R	1–16
Ps. aeruginosa	2	4	32	2	64	16–32	32	R
B. fragilis	16	8	16	8	16	16	ND	R

R, resistant (MIC ≥ 128 mg/l). ND, No data.

GROUP 5: PENICILLINS ACTIVE AGAINST *PS. AERUGINOSA*

Certain derivatives of benzylpenicillin or ampicillin exhibit useful activity against *Ps. aeruginosa*. Three derivatives of benzylpenicillin possessing an acidic group in the acyl side chain are in clinical use: carbenicillin and ticarcillin are α-carboxypenicillins, and the third, sulbenicillin, possesses a sulfonic acid group in the side chain. The acyl derivatives of ampicillin active against *Ps. aeruginosa* include the acylureidopenicillins: azlocillin, mezlocillin and piperacillin. Apalcillin and aspoxicillin are also acylaminopenicillins, with properties generally similar to the ureidopenicillins, but lack the ureido group in the side chain.

In addition, two prodrug forms of carbenicillin are available for oral use: the phenyl ester, carfecillin, and the indanyl ester, carindacillin. Unlike ampicillin esters, these compounds are esterified at the side-chain carboxyl group and, since the carboxyl of the penicillin nucleus is free, they exhibit antibacterial activity in vitro which differs in some respects from that of the parent compound. This is of academic interest only because in the body they are rapidly hydrolyzed to carbenicillin, to which they owe their therapeutic activity. Carbenicillin and ticarcillin exist as pairs of diastereoisomers (R and S epimers), which interconvert in aqueous solutions at rates that depend on temperature, pH and ionic strength. The epimers show differences in detail in their antimicrobial activity and pharmacokinetic behavior, but this is considered not to influence the clinical efficacy of the mixtures.

ANTIMICROBIAL ACTIVITY

The acylureidopenicillins and the carboxypenicillins display similar antibacterial spectra, but the ureidopenicillins are more active against streptococci and enterococci (Table 16.4). Both groups are as active as ampicillin against susceptible Gram-negative bacteria and exhibit moderate to good activity against many ampicillin-resistant strains of Enterobacteriaceae possessing class C chromosomally mediated β-lactamases (p. 263–264), including nosocomial pathogens such as *Citrobacter, Enterobacter, Morganella, Providencia* and *Serratia* spp. However, strains producing elevated amounts of β-lactamase, such as those organisms with derepressed β-lactamase production, are resistant. Particular interest in these penicillins lies in their activity against *Ps. aeruginosa*. Apalcillin, azlocillin and piperacillin display greater activity in vitro than the carboxypenicillins. However, the ureidopenicillins are not stable to the chromosomally mediated AmpC β-lactamase of *Ps. aeruginosa*, and activity is greatly reduced in tests with high bacterial inocula. The superior activity of the ureidopenicillins against *Ps. aeruginosa* may be due to a combination of better penetration characteristics and greater affinity for PBPs. All these compounds exhibit reduced activity against *Bacteroides* spp.

ACQUIRED RESISTANCE

Resistance in clinical isolates is due primarily to their hydrolysis by plasmid-mediated β-lactamases. Activity can often be restored by combinations with β-lactamase inhibitors; fixed combinations of ticarcillin with clavulanic acid (p. 274) and piperacillin with tazobactam (p. 277) have been developed for clinical use.

PHARMACOKINETICS

None of the compounds is orally absorbed, but two esters of carbenicillin are available for oral use. After parenteral administration the plasma half-lives of carbenicillin and ticarcillin are approximately 1 h and the compounds are predominately excreted unchanged by tubular secretion, only small amounts appearing in the bile.

The acylureidopenicillins produce peak plasma levels that are lower than those obtained with the carboxypenicillins. The half-lives and volumes of distribution of the ureidopenicillins are generally similar and increase with larger doses. Elimination from the body is largely by the renal route and most of the drug appears unchanged in the urine, but comparatively high concentrations appear in bile.

Apalcillin differs from the ureidopenicillins in being largely eliminated via the liver; this is related to high molecular weight and high protein binding, and only about 20% of the drug appears in the urine, some in the form of penicilloic acid.

CLINICAL USE

A major role of these compounds is the treatment of established pseudomonal infection, but they are also active against other penicillin-resistant Gram-negative bacilli, including *Enterobacter* spp., indole-positive *Proteus* and *Morganella* spp. They are also used in the treatment and prophylaxis of anaerobic and mixed infections. A special role has been claimed, particularly for the acylureidopenicillins in providing broad prophylactic cover, notably in bowel surgery (Ch. 42). An advantage claimed for acylureidopenicillins over carboxypenicillins is that they are mono- rather than di-sodium salts. They therefore present substantially less sodium load, but the clinical importance of this is not clear.

There is no reason to believe that these compounds are adequate when used alone for the treatment of patients with severe undiagnosed sepsis. In neutropenic patients they should be combined with an aminoglycoside. However, it should be noted that penicillins and aminoglycosides should not be mixed in infusion fluids because of the possibility of mutual degradation (p. 159).

Combination therapy with an aminoglycoside is recommended in *Ps. aeruginosa* pneumonia, although the penicillins alone are more effective than aminoglycosides alone. Soft-tissue and burn wound infections usually respond, but infections requiring treatment with these agents generally arise in patients with underlying disorders, and suppression rather than eradication of infection is often the best result obtainable. Good examples of such 'control' are provided by:

- Cystic fibrosis (where accelerated elimination of the drugs requires high dosage).
- Osteomyelitis.
- Urinary tract infection in catheterized patients.
- The grave necrotizing otitis externa of diabetes.

With all these agents, treatment failures are often due to the emergence of resistant variants.

 Further information

Tan JS, File TM Jr. 1995 Antipseudomonal penicillins. *Medical Clinics of North America* 79: 679–693.

 AZLOCILLIN

Molecular weight (free acid): 461.5; (sodium salt): 483.5.

A semisynthetic acylureidopenicillin supplied as the sodium salt for parenteral administration.

Antimicrobial activity

Azlocillin is distinguished mainly by its activity against *Ps. aeruginosa* (Table 16.4), including some carbenicillin-resistant strains; most strains are inhibited by 4–8 mg/l, although activity is inoculum dependent. It is active against a wide range of other Gram-negative bacteria, including *Enterobacter* spp., *Pr. vulgaris*, *Morganella morganii*, *Providencia* spp. and *Ser. marcescens*, but is less active than mezlocillin and piperacillin against most Enterobacteriaceae. *B. fragilis* and other anaerobes are moderately susceptible. Like other ureidopenicillins, azlocillin is active against Gram-positive cocci, *H. influenzae* and *N. gonorrhoeae*. Because it can be hydrolyzed by most β-lactamases, β-lactamase-producing isolates are resistant.

Pharmacokinetics

Oral absorption	Negligible
C_{max} 3 g intravenous infusion (15–30 min)	250 mg/l
Plasma half-life	0.9–1.1 h
Volume of distribution	0.2 l/kg
Plasma protein binding	20–30%

Distribution
There is evidence of dose-dependent pharmacokinetics. Concentrations of 0.5–4 mg/kg were detected in the sputum of about a third of patients receiving 40 mg/kg intravenously over 10 min, 4-hourly. Concentrations in amniotic fluid and cord serum were 2.9–7.6 and 12–18 mg/l, respectively, when the maternal serum concentrations following 2 g by intravenous bolus were 48–69 mg/l.

Metabolism and excretion
Up to 60% of the dose is recoverable from the urine, mostly unchanged, although some hydrolysis of the β-lactam ring takes place in the body. The plasma half-life rises to 6 h when the creatinine clearance is less than 10 ml/3 min.

Toxicity and side effects

Reactions similar to those associated with carboxypenicillins occur, including hypersensitivity, increase of bleeding time and abnormalities of liver enzymes. Reversible neutropenia has been encountered relatively frequently in patients treated for more than 2 weeks. A mean fall in serum uric acid from 6.4 to 2.3 mg/dl has been observed in treated patients, indicating a probenecid-like effect.

Clinical use

Serious infection with susceptible organisms, including lower respiratory tract, intra-abdominal, urinary tract and gynecological infections.

Preparations and dosage

Proprietary name: Securopen.

Preparation: Injection.

Dosage: Adults, 2–5 g every 8 h depending on severity of infection. Children 1–14 years, 75 mg/kg every 8 h. Premature infants, 50 mg/kg every 12 h; neonates, 100 mg/kg every 12 h; infants 7 days to 1 year, 100 mg/kg every 8 h.

No longer widely available.

Further information

Anonymous 1999 Azlocillin sodium. In: Dollery C (ed.) *Therapeutic Drugs* 2nd edn. Churchill Livingstone, Edinburgh, pp. A265–A267.

Drusano GL, Schimpff SC, Hewitt WL 1984 The acylampicillins: mezlocillin, piperacillin and azlocillin. *Reviews of Infectious Diseases* 6: 13–32.

Jacobs JY, Livermore DM, Davy KWM 1984 Pseudomonas aeruginosa beta-lactamase as a defence against azlocillin, mezlocillin and piperacillin. *Journal of Antimicrobial Chemotherapy* 14: 221–229.

Lander RD, Henderson RP, Pyszcynski DR 1989 Pharmacokinetic comparison of 5 g of azlocillin every 8 h and 4 g every 6 h in healthy volunteers. *Antimicrobial Agents and Chemotherapy* 33: 710–713.

Symposium 1983 Azlocillin – an antipseudomonas penicillin. *Journal of Antimicrobial Chemotherapy* 11 (Suppl. B): 1–239.

Wenk M, Follath F 1986 Azlocillin serum levels on repetitive dosage in patients with normal and abnormal renal function. *Chemotherapy* 32: 205–208.

White AR, Comber KR, Sutherland R 1980 Comparative bactericidal effects of azlocillin and ticarcillin against *Pseudomonas aeruginosa*. *Antimicrobial Agents and Chemotherapy* 18: 182–189.

 MEZLOCILLIN

Molecular weight (free acid): 539.6; (sodium salt): 561.6.

A semisynthetic acylureidopenicillin supplied as the sodium salt for parenteral administration.

Antimicrobial activity

Activity against common pathogenic bacteria is shown in Table 16.4. Ampicillin-susceptible strains of *H. influenzae* and *Neisseria* spp. are very susceptible. β-Lactamase-producing organisms are usually resistant, because these enzymes hydrolyze mezlocillin. It is less active than azlocillin and piperacillin against *Ps. aeruginosa* and its activity is inoculum dependent. Activity against *B. fragilis* is variable, and is usually related to β-lactamase production.

Mezlocillin exhibits typical β-lactam synergy with aminoglycosides against *Ps. aeruginosa* and enterobacteria. In combination with cefoxitin, antagonism is observed in tests against *Enterobacter*, *Serratia* and *Pseudomonas* spp. as a result of β-lactamase induction by cefoxitin.

Pharmacokinetics

Oral absorption	Negligible
C_{max} 2 g (2–5 min intravenous injection)	250 mg/l after 5 min
Plasma elimination half life	55 min
Volume of distribution	0.38–0.55 l/kg
Plasma protein binding	20–30%

Although the rate of elimination is dose dependent there is a loss of dose linearity at higher doses, probably due to saturation of non-renal clearance. Up to 60% is recoverable unchanged from the urine. The elimination half-life rises with decline in renal function and urinary excretion falls to 5% or less, but non-renal clearance is appreciable and no change in dosage is indicated until the glomerular filtration rate falls to less than 10%. Up to 2.5% is excreted in the bile, producing concentrations around 300 mg/l after a 1 g intravenous injection. Plasma clearance is inversely related to serum alkaline phosphatase and total bilirubin.

Toxicity and side effects

Untoward reactions are similar to those associated with carboxypenicillins, including hypersensitivity, prolongation of bleeding time (less than with carbenicillin), reversible neutropenia and abnormalities of liver enzymes. False reactions for urinary protein may occur.

Clinical use

Serious infection with susceptible organisms, including lower respiratory tract, intra-abdominal, urinary tract and gynecological infections.

Preparations and dosage

Proprietary name: Baypen; Mezlin.

Preparation: Injection.

Dosage: Adults, i.v., 2–4 g every 6 h depending on severity of infection; maximum daily dose 24 g. Children, i.v., 150–300 mg/kg/day in divided doses.

Limited availability.

Further information

Anonymous 1999 Mezlocillin. In: Dollery C (ed.) *Therapeutic Drugs* 2nd edn. Churchill Livingstone, Edinburgh, pp. M158–M161.

Colaizzi PA, Coniglio AA, Poynor WJ, Vishniavsky N, Karnes HT, Polk RE 1986 Comparative pharmacokinetics of two multiple-dose mezlocillin regimens in normal volunteers. *Antimicrobial Agents and Chemotherapy* 30: 675–678.

Esposito S, Galante D, Barba D 1986 In vitro microbiological properties of mezlocillin compared with four cephalosporins. *Chemioterapia* 5: 273–277.

Flaherty JF, Barriere SL, Mordenti J, Gambertoglio JG 1987 Effect of dose on pharmacokinetics and serum bactericidal activity of mezlocillin. *Antimicrobial Agents and Chemotherapy* 31: 895–898.

Symposium 1983 Mezlocillin – a broad spectrum penicillin. An update. *Journal of Antimicrobial Chemotherapy* 11 (Suppl. C): 1–108.

PIPERACILLIN

Molecular weight (free acid): 517.6; (sodium salt): 539.6.

A semisynthetic acylureidopenicillin supplied as the sodium salt for parenteral administration. A formulation with tazobactam is also available (p. 277).

Antimicrobial activity

The activity against common bacterial pathogens is shown in Table 16.4. It displays good activity against penicillin-susceptible strains of *Staph. aureus* and *N. gonorrhoeae*, and ampicillin-susceptible *H. influenzae*, but β-lactamase-producing strains are resistant. It is the most active of the commonly used antipseudomonal penicillins against *Ps. aeruginosa*. Because it is less labile than many other penicillins to hydrolysis by plasmid-encoded β-lactamases, it is active against a number of Enterobacteriaceae, including some ampicillin-resistant species such as *Citrobacter*, *Enterobacter*, *Morganella*, *Providencia* and *Ser. marcescens*. *B. fragilis* and many other anaerobes are susceptible, but differences between MIC_{50} and MIC_{90} values can be considerable owing to variable levels of β-lactamase production.

It is only slowly bactericidal, with the possibility for wide divergence between the MIC and MBC; some susceptible strains are not killed by 256 mg/l. Synergy with aminoglycosides has been demonstrated against many strains of Enterobacteriaceae and *Ps. aeruginosa*.

Acquired resistance

There is complete cross-resistance with other ureidopenicillins, but strains of *Ps. aeruginosa* moderately resistant to carbenicillin and ticarcillin are often susceptible. Because it is hydrolyzed by most β-lactamases, many β-lactamase-producing isolates are resistant unless it is protected by β-lactamase inhibitors.

Monotherapy of *Ps. aeruginosa* infections has resulted in the development of resistance during treatment, often due to the concomitant production of elevated amounts of chromosomal β-lactamase in association with altered permeability. Piperacillin-resistant strains of *B. fragilis* and other *Bacteroides* spp. are common. The spread of plasmid-mediated β-lactamases among Gram-negative bacilli has led to increased resistance to piperacillin and corresponding interest in the combination with the β-lactamase inhibitor tazobactam.

Pharmacokinetics

Oral absorption	Negligible
C_{max} 2 g (2–3 min intravenous injection)	305 mg/l after 5 min
Plasma elimination half life	0.9 h
Volume of distribution	16–24 l/1.73 m²
Plasma protein binding	16%

Serum levels lack dose proportionality. In patients with meningitis, mean CSF penetration of 30% has been found. The urine is the principal route of excretion, 50–70% of the dose appearing over 12 h, most in the first 4 h. Most is excreted via the tubules, 75–90% in active form. The half-life is prolonged in renal failure but much less than is the case with carboxypenicillins. Neither serum half-life nor clearance is correlated with creatinine clearance, indicating significant non-renal elimination. There is substantial biliary excretion, levels in common duct bile after a 1 g intravenous dose commonly reaching 500 mg/l or more. During hemodialysis the plasma half-life remains elevated and only 10–15% of the dose is removed.

Toxicity and side effects

Piperacillin is generally well tolerated, with mild to moderate pain on injection, thrombophlebitis and diarrhea in some patients. It otherwise exhibits side effects common to the group, including hypersensitivity, leukopenia and abnormalities of platelet aggregation without coagulation defect, except on prolonged treatment.

Clinical uses

Serious infection with susceptible organisms, including lower respiratory tract, intra-abdominal, urinary tract and gynecological infections.

Preparations and dosage

Proprietary names: Pipril; Pipracil; Tazocin, Zosyn (with tazobactam).

Preparation: Injection.

Dosage: Piperacillin, adults, i.m., i.v., 100–150 mg/kg per day in divided doses, increased to 200–300 mg/kg per day in severe infections; in life-threatening infections a dose of not less than 16 g/day is recommended. Children 2 months to 12 years, 100–300 mg/kg per day in 3–4 divided doses; neonates and infants <2 months, 150–300 mg/kg per day in 2–3 equally divided doses. Piperacillin with tazobactam, adults and children >12 years, i.v., 2.25–4.5 g every 6–8 h.

Widely available.

Further information

Anonymous 1999 Piperacillin (sodium). In: Dollery C (ed.) *Therapeutic Drugs* 2nd edn. Churchill Livingstone, Edinburgh, pp. P133–P136.

Daschner FD, Just M, Spillner G, Schlosser V 1982 Penetration of piperacillin into cardiac valves, subcutaneous and muscle tissue of patients undergoing open-heart surgery. *Journal of Antimicrobial Chemotherapy* 9: 489–492.

Dickinson GM, Droller DG, Greenman RL, Hoffman TA 1981 Clinical evaluation of piperacillin with observation on penetrability into cerebrospinal fluid. *Antimicrobial Agents and Chemotherapy* 20: 481–486.

Giron JA, Meyers BR, Hirschmann SZ 1981 Biliary concentration of piperacillin in patients undergoing cholecystectomy. *Antimicrobial Agents of Chemotherapy* 19: 309–311.

Holmes B, Richards DM, Brogdeb RN, Heel RC 1984 Piperacillin. A review of its antibacterial activity, pharmacokinetic properties and therapeutic use. *Drugs* 28: 375–425.

Lee M, Stobnicki M, Sharifi R 1986 Haemorrhagic complications of piperacillin therapy. *Journal of Urology* 136: 454–455.

Stefani S, Russo G, Nicolosi VM, Nicoletti G 1987 Enterococci and aminoglycosides: evaluation of susceptibility and synergism of their combination with piperacillin. *Chemioterapia* 6: 12–16.

Symposium 1982 From penicillin to piperacillin. *Journal of Antimicrobial Chemotherapy* 9 (Suppl. B): 1–101.

Symposium 1993 Piperacillin/tazobactam; a new β-lactam/β-lactamase inhibitor combination. *Journal of Antimicrobial Chemotherapy* 31 (Suppl. A): 1–124.

Tartaglione TA, Nye I, Vishniavsky N, Poynor W, Polk RE 1986 Multiple dose pharmacokinetics of piperacillin and azlocillin in 12 healthy volunteers. *Clinical Pharmacology* 5: 911–916.

Thrumoorthi MC, Asmar BI, Buckley JA, Bollinger RO, Kauffman E, Dajani AS 1983 Pharmacokinetics of intravenously administered piperacillin in pre-adolescent children. *Journal of Pediatrics* 102: 941–946.

Welling PG, Craig WA, Buntzen RW, Kwok FW, Gerber AU, Matsen PO 1983 Pharmacokinetics of piperacillin in subjects with various degrees of renal failure. *Antimicrobial Agents and Chemotherapy* 23: 881–887.

TICARCILLIN

Molecular weight (free acid): 384.4; (disodium salt): 428.4.

A semisynthetic carboxypenicillin supplied as the disodium salt for parenteral use. A formulation with clavulanic acid is also available (p. 274).

Antimicrobial activity

The activity against common bacterial pathogens is shown in Table 16.4. Because it is hydrolyzed less rapidly than ampicillin, it displays activity against Enterobacteriaceae, including some ampicillin-resistant species such as *Citrobacter*, *Enterobacter*, *M. morganii*, *Providencia* spp. and *Ser. marcescens*. β-Lactamase-negative strains of *H. influenzae* and *N. gonorrhoeae* are highly susceptible. Most aerobic and anaerobic Gram-positive bacteria are susceptible, with the exception of *E. faecalis* and β-lactamase-producing *Staph. aureus*. Anaerobic Gram-negative bacteria including *B. fragilis* are usually susceptible. Bactericidal synergy with aminoglycosides is demonstrable against *Ps. aeruginosa* and enterobacteria.

Acquired resistance

Ticarcillin is generally cross-resistant with carbenicillin. It is comparatively stable to the AmpC chromosomally mediated β-lactamases of Gram-negative bacilli, but can be hydrolyzed by most other chromosomally and plasmid-mediated enzymes unless protected by a β-lactamase inhibitor.

Pharmacokinetics

Oral absorption	Negligible
C_{max} 1 g intramuscular	35 mg/l after 1 h
Plasma half-life	1.3 h
Volume of distribution	0.21 l/kg
Plasma protein binding	50–60%

Absorption

It is not orally absorbed. On coadministration with gentamicin, the plasma concentration of ticarcillin is unaffected, but the concentration of gentamicin is lowered. Doubling the dose approximately doubles the mean peak concentration. There is no evidence of dose-dependent pharmacokinetics at doses between 50 and 80 mg/kg.

Distribution

Ticarcillin is distributed in the extracellular fluid. Plasma levels are reduced when the extracellular volume is increased. It enters the serous fluids, providing concentrations up to 60% of those of the plasma. Concentrations can reach 25% of those of the plasma in sputum and in skin window fluid. It does not cross the normal meninges but levels of up to 50% of those of the plasma can be found in meningitis. On co-administration with clavulanic acid, there is preservation of the ratio to serum concentration in lymph and in peritoneal fluid, with peak concentrations of 70% and 67% of the plasma concentrations of ticarcillin and clavulanic acid, respectively, declining in parallel with the plasma concentrations.

Metabolism

Up to 15% is excreted as penicilloic acid, a higher fraction than for carbenicillin (up to 5%).

Excretion

Some is excreted in the bile, producing levels 2–3 times those in the plasma, but the main route of excretion is through the kidneys (80%), principally as unchanged drug, appearing in the urine in the first 6 h, producing concentrations of 650–2500 mg/l after doses of 3 g intravenously. Peak plasma levels are elevated and prolonged by probenecid and the half-life is prolonged in the newborn and in renal failure. Some further prolongation occurs in the presence of hepatic failure. It is more rapidly disposed of in children with cystic fibrosis.

Toxicity and side effects

As with all penicillins, hypersensitivity reactions may occur, but are less frequent and severe than those associated with benzylpenicillin. Rashes and eosinophilia occur; reversible neutropenia, dose-related platelet abnormalities (occasionally leading to hemorrhage) and interstitial nephritis are rarely encountered. In volunteers receiving 100–300 mg/kg per day for 3–10 days coagulation was unaffected, but platelet function was impaired. Petechiae, ecchymoses and epistaxis are reported in patients with impaired renal function who received normal dosages. Reversible abnormalities of liver function can develop. Since large doses of the drug have to be used, convulsions can occur, as with other penicillins, and being a disodium salt, electrolyte disturbances can result from the sodium load and from loss of potassium.

Clinical use

Serious infection, including septicemia, respiratory tract infections, genitourinary tract infections and skin and soft-tissue infections caused by susceptible bacteria.

Because of the increasing prevalence of bacteria possessing class A β-lactamases it is now more commonly used in combination with clavulanic acid.

Preparations and dosage

Proprietary names: Ticar, Timentin (with clavulanic acid).

Preparation: Injection.

Dosage: Ticarcillin, adults, i.v., 15–20 g/day in divided doses. Children, 200–300 mg/kg per day in divided doses. Ticarcillin with clavulanic acid, adults, i.v., 3.2 g every 6–8 h increased to every 4 h in more severe infections. Children, 80 mg/kg every 6–8 h; neonates, 80 mg/kg every 12 h.

Widely available.

Further information

Anonymous 1999 Ticarcillin (disodium). In Dollery C (ed.) *Therapeutic Drugs* 2nd edn. Churchill Livingstone, Edinburgh, pp. T106–T109.

Brogden RN, Heel RC, Speight TM, Avery GS 1980 Ticarcillin: a review of its pharmacological properties and therapeutic efficacy. *Drugs* 20: 325–352.

Guenthner SH, Chao HP, Wenzel RP 1986 Synergy between amikacin and ticarcillin or mezlocillin against nosocomial blood-stream isolates. *Journal of Antimicrobial Chemotherapy* 18: 550–552.

Gugliemo BJ, Flaherty JF, Batman R, Barriere SL, Gambertoglio JG 1986 Comparative pharmacokinetics of low- and high-dose ticarcillin. *Antimicrobial Agents and Chemotherapy* 30: 359–360.

Symposium 1978 Ticarcillin (BRL 2288). International Congress Series No. 445. Excerpta Medica, Oxford, pp. 3–163.

OTHER GROUP 5 PENICILLINS

Apalcillin

A semisynthetic acyaminopenicillin supplied as the sodium salt for parenteral administration. The antibacterial spectrum is similar to that of the acylureidopenicillins (Table 16.4). It is relatively labile to many β-lactamases, including the common TEM plasmid-mediated enzyme.

Apalcillin is 80–90% bound to plasma protein and its activity in vitro is reduced in the presence of plasma. A 30-min intravenous infusion of 30 mg/kg achieves a concentration of around 85 mg/l. Mean concentrations in bronchial secretions in patients receiving 3 g intravenously were 5.8 mg/l. Following similar doses, concentrations in normal CSF did not exceed 1.75 mg/l, but in the presence of inflammation reached 5–30 mg/l.

The plasma elimination half life is about 1–2 h. Only 20% of the dose appears in the urine, mostly as two inactive penicilloic acids. It is mainly eliminated via the liver, concentrations of active drug in the common duct bile reaching 2–4 g/l, accounting for about 12% of the dose. The remainder is eliminated as metabolites; there is no significant enterohepatic recirculation.

Apalcillin is generally well tolerated but maculopapular rashes, which resolve on cessation of treatment, are relatively common. In volunteers receiving 75–225 mg/kg, abnormal platelet aggregation developed and there was a consistent and major fall in antithrombin III activity, however, plasma coagulation and fibrinogen were not affected.

Its uses are those of group 5 penicillins (p. 250).

Preparations and dosage

Dosage: Adults, i.v., 2–3 g three times daily.

Available in Germany.

Further information

Bergogne-Berezin E, Pierre J, Chastre J, Gilbert C, Heinzel G, Akbaraly JP 1984 Pharmacokinetics of apalcillin in intensive-care patients: study of penetration into the respiratory tract. *Journal of Antimicrobial Chemotherapy* 14: 67–73.

Hoffler U 1986 Efficacy of apalcillin alone and in combination with four aminoglycoside antibiotics against *Pseudomonas aeruginosa. Chemotherapy* 32: 255–259.

Neu HC, Labthavikul P 1982 In vitro activity of apalcillin compared with that of other new penicillins and antipseudomonas cephalosporins. *Antimicrobial Agents and Chemotherapy* 21: 906–911.

Raoult D, Gallias H, Casanova P, Bedjaoui A, Akbaraly R, Auzerie J 1985 Meningeal penetration of apalcillin in man. *Journal of Antimicrobial Chemotherapy* 15: 123–125.

Aspoxicillin

An acylaminopenicillin, synthesized from amoxicillin. It has a broad antibacterial spectrum against Gram-positive and Gram-negative aerobes and anaerobes. It is more active than carbenicillin against *Ps. aeruginosa* and is less active than piperacillin against *Staph. aureus, H. influenzae, Esch. coli, K. pneumoniae* and *Ps. aeruginosa*. It is not absorbed when dosed orally; the plasma half-life is 87 min after intravenous infusion.

Aspoxicillin is reported to be more efficacious against experimental infections than would be predicted from its in-vitro activity. It has been used in the treatment of respiratory, skin and soft tissue and urinary infections in adults and children, and, in combination with aminoglycosides, against gynecological infections and infections in patients with hematological disorders.

Further information

Geyer J, Hoffler D, Koeppe P 1988 Pharmacokinetics of aspoxicillin in subjects with normal and impaired renal function. *Arzneimittelforschung* 11: 1635–1639.

Wagatsuma M, Seto M, Miyagishima T, Kawazu M, Yamagushi T, Ohshima S 1983 Synthesis and antibacterial activity of asparagine derivatives of aminobenzylpenicillin. *Journal of Antibiotics* 36: 147–154.

Carbenicillin

α-Carboxybenzylpenicillin; the first antipseudomonal penicillin to be developed. A semisynthetic carboxypenicillin supplied as the disodium salt for parenteral administration. Two esterified prodrug formulations, carindacillin (carbenicillin indanyl sodium) and carfecillin (carbenicillin carboxyphenyl ester) have been developed for oral administration.

Antimicrobial activity

Carbenicillin is the least active of the group 5 agents (Table 16.4, p. 249), with a notable reduction in activity against Gram-positive cocci compared to benzylpenicillin. *E. faecalis* and β-lactamase-producing strains of *Staph. aureus* are resistant. It is labile to many plasmid-mediated β-lactamases, but is comparatively stable to class C chromosomal β-lactamases (p. 263–264). Synergy is demonstrable with aminoglycosides against *Ps. aeruginosa* and other Gram-negative bacteria.

Pharmacokinetics

Carbenicillin is not orally absorbed, except in esterified form (*see below*). A 1 g intramuscular injection achieves a plasma peak concentration of 20–30 mg/l after 0.5–1.5 h. The half-life is around 1 h. Plasma protein binding is 50–60%.

The drug is distributed in the extracellular fluid, providing concentrations up to 60% of those of the plasma. Concentrations can reach 25% of those of the plasma in sputum, but in patients with cystic fibrosis these may not reach inhibitory levels for *Ps. aeruginosa*. It does not cross the normal meninges but levels of up to 50% of those of the plasma can be found in patients with meningitis.

Around 80% of the dose appears as unchanged drug in the urine, producing very high levels (2–4 g/l). Excretion is by both glomerular filtration and tubular secretion, which accounts for about 40%. It is more rapidly disposed of in patients with cystic fibrosis.

Toxicity and side effects

As with all penicillins, hypersensitivity reactions may occur, but these are less frequent and severe than those associated with benzylpenicillin. High blood levels sometimes cause a coagulation defect, manifested by prolonged bleeding time due to an action on platelets. Purpura and mucosal bleeding has occasionally progressed to life-threatening bleeding. The effect is dose dependent and most likely to be seen in patients with impaired excretion while receiving 500 mg/kg per day or more.

Reversible abnormalities of liver function can occur, apparently more commonly than with other antipseudomonal penicillins. Since large doses of the drug have to be used, convulsions can occur (as with other penicillins; p. 227) and, being administered as the disodium salt, electrolyte disturbances can result.

Clinical use

Treatment of serious infections, especially those involving *Ps. aeruginosa*.

Preparations and dosage

Proprietary name: Pyopen.

Preparation: Injection.

Dosage: Adults, i.v., 5 g every 4–6 h; i.m., 2 g every 6 h. Children, i.v., 250–400 mg/kg per day in divided doses; i.m., 50–100 mg/kg per day in divided doses.

No longer widely available.

Further information

Godfrey AJ, Bryan LE, Rabin HR 1981 Beta-lactam-resistant *Pseudomonas aeruginosa* with modified penicillin-binding protein emerging during cystic fibrosis treatment. *Antimicrobial Agents and Chemotherapy* 19: 705–711.

Sattler FR, Weitekamp MR, Sayegh A, Ballard JO 1988 impaired hemostasis caused by beta-lactam antibiotics. *American Journal of Surgery* 155 (5A): 30–39.

Symposium 1970 Symposium on carbenicillin: a clinical profile. *Journal of Infectious Diseases* 122 (suppl) S1–S116.

Williams RJ, Lindridge MA, Said AA, Livermore DM, Williams JD 1984 National survey of antibiotic resistance in *Pseudomonas aeruginosa*. *Journal of Antimicrobial Chemotherapy* 14: 9–16.

Carbenicillin esters

Carfecillin

Carfecillin is esterified on the side chain and, because the carboxyl group of the nucleus is free, exhibits greater activity in vitro than carbenicillin against Gram-positive cocci. In vivo it is rapidly de-esterified to yield carbenicillin and phenol, which is rapidly detoxified by conjugation and excreted in the urine. In-vivo activity and toxicity are primarily due to liberated carbenicillin. Only trace amounts of the ester are found in the serum. A 1 g oral dose achieves levels of 5 mg/l after 1–2 h. About 30–35% of the dose is excreted over 6 h in the urine, producing concentrations following an oral dose of 1 h around 500–1000 mg/l. The liberated phenol moiety is excreted as glucuronide and sulfate. Because of its antibacterial activity, unabsorbed ester may affect the gut flora.

Its sole use is in the treatment of urinary tract infection due to *Ps. aeruginosa* and other resistant organisms.

Preparations and dosage

Proprietary name: Uticillin.

Preparation: Tablets.

Dosage: Adults, oral, 0.5–1 g three times daily. Children 2–10 years, half the adult dose.

Limited availability.

Further information

O'Grady F (ed.) 1979 *Carfecillin*. International Congress Series No. 467. Excerpta Medica, Oxford.

Carindacillin

The indanyl ester of carbenicillin supplied as the sodium salt. As with carfecillin, it shows activity independent of that of carbenicillin in vitro but not in vivo.

After absorption carindacillin is rapidly hydrolyzed to carbenicillin and indanol, which is excreted in the urine. The peak blood level after a dose of 1 g is only about 10 mg/l, but high concentrations are attained in the urine. A bitter aftertaste (and sometimes vomiting) occur and doses adequate to achieve a systemic effect are impracticable.

Preparations and dosage

Proprietary name: Carindacillin; Geocillin.

Preparation: Tablets.

Dosage: Adults, oral, 382–764 mg four times daily.

Limited availability.

Further information

English AR, Retsema JA, Ray VA, Lynch JE 1972 Carbenicillin indanyl sodium, an orally active derivative of carbenicillin. *Antimicrobial Agents and Chemotherapy* 1: 185–191.

Knirsch AK, Hobbs DC, Korst JJ 1973 Pharmacokinetics, toleration and safety of indanyl carbenicillin in man. *Journal of Infectious Diseases* 127 (Suppl.): S105–S110.

Sulbenicillin

α-Sulfobenzylpenicillin, a semisynthetic penicillin supplied as the disodium salt. Its antimicrobial spectrum (Table 16.4, p. 249) and pharmacokinetic behavior closely resemble those of carbenicillin. Following intravenous administration of 4 g, the mean plasma concentration at 1 h was approximately 160 mg/l, with a plasma elimination half-life around 70 min. It is largely excreted in the urine, about 80% of the dose appearing in the first 24 h, less than 5% as the penicilloic acid. There is an inverse correlation between creatinine clearance and plasma half-life.

It has been noted that the penicilloic acid causes much stronger platelet aggregation than its parent.

Preparations and dosage

Preparation: Injection.

Dosage: Adults, i.m., i.v., 2–4 g/day in divided doses. Doses can be increased in severe infections.

Very limited availability. Available in Japan.

Further information

Eftimiadi C, DeLeo C, Schito GC 1985 Antibacterial activity in vitro of sulbenicillin against mucoid and non-mucoid strains of *Pseudomonas aeruginosa*, *Drugs under Experimental and Clinical Research* 11: 241–245.

Hansen I, Jacobsen E, Weiss J 1975 Pharmacokinetics of sulbenicillin, a new broad-spectrum semisynthetic penicillin. *Clinical Pharmacology and Therapeutics* 17: 339–347.

Ikeda Y, Kikuchi M, Matsuda S et al 1978 Inhibition of platelet function by sulbenicillin and its metabolite. *Antimicrobial Agents and Chemotherapy* 13: 881–883.

GROUP 6: β-LACTAMASE-RESISTANT PENICILLINS

The introduction of substituents into the 6-α-position of the penicillin nucleus generally results in loss of antibacterial activity, but the 6-α-methoxy derivative of ticarcillin, temocillin, possesses useful antibacterial and pharmacokinetic properties and has attained clinical status. Like the cephamycins (p. 260), which also contain an α-methoxy group on the β-lactam nucleus, it is highly resistant to most bacterial β-lactamases. It is not absorbed by the oral route, but it has a long serum half-life after parenteral administration. The *o*-methylphenyl ester produced substantial serum concentrations after oral dosing to human volunteers, but has not progressed to clinical trial.

 TEMOCILLIN

Molecular weight (free acid): 414.4; (disodium salt): 458.4.

A semisynthetic 6-α-methoxylpenicillin supplied as the disodium salt for parenteral administration.

Antimicrobial activity

Activity against common pathogenic bacteria is shown in Table 16.4 (p. 249). The introduction of the 6-α-methoxy group has resulted in loss of activity against Gram-positive cocci and anaerobic Gram-negative bacilli, but it is active against enterobacteria (MIC 1–8 mg/l), *H. influenzae* and *M. catarrhalis*. In most cases, β-lactamase-positive and negative strains are equally susceptible. In contrast to the structurally related ticarcillin, it is inactive against *Ps. aeruginosa*, but *Burkholderia cepacia*, *Ps. acidovorans* and *Aeromonas* spp. are susceptible (MIC 4 mg/l). Most *Acinetobacter* spp. are resistant, and *Ser. marcescens* exhibits variable susceptibility.

Temocillin is bactericidal at concentrations 2–4 times the MIC; filaments formed at lower concentrations slowly lyse at higher drug levels. Temocillin consists of diastereoisomers. The naturally predominant *R* epimer is more rapidly bactericidal than the *S* epimer. It is highly resistant to most bacterial β-lactamases, including the extended-spectrum β-lactamases that confer resistance to extended-spectrum cephalosporins, and, as a result, there is no inoculum effect with most β-

lactamase-producing bacteria. It is hydrolyzed by β-lactamases produced by *Flavobacterium* spp. and by those of *Bacteroides* spp.

Pharmacokinetics

Oral absorption	Negligible
C_{max} 1 g intramuscular injection	70 mg/l
1 g rapid intravenous infusion	172 mg/l after 5 min
Plasma elimination half life	4.3–5.4 h
Plasma protein binding	85%

Distribution

Relatively high protein binding, together with its distribution in a volume less than the extracellular fluid, accounts for its relatively low renal clearance. In artificial blister fluid and peritoneal fluid concentrations reach 50% of the peak plasma level, and in lymph concentrations reach 25–60% of the simultaneous plasma level, with a similar half-life. The *R* epimer differs from the *S* epimer in lower protein binding, a 25% greater volume of distribution and a 60% shorter half-life.

Metabolism and excretion

Elimination is principally in the glomerular filtrate, with 80% of the dose appearing in the urine in the first 24 h. A small amount is disposed of in the bile and by degradation. Following a 2 g dose, concentrations in the bile of 300–1200 mg/l have been found. Elimination declines in parallel with renal function, the half-life reaching 30 h in patients with creatinine clearance below 5%.

Toxicity and side effects

As with all penicillins, hypersensitivity reactions, including serious anaphylactic responses, may occur. Temocillin is generally well tolerated and administration of 4 g intravenously 12-hourly produced no significant effect on template bleeding time, prothrombin time or ADP-induced platelet aggregation.

Clinical use

- Severe infection with susceptible bacteria, including urinary and respiratory tract infections, peritonitis and septicemia.

Preparations and dosage

Proprietary name: Temopen.

Preparation: Injection.

Dosage: Adults, i.m., i.v., 1–2 g every 12 h.

Very limited availability, not available in the UK.

Further information

Brown RM, Wise R, Andrews JM 1982 Temocillin, in-vitro activity and the pharmacokinetics and tissue penetration in healthy volunteers. *Journal of Antimicrobial Chemotherapy* 10: 295–302.

Guest EA, Horton R, Mellows G, Slocombe B, Swaisland AJ, Tasker TCG 1985 Human pharmacokinetics of temocillin (BRL 17421) side chain epimers. *Journal of Antimicrobial Chemotherapy* 15: 327–336.

Jules K, Neu HC 1982 Antibacterial activity and beta-lactamase stability of temocillin. *Antimicrobial Agents and Chemotherapy* 22: 453–460.

Lode H, Verbist L, Williams JD, Richards DM 1985 First international workshop on temocillin. *Drugs* 29 (Suppl. 5): 1–243.

Spencer RC 1990 Temocillin. *Journal of Antimicrobial Chemotherapy* 26: 735–737.

17 Other β-lactam antibiotics

K. Bush

In the penicillins and cephalosporins, the β-lactam ring is fused to a five- and six-membered ring, respectively, but monocyclic and tricyclic β-lactam compounds also exist. Indeed, the situation has become so complicated that it is necessary to group the divergent β-lactams according to their chemical structure. There are nine chemical skeletons other than penicillins or cephalosporins which support β-lactam-containing agents that have current or potential therapeutic use. Although many of these novel β-lactam structures are based on natural products, classes of agents such as the penems, the oxacephems and tribactams are purely synthetic molecules that have relied on previous knowledge of β-lactam properties to design agents with broad spectrum antibacterial activity. Characteristics of each of the various classes are listed below.

- **Penams (penicillins)** *N*-acylated derivatives of 6-β-aminopenicillanic acid. In these compounds the β-lactam ring is fused with a saturated five-membered thiazolidine ring containing sulfur.
- **Penicillanic acid sulfones** Penams that lack a 6-amino substituent and in which the sulfur is oxidized synthetically to a sulfone to yield β-lactamase inhibitors such as sulbactam or tazobactam.
- **Penems** These differ from penams by the presence of a double bond between C-2 and C-3.
- **Carbapenams and carbapenems** Compounds in which CH_2 replaces sulfur in the five-membered ring. Many natural and synthetic members of the group have been described, of which the most interesting therapeutically are the natural product thienamycin and its analogs.

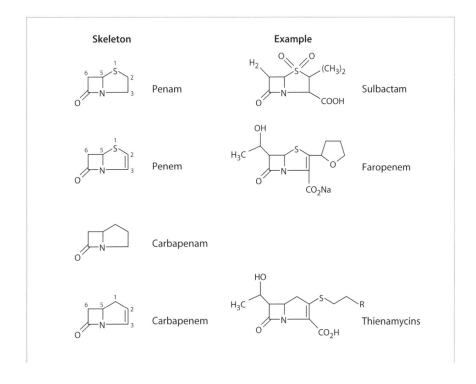

- **Cephems (cephalosporins)** N-acylated derivatives of 7-β-aminocephalosporanic acid. In these compounds, the β-lactam ring is fused with a six-membered dihydrothiazine ring containing sulfur and a double bond. Closely related are: cephamycins, which are substituted at the 7-position with an α-methoxy group; oxacephems, notably latamoxef, in which the sulfur of cephalosporins is replaced by oxygen; and carbacephems, including loracarbef, in which the sulfur is replaced by carbon.
- **Clavams** Compounds that differ from penams in the substitution of oxygen for sulfur. The only notable member of the clavam family at present is clavulanic acid, a compound that has only modest antibacterial activity and owes its therapeutic place to its ability to inhibit class A (functional group 2) bacterial β-lactamases.
- **Monobactams** β-Lactam compounds with no fused secondary ring. The monocyclic β-lactam antibiotics are most prominently represented by aztreonam and carumonam, but the group also contains the nocardicins.
- **Tribactams** Compounds closely related to the carbapenems, but with a fused tricyclic skeleton. This type of molecule is currently at the investigational stage in an attempt to provide a broad-spectrum β-lactam agent.

The penicillins are considered in Chapter 16, and the cephalosporins and their close relatives, the cephamycins, oxacephems and carbacephems, in Chapter 15. This chapter deals with the remaining agents: the penems, carbapenems, monobactams and tribactams, which are notable for their antibacterial activity; and clavulanic acid, and the penicillanic acid sulfones, which are primarily of interest as inhibitors of β-lactamases. The antibacterial activity of these inhibitors is associated with the synergistic activity seen with the accompanying penicillin in a β-lactamase inhibitor combination.

In-vitro activity of agents in each of these classes is highly dependent upon the chemical class to which it belongs. For example, carbapenems and β-lactamase inhibitor combinations tend to have broad-spectrum activity covering Gram-positive and Gram-negative anaerobic and aerobic organisms, whereas the monobactams lack useful activity against Gram-positive bacteria and anaerobes. Penems and tribactams tend to have profiles similar to those for the carbapenems.

Resistance to β-lactam agents is most frequently associated with production of enzymes that hydrolyze the β-lactam ring and since these novel compounds are all characterized by resistance to at least some β-lactamases, the classification of these enzymes is also dealt with in this chapter.

 ## Further information

Demain AL, Elander RP 1999 The β-lactam antibiotics: past, present, and future. *Antonie van Leeuwenhoek* 75: 5–19.

Edwards JR, Betts MJ 2000 Carbapenems: the pinnacle of the β-lactam antibiotics or room for improvement? *Journal of Antimicrobial Chemotherapy* 45: 1–4.

Frere JM, Joris B, Varetto L, Crine M 1988 Structure-activity relationships in the β-lactam family: an impossible dream. *Biochemical Pharmacology* 37: 125–132.

Rolinson GN 1998 Forty years of β-lactam research. *Journal of Antimicrobial Chemotherapy* 41: 589–603.

Schofield CJ, Walter MW 1999 β-Lactam chemistry. *Amino Acids, Peptides, Proteins* 30: 335–397.

Southgate R 1994 The synthesis of natural β-lactam antibiotics. *Contemporary Organic Synthesis* 1: 417–431.

Sykes RB, Koster WH, Bonner DP 1988 The new monobactams: chemistry and biology. *Journal of Clinical Pharmacology* 28: 113–119.

β-LACTAMASES

Even before penicillin was widely used clinically, bacteria such as *Escherichia coli* and *Staphylococcus aureus* were reported to have the capability of degrading this agent. The bacterial enzyme shown to hydrolyze the β-lactam ring was initially called 'penicillinase', and penicillinase-producing *Staph. aureus* became of great importance in outbreaks of hospital infection in the 1950s. Since that time, similar enzymes have become increasingly important as a cause of resistance in many pathogenic Gram-positive and Gram-negative bacteria, and even in legionellae, mycobacteria and nocardia. Because of their collective ability to destroy a wide range of β-lactam agents, the enzymes have been renamed β-lactamases. In the case of the penicillins the products are stable penicilloates, but in the case of cephalosporins the 'cephalosporoates' may rapidly undergo further degradation, liberating a variety of fragments depending on the C-3 substituent. Virtually every β-lactam, including monobactams, β-lactamase inhibitors and carbapenems, can be inactivated by an appropriate β-lactamase.

β-Lactam antibiotics can be attacked at other chemical sites by microbial acylases and esterases, but these enzymes, which have important uses in semisynthetic processes, are of no significance as a cause of clinical resistance. The presence of esterases in mammalian tissues is exploited in the cleavage of oral prodrug esters of penicillins and cephalosporins with liberation of the active parent compound. Some penems and carbapenems can also be hydrolyzed by mammalian dehydropeptidases (see below).

GENERAL PROPERTIES

With the advent in the early 1960s of the broad-spectrum penicillins ampicillin and carbenicillin, it became evident that the resistance of Gram-negative bacilli to these agents was most often associated with β-lactamase production. Most aerobic and anaerobic Gram-negative bacilli were discovered to produce chromosomally mediated β-lactamases characteristic of each species, which accounted for the intrinsic resistance of organisms such as *Bacteroides fragilis*, *Klebsiella pneumoniae* and other enterobacteria to benzylpenicillin and ampicillin. The discovery in 1965 that β-lactamases could be encoded by plasmids and readily transferred by conjugation among Gram-negative bacilli raised the specter of widespread dissemination among Gram-negative bacteria, including species not previously known to possess these enzymes. This prediction has been largely fulfilled, and plasmid-mediated β-lactamase-producing isolates of Gram-negative bacilli are currently a major and increasing clinical problem. In addition, β-lactamase-producing strains of *Haemophilus influenzae*, *Moraxella catarrhalis* and *Neisseria gonorrhoeae*, which were unknown before the mid-1970s, are now common causes of infection. The increase in β-lactamase dissemination and the identification of new β-lactamase entities has often followed the development and use of new β-lactam-containing agents that have served as the selecting agents for the next generation of enzymes.

Bacterial β-lactamases may also be chromosomally encoded, with inducible or constitutive production; only rare reports of inducible plasmid-encoded enzymes have been documented. The β-lactamase genes may be translocated from or into the chromosome or into another plasmid by transposons (Ch. 3). Transfer within and between species or genera explains the successful spread of resistance mediated by these enzymes. For instance, the TEM-1 β-lactamase has been identified in virtually every genus of Enterobacteriaceae. Plasmid-encoded cephalosporinases derived from common class C chromosomal cephalosporinases are being identified more frequently. Most seriously, plasmid-encoded metallo-β-lactamases are now being identified that are capable of hydrolyzing almost all classes of β-lactam agent and which are refractory to inhibition by commercially available β-lactamase inhibitors.

Those β-lactamases found in Gram-positive organisms are often extracellular enzymes, but Gram-negative β-lactamases are almost inevitably confined to the periplasmic space. Because the outer membrane of Gram-negative bacteria generally restricts transport of large molecules, little β-lactamase activity is detected extracellularly. Quantitative measurement of β-lactamase activity in intact cells can be difficult, depending upon the permeability properties of the specific outer membrane of an organism, so that the enzymes are usually studied in extracts after disruption of the cell.

CLASSIFICATION

β-Lactamases are usually characterized on the basis of one of two properties: molecular characteristics, which now routinely include a full nucleotide or amino acid sequence; or functional characteristics, including substrate and inhibition profiles (Table 17.1). Numerous classification schemes have been proposed. The three most cited schemes are that of Ambler, who proposed a classification based upon molecular structure, that of Richmond and Sykes, who divided the β-lactamases produced by Gram-negative bacteria according to functional properties, and that of Bush, who combined the functional properties with the known molecular sequences of β-lactamases from both Gram-positive and Gram-negative bacteria. Bush's scheme was expanded in collaboration with Jacoby and Medeiros to include 190 unique β-lactamases in a functional classification that has been correlated with their molecular classification. The number of enzymes classified in this scheme numbered at least 350 in 2001.

Hydrolytic activity is customarily defined by comparison with benzylpenicillin or cephaloridine, with rates of hydrolysis normalized to 100 for the reference compound. Inhibitory properties deemed to be significant include inhibition by clavulanic acid, (a good inhibitor of many β-lactamases that contain an active site serine), and inhibition by the chelating agent ethylenediaminetetraacetic acid (EDTA), which is used to identify the zinc-containing metallo-β-lactamases. Characteristics of representative β-lactamases from each class are shown in Table 17.2.

Molecular classification of β-lactamases requires sequence determinations of either the gene encoding the enzyme or the amino acid sequence of the protein. Class A, C, and D β-lactamases are all enzymes that require an active site serine to acylate the β-lactam substrate during the hydrolysis reaction. Class C β-lactamases tend to have higher molecular weights than the other classes. Class B β-lactamases contain at least one functional Zn^{2+} atom at the active site that participates in the hydrolytic process. A number of characteristic amino acid sequences have been identified to differentiate the various molecular classes.

Functional (Bush et al) groups are identified according to inhibitory properties based primarily upon clavulanic acid and EDTA. For many enzymes, the inhibitory activities of clavulanic acid and tazobactam are similar. Additional subgroups are identified according to substrate hydrolysis profiles. The easiest group to identify is that containing the group 3 metallo-β-lactamases, which were not included in earlier functional classification schemes. These enzymes are readily distinguished from all other β-lactamases because they can hydrolyze carbapenems and they are not inhibited by clavulanic acid, but are inhibited by chelators such as EDTA.

Functional group 1 cephalosporinases include the chromosomal β-lactamases from Enterobacteriaceae that are not inhibited well by clavulanic acid. A second cephalosporinase class was segregated into group 2e due to high affinity for clavulanic acid, a good inhibitor of these enzymes. Sequencing data have shown that functional group 1 enzymes belong to molecular class C, whereas the functional group 2e

Table 17.1 Classification of bacterial β-lactamases

Functional group	Molecular class	Preferred substrates	Inhibited by		Representative enzymes
			CA	EDTA	
1	C	Ceph	–	–	AmpC, plasmid-encoded cephalosporinases (Gram-negative bacteria), CMY-1
2a	A	Pen	+	–	Penicillinases from Gram-positive bacteria
2b	A	Pen, ceph	+	–	TEM-1, TEM-2, SHV-1
2be	A	Pen, ceph, extended-spectrum ceph, monobactam	+	–	TEM-3 … TEM-105, SHV-2 … SHV-39
2br	A	Pen	+/–	–	TEM-30 … TEM-39 … (IRT 1 – IRT-26), SHV-10
2c	A	Pen, carbenicillin	+	–	PSE-1, PSE-3, PSE-4
2d	D	Pen, cloxacillin	+/–	–	OXA-1 … OXA-40, OXA-10 = PSE-2
2e	A	Ceph	+	–	Inducible cephalosporinases from *Pr. vulgaris*, SFO-1
2f	A	Ceph, pen, carbapenems	+	–	NMC-A, SME-1, IMI-1
3	B	Carbapenems. Often, all ceph, pen. No monobactam	–	+	L1 from *S. maltophilia*, CfiA/CcrA from *B. fragilis*, VIM-1, IMP-1 … IMP-9
4	Not determined	Pen	–	–	Penicillinase from *Burk. cepacia*

Pen, penicillin; ceph, cephalosporin; CA, clavulanic acid; EDTA, ethylenediaminetetraacetic acid.
Based on Bush K, Jacoby GA, Medeiros AA 1995 *Antimicrobial Agents and Chemotherapy* 39: 1211–1233, and Bush K 2001 *Clinical Infectious Diseases* 32: 1085–1089.

Table 17.2 Characteristics of selected bacterial β-lactamases

β-Lactamase	Functional group	Molecular class	Molecular mass (kDa)	Relative hydrolysis of major substrates compared to benzylpenicillin as 100					Clavulanic acid IC$_{50}$ (μmol)
				Amp	Lor	Ctx	Caz	Imp	
Enterobacteria cloacae P99	1	C	40	0.3	6700	<7	<0.7	<0.7	>100
Staphylococcus aureus PC1	2a	A	27	180	1.1	<0.1	No data	No data	0.03
TEM-1	2b	A	29	110	140	0.07	0.01	<0.01	0.09
TEM-3	2be	A	29	110	120	170	8.3	0.01	0.03
TEM-10	2be	A	29	130	77	1.6	68	<0.02	0.03
SHV-1	2b	A	29	150	48	0.18	0.02	<0.01	0.03
SHV-5	2be	A	29	240	140	130	49	<1	0.01
TEM-31 (IRT-1)	2br	A	29	250	13	<1	<1	<1	9.4
PSE-4 (Dalgleish)	2c	A	32	88	40	0.02	0.02	0.01	0.15
OXA-10 (PSE-2)	2d	A	28	270	32	1	0.12	0.05	0.81
Proteus vulgaris	2e	A	28	100	3000	13	0.17	No data	0.35
Serratia marcescens SME-1	2f	A	29	1300	5100	<5	<0.5	530	0.28
Bacteroides fragilis CfiA/CcrA	3	B	26	98	22	51	68	100	>500*
Pseudomonas paucimobilis	4	No data	30	62	3.9	No data	<0.1	<0.1	19

Amp, ampicillin; Lor, cephaloridine; Ctx, cefotaxime; Caz, ceftazidime; Imp, imipenem.
Data from Bush K, Jacoby GA, Medeiros AA 1995 *Antimicrobial Agents and Chemotherapy* 39: 1211–1233.
*Inhibited by EDTA.

enzymes are all members of molecular class A, like most group 2 β-lactamases.

Other group 2 enzymes are generally inhibited by clavulanate, with the exception of the rare TEM-1 β-lactamase derivatives – the inhibitor-resistant TEM (IRT) enzymes – which have reduced affinity for the inhibitor. Group 2a enzymes are penicillinases; group 2b enzymes have a broader spectrum of activity, hydrolyzing penicillins and cephalosporins almost equally well. Group 2be enzymes, the extended-spectrum β-lactamases (ESBL), are often derived from group 2b enzymes, but exhibit enhanced hydrolytic properties that enable them to hydrolyze extended-spectrum cephalosporins and monobactams. Group 2c enzymes hydrolyze carbenicillin, and group 2d enzymes hydrolyze the isoxazolyl penicillins such as cloxacillin or oxacillin. The 2d enzymes are the only β-lactamases that belong to molecular class D rather than class A. The 2f enzymes are carbapenem-hydrolyzing enzymes that are class A serine β-lactamases rather than metalloenzymes.

STAPHYLOCOCCUS AUREUS β-LACTAMASE

Today at least 90% of *Staph. aureus* causing infections in community and hospital practice are β-lactamase-producing strains. The enzyme produced occurs in four serologically distinct forms that are closely related on a molecular level. Production may be plasmid-encoded or chromosomal. The chromosomal enzymes can be induced by penicillins such as methicillin or by the β-lactamase inhibitor sulbactam. The enzymes are predominantly active against penicillins, but can be differentiated on the basis of hydrolysis of cephalosporins including cefaloridine, nitrocefin and cefazolin.

CHROMOSOMAL CEPHALOSPORINASES OF GRAM-NEGATIVE BACTERIA

Most Gram-negative bacteria elaborate chromosomally mediated enzymes, most of which fall into group 1. These hydrolyze cephalosporins up to 1000 times more rapidly than penicillins, some of which (e.g. cloxacillin) may inhibit them. Traditional β-lactamase-inhibitors work poorly against these enzymes, but monobactams such as aztreonam bind tightly and act like potent inactivators.

In some species, including *Acinetobacter, Citrobacter, Enterobacter, Morganella, Pseudomonas* and *Serratia*, group 1 cephalosporinases are inducible and often species specific. Plasmid-encoded forms of these enzymes, such as those designated FOX-1, LAT-1, MIR-1 and MOX-1, have appeared, particularly in *K. pneumoniae* strains that have an additional β-lactamase. Sequence data indicate high homology with the AmpC cephalosporinases from *Pseudomonas aeruginosa, Serratia marcescens, Enterobacter cloacae* or *Citrobacter freundii*.

Induction is a clinically relevant phenomenon when the inducing molecule is a substrate that can be hydrolyzed by the enzyme, such as ampicillin or amoxicillin. Many good inducers, such as cefoxitin and imipenem, are not good substrates for these enzymes, and pose problems primarily when they are coadministered with a second β-lactam agent. Because induction is a transient event, the producing organisms revert to their original low basal production of β-lactamase on removal of the inducer. A more serious problem occurs if there is selection for a permanently altered organism with derepressed production of the chromosomal β-lactamase. Enterobacteria that hyperproduce group 1 cephalosporinases are sometimes responsible for clinical failures of cephalosporins. Interestingly, β-lactam compounds that are good inducers rarely select for derepressed hyperproducing mutants.

PLASMID-ENCODED β-LACTAMASES

Plasmid-encoded enzymes account for perhaps the most important β-lactamase-related resistance mechanisms. The most common β-lactamase in Gram-negative organisms is the TEM-1 β-lactamase, responsible for transferable ampicillin resistance among Enterobacteriaceae worldwide. In *K. pneumoniae*, the broad-spectrum SHV-1 β-lactamase predominates. Other important families of plasmid-mediated β-lactamases include the OXA enzymes that hydrolyze oxacillin and the PSE enzymes, a group originally believed to be confined to pseudomonads.

In the mid-1980s, plasmid-encoded β-lactamases that conferred resistance to oxyimino β-lactam agents (notably cefotaxime), and/or ceftazidime and aztreonam, began to appear in central Europe. The major families of expanded-spectrum β-lactamases (functional group 2be) include numerous variants of TEM-1 and SHV-1 that are now numbered through at least TEM-105 and SHV-39. It should be noted that the sequential numbers of each family include at least five sequences that have been withdrawn, and approximately 24 inhibitor-resistant TEM enzyme sequences.

Organisms elaborating extended-spectrum β-lactamases may remain susceptible to cefoxitin and imipenem, or piperacillin–tazobactam. The enzymes are readily inhibited by clavulanic acid, sulbactam or tazobactam. They differ from their parent TEM and SHV enzymes by selected point mutations; two or more amino acid substitutions often lead to high-level resistance (cephalosporin MICs >32 mg/l), especially if the organisms also have porin mutations. Such organisms have spread rapidly within localized metropolitan areas to cause hospital outbreaks and colonization in nursing homes. TEM variants resistant to β-lactamase inhibitors have also become a community problem in Europe. Infections caused by organisms producing these enzymes do not respond to clavulanic acid or sulbactam inhibitor combinations, but are often susceptible to early cephalosporins.

METALLO-β-LACTAMASES

Perhaps the most formidable β-lactamases known are the metallo-β-lactamases, which rapidly hydrolyze most β-lactam agents, especially the carbapenems, but not the monobactams, and are resistant to β-lactamase inhibitors. These enzymes were originally confined to a few isolated strains of *B. fragilis* and *Bacillus cereus* as chromosomal enzymes, but were then identified in Japan on plasmids found in *B. fragilis, Ser. marcescens, K. pneumoniae* and *Ps. aeruginosa*. Such strains appear to be confined to localized areas, but have now been identified in most parts of the world. Because of the low catalytic efficiencies of these enzymes, they are almost always produced in combination with at least one other β-lactamase of a different class, thus expanding the hydrolytic repertoire for the organism.

 ## Further information

Ambler RP 1980 The structure of β-lactamases. *Philosophical Transactions of the Royal Society of London, Series B* 289: 321–331.

Bush K, Jacoby GA, Medeiros AA 1995 A functional classification scheme for β-lactamases and its correlation with molecular structure. *Antimicrobial Agents and Chemotherapy* 39: 1211–1233.

Bush K, Mobashery S 1998 How β-lactamases have driven pharmaceutical drug discovery: From mechanistic knowledge to clinical circumvention. *Advances in Experimental and Medical Biology* 456: 71–98.

Chaibi EB, Sirot D, Paul G, Labia R 1999 Inhibitor-resistant TEM β-lactamases: phenotypic, genetic and biochemical characteristics. *Journal of Antimicrobial Chemotherapy* 43: 447–458.

Jacoby GA 1997 Extended-spectrum β-lactamases and other enzymes providing resistance to oxyimino-β-lactams. *Infectious Diseases Clinics of North America* 11: 875–87.

Livermore D 1998 β-Lactamase-mediated resistance and opportunities for its control. *Journal of Antimicrobial Chemotherapy* 41 (Suppl. D): 25–41.

Medeiros AA 1997 Evolution and dissemination of β-lactamases accelerated by generations of β-lactam antibiotics. *Clinical Infectious Diseases* 24: S19–S45.

Payne DJ 1993 Metallo-β-lactamases – a new therapeutic challenge. *Journal of Medical Microbiology* 39: 93–99.

Philippon A, Dusart J, Joris B, Frère J-M 1998 The diversity, structure, and regulation of β-lactamases. *Cellular and Molecular Life Sciences* 54: 341–346.

Rasmussen BA, Bush K 1997 Carbapenem-hydrolyzing β-lactamases. *Antimicrobial Agents and Chemotherapy* 41: 223–232.

Sanders CC 1987 Chromosomal cephalosporinases responsible for multiple resistance to newer β-lactam antibiotics. *Annual Review of Microbiology* 41: 573–593.

Zygmunt DJ, Stratton CW, Kernodle DS 1992 Characterization of four β-lactamases produced by *Staphylococcus aureus*. *Antimicrobial Agents and Chemotherapy* 36: 440–445.

CARBAPENEMS

More than 40 carbapenems have been isolated from fermentation products of various streptomycetes. Their nomenclature has been complicated by the use of multiple generic names to describe the same class of compounds, including thienamycins, olivanic acids, carpetimycins, asparenomycins and pluracidomycins. Their interest lies in their potent activity against a broad range of Gram-positive and Gram-negative bacteria and in their resistance to hydrolysis by β-lactamases. Some are also β-lactamase inhibitors. The most active of the natural compounds, thienamycin, is produced by *Streptomyces cattelya* although concentration-related instability precludes its clinical use.

A search for more stable derivatives that retain potent antibacterial activity led to the development of *N*-formimidoyl-thienamycin, imipenem. This compound is stable to practically all bacterial β-lactamases other than the metalloenzymes, but it is rapidly degraded by the mammalian renal dipeptidase, dehydropeptidase I. This enzyme hydrolyzes carbapenems and penems but not aztreonam, benzylpenicillin or cephaloridine. Various potential inhibitors of dehydropeptidase have been investigated for coadministration with imipenem and one of these, cilastatin, is included in therapeutic formulations. Coincidentally, cilastatin also acts as a nephroprotectant when administered with imipenem.

Addition of a 1-β-methyl substituent on the carbapenem ring confers stability to hydrolysis by dehydropeptidase. As a result, semisynthetic carbapenems such as meropenem, ertapenem and biapenem have been developed. These compounds retain broad-spectrum antimicrobial activity and β-lactamase stability, and do not need to be administered with a dehydropeptidase inhibitor.

 ## BIAPENEM

A semisynthetic carbapenem with a 2-substituted triazolium moiety. It has broad-spectrum activity against most aerobic and anaerobic Gram-positive and Gram-negative organisms. It is equivalent to, or slightly more active than, imipenem against Gram-negative aerobic bacteria and slightly less active than imipenem against Gram-positive organisms. The methyl group at C-1 confers stability to hydrolysis by dehydropeptidase from various sources, including human kidney. Efficacy in animal infections is equivalent to, or better than, that of imipenem plus cilastatin. It is not hydrolyzed by most serine β-lactamases, but like all carbapenems and penems is readily hydrolyzed by metallo-β-lactamases. The potential for neurotoxicity is less than that of imipenem.

 ## Further information

Hikida M, Masukawa Y, Nishiki K, Inomata N 1993 Low neurotoxicity of LJC 10,627, a novel 1-β-methyl carbapenem antibiotic inhibition of γ-aminobutyric acid$_A$, benzodiazepine, and glycine receptor binding in relation to lack of central nervous system toxicity in rats. *Antimicrobial Agents and Chemotherapy* 37: 199–202.

Petersen PJ, Jacobus NV, Weiss WJ, Testa RT 1991 In vitro and in vivo activities of LJC10,627, a new carbapenem with stability to dehydropeptidase 1. *Antimicrobial Agents and Chemotherapy* 35: 203–207.

Ubukata K, Hikida M, Yoshida M et al 1990 In vitro activity of LJC10,627, a new carbapenem antibiotic with high stability to dehydropeptidase 1. *Antimicrobial Agents and Chemotherapy* 34: 994–1000.

Yang Y, Bhachech N, Bush K 1995 Biochemical comparison of imipenem, meropenem and biapenem: permeability, binding to penicillin-binding proteins and stability to hydrolysis by β-lactamases. *Journal of Antimicrobial Chemotherapy* 35: 75–84.

 ## ERTAPENEM

Molecular weight (monosodium salt): 497.5.

A 1-β-carbapenem, formulated as the sodium salt for parenteral administration. It is stable to renal dehydropeptidase and can be administered as a single agent.

Antimicrobial activity

Activity against aerobic and anaerobic pathogens is comparable to that of imipenem (Table 17.3): MIC values for Gram-negative bacilli (with the exception of *Ps. aeruginosa*) are generally lower and those for Gram-positive cocci higher.

Ertapenem is stable to most serine β-lactamases, but is hydrolyzed by metallo-β-lactamases.

Pharmacokinetics

C_{max} 1 g intramuscular	*c.* 65 mg/l after 2 h
1 g intravenous infusion (30 min)	*c.* 150 mg/l end infusion
Plasma half-life	*c.* 4 h
Volume of distribution	*c.* 8 l (steady state)
Plasma protein binding	85–95%

Absorption after intramuscular injection is essentially complete. The modestly extended plasma half-life allows once daily dosing.

Excretion is predominantly by the renal route, about 80% being recovered in the urine within 24 hours. About 40% is

Table 17.3 Activity of the carbapenems ertapenem, imipenem and meropenem, and the monobactam, aztreonam against common bacterial pathogens: MIC (mg/l)*

Organism	Ertapenem	Imipenem	Meropenem	Aztreonam
Staph. aureus (MSSA)	0.12	0.03	0.12	R
Staph. aureus (MRSA)	2.0	0.5	2.0	R
Str. pyogenes	≤0.03	≤0.01	≤0.01	8
Str. pneumoniae				
penicillin-susceptible	≤0.03	0.008	0.008	R
penicillin-resistant	1.0	0.03	0.12	No data
E. faecalis	16	1.0	4.0	R
H. influenzae	≤0.03	1.0	0.06	≤0.1
Neisseria spp.	≤0.03	≤0.25	≤0.03	≤0.1
Esch. coli	≤0.03	0.12	0.03	≤0.1
K. pneumoniae	≤0.03	≤0.25	0.03	≤0.1
Ps. aeruginosa	4.0	4.0	4.0	8
B. fragilis	0.25	0.25	0.12	32
Chlamydia spp.	No data	No data	No data	≤0.25

R, resistant (MIC >32 mg/l). *MIC against 50% of strains.

eliminated unchanged; the rest as a biologically-inactive ring-opened metabolite. Dosage should be reduced in severe renal impairment.

Toxicity and side effects

Clinical experience is presently limited, but ertapenem appears to be generally well tolerated. Various adverse events, most notably nausea and diarrhea have been noted in early studies. Seizures have occasionally been reported in patients with a history of disorders of the central nervous system.

Clinical use

- Serious infections caused by multiresistant Gram-negative bacilli.

Further information

Fuchs PC, Barry AL, Brown SD 1999 In-vitro antimicrobial activity of a carbapenem, MK-0826 (L-749,345) and provisional interpretive criteria for disc tests. *Journal of Antimicrobial Chemotherapy* 43: 703–706.

Gill CJ, Jackson JJ, Gerckens LS et al 1998 In vivo activity and pharmacokinetic evaluation of a novel long-acting carbapenem antibiotic, MK-826 (L-749,345). *Antimicrobial Agents and Chemotherapy* 42: 1996–2001.

Graham DR, Lucasti C, Malafaia O, et al. 2002 Ertapenem once daily versus piperacillin-tazobactam 4 times per day for treatment of complicated skin and skin-structure infections in adults: results of a prospective, randomized, double-blind multicenter study. *Clinical Infectious Diseases* 34: 1460–1468.

Odenholt I 2001 Ertapenem: a new carbapenum. *Expert Opinion on Investigational Drugs*. 10: 1157–1166.

Preparations and dosage

Proprietary name: Invanz.

Preparations: Lyophilized powder for reconstitution for i.m. injection (with 1% lidocaine) or i.v. infusion over 30 min.

Dosage: Adults: 1 g intramuscularly or by intravenous infusion once daily for 3–14 days depending on severity of infection. Not recommended for use in children.

Available in USA

IMIPENEM

N-formimidoylthienamycin. Molecular weight (monohydrate): 317.37.

A semisynthetic carbapenem available as the monohydrate; formulated in a 1:1 ratio with the dehydropeptidase inhibitor, cilastatin sodium (molecular weight [monosodium salt] 380.43) for intramuscular and intravenous administration.

It is stable in the solid state for 6 months at 37°C. In aqueous solution at room temperature it decays at 10%/h.

Antimicrobial activity

Imipenem shows potent activity against a very wide range of Gram-positive and Gram-negative aerobes and anaerobes, including many resistant to other agents. Its activity against common pathogenic organisms is shown in Table 17.3. Concentrations (mg/l) inhibiting 50% of strains of other organisms are: *Listeria monocytogenes*, 0.03; *Legionella pneumophila*, 0.03; *Enterococcus faecium*, 4; *Yersinia* spp., 0.06. *Mycobacterium fortuitum* is inhibited by 6.25 mg/l. Imipenem is active against most *Pseudomonas* species, but not *Stenotrophomonas maltophilia*. It is active against most anaerobes, with the exception of *Clostridium perfringens*, which is only moderately susceptible. There is usually little effect of inoculum size up to 10^7 colony-forming units (cfu)/ml; of pH up to 8; or the presence of serum. However, marked inoculum effects have been described with strains of *Haemophilus influenzae*, *Enterococcus faecalis* and methicillin-resistant *Staphylococcus aureus*, in which resistance to β-lactam antibiotics is due not to β-lactamase production but to poor affinity for specific target penicillin-binding proteins. It is bactericidal at 2–4 times the minimum inhibitory concentration (MIC) for most species, but some strains of *Staph. aureus* exhibit 'tolerance' (see p. 15). Bactericidal synergy with aminoglycosides, glycopeptides, fosfomycin and rifampicin has been observed against many strains of *Staph. aureus* and enterococci.

Antibacterial activity is unaffected by the presence of cilastatin, which is itself devoid of antimicrobial activity.

Imipenem is stable to hydrolysis by most serine β-lactamases, with the exception of the rare group 2f carbapenem-hydrolyzing enzymes (see above). It is a potent inhibitor of group 1 β-lactamase from *Ps. aeruginosa* and the group 2a penicillinase from *Bacillus cereus*, acting like a poor substrate that is released slowly. It can be hydrolyzed by the TEM-1 and TEM-2 β-lactamases, but so slowly that producing organisms remain susceptible. β-Lactamase-producing strains of *H. influenzae* and *N. gonorrhoeae* are generally as susceptible as β-lactamase-negative strains. Strains of *B. fragilis*, *Aeromonas* spp. and *Sten. maltophilia* can produce metallo-β-lactamases that hydrolyze the drug rapidly. These strains, in addition to occasional strains of enterobacteria and *Ps. aeruginosa*, show variable resistance to imipenem depending upon the level of carbapenem-hydrolyzing activity and the presence or absence of imipenem-specific porins. Efflux pumps also exist that may extrude imipenem from Gram-negative bacteria.

Acquired resistance

Some strains of *Citrobacter*, *Enterobacter*, *Proteus vulgaris*, *Providencia*, *Ps. aeruginosa* and *Serratia* spp. that elaborate high levels of β-lactamases may be resistant to imipenem and other β-lactam agents, often because of the selection of stably derepressed mutants expressing high levels of group 1 β-lactamases. These cephalosporinases can hydrolyze imipenem and extended-spectrum cephalosporins very slowly, but the mutants usually also exhibit decreased permeability; they are resistant to all β-lactam agents, but imipenem is usually affected less than aminothiazolyloxyimino cephalosporins and aztreonam.

Induction of class 1 β-lactamases by imipenem in strains of *Aeromonas*, *Pseudomonas* and *Serratia* spp. is responsible for antagonism of β-lactamase-labile β-lactam agents in vitro. Resistance in *Ps. aeruginosa* has also been documented following selection by imipenem of mutants that hyperproduce the group 1 cephalosporinase and which are also deficient in an outer membrane protein (OprD or D2) which specifically transports imipenem and other carbapenems, but not cephalosporins or monobactams.

Pharmacokinetics

C_{max} 500 mg intravenous (15–30 min infusion)	*c.* 20 mg/l end infusion
Plasma half-life	1 h
Volume of distribution	*c.* 0.2 l/kg
Plasma protein binding	20%

Absorption

Imipenem is not absorbed by the oral route. In volunteers receiving 2 g of the combination with cilastatin intravenously over 30 min, every 6 h for 40 doses, serum concentrations of imipenem at the end of infusion were around 19 mg/l after the first dose and 23 mg/l after the last.

Distribution

In patients with bacterial meningitis receiving 1 mg/kg intravenously over 20 min, cerebrospinal fluid (CSF) concentrations of 0.5–11 mg/l have been found. The plasma clearance of cilastatin was about one-quarter that of imipenem but its urinary concentration was approximately double. There was marked intersubject variation, especially in the handling of cilastatin.

Metabolism

In the absence of cilastatin, imipenem is slowly hydrolyzed, with a half-life of 0.7 h in serum in vitro; at the end of intravenous infusion over 20 min about 9% of the labelled drug is in the form of the open-ring metabolite. Most destruction, however, occurs in the kidney and only 5–40% of the drug is recovered in the urine, where 80–90% is in the open-ring form. When imipenem is administered with cilastatin in a 1:1 ratio, urinary recovery of imipenem rises to 65–75%, with only 20% in the open-ring form.

One source of intersubject variation described in adults may be in the ability to metabolize the drug. The inhibitor has more effect in 'high metabolizers' – those in whom less than 16% of the dose appears in the urine.

Excretion

In volunteers receiving 2 g of the mixture intravenously over 30 min, every 6 h for 40 doses, half-lives were 0.9 h after the first dose and 0.8 h after the last. Renal excretion was 55–60%.

Probenecid has little effect on the plasma half-life, but markedly increases urinary recovery. Renal excretion of cilastatin closely follows that of imipenem, 75% being excreted unchanged in the urine over 6 h, with about 12% as the *N*-acetyl metabolite.

In patients with chronic renal failure, about 75% of the mixture was eliminated by 3 h hemofiltration. The half-lives of the two components differed markedly: around 3.4 h for imipenem and 16 h for cilastatin.

Toxicity and side effects

Central nervous system (CNS) effects such as confusional states and seizures have been reported, especially when recommended doses were exceeded, and in patients with renal failure or creatinine clearances of ≤ 20 ml/min/1.73 m^2. Generalized seizures have been observed in patients who have received ganciclovir concomitantly.

Other reactions include phlebitis/thrombophlebitis (3.1%), nausea (2.0%), diarrhea (1.8%), and vomiting (1.5%). Increased hepatic enzymes may be seen in adults and children. Superinfection with *Aspergillus*, *Candida* and resistant *Pseudomonas* spp. have been described and pseudomembranous colitis has been reported.

Patients with a history of hypersensitivity reactions to penicillins, cephalosporins or other β-lactam antibiotics should be treated cautiously with carbapenems.

Clinical use

- Lower respiratory tract infections.
- Urinary tract infections (complicated and uncomplicated).
- Intra-abdominal infections.
- Gynecological infections.
- Bacterial septicemia.
- Bone and joint infections.
- Skin and skin structure infections.
- Endocarditis.
- Polymicrobial infections.

Preparations and dosage

Proprietary names: Primaxin.

Preparation: i.v. or i.m.

Dosage: Adults, deep i.m. injection, 500–750 mg every 12 h, depending on the severity of the infection; gonococcal urethritis or cervicitis, 500 mg as a single dose.

Adults, i.v., 1–2 g/day in 3–4 equally divided doses (maximum dose 4 g per day); the dose is determined by the severity of the infection and the condition of the patient. Children 3 months (< 40 kg body weight), 15 mg/kg per dose four times daily, with a maximum daily dose of 60 mg/kg (2 g daily).

Widely available.

Further information

Alarabi AA, Cars O, Danielson BG, Salmonson T, Wikstrom B 1990 Pharmacokinetics of intravenous imipenem/cilastatin during intermittent haemofiltration. *Journal of Antimicrobial Chemotherapy* 26: 91–98.

Bint AJ, Speller DCE, Williams RJ (eds) 1986 Imipenem – assessing its clinical role. *Journal of Antimicrobial Chemotherapy* 18 (Suppl. E): 1–210.

Clissold SP, Todd PA, Campoli-Richards DM 1987 Imipenem/cilastatin: a review of its antibacterial activity, pharmacokinetic properties and therapeutic efficacy. *Drugs* 33: 183–241

Geddes AM, Stille W (eds) 1985 Imipenem: the first thienamycin antibiotic. *Reviews of Infectious Diseases* 7 (Suppl. 3): S353–S356.

Livermore D 1992 Interplay of impermeability and chromosomal β-lactamase activity in imipenem-resistant *Pseudomonas aeruginosa*. *Antimicrobial Agents and Chemotherapy* 36: 2046–2048.

Luthy R, Neu HC, Phillips I (eds) 1983 A perspective of imipenem, *Journal of Antimicrobial Chemotherapy* 12 (Suppl. D): 1–153.

Remington JS (ed) 1985 Carbapenems: a new class of antibiotics (Symposium on imipenem – cilastatin). *American Journal of Medicine* 78 (Suppl. 6A): 1–167.

Saxon A, Adelman DC, Patel A, Hajdu R, Calandra GB 1988 Imipenem cross-reactivity with penicillin in humans. *Journal of Allergy and Clinical Immunology* 82: 213–217.

Trias J, Nikaido, H 1990 Outer membrane protein D2 catalyzes facilitated diffusion of carbapenems and penems through the outer membrane of *Pseudomonas aeruginosa*. *Antimicrobial Agents and Chemotherapy* 34: 52–57.

MEROPENEM

Molecular weight (trihydrate): 437.52.

A semisynthetic carbapenem formulated as the trihydrate for intravenous infusion. It is soluble in 5% monobasic potassium phosphate solution, sparingly soluble in water, very slightly soluble in hydrated ethanol, and practically insoluble in acetone or ether. The β-methyl group at C-1 confers increased stability to hydrolysis by most mammalian dehydropeptidase I enzymes (excluding rodents), thereby eliminating the need for a dehydropeptidase inhibitor in the dosing regimen.

Antimicrobial activity

The unique side-chain at C-2 is associated with increased activity against Gram-negative bacteria, including *H. influenzae*. It is slightly less active than imipenem against Gram-positive organisms (Table 17.3). It is quite active against anaerobes and more active against some strains that are moderately resistant (but not those that are fully resistant) to imipenem. Its excellent activity against Gram-negative organisms is due to high affinity for multiple penicillin-binding proteins (PBPs; see p. 14). Activity is little affected by inoculum size or the presence of serum. It is bactericidal at concentrations close to the MIC.

Stability to β-lactamases is similar to that of other carbapenems: it is highly resistant to most serine β-lactamases, including extended-spectrum enzymes, but can be hydrolyzed by metallo-β-lactamases and by rare carbapenem-hydrolyzing group 2f serine β-lactamases. It induces, but is not degraded by, chromosomally mediated group 1 enzymes (see p. 264).

Pharmacokinetics

C_{max} 500 mg intravenous (30 min infusion)	23 mg/l end infusion
1 g intravenous (30 min infusion)	49 mg/l end infusion
Plasma half-life	1 h
Volume of distribution	c. 0.3 l/kg
Plasma protein binding	2%

Absorption

Meropenem is not absorbed after oral administration.

Distribution

It penetrates well into most body fluids and tissues, including CSF, achieving concentrations matching or exceeding those required to inhibit most susceptible bacteria. Concentrations in CSF are directly related to the degree of meningeal inflammation. In patients with inflamed meninges it achieves CSF levels of 0.9–6.5 mg/l after a single intravenous infusion over 30 min. The CSF:plasma concentration ratio is 0.02–0.5. After a single intravenous dose, the highest mean concentrations of meropenem were found in tissues and fluids at 1 h (0.5–1.5 h) after the start of infusion.

Metabolism

The mean recovery of unchanged meropenem is 65–79%, attesting to its stability to human dehydropeptidase. The remainder of the material was identified as the microbiologically inactive open-ring form, produced by chemical hydrolysis, by the action of dehydropeptidase or by other metabolic enzymes.

Excretion

Renal excretion is greater than 70% of the plasma clearance. Coadministration with probenecid significantly prolongs the half-life by around 33% and increases the area under the curve (AUC) by about 56%, but peak concentrations are not greatly affected. The half-life of meropenem and its metabolite increase proportionately to the degree of renal impairment and the dose should be adjusted accordingly. Parent drug and metabolite are removed by hemodialysis.

Toxicity and side effects

Seizures and other CNS adverse experiences have been reported in <0.5% of all adult patients, most commonly in patients with CNS disorders or with bacterial meningitis and/or renal impairment. Pseudomembranous colitis has been reported.

Other reactions include diarrhea (5.0%), nausea and vomiting (3.9%), inflammation at the site of injection (3.0%), headache (2.8%), rash (1.7%), pruritus (1.6%), apnea (1.2%), constipation (1.2%), phlebitis/thrombophlebitis (1.2%), and injection site reaction (1.1%). Increased hepatic enzymes, hematological effects, and increased creatinine and blood urea nitrogen are seen in <0.2–1.0% of patients. Moniliasis occurs in 2.0–3.5% of pediatric patients.

Patients with a history of hypersensitivity reactions to other β-lactam agents should be treated cautiously.

Clinical use

- Intra-abdominal infections.
- Bacterial meningitis (pediatric patients ≥3 months).

Preparations and dosage

Proprietary names: Merrem, Meronem.

Preparation: Intravenous.

Dosage: Adults, i.v., 0.5–1 g every 8 h or 2 g every 8 h for meningitis. Children ≥3 months, 10–20 mg/kg every 8 h for intra-abdominal infections or 40 mg/kg every 8 h for meningitis.

Widely available.

Further information

Conference 1989 Meropenem (SM 7338) – a new carbapenem. *Journal of Antimicrobial Chemotherapy* 24 (Suppl. A): 1–320.

Craig WA 1997 The pharmacology of meropenem, a new carbapenem antibiotic. *Clinical Infectious Diseases* 24(Suppl. 2): S266–275.

Dagan R, Velghe L, Rodda JL, Klugman KP 1994 Penetration of meropenem into the cerebrospinal fluid of patients with inflamed meninges. *Journal of Antimicrobial Chemotherapy* 34: 175–179.

Davey P, Davies A, Livermore D, Speller D, Daly PJ (eds) 1989 Meropenem (SM7338) – a new carbapenem. *Journal of Antimicrobial Chemotherapy* 24 (Suppl. A): 1–320.

Fukasawa M, Sumita Y, Harabe ET et al 1992 Stability of meropenem and effect of 1β-methyl substitution on its stability in the presence of renal dehydropeptidase I. *Antimicrobial Agents and Chemotherapy* 36: 1577–1579.

Lowe MN, Lamb HM 2000 Meropenem: a review of its use in patients in intensive care. *Drugs* 59: 653–680.

PANIPENEM

A 3-acetimidoylpyrrolidinyl-substituted carbapenem with no methyl group at the C-1 position. It has broad-spectrum antibacterial activity against Gram-positive and Gram-negative organisms. It is coadministered with betamipron (N-benzoyl-β-alanine) in a ratio of 1:1. Betamipron is a renal anion transport inhibitor that decreases nephrotoxicity caused by high doses of the carbapenem by inhibiting its accumulation in the renal cortex. Panipenem is slightly more stable to hydrolysis by dehydropeptidase than imipenem, but not as stable as meropenem or biapenem. It is hydrolyzed by metallo-β-lactamases.

Antimicrobial activity

Its activity is very similar to that of other carbapenems.

Pharmacokinetics

Mean maximum blood concentrations following intravenous infusion of 0.5 g and 0.75 g of each component were 37 and 61 mg/l for panipenem and 24 and 39 mg/l for betamipron. Following intravenous infusion in children (10 mg or 20 mg of each component per kg), the half-life of panipenem was about 1.2 h, the half-life of betamipron was about 0.9 h. Drug levels in the CSF were at least 8-fold lower than serum concentrations.

Toxicity and side effects

Side effects are similar to those reported for other carbapenems (incidence <10%) and are generally mild. Occasional transient elevations of transaminases and other hepatic markers have been reported. Patients with a history of previous hypersensitivity reactions to penicillins, cephalosporins or other β-lactam antibiotics should be treated cautiously.

Clinical use

Adults
- Urinary tract infections.
- Skin and soft-tissue infections.
- Surgical infections.

Children
- Respiratory infections.
- Otitis media.
- Sepsis.

 Further information

Panipenem/betamipron 1991 In: *Chemotherapy (Tokyo)* S-3: 1–813.
Shimada K 1994 Panipenem/betamipron. *Japanese Journal of Antibiotics* 47: 219–244.
Shimada J, Kawahara Y 1994 Overview of a new carbapenem panipenem/betamipron. *Drugs under Experimental and Clinical Research* 20: 241–245.

Available in Japan.

MONOBACTAMS

Study of the structural basis of activity of early β-lactam compounds led to the expectation that compounds in which the β-lactam ring was not strained by fusion to another ring would be inactive as antimicrobial agents. It came as a surprise, therefore, to find active natural monocyclic β-lactam antibiotics, nocardicins and monobactams.

Nocardicin A, the most potent of the seven nocardicin analogs, attracted interest principally for its activity against *Ps. aeruginosa* and for an apparently beneficial interaction with host defences, but it has been overtaken by more active compounds and was not further developed.

The antibacterial monocyclic β-lactam-1-sulfonic acids, originally called 'sulfazecins' and later 'monobactams', are produced by bacteria, in contrast to penicillins and cephalosporins, which are commonly produced by fungi and actinomycetes. In the naturally occurring monobactams the β-lactam ring may carry an α-methoxy group, a feature which is responsible for β-lactamase stability in cephamycins. Because of their simplicity of structure, they can be obtained by total synthesis. The compound which first came into therapeutic use, and has been the only monobactam to achieve even modest commercial acceptability, is aztreonam, which incorporates an unnatural aminothiazoleoxime substituent in the 3-position.

Monobactams exhibit no useful activity against Gram-positive organisms or strict anaerobes because of poor binding to PBPs (p. 14). Activity against Gram-negative bacteria, including *Ps. aeruginosa*, is due to tight binding to PBP3 in *Esch. coli* and analogous PBPs in other Gram-negative organisms. The effect is manifested predominantly by conversion of the organisms to filaments, which slowly lyse.

Monobactams are hydrolyzed poorly by many serine β-lactamases and all metallo-β-lactamases tested to date, but can be hydrolyzed by the extended-spectrum β-lactamases. Group 1 cephalosporinases have high affinities for non-methoxylated monobactams, whereas group 2 β-lactamases generally bind aztreonam poorly. They are generally not inducers of the group 1 chromosomal cephalosporinases of Gram-negative bacteria.

 AZTREONAM

Molecular weight: 435.43.

A synthetic analog of a monobactam antibiotic from the bacterium *Chromobacterium violaceum*. Now obtained by chemical synthesis and available for intramuscular or intravenous administration. Aqueous solutions have a pH of 4.5–7.5 and can be maintained at room temperature for up to 48 h.

Antimicrobial activity

Its activity against common pathogenic organisms is shown in Table 17.3 (p. 266). Concentrations (mg/l) inhibiting 50% of other organisms are: *Aeromonas* spp., 0.1; *Acinetobacter* spp., 16; *M. catarrhalis*, 0.1; *Burkholderia cepacia*, 2; *Sten. maltophilia*, 128; and *Yersinia* spp., 0.1. An inoculum effect may be observed in Enterobacteriaceae when tested at 10^7 cfu, perhaps due to selection of variants exhibiting derepressed production of chromosomal cephalosporinases together with decreased outer membrane permeability. Synergy has been shown with gentamicin, tobramycin and amikacin against 52–89% of strains of *Ps. aeruginosa* and gentamicin-resistant Gram-negative bacteria. Aztreonam does not inactivate and is not inactivated by gentamicin.

Pharmacokinetics

C_{max} 1 g intravenous	90 mg/l end-infusion
1 g intramuscular	46 mg/l after 1 h
Plasma half-life	1.7 h
Volume of distribution	0.18 l/kg
Plasma protein binding	50%

Absorption

Bioavailability by the intramuscular route is 100%. Oral bioavailability is less than 1%. It is not accumulated in adults with normal renal clearance.

Distribution

Peak concentrations above the median MIC against most targeted Gram-negative pathogens are achieved in sputum, bronchial secretions, cantharides blister fluid, synovial fluid, cancellous bone and prostate tissue after 1 g intramuscular or intravenous doses.

In patients receiving 2 g intravenously over 5 min, concentrations in the CSF in the absence of inflammation were 0.5–0.9 mg/l at 1.2–8 h; in the presence of inflammation 2.0–3.2 mg/l and in patients with bacterial meningitis 0.8–16 mg/l. In children receiving 30 mg/kg intravenously in a single dose, CSF concentrations of 2–20 mg/l were found, depending on the time of sampling and disease state. In patients receiving 1 or 2 g intravenously, concentrations in the aqueous humor were 2.1–12.5 mg/l.

Metabolism

It is not extensively metabolized, the most prominent product, that results from opening the β-lactam ring, being scarcely detectable in the serum and accounting for about 7% of the dose in the urine and 3% in the feces. Its half-life is much longer than that of the parent compound.

Excretion

It is predominantly eliminated in the urine, where 58–72% appears within 24 h. The mean plasma clearance correlates well with creatinine clearance corrected for sex and age, the elimination half-life rising to 6 h in severe renal failure, with recovery in the urine falling to 1.4%. Less than 1% is eliminated unchanged in the feces, suggesting low biliary excretion.

Toxicity and side effects

Emergence of *Candida* and staphylococci has been observed in some patients. Rare cases of toxic epidermal necrolysis have been described in patients undergoing bone marrow transplant with multiple risk factors. Pseudomembranous colitis has been reported.

Local reactions include injection site reaction (2.4%) and phlebitis/thrombophlebitis (1.9%). Systemic reactions include diarrhea, nausea and/or vomiting and rash (1–1.3%). Neutropenia was seen in 11.3% of the pediatric patients younger than 2 years.

There are no reactions in patients with immunoglobulin E (IgE) antibodies to benzylpenicillin or penicillin moieties. It is rarely cross-reactive with other β-lactam antibiotics and is weakly immunogenic.

Clinical use

- Urinary tract infections, including pyelonephritis and cystitis.
- Lower respiratory tract infections, including pneumonia and bronchitis caused by Gram-negative bacilli.
- Septicemia.
- Skin and skin-structure infections, including postoperative wounds, ulcers and burns.
- Intra-abdominal infections, including peritonitis.
- Gynecological infections, including endometritis and pelvic cellulitis.

 Preparations and dosage

Proprietary name: Azactam.

Preparation: Injection.

Dosage: Adults, i.m., i.v., i.v. infusion, 1–8 g/day in equally divided doses. The route and dose is determined by the severity of the infection and the condition of the patient. Children, 30 mg/kg every 6–8 h; the total daily dose is 120 mg/kg/day. In severe infections (>2 years old) 50 mg/kg every 6–8 h (maximum dose 8 g per day).

Widely available, including UK and USA.

 Further information

Acar JF, Neu HC (eds) 1985 Gram-negative aerobic bacterial infections: a focus on directed therapy with special reference to aztreonam. *Reviews of Infectious Diseases* 7 (Suppl. 4): S537–S843.

Brogden RN, Heel RC 1986 Aztreonam: a review of its antibacterial activity, pharmacokinetic properties and therapeutic use. *Drugs* 31: 96–130.

Swabb EA 1985 Review of the clinical pharmacology of the monobactam antibiotic aztreonam. *American Journal of Medicine* 78 (2A): 11–18.

Sykes RB, Phillips I (eds) 1981 Azthreonam, a synthetic monobactam. *Journal of Antimicrobial Chemotherapy* 8 (Suppl. E): 1–146.

CARUMONAM

A synthetic monobactam.

Antimicrobial activity

Activity against common pathogenic organisms is similar to that of aztreonam: MICs generally differ no more than two-fold, except for strains of *Klebsiella* that produce an aztreonam-hydrolyzing enzyme. As with aztreonam, the principal biochemical target is PBP3 of Gram-negative bacteria.

It is resistant to hydrolysis by the common plasmid and chromosomal β-lactamases, but it can be hydrolyzed by extended-spectrum β-lactamases. It inhibits but does not induce chromosomal cephalosporinases.

Pharmacokinetics

C_{max} 1 g intravenous (20 min infusion)	78 mg/l end-infusion
Plasma half-life	1.7 h
Plasma protein binding	18–28%

A linear correlation has been found between the dose and AUC. In blister fluid a peak concentration of 61 mg/l was found 1.5 h after an intravenous infusion of 2 g over 20 min, with a half-life identical to that in serum.

Carumonam is almost entirely eliminated in the glomerular filtrate, probenecid having no effect on excretion; 96% of labelled compound is found in the urine, with 3% in the feces. Between 68% and 91% of the dose appears in the urine within 24 h. In patients with renal failure whose creatinine clearance was less than 10 ml/min the half-life rose to 11 h.

Side effects and clinical use

Similar to those of aztreonam.

 ### Preparations and dosage

Preparation: Injection.

Dosage: Adult, i.m., i.v., 1–2 g per day in two divided doses.

Available in Japan. Not available in Europe or the USA.

 ### Further information

Imada A, Kondo M, Okonogi K, Yukishige K, Kuno M 1985 In vitro and in vivo antibacterial activities of carumonam (AMA-1080), a new *N*-sulfonated monocyclic β-lactam antibiotic. *Antimicrobial Agents and Chemotherapy* 27: 821–827.

McNulty CA, Garden GM, Ashby J, Wise R 1985 Pharmacokinetics and tissue penetration of carumonam, a new synthetic monobactam. *Antimicrobial Agents and Chemotherapy* 28: 425–427.

Neu HC, Chin NX, Labthavikul P 1986 The in vitro activity and β-lactamase stability of carumonam. *Journal of Antimicrobial Chemotherapy* 18: 35–44.

Patel JH, Soni PP, Portmann R, Suter K, Banken L, Weidekamm E 1989 Multiple intravenous dose pharmacokinetic study of carumonam in healthy subjects. *Journal of Antimicrobial Chemotherapy* 23: 107–111.

β-LACTAMASE INHIBITORS

Because β-lactamase production is the predominant cause of clinically important resistance to β-lactam antibiotics in most bacteria, an attractive approach to the therapy of infections caused by such organisms is to coadminister an agent capable of inhibiting the enzyme together with the labile antibiotic. Implicit in this approach, however, are some demanding requirements:

- the inhibitor must be active against a wide range of β-lactamases, since tests for differential activity as a guide to therapy are not practicable in the diagnostic laboratory;
- the absorption, distribution and excretion characteristics of the inhibitor must match closely those of the β-lactam agent with which it is to be paired;
- its use must not add materially to the toxicity.

The ability of certain natural and semisynthetic β-lactam agents to inhibit selected β-lactamases has been known for a long time. Cephalosporin C, some semisynthetic cephalosporins and isoxazolyl penicillins all show limited inhibitory activity against a relatively narrow range of enzymes. A wide search for more potent compounds resulted in the discovery of carbapenems and clavulanic acid from natural products, and the subsequent synthesis of the sulfones, sulbactam and tazobactam. The β-lactamase inhibitors in therapeutic use have poor antimicrobial activity and act synergistically in combination with β-lactamase-labile penicillins. None is effective against metallo-β-lactamases. In some organisms these inhibitors may act as inducers of β-lactamase activity.

The penicillins, cephalosporins, carbapenems, and monobactams are primarily competitive inhibitors, or, more specifically, competitive substrates, with monobactams exhibiting inhibitory activity of group 1 cephalosporinases at nanomolar concentrations. Their action is often reversible, leaving the enzyme intact, because they simply act as poor substrates that are bound tightly to the β-lactamase and are hydrolyzed slowly. The most effective inhibitors that have been developed commercially are irreversible. The enzyme and inhibitor interact competitively initially and then progressively form a complex in which both enzyme and inhibitor are inactivated: progressive or 'suicide' inhibitors. Inactivation usually occurs after a fixed amount of inhibitor has been hydrolyzed like a normal substrate. Clavulanic acid, sulbactam, and tazobactam are all of this form, although the precise nature, rate and degree of inactivation differ considerably among the various combinations of agents and enzymes.

 ### Further information

Farmer TH, Reading C 1988 The effects of clavulanic acid and sulbactam on β-lactamase biosynthesis. *Journal of Antimicrobial Chemotherapy* 22: 105–111.

Knowles JR 1985 Penicillin resistance: the chemistry of β-lactamase inhibition. *Accounts of Chemical Research* 18: 97–104.

Muratani T, Yokota E, Nakane T, Inoue E, Mitsuhashi S 1993 In-vitro evaluation of the four β-lactamase inhibitors: BRL-42715, clavulanic acid, sulbactam, and tazobactam. *Journal of Antimicrobial Chemotherapy* 32: 421–429.

Payne DJ, Cramp R, Winstanley DJ, Knowles DJC 1994 Comparative activities of clavulanic acid, sulbactam, and tazobactam against clinically important β-lactamases. *Antimicrobial Agents and Chemotherapy* 38: 767–772.

Rolinson GN 1994 A review of the microbiology of amoxycillin/clavulanic acid over the 15 year period 1978–1993. *Journal of Chemotherapy* 6: 283–318.

Sirot D, Chanal C, Henquell C, Labia R, Sirot J, Cluzel R 1994 Clinical isolates of *Escherichia coli* producing multiple TEM mutants resistant to β-lactamase inhibitors. *Journal of Antimicrobial Chemotherapy* 33: 1117–1126.

Weber DA, Sanders CC 1990 Diverse potential of β-lactamase inhibitors to induce class I enzymes. *Antimicrobial Agents and Chemotherapy* 34: 156–158.

Wexler HM, Molitoris E, Finegold SM 1991 Effect of β-lactamase inhibitors on the activities of various β-lactam agents against anaerobic bacteria. *Antimicrobial Agents and Chemotherapy* 35: 1219–1224.

Williams JD 1999 β-Lactamases and β-lactamase inhibitors. *International Journal of Antimicrobial Agents* 12 (Suppl. 1): S3–7.

CLAVULANIC ACID

Molecular weight (potassium salt): 237.25.

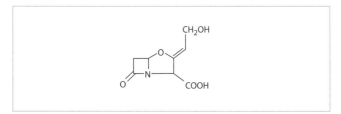

An oxapenam (clavam) produced by *Streptomyces clavuligerus*. It is available as the potassium salt for oral and intravenous use in fixed-ratio combination with amoxicillin and for intravenous use in combination with ticarcillin. It is freely soluble in water.

Antimicrobial activity

It exhibits broad-spectrum but low intrinsic activity, most MICs being in the range 16–128 mg/l. Enterobacteriaceae and *Staph. aureus* are at the lower end of the range and *Ps. aeruginosa* at the upper. MICs of 8 mg/l against *H. influenzae* and 0.1–4 mg/l for penicillinase-producing *N. gonorrhoeae* are notable.

β-Lactamase inhibitory activity

Clavulanic acid is a potent, progressive inhibitor of most group 2 β-lactamases, with the exception of some TEM variants. It is particularly active against many of the plasmid-mediated enzymes that include broad-spectrum TEM and SHV enzymes as well as their extended-spectrum variants PSE-2, and PSE-4. It is very active against the *K. pneumoniae* K1 (group 2be) enzyme, the group 2e chromosomal enzymes produced by *Pr. vulgaris* and *B. fragilis*, both enzymes produced by *M. catarrhalis* and the group 2a penicillinases from *Staph. aureus*. It does not effectively inhibit the group 1 chromosomal cephalosporinases from Enterobacteriaceae or the group 3 metallo-β-lactamases.

In the presence of low concentrations of clavulanic acid (0.5–1 mg/l) the MICs of amoxicillin and ticarcillin for many β-lactamase-producing *Staph. aureus*, *M. catarrhalis*, *N. gonorrhoeae*, *H. influenzae*, enterobacteria and *B. fragilis* strains are reduced 8- to 64-fold. Both inhibitory and bactericidal activity are enhanced. In *B. fragilis* strains resistant to penicillin, the addition of clavulanic acid renders most of the strains susceptible to amoxicillin or ticarcillin. Susceptibility of methicillin-resistant strains of *Staph. aureus* is unaffected by the presence of clavulanic acid.

Resistance that develops during therapy is generally due to overproduction of the sensitive β-lactamase, e.g., TEM-1 or SHV-1, which is no longer effectively inhibited by a limited quantity of clavulanic acid. Occasional 'inhibitor-resistant' β-lactamases have been identified, most often derived from the TEM broad-spectrum β-lactamases as a result of one or two amino acid modifications.

AMOXICILLIN–CLAVULANIC ACID

Co-amoxiclav. A mixture of potassium clavulanate and amoxicillin trihydrate (oral formulations) or amoxicillin sodium (parenteral formulations). The ratio of amoxicillin to clavulanic acid in the commercially available oral preparations is 2:1, 4:1, 7:1 or 14:1; it is 5:1 in the intravenous formulation.

Antimicrobial activity

Activity is that of amoxicillin (p. 242), the role of the inhibitor being to restore the activity against β-lactamase-producing strains that would otherwise hydrolyze the drug.

Pharmacokinetics

	Amoxicillin	Clavulanic acid
Oral absorption	*c.* 90%	*c.* 90%
C$_{max}$ 500 mg amoxicillin + 250 mg clavulanic acid oral	10 mg/l after 1 h	6 mg/l after 1 h
400 mg amoxicillin + 57 mg clavulanic acid oral	6.9 mg/l	1.1 mg/l
Plasma half-life	1.3 h	1.0 h
Plasma protein binding	18%	25%

Absorption

There is little effect on the pharmacokinetics of each agent from the presence of the other, although clavulanic acid is marginally better absorbed in the presence of amoxicillin. There is no significant effect of food on absorption. There is wide individual variation in bioavailability of (30–99%).

Distribution

Effective levels are found in bile, middle ear fluid, tonsil tissue, wound pus and amniotic fluid. Penetration into peritoneal fluid is 66% (the half-life similar to that in serum), 55% into cantharides blister fluid, and 46–91% into pleural fluid. In patients with bacterial meningitis receiving 0.2 g clavulanate plus 2 g amoxicillin by intravenous infusion over 30 min, concentrations of the drugs in the CSF were highest in patients with moderate to severe inflammation: around 0.25 mg/l for clavulanate and over 2 mg/l for amoxicillin at about 2 h. Total penetration into the CSF was 8% and 6% of the corresponding plasma values for clavulanate and amoxicillin, respectively. Clavulanate penetrates poorly into sputum after oral dosing.

Metabolism

Clavulanic acid appears to be metabolized extensively, with metabolites eliminated via the urine, bile, feces and lungs. Variation in bioavailability may be related to differences in first-pass effects through those organs.

Excretion

Approximately 50–70% of the administered amoxicillin and 25–40% of clavulanic acid are recovered intact from the urine. After a dose of 250 mg amoxicillin plus 125 mg clavulanate the mean recovery of clavulanate was 37%, falling to 30% when the mixture was taken with food, while that of amoxicillin was 70%. Most renal excretion occurs in the first 6 h and is unaffected by probenecid, although probenecid prolongs the renal excretion of amoxicillin. In renal failure, the volume of distribution and systemic availability are unaffected after oral or intravenous administration, but clearance is progressively depressed with renal function.

Toxicity and side effects

Cholestatic jaundice is much more common with co-amoxiclav than with amoxicillin alone and the combination should be used with caution in patients with evidence of hepatic dysfunction. Hepatotoxicity is more common in elderly men and is usually reversible.

Other common side effects are diarrhea (9%), nausea (3%), skin rashes and urticaria (3%), vomiting (1%) and vaginitis (1%). The overall incidence of side effects, and in particular diarrhea, increases with the higher recommended dose. Pseudomembranous colitis has been reported.

For side effects attributable to amoxicillin see p. 243.

Clinical use

- Lower respiratory tract infections.
- Otitis media.
- Sinusitis.
- Skin and skin structure infections.
- Urinary tract infections.

It is usually reserved for use against amoxicillin-resistant organisms if the susceptibility status is known.

Preparations and dosage

Proprietary name: Augmentin.

Preparations: Tablets, suspension, injection.

Dosage: Adults, oral, 250/62.5 or 250/125 or 500/125 mg every 8 h, or 500/125 or 875/125 mg every 12 h. Children, the dose varies according to age and severity of infection.

Adults, i.v., 1 g every 6–8 h, depending on severity of infection. Infants ≤ 3 months, 25 mg/kg every 8 h (every 12 h in the perinatal period and premature infants); children 3 months to 12 years, 25 mg/kg every 6–8 h depending on severity of infection.

Widely available.

TICARCILLIN–CLAVULANIC ACID

A mixture of potassium clavulanate and ticarcillin disodium in a 1:15 or 1:30 ratio for parenteral administration.

Antimicrobial activity

Activity is that of ticarcillin (p. 253), the role of the inhibitor being to restore the activity against β-lactamase-producing strains that would otherwise hydrolyze the drug.

Pharmacokinetics

	Ticarcillin	Clavulanic acid
C_{max} 3 g ticarcillin + 100 mg clavulanate intravenous infusion	320 mg/l end infusion	8 mg/l end infusion
Plasma half-life	1.1 h	1.1 h
Plasma protein binding	45%	25%

The pharmacokinetics of the two agents are mutually unaffected by coadministration. Ticarcillin can be detected in tissues and interstitial fluid following parenteral administration. Penetration into bile, peritoneal fluid and pleural fluid has been demonstrated. Concentrations in blister fluid were significantly lower than those in serum.

Around 60–70% of ticarcillin and 35–45% of clavulanic acid are excreted unchanged in urine during the first 6 hours after administration of a single dose of the mixture.

Toxicity and side effects

Adverse reactions associated with ticarcillin occur (see p. 253). As with co-amoxiclav, there is a risk of cholestatic jaundice (see above). Pseudomembranous colitis has been reported.

Clinical use

- Septicemia, including bacteremia.
- Lower respiratory infections.
- Bone and joint infections.
- Skin and skin structure infections.
- Urinary tract infections (complicated and uncomplicated).

- Gynecological infections, endometritis
- Intra-abdominal infections, peritonitis.

Its main use is in infections in which *Ps. aeruginosa* is suspected or proven.

Preparations and dosage

Proprietary name: Timentin.

Preparation: Injection.

Dosage: Adults, i.v. infusion, 3.1 g (or 3.2 g) every 4–8 h. Children under 60 kg, 150–300 mg/kg per day in 4–6 divided doses, 60 kg, 3.1 g (or 3.2 g) every 4–8 h depending on severity.

Widely available.

Further information

Allen GD, Coates PE, Davies BE 1988 On the absorption of clavulanic acid. *Biopharmaceutics and Drug Disposition* 9: 127–136.

Bakken JS, Bruun JN, Gaustad P, Tasker TC 1986 Penetration of amoxicillin and potassium clavulanate into the cerebrospinal fluid of patients with inflamed meninges. *Antimicrobial Agents and Chemotherapy* 30: 481–484.

Bolton GC, Allen GD, Davies BE, Filer CW, Jeffery DJ 1986 The disposition of clavulanic acid in man. *Xenobiotica* 16: 853–863.

Ferslew KE, Daigneault GA, Aten RM, Roseman RM 1984 Pharmacokinetics and urinary excretion of clavulanic acid after oral administration of amoxicillin and potassium clavulanate. *Journal of Clinical Pharmacology* 24: 452–456.

Jones AE, Barnes ND, Tasker TCG, Horton R 1989 Pharmacokinetics of intravenous amoxycillin and potassium clavulanate in seriously ill children. *Journal of Antimicrobial Chemotherapy* 25: 269–274.

Leigh DA, Robinson OPW (eds) 1982 Augmentin: clavulanate-potentiated amoxycillin. Excerpta Medica, Amsterdam, p 1–244.

Leigh DA, Phillips I, Wise R (eds) 1986 Timentin–ticarcillin plus clavulanic acid: a laboratory and clinical perspective. *Journal of Antimicrobial Chemotherapy* 17 (Suppl. C): 1–240.

Neu HC 1985 β-Lactamase inhibition: therapeutic advances (Symposium on ticarcillin–clavulanate). *American Journal of Medicine* 79 (Suppl. 5B): 1–196.

Sanders CC, Jaconis JP, Bodey GP, Samonis G 1988 Resistance to ticarcillin-potassium clavulanate among clinical isolates of the family Enterobacteriaceae: the role of PSE-1 β-lactamase and high levels of TEM-I and SHV-I and problems with false susceptibility in disk diffusion tests. *Antimicrobial Agents and Chemotherapy* 32: 1365–1369.

Speller DCE, White LO, Wilkinson PJ (eds) 1989 Clavulanate/β-lactam antibiotics: further experience. *Journal of Antimicrobial Chemotherapy* 24 (Suppl. B): 1–226.

SULBACTAM

Molecular weight (sodium salt): 255.22.

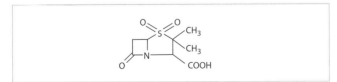

A penicillanic acid sulfone available as the sodium salt. Formulations combining ampicillin or cefoperazone with sulbactam in a 2:1 ratio are available for parenteral use. A methylene-linked double ester of penicillin and sulbactam, sultamicillin, is used for oral administration.

Antimicrobial activity

Sulbactam has very weak antimicrobial activity against most bacteria. Its only notable activity is against *N. gonorrhoeae*, *N. meningitidis* and *Acinetobacter baumanii*.

β-Lactamase-inhibitory activity

It inhibits a wide range of group-2 β-lactamases, including those from *Staph. aureus*, *K. pneumoniae* and *B. fragilis*. It is a good-to-moderate inhibitor of the TEM enzymes of groups 2b and 2be but has little effect on group 1, group 2br or group 3 β-lactamases. It does not induce the activity of cephalosporinases from Gram-negative bacteria but is a weak inducer of penicillinases from *Staph. aureus*. Inhibitory effects are dependent upon the amount of enzyme in the organism, so increased β-lactamase production results in lower efficacy for sulbactam-β-lactam combinations.

A concentration of 4–8 mg/l restores the activity of ampicillin for many β-lactamase-producing strains of *Staph. aureus*, *H. influenzae*, *M. catarrhalis*, enterobacteria and *B. fragilis*, but there is a large inoculum effect. The combination is bactericidal at concentrations that are usually no more than double the MICs. Resistance may arise due to hyperproduction of a sensitive β-lactamase or due to relatively rare 'inhibitor-resistant' TEM or SHV-derived variants.

Clinical use

Sulbactam has been used alone in the treatment of uncomplicated gonorrhea, for which it is not satisfactory. Ampicillin–sulbactam was successfully used in an outbreak of infection with *A. baumanii* in which the inhibitor was shown to be responsible for the antimicrobial activity of the combination.

Preparations

Preparation: Injection.

Not available in the UK or USA.

AMPICILLIN–SULBACTAM

Antimicrobial activity

Activity is that of ampicillin (p. 243), the role of the inhibitor being to restore the activity against β-lactamase-producing strains that would otherwise hydrolyze the drug.

Pharmacokinetics

	Ampicillin	Sulbactam
Oral absorption (sultamicillin)	>80%	>80%
C_{max} ampicillin 2 g + sulbactam 1 g intravenous 750 mg oral (sultamicillin)	109–150 mg/l end infusion 9.1 mg/l after 1 h	48–88 mg/l end infusion 8.9 mg/l after 1 h
Plasma half-life	1 h	1 h
Plasma protein binding	30%	38%

Absorption

The sodium salt of sulbactam is poorly absorbed orally, but the linked prodrug sultamicillin is well absorbed; it undergoes first-pass hydrolysis to liberate equimolecular proportions of the components.

Ampicillin–sulbactam is completely bioavailable after intramuscular injection, doses of 0.5 and 1 g producing mean peak plasma levels around 13 and 28 mg/l, respectively. Coadministration of sulbactam with ampicillin, benzylpenicillin or cefoperazone has no effect on the pharmacokinetics of either agent.

Distribution

After intravenous administration both drugs penetrate peritoneal fluid, blister fluid (cantharides-induced), tissue fluid, and intestinal mucosa and appendix to provide concentrations ≥8 mg/l. Penetration of both ampicillin and sulbactam into CSF in the presence of inflamed meninges has been demonstrated.

Metabolism

Sulbactam is not metabolized. Ampicillin metabolism is described on p. 244.

Excretion

In normal volunteers 75–85% of both ampicillin and sulbactam are excreted unchanged in the urine during the first 8 h after administration.

Toxicity and side effects

Local adverse reactions include pain at the injection site (intramuscular 16%, intravenous 3%) and thrombophlebitis (3%). Systemic adverse reactions include diarrhea (3%) and rash (<2%). Pseudomembranous colitis has been reported. For side effects attributable to ampicillin see p. 244.

Clinical use

- Skin and skin structure infections.
- Intra-abdominal infections.
- Gynecological infections.

Preparations and dosage

Preparation: Injection.

Dosage: Adult, i.m., i.v., 1.5–3 g every 6 h; Children, 150–300 mg/kg per day in 3–4 divided doses.

Available in the USA. Not available in the UK. Sulbactam–cefoperazone and sultamicillin are available in Japan.

Further information

Campoli-Richards DM, Brogden RN 1987 Sulbactam/ampicillin. A review of its antibacterial activity, pharmacokinetic properties and therapeutic use. *Drugs* 33: 577–609.

Foulds G, McBride TJ, Knirsch AK, Rodriguez WJ, Khan WN 1987 Penetration of sulbactam and ampicillin into cerebrospinal fluid of infants and young children with meningitis. *Antimicrobial Agents and Chemotherapy* 31: 1703–1705.

Frieder HA, Campoli-Richards DM, Goa KL 1989 Sultamicillin. A review of its antibacterial activity, pharmacokinetic properties and therapeutic use. *Drugs* 37: 491–522.

Symposium 1986 Enzyme-mediated resistance to β-lactam antibiotics. A symposium on sulbactam/ampicillin. *Reviews of Infectious Diseases* 8 (Suppl. 5): S465–S650.

Symposium 1988 Sulbactam-ampicillin in clinical practice. *Drugs* 35 (Suppl. 7): 1–94.

Urban C, Go E, Mariano N et al 1993 Effect of sulbactam on infections caused by imipenem-resistant *Acinetobacter calcoaceticus* biotype *anitratus*. *Journal of Infectious Diseases* 167: 448–451.

TAZOBACTAM

Molecular weight (sodium salt): 322.3.

A synthetic penicillanic acid sulfone available as the sodium salt. It is formulated with piperacillin in a piperacillin:tazobactam ratio of 8:1

Antimicrobial activity

Tazobactam exhibits little useful antimicrobial activity, although activity against *Acinetobacter* spp. and *Borrelia burgdorferi* has been reported.

β-Lactamase inhibitory activity

Tazobactam inhibits a wide range of β-lactamases, including the group 2 penicillinases from *Staph. aureus*, the broad-spectrum TEM and SHV-1 β-lactamases, most extended-spectrum enzymes in the TEM and SHV families, and the common group 2e cephalosporinases of *B. fragilis*. Against the group 1 cephalosporinases, activity is strongly influenced by the amount of enzyme produced. Diminished inhibition of the inhibitor-resistant group 2br TEM β-lactamases is seen; group 3 metallo-β-lactamases are not inhibited at clinically useful levels. It is a poor inducer of β-lactamases of Gram-positive and Gram-negative organisms.

At a concentration of 4 mg/l it markedly reduces the MIC and enhances the bactericidal activity of piperacillin against most β-lactamase-producing organisms, but only moderately against those elaborating group 1 cephalosporinases. It enhances activity against β-lactamase-producing *Staph. aureus*, *H. influenzae*, *M. catarrhalis*, most of the *B. fragilis* group, *Acinetobacter* spp., many enterobacteria, especially *Pr. mirabilis* and *Morganella morganii*, and occasional *Enterobacter* spp. and *C. freundii*.

PIPERACILLIN–TAZOBACTAM

Antimicrobial activity

Activity is that of piperacillin (p. 252), the role of the inhibitor being to restore the activity against β-lactamase producing strains that would otherwise hydrolyze the drug. Although the activity of piperacillin against *Ps. aeruginosa* is not enhanced, it remains the most active combination in vitro against *Ps. aeruginosa* (MIC of piperacillin 4 mg/l in the presence of tazobactam 4 mg/l).

Pharmacokinetics

	Piperacillin	Tazobactam
C_{max} 2 g piperacillin + 250 mg tazobactam intravenous infusion	134 mg/l end infusion	15 mg/l end infusion
Plasma half-life	1 h	1.1 h
Plasma protein binding	25%	25%

Absorption

Coadministration of tazobactam does not affect the pharmacokinetics of piperacillin, but the pharmacokinetics of tazobactam are altered: peak serum concentrations after an intravenous dose of 0.5 g increased from 24 mg/l to 27 mg/l when piperacillin was given simultaneously; the mean serum level at 4 h doubled from 0.6 to 1.2 mg/l. Pharmacokinetic properties of piperacillin and tazobactam were altered less than 14% when given with tobramycin. Coadministration of piperacillin and tazobactam with vancomycin resulted in a <7% increase in AUC for piperacillin, and no other change in pharmacokinetic properties.

Distribution

The combination has good tissue distribution, as judged by penetration into blister fluid. Mean maximum concentrations of tazobactam in the inflammatory exudate were 6.4 mg/l when 0.5 g was given alone and 11.3 mg/l when administered with piperacillin. Both agents are found in most tissues, including bronchial secretions, prostatic secretions and tissue in elderly patients, and in uterine, ovarian and fallopian tube tissue.

Metabolism

A small amount of piperacillin is metabolized to a microbiologically active desethyl metabolite, and some undergoes cleavage of the β-lactam ring. Tazobactam is metabolized to a ring-opened compound that further degrades to a butanoic acid derivative devoid of pharmacological activity.

Excretion

Renal clearance of both drugs occurs by glomerular filtration and tubular secretion. Urinary excretion of piperacillin is 68%, whereas tazobactam and its metabolite are eliminated primarily by renal excretion (80%). Biliary secretion of piperacillin, tazobactam, and desethyl piperacillin are also observed.

A decrease in renal clearance of tazobactam from 279 to 164 ml/min was seen when it was coadministered with piperacillin. A decrease in systemic clearance of the two agents is seen in cirrhotic subjects.

Toxicity and side effects

Most adverse events are mild to moderate, and transient. Most common are diarrhea (11.3%), headache (7.7%), constipation (7.7%), nausea (6.9%), insomnia (6.6%), rash (4.2%). Pseudomembranous colitis has been reported.

For side effect attributable to piperacillin, see p. 252.

Clinical use

- Uncomplicated and complicated skin and skin structure infection.
- Postpartum endometritis or pelvic inflammatory disease.
- Community-acquired pneumonia (moderate severity).
- Nosocomial pneumonia (moderate to severe).
- Appendicitis and peritonitis.

Preparations and dosage

Proprietary name: Tazocin, Zosyn.

Preparation: Injection.

Dosage: Adults and children over 12 years, by i.v. injection, usually 2.25–4.5 g every 6–8 h (up to 16 g piperacilllin – 2 g tazobactam sodium daily); may be dosed 3.375 g every 4 h plus an aminoglycoside for patients with nosocomial pneumonia. Children <50 kg with neutropenia, 90 mg/kg every 6 h.

Widely available.

Further information

Anonymous 1999 Tazobactam. In: Dollery C (ed.) *Therapeutic Drugs* 2nd edn. Churchill Livingstone, Edinburgh, pp. T16–T20.

Bush K, Macalintal C, Rasmussen BA, Lee VJ, Yang Y 1993 Kinetic interactions of tazobactam with β-lactamases from all major structural classes. *Antimicrobial Agents and Chemotherapy* 37: 851–858.

Greenwood D, Finch RG (eds) 1993 Piperacillin/tazobactam: a new β-lactam/β-lactamase inhibitor combination. *Journal of Antimicrobial Chemotherapy* 31 (Suppl. A): 1–124.

Kuck NA, Jacobus NV, Petersen PJ, Weiss WJ, Testa RT 1989 Comparative in vitro and in vivo activities of piperacillin combined with the β-lactamase inhibitors tazobactam, clavulanic acid, and sulbactam. *Antimicrobial Agents and Chemotherapy* 33: 1964–1969.

Kuye O Teal J, DeVries VG, Morrow CA, Tally FP 1993 Safety profile of piperacillin/ tazobactam in phase I and III clinical studies. *Journal of Antimicrobial Chemotherapy* 31 (Suppl. A): 113–124.

Murray PR, Cantrell HF, Lankford RB, In vitro Susceptibility Surveillance Group 1994 Multicenter evaluation of the in vitro activity of piperacillin-tazobactam compared with eleven selected β-lactam antibiotics and ciprofloxacin against more than 42,000 aerobic Gram-positive and Gram-negative bacteria. *Diagnostic Microbiology and Infectious Disease* 19: 111–120.

Shlaes DM, Baughman R, Boylen CT et al 1994 Piperacillin/tazobactam compared with ticarcillin/clavulanate in community-acquired bacterial lower respiratory tract infection. *Journal of Antimicrobial Chemotherapy* 34: 565–577.

Tan JS, Wishnow RM, Talan DA, Duncanson FP, Norden CW 1993 Treatment of hospitalized patients with complicated skin and skin structure infections: double-blind, randomized, multicenter study of piperacillin – tazobactam versus ticarcillin – clavulanate. *Antimicrobial Agents and Chemotherapy* 37: 1580–1586.

Wise R, Logan M, Cooper M, Andrews JM 1991 Pharmacokinetics and tissue penetration of tazobactam administered alone and with piperacillin. *Antimicrobial Agents and Chemotherapy* 35: 1081–1084.

OTHER NOVEL β-LACTAM COMPOUNDS

Many novel molecules containing a β-lactam ring have been investigated, but few have survived the early stages of development. Prominent among those that have are the penems and tribactams (trinems), which are synthetic, not natural compounds. Many penems have been synthesized. Despite their broad spectrum and potent antibacterial activity only one, faropenem, has entered limited clinical use. Among tribactams, most interest has centered on sanfetrinem.

 ## FAROPENEM

An orally active penem with a broad spectrum of antibacterial activity, including activity against selected anaerobic pathogens (Table 17.4). Although it is active against most enterobacteria, it has reduced activity against *Ser. marcescens*, *Enterobacter* spp. and some *Providencia* spp. It has no useful

Table 17.4 Activity of the penem faropenem and the tribactam sanfetrinem against common bacterial pathogens: MIC (mg/l)

Organism	Faropenem	Sanfetrinem
Staph. aureus	0.06	0.06
Staph. aureus (MRSA)	2.0	4.0
Str. pyogenes	0.015	0.007
Str. pneumoniae penicillin-susceptible	0.06	0.003
penicillin-resistant	0.5	No data
E. faecalis	1.0	2.0
H. influenzae	≤2.0	0.06
Neisseria spp.	≤0.03	≤0.015
Esch. coli	0.5	0.5
K. pneumoniae	0.5	1.0
Ps. aeruginosa	R	>16
B. fragilis	1.0	0.06

R, resistant (MIC>32 mg/l).

activity against *Ps. aeruginosa*. It generally retains activity against many Gram-positive organisms. MIC$_{50}$ values suggest possible utility against MRSA, although MICs shift to at least 8 mg/l in the presence of serum, and many strains for which the MIC of faropenem is >16 mg/l have been identified. It has reduced activity against *E. faecium* and some strains of coagulase-negative staphylococci. It is stable to hydrolysis by extended spectrum β-lactamases, but is hydrolyzed by metallo-β-lactamases.

 ## Further information

Fuchs P, Barry AL, Sewell DL 1995 Antibacterial activity of WY-49605 compared with those of six other oral agents and selection of disk content for disk diffusion susceptibility testing. *Antimicrobial Agents and Chemotherapy* 39: 1472–1479.

Woodcock JM, Andrews JM, Brenwald NP, Ashby JP, Wise R 1997 The in-vitro activity of faropenem, a novel oral penem. *Journal of Antimicrobial Chemotherapy* 39: 35–43

Available in Japan.

 ## SANFETRINEM

The first member of the tribactam (trinem) class of antibiotics to be selected for clinical development. It has broad-spectrum activity that includes both aerobic and anaerobic bacteria (Table 17.4). Its antibacterial spectrum of activity is similar to that of the carbapenems with the exception of its lack of activity against *Ps. aeruginosa*. It is stable to hydrolysis by renal dehydropeptidase and most β-lactamases, with the exception of the metallo-β-lactamases.

It is administered as the oral prodrug, sanfetrinem hexetil. A peak concentration of around 2.5 mg/l is achieved 1.1 h after an oral 500 mg dose. The plasma half-life is 1.7 h and plasma protein binding 20%. About 24% of the drug is recovered in the urine following a 500 mg oral dose.

 ## Further information

Di Modugno E, Erbetti I, Ferrari L, Galassi G, Hammond SM, Xerri L 1994 In vitro activity of the tribactam GV104326 against gram-positive, gram-negative, and anaerobic bacteria. *Antimicrobial Agents and Chemotherapy* 38: 2362–2368.

Singh KV, Coque TM, Murray BE 1996 In vitro activity of the trinem sanfetrinem (GV104326) against gram-positive organisms. *Antimicrobial Agents and Chemotherapy* 40: 2142–2146.

Wise R, Andrews JM, Da Ros L, Child J, Mortiboy D 1997 A study to determine the pharmacokinetics and inflammatory fluid penetration of two doses of a solid formulation of the hexetil prodrug of a trinem, sanfetrinem (GV 104236) *Antimicrobial Agents and Chemotherapy* 42: 1761–1764.

18 Chloramphenicol and thiamphenicol

M. H. Wilcox

Chloramphenicol was the first broad-spectrum antibiotic to be discovered. It was isolated independently from streptomycetes from soil in Venezuela and a compost heap in Illinois. The commercial product is manufactured synthetically. There are four isomers, all of which have been synthesized, but none has greater activity than the natural compound. The major drawback is a rare, idiosyncratic, often fatal aplastic anemia, and numerous attempts have been made to manufacture related agents which retain the spectrum of activity and pharmacokinetics of the parent compound, but not the toxicity. The only derivative to come into commercial use in which this is believed to have been achieved is thiamphenicol, in which the nitro group of chloramphenicol is replaced by a sulfomethyl group. However, compounds in which the nitro group is replaced are all less active than the parent compound.

Substitution of the 3'-OH group or fluorine for chlorine has produced analogs of chloramphenicol and thiamphenicol that are active against strains of bacteria that owe their resistance to chloramphenicol acetylation, but not against organisms with reduced permeability. Fluorinated derivatives are not marketed for human use, but florfenicol is available in veterinary practice and aquaculture in some countries.

Further information

Fuglesang J, Bergan T 1982 Chloramphenicol and thiamphenicol. *Antibiotics and Chemotherapy* 31: 1–21.
Holt D, Harvey D, Hurley R 1993 Chloramphenicol toxicity. *Adverse Drug Reactions and Toxicology Reviews* 12: 83–95.
Prescott JF, Baggot JD, Walker RD 2000 *Antimicrobial Therapy in Veterinary Medicine*, 3rd edn. Iowa State University Press, Ames, Iowa.
Vining LC, Stuttard C 1995 Chloramphenicol. *Biotechnology* 28: 505–530.

 CHLORAMPHENICOL

Molecular weight: 323.1.

$$O_2N - \underset{OH \ H}{\overset{H \ NHCOCHCl_2}{C - C}} - CH_2OH$$

A fermentation product of *Streptomyces venezualae*. Commercially manufactured synthetically. Formulated as the free compound (which is extremely bitter) or as the palmitate ester for oral administration; as the free compound for topical use; and as the sodium succinate for injection. Aqueous solutions are extremely stable, but some hydrolysis occurs on autoclaving.

Antimicrobial activity

Chloramphenicol is active against a very wide range of organisms. The susceptibility of common pathogenic bacteria is shown in Table 18.1. Minimum inhibitory concentrations (MICs) (mg/l) for other organisms are: *Staphylococcus epidermidis*, 1–8; *Corynebacterium diphtheriae*, 0.5–2; *Bacillus anthracis*, 1–4; *Clostridium perfringens*, 2–8; *Mycobacterium tuberculosis*, 8–32; *Legionella pneumophila*, 0.5–1; *Bordetella pertussis*, 0.25–4; *Brucella abortus*, 1–4; *Campylobacter fetus*, 2–4; *Pasteurella* spp., 0.25–4; *Serratia marcescens*, 2–8; *Burkholderia pseudomallei*, 4–8. Most Gram-negative bacilli are susceptible, but *Pseudomonas aeruginosa* is resistant. *Leptospira* spp., *Treponema pallidum*, chlamydiae, mycoplasmas and rickettsiae are all susceptible, but *Nocardia* spp. are resistant. It is widely active against anaerobes, including *Actinomyces israelii* (MIC 1–4 mg/l), *Peptostreptococcus* spp. (MIC 0.1–8 mg/l), and *Fusobacterium* spp. (MIC 0.5–2 mg/l), but *Bacteroides fragilis* is only moderately susceptible (MIC about 8 mg/l).

Chloramphenicol is strictly bacteristatic against almost all bacterial species, but exerts a bactericidal effect at 2–4 times

Table 18.1 Activity of chloramphenicol and thiamphenicol: MIC (mg/l)

	Chloramphenicol	Thiamphenicol
Staphylococcus aureus	2–8	4–32
Streptococcus pyogenes	2–4	1–2
Streptococcus pneumoniae	1–4	2–4
Enterococcus faecalis	4–16	8–32
Neisseria gonorrhoeae	0.5–2	0.5–2
Neisseria meningitidis	0.5–2	0.5–2
Haemophilus influenzae	0.25–0.5	0.1–2
Escherichia coli	2–8	4–64
Klebsiella pneumoniae	0.5–32	4–32
Salmonella enterica	0.5–8	0.5–8
Shigella spp.	1–8	2–8
Pseudomonas aeruginosa	32–R	16–R
Bacteroides spp.	1–8	0.5–32

R, resistant (MIC >64 mg/l).

the MIC against some strains of Gram-positive cocci, *H. influenzae* and *Neisseria* spp. The minimum bactericidal concentrations (MBCs) of chloramphenicol for penicillin-resistant pneumococci are often significantly higher than those for penicillin-susceptible strains, although this cannot be detected by conventional disk susceptibility testing or MIC determination. Its bacteristatic effect may inhibit the action of penicillins and other β-lactam antibiotics against *Klebsiella pneumoniae* and other enterobacteria in vitro, but the clinical significance of this is doubtful. The presence of ampicillin does not affect the bactericidal effect of chloramphenicol on *H. influenzae*.

Acquired resistance

Resistance is seen in many Gram-positive and Gram-negative organisms and the prevalence of resistant strains often reflects usage of the antibiotic. Over-the-counter sales are believed to have compounded the problem in some countries. For example, chloramphenicol has long been the drug of choice for the treatment of typhoid and paratyphoid fevers, but its widespread use led to a high prevalence of resistant *Salmonella enterica* serotype Typhi. Outbreaks of infection caused by chloramphenicol-resistant *S.* Typhi have been seen since the early 1970s. The prescription of alternative antibiotics, such as co-trimoxazole and fluoroquinolones, has in turn resulted in a decline in chloramphenicol resistance in some typhoid endemic areas. Many hospital outbreaks caused by multiresistant strains of enterobacteria, notably *Enterobacter*, *Klebsiella* and *Serratia* spp., have been described.

Plasmid-borne resistance was first noted in shigellae in Japan and subsequently spread widely in Central America to Mexico, where *S.* Typhi acquired the same resistance and was responsible for a huge outbreak. Strains of *S.* Typhi resistant to many antibiotics including chloramphenicol are now par-

ticularly common in the Indian subcontinent. Resistance in shigella is also relatively common in some parts of the world. Resistant strains of *H. influenzae* (some also resistant to ampicillin), *Staph. aureus* and *Str. pyogenes* are also encountered. Most *Neisseria meningitidis* strains remain susceptible, but high-level resistance (MIC ≥64 mg/l) due to the production of chloramphenicol acetyltransferase (p. 28) has been described. In this case the nucleotide sequence of the resistance gene was indistinguishable from that found on a transposon in *Cl. perfringens*. Resistance in *H. influenzae* is particularly common in Spain. Resistant strains of *Enterococcus faecalis* are relatively common, and resistance to chloramphenicol is found in the multiresistance of some South African strains of pneumococci.

Resistance in *Staph. aureus* is caused by an inducible acetyltransferase. In *Esch. coli*, the capacity to acetylate chloramphenicol (at least three enzymes are involved) is carried by R factors. Replacement of the 3-OH group, which is the target of acetylation, accounts for the activity of fluorinated analogs against strains resistant to chloramphenicol and thiamphenicol. The resistance of *B. fragilis* and some strains of *H. influenzae* is also due to elaboration of a plasmid-encoded acetylating enzyme; in others it is due to reduced permeability resulting from loss of an outer membrane protein. Some resistant bacteria reduce the nitro group or hydrolyze the amide linkage. Resistance of *Ps. aeruginosa* is partly enzymic and partly due to impermeability.

Pharmacokinetics

Oral absorption	80–90%
C_{max} 500 mg oral	10–13 mg/l after 1–2 h
Plasma half-life	1.5–3.5 h
Volume of distribution	0.25–2 l/kg
Plasma protein binding	*c.* 25–60%

Absorption

The plasma concentration achieved is proportional to the dose administered. Suspensions for oral administration to children contain chloramphenicol palmitate, a tasteless and bacteriologically inert compound, which is hydrolyzed in the gut to liberate chloramphenicol. Following a dose of 25 mg/kg peak plasma levels around 6–12 mg/l are obtained, but there is much individual variation.

Pancreatic lipase is deficient in neonates and, because of poor hydrolysis, the palmitate should be avoided. In very young infants, deficient ability to form glucuronides and low glomerular and tubular excretion ability greatly prolong the plasma half-life.

For parenteral use, chloramphenicol sodium succinate, which is freely soluble and undergoes hydrolysis in the tissues with the liberation of chloramphenicol, can be injected intravenously or in small volumes intramuscularly. The plasma concentrations after administration by these routes are unpredictable, and approximate to only 30–70% of those obtained after the same dose by the oral route. Protein binding is reduced in cirrhotic patients and neonates, with correspondingly elevated concentrations of free drug.

Distribution

Free diffusion occurs into serous effusions. Penetration occurs into all parts of the eye, the therapeutic levels in the aqueous humor being obtained even after local application of 0.5% ophthalmic solution. Concentrations obtained in cerebrospinal fluid (CSF) in the absence of meningitis are 30–50% of those of the blood and greater in brain. It crosses the placenta into the fetal circulation and appears in breast milk.

Metabolism

Chloramphenicol is largely inactivated in the liver by conjugation with glucuronic acid or by reduction to inactive arylamines; clearance of the drug in patients with impaired liver function is depressed in relation to the plasma bilirubin level. It has been suggested that genetically determined variance of hepatic glucuronyl transferase might determine the disposition and toxicity of the drug.

Excretion

It is excreted in the glomerular filtrate and in the newborn its elimination may be impaired by the concomitant administration of benzylpenicillin, which is handled early in life by the same route. Its inactive derivatives are eliminated partly in the glomerular filtrate and partly by active tubular secretion. Over 24 h, 75–90% of the dose appears in the urine, 5–10% in the biologically active forms and the rest as metabolites, chiefly as a glucuronide conjugate. Excretion diminishes linearly with renal function and at a creatinine clearance of less than 20 ml/min, maximum urinary concentrations are 10–20 mg/l rather than the 150–200 mg/l found in normal subjects. Because of metabolism, blood levels of active chloramphenicol are only marginally elevated in renal failure, but microbiologically inactive metabolites accumulate. The plasma half-life of the products in the anuric patient is around 100 h, and little is removed by peritoneal or hemodialysis. Dosage modification is normally unnecessary in renal failure as the metabolites are less toxic than the active parent compound. About 3% of the administered dose is excreted in the bile, but only 1% appears in the feces, and this mostly in inactive forms.

Interactions

Induction of liver microsomal enzymes, for example by phenobarbitone or rifampicin, diminishes blood levels of chloramphenicol; conversely, chloramphenicol, which inhibits hepatic microsomal oxidases, potentiates the activity of dicoumerol, phenytoin, tolbutamide and those barbiturates which are eliminated by metabolism. It also depresses the action of cyclophosphamide, which depends for its cytotoxicity on transformation into active metabolites. It is uncertain whether this interaction may lead to a clinically significant level of inhibition of the activity of cyclophosphamide. The half-life of chloramphenicol is considerably prolonged if paracetamol (acetaminophen) is given concurrently, and coadministration of these drugs should therefore be avoided.

Toxicity and side effects

Glossitis, associated with overgrowth of *Candida albicans*, is fairly common if the course of treatment exceeds 1 week. Stomatitis, nausea, vomiting and diarrhea may occur, but are uncommon. Hypersensitivity reactions are very uncommon. Jarisch–Herxheimer-like reactions have been described in patients treated for brucellosis, enteric fever and syphilis.

Bone marrow effects

Chloramphenicol exerts a dose-related but reversible depressant effect on the marrow of all those treated, resulting in vacuolization of erythroid and myeloid cells, reticulocytopenia and ferrokinetic changes indicative of decreased erythropoiesis. Evidence of bone-marrow depression is regularly seen if the plasma concentration exceeds 25 mg/l, and leukopenia and thrombocytopenia may be severe. There is no evidence that this common marrow depression is the precursor of potentially fatal aplasia, which differs in that it is fortunately rare, late in onset, usually irreversible and may follow the smallest dose. Aplasia can follow systemic, oral and even ophthalmic administration and may be potentiated by cimetidine. Liver disease, uremia and pre-existing bone-marrow dysfunction may increase the risk. It is unusual for manifestations to appear during treatment, and the interval between cessation of treatment and onset of dyscrasia can be months. A few patients survive with protracted aplasia, and myeloblastic leukemia then often supervenes.

It is thought that the toxic agent is not chloramphenicol itself but an as yet unidentified metabolite. Chloramphenicol is partially metabolized to produce oxidized, reduced and conjugated products. The toxic metabolite may be a short-lived product of reduction of the nitro group, which damages DNA by helix destabilization and strand breakage. Predisposition to aplasia may be explained by genetically determined differences in metabolism of the agent. Risk of fatal aplastic anemia has been estimated to increase 13-fold on average treatment with 4 g of chloramphenicol. Corresponding increases are 10-fold in patients treated with mepacrine (quinacrine) and 4-fold in patients treated with oxyphenbutazone.

Children

Infants given large doses of chloramphenicol may develop exceedingly high plasma levels of the drug because of their immature conjugation and excretion mechanisms. A life-threatening disorder called the 'gray baby' syndrome, characterized by vomiting, refusal to suck and abdominal distension followed by circulatory collapse, may appear when the plasma concentration exceeds 20 mg/l. If concentrations reach 200 mg/l, the disorder can develop in older children or even adults.

Optic neuritis has been described in children with cystic

fibrosis receiving prolonged treatment for pulmonary infection. Most improve when the drug is discontinued, but central visual acuity can be permanently impaired. There is some experimental evidence that ear drops containing 5% chloramphenicol sodium succinate can damage hearing. One study identified an increased risk of acute leukemia following childhood administration of chloramphenicol, particularly for durations exceeding 10 days.

Clinical use

- Typhoid fever and other severe infections due to salmonellae.
- Rickettsial infections.
- Meningitis.
- Invasive infection caused by *H. influenzae*.
- Destructive lung lesions involving anaerobes.
- Eye infections (topical).

Reference is made to its use in cholera (p. 673), plague, tularemia and bartonellosis (pp. 866–868), melioidosis, Whipple's disease (p. 677) and relapsing fever. Treatment for other serious infections should be restricted to those organisms (now very uncommon) that are resistant or much less susceptible to other antibiotics. It has been used, with varying success, to treat infections caused by glycopeptide-resistant enterococci. Meningitis caused by penicillin-resistant pneumococci responds poorly, apparently due to failure to achieve bactericidal concentrations in CSF. It should never be given systemically for minor infections. Topical use in the treatment of eye infections is extremely controversial given the unsubstantiated risk of bone marrow aplasia.

The daily dose should not normally exceed 2 g, and the duration of the course should be limited (e.g. 10 days). Although patients may show toxic manifestations after receiving very little of the drug, the danger is almost certainly increased by excessive or repeated dosage or by the treatment of patients with impaired hepatic or renal function, including those at the extremes of life. The wide pharmacokinetic variability of the antibiotic in neonates makes monitoring of serum concentrations advisable. Determination of full blood counts should be carried out twice weekly.

Preparations and dosage

Proprietary names: Chloromycetin, Kemicetine.

Preparations: Capsules, suspension, injection.

Dosage: Adults, oral, i.v., 50 mg/kg per day in four divided doses; the dose may be doubled for severe infections and reduced as soon as clinically indicated. Children, 50–100 mg/kg per day in divided doses; infants <2 weeks, 25 mg/kg per day in four divided doses; infants 2 weeks to 1 year, 50 mg/kg per day in four divided doses.

Widely available.

Further information

Anonymous 1999 Chloramphenicol. In Dollery C (ed.) *Therapeutic Drugs*, 2nd edn. Churchill Livingstone, Edinburgh, pp. C168–C172.

Doona M, Walsh JB 1995 Use of chloramphenicol as topical eye medication: time to cry halt? *BMJ* 310: 1217–1218.

Friedland IR, Klugman KP 1992 Failure of chloramphenicol therapy in penicillin-resistant pneumococcal meningitis. *Lancet* 339: 405–408.

Friedland IR, Shelton S, McCracken GH 1992 Chloramphenicol in penicillin-resistant pneumococcal meningitis. *Lancet* 342: 240–241.

Galimand M, Gerbaud G, Guibourdenche M, Riou JY, Courvalin P 1998 High-level chloramphenicol resistance in *Neisseria meningitidis*. New England Journal of Medicine 339: 868–874.

Holt DE, Hurley R, Harvey D 1995 A reappraisal of chloramphenicol metabolism: detection and quantification of metabolites in the sera of children. *Journal of Antimicrobial Chemotherapy* 35: 115–127.

Lautenbach E, Schuster MG, Bilker WB, Brennan PJ 1998 The role of chloramphenicol in the treatment of bloodstream infection due to vancomycin-resistant *Enterococcus*. *Clinical Infectious Diseases* 27: 1259–1265.

Mirza SH, Beeching NJ, Hart CA 1996 Multi-drug resistant typhoid: a global problem. *Journal of Medical Microbiology* 44: 317–319.

Ramilo O, Kinane BT, McCracken GH 1988 Chloramphenicol neurotoxicity. *Pediatric Infectious Diseases Journal* 7: 358–359.

West BC, De Vault GA, Clement JC, Williams DM 1988 Aplastic anemia associated with parenteral chloramphenicol: review of 10 cases, including the second case of possible increased risk with cimetidine. *Reviews of Infectious Diseases* 10: 1048–1051.

Wiholm BE, Kelly JP, Kaufman D et al 1998 Relation of aplastic anaemia to use of chloramphenicol eye drops in two international case-control studies. *BMJ* 316: 666.

THIAMPHENICOL

Molecular weight: 356.2.

$$CH_3SO_2 - \text{(benzene ring)} - \underset{\underset{OH}{|}}{\overset{\overset{H}{|}}{C}} - \underset{\underset{H}{|}}{\overset{\overset{NHCOCHCl_2}{|}}{C}} - CH_2OH$$

A chloramphenicol analog in which a sulfomethyl group is substituted for the *p*-nitro group. Also available as the glycinate hydrochloride (1.26 g approximately equivalent to 1 g thiamphenicol). Aqueous solutions are very stable.

Antimicrobial activity

It is generally less active than chloramphenicol (Table 18.1), but is equally active against *Str. pyogenes*, *Str. pneumoniae*, *H. influenzae* and *N. meningitidis*, including some strains resistant to chloramphenicol. It is more actively bactericidal against *Haemophilus* and *Neisseria* spp.

Acquired resistance

There is complete cross-resistance with chloramphenicol in those bacteria which elaborate acetyltransferase, although the affinity of the enzyme for thiamphenicol is lower. Organisms that owe their resistance to other mechanisms may be susceptible.

Pharmacokinetics

An oral dose of 500 mg produces a peak plasma level of 3–6 mg/l after about 2 h. The plasma half-life is 2.6–3.5 h. It is said to reach the bronchial lumen in concentrations sufficient to exert a bactericidal effect on *H. influenzae*. Disposal of the drug is different from that of chloramphenicol: it is not a substrate for hepatic glucuronyl transferase, it is not eliminated by conjugation, and its half-life is not affected by phenobarbitone induction.

About 50% of the dose can be recovered in an active form in the urine within 8 h and 70% over 24 h. The drug is correspondingly retained in the presence of renal failure, and in anuric patients the plasma half-life has been reported to be 9 h, a value not significantly affected by peritoneal dialysis. Biliary excretion is believed to account for removal of the antibiotic in anuric patients. The plasma concentration is elevated and half-life prolonged in patients with hepatitis or cirrhosis.

Toxicity and side effects

There are no reports of irreversible bone-marrow toxicity. This has been related to the absence of the nitro group, and hence its reduction products, and differences in the details of the biochemical effects of thiamphenicol and chloramphenicol on mammalian cells. Thiamphenicol induces dose-dependent reversible depression of hemopoiesis and immunogenesis to a greater extent than does chloramphenicol, and has been used for its immunosuppressive effect. Therapeutic doses (1–1.5 g) are likely to depress erythropoiesis in the elderly or others with impaired renal function.

Clinical use

Similar to that of chloramphenicol.

 Preparations and dosage

Preparations: Oral, injection.

Dosage: Adults, i.m., oral, 1.5–3 g per day in divided doses depending on severity of infection. Children, 30–100 mg/kg per day in divided doses.

Limited availability in continental Europe and Japan. Not available in the UK or USA.

 Further information

Franceschinis R (ed.) 1984 International symposium on thiamphenicol and sexually transmitted diseases. *Sexually Transmitted Diseases* 11 (Suppl. 4): 333–469.

Goris H, Loeffler M, Bungart B, Schmitz S, Nijhof W 1989 Hemopoiesis during thiamphenicol treatment. *Experimental Hematology* 17: 957–961, 962–967.

Ravizzola G 1984 In vitro antibacterial activity of thiamphenicol. *Chemioterapia* 3: 163–166.

19 Diaminopyrimidines

R. L. Then

This group of agents comprises mainly 5-substituted 2,4-diamino-pyrimidines, such as trimethoprim, tetroxoprim, cycloguanil and pyrimethamine, which have antibacterial or antiprotozoal activity. The diaminopyrimidine moiety can also be part of a pteridine or quinazoline ring system, as in the antineoplastic agents methotrexate and trimetrexate.

They are potent inhibitors of the enzyme dihydrofolate reductase (*see* Ch. 2) and are generally termed antifolates.

Trimethoprim and pyrimethamine emerged from an antimetabolite program initiated in the early 1940s by G.H. Hitchings and colleagues. Exploitation of species differences in activity later led to compounds such as diaveridine and ormetoprim used as coccidiostats in veterinary medicine. Several trimethoprim analogs were subsequently synthesized, including tetroxoprim, brodimoprim and epiroprim as well as the veterinary agents, aditoprim and baquiloprim.

Clinical development of trimethoprim concentrated on a synergistic combination with sulfamethoxazole. The biochemical basis is the sequential blockade of two steps in the biosynthesis of reduced folates. This double blockade results in greatly enhanced antibacterial activity, extends the antibacterial spectrum, slows down resistance development (at least under laboratory conditions) and increases the bactericidal potency.

Soon after the introduction of co-trimoxazole in 1969 the combination produced impressive clinical results and became very successful. However, the practice of applying a potent agent such as trimethoprim exclusively in combination with a sulfonamide was disputed on several grounds.

- Although the pharmacokinetic properties of trimethoprim and sulfamethoxazole match fairly well in the plasma, conditions far from those optimal for synergy prevail in different body compartments.

- Synergy is relevant only at sites in which concentrations fall below levels effective alone, whereas the combination is administered at doses that produce plasma levels of both components above the MIC.

- Resistance to sulfonamides was already widespread at the time of launch of the combination, and hence trimethoprim alone is the active component against such strains.

- The sulfonamide component, which is in five-fold excess over trimethoprim, is responsible for many of the undesirable side effects.

- The high concentrations of trimethoprim reached in urine are sufficient to treat uncomplicated cystitis and other infections of the urinary tract.

These considerations led to the clinical use of trimethoprim alone, first in Finland in 1972, and then in many other countries. The use of trimethoprim alone is, however, mainly restricted to urinary tract infections and on a global scale only a small fraction of all trimethoprim is used as a single agent, the bulk being used as a fixed combination with sulfonamides, usually sulfamethoxazole.

The Medicines Control Agency in the UK has imposed restrictions on the use of co-trimoxazole, confining it to the treatment and prophylaxis of *Pneumocystis carinii* pneumonia and certain other infections, in which there are good grounds for preferring the combination over trimethoprim alone.

In view of increasing resistance to trimethoprim and its sulfonamide combinations there is a strong tendency to replace these agents by fluoroquinolones, macrolides or ketolides, but there remain a number of important indications in which these drugs remain of great importance.

Further information

Anonymous 1995 Co-trimoxazole use restricted. *Drug and Therapeutics Bulletin* 33: 92–93.

Baccanari DP, Kuyper LF 1993 Basis of selectivity of antibacterial diaminopyrimidines. *Journal of Chemotherapy* 5: 393–399.

Periti P (ed.) 1993 Seminar on bacterial dihydrofolate reductase inhibitors in antimicrobial chemotherapy. *Journal of Chemotherapy* 5: 357–566.

Talan DA, Stamm WE, Hooton TM et al 2000 Comparison of ciprofloxacin (7 days) and trimethoprim-sulphamethoxazole (14 days) for uncomplicated pyelonephritis in women: a randomized trial. *Journal of the American Medical Association* 283: 1583–1590.

Tauchnitz C 1997 Stellung der Trimethoprim-Sulfonamid-Kombination heute. *Chemotherapie Journal* 6: 17–20.

Then RL 1993 History and future of antimicrobial diaminopyrimidines. *Journal of Chemotherapy* 5: 361–368.

Winkler FK, D'Arcy A, Müller K et al 1990 Comparison between human and bacterial dihydrofolate reductase structures. In: Curtius HC, Ghisla S, Blau N (eds). *Chemistry and Biology of Pteridines* Walter de Gruyter Berlin, New York, pp. 702–707.

PYRIMETHAMINE

2,4-Diamino-5-(p-chlorophenyl)-6-ethylpyrimidine. Molecular weight: 248.717.

A synthetic diaminopyrimidine. Extremely insoluble. Available as a single agent (Daraprim) or in fixed combination with sulfadoxine (Fansidar), dapsone (Maloprim) or triple combination with mefloquine and sulfadoxine (Fansimef).

Antimicrobial activity

Most notable activity is against *Plasmodium* spp., *Toxoplasma gondii* and *Pneumocystis carinii*. Its activity against plasmodial dihydrofolate reductase is about 1000 times that against the human enzyme. It has no useful antibacterial activity. Slow growing bradyzoite forms of *Tox. gondii* in tissue cysts are less sensitive than the intracellular tachyzoites. It is strongly recommended that it is used together with a sulfonamide for the treatment of malaria and toxoplasmosis, since the mixture lowers the ED_{50} and clinically curative dose approximately ten-fold.

Acquired resistance

Resistant plasmodia are rapidly selected during treatment or prophylaxis with pyrimethamine alone, but much less so with the combinations. A common reason for resistance is a point mutation (Ser-108-Asn) in the plasmodial dihydrofolate reductase. Several point mutations are associated with increasing levels of resistance to pyrimethamine, but to a much lesser extent to the related antifolate drug cycloguanil. Resistance to pyrimethamine is widespread in Africa and Latin America.

Sequence variations are also the reason for resistance of *P. falciparum* to sulfadoxine. The multidrug resistance transporter *pfmdr1* may also be involved in resistance to pyrimethamine and sulfadoxine.

Pharmacokinetics

Oral absorption	Well absorbed
C_{max} (25 mg oral)	0.13–0.4 mg/l after 2–6 h
Plasma half-life	111 (54–148) h
Volume of distribution	0.68 l/kg
Plasma protein binding	87%

Absorption

Pyrimethamine is well absorbed by mouth. The long plasma half-life is unaffected in the presence of dapsone or sulfadoxine. Considerable variation of pyrimethamine disposition has been found in AIDS patients.

Distribution

Levels in cerebrospinal fluid (CSF) are around 10–25% of the simultaneous plasma level. A substantial part of the dose appears in maternal milk, the ratio of milk:serum area under the curve (AUC) being 0.46–0.66, so that an infant might ingest almost half the maternal dose over 9 days. There is placental transfer of pyrimethamine, resulting in 50–100% of the maternal plasma concentrations in the neonate.

Metabolism and excretion

Plasma clearance is 15.9 ml/h/kg and elimination is mainly by hepatic metabolism. More than 16 metabolites are found in urine.

Toxicity and side effects

When administered with a sulfonamide or dapsone, all major side effects of these agents (including Stevens–Johnson syndrome) may occur, particularly hypersensitivity reactions. The principal toxic effect of pyrimethamine is on the bone marrow, producing megaloblastic anemia, leukocytopenia, thrombocytopenia or pancytopenia. This is particularly seen on prolonged administration and with the high doses used for *Toxoplasma* therapy. Very large doses in children have produced vomiting, convulsions, respiratory failure and death. Aggravation of subclinical folate deficiency may be alleviated by folinic acid. Pyrimethamine is teratogenic in animals and produces significant abnormalities. It should be used in pregnant women only after thoroughly weighing the risk–benefit for mother and child.

Clinical use

- Malaria (usually in combination with sulfadoxine, sulfalene [sulfametopyrazine] or dapsone).
- Toxoplasmosis (usually in combination with sulfadiazine).
- *Pneumocystis* pneumonia (usually in combination with dapsone).

Preparations and dosage

Proprietary names: Daraprim, Fansidar (with sulfadoxine), Maloprim (with dapsone), Fansimef (with mefloquine and sulfadoxine).

Preparation: Tablets.

Dosage: Depends on indication. For acute malaria treatment 2–3 tablets (25 mg, plus sulfonamide) is the usual dose. Children 9–14 years, two tablets; 4–8 years, one tablet; under 4 years half a tablet. For prophylaxis (no longer recommended), adult dose one tablet per week, children 5–10 years half a tablet per week. For toxoplasmosis the starting dose is 50–75 mg of pyrimethamine daily, with 1–4 g of a sulfonamide.

Widely available as combination, limited availability of pyrimethamine alone.

Further information

Almond DS, Szwandt ISF, Edwards G et al 2000 Disposition of intravenous pyrimethamine in healthy volunteers. *Antimicrobial Agents and Chemotherapy* 44: 1691–1693.

Basco LK, Tahar R, Keundjian A, Ringwald P 2000 Sequence variation in the genes encoding dihydropteroate synthase and dihydrofolate reductase and clinical response to sulfadoxine-pyrimethamine in patients with acute uncomplicated falciparum malaria. *Journal of Infectious Diseases* 182: 624–628.

Duombo OK, Kayentao K, Djimde A et al 2000 Rapid selection of *Plasmodium falciparum* dihydrofolate reductase mutants by pyrimethamine prophylaxis. *Journal of Infectious Diseases* 182: 993–996.

Duraisingh MT, Roper C, Walliker D, Warhurst DC 2000 Increased sensitivity to the antimalarials mefloquine and artemisinin is conferred by mutations in the *pfmdr1* gene in *Plasmodium falciparum. Molecular Microbiology* 36: 955–961.

Edstein MD, Rieckmann KH, Veenendaal JR 1990 Multiple-dose pharmacokinetics and in vitro antimalarial activity of dapsone plus pyrimethamine (Maloprim) in man. *British Journal of Clinical Pharmacology* 30: 259–265.

Girard PM, Landman R, Gaudebout C et al 1993 Dapsone–pyrimethamine compared with aerosolized pentamidine as primary prophylaxis against *Pneumocystis carinii* pneumonia and toxoplasmosis in HIV infection. *New England Journal of Medicine* 328: 1514–1520.

Peytavin, G, Leng JJ, Forestier F et al 2000 Placental transfer of pyrimethamine studied in an ex vivo placental perfusion model. *Biology of the Neonate* 78: 83–85.

Winstanley P, Khoo S, Szwandt S et al 1995 Marked variation in pyrimethamine disposition in AIDS patients treated for cerebral toxoplasmosis. *Journal of Antimicrobial Chemotherapy* 36: 435–439.

TETROXOPRIM

2,4-Diamino-5-3,5-dimethoxy-4-(2-methoxyethoxy)-benzylpyrimidine. Molecular weight: 334.38.

A close analog of trimethoprim, in which the 3′-methoxy-group is replaced by $O.CH_2.CH_2.O.CH_3$. It has a lower affinity than trimethoprim for *Esch. coli* dihydrofolate reductase and this correlates with a generally weaker in-vitro activity against various bacteria. Tetroxoprim is exclusively used in combination with sulfadiazine (co-tetroxazine). MIC values for co-tetroxazine are generally higher than for co-trimoxazole. Published information on this compound is sparse and no advantages over co-trimoxazole have been demonstrated clinically.

Preparations and dosage

Proprietary name: Sterinor.

Preparations: Tablets (250 mg sulphadiazine plus 100 mg tetroxoprim), oral suspension for adults, children.

Dosage: Adults: one tablet every 12 h.

Not widely available.

Further information

Wise R, Reeves DS eds 1979 Advances in therapy with antibacterial folate inhibitors. Proceedings of a symposium held at the Royal College of Physicians, London, 22 to 23 March 1979. *Journal of Antimicrobial Chemotherapy* 5: Suppl. B.

TRIMETHOPRIM

2,4-Diamino-5-(3,4,5-trimethoxybenzyl)-pyrimidine. Molecular weight: 290.323.

The most frequently used synthetic diaminopyrimidine. It is poorly soluble in water and has a very bitter taste. It is available in oral formulations or, as trimethoprim lactate, as an injectable preparation.

Antimicrobial activity

Trimethoprim is a broad-spectrum agent (Table 19.1). It is active against Gram-positive bacilli and cocci, including *Staphylococcus aureus*, irrespective of β-lactamase production or methicillin-resistance. In vitro, folinic acid antagonizes the activity of trimethoprim and sulfamethoxazole against *Enterococcus faecalis*, which is unusual in being able to utilize preformed folinic acid, thymine and thymidine. The clinical efficacy of trimethoprim in enterococcal infections is thus controversial and there are no conclusive clinical studies.

Table 19.1 Representative minimum inhibitory concentrations of trimethoprim and co-trimoxazole for common pathogenic bacteria* (mg/l)

Organism	Trimethoprim	Co-trimoxazole†
Staphylococcus aureus	0.2–2	0.03–0.06
Streptococcus pneumoniae	0.5–2	0.06–2
Streptococcus pyogenes	0.5–1	0.03–2
Enterococcus faecalis	0.15–0.5	0.015–0.4
Haemophilus influenzae	0.02–1	0.02–16
Neisseria gonorrhoeae	8–R	0.15–4
Neisseria meningitidis	4–32	0.01–2
Escherichia coli	0.05–R	0.25–64
Klebsiella pneumoniae	0.5–8	0.5–4
Pseudomonas aeruginosa	R	R
Bacteroides fragilis	8–16	>4

*Data from various studies; a broad range indicates that resistant strains were included.

†Tested as a 1 + 19 fixed combination of trimethoprim with sulfamethoxazole. R: resistant (MIC >64 mg/l).

Haemophilus spp., including β-lactamase-producing strains and *Haemophilus ducreyi* (MIC 0.03–0.6 mg/l) are susceptible. Most enterobacteria are susceptible, as are *Bordetella*, *Legionella*, *Pasteurella* and *Vibrio* spp. Pseudomonads, with the exception of *Burkholderia cepacia* (MIC 1–2 mg/l) are resistant. Nocardiae, *Neisseria* spp. and *Brucella* spp. are relatively resistant, owing to their species-specific dihydrofolate reductase sensitivities, although they are susceptible to trimethoprim-sulfonamide combinations.

Most anaerobes are resistant, as are *Chlamydia*, *Coxiella*, *Leptospira*, *Mycoplasma*, *Rickettsia* and *Treponema* spp. *Mycobacterium tuberculosis* is resistant, but *M. marinum* (MIC 16 mg/l) and *M. smegmatis* (MIC 4 mg/l) are susceptible, as are *Listeria* spp.

Among non-bacterial organisms *Naegleria* spp, *Plasmodium* spp, *Pn. carinii*, and *Tox. gondii* exhibit some sensitivity to trimethoprim, which can often be potentiated by a sulfonamide. Its differential activity is such that it can also be used in selective media for the isolation of *N. gonorrhoeae* and group A streptococci. Depending on the concentration, test medium and the particular organism trimethoprim can be bacteristatic or bactericidal.

Acquired resistance

The prevalence of trimethoprim resistance varies among different geographic regions and between hospitals and hospital units. Resistance can be due to a variety of mechanisms. Chromosomal mutations in the structural gene for dihydrofolate reductase or in its promoter can result in modification or overproduction of the target enzyme. As well as these mutations, alterations in the metabolic pathway, or changes that affect the permeability of the cell or efflux pumps generally, confer moderate degrees of resistance. More than one mechanism can occur in the same cell, leading to higher resistance levels.

Plasmid-encoded resistance, often encoded by genes found on class I integrons, is widespread, especially in enteric Gram-negative bacilli including *Esch. coli*, *Salmonella enterica* serotypes. and *Acinetobacter* spp. It usually results in the synthesis of an additional, trimethoprim-resistant dihydrofolate reductase and confers high levels of resistance. Currently there are more than 16 distinct enzymes known in Gram-negative bacteria and their number is growing steadily. In no case is the origin of the new enzyme known. Only a few of these enzymes have so far been described in Gram-positive bacteria, mainly in staphylococci but also in enterococci and *Listeria*.

Campylobacter jejuni, which was previously thought to be intrinsically resistant to trimethoprim, owes its high level resistance to acquired *dfr1* and *dfr9* genes. In contrast, trimethoprim resistance in *H. influenzae* seems to be frequently caused by mutations in the *dfr* promoter region or the trimethoprim-binding domains of the structural gene.

The prevalence of the various *dfr* genes varies with geographic region. Most frequently found are the enzyme types Ib, VIII, V and Ia. The most prevalent type in staphylococci around the world is the S1 enzyme, which is coded for by transposon Tn *4003* and probably originated in *Staph. epidermidis*. Other genes for trimethoprim resistance have been detected in *Staph. haemolyticus* and *E. faecalis*.

In *Ps. aeruginosa* intrinsic resistance to trimethoprim and sulfamethoxazole may be mediated by the multidrug efflux system mexABoprM.

Since thymidine can supply the metabolic requirement imposed by trimethoprim blockade, thymine-requiring bacteria are resistant to trimethoprim. Such organisms have rarely been implicated in infection, either because tissues generally fail to provide the necessary thymidine or because they escape detection owing to their slow growth on conventional media, which are low in thymine and thymidine. Infection with trimethoprim-resistant, thymine-requiring mutants has occasionally been observed in patients treated for prolonged periods with co-trimoxazole. Under certain pathological conditions these mutants seem to rescue enough thymidine from body fluid.

Pharmacokinetics

Oral absorption	95–100%
C_{max} (100 mg orally)	c. 1 mg/l after 1.5–3.5 h
Plasma half-life	8–11 h
Volume of distribution	69–133 l
Plasma protein binding	42–46%

Absorption

Absolute bioavailability of trimethoprim has not well been studied, but it is rapidly absorbed from the gut after oral administration.

Distribution

Plasma levels increase in a dose-proportional fashion. It is widely distributed in tissues and body fluids, including CSF, in which concentrations around half the simultaneous plasma level are achieved. Trimethoprim passes the placental barrier and is excreted in breast milk.

Metabolism

About 10–20% of trimethoprim is metabolized, primarily in the liver. The remainder is excreted unchanged in the urine. Main metabolites are the 1- and 3-oxides, and the 3′- and 4′-hydroxy derivatives.

Excretion

Elimination of trimethoprim is mainly through glomerular filtration and tubular secretion. High concentrations are found in urine, reaching 30–160 mg/l within 4 h of a single 100 mg oral dose, and declining to 18–91 mg/l during the following 8–24 h. About 70% is excreted in the first 24 h, but detectable levels are present in the urine for 4–5 days, during which time about 90% of the dose can be recovered. The renal clearance of trimethoprim in normal subjects is 19–148 ml/min, the wide variation largely being accounted for by the influence of pH. Trimethoprim is a weak base, and urinary excretion rises sharply with falling pH as the drug ionizes and non-ionic back diffusion in the tubules decreases. In patients with severely impaired renal function the half-life increases and a dose adjustment is needed.

Toxicity and side effects

- Rash, pruritus (2.9–6.7%).
- Nausea, vomiting, glossitis.

Hypersensitivity reactions (exfoliative dermatitis, erythema multiforme, Stevens–Johnson syndrome, Lyell's syndrome, anaphylaxis, aseptic meningitis) are rare, as are hematological side effects.

A foreseeable mechanism-related side effect, the induction of folate deficiency and interference with hematopoiesis, is rarely observed even after high doses or prolonged administration. Trimethoprim should, however, be given with caution to pregnant women and to patients with possible folate deficiency. Reduced folates can be administered without interfering with the antibacterial action of trimethoprim.

Mutagenicity tests have been uniformly negative. Teratogenic effects have been observed in rats and rabbits only at doses far exceeding those used in humans.

Trimethoprim may inhibit the hepatic metabolism of phenytoin. Common clinical doses increased the phenytoin half-life by 51% and lowered the metabolic clearance rate by 30%.

Clinical use

- Urinary tract infections.
- Enteric fever.

Topical preparations have been used in the treatment of burns and, combined with polymyxin, as eye drops to treat infective conjunctivitis.

Preparation and dosage

Proprietary names: Ipral, Monotrim, Solotrim, Trimpex.

Preparations: Tablets, suspension, injection.

Dosage: Oral: Adults acute infections 100 mg twice a day, 200 mg once or twice a day.

Children 6–12 years, 100 mg twice a day, 6 months to 5 years, 50 mg twice a day, 6 weeks to 5 months, 25 mg twice a day (approx. 8 mg/kg daily). Long-term and prophylaxis: Adults, 100 mg at night. Children 6–12 years, 50 mg at night, 6 months to 5 years, 25 mg at night.

Intravenous injection: Adults: 150–250 mg every 12 h. Children under 12 years, 6–9 mg/kg daily in two or three divided doses.

Widely available.

Further information

Brogden RN, Carmine AA, Heel RC et al 1982 Trimethoprim: a review of its antibacterial activity, pharmacokinetics and therapeutic use in urinary tract infections. *Drugs* 23: 405–430.

Coque TM, Singh KV, Weinstock GM, Murray BE 1999 Characterization of dihydrofolate reductase genes from trimethoprim-susceptible and trimethoprim-resistant strains of *Enterococcus faecalis*. *Antimicrobial Agents and Chemotherapy* 43: 141–147.

DeGroot R, Sluijter M, deBruyn A et al 1996 Genetic characterization of trimethoprim resistance in *Haemophilus influenzae*. *Antimicrobial Agents and Chemotherapy* 40: 2131–2136.

Gibreel A, Sköld O 1998 High-level resistance to trimethoprim in clinical isolates of *Campylobacter jejuni* by acquisition of foreign genes (*dfr1* and *dfr9*) expressing drug-insensitive dihydrofolate reductases. *Antimicrobial Agents and Chemotherapy* 42: 3059–3064.

Hamilton-Miller JMT 1988 Reversal of activity of trimethoprim against Gram-positive cocci by thymidine, thymine and 'folates'. *Journal of Antimicrobial Chemotherapy* 22: 35–39.

Huovinen P, Sundström L, Swedberg G, Sköld O 1995 Trimethoprim and sulfonamide resistance. *Antimicrobial Agents and Chemotherapy* 39: 279–289.

Köhler T, Kok M, Michea-Hamzehpour M et al 1996 Multidrug efflux in intrinsic resistance to trimethoprim and sulfamethoxazole in *Pseudomonas aeruginosa*. *Antimicrobial Agents and Chemotherapy* 40: 2288–2290.

Kresken M, Hafner D and study group 2000 Resistenzsituation bei klinisch wichtigen Infektionserregern gegenüber Chemotherapeutika in Mitteleuropa. *Chemotherapie Journal* 9: 51–86.

Then RL 1982 Mechanisms of resistance to trimethoprim, the sulphonamides, and trimethoprim-sulphamethoxazole. *Reviews of Infectious Diseases* 4: 261–269.

Then RL 1980 Role of thymidine for the activity of trimethoprim, sulfonamides and their combinations. *Zentralblatt für Bakteriologie und Hygiene I. Abteilung Original* A247: 483–494.

Thomson CJ 1993 Trimethoprim and brodimoprim resistance of Gram-positive and Gram-negative bacteria. *Journal of Chemotherapy* 5: 458–464.

TRIMETREXATE

5-methyl-6-[[(3,4,5-trimethoxyphenyl)amino]methyl]2,4-quinazolinediamine. Molecular weight 369.42; trimetrexate glucuronate: 563.56.

A synthetic 2,4-diaminoquinazoline, structurally related to the anticancer drug methotrexate. Formulated as the glucuronate. It is a non-specific inhibitor of dihydrofolate reductase. It is more lipophilic than methotrexate and uses different routes for cellular uptake.

Antimicrobial activity

Although trimetrexate exhibits non-specific activity against dihydrofolate reductases it is a much more potent inhibitor of the *Pn. carinii* (and mammalian) dihydrofolate reductase than trimethoprim: the 50% inhibitory concentration is 26 nmol/l, compared with 43 μmol/l for trimethoprim. The high affinity for the mammalian enzyme would produce severe neutropenia and has to be circumvented by the concurrent administration of leucovorin (folinic acid), which *Pn. carinii* lacks the ability to take up.

Pharmacokinetics

The pharmacokinetic properties of trimetrexate are not yet completely established.

Absorption
After intravenous infusion of 30 mg/m² to adult patients with AIDS, concentrations of trimetrexate were around 2 μmol/l at 4 h. Although the drug is usually administered by intravenous infusion, oral bioavailability is about 44% and concentrations comparable to those achieved by an intravenous infusion of 30 mg/m² were achieved 2 h after an oral dose of 60 mg/m².

Distribution
Elimination half-lives varied from 8.3 to 10 h for the early or late phase of a treatment course and terminal elimination half-lives were as long as 15–16 h. Protein binding is >95%.

Metabolism and excretion

The metabolism of trimetrexate involves oxidative demethylation, followed by glucuronidation. Some of the metabolites seem to be biologically active. Excretion is largely by the renal route. 10–20% of the dose is found in urine after 24–48 h and a substantial proportion of the dose is excreted as metabolites.

Toxicity and side effects

As might be expected from its anticancer activity, it is extremely toxic unless administered with leucovorin (*see above*). Important hematological side effects include neutropenia, thrombocytopenia, bone marrow suppression and anemia. Other adverse reactions are ulceration of the oral and gastric mucosa, and impairment of hepatic and renal function. Administration of leucovorin should be continued for 72 h after the last dose of trimetrexate in order to minimize these complications.

Clinical use

Trimetrexate glucuronate is indicated in moderate to severe *Pn. carinii* pneumonia in patients who are intolerant of or refractory to co-trimoxazole, or those in whom co-trimoxazole is contraindicated. It must always be administered together with folinic acid.

 Preparation and dosage

Proprietary name: Neutrexin.

Preparations: Lyophilizate for i.v. infusion, 25 mg.

Dosage: 45 mg/m² once daily by intravenous infusion over 60–90 min. Leucovorin, 20 mg/m² intravenously over 5–10 min, or orally every 6 h. Leucovorin must be continued for 72 h after the last dose of trimetrexate. Recommended course of therapy 21 days (24 days of leucovorin).

Available in the USA, UK and elsewhere.

Further information

Fulton B, Wagstaff A, McTavish D 1995 Trimetrexate: a review of its pharmacodynamic and pharmacokinetic properties and therapeutic potential in the treatment of *Pneumocystis carinii* pneumonia. *Drugs* 49: 563–576.

Koda RT, Dubé MP, Li WY et al 1999 Pharmacokinetics of trimetrexate and dapsone in AIDS patients with *Pneumocystis carinii* pneumonia. *Journal of Clinical Pharmacology* 39: 268–274.

Ramanathan RK, Lipsitz S, Asbury RF et al 1999 Phase II trial of trimetrexate for patients with advanced gastric carcinoma: an Eastern Cooperative Oncology Group Study (E1287). *Cancer* 86: 572–576.

Rogers P, Allegra CJ, Murphy RF et al 1988 The bioavailability of oral trimetrexate in patients with acquired immunodeficiency syndrome. *Antimicrobial Agents and Chemotherapy* 32: 324–326.

Then RL, Hartman PG, Kompis I, Santi, D 1993 Selective inhibition of dihydrofolate reductase from problem human pathogens. In: Ayling JE, Nair MG, Baugh CM (eds) *Chemistry and Biology of Pteridines and Folates.* Plenum Press, New York, pp. 533–536.

OTHER DIAMINOPYRIMIDINES AND RELATED STRUCTURES

Methotrexate is a powerful, but unselective inhibitor of dihydrofolate reductases. It is used parenterally for the treatment of certain cancers and of rheumatoid arthritis. It has no useful antibacterial activity, since the charged molecule is not taken up by most pathogenic bacteria.

Brodimoprim is a trimethoprim analog in which bromine replaces methoxy at position 4 of the phenyl substituent. It is used as a single agent for the oral treatment of bacterial infections of the respiratory tract, but has been withdrawn from most markets. Its antibacterial and toxicological properties are similar to those of trimethoprim, but its pharmacokinetic behavior is distinctly different. It has a long elimination half-life of 32–35 h, allowing once-daily dosing.

Epiroprim is more lipophilic than trimethoprim. It showed encouraging activities either alone or in combination with sulfonamides or dapsone against bacteria, *Pn. carinii* and *Toxoplasma*, but was not further developed.

Piritrexim is a lipophilic dihydrofolate reductase inhibitor, which is being studied as a cytostatic agent in certain cancers.

Cycloguanil, a 2,4-diamino-triazine inhibitor of plasmodial dihydrofolate reductase, is the major human metabolite of proguanil (*see* p. 461).

Further information

Locher HH, Schlunegger H, Hartman PG et al 1996 Antibacterial activities of epiroprim, a new dihydrofolate reductase inhibitor, alone and in combination with dapsone. *Antimicrobial Agents and Chemotherapy* 40: 1376–1381.

Periti P (ed.) 1993 Seminar on bacterial dihydrofolate reductase inhibitors in antimicrobial chemotherapy. Proceedings. *Journal of Chemotherapy* 5: 357–566.

Takimoto CH 1996 New antifolates: Pharmacology and clinical applications. *Oncologist* 1: 68–81.

Then RL, Hartman PG, Kompis I et al 1994 Epiroprim. *Drugs of the Future* 19: 446–449.

DIAMINOPYRIMIDINE-SULFONAMIDE COMBINATIONS

Several fixed ratio combinations have so far come into use:

- Co-trimoxazole: a 1:5 mixture of trimethoprim and sulfamethoxazole.
- Co-trimazine: a 1:5 mixture of trimethoprim and sulfadiazine.
- Co-trifamole: a 1:5 mixture of trimethoprim and sulfamoxole.
- Co-soltrim: a 1:5 mixture of trimethoprim with sulfametrole
- Co-tetroxazine: a 1:2.5 mixture of tetroxoprim and sulfadiazine.
- A 1:1.5 ratio mixture of trimethoprim and sufamerazine.
- A 4:5 ratio mixture of trimethoprim and sulfamethoxypyridazine.

In addition to these mainly antibacterial preparations, the antiprotozoal agent pyrimethamine is used in combination with dapsone or sulfonamides (*see* Ch. 64). Proguanil, the metabolic precursor of cycloguanil, is used in combination with atovaquone (p. 462).

These combinations exhibit the activity of, and synergistic interaction between, the two components. They may also mutually cross-suppress the emergence of resistance. Maximum potentiation occurs when the drugs are present in the ratio of their MICs. For example, an organism susceptible to 1 mg trimethoprim/l and 20 mg sulfonamide/l will show maximum inhibition when exposed to a 1:20 mixture. This is the optimum ratio for many organisms, but for others proportionally more trimethoprim is required. Important examples are neisseriae and *Pn. carinii*, which are more susceptible to sulfonamide than trimethoprim; for optimum synergy the mixture must contain more trimethoprim than sulfonamide. Synergy is most impressive against those organisms that arc only moderately susceptible to one of the components alone. In the case in neisseriae, nocardiae and *Pn. carinii* in-vitro synergy also clearly translates into clinical synergy. In addition to lowering the concentration required to inhibit growth, the mixture is often bactericidal, whereas the individual components are bacteristatic. In some cases synergy may be so marked that organisms that are conventionally regarded as resistant to one or the other agent are rendered susceptible to the combination.

The pharmacokinetic behavior of the different mixtures is that of the components, there being no significant interactions between them. The efficacies of the different mixtures have not been compared in detail, so that no clear differences have emerged in their therapeutic utility. By far the most widely used combination is co-trimoxazole, which is sold worldwide in approximately 100 different generic brands. The use of the other combinations is much more geographically limited.

Rifampicin and polymyxin also act synergistically with both sulfonamides and trimethoprim against Gram-negative bacilli. Formulations of trimethoprim with polymyxin B are widely available for topical use in eye drops and ointment. The triple mixture of sulfamethoxazole, trimethoprim and colistin may be more active than any pair of these agents against some organisms, including multiresistant *Serratia*.

 ## CO-TRIMAZINE

A fixed-ratio (1:5) combination of trimethoprim and sulfadiazine.

Its antimicrobial activity is that of its components and synergistic interaction between them. Following a dose of 1 g, mean peak serum concentrations of sulfadiazine are around 25 mg/l, with a plasma elimination half life of 9.3 h. Untoward effects resemble those of co-trimoxazole, and its clinical uses are similar.

 ### Preparation and dosage

Proprietary names: Sulfatrim; Triglobe.

Preparations: Tablets (820 mg sulfadiazine plus 180 mg trimethoprim) and suspension.

Dosage: Adults, oral, 1 g/day as a single dose or in two divided doses. Infants >3 months and children, 7 mg of sulfadiazine plus 1.5 mg of trimethoprim per kg every 12 hours.

Limited availability, not available in the UK or USA.

Further information

Bergan T, Allgulander S, Fellner H 1986 Pharmacokinetics of co-trimazine (sulfa-diazine plus trimethoprim) in geriatric patients. *Chemotherapy* 32: 478–485.

Bergan T, Ortengan B, Westerlund D 1986 Clinical pharmacokinetics of co-tri-mazine. *Clinical Pharmacokinetics* 11: 372–386.

Ekström B, Marget W (eds) 1979 Studies on trimethoprim/sulphonamide develop-ments. Proceedings of a symposium. 19–23 September, 1978, Corfu, Greece. *Infection* (Suppl. 4) S307–S420.

Jodal U, Fellner H 1988 Plasma and urine concentrations of trimethoprim–sulpha-diazine (Co-trimazine) in children given one dose per day. *Scandinavian Journal of Infectious Diseases* 20: 91–95.

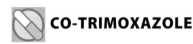

CO-TRIMOXAZOLE

A fixed-ratio (1:5) combination of trimethoprim and sulfa-methoxazole.

Antimicrobial activity

The antimicrobial spectrum covers pathogens susceptible to the individual agents and is expanded by synergistic inter-action. Some organisms that are refractory to many other antibiotics remain susceptible to co-trimoxazole. These include *Acinetobacter* spp, *B. cepacia*, *Stenotrophomonas maltophilia* and some fast-growing mycobacteria such as *M. marinum* and *M. kansasii*.

Acquired resistance

Resistance has increased over the years, but there are large regional differences and differences between hospitals and wards. A study of methicillin-resistant *Staph. aureus* isolates in 20 European hospitals found 71% to be susceptible to co-tri-moxazole; similar rates have been reported elsewhere. Large regional variations have been found for co-trimoxazole resis-tance in pneumococci, ranging from 8.6% in the Czech Republic in 1997 to 79.6% in Hong Kong. Resistance is lowest in penicillin-susceptible pneumococci and highest in penicillin-resistant pneumococci. It has been suggested that the use of sulfadoxine-pyrimethamine in malaria may select for co-tri-moxazole-resistant pneumococci.

Among Gram-negative organisms, a large study of blood-stream isolates from the USA, Canada and Latin America in 1998 reported susceptibility to co-trimoxazole in 47.5–77.9% of *Esch. coli* isolates; 81–87.7% of *Klebsiella* spp.; and 69.8–83.1% of *Enterobacter* spp.

Emergence of resistance in the course of treatment is not usually a problem.

Pharmacokinetics

	Trimethoprim	Sulfamethoxazole
Oral absorption	>95%	85%
C_{max} 160 mg trimethoprim + 800 mg sulfamethoxazole) orally	1–2 mg/l after 2 h	40–60 mg/l after 4 h
Plasma half-life	c. 11 h	c. 10 h
Volume of distribution	100–120 l	12–18 l
Plasma protein binding	c. 44%	c. 70%

Absorption

Trimethoprim is usually absorbed more rapidly than sulfa-methoxazole when given as a single oral dose of the combina-tion. After twice-daily administration of one tablet the steady state is reached in adults after 2–3 days; the steady state peak serum concentrations are approximately 50% greater than the peak levels after a single dose. Elderly patients behave as normal adults.

Distribution

Because of unequal distribution there is a wide range of con-centration ratios of the two drugs in body tissues and fluids. The concentration of trimethoprim is equal to or greater than the simultaneous plasma level in saliva, intracellular fluid, breast milk, prostatic tissue, sputum, lung tissue, vaginal secretions, bile and urine. Concentrations of sulfamethoxazole in all these tissues and fluids, except urine, are lower than in plasma. Concentrations of trimethoprim in prostatic fluid are twice as high as in the plasma in elderly men. Trimethoprim and sulfa-methoxazole both cross the human placenta and penetrate into the cerebrospinal fluid, where concentrations around half of the simultaneous plasma levels are usually reached.

Metabolism and excretion

Metabolism and excretion of the components of co-trimoxa-zole are described on pp. 288 and 389. The excretion of trimethoprim increases in acid urine, while that of the sulfon-amide is unchanged; in alkaline urine the excretion of trimetho-prim is depressed and that of sulfamethoxazole enhanced. As a result, the ratio of the urinary concentrations of active sul-fonamide to trimethoprim is around 1 in acid urine and around 5 in alkaline urine. When the creatinine clearance falls below 30 ml/min the elimination half-lives of both drugs can increase up to 45–60 h and the quantity of the drug cleared by the kidney decreases.

Toxicity and side effects

Side effects are those described for the two components (*see* pp. 288 and 389); most adverse reactions are usually attrib-uted to the sulfonamide. Serious toxicity is uncommon, but the increased risks of co-trimoxazole compared with trimetho-prim alone, particularly in the elderly, have been sufficient to limit the licensed indications for the combination. Co-trimoxazole is less well tolerated in HIV-positive patients than in other patient groups. The production of a toxic hydroxylamine metabolite of sulfamethoxazole by the cytochrome P_{450} pathway is suspected to be the underlying reason for this.

Administration of co-trimoxazole (or trimethoprim alone) results in marked depression of fecal enterobacteria with little or no effect on fecal anaerobes. Corresponding clearance of enterobacteria from the perineal area is believed to be an important feature of the value of the drug in the control of recurrent urinary tract infection (Ch. 57). While intrinsically resistant species, including *Ps. aeruginosa*, have naturally persisted, major overgrowth has not been a troublesome feature.

In the rat, doses greater than 200 mg/kg daily are teratogenic, but complete protection is afforded by folinic acid or dietary folate supplements. No abnormalities were produced in the rabbit or infants born to treated mothers, but use of the drug in pregnancy is not recommended.

Hyperkalemia is a well described complication of therapy with high-dose trimethoprim (20 mg/kg body weight daily) in patients with AIDS and may also develop in about 20% of patients under standard therapy with co-trimoxazole, especially in patients with renal insufficiency.

Clinical use

- Treatment and prophylaxis of *Pn. carinii* pneumonia.
- Nocardiasis.
- Urinary tract infections.
- Acute exacerbations of chronic bronchitis.
- Acute otitis media.
- Shigellosis.
- Other infections caused by pathogens susceptible to co-trimoxazole.

Co-trimoxazole has been used for infections as diverse as acne, listeriosis, nocardiasis, gonorrhea, brucellosis, endocarditis, severe enterobacterial infections (including enteric fever and cholera), plague, meningitis (since both components penetrate well into the CSF), chancroid, melioidosis, Whipple's disease, Wegener's granulomatosis, and granuloma inguinale. In some of these indications co-trimoxazole has been replaced by the fluoroquinolones.

The only first-line indication in the UK is the treatment and prophylaxis of *Pn. carinii* pneumonitis. It can also be used in toxoplasmosis, nocardiasis and in certain other conditions in which there is microbiological evidence of sensitivity to the combination and good reason to prefer the combination to trimethoprim alone. Leucovorin is sometimes used to reduce the incidence of neutropenia; this may, however, interfere with the efficacy of co-trimoxazole against *Pn. carinii*.

Co-trimoxazole has some activity against protozoa. It has been used in malaria and toxoplasmosis, especially in AIDS patients, but is much inferior to pyrimethamine combinations. It is recommended for treatment of *Isospora belli* and *Cyclospora cayetanensis* infections in humans.

Preparation and dosage

Proprietary names: Bactrim, Septrin, Cotrim and others.

Preparations: Tablets (400 mg sulfamethoxazole plus 80 mg trimethoprim or double-strength tablet: 800 mg sulfamethoxazole plus 160 mg trimethoprim), injections, pediatric suspension.

Dosage: Adults: oral 960 mg every 12 h, increased to 1.44 g every 12 h in severe infections.

Children >12 years, as for adults; 6 weeks to 5 months, 120 mg every 12 h; 6 months to 5 years, 240 mg every 12 h; 6–12 years, 480 mg every 12 h.

High dose therapy for *P. carinii* infections: 120 mg/kg per day, divided into 2–4 doses for 14 days.

P. carinii prophylaxis: 1 double-strength tablet per day. Adults, intramuscular or intravenous infusion, 960 mg every 12 h increased to 1.44 g every 12 h for severe infections. Children, intravenous infusion 36 mg/kg per day in two divided doses, increased to 54 mg/kg per day in severe infections.

Widely available.

Further information

Alappan R, Perazella MA, Buller GK 1996 Hyperkalemia in hospitalized patients treated with trimethoprim-sulphamethoxazole. *Annals of Internal Medicine* 124: 316–320.

Diekema DJ, Pfaller MA, Jones RN et al 1999 Survey of blood stream infections due to Gram-negative bacilli: frequency of occurrence and antimicrobial susceptibility of isolates collected in the United States, Canada, and Latin America for the SENTRY antimicrobial surveillance program, 1997. *Clinical Infectious Diseases* 29: 595–607.

Diekema DJ, Pfaller MA, Jones RN et al 2000 Trends in antimicrobial susceptibility of bacterial pathogens isolated from patients with blood stream infections in the USA, Canada and Latin America. *International Journal of Antimicrobial Agents* 13: 257–271.

Feikin DR, Dowell SF, Nwanyanwu OC et al 2000 Increased carriage of trimethoprim/sulphamethoxazole resistant *Streptococcus pneumoniae* in Malawian children after treatment for malaria with sulfadoxine/pyrimethamine. *Journal of Infectious Diseases* 181: 1501–1505.

Felmingham D, Grüneberg RN 2000 The Alexander Project 1996–1997: latest susceptibility data from this international study of bacterial pathogens from community-acquired lower respiratory tract infections. *Journal of Antimicrobial Chemotherapy* 45: 191–203.

Jick H, Derby LE 1995 Is co-trimoxazole safe? *Lancet* 345: 1118–1119.

Jones RN, Croco MAT, Kugler KC et al 2000 Respiratory tract pathogens isolated from patients hospitalized with suspected pneumonia: frequency of occurrence and antimicrobial susceptibility patterns from the SENTRY antimicrobial surveillance program (United States and Canada, 1997). *Diagnostic Microbiology and Infectious Diseases* 37: 115–125.

Lee BL 1996 Adverse reactions to trimethoprim-sulfamethoxazole. *Clinical Reviews in Allergy and Immunology* 14: 451–455.

Razavi B, Lund B, Allen BL, Schlesinger L 2002 Failure of trimethoprim/sulfamathoxazole prophylaxis for *Pneumocystis carinii* pneumonia with concurrent leucovorin use. *Infection* 30: 41–42.

Schmitz FJ, Krey A, Geisel R et al 1999 Susceptibility of 302 methicillin-resistant *Staphylococcus aureus* isolates from 20 European university hospitals to vancomycin and alternative antistaphylococcal compounds. *European Journal of Clinical Microbiology and Infectious Diseases* 18: 528–530.

Torre D, Speranza F, Martegani R et al 1998 A retrospective study of treatment of cerebral toxoplasmosis in AIDS patients with trimethoprim-sulphamethoxazole. *Journal of Infection* 37: 15–18.

Wacker P, Ozsahin H, Groll AH et al 2000 Trimethoprim-sulfamethoxazole salvage for refractory listeriosis during maintenance chemotherapy for acute lymphoblastic leukemia. *Journal of Pediatric Hematology/Oncology* 22: 340–343.

Williams L, Bender BS 1994 Trimethoprim–sulphamethoxazole. In: Yoshikawa TT, Norman DC (eds). *Antimicrobial therapy in the elderly patient*. M. Dekker, New York, pp. 169–181.

Preparation and dosage of other trimethoprim–sulfonamide combinations

 Preparation and dosage

Proprietary names: Lidaprim; Lidatrim (trimethoprim plus sulfametrole 1:5)

Preparations: Tablet (800 mg sulfametrole + 160 mg trimethoprim).

Dosage: As with co-trimoxazole.

Not widely available.

Proprietary name: Berlocombin (trimethoprim + sulfamerazine 1 + 1.5).

Preparations: Tablet (80 mg trimethoprim + 120 mg sulfamerazine)

Dosage: Adults, Initial 2–3 tablets, followed by 1.5–2 tablets every 12 h.

Not widely available.

20 Fosfomycin and fosmidomycin

D. Greenwood

Fosfomycin (originally called phosphonomycin) was discovered in Spain in 1969 and jointly developed in Spain and the USA. Fosmidomycin was synthesized in Japan a decade later. They are phosphonic acid derivatives, with unique structures that set them apart from other antimicrobial agents and, probably, from each other.

Uptake of these compounds in many Gram-negative bacteria, notably *Escherichia coli*, is induced by glucose 6-phosphate and this substance greatly potentiates the activity in vitro. Glucose 6-phosphate is present in places where glycolysis takes place, but the tissue content generally is low and located intracellularly. It is not present in the serum or cerebrospinal fluid (CSF) and is probably suboptimal at sites of infection, since the efficacy of the agents in experimental infection is increased by coadministration of glucose 6-phosphate. None the less, the correlation between their in-vivo and in-vitro activity is better when tested in the presence of the inducer.

Synergy with aminoglycosides and with other cell wall active agents, notably β-lactam antibiotics, has been demonstrated against some organisms.

Resistant mutants, typically exhibiting loss of the hexose phosphate transport system induced by glucose 6-phosphate, arise in vitro with relatively high frequency (10^{-4}–10^{-5}). Resistance that emerges in vivo is generally associated with deletion of the α-glycerophosphate transport mechanism. Plasmid-encoded resistance to fosfomycin also occurs in some species and such strains may remain susceptible to fosmidomycin.

 Further information

Neuman M 1984 Recent developments in the field of phosphonic acid antibiotics. *Journal of Antimicrobial Chemotherapy* 14: 309–311.

Kanimoto Y, Greenwood D 1987 Comparison of the response of *Escherichia coli* to fosfomycin and fosmidomycin. *European Journal of Clinical Microbiology* 6: 386–391.

 FOSFOMYCIN

cis-1,2-Epoxypropylphosphonic acid. Molecular weight: 138.

$$\text{H}_3\text{C}\underset{O}{\overset{\overset{\displaystyle H\quad H}{\underset{\displaystyle C-C}{}}}{}}\text{PO}_3\text{H}_2$$

A fermentation product of *Streptomyces fradiae*, *Streptomyces viridochromogenes* and *Streptomyces wedmorensis*. Commercially produced synthetically. It is stable for several years in powder form and for 48 h in aqueous solution. Fosfomycin tromethamine (*syn*: trometamol; tris(hydroxymethyl) aminomethane) and the much less soluble calcium salt are used in oral preparations; the very soluble sodium and disodium salts are used for parenteral administration.

Antimicrobial activity

Fosfomycin is moderately active against a wide range of pathogens, but its activity in vitro is reduced at an alkaline pH and in the presence of glucose, phosphates or sodium chloride. Consequently, different results may be obtained depending on the medium used: inhibitory concentrations observed in simple nutrient broth or agar are usually lower than those in Mueller–Hinton medium. Addition of glucose-6-phosphate (25 mg/l) to the medium enhances the activity of the drug against most enterobacteria. Its activity against common pathogens (in the presence of glucose-6-phosphate) is shown in Table 20.1. It is, in general, more active against Gram-negative bacilli than Gram-positive cocci, although most strains of *Staphylococcus aureus* (including methicillin-resistant strains) are susceptible and *Pseudomonas aeruginosa* is usually resistant. Synergy with a variety of β-lactam antibiotics, aminoglycosides and other agents has been exhibited against some enterococci, methicillin-resistant *Staph. aureus* and enterobacteria. The tromethamine salt exhibits half the activity of other derivatives

Table 20.1 Activity of fosfomycin and fosmidomycin, in the presence of glucose 6-phosphate against common pathogenic bacteria: MIC (mg/l)

	Fosfomycin	Fosmidomycin
Staphylococcus aureus	2–32	R
Streptococcus pyogenes	8–64	R
Streptococcus pneumoniae	8–64	R
Enterococcus faecalis	64	R
Haemophilus influenzae	4	0.5–R
Neisseria spp.	32–64	R
Escherichia coli	1–4	1
Klebsiella pneumoniae	2–64	0.5
Enterobacter spp.	2–R	0.1
Pseudomonas aeruginosa	4–R	2–R
Bacteroides fragilis	R	R

R, resistant (MIC >64 mg/l).

in tests in vitro since the tromethamine component has a molecular weight similar to that of fosfomycin itself.

Acquired resistance

Bacterial populations contain variants that are resistant to the drug, but these are not highly prevalent even in those countries in which it has been widely used. There is no cross-resistance with other antibiotics, and it is active against many strains resistant to other agents. A type of enzyme-mediated resistance in which the epoxide ring is opened in the presence of glutathione is transferred by plasmids and may be associated with multidrug resistance.

Pharmacokinetics

Oral absorption	
calcium salt	c. 30–40%
tromethamine salt	c. 60%
C_{max} calcium salt 1 g oral	7 mg/l after 4 h
tromethamine salt 50 mg/kg oral	32 mg/l after 2 h
sodium salt 1 g intramuscular	28 mg/l after 1 h
sodium salt 20 mg/kg intravenous	130 mg/l end infusion
Plasma half-life	2–5 h
Volume of distribution	20–22 l
Plasma protein binding	<3%

Absorption

Absorption of the tromethamine salt is dose dependent, the fraction recovered from the urine falling from about a half after 2 g to a fifth after 5 g. The effect of food is variable, but generally depresses absorption. The sodium salt causes gastric irritation and is used only for parenteral administration. There is some accumulation after repeated doses given 6-hourly. Constant intravenous infusion of 500 mg/h produced a steady-state blood level of about 60 mg/l.

Distribution

Fosfomycin diffuses freely into interstitial fluid and tissues. Diffusion into CSF is modest, but improves with meningeal inflammation. In patients with acute meningitis, CSF levels were 10.9 mg/l when the serum level was 65.2 mg/l. In patients with pleural effusions given 30 mg/kg as an intravenous bolus, average peak concentrations in pleural fluid around 43 mg/l were found at 3.7 h; clearance was slower than from plasma. Relatively high concentrations have been found in fetal blood (17.6 mg/l) and amniotic fluid (45 mg/l). Concentrations in breast milk are about 10% of the mother's plasma levels.

Metabolism and excretion

Fosfomycin is not metabolized in humans. The drug is excreted into urine by glomerular filtration. About 80% of an intravenous dose is recoverable in urine in the first 24 h, achieving a peak concentration in excess of 1000 mg/l. Less than 20% of an oral dose of the calcium salt finds its way into urine, but a single 50 mg/kg dose of the tromethamine salt provides a urinary concentration that remains above 1000 mg/l for 12 h. Renal impairment increases the half-life proportional to the fall in creatinine clearance, reaching around 50 h as the creatinine clearance level falls below 10 ml/min. Most of the drug is removed by hemodialysis. Fosfomycin is excreted into bile, but is returned to the circulation by enterohepatic recycling.

Toxicity and side effects

Adverse reactions have been observed in about 10–17% of patients, mostly slight gastrointestinal disorders. There may be a transient rise in transaminase levels.

Clinical use

Sodium salt
- Respiratory, gastrointestinal, generalized and genitourinary infections.

Tromethamine salt
- Single-dose treatment of cystitis.
- Prophylaxis in transurethral surgery.

 Preparations and dosage

Fosfomycin tromethamine
Proprietary names: Monuril, Monurol.

Preparation: Granules in 3 g sachets, injection.

Dosage: Urinary tract infection: Adults, oral, 3 g as a single dose. Children >5 years, 2 g as a single dose. Surgical prophylaxis: 3 g preoperatively; 3 g after 24 h. Injection, 2–4 g per day in divided doses (maximum 20 g per day).

Widely available.

Fosfomycin sodium
Limited availability; not USA or UK.

Further information

Greenwood D, Jones A, Eley A 1986 Factors influencing the activity of the trometa-mol salt of fosfomycin. *European Journal of Clinical Microbiology* 5: 29–34.

Kuhnen E, Pfeifer G, Frenkel C 1987 Penetration of fosfomycin into cerebrospinal fluid across non-inflamed and inflamed meninges. *Infection* 15: 422–424.

Patel SS, Balfour JA, Bryson HM 1997 Fosfomycin tromethamine. A review of its antibacterial activity, pharmacokinetic properties and therapeutic efficacy as a single-dose oral treatment for uncomplicated lower urinary tract infections. *Drugs* 53: 637–656.

Reeves DS 1994 Fosfomycin trometamol. *Journal of Antimicrobial Chemotherapy* 34: 853–858.

Suárez JE, Mendoza MC 1991 Plasmid-encoded fosfomycin resistance. *Antimicrobial Agents and Chemotherapy* 35: 791–795.

 FOSMIDOMYCIN

Sodium hydrogen-3 (*N*-hydroxyformamido) propyl phosphate. Molecular weight (sodium salt): 191.

Antimicrobial activity

Fosmidomycin is active against a broad range of enterobacteria, but not against Gram-positive organisms or anaerobes (Table 20.1). Activity is affected by medium composition and enhanced by glucose 6-phosphate. It is slowly bactericidal at concentrations close to the minimum inhibitory concentration and shows synergy with aminoglycosides and β-lactam antibiotics. Bacteria resistant to fosfomycin are usually, but not always, cross-resistant to fosmidomycin.

Interest in fosmidomycin has been revived by demonstration of antimalarial activity: malaria parasites, as well as some Gram-negative bacilli share a vulnerable isoprenoid biosynthetic pathway (*see* p. 12).

Pharmacokinetics

Oral absorption	c. 25%
C_{max} 500 mg oral	2.3 mg/l after 2.4 h
7.5 mg/kg intramuscular	11 mg/l after 1 h
30 mg/kg intravenous	160 mg/l end infusion
Plasma half-life	1.6–1.8 h
Plasma protein binding	<5%

It is not metabolized and there is no evidence of accumulation after multiple dosing. Elimination is almost entirely renal: mean urinary recoveries in the first 24 h after oral, intramuscular and intravenous administration are around 25%, 65%, and 85%, respectively.

Toxicity, side effects and clinical use

Fosmidomycin appears to be well tolerated. Uses are similar to those of fosfomycin against Gram-negative organisms. Better-absorbed prodrug formulations of a derivative of fosmidomycin, FR900098, are being investigated as potential antimalarial agents.

 Further information

Kuemmerle HP, Murakawa T, De Santis F 1987 Pharmacokinetic evaluation of fosmidomycin, a new phosphonic acid antibiotic. *Chemiotherapia* 6: 113–119.

Jomaa H, Wiesner J, Sanderbrand S et al 1999 Inhibitors of the nonmevalonate pathway of isoprenoid biosynthesis as antimalarial agents. *Science* 285: 1573–1576.

Neu HC, Kamimura T 1981 In vitro and in vivo antibacterial activity of FR-31564, a phosphonic acid antimicrobial agent. *Antimicrobial Agents and Chemotherapy* 19: 1013–1023.

Reichenberg A, Wiesner J, Wiedemeyer C et al 2001 Diaryl ester prodrugs of FR900098 with improved in vivo antimalarial activity. *Bioorganic and Medicinal Chemistry Letters* 11: 833–855.

Ridley RG 1999 Planting the seeds of new antimalarial drugs. *Science* 285: 1502–1503.

21 Fusidanes

D. Greenwood

The fusidanes are steroid-like antibiotics with a basic cyclopentanophenanthrene structure. Their stereochemistry differs from that of metabolically active steroids and they do not exert any hormonal or anti-inflammatory activity. The group includes helvolic acid, cephalosporin P₁ and fusidic acid. Helvolic acid, a product of *Aspergillus fumigatus*, attracted some early attention because of its weak antimycobacterial activity; cephalosporin P₁ was a component of the antibiotic complex of the mold that also yielded the first true cephalosporin.

Fusidic acid, is much the most active member of the group and is the only one commercially available. It was discovered in Denmark in 1960 as a product of a fungus originally isolated in Japan from monkey dung. The principal interest of fusidic acid lies in its antistaphylococcal activity.

 FUSIDIC ACID

Molecular weight (sodium salt): 538.7.

A fermentation product of *Fusidium coccineum*. Supplied as the sodium salt, which is readily soluble in water, or suspension of the acid. Intravenous preparations (sodium or diethanolamine salt) are dissolved in phosphate–citrate buffer. Several formulations are available for topical application. The dry powder is stable for 3 years.

Antimicrobial activity

Fusidic acid is active against most Gram-positive bacteria, but all aerobic Gram-negative negative bacilli are resistant (Table 21.1). Streptococci and pneumococci are much less susceptible than staphylococci. *Bacteroides fragilis, Nocardia asteroides* (MIC 0.5–4 mg/l) and *Corynebacterium diphtheriae* (MIC <0.01 mg/l), *Clostridium* spp. (MIC 0.01–0.5 mg/l) are susceptible. It is moderately active against many mycobacteria, including *Mycobacterium tuberculosis, Mycobacterium bovis, Mycobacterium malmoense* and *Mycobacterium leprae*, but other mycobacteria are resistant. Fusidic acid shows some activity against certain protozoa, including *Giardia lamblia* and *Plasmodium falciparum*.

In 50% serum, the MIC may double and it is slightly more effective at pH 6–7 than at pH 8. It is bactericidal in concentrations close to the MIC.

Interaction with penicillins is complex. Against some strains of staphylococci synergy occurs, but others show two-way antagonism or 'indifference'. There is no useful synergy with other antistaphylococcal agents.

Table 21.1 Activity of sodium fusidate against some common pathogenic bacteria

Species	MIC (mg/l)
Staphylococcus aureus	0.03–0.1
Streptococcus pyogenes	4–16
Streptococcus pneumoniae	2–16
Enterococcus faecalis	1–4
Neisseria spp.	0.03–1
Escherichia coli	R
Klebsiella pneumoniae	R
Pseudomonas aeruginosa	R
Bacteroides fragilis	2
Mycobacterium tuberculosis	8–32

R, resistant (MIC >64 mg/l)

Acquired resistance

Large inocula of most strains of *Staph. aureus* contain a small number of resistant mutants, which emerge rapidly in vitro and sometimes during therapy. The growth rate, coagulase, hemolysin and β-lactamase production of these mutants appear to be unimpaired. Despite the ease of emergence of resistance in vitro, resistance remains rare in clinical isolates (1–2%) and is mostly plasmid mediated. Although topical applications are liable to facilitate the emergence of resistant mutants, extensive use of the drug on the skin does not seem to have added significantly to the pool of resistant strains in circulation.

Resistance in staphylococci is usually due to chromosomal mutation, which results in a change at the target site (elongation factor G). Plasmid-mediated resistance also occurs and appears to be associated with drug exclusion. Genes for β-lactamase and sodium fusidate resistance are commonly carried on the same plasmid.

Antistaphylococcal penicillins prevent the emergence of fusidic acid-resistant mutants of *Staph. aureus*. In addition, the effect of fusidic acid on protein synthesis may prevent generation of sufficient β-lactamase to destroy penicillin.

Pharmacokinetics

Oral absorption: sodium salt	>90%
suspension	70%
C_{max}: 500 mg oral	30 mg/l after 2–3 h
500 mg i.v.	50 mg/l end-infusion
Plasma half-life	*c*. 9 h
Volume of distribution	*c*. 12 l
Plasma protein binding	97%

Absorption

Fusidic acid suspension is less well absorbed than the sodium salt of the tablet formulation. In children absorption is more rapid than in adults. Milk appears to delay absorption, peak concentrations not being reached for 4–8 h. Because of slow elimination, considerable accumulation of the drug occurs on repeated administration of both oral and intravenous formulations.

Distribution

Sodium fusidate is well distributed in the tissues and most organs of the body. It does not reach the cerebrospinal fluid, but penetrates into cerebral abscesses. Inhibitory levels are obtained in muscle, kidney, lungs and pleural exudate. Bone concentrations in samples taken at operation from patients with chronic osteomyelitis treated for at least 5 days were 1.7–14.9 mg/g in patients receiving 1.5 g/day and 3.4–14.8 mg/g in patients receiving 3 g/day.

Levels in excess of 7 mg/l have been found in aspirated synovial fluid from patients with osteo- or rheumatoid arthritis after 3–7 days' treatment with 0.75 or 1.5 g/day. The drug has been detected in brain, milk and placenta, which it crosses to reach the fetus. In patients treated with 1.5 g/day, levels of 0.08–0.84 mg/l were found in the aqueous humor after 1 day and 1.2–2.0 mg/l after 3 days' treatment. In the post-distribution phase, about half of the drug is in the peripheral compartment, in keeping with the known ability of sodium fusidate to penetrate into tissues including bone.

Metabolism and excretion

It is extensively metabolized in the liver and is excreted in the bile in the form of glucuronides and various other metabolites. Only about 2% of the administered dose can be recovered in active form in the feces. Less than 1% of active antibiotic is excreted in the urine. Very little of the drug is removed by dialysis.

Toxicity and side effects

Oral sodium fusidate has been administered for prolonged periods for the control of chronic staphylococcal sepsis without mishap. Mild gastrointestinal disturbance and occasional rashes have been reported. Some patients develop abnormalities in liver function tests and jaundice which resolve on withdrawal of therapy. Jaundice is less common with oral than with parenteral therapy. The drug is not recommended in hepatic insufficiency. Rapid infusion of diethanolamine fusidate may lead to venospasm or thrombosis, and occasionally to hypocalcemia, possibly as an effect of the buffer.

Clinical use

Systemic formulations
- Severe staphylococcal infections, particularly bone and joint infections (in combination with penicillins, erythromycin or clindamycin).
- Infection with methicillin-resistant staphylococci (including endocarditis).
- Prosthetic valve endocarditis due to 'diphtheroids' (in combination with erythromycin).

Topical formulations
- Skin infections, principally those involving staphylococci, but including erythrasma.
- Acute staphylococcal conjunctivitis.

In addition to its antibacterial activity, fusidic acid possesses immunomodulatory properties by stimulation of T cells and interference with cytokine production. This has led to the suggestion that it might be of value in the treatment of several non-bacterial conditions, including Crohn's disease and autoimmune diabetes.

Preparations and dosage

Proprietary name: Fucidin.

Preparations: Tablets, suspension, injection, topical preparations.

Dosage: Adults, oral (as sodium fusidate): 500 mg every 8 h, doubled for severe infections. Children (as fusidic acid) ≤1 year, 50 mg/kg per day in three divided doses; 1–5 years, 250 mg every 8 h; 5–12 years, 500 mg every 8 h.

Intravenous infusion (as sodium fusidate): adults >50 kg, 500 mg three times daily; adult <50 kg and children, 6–7 mg/kg three times daily.

Widely available (not USA).

 Further information

Franzblau SG, Biswas AN, Harris EB 1992 Fusidic acid is highly active against extracellular and intracellular *Mycobacterium leprae*. *Antimicrobial Agents and Chemotherapy* 36: 92–94.

Nicoletti F, Di Marco R, Conget I et al 2000 Sodium fusidate ameliorates the course of diabetes induced in mice by multiple low doses of streptozotocin. *Journal of Autoimmunity* 15: 395–405.

Reeves DS 1987 The pharmacokinetics of fusidic acid. *Journal of Antimicrobial Chemotherapy* 20: 467–476.

Various authors 1990 Fusidic acid: a reappraisal. *Journal of Antimicrobial Chemotherapy* 25 (Suppl. B): 1–60.

Various authors 1999 Fusidic acid. *International Journal of Antimicrobial Agents* 12 (Suppl. 2): S1–S93.

D. Greenwood

The glycopeptides are a group of chemically complex antibacterial compounds obtained originally from various species of soil actinomycetes. They all contain a core heptapeptide to which are attached sugar moieties, some of which are unique. Vancomycin and ristocetin were discovered in the mid-1950s and developed for the treatment of serious infection caused by Gram-positive bacteria, particularly *Staphylococcus aureus*. However, ristocetin was withdrawn soon afterwards because of bone marrow and platelet toxicity. Teicoplanin, the only other glycopeptide presently in clinical use, was first described in 1978.

Among other glycopeptides, avoparcin and actaplanin have been used as animal feed additives, while actinoidin, like ristocetin, has been used as an investigational aid in the diagnosis of von Willebrand's disease and platelet aggregation dysfunction.

Characterization of naturally occurring and chemically derived analogs of vancomycin, including the synmonicins, orienticins, chloro-orienticins and eremomycin, has allowed a better understanding of structure–activity relationships among the glycopeptides. Particularly interesting is the observation that *N*-alkylization of the vancosamine sugar of vancomycin imparts activity against vancomycin-resistant strains of Gram-positive cocci. A semisynthetic derivative of this type, oritavancin (LY333328), is presently in clinical trial. Semisynthetic derivatives of the teicoplanin complex have also been produced. An amide derivative of the teicoplanin complex, BI 397, is 2–4 times more active than teicoplanin against most Gram-positive organisms; it is also active against the more resistant isolates of coagulase-negative staphylococci, but not against vancomycin-resistant enterococci.

A naturally occurring lipoglycodepsipeptide, ramoplanin, shares many of the microbiological properties of vancomycin and teicoplanin. It is, however, chemically distinct and has a different mode of action. It is more potent against staphylococci and is active against glycopeptide-resistant enterococci. It is too toxic for systemic use, but is under investigation as a topical agent, as a component of oral gut decontamination regimens, and for the oral therapy of antibiotic-associated colitis.

ANTIMICROBIAL ACTIVITY

The activity of glycopeptides is essentially restricted to Gram-positive organisms, notably staphylococci and streptococci of all kinds. However, *Lactobacillus*, *Leuconostoc*, *Pediococcus* and *Erysipelothrix* spp. are inherently resistant. They act on bacterial cell wall synthesis (*see* p. 13), although ramoplanin acts at a slightly earlier stage than true glycopeptides. Their large molecular size prevents them from penetrating the Gram-negative outer membrane and, with rare exceptions (e.g. some *Prevotella* and *Porphyromonas* spp.), they are inactive against Gram-negative bacteria.

ACQUIRED RESISTANCE

ENTEROCOCCI

Five distinct resistance phenotypes are recognized, of which the first two are most prevalent, especially in *Enterococcus faecium* (*see also* p. 32).

- VanA resistance is associated with the substitution of D-alanyl-D-lactate for D-alanyl-D-alanine at the carboxy terminus of the pentapeptide side chain of *N*-acetylmuramic acid (*see* p. 13), with a consequent loss of binding affinity for both vancomycin and teicoplanin. The modification is inducible and is brought about by the functioning of a cluster of genes that are on a transposable element and may be present on a transferable plasmid.
- VanB resistance also results from a D-lac substitution that is inducible by vancomycin but not by teicoplanin, to which susceptibility is retained. It is usually chromosomally mediated and transferability has been shown in some cases.
- VanC resistance is characteristic of *Enterococcus gallinarum* and some other enterococci that are infrequently encountered as pathogens. It is chromosomally mediated, con-

stitutively expressed and is characterized by low-level resistance to vancomycin alone.

- VanD resistance has been found in a few strains of *E. faecium*. It confers non-transferable resistance to vancomycin and reduced susceptibility to teicoplanin.
- VanE resistance has been described in a strain of *E. faecalis* that displayed reduced susceptibility to vancomycin alone.

STAPHYLOCOCCI

Low-level resistance is described in clinical isolates of staphylococci, including *Staph. aureus*, *Staph. epidermidis* and *Staph. haemolyticus*. Such resistance has been variously attributed to alterations in cell wall structure, overproduction of the cell wall peptidoglycan and binding to cell wall sites other than the primary target. Resistance associated with the production of a 39-kDa cell wall protein has also been demonstrated in laboratory derivatives of *Staph. aureus*, but clinical isolates of this type have not so far been described. Further work is necessary to elucidate fully the mechanisms of resistance among the different phenotypes.

DETECTION OF GLYCOPEPTIDE RESISTANCE

The routine detection of glycopeptide resistance may present problems, especially with strains exhibiting low-level resistance, such as glycopeptide-intermediate *Staph. aureus*. In general, quantitative methods are recommended for accurate determination of inhibitory concentrations whenever possible.

 Further information

Arthur M, Courvalin P 1993 Genetics and mechanisms of glycopeptide resistance in enterococci. *Antimicrobial Agents and Chemotherapy* 37: 1563–1571.

Biavasco F, Vignaroli C, Varaldo PE 2000 Glycopeptide resistance in coagulase-negative staphylococci. *European Journal of Clinical Microbiology and Infectious Diseases* 19: 403–417.

Cetinkaya Y, Falk P, Mayhall CG 2000 Vancomycin-resistant enterococci. *Clinical Microbiology Reviews* 13: 686–707.

Jones RN, Barrett MS, Erwin ME 1997 In vitro activity and spectrum of LY333328, a novel glycopeptide derivative. *Antimicrobial Agents and Chemotherapy* 41: 488–493.

Jones RN Biedenbach DJ, Johnson DM, Pfaller MA 2001 *In vitro* evaluation of BI 397, a novel glycopeptide antimicrobial agent. *Journal of Chemotherapy* 13: 244–254.

Sanyal D, Johnson AP, George RC, Edwards R, Greenwood D 1993 In-vitro characteristics of glycopeptide resistant strains of *Staphylococcus epidermidis* isolated from patients on CAPD. *Journal of Antimicrobial Chemotherapy* 32: 267–278.

Tenover FC, Biddle JW, Lancaster MV 2001 Increasing resistance to vancomycin and other glycopeptides in *Staphylococcus aureus*. *Emerging Infectious Diseases* 7: 327–332.

Woodford N, Johnson AP, Morrison D, Speller DCE 1995 Current perspectives on glycopeptide resistance. *Clinical Microbiology Reviews* 8: 585–615.

Woodford N 1998 Glycopeptide-resistant enterococci: a decade of experience. *Journal of Medical Microbiology* 47: 849–862.

 TEICOPLANIN

Molecular weight: (A$_2$-1): 1877.7; (A$_2$-2 and A$_2$-3): 1879.7; (A$_2$-4 and A$_2$-5): 1893.7.

A complex of several molecules of similar antibiotic potency produced by *Actinoplanes teichomyceticus*. An aglycone backbone consisting of a linear heptapeptide of linked aromatic amino acids is substituted with two sugars, D-mannose and *N*-acetylglucosamine. The five components (A$_2$-1, A$_2$-2, A$_2$-3, A$_2$-4 and A$_2$-5) are differentiated from each other by the acyl-aliphatic side-chain substitutions present on the additional sugar. It is formulated as the sodium salt for intramuscular or intravenous administration.

Antimicrobial activity

In general, teicoplanin is 2–4 times more active than vancomycin against susceptible strains (Table 22.1). Against some coagulase-negative staphylococci, especially *Staph. haemolyticus*, it may be less active (minimum inhibitory concentration (MIC) 16–64 mg/l compared with ≤4 mg vancomycin/l). For these strains, the MIC of teicoplanin, but not vancomycin, is greatly affected by the composition of the medium, including the presence of lysed horse blood, and the bacterial inoculum density. Isolates inhibited by ≤8 mg/l are usually considered susceptible. Bactericidal activity is similar to that of vancomycin.

Acquired resistance

Vancomycin-resistant enterococci of the VanA type are resistant; VanB strains are usually susceptible, although mutation to resistance may develop. Coagulase-negative staphylococci

Table 22.1 Comparative in vitro activity of glycopeptides against some common pathogenic bacteria: MIC (mg/l)

Species	Vancomycin	Teicoplanin
Staph. aureus	1–2	0.12–1
Str. pyogenes	0.12–0.25	0.03–0.12
Str. pneumoniae	0.12–0.25	0.03–0.12
E. faecalis	1–4	0.12–0.5
H. influenzae	16–R	R
Neisseria spp.	8–32	No data
Esch. coli	R	R
K. pneumoniae	R	R
Ps. aeruginosa	R	R
Cl. difficile	0.06–1	0.03–0.25
B. fragilis	R	R

R, resistant (MIC >32 mg/l).

exhibiting low-level glycopeptide resistance are often more resistant to teicoplanin than vancomycin even when they emerge during vancomycin therapy.

Pharmacokinetics

Oral absorption	Very low
C$_{max}$ 400 mg intravenous bolus 6 mg/kg intramuscular	25–40 mg/l after 1 h *c.* 10 mg/l after 2 h
Plasma half-life (terminal)	90 h (mean)
Volume of distribution (steady state)	0.9–1.6 l/kg
Plasma protein binding	>90%

Absorption

Bioavailability after intramuscular administration is about 90%. The area under the concentration–time curve (AUC) is similar after intravenous or intramuscular administration. In children a daily dose of 6 mg/kg body weight produced a mean trough concentration of 4.6 mg/l and a peak concentration of 19.1 mg/l. After a dose of 10 mg/kg the corresponding concentrations were 15.8 and 36.9 mg/l, respectively.

Distribution

Teicoplanin is widely distributed and penetrates readily into tissues, peritoneal fluid, synovial fluid and bone. It crosses the placenta, but not the blood–brain barrier.

Metabolism and excretion

No metabolic products have been identified. The drug is removed from the body almost entirely by glomerular filtration. The terminal half-life ranges from 33 to 190 h or longer, depending upon the pharmacokinetic model used for analysis and the last sampling time. The half-life may be shorter in children and is substantially altered in patients with renal failure (and the elderly), so that adjustment of dosage may be necessary. It is not removed during hemodialysis or hemofiltration

and clearance by peritoneal dialysis is less than 20% of total body clearance. In all three procedures, management of plasma concentration is best achieved by giving a loading dose followed by monitoring at appropriate intervals.

Toxicity and side effects

Unlike vancomycin, teicoplanin does not cause significant histamine release and the 'red-man' syndrome is very seldom seen. Nephrotoxicity is uncommon and, when it does occur, is not related to dose, plasma concentration or concomitant therapy with an aminoglycoside. Ototoxicity has been reported rarely and is not dose related.

Other, reversible, adverse effects include allergy, local intolerance, fever and altered liver function. Thrombocytopenia has been seen in patients with raised trough levels (about 60 mg/l). None of these effects occur with a frequency greater than 3%. Teicoplanin should be used with caution in patients with a history of hypersensitivity to vancomycin.

Safety in pregnancy has not been established. Accidental overdosing in two children, in whom plasma levels in excess of 300 mg/l were found, was not associated with symptoms or laboratory abnormalities.

Clinical use

- Infections caused by *Staph. aureus* and other Gram-positive pathogens (especially those caused by methicillin-resistant staphylococci and in patients hypersensitive to β-lactam antibiotics).
- Treatment of vancomycin-resistant enterococci (other than VanA strains).
- Treatment and prophylaxis of endocarditis caused by Gram-positive species (often in combination with an aminoglycoside).
- Peritonitis associated with continuous ambulatory peritoneal dialysis (intraperitoneal).

 Preparations and dosage

Proprietary name: Targocid.

Preparation: Injection.

Dosage: Adults, i.v., 400 mg initial loading dose on day 1 then 200 mg/day; severe infections, 400 mg loading dose every 12 h for the first three doses, then 400 mg/day. Children ≥2 months, 10 mg/kg every 12 h for three doses then 6 mg/kg daily; severe infections, 10 mg/kg every 12 h for three doses, then 10 mg/kg daily. Neonates, 16 mg/kg initial loading dose on day 1, subsequently 8 mg/kg daily.

Widely available.

 Further information

Anonymous 1999 Teicoplanin. In Dollery C (ed.) *Therapeutic Drugs* 2nd ed. Churchill Livingstone, Edinburgh, pp. T20–T24.

Brogden RN, Peters DH 1994 Teicoplanin. A reappraisal of its antimicrobial activity, pharmacokinetic properties and therapeutic efficacy. *Drugs* 47: 823–854.

Parenti F, Schito GC, Courvalin P 2000 Teicoplanin chemistry and microbiology. *Journal of Chemotherapy* 12: 5–14.

Rybak MJ, Lerner SA, Levine DP et al 1991 Teicoplanin pharmacokinetics in intravenous drug abusers being treated for bacterial endocarditis. *Antimicrobial Agents and Chemotherapy* 35: 696–700.

Wilson APR 2000 Clinical pharmacokinetics of teicoplanin. *Clinical Pharmacokinetics* 39: 167–183.

Wood MJ 2000 Comparative safety of teicoplanin and vancomycin. *Journal of Chemotherapy* 12: 21–25.

 VANCOMYCIN

Molecular weight (free base): 1449; (hydrochloride): 1485.7.

A tricyclic glycopeptide isolated from the fermentation products of the actinomycete, *Amycolatopsis orientalis* (formerly *Streptomyces orientalis*). Two chlorinated β-hydroxytyrosine molecules, three substituted phenylglycine systems, *N*-methylleucine and aspartic acid amide form the basic heptapeptide chain. A disaccharide, made up of glucose and the unique amino sugar vancosamine, is attached to one of the phenylglycine residues. It is formulated as the water-soluble hydrochloride for intravenous infusion or oral administration.

Antimicrobial activity

The antibacterial activity is essentially restricted to Gram-positive species (Table 22.1), including methicillin-resistant strains of staphylococci. Viridans streptococci, *Listeria monocytogenes*, *Propionibacterium acnes* and corynebacteria are all susceptible (MIC 0.25–2 mg/l), as are Gram-positive anaerobes, including *Clostridium difficile* (MIC 0.06–1 mg/l) and *C. perfringens* (MIC 0.12–0.5 mg/l). Mycobacteria are resistant.

Vancomycin is slowly bactericidal for most susceptible bacteria (≥99.9% reduction in viability after 6–12 h exposure of the inoculum to eight times the MIC). However, against isolates of *Enterococcus* spp., some viridans streptococci and *Staph. haemolyticus*, vancomycin is effectively bacteristatic. Gentamicin enhances the bactericidal effect.

Acquired resistance

Resistance is uncommon, except in enterococci, in which resistance has emerged in response to widespread use in hospitals. The use of avoparcin as a growth promoter in animal husbandry may also have played a part in encouraging resistance.

Low-level resistance (MIC 8–32 mg/l) has been described in coagulase-negative staphylococci, usually *Staph. epidermidis* or *Staph. haemolyticus*, sometimes emerging during protracted treatment. Strains of *Staph. aureus* exhibiting reduced susceptibility (MIC 4–8 mg/l) were first reported from Japan in 1997 and have since been found in other countries. The prevalence of these strains, most of which exhibit heteroresistance, appears to be very low, though there are difficulties in detecting them in vitro.

Pharmacokinetics

Oral absorption	Very low
C_{max} 500 mg slow intravenous infusion (>1 h)	10–25 mg/l 1 h after end infusion
1 g slow intravenous infusion (>1 h)	20–50 mg/l 1 h after end infusion
Plasma half-life	5–11 h
Volume of distribution	0.6 l/kg
Plasma protein binding	*c.* 55%

Rapid infusion (<1 h) or bolus administration is dangerous. The intramuscular route of administration causes pain and necrosis and is not used. Slow intravenous infusion over at least 100 min is recommended. Dosage should be adjusted to give a peak concentration of 25–40 mg/l and a trough of 5–10 mg/l.

Absorption

Vancomycin is very poorly absorbed from the gastrointestinal tract and large concentrations of unaltered drug are found in the feces after oral administration.

Distribution

After slow intravenous infusion vancomycin is distributed widely, reaching therapeutic concentrations in most body compartments. It does not penetrate appreciably into the cerebrospinal fluid of subjects with normal meninges, although levels in patients with meningitis may approach therapeutic concentrations.

Metabolism and excretion

Vancomycin is not metabolized and 90% of an intravenous dose is eliminated in the urine, almost exclusively by glomerular filtration. The elimination half-life in patients with normal renal function is usually 6–8 h, but is altered substantially in patients with impaired renal function, necessitating dosage modification. This can be predicted to some extent by creatinine clearance values but adequately optimized only by monitoring plasma concentrations.

Renal clearance may be more rapid in intravenous drug abusers and children (with the exception of neonates in whom the half-life may be prolonged), and plasma monitoring is indicated in such patients, particularly those receiving therapy for endocarditis or other life-threatening sepsis. A prolonged half-life has been observed in some patients with hepatic failure. Plasma monitoring is also indicated in these patients.

It is not removed efficiently by hemodialysis or hemofiltration. Patients undergoing these procedures should be given an appropriate loading dose and the frequency and size of further doses determined by monitoring plasma concentrations. Vancomycin crosses the peritoneal membrane in both directions with a transfer half-life of about 3 h, resulting in about 75% equilibration over a 6-h dialysis period. Because of the large dilution effect, many exchanges may be required before the plasma concentration reaches that of the dialyzate, and to achieve rapid equilibration a loading dose of about three times the maintenance dose has been suggested. Thus, in patients on continuous ambulatory peritoneal dialysis, incorporation of 50 mg vancomycin/l of dialyzate eventually produces plasma concentrations of 5–20 mg/l. Alternatively, a loading dose of 0.5 g vancomycin, administered by intravenous infusion, followed by 7.5 mg/l dialyzate with 4–6-hourly exchange, produces plasma concentrations of 6.5–37 mg/l.

Interactions

Gentamicin and furosemide (frusemide) or other loop diuretics may increase the potential for nephrotoxicity and ototoxicity. Owing to the acidic nature of solutions, vancomycin is incompatible in vitro with various agents, including β-lactam antibiotics, aminophylline and heparin.

Toxicity and side effects

Rapid administration (<60 min) may result in release of histamine from basophils and mast cells, leading to the so-called 'red-man' or 'red-neck' syndrome, characterized by one or more of pruritus, erythema, flushing of the upper torso, anaphylactoid reaction, angioedema and, rarely, cardiovascular depression and collapse.

Vancomycin is potentially nephrotoxic and ototoxic, although the highly purified drug preparations in current use are safer. Increased risk of nephrotoxicity has been associated with treatment for longer than 3 weeks, trough plasma concentrations continually in excess of 10 mg/l, and concurrent therapy with an aminoglycoside or a loop diuretic. Ototoxicity, often irreversible, used to be seen particularly in elderly patients and in patients receiving excessive dosage, but is unusual with the more highly purified preparations. The risk of ototoxicity is minimized if the peak serum level is kept below 50 mg/l and is very unusual if the level is less than 30 mg/l, unless the patient has prior auditory nerve damage or is receiving another potentially ototoxic drug. Reversible neutropenia

and/or thrombocytopenia, which can be profound, may occur, notably in patients with renal impairment.

Clinical use

- Infections caused by *Staph. aureus* and other Gram-positive pathogens (especially those caused by methicillin-resistant staphylococci and in patients hypersensitive to β-lactam antibiotics).
- Empirical therapy of febrile and profoundly neutropenic patients (in combination with other agents).
- Treatment and prophylaxis of endocarditis caused by Gram-positive species (often in combination with an aminoglycoside).
- Peritonitis associated with continuous ambulatory peritoneal dialysis (intraperitoneal).
- Antibiotic-associated colitis (oral).
- Suppression of bowel flora in neutropenic patients (oral; in combination with other agents).

Preparations and dosage

Proprietary name: Vancocin.

Preparations: Injection, capsules.

Dosage: Adults, oral, 125 mg every 6 h for 7–10 days, up to 2 g per day in severe infections; i.v., 500 mg every 6 h or 1 g every 12 h. Children, oral, 5–10 mg/kg every 6 h; >5 years, half the adult dose. Children, i.v., >1 month, 10 mg/kg every 6 h; infants 1–4 weeks, 15 mg/kg initially then 10 mg/kg every 8 h; neonates up to 1 week, 15 mg/kg initially then 10 mg/kg every 12 h.

Widely available.

Further information

Anonymous 1999 Vancomycin (hydrochloride). In: Dollery C (ed.) *Therapeutic Drugs* 2nd edn. Churchill Livingstone, Edinburgh, pp. V6–V10.

Aucken HM, Warner M, Ganner M et al. 2000 Twenty months of screening for glycopeptide intermediate *Staphylococcus aureus. Journal of Antimicrobial Chemotherapy* 46: 639–640.

Gold HS 2001 Vancomycin-resistant enterococci: mechanisms and clinical observations. *Clinical Infectious Diseases* 33: 210–219.

Hiramatsu K, Hanaki H, Ino T, Yabuta K, Oguri T, Tenover FC 1997 Methicillin-resistant *Staphylococcus aureus* clinical strain with reduced vancomycin susceptibility. *Journal of Antimicrobial Chemotherapy* 40: 135–136.

Levine JF 1987 Vancomycin: a review. *Medical Clinics of North America* 71: 1135–1145.

Rice LB 2001 Emergence of vancomycin-resistant enterococci. *Emerging Infectious Diseases* 7: 183–187.

Rybak MJ, Albrecht LM, Berman JR, Warbasse LH, Svensson CK 1990 Vancomycin pharmacokinetics in burn patients and intravenous drug abusers. *Antimicrobial Agents and Chemotherapy* 34: 792–795.

Rybak MJ, Albrecht LM, Boike SC, Chandreesekar PH 1990 Nephrotoxicity of vancomycin, alone and with an aminoglycoside. *Journal of Antimicrobial Chemotherapy* 25: 679–687.

Wilcox M, Fawley W 2001 Extremely low prevalence of UK *Staphylococcus aureus* with reduced susceptibility to vancomycin. *Journal of Antimicrobial Chemotherapy* 48: 144–145.

Wilhelm MP, Estes L 1999 Symposium on antimicrobial agents Part XII. Vancomycin. *Mayo Clinic Proceedings* 74: 928–935.

CHAPTER

23 Lincosamides

D. Greenwood

The lincosamides are a small group of agents with a novel structure unlike that of any other antibiotic. The naturally occurring members of the group are lincomycin and the much less active celesticetin. Attempts to prepare semisynthetic derivatives with improved properties have been largely unsuccessful, with the important exception of the chlorinated derivative, clindamycin. Pirlimycin, a clindamycin analog that appears to be less extensively metabolized, is used in animal husbandry.

Lincosamides have an unusual antimicrobial spectrum, being widely active against Gram-positive bacteria and most anaerobes, but not Gram-negative aerobes. They are also active against some mycoplasmas and protozoa. Their principal therapeutic indications are penicillin-susceptible infections in allergic patients, staphylococcal infections, particularly of bones and joints, and anaerobic infections, including mixed infections for which they must be combined with an agent active against aerobic Gram-negative bacilli. They are moderately well absorbed when administered by mouth and distributed widely to tissues, including penetration into cells and bone. They are generally well tolerated, except for the relative frequency with which they have been associated with severe diarrhea, including *Clostridium difficile*-associated pseudomembranous colitis.

 Further information

Phillips I, Wise R (eds) 1985 Macrolides-lincosamides-streptogramins. *Journal of Antimicrobial Chemotherapy* 16 (Suppl. A): 1–226.
Steigbigel NH 2000 Macrolides and clindamycin. In: Mandell GL, Bennett J RE, Dolin R (eds). *Principles and Practice of Infectious Diseases*. Churchill Livingstone, Edinburgh, pp. 366–382.

 CLINDAMYCIN

7-Chloro-7-deoxylincomycin. Molecular weight (anhydrous free base): 425.

A semisynthetic derivative of lincomycin. Aqueous suspensions are stable for up to 2 weeks at room temperature. Several formulations are in use. Capsules contain clindamycin hydrochloride, which has a very bitter taste, detectable in concentrations as low as 8 mg/l; the syrup contains a suspension of the ester, clindamycin palmitate, which is palatable for children. Clindamycin hydrochloride is poorly soluble at neutral pH and too irritating for parenteral use, so clindamycin phosphate is used for this purpose. Clindamycin palmitate and clindamycin phosphate are both inactive in vitro and must be hydrolyzed to liberate clindamycin.

Antimicrobial activity

The spectrum includes most Gram-positive organisms, notably staphylococci (including methicillin-resistant strains) and streptococci, but not enterococci (Table 23.1). An effect on streptococcal toxin expression has been proposed as a reason for superior performance in severe cellulitis. Aerobic Gram-negative rods are uniformly resistant, but most anaerobic bacteria are highly susceptible. Typical minimum inhibitory concentrations (MICs) are: *Prevotella* and *Porphyromonas* spp., 0.1–2 mg/l; *Fusobacterium* spp., <0.5 mg/l; *Peptostreptococcus* spp., 0.1–0.5 mg/l. Clostridia, with the notable exception of *Clostridium perfringens* (MIC <0.1–8 mg/l) are less susceptible. Corynebacteria, *Bacillus anthracis*, and *Nocardia asteroides* are

Table 23.1 Susceptibility of common pathogenic bacteria: MIC (mg/l)

	Clindamycin	Lincomycin
Staphylococcus aureus	0.1–1	0.5–2
Streptococcus pyogenes	0.01–0.25	0.05–1
Streptococcus pneumoniae	0.05	0.1–1
Enterococcus faecalis	4–R	2–R
Haemophilus influenzae	0.5–16	4–16
Neisseria spp.	0.5–4	8–64
Escherichia coli	R	R
Klebsiella pneumoniae	R	R
Pseudomonas aeruginosa	R	R
Bacteroides fragilis	0.02–2	2–4

R, resistant (MIC >64 mg/l).

all susceptible, but mycobacteria are resistant. The MIC for *Chlamydia trachomatis* is 16 mg/l, that for *Mobiluncus* spp. is 0.5 mg/l, and that for *Gardnerella vaginalis* is 0.03 mg/l. *Mycoplasma hominis* is susceptible (MIC <1 mg/l), *M. pneumoniae* somewhat less so (MIC 1–4 mg/l), but ureaplasmas are resistant. Clindamycin is active against some protozoa, including *Toxoplasma gondii*, *Plasmodium falciparum* and *Babesia* spp.

Various types of interaction with other antimicrobial agents have been described, including interference with the bactericidal activity of aminoglycosides against Gram-negative bacilli. The combination with primaquine showed enhanced activity in experimental infections with *Pneumocystis carinii*.

Acquired resistance

Clindamycin-resistant staphylococci, streptococci (including pneumococci) and *Bacteroides* spp. are found with variable frequency throughout the world and these strains are commonly also resistant to erythromycin. Resistance may be caused by changes in a ribosomal protein or, less commonly, by enzymic inactivation of clindamycin. There is complete cross-resistance with lincomycin. A form of resistance that embraces macrolides, lincosamides and type B streptogramins is associated with methylation of adenine residues at a common binding site. The methylase is inducible by macrolides, but not lincosamides (or streptogramins), which consequently remain active in the absence of macrolides.

Pharmacokinetics

Oral absorption	80–90%
C_{max}: hydrochloride 300 mg oral	3.6 mg/l after 1–2 h
palmitate 300 mg oral	1.4–4.2 mg/l after 1 h
phosphate 300 mg intramuscular	4–5 mg/l after 2 h
phosphate 300 mg intravenous	5–6 mg/l end infusion
Plasma half-life	c. 2–3 h
Volume of distribution	43–74 l/m²
Plasma protein binding	94%

Absorption

The presence of food does not depress or delay oral absorption. The palmitate is rapidly and completely hydrolyzed in the gut. In contrast, clindamycin phosphate is absorbed intact after intramuscular injection and relatively slowly hydrolyzed by alkaline phosphatases. A substantial amount of unhydrolyzed clindamycin phosphate (1–2 mg/l) has been detected in the serum at 30–60 min and up to 10% of the dose may still be present as phosphate after 8 h. The bioavailability in relation to dose is linear, but not proportional.

Plasma levels in pregnant women following a single oral dose of 450 mg (3.4–9 mg/l) were similar to those found in non-pregnant women. After intravaginal administration of 5 ml of 2% clindamycin phosphate cream (100 mg) to healthy women and women suffering from bacterial vaginosis, less than 5% of the dose was subsequently found in the plasma.

Distribution

After hydrolysis in the serum, clindamycin phosphate is rapidly and widely distributed, but CSF concentrations are low (0.14–0.46 mg/l, following a single dose of 150 mg) and levels in brain are low or absent.

The drug is excreted in breast milk and crosses the placenta. In patients undergoing caesarean section, mean peak fetal plasma concentrations of about 3 mg/l (46% maternal level) have been found after a 600 mg intravenous dose of clindamycin phosphate.

Therapeutic concentrations are achieved in both cancellous and cortical bone. The tissue:serum concentration ratio has been found to be 1.0 in bone marrow, 0.5–0.75 in spongy and 0–0.15 in compact bone. Hydroxyapatite binds clindamycin and probably also the ester.

Uptake of clindamycin phosphate into neutrophils is rapid, temperature dependent, saturable and depressed by acid pH. Clindamycin is accumulated by lysosomes to active concentrations around 40 times those of the extracellular fluid. After an initially high rate of hydrolysis by intracellular alkaline phosphatase, enzyme activity declines and after 4 h, around half of the drug is still unhydrolyzed. Similar product inhibition may prevent the complete hydrolysis of the phosphate in pus where alkaline phosphatase is liberated from neutrophils.

Metabolism

Clindamycin is extensively metabolized in the liver to clindamycose, desmethyl clindamycin, and sulfoxide derivatives of clindamycin and desmethyl clindamycin. Desmethyl clindamycin and clindamycin sulfoxide retain antibacterial activity, but clindamycose and desmethyl clindamycin sulfoxide are much less active than the base.

Excretion

Only about 13% of an oral dose is excreted unchanged in urine, somewhat less after a parenteral dose of clindamycin phosphate. Bioactivity persists in the urine for up to 4 days, suggesting slow release of the drug or its active metabolites from tissues or body fluids. In patients with severe renal disease, plasma levels may be 3–4 times normal and persist for over 24 h. Urinary recovery of the drug can fall below 1% in severe renal failure. Clindamycin is not removed by hemodialysis or peritoneal dialysis.

The liver plays a significant part in the metabolism and elimination of the drug. High concentrations have been found in the bile of patients with patent common ducts undergoing biliary tract surgery, most of the activity being due to the desmethyl metabolite. The concentrations in gallbladder bile, common duct bile, gallbladder wall and liver were 2–3 times those in serum. Where the common duct was obstructed, none could be detected in bile and the level was lower in gall-bladder wall, but the concentration in liver was slightly higher than in those without obstruction. The ranges found when the serum concentration was 10–30 mg/l were: gall-bladder bile 8–100 mg/l; common duct bile 15–170 mg/l; and gall-bladder wall 5–45 mg/kg. Patients with proven hepatic cirrhosis show significant impairment of clindamycin elimination. Clindamycin phosphate may be slowly converted to the base in patients with hepatic impairment. Less than 5% of an oral dose can be recovered from the feces, but excretion of bioactive drug persists for several days and may continue to affect the normal gut flora.

The plasma half-life in premature infants (8.7 h) is significantly longer than in term infants (3.6 h).

Toxicity and side effects

Up to 30% of patients experience diarrhea, especially when taking the drug orally. This is often due to *Clostridium difficile* toxins and in a small proportion of cases leads to pseudomembranous colitis. Diarrhea is more common in women, and in patients over 60 years of age. Diarrhea may abate if treatment is continued, but because of the risk of pseudomembranous colitis administration of the drug should be stopped.

Parenteral administration can cause elevation of transaminases and serum alkaline phosphatase, but these are generally reversible. Intravenous administration may be complicated by thrombophlebitis.

Rashes occur in about 10% of patients, but severe eruptions are rare. Isolated episodes of toxic epidermal necrolysis, blood dyscrasias and erythema multiforme have been reported and there is a single report of prolonged neuromuscular blockade after an accidental intravenous overdose (2.4 g instead of 600 mg).

Clinical use

- Staphylococcal soft tissue, bone and joint infection.
- Streptococcal infection (as a penicillin substitute in allergic patients, including prophylaxis of endocarditis in special risk patients undergoing dental procedures).
- Prophylaxis and treatment of anaerobic infections (with appropriate agents where the infection is likely to include aerobic Gram-negative rods).

- Bacterial vaginosis.
- Acne.
- Toxoplasmosis.
- Babesiosis (in combination with quinine).
- *Pneumocystis carinii* pneumonia (in combination with primaquine).

Preparations and dosage

Proprietary names: Dalacin C, Dalacin T.

Preparations: Capsules, suspension, injection.

Dosage: Adults, oral, 150–300 mg every 6 h, increased to 450 mg every 6 h for severe infections. Children, oral, 3–6 mg/kg every 6 h. Adults, i.m., i.v., 600 mg to 1.2 g daily in 2–4 equal doses; more severe infections, 1.2–2.7 g/day in 2–4 equal doses; life-threatening infections, up to 4.8 g/day. Children >1 month, i.m., i.v., 15–25 mg/kg per day in 3–4 divided doses; severe infections, 25–40 mg/kg per day in 3–4 divided doses; in severe infections it is recommended that children are given no less than 300 mg/day, regardless of body weight. Neonates have been given 15–20 mg/kg per day in 3–4 divided doses.

Widely available.

Further information

Ahmed Jushuf IH, Shahmanesh M, Arya OP 1995 The treatment of bacterial vaginosis with a 3 day course of 2% clindamycin cream: results of a multicentre, double blind, placebo controlled trial. *Genitourinary Medicine* 71: 254–256.

Anonymous 1999 Clindamycin (hydrochloride). In: Dollery C (ed). *Therapeutic Drugs*, 2nd edn. Churchill Livingstone, Edinburgh. pp. C 257–C 261.

Bell MJ, Shackelford P, Smith R, Schroeder K 1984 Pharmacokinetics of clindamycin phosphate in the first year of life. *Journal of Paediatrics* 105: 482–486.

Blais J, Tardif C, Chamberland S 1993 Effect of clindamycin on intracellular replication, protein synthesis, and infectivity of *Toxoplasma gondii*. *Antimicrobial Agents and Chemotherapy* 37: 2571–2577.

Dajani AS, Taubert KA, Wilson W et al 1997 Prevention of bacterial endocarditis. Recommendations by the American Heart Association. *Journal of the American Medical Association* 277: 1794–1801.

Easmon CSF, Crane JP 1984 Cellular uptake of clindamycin and lincomycin. *British Journal of Experimental Pathology* 65: 725–730.

Falagas ME, Gorbach SL 1995 Clindamycin and metronidazole. *Medical Clinics of North America* 79: 845–867.

Joesoef MR, Schmid GP, Hiller SL 1999 Bacterial vaginosis: review of treatment options and potential clinical indications for therapy. *Clinical Infectious Diseases* 28 (Suppl. 1): S57–S65.

Kremsner PG, Radloff P, Metzger W et al 1995 Quinine plus clindamycin improves chemotherapy of severe malaria in children. *Antimicrobial Agents and Chemotherapy* 39: 1603–1605.

Oleske JM, Phillips I (eds) 1983 Clindamycin: bacterial virulence and host defence. *Journal of Antimicrobial Chemotherapy* 12 (Suppl. C): 1–122.

Paquet P, Schaaf-Lafontaine N, Piérard GE 1995 Toxic epidermal necrolysis following clindamycin treatment. *British Journal of Dermatology* 132: 665–666.

Plaisance KI, Drusano GL, Forrest A, Townsend RJ, Standiford HC 1989 Pharmacokinetic evaluation of two dosage regimens of clindamycin phosphate. *Antimicrobial Agents and Chemotherapy* 33: 618–620.

Warren E, George S, You J, Kazanjian P 1997 Advances in the treatment and prophylaxis of *Pneumocystis carinii* pneumonia. *Pharmacotherapy* 17: 900–916.

LINCOMYCIN

Molecular weight (hydrochloride monohydrate): 461.

A fermentation product of *Streptomyces lincolnensis* var. *lincolnensis* supplied as the hydrochloride. The dry crystalline hydrochloride is very soluble in water and very stable.

Antimicrobial activity

The spectrum closely resembles that of clindamycin, but it is generally less potent (Table 23.1).

Acquired resistance

There is complete cross-resistance between clindamycin and lincomycin. Clinical isolates of streptococci and enterococci are commonly cross-resistant to erythromycin. A transposon carrying a lincomycin resistance gene similar to that found in *Staph. aureus* has been reported in *Bacteroides* strains.

Pharmacokinetics

Oral absorption (fasting)	20–35%
T_{max} 500 mg oral	2–3 mg/l after 2–4 h
600 mg intramuscular	8–18 mg/l after 1–2 h
600 mg intravenous	18–20 mg/l end infusion
Plasma half-life	4–6 h
Plasma protein binding	72%

Absorption

It is less well absorbed than clindamycin. Food significantly delays and decreases absorption, the mean peak plasma level from a dose given immediately after a meal being only about half the fasting levels.

Distribution

It is widely distributed in a volume approximating to the total body water. Levels in normal CSF are low, but in the presence of inflammation, CSF:serum concentration ratios around 0.4 have been found. Penetration occurs into cerebral abscesses. Concentrations in saliva and sputum approximate to the simultaneous serum level. Concentrations of 1.5–6.9 mg/l have been found in cord serum or amniotic fluid after the mother received 600 mg intramuscular and 0.5–2.4 mg/l in human milk after the second of two maternal 500 mg doses.

In patients undergoing total hip replacement given 600 mg lincomycin intramuscularly 6 h preoperatively, and again by intravenous infusion perioperatively, mean concentrations achieved were: capsule 9.4 mg/kg; synovial fluid 5.4 mg/l; cancellous bone 7.2 mg/kg; cortical bone 5.4 mg/kg.

Peak concentrations of 30–135 mg/l were found in the aqueous humor 1–2 h after subconjunctival injection of 75 mg in all but one case; plasma levels were around 2–3 mg/l within 10 min.

Metabolism and excretion

Like clindamycin, lincomycin is metabolized in the liver and excreted in the bile. About 40% of an oral dose can be recovered from the feces. In patients with severe hepatic dysfunction the plasma half-life is approximately doubled and the proportion of the dose appearing in the urine increases.

Less than 5% of an oral dose appears in the urine over 24 h, but up to 60% after intravenous administration, mostly in the first 4 h. It appears to be virtually non-dialyzable, since its plasma half-life in dialyzed and undialyzed azotemic patients is approximately the same.

Toxicity and side effects

Nausea, vomiting and abdominal cramps may occur, but there are usually no side effects apart from diarrhea, which affects at least 10% of patients. Diarrhea can occur after oral or parenteral administration, usually within a few days of the institution of therapy. It is more common in older patients and uncommon in children. Symptoms range from watery diarrhea without fever or leukocytosis to severe, often bloody, diarrhea, with abdominal pain progressing to profound shock and dehydration with high mortality.

Hypersensitivity reactions are rare. Transient changes occur in liver function tests, probably due to interference with the tests, since abnormalities in specific enzyme tests and clinical evidence of hepatic dysfunction are rare.

In some patients receiving large doses by rapid intravenous injection, the blood pressure had fallen precipitately with nausea, vomiting, arrhythmias and, exceptionally, cardiac arrest. It can transiently depress neuromuscular transmission and might depress respiration after anesthesia, but the effect is much weaker than that of neomycin.

There is no evidence of risk in pregnancy.

Clinical use

Uses are similar to those of clindamycin, by which it has been generally superseded.

Preparations and dosage

Proprietary name: Lincoain.

Preparations: Capsules, syrup, injection.

Dosage: Adults, oral, 500 mg, 3–4 times daily; i.m., 600 mg, 1–2 times daily; i.v. infusion, 600 mg to 1 g, 2–3 times daily, up to 8 g daily in severe infections. Children >1 month, oral, 30–60 mg/kg per day in divided doses; i.m., i.v., 10–20 mg/kg per day in divided doses.

Limited availability; available in USA, but not in the UK.

Further information

Gwilt PR, Smith RB 1986 Protein binding and pharmacokinetics of lincomycin following intravenous administration of high doses. *Journal of Clinical Pharmacology* 26: 87–90.

Mickal A, Panzer JD 1975 The safety of lincomycin in pregnancy. *American Journal of Obstetrics and Gynecology* 121: 1071–1074.

Parsons RL, Beavis JP, Hossack GA, Paddock GM 1977 Plasma, bone, hip capsule synovial and drain fluid concentration of lincomycin during total hip replacement. *British Journal of Clinical Pharmacology* 4: 433–437.

Rosato A, Vicarini H, Leclerc R 1999 Inducible or constitutive expression of resistance in clinical isolates of streptococci and enterococci cross-resistant to erythromycin and lincomycin. *Journal of Antimicrobial Chemotherapy* 43: 559–562.

Smith RB, Lummis WL, Monovich RE, DeSante KA 1981 Lincomycin serum and saliva concentrations after intramuscular injection of high doses. *Journal of Clinical Pharmacology* 21: 411–417.

Wang J, Shoemaker NB, Wang GR, Salyers AA 2000 Characterization of a Bacteroides mobilizable transposons, NBU2, which carries a functional lincomycin resistance gene. *Journal of Bacteriology* 182: 3559–3571.

24 Macrolides

A. Bryskier and J.-P. Butzler

The macrolides form a large group of closely related antibiotics produced mostly by *Streptomyces* and related species. They are characterized by a macrolactone ring (to which they owe their generic name), to which typically two sugars, one an amino sugar, are attached. The original macrolide complex, erythromycin, was isolated in 1952 as a natural product of *Streptomyces erythreus* (now *Saccharopolyspora erythraea*). Interest in the group has been greatly stimulated by the activity of erythromycin A against emergent pathogens, such as the *Mycobacterium avium* complex, *Campylobacter* spp, *Legionella* spp and *Chlamydia* spp. Focusing on erythromycin A has emphasized both its desirable properties and its deficiencies, and stimulated the search for analogs with extended antibacterial spectrum, notably against fastidious Gram-negative pathogens, improved pharmacokinetic properties, such as increased acid stability, and reduced gastrointestinal intolerance.

Through a Beckman reaction an endocyclic 9a-methyl nitrogen was inserted into the erythronolide A ring of erythromycin A, yielding a chemical subclass known as azalides. Azithromycin is the first azalide to reach clinical use. It shares the antibacterial spectrum and clinical indications of other macrolide antibiotics, but exhibits increased potency against fastidious Gram-negative bacteria, and a longer apparent half-life.

To overcome erythromycin A resistance within Gram-positive cocci, ketolides – semisynthetic derivatives of erythromycin A lacking α-L cladinose at position 3 of the erythronolide A ring – have been synthesized. Their main characteristics are high stability even at pH 1.0, activity against isolates resistant to erythromycin A due to methylation or efflux and inability to induce resistance to macrolides due to methylation. One such compound, telithromycin, is clinically available. A further derivative, ABT 773, is currently in clinical development.

Three macrolides, tylosin, mycinamycin and tilmicosin (a derivative of tylosin) are used only in veterinary medicine and are not discussed further here.

CLASSIFICATION

The most important therapeutic macrolides are characterized by a 14-, 15- or 16-membered lactone ring. Members of the group with a 12-membered ring are also known, but are only research compounds. In the group that includes erythromycin A and oleandomycin the lactone ring contains 14 atoms and one or two sugar groups are attached by α- or β-glycosidic linkages to the aglycone. In the 16-membered-ring macrolides, two sugars are linked together and attached to the lactone ring through the amino sugar.

Chemically, azalides are semisynthetic erythromycin A derivatives with the macrolactone ring expanded to 15 atoms by the insertion of nitrogen. All ketolides share a comparable chemical structure: a 3-keto function, a C11–C12 carbamate side chain and a 6-OH substituted chain.

ANTIBACTERIAL ACTIVITY

The 14-, 15- and 16-membered-ring macrolides share the same antibacterial spectrum, including most Gram-positive organisms, *Neisseria* spp., *Haemophilus* spp., *Bordetella pertussis*, *Moraxella catarrhalis* and both Gram-positive and Gram-negative anaerobes. Activity against common pathogen bacteria

Group 1 14-membered ring compounds	Group 2 16-membered ring compounds	Group 3 Azalides (15-membered ring)	Group 4 Ketolides (14-membered ring)
Clarithromycin*	Josamycin,	Azithromycin*	Telithromycin*
Dirithromycin*	Kitasamycin (leucomycin)		
Erythromycin A	Midecamycin		
Flurithromycin*	Miokamycin*		
Oleandomycin	Rokitamycin*		
Roxithromycin*	Spiramycin		

*Semi-synthetic compounds

Table 24.1 Susceptibility (MIC range: mg/l) of some common pathogenic bacteria to macrolides

	Azithromycin	Erythromycin A	Josamycin	Midecamycin	Miokamycin	Oleandomycin	Roxithromycin	Spiramycin	Telithromycin
Staph. aureus	0.25–1	0.1–1	0.25–4	0.5–2	0.5–1	0.25–4	0.1–2	0.25–1	0.12–0.25
Str. pyogenes	0.03–0.1	0.01–0.25	0.06–0.5	0.1–2	0.5–2	0.1–1	0.06–0.25	0.1–2	0.01–0.06
Str. pneumoniae	0.03–0.25	0.01–0.25	0.03–0.5	–	0.1–2	0.1–0.25	0.01–4	–	0.004–0.06
E. faecalis	0.5–R	0.5–4	0.5–4	1–4	0.5–R	2–4	0.5–8	2–4	–
N. gonorrhoeae	0.03–2	0.03–0.5	0.5–2	–	–	2–4	0.03–2	2–4	–
N. meningitidis	0.01–0.06	0.03–1	0.06–2	–	0.03–4	2–4	0.03–2	–	0.03–0.25
H. influenzae	0.25–2	0.5–8	2–16	1–4	0.25–32	0.1–2	0.5–16	2–8	0.5–4
Esch. coli	0.5–2	8–32	R	R	R	R	R	32	–
Ps. aeruginosa	R	R	R	R	R	R	R	R	–
B. fragilis	0.5–16	0.1–16	0.06–1	2–32	0.5–2	–	0.25–64	–	–

R, resistant (MIC ≥64 mg/l); –, no data.

is shown in Table 24.1. They are inactive or poorly active against Enterobacteriaceae and non-fermentative Gram-negative bacteria such as *Pseudomonas aeruginosa*.

The semisynthetic macrolides do not provide a significant advantage over erythromycin A against staphylococci and streptococci, and are poorly active against enterococci. They are active against *Moraxella catarrhalis*, *Bordetella pertussis*, *Neisseria gonorrhoeae*, *Campylobacter jejuni*, *Rhodococcus equi*, *Haemophilus ducreyi*, *Gardnerella vaginalis*, *Mobiluncus* spp., *Propionibacterium acnes*, *Borrelia burgdorferi* and *Treponema pallidum*. The minimum inhibitory concentrations (MICs) against *Haemophilus influenzae* range from 0.25 to 8 mg/l, azithromycin being the most active. Variable susceptibilities are reported for *Bordetella bronchiseptica*, *Listeria monocytogenes*, *Corynebacterium jeikeium*, *Eikenella corrodens*, *Pasteurella multocida*, *Bacteroides fragilis*, *Prevotella melaninogenica*, *Fusobacterium* spp. and *Clostridium perfringens*.

In-vitro activity against common respiratory pathogens is shown in Table 24.2. Telithromycin (a ketolide) is the most active compound and retains activity against erythromycin A-resistant strains.

The semisynthetic macrolides exert important activity against intracellular pathogens, including *Chlamydia trachomatis* (MIC_{50} clarithromycin 0.007 mg/l; azithromycin 0.125 mg/l; roxithromycin, 0.06 mg/l), *Chlamydophila* (formerly *Chlamydia*) *pneumoniae*, *Legionella pneumophila* and other *Legionella* spp., the *Mycobacterium avium* complex (MIC: clarithromycin 0.25–4.0 mg/l; azithromycin and roxithromycin 4–32 mg/l), *M. leprae* and *Rickettsia* spp. (MIC: 1–2 mg/l). Azithromycin appears to be the most active of the compounds against *Brucella melitensis* and atypical pathogens such as *Ureaplasma urealyticum* and *Mycoplasma* spp.

ACQUIRED RESISTANCE

Widespread use of erythromycin and semisynthetic analogs has led to the emergence of resistance in *Staph. aureus* and in Lancefield group A streptococci (*Str. pyogenes*). Resistance to erythromycin A is of both chromosomal and plasmid origin, and can be inducible or constitutive. Intrinsic resistance of Gram-negative bacilli to macrolides is probably due to the relative impermeability of the outer membrane to the hydrophobic compounds and/or to an efflux mechanism of resistance. However, in azithromycin, introduction of the endocyclic nitrogen into the lactone ring contributes to enhanced activity against fastidious Gram-negative bacilli – in particular *Haemophilus influenzae*.

Acquired resistance to macrolides involves three mechanisms: modification of the target, active efflux or inactivation. In the first type of resistance, a single alteration in 23S ribosomal RNA confers cross-resistance to macrolides, azalides, lincosamides and streptogramin-B-type antibiotics (the so-called MLS_B phenotype), whereas the two other types confer resistance to structurally related antibiotics only.

Modification of the ribosomal targets is a complex mechanism. Several types have been described:

- Monomethylation of adenine-2058 located in domain V of the 23S rRNA, resulting in a blockade of the N^6 amino group of adenine and inhibition of binding of erythromycin A or its derivatives. The phenomenon can be induced by 14-membered-ring macrolides and azalides, but not by 16-membered-ring macrolides or ketolides. Monomethylation or bimethylation of adenine 2058 or 2059 may be constitutive and affects all available macrolides. Monomethylation does not affect telithromycin.
- Mutation of adenine 2058 to guanine has been described in many bacterial species, such as staphylococci, streptococci (including *Str. pneumoniae* and *Str. pyogenes*), *H. pylori*, the *M. avium* complex and *T. pallidum*. Other point mutations on the peptidyltransferase site, such as adenine 2611 to guanine, lead to resistance to 14- and 15-membered-ring macrolides.
- Mutations at ribosomal proteins L4 and L22, which are close to the exit channel, have been reported in clinical isolates of *Str. pneumoniae*, *Str. oralis* and *Str. pyogenes*.

An efflux pump, Mef, encoded by a *mef* gene, accounts for resistance in over 50% of *Str. pneumoniae* or *Str. pyogenes* isolates in certain geographic areas. Other pumps involved in macrolide resistance include Msr A/B in staphylococci, Acr-like in *H. influenzae* and Mre A in *Str. agalactiae*. The Mef group has been described in all streptococci, including the viridans group streptococci.

Macrolide-inactivating enzymes include esterases that

Table 24.2 In vitro activity of selected macrolides against respiratory pathogens: MIC_{50} (mg/l)

	Erythromycin A	Azithromycin	Clarithromycin	Dirithromycin	Roxithromycin	Telithromycin
Str. pneumoniae	0.06	0.06	0.015	0.06	0.06	0.008
Str. pyogenes	0.06	0.06	0.015	0.12	0.12	0.01
H. influenzae	4	1	4	8	8	1
Mor. catarrhalis	0.12	0.03	0.06	0.12	0.25	0.06
M. pneumoniae	0.01	0.004	0.004	0.03	0.03	0.001
C. pneumoniae	0.03	0.06	0.03	1	0.06	0.01
L. pneumophila	0.25	0.12	0.03	1	0.12	0.03

hydrolyze the lactone ring and which are found mainly in *Esch. coli*, and enzymes that fix either a glucose or a phosphate at the 2′ OH group of D-desosamine. Among clinical bacterial species, those mechanisms have been reported in *Nocardia* spp., which are resistant to all macrolides having a D-desosamine. The same mechanisms of inactivation have been reported in the 16-membered-ring macrolides.

PHARMACOKINETICS

Erythromycin, the first macrolide antibiotic to be available in clinical practice, is characterized by poor water solubility and rapid inactivation by stomach acidity, which results in widely varying bioavailability after oral administration. Structural alterations of erythromycin A have resulted in improved pharmacokinetic properties, including bioavailability, gastro-intestinal tolerance, higher peak plasma levels, longer apparent elimination plasma half-lives and improved tissue concentrations.

Macrolides are mainly given orally, but oral absorption and bioavailability vary from one drug to the next, partly reflected in differences in daily dosage. Oral absorption is rapid, with plasma peaks varying between 0.4 mg/l (azithromycin) and 11 mg/l (roxithromycin). Maximum concentrations are reached between 0.5 h (rokitamycin) and 3 h (clarithromycin) and are dose dependent.

The apparent elimination half-life varies from 1 h (miokamycin) to 44 h (dirithromycin); the absolute bioavailability varies between 10% (dirithromycin) and 55–60% (roxithromycin, clarithromycin). The absolute bioavailability of azithromycin is about 37%. The main elimination route is via the bile and feces; a proportion of clarithomycin is excreted via the intestinal mucosa. A substantial part of the administered dose of clarithromycin is eliminated in urine. The long apparent elimination half-lives of roxithromycin, azithromycin and dirithromycin allow them to be administered as single daily oral doses.

Table 24.3 Uptake of macrolides into polymorphonuclear neutrophils

Macrolide	Uptake*	Efflux†	Percentage in granule
Azithromycin	>300	≤20	60
Clarithromycin	9–100	80	30
Dirithromycin	60–80	52	73
Erythromycin A	4–18	80	35
Erythromycylamine	25	63	45
Flurithromycin	>10	–	–
Josamycin	21	>20	13
Rokitamycin	30	>70	–
Roxithromycin	40–100	80	49
Telithromycin	348	45	56–75

*Ratio of intracellular: extracellular concentration; †Over 60 min.

Table 24.4 Concentration of macrolides in respiratory tissue

Macrolide	Dose (mg)	Plasma (mg/l)	Bronchial mucosa (mg/kg)	Tonsils (mg/kg)
Azithromycin	500 (S)	–	3.9	–
Clarithromycin	500 (R)	2.5	–	1.9
Dirithromycin	500 (R)	0.22	1.9	3.5
Erythromycin	500 (R)	3.08	7.2	2.9
Josamycin	1000 (R)	0.39	–	21.4
Oleandomycin	2000 (S)	–	–	4.1
Miokamycin	600 (R)	2.3	–	3.2
Roxithromycin	150 (R)	6.3	–	2.9
Spiramycin	2000 (R)	2.4	13–36	21.5–40
Telithromycin	800 (S)	1.9–2.7	0.7–3.9	0.7–3.95

S, single dose; R, repeated dose.

INTRACELLULAR CONCENTRATION

Macrolide antibiotics concentrate within cells and are active against intracellular pathogens. The rates of uptake and efflux vary for each compound (Table 24.3). Azithromycin concentrates progressively, with a high concentration after 3 h. The same pattern is described for dirithromycin and telithromycin. Macrolides usually concentrate in the granule zone of polymorphonuclear neutrophils. Macrolides are highly concentrated in the bronchial mucosa and tonsils (Table 24.4).

INTERACTIONS

Erythromycin A and oleandomycin (14-membered-ring macrolides) induce hepatic microsomal enzymes and interfere via the cytochrome P_{450} system with clearance of other drugs such as theophylline, antipyrine and carbamazepine, increasing their plasma levels. The induced isoenzymes of cytochrome P_{450} rapidly demethylate and oxidize macrolides to nitrosoalkanes, which combine with the iron of the enzymes, thereby inactivating them. The 16-membered-ring macrolides such as josamycin and spiramycin have no such effect. Erythromycin base, estolate and stearate and a metabolite of triacetyloleandomycin all form stable complexes with cytochrome P_{450}. Josamycin base forms an unstable complex, and josamycin propionate, spiramycin base and adipate do not bind.

TOXICITY AND SIDE EFFECTS

Macrolides are generally safe drugs and serious adverse events are rare. A notable exception is erythromycin estolate, which is hepatotoxic and may cause severe hepatitis, probably as a result of the mixture of lauryl sulfate and the 2′-propionyl ester. Gastrointestinal complaints (nausea, vomiting, abdominal pain or, more infrequently, diarrhea) are the most common adverse events. These reactions present a problem mainly when erythromycin doses are higher than those recommended and are partly due to the hemiketal degradation product, which acts on motilin, an intestinal endopeptide.

The semisynthetic 14- and 15-membered-ring macrolides are more acid stable than erythromycin and are better tolerated. Some macrolides, depending on their chemical structures, can interact with several other drugs, markedly changing their pharmacokinetics.

CLINICAL USE

The macrolides retain the classic clinical applications of erythromycin, including activity against Gram-positive cocci and intracellular pathogens such as *Legionella*, *Chlamydia* and *Rickettsia* spp. The improved pharmacokinetic properties and tissue distribution of some semisynthetic compounds may prove useful in more unusual settings such as infections due to mycobacteria (*M. avium* complex) and protozoa (e.g. *Toxoplasma gondii*, *Entamoeba histolytica*, *Plasmodium falciparum*). Other target infections are chronic gastritis (*Helicobacter pylori*) and borreliosis (*Borrelia burgdorferi*).

 Further information

Bryskier A 1992 Newer macrolides and their potential target organisms. *Current Opinion in Infectious Diseases* 5: 764–772.

Bryskier A 1997 Novelties in the field of macrolides. *Expert Opinion on Investigational Drugs* 6: 1697–1709.

Bryskier A 1999 *Antibiotiques et agents antibactériens et antifongiques.* Ellipses, Paris.

Bryskier A, Agouridas C, Chantot JF 1993 Acid stability of new macrolides. *Journal of Chemotherapy* 5 (Suppl. A): 158–159.

Bryskier A, Agouridas C, Chantot JF 1995 New insights into the structure-activity relationship of macrolides and azalides. In: Zinner SH, Young LS, Acar JF, Neu HC (eds). *New macrolides, azalides and streptogramins in clinical practice.* Marcel Dekker, Inc., New York, pp. 3–30.

Bryskier A, Agouridas C, Chantot JF 1997 Ketolides: new semisynthetic 14-membered ring macrolides. In: Zinner SH, Young LS, Acar JF, Neu HC (eds) *Expanding indications for the new macrolides, azalides, and streptogramins.* Marcel Dekker, Inc., New York, pp. 39–50.

Bryskier A, Agouridas C 1993 Azalides, a new medicinal chemical entity? *Current Opinion on Investigational Drugs* 2: 687–694.

Bryskier A, Labro MT 1994 Macrolides–Nouvelles perspectives thérapeutiques. *Presse Médicale* 23: 1762–1766.

Bryskier A, Butzler JP, Neu HC (eds) 1993 *Macrolides: chemistry, pharmacology and clinical uses.* Blackwell-Arnette, Paris, p. 698.

Butzler JP, Kobayashi H 1985 Macrolides: a review with outlook on future development. Excerpta Medica, Amsterdam, p. 157.

Hardy DJ, Hensey DM, Beyer JM, Vojkko C, McDonald EJ, Fernandes PB 1988 Comparative in vitro activity of new 14-, 15-, and 16-membered macrolides. *Antimicrobial Agents and Chemotherapy* 32: 1710–1719.

Kirst HA 1992 New macrolides: expanded horizons for an old class of antibiotic. *Journal of Antimicrobial Chemotherapy* 28: 787–790.

Kirst HA, Sides GD 1989 New directions for macrolide antibiotics: pharmacokinetics and clinical efficacy. *Antimicrobial Agents and Chemotherapy* 33: 1419–1422.

Neu HC, Young LS, Zinner SH 1993 The new macrolides, azalides and streptogramins. In: Pharmacology and clinical applications. Marcel Dekker, New York, p. 228.

Phillips I, Williams JD 1985 Macrolides, lincosamides, streptogramins. *Journal of Antimicrobial Chemotherapy* 16 (Suppl. A).

Williams JD, Sefton AM 1993 Comparison of macrolide antibiotics. *Journal of Antimicrobial Chemotherapy* (Suppl. C): 11–26.

GROUP 1: 14-MEMBERED RING MACROLIDES

 ## CLARITHROMYCIN

Molecular weight: 748.

A semisynthetic erythromycin A derivative (6-*O*-methyl-erythromycin A) formulated for oral and intravenous use.

Antibacterial activity

Clarithromycin is two of four times more active than erythromycin A against susceptible common pathogens (Table 24.1). Most respiratory pathogens are inhibited at a concentration of ≤0.25 mg/l, with the exception of *H. influenzae* (MIC 1–8 mg/l). It is twice as active as erythromycin A against *Str. pyogenes* (MIC_{50} 0.015 mg/l), but the 14-OH metabolite is equivalent in activity (MIC_{50} 0.03 mg/l). Comparable activity is found against *Str. pneumoniae*. Clarithromycin inhibits *Mycoplasma pneumoniae* at 0.004 mg/l and *Mor. catarrhalis* at 0.06 mg/l. It is eight times more active than erythromycin A against *Legionella* spp, *C. trachomatis* and *C. pneumoniae*. Against anaerobic species activity is similar to that of erythromycin A. Against *H. influenzae* the 14-hydroxy metabolite is twice as active as the parent compound.

Pharmacokinetics

Oral absorption	55%
C_{max} 250 mg oral	0.75 mg/l after 1.7 h
500 mg oral	1.65 mg/l after 2 h
Plasma half-life	2.7–3.5 h
Volume of distribution	250 l
Plasma protein binding	80%

Absorption

Clarithromycin is more stable to gastric acid than erythromycin, but internal ketalization between the 9-keto group and the C-12 hydroxyl group has been described resulting in an inactive product: pseudo clarithromycin. It is rapidly absorbed orally and absorption is not affected by food.

Distribution

The drug penetrates the tissue of the respiratory tract, giving concentrations in tonsil and lung tissues that exceed the simultaneous plasma level two-fold and four-fold, respectively.

Metabolism

The primary metabolic pathway in humans is *N*-demethylation of the D-desosamine and stereospecific hydroxylation at the 14-position of the erythronolide A ring. Metabolism to the 14-hydroxy derivative is saturable above 800 mg. The apparent elimination half-life of the 14-hydroxy metabolite is around 7 h.

Excretion

Around 20–40% of the administered dose is eliminated in urine. The parent compound and its principal metabolite are retained in renal impairment, resulting in long apparent elimination half-lives, exceeding 30 and 45 h, respectively, in patients whose creatinine clearance is less than 30 ml/min.

Toxicity and side effects

Clarithromycin is well tolerated, producing little gastrointestinal disturbance and only transient changes in some liver function tests.

Clinical use

- Upper and lower respiratory tract infections, including streptococcal pharyngitis, acute bacterial maxillary sinusitis, bacterial exacerbations of chronic bronchitis and community-acquired pneumonia.
- Skin and soft-tissue infections.
- *Helicobacter pylori* infection (in combination with other agents).

 ## Preparations and dosage

Proprietary name: Kloricid, Biacin.

Preparations: Tablets, suspension, granules, injection.

Dosage: Adults, oral, 250–500 mg every 12 h for 7–14 days, depending on severity of infection. Children, oral, body weight <8 kg, 7.5 mg/kg twice daily; body weight 8–11 kg, 62.5 mg twice daily; body weight 12–19 kg, 125 mg twice daily; body weight 20–29 kg, 187.5 mg twice daily; body weight 30–40 kg, 250 mg twice daily. Adults, i.v. infusion, 500 mg twice daily.

Widely available.

 ## Further information

Anonymous 1999 Clarithromycin. In: Dollery C (ed.) *Therapeutic Drugs* 2nd edn. Churchill Livingstone, Edinburgh, pp. C248–C253.
Finch RG, Speller DCE, Daly PJ 1991 Clarithromycin: new approaches to the treatment of respiratory tract infections. *Journal of Antimicrobial Chemotherapy* 27 (Suppl. A).

DIRITHROMYCIN

Molecular weight: 835.

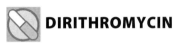

A prodrug of erythromycylamine, a semi-synthetic erythromycin A derivative, formulated for oral administration.

Antibacterial activity

Dirithromycin and erythromycylamine share the same antibacterial spectrum as other 14-membered-ring macrolides, but are less active than erythromycin A. The MIC of dirithromycin for Gram-positive bacteria is the same or twice that of erythromycylamine, which is usually 4- to 8-fold less active than erythromycin A. Activity against respiratory pathogens is shown in Table 24.2. Against *B. pertussis*, *H. pylori* and *C. jejuni*, dirithromycin and erythromycylamine show the same antibacterial activity. Activity against anaerobes is poor.

Pharmacokinetics

The long apparent elimination half-life allows once-daily administration. It achieves a greater cellular:extracellular concentration ratio than erythromycin A and a higher concentration in some tissues. The intracellular:extracellular ratio in polymorphonuclear leukocytes is time dependent, reaching 60–80 after 120 min.

Dirithromycin is rapidly hydrolyzed to erythromycylamine: 60–90% of a dose is converted to erythromycylamine within 35 min after intravenous administration. After oral administration of single doses of 500, 750 and 1000 mg to healthy volunteers, the peak plasma concentrations ranged between 0.29 and 0.64 mg/l 4–5 h after administration. The AUC values were 3.37–6.45 mg.h/l, with an apparent elimination half-life of 30–44 h. The total clearance was 250–500 ml/min.

The absolute bioavailability of dirithromycin after oral administration is about 10% of the given dose. After a 500 mg single oral dose, the mean peak biliary concentration was 139 mg/l. In elderly patients, there was a trend toward an increase in AUC but not in the plasma peak. Renal and non-renal clearance was lower in patients with biliary disease than in other patients or healthy volunteers.

Between 62% and 81% of an oral dose and 81–97% of an intravenous dose are eliminated in the feces, predominantly as erythromycylamine. Urinary recovery accounted for 1.2–2.9% of the orally administered dose. Dosage adjustments do not appear necessary in patients with mild or moderate hepatic, biliary or renal impairment. Negligible amounts of the drug were removed during hemodialysis.

Toxicity and side effects

The frequency and nature of adverse events are similar to those experienced by patients receiving other macrolides. Gastrointestinal events are most common, and include abdominal pain (5.6% and 4.7% of patients receiving dirithromycin and comparator agents, respectively), diarrhea (5.0% and 5.5%) and nausea (4.9% and 5.1%).

Clinical use

- Community-acquired infections of the respiratory tract
- Skin and soft-tissue infections.

Preparations and dosage

Proprietary name: Dynabac.
Preparation: 250 mg tablets.
Dosage: Adults, oral, 500 mg once daily.
Available in continental Europe and the USA.

Further information

Brogden RN, Peters DH 1994 Dirithromycin – a review of its antimicrobial activity, pharmacokinetic properties and therapeutic efficacy. *Drugs* 48: 599–616.
Finch RG, Hamilton-Miller JMT, Lovering AM, Daly PJ 1993 Dirithromycin: a new once-daily macrolide. *Journal of Antimicrobial Chemotherapy* 31 (Suppl. C).

 ERYTHROMYCIN

Molecular weight (erythromycin A base): 733.9; (ethyl succinate): 862.1; (stearate): 1018.4; (estolate): 1056.4.

A natural antibiotic produced as a complex of six components (A–F) by *Saccharopolyspora erythraea*. Only erythromycin A has been developed for clinical use. It is available in a large number of forms for oral administration: the base compound (enteric- or film-coated to prevent destruction by gastric acidity); 2′-propionate and 2′-ethylsuccinate esters; a stearate salt; estolate and acistrate salts of 2′-esters. The 2′-esters and their salts have improved pharmacokinetic and pharmaceutical properties and are less bitter than erythromycin. It is also formulated as the lactobionate and gluceptate for parenteral use.

Antibacterial activity

Activity against common bacterial pathogens is shown in Table 24.1 (p. 311). Gram-positive rods, including *Clostridium* spp (MIC_{50} 0.1–1 mg/l), *C. diphtheriae* (MIC_{50} 0.1–1 mg/l), *L. monocytogenes* (MIC_{50} 0.1–0.3 mg/l) and *B. anthracis* (MIC_{50} 0.5–1.0 mg/l), are generally susceptible. Most strains of *Mycobacterium scrofulaceum* and *Mycobacterium kansasii* are susceptible (MIC_{50} 0.5–2 mg/l), but *Mycobacterium intracellulare* is often and *Mycobacterium fortuitum* regularly resistant. *Nocardia* isolates are resistant. *H. ducreyi*, *B. pertussis* (MIC_{50} 0.03–0.25 mg/l), some *Brucella*, *Flavobacterium*, *Legionella* (MIC_{50} 0.1–0.5 mg/l) and *Pasteurella* spp. are susceptible. *H. pylori* (MIC 0.06–0.25 mg/l) and *C. jejuni* are usually susceptible, but *C. coli* may be resistant. Most anaerobic bacteria, including *Actinomyces* and *Arachnia* spp., are susceptible or moderately so, but *B. fragilis* and *Fusobacterium* spp. are resistant. *T. pallidum* and *Borrelia* spp. are susceptible, as are *Chlamydia* spp. (MIC ≤0.25 mg/l), *M. pneumoniae* and *Rickettsia* spp. *M. hominis* and *Ureaplasma* spp. are resistant. Enterobacteriaceae are resistant, although some strains of *Escherichia coli* are inhibited and killed by as little as 8 mg/l.

Inoculum size or the presence of serum has only a small effect on the MIC, but activity increases with increasing pH up to 8.5. Incubation in an atmosphere containing 5–6% CO_2

raises the MIC for *H. influenzae* from 0.5–8 to 4–32 mg/l, and MICs against *B. fragilis*, *Str. pneumoniae* and *Str. pyogenes* also rise steeply. Activity is predominantly bacteristatic.

Acquired resistance

Acquired resistance is a worldwide problem within streptococci. In Europe, the USA and other countries the incidence of erythromycin A resistance ranged from 5% to over 60% for *Str. pneumoniae*. The percentage of resistant isolates is greater in *Str. pneumoniae* strains resistant or intermediately susceptible to penicillin G, with reported resistance rates above 80%.

Worldwide, increasing and alarming reports of resistance in clinical isolates of *Str. pyogenes* have been reported, threatening its use as an alternative to penicillin G in allergic patients.

Lower rates of resistance have been reported in other bacterial species, including methicillin-resistant *Staph. aureus*, coagulase-negative staphylococci, *Str. agalactiae*, Lancefield group C and G streptococci, viridans group streptococci, *H. pylori*, *T. pallidum*, *C. diphtheriae* and *N. gonorrhoeae*.

Pharmacokinetics

Oral absorption	Variable
C_{max}	
base 250 mg oral	1.3 mg/l after 3–4 h
500 mg oral	2 mg/l after 2–4 h
1000 mg oral	1.3–1.5 mg/l after 4 h
stearate 250 mg oral (fasting)	0.88 mg/l after 2.2 h
500 mg oral (fasting)	2.4 mg/l after 2–4 h
500 mg oral (after food)	0.1–0.4 mg/l after 2–4 h
2′-propionate 500 mg oral (fasting)	0.4–1.9 mg/l after 2–4 h
500 mg oral (after food)	0.3–0.5 mg/l after 4 h
2′-estolate 250 mg oral (fasting)	0.36–3 mg/l after 2–4 h
500 mg oral (fasting)	1.4–5 mg/l after 1–2 h
250 mg oral (after food)	1.1–2.9 mg/l after 2–4 h
500 mg oral (after food)	1.8–5.2 mg/l after 2–4 h
lactobionate 500 mg intravenous	11.5–30 mg/l end infusion
gluceptate 250 mg intravenous	3.5–10.7 mg/l end infusion
Plasma half-life:	
base	1.6–2 h
stearate	1.6–4 h
2′-propionate	3–5 h
2′-estolate	2–4 h
lactobiobate/gluceptate	1–2 h
Volume of distribution	0.75 l/kg
Plasma protein binding:	
base	70%
propionate	93%

Absorption and metabolism

The acid lability of erythromycin base necessitates administration in a form giving protection from gastric acid. In acid media it is rapidly degraded (10% loss of activity at pH 2 in less than 4 s) by intramolecular dehydrogenation to a hemiketal and hence to anhydroerythromycin A, neither of which exert antibacterial activity. Delayed and incomplete absorption is obtained from coated tablets and there is an important inter- and intra-individual variation, adequate levels not being attained at all in a few subjects. Food delays absorption of erythromycin base. After 500 mg of the 2′-ethylsuccinyl ester, mean peak plasma levels at 1–2 h were 1.5 mg/l. In subjects given 1 g of the 2′-ethylsuccinate 12-hourly for seven doses, the mean plasma concentration 1 h after the last dose was around 1.4 mg/l. Intra- and inter-subject variation and delayed and erratic absorption in the presence of food has not yet been eliminated by new formulations. Improved 500 mg preparations of erythromycin stearate are claimed to produce peak plasma levels of 0.9–2.4 mg/l that are little affected by the presence of food. 2′-Esters of erythromycin are partially hydrolyzed to erythromycin; 2′-acetyl erythromycin is hydrolyzed more rapidly than the 2′-propionyl ester, but more slowly than the 2′-ethylsuccinate.

The stoichiometric mixture with stearate does not adequately protect erythromycin from acid degradation. After an oral dose of erythromycin stearate, equivalent concentrations of erythromycin and its main degradation product, anhydroerythromycin, could be detected.

Doses of 10 mg/kg produced mean peak plasma concentrations around 1.8 mg/l in infants weighing 1.5–2 kg and 1.2 mg/l in those weighing 2–2.5 kg. In infants less than 4 months old, 6-hourly doses of 10 mg/kg of the 2′-ethylsuccinate produced steady state plasma levels of around 1.3 mg/l. The apparent elimination half-life was 2.5 h. In children given 12.5 mg/kg of erythromycin 2′-ethylsuccinate 6-hourly, the concentration in the plasma 2 h after the fourth dose was around 0.5–2.5 mg/l.

Distribution

Only very low levels are obtained in cerebrospinal fluid (CSF), even in the presence of meningeal inflammation, and are not raised to therapeutic levels by parenteral administration of the drug. Levels of 0.1 mg/l in aqueous humor were found when the serum level was 0.36 mg/l, but there was no penetration into the vitreous. In children with otitis media given 12.5 mg/kg of erythromycin 2′-ethylsuccinate 6-hourly, concentrations in middle ear exudate were 0.25–1 mg/l. In patients with chronic serous otitis media given 12.5 mg/kg up to a maximum of the equivalent of 500 mg, none was detected in middle ear fluid, but on continued treatment levels up to 1.2 mg/l have been described. Penetration also occurs into peritoneal and pleural exudates. Mean concentrations of 2.6 mg/l have been found in sputum in patients receiving 1 g of erythromycin lactobionate intravenously 12-hourly and 0.2–2 mg/l in those receiving an oral stearate formulation. Levels in prostatic fluid are about 40% of those in the plasma. Salivary levels of around 4 mg/l were found in subjects receiving 0.5 g doses 8-hourly at 5 h after a dose, when the plasma concentration was around 5.5 mg/l. Intracellular: extracellular ratios of 4–18 have been found in polymorphonuclear neutrophils.

Fetal tissue levels are considerably higher after multiple doses; when the mean peak maternal serum level was 4.94

(0.66–8) mg/l, the mean concentration in fetal blood was 0.06 (0–0.12) mg/l and in amniotic fluid 0.36 (0.32–0.39) mg/l. Concentrations were more than 0.3 mg/l in most other fetal tissues, but the concentrations were variable and unmeasurable in some. Erythromycin appears to be concentrated by fetal liver.

Excretion

Erythromycin is excreted both in urine and in the bile but only a fraction of the dose can be accounted for in this way. Only about 2.5% of an oral dose or 15% of an intravenous dose is recovered unchanged in the urine. Urinary concentrations in patients receiving 1 g of erythromycin base daily have been reported to be 13–46 mg/l. It is not removed to any significant extent by peritoneal dialysis or hemodialysis. Reported changes in apparent elimination half-life in renal impairment may be related to the saturable nature of protein binding. Fairly high concentrations (50–250 mg/l) are found in the bile, the bile: serum concentration ratio in those receiving the base being about 30. In cirrhotic patients receiving 500 mg of the base, peak plasma levels were higher and earlier than in healthy volunteers (2.0 and 1.5 mg/l at 4.6 and 6.3 h, respectively). The apparent elimination half-life was 6.6 h. It is possible that the smaller excretion of the 2′-propionyl ester in the bile in comparison to the base accounts in part for its better-maintained serum levels. There is some enterohepatic recycling, but some of the administered dose is lost in the feces, producing concentrations of around 0.5 mg/g.

Interactions

Interaction with the hepatic metabolism of other drugs can result in clinically significant potentiation of the action of carbamazepine, cyclosporin, methylprednisolone, theophylline, midazolam, terfenadine and warfarin and in adverse responses to digoxin and ergot alkaloids.

Toxicity and side effects

Oral administration, especially of large doses, commonly causes epigastric distress, nausea and vomiting, which may be severe. Solutions are very irritant: intravenous infusions almost invariably produce thrombophlebitis. Cholestatic hepatitis occurs rarely. Transient auditory disturbances have been described after intravenous administration of the lactobionate salt, and occasionally in patients with renal and hepatic impairment in whom oral dosage has produced high plasma levels. Sensorineural hearing impairment can occur and, although this is usually a reversible effect which occurs at high dosage, can be permanent. Prolongation of the apparent elimination half-life of carbamazepine, due to inhibition of its conversion to the epoxide, usually results in central nervous system (CNS) disturbances. Nightmares are troublesome in some patients. Allergic effects occur in about 0.5% of patients.

The estolate is particularly prone to give rise to liver abnormalities. These consist of upper abdominal pain, fever, hepatic enlargement, a raised serum bilirubin, with or without actual jaundice, pale stools and dark urine and eosinophilia. The condition, which is rare and usually seen 10–20 days after the initiation of treatment, may mimic viral hepatitis, cholecystitis, pancreatitis or cardiac infarction, and on stopping the drug recovery has been complete. Once patients have recovered, recurrence of symptoms can be induced by giving the estolate but not by giving the base or stearate. There is evidence that erythromycin estolate is more toxic to isolated liver cells than is the 2′-propionate or the base, and it is suggested that the essential molecular feature responsible for toxicity is the propionyl–ester linkage. The relative frequency of the reaction and its rapidity of onset (within hours) after second courses of the drug, peripheral eosinophilia and other evidence of hypersensitivity, and the histological appearance suggest a mixture of hepatic cholestasis, liver cell necrosis and hypersensitivity. Abnormal liver function tests in patients receiving the estolate must be interpreted with caution, since increased level of transaminases is often the only abnormality and some metabolites of the estolate can interfere with the measurement commonly used. Elevated levels of transaminases return to normal after cessation of treatment. Serum bilirubin is generally unchanged in these patients, but γ-glutamyl transpeptidase may also be affected.

Clinical use

- Lower and upper respiratory tract infections (including those caused by atypical and intracellular pathogens).
- Legionellosis (alone or in combination with rifampicin).
- Skin and soft-tissue infections.
- *Campylobacter* infection.
- Syphilis (penicillin-allergic patients).
- Whooping cough.
- Diphtheria (including treatment of carriers).

Concentrations found in middle ear exudate are unlikely to be sufficient to inhibit *H. influenzae* isolates, which is a common cause of otitis media in children.

Preparations and dosage

Proprietary names: Erythrocin, Ilosone and many generic forms.

Preparations: Tablets film coated (as ethyl succinate and stearate), suspension (as ethyl succinate), capsules, injection (as lactobionate).

Dosage: Adults and children >8 years, oral, 250–500 mg every 6 h or 0.5–1 g every 12 h, up to 4 g/day for severe infections. Children up to 2 years, oral, 125 mg every 6 h; 2–8 years, 250 mg every 6 h; doses doubled for severe infection. Adults, children, i.v., 50 mg/kg per day by continuous i.v. infusion or in divided doses every 6 h for severe infections; 25 mg/kg per day for mild infections when oral treatment is not possible.

Widely available.

Further information

Anonymous 1999 Erythromycin. In: Dollery C (ed.) *Therapeutic Drugs* 2nd edn. Churchill Livingstone, Edinburgh, pp. E50–E54.

Barre J, Mallatt A, Rosembaum J et al 1987 Pharmacokinetics of erythromycin in patients with severe cirrhosis. Respective influence of decreased serum binding and impaired liver metabolic capacity. *British Journal of Clinical Pharmacology* 23: 753–757.

Brummett RE, Fox KE 1989 Vancomycin- and erythromycin-induced hearing loss in humans. *Antimicrobial Agents and Chemotherapy* 33: 791–796.

Carter BL, Woodhead JC, Cole KJ, Milavetz G 1987 Gastrointestinal side effects with erythromycin preparations. *Drug Intelligence and Clinical Pharmacy* 21: 734–738.

Descotes J, Andre P, Evreux JC 1985 Pharmacokinetic drug interactions with macrolide antibiotics. *Journal of Antimicrobial Chemotherapy* 15: 659–664.

Eady EA, Ross JJ, Cove JH 1990 Multiple mechanisms of erythromycin resistance. *Journal of Antimicrobial Chemotherapy* 26: 461–465.

Gupta SK, Bakran A, Johnson RW, Rowland M 1989 Cyclosporin-erythromycin interaction in renal transplant patients. *British Journal of Clinical Pharmacology* 27: 475–481.

Inman WAW, Rawson NSB 1983 Erythromycin estolate and jaundice. *British Medical Journal* 286(1): 1954–1957.

Kanfer A, Stamatakis G, Torlotin JC, Fredt G, Kenouch S, Mery JP 1987 Changes in erythromycin pharmacokinetics induced by renal failure. *Clinical Nephrology* 27: 147–150.

Larrey D, Funck-Bretano C, Brell P et al 1983 Effects of erythromycin on hepatic drug metabolising enzymes in humans. *Biochemical Pharmacology* 32: 1063–1068.

Miles MV, Tennison MB 1989 Erythromycin effects on multiple-dose carbamazepine kinetics. *Therapeutic Drug Monitoring* 11: 47–52.

Paulsen O, Hoglund P, Nilsson LG, Bengtsson HI 1987 The interaction of erythromycin with theophylline. *European Journal of Clinical Pharmacology* 32: 493–498.

Peeters T, Matthijs G, Depoortere I, Cachet T, Hoogmartens J, Vantrappen G 1989 Erythromycin is a motilin receptor agonist. *American Journal of Physiology* 257: G470–474.

Scott RJ, Naidoo J, Lightfoot NF, George RC 1989 A community outbreak of group A beta haemolytic streptococci with transferable resistance to erythromycin. *Epidemiology and Infection* 102: 85–91.

Umstead GS, Neumann KH 1986 Erythromycin ototoxicity and acute psychotic reaction in cancer patients with hepatic dysfunction. *Archives of Internal Medicine* 146: 897–899.

Weisblum B 1984 Inducible erythromycin resistance in bacteria. *British Medical Bulletin* 40: 47–53.

ROXITHROMYCIN

Molecular weight: 837.04.

A semisynthetic derivative of erythromycin A formulated for oral use.

Antibacterial activity

Its activity against common pathogens is shown in Table 24.1 (p. 311). The antibacterial spectrum is comparable to that of erythromycin. It is inactive against Enterobacteriaceae and *Pseudomonas* spp. It is active against *L. monocytogenes*, *C. jejuni*, *H. ducreyi*, *G. vaginalis*, *Bord. pertussis*, *C. diphtheriae*, *B. burgdorferi*, *H. pylori*, the *M. avium* complex, *Chlamydia* spp., and *U. urealyticum*. Its activity against respiratory pathogens is shown in Table 24.2 (p. 312).

Pharmacokinetics

Oral absorption	50–55%
C_{max} 150 mg oral	7.9 mg/l after 1.9 h
300 mg oral	10.8 mg/l after 1.5 h
Plasma half-life	10.5–11.9 h
Protein binding	c. 90%

Absorption

Absorption is not affected by food. Oral administration with antacids or H_2-receptor antagonists does not significantly affect bioavailability. In a direct comparison, the AUC produced by a 150 mg dose was 16.2 times greater than that produced by 250 mg erythromycin A. Multiple doses produced similar differences.

Behavior in children is broadly similar to that in adults, repeated doses of 2.5 mg/kg producing age-independent mean peak plasma concentrations around 10 mg/l at 1–2 h, but the apparent elimination half-life was longer (approximately 20 h).

Roxithromycin is saturably bound to α_1-acid glycoprotein in plasma. The plasma clearance appears to be dose dependent or plasma concentration dependent.

Distribution

It is widely distributed, but does not reach the CSF. Concentrations close to the simultaneous serum level have been found in tonsillar, lung and prostatic tissue, myometrium, endometrium and synovial fluid. It achieves high levels in skin.

Excretion

Less than 5% of the administered dose is eliminated as degradation products. Rather more than half the dose appears in the feces and only 7–10% (including metabolites) in the urine; up to 15% is eliminated via the lungs. Renal clearance increased in volunteers as the dose was raised from 150 to 450 mg, and is decreased in elderly subjects. In patients in whom the creatinine clearance was <10 ml/min, the apparent elimination half-life rose to around 15.5 h and total body clearance was significantly reduced. The apparent elimination half-life was somewhat increased in patients with hepatic cirrhosis.

Interactions

The half-life of simultaneously administered theophylline is increased by about 10%, but there is no effect on that of carbamazepine and no interaction with warfarin or cyclosporin.

Toxicity and side effects

Roxithromycin is generally well tolerated, adverse effects being described in 3–4% of patients, mostly gastrointestinal disturbance (notably abdominal pain, nausea and diarrhea). Headache, weakness, dizziness, rash and reversible changes in liver function tests and increased eosinophils and platelets have also been described.

Clinical use

- Upper and lower respiratory tract infections.
- Skin and soft-tissue infections.
- Urogenital infections.
- Orodental infections.

Preparations and dosage

Proprietary name: Rulid, Surlid.

Dosage: Adults, oral, 150 mg twice daily or 300 mg once daily. Children, oral, 2.5–5 mg/kg twice daily.

Available in Europe, Japan, Africa, Latin America, South East Asia, Middle-East, Indian subcontinent.

Further information

Bryskier A 1998 Roxithromycin: review of its antimicrobial activity *Journal of Antimicrobial Chemotherapy* 41: 1–21.

Phillips I, Péchère J-C, Speller D 1987 Roxithromycin: a new macrolide. *Journal of Antimicrobial Chemotherapy* 21 (Suppl. B).

Young LS, Lode H 1995 Roxithromycin: first of a new generation of macrolides: update and perspectives. *Infection* 23 (Suppl. 1).

OTHER GROUP 1 MACROLIDES

Flurithromycin

A semisynthetic derivative of erythromycin A, supplied for oral administration. It was first isolated when (*S*)-8-fluoroerythronolide A was added to the fermentation broth of a blocked mutant of an erythromycin-producing strain of *Saccharopolyspora erythraea*. Flurithromycin is also obtained by fluorination of 8,9-anhydroerythromycin-6,8-hemiketal *N*-oxide. It is stable at acid pH due to the presence of the fluorine atom at C-8 of the erythronolide A ring.

Antibacterial activity

The drug is active against most streptococci, including *Str. pneumoniae* and *Str. agalactiae* (MIC$_{50}$ 0.03 mg/l). It has little or no activity against *H. influenzae*. It is active against *Mor. catarrhalis*, *N. gonorrhoeae* (MIC$_{50}$ 0.04 mg/l), *C. trachomatis* (MIC 0.06–0.125 mg/l), *M. genitalium* (MIC$_{50}$ 0.007 mg/l), and *U. urealyticum* (MIC$_{50}$ 0.03 mg/l). It is inactive against *Mycoplasma. hominis*. Activity against anaerobes is similar to that of erythromycin A. It displays cross-resistance with erythromycin A.

Pharmacokinetics

A single 500 mg oral dose achieved a mean peak plasma concentration of 1.2–2 mg/l after 1–2 h; the AUC was 16.2 mg.h/l. The apparent elimination half-life was 8 h and the volume of distribution 5.5 l/kg. With repeated doses (500 mg orally three times daily for 10 doses), plasma concentrations were 0.72 mg/l immediately before and 0.67 mg/l at 4 h after the last dose. Absorption is not significantly affected by food. After administration of a single 375 mg tablet of flurithromycin ethylsuccinate, the mean serum levels at 0.5 h were 0.43 ± 0.35 mg/l. The mean peak serum concentration (1.41 ± 0.49 mg/l) was achieved at 1 h. At 8 and 12 h, the serum levels were 0.14 (±0.05) and 0.04 (± 0.04) mg/l, respectively. The apparent elimination half-life is 3.94 (±1.42) h. The apparent half-life in artificial gastric juice was about 40 min.

Flurithromycin is generally well tolerated and has been used successfully for the treatment of lower respiratory tract infections.

Proprietary name: Flurizic, Mizar, Ritro.

Limited availability.

Further information

Bariffi F, Clini V, Ginesu F, Mangiarotti P, Romoli L, Gialdroni-Grassi G 1994 Flurithromycin ethylsuccinate in the treatment of lower respiratory tract bacterial infections. *Infection* 22: 226–230.

Benonl G, Cuzzolin L, Leone R et al 1988 Pharmacokinetics and human tissue distribution of flurithromycin. *Antimicrobial Agents and Chemotherapy* 32: 1875–1878.

Cocuza CE, Mattina R, Lanzafame A, Romoli L, Lepore AM 1994 Serum levels of flurithromycin ethylsuccinate in healthy volunteers. *Chemotherapy* 40: 157–160.

Nord CE, Lindmark A, Persson I 1988 Comparative antimicrobial activity of the new macrolide flurithromycin against respiratory pathogens. *European Journal of Clinical Microbiology and Infectious Diseases* 7: 71–73.

Oleandomycin

A natural 14-membered-ring macrolide produced by *Streptomyces antibioticus*. It is stable in acid conditions.

Oleandomycin is less active than erythromycin A in vitro, but four times more active than spiramycin (Table 24.1;

p. 311). Several attempts have been made to improve its potency by chemical modification while retaining its relative acid stability.

It is incompletely absorbed, but an ester, triacetyloleandomycin, gives improved plasma levels. Following doses of 0.5 g, mean peak serum levels around 0.8 mg/l were reached by the base and 2 mg/l by the triacetyl ester. A single oral dose of 1 g of the ester produced a mean plasma oleandomycin concentration of 4.0 mg/l at 1 h after dosing, with an AUC of 14 mg.h/l. The apparent elimination half-life was 4.2 h. Significant quantities of mostly inactivated compound are eliminated in the bile. About 10% of the dose appears in the urine after administration of the base and about 20% after the ester.

Nausea, vomiting and diarrhea are common. Like erythromycin estolate, triacetyloleandomycin can cause liver damage. Abnormal liver function tests were found in about a third of patients treated for 2 weeks. Hepatic dysfunction resolved when treatment was discontinued. The action of drugs eliminated via the cytochrome P_{450} system may be potentiated.

Its uses are similar to those of erythromycin.

Proprietary name: TAO.

 Further information

Koch R, Asay LD 1958 Oleandomycin, a laboratory and clinical evaluation. *Journal of Pediatrics* 53: 676–682.

Ticktin HE, Zimmerman HJ 1962 Hepatic dysfunction and jaundice in patients receiving triacetyloleandomycin. *New England Journal of Medicine* 267: 964–968.

GROUP 2: 16-MEMBERED-RING MACROLIDES

 ## SPIRAMYCIN

Molecular weight (spiramycin 1): 843.

A fermentation product of *Streptomyces ambofaciens*, composed of several closely related compounds. Spiramycin 1 is the major component (*c.* 63%); spiramycins 2 and 3 are the acetate and monoproprionate esters, respectively. It is available for oral administration and as spiramycin adipate for intravenous infusion. Spiramycins are relatively stable in acid conditions.

Antibacterial activity

Its activity against common pathogens is shown in Table 24.1 (p. 311). *L. pneumophila* is inhibited by 1–4 mg/l and *Campylobacter* spp. by 0.5–16 mg/l. Enterobacteriaceae are resistant. Spiramycin is active against anaerobic species also: *Actinomyces israelii* (MIC 2–4 mg/l), *C. perfringens* (MIC 2–8 mg/l) and *Bacteroides* spp (MIC 4–14 mg/l). It is also active against *Toxoplasma gondii*.

Pharmacokinetics

Oral absorption	Variable
C_{max} 1 g oral	2.8 mg/l after 2 h
Plasma half-life	4–8 h
Volume of distribution	383 l
Plasma protein binding	15%

In healthy volunteers given 2 g orally followed by 1 g 6-hourly, peak plasma levels were 1.0–6.7 mg/l. After 1 g orally the AUC was 10.8 mg.h/l, with an apparent elimination half-life of 2.8 h. It is widely distributed in the tissues. It does not reach the CSF. Levels 12 h after a dose of 1 g were 0.25 mg/l in serum, 5.3 mg/l in bone and 6.9 mg/l in pus. Levels of 10.6 mg/l have been found 4 h after dosing in saliva, and concentrations at least equal to those in the serum are seen in bronchial secretions. A concentration of 27 mg/g was found in prostate tissues after repeated dosage. Only 5–15% is recovered from the urine. Most is metabolized, but significant quantities are eliminated via the bile, in which concentrations up to 40 times those in the serum may be found.

Toxicity and side effects

Spiramycin is generally well tolerated, the most common adverse reactions being gastrointestinal disturbances, notably abdominal pain, nausea and vomiting, rashes and sensitization following contact.

Clinical use

- Respiratory tract infections.
- Toxoplasmosis (especially in pregnancy).

Preparations and dosage

Proprietary name: Rovamycine.

Preparations: Tablets, capsules; intravenous formulation (spiramycin adipate).

Dosage: Adults, oral, 2–4 g/day in two divided doses; i.v., 0.5–1 g every 8 h. Children, oral, 50–100 mg/kg per day in divided doses.

Limited availability.

Further information

Anonymous 1999 Spiramycin. In: Dollery C (ed.) *Therapeutic Drugs* 2nd edn. Churchill Livingstone, Edinburgh, pp. S85–S88.
Davey P, Speller D, Daly PJ 1988 Spiramycin reassessed. *Journal of Antimicrobial Chemotherapy* 22 (Suppl. B).
Shah P, Simon C 1990 Neue Makrolide. *Fortschritte der Antimikrobiellen und Antineoplastichen Chemotherapie* (Suppl.): 9–1.
Symposium 1988 Spiramycin reassessed. *Journal of Antimicrobial Chemotherapy* 22 (Suppl. B): 1–210.
Vernillet L, Bertault-Peres P, Berland Y, Barradas J, Durand A, Olmer M 1989 Lack of effect of spiramycin on cyclosporin pharmacokinetics. *British Journal of Clinical Pharmacology* 27: 789–794.

OTHER GROUP 2 MACROLIDES

Josamycin

A naturally occurring antibiotic produced by *Streptomyces narbonensis* var. *josamyceticus* and belonging to the leucomycin group of macrolides. It is formulated for oral administration.

Activity is comparable to that of erythromycin A (Table 24.1; p. 311), susceptible organisms being inhibited by ≤2 mg/l. Many Gram-positive and Gram-negative anaerobes are susceptible, including *Peptostreptococcus* spp., *Propionibacterium* spp., *Eubacterium* spp. and *Bacteroides* spp.

After a single 1 g oral dose, a peak serum concentration of 2.74 mg/l was achieved 0.75 h after dosing. The AUC was 4.2 mg.h/l, and the apparent elimination half-life 1.5 h. Several inactive metabolites could be detected. Josamycin penetrates into saliva, tears and sweat, and achieves high levels in bile and lungs. It is mostly metabolized and excreted in the bile in an inactive form. Less than 20% of the dose appears in the urine, producing levels of around 50 mg/l.

The drug is generally well tolerated, producing only mild gastrointestinal disturbance. Its uses are similar to those of erythromycin.

Preparations and dosage

Proprietary name: Josacine

Dosage: Adults, oral, 1–2 g/day in two or more divided doses. Children, oral, 30–75 mg/kg/day in 2–4 divided doses.

Available in some European countries and Japan.

Further information

Chabbert YA, Modai J 1985 Perspectives josamycine – Symposium International du 16–18 mai 1985, Lisbones. *Médicine et Maladies Infectieuses* (Suppl.).
Maskell JP, Sefton AM, Cannell H et al 1990 Predominance of resistant oral streptococci in saliva and the effect of a single course of josamycin or erythromycin. *Journal of Antimicrobial Chemotherapy* 26: 539–548.

Kitasamycin (leucomycin)

A naturally occurring product of *Streptomyces kitasatoensis*, available in Japan for parenteral and oral use, and as acetyl-kitasamycin for topical application. Elsewhere it is chiefly used in veterinary medicine.

Midecamycin

A naturally occurring metabolite of *Streptomyces mycarofaciens*, supplied as the native compound and as midecamycin acetate for oral administration.

The antibacterial spectrum is comparable to that of erythromycin A, but it is less active (Table 24.1; p. 311). It is rapidly and extensively metabolized and is said to exhibit less toxicity than earlier macrolides.

Preparations and dosage

Proprietary names: Mosil, Aboren, Macropen, Medemycin, Midecin, Miocamen.

Dosage: Adults, oral, 0.8–1.6 g/day in divided doses.

Available in Japan, Italy and France.

Further information

Neu HC 1983 In vitro activity of midecamycin, a new macrolide antibiotic. *Antimicrobial Agents and Chemotherapy* 24: 443–444.

Miokamycin

A semisynthetic diacetyl derivative of midecamycin A₁, it exhibits a bimodal distribution of MICs for *H. influenzae* and *E. faecalis* (Table 24.1; p. 311). It is rapidly and extensively metabolized (about 12 metabolites, some of which exhibit good antibacterial activity).

Absorption of dry formulations of miokamycin is unaffected by food, whereas absorption of the oral suspension is delayed. In various studies the peak plasma concentration was 1.65, 1.31–3 and 1.3–2.7 mg/l after doses of 400, 600 and 800 mg, respectively.

Miokamycin is said to exhibit less toxicity than earlier macrolides. Attention has been paid to its interaction with theophylline, which resembles that of other macrolides.

Preparations and dosage

Proprietary name: Merced.

Preparations: Tablets, granules, sachets.

Dosage: Adults, oral, 0.9–1.8 g/day in two or three divided doses. Children > 1 year, oral, 35–55 mg/kg/day in two or three divided doses.

Available in some European countries.

Further information

Lacey RW, Lord VL, Howson GL 1984 In vitro evaluation of miokamycin bactericidal activity against streptococci. *Journal of Antimicrobial Chemotherapy* 13: 5–13.

Obadia L 1985 Results obtained with miocamycin in the treatment of pyodermas in children. *Recent Advances in Chemotherapy* 2: 1461–1462.

Principi N, Onorato J, Giuliani MG, Vigano A 1987 Effect of miokamycin on theophylline levels in children. *European Journal of Clinical Pharmacology* 31: 701–704.

Rimoldi R, Bandera M, Fioretti M, Giorcelli R 1986 Miokamycin and theophylline blood levels. *Chemiotherapia* 5: 213–216.

Rokitamycin

3″-Propionyl leucomycin A$_5$. A semisynthetic macrolide. Unstable in acid media.

The antibacterial spectrum is identical to that of erythromycin A, but it is less active against Gram-positive cocci. It is active against *Staph. aureus* (MIC$_{50}$ 0.5 mg/l), *Str. pyogenes* (MIC$_{50}$ < 0.05 mg/l), *Str. pneumoniae* (MIC$_{50}$ 0.25 mg/l) and *E. faecalis* (MIC$_{50}$ 0.5 mg/l). It is poorly active against *H. influenzae* (MIC$_{50}$ 8 mg/l) and *Mor. catarrhalis* (MIC$_{50}$ 4 mg/l). It displays good activity against *Campylobacter* spp. (MIC$_{50}$ 0.1 mg/l), *L. pneumophila* (MIC$_{50}$ 0.1 mg/l) and *Mycoplasma. pneumoniae* (MIC$_{50}$ 0.003 mg/l). It is active against anaerobes, including *Peptostreptococcus* spp. (MIC$_{50}$ < 0.05 mg/l) and some species of the *Bacteroides* group (MIC$_{50}$ < 0.05 mg/l).

After a single oral dose of 600 mg, the peak plasma concentration was 1.9 mg/l after 0.6 h. The AUC is 3.72 mg.h/l, with an apparent elimination half-life of 2.0 h. Oral doses of 5, 10 and 15 mg/kg of a syrup formulation given to children achieved plasma concentrations of 0.26, 0.55 and 0.79 mg/l respectively after about 40 min; the half-life was around 2 h.

Rokitamycin is mainly eliminated in the bile and only about 2% appears in the urine. Its major metabolites are leucomycin A$_7$ 10″-OH-rokitamycin (which show some antibacterial activity) and leucomycin V. In healthy adult volunteers, the proportions of rokitamycin and its metabolites in serum 30 min after a single oral dose of 1200 mg were 18% (leucomycin A$_7$), 33% (10″-OH-rokitamycin) and 9% (leucomycin V). The pharmacokinetic behavior is not altered in patients with liver cirrhosis.

Preparations and dosage

Proprietary names: Paidocin, Ricamycin, Rokital.

Preparations: Tablets, granules.

Dosage: Adults, oral, 400 mg twice daily. Children, oral, 20–40 mg/kg/day in two divided doses.

Available in Italy and Japan.

GROUP 3: AZALIDES

AZITHROMYCIN

Molecular weight (dihydrate): 785.

A semisynthetic derivative of erythromycin A, supplied as the dihydrate for oral administration.

Antibacterial activity

Activity in vitro against common bacterial pathogens is shown in Table 24.1 (p. 311). It is less potent than erythromycin A against Gram-positive isolates, but is more active against Gram-negative bacteria. It is four times more potent than erythromycin A against *H. influenzae*, *N. gonorrhoeae* and *Campylobacter* spp., and twice as active against *Mor. catarrhalis*. It also exhibits superior potency against all of the Enterobacteriaceae, notably *Esch. coli*, *Salmonella enterica* serotypes, and *Shigella* spp. It is active against *Mycobacteria*, notably the *M. avium* complex and against intracellular microorganisms such as *Legionella* and *Chlamydia* spp.

Pharmacokinetics

Oral absorption	37%
C$_{max}$ 250 mg oral	0.17 mg/l after 2.2 h
500 mg oral	0.4 mg/l after 2 h
Plasma half-life (terminal)	11–40 h
Volume of distribution	31 l/kg
Plasma protein binding	7–50%

Chemical modification at the 9 position of the erythronolide A ring of erythromycin A blocks the internal ketalization and markedly improves acid stability. At pH 2, loss of 10% activity occurred in less than 4 s with erythromycin A, but took 20 min with azithromycin. The AUC at 0–24 h is 4.5 mg.h/l. The level is only slightly increased on repeated dosing.

Binding to plasma protein varies with the concentration, from around 50% at 0.05 mg/l to 7.1% at 1 mg/l. The apparent elimination half-life is dependent upon sampling interval: between 8 and 24 h it ranged from 11 to 14 h; between 24 h and 72 h it was 35–40 h.

Azithromycin rapidly penetrates the tissues, reaching levels that approach, or in some cases, exceed, the simultaneous plasma levels and persist for 2–3 days. Only about 6% of the dose was recovered from the urine in the first 24 h.

Toxicity and side effects

Azithromycin is well tolerated with little gastrointestinal disturbance.

Clinical use

- Lower and upper respiratory tract infections.
- Skin and soft-tissue infections.
- Uncomplicated urethritis/cervicitis associated with *N. gonorrhoeae*, *C. trachomatis* or *U. urealyticum*.
- Trachoma.

Preparations and dosage

Proprietary name: Zithromax.

Preparations: Capsules, tablets, suspension.

Dosage: Adults, oral, 500 mg/day for 3 days. Children >6 months, 10 mg/kg once daily for 3 days; body weight 15–25 kg, 200 mg/day for 3 days; body weight 26–35 kg, 300 mg/day for 3 days; body weight 36–45 kg, 400 mg/day for 3 days.

Widely available.

Further information

Anonymous 1999 Azithromycin. In: Dollery C (ed.) *Therapeutic Drugs* 2nd edn. Churchill Livingstone, Edinburgh, pp. A261–A265.

Leigh DA, Ridgway GL, Leeming JP, Speller DCE 1990 Azithromycin (CP 62,993): the first azalide antimicrobial agent. *Journal of Antimicrobial Chemotherapy* 25 (Suppl. A).

GROUP 4: KETOLIDES

TELITHROMYCIN

Molecular weight: 812.

A 14-membered-ring ketolide, obtained by semisynthesis from erythromycin A. Formulated for oral administration.

Antibacterial activity

The activity against common bacterial pathogens is shown in Table 24.1 (p. 311). The spectrum covers Gram-positive and Gram-negative cocci, Gram-positive bacilli, fastidious Gram-negative bacilli, atypical mycobacteria, *M. leprae*, *H. pylori*, anaerobes, *T. pallidum*, intracellular pathogens and atypical organisms.

Telithromycin exhibits bactericidal activity in vitro against isolates of *Str. pneumoniae* regardless of the underlying resistance to penicillin G, erythromycin A and other agents. It is two to four times more active than clarithromycin against erythromycin A-susceptible isolates of *Str. pneumoniae* and other streptococci. Against *H. influenzae* the MIC range is 1–4 mg/l. It also exhibits good in-vitro activity against *Coxiella burnetii* (MIC 1 mg/l) and various Gram-positive species, including viridans streptococci (MIC ≤ 0.015–0.25 mg/l), *C. diphtheriae* (MIC 0.004–0.008 mg/l) and *Listeria* spp. (MIC 0.03–0.25 mg/l).

Unlike macrolides, it inhibits protein synthesis by acting in two parts of the peptidyl transferase loop and by inhibiting the formation of ribosomal subunits.

Acquired resistance

Telithromycin retains activity against isolates resistant to erythromycin A. *Str. pneumoniae* and *Str. pyogenes* isolates for which the MIC of telithromycin is above the resistance breakpoint of 2.0 mg/l are presently rare. It is not active against *Staph. aureus* isolates that owe their resistance to erythromycin to constitutive methylation of adenine 2058 on domain V of the peptidyl transferase loop.

Pharmacokinetics

Oral absorption	90%
C_{max} 800 mg oral	1.9–2.27 mg/l (steady state after 2–3 days)
Plasma half-life	10–12 h
Volume of distribution	210 l
Plasma protein binding	60–70%

After oral administration the absolute bioavailability is 57% in both young and elderly subjects. The rate and extent of absorption are not influenced by food. In a study of ascending doses administered to healthy volunteers, peak plasma concentration ranged from 0.8 mg/l (400 mg dose) to 6 mg/l (2400 mg). The peak plasma concentration was reached after 1–2 h. The apparent elimination half-lives ranged from 10–14 h, with an AUC of 2.6 mg.h/l (400 mg) to 43.3 mg.h/l (2400 mg). After oral repeated doses the ratios between day 1 and day 10 ranged from 1.3 to 1.5. After once-daily oral dosing with 800 mg, the AUC is 8.25 mg.h/l. Concentrations in alveolar macrophages, epithelial lining fluid, and bronchial tissue are shown in Table 24.5.

Table 24.5 Telithromycin concentration in respiratory tissue (800 mg oral daily dose)

	Mean concentrations (mg/l)			
	2–3 h	6–8 h	12 h	24 h
Epithelial lining fluid	5.4–14.9	4.2	3.3	0.8–1.2
Alveolar macrophages	65–69	100	3.8	41–162
Bronchial tissues	0.68–3.9	2.2	1.4	0.7
Tonsils	3.95	–	0.9	0.7

Toxicity and side effects

Telithromycin was well tolerated during clinical trials. The main adverse event was diarrhea.

Clinical use

- Lower and upper respiratory tracts infections in adult patients (community-acquired pneumonia, acute exacerbations of chronic bronchitis, acute bacterial maxillary sinusitis and pharyngitis).

Preparations and dosage

Proprietary name: Ketek.

Preparation: Tablet (400 mg).

Dosage: Adults, oral, 800 mg once daily.

Available (2002) in Europe, Latin America, Australia.

Further information

Bryskier A 2001 Telithromycin – an innovative ketolide antimicrobial. *Japanese Journal of Antibiotics* 54 (Suppl. A): 64–69.

Champney WS, Tober CL 1998 Inhibition of translation and 50 S ribosomal subunit formation in *Staphylococcus aureus* cells by 11 different ketolide antibiotics. *Current Microbiology* 37: 418–425.

Denis A, Agouridas C et al 1999 Synthesis and antibacterial activity of HMR 3647, a new ketolide highly potent against erythromycin-resistant and -susceptible pathogens. *Bioorg Med Chem Lett* 9: 3075–3080.

Hansen LH, Mauvais P, Douthwaite S 1999 The macrolide-ketolide antibiotic binding site is formed by structures in domain II and V of 23S ribosomal RNA. *Molecular Microbiology* 31: 623–631.

Vazifeh D, Preira A, Bryskier A, Labro MT 1998 Interactions between HMR 3647, a new ketolide, and human polymorphonuclear neutrophils. *Antimicrobial Agents and Chemotherapy* 42: 1944–1951.

OTHER KETOLIDES

ABT 773

A semisynthetic derivative of erythromycin A. It is a C11–C12 carbamate ketolide and has an unsaturated chain with a quinoline ring at the C-6 position. It has the same antibacterial spectrum as telithromycin. Typical MIC values are: 0.016–0.06 mg/l (*Str. pneumoniae*); 0.015–0.015 mg/l (*Str. pyogenes*); 2.0–4.0 mg/l (*H. influenzae*, irrespective of β-lactamase production); 0.03–0.12 mg/l (*Mor. catarrhalis*); 2.0–4.0 mg/l 0.03–0.06 mg/l; 0.015–0.015 mg/l (*Chlamydophila pneumoniae*); 0.016–0.064 mg/l (*Legionella* spp.) (*Staph. aureus*, susceptible or resistant to methicillin).

The apparent elimination half-life ranges from 3.6 to 6.7 h. In an escalating oral dose study, the peak plasma concentration ranged from 0.14 mg/l (100 mg dose) to 1.2 mg/l (1200 mg) after 0.5–5.1 h. The AUC ranged from 0.63 mg.h/l (100 mg) to 11.0 mg.h/l (1200 mg) with a total clearance of 183–254 l/h.

Clinical efficacy in respiratory tract infections is currently under investigation.

Further information

Barry AL, Fuchs PC, Brown SD 2001 In vitro activity of ABT 773. *Antimicrobial Agents and Chemotherapy* 45: 2922–2924.

Brueggemann AB, Doern GV, Huynh HK, Wingert EM, Rhomberg PR 2000 In vitro activity of ABT 773, a new ketolide, against recent clinical isolates of *Streptococcus pneumoniae*, *Haemophilus influenzae* and *Moraxella catarrhalis*. *Antimicrobial Agents and Chemotherapy* 44: 447–449.

Davies TA, Ednie LM, Hoellman DM, Panduch GA, Jacob MR, Appelbaum PC 2000 Antipneumococcal activity of ABT-773 compared to those of 10 other agents. *Antimicrobial Agents and Chemotherapy* 44: 1894–1899.

Edelstein PH, Higa F, Edelstein MAC 2001 In vitro activity of ABT 773 against *Legionella pneumophila*, its pharmacokinetics in guinea pigs, and its use to treat guinea pigs with *Legionella pneumonia*. *Antimicrobial Agents and Chemotherapy* 45: 2685–2690.

Strigl S, Roblin PM, Reznik T, Hammerschlag MR 2000 In vitro activity of ABT 773, a new ketolide antibiotic, against *Chlamydia pneumoniae*. *Antimicrobial Agents and Chemotherapy* 44: 1112–1113.

25 Mupirocin

M. W. Casewell

A fermentation product of *Pseudomonas fluorescens* formerly called 'pseudomonic acid'. It is supplied as the calcium salt or, for the ointment, as the free acid. It is structurally unlike any other antimicrobial agent, and contains a unique hydroxynonanoic moiety linked to monic acid.

There are four pseudomonic acids (A, B, C and D) of which that available commercially is A:

Antimicrobial activity

Activity against common bacterial pathogens is shown in Table 25.1. Other susceptible organisms include *Mycoplasma* spp. and some dermatophytes. *Enterococcus faecium* is usually

Table 25.1 Activity of mupirocin against some common pathogenic bacteria: MIC (mg/l)

Species	MIC
Staphylococcus aureus (including MRSA)	0.01–0.25
Coagulase-negative staphylococci	0.01–4.0
Streptococcus pyogenes	0.06–0.5
Streptococcus pneumoniae	0.06–0.5
Enterococcus faecalis	16–R
Enterococcus faecium	1.0–4.0
Neisseria gonorrhoeae	0.03–0.25
Neisseria meningitidis	0.03–0.25
Haemophilus influenzae	0.003–0.25
Enterobacter spp.	R
Pseudomonas aeruginosa	R
Bacteroides fragilis	R

R, resistant (MIC >64 mg/l).

susceptible in contrast to *Enterococcus faecalis*, which is resistant. It is slowly bactericidal. Activity against *Staphylococcus aureus* (including methicillin-resistant *Staph. aureus*; MRSA) is much affected by inoculum size and pH, with enhanced activity at the acid pH (5.5) of the skin. In the anterior nares its anti-staphylococcal activity is not decreased by nasal secretions.

Acquired resistance

Before the introduction of mupirocin, naturally resistant strains of *Staph. aureus* were rare, occurring in most studies with a frequency of 1 in 10^9. Low-level resistance (MIC 8–256 mg/l) in *Staph. aureus* is of dubious clinical significance and can be produced in vitro by passage in the presence of mupirocin and in patients by prolonged topical treatment of the anterior nares during MRSA outbreaks. High-level transferable resistance (MIC >256 mg/l), for which coagulase-negative staphylococci may be the source, has been observed following prolonged topical use for dermatological conditions or nasal application in some prolonged hospital outbreaks of MRSA.

Pharmacokinetics

On parenteral injection, it is rapidly de-esterified by non-specific esterases (possibly in renal or liver tissues since it is reasonably stable in blood) to inactive monic acid and its conjugates. It is strongly bound to protein. About 0.25% is absorbed from intact skin. The skin ointment, but not the cream, contains polyethylene glycol, which may be absorbed significantly when applied to open wounds or to damaged skin such as burns.

Toxicity and side effects

Topical applications are well tolerated. It may cause irritation if applied to the conjunctiva, which is therefore contraindicated. Trivial complaints of irritation and taste have been recorded for very few patients following nasal application.

Polyethylene glycol from the ointment base may, if absorbed from application to open wounds or damaged skin, cause nephrotoxicity.

Clinical use

Nasal ointment
- Elimination of nasal carriage of MRSA (hospital patients and staff).

Ointment
- Staphylococcal and streptococcal infection of the skin (impetigo, infected eczema, wounds and burns).

It is more effective than topical bacitracin, fusidic acid or chlorhexidine in eliminating nasal carriage of MRSA in the absence of high-level mupirocin resistance.

There is evidence to suggest that the perioperative elimination of nasal *Staph. aureus* with mupirocin reduces the rate of staphylococcal infection in cardiothoracic surgery and that intermittent nasal application in hemodialysis patients reduces the rate of bacteremia caused by *Staph. aureus*.

Topical application in skin infection is increasingly associated with the emergence of high-level resistance, and prolonged use is best avoided.

Preparations and dosage

Proprietary name: Bactroban.

Preparations: 2% mupirocin as ointment, cream or nasal ointment.

Dosage: Topical application, up to three times daily for a maximum of 10 days. Nasal application, up to three times daily for 3–5 days.

Widely available.

Further information

Casewell MW (ed.) 1998 New advances in preventing serious infections with *Staphylococcus aureus* during surgery and dialysis. *Journal of Hospital Infection* 40 (Suppl. B): S1–S47.

Casewell MW, Hill RLR 1986 Elimination of nasal carriage of *Staphylococcus aureus* with mupirocin ('pseudomonic acid') – a controlled trial. *Journal of Antimicrobial Chemotherapy* 17: 365–372.

Cookson BD 1998 The emergence of mupirocin resistance: a challenge to infection control and antibiotic prescribing practice. *Journal of Antimicrobial Chemotherapy* 41: 11–18.

Hill RLR, Duckworth GD, Casewell MW 1988 Elimination of nasal carriage of methicillin-resistant *Staphylococcus aureus* with mupirocin during a hospital outbreak. *Journal of Antimicrobial Chemotherapy* 22: 377–384.

Hudson I 1994 The efficacy of mupirocin in the prevention of staphylococcal infections: a review of recent experience. *Journal of Hospital Infection* 27: 81–98.

Working Party Report 1998 Revised guidelines for the control of methicillin-resistant *Staphylococcus aureus* infection in hospitals. *Journal of Hospital Infection* 39: 253–290.

26 Nitrofurans

J. M. T. Hamilton-Miller

The antimicrobial activity of the nitrofurans was first discovered in the early 1940s as a result of chemical synthesis and microbiological testing in the USA and Germany. The findings, made at a time when virtually no other antibacterial compounds were available, encouraged pharmaceutical companies to produce thousands of variations on the nitrofuran theme. Several of these were introduced into medical and veterinary practice, and 30 years ago four were available in the UK: nitrofurantoin, nitrofurazone, nifuratel and furazolidone. Now, however, only nitrofurantoin is used in human medicine in the UK, although others (e.g. nifuroxime, nifurtoinol, nifurtimox) are available elsewhere. One nitrofuran, nifuroquine, is used exclusively in veterinary medicine and is not dealt with here. The relatively small use of this class of compounds has been due to a lack of interest rather than any problems of treatment failure or adverse events resembling those surrounding the withdrawal of furaltadone 40 years ago.

These agents are unusual in that their activity depends largely on their being metabolized to highly reactive and in some cases short-lived intermediates, a process that also involves the production of superoxide. This has an important bearing on their mode of action (see Ch. 2), acquisition and mechanism of resistance, and pharmacokinetic properties.

As the compounds in use today were discovered and licensed many years ago, the amount of fundamental research and the numbers of comparative clinical trials carried out are less than are available for more recently introduced drugs. There are thus gaps in our knowledge and disagreements as to detail that are unlikely to be resolved.

CHEMISTRY

Antimicrobial nitrofurans are based on the 5-nitro-2-furaldehyde molecule:

As 2-furaldehyde has the trivial name furfural, these compounds can also be described as 5-nitrofurfuryl derivatives.

Antimicrobial activity requires the 5-nitro group, while substitutions may be made on the aldehyde at the 2 position. This produces a large number of different compounds with varying activities and pharmacokinetic properties. Many are aldimines (Schiff bases), and most contain a nitrogen heterocycle (hydantoin, oxazolidinone, thiazine). They are yellow or orange compounds and are relatively easy to synthesize. They are poorly soluble in water, but often dissolve well in aprotic solvents such as dimethyl sulfoxide or dimethylformamide.

ANTIMICROBIAL ACTIVITY

Nitrofurans are active in vitro against a wide range of bacteria, including staphylococci, streptococci, enterococci, corynebacteria, clostridia and many species of enterobacteria (Table 26.1). Staphylococci are considerably more sensitive than micrococci, and testing with a 100-μg disk of furazolidone helps to differentiate these genera. *Serratia marcescens*, *Pseudomonas aeruginosa* and members of the Proteae tribe are resistant. They are less active under alkaline conditions, but this phenomenon is not associated with urease production by the target organisms.

They are active against the increasing numbers of strains of *Helicobacter pylori* that have acquired resistance to metronidazole, but it is not yet clear whether this reflects therapeutic efficacy.

PHARMACOKINETICS

The pharmacokinetics of this group are not fully understood, due to a lack of realization of the importance of such properties at the time they were developed, the large degree of metabolism that occurs, and the existence of several assay methods measuring different parameters. Many metabolites are found in vivo (e.g. reduction, oxidation and open ring products), depending upon the animal species, and not all have been fully characterized. It seems probable that most lack antibacterial activity, but they may be responsible for certain adverse reactions.

TOXICITY AND SIDE EFFECTS

Many nitrofurans are mutagenic, and some are said to be cocarcinogenic. Had these findings been available at the time the therapeutically available compounds were under investigation, further work on the entire group would doubtless have been stopped. However, therapeutic use of nitrofurans over many years has shown no evidence of long-term harmful effects, and indeed nitrofurantoin is regarded by many as the antibiotic of choice for treating bacteriuria in pregnancy. Following the withdrawal of furaltadone in 1961 on grounds of neurotoxicity, intensive post-marketing surveillance has been carried out on nitrofurantoin, nitrofurazone and furazolidone, allowing the accumulation of perhaps the largest database of adverse events for any group of antimicrobial compounds.

Nitrofurans share a class side effect of causing nausea. They may also bring about hemolysis in patients with a deficiency of glucose-6-phosphate dehydrogenase.

 Further information

Chamberlain RE 1976 Chemotherapeutic properties of prominent nitrofurans. *Journal of Antimicrobial Chemotherapy* 2: 325–336.

Debnath AK, Hansch C, Kim KH, Martin YC 1993 Mechanistic interpretation of the genotoxicity of nitrofurans (antibacterial agents) using quantitative structure-activity relationships and comparative molecular field analysis. *Journal of Medicinal Chemistry* 36: 1007–1016.

Rozenski J, De Ranter CJ, Verplanken H 1995 Quantitative structure-activity relationships for antimicrobial nitroheterocyclic drugs. *Quantitative Structure–Activity Relationships* 14: 134–141.

 FURAZOLIDONE

Molecular weight: 225.2.

A non-ionic synthetic compound, available for oral use only. It is poorly soluble in water (40 mg/l) and ethanol (90 mg/l), dissolves well in dimethylformamide (10 g/l). It decomposes in the presence of alkali.

Antimicrobial activity

Activity against common bacterial pathogens is shown in Table 26.1. It is active against a wide range of enteric pathogens, including *Salmonella enterica*, *Shigella* spp., enterotoxigenic *Esch. coli*, *Campylobacter jejuni*, *Aeromonas hydrophila*, *Plesiomonas shigelloides*, *Vibrio cholerae* and *Vibrio parahaemolyticus*. *Yersinia enterocolitica* is intrinsically resistant. Furazolidone is also active against the protozoa *Giardia lamblia* and *Trichomonas vaginalis*.

Acquired resistance

Unlike the situation with nitrofurantoin, acquired resistance has been observed, for example in *V. cholerae* O1 and O139, *S. enterica* serotypes Typhi and Enteritidis (especially strains of phage type 4), *A. hydrophila* and to smaller extent in *Shigella* spp. Such resistance may be transferable, and there is cross-resistance with nitrofurantoin. Many of these reports come from the Indian subcontinent, where furazolidone is used widely for treating diarrheal diseases.

Pharmacokinetics

There is a wide misconception that furazolidone is poorly absorbed from the intestine. In fact, there is substantial absorp-

Table 26.1 Activity of nitrofurans against common pathogenic bacteria (MIC, mg/l)

	Furazolidone	Nitrofurazone	Nitrofurantoin
Staphylococcus aureus	2–8	8–16	4–32
Streptococcus pyogenes	4–8	8–64	4–16
Enterococcus faecalis	8–32	32–128	4–128
Neisseria gonorrhoeae	No data	0.1–8	0.25–2
Escherichia coli	<0.5–4	4–16	0.5–R
Proteus spp.	32–128	8–128	8–R
Klebsiella pneumoniae	2–8	8–128	32–R
Salmonella enterica	0.25–2	4–16	4–128
Shigella spp.	0.25–4	4–32	4–128
Pseudomonas aeruginosa	R	R	R
Bacteroides fragilis	8–16	4–32	8–16
Helicobacter pylori	0.06–0.25		8–32

R, resistant (MIC >128 mg/l).

tion (65–70%) after oral administration, but the drug is heavily metabolized to, among others, 5-amino and 4-hydroxy derivatives, so that only about 5% of the material excreted is microbiologically active. A dose of 5 mg/kg achieves a maximum plasma concentration around 1 mg/l. Protein binding is about 30%. Intact drug can be found in various body fluids in concentrations approximating to the MIC for various intestinal pathogens. Less than 1% of the drug is excreted into urine.

Toxicity and side effects

A review covering 10 443 treated patients reported in 191 publications found the most common side effects to be gastrointestinal (mainly nausea and vomiting), experienced by 8% of patients. Other adverse events included neurological reactions (mainly headache; 1.3% of patients), 'systemic' reactions such as fever and malaise (0.6%) and skin rashes (0.54%).

Administration of furazolidone may give rise to inhibition of monoamine oxidase, and disulfiram-like reactions have been reported. Most of the reported side effects are mild and only rarely cause discontinuation of treatment.

Clinical use

Furazolidone is used in gastrointestinal infections and vaginitis.

It is used more commonly in developing countries, where diarrheal diseases of varying etiology present an enormous problem. There are a few reports of its successful use in acute typhoid fever.

Preparations and dosage

Preparations: Tablets, suspension.

Dosage: Adults, oral, 100 mg, four times daily for 7–10 days.

Children, 1.25 mg/kg, four times daily (suspension available).

Limited availability in continental Europe and USA.

Further information

DuPont HI (ed) 1989 Recent developments in the use of furazolidone and other antimicrobial agents in typhoid fever and infectious diarrheal diseases. *Scandinavian Journal of Gastroenterology* 24: (Suppl. 169): 1–80.

Phillips KF, Haley FJ 1986 The use of Furoxone: a perspective. *Journal of International Medical Research* 14: 19–29.

NIFURATEL

Molecular weight: 285.3.

A synthetic compound available as tablets and vaginal preparations. It is poorly soluble in water and acetone. Readily soluble in dimethylformamide.

Antimicrobial activity

The activity is similar to that of nitrofurantoin but it is more active, especially against Gram-negative anaerobes. It also has modest, but clinically useful, activity against *Candida albicans*.

Pharmacokinetics

Oral absorption	Not known
C_{max} 200 mg oral	0.005–0.02 mg/l after 2 h
Plasma half-life	2.75 h
Volume of distribution	15 l
Plasma protein binding	30%

Little is known about the pharmacokinetics. It structurally resembles furazolidone, and may undergo a similar degree of metabolism in humans, which would be consistent with the animal data. It seems likely that the antibacterial activity in urine is due to active metabolites. There is little or no systemic absorption when vaginal suppositories are used.

Toxicity and side effects

Side effects are said to be minimal and, as with other members of the group, mostly associated with the upper gastrointestinal tract.

Clinical use

Nifuratel is used to treat urinary infections and vaginal candidiasis.

Preparations and dosage

Preparations: Tablets and vaginal pessaries.

Dosage: Adults, oral, 200–400 mg three times daily. A 250 mg vaginal pessary may be used concurrently once a day for 10 days.

Available in some countries in continental Europe.

NIFUROXIME

Molecular weight: 156.1

A synthetic compound formulated as a topical agent, sometimes in combination with furazolidone. It is moderately soluble in water (1 g/l), better in ethanol (4 g/l), and very soluble in dimethylformamide.

Antimicrobial activity

The main activity is against yeasts and fungi. It has also been reported to be active in vitro against *Trypanosoma cruzi* and *T. brucei*.

Clinical use

The drug is used in treatment of vaginal candidiasis.

Preparations and dosage

Preparations: Suppositories and powder.

Available in Italy and USA.

Further information

Blumenstiel K, Schoneck R, Yardley V, Croft SL, Krauth-Siegel RL 1999 Nitrofuran drugs as common subversive substrates of *Trypanosoma cruzi* lipoamide dehydrogenase and trypanothione reductase. *Biochemical Pharmacology* 58: 1791–1799.

NIFURTIMOX

Molecular weight: 287.3.

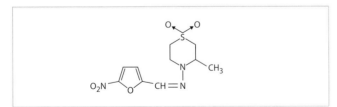

A synthetic compound available for oral use. It is soluble in water, acetone and alcohol.

Antimicrobial activity

It exhibits antibacterial activity typical of the group, but its most notable property is its activity against trypanosomes, especially *Trypanosoma cruzi*. This parasite lacks catalase and has only low levels of reduced glutathione, rendering it particularly susceptible to attack by free radicals.

Pharmacokinetics

Oral absorption	Good
C_{max} 15 mg/kg oral	0.5–1 mg/l after *c.* 2 h
Plasma half-life	2–4 h
Volume of distribution	*c.* 750 l
Plasma protein binding	Not known

In common with other nitrofurans, nifurtimox is rapidly and extensively metabolized, so that urinary excretion of the intact molecule amounts to less than 1% of the administered dose. In renal failure, clearance is somewhat reduced but the half-life is unchanged.

Toxicity and side effects

Adverse events are common. Many patients experience anorexia, which may be combined with vomiting and abdominal pain. There may also be neurological reactions such as restlessness, insomnia, headache and disorientation.

Clinical use

Chagas' disease (South American trypanosomiasis).

Preparations and dosage

Preparation: Oral.

Dosage: Adults, oral, 8–10 mg/kg per day in divided doses. Children: 1–10 years, 15–20 mg/kg per day in divided doses; 11–16 years, 12.5–15 mg/kg per day in divided doses. Treatment should last 60–120 days.

Available in South America.

Further information

Anonymous 1999 Nifurtimox. In: Dollery C (ed.) *Therapeutic Drugs* 2nd edn. Churchill Livingstone, Edinburgh, pp. N91–N95.

Gonzales-Martin G, Thambo S, Paulos C, Vasquez I, Paredes J 1992 The pharmacokinetics of nifurtimox in chronic renal failure. *European Journal of Clinical Pharmacology* 42: 671–673.

Kirchhoff LV 1993 Chagas disease. American trypanosomiasis. *Infectious Disease Clinics of North America* 7: 487–502.

Paulos C, Paredes J, Vasquez I, Thambo S, Arancibia A, Gonzales-Martin G 1989 Pharmacokinetics of a nitrofuran compound, nifurtimox, in healthy volunteers. *International Journal of Clinical Pharmacology, Therapy and Toxicology* 27: 454–457.

NIFURTOINOL

Molecular weight: 268.2.

The hydroxymethyl derivative of nitrofurantoin, formulated for oral administration. It is slightly soluble in water and very soluble in dimethylformamide.

Antimicrobial activity

The activity is similar to that of nitrofurantoin.

Pharmacokinetics

Little is known about the pharmacokinetic behavior. It is said to be more rapidly absorbed than nitrofurantoin and excreted into the urine to a greater extent.

Clinical use

Urinary tract infection.

Preparations and dosage

Dosage: Adults, oral, up to 300 mg per day by mouth.

Available in some countries in continental Europe.

NITROFURANTOIN

Molecular weight: 238.2.

A synthetic compound available only for oral administration. There are three formulations, differing in their crystalline nature: microcrystalline; macrocrystalline; and a delayed-release preparation containing a combination of the two. The macrocrystalline form is said to be released in a steadier and more predictable manner, and so is less liable to give rise to the most common adverse event, nausea. However, pharmacokinetic and clinical trial evidence for this assertion is not very strong.

Nitrofurantoin has an ionizable secondary amino group

($p\text{K}_a = 7$). It is slightly soluble in water (c. 200 mg/l), but more so in dilute alkali. Solubility in ethanol is modest (500 mg/l), but the compound dissolves very well in dimethylformamide (80 g/l) or acetone (5 g/l). If packaged in light-resistant containers and kept at room temperature, it is stable for more than 5 years. The yellow solution should be kept in the dark.

Antimicrobial activity

Activity against common bacterial pathogens is shown in Table 26.1 (p. 329). It is active against almost all the common urinary pathogens, except *Proteus mirabilis*. It is bactericidal. A postantibiotic effect of 1.5 h has been found after *Esch. coli* was exposed to $2 \times \text{MIC}$ for 1 h.

It antagonizes the activity of nalidixic acid and other quinolones in vitro, but this combination is unlikely to be used clinically.

Acquired resistance

In marked contrast to the situation with other agents and for bacteria that cause intestinal infections (*see above*), nitrofurantoin remains as active against organisms causing urinary infections as it was when first introduced. However, the position is not entirely clear owing to several factors, especially the use of differing breakpoints (32 mg/l in the UK, 64 mg/l in the Netherlands and 128 mg/l in the USA) in susceptibility testing.

R-factor-mediated resistance has been reported on at least two occasions, but this appears to be very unusual. The mechanism of resistance seems to be a decreased nitroreductase activity in the target organism.

There is cross-resistance within the nitrofuran group, but none with antibiotics of other chemical classes.

Pharmacokinetics

Oral absorption	>95%
C_{max} 100 mg oral	<2 mg/l after 1–4 h
Plasma half-life	0.5–1 h
Volume of distribution	0.6 l/kg
Plasma protein binding	60–70%

Absorption

It is absorbed mainly from the proximal small intestine, which explains why the plasma peak concentration may not be achieved for as long as 4 h. There are varying opinions concerning the effect of food. The recommendation to take the drug with food may be motivated by reducing the incidence of nausea rather than increasing bioavailability.

Bioavailability varies widely between different brands and this may not be apparent from results of standard in-vitro pharmaceutical tests. Therefore, different brands should not be substituted unless therapeutic equivalence has been formally established.

Distribution

Serum levels are low, presumably due to extensive metabolism and the short plasma half-life. Tissue concentrations are too low for adequate treatment of systemic infection, including pyelonephritis, although good results were obtained with an intravenous preparation that was formerly available. Negligible concentrations are found in breast milk and only a small amount crosses the placenta.

Metabolism and excretion

About 20% of the dose is excreted in microbiologically active form in the urine. This is sufficient to give inhibitory concentrations against urinary pathogens for up to 6 h. A further 17% is excreted as an inactive reduction product, aminofurantoin. In the event of reduced renal function (creatinine clearance <60 ml/min), urinary excretion falls, and virtually ceases when creatinine clearance is below 20 ml/min. This gives rise to the risk of accumulation in the blood and inadequate urine levels. With this proviso, it can be given to elderly patients. Infants over the age of 3 months may also be treated, but in the absence of a suitable suspension, and at the recommended dosage, a 6-month baby would require to be given one-tenth of a standard 50 mg tablet.

Toxicity and side effects

The most common adverse event is nausea, which may be combined with anorexia or vomiting, or both. This occurs in about 30% of patients taking the microcrystalline form, causing about 10% to stop treatment. The frequency of nausea appears to be approximately halved when the macrocrystalline form is taken. Nausea is due to a direct effect on the vomiting center; it occurs early in the course, and its incidence may be reduced by taking the medication with food or milk.

Side effects calculated from 128 million courses of treatment prescribed worldwide have revealed the following incidences: pulmonary 0.001%; hepatic 0.0003%; neurological 0.0007%; hematological 0.0004%. Most of these have the characteristics of hypersensitivity reactions. Fatalities have been extremely rare. Members of the Nordic races appear to be predisposed to such adverse reactions.

There are two kinds of pulmonary reaction. Acute reactions are the more common, starting within 5–10 days of the first dose, or within a few hours on re-challenge. Symptoms may resemble those found in asthma, tracheobronchitis or pneumonia, and usually resolve permanently within 2 days. There may be an eosinophilia. Subacute or chronic reactions, often referred to as pneumonitis, are of more gradual onset, and resolve only slowly when the drug is stopped. Prolonged dyspnea and cough may be accompanied by fibrosis.

Hepatic reactions are usually chronic, manifesting as chronic active hepatitis, sometimes with cirrhosis, and follow prolonged drug usage. The prognosis is good, but recovery may take months.

Peripheral neuropathy has been reported mainly in patients with pre-existing impaired renal function. The prognosis

depends upon the severity of the symptoms. Unlike hepatic and pulmonary effects, for which immunological phenomena seem to be responsible, neurological events have been attributed to a direct toxic effect of the drug, one of its metabolites or the superoxide generated in vivo.

In common with other members of this chemical class, nitrofurantoin may cause hemolysis in patients whose erythrocytes lack glucose-6-phosphate dehydrogenase.

Clinical use

- Acute dysuria and frequency.
- Bacteriuria in pregnancy.
- Prophylaxis of recurrent cystitis (reduced dosage).

Preparations and dosage

Proprietary names: BPC, Furadantin (microcrystalline); Macrodantin (macrocrystalline); Macrobid (mixture).

Preparations: Tablets, capsules, suspension.

Dosage: Adults, oral, 50 or 100 mg four times daily for 5 or 7 days for acute infection; 50–100 mg at night for prophylaxis. Children >3 months, 3 mg/kg per day, in four divided doses; 1 mg/kg at night for prophylaxis.

Widely available.

Further information

Anonymous 1990 Nitrofurantoin. *IARC Monographs* 50: 211–231.

Anonymous 1999 Nitrofurantoin. In Dollery C (ed.) *Therapeutic Drugs* 2nd edn. Churchill Livingstone, Edinburgh, pp. N114–N117.

Brumfitt W, Hamilton-Miller JMT 1998 Efficacy and safety profile of long-term nitrofurantoin in urinary infections: 18 years' experience. *Journal of Antimicrobial Chemotherapy* 42: 363–371.

Christensen B 2000 Which antibiotics are appropriate for treating bacteriuria in pregnancy? *Journal of Antimicrobial Chemotherapy* 46 (Suppl. S1): 29–34.

Cunha BA 1988 Nitrofurantoin – bioavailability and therapeutic equivalence. *Advances in Therapy*, 5: 54–63.

D'Arcy PF 1985 The comparative safety of therapies for urinary tract infection, with special reference to nitrofurantoin. In Schroder FH (ed.) *Recent Advances in the Treatment of Urinary Tract Infections*. Royal Society of Medicine International Congress and Symposium Series, London no 97, pp 45–59.

Kahlmeter G 2000 The ECO.SENS Project: a prospective, multinational, multicentre epidemiological survey of the prevalence and antimicrobial susceptibility of urinary tract pathogens – interim report. *Journal of Antimicrobial Chemotherapy* 46 (Suppl. S1): 5–22.

Naber KG 2000 Survey on antibiotic usage in the treatment of urinary tract infections. *Journal of Antimicrobial Chemotherapy* 46 (Suppl. S1): 49–52.

Penn RG, Griffin JP 1982 Adverse reactions to nitrofurantoin in the United Kingdom, Sweden and Holland. *British Medical Journal* 284: 1440–1442.

Shah RR, Wade G 1989 Reappraisal of the risk/benefit of nitrofurantoin: review of toxicity and efficacy. *Adverse Drug Reactions* 8: 183–201.

NITROFURAZONE

Molecular weight: 198.1.

A synthetic compound formulated for topical use. It is slightly soluble in water (0.25 g/l), more so in alcohol (1.7 g/l) and soluble in dimethylformamide.

Antimicrobial activity

Activity against the common bacterial pathogens is shown in Table 26.1 (p. 329). The spectrum is sufficient to cover, in topical use, most pathogens that cause infections of burns and wounds, with the important exception of *Ps. aeruginosa*. Attention has been drawn to its activity against methicillin-resistant *Staph. aureus*, and its use in clearing carriage has been suggested.

Pharmacokinetics

Slight absorption occurs from intact skin (*c.* 1%) and burned skin (5%). Good penetration into burn eschar has been reported.

Toxicity and side effects

A review of 136 published studies reported 176 cases of skin reactions in 15 162 patients treated (1.2%). It is neither a primary irritant nor a sensitizer, but some preparations contain polyethylene glycol as a vehicle, and absorption can cause problems in patients with reduced renal function.

Clinical use

The drug is used in topical treatment of wounds and burns and as an instillation for bladder washout.

 Preparations and dosage

Preparations: Creams and ointments (usually 0.2%), soluble dressings.

Dosage: Apply topically.

Not available in the UK, but widely elsewhere.

Further information

Anonymous 1990 Nitrofural (nitrofurazone). *IARC Monographs* 50: 195–209.

Hooper G, Covarrubias J 1983 Clinical use and efficacy of Furacin: a historical perspective. *Journal of International Medical Research* 11: 289–293.

27 Nitroimidazoles

D. I. Edwards

The history of the nitroimidazoles as agents for clinical disease began with the recognition in 1953 that vaginitis was caused by the protozoon *Trichomonas vaginalis*. This led to an intensive search for a drug that would provide an effective treatment.

In 1955, at the research laboratories of Rhône Poulenc, Paris, a crude extract of a streptomycete isolated from a soil sample collected from the island of Réunion in the Indian Ocean was found to produce three antibiotics, one of which had activity against *T. vaginalis*. The active compound was subsequently found to be azomycin (2-nitroimidazole), an antibiotic discovered by Japanese researchers 2 years earlier. This led to the synthesis of several hundred related compounds, one of which had optimal activity against the parasite and acceptable animal toxicity. This compound, first synthesized in 1957, was called metronidazole. The results of the first clinical trial were reported in 1959 and the drug entered the French and UK markets for trichomonal vaginitis in 1960.

The imidazole ring is an important feature of many natural compounds with a wide range of biological activities including the amino acid L-histidine and the purine nucleotides adenine and guanine. The ring also appears as part of a much larger structure in the vitamin biotin and in the antitumor antibiotics of the bleomycin group.

Nitration of imidazoles was first reported in 1892 and again in 1909, but the first patent application for a nitroimidazole was filed in 1961, since when thousands have been synthesized. 2-Nitroimidazoles, halogenated-, dinitro- and aziridine derivatives have been examined as possible radiosensitizers for the treatment of hypoxic tumors. In general, the nitration of imidazole by conventional methods leads the nitro group into the 4- or 5-position. These are equivalent if the imine nitrogen (*N*-1) is unsubstituted but if it is substituted, isomers are formed and the nitro group can enter either the 4- or 5-position, although those in the 4-position predominate.

Among 5-nitroimidazoles, metronidazole, tinidazole and ornidazole are in widespread clinical use; others include secnidazole and nimorazole. Carnidazole, dimetridazole, ipronidazole and ronidazole are used in veterinary medicine and are not discussed further here. Flexinidazole, panidazole and satranidazole, are used experimentally, but are not marketed.

ANTIMICROBIAL ACTIVITY

Nitroimidazole drugs have an unusual spectrum of activity which transcends the taxonomic boundaries typical of other antibiotics. No other family of compounds has useful activity against bacteria, protozoa and some helminths, as well as potential for the treatment of hypoxic tumors.

However, it is the ability to kill organisms that inhabit a low redox environment and are thus capable of anaerobic metabolism that has proved most useful. The 5-nitroimidazoles exhibit excellent potency against common anaerobic pathogens (Table 27.1) as well as several microaerophilic species, including *Helicobacter pylori*, and *Gardnerella vaginalis*. Susceptible protozoa including *T. vaginalis*, *Giardia lamblia* (*Giardia intestinalis*), *Entamoeba histolytica*, *Balantidium coli* and *Blastocystis hominis*. The spectrum of the related 2-nitroimidazole, benznidazole, is restricted to *Trypanosoma cruzi*.

Synergy has been described between metronidazole, its hydroxy metabolite and amoxicillin against the capnophilic Gram-negative bacillus *Actinobacillus actinomycetemcomitans*,

Table 27.1 Activity of nitroimidazoles against anaerobic bacteria: MIC (mg/l)

	Metronidazole	Ornidazole	Tinidazole
B. fragilis	0.25–4	<0.1–4	0.1–4
B. melaninogenicus	<0.1	<0.1	<0.1
Fusobacterium spp.	<0.1–1	<0.1–1	0.1–2
C. perfringens	0.25–2	0.25–2	0.25–2
Peptococcus and *Peptostreptococcus* spp.	<0.1–4	<0.1–2	<0.1–2
Veillonella spp.	1–2	0.5–1	0.5–2
Eubacterium spp.	0.5–2	0.5–1	0.5–2
Propionibacterium spp.	R	R	R

R, resistant (MIC >16 mg/l).

which plays a major role in periodontal disease. Both metronidazole and ornidazole have been found to interact with fleroxacin in mixed anaerobe–aerobe cultures, but it remains to be established whether this is a general property of the nitroimidazole group of drugs.

FACTORS AFFECTING ACTIVITY IN VITRO

All nitroimidazoles exert their antimicrobial effect via reduction of the nitro group, which occurs at reduction potentials that are generated only in anaerobes. The major factor affecting in-vitro activity is the failure to achieve anaerobic conditions, which can lead to resistance. The presence of traces of oxygen may inhibit or reverse reduction of the drug – an effect known as the 'futile' cycle. It is essential, therefore, to check that fully anaerobic conditions are maintained during susceptibility testing.

All nitroimidazoles are capable of being photodegraded and should be protected from light.

ACQUIRED RESISTANCE

T. VAGINALIS AND G. LAMBLIA

Although resistance rates of T. vaginalis and G. lamblia are low, millions of cases of infection occur each year and the number of treatment failures due to resistance is significant. The earliest studies on clinical failure of trichomonal vaginitis treated with metronidazole revealed the presence of fully susceptible trichomonads. This led to the observation that aerobic or microaerophilic bacteria in the vagina could 'absorb' the drug without loss of viability, thus decreasing the drug concentration available to kill the protozoon. However, the MIC of metronidazole for strains of T. vaginalis from refractory vaginitis is frequently 3–8 times the value for susceptible strains.

In Trichomonas spp. resistance to metronidazole and other nitroimidazoles is characterized by a tolerance to oxygen, which results in decreased susceptibility under both anaerobic and aerobic conditions, suggesting that the organism is resistant to oxygen in the environment.

Anaerobic and aerobic types of resistance are recognized in T. vaginalis. In susceptible cells, metronidazole is reduced by an intracellular pyruvate ferredoxin oxidoreductase (PFOR) system unique to anaerobes. In trichomonads exhibiting the anaerobic type of resistance this system is decreased and in fully resistant strains in vitro it is absent. The consequences of this are that pyruvate oxidation in the hydrogenosome is diverted to alternative pathways which favor the formation of lactate (in T. vaginalis) or ethanol (in Trichomonas fetus). This mechanism of resistance appears to dominate in resistant organisms cultured anaerobically or microaerophilically.

'Aerobic' resistance is shown by some strains that occur clinically. Trichomonads, which are now regarded as microaerophiles rather than anaerobes, have evolved at least four oxidases capable of scavenging oxygen. In aerobically resistant strains, the hydrogenosomal oxidases are defective and have a much reduced affinity for oxygen. Thus more is available to a process known as 'futile' cycling, in which reduced drug (the nitro group is reduced to a nitro radical anion) is oxidized by oxygen reforming the original drug and reducing oxygen to superoxide.

Other resistance mechanisms include decreased transcription of the ferredoxin gene resulting in decreased levels of a functional PFOR system. Rare resistance in G. lamblia is also due to decreased levels of the PFOR system.

BACTEROIDES AND CLOSTRIDIUM SPP.

Reduced susceptibility to metronidazole and other nitroimidazoles has been described in B. fragilis, B. distasonis and B. bivius. In those strains in which the resistance mechanism has been studied, decreased levels of the PFOR system have been found. There have been reports that the gene(s) for resistance are borne on a 7.7 kb plasmid and transferable by conjugation, but the gene product is not known.

Metronidazole-resistant strains of clostridia have not been reported clinically, but a laboratory strain of Clostridium perfringens made resistant by mutation possessed decreased levels of PFOR.

MOBILUNCUS SPP.

In one study, all isolates of Mobiluncus curtisii (Gardnerella mobiluncus) were resistant to metronidazole and to its hydroxy metabolite. About half of all strains of Mobiluncus mulieris were resistant and about 20% were also resistant to the hydroxy metabolite. Acquired resistance in Mobiluncus spp. does not appear to be a problem at present.

HELICOBACTER SPP.

H. pylori is a microaerophile requiring about 5% oxygen. Resistance is a consequence of the environment, since all strains are susceptible when cultured anaerobically. The amount of metronidazole taken up by Helicobacter spp. depends on the oxygen tension and cell density: high microaerophilic levels decrease the rate of drug entry into the cell and hence the amount available to kill the cell, resulting in apparent resistance. This has led to the proposal that H. pylori maintains an anaerobic microenvironment by scavenging oxygen using NADH and NADPH oxidases. In metronidazole-resistant strains (MIC 8–32 mg/l) NADH oxidase levels are significantly decreased, thus allowing 'futile' cycling to occur (see above); this may be significant at normal oxygen levels.

H. pylori possesses a pyruvate-linked flavodoxin oxidoreductase system (PflOR) similar to the PFOR system typical of anaerobes, but which is absent in aerobes. Null mutations (those that produce neither a transcriptional nor a protein product) in the *rdxA* gene that codes for an oxygen-insensitive NADPH nitroreductase result in metronidazole resistance in *H. pylori*.

Other mechanisms of resistance may exist. One group has shown that the activity of NADH oxidase resides within the catalase gene and that resistant strains of *H. pylori* lacked this activity. It is suggested that susceptible strains possess a bifunctional catalase (having catalase and NADH oxidase activity) and resistant strains have a monofunctional enzyme (catalase only). Mutations in the catalase gene responsible for this occur outside the *Kat A* core.

PHARMACOKINETICS

Nitroimidazoles are generally well absorbed and widely distributed in body tissues. Binding to proteins is low. They give peak plasma levels 1–2 h after oral dosing. The decay from the peak is exponential, with the rate depending on the half-life of the drug.

METABOLISM

5-Nitroimidazoles with a 2-methyl group (except nimorazole) are metabolized to the corresponding methoxy derivative and those with an alcohol side chain are metabolized to the corresponding acid metabolite. All can form glucuronide conjugates and, occasionally, the ethereal sulfate conjugate. The nitro group of benznidazole, a 2-nitroimidazole, undergoes reduction to the amine and hydrolysis to the hydroxy derivative.

TOXICITY AND SIDE EFFECTS

These are not generally a problem, although some degree of gastrointestinal disturbance is fairly common, as is a metallic taste in the mouth. Nitroimidazoles may interact with alcohol to give a disulfiram-like effect. Prolonged or high doses, particularly when used to eradicate hypoxic cells in tumors, may give peripheral and central neurotoxicity. Although concern has been expressed about their long-term safety, particularly since their mechanism of action has DNA as a major target, there is no evidence that they are carcinogenic in humans.

CLINICAL USE

These drugs are used in amebiasis, giardiasis, balantidiasis and in mixed anaerobic infections such as are found in Vincent's stomatitis, Melaney's gangrene and synergistic and necrotizing fasciitis. They are routinely used to prevent postoperative sepsis. Metronidazole and tinidazole are used as components of multidrug regimens for the treatment of gastroduodenal

ulcers caused by *H. pylori*. In the treatment of bacterial vaginosis or non-specific vaginitis caused by the microaerophile *Gard. vaginalis*, single-dose therapy with metronidazole (or its hydroxy metabolite) appears to allow the vaginal lactobacilli to recolonize, thus restoring the normal vaginal pH.

Benznidazole (a 2-nitroimidazole) is used for the treatment of *T. cruzi* infections (Chagas' disease) and for the experimental treatment of radioresistant hypoxic tumors.

 Further information

Edwards DI 1993 Nitroimidazole drugs – action and resistance mechanisms. I Mechanisms of action. *Journal of Antimicrobial Chemotherapy* 31: 9–20.

Edwards DI 1993 Nitroimidazole drugs – action and resistance mechanisms. II Mechanisms of resistance. *Journal of Antimicrobial Chemotherapy* 31: 201–210.

Edwards DI 1997 Resistance to nitroimidazoles in anaerobes. In: Eley AR, Bennett KW (eds) *Anaerobic Pathogens*, Sheffield, Sheffield University Press, pp. 437–448.

Pavicic MJAMP, van Winkelhoff AJ, de Graaff J 1991 Synergistic effects between amoxycillin, metronidazole and the hydroxy metabolite of metronidazole against *Actinobacillus actinomycetemcomitans*. *Antimicrobial Agents and Chemotherapy* 35: 961–966.

 BENZNIDAZOLE

Molecular weight: 260.26.

A synthetic 2-nitroimidazole, formulated for oral administration. Solubility in water 400 mg/l.

Antimicrobial activity

It exhibits antiprotozoal activity, particularly against *Trypanosoma cruzi*.

Pharmacokinetics

Oral absorption	Good
C_{max} 100 mg oral	2.2–2.8 mg/l after 3–4 h
Plasma half-life	10.5–13.6 h
Volume of distribution	c. 0.56 l/kg
Plasma protein binding	c. 44%

Metabolic studies have revealed an amine and hydroxy metabolite, both in the C-2 position, indicating reduction of the nitro group and hydrolysis or an oxidative deamination of the amine metabolite.

Toxicity and side effects

Adverse effects include nausea, vomiting, abdominal pain, peripheral neuropathy and severe skin reactions.

Clinical use

Benznidazole is used in treatment of South American trypanosomiasis (Chagas' disease).

Preparations and dosage

Preparation: Tablets.

Dosage: Adults, oral, 5–10 mg/kg per day, for 30–60 days. Children, oral, 5–10 mg/kg per day for 30–60 days.

Available in South America.

Further information

Apt W 1986 Clinical trial of benznidazole and an immunopotentiator against Chagas' disease in Chile. *Transactions of the Royal Society of Tropical Medicine and Hygiene* 80: 1010.

Gutteridge WE 1985 Existing chemotherapy and its limitations. *British Medical Bulletin* 41: 162–168.

WHO 1991 Control of Chagas' disease: report of a WHO expert committee. WHO Technical Report Series NO 811. Geneva: WHO.

METRONIDAZOLE

Molecular weight (free compound): 171.16; (hydrochloride): 207.6; (benzoate): 275.3.

A 5-nitroimidazole available for oral administration or as a suppository; also formulated as the hydrochloride for intravenous use, and as the benzoate in an oral suspension and a dental gel. Aqueous solubility: 10 g/l at 20°C. Soluble in dilute acids. It is photolabile and preparations should be protected from light. Metronidazole hydrochloride has a low pH (0.5–2.0) when reconstituted, and reacts with aluminum in equipment, including needles, to produce a reddish-brown discoloration. It is incompatible with several agents and other drugs should not be added to intravenous solutions.

Antimicrobial activity

It is a potent inhibitor of obligate anaerobic bacteria (Table 27.1) and protozoa, but not of any organism that is aerobic or incapable of anaerobic metabolism. Susceptible protozoa include *T. vaginalis*, *G. lamblia*, *E. histolytica*, *Bal. coli* and *Blast. hominis*, which are inhibited by concentrations of 0.2–0.25 mg/l. *Clostridium* spp. (including *Clostridium difficile*) are inhibited at concentrations of 0.1–8 mg/l. It is also active against the microaerophilic *H. pylori* (MIC for susceptible strains <1–2 mg/l). The 2-methoxy metabolite of metronidazole is more active (MIC about 0.3 mg/l), but the acid metabolite shows less activity than the parent drug (MIC about 3 mg/l). *Gard. vaginalis* shows similar susceptibility (MIC 1–8 mg/l). The methoxy metabolite is more active (MIC 0.02–2 mg/l).

Although metronidazole is inactive against aerobes, a recent report indicates that the drug is bactericidal to dormant cells of *Mycobacterium tuberculosis*, indicating that the dormant phase is primarily anaerobic.

Acquired resistance

Although resistance in *Bacteroides* spp. and *T. vaginalis* is well documented, it is uncommon. Resistance occurs more frequently in *H. pylori* and failure of treatment with triple drug regimens may be associated with resistance to the metronidazole component.

Pharmacokinetics

Oral absorption	>90%
C_{max} 500 mg oral	*c.* 12 mg/l after 20 min to 3 h
Plasma half-life	6–11 h
Volume of distribution	0.6–1.1 l/kg
Plasma protein binding	<20%

Absorption

Peak plasma concentrations after oral administration are proportional to the dose. There is no difference between the bioavailability of the drug in men and women, but because of weight differences plasma levels are usually lower in men. In patients treated intravenously with a loading dose of 15 mg/kg followed by 7.5 mg/kg every 6 h, peak steady state plasma concentrations averaged 25 mg/l with minimum trough concentrations averaging 18 mg/l.

The bioavailability of metronidazole in suppositories is 60–80%. Effective blood concentrations occur 5–12 h after the first suppository and are maintained by an 8 h regimen.

There are conflicting data on the effects of age on absorption. One study, which did not distinguish between metronidazole and its metabolites, indicated that the area under the curve (AUC) for plasma was almost doubled in the elderly. However, the general consensus is that there is no requirement for a decreased dosage for the elderly, unless there is overt renal insufficiency.

Distribution

The drug is widely distributed in body tissues and distribution is similar for oral and intravenous forms. It appears about 90 min after an oral dose in cerebrospinal fluid (CSF), saliva and breast milk in concentrations similar to those found in plasma, and in vaginal secretions, pleural and prostatic fluid at levels about 40% of those of the plasma. In patients receiving 500 mg twice daily or 1 g 6-hourly, CSF levels of up to 2 and 8 mg/l, respectively, have been found. Bactericidal concentrations of metronidazole have been found in pus from hepatic abscesses. Concentrations in placenta and fetal tissue are related to the corresponding maternal plasma levels: concentrations of 3.5 mg/kg (placenta) and 9 mg/kg (fetus) have been found when the plasma concentration was 13.5 mg/l.

Metabolism

Metronidazole is metabolized in the human liver by side-chain oxidation and glucuronide formation, although some dispute this because the metabolic pattern is not changed in cirrhosis. There are two principal oxidative metabolites: the acid and hydroxy derivatives. The acid metabolite is produced by oxidation of the N-1 ethanol side-chain to the corresponding acetic derivative. This metabolite is microbiologically inactive and appears in the urine because of its high water solubility. The hydroxy derivative, which is as active as the parent drug against *Gard. vaginalis*, is formed by oxidation of the methyl group on C-2 of the imidazole ring first to the hydroxymethyl derivative and subsequently, and less significantly, to the carboxylic acid. Both metronidazole itself and the hydroxymethyl metabolite can form sulfate or glucuronide conjugates, and the acid metabolite may be excreted as the glycine conjugate.

Small amounts of metabolites derived from reduction of the nitro group, notably the oxamic acid and acetamide, have been detected in urine and are assumed to be formed by the intestinal flora. This is indicative of fragmentation of the imidazole ring. There is no evidence for the reduction of the nitro group to the amine, which is known to be highly unstable.

Excretion

The major route of elimination is renal with 60–80% of the dose appearing in the urine; fecal excretion accounts for 6–15%. The hydroxy metabolite and the acid metabolite are also excreted in the urine. Conjugation of the unchanged drug with glucuronide accounts for approximately 20% of the total. Renal clearance is approximately 10 ml/min per 1.73 m². Decreased renal function does not alter the single-dose kinetics, but plasma clearance is decreased in patients with impaired liver function. Newborn infants appear to possess a decreased capacity to eliminate metronidazole. In one study, the elimination half-life measured during the first 3 days of life was inversely related to gestational age. In infants whose gestational ages were between 28 and 40 weeks, the corresponding half-life elimination rates ranged from 10.9 to 22.5 h.

Toxicity and side effects

Precautions

Alcohol should not be taken during metronidazole therapy and for 48 h after because of a possible disulfuram-like reaction; neither should the drug be combined with formulations containing alcohol. It should not be given in cases of known hypersensitivity to nitroimidazoles.

Metronidazole enhances the anticoagulant effect of warfarin and may impair the clearance of phenytoin and lithium. Phenytoin may increase the metabolism of metronidazole. Plasma concentrations are decreased by the concomitant administration of phenobarbitone. The drug may also mask the immunological response of untreated early syphilis cases because of its antitreponemal activity.

Metronidazole should be used with care in patients with blood dyscrasias or with any central nervous system (CNS) disease. If any peripheral neuropathy or CNS toxicity occurs, which is more likely in patients treated for 10 days or more, treatment should be discontinued. The coadministration of cimetidine increases plasma levels of metronidazole and may increase the risk of neurological side effects.

The drug should be avoided in pregnancy, especially during the first trimester and particularly if high doses are being administered. Use during the second and third trimesters may be acceptable if alternative therapies for trichomoniasis have failed, but single-dose (2 g oral) therapy should be avoided. The drug may cause the breast milk to taste bitter. Breast feeding should be discontinued until 24 h after the last dose to allow excretion of the drug. It appears safe when given to nursing mothers at doses of up to 400 mg three times daily.

Adverse effects

The adverse effects are dose related.

NERVOUS SYSTEM

Convulsive seizures and peripheral neuropathy have been reported in patients treated with the intravenous preparation. Use of the intravenous preparation has also caused headache, dizziness, syncope, ataxia and confusion. Convulsive seizures, peripheral neuropathy, dizziness, vertigo, incoordination, ataxia, confusion, irritability, depression, weakness and insomnia have been reported in association with oral preparations.

Peripheral neuropathy was found in 11 of 13 patients aged 12–22 years treated for Crohn's disease. The symptoms disappeared when the dose was discontinued or markedly reduced. A patient receiving 2 g daily for 50 days, again for Crohn's disease, developed persistent peripheral neuropathy.

GASTROINTESTINAL

Gastrointestinal disturbances include nausea, vomiting, abdominal discomfort and diarrhea, have been noted with both intravenous and oral preparations. Pseudomembranous colitis is also reported, but with its increasing use in the treatment of gastroduodenal ulcer it is perhaps surprising that more reports are not known.

HEMATOPOIETIC

Reversible neutropenia (leukopenia) has been reported after administration of both intravenous and oral preparations. Bone-marrow aplasia and reversible thrombocytopenia have also been rarely reported. A hemolytic–uremic syndrome was reported in six children who had been given metronidazole for non-specific diarrhea or for prophylaxis after bowel surgery.

MOUTH

An unpleasant sharp, metallic taste is not unusual. Furry tongue, glossitis and stomatitis have occurred; stomatitis may be associated with overgrowth of *Candida* spp. during treatment.

DERMATOLOGICAL

Erythematous rash and pruritus have been reported after use of the intravenous preparation, as has thrombophlebitis. The latter can be minimized by avoiding prolonged indwelling catheters for intravenous infusion.

OTHER REACTIONS

Flattening of the T-wave may be seen in electrocardiographic tracings. A number of cases of deafness have been reported. Myopia related to 11 days' oral treatment for trichomoniasis disappeared 4 days after treatment was stopped, but returned when treatment was resumed. There have been two reports of pancreatitis. Gynecomastia has been reported in a 36-year-old man who took metronidazole for about a month for ulcerative colitis.

Mutagenicity and carcinogenicity

Metronidazole and some of its metabolites in human urine are weakly mutagenic by the Ames histidine reversion test, but only under anaerobic or microaerophilic conditions that lead to reduction of the nitro group, an essential prerequisite for its bactericidal action. The microsomal fraction added to activate drugs in the Ames test has a high oxygen demand and can rapidly deplete the preparation of oxygen, resulting in the creation of anaerobiosis in a seemingly aerobic environment. Other mutagenicity and genotoxicity studies in experimental animals and in-vitro tests of human cells have proved negative.

Reports of metronidazole-induced carcinogenicity are conflicting and confused. Some studies indicated that high-doses of metronidazole caused lung tumors in mice, lymphoreticular neoplasms in female mice only and hepatomas and mammary tumors in rats. Other studies show lung tumors in male mice only, or in both sexes, while one study in female rats proved negative and another non-significant. Two studies in hamsters have failed to show carcinogenicity. Some studies have been criticized on the grounds that overfeeding of animals may lead to the development of cancers.

A retrospective studies of 771 patients given metronidazole for trichomoniasis, and another involving 2460 patients, found no increase in the incidence of cancer. A subsequent 15–25 year follow-up study reporting to 1984 also showed no increase in cancers or cancer-related morbidity or mortality.

Clinical use

- Trichomonal vaginitis.
- Anaerobic infections, including those caused by *Clostridium* or *Bacteroides* spp.
- Acute necrotizing ulcerative gingivitis (Vincent's stomatitis).
- Bacterial vaginosis (non-specific vaginitis).
- *Cl. difficile*-related pseudomembranous colitis.
- Gastroduodenal ulcers caused by *H. pylori* (in combination with other agents, see pp. 677–678).
- Surgical prophylaxis (abdominal and gynecological).

T. vaginalis infections resistant to the usual dosage require special treatment (p. 900). Metronidazole is also used in rosacea and Guinea worm infection. It is not generally indicated in Crohn's disease, despite reports of its success in treating the condition.

Preparations and dosage

Proprietary names: Flagyl and numerous generic preparations.

Preparations: Tablets, suppositories, topical gel and cream, i.v. infusion, oral suspension.

Dosage:

Trichomonal vaginitis: Adults: a single 2 g oral dose or a 7-day course of 200–250 mg three times a day, or 400 mg twice daily. Alternatively, 800 mg in the morning and 1200 mg in the evening for 2 days. All sexual partners should be treated concomitantly. Children aged 1–3 years: 50 mg three times daily for 7 days; aged 3–7 years: 100 mg twice daily; 7–10 years: 100 mg three times daily. Alternatively, 15 mg/kg orally, daily in divided doses for 7 days.

Anaerobic bacterial infections: Adults: an initial dose of 800 mg orally followed by 400 mg every 8 h, for about 7 days. If oral therapy is not possible 500 mg intravenous infusion as 100 ml of a 5 mg/ml solution at a rate of 5 ml/min every 8 h.

Children: 7.5 mg/kg 8 hourly orally, rectally, or intravenously. Alternatively, a 1 g suppository every 8 h for 3 days, then every 12 h. Children aged 5–10 years should receive a 500 mg suppository and the adult schedule followed; those of 1–5 years should receive a 250 mg suppository as per the adult schedule and infants under 1 year should receive 125 mg suppository according to the adult schedule. In all cases of treatment by suppository oral medication should replace it as soon as feasible.

In the US: Adults 7.5 mg/kg every 6 h orally or 15 mg/kg by intravenous 1 h infusion, followed by 7.5 mg/kg every 6 h. No more than 4 g in 24 h.

Surgical prophylaxis. Adults: 400 mg orally every 8 h in the 24 h preceding surgery, followed postoperatively by intravenous or rectal administration until oral therapy is possible. Alternatively, 500 mg intravenously shortly before surgery and repeated every 8 h until substitution of oral medication. Children: 7.5 mg/kg (1.5 ml/kg) 8 hourly. Oral doses of 400 mg every 8 h should be substituted as soon as possible. Alternatively, 1 g rectally 2 h before surgery and then every 8 h. Children 5–10 years should be given 500 mg 8 hourly until oral medication becomes possible, or 7.5 mg/kg every 8 h. *In the US:* Adults undergoing colorectal surgery, 15 mg/kg by intravenous infusion over 30–60 min and completed about 1 h before surgery, followed by two further intravenous doses of 7.5 mg/kg infused at 6 and 12 h after the initial dose.

Cl. difficile overgrowth: 250 mg orally, four times daily for up to 2 weeks, or 400 mg three times daily.

Intestinal amebiasis: Adults: 800 mg three times daily orally for 5 days (10 days in the USA). Children aged 1–3 years: 200 mg three times daily for 5 days; aged 3–7 years: 200 mg four times daily; aged 7–10 years: 400 mg three times daily for 5 days.

Extra-intestinal amebiasis: Adults: 400 mg three times daily for 5 days. Children aged 1–3 years: 100 mg three times daily for 5 days; aged 3–7 years: 100 mg four times daily for 5 days; aged 7–10 years: 200 mg three times daily for 5 days.

Symptomless cyst passers: Adults: 400–800 mg three times daily for 5–10 days. Children aged 1–3 years: 100–200 mg three times daily for 5–10 days; aged 3–7 years: 100–200 mg four times daily for 5–10 days; aged 7–10 years: 200–400 mg three times daily for 5–10 days. Similar doses to those given for amebiasis may be used for balantidiasis and *Blastocystis hominis* infections.

Giardiasis: Adults: 2 g metronidazole daily, orally, as a single dose for 3 days. Alternatively, 250 mg three times a day for 5–7 days for adults. Children aged 1–3 years: 500 mg once daily for 3 days; aged 3–7 years: 600–800 mg once daily for 3 days; aged 7–10 years 1 g once daily for 3 days.

Acute ulcerative gingivitis: Adults: 200 mg orally, three times daily for 3 days. Children aged 1–3 years: 50 mg three times a day for 3 days; aged 3–7 days: 100 mg twice daily for 3 days; aged 7–10 years: 100 mg three times daily for 3 days.

Bacterial vaginosis: 500 mg twice daily or 250 mg three times daily orally for 7 days; or a single 2 g tablet repeated after 48 h. Alternatively, 400 mg or 500 mg orally, twice daily for 7 days; or a 500 mg vaginal pessary each evening for 7 days.

Gastroduodenal ulcers (H. pylori): 400 mg twice daily for 7 days (in combination with other agents)

Widely available.

 ## Further information

Anonymous 1991 Drug-induced ototoxicity. *WHO Drug Information* 5: 12–16.
Anonymous 1999 Metronidazole. In: Dollery C (ed.) *Therapeutic Drugs* 2nd edn. Churchill Livingstone, Edinburgh, pp. M146–M151.
Calam J 1996 Clinicians Guide to *Helicobacter pylori*. London, Chapman & Hall.
Cederbrant G, Kahlmeter G, Ljungh A 1992 Proposed mechanisms for metronidazole resistance in *Helicobacter pylori*. *Journal of Antimicrobial Chemotherapy* 29: 115–120.
Edwards DI 1993 Nitroimidazole drugs – action and resistance mechanisms. I. Mechanisms of action. *Journal of Antimicrobial Chemotherapy* 31: 9–20.
Edwards DI 1993 Nitroimidazole drugs – action and resistance mechanisms. II. Mechanisms of resistance. *Journal of Antimicrobial Chemotherapy* 31: 201–210.
Ellis JE, Cole D, Lloyd D 1992 Influence of oxygen on the fermentative metabolism of metronidazole-sensitive and resistant strains of *Trichomonas vaginalis*. *Molecular and Biochemical Parasitology* 56: 79–88.
Jenks PJR, Ferrero L, Labigne A 1999 The role of the *rdxA* gene in the evolution of metronidazole resistance in *Helicobacter pylori*. *Journal of Antimicrobial Chemotherapy* 43: 753–758.
Johnson PJ 1993 Metronidazole and drug resistance. *Parasitology Today* 9: 183–186.
Lossick JG 1990 Treatment of sexually transmitted vaginosis/vaginitis. *Reviews of Infectious Diseases* 12 (Suppl. 6): S665–S681.
Quon DVK, D'Oliveira CE, Johnson PJ 1992 Reduced transcription of the ferredoxin gene in metronidazole-resistant *Trichomonas vaginalis*. *Proceedings of the National Academy of Sciences USA* 89: 4402.
Smith MA, Edwards DI 1997 Oxygen scavenging, NADH oxidase and metronidazole resistance in *Helicobacter pylori*. *Journal of Antimicrobial Chemotherapy* 39: 347–353.
Tachezy J, Kulda K, Tomkova E 1993 Aerobic resistance of *Trichomonas vaginalis* to metronidazole induced in vitro. *Parasitology* 106: 31–37.
Wayne LG, Sramek H 1994 Metronidazole is bactericidal to dormant cells of *Mycobacterium tuberculosis*. *Antimicrobial Agents and Chemotherapy* 38: 2054–2058.

 # NIMORAZOLE

Nitrimidazine. Molecular weight: 226.23.

Antimicrobial activity

Nimorazole is active against *T. vaginalis*, *G. lamblia*, *E. histolytica*, anaerobic bacteria and *Gard. vaginalis*. Activity against *B. fragilis* and *Fusobacterium* spp. is similar to or slightly less than that of metronidazole (mean MIC 0.25–1 mg/l).

Pharmacokinetics

It is absorbed from the intestine. A peak blood concentration of about 32 mg/l occurs within 2 h of a 500 mg oral dose. High concentrations are achieved in saliva and vaginal secretions. Excretion is principally via the urine where the drug appears as metabolites which also display antimicrobial and antiprotozoal activity, but less so than that of the parent drug.

Toxicity and side effects

It is generally well tolerated even at the high doses required in conjunction with radiotherapy for the treatment of head and neck tumors. Adverse effects are the same as those of metronidazole. Disulfiram-like reactions appear to be rare.

Clinical use

- Trichomonal vaginitis (single-dose treatment).
- Giardiasis.
- Intestinal amebiasis.
- Vincent's stomatitis.

It is also used in the conjunctive therapy of hypoxic tumors.

A 5-nitroimidazole available for oral administration. It is slightly soluble in water at room temperature, soluble in alcohols, acetone and chloroform.

Preparations and dosage

Proprietary names: Esclama; Naxogin; Naxogyn.

Preparation: Tablets.

Dosage:

Trichomoniasis: 2 g as a single oral dose with a main meal, can be repeated after 1 month. Sexual partners should be treated concomitantly.

Giardiasis or amebiasis: adults, oral, 500 mg to 1 g twice daily for 5 days. Children >10 kg body weight, 500 mg/day for 5 days; <10 kg body weight, 250 mg/day for 5 days.

Ulcerative gingivitis: 500 mg twice daily for 2 days.

Available in continental Europe and South Africa.

Further information

Mohanty KC, Deighton R 1987 Comparison of 2 g single dose of metronidazole, nimorazole and tinidazole in the treatment of vaginitis associated with *Gardnerella vaginalis*. *Journal of Antimicrobial Chemotherapy* 19: 393–399.

Overgaard J, Hansen HS, Lindelov B et al 1991 Nimorazole as a hypoxic radiosensitizer in the treatment of supraglottic larynx and pharynx carcinoma. First report from the Danish Head and Neck Cancer Study (DAHANCA) protocol 5–85. *Radiotherapy and Oncology* 20 (Suppl.): 143–149.

Pamba HO 1990 Comparative study of aminosidine etophamide and nimorazole alone or in combination in the treatment of intestinal amoebiasis in Kenya. *European Journal of Clinical Pharmacology* 39: 353–357.

ORNIDAZOLE

Molecular weight 219.6.

A 5-nitroimidazole available for oral administration, intravenous infusion and as a vaginal pessary.

Antimicrobial activity

Its activity closely parallels that of metronidazole and tinidazole (Table 27.1; p. 335).

Pharmacokinetics

Ornidazole is readily absorbed from the intestinal tract; peak plasma levels reach 30 mg/l within 2 h of a single oral dose of 1.5 g. After a 750 mg oral dose, peak plasma concentrations reach 11 mg/l at 2–4 h. The half-life is 12–14 h. It is also well absorbed from the vagina, with peak plasma concentrations of 5 mg/l being reached 12 h after the insertion of a 500 mg vaginal pessary. After a single 1 g intravenous infusion for colorectal surgery, serum levels reached about 24 mg/l after 15 min and about 6 mg/l after 24 h. It has wide tissue distribution, including CSF.

Metabolism of the drug occurs in the liver. The plasma clearance rate decreases in hepatic failure because of reduced liver metabolism and decreased biliary elimination. About 60% of an oral dose is recovered in the urine and 20% in the feces. During hemodialysis, ornidazole is removed and there is no clear indication as to whether the drug should be given before or after such dialysis.

Toxicity and side effects

These are similar to those of metronidazole and tinidazole.

Clinical use

- Trichomonal vaginitis.
- Giardiasis.
- Intestinal amebiasis and amebic liver abscess.
- Treatment and prophylaxis of anaerobic bacterial infections.
- Bacterial vaginosis.

Preparations and dosage

Preparations: Tablets, vaginal pessary, i.v. infusion.

Dosage:

Amebiasis: Adults, oral, 500 mg twice daily for 5–10 days; 1.5 g as a single dose for 3 days for amebic dysentery. Children: 25 mg/kg body weight per day as a single dose for 5–10 days; 40 mg/kg per day in amebic dysentery. In severe cases of amebic dysentery or severe amebic liver abscess 0.5 g–1 g intravenously over 15–30 min, followed by 500 mg every 12 h for 3–6 days. Children: 20–30 mg/kg per day.

Giardiasis: Adults, oral, 1–1.5 g as a single daily dose for 1–2 days; children: 30–40 mg/kg per day.

Trichomonal vaginitis: Adults, oral, a single 1.5 g tablet, or 1 g orally, together with 500 mg vaginally; alternatively, 500 mg twice daily for 5 days with or without a 500 mg vaginal pessary. Children: 25 mg/kg per day.

Anaerobic bacterial infections: Adults, an initial dose of 0.5–1.0 g intravenously, followed by 500 mg every 12 h for 5–10 days. Oral therapy with 500 mg every 12 h should be substituted as soon as possible. Children, 10 mg/kg every 12 h.

Surgical prophylaxis: 1 g intravenously about 30 min before surgery.

Available widely. Not in UK.

Further information

Bourget P 1988 Ornidazole pharmacokinetics in several hepatic diseases. *Journal de Pharmacologie Clinique* 7: 25–32.

Horber FF, Maurer O, Probst PJ, Heizman E, Frey FJ 1989 High haemodialysis clearance of ornidazole in the presence of a negligible renal clearance. *European Journal of Clinical Pharmacology* 36: 389–393.

Martin C, Bruguerolle B, Mallet MN, Condomines M, Sastre B, Gouin F 1990 Pharmacokinetics and tissue penetration of a single dose of ornidazole (1000 milligrams intravenously) for antibiotic prophylaxis in colorectal surgery. *Antimicrobial Agents and Chemotherapy* 34: 1921–1924.

Meech RJ, Loutit J 1985 Non-specific vaginitis: diagnostic features and response to imidazole therapy (metronidazole, ornidazole). *New Zealand Medical Journal* 98: 389–391.

Merjian H, Baumelou A, Diquet B, Chick O, Singlas E 1985 Pharmacokinetics of ornidazole in patients with renal insufficiency: influence of haemodialysis and peritoneal dialysis. *British Journal of Clinical Pharmacology* 19: 211–217.

Taburet AM, Attili P, Bourget P, Etienne JP, Singlas E 1989 Pharmacokinetics of ornidazole in patients with acute viral hepatitis, alcoholic cirrhosis and extrahepatic cholestasis. *Clinical Pharmacology and Therapeutics* 45: 373–379.

Turcant A, Granry JC, Allain P, Cavellat M 1987 Pharmacokinetics of ornidazole in neonates and infants after a single intravenous infusion. *European Journal of Clinical Pharmacology* 32: 111–113.

SECNIDAZOLE

Molecular weight: 185.2.

Its properties are similar to those of metronidazole, but it is distinguished by having the longest plasma half-life (18 h) of clinically used nitroimidazole drugs. It is used in the treatment of intestinal amebiasis and giardiasis, and has been used in trichomoniasis.

Preparations and dosage

Proprietary name: Flagentyl.

Dosage: Adults, oral, 2 g as a single dose; children, 30 mg/kg as a single dose. In invasive amebiasis, 1.5 g per day for 5 days. Children, 30 mg/kg per day for 5 days.

Available in France.

Further information

Soedin K 1985 Comparison between the efficacy of a single dose of secnidazole with a 5-day course of tetracycline and clioquinol in the treatment of acute intestinal amoebiasis. *Pharmatherapeutica* 4: 251–254.

Develoux M 1990 Traitement de la giardiase par une dose unique de 30 mg/kg de secnidazole. *Médecine d'Afrique Noire* 37: 412–413.

TINIDAZOLE

Molecular weight: 247.3.

A 5-nitroimidazole available for oral administration and, in some countries, for intravenous infusion.

Antimicrobial activity

Its antibacterial and antiprotozoal activity is similar to that of metronidazole. Activity against the common anaerobic bacterial pathogens is shown in Table 27.1 (p. 335). The MIC against *Gard. vaginalis* is 0.2–2 mg/l; the hydroxy metabolite is significantly more active than that of metronidazole. *H. pylori* is inhibited by 0.5 mg/l. Tinidazole inhibits *T. vaginalis* and *T. fetus* at 2.5 mg/l and *E. histolytica* at about 0.3–2.5 mg/l.

Pharmacokinetics

Oral absorption	>95%
C_{max} 2 g oral	40 mg/l after 2 h (*c.* 10 mg/l at 24 h; 2.5 mg/l at 48 h)
Plasma half-life	12–14 h
Volume of distribution	0.64 l/kg
Plasma protein binding	12%

Six minutes after the end of infusion of 800 mg over 30 min, the mean plasma concentration was 12 mg/l. Daily doses of 1 g maintain plasma levels in excess of 8 mg/l, irrespective of whether the dose is oral or intravenous.

Distribution

Tissue distribution is widespread, with concentrations in bile, CSF, breast milk and saliva similar to those reached in plasma. The drug readily crosses the placenta. In women undergoing first trimester abortion, concentrations of 4.9 mg/kg (placenta) and 7.6 mg/kg (fetus) were found when the plasma concentration was 13.2 mg/l.

Metabolism

Metabolism in mammals forms the 2-hydroxymethyl derivative, its glucuronide and two minor and unidentified metabolites. In urine about half the drug remains unmetabolized.

Excretion

Tinidazole and its metabolites are excreted primarily in the urine and to a minor extent in the feces. The clearance rate is about 0.73 ml/min per kg and the urinary excretion is about

21% of the dose. Total clearance of the drug is 51 ml/min, renal clearance 10 ml/min. In healthy volunteers given an intravenous infusion of 800 mg [^{14}C]tinidazole over 30 min, a mean of 44% of the dose was excreted in the urine during the first 24 h. This increased to 63% of the dose over 5 days. Only 12% of the dose appeared in the feces, indicating a possible role for biliary excretion. Unchanged tinidazole comprised 32% of urinary ^{14}C in 0–12 h urine. The 2-hydroxymethyl metabolite accounted for about 9% of the urinary ^{14}C and was also present in plasma.

In renal failure the pharmacokinetics are not significantly different from those in healthy individuals, but because the drug is rapidly removed by hemodialysis it is recommended that the normal dosage be given after each dialysis, or that if treatment precedes dialysis a half dose be infused after the end of hemodialysis.

Toxicity and side effects

Tinidazole is generally well tolerated. Infrequent and transient effects include nausea, vomiting, diarrhea and a metallic taste. Disulfiram-like reactions may occur and rare neurological disturbances and transient leukopenia have been described. Rash, which may be severe, urticaria and angioneurotic edema can occur.

Clinical use

- Anaerobic bacterial infections (prophylaxis and treatment).
- Trichomoniasis.
- Giardiasis (single dose).
- Amebiasis (including amebic liver abscess).
- Bacterial vaginosis.
- Gastroduodenal ulcers (in combination with other agents).

Preparations and dosage

Proprietary names: Fasigin, Fasigyn, Fasigyne Simplotan, Sorquetan, Tricolam.

Preparations: Tablets, intravenous infusion.

Dosage:

In general, tinidazole in tablet form is taken with or after food.

Trichomoniasis, giardiasis, bacterial vaginosis and acute necrotizing gingivitis: Adults, a single oral 2 g dose. In trichomoniasis all sexual partners should be treated. Children, 50–75 mg/kg body weight, repeating the dose once if necessary.

Anaerobic bacterial infection: 2 g orally, then 1 g daily as a single dose or two divided doses for 5–6 days. Intravenous infusion: 800 mg as 400 ml of a 2 mg/ml solution at 10 ml/min, followed by 800 mg daily or 400 mg twice daily until oral therapy can be substituted.

Surgical prophylaxis: 2 g orally about 12 h before surgery; alternatively 1.6 g as a single intravenous infusion before surgery, or in two divided doses, one just before surgery, the other during or not longer than 12 h after surgery.

Intestinal amebiasis: Adults, a single 2 g dose for 2–3 days. Children, 50–60 mg/kg as a single daily dose for 3 days.

Liver amebiasis: Adults, 1.5–2 g as a single daily dose for 3–6 days. Children, 50–60 mg/kg as a single daily dose for 5 days.

Gastroduodenal ulcers (H. pylori): 500 mg twice daily for 7 days in combination with other drugs.

Available widely in continental Europe, including the UK. Not available in USA.

Further information

Anonymous 1988 Critical care requirements after elective surgery of the alimentary tract. *Current Medical Research Opinions* 11: 196–204.

Bannatyne RM, Jackowski J, Karmali MA 1987 Susceptibility of *Campylobacter* species to metronidazole, its bioactive metabolites and tinidazole. *Infection* 15: 457–458.

Boreham PFL, Philips RE, Shepherd RWA 1985 A comparison of the in-vitro activity of some 5-nitroimidazoles and other compounds against *Giardia intestinalis*. *Journal of Antimicrobial Chemotherapy* 16: 589–595.

Edwards DI 1993 Nitroimidazole drugs – action and resistance mechanisms. I. Mechanisms of action. *Journal of Antimicrobial Chemotherapy* 31: 9–20.

Edwards DI 1993 Nitroimidazole drugs – action and resistance mechanisms. II. Mechanisms of resistance. *Journal of Antimicrobial Chemotherapy* 31: 201–210.

Evaldson GR, Lindgren S, Nord CE, Rane AT 1985 Tinidazole milk excretion and pharmacokinetics in lactating women. *British Journal of Clinical Pharmacology* 13: 503–507.

Lossick JG 1990 Treatment of sexually transmitted vaginosis/vaginitis. *Reviews of Infectious Diseases* 12 (Suppl. 6): S665–S681.

Lossick JG, Kent HL 1991 Trichomoniasis: trends in diagnosis and management. *American Journal of Obstetrics and Gynecology* 165: 1217–1222.

Wood SG, John BA, Chasseaud LF et al 1986 Pharmacokinetics and metabolism of ^{14}C-tinidazole in humans. *Journal of Antimicrobial Chemotherapy* 17: 801–809.

28 Oxazolidinones

U. Ni Riain and A. P. MacGowan

The oxazolidinones are a novel class of synthetic antimicrobial agents unrelated to any existing class. The first members of the group were developed in the 1970s by E.I. DuPont de Nemours and Co. for control of bacterial and fungal disease in plants. Subsequently two 5(S)-acetamidomethyl-2-oxazolidinones, DuP 721 and DuP 105, emerged as potential candidates for clinical use. These early compounds exhibited potent activity against Gram-positive organisms, including strains resistant to many other classes of antibiotics, such as methicillin-resistant *Staphylococcus aureus*. However, due to toxicity associated with DuP 721, demonstrated in animal models, these agents were not developed for human use.

In the 1990s Pharmacia and Upjohn developed two further oxazolidinones, eperezolid (U-100592), a piperazine derivative, and linezolid (U-100766), a morpholine derivative. Preliminary studies indicated that their in vitro spectrum of activity was similar to that of the earlier agents, but they were less toxic in animals. In phase I clinical trials, linezolid was found to have the more favorable pharmacokinetic profile, and it has since proceeded successfully through phase II and III clinical trials to become the first member of this drug class licensed for human use (in 2000 in the USA and in 2001 in the UK).

Numerous chemical analogs have been screened in a search for compounds with enhanced potency or a broader spectrum of activity. Several promising candidates have been described, but to date, linezolid remains the only oxazolidinone licensed for human use.

These drugs inhibit protein synthesis (*see* p. 17) and exhibit potent activity against aerobic Gram-positive organisms including methicillin-resistant *Staph. aureus*, penicillin-resistant pneumococci and vancomycin-resistant enterococci. They are inactive against most Gram-negative species. They have potentially useful activity against mycobacteria. Resistance has not been detected in wild strains and so far only rarely during therapy.

Further information

Brickner SJ, Hutchinson DK, Barbachyn MR et al 1996 Synthesis and antibacterial activity of U-100592 and U-100766, two oxazolidinone antibacterial agents for the potential treatment of multidrug-resistant Gram-positive bacterial infections. *Journal of Medicinal Chemistry* 39: 673–679.

Diekema DJ, Jones RN 2000 Oxazolidinones. *Drugs* 59: 7–16.

Dresser LD, Rybak MD 1998 The pharmacologic and bacteriologic properties of oxazolidinones, a new class of synthetic antimicrobials. *Pharmacotherapy* 18: 456–462.

Ford C, Hamel JC, Stapert D et al 1997 Oxazolidinones: new antibacterial agents. *Trends in Microbiology* 5: 196–200.

Zurenko GE, Yagi BH, Schaadt RD et al 1996 In vitro activities of U-100592 and U-100766, novel oxazolidinone antibacterial agents. *Antimicrobial Agents and Chemotherapy* 40: 839–845.

LINEZOLID

Molecular weight: 337.35.

A synthetic oxazolidinone available for oral or intravenous administration. Soluble in water at a pH range of 5–9. Aqueous solutions (2 g/l) are stable at 25°C, 4°C and −20°C for at least 3 months.

Antimicrobial activity

The in-vitro activity against common pathogenic bacteria is shown in Table 28.1. It exhibits potent activity against a wide range of Gram-positive organisms, including those that are resistant to other antimicrobial agents. Methicillin-resistant *Staph. aureus* and coagulase-negative staphylococci are susceptible, as are enterococci, including vancomycin-resistant *Enterococcus faecalis* and *Enterococcus faecium*. Penicillin-sensitive and resistant isolates of *Streptococcus pneumoniae* are equally susceptible. Less common Gram-positive pathogens are also susceptible; the MICs for *Bacillus* spp., *Corynebacterium* spp., *Listeria monocytogenes* and *Rhodococcus equi* are all ≤4 mg/l.

All enterobacteria, *Pseudomonas* spp. and other non-fermentative aerobic Gram-negative bacilli, including

Table 28.1 Activity of linezolid against common pathogenic bacteria: MIC (mg/l)

	MIC
Staph. aureus (methicillin susceptible)	0.06–4
(methicillin resistant)	0.12–4
Coagulase-negative staphylococci	0.5–2
Str. pyogenes	0.5–4
Str. pneumoniae (penicillin susceptible)	0.12–4
(penicillin resistant)	0.5–4
E. faecalis (vancomycin susceptible)	0.5–4
(vancomycin resistant)	1–4
E. faecium (vancomycin susceptible)	1–4
(vancomycin resistant)	0.5–4
H. influenzae	8–16
N. gonorrhoeae	4–>16
Esch. coli	R
K. pneumoniae	R
Ps. aeruginosa	R
B. fragilis	1–8

R, resistant (MIC >32 mg/l).

Acinetobacter spp. are resistant. *Moraxella catarrhalis*, *Legionella* spp., *Mycoplasma* spp. and *Chlamydia* spp. are inhibited by 4–8 mg/l. Activity against *Haemophilus influenzae* is modest.

Among anaerobes, *Clostridium perfringens* and *Peptostreptococcus* spp. are inhibited by <2 mg/l. Typical MICs (mg/l) for Gram-negative anaerobes include: *Bacteroides* spp., 4–8; *Prevotella* spp., 1–4; *Fusobacterium* spp., 0.125–1. Data regarding the activity against *Mycobacterium* spp. are limited, but among the small number of isolates of *Mycobacterium tuberculosis* that have been tested the MICs were ≤2 mg/l, for sensitive and multidrug-resistant strains.

Activity is bacteristatic against most susceptible species, but bactericidal activity has been demonstrated against some strains of *Str. pneumoniae*, *C. perfringens* and *Bacteroides fragilis*. Inhibition of toxin production by staphylococci and streptococci in the presence of sub-MIC concentrations has been described.

Information on interactions with other antibacterial agents is limited, but no evidence of synergy has been found in various experimental systems with gentamicin against vancomycin-resistant *Enterococcus* spp. or with several other antibacterial agents against methicillin-resistant *Staph. aureus*.

Acquired resistance

In laboratory attempts to induce resistance in *Staph. aureus* no resistant mutants were found at 2, 4 or 8 times the MIC, yielding a spontaneous mutation frequency of $<8 \times 10^{-11}$. Isolates of *Staph. aureus* and *E. faecalis*, with stably elevated MICs have been obtained in vitro following serial exposure to gradients of linezolid. However, induction of resistance appears very difficult, requiring multiple passages over several weeks. Resistance

in these laboratory mutants is associated with modifications of the 23S rRNA gene – specifically, substitution of uridine for guanine at bases 2447(G2447U) and 2528(G2528U) of the 16S rRNA gene in *Staph. aureus* and *E. faecalis*, respectively. Among *Staph. aureus* isolates for which the MIC of linezolid ranged from 4 to 64 mg/l, those for which the MIC was at the higher end of the range had more mutations in 23S rRNA genes.

Emergence of resistance during therapy has so far been reported very rarely. The resistant isolates were primarily associated with prolonged use of the drug in the presence of irremovable indwelling devices, or, with low-dose therapy for infections caused by vancomycin-resistant enterococci or methicillin-resistant *Staph. aureus*.

To date, bacterial strains resistant to macrolides, lincosamides, chloramphenicol and other agents have not been observed to exhibit reduce susceptibility to linezolid.

Pharmacokinetics

Oral absorption	>95%
C_{max} 400 mg oral	11–12 mg/l after 1–2 h
600 mg oral	18–21 mg/l after 1–2 h
600 mg intravenous	>15 mg/l after 1 h
Plasma half-life	c. 5.5 h
Volume of distribution	45–50 l
Plasma protein binding	31%

Absorption

Bioavailability after oral administration is almost complete. Plasma trough concentrations following oral doses of 400 mg and 600 mg given 12-hourly are >3.0 and >4.0 mg/l, respectively. With the higher dose, administered orally or intravenously, plasma concentrations remain above the MIC for most susceptible species throughout a 12 h dosage interval. After administration with high fat content food the maximum serum concentration achieved is lower and the peak delayed, but the area under the time–concentration curve (AUC), is unaltered.

Distribution

Linezolid is distributed widely in tissues and fluids. Studies with human volunteers have indicated good concentrations in pulmonary alveolar fluid with a mean fluid to plasma ratio of 3.2:1. Other sites where local concentrations exceed corresponding plasma concentrations, based on animal studies, include kidney, adrenal, liver and gastrointestinal tract. In human volunteers, maximum concentrations in inflammatory blister fluid averaged over 16 mg/l, with a mean penetrancy of 104%. In a rat model of endocarditis, heart valve tissue and plasma concentrations were approximately equivalent. When the meninges are not inflamed, the concentration in cerebrospinal fluid (CSF) is lower than that of plasma, with a CSF:plasma ratio of approximately 0.7:1. The concentration in sweat is about half that of plasma.

Pharmacokinetic properties are unaltered in elderly patients, and dose adjustment is unnecessary. Single-dose pharmacokinetic studies indicate that plasma clearance and volume of distribution are greater in children than in adults, while peak and trough serum concentrations are lower.

Metabolism

Linezolid undergoes non-renal as well as renal metabolism. Non-renal metabolism is by slow chemical oxidation in a process that does not discernibly interact with the hepatic cytochrome P_{450} system. The oxidants contributing to metabolism of the drug have not been fully elucidated, but in-vivo studies suggest the process is mediated by reactive oxygen species produced throughout the body. The metabolites produced following non-renal metabolism are an aminoethoxyacetic acid and a hydroxyethyl glycine metabolite, neither of which has any significant antimicrobial activity. Non-renal clearance rates are 120 ml/min and account for almost 65% of total body clearance. Since it does not appear to act as an inducer or inhibitor of cytochrome P_{450} enzymes, interactions with drugs metabolized by these enzymes are unlikely to occur.

Excretion

Renal clearance accounts for approximately 50 ml/min of the total body clearance of 170 ml/min. Under steady-state conditions, approximately 30% of the dose is excreted unchanged in the urine.

In populations with varying degrees of renal function (creatinine clearance range of 10–>80 ml/min) there was no evidence of alteration in total body clearance, and adjustment of dose in patients with renal insufficiency is not thought to be necessary. However, accumulation of metabolites may occur in patients with severe renal impairment; the clinical significance of this is not yet known. There is an 80% increase in clearance on hemodialysis, suggesting the need to defer a due dose, or to administer an additional dose, after dialysis. Data for patients undergoing peritoneal dialysis are not currently available.

In patients with mild to moderate hepatic impairment there was no significant change to the pharmacokinetic profile. Accordingly, dosage adjustment is not recommended in patients with mild to moderate liver disease.

Pharmacodynamics

In mouse and rat models of infection with *Str. pneumoniae*, the parameter that best correlated with efficacy was the time the drug concentration remained above the MIC. In over 240 patients with significant infection caused by Gram-positive organisms, optimal efficacy was observed when plasma concentrations remained above the MIC for ≥ 85% of the dosage interval, or when the AUC:MIC ratio was ≥100.

A postantibiotic effect, which was more prolonged at 4 × MIC than at 1 × MIC, has been demonstrated for staphylococci and enterococci in vitro. A postantibiotic effect of 3–4 h

against *Staph. aureus* and *Str. pneumoniae* has been described in a mouse thigh model of infection.

Toxicity and side effects

Most reported adverse events have been mild or moderate, with reactions severe enough to lead to withdrawal of therapy occurring in less than 3% of patients. The most common adverse events are shown in Table 28.2. Overall, the most frequent side effects are gastrointestinal disturbances (diarrhea, nausea, vomiting and taste alteration) and headache. The reported incidence of *Clostridium difficile* complications is 0.2%.

Skin reactions, including rashes and dermatitis, were relatively common in phase I clinical trials, but occurred in <1% of patients in cumulative phase III trials.

Table 28.2 Common adverse drug reactions to linezolid

Adverse event	Frequency (%)
Diarrhea	4.3
Nausea	3.4
Headache	2.2
Vaginal candidiasis	1.2
Taste alteration (metallic taste)	1.2
Vomiting	1.1
Abnormal liver function tests	1.0

Mild and transient abnormalities of liver function tests (elevation of transaminases and/or alkaline phosphatase) have been observed in 1% of patients.

Reversible thrombocytopenia and fall in hemoglobin have been documented. Limited information from compassionate use programs indicates that the effect may be related to duration of therapy and may occur more frequently in patients with severe renal insufficiency. Monitoring of full blood count is recommend for patients with pre-existing anemia or thrombocytopenia, those receiving concomitant drugs which may cause anemia or thrombocytopenia, patients with severe renal insufficiency and patients treated for more than 10–14 days.

Although linezolid is a weak, reversible monoamine oxidase inhibitor in vitro, adverse events due to such inhibition have not yet been reported. However, because of the potential interaction, linezolid therapy is contraindicated for patients who are taking monoamine oxidase inhibitors concomitantly, or within 2 weeks of completing such therapy. Similarly, the drug should be administered to patients on concomitant therapy with sympathomimetics, vasopressors, tricyclic antidepressants or dopaminergic agents only under conditions where close observation and monitoring of blood pressure is available.

Clinical use

- Community- and hospital-acquired pneumonia caused by Gram-positive pathogens.
- Gram-positive skin and soft-tissue infections.
- Other serious infections caused by resistant Gram-positive organisms (currently outside the licensed indications in the UK).

Linezolid is primarily used for the treatment of infections caused, or likely to be caused, by methicillin-resistant *Staph. aureus*, vancomycin-resistant enterococci and penicillin-resistant *Str. pneumoniae*.

Preparations and dosage

Proprietary name: Zyvox.

Preparations: Tablets, suspension, injection.

Dosage: Adults, oral 400–600 mg every 12 h; i.v., 600 mg every 12 h. Not currently licensed for use in children.

Limited availability.

Further information

Bowersock TL, Salmon SA, Portis ES et al 2000 MICs of oxazolidinones for *Rhodococcus equi* strains isolated from humans and animals. *Antimicrobial Agents and Chemotherapy* 44: 1367–1369.

Clemett D, Markham A 2000 Linezolid. *Drugs* 59: 815–827.

Corti G, Cinelli R, Paradisi F 2000 Clinical and microbiologic efficacy and safety profile of linezolid, a new oxazolidinone antibiotic. *International Journal of Antimicrobial Agents* 16: 527–530.

Eliopoulos GM, Wennersten CB, Gold HS et al 1996 In vitro activities of new oxazolidinone antimicrobial agents against enterococci. *Antimicrobial Agents and Chemotherapy* 40: 1745–1747.

Ford CW, Hamel JC, Wilson DM et al 1996 In vivo activities of U-100592 and U-100766, novel oxazolidinone antimicrobial agents, against experimental bacterial infections. *Antimicrobial Agents and Chemotherapy* 40: 1508–1513.

Gee T, Ellis R, Marshall G et al 2001 Pharmacokinetics and tissue penetration of linezolid following multiple oral doses. *Antimicrobial Agents and Chemotherapy* 45: 1843–1846.

Goldstein EJ, Citron DM, Merriam CV 1999 Linezolid activity compared to those of selected macrolides and other agents against aerobic and anaerobic pathogens isolated from soft tissue bite infections in humans. *Antimicrobial Agents and Chemotherapy* 43: 1469–1474.

Hamel JC, Stapert D, Moerman JK et al 2000 Linezolid, critical characteristics. *Infection* 28: 60–64.

Hendershot PE, Jungbluth GL, Cammarata SK et al 1999 Pharmokinetics of linezolid in patients with liver disease. *Journal of Antimicrobial Chemotherapy* 44 (Suppl. A): 55.

Henwood CJ, Livermore DM, Johnson AP et al 2000 Susceptibility of Gram-positive cocci from 25 UK hospitals to antimicrobial agents including linezolid. *Journal of Antimicrobial Chemotherapy* 46: 931–940.

Johnson AP, Warner M, Livermore DM 2000 Activity of linezolid against multi-resistant Gram-positive bacteria from diverse hospitals in the United Kingdom. *Journal of Antimicrobial Chemotherapy* 45: 225–230.

Jones ME, Visser MR, Klootwijk M et al 1999 Comparative activities of clinafloxacin, grepafloxacin, levofloxacin, moxifloxacin, ofloxacin, sparfloxacin, and trovofloxacin and nonquinolones linezolid, quinupristin-dalfopristin, gentamicin and vancomycin against clinical isolates of ciprofloxacin-resistant and -susceptible *Staphylococcus aureus* strains. *Antimicrobial Agents and Chemotherapy* 43: 421–423.

Jones RN, Johnson DM, Erwin ME 1996 In vitro antimicrobial activities and spectra of U-100592 and U100766, two novel fluorinated oxazolidinones. *Antimicrobial Agents and Chemotherapy* 40: 720–726.

Kearns GL, Abdel-Rahman SM, Blumer JL et al 2000 Single dose pharmacokinetics of linezolid in infants and children. *Pediatric Infectious Disease Journal* 19: 1178–1184.

Mason EO, Lamberth LB, Kaplan SL 1996 In vitro activities of oxazolidinones U-100592 and U-100766 against penicillin-resistant and cephalosporin-resistant strains of *Streptococcus pneumoniae*. *Antimicrobial Agents and Chemotherapy* 40: 1039–1040.

Perry CM, Jarvis B 2001 Linezolid: a review of its use in the management of serious gram-positive infection. *Drugs* 61: 525–551.

Rybak MJ, Cappelletty DM, Moldovan T et al 1998 Comparative *in vitro* activities and postantibiotic effects of the oxazolidinone compounds eperezolid (PNU-100592) and linezolid (PNU-100766) versus vancomycin against *Staphylococcus aureus*, coagulase-negative staphylococci, *Enterococcus faecalis*, and *Enterococcus faecium*. *Antimicrobial Agents and Chemotherapy* 42: 721–724.

Schulin T, Wennersten CB, Ferraro MJ et al 1998 Susceptibilities of *Legionella* spp. to newer antimicrobials in vitro. *Antimicrobial Agents and Chemotherapy* 42: 1520–1523.

Stevens DL, Smith LG, Bruss JB et al 2000 Randomized comparison of linezolid (PNU-100766) versus oxacillin-dicloxacillin for treatment of complicated skin and soft tissue infections. *Antimicrobial Agents and Chemotherapy* 44: 3408–3413.

Wise R, Andrews JM, Boswell FJ et al 2000 The in vitro activity of linezolid (U-100766) and tentative breakpoints. *Journal of Antimicrobial Chemotherapy* 42: 721–728.

Wynalda MA, Hauer MJ, Wiwnkers LC 2000 Oxidation of the novel oxazolidinone antibiotic linezolid in human liver microsomes. *Drug Metabolism and Disposition* 28: 1014–1017.

Zurenko GE, Yagi BH, Schaadt RD et al 1996 In vitro activities of U-100592 and U-100766, novel oxazolidinone antibacterial agents. *Antimicrobial Agents and Chemotherapy* 40: 839–845.

29 Quinolones

Vincent T. Andriole

The quinolones comprise a large and expanding group of synthetic compounds based on the 4-quinolone nucleus:

A dual-ring structure with nitrogen at position 1, a carbonyl group at position 4 and a carboxyl group at position 3 of the first ring characterize all such compounds. X may be CH or N and ring closure can occur between R_1/R_2 and R_3/R_4, thereby giving rise to compounds that are structurally diverse, but in which the properties of the quinolone nucleus are preserved and may be enhanced. Quinolones have a carbon atom whereas naphthyridones have a nitrogen atom at position 8 of the second ring.

The first of the 4-quinolones, nalidixic acid (a 1,8-naphthyridine) was introduced for clinical use in 1962. Several others, including oxolinic acid and cinoxacin, quickly followed. The antimicrobial activity and pharmacokinetics of the original quinolones limited their clinical use. However, several key discoveries have led to better compounds with superior properties:

- the addition of a fluorine atom at position C-6 enhances antibacterial potency and provides activity against staphylococci;
- addition of a piperazine group at C-7 results in improved activity against aerobic Gram-negative bacteria and staphylococci;
- addition of a second fluorine group at C-8 increases absorption and results in a longer half-life, but also increases phototoxicity;
- ring alkylation improves anti-Gram-positive activity and half-life;
- addition of a cyclopropyl group at N-1, an amino group at C-5, and a fluorine group at C-8 increases activity against mycoplasmas and chlamydiae;
- addition of a methoxy group at C-8 targets both topoisomerase II and IV (*see* p. 18) and probably decreases development of quinolone resistance.

Application of these findings has led to numerous derivatives appearing on the world market and more are in development.

CLASSIFICATION

Like the cephalosporins, quinolones defy any rigid categorization, but presently available compounds can be classified into four broad groups:

Group 1: Older compounds with a spectrum of useful activity largely confined to *Escherichia coli* and other enterobacteria.

Group 2: Compounds developed in the 1980s with much improved activity against enterobacteria and an enhanced spectrum that included *Pseudomonas aeruginosa* and many Gram-positive cocci. Such compounds are characterized by 6-fluoro and 7-piperazinyl groups and became known as *fluoroquinolones*.

Group 3: Later compounds with further improvements in the spectrum, notably to include useful activity against *Streptococcus pneumoniae* and some other Gram-positive cocci, and, in some cases, improved pharmacological properties.

Group 4: The most recent compounds characterized by enhanced activity against Gram-positive cocci, including pneumococci, and anaerobes.

Compounds in groups 3 and 4 are also fluoroquinolones, but exhibit further structural modifications that contribute to their properties.

Some promising compounds (temafloxacin, grepafloxacin, and clinafloxacin) have been withdrawn from clinical use because of serious toxicity. Others, including danofloxacin, difloxacin, enrofloxacin, marbofloxacin, orbifloxacin and sarafloxacin, have been approved only for veterinary use. These compounds are not discussed further here, though there is debate about the contribution of veterinary quinolones to the development and spread of resistance.

Group 1	Group 2	Group 3	Group 4
Acrosoxacin	Ciprofloxacin	Gatifloxacin	Gemifloxacin
Cinoxacin	Enoxacin	Pazufloxacin	Moxifloxacin
Flumequine	Fleroxacin	Sparfloxacin	Sitafloxacin
Nalidixic acid	Levofloxacin	Tosufloxacin	Trovafloxacin
Oxolinic acid	Lomefloxacin		
Pipemidic acid	Norfloxacin		
Piromidic acid	Ofloxacin		
	Pefloxacin		
	Rufloxacin		

ANTIMICROBIAL ACTIVITY

Group 1 quinolones exhibit moderate activity against a wide range of enterobacteria, as well as *Haemophilus influenzae* and *Neisseria* spp. They have little or no activity against *Ps. aeruginosa*, anaerobes or Gram-positive bacteria (Table 29.1).

Manipulation of the chemical structure of the early quinolones produced compounds with greater potency and a much broader spectrum of activity (Table 29.2). Minimum inhibitory concentrations (MICs) of the group 2 fluoroquinolones are up to 100-fold lower than those of group 1 compounds for enterobacteria, *Aeromonas* spp., *Campylobacter* spp., *Yersinia* spp., *H. influenzae*, *Neisseria* spp. and *Moraxella catarrhalis*. Unlike non-fluorinated quinolones, they also exhibit useful activity against *Ps. aeruginosa*, and the most potent compounds are active against non-aeruginosa pseudomonads, *Acinetobacter* spp. and *Stenotrophomonas maltophilia*.

Fluoroquinolones have some activity against methicillin-resistant *Staphylococcus aureus* and *Staphylococcus epidermidis*, but greater activity against methicillin-susceptible strains.

Activity of the group 2 fluoro derivatives against *Str. pneumoniae* is poor, but some compounds of groups 3 and 4, including trovafloxacin, gatifloxacin and moxifloxacin, are very potent; they are less active against *Enterococcus* spp. and *Listeria monocytogenes*. Some group 3 (tosufloxacin, sparfloxacin) and group 4 (moxifloxacin, gemifloxacin, trovafloxacin) compounds also exhibit much improved activity against anaerobes.

Most fluoroquinolones exhibit activity against mycoplasmas, ureaplasmas and *Brucella* spp., as well as important intracellular pathogens including *Legionella* spp., *Chlamydophila* (formerly *Chlamydia*) *pneumoniae*, *Chlamydia trachomatis* and *Coxiella burnetii*. Some are also active against *Mycobacterium tuberculosis*. Other mycobacteria, including organisms of the *M. avium* complex are less susceptible.

The quinolones are rapidly bactericidal against most susceptible species at concentrations typically exceeding the MIC by no more than four-fold. However, there is usually an optimal bactericidal concentration above which the lethal action is diminished. This paradoxical effect is probably caused by dose-dependent inhibition of RNA synthesis.

Table 29.1 Activity of selected group 1 quinolones against common pathogenic bacteria: MIC (mg/l)

Species	Cinoxacin	Nalidixic acid	Pipemidic acid
Staph. aureus	64–R	R	R
Str. pyogenes	R	R	R
Str. pneumoniae	R	R	R
E. faecalis	R	R	R
N. gonorrhoeae		1	
H. influenzae	1	1	2
Esch. coli	1–4	4–8	2
K. pneumoniae	2–32	8–16	
Ps. aeruginosa	R	R	8–32
Acinetobacter spp.	R	R	
B. fragilis	R	R	32–R

R, resistant (MIC>64 mg/l).

Table 29.2 Activity of group 2 fluoroquinolones against common pathogenic bacteria: MIC (mg/l)

	Ciprofloxacin	Enoxacin	Fleroxacin	Levofloxacin	Lomefloxacin	Norfloxacin	Ofloxacin	Pefloxacin	Rufloxacin
Staph. aureus	0.25–1	2	1–2	0.25	1–2	1	0.12–1	0.5–1	2
Str. pyogenes	0.5–2	8–16	4–16	0.5	4–8	4	2	4–8	16
Str. pneumoniae	1–4	8–16	4–16	2	2–8	8	1–4	8	32
E. faecalis	0.5–2	≥8	4–16	2	8–16	8	2–4	4	32
Neisseria spp.	≥0.06	0.12	<0.06–0.5	<0.06	<0.06–0.12	≥0.06	≥0.06	≥0.06	0.12
H. influenzae	≥0.06	0.12	<0.06–0.25	<0.06	≥0.06–0.25	≥0.06	≥0.06	≥0.06	0.5
Esch. coli	≥0.06	0.25	0.12–0.5	0.25	0.25	0.25	0.06–0.25	0.25	2
K. pneumoniae	0.06–0.25	0.25	0.12–2	0.5	0.25	0.5	0.25	0.5	32
Ps. aeruginosa	0.25–2	2–8	1–8	1	0.25–4	1–2	2–4	2–4	8
B. fragilis	4–16	≥32	8–64	1	8–64	8–32	8	16	32
C. trachomatis	0.5–2	0.5–2	No data	0.25–1	0.5–2	4–16	0.5–2	2–8	4–8
M. tuberculosis	0.25–4	>4	>4	0.25	>4	2–8	0.5–2	>4	No data

ANTIMICROBIAL INTERACTIONS

Synergy or antagonism between quinolones and other antibacterial agents has been observed only rarely. Combinations of ciprofloxacin with imipenem or azlocillin have been found to be synergistic in vitro, particularly against *Ps. aeruginosa*. Rifampicin and fusidic acid have both been shown to antagonize the bactericidal activities of ciprofloxacin and pefloxacin against strains of *Staph. aureus*. However, these observations must be viewed with caution as conflicting results have been obtained with different in-vitro methods and with in-vivo tests.

INTERACTIONS WITH HOST DEFENCES

The fluoroquinolones rapidly accumulate in polymorphs and mononuclear cells, partly because of their lipid solubility. The ratio of cellular to extracellular concentrations range from 2:1 to 10:1, depending on the drug, the cell type and the bacterial species. Quinolones are also active intracellularly, exhibiting intraphagocytic cidal activities against a number of pathogens. They have no effect on chemotaxis, but preincubation of some pathogens in the presence of subinhibitory concentrations results in enhanced phagocytic killing. Subinhibitory concentrations of quinolones have also been shown to antagonize the adherence of both Gram-positive and Gram-negative bacteria to buccal and urinary tract epithelium and to fibrin-platelet matrices; this may be attributed to diminished production of bacterial adhesins, alterations to outer membrane proteins or changes in the surface properties of the host cells.

ACQUIRED RESISTANCE

MECHANISMS

The frequency with which bacteria develop resistance to the quinolones is much lower for the fluoroquinolones (10^{-12}) than for non-fluorinated compounds such as nalidixic acid (10^{-8}). Moreover, Gram-positive bacteria mutate to quinolone resistance at higher frequencies than Gram-negative organisms. Single-step mutations generally lead to two- to eight-fold increases in MICs and mutational resistance to one quinolone tends to confer some degree of resistance to all the other drugs in the group. The species that are most likely to become resistant to group 2 fluoroquinolones in a single mutational step are those of borderline susceptibility (e.g. *Ps. aeruginosa*, *Serratia* spp., *Acinetobacter* spp., *Staphylococcus* spp.). Organisms that are highly susceptible to fluoroquinolones remain within the susceptible range after single-step mutations and require multiple mutations before resistance becomes apparent.

Mutational resistance to quinolones usually occurs by chromosomal mutation in topoisomerases II (DNA gyrase) and IV (*see* p. 33). In addition, active efflux, a mechanism found in many clinically relevant bacteria, is responsible for low-level resistance that might act as a first step in resistance selection. Mutations that result in diminished production of outer membrane proteins, particularly OmpF, may also contribute to resistance by reducing uptake of quinolones in some species. However, the role of outer membrane proteins in acquired resistance remains unclear because porin mutations do not significantly alter quinolone MICs.

Apart from two unconfirmed reports of plasmid-mediated nalidixic acid resistance in *Shigella dysenteriae*, neither plasmid- nor transposon-mediated resistance to the 4-quinolones has been described to date in clinical isolates; indeed, these drugs have been used as plasmid-curing agents.

EPIDEMIOLOGY

In a UK study between 1971 and 1992, the percentage of urinary pathogens susceptible to nalidixic acid fell from 91 to 78 among community isolates and from 85 to 63 among hospital isolates.

Surveys of susceptibility to group 2 fluoroquinolones have

not detected large increases in the levels of resistance among species that are normally highly susceptible, despite the extensive use of these agents. However, clinically significant resistance has been found among bacterial species of otherwise borderline susceptibility, including *Ps. aeruginosa*, *Staph. aureus* (particularly methicillin-resistant strains, for which resistance rates of up to 80% have been reported), coagulase-negative staphylococci and *Acinetobacter* spp. Strains of *Neisseria gonorrhoeae* with reduced susceptibilities to fluoroquinolones have been isolated and are common in some countries of the world.

EFFECT OF TREATMENT

The emergence of resistance during treatment with quinolones is most likely to occur where large numbers of organisms are present at the sites of infection or where antibiotic concentrations at these sites are subinhibitory, either because of inadequate dosage or because antibiotic penetration is impaired. Such situations arise during prolonged or repeated courses of treatment in patients with chronic infections (e.g. acute exacerbations in patients with cystic fibrosis), when vascularity is compromised (e.g. infected leg ulcers), when large numbers of pathogens are sequestered in tissues where antibiotic penetration is poor (e.g. inadequately drained abscesses and osteomyelitis) and in the presence of foreign bodies.

The emergence and spread of resistant strains reflect the selective pressures of excessive use, hospitals in which fluoroquinolone prescribing is restricted reporting lower rates of resistance than those in which it is uncontrolled.

PHARMACOKINETICS

ABSORPTION

Most quinolones are rapidly absorbed when given by mouth, although there is considerable individual variation among different compounds. Absorption is inhibited by coadministration with antacids containing divalent metals, such as magnesium, calcium and iron, with which they form insoluble chelates. The pharmacokinetics of the fluoroquinolones that can be administered intravenously are similar to those following oral administration.

DISTRIBUTION

Protein binding of fluoroquinolones is low and they have large volumes of distribution. Concentrations approximating those in the plasma are found in tissue fluid and they penetrate into bone and prostate. Concentrations in the bronchial mucosa, lung epithelial lining fluid, and alveolar macrophages are usually higher than in plasma, and they are taken up by neutrophils and macrophages.

Concentrations of quinolones in cerebrospinal fluid (CSF) are about a third to a half the corresponding plasma level; the presence of inflammation does not appear to enhance penetration significantly.

ELIMINATION

The plasma half-life differs considerably among the different compounds. Most fluoroquinolones are eliminated primarily by hepatic metabolism and renal excretion. Ciprofloxacin, levofloxacin, gatifloxacin and gemifloxacin are highly dependent on renal elimination. Glomerular filtration and active tubular secretion represent major renal excretion pathways. Renal elimination of ciprofloxacin, levofloxacin and gatifloxacin are blocked by probenecid. These renally eliminated quinolones have significantly longer half-lives in patients with reduced renal function and dosing should be adjusted appropriately. Moxifloxacin, pefloxacin and trovafloxacin are not primarily dependent on renal elimination but are metabolized to varying degrees by the liver. In patients with mild to moderate hepatic failure, the pharmacokinetics of ofloxacin are unaltered, while those of ciprofloxacin are only slightly modified and those of pefloxacin and trovafloxacin are significantly modified, with an increased plasma half-life and area under the curve (AUC).

Changes in pharmacokinetics in the elderly are variable and usually small. Dosage modification is therefore not usually needed on the basis of age alone.

There is some excretion in the bile and high concentrations are found in the feces with resulting marked suppression of the aerobic Gram-negative flora. The flora returns to normal after cessation of treatment. Effects on the Gram-positive flora are less marked and the anaerobic flora is unaffected. Effects on the oropharyngeal flora are minimal, only *Neisseria* spp. being noticeably affected.

TOXICITY AND SIDE EFFECTS

The frequency of adverse events in patients receiving quinolones is comparable to that seen with other commonly used antibacterial agents. Rates of 6–10% have been described, with less than 1% of adverse events being recorded as serious. Although the frequency and severity of the various types of adverse events vary between individual quinolones, the nature of the events is similar for all congeners. Adverse events related to the gastrointestinal tract are by far the most common (about 5%), while those related to the CNS (about 1–2%) and the skin (0.5–1.5%) are less frequent. Most adverse events resolve without sequelae on stopping the drug.

GASTROINTESTINAL SYMPTOMS

Adverse events include nausea, diarrhea, dyspepsia, abdominal pain and anorexia; vomiting has been reported less frequently. Antibiotic-associated colitis or the asymptomatic excretion of *Clostridium difficile* toxin has been only rarely observed.

CENTRAL NERVOUS SYSTEM

Mild reactions such as headache, dizziness, tiredness or sleeplessness may occur; some patients experience abnormal vision, restlessness or unpleasant dreams. Severe side effects are rare (<0.5%) but have occurred with most quinolones and include psychotic reactions, hallucinations, depression, and grand mal convulsions. These reactions generally begin after a few days of therapy and end when therapy is stopped. Benign intracranial hypertension has been well described with nalidixic acid and has also been reported with pipemidic acid and ciprofloxacin. The mechanism of CNS effects is thought to be the blockade of synaptic inhibition by γ-aminobutyric acid.

SKIN REACTIONS

The most common skin reactions are erythema, pruritus, urticaria, rash and other cutaneous reactions. Phototoxic risks are high with C-8 halogen derivatives (fleroxacin, lomefloxacin and sparfloxacin) and low with C-8 methoxy derivatives (moxifloxacin and gatifloxacin). Phototoxicty can occur up to several weeks after stopping therapy and is unrelated to dosage.

HEMATOLOGICAL SYSTEM

Thrombocytopenia, leukopenia and anemia have been described. In one patient given norfloxacin a leukoagglutinin was detected, implying an immunological mechanism. An immunological mechanism has been ascribed to the hemolytic anemia rarely seen with nalidixic acid.

GENERAL IMMUNOLOGICAL REACTIONS

Very rare anaphylactoid reactions, including hypotension, bronchospasm and angioedema, have been reported. Onset is virtually immediate, suggesting a pre-existing allergy. The use of quinolones should be avoided in patients with a history of allergy to any quinolone. Patients with HIV infection appear to be particularly prone to such reactions.

NEPHROTOXICITY

Rare cases of acute interstitial nephritis or nephrotoxic reactions resulting from crystalluria with elevated plasma creatinine levels have occurred with fluoroquinolone therapy and are associated with alkaline urine. These lesions resolved on stopping therapy.

ARTHROPATHY

Arthralgia has been described in 1.5% of treatment courses in children with cystic fibrosis treated with ciprofloxacin and in 14% of adolescents treated with pefloxacin but, unlike the joint damage seen in young dogs, resolved on stopping treatment. Arthropathy has been described in older patients given nalidixic acid or norfloxacin. Tendonitis and Achilles' tendon rupture has been associated most frequently with pefloxacin therapy, and very rarely with ciprofloxacin, ofloxacin, levofloxacin, norfloxacin and enoxacin.

CARDIOVASCULAR EFFECTS

Hypertension and tachycardia have been seen during therapy with most quinolones, but their cardiotoxic potential varies. Sparfloxacin and grepafloxacin have the highest potential to induce QTc prolongation and arrhythmias including torsade de pointes; such complications have also been described infrequently in patients treated with levofloxacin or ofloxacin, but not so far in patients treated with moxifloxacin. Fluoroquinolones, however, are not recommended for use in patients receiving Class IA drugs that have Class III properties (e.g. quinidine, procainamide) or Class III (e.g. amiodarone, sotalol) anti-arrhythmic agents.

DRUG INTERACTIONS

The metabolized compounds can depress the hepatic cytochrome P_{450} isoform CYPIA2 enzyme system, resulting in reduced elimination of drugs which are handled similarly (e.g. some quinolones, particularly enoxacin and methylxanthines). Inhibition of the metabolism of theophylline and other xanthine derivatives increases their blood concentrations to toxic levels if dosage is not moderated. Serious manifestations of toxicity have included hallucinations, seizures, supraventricular tachycardia and atrial fibrillation.

The quinolones may interact to varying degrees with other drugs, including warfarin, H_2-receptor antagonists, cyclosporine, rifampicin, and non-steroidal anti-inflammatory drugs (NSAIDs). Concomitant administration of an NSAID with a quinolone may increase the risk of CNS stimulation and convulsive seizures.

Disturbances of blood glucose, including symptomatic hyper- and hypoglycemia, have been reported, usually in diabetic patients receiving concomitant treatment with an oral hypoglycemic or insulin. In these patients, careful monitoring of blood glucose is recommended, and the quinolone should be discontinued if a hypoglycemic reaction occurs.

CLINICAL USE

GROUP 1 QUINOLONES

The narrow Gram-negative spectrum of group 1 quinolones makes them suitable for the treatment of urinary tract infection. However, the readiness with which resistance develops in catheterized patients and those with complicated infections has restricted their use chiefly to the treatment of lower tract infection in domiciliary practice. They have also been used in some countries for enteric infections, notably severe *Shigella* dysentery.

FLUOROQUINOLONES (GROUPS 2–4)

Although some fluoroquinolones are available in both oral and parenteral formulations many infectious diseases can be treated successfully with oral therapy. The following are among common indications.

- Respiratory infections (i.e. acute bacterial exacerbations of chronic bronchitis, community-acquired pneumonia and sinusitis).
- Uncomplicated and some complicated urinary tract infections.
- Bacterial prostatitis.
- Skin and soft tissue infections.
- Bone and joint infections.
- Gastrointestinal infections, particularly infectious diarrhea caused by toxigenic *Esch. coli*, *Salmonella enterica* (including typhoid and paratyphoid fevers, and the chronic *Salmonella* carrier state), *Shigella*, *Campylobacter*, *Aeromonas*, and *Vibrio* species, as well as *Plesiomonas shigelloides*.
- Sexually transmitted diseases (gonococcal and chlamydial infections; chancroid) and pelvic infections.

However, not all fluoroquinolones have been approved for use in all of the infections mentioned above and individual compounds should only be used for approved indications. Use of trovafloxacin has been severely restricted in the US and withdrawn from use in other countries because of rare but severe hepatotoxicity. Quinolones are not recommended for use in pregnant or lactating women or in children unless there are overriding reasons for their use.

Urinary tract infections

Many quinolones are effective in uncomplicated cystitis; fluoroquinolones are also effective in pyelonephritis, complicated urinary tract infection, and as long-term, low-dosage prophylaxis. Single oral doses of these drugs are often curative in patients with uncomplicated infections, but 3-day regimens result in the highest cure rates. Despite their effectiveness, some believe fluoroquinolones should be reserved for infec-

tions caused by organisms resistant to standard therapeutic agents.

Group 2 fluoroquinolones, administered for 4–6 weeks, have been effective in episodes of prostatitis caused by *Esch. coli* and other enterobacteria. However, treatment failures are common in patients infected with *Ps. aeruginosa*, enterococci, staphylococci and *C. trachomatis*.

Sexually transmitted diseases

Single oral doses of most fluoroquinolones produce cure rates in excess of 97% in uncomplicated gonococcal infections. Although single-dose regimens have not been as effective in infections caused by *C. trachomatis*, 7-day courses of ofloxacin, fleroxacin, trovafloxacin, grepafloxacin or sparfloxacin have been associated with response rates of 97–100%, comparable to those achieved with doxycycline; in contrast, the failure rates with norfloxacin, enoxacin, pefloxacin and ciprofloxacin have been unacceptably high. Three-day courses of ciprofloxacin, ofloxacin, enoxacin or fleroxacin have been highly successful in patients with chancroid.

Respiratory tract infections

Clinical response rates equivalent or superior to those achieved with established agents have been achieved with fluoroquinolones in patients with acute bacterial exacerbations of chronic bronchitis, community- and hospital-acquired pneumonia, bronchiectasis and acute bacterial sinusitis. Remarkably high bacteriological eradication rates with the newer quinolones have been reported for *Str. pneumoniae*, *H. influenzae*, *Mor. catarrhalis* and enterobacteria, but there have been failures in patients infected with *Ps. aeruginosa*. Group 3 and group 4 fluoroquinolones are effective in penicillin-resistant pneumococcal infections and may be the therapy of choice in areas in which these organisms are prevalent.

For nosocomial pneumonia caused by Gram-negative bacilli, intravenous followed by oral quinolones have been effective, but patients with infections caused by *Ps. aeruginosa* may not respond and resistance can be expected to arise in a high percentage of strains.

Ciprofloxacin has been widely used in pediatric cystic fibrosis patients and is at least as effective as combination therapy with intravenous antipseudomonal β-lactam agents and aminoglycosides in improving pulmonary function. It is well tolerated and oral therapy reduces hospital stay. However, in common with other regimens, it does not eradicate *Ps. aeruginosa* from sputum. Development of ciprofloxacin resistance of *Ps. aeruginosa* is rare and usually transient. Ofloxacin and pefloxacin have also been used, but experience is much less. Ciprofloxacin has also been found to be effective in patients with proven *Legionella* infections, including those who were unresponsive to erythromycin.

Some quinolones (sparfloxacin, ciprofloxacin, ofloxacin), as part of multidrug regimens, have produced clinical and bacteriological cures in AIDS and non-AIDS patients infected with multidrug resistant strains of *M. tuberculosis* and in those with disseminated infections caused by organisms of the *M. avium* complex.

Skin and soft-tissue infections

Many fluoroquinolones are effective in cellulitis, subcutaneous abscesses, postoperative and post-traumatic wound infections, infected decubitus, ischemic and diabetic ulcers, polymicrobial deep foot infections and infected burns. Although the need to treat anaerobic bacteria in diabetic foot infections is controversial, if a quinolone is used to treat severe limb-threatening infected foot ulcers in diabetics, addition of a second antibiotic effective against anaerobes is prudent.

Quinolones should not be used as monotherapy where anaerobic bacteria might be present and they should not be used as first-line, empirical therapy for infections caused by methicillin-resistant *Staph. aureus*. In patients colonized or infected with methicillin-resistant *Staph. aureus*, quinolone treatment has resulted in low rates of eradication, high rates of recolonization and frequent emergence of quinolone-resistant strains. Quinolones are not recommended for severe β-hemolytic streptococcal infections, such as necrotizing fasciitis.

Osteomyelitis and septic arthritis

Until quinolones can be confirmed to be at least as effective as standard antistaphylococcal drugs, they should not be prescribed for bone infections caused by this pathogen. In all other types of osteomyelitis clinical and bacteriological cure rates achieved by fluoroquinolones have been similar to, or better than, those following standard parenteral therapy. The emergence of resistant strains during therapy has been observed most notably with *Ps. aeruginosa* and has been almost invariably associated with the presence of a prosthesis. This may be limited by administering a β-lactam antibiotic and/or an aminoglycoside for a brief initial period.

Enteric infections

Group 2 fluoroquinolones are now regarded as first-choice treatment of severely ill patients with gastroenteritis of suspected or proven bacterial etiology. Clinical cure rates in infections caused by *Salmonella enterica* serotypes Typhi and Paratyphi are superior to those produced by all other regimens. Owing to the high concentrations attained in the liver, bile and gall-bladder, fluoroquinolones are also more effective than conventional therapy in eradicating the chronic carrier state.

In the treatment of diarrhea caused by salmonellae, shigellae or campylobacter, fluoroquinolones are significantly better than placebo or older antibiotics in shortening the duration of fever and diarrhea, as well as in eradicating the pathogens from feces. Administration for periods as short as 3 days, is as effective as tetracycline in patients with moderate to severe cholera. Quinolones, in particular ciprofloxacin, have also been used successfully to eliminate *Salmonella* carriage in institutional outbreaks where there are high risks of person-to-person spread. However, both persistence and relapse have been described, particularly in patients with AIDS, despite prolonged administration.

Several quinolones reduce both the duration (by 1–3 days) and intensity of travellers' diarrhea. Reports of the emergence of resistant strains of enteric pathogens (other than *Campylobacter* spp.) during therapy have so far been rare.

Infection in the neutropenic patient

In neutropenic patients receiving cytotoxic therapy, prophylactic administration of ciprofloxacin, ofloxacin and pefloxacin has been associated with reductions in the incidence of bacteremias caused by enterobacteria, but not those caused by Gram-positive bacteria. Indeed, quinolone prophylaxis has contributed to the emergence of these latter organisms as the predominant pathogens in the neutropenic patient. The strategy of combining a quinolone with benzylpenicillin, rifampicin (rifampin) or a macrolide has been successful in some, but not all, trials, but did not reduce overall morbidity. Of concern in patients receiving quinolone chemoprophylaxis is the development of quinolone-resistant strains of *Esch. coli*, *Ps. aeruginosa* and non-aeruginosa pseudomonads.

Monotherapy with group 2 quinolones should not be used empirically for febrile neutropenic patients and should not replace a standard β-lactam/aminoglycoside regimen unless the latter is contraindicated, in which case the quinolone should be combined with an agent that has greater activity against Gram-positive pathogens. Although, ciprofloxacin in combination with benzylpenicillin, an aminoglycoside, a glycopeptide or an extended-spectrum penicillin seems to be at least as effective as other standard regimens such combinations have not been thoroughly evaluated.

Meningitis

Fluoroquinolones penetrate into CSF in concentrations that are bactericidal for *H. influenzae*, *N. meningitidis* and many Gram-negative rods, but the concentrations of the older drugs, even following intravenous administration, are unlikely to exceed the MIC_{90} for *Str. pneumoniae*. However, fluoroquinolones of groups 3 and 4 have much better activity against *Str. pneumoniae*, making them attractive alternatives in the era of drug-resistant pneumococci.

Quinolones of groups 2 and 3 have been used sporadically in treating bacterial meningitis. Their major role has been in patients with multiresistant Gram-negative bacillary meningitis, most of whom were cured with intravenous therapy. Trovafloxacin, given orally or intravenously, was found to be as effective as ceftriaxone during an epidemic of meningococcal meningitis in Nigeria.

Group 2 quinolones are inappropriate for patients with CSF shunt infections in whom the predominant pathogens are coagulase-negative staphylococci and the degree of meningeal inflammation is usually minimal. However, they may be life-saving alternatives to standard agents in patients with infections caused by multiresistant Gram-negative rods, including *Ps. aeruginosa*.

Ciprofloxacin, in a single dose or twice daily for 2 days, is highly effective (93–96%) at eradicating nasopharyngeal carriage of *N. meningitidis* and is an appropriate alternative to rifampicin for this purpose and as prophylaxis in close contacts of patients with meningococcal disease.

Miscellaneous use

In patients receiving continuous ambulatory peritoneal dialysis (CAPD), the relative lack of efficacy of quinolones as treatment of episodes of peritonitis caused by Gram-positive cocci, particularly staphylococci, the chelation of these drugs with coadministered oral bivalent and trivalent metal ions (frequently given to patients with end-stage renal disease) and the variable bioavailabilities of oral formulations combine to restrict the use of fluoroquinolones to the treatment of exit-site infections.

Fluoroquinolones are highly effective as therapy of malignant otitis externa (caused primarily by *Ps. aeruginosa*) and might be used empirically in place of standard antipseudomonal regimens. Topical preparations have also been used successfully to treat bacterial conjunctivitis and blepharitis.

Prophylaxis

Ciprofloxacin is effective in preventing genitourinary tract infections following transurethral prostatectomy and as prophylaxis in patients undergoing biliary tract, orthopedic implant, cardiac and vascular surgery. Advantages of quinolones over alternative regimens are most apparent in prostatic and biliary surgery, particularly if they are administered by the oral route.

Quinolones prevent bacterial infections in patients following liver transplantation, in those with acute hepatic failure and in cirrhotic patients with gastrointestinal tract hemorrhage. When a quinolone (norfloxacin) was used alone or in place of an aminoglycoside for selective digestive tract decontamination in patients in intensive care units, the incidence of nosocomial infections was reduced. Nonetheless, there are justifiable concerns about the use of quinolones for this purpose.

 Further information

Ackerman G, Schaumann R, Pless B et al 2000 Comparative activity of moxifloxacin in vitro against obligately anaerobic bacteria. *European Journal of Clinical Microbiology and Infectious Diseases* 19: 229–232.

Andriole VT (ed.) 2000 *The Quinolones*, 3rd edn. Academic Press, San Diego, CA.

Carratala J, Fernandez-Sevilla A, Tubau F, Callis M, Gudiol F 1995 Emergence of quinolone-resistant *Escherichia coli* bacteremia in neutropenic patients with cancer who have received prophylactic norfloxacin. *Clinical Infectious Diseases* 20: 557–560.

Courvalin P 1990 Plasma-mediated 4-quinolone resistance; a real or apparent absence? *Antimicrobial Agents and Chemotherapy* 34: 681–684.

Cruciani M, Bassetti D 1994 The fluoroquinolones as treatment for infections caused by Gram-positive bacteria. *Journal of Antimicrobial Chemotherapy* 33: 403–417.

Dembry LM, Farrington JM, Andriole VT 1999 Fluoroquinolone antibiotics: Adverse effects and safety profiles. *Infectious Diseases in Clinical Practice* 8: 9–16.

Dong Y, Xu C, Zhao X, et al 1998 Fluoroquinolone action against mycobacteria: Effects of C-8 substituents on growth, survival and resistance. *Antimicrobial Agents and Chemotherapy* 42: 2978–2984.

Harnett N, McLeod S, Au Yong Y, Hewitt C, Vearncombe M, Krishnan C 1995 Quinolone resistance in clinical strains of *Campylobacter jejuni* and *Campylobacter coli*. *Journal of Antimicrobial Chemotherapy* 36: 269–270.

Smith JT, Lewin CS 1988 Chemistry and mechanism of action of the quinolone antibacterials. In: Andriole VT (ed.) *The Quinolones*, 2nd edn. Academic Press, London, pp. 23–81.

Zhanel GG, Walkty A, Vercaigne L et al 1999 The new fluoroquinolones: a critical review. *Canadian Journal of Infectious Diseases* 10: 207–238.

GROUP 1 QUINOLONES

 CINOXACIN

Molecular weight: 262.2.

A cinnoline derivative available for oral administration.

Antimicrobial activity

The activity against common pathogens is shown in Table 29.1 (p. 350). It is active against most enterobacteria, but *Ps. aeruginosa*, Gram-positive bacteria and anaerobes are resistant.

Acquired resistance

Resistant mutants are relatively easily selected by serial passage in the presence of the drug and have emerged during courses of treatment.

Pharmacokinetics

Oral absorption	95%
C_{max} 500 mg oral	c. 15 mg/l after 1–3 h
Plasma half-life	1–1.5 h
Volume of distribution	c. 0.25 l/kg
Plasma protein binding	60–70%

Absorption and distribution

Administration with food reduces the peak concentration by about a third, but the area under the curve (AUC) remains unchanged. Concentrations in prostatic and bladder tissues reach 60% and 80%, respectively, of the simultaneous serum concentrations.

Metabolism and excretion

It is almost entirely excreted in the urine, about 40–60% as unchanged drug and the rest as metabolites, most of which have no antimicrobial activity. Urinary concentrations of active drug in the first 2 h after administration of a dose are 100–500 mg/l. Elimination is reduced by probenecid and by renal impairment, the half-life rising to about 12 h in end-stage renal failure.

Toxicity and side effects

It is generally well tolerated, adverse reactions that are common to the group (p. 352) being reported in 4–5% of patients; these are primarily gastro-intestinal tract disturbances, but rashes occur in up to 3% and CNS disturbances in less than 1%.

Clinical use

- Uncomplicated urinary tract infection.

Preparations and dosage

Proprietary name: Cinobac.

Preparation: Capsules.

Dosage: 500 mg every 6–12 h; prophylaxis 250–500 mg/day.

Widely available, not UK.

Further information

Anonymous 1999 Cinoxacin. In: Dollery C (ed.) *Therapeutic Drugs* 2nd edn. Churchill Livingstone, Edinburgh, pp. C224–C226.
Sisca TS, Heel RC, Romakiewicz JA 1983 Cinoxacin. A review of its pharmacological properties and therapeutic efficacy in the treatment of urinary tract infections. *Drugs* 25: 544–569.

NALIDIXIC ACID

Molecular weight: 232.2.

A naphthyridine derivative available for oral administration.

Antimicrobial activity

Its activity against common pathogenic organisms is shown in Table 29.1 (p. 350). It is active in vitro against a wide range of enterobacteria, including many strains that are resistant to β-lactam antibiotics and other drugs. *Ps aeruginosa*, Gram-positive bacteria and anaerobes are resistant.

Acquired resistance

Resistance develops readily following serial passage in the presence of nalidixic acid, although primary resistance among urinary pathogens is unusual. The development of resistance is observed more frequently with *Proteus*, *Klebsiella* and *Enterobacter* spp. than with *Esch. coli*. The emergence of resistance during treatment sometimes occurs, especially in patients with complicated urinary tract infections.

Pharmacokinetics

Oral absorption	>90%
C_{max} 1 g oral	c. 25 mg/l
Plasma half-life	c. 1.5 h
Volume of distribution	0.4 l/kg
Plasma protein binding	93%

Absorption and distribution

The plasma concentrations achieved in individual subjects after oral administration vary widely. In infants with acute shigellosis, absorption is much impaired by diarrhea. Administration with an alkaline compound leads to higher plasma concentrations, partly as the result of enhanced dissolution (nalidixic acid is much more soluble at higher pH) and absorption and partly because of reduced tubular reabsorption.

Metabolism and excretion

It is rapidly metabolized, principally to the hydroxy acid, which is microbiologically active, and glucuronide conjugates, which are not. Virtually all of a dose appears in the urine over 24 h. Excretion is reduced by probenecid. In the presence of renal impairment there is little accumulation of the active compound because it continues to be metabolized. However, elimination of metabolites is progressively delayed as renal function declines. About 4% of a dose appears in the feces.

Toxicity and side effects

Adverse reactions are generally those common to all quinolones (p. 352), i.e. gastrointestinal tract and CNS disturbances and skin rashes, including eruptions related to photosensitivity. About half of the reported CNS reactions involve visual disturbances, hallucinations or disordered sensory perception. Severe excitatory states, including acute psychoses and convulsions, are usually observed in patients receiving high dosages. The drug should be avoided in patients with psychiatric disorders or epilepsy.

Acute intracranial hypertension has been observed in children, some of whom have also manifested cranial nerve palsies. Hemorrhage has occurred in patients who were also receiving warfarin, presumably due to displacement of the anticoagulant from its protein binding sites by the nalidixic acid. Hemolytic anemia has been described several times in infants with or without glucose-6-phosphate dehydrogenase deficiency; in adults, death has occurred from autoimmune hemolytic anemia. Arthralgia and severe metabolic acidosis have been reported rarely.

Clinical use

- Urinary tract infection.
- Prophylaxis in patients undergoing transurethral surgery.
- Treatment of acute shigellosis.

Preparations and dosage

Proprietary names: Mictral, Negram, Uriben.

Preparations: Tablets, suspension.

Dosage: Adults, oral, 1 g every 6 h for 7 days; for chronic infections, 500 mg every 6 h. Children >3 months, oral, 50 mg/kg per day in divided doses; reduced in prolonged therapy to 30 mg/kg per day.

Widely available.

Further information

Andriole, VT (ed.) 2000 *The Quinolones* 3rd edn. Academic Press, San Diego.

Anonymous 1999 Nalidixic acid. In: Dollery C (ed.) *Therapeutic Drugs* 2nd edn. Churchill Livingstone, Edinburgh, pp. N17–20.

Barbeau G, Belanger P-M 1982 Pharmacokinetics of nalidixic acid in old and young volunteers. *Journal of Clinical Pharmacology* 22: 490–496.

Gleckman R, Alvarez S, Joubert DW, Matthews SJ 1979 Drug therapy reviews: nalidixic acid. *American Journal of Hospital Pharmacy* 36: 1071–1076.

Islam MR, Alam AN, Hossain MS, Mahalanabis D, Hye HK 1994 Double-blind comparison of oral gentamicin and nalidixic acid in the treatment of acute shigellosis in children. *Journal of Tropical Pediatrics* 40: 320–325.

Schaad UB, Wedgwood-Krucko J 1987 Nalidixic acid in children: retrospective matched controlled study for cartilage toxicity. *Infection* 15: 165–168.

PIPEMIDIC ACID

Molecular weight: 302.3.

A pyridopyrimidine, available for oral administration.

Antimicrobial activity

The piperazine substitution at C-7 increases in-vitro activity against *Ps. aeruginosa*. It exhibits no useful activity against Gram-positive bacteria or anaerobes (Table 29.1; p. 350). Resistant mutants develop readily and can emerge during courses of treatment.

Pharmacokinetics

Oral absorption	>90%
C_{max} 500 mg oral	3–4 mg/l after 1–2 h
Plasma half-life	*c.* 3.5 h
Plasma protein binding	15–40%

The drug is rapidly metabolized, primarily to acetyl, formyl and oxo derivatives, which exhibit 10–30% of the antimicrobial activity of the parent compound.

It is excreted in the urine, 50–85% of a dose appearing over the first 24 h, less than 2% as inactive metabolites. Non-renal clearance accounts for 10–40% of a dose in the young, rising to 40–70% in the elderly and thereby compensating for renal insufficiency. No dosage adjustment is necessary in patients with mild renal insufficiency. Some of the drug is eliminated in the bile and a significant portion of a dose appears in the feces.

Toxicity and side effects

Nausea and vomiting are common; dizziness, weakness and grand mal seizures have been observed, principally in the elderly. A number of reactions have been sufficiently severe to require discontinuation of therapy.

Clinical use

- Urinary tract infection.

Preparations and dosage

Dosage: Adults, oral, 400 mg twice daily.

Widely available in continental Europe and Japan.

Further information

Klinge E, Mannisto PT, Mantyla R, Mattila J, Hanninen U 1984 Single- and multiple-dose pharmacokinetics of pipemidic acid in normal human volunteers. *Antimicrobial Agents and Chemotherapy* 26: 69–73.

Mannisto P, Solkinen A, Mantyla R et al 1984 Pharmacokinetics of pipemidic acid in healthy middle-aged volunteers and elderly patients with renal insufficiency. *Xenobiotica* 14: 339–347.

OTHER GROUP 1 QUINOLONES

Acrosoxacin (rosoxacin)

The antimicrobial spectrum and potency resemble those of other members of the group, but it is particularly active against *N. gonorrhoeae* (MIC 0.06–0.01 mg/l), including β-lactamase producers.

A single oral dose of 300 mg produces a mean peak plasma concentration of 4–5 mg/l at about 2–4 h, with a plasma elimination half-life of about 6 h. Excretion in the urine is partly as the *N*-oxide metabolite and the glucuronides of this metabolite.

Side effects are those common to the quinolones (p. 352), notably gastrointestinal tract and CNS disturbances. About 50% of patients treated with single oral doses of 100–400 mg developed dizziness, drowsiness, altered visual perception and other CNS effects, none of which was clearly dose-related.

It is effective as single-dose treatment of patients with urethral and anorectal gonorrhea, but coexistent *C. trachomatis* infection is not eliminated from most patients and postgonococcal urethritis develops in up to 30%.

Preparations and dosage

Proprietary name: Eradacin.
Preparation: Capsules.
Dosage: Adult, oral, 300 mg as a single dose.
Limited availability.

Further information

Handsfield HH, Judson FN, Holmes KK 1981 Treatment of uncomplicated gonorrhoea with rosoxacin. *Antimicrobial Agents and Chemotherapy* 20: 625–629.
Park GB, Saneski J, Weng T, Edelson J 1982 Pharmacokinetics of rosoxacin in human volunteers. *Journal of Pharmaceutical Sciences* 71: 461–462.
Romanowski B, Austin TW, Pattison FLM et al 1984 Rosoxacin in the therapy of uncomplicated gonorrhoea. *Antimicrobial Agents and Chemotherapy* 25: 445–457.

Flumequine

A 6-fluoroquinolone with activity similar to that of nalidixic acid, although it is somewhat more active against some enterobacteria. Resistant strains that are cross-resistant to nalidixic and oxolinic acids have emerged during treatment.

Following oral doses of 400, 800 or 1200 mg mean peak plasma concentrations, obtained at about 2 h, are 13.5, 23.8 and 31.9 mg/l, respectively. The plasma elimination half-life is about 7 h. The principal metabolite, hydroxyflumequine, is much more rapidly eliminated. About 60% of a dose appears in the urine, mostly in the form of conjugates. Urinary concentrations following an 800 mg dose are 10–35 mg/l, with a peak of 105 mg/l. It has no effect on the pharmacokinetics of theophylline.

Flumequine is generally well tolerated, side effects being mainly mild gastrointestinal tract disturbances, rashes, dizziness and confusion.

It is principally used in uncomplicated urinary tract infection.

Preparations and dosage

Dosage: Adult, oral, 400 mg two to three times daily.
Limited availability in continental Europe.

Further information

Schuppan D, Harrison LI, Rohlfing SR et al 1985 Plasma and urine levels of flumequine and 7-hydroxyflumequine following single and multiple oral dosing. *Journal of Antimicrobial Chemotherapy* 15: 337–343.

Oxolinic acid

An oral 4-quinolone with a cyclized 6,7-methylenedioxy structure.

Its spectrum is very similar to that of nalidixic acid, but it is more active against enterobacteria (MIC 0.25–2 mg/l). It also has some activity against *Staph. aureus* (MIC 4–16 mg/l), but other Gram-positive bacteria, *Ps. aeruginosa* and anaerobes are resistant. Bacteria readily acquire resistance. In some series, the emergence of resistant strains has been a notable cause of treatment failure.

It is erratically absorbed when administered by mouth. In patients receiving 750 mg twice daily, mean plasma concentrations are initially very low, but by the third day rise to around 3.5 mg/l. Administration with food delays absorption. Binding to plasma protein is about 80%. It undergoes complex biotransformation, and enterohepatic recycling may account for the increase in the plasma elimination half-life from 4 to 15 h over 7 days of treatment and for the 20% of a dose which can be recovered from the feces. About 50% of a dose appears in the urine in the first 24 h, partly in the form of metabolites, some of which are microbiologically active.

Side effects common to the 4-quinolones (p. 352) occur frequently. Of patients treated with a dosage regimen of 750 mg twice daily, about a quarter suffered nausea and vomiting or restlessness and insomnia. Its only use is in the treatment of patients with lower urinary tract infections, where its efficacy is undermined by irregular absorption and the frequency of side effects.

Preparations and dosage

Dosage: Adults, oral, 750 mg every 12 h. Children, 50–600 mg every 12 h (age dependent).
Widely available in continental Europe.

Further information

Gleckman R, Alvarez S, Joubert DW, Matthews SJ 1979 Drug therapy reviews: oxolinic acid. *American Journal of Hospital Pharmacy* 36: 1077–1010.

Piromidic acid

A pyrimidopyrimidine with properties similar to those of pipemidic acid. Its antimicrobial activity is no better than that of nalidixic acid and there have been suspicions of renal toxicity. More potent compounds have overtaken it, but it is still available in some countries, including Japan.

GROUP 2 QUINOLONES

CIPROFLOXACIN

Molecular weight (free base): 331.4.

A 6-fluoro, 7-piperazinyl quinolone formulated as the hydrochloride for oral administration and as the lactate for intravenous use.

Antimicrobial activity

Activity against common bacterial pathogens is shown in Table 29.2 (p. 351). It exhibits potent activity against most enterobacteria, including many strains resistant to unrelated agents. *Acinetobacter* spp. (MIC 0.25–1 mg/l), *Mor. catarrhalis* (MIC 0.06–0.25 mg/l) and *Campylobacter jejuni* (MIC 0.12 mg/l) are all sensitive. *Ps. aeruginosa*, other non-fermenting Gram-negative bacilli, *Staph. aureus* (including methicillin-resistant strains), coagulase-negative staphylococci, *Str. pyogenes*, *Str. pneumoniae* and enterococci are less susceptible (MIC c. 0.5–2 mg/l). It has poor activity against anaerobes, but useful activity against *M. tuberculosis* and other *Mycobacterium* spp. *Mycoplasma* spp. and intracellular pathogens such as *Chlamydia* and *Legionella* are also susceptible.

Acquired resistance

Resistant mutants can be selected by passage in the presence of increasing concentrations of the drug and have emerged during courses of treatment of some patients, particularly those infected with *Ps. aeruginosa* or methicillin-resistant strains of *Staph. aureus* or coagulase-negative staphylococci. In such cases, there is cross-resistance with other fluoroquinolones.

There have been several reports of large increases in the prevalence of resistance in *Staph. aureus* in hospitals in which ciprofloxacin has been extensively used.

Pharmacokinetics

Oral absorption	50–80%
C_{max} 500 mg oral	1.5–2 mg/l after 1–2 h
200 mg intravenous (15 min infusion)	3.5 mg/l end infusion
Plasma half-life	3–4 h
Volume of distribution	3–4 l/kg
Plasma protein binding	20–40%

Absorption

Mean peak plasma concentrations increase proportionately with dose. Some accumulation occurs with 500 mg oral doses or 200 mg intravenous doses twice daily and the plasma half-life has been reported to rise to about 6 h after a regimen of 250 mg twice daily for 6 days. Absorption is delayed, but otherwise unaffected by food and, in common with other quinolones, is depressed by certain antacids. Coadministration of sucralfate reduced the peak plasma concentrations of ciprofloxacin to undetectable levels in a number of subjects and the mean value from 2 to 0.2 mg/l. The AUC was reduced to 12% of the value obtained when ciprofloxacin was administered alone. Ferrous sulfate and multivitamin preparations containing zinc significantly reduce absorption, which is also impaired in patients receiving cytotoxic chemotherapy for hematological malignancies. Calculated total bioavailability is 60–70%.

Distribution

The drug is widely distributed in body water, concentrations in most tissues and in phagocytic cells approximating those in plasma. Concentrations in the CSF, even in the presence of meningitis, are about half the simultaneous plasma levels. In patients with hydrocephalus without meningeal inflammation who received 200 mg twice daily by intravenous infusion over 30 min, CSF concentrations reached 0.04–0.2 mg/l and did not significantly increase as the course of treatment proceeded. In the prostate, and particularly in the lung, concentrations can exceed those in plasma by many-fold.

Metabolism

Ciprofloxacin is partly metabolized to four products, all but one of which (desethylciprofloxacin) are microbiologically active.

Excretion

About 95% of a dose can be recovered from the feces and urine. Around 40% of an oral and 75% of an intravenous dose appear in the urine over 24 h. Excretion is by both glomerular filtration and tubular secretion (60–70%) and is depressed by concurrently administered probenecid and by renal insufficiency. Other organic acids can compete for elimination, and administration with azlocillin results in reduced clearance and significantly elevated and prolonged plasma concentrations of ciprofloxacin, without any change in the pharmacokinetics of azlocillin. It is poorly removed by hemodialysis. Some is excreted in the bile, and enterohepatic recirculation evidently plays some part in prolonging the half-life, although most of the drug detected in the feces is unabsorbed. Small quantities of the four metabolites are present in the urine and feces where concentrations of active agent after conventional dosages have been around 100–200 mg/l and 200–2000 mg/kg, respectively.

Toxicity and side effects

Untoward reactions are uncommon, those encountered being typical of the group (p. 352). Reactions severe enough to require withdrawal of treatment have occurred in less than 2% of patients. The most common reactions, gastrointestinal tract disturbances, have been seen in 5% of patients and rashes (rarely photosensitive) in about 1%. CNS disturbances typical of quinolones have been reported in 1–2% of patients. Potentiation of the action of theophylline and other drugs metabolized by microsomal enzymes can occur. Crystalluria and transient arthralgia have been rarely reported. In volunteers, dosages of up to 750 mg produced no change in the numbers of fecal streptococci and anaerobes, but a $2.5 \times \log_{10}$ decline in the numbers of enterobacteria, which lasted 1 week. There was no change in the MICs of the affected organisms and no overgrowth by resistant strains. As with other quinolones, ciprofloxacin is not recommended for use in children or in pregnant or lactating women.

Clinical use

- Urinary tract infections (especially pathogens resistant to standard agents).
- Prostatitis.
- Uncomplicated urogenital and rectal gonorrhea (single dose).
- Purulent bronchitis, bronchopneumonia, acute exacerbations of chronic obstructive airways disease, pneumonia (other than pneumococcal pneumonia) and bronchiectasis; pulmonary exacerbations in cystic fibrosis; legionellosis.
- Osteomyelitis caused by Gram-negative bacteria
- Enteric fever (including chronic carriage); severe bacterial gastroenteritis; cholera.
- Mycobacterial infections caused by multidrug resistant *M. tuberculosis* or *M. avium* complex (in combination with other agents).
- Eradication of nasopharyngeal carriage of *N. meningitidis*.

The drug should be avoided in suspected or confirmed infections caused by *Str. pneumoniae*. It is inferior to conventional agents and some other fluoroquinolones in the treatment of genital tract infections caused by *C. trachomatis*.

Ciprofloxacin has also been shown to be effective in the treatment of patients with malignant otitis externa or cat-scratch disease, the prevention of infection in patients undergoing biliary tract surgery and the treatment of infections of the biliary tract. A topical preparation of ciprofloxacin for use in the treatment of ocular infections is available, but is neither more effective nor safer than established topical agents; it may be indicated for superficial eye infections caused by pathogens resistant to conventional drugs or in patients unable to tolerate standard therapeutic agents.

Preparations and dosage

Proprietary name: Ciproxin.

Preparations: Tablets, oral suspension, injection, ophthalmic.

Dosage: Adults, oral, 250–750 mg twice daily; i.v. infusion, 100–400 mg twice daily. Children, where the benefits outweigh the risks, oral, 7.5–15 mg/kg per day in two divided doses; i.v., 5–10 mg/kg per day in two divided doses. Higher doses needed in pseudomonal lower respiratory tract infection in cystic fibrosis.

Widely available.

Further information

Andriole VT (ed.) 2000 *The Quinolones* 3rd edn. Academic Press, San Diego.

Anonymous 1999 Ciprofloxacin (hydrochloride). In: Dollery C (ed.) *Therapeutic Drugs* 2nd edn. Churchill Livingstone, Edinburgh, pp. C230–C235.

Wilson APR, Gruneberg RN 1997 Ciprofloxacin. Ten years clinical experience. Maxim Medical, Oxford, England.

Garretts JC, Godley PJ, Peterie JD, Gerlach EH, Yakshe CC 1990 Sucralfate significantly reduces ciprofloxacin concentrations in serum. *Antimicrobial Agents and Chemotherapy* 34: 931–933.

Hirata CAI, Guay DRP, Awni WM, Stein DJ, Peterson PK 1989 Steady-state pharmacokinetics of intravenous and oral ciprofloxacin in elderly patients. *Antimicrobial Agents and Chemotherapy* 33: 1927–1931.

Jacobs F, Marchal M, de Francquen P, Kains J-P, Ganji D, Thys J-P 1990 Penetration of ciprofloxacin into human pleural fluid. *Antimicrobial Agents and Chemotherapy* 34: 934–936.

Lettieri JT, Rogge MC, Kaiser K, Echols RM, Meller AN 1992 Pharmacokinetic profile of ciprofloxacin after single intravenous and oral doses. *Antimicrobial Agents and Chemotherapy* 36: 993–996.

Nau R, Prange HW, Martell J, Sharifi S, Kolenda H, Bircher J 1990 Penetration of ciprofloxacin into the cerebrospinal fluid of patients with uninflamed meninges. *Journal of Antimicrobial Chemotherapy* 25: 956–973.

Oppenheim BA, Hartley JW, Lee W, Burnie JP 1989 Outbreak of coagulase negative staphylococcus highly resistant to ciprofloxacin in a leukaemia unit. *British Medical Journal* 299: 294–297.

Polk RE, Healy DP, Sahai J, Orwal L, Racht E 1989 Effect of ferrous sulfate and multivitamins with zinc on absorption of ciprofloxacin in normal volunteers. *Antimicrobial Agents and Chemotherapy* 33: 1841–1844.

Raviglione MC, Boyle JF, Mariuz P, Pablos-Mendez A, Cortes H, Merlo A 1990 Ciprofloxacin-resistant methicillin-resistant *Staphylococcus aureus* in an acute-care hospital. *Antimicrobial Agents and Chemotherapy* 34: 2050–2054.

Smith DM, Eng RHK, Bais P, Fan-Havard P, Tecson-Tumang F 1990 Epidemiology of ciprofloxacin resistance among patients with methicillin-resistant *Staphylococcus aureus*. *Journal of Antimicrobial Chemotherapy* 26: 567–572.

ENOXACIN

Molecular weight: 321.3.

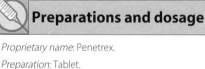

A 6-fluoro, 7-piperazinyl naphthyridine available for oral administration.

Antimicrobial activity

Activity against common bacterial pathogens is shown in Table 29.2 (p. 351). *Mor. catarrhalis* and *Campylobacter* spp. are susceptible, *Ps. aeruginosa*, *Serratia* and *Citrobacter* spp. less so and *Acinetobacter* spp. resistant. It has poor activity against *L. monocytogenes*, *Nocardia* spp. and *Mycobacterium* spp. Anaerobes and *Chlamydia* and *Ureaplasma* spp. are all moderately resistant.

Acquired resistance

Resistant mutants are selected following serial passage in the presence of the drug and have occasionally emerged during courses of treatment. There is cross-resistance with other quinolones, but not with unrelated agents.

Pharmacokinetics

Oral absorption	*c*. 80%
C_{max} 400 mg oral	2–3 mg/l after 1–2 h
Plasma half-life	3–6 h
Volume of distribution	2.5–3 l/kg
Plasma protein binding	35%

Absorption

With a regimen of 400 mg twice daily for 14 days, mean peak plasma concentrations reach 3.5–4.5 mg/l, a steady state being achieved in 3–4 days. Absorption is not significantly affected by food, but ranitidine, sucralfate, some antacids and some mineral supplements may interfere with absorption.

Distribution

It is widely distributed; concentrations close to, or exceeding by up to two-fold, those in plasma are found in saliva, sputum, prostatic fluid, bone and blister fluid. Very high concentrations (>100 mg/kg) have been detected in lung tissue after a dose of 400 mg twice daily for 5 days.

Metabolism and excretion

About 40–60% of a dose is excreted unchanged in the urine with less than 10% as the 3-oxo metabolite, which is 10–20 times less active microbiologically. In renal failure, the plasma elimination half-life rises to >20 h, with marked reduction in the elimination of the oxo metabolite. Hemodialysis removes insignificant amounts of both compounds. Some is excreted in bile, where concentrations of 4.5–25 mg/l have been found when the corresponding serum levels were 0.5–2 mg/l.

Toxicity and side effects

About 6% of patients experience mild and transient effects typical of the quinolones: gastrointestinal tract disturbances, rashes, headaches and dizziness. Epileptiform and asthmatic attacks have occurred, but serious effects have been rare. In patients also receiving theophylline, concentrations of this compound are raised.

Clinical use

- Urinary tract infection

In lower respiratory tract infection good clinical response rates have been reported, but bacteriological eradication rates for *Str. pneumoniae* were significantly lower than those for Gram-negative bacteria such as *H. influenzae*.

It is inferior to other fluoroquinolones in urogenital or anorectal gonorrhea. It has been used successfully to treat chancroid, but it has frequently failed to cure patients with infections caused by *C. trachomatis* or genital mycoplasmas.

 Preparations and dosage

Proprietary name: Penetrex.

Preparation: Tablet.

Dosage: Adults, oral, 200–400 mg twice daily.

Available in the USA and continental Europe.

Further information

Henwood JM, Monk JP 1988 Enoxacin. A review of its antibacterial activity, pharmacokinetic properties and therapeutic use. *Drugs* 36: 32–66.

Jaber LA, Bailey EM, Rybak MJ 1989 Enoxacin: a new fluoroquinolone. *Clinical Pharmacy* 8: 97–107.

Koup JR, Toothaker RD, Posvar E, Sedman AJ, Colburn WA 1990 Theophylline dosage adjustment during enoxacin co-administration. *Antimicrobial Agents and Chemotherapy* 34: 803–807.

Van der Auwera P, Stolear JC, George B, Dudley MN 1990 Pharmacokinetics of enoxacin and its oxometabolite following intravenous administration in patients with different degrees of renal impairment. *Antimicrobial Agents and Chemotherapy* 34: 1491–1497.

FLEROXACIN

Molecular weight: 369.4.

A trifluorinated quinolone formulated as the hydrochloride for oral use.

Antimicrobial activity

The spectrum and activity are similar to those of norfloxacin and ofloxacin (Table 29.2; p. 351).

Pharmacokinetics

Oral absorption	>90%
C_{max} 400 mg oral	6 mg/l after 1–2 h
Plasma half-life	9–12 h
Volume of distribution	1.43 l/kg
Plasma protein binding	30%

Absorption and distribution
Absorption is not affected by food. Bioavailability is virtually complete and binding to plasma protein is around 30%. Steady-state plasma concentrations in subjects receiving 200 or 400 mg twice daily are 2–4 and 4–9 mg/l, respectively. Accumulation occurs following multiple dosing of 800 mg or more over 10 days. It is widely distributed with tissue or fluid:plasma ratios of 0.6 in saliva, 0.3–2 in prostate and 1.7 in seminal fluid.

Metabolism and excretion
About 50% of a dose appears in the urine as unchanged drug and about 5% as each of the principal (desmethyl and *N*-oxide) metabolites, giving urinary concentrations of the active compound of around 150–300 mg/l. The dosage interval (normally 24 h) should be increased in renal failure. Concentrations in T-tube bile are 2–3 times those in plasma. About 3% of a 400 mg oral dose appears in the feces, producing concentrations of 100–150 mg/g.

Toxicity and side effects

Untoward effects are those typical of the group (p. 354). Gastrointestinal tract, CNS disturbances (particularly insomnia and bad dreams) and phototoxicity occur most frequently.

Clinical use

- Simple or complicated urinary tract infections.
- Uncomplicated gonococcal infections; chlamydial genital tract infections; chancroid.
- Bacterial enteritis; typhoid fever.

Fleroxacin is effective in patients with respiratory tract infections, including acute bacterial exacerbations of chronic bronchitis and pneumonia, but in common with other group 2 fluoroquinolones, its use should be avoided in infections that are known or suspected to be caused by *Str. pneumoniae*. Limited data suggest it is effective in osteomyelitis and biliary tract infections.

 Preparations and dosage

Proprietary name: Quinodis.

Preparations: Tablet, injection.

Dosage: Adult, oral and i.v., 200–400 mg once daily, increased to twice daily in severe infections.

Available in Japan and continental Europe.

 Further information

Andriole, VT (ed.) 2000 *The Quinolones* 3rd edn. Academic Press, San Diego.

Balfour JA, Todd PA, Peters DH 1995 Fleroxacin. A review of its pharmacology and therapeutic efficacy in various infections. *Drugs* 49: 794–850.

DeLepeleire I, Van Hecken A, Verbesselt R, Tjandra-Maga TB, DeShepper PJ 1988 Comparative oral pharmacokinetics of fleroxacin and pefloxacin. *Journal of Antimicrobial Chemotherapy* 22: 197–202.

Singlas E, Leroy A, Sultan E et al 1990 Disposition of fleroxacin, a new trifluoroquinolone, and its metabolites. Pharmacokinetics in renal failure and influence of haemodialysis. *Clinical Pharmacokinetics* 19: 67–79.

Symposium 1988 Fleroxacin, a long acting fluoroquinolone with broad spectrum activity. *Journal of Antimicrobial Chemotherapy* 22 (Suppl. D): 1–230.

 LEVOFLOXACIN

Molecular weight and structure: see ofloxacin (p. 366). Levofloxacin is the L-isomer of ofloxacin.

Antimicrobial activity

Levofloxacin is generally twice as active as ofloxacin (Table 29.2; p. 351). It exhibits excellent activity against enterobacteria and *Mor. catarrhalis*, but only moderate activity against *Ps. aeruginosa* and *Acinetobacter* spp. It has only modest activity against Gram-positive bacteria (*Staph. aureus* being the most susceptible), *C. trachomatis* and *B. fragilis*. It has some activity against *M. tuberculosis*.

Pharmacokinetics

Oral absorption	>95%
C_{max} 500 mg oral	c. 5 mg/l after 3 h
500 mg intravenous (1 h infusion)	c. 6 mg/l end infusion
Plasma half-life	6–8 h
Volume of distribution	0.6–0.8 l/kg
Plasma protein binding	<25%

Coadministration with antacids, calcium, sucralfate and heavy metals decreases bioavailability and AUC. It undergoes limited metabolism in humans and is excreted primarily unchanged in urine by both glomerular filtration and tubular secretion. Concomitant administration of either cimetidine or probenecid reduces renal clearance by approximately one-third. Clearance is reduced and half-life is prolonged in patients with impaired renal function.

Toxicity and side effects

Serious and sometimes fatal events have been reported rarely. Side effects have been reported in 6–7% of patients and include fever, rash and other side effects common to the group (p. 352).

Clinical use

- Acute maxillary sinusitis.
- Acute bacterial exacerbations of chronic bronchitis; community-acquired pneumonia.
- Uncomplicated skin and skin structure infections.
- Uncomplicated and complicated urinary infections including acute pyelonephritis.

Preparation and dosage

Proprietary name: Levoquin.

Preparations: Tablets and injection.

Dosage: Adults, oral, 250–500 mg/day; IV, 250–500 mg/day. Community acquired pneumonia, up to 500 mg twice daily.

Widely available.

Further information

Andriole VT (ed.) 2000 *The Quinolones*. Academic Press, San Diego.

Yew WW, Piddock LJV, Li MSK, Lyon D, Chan CY, Cheng AFB 1994 In-vitro activity of quinolones and macrolides against mycobacteria. *Journal of Antimicrobial Chemotherapy* 34: 343–351

LOMEFLOXACIN

Molecular weight (free base): 351.4.

A difluoropiperazinyl quinolone formulated as the hydrochloride for oral administration.

Antimicrobial activity

The spectrum and activity of lomefloxacin are typical of those of other members of the group (Table 29.2; p. 351). It is active against *Mor. catarrhalis* and *L. pneumophila*. Less susceptible are *Campylobacter* spp., *Ps. aeruginosa*, *Acinetobacter* and *Chlamydia* spp. Lomefloxacin has reduced activity against staphylococci and poor activity against streptococci (including *Str. pneumoniae* and enterococci), *L. monocytogenes*, anaerobes and *Mycobacterium* spp.

Pharmacokinetics

Oral absorption	>95%
C_{max} 400 mg oral	3–5 mg/l after 1–1.5 h
Plasma half-life	7–8 h
Volume of distribution	1.8 l/kg
Plasma protein binding	c. 10%

Absorption and distribution

In volunteers the AUC was essentially proportional to the dosage, the mean plasma concentrations following 100, 400 and 800 mg doses being around 1.1, 4.7 and 7.5 mg/l, respectively. Some accumulation occurred in volunteers receiving 200 mg twice daily for 5 days, with a 20% increase in the AUC. Blister fluid contains around 3.5 mg/l 2.7 h after an oral dose of 400 mg. The drug is concentrated in various tissues.

Metabolism and excretion

Several metabolites have been described, but they account for <5% of the oral dose. Excretion is principally by the kidneys and 50–70% of a dose appears in the urine over 24 h. In patients with impaired renal function given 400 mg orally, the plasma elimination half-life ranged from 8 to 44 h, depending on the degree of renal failure. Non-renal clearance was also impaired, but there was no significant change in other pharmacokinetic parameters. Mean urinary excretion of the drug and its glucuronide fell from 60% to 1% over 48 h. The daily dosage (normally 400 mg) should be reduced to 280 mg when the creatinine clearance falls below 30 ml/min. Hemodialysis has no effect on the plasma concentration. The effect of lomefloxacin on the plasma concentration of theophylline is clinically insignificant and no dosage adjustment is required.

Toxicity and side effects

Adverse events occur in about 10% of patients, mainly diarrhea, abdominal pain, skin reactions (chiefly phototoxicity) and CNS effects (dizziness, headache and sleeplessness).

Clinical use

- Urinary tract infection.
- Transurethral surgery (prophylaxis).
- Acute exacerbations of chronic bronchitis.

Preparations and dosage

Proprietary name: Maxaquin.

Preparation: Tablets, ophthalmic.

Dosage: Adults, oral, 400 mg once daily.

Available in the USA and Japan; not available in the UK.

Further information

Andriole VT (ed.) 2000 *The Quinolones* 3rd edn. Academic Press, San Diego.

Anonymous 1999 Lomefloxacin (hydrochloride). In: Dollery C (ed.). *Therapeutic Drugs* 2nd edn. Churchill Livingstone, Edinburgh, pp. L80–L86.

Blum RA, Schultz RW, Schentag JJ 1990 Pharmacokinetics of lomefloxacin in renally compromised patients. *Antimicrobial Agents and Chemotherapy* 34: 2364–2368.

Freeman CD, Nicolan DP, Belliveau PP, Nightingale CH 1993 Lomefloxacin clinical pharmacokinetics. *Clinical Pharmacokinetics* 25: 6–19.

Nix DE, Norman A, Schentag JJ 1989 Effect of lomefloxacin on theophylline pharmacokinetics. *Antimicrobial Agents and Chemotherapy* 33: 1006–1008

NORFLOXACIN

Molecular weight: 319.3.

A 6-fluoro, 7-piperazinyl quinolone available for oral administration and as an ophthalmic ointment.

Antimicrobial activity

The activity against common bacterial pathogens is shown in Table 29.2 (p. 351). It is active against a wide range of Gram-negative bacteria, including *Campylobacter* spp. Gram-positive bacteria particularly pneumococci and enterococci, *Ps. aeruginosa* and *Acinetobacter*, *Serratia* and *Providencia* spp. are less susceptible (and often resistant). It has no useful activity against important anaerobes, *Chlamydia*, *Mycoplasma* and *Mycobacterium* spp.

Acquired resistance

Less than 5% of strains of enterobacteria causing urinary tract infections are currently resistant. There is complete cross-resistance with other quinolones but none with unrelated agents.

Pharmacokinetics

Oral absorption	50–70%
C_{max} 400 mg oral	1.5 mg/l after 1–1.5 h
Plasma half-life	3–4 h
Volume of distribution	2.5–3.1 l/kg
Plasma protein binding	15%

Absorption and distribution

Doubling the dosage approximately doubles the peak plasma concentration. There is no significant accumulation with the recommended dosage of 400 mg twice daily. Food slightly delays but does not otherwise impair absorption. Antacids reduce absorption. It is widely distributed, but concentrations in tissues other than those of the urinary tract are low; levels in the prostate are around 2.5 mg/g.

Metabolism and excretion

Six or more metabolites are produced, most being microbiologically inactive. Around 30% of a dose appears as unchanged drug in the urine and less than 10% as metabolites, producing peak concentrations of microbiologically active drug of around 100–400 mg/l. Urinary recovery is halved by probenecid, with little effect on the plasma concentration. The plasma elimination half-life increases with renal impairment, rising to around 8 h in the anuric patient. Some of the drug appears in the bile where concentrations three- to seven-fold greater than the simultaneous plasma levels are achieved, but this is not a significant route of elimination and hepatic impairment is without effect. Very variable quantities, averaging 30% of a dose, appear in the feces, producing concentrations of active agent of around 200–2000 mg/kg.

Toxicity and side effects

Untoward reactions are those common to the fluoroquinolones (p. 352). Gastrointestinal tract disturbances, which are generally mild, have been reported in 2–4% of patients. CNS disturbances have largely been limited to headache, drowsiness and dizziness. Coadministration with theophylline results in increased plasma theophylline levels.

Clinical use

- Simple or complicated urinary tract infections (including prophylaxis in recurrent infections); prostatitis.
- Uncomplicated gonorrhea.
- Gastroenteritis caused by *Salmonella*, *Shigella* and *Campylobacter* spp. *V. cholerae*.
- Conjunctivitis (ophthalmic preparation).

Preparations and dosage

Proprietary name: Utinor.

Preparations: Tablets, ophthalmic.

Dosage: Adults, oral, 400 mg twice daily for 7–10 days; uncomplicated lower urinary tract infections, 400 mg twice daily for 3 days; chronic relapsing urinary tract infections, 400 mg twice daily for 12 weeks, reduced to 400 mg/day if adequate suppression within first 4 weeks.

Widely available.

Further information

Andriole VT (ed.) 2000 *The Quinolones* 3rd edn. Academic Press, San Diego.

Anonymous 1999 Norfloxacin. In: Dollery C (ed.) *Therapeutic Drugs* 2nd edn. Churchill Livingstone, Edinburgh, pp. N137–N141.

Holmes B, Brogden RN, Richards DM 1985 Norfloxacin. A review of its antibacterial activity, pharmacokinetic properties and therapeutic use. *Drugs* 30: 482–513.

Symposium 1987 Norfloxacin: a fluoroquinolone carboxylic acid antimicrobial agent. *American Journal of Medicine* 82 (Suppl. 6B): 1–92.

OFLOXACIN

Molecular weight: 361.38.

A 6-fluoro, 7-piperazinyl quinolone with a methyl-substituted oxazine ring. The methyl group can be in the D- or L-configurations and pharmaceutical preparations formulated for oral, intravenous or ophthalmic use are mixtures of the two isomers.

Antimicrobial activity

Activity against the common bacterial pathogens is shown in Table 29.2 (p. 351). It exhibits potent activity against a wide range of enterobacteria, including strains resistant to nalidixic acid, as well as against *Aeromonas*, *Campylobacter*, *Vibrio* and *Mor. catarrhalis*. Staphylococci are more susceptible than streptococci, including pneumococci and enterococci, against which activity is limited. Most anaerobes are either moderately or completely resistant. It is active against *L. pneumophila*, *C. pneumoniae*, *C. trachomatis*, mycoplasmas and ureaplasmas. *M. tuberculosis*, *M. fortuitum*, *M. kansasii* and *M. chelonei* are moderately susceptible; the *M. avium* complex less so.

Acquired resistance

Resistant mutants can be generated by a single passage in the presence of 4–8 times the MIC of the agent: *Staph. aureus* and *Esch. coli* with a frequency of *c.* 10^{-10} and *Ps. aeruginosa* with a frequency of *c.* 10^{-8}. There is complete cross-resistance with other quinolones, but not with unrelated agents.

Pharmacokinetics

Oral absorption	*c.* 95%
C_{max} 400 mg oral	3–5 mg/l after 1–1.5 h
200 mg intravenous (30 min infusion)	1.8 mg/l 1 h after end infusion
Plasma half-life	5–7 h
Volume of distribution	1–2.5 l/kg
Plasma protein binding	*c.* 25%

Absorption

There is no significant interference with absorption by magnesium-aluminum hydroxide or calcium carbonate compounds that normally impair quinolone absorption, providing administration is separated by at least 2 h. In patients receiving repeated 200 mg doses, the mean peak plasma concentration rises from 2.7 mg/l after the first dose to 3.4 mg/l after the seventh.

Distribution

It is widely distributed, achieving concentrations in many tissues, including lung and bronchial secretions, of 50% or more of the simultaneous plasma concentrations. In cantharides and suction blisters the peak concentrations exceed those in plasma, while the elimination half-life is similar. In patients with non-inflamed meninges, 200 mg administered orally or by intravenous infusion over 30 min produced CSF concentrations of around 0.4–1 mg/l at 2–4 h when the plasma concentration was 1.7–4 mg/l; a 400 mg intravenous infusion yielded a CSF concentration of 2 mg/l, which is adequate for some Gram-negative bacteria, but not for Gram-positive bacteria or *Ps. aeruginosa*.

Metabolism and excretion

There is limited metabolism to the desmethyl and *N*-oxide derivatives, only about 20% of a dose being eliminated by non-renal routes. There is a very slight effect on cytochrome-P_{450}-related isoenzymes and no significant effect on the metabolism of theophylline in dosages of up to 800 mg.

About 60% of a dose appears in the urine over 12 h; 80–90% over 48 h. The plasma elimination half-life is prolonged in renal failure, reaching 30–50 h in anuria, and therefore necessitating a dosage reduction. The desmethyl metabolite accumulates in all patients and the *N*-oxide in 50%. Absorption and distribution are not affected by renal failure. Significant amounts of the drug appear in the feces, producing very variable concentrations up to 100 mg/kg.

Toxicity and side effects

Untoward reactions have been described in 2.5–7.5% of patients, and are those common to the group: gastrointestinal tract disturbances, rashes and insomnia. More dramatic CNS effects in some patients have included hallucinations, mostly visual, and psychotic reactions. In some patients, influenza-like symptoms have been described.

The presence of the drug in feces results in rapid and virtually complete elimination of enterobacteria, with some increase in the numbers of streptococci, but no effect on the numbers of anaerobes. The fecal flora returns to normal 3–26 days after discontinuing treatment.

Clinical use

- Simple and complicated infections of the urinary tract; chronic prostatitis.
- Uncomplicated urogenital and anorectal gonorrhea (single-dose); chancroid (3-day course); genital chlamydial infections (7-day course).
- Respiratory tract infections, including bronchopneumonia, community-acquired pneumonia (except pneumococcal pneumonia), acute bacterial exacerbations of chronic bronchitis and bronchiectasis.
- Enteric fever, including the chronic carrier state; gastroenteritis caused by enterotoxigenic *Esch. coli* and *Salmonella*, *Shigella* and *Campylobacter* spp.
- Other infections caused by susceptible organisms.
- Ocular infections (ophthalmic preparation).

 Preparations and dosage

Proprietary name: Tarivid.

Preparations: Tablets, injection, ophthalmic.

Dosage: Adults, oral, 200–400 mg/day, increased to 400 mg twice daily in severe infections; i.v., 200–400 mg once or twice a day depending on severity of infection.

Widely available.

 Further information

Andriole VT (ed.) 2000 *The Quinolones* 3rd edn. Academic Press, San Diego.

Anonymous 1999 Ofloxacin. In: Dollery C (ed.) *Therapeutic Drugs* 2nd edn. Churchill Livingstone, Edinburgh, pp. O7–O12.

Flors S, Guay DRP, Opsahl JA, Tack K, Matzke GR 1990 Effects of magnesium-aluminium hydroxide and calcium carbonate antacids on bioavailability of ofloxacin. *Antimicrobial Agents and Chemotherapy* 34: 2436–2438.

Guay DRP, Opsahl JA, McMahon FG, Vargas R, Matzke GR, Flor S 1992 Safety and pharmacokinetics of multiple doses of intravenous ofloxacin in healthy volunteers. *Antimicrobial Agents and Chemotherapy* 36: 308–312.

Navarro AS, Lanao JM, Recio MMS et al 1990 Effect of renal impairment on distribution of ofloxacin. *Antimicrobial Agents and Chemotherapy* 34: 455–459.

Symposium 1990 Ofloxacin – developments in therapy. *Journal of Antimicrobial Chemotherapy* 26 (Suppl. D): 1–142.

 PEFLOXACIN

Molecular weight 333.3.

A 6-fluoro, 7-piperazinyl quinolone available for oral and intravenous administration.

Antimicrobial activity

The activity of pefloxacin is very similar to that of norfloxacin, which it closely resembles. (Table 29.2; p. 351). It is active against *Mor. catarrhalis*, *H. ducreyi*, *Vibrio cholerae* and *Legionella* spp. *Campylobacter* and *Acinetobacter* spp. and pseudomonads are only moderately susceptible. It has poor activity against mycobacteria, chlamydiae, mycoplasmas and ureaplasmas. *L. monocytogenes*, *Nocardia* spp. and anaerobes are resistant.

Pharmacokinetics

Oral absorption	>90%
C_{max} 400 mg oral	4.5–6 mg/l after 1–1.5 h
400 mg intravenous	5.8 mg/l
Plasma half-life	8.5–13 h
Volume of distribution	1.9 l/kg
Plasma protein binding	20–30%

The plasma elimination half-life rises to 15 h after multiple dosing, when the steady-state concentration is achieved in less than 48 h. It is widely distributed, concentrations in bone, brain, blister fluid, CSF, saliva, sputum and prostate all approximating, and in some cases exceeding, the simultaneous plasma concentration. It is extensively metabolized to the desmethyl (= norfloxacin) and *N*-oxide derivatives. Some 60–70% of a dose, only about 10% of which is unchanged, appears in the urine; 25% of a dose appears in the feces, a small part contributed by excretion in the bile.

The half-life also increases with hepatic impairment, but is virtually unaffected by renal failure. In patients on CAPD given 800 mg followed by 400 mg twice daily for 10–12 days, there was no significant accumulation of pefloxacin or its metabolite, norfloxacin, but concentrations of pefloxacin *N*-oxide rose continuously in plasma and dialysate; all concentrations fell rapidly when treatment was discontinued.

Toxicity and side effects

Adverse reactions are those common to the group (p. 352). Most common are gastrointestinal tract disturbances, although some typical CNS reactions have been encountered. Skin eruptions (some photosensitive) occur and rashes appeared in about one-third of a group of patients who were given long-term therapy.

Clinical use

- Simple or complicated urinary tract infections.
- Chronic prostatitis.
- Uncomplicated gonococcal infections.
- Respiratory tract infections, including acute bronchitis, acute bacterial exacerbations of chronic bronchitis and pneumonia (except severe pneumococcal infections).
- Other infections caused by susceptible organisms.

 Preparations and dosage

Preparations: Tablets, injection.

Dosage: Adults, oral, i.v., 400 mg twice daily.

Available in continental Europe.

 Further information

Andriole VT (ed) 2000 *The Quinolones* 3rd edn. Academic Press, San Diego.

Gonzalez JP, Henwood JM 1989 Pefloxacin: a review of its antibacterial activity, pharmacokinetic properties and therapeutic use. *Drugs* 37: 628–668.

Jones RN 1989 Antimicrobial activity and interaction of pefloxacin and its principal metabolites. Collaborative Antimicrobial Susceptibility Testing Group. *European Journal of Clinical Microbiology and Infectious Diseases* 8: 551–556.

Rose TF, Bremner DA, Collins J et al 1990 Plasma and dialysate levels of pefloxacin and its metabolites in CAPD patients with peritonitis. *Journal of Antimicrobial Chemotherapy* 25: 657–664.

Symposium 1990 Pefloxacin in clinical practice. *Journal of Antimicrobial Chemotherapy* 26 (Suppl. B): 1–229.

 RUFLOXACIN

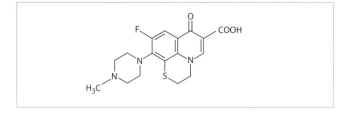

A 6-fluoro, 7-piperazinyl quinolone formulated for oral use.

Antimicrobial activity

Activity against common bacterial pathogens is shown in Table 29.2 (p. 351). It is less active than other group 2 quinolones against most bacteria within the spectrum.

Pharmacokinetics

Oral absorption	Good
C_{max} 400 mg oral	3.5–4.5 mg/l after 2–4 h
Plasma half-life	30–45 h
Volume of distribution	1.43 l/kg
Plasma protein binding	57%

Absorption and distribution

Rufloxacin is rapidly and well absorbed after oral administration. It is widely distributed in tissues where it is found in therapeutic concentrations. In bronchial mucosa, alveolar macrophages and lung epithelial lining fluid, and in prostatic tissue and secretions, concentrations exceed those in the plasma.

Metabolism and excretion

It undergoes extensive metabolism to the active *N*-desmethyl metabolite, the plasma concentrations of which are about double those of the parent drug. In 72 h about 27% of a dose is recovered in the urine and 1% in the bile; biliary concentrations are sufficiently high to suggest utility in treating biliary infections. Urinary concentrations (30–50 mg/l) exceed the MICs for susceptible pathogens, and concentrations of about 20 mg/l can still be found 3 days after dosing.

The renal clearance diminishes with falling renal function, but the plasma half-life does not increase greatly. It has been suggested that the dosage interval should be doubled to 48 h in patients with creatinine clearances of <30 ml/min per 1.73 m^2.

Toxicity and side effects

Side effects are those common to other quinolones (p. 352).

Clinical use

- Urinary tract infection.
- Chronic prostatitis.

Clinical experience is limited.

Preparations

Proprietary name: Qari.

Dosage: Adults, oral, 400 mg on day 1, followed by 200 mg/day.

Available in Italy.

Further information

Andriole VT (ed.) 2000 *The Quinolones* 3rd edn. Academic Press, San Diego.

Boerema JBJ, Bischoff W, Focht J, Naber KG 1991 An open multicentre study on the efficacy and safety of rufloxacin in patients with chronic bacterial prostatitis. *Journal of Antimicrobial Chemotherapy* 28: 587–597.

Mattina R, Bonfiglio G, Cocuzza CE, Gulisano G, Cesana M, Imbimbo BP 1991 Pharmacokinetics of rufloxacin in healthy volunteers after repeated oral doses. *Chemotherapy* 37: 389–397.

GROUP 3 QUINOLONES

GATIFLOXACIN

Molecular weight: 375.4.

An 8-methoxy, 7-piperazinyl, 6-fluoroquinolone formulated for oral and intravenous administration.

Antimicrobial activity

Activity against common bacterial pathogens is shown in Table 29.3. It exhibits excellent in-vitro activity against many Gram-positive and Gram-negative bacteria, including *Mor. catarrhalis*, *Acinetobacter* spp. and *Aeromonas* spp. but is not very active against *Pseudomonas aeruginosa* and other non-fermenting Gram-negative rods. It is more active against methicillin-susceptible strains of staphylococci than methicillin-resistant strains. It is also active against *Chlamydia*, *Mycoplasma* and *Legionella* spp. and has some activity against anaerobes.

Acquired resistance

Resistant mutants develop slowly in vitro and require multiple-step mutations. The C-8 moiety appears to discourage the selection of resistant mutants of Gram-positive bacteria. Although cross-resistance with other fluoroquinolones occurs, some bacteria resistant to other fluoroquinolones remain susceptible to gatifloxacin.

Pharmacokinetics

Oral absorption	>95%
C_{max} 400 mg oral	3.4–3.8 mg/l after 1–2 h
Plasma half-life	6–8 h
Volume of distribution	1.5–2.0 l/kg
Plasma protein binding	20%

Absorption and distribution

Gatifloxacin is almost completely absorbed when given orally. The oral and intravenous routes are interchangeable when equal doses are given. It is widely distributed throughout the body into many body tissues and fluids. Rapid distribution of

Table 29.3 Activity of group 3 and group 4 fluoroquinolones against common pathogenic bacteria: MIC (mg/l)

	Gatifloxacin	Moxifloxacin	Sparfloxacin	Tosufloxacin	Trovafloxacin
Staph. aureus	0.125	0.06	0.12–4	0.12	0.03–2
Str. pyogenes	0.5	0.5	0.5	0.25	0.12
Str. pneumoniae	1	0.25	0.5	0.5	0.12
E. faecalis	2	0.5	1	1	0.5
Neisseria spp.	0.016	0.016	0.004	0.06	0.015
H. influenzae	0.016	0.06	0.025	0.06	0.03
Esch. coli	0.06	0.06	0.05	0.5	0.12
K. pneumoniae	1	0.5	0.12	0.5	0.5
Ps. aeruginosa	32.0	8	8	8	8
B. fragilis	1	2	8	2	4
C. trachomatis	0.06–0.25	0.03–0.125	0.06	0.25	1
M. tuberculosis	0.12	0.25–1.0	0.5	No data	>8

the drug into tissues results in higher concentrations in most target tissues than in serum.

Metabolism and excretion

The drug undergoes limited metabolism (less than 1%) and does not inhibit cytochrome P_{450} isoenzymes so that it is unlikely to alter the pharmacokinetics of drugs metabolized by these enzymes. More than 70% of the drug is excreted unchanged in the urine. It undergoes both glomerular filtration and tubular secretion and probenecid decreases renal elimination. Renal clearance of gatifloxacin is reduced by 57% in moderate renal insufficiency, and by 77% in severe renal insufficiency. A reduced dosage is recommended in patients with creatinine clearances <40 ml/min including patients who require hemodialysis or continuous ambulatory peritoneal dialysis.

Toxicity and side effects

Adverse events are uncommon and similar to those for other fluoroquinolones. Gastrointestinal reactions are most common; CNS disturbances, primarily headache and dizziness may occur as well as allergic reactions, chills, fevers, and rash. Rarely, serious and occasionally fatal hypersensitivity or anaphylactic reactions have been reported, usually following the first dose. Gatifloxacin has the potential to prolong QTc interval in some patients.

Clinical use

- Acute bacterial sinusitis.
- Acute bacterial exacerbations of chronic bronchitis, community-acquired pneumonia.
- Uncomplicated and complicated urinary infections, pyelonephritis.
- Uncomplicated urethral and cervical gonorrhea.

 Preparation and dosage

Proprietary name: Tequin.

Preparations: Tablets and intravenous infusion.

Dosage: Adults oral, 200 and 400 mg tablets once daily; infusion 200 and 400 mg vials once daily.

Limited availability.

 Further information

Andriole VT (ed.) 2000 The quinolones: Prospects. In: *The Quinolones* 3rd edn. Academic Press, San Diego, p. 477.

Dembry LM, Farrington JM, Andriole VT 1999 Fluoroquinolone antibiotics: Adverse effects and safety profiles. *Infectious Diseases in Clinical Practice* 8: 9–16.

Fogarty C, Dowell M, Ellison T, Vrooman P, White B, Mayer H 1999 Treating community-acquired pneumonia in hospitalised patients: Gatifloxacin vs. ceftriaxone/clarithromycin. *Journal of Respiratory Diseases* 20 (Suppl.): S60–S69.

Hosaka M, Kinoshita S, Royama A, Otsuki M, Nishino T 1995 Antibacterial properties

of AM-1155, a new methoxy quinolone. *Journal of Antimicrobial Chemotherapy* 36: 293–301.

Iannini P, Niederman MS, Andriole VT 2000 Treatment of respiratory infections with quinolones. In: Andriole VT (ed.) *The Quinolones* 3rd edn. Academic Press, San Diego, p. 255.

Ramirez A, Molina J, Dolmann A et al 1999 Gatifloxacin treatment in patients with acute exacerbations of chronic bronchitis: Clinical trial result. *Journal of Respiratory Diseases* 20 (Suppl.) S30–S39.

Sullivan J, McElroy A, Honsinger R et al 1999 Treating community-acquired pneumonia with once-daily gatifloxacin vs once-daily levofloxacin. *Journal of Respiratory Diseases* 20 (Suppl.), S49–S59.

 SPARFLOXACIN

Molecular weight: 393.4.

A dimethylpiperazinyl difluoroquinolone formulated for oral use.

Antimicrobial activity

Activity against common bacterial pathogens is shown in Table 29.3. It is highly active against most aerobic Gram-positive cocci and Gram-negative bacilli, including *Mor. catarrhalis*, *Acinetobacter* spp., *Campylobacter* spp. and *Legionella* spp.; *Ps. aeruginosa* is less susceptible. Its activity also extends to the genital mycoplasmas, and *Mycobacterium* spp., including *M. avium* complex strains. It is moderately active against some anaerobes (including the *B. fragilis* group); *L. monocytogenes* is resistant.

Pharmacokinetics

Oral absorption	*c*. 90%
C_{max} 200 mg oral	0.7 mg/l after 4.5 h
400 mg oral	1–1.5 mg/l after 4.5 h
Plasma half-life	15–20 h
Volume of distribution	5 l/kg
Plasma protein binding	37%

Absorption and distribution

Absorption is decreased in the presence of antacids due to the formation of chelates with metallic ions. Concentrations in many tissues, including lung, exceed those in plasma. The drug accumulates rapidly in macrophages, polymorphonuclear cells and fibroblasts. CSF penetration is limited, with CSF concentrations <0.1 mg/l after a single 200 mg oral dose.

Metabolism and excretion

Around 5–10% of a dose is excreted unchanged in the urine, with about 30% appearing as the glucuronide. Total clearance is 10–15 l/h. The plasma half-life increases only modestly in renal failure to 30–40 h. About 50–60% of the dose appears as unchanged drug in the feces with biliary excretion, mainly as the glucuronide, accounting for 10–20% of a dose.

Toxicity and side effects

Adverse events are those common to fluoroquinolones (p. 352), in particular, gastrointestinal tract disturbances, CNS effects (mainly headache and insomnia) and rashes. Photosensitivity reactions have been observed in 2–11% of patients. It can prolong the QTc interval. It does not potentiate the toxicity of theophylline.

Clinical use

- Bronchopneumonia, acute bacterial exacerbations of chronic bronchitis and community-acquired pneumonia, including those infections due to *Str. pneumoniae* and atypical pathogens.
- Gonococcal and chlamydial genital tract infections.
- Urinary tract infection.
- Other infections caused by susceptible bacteria.

 Preparations and dosage

Proprietary name: Zagam.

Preparation: Tablets.

Dosage: Adult, oral, 400 mg on day 1; 200 mg daily thereafter.

Available in the USA and continental Europe.

 Further information

Andriole VT (ed.) 2000 *The Quinolones* 3rd edn. Academic Press, San Diego. Canton N, Peman J, Jimenez MT, Ramon MS, Gobemado M 1992 In vitro activity of sparfloxacin compared with those of five other quinolones. *Antimicrobial Agents and Chemotherapy* 36: 558–565.

Nakata K, Maeda H, Fujii A, Arakawa S, Umeza K, Kamidono S 1992 In vitro and in vivo activities of sparfloxacin, other quinolones, and tetracyclines against *Chlamydia trachomatis*. *Antimicrobial Agents and Chemotherapy* 36: 188–190.

Rastogi N, Goh KS 1991 In vitro activity of the new difluorinated quinolone sparfloxacin (AT-4140) against *Mycobacterium tuberculosis* compared with activities of ofloxacin and ciprofloxacin. *Antimicrobial Agents and Chemotherapy* 35: 1933–1936.

Shimada J, Nogita T, Ishibashi Y 1993 Clinical pharmacokinetics of sparfloxacin. *Clinical Pharmacokinetics* 25: 358–369.

 TOSUFLOXACIN

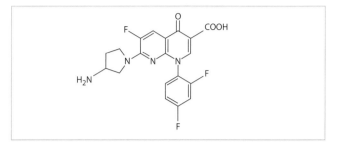

A naphthyridine derivative with a pyrrolidinyl substituent at position 7. Formulated for oral administration.

Antimicrobial activity

Activity against the common bacterial pathogens is shown in Table 29.3. It is highly active against a wide range of Gram-positive and Gram-negative bacteria, including *Mor. catarrhalis*, *Acinetobacter* spp. *L. pneumophila* and *Campylobacter* spp. Unlike many quinolones, the drug is moderately active against *L. monocytogenes*. *C. trachomatis* is also moderately susceptible. It is active against some anaerobes, including the *B. fragilis* group. Activity against *Mycobacterium* spp. is limited.

Pharmacokinetics

Oral absorption	Good
C_{max} 300 mg oral	1 mg/l after 4 h
Plasma half-life	6–7 h
Plasma protein binding	*c*. 35%

Around 30–35% of the dose is excreted in the urine. The concentration in prostatic tissue is similar to that seen in plasma.

Clinical use

Clinical experience is limited, but high clinical and bacteriological cure rates have been obtained in patients with skin and soft-tissue infections.

 Preparations and dosage

Proprietary names: Ozex; Tosuxacin.

Dosage: Adult, oral, 150 mg three times daily.

 Further information

Barry AL, Fuchs PC 1991 In vitro activities of sparfloxacin, tosufloxacin, ciprofloxacin and fleroxacin. *Antimicrobial Agents and Chemotherapy* 35: 955–960.

GROUP 4 QUINOLONES

 MOXIFLOXACIN

Molecular weight: 401.4.

An 8-methoxy, 7-diazabicyclononyl fluoroquinolone, formulated as the hydrochloride for oral or intravenous use.

Antimicrobial activity

The activity against common bacterial pathogens is shown in Table 29.3 (p. 369). It has excellent in-vitro activity against a wide range of Gram-positive and Gram-negative micro-organisms, including *Mor. catarrhalis*, *Acinetobacter* spp, *Aeromonas* spp and *Stenotrophomonas maltophilia*; it is less active against *Ps. aeruginosa* and other non-fermenting Gram-negative rods. The spectrum encompasses all species of staphylococci and streptococci although it exhibits less potent activity against enterococci. It is very active against *Chlamydia*, *Mycoplasma* and *Legionella* spp. and has good activity (>90% of strains) against anaerobes including *B. fragilis*. It also has activity against *M. tuberculosis*, but is less active against *M. avium* complex, *M. intracellulare*, *M. chelonei* and *M. fortuitum*.

Acquired resistance

Resistance develops in Gram-negative organisms by alterations in topoisomerase II. Cross-resistance with other fluoroquinolones has been observed in Gram-negative bacteria, but the C-8 methoxy moiety contributes to enhanced activity and lower selection of resistant mutants of Gram-positive bacteria so that strains resistant to other fluoroquinolones may remain susceptible to moxifloxacin.

Pharmacokinetics

Oral absorption	86–92%
C_{max} 400 mg oral	3.1–4.5 mg/l after 1–2 h
Plasma half-life	12–13 h
Volume of distribution	1.84 l/kg
Plasma protein binding	30–50%

Absorption and distribution

Moxifloxacin is widely distributed throughout the body and into many tissues in concentrations exceeding those in plasma.

Approximately 50–80% of plasma concentrations penetrate into CSF if the meninges are inflamed. The rate of elimination from tissues parallels the elimination from plasma. Pharmacokinetic behavior after administration by the oral and intravenous routes is very similar when equal doses are given.

Metabolism and excretion

It is metabolized via glucuronide and sulfate conjugation. The cytochrome P_{450} system is not involved, so that it is unlikely to alter the pharmacokinetics of drugs metabolized by these enzymes.

Approximately 45% of an oral or intravenous dose is excreted unchanged in urine and feces. The pharmacokinetics are not significantly altered in renal insufficiency so that dosage adjustments are not necessary. Also, no dosage adjustment is necessary in patients with mild or moderate hepatic insufficiency; the pharmacokinetics have not been studied in patients with severe hepatic insufficiency.

Toxicity and side effects

Adverse events are uncommon and are similar to those for other fluoroquinolones. Gastrointestinal side effects are the most common, particularly nausea, diarrhea, abdominal pain and vomiting. Dizziness and headache may occur as well as allergic reactions. Moxifloxacin has the potential to prolong QTc interval in some patients.

Clinical use

- Acute bacterial exacerbations of chronic bronchitis and community-acquired pneumonia.
- Acute bacterial sinusitis.

 Preparation and Dosage

Proprietary name: Avalox.

Preparations: Tablets.

Dosage: Adults, oral, 400 mg tablets once daily.

Widely available.

Further information

Chodosh S, DeAbate C, Haverstock D, Aneiro L, Church D and the Bronchitis Study Group 2000 Short-course moxifloxacin therapy for treatment of acute bacterial exacerbations of chronic bronchitis. *Respiratory Medicine* 94: 18–27.

Church D, Haverstock D, Andriole VT 2000 Moxifloxacin: A review of its safety profile based on worldwide clinical trials. *Today's Therapeutic Trends* 18: 205–223.

Iannini, PB, Niederman MS, Andriole, VT 2000 Treatment of respiratory infections with quinolones. In: Andriole VT (ed.) *The Quinolones*. 3rd edn. Academic Press, San Diego, p. 255.

Niederman M, Church D, Haverstock M, Springsklee M 2000 Does appropriate antibiotic therapy influence outcome in community-acquired pneumonia (CAP) and acute exacerbations of chronic bronchitis (AECB). Abstract A14. *Respiratory Medicine* 94 (Suppl. A), p. E23.

Wilson R, Kubin R, Ballin I et al 1999 Five day moxifloxacin therapy compared with 7 day clarithromycin therapy for the treatment of acute exacerbations of chronic bronchitis. *Journal of Antimicrobial Chemotherapy* 44: 501–513.

 # TROVAFLOXACIN

Molecular weight (trovafloxacin): 416.4; alatrofloxacin: 558.6.

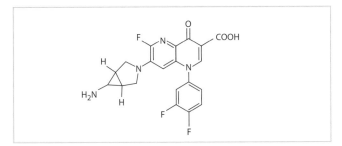

A trifluoroquinolone, formulated as the mesylate for oral administration and as the more soluble prodrug, alatrofloxacin mesylate, for intravenous use.

Antimicrobial activity

Activity against the common bacterial pathogens is shown in Table 29.3 (p. 369). It exhibits excellent potency against a wide range of Gram-positive and Gram-negative micro-organisms, including *Mor. catarrhalis* (MIC 0.015 mg/l), *Legionella pneumophila* (MIC 0.004 mg/l) and *L. monocytogenes* (MIC 0.25 mg/l). It is less activity against pseudomonads, including *Sten. maltophilia* and *Burk. cepacia* (MIC 0.5–8 mg/l). Most anaerobes are inhibited by 0.5–1 mg/l, but *Cl. difficile* is less susceptible.

Pharmacokinetics

Oral absorption	*c.* 90%
C_max 200 mg oral	2–3 mg/l after 1.1 h
300 mg intravenous (60 min infusion)	3.6 mg/l
Plasma half-life	11 h
Volume of distribution	1.2 l/kg
Plasma protein binding	73%

Toxicity and side effects

Common side effects are those experienced with other quinolones (p. 352). Hepatotoxicity, sometimes with clinical jaundice and acute liver failure has been sufficiently frequent to have led to restrictions on the licensed indications.

Clinical use

- Severe infections, including life-threatening pneumonia and intra-abdominal infections.

 ## Preparations and dosage

Proprietary name: Trovan.

Dosage: Adult, 200–300 mg intravenous infusion once daily. Oral, 100–200 mg once daily.

Available in the USA. Not available in Europe.

 ## Further information

Algahasham AA, Nahata MC 1999 Trovafloxacin: a new fluoroquinolone. *Annals of Pharmacotherapy* 33: 48–60.
Garey KW, Amsden GW 1999 Trovafloxacin: an overview. *Pharmacotherapy* 19: 21–34.
Haria M, Lamb HM 1997 Trovafloxacin. *Drugs* 54: 435–445.

OTHER NOVEL QUINOLONES

Current interest in quinolones is so great that it would be impossible to mention all those that are in various stages of development around the world. Those in late development at the time of writing include the following.

- **Gemifloxacin**. A group 4 compound with excellent activity against Gram-positive cocci, including multiresistant strains of *Staph. aureus* and *Str. pneumoniae*. It is less active than some other Group 4 compounds against anaerobes.
- **Nadifloxacin**. A fluoroquinolone similar in structure to ofloxacin, but with a hydroxyl replacing the methyl group on the piperazine ring and a simple ring lacking an oxygen atom between the N-1 and C-8 positions. It is active against many Gram-positive skin bacteria, including *Propionibacterium acnes*, and appears to inhibit the generation of reactive oxygen species by neutrophils. The sodium salt is marketed in Japan as a cream for use in acne and other skin conditions.
- **Pazufloxacin**. A group 3 compound that appears to be similar to tosufloxacin in its antibacterial and pharmacokinetic properties. An injectable formulation, pazufloxacin mesylate, is under development.
- **Sitafloxacin**. A group 4 compound with activity similar to or better than that of moxifloxacin. It has a chloro substitution at the C-8 position, a feature that is suspected to be associated with phototoxicity.

The search for new quinolones with further improved properties – including activity outside the antibacterial field – continues unabated. Enthusiasm has been tempered somewhat by unexpected toxicity among some otherwise promising compounds, but new insights into structure–activity relationships suggests that progress will continue to be made.

30 Rifamycins

F. Parenti and G. Lancini

The rifamycins are a family of antibiotics produced by an actinomycete originally named *Streptomyces mediterranei*, later reclassified as *Nocardia mediterranea* and then as *Amycolatopsis mediterranei*. All the therapeutically useful rifamycins are semisynthetic derivatives of rifamycin B, a fermentation product that is poorly active, but easily produced and readily converted chemically into rifamycin S, from which most active derivatives are prepared. They all share the general structure:

Natural products, like rifamycins, which are characterized by an aromatic ring spanned by an aliphatic bridge (ansa) are called 'ansamycins'. To this class belong the streptovaricins and the tolypomycins (chemically and biologically similar to rifamycins) and geldanamycin and the maytansines, which have quite different, antiblastic, biological activities. Among the vast number of rifamycin derivatives investigated, rifampicin (rifampin) is by far the most important and most widely used. Rifabutin and rifapentine are also used in mycobacterial disease. Rifamycin SV (also produced naturally by some strains of *A. mediterranei*), rifaximin and rifamide are used in a few countries only.

Interest in these antibiotics is centered on their potent activity against pathogenic Gram-positive cocci and mycobacteria. They were the first substances encountered with minimum inhibitory concentrations below 0.01 mg/l. *Neisseria* and some other Gram-negative organisms are susceptible, but activity against enterobacteria is poor.

Knowledge of the general properties of the group is largely based on extensive study and use of rifampicin but, insofar as they have been investigated, the main features are exhibited also by the other congeners:

- action through inactivation of bacterial DNA-dependent RNA polymerase;
- bactericidal effect;
- relatively high frequency of resistant mutants;
- stimulation of hepatic metabolism and significant biliary excretion.

However, the different congeners differ substantially in their pharmacokinetic behavior. Several rifamycins inhibit eukaryotic DNA and RNA polymerases and viral reverse transcriptase; some also exert an immunosuppressive effect in animals. These effects have no clinical significance.

Rifampicin proved so important in the treatment of tuberculosis, where its potent action allowed the introduction of short-course therapy, that in many countries its use was restricted to that indication for fear that more widespread use would encourage the emergence of resistant *Mycobacterium tuberculosis*. Those fears have proven to be exaggerated (the frequency of resistant mutants in sensitive bacterial populations is high, but resistance is not transferable) and, increasingly, interest has been refocused on what was originally anticipated to be an important use: treatment of severe Gram-positive infections. To prevent emergence of resistance coadministration of another effective agent is required.

📖 Further information

Lancini GC, Zanichelli W 1977 Structure–activity relationships in rifamycins. In: Perlman D (ed.) *Structure-activity relationships among the semisynthetic antibiotics.* Academic Press, San Francisco, pp. 531–600.

Sensi P, Lancini GC 1990 Inhibitors of transcribing enzymes: rifamycins and related agents. In: Hansch C, Sammes PG, Taylor JB (eds) Comprehensive medicinal chemistry vol 2. Pergamon, Oxford, pp. 793–811.

Riva S, Silvestri G 1972 Rifamycins: a general view. *Annual Review of Microbiology* 26: 199–224.

RIFABUTIN

Rifabutine; ansamycin; Molecular weight: 847.02.

A semisynthetic spiropiperidyl derivative of rifamycin S, available for oral administration. It is slightly soluble in water and soluble in organic solvents.

Antimicrobial activity

The activity is similar to that of rifampicin, but it is somewhat more active against the *Mycobacterium avium* complex (MIC 0.01–2 mg/l) (Table 30.1).

Table 30.1 The activity of rifabutin and rifampicin on *M. avium* complex strains

Rifampicin MIC (mg/l)	Number of strains	Percentage of strains resistant to rifabutin 1 mg/l
<1 (susceptible)	30	0
1–4	163	0
5–9	105	2.9
≥10.0	225	19.6

Rifabutin inhibits the replication of human immunodeficiency virus 1 (HIV-1) in concentrations (10 mg/l) that are not toxic to lymphoid cells, but no efficacy on HIV infections has been demonstrated.

Acquired resistance

Although the mechanism of resistance is the same as for all rifamycins, the frequency of spontaneously resistant strains in several bacterial species, including *M. tuberculosis*, *M. leprae*, *Staphylococcus aureus* and *Chlamydia trachomatis*, is somewhat lower than with rifampicin.

Pharmacokinetics

Oral absorption	12–20%
C_{max} 300 mg oral	0.38 mg/l after 3.3 h
Plasma half-life	16 h
Volume of distribution	9.3 l/kg
Plasma protein binding	85%

Absorption
Oral absorption is rapid but incomplete, with considerable interpatient variation.

Distribution
Rifabutin is well distributed, concentrations in many organs being higher than that in plasma. The average concentration in lungs is 6.5 times the simultaneous plasma concentration.

Metabolism and excretion
Rifabutin is mainly metabolized to the active desacetyl derivative, although several other oxidation products have been detected in urine, where some 10% of the dose is eliminated. About 30–50% of the dose can be recovered from the feces. Elimination from plasma is biphasic, with a terminal half-life of 45 h. The drug is a weak inducer of hepatic enzymes. The rate of metabolism increases, and the plasma area under the curve (AUC) declines as the treatment continues.

Interactions

Pharmacokinetic interaction with other drugs used in AIDS treatment has been demonstrated: both clarithromycin and ritonavir inhibit cytochrome P_{450}, resulting in decreased metabolism and increased plasma levels of rifabutin when the drugs are used together. Association with delavirdine should be avoided.

Toxicity and side effects

Rash (4% of patients), gastrointestinal intolerance (3%) and neutropenia (2%) are fairly common and may require discontinuation of treatment. Uveitis and general arthralgia are rare with a 300 mg dosage, but frequent with higher dosages, especially with concomitant use of fluconazole or macrolide antibiotics.

Clinical use

- Prevention of infections with *M. avium* complex in AIDS patients.
- Treatment of non-tuberculous mycobacterial disease (in combination with other agents).

Although some efficacy has been observed in the treatment of tuberculosis, its use for this condition is not recommended.

Preparations and dosage

Proprietary name: Mycobutin.

Preparation: Capsules.

Dosage: Adults, oral, prophylaxis of *M. avium* complex infections in immunocompromised patients with low CD4 count, 300 mg/day as a single dose. Treatment of non-tuberculous mycobacterial disease, in combination with other drugs, 450–600 mg/day as a single dose for up to 6 months after cultures become negative. Treatment of pulmonary tuberculosis, in combination with other drugs, 150–450 mg/day as a single dose for at least 6 months.

Widely available, including UK and USA.

Further information

Griffith DE, Brown BA, Girard WM, Wallace RJ 1995 Adverse events associated with high dose rifabutin in macrolide containing regimens for the treatment of *Mycobacterium avium* complex lung disease. *Clinical Infectious Diseases* 21: 594–598.

Klemens SP, Grossi MA, Cynamon MH 1994 Comparative in vivo activities of rifabutin and rifapentine against *Mycobacterium avium* complex. *Antimicrobial Agents and Chemotherapy* 38: 234–237.

Kuper JJ, D'Aprile M 2000 Drug–drug interactions of clinical significance in the treatment of patients with *Mycobacterium avium* disease. *Clinical Pharmacokinetics* 39: 203–214.

Nightingale SD, Cameron DW, Gordin FM et al 1993 Two controlled trials of rifabutin prophylaxis against *Mycobacterium avium* complex infection in AIDS. *New England Journal of Medicine* 329: 828–833.

O'Brien RJ, Lyle MA, Snider DE 1987 Rifabutin (Ansamycin LM 427): a new rifamycin S derivative for the treatment of mycobacterial diseases. *Reviews of Infectious Diseases* 9: 519–530.

Skinner MH, Hsieh M, Torseth J et al 1989 Pharmacokinetics of rifabutin. *Antimicrobial Agents and Chemotherapy* 33: 1237–1241.

 RIFAMIDE

Molecular weight: 810.94. The diethyl amide of rifamycin B, formulated as the sodium salt for parenteral administration.

Antimicrobial activity

Rifamide exhibits high activity against Gram-positive organisms and *M. tuberculosis* typical of the group. MICs for Gram-negative bacilli are of the order of 20–50 mg/l.

Pharmacokinetics

It is absorbed orally and is rapidly eliminated through the bile, achieving concentrations sufficient to inhibit Gram-negative bacilli. In contrast to rifampicin, it can be administered as the sodium salt by intramuscular injection. A dose of 150 mg produces mean plasma levels of about 1 mg/l. The plasma half-life is about 2 h.

Toxicity and side effects

Similar to those of other rifamycins.

Clinical use

- Staphylococcal infections.
- Infections of the biliary tract.

The drug is unsuitable for the treatment of tuberculosis because of insufficient distribution to the tissues.

Preparations and dosage

Preparations: Parenteral injection, i.m., i.v., topical.

Dosage: i.m., 250 mg three times daily; i.v. infusion (slow), up to 750 mg every 12 h.

Limited availability.

Further information

Khan GA, Scott AG 1967 The place of rifamycin B diethylamide in the treatment of cholangitis complicating biliary obstructions. *British Journal of Pharmacology and Chemotherapy* 31: 506–512.

Pallanza R, Füresz S, Timbal MT, Carniti G 1965 In vitro bacteriological studies on rifamycin B diethylamide (rifamide). *Arzneimittelforschung* 15: 800–802.

 RIFAMPICIN

Rifampin (USAN). Molecular weight: 822.95.

A semisynthetic derivative of rifamycin SV, available for oral administration or intravenous infusion and in several combined formulations with other antimycobacterial drugs. It is poorly soluble in water, but soluble in organic solvents.

Antimicrobial activity

The activity against common bacterial pathogens is shown in Table 30.2. It exhibits potent activity in vitro against Gram-positive cocci, including methicillin-resistant staphylococci (MIC <0.025–0.5 mg/l) and penicillin-resistant pneumococci.

Table 30.2 Activity of rifampicin against common pathogenic bacteria

Organism	MIC (mg/l)
Staph. aureus	0.008–0.06
Str. pyogenes	0.03–0.1
Str. pneumoniae	0.06–4
E. faecalis	1–4
M. tuberculosis	0.1–1
N. gonorrheae	0.06–0.5
N. meningitidis	0.01–0.5
H. influenzae	0.5–1
Esch. coli	8–16
K. pneumoniae	16–32
Ps. aeruginosa	32–64

Enterococci are less susceptible. Gram-positive bacilli including *Bacillus* spp., *Clostridium difficile*, *Corynebacterium* spp. and *Listeria monocytogenes* are highly susceptible (MIC 0.025–0.5 mg/l). The pathogenic *Neisseria* and *Moraxella* spp. are also highly susceptible.

Enteric Gram-negative bacteria are generally less sensitive (MIC 1–32 mg/l), but *Bacteroides fragilis* is highly susceptible. Among other Gram-negative bacilli, *Haemophilus influenzae*, *Haemophilus ducreyi*, *Flavobacterium meningosepticum* and *Legionella* spp. are highly susceptible (MIC <0.025–2 mg/l). *Chlamydia trachomatis* and *C. psittaci* are inhibited by low concentrations (0.025–0.5 mg/l).

Most strains of *M. tuberculosis*, *M. kansasii* and *M. marinum* are inhibited by <0.01–0.1 mg/l, but *M. fortuitum* and members of the *M. avium* complex are resistant. *M. leprae* is highly sensitive.

Rifampicin is active against some eukaryotic parasites through unknown mechanisms, although inhibition of the prokaryote-like polymerase of kinetoplasts or mitochondria has been postulated. Maturation of *Plasmodium falciparum* is inhibited by 2–10 mg/l; at higher concentrations *Leishmania* spp. are also inhibited.

High concentrations inhibit growth of a variety of poxviruses by interference with viral particle maturation; viral reverse transcriptase is unaffected.

Antimicrobial interactions

Because of the relative ease with which resistant mutants emerge, rifampicin is normally used in combination with unrelated antibiotics. Suppression of the emergence of resistant mutants is the principal value of the addition of the unrelated agent.

Combination with β-lactam agents or glycopeptides (vancomycin and teicoplanin) in vitro usually results in antagonism or indifference, but synergy with penicillins is found in some strains of *Staph. aureus* and the combination has proved effective in some cases in vivo. Rifampicin antagonizes the bactericidal effect of ciprofloxacin against *Staph. aureus*. Synergy with aminoglycosides occurs in vitro against *Esch. coli* and with polymyxin B against multiresistant *Serratia marcescens*. Synergy with trimethoprim against enterobacteria, streptococci and staphylococci has been reported, but others have found indifference, or sometimes antagonism, and there appears to be substantial individual strain variation. Synergy with erythromycin, clindamycin and other antistaphylococcal agents has been demonstrated against some strains of *Staph. aureus*.

In-vitro activity against *M. tuberculosis* is increased in the presence of streptomycin and isoniazid, but not ethambutol. Synergy with amphotericin B against *Candida albicans* and against the mycelial, but not the spherule-endospore, phase of *Coccidioides immitis* is seen in vitro. However, this is not a clinically useful interaction.

Acquired resistance

Most large bacterial populations contain resistant mutants, which readily emerge in the presence of the drug and can emerge during treatment. The mutation rate to resistance in *Staph. aureus*, *Str. pyogenes*, *Str. pneumoniae*, *Esch. coli* and *Proteus mirabilis* is about 10^{-7} and that to *M. tuberculosis* and *M. marinum* 10^{-9}–10^{-10}. Primary resistance in *M. tuberculosis* remained low for many years, but is now increasing.

Resistance is of the one-step type, and several classes of mutants exhibiting different degrees of resistance can be selected by exposing a large population to a relatively low concentration of the drug. Some of these mutants may be susceptible to other rifamycin derivatives.

Resistance is not due to enzymic destruction and is not transferable. It is due to a change in a single amino acid of the β subunit of DNA-dependent RNA polymerase, which no longer forms a stable complex with rifampicin. There is no cross-resistance with any other class of antibiotics presently in clinical use. The susceptible strains of the gastrointestinal flora become rapidly resistant during rifampicin treatment without alteration in the flora composition, and revert to susceptibility within a few weeks of cessation of treatment.

Pharmacokinetics

Oral absorption	>90%
C_{max} 300 mg oral	4 mg/l after 2 h
600 mg oral	10 mg/l after 2 h
Plasma half-life	2.5 h
Volume of distribution	1.5 l/kg
Plasma protein binding	80%

Absorption

Rifampicin is virtually completely absorbed when administered orally, but substantial differences in blood levels have been reported in comparisons of capsules or tablets from different manufacturers. Peak plasma levels differ noticeably between individuals. Food affects absorption, the peak plasma levels being delayed and about 2 mg/l lower after a meal. Although the AUC and the length of time for which effective antibacterial levels are maintained are little affected, it is preferable that patients take the drug before meals.

Intravenous administration produces AUCs and elimination half-lives similar to those obtained after oral doses.

Distribution

The lipid solubility of the drug facilitates its distribution. It is widely distributed in the internal organs, bones, and fluids, including tears, saliva, ascitic fluid, and abscesses. It penetrates into cells, and is active against intracellular bacteria. Low concentrations are found in the cerebrospinal fluid (CSF), but these are substantially higher when the meninges are inflamed. Concentrations around 60% of the simultaneous plasma value were found in the heart valves of patients receiving a 600 mg dose before surgery.

Metabolism

Rifampicin is metabolized principally to its desacetyl derivative, which is also antimicrobially active, and this process is accelerated by its stimulatory effect on hepatic microsomal enzymes. As a consequence, hepatic clearance increases on continuous administration and, especially with high doses, the serum half-life becomes shorter after a few days of treatment.

Excretion

The main route of elimination is secretion into the bile, a process that is dose dependent, being efficient at low dosage but limited at high dosage. As a result, the dose determines the proportion excreted via the bile or passing the liver to be excreted in the urine. Because there is a limit to the rate at which the liver can deliver the drug to the bile the elimination half-life after a 600 mg dose rises to 3 h, and may be as long as 5 h with a 900 mg dose.

The desacetyl compound is mainly found in the bile, where the parent compound accounts for only 15% of the total. Plasma levels are increased by hepatic insufficiency, biliary obstruction and by probenecid, which depresses hepatic uptake. The drug escaping biliary excretion appears in the urine, to which it imparts an orange–red color, the parent compound and the desacetyl metabolites being present in about equal proportions. The plasma concentration and half-life are not significantly affected by renal failure. The drug is not removed by hemodialysis.

Drug interactions

The antibiotic is a potent inducer of hepatic cytochrome P_{450} microsomal enzymes, and this leads not only to more rapid self-elimination but also to enhanced metabolism of other agents handled by the same process. The effect is selective and it is not possible to predict which drugs may be affected. The most important are warfarin, the anticoagulant effect of which is thereby diminished, and oral contraceptives, with possible breakthrough bleeding and unwanted pregnancy. Addisonian crises have been described, and adjustments to steroid dosage in patients with Addison's disease may be necessary. Plasma concentrations of a number of other drugs may be affected, including digoxin, quinidine, methadone, hypoglycemic agents and barbiturates, with corresponding pharmacological effects.

Among antiretroviral drugs, use in combination with indinavir and its congeners is not recommended, but it can be used with ritonavir or nevirapine.

Toxicity and side effects

Rifampicin is relatively non-toxic, even when administered for a long period (as in the treatment of tuberculosis). However, several unwanted effects, including pink staining of soft contact lenses, are associated with its use. Other reactions can be divided into those associated with daily or intermittent administration, and those found only with intermittent therapy.

Adverse events associated with daily or intermittent therapy

Most common are skin reactions (mostly flushing with or without rash, and often transient even when therapy is continued), gastrointestinal disturbances (usually mild and most common in the early weeks of treatment) and disturbance of hepatic function. Transient abnormalities of liver function, especially a rise in serum transaminases (and, less often, a raised bilirubin level), are common, and clinical hepatitis, usually of mild degree, also occurs. Hepatitis was commonly recorded in some early studies, but the incidence in short-course regimens appears to be low. Earlier suggestions that hepatic damage was more common in rapid acetylators when given in combination with isoniazid were not borne out by subsequent studies.

Thrombocytopenia, associated with complement-fixing serum antibodies, is an uncommon adverse reaction. The platelet count falls within a few hours, returning to normal within a day or two. Rifampicin administration should be discontinued at once. Thrombocytopenia is more common with intermittent schemes, but is also encountered in patients receiving daily treatment.

Adverse events confined to patients receiving intermittent therapy

The most important is the 'flu' syndrome, with fever, chills and malaise usually developing after 3–6 months of treatment. Its incidence is less with frequent than infrequent dosage; less with lower than higher doses; and less when intermittent therapy is preceded by an initial phase of daily treatment. It was not, however, prevented by a daily supplement of 25 mg in an intermittent regimen. Circulating immunoglobulin M (IgM) antibodies to rifampicin are found in serum, and the 'flu' syndrome may be caused by resulting complement activation.

Other rare syndromes associated with intermittent administration are acute renal failure, sometimes associated with acute hemolysis. Shortness of breath, wheezing and fall of blood pressure have occasionally been recorded.

There is considerable evidence that rifampicin has immuno-suppressive properties, demonstrable in a number of experimental systems, but no effect in humans resulting from these properties has been demonstrated.

Clinical use

- Tuberculosis (in combination with other antituberculosis agents; *see* Ch. 61).
- Leprosy (in combination with other antileprotic agents; *see* Ch. 60).
- Serious infection with multiresistant staphylococci and pneumococci (in combination with a glycopeptide).
- Elimination of nasopharyngeal carriage of *Neisseria meningitidis* and *H. influenzae*.

Reference is made to its use in legionellosis (Ch. 48), meningitis (Ch. 53) and brucellosis (Ch. 63).

Preparations and dosage

Proprietary names: Rifadin, Rimactane. In combination with isoniazid: Rifinah, Rimactazid. In combination with isoniazid and with pyrazinamide: Rifater.

Preparations: Capsules, syrup, i.v. infusion.

Dosage: Adults, oral, 450–600 mg/day as a single dose, based on approx. 10 mg/kg daily. Children, up to 20 mg/kg daily as a single dose, to a maximum of 600 mg as a single dose. Premature and newborn infants, 10 mg/kg once daily; treat only in cases of emergency and with extreme caution because their liver enzyme system may not be fully developed. Adults, i.v. infusion, 450–600 mg/day as a single dose, based on approx. 10 mg/kg daily. Lower doses are recommended for small or frail patients. Children, 20 mg/kg daily, with a maximum daily dose of 600 mg. Premature and newborn infants, 10 mg/kg daily with caution, as for oral dose. Chemoprophylaxis of meningococcal meningitis: adults, oral, 600 mg every 12 h (twice daily) for 2 days; children 1–12 years, 10 mg/kg every 12 h for 2 days; infants up to 1 year, 5 mg/kg every 12 h for 2 days.

Widely available.

Further information

Bemer-Melchior P, Bryskier A, Drugeon HB 2000 Comparison of in vitro activities of rifapentine and rifampicin against *Mycobacterium tuberculosis* complex. *Journal of Antimicrobial Chemotherapy* 46: 571–576.

Ellard GA, Fourie PB 1999 Rifampicin bioavailability: a review of its pharmacology and the chemotherapeutic necessity for ensuring optimal absorption. *International Journal of Tuberculosis and Lung Disease* 3 (Suppl 3:) 301S–308S.

Havlir DV, Barnes PF 1999 Tuberculosis in patients with human immunodeficiency virus infection. *New England Journal of Medicine* 340: 367–73.

Lester W 1972 Rifampin: a semisythetic derivative of rifamycin – A prototype for the future. *Annual Review of Microbiology* 26: 85–102.

Loeffler AM 1999 Uses of rifampin for infections other than tuberculosis. *Pediatric Infectious Diseases* 18: 631–632.

Martinez E, Collazos J, Mayo J 1999 Hypersensitivity reactions to rifampin. Pathogenic mechanisms, clinical manifestations, management strategies, and review of anaphylactic-like reactions. *Medicine (Baltimore)* 78: 361–369.

Morris AB, Brown RB, Sands M 1993 Use of rifampin in nonstaphylococcal, non-mycobacterial disease. *Antimicrobial Agents and Chemotherapy* 37: 1–7.

Venkatesan K 1992 Pharmacokinetic drug interactions with rifampicin. *Clinical Pharmacokinetics* 22: 47–65.

RIFAMYCIN SV

Molecular weight: 697.77.

The simplest rifamycin in clinical use, obtained by elimination of a glycolic moiety from rifamycin B. Formulated as sodium salt for parenteral administration. Also available for topical use.

Its activity, pharmacokinetic properties and clinical uses are very similar to those of rifamide (*see above*). It is orally absorbed and excreted mainly in the bile. Intramuscular doses of 250 mg produce mean plasma levels of about 2 mg/l. The plasma half-life is around 2 h.

A topical preparation has been used for application to wounds and bedsores.

Preparations and dosage

Proprietary names: Chibro-Rifamycin, Otofa, Rifocine.

Preparations: Parenteral injection, i.m., i.v., topical.

Dosage: I.m., 250 mg three times daily; i.v. infusion (slow), up to 750 mg every 12 h.

Available in Italy, Switzerland, Germany.

Further information

Bergamini G, Fowst G 1965 Rifamycin SV. A review. *Arzneimittelforschung* 15: 951–1002.

RIFAPENTINE

Molecular weight: 877.04.

An analog of rifampicin in which a cyclopentyl group is substituted for a methyl group on the piperazine ring. It is available for oral administration.

Antimicrobial activity

Activity against most bacterial pathogens is similar to that of rifampicin, but it is more active against atypical mycobacteria, especially the *M. avium* complex (MIC <0.06–0.5 mg/l). Rifapentine has good activity on staphylococci and streptococci (MIC 0.01–0.5 mg/l), *L. monocytogenes* and *Brucella* spp.; less against *E. faecalis* (MIC 1–4 mg/l). *Bacteroides* spp. are inhibited by 0.5–2 mg/l. Gram-negative cocci are susceptible, and some Gram-negative bacilli are inhibited by 4–32 mg/l, but most are resistant.

Pharmacokinetics

Oral absorption	c. 70%
C_{max} 600 mg oral	12 mg/l after 5 h
Plasma half-life	13 h
Volume of distribution	1.5 l/kg
Plasma protein binding	97%

Absorption

The absolute oral bioavailability of rifapentine has not been determined. The relative bioavailability of capsules (with an oral solution as reference) is 70%. Food increases absorption: a 600 mg dose taken after a meal gives a C_{max} value 44% and an AUC 43% higher than under fasting conditions. The extended half-life provides therapeutic concentrations for at least 72 h after administration, thus allowing less frequent dosing.

Distribution

Animal data suggest that it is well distributed in the body, with tissue concentrations exceeding the plasma concentration, except in bone, testes and brain. The ratio of intracellular:extracellular concentration in macrophages was estimated as 24:1.

Metabolism

The main metabolite is an antimicrobially active 25-desacetyl derivative. Although it induces liver cytochromes it is not an inducer of its own metabolism, which is mediated by an esterase. The peak concentration of 25-desacetyl rifapentine is about one-third of that of the unchanged drug, and is attained after about 11 h.

Excretion

The main route of elimination is through the bile. In healthy volunteers about 70% of a 600 mg dose of ^{14}C rifapentine was recovered in the feces, and less than 17% in the urine. There is evidence of enterohepatic recycling in humans.

Drug interactions

The metabolism of several drugs concurrently administered can be substantially accelerated and adjustment of their dosage may be necessary. In particular, treatment of AIDS patients with rifapentine resulted in a 70% reduction in the AUC of indinavir. It should be used with extreme caution, if at all, in patients who are also taking protease inhibitors.

Toxicity and side effects

Signs of teratogenic effects and fetal toxicity have been observed when administered during pregnancy to rats and rabbits. Rifapentine should be used during pregnancy only if the potential benefit justifies the potential risk to the fetus.

Adverse events observed in clinical trials in combination with other antimycobacterial agents found the most common effect to be hyperuricemia, most probably due to pyrazinamide. Effects likely to be due to rifapentine were neutropenia (3.7% of patients) and hepatitis (increased transaminases in 1.6% of patients).

Clinical use

- Tuberculosis (in combination with other antituberculosis drugs)

Preparations and dosage

Proprietary name: Priftin.

Preparation: 150 mg tablets.

Dosage: Adults, oral, 600 mg (4 tablets) twice a week during the 2 month intensive phase treatment. 600 mg once a week in the 4 month continuation phase.

Available in the USA.

Further information

Heifets LB, Lindholm-Levy P, Flory M 1990 Bactericidal activity in vitro of various rifamycins against *Mycobacterium avium* and *Mycobacterium tuberculosis*. *American Reviews of Respiratory Disease* 141: 626–630.

Jarvis B, Lamb MM 1998 Rifapentine. *Drugs* 56: 607–616.

Keung AC-F, Owens RC, Eller MG, Weir SJ, Nicolau DP, Nightingale CH 1999 Pharmacokinetics of rifapentine in subjects seropositive for the human immunodeficiency virus: a phase 1 study. *Antimicrobial Agents and Chemotherapy* 43: 1230–1233.

Mor N, Simon B, Mezo N, Heifets LB 1995 Comparison of activities of rifapentine and rifampin against *Mycobacterium tuberculosis* residing in human macrophages. *Antimicrobial Agents and Chemotherapy* 39: 2073–2077.

Rastogi N, Goh KS, Berchel M, Bryskier A 2000 Activity of rifapentine and its metabolite 25-O-desacetylrifapentine compared with rifampicin and rifabutin against *Mycobacterium tuberculosis, Mycobacterium africanum, Mycobacterium bovis* and *M. bovis* BCG. *Journal of Antimicrobial Chemotherapy* 46: 565–570.

Temple ME, Nahata MC 1999 Rifapentine: its role in treatment of tuberculosis. *Annals of Pharmacotherapy* 33: 1203–1210.

RIFAXIMIN

A semisynthetic derivative of rifamycin S formulated for oral administration.

The spectrum of activity is similar to that of the other rifamycins. It is poorly absorbed from the gastrointestinal tract, where the high concentrations are effective against a variety of gastrointestinal pathogens. It is used in the treatment of gastrointestinal infections. It has been also proposed for the treatment of chronic hepatic encephalopathy and for topical treatment of bacterial vaginitis.

 Preparations and dosage

Proprietary names: Normix, Rifacol.

Preparations: Tablets, granules, topical.

Dosage: Adults, oral, 10–15 mg/kg per day. Children, oral, 20–30 mg/kg per day.

Available in Italy.

 Further information

Corazza GR, Ventrucci M, Strocchi A et al 1988 Treatment of small intestine bacterial overgrowth with rifaximin, a non-absorbable rifamycin. *Journal of International Medical Research* 16: 312–316.

Festi D, Mazzella G, Orsini M et al 1993 Rifaximin in the treatment of chronic hepatic encephalopathy; results of a multicenter study of efficacy and safety. *Current Therapy Research* 54: 598–609.

Ripa S, Mignini F, Prenna M, Falcioni E 1987 In vitro antibacterial activity of rifaximin against *Clostridium difficile*, *Campylobacter jejuni* and *Yersinia* spp. *Drugs under Experimental and Clinical Research* 13: 483–488.

31 Streptogramins

J. C. Pechère

The streptogramins are a very large group of natural cyclic peptides. They are unique in that they consist of two groups (A and B) of structurally unrelated molecules that act synergistically against susceptible bacteria. Group A streptogramins are polyunsaturated macrolactones which contain lactam and lactone linkages and incorporate an oxazole ring. The main compounds of this group are pristinamycin II$_A$ (virginiamycin M$_I$), madumycin and griseoviridin. Group B molecules are cyclic hexadepsipeptides, the two principal products being pristinamycin I$_A$ and virginiamycin S$_I$. Group B components share in the plasmid-borne variety of resistance to macrolides and lincosamides, which is induced by erythromycin (p. 312).

Synergy between groups A and B renders the combination bactericidal to a wide variety of Gram-positive bacteria and reduces the number of resistant strains. Typically, the in-vitro antibacterial activity of the mixture of A and B compounds is at least 10 times greater than the sum of the activities of the individual components.

In spite of their antibacterial potency, the earlier streptogramins were not used much in clinical practice because of the lack of a parenteral form to treat the most severe infections. Until recently, only two oral drugs were developed commercially: virginiamycin (which is also used as an animal feed additive) and pristinamycin, which has been used almost exclusively for the oral treatment of staphylococcal infections. Intensive work has resulted in the synthesis of water-soluble derivatives of the two groups, allowing the development of an injectable semisynthetic streptogramin, quinupristin/dalfopristin. Oral formulations represented by RPR-106972 are under development.

Further information

Bonfiglio G, Furneri PM 2001 Novel streptogramin antibiotics. *Expert Opinion on Investigational Drugs* 10: 185–198.

QUINUPRISTIN/DALFOPRISTIN

Molecular weight quinupristin: 1022; dalfopristin: 690.

A fixed combination of two purified water-soluble compounds derived from natural pristinamycin I$_A$ and II$_B$, respectively. Both compounds are formulated as the mesylate for intravenous infusion.

Antimicrobial activity

The mixture is active against a wide range of aerobic and anaerobic Gram-positive organisms, notably staphylococci and enterococci, and against a limited number of Gram-negative bacteria (Table 31.1). The MIC for *Streptococcus agalactiae* is

Table 31.1 Susceptibility of common pathogenic bacteria to quinupristin/dalfopristin: MIC (mg/l)

Staph. aureus	
Methicillin susceptible	0.03–2
Methicillin resistant	0.03–4
Erythromycin susceptible	0.06–1
Erythromycin resistant	0.12–2
Staph. epidermidis	
Methicillin susceptible	0.03–4
Methicillin resistant	0.03–4
Str. pyogenes	0.06–0.5
Str. pneumoniae	
Erythromycin susceptible	0.12–0.5
Erythromycin resistant	0.25–1
E. faecalis	1–8
E. faecium	0.25–8
H. influenzae	1–8
N. gonorrhoeae	0.25–1
N. meningitidis	≤0.12–1
Enterobacteria	R

R, resistant (MIC >32 mg/l)

0.03–0.5 mg/l and for viridans streptococci is 0.25–1 mg/l. *Listeria monocytogenes* strains are inhibited by 2–16 mg/l, most Gram-positive anaerobic bacteria by 0.125–0.5 mg/l, *Legionella pneumophila* by 0.03–3 mg/l and *Moraxella (Branhamella) catarrhalis* by ≤0.12–1 mg/l.

The combined preparation exerts rapid bactericidal activity against most susceptible strains; it is as active at pH 6 as at pH 7 and there is no appreciable inoculum effect. A post-antibiotic effect (2.4 h at the MIC; >5 h at 10 × MIC) has been observed against *Staphylococcus aureus* and enterococci.

Acquired resistance

Several mechanisms of resistance have been described.

- Modifications of the drug target (post-transcriptional modifications of rRNAs, some mutations in rRNA).
- Drug inactivation by actyltransferases, hydrolases or lactonases.
- VgA efflux, found only in staphylococci and conferring resistance to streptogramin A.

Activity is not affected by several mechanisms of staphylococcal resistance to macrolides, including those of target modification (genotypes ermA and ermC), active efflux (erpA or msrA) and lincosamide nucleotidylation.

Pharmacokinetics

	Quinupristin	Dalfopristin
C_{max} 7.5 mg/kg intravenous infusion (1 h)	3.2 mg/l	7.96 mg/l
Plasma half-life	3.07 h	1.04 h
Volume of distribution	0.45 l/kg	0.24 l/kg
Plasma protein binding	*c.* 90%	*c.* 90%

Absorption, distribution and metabolism

Oral formulations are not available. After intravenous infusion both components are converted to several active metabolites, occurring by non-enzymatic reactions independent of cytochrome-P_{450} or glutathione-transferase enzyme activities. After administration of 7.5 mg/kg 8 hourly, the area under the time–concentration curve (AUC) was 7.2 mg.h/ml for quinupristin and metabolites, and 10.57 mg.h/ml for dalfopristin and metabolites, respectively. The two components penetrate and accumulate in macrophages, the cellular:extracellular concentration ratios in vitro being 34 and 50, respectively. In cardiac vegetations of experimental endocarditis, quinupristin was homogeneously distributed, whereas dalfopristin showed a gradient of concentration, the diffusion of component I being about 2–4 times that of component II. The compounds do not penetrate into the cerebrospinal fluid or cross the placenta.

Excretion

Parent compounds and metabolites are primarily excreted in the bile, with less than 20% being found in urine. The clearances of unchanged quinupristin and dalfopristin are similar at 0.72 l/h/kg. Adjustment of dosage is unnecessary in patients with impaired renal function, but may be required in hepatic impairment.

Interactions

Quinupristin/dalfopristin can inhibit the metabolism of drugs metabolized by the cytochrome P_{450} system and caution is required if coadministered with such agents.

Toxicity and side effects

It is generally well tolerated, but shared allergy to streptogramins has been encountered. Various gastrointestinal and other side effects have been reported, but appear to be uncommon. Infusion site reactions may be a problem.

Clinical use

Serious infections with susceptible organisms, especially vancomycin-resistant *E. faecium* and multiresistant strains of staphylococci and pneumococci.

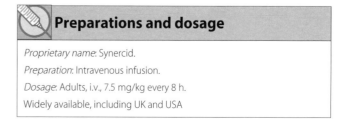

Preparations and dosage

Proprietary name: Synercid.

Preparation: Intravenous infusion.

Dosage: Adults, i.v., 7.5 mg/kg every 8 h.

Widely available, including UK and USA

Further information

Allington DR, Rivey MP 2001 Quinupristin/dalfopristin: a therapeutic review. *Clinical Therapeutics* 23: 24–44.

Bryson H, Spencer C 1996 Quinupristin-dalfopristin. *Drugs* 52: 406–415.

Delgado G, Neuhauser MM, Bearden DT, Danziger LH 2000 Quinupristin-dalfopristin: an overview. *Pharmacotherapy* 20: 1469–1485.

Desnottes JF, Diallo N 1992 Cellular uptake and intracellular bactericidal activity of RP 59500 in murine macrophages. *Journal of Antimicrobial Chemotherapy* 30 (Suppl. A): 25–28.

Fagon JY, Patrick H, Haas DW 2000 Treatment of Gram-positive nosocomial pneumonia: prospective randomised comparison of quinupristin/dalfopristin versus vancomycin. *American Journal of Respiratory Critical Care Medicine* 161: 753–762.

Fantin B, Leclercq R, Ottaviani M et al 1994 In vitro activities and penetration of the two component of the streptogramin RP 59500 in cardiac vegetation of experimental endocarditis. *Antimicrobial Agents and Chemotherapy* 38: 432–437.

Leclercq R, Nantas L, Soussy CJ, Duval J 1992 Activity of RP 59500, a new parenteral semisynthetic streptogramin, against staphylococci with various mechanisms of resistance to macrolide–linocomycin–streptogramin antibiotics. *Journal of Antimicrobial Chemotherapy* 30 (Suppl. A): 67–75.

Low DE 1995 Quinupristin/dalfopristin: spectrum of activity, pharmacokinetics and initial clinical experience. *Microbial Drug Resistance* 1: 223–234.

Moellering RC 1999 Quinupristin/dalfopristin: therapeutic potential for vancomycin-resistant enterococcal infections. *Journal of Antimicrobial Chemotherapy* 44 (Topic A): 25–30.

Nougayrede A, Berthaud N, Bouanchaud DH 1992 Post-antibiotic effects of RP 59500 with *Staphylococcus aureus*. *Journal of Antimicrobial Chemotherapy* 30 (Suppl. A): 101–106.

Pechère J-C 1992 In-vitro activity of RP 59500, a semisynthetic streptogramin, against staphylococci and streptococci. *Journal of Antimicrobial Chemotherapy* 30 (Suppl. A): 15–18.

Vannufel P, Di Giambattista M, Cocito C 1992 The role of rRNA bases in the interaction of peptidyltransferase inhibitors with bacterial ribosomes. *Journal of Biological Chemistry* 267: 16114–16120.

Verbist L, Verhaegen J 1992 Comparative activity of RP 59500. *Journal of Antimicrobial Chemotherapy* 30 (Suppl. A): 39–44.

OTHER STREPTOGRAMINS

PRISTINAMYCIN

A naturally occurring antibiotic isolated from *Streptomyces pristinaespiralis*. It includes two major components: pristinamycin I_A and pristinamycin I_B. The activity is very similar to that of quinupristin/dalfopristin (Table 31.1). It is available in some countries for the oral treatment of upper respiratory, dental, bronchopulmonary, skin, genital and bone infections caused by susceptible organisms.

Preparations and dosage

Preparation: Tablets (250 mg).

Dosage: Adults, oral, 2–4 g/day, in three equal doses, with meals. Children, 50–100 mg/kg per day in three equal doses, with meals.

Available in Belgium and France.

VIRGINIAMYCIN

A natural product of *Streptomyces virginiae*. Antimicrobial activity is similar to that of other streptogramins. It has chiefly been used as an animal feed additive, but is available in some countries for oral administration and in topical preparations.

Preparations and dosage

Preparations: Tablets, ointment, powder.

Dosage: Adults, oral, 2–3 g daily in divided doses. Children, 50–100 mg/kg daily in divided doses.

Available in Belgium and France.

32 Sulfonamides

D. Greenwood

The original sulphonamide, sulphanilamide, was the active principle of Prontosil, which holds a special place in medicine as the first agent to exhibit broad-spectrum activity against systemic bacterial disease.

$$H_2N \underset{}{\longrightarrow} SO_2NH_2$$

Introduction of this agent in 1935 had an immediate profound effect on mortality from many infections, notably puerperal fever (*see* Ch. 1).

Within a few years of the introduction of Prontosil, numerous sulfonamide derivatives were synthesized. Advances included increased antibacterial potency, decreased toxicity, and the introduction of compounds with special properties such as high or low solubility and prolonged duration of action. Most have since been discarded, as safer and more active antibacterial agents have overtaken them but a few are still in use for particular purposes, often in combination with diaminopyrimidines (*see* Ch. 19). Some survive in topical preparations, often in multi-ingredient formulations. Discussion here is limited to the most important sulfonamides that are still widely available; a short description is included of some of the many other compounds that are of more restricted availability.

ANTIBACTERIAL ACTIVITY

Sulfonamides exhibit broad-spectrum activity against common Gram-positive and Gram-negative pathogens, although the potency against many bacteria within the spectrum is modest by present standards. Meningococci are generally much more susceptible than gonococci. Other organisms commonly susceptible include *Bordetella pertussis*, *Yersinia pestis*, *Actinomyces* spp., *Nocardia* spp., *Bacillus anthracis*, *Corynebacterium diphtheriae*, *Legionella pneumophila*, *Brucella* spp. and several important causes of sexually transmitted diseases (*Chlamydia trachomatis*, *Haemophilus ducreyi* and *Calymmatobacterium granulomatis*). Activity against anaerobes is generally poor. *Pseudomonas aeruginosa* is usually resistant, as are *Leptospira*, *Treponema* and *Borrelia* spp., rickettsiae, *Coxiella burnetii* and

mycoplasmas. Mycobacteria are resistant, although the related sulfone, dapsone, exhibits good activity against *M. leprae* (*see* p. 433) and *p*-aminosalicylic acid, which is structurally similar, was formerly widely used in tuberculosis (p. 430). Sulfonamides act synergistically with certain diaminopyrimidines against many bacteria and some protozoa, including plasmodia and *Toxoplasma gondii* (Chapter 19).

In-vitro tests are markedly influenced by the composition of the culture medium and the size of the inoculum. The different derivatives vary somewhat in antibacterial activity (Table 32.1). Among those that are still fairly widely available as antibacterial agents, sulfadimidine shows comparatively low activity, whereas sulfadiazine, sulfisoxazole (sulphafurazole) and sulfamethoxazole, the sulfonamide commonly combined with trimethoprim (p. 291), are relatively more active.

ACQUIRED BACTERIAL RESISTANCE

Resistance is now widespread and there is complete cross-resistance among sulfonamides. Plasmid-mediated resistance in all enterobacteria is common. Resistance is found in 25–40% of strains of *Escherichia coli* and other enterobacteria infecting the urinary tract. Many strains of meningococci and *H. ducreyi* are now resistant.

PHARMACOKINETICS

Most sulfonamides are well absorbed after oral administration, reaching a peak concentration in the blood of 50–100 mg/l 2–4 h after a dose of 2 g. After absorption, the behavior of the individual compounds varies widely, depending on the extent of protein-binding and metabolization. The main metabolic pathway is conjugation by acetylation in the liver, although glucuronidation and oxidation also occur. Sulfonamide acetylation shows a bimodal distribution in the population, rapid and slow inactivators corresponding with rapid and slow inactivators of isoniazid (p. 437). The conjugates are inactive anti-

Table 32.1 Activity of selected sulfonamides against common pathogenic bacteria: MIC (mg/l)

	Sulfadiazine	Sulfadimidine	Sulfamethoxazole	Sulfisoxazole
Staph. aureus	16–32	32–R	4–32	4–16
Str. pyogenes	0.5–64	1–64	0.25–16	0.25–4
Str. pneumoniae	8–64	4–64	4–64	2–16
E. faecalis	R	R	R	R
H. influenzae	2–4	8–16	2–4	0.5–2
N. gonorrhoeae	1–32	16–R	1–32	1–64
N. meningitidis	0.12–1	0.5–8	0.12–1	0.12–0.5
Esch. coli	4–16	16–64	4–8	8–16
K. pneumoniae	8–16	64–R	4–16	8–16
Ps. aeruginosa	64	R	R	R

R, resistant (MIC >64 mg/l).

bacterially and the low solubility of the acetyl conjugates of some of the earlier compounds may give rise to renal toxicity.

A proportion, varying considerably with different compounds, is contained in the red cells, some is free in the plasma and some is bound to plasma albumin. Protein binding varies widely, the highest levels being seen with long-acting sulfonamides such as sulfadoxine. The degree of binding depends on the serum albumin concentration and on the total drug concentration in the blood, the proportion of protein-bound drug decreasing as the total drug concentration rises.

Sulfonamides can be displaced from their protein binding sites by a variety of compounds, the most important clinically being oral anticoagulant drugs. Simultaneous administration of these compounds with sulfonamides potentiates the anticoagulant effect and produces higher concentrations of diffusible sulfonamide. Competition for plasma albumin binding sites causes sulfonamides to displace albumin-bound bilirubin.

Sulfonamides are distributed throughout the body tissues. Access to the cerebrospinal fluid (CSF) is normally limited to the unbound drug, but with increasing capillary permeability and the passage of protein into the CSF in inflammation, protein-bound sulfonamide enters and the total concentration of drug in the CSF rises. The concentration of short-acting sulfonamides in CSF varies between 30% and 80% of the corresponding plasma concentration. Sulfonamides also enter other body fluids, including the eye. They pass readily through the placenta into the fetal circulation and also reach the infant via the breast milk.

Sulfonamides are excreted mainly in the urine, the free drug and its conjugates being frequently excreted at different rates and by different mechanisms. As a result, the peak plasma concentrations of free drug and conjugate may occur at different times and the proportion of free drug to conjugate may be very different in the plasma and urine. Excretion is partly by glomerular filtration and partly by tubular secretion, during which some of the drug is reabsorbed. The extent of these processes differs among the sulfonamides and may differ markedly for the free drug and its conjugates. As a result, the plasma clearance values vary from 10 to >200 ml/min.

Substances with high clearances (e.g. sulfisoxazole) are rapidly eliminated from the plasma and achieve high concentrations in the urine. Substances with low clearances are slowly excreted, plasma levels are maintained for long periods, and low concentrations appear in the urine. If renal function is impaired, excretion may be delayed still further and therapeutic levels may persist for considerably longer; if the drugs are given repeatedly, high and possibly toxic levels may develop. Less than 1% of the dose of the older sulfonamides is excreted in the bile, but the proportion is greater (2.4–6.3%) for the long-acting compounds.

TOXICITY AND SIDE EFFECTS

With proper attention to dosage, side effects are relatively uncommon, but some are serious. Crystals of less soluble compounds, such as sulfadiazine, or of less soluble conjugates may deposit in the urine and block the renal tubules or the upper orifice of the ureter. Hematuria is a common early sign. However, renal damage during sulfonamide therapy is often due to a hypersensitivity reaction, rather than to tubular blockage, with changes of tubular necrosis or vasculitis. Renal failure has been recorded in several patients after treatment with sulfamethoxazole, as a component of co-trimoxazole.

Hypersensitivity reactions usually occur as moderate fever with a rash on about the ninth day of a course of treatment. Repetition after an interval elicits the reaction immediately. Rashes are commonly erythematous, maculopapular or urticarial, and recur if the drug is given again. Well documented, but uncommon, is a severe serum-sickness-like reaction with fever, urticarial rash, polyarthropathy and eosinophilia. Eosinophilia may occur without other allergic manifestations.

Stevens–Johnson syndrome is a rare, but potentially fatal complication (one estimate puts the risk at 1–2 cases per 10 million doses). The relative risks of different sulfonamides are not known accurately, but there are many reports of this complication following the use of long-acting sulfonamides. The time of onset varies from 2 to 24 days, and sometimes as long as 6 weeks after discontinuing the drug. Toxic epidermal necrolysis (Lyell's syndrome) has also been recorded after administration of long-acting sulfonamides.

Drug fever without other features may occur. A special problem of hypersensitivity to the sulfonamide component of co-trimoxazole is its frequency in the treatment of acquired immune deficiency syndrome (AIDS). Sulfonamides are among the compounds reported to provoke systemic lupus erythematosus. An intractable type of sensitization may result from local applications.

In patients with inherited glucose-6-phosphate dehydrogenase deficiency, intravascular hemolysis and hemoglobinuria may occur. Hemolysis may also occur as part of a generalized sensitivity reaction. Agranulocytosis, aplastic anemia and thrombocytopenia have been occasionally reported, especially with earlier sulfonamides. Liver injury is rare.

Interference with bilirubin transport in the fetus by sulfonamide administered to the mother may increase the free plasma bilirubin level and result in kernicterus. Many other interactions arise as a result of competition for plasma albumin binding sites. Those of greatest potential clinical importance are increases in the actions of oral anticoagulants and sulfonylureas (but not biguanides) and increased toxicity of methotrexate.

CLINICAL USE

Absolute indications for the use of sulfonamides are very few and have been further constrained by the prevalence of resistance. They were formerly much used, alone or in combination with trimethoprim, for the treatment of urinary tract infection, but are no longer recommended because of potential adverse reactions. Use in the treatment of respiratory infections is now confined to a few special problems, notably nocardiasis (and also for cerebral nocardiasis) and, in combination with trimethoprim, in the prevention and treatment of *Pneumocystis carinii* pneumonia. The value of sulfonamides in the prophylaxis and treatment of meningococcal infection is now greatly reduced by bacterial resistance. Sulfonamides are sometimes used for chlamydial infections and chancroid but are unreliable. Some formulations are used topically in eye infections and bacterial vaginosis. Combined preparations with pyrimethamine are used in the treatment of drug-resistant malaria and for toxoplasmosis (Chs 64 and 65).

 Further information

Gruchalla RS 1999 Diagnosis of allergic reactions to sulfonamides *Allergy* 54 (Suppl. 58): 28–32.

Smith CL, Powell KR 2000 Review of the sulfonamides and trimethoprim. *Pediatrics in Review* 21: 368–371.

Vree TB, Hekster YA 1987 Clinical pharmacokinetics of sulphonamides and their metabolites. *Antibiotics and Chemotherapy* 37: 1–208.

 SULFADIAZINE

2-Sulfanilamidopyrimidine. Molecular weight: 250.3.

$$H_2N - \text{(benzene ring)} - SO_2 - \underset{H}{N} - \text{(pyrimidine ring)}$$

Sulfadiazine is almost insoluble in water and unstable on exposure to light. It is administered orally or, as the sodium salt, by intravenous injection. It is a component of several multi-ingredient preparations. Its low solubility in urine led to its general replacement by other compounds, but it remains one of the few sulfonamides available for intravenous injection on the rare occasions when this is indicated; the solution is highly alkaline and should not be given by any other route.

Antimicrobial activity

Sulfadiazine exhibits relatively high potency compared with other sulphonamides (Table 32.1).

Pharmacokinetics

Oral absorption	Very good
C_{max} 3 g oral	c. 50 mg/l after 3–4 h
Plasma half-life	7–12 h
Volume of distribution	0.36 l/kg
Plasma protein binding	c. 40%

Absorption and distribution

Adequate blood concentrations are easily achieved and maintained after oral administration. It is well distributed and penetrates in therapeutic concentrations into the CSF. For this reason sulfadiazine was often the sulfonamide of choice in meningitis, before drug resistance rendered it ineffective. It crosses the placenta and enters breast milk to achieve concentrations around 20% of plasma levels.

Metabolism and excretion

Sulfadiazine is subject to acetylation in the liver. The acetyl derivative lacks antibacterial activity and is excreted more slowly (half-life 8–18 h). Parent compound and metabolite are both excreted mainly by glomerular filtration.

Toxicity and side effects

In addition to side effects common to the group, sulfadiazine inhibits the metabolism of phenytoin. The risk of crystalluria can be reduced by high fluid intake and alkalization of the urine.

Clinical use

- Urinary tract infection.
- Nocardiasis.
- Chancroid.
- Toxoplasmosis (in combination with pyrimethamine).
- Meningococcal infections.
- Prophylaxis of rheumatic fever.

Preparations and dosage

Preparations: Tablets, 4 ml ampoules, each containing 1 g for i.v. injection.

Dosage: Adult, 1–1.5 g, 4-hourly for 2 days, then oral.

Available in the UK, the USA, Canada, Belgium and Australia. Widely available in multi-ingredient preparations.

Further information

Anonymous 1999 Sulfadiazine. In: Dollery C (ed.) *Therapeutic Drugs* 2nd ed. Churchill Livingstone, Edinburgh, pp. S126–S129.

SULFADIMIDINE

2-Sulfanilamido-4,6-methylpyrimidine; sulphamethazine, sulfamezathine. Molecular weight: 278.3.

Sulfadimidine is soluble in water and unstable on exposure to light. It is usually administered by mouth and is a component of some triple sulfonamide combinations.

Antimicrobial activity

The spectrum is typical of the group, but sulfadimidine exhibits relatively low potency (Table 32.1).

Pharmacokinetics

Oral absorption	Very good
C_{max} 1 g oral	*c.* 50 mg/l after 3–4 h
Plasma half-life	1.5–5 h
Volume of distribution	0.61 l/kg
Plasma protein binding	90%

Sulfadimidine is well absorbed after oral administration. It is extensively metabolized, predominantly by acetylation. The mean plasma half-life varies with acetylator status.

Toxicity and side effects

Toxic effects and sensitivity reactions are uncommon. In addition to side effects common to the group a serious interaction between cyclosporin A and sulfadimidine, leading to reduced cyclosporin levels, has been reported.

Clinical use

- Urinary tract infection.
- Meningococcal meningitis.

Preparations and dosage

Preparations: Tablets, injection.

Dosage: Adults, oral, 2 g initially, then 0.5–1 g every 6–8 h; i.m., i.v., 3 g initially, then 1.5 g every 6 h

Widely available in multi-ingredient preparations, limited availability in tablet and injectable forms. No longer available in the UK.

Further information

Anonymous 1999 Sulfadimidine. In: Dollery C. (ed.) *Therapeutic Drugs* 2nd ed. Churchill Livingstone, Edinburgh, pp. S130–S132.

SULFADOXINE

4-Sulfanilamido-5,6-dimethoxypyrimidine. Molecular weight: 310.3.

Sulfadoxine is an ultra-long-acting sulfonamide. It is no longer prescribed alone, but is used in combination with pyrimethamine as the antimalarial agent Fansidar (*see* Ch. 64). It is poorly soluble in water.

Antimicrobial activity

In terms of antibacterial activity it is among the least potent of sulfonamides. Used alone it has a slow and uncertain effect against malaria parasites. Resistance of malaria parasites to the combination with pyrimethamine is common in many endemic areas.

Pharmacokinetics

Oral absorption	Extensive
C_{max} 500 mg oral	c. 60 mg/l after 3–4 h
Plasma half-life	c. 6 days
Volume of distribution	0.13 l/kg
Plasma protein binding	94%

The extremely long half-life allows administration at weekly intervals. The acetyl metabolite has a similarly long half-life, but sulfadoxine is less extensively metabolized than many other sulfonamides.

Toxicity and side effects

Side effects are those common to the group. There have been many reports of Stevens–Johnson syndrome following its use and the combination with pyrimethamine is no longer recommended for the prophylaxis of malaria.

Clinical use

Sulfadoxine is used only in combination with pyrimethamine.

Preparations and dosage

Proprietary names: Fansidar, Fanasil, in combination with pyrimethamine.

Preparations: Tablets containing 500 mg sulfadoxine and 25 mg pyrimethamine.

Dosage: Adults, oral, three tablets as a single dose. Children 10–14 years, two tablets; 7–9 years, 1½> tablets; 4–6 years, one tablet; under 4 years, half a tablet.

Very limited availability as a single agent; widely available in combination with pyrimethamine as Fansidar.

Further information

Anonymous 1999 Sulfadoxine. In: Dollery C (ed.) *Therapeutic Drugs* 2nd ed. Churchill Livingstone, Edinburgh, pp. S132–S135.

Hellgren U, Rombo L, Berg B, Carlson J, Wilholm B-E 1987 Adverse reactions to sulphadoxine-pyrimethamine in Swedish travellers. Implications for prophylaxis. *British Medical Journal* 295: 365–366.

Selby CD, Ladusans EJ, Smith PG 1985 Fatal multisystem toxicity associated with prophylaxis with pyrimethamine and sulfadoxine (Fansidar). *British Medical Journal* 290: 113–114.

SULFAMETHOXAZOLE

5-Methyl-3-sulfanilamidoisoxazole. Molecular weight: 253.2.

This is the sulfonamide component of co-trimoxazole (p. 291). It is slightly soluble in water.

Antimicrobial activity

The intrinsic activity is similar to that of sulfadiazine (Table 32.1).

Pharmacokinetics

Oral absorption	85%
C_{max} 800 mg oral	c. 50 mg/l after 3–6 h
Plasma half-life	6–20 h
Volume of distribution	12–18 l
Plasma protein binding	65%

Penetration of extravascular sites, including the CSF, is good. It crosses the placenta and achieves levels in breast milk of about 10% the simultaneous plasma concentration. It is extensively metabolized, but about 30% of the dose is excreted unchanged in urine so that high concentrations are achieved.

Toxicity and side effects

Unwanted effects are those common to sulfonamides. In addition, benign intracranial hypertension has been reported in children. Most side effects of co-trimoxazole are thought to be attributable to the sulfonamide component.

Clinical uses

Sulfamethoxazole is used only in combination with the diaminopyrimidine trimethoprim (*see* p. 291).

Preparations

Very limited availability as a single agent.

Further information

Anonymous 1999 Sulfamethoxazole and trimethoprim combination. In: Dollery C (ed.) *Therapeutic Drugs*, 2nd ed. Churchill Livingstone, Edinburgh, pp. S136–S140.

SULFISOXAZOLE

3,4-Dimethyl-5-sulfanilamidoisoxazole; sulphafurazole.
Molecular weight: 243.

Sulfisoxazole is highly soluble, even in acid urine.

Antimicrobial activity

The spectrum and potency are typical of the group (Table 32.1; p. 386).

Pharmacokinetics

Oral absorption	Very good
C_{max} 2 g oral	c. 20 mg/l after 3–4 h
Plasma half-life	3–7 h
Plasma protein binding	90%

Toxicity and side effects

Side effects are those common to other sulfonamides. It has good solubility and is less prone than some other members of the group to cause renal problems.

Clinical use

Its principal use is in urinary tract infection.

Preparations and dosage

Preparations: Tablets, suspension, ophthalmic preparations.

Dosage: Adults, oral, 2–4 g initially, then 4–8 g/day in divided doses every 4–6 h.

Children, oral, 75 mg/kg initially, then 150 mg/kg/day in divided doses (maximum 6 g per day).

Limited availability; not available in the UK.

OTHER SULFONAMIDES

Sulfacetamide

N-acetylsulfanilamide. It is very soluble in water and was formerly used in urinary tract infection. It is available in some countries in ophthalmic preparations and as a component (with sulfathiazole and sulfabenzamide) of a triple sulfonamide cream for the topical treatment of bacterial vaginosis.

Sulfacetamide is one of the least active sulfonamides. It is well absorbed when given orally and is excreted into the urine with a half life of around 9 h. About 70% is excreted unchanged, the remainder being present as the acetyl metabolite. Adverse reactions are those common to the group. Stevens–Johnson syndrome has been reported several times after topical use in conjunctivitis.

Preparations

Proprietary name: Albucid, Ocusulf etc.

Sultrin, Triple sulpha cream containing sulfathiazole 3.42% sulfacetamide 2.86% and sulfabenzamide 3.7% w/v.

Limited availability.

Sulfadimethoxine

2,4-Dimethoxy-6-sulfanilamido-1,3-diazine. A rapidly absorbed compound with a long half-life (38–40 h), and a high degree of protein binding (98%). Renal clearance is very slow, and daily dosage maintains adequate plasma levels.

Preparations and dosage

Proprietary name: Madribon.

Preparation: Tablets.

Dosage: Adults, oral, 1–2 g followed by 0.5–1.0 g/day.

Fairly widely available in Europe, Japan, South America and South Africa.

Sulfaguanidine

1-Sulfanilylguanidine. A poorly absorbed compound, less potent than succinylsulfathiazole but with similar uses. Blood concentrations of 15–40 mg/l have been found after single doses of 1–7 g. Excretion in the urine is rapid.

Preparations

Available in multi-ingredient preparations; not available in the UK.

Sulfaloxate

A poorly absorbed compound formulated as the calcium salt. About 5% is absorbed from the gastrointestinal tract. Formerly used to treat intestinal infections.

Preparations

Preparation: Tablets.

Very limited availability.

Sulfamerazine

2-Sulfonamido-4-methylpyrimidine. A component of some triple sulfa combinations. Plasma half-life is *c.* 24 h and protein binding *c.* 75%. It is less active than sulfadiazine.

Sulfamethizole

2-Sulfanilamido-5-methyl-1,3,4-thiodiazole. A short-acting sulfonamide (plasma half-life 2.5 h). Protein binding is *c.* 85%. About 60% is excreted in the urine within 5 h.

 Preparations and dosage

Proprietary name: Urolucosil.
Preparation: Tablets.
Dosage: Adult, oral, 1.5–4 g/day in 3–4 divided doses. Children >2 months, oral, 30–45 mg/kg/day in four divided doses.
Widely available; not available in the UK.

Sulfamethoxypyridazine

2-sulfanilamido-5-methoxypyrimidine. A long-acting compound with activity similar to that of sulfadiazine. Binding to plasma proteins is about 75%.

 Preparations and dosage

Proprietary name: Durenate.

Sulfamethoxypyridazine

3-Sulfanilamido-6-methoxypyridazine.

Properties are similar to those of sulfadimethoxine: A rapidly absorbed, long-acting compound (half-life 38 h) with a high degree of protein binding (96%). A 1 g oral dose achieves a peak plasma concentration of around 100 mg/l after 5 h. It use has been largely discontinued because of frequent adverse effects, but there are reports of benefit in dermatitis herpetiformis. It has been used in combination with trimethoprim.

 Preparations

Preparation: Tablets.
Very limited availability in Continental Europe.

Sulfametopyrazine

2-Sulfanilamido-3-methoxypyrazine; sulfalene.

A very long-acting compound (plasma half-life 60 h). Adequate blood levels can be maintained by giving a dose of 2 g once weekly. The protein binding is *c.* 70%. It has been successfully used in the single-dose treatment of urinary tract infection. As with other long-acting compounds sulfametopyrazine has been associated with an increased incidence of erythema multiforme.

 Preparations and dosage

Proprietary name: Kelfizine W.
Preparation: Tablets.
Dosage: Adults, oral, 2 g once weekly.
Limited availability; available in the UK.

Sulfathiazole

2-Sulfanilamidothiazole.

A short-acting compound (half-life *c.* 4 h) with relatively high activity. Protein binding is *c.* 75%. Its use has declined because of a high incidence of side effects. It is one of the constituents of triple sulfonamide mixtures, of which local preparations are still available.

Two compounds, pthalylsulfathiazole (sulfathalidine) and succinylsulfathiazole (sulfasuxidine) owe their activity to the slow liberation of sulfathiazole in the bowel. They are poorly soluble and very little is absorbed after oral administration. They were formerly used in the treatment of intestinal infections and in bowel preparation before surgery. They are available in multi-ingredient preparations in some countries.

 Preparations

Tablets, 0.5 g
Cream (*see under sulfacetamide*).
Widely available in multi-ingredient preparations.

Sulfisomidine

6-Sulfanilamido-2,4-dimethylpyrimidine; sulphasomidine.

A highly soluble sulfonamide with a plasma half-life of 6–8 h. Protein binding is about 90%. Activity is similar to that of sulfadiazine. It is less extensively metabolized than most other sulfonamides and is largely excreted unchanged in the urine.

 Preparations and dosage

Proprietary name: Elkosin.
Preparations: Tablets, topical preparations.
Available in some European countries, Mexico, Japan and South Africa.

SULFONAMIDES FOR SPECIAL PURPOSES

Mafenide

p-Aminomethylbenzene sulfonamide; Sulfamylon.

A topical agent formerly used extensively in burns, especially for its action in suppressing *Ps. aeruginosa*. It is rapidly absorbed through burned skin and is unusual in that it is not neutralized by *p*-aminobenzoic acid or by tissue exudates. Disadvantages of its use are local pain and burning, a variety of allergic reactions including erythema multiforme and its capacity to inhibit carbonic anhydrase, necessitating careful observation to detect the development of metabolic acidosis. Its metabolite, *p*-carboxybenzene sulfonamide, also inhibits carbonic anhydrase but has no antibacterial activity. Mafenide propionate was formerly used in ophthalmic preparations.

Silver sulfadiazine

Silver sulfadiazine is extremely insoluble. In addition to the usual activity of sulfonamides it exhibits activity – almost certainly attributable to the silver component – against *Ps. aeruginosa* and some fungi.

It is variably absorbed after topical application depending on the integrity of the skin. Toxic concentrations may be achieved in patients with extensive burns. It is used topically, mainly for burns, pressure sores and leg ulcers. Other suggested uses include the prevention of infection in skin graft donor sites and cord care in newborn infants.

 Preparations

Proprietary name: Flamazine.

Preparation: Topical cream containing 1% w/w silver sulfadiazine.

Widely available.

 Further information

Anonymous 1999 Silver sulfadiazine. In: Dollery C. (ed.) *Therapeutic Drugs* 2nd edn. Churchill Livingstone, Edinburgh, pp. S32–S35.

Sulfasalazine

One of the earliest and most successful sulfonamides to be developed was sulfapyridine, which fell into disuse because of unwanted effects such as crystalluria. Later, a number of salicylazosulfonamides, developed because of their increased water solubility, showed anti-inflammatory properties; one of them, sulfasalazine (salicylazosulfapyridine), has come into general use for ulcerative colitis.

After oral administration, some intact compound is absorbed from the upper gastrointestinal tract, appearing in the blood in 1–2 h, but most is cleaved by colonic bacteria to yield sulfapyridine and 5-aminosalicylic acid (mesalamine, mesalazine). Controlled trials have confirmed the efficacy of 5-aminosalicylic acid alone in ulcerative colitis, the sulfonamide component merely acting as a carrier. Thus, in remarkable extension of the good fortune that attended the discovery of sulfanilamide as the unexpected active principle of Prontosil (*see* Ch. 1), a cleavage product appears to be responsible for the beneficial effect of sulfasalazine. Since most of the side effects associated with sulfasalazine are attributable to sulfapyridine there seems little reason, other than cost, to use it in preference to mesalamine.

Sulfasalazine is also of benefit in Crohn's disease and rheumatoid arthritis, but the role, if any, of sulfapyridine in the overall effect is unclear.

 Preparations

Proprietary name: Salazopyrin.

Preparations: Tablets, enema, suppositories, suspension.

Widely available.

 Further information

Anonymous 1999 Sulfasalazine. In: Dollery C (ed.) *Therapeutic Drugs*, 2nd edn. Churchill Livingstone, Edinburgh, pp. S140–S144.

Anonymous 1999 Mesalamine. In: Dollery C (ed.) *Therapeutic Drugs* 2nd edn. Churchill Livingstone, Edinburgh, pp. M61–M65.

Azad Khan AK, Piris J, Truelove SC 1977 An experiment to determine the active moiety of sulphasalazine. *Lancet* ii: 892–895.

Box SA, Pullar T 1997 Sulphasalazine in the treatment of rheumatoid arthritis. *British Journal of Rheumatology* 36: 382–386.

Steinhart AH, Hemphill D, Greenberg GR 1994 Sulfasalazine and mesalamine for the maintenance therapy of Crohn's disease: a meta-analysis. *American Journal of Gastroenterology* 89: 2116–2124.

33 Tetracyclines

I. Chopra

A group of natural products derived from *Streptomyces* spp. and their semisynthetic derivatives. The minimum pharmacophore is a linear fused tetracyclic molecule, 6-deoxy-6-demethyltetracycline:

In the various members of the class a variety of functional groups are attached to the rings designated A, B, C and D. Natural products include chlortetracycline, oxytetracycline, tetracycline and demeclocycline (demethychlortetracycline). Semisynthetic derivatives include methacycline, doxycycline, minocycline, lymecycline, rolitetracycline and the glycylcycline, tigecycline (GAR-936), which has been developed to overcome problems of bacterial resistance to earlier tetracyclines and is under trial at the time of writing.

ANTIMICROBIAL SPECTRUM

Tetracyclines are broad-spectrum, essentially bacteristatic agents. Hydrophilic analogs (e.g. tetracycline) are generally less active than lipophilic analogs (e.g. minocycline and doxycycline).

They are active against many Gram-positive and Gram-negative bacteria, chlamydiae, mycoplasmas, rickettsiae, coxiellae, spirochaetes and some mycobacteria. Most streptococci are sensitive, except *Streptococcus agalactiae*, and enterococci. Susceptible Gram-positive bacilli include *Actinomyces israelii*, *Arachnia propionica*, *Listeria monocytogenes*, most clostridia and *Bacillus anthracis*. Nocardia are much less susceptible, minocycline demonstrating the greatest activity against them.

Among Gram-negative bacteria most enterobacteria and most strains of *Moraxella catarrhalis*, *Neisseria meningitidis* and *Haemophilus influenzae* are sensitive. Legionellae, brucellae,

Francisella tularensis, *Vibrio cholerae*, *Campylobacter* spp., *Helicobacter pylori*, *Plesiomonas shigelloides* and *Aeromonas hydrophila* are all susceptible. Many anaerobic bacteria are susceptible, doxycycline and minocycline being the most active members of the class. Rickettsiae are generally sensitive, especially to doxycycline, minocycline and tetracycline. None of the tetracyclines is active against *Pseudomonas aeruginosa*, *Proteus* spp. or *Providencia* spp., but *Burkholderia pseudomallei* and *Stenotrophomonas maltophilia* are usually susceptible.

Tetracylines are generally inactive against fungi, although minocycline shows some activity against *Candida albicans*. They show useful activity against *Entamoeba histolytica* and plasmodia.

ACQUIRED RESISTANCE

Resistance to the class has emerged in an ever-increasing number of bacterial species. Although some strains of *Staphylococcus aureus* remain sensitive, the prevalence of resistance in hospital isolates is now substantial. Resistance in Gram-negative bacteria continues to increase. Most strains of *Bacteroides* are now resistant. Although chlamydiae generally remain susceptible, there have been reports of resistance in *Chlamydia trachomatis* isolates that have led to therapeutic failures.

Resistance arises primarily from acquisition of genes encoding proteins that either confer the capacity to eliminate the drug from the cell or protect the ribosome from inhibition. In some cases resistance has arisen by point mutation in ribosomal RNA (e.g. in propionibacteria), or through the activity of innate (endogenous) bacterial efflux proteins that confer resistance to a number of structurally unrelated biocides and antibiotics, as well as tetracyclines. However, the most important clinical mechanisms of resistance result from acquisition of genetically mobile tetracycline resistance genes, a large number of which have been identified in bacteria.

CLASSIFICATION OF RESISTANCE GENES

Twenty-seven different tetracycline resistance (*tet*) genes, three oxytetracycline resistance (*otr*) genes and a gene designated *tcr*3 have been characterized (Table 33.1). Seventeen *tet* genes, one *otr* gene and *tcr*3 code for transport proteins that mediate energy-dependent efflux of tetracyclines from the bacterial cell. Eight *tet* genes and one of the *otr* genes, *otr*(A), code for ribosomal protection proteins. The presence of *tet* genes in pathogenic and commensal bacteria with efflux or ribosomal protection mechanisms similar to those encoded by *otr* genes found in streptomycetes is consistent with lateral gene transfer from the tetracycline-producing streptomycetes to other bacteria.

Table 33.1 Characterized tetracycline resistance genes (*tet* and *otr*) and the mechanisms of resistance they encode

Efflux	Ribosomal protection	Enzymatic	Unknown[a]
tet (A), (B), (C), (D), (E)	*tet* (M)	*tet* (X)	*tet* (U)
tet (G), (H), (I), (J)	*tet* (O)		*otr* (C)
tet (K), (L)	*tet* (Q), (S), (T)		
tet (V)	*tet* (W)		
tet (Y), (Z)	*tet*[b]		
*tcr*3[b]	*otr* (A)		
tet (30), (31)	*tet* P(B)[c]		
otr (B)			
tet P(A)			

Letters and numbers in brackets refer to sequential designations as new genes are discovered; numbers replaced letters after Z was reached.
[a] *tet* (U) has been sequenced but does not appear to be related to either efflux or ribosomal protection proteins; *otr* (C) has not been sequenced.
[b] These genes have not been given new designations.
[c] Does not independently confer tetracycline resistance when separated from *tet*P (A).

The *otr*(C) gene has not been sequenced, and the *tet*(U) sequence is unrelated to tetracycline efflux, ribosomal protection, or enzymatic proteins. The *tet*(I) gene has not been sequenced but phenotypic studies suggest it encodes an efflux pump. The *tet*(X) gene encodes an enzyme which modifies and inactivates tetracyclines. However, its clinical relevance is doubtful since it requires oxygen to function and the gene has been found only in strict anaerobes.

DISTRIBUTION OF *tet* GENES

Many tetracycline resistance genes are associated with mobile plasmids, transposons, conjugative transposons and integrons (gene cassettes). These have enabled the resistance genes to move from species to species and into a wide range of genera by conjugation.

The *tet*(A–E), *tet*(G–J), *tet*(Y), *tet*(30) and *tet*(31) genes are found exclusively in Gram-negative genera. Although many were first described in enterobacteria, they have now been found in pseudomonads and in *Neisseria*, *Haemophilus*, *Treponema* and *Vibrio* spp. and in *Mannheimia* (formerly *Pasteurella*) *haemolytica*. The *tet*(B) gene has been identified in 20 Gram-negative genera, whereas the distribution of *tet*(E) *tet*(I), *tet*(J), *tet*(30), and *tet*(31) is more restricted. To date, no naturally occurring ribosomal protection genes have been found in the enterobacteria, although *tet*(M), *tet*(O), *tet*(Q), and *tet*(W) occur naturally in other Gram-negative species. Carriage of multiple *tet* genes of different classes is common in Gram-positive bacteria, but uncommon in Gram-negative bacteria, especially enteric species. The reason for this is unknown, but a similar situation exists for the carriage of other antibiotic resistance genes.

Naturally occurring tetracycline efflux genes of Gram-negative bacteria do not appear to have spread to Gram-positive species, probably because they have higher G+C contents (>40%) than those of Gram-positive origin and do not express well if moved into Gram-positive species. Gram-positive *tet* genes have relatively low G+C contents (≤35%). These genes are found in an increasing number of Gram-negative species, including anaerobes. The *tet*(M) ribosomal protection gene has been identified in clinical isolates from eight Gram-negative and 18 Gram-positive genera.

INCIDENCE OF RESISTANCE

Rates of tetracycline resistance vary widely on the basis of geographical locale and year of isolation. In some locations resistance rates have been very high. For instance, in a Boston Hospital in 1969, 38% of *Staph. aureus*, 61% of *Esch. coli* and 62% of *Klebsiella* spp. were resistant. Comparable high rates of resistance were also recorded in *B. fragilis* and *H. influenzae* in the early 1980s, in both the USA and Europe.

Multidrug resistance, which includes resistance to tetracyclines, is also common. A Brazilian study in the period 1988–1993 showed that over 60% of *Shigella flexneri* strains were resistant to tetracycline, streptomycin, and chloramphenicol. Many isolates of *Salmonella enterica* serovar Typhimurium DT104 carry a class 1 integron containing a variety of different antibiotic resistance genes including tetracycline. In a Canadian study ten human and eight non-human isolates carried *tet*(G) along with genes conferring resistance to one or more other antibiotics, including ampicillin, chloramphenicol, streptomycin, spectinomycin and sulfonamide. One human isolate carried the *tet*(A) gene and three carried *tet*(B) in place of *tet*(G).

Related events have occurred in Gram-positive species. A study in 1994 found that approximately 90% of methicillin-resistant *Staph. aureus* (MRSA), 70% of *Str. agalactiae*, 70% of multiresistant *E. faecalis* and 60% of multiresistant *Str. pneumoniae* were resistant to tetracyclines.

PHARMACOKINETICS

ABSORPTION

Tetracyclines are usually administered by mouth. However, tetracycline, oxytetracycline, lymecycline, rolitetracycline, doxycycline and minocycline have all been prepared in forms suitable for injection. Absorption occurs largely in the proximal small bowel, but may be diminished by the simultaneous presence of food, milk or cations, which form non-absorbable tetracycline chelates. Cimetidine and presumably other H_2-receptor antagonists also impair absorption of tetracyclines by interfering with their dissolution, which is pH dependent.

The absorption problems of earlier compounds have been essentially overcome in the later tetracyclines. Improved absorption is claimed for lymecycline, demeclocycline and methacycline, but is best established for doxycycline and minocycline, which may be administered with food and for which the proportion of administered dose absorbed is more than 90%.

DISTRIBUTION

Peak plasma concentrations follow 1–3 h after ingestion. The plasma concentration curve is plateau shaped, having a small rise and a still slower fall. Factors contributing to this are continued absorption, biliary recirculation and protein binding, which varies from 20–35% for oxytetracycline to 80–90% for demeclocycline, doxycycline and minocycline. Blood levels achieved after normal oral dosage are of the order of 1.5–4.0 mg/l. Most tetracyclines must be given four times daily to maintain therapeutic concentrations in the blood, but demeclocycline and minocycline can be administered twice daily and doxycycline once daily.

Tetracyclines penetrate moderately well into body fluids and tissues. This is reflected in their large volumes of distribution, which in most cases exceeds 100 l. Tissue concentrations are related to lipid solubility, which is in the order minocycline > doxycycline > older tetracyclines. Concentrations in the cerebrospinal fluid (CSF) are about 10–25% of those in the blood. A unique feature is deposition and persistence in areas where bone and teeth are being laid down.

The mean sputum level, about 20% of that in serum, is high enough to inhibit tetracycline-susceptible pneumococci and *H. influenzae*, the penetration of tetracycline and minocycline being superior to that of doxycycline. They also penetrate into the sebum and are excreted in perspiration, properties which contribute to their usefulness in the management of acne. They are found in substantial concentrations in the eye.

EXCRETION

The main excretory route is the kidney, but they are also eliminated in the feces. Fecal excretion occurs even after parenteral administration as a result of passage of the drug into the bile. The concentrations obtained in bile are 5–25 times those in the blood, doxycycline attaining especially high levels. These concentrations are lowered in the presence of biliary obstruction. The proportion of administered dose found in the urine is, for most tetracyclines, in the range 20–60%, but is less for chlortetracycline and doxycycline and least for minocycline. Glomerular filtration is the main determinant of renal excretion, with the exception of doxycycline. Tetracyclines are removed slowly by hemodialysis and minimally by peritoneal dialysis.

TOXICITY AND SIDE EFFECTS

The most important adverse effect is gastrointestinal intolerance, which is dose dependent. Allergic reactions are uncommon. Photosensitivity is a class phenomenon and is most marked for demeclocycline. Deposition in developing bones and teeth precludes their use in young children and during late pregnancy. Most compounds show antianabolic effects and accumulate in renal failure, with the notable exception of doxycycline.

Gastrointestinal disturbances are more common when larger doses (2 g or more) are given. Nausea and vomiting are presumed to be due to a direct irritant effect of the drug on the gastric mucosa, but diarrhea is probably the result of disturbance of the normal flora. The frequency and nature of superinfection with resistant organisms depends much on local ecology. Pseudomembranous colitis has been associated with tetracyclines, but they do not appear to be a particularly common precursor of that complication. Other organisms that often become dominant in the fecal flora after administration of tetracyclines are *Candida*, *Proteus* or *Pseudomonas* spp. Some serious consequences of superinfection are well documented, including *Staph. aureus* enterocolitis, which was much more common in hospital when the tetracyclines were more widely prescribed.

Glossitis and pruritus ani, vulvitis and vaginitis are well recognized; less common side effects include esophageal ulceration and acute pancreatitis. Changes occur in the surface lipids of the skin, notably a decrease in fatty acids and reciprocal increase in triglycerides that probably results from inhibition of extracellular bacterial lipase production by *Propionibacterium acnes*.

In patients with impaired renal function, treatment may lead to biochemical deterioration and even to irreversible renal failure. The changes are proportional to the degree of renal impairment and to the dose and duration of therapy. The maximal effects are often reached some days after the course of treatment has finished. An exception to this is doxycycline, for which an alternative path of elimination exists.

Tetracyclines are deposited in teeth and bone during the early stages of calcification. This may occur in utero if the mother is treated after the fifth month, when calcification of the deciduous teeth begins, or be produced by treatment of the child after birth. Treatment is therefore to be avoided in early childhood up to the age of 8 years, except for imperative indications or unless a short course will suffice. Direct ill-effects on teeth are compounded by the use in children of liquid preparations containing sucrose, which are associated with increased risk of dental caries. Pediatric formulations of tetracyclines have been discontinued in some countries, including the USA and UK.

Deaths have been reported in pregnant women given tetracycline in large intravenous doses (>1 g/day) usually for the treatment of pyelonephritis. The main lesion found at autopsy was diffuse fatty degeneration of the liver, which may also involve the pancreas, kidneys and brain. Mild derangements of liver enzyme function are not uncommon, although tetracycline and oxytetracycline have a lower incidence than other tetracyclines.

A number of infants treated with tetracyclines have developed bulging of the anterior fontanelle; benign intracranial hypertension has also been described in older children and even in adults, with headache, photophobia and papilledema. Symptoms disappear quickly after the drug is withdrawn, but papilledema may persist in some patients for many months or reappear when tetracycline is given again. The mechanism is unknown.

Hypersensitivity rashes, including exfoliation, occasionally occur, but skin reactions are more often manifestations of photosensitivity. A reaction may occur after administration of any tetracycline, but is especially associated with demeclocycline and may be less common with doxycycline and minocycline. Fixed drug eruptions, onycholysis and nail and thyroid pigmentation have also been reported. Angiedema and ana-

phylaxis are rare. Hypersensitivity reactions to one tetracycline generally infer cross-hypersensitivity to the other agents. Reported inhibitory effects on several human polymorphonuclear leukocyte and lymphocyte functions in vitro have yet to be shown to have any therapeutic significance.

Drug interactions include complexes with divalent and trivalent cations together with chelation by iron-containing preparations. The anticonvulsants carbamazepine, phenytoin and barbiturates decrease the half-life of doxycycline through enzyme induction. The anesthetic methoxyflurane has been reported to cause nephrotoxicity when coadministered with tetracyclines. The efficiency of oral contraceptives is reduced, as with many other broad-spectrum antibiotics.

CLINICAL USE

The use of tetracyclines has significantly declined in most countries as the incidence of bacterial resistance has increased and more active and better tolerated antimicrobial agents have been introduced. However, some new applications have emerged, such as their use as part of multidrug regimens for the management of gastritis and peptic ulcer disease associated with *H. pylori*. Their activity against malaria has become important for prophylaxis following the rapid increase of chloroquine and mefloquine-resistant *Plasmodium falciparum*.

Current anti-infective applications of the tetracyclines in humans are summarized in Table 33.2. Fortunately, resistance has not yet become a problem for those infections in which they are still the drugs of choice.

Table 33.2 Current applications of the tetracyclines for therapy and prophylaxis of infections in human beings

Type of infection	First choice	Acceptable alternative to other agents
Respiratory	Atypical pneumonia due to *Mycoplasma pneumoniae*, *Chlamydophila* (formerly *Chlamydia*) *pneumoniae*, *C. psittaci*	Community-acquired pneumonia[a] Infective exacerbations of chronic bronchitis[a] Legionellosis (doxycycline)
Bowel	Cholera Prophylaxis of travellers' diarrhea	
Genital	Non-gonococcal urethritis; cervicitis Lymphogranuloma venereum Pelvic inflammatory disease Granuloma inguinale	Syphilis Epididymitis Prostatitis
Other infections	Rocky Mountain spotted fever Endemic and epidemic typhus Trachoma (topical or oral) Q fever Brucellosis[c] Lyme disease Relapsing fever Periodontal infection (topical tetracycline or minocycline) Acne vulgaris (topical and systemic treatment) Prophylaxis of drug-resistant *Plasmodium falciparum* malaria	MRSA, MRSE (minocycline[b]) Plague Tularemia Bartonellosis Leptospirosis Whipple's disease Cutaneous *Mycobacterium marinum* infections Ocular *M. chelonei* infections[c] *Helicobacter pylori* infections[c]

MRSA, methicillin-resistant *Staphylococcus aureus*; MRSE; methicillin-resistant *Staphylococcus epidermidis*.
[a]Except in situations where there is a high rate of resistance among pneumococci and/or *H. influenzae*.
[b]When vancomycin or other agents inappropriate.
[c]In combination with other agents.

Further information

Agalar C, Usubutun, S, Turkyilmaz 1999 Ciprofloxacin and rifampicin versus doxycycline and rifampicin in the treatment of brucellosis. *European Journal of Clinical Microbiology and Infectious Diseases* 18: 535–538.

Chopra I, Hawkey PM, Hinton M 1992 Tetracyclines, molecular and clinical aspects. *Journal of Antimicrobial Chemotherapy* 29: 245–277.

Chopra I, Roberts M 2001 Tetracycline antibiotics: mode of action, applications, molecular biology and epidemiology of bacterial resistance. *Microbiology and Molecular Microbiology Reviews* 65: 232–260.

Davey PG, Bax RP, Newey J et al 1996 Growth in the use of antibiotics in the community in England and Scotland in 1980–93. *British Medical Journal* 312: 613.

Doern GV, Brueggemann AB, Huynh H et al 1999 Antimicrobial resistance with *Streptococcus pneumoniae* in the United States, 1997–98. *Emerging Infectious Diseases* 5: 757–765.

Felmingham D, Gruneberg RN and the Alexander Project Group 2000 The Alexander Project 1996–1997: latest susceptibility data from this international study of bacterial pathogens from community-acquired lower respiratory tract infections. *Journal of Antimicrobial Chemotherapy* 45: 191–203.

Graeme KA, Pollack CV, 1996 Antibiotic use in the emergency department. II. The aminoglycosides, macrolides, tetracyclines, sulfa drugs and urinary antiseptics. *Journal of Emergency Medicine* 14: 361–371.

Humbert P, Treffel P, Chapius J-F et al 1991 The tetracyclines in dermatology. *Journal of the American Academy of Dermatology* 25: 691–697.

Klein NC, Cunha BA 1995 Tetracyclines. *Medical Clinics of North America* 79: 789–801.

Maurin M, Raoult D, 1999 Q fever. *Clinical Microbiology Reviews* 12: 518–553.

McCaig LF, Hughes JM 1995 Trends in antimicrobial drug prescribing among office-based physicians in the United States. *Journal of the American Medical Association* 273: 214–219.

Ross JI, Eady EA, Cove JH et al 1998 16S rRNA mutation associated with tetracycline resistance in a Gram-positive bacterium. *Antimicrobial Agents and Chemotherapy* 42: 1702–1705.

Roberts MC 1996 Tetracycline resistant determinants: mechanisms of action, regulation of expression, genetic mobility and distribution. *FEMS Microbiology Reviews* 19: 1–24.

Schnappinger D, Hillen W 1996 Tetracyclines: antibiotic action, uptake, and resistance mechanisms. *Archives of Microbiology* 165: 359–369.

Smilack JD 1999 The tetracyclines. *Mayo Clinic Proceedings* 74: 727–729.

Somani J, Bhullar VB, Workowski A et al 2000 Multiple drug-resistant *Chlamydia trachomatis* associated with clinical treatment failure. *Journal of Infectious Diseases* 181: 1421–1427.

Urquhart E, Addy M 1995 Topical antimicrobials: new horizons for management of periodontal disease in general practice? *Dental Update* April: 104–111.

Van der Hulst RWM, Keller JJ, Rauws EAJ, Tytgat GNJ 1996 Treatment of *Helicobacter pylori* infection: a review of the world literature. *Helicobacter* 1: 6–19.

Van Steenberghe D, Rosling B, Soder PO et al 1999 A 15-month evaluation of the effects of repeated subgingival minocycline in chronic adult periodontitis. *Journal of Periodontology* 70: 657–667.

Welsh LE, Gaydos CA, Quinn TC 1992 In vitro evaluation of activities of azithromycin, erythromycin and tetracycline against *Chlamydia trachomatis* and *Chlamydia pneumoniae*. *Antimicrobial Agents and Chemotherapy* 36: 291–294.

Wright AL, Colver GB 1988 Tetracyclines – how safe are they? *Clinical and Experimental Dermatology* 13: 57–61.

CHLORTETRACYCLINE

Molecular weight (free base): 478.9; (hydrochloride): 515.3.

7-Chlortetracycline. A fermentation product of certain strains of *Streptomyces aureofaciens*. Formulated as the hydrochloride or the free base for oral or topical application.

Antimicrobial activity

The activity against a range of pathogenic bacteria is shown in Table 33.3. It is slightly less active than tetracycline against many bacteria, with the exception of Gram-positive organisms.

Table 33.3 Activity of tetracyclines against common pathogenic bacteria: MIC (mg/l). Data compiled from a variety of sources

Organism	Chlortetracycline	Demeclocycline	Doxycycline	Methacycline	Minocycline	Oxytetracycline	Tetracycline	Tigecycline
Staph. aureus	0.5–R	1–R	0.5–16	0.5–R	0.5–16	2–R	2–R	0.25–2
Str. pyogenes	0.1–32	0.25–32	0.1–16	0.1–32	0.1–16	0.25–32	0.25–32	0.06–0.25
Str. pneumoniae	No data	No data	0.06–32	No data	0.06–16	No data	0.12–R	0.03–0.25
E. faecalis	4–R	2–R	2–R	4–R	2–R	8–R	8–R	0.12–1
N. gonorrhoeae	0.25–>8	0.5–>8	0.1–>8	0.1–>8	0.25–8	1–>8	0.5–>8	0.008–0.12
N. meningitidis	No data	No data	No data	No data	0.06–0.12	No data	0.06–0.25	0.015–0.12
H. influenzae	1–>8	2–>8	1–2	1–>8	0.12–2	4–16	0.25–>8	1–4
Esch. coli	8–16	4–16	2–16	4–16	4–8	2–16	2–16	0.12–0.25
K. pneumoniae	8–R	8–R	8–R	8–R	4–32	16–R	4–R	0.5–4
Pr. mirabilis	R	32–R	R	R	R	R	32–R	2–R
Ser. marcescens	R	R	R	R	32	R	4–16	1–8
Ps. aeruginosa	R	32–R	32–R	R	R	R	32–R	4–>8
B. fragilis	No data	No data	No data	No data	0.25–R	0.5–R	No data	1–32

R, resistant (MIC >32 mg/l).

Pharmacokinetics

Oral absorption	30–60%
C_{max} 500 mg oral	2.5–7 mg/l
Plasma half-life	5–6 h
Volume of distribution	c. 2 l/kg
Plasma protein binding	47–65%

Absorption is relatively poor compared with other tetracyclines. It undergoes rapid metabolism and is largely eliminated by biliary excretion, with only a small proportion eliminated via the kidney. Despite this, chlortetracycline is not recommended for patients in renal failure, since accumulation occurs as a consequence of the half-life increase to approximately 7–11 h.

Toxicity and side effects

Side effects are typical of the group (p. 395). Contact hypersensitivity has been reported with topical application to abraded skin and varicose ulcers.

Clinical use

Its uses are those common to the group (Table 33.2). It has also been used topically in the management of recurrent aphthous ulcers of the mouth, but experience is limited and the mechanism of action is unknown.

Preparations and dosage

Proprietary name: Aureomycin.

Preparations: Topical, ophthalmic, capsules.

Dosage: Adults, oral, 250–500 mg, four times daily.

Widely available; oral preparation not available in the UK.

Further information

Anonymous 1999 Chlortetracycline (hydrochloride). In: Dollery C (ed.) *Therapeutic Drugs* 2nd edn. Churchill Livingstone, Edinburgh, pp. C199–C201.

DEMECLOCYCLINE

Molecular weight (free base): 464.9; (hydrochloride): 501.3.

6-Demethyl-7-chlortetracycline. A fermentation product of a mutant strain of *Streptomyces aureofaciens* formulated as the hydrochloride for oral administration.

Antimicrobial activity

Activity against a range of pathogenic bacteria is shown in Table 33.3. Occasional strains of viridans streptococci, *N. gonorrhoeae* and *H. influenzae* are more susceptible than to tetracycline. It is the most active tetracycline against *Brucella* spp.

Pharmacokinetics

Oral absorption	60–70%
C_{max} 300 mg oral	2 mg/l after 3–6 h
Plasma half-life	c. 12 h
Volume of distribution	c. 1.7 l/kg
Plasma protein binding	90%

Absorption

It is promptly yet incompletely absorbed by mouth, giving mean peak plasma levels after a single dose that are slightly higher than those produced by oxytetracycline and chlortetracycline, but lower than those achieved by tetracycline. However, with repeat dosing, steady-state concentrations exceed those for tetracycline. Simultaneous administration of antacids markedly depresses blood levels.

Distribution and excretion

It is widely distributed, achieving concentrations in pleural exudates similar to those of blood. CSF penetration is poor, especially in the absence of inflammation. Biliary concentrations are 20–30 times higher than those of plasma, and 40–50% of the drug can be recovered from feces. The other route of elimination is via glomerular filtration without reabsorption and accumulation occurs in renal failure.

Toxicity and side effects

Untoward reactions, notably gastrointestinal intolerance, are generally those typical of the group (p. 395). Occasional patients develop transient steatorrhea.

Of particular note is the occurrence of nephrogenic diabetes insipidus with development of vasopressin-resistant polyuria. The effect is dose dependent and occurs with daily doses in excess of 1.2 g. The drug inhibits activation of adenylate cyclase and protein kinase, which are both important in the interaction of antidiuretic hormone (ADH) with receptors within the renal tubule, thus decreasing the effect of ADH on the kidney. As a result, it has found a place in the treatment of inappropriate ADH secretion.

Renal failure may occur, particularly if prescribed for those with advanced liver cirrhosis. The mechanism is uncertain but may in part be related to the antianabolic effect of the tetracyclines as well as a direct toxic effect.

Photosensitivity may be severe and accompanied by vesiculation, edema and onycholysis. It is largely restricted to exposed skin; patients should avoid prolonged exposure to sunlight.

Clinical use

Its uses are those common to the group (Table 33.2). It has been extensively used in the management of the syndrome of inappropriate ADH secretion in a dose of at least 1.2 g/day; therapeutic response may take several days, but is superior to that of lithium. It has also found occasional use in patients with water retention as a result of congestive cardiac failure and in those with alcoholic cirrhosis and water and electrolyte retention.

Preparations and dosage

Proprietary name: Declomycin

Preparations: Capsules, tablets.

Dosage: Adults, oral, 150 mg every 6 h, or 300 mg every 12 h.

Widely available.

Further information

Anonymous 1999 Demeclocycline (hydrochloride). In: Dollery C (ed.) *Therapeutic Drugs* 2nd edn. Churchill Livingstone, Edinburgh, pp. D29–D31.

de Troyer A 1977 Demeclocycline treatment for syndrome of inappropriate antidiuretic hormone secretion. *Journal of the American Medical Association* 237: 2723–2726.

Geheb M, Cox M 1980 Renal effects of demeclocycline. *Journal of the American Medical Association* 243: 2519–2520.

Miller PD, Linas SL, Schrier RW 1980 Plasma demeclocycline levels and nephrotoxicity. Correlation in hyponatremic cirrhotic patients. *Journal of the American Medical Association* 243: 2513–2515.

DOXYCYCLINE

Molecular weight (free base): 444.5; (hyclate): 512.9.

![structure](CH3 OH N(CH3)2 OH OH O OH O CONH2)

6-Deoxy-5 β-hydroxytetracycline. A semisynthetic product supplied as the hyclate, calcium salt or the hydrochloride for oral and intravenous administration.

Antimicrobial activity

Its activity and spectrum are typical of the group (Table 33.3). It is active against some tetracycline-resistant *Staph. aureus* and is more active than other tetracyclines against *Str. pyogenes*, enterococci and *Nocardia* spp. *Mor. catarrhalis* (MIC 0.5 mg/l), *Legionella pneumophila* and most strains of *Ureaplasma urealyticum* (MIC 0.5 mg/l) are susceptible.

Pharmacokinetics

Oral absorption	90%
C_{max} 100–200 mg oral	1.7–5.7 mg/l after 2–3.5 h
100 mg intravenous infusion (1 h)	2.5 mg/l end infusion
Plasma half-life	18 h
Volume of distribution	0.9–1.8 l/kg
Plasma protein binding	90%

Absorption

Doxycycline is rapidly absorbed from the upper gastrointestinal tract and absorption appears to be linearly related to the administered dose. Food, especially dairy products, reduces peak serum concentrations by 20%. Alcohol also delays absorption. As with other tetracyclines, divalent and trivalent cations, as in antacids and ferrous sulfate, form chelates which reduce absorption.

Distribution

The greater lipophilicity of doxycycline is responsible for its widespread tissue distribution. Concentrations in liver, biliary system, kidneys and the digestive tract are approximately twice those in plasma. Within the respiratory tract, it achieves concentrations of 2.3–6.7 mg/kg in tonsils and 2.3–7.5 mg/kg in maxillary sinus mucosa. In bronchial secretions concentrations are about 20% of plasma levels, increasing to 25–35% in the presence of pleurisy. Gall-bladder concentrations are approximately 75% those of plasma, and prostate concentrations 60–100%. It penetrates well into the aqueous humor. CSF concentrations range from 11 to 56% of plasma levels and are not affected by inflammation. In the elderly, tissue concentrations are 50–100% higher than in young adults. The half-life remains unaltered and one explanation is reduced fecal elimination.

Metabolism and excretion

Doxycycline is largely excreted unchanged. Around 35% is eliminated through the kidneys and the remainder through the digestive tract. Renal clearance ranges from 1.8 to 2.1 l/h, and is largely via glomerular filtration, with approximately 70% tubular reabsorption. Alkalinization enhances renal clearance. Fecal elimination partly reflects biliary excretion but also includes diffusion across the intestinal wall. Provided the drug is not chelated, reabsorption occurs with enterohepatic recycling. The elimination half-life is long (15–25 h).

The half-life and area under the curve (AUC) are little altered in renal insufficiency, with no evidence of accumulation after repeat dosing, even in anuric patients, evidently as a result of increased clearance through the liver or gastrointestinal tract, since biliary and fecal concentrations increase in renal failure. Although the plasma elimination half-life is unchanged, the drug appears to accumulate in tissues with increasing renal failure, and it has been suggested that less drug is bound to plasma protein and red cells through competition with other metabolites, which in turn increases hepatic elimination. Pharmacokinetics are unaltered by hemodialysis or peritoneal dialysis. Clearance is decreased by about half in patients with type IIa and type IV hyperlipidemia.

The plasma elimination half-life is shortened by a variety of antiepileptic agents including phenytoin, barbiturates and carbamazepine, presumably as a result of liver enzyme induction, although there is also evidence for some interference with the protein binding of doxycycline.

Toxicity and side effects

Untoward reactions are generally those typical of the group (p. 395) but gastrointestinal side effects are less common than with other tetracyclines due to the lower total dosage and the ability to administer the drug with meals. As with other tetracyclines, esophageal ulceration as a result of capsule impaction has been reported. Dental and bone deposition appear to be less common than with other tetracycline derivatives. Other adverse phenomena include occasional vestibular toxicity.

Hypersensitivity reactions include photosensitivity and eosinophilia, but rarely anaphylaxis. In common with demeclocycline and chlortetracycline it may be a more powerful sensitizer than other tetracyclines. It is contraindicated in patients with acute porphyria because it has been demonstrated to be porphyrinogenic in animals.

Clinical use

Uses are those common to the group (Table 33.2; p. 396). Its once-daily administration and safety in renal insufficiency make it one of the most widely used tetracyclines. It is used in the prophylaxis and treatment of malaria in areas in which resistance to conventional antimalarial agents is common.

 Preparations and dosage

Proprietary name: Vibramycin.

Preparations: Capsules, tablets, suspension.

Dosage: Adults, oral, 200 mg on day 1 then 100 mg per day; severe infections, 200 mg per day; acne, 50 mg per day for 6 weeks or longer.

Widely available.

 Further information

Anonymous 1999 Doxycycline hyclate. In: Dollery C (ed.) Therapeutic Drugs 2nd edn. Churchill Livingstone, Edinburgh, pp. D229–D232.
Cunha BA 1999 Doxycycline re-visited. *Archives of Internal Medicine* 159: 1006–1007.
Houin G, Brunner F, Nebout Th et al 1983 The effects of chronic renal insufficiency on the pharmacokinetics of doxycycline in man. *British Journal of Clinical Pharmacology* 16: 245–252.
Joshi N, Miller DQ 1997 Doxycycline revisited. *Archives of Internal Medicine* 157: 1421–1428.
Wojcicki J, Kalinowski W, Gawronska-Szlarz B 1985 Comparative pharmacokinetics of doxycycline and oxytetracycline in patients with hyperlipidemia. *Arzneimittelforschung* 35: 991–993.

 # LYMECYCLINE

2-N-lysinomethyl-tetracycline.

A water-soluble prodrug of tetracycline available for oral administration.

Its antimicrobial activity is due to the tetracycline content. Lymecycline is lipophilic, rapidly absorbed from the gastrointestinal tract and widely distributed. In maxillary sinus tissue concentrations around 1 mg/kg have been found some 3 h after administration of a conventional dose. The half-life is 7–14 h. Approximately 30% of an orally administered dose is excreted as active drug in the urine, where it achieves concentrations of 300 mg/l.

Its untoward effects and clinical uses are those of tetracycline, although it is claimed to be better tolerated.

 Preparations and dosage

Proprietary name: Tetralysal 300.

Preparation: Capsules.

Dosage: Adults, oral, 408 mg every 12 h. In severe infections, up to 3–4 capsules per day in divided doses; acne, 408 mg per day for 8 weeks or longer.

Available in the UK and continental Europe.

 Further information

Bergholm AM 1987 Studies of the penetration of lymecycline into paranasal sinus in man. *Acta Oto-Rhino-Laryngologia Belgica* 37: 649–653.
Forsberg GS, Hermansson J 1984 Comparative bioavailability of tetracycline and lymecycline. *British Journal of Pharmacology* 18: 529–533.

METHACYCLINE

6-Methylene-5-hydroxy-tetracycline. Molecular weight (free base): 442.5.

A semisynthetic derivative supplied as the hydrochloride for oral administration.

Its activity against common pathogenic bacteria is shown in Table 33.3 (p. 397).

Methaycline is absorbed by mouth, mean peak plasma concentrations of 2–6 mg/l being found about 4 h after a 300 mg dose. Food or milk reduces uptake by half. Protein binding is 80–90%. The plasma elimination half-life varies between 7 and 15 h and increases to 44 h in severe renal impairment. It is widely distributed, producing lung concentrations similar to, or greater than, the simultaneous plasma concentration. About a third is excreted in the urine.

Untoward reactions are generally those common to the group (p. 395), although gastrointestinal intolerance is reported to be less frequent than with other tetracyclines, largely because of the lower dosages used. There are no unique adverse drug reactions, although skin and conjunctival pigmentation have been reported.

Its clinical uses are those common to the group (Table 33.2; p. 396).

Preparations and dosage

Proprietary name: Rondomycin.

Preparation: Capsules.

Dosage: Adults, oral, 600 mg per day in two or four divided doses.

Widely available in continental Europe.

Further information

Wright AL, Colver GB 1988 Tetracyclines – how safe are they? *Clinical and Experimental Dermatology* 13: 57–61.

MINOCYCLINE

7-Dimethylamino-6-demethyl-6-deoxy-tetracycline. Molecular weight (free base): 457.5; (hydrochloride): 493.9.

A semisynthetic tetracycline derivative supplied as the hydrochloride for oral administration.

Antimicrobial activity

Activity against common bacterial pathogens is shown in Table 33.3 (p. 397). It exhibits the broad-spectrum activity typical of the group, but it is more active than other tetracyclines against *Staph. aureus*, including strains resistant to other tetracyclines. It is the most active tetracycline against β-hemolytic streptococci and is active against some tetracycline-resistant pneumococci.

It is also active against some enterobacteria resistant to other tetracyclines, probably because some Gram-negative efflux pumps remove minocycline less effectively than other tetracyclines. Some strains of *H. influenzae* resistant to other tetracyclines are susceptible. *Sten. maltophilia* is susceptible, as are most strains of *Acinetobacter* spp. and *L. pneumophila*.

It is notable for its activity against *Bacteroides* and *Fusobacterium* spp., and is more active than other tetracyclines against *C. trachomatis*, brucellae and nocardiae. It inhibits *Mycobacterium tuberculosis*, *M. bovis*, *M. kansasii* and *M. intracellulare* at 5–6 mg/l. *Candida albicans* and *C. tropicalis* are also slightly susceptible.

Pharmacokinetics

Oral absorption	95–100%
C_{max} 150 mg oral	2 mg/l after 2 h
300 mg oral	4 mg/l after 2 h
Plasma half-life	12–24 h
Volume of distribution	80–115 l
Plasma protein binding	76%

Absorption

Food does not significantly affect absorption, which is depressed by coadministration with milk. It is chelated by metals and suffers the effects of antacids and ferrous sulfate common to tetracyclines. On a regimen of 100 mg 12-hourly, steady-state concentrations ranged between 2.3 and 3.5 mg/l.

Distribution

The high lipophilicity of minocycline provides wide distribution and tissue concentrations that often exceed those of the plasma. The tissue:plasma ratio in maxillary sinus and tonsillar tissue is 1.6; that in lung is 3–4. Sputum concentrations may reach 37–60% of simultaneous plasma levels. In bile, liver and gall-bladder the ratios are 38, 12 and 6.5, respectively.

Prostatic and seminal fluid concentrations range from 40 to 100% of those of serum. CSF penetration is poor, especially in the non-inflamed state. Concentrations in tears and saliva are high, and may explain its beneficial effect in the treatment of meningococcal carriage.

Metabolism

Biotransformation to three microbiologically inactive metabolites occurs in the liver; the most abundant is 9-hydroxy-minocycline.

Excretion

Only 4–9% of administered drug is excreted in the urine, and in renal failure elimination is little affected. Neither hemodialysis nor peritoneal dialysis affects drug elimination. Fecal excretion is relatively low and evidence for enterohepatic recirculation remains uncertain. Despite high hepatic excretion, dose accumulation does not occur in liver disease, such as cirrhosis. Type IIa and type IV hyperlipidemic patients show a decreased minocycline clearance of 50%, suggesting that dose modification may be necessary.

Toxicity and side effects

Minocycline shares the untoward reactions common to the group (p. 395) with gastrointestinal side effects being most common, and more prevalent in women. Diarrhea is less common than with other tetracyclines, presumably as a result of its lower fecal concentrations. Hypersensitivity reactions, including rashes, interstitial nephritis and pulmonary eosinophilia, are occasionally seen.

Staining of the permanent dentition is common to all tetracyclines; a side effect that appears to be unique to minocycline is that of tissue discoloration and skin pigmentation. Tissues that have become pigmented include the skin, skull and other bones and the thyroid gland, which at autopsy appears blackened. The pigmentation tends to resolve slowly with discontinuation of the drug and is related to the length of therapy. Three types of pigmentation have been identified.

- A brown macular discoloration ('muddy skin syndrome'), which occurs in sun-exposed parts and is histologically associated with melanin deposition.
- Blue–black macular pigmentation occurring within inflamed areas and scars associated with hemosiderin deposition.
- Circumscribed macular blue–grey pigmented areas occurring in sun-exposed and unexposed skin, which appears to be linked to a breakdown product of minocycline.

CNS toxicity has been prominent; notably benign intracranial hypertension, which resolves on discontinuation of the drug and, more commonly, dizziness, ataxia, vertigo, tinnitus,

nausea and vomiting, which appear to be more frequent in women. These primarily vestibular side effects have ranged in frequency from 4.5 to 86%. They partly coincide with plasma concentration peaks, but their exact pathogenesis has yet to be determined.

Clinical use

Its uses are those common to the group (Table 33.2; p. 396) and there appear to be few situations in which it has a unique therapeutic advantage. Its use has been tempered by the high incidence of vestibular side effects.

Although used in the long-term management of acne, the potential for skin pigmentation must be considered. Because of its high tissue concentrations, it may occasionally provide a useful alternative to other agents for the treatment of chronic prostatitis. It has a role in the treatment of sexually transmitted chlamydial infections.

Preparations and dosage

Proprietary name: Minocin MR.

Preparations: Tablets, capsules.

Dosage: Adults, oral, 100 mg twice daily; acne, 100 mg per day as a single or two divided doses.

Widely available.

Further information

Anonymous 1999 Minocycline (hydrochloride). In: Dollery C ed. *Therapeutic Drugs* 2nd edn. Churchill Livingstone, Edinburgh, pp. M187–M190.

Basler RSW 1985 Minocycline-related hyperpigmentation. *Archives of Dermatology* 121: 606–609.

Dykhuizen RS, Zaidi AM, Godden DJ, Jegarajah S, Legge JS 1995 Minocycline and pulmonary eosinophilia. *British Medical Journal* 310: 1520–1521.

Freeman CD, Nightingale CH, Quintiliani R 1994 Minocycline: old and new therapeutic uses. *International Journal of Antimicrobial Agents* 4: 325–335.

Nelis HJCF, De Leenheer AP 1982 Metabolism of minocycline in humans. *Drug Metabolism and Disposition* 10: 142–146.

Okada N, Moriya K, Nishida K et al 1989 Skin pigmentation associated with minocycline therapy. *British Journal of Dermatology* 121: 247–257.

Pearson MG, Littlewoods SM, Bowden AN 1981 Tetracycline and benign intracranial hypertension. *British Medical Journal* 282: 568–569.

Poliak SC, D'Giovanna JJ, Gross EG et al 1985 Minocycline-associated tooth discoloration in young adults. *Journal of the American Medical Association* 254: 2930–2932.

Ridgway HA, Sonnex TS, Kennedy CT et al 1982 Hyperpigmentation associated with oral minocycline. *British Journal of Dermatology* 107: 95–102.

Saivin S, Houin G 1988 Clinical pharmacokinetics of doxycycline and minocycline. *Clinical Pharmacokinetics* 15: 355–366.

Simon C 1981 Penetration of various antibiotics into sputum. In: Van Furth R (ed.) *Developments in antibiotic treatment of respiratory infections*. Martinus Njhoff, The Hague, p 86–97.

Tsukamura M 1980 In vitro antimycobacterial activity of minocycline. *Tubercule* 61: 37–38.

Wilkinson SP, Stewart WK, Spiers EM, Pears J 1989 Protracted systemic illness and interstitial nephritis due to minocycline. *Postgraduate Medical Journal* 65: 53–56.

OXYTETRACYCLINE

5-Hydroxytetracycline. Molecular weight (free base): 460.4; (dihydrate): 496.5.

A fermentation product of certain strains of *Streptomyces rimosus*, supplied as the dihydrate or hydrochloride for oral or parenteral administration.

Antimicrobial activity

Its spectrum and activity are typical of the group (Table 33.3; p. 397). It is slightly less active than other tetracyclines against most common pathogenic bacteria.

Pharmacokinetics

Oral absorption	c. 60%
C_{max} 500 mg oral	3–4 mg/l after 2–4 h
Plasma half-life	c. 9 h
Volume of distribution	c. 1.8 l/kg
Plasma protein binding	20–35%

Oxytetracycline is moderately well absorbed from the upper gastrointestinal tract. Food decreases plasma levels by approximately 50%. Although widely distributed in the tissues, it achieves lower concentrations than related agents such as minocycline. Sputum concentrations of 1 mg/l have been recorded on a daily dosage of 2 g. Approximately 60% is excreted in the urine and the half-life is prolonged in renal insufficiency.

Toxicity and side effects

Gastrointestinal intolerance is responsible for most side effects, and tends to be more severe than with other tetracyclines. Esophageal irritation may result from the local effects of the swallowed drug. Potentially serious adverse reactions have included neuromuscular paralysis following intravenous administration to patients with myasthenia gravis. Thrombocytopenic purpura and lupus erythematosus syndrome have been reported, although a direct role for the drug in the latter remains uncertain. Apart from the effect on nitrogen balance common to many tetracyclines, a metabolic effect on glucose homeostasis has been noted in type 1 diabetes mellitus. Allergic contact sensitivity reactions have also been reported.

Clinical use

Its uses are those common to the group (Table 33.2; p. 396). It offers no unique therapeutic advantages, although it is one of the cheaper preparations.

Preparations and dosage

Proprietary name: Terramycin.

Preparations: Tablets, capsules.

Dosage: Adults, oral, 250–500 mg every 6 h; acne, 250 mg–1 g per day as a single or two divided doses.

Widely available.

Further information

Anonymous 1999 Oxytetracycline (dihydrate). In: Dollery C (ed.) Therapeutic Drugs 2nd edn. Churchill Livingstone, Edinburgh, pp. O55–O58.

Snaveley SR, Hodges GR 1984 The neurotoxicity of antibacterial agents. *Annals of Internal Medicine* 101: 92–104.

Wright AL, Colver GB 1988 Tetracyclines – how safe are they? *Clinical and Experimental Dermatology* 13: 57–61.

ROLITETRACYCLINE

2-N-pyrrolidinomethyl-tetracycline. Molecular weight (free base): 564.

A semisynthetic derivative of tetracycline supplied as the nitrate sesquihydrate for parenteral use.

Antimicrobial activity

Activity and spectrum are typical of the group (p. 393).

Pharmacokinetics

Rolitetracycline is not absorbed from the gastrointestinal tract. It is highly soluble and therefore can be administered parenterally. Peak plasma concentration of 4–6 mg/l occur at 0.5–1 h after 350 mg intravenously. The plasma elimination half-life is 5–8 h. About 50% of the dose is excreted in the urine producing high concentrations.

Toxicity and side effects

Intravenous administration is occasionally accompanied by abnormal taste, shivering and rigors, hot flushes, facial reddening, dizziness and, rarely, circulatory collapse. Symptoms of myasthenia gravis have occasionally been exacerbated.

Clinical use

Uses are those common to the group (Table 33.2; p. 396).

Preparations and dosage

Proprietary name: Reverin.

Preparation: Injection.

Dosage: Adults, i.m., 350 mg per day, i.v., 275 mg per day. In severe infections, 275 mg up to three times daily.

Limited availability in continental Europe.

TETRACYCLINE

Molecular weight (free base): 444.4; (hydrochloride): 480.9.

A fermentation product of *Streptomyces aureofaciens*, also produced from chlortetracycline. Available as the hydrochloride for oral and topical use.

Antimicrobial activity

Its activity against common pathogenic bacteria is shown in Table 33.3 (p. 397). It is also active against *V. cholerae*, chlamydiae, rickettsiae and spirochaetes.

Pharmacokinetics

Oral absorption	*c.* 75%
C_{max} 500 mg oral	2–4 mg/l
Plasma half-life	8.5 h
Volume of distribution	*c.* 1.3 l/kg
Plasma protein binding	*c.* 50–60%

Absorption

When taken with food, absorption is reduced by approximately 50%. Steady-state plasma concentrations of 4–5 mg/l occur after oral doses of 500 mg, 6-hourly. Women appear to produce higher concentrations than men. Divalent and trivalent cations such as calcium and aluminum present in antacids and milk interfere with absorption through chelation, as does ferrous sulfate. H_2-receptor antagonists, by raising gastric pH, also interfere with absorption through impaired drug dissolution. Despite the effect of gastric pH, oral absorption is not affected in elderly patients with achlorhydria.

Distribution

Tetracycline is widely distributed in the body tissues. In particular, it penetrates well into the prostate, uterus, ovary and bladder, and also appears to be preferentially taken up by the gastrointestinal tract. It is also detectable within reticuloendothelial cells of the liver, spleen and bone marrow.

Protein binding is reduced in states of malnutrition. It is also bound to bone, dentine and tooth enamel of unerupted teeth. Sputum concentrations of 0.4–2.6 mg/l have been detected after 250 mg oral dosage, three times daily. Maxillary sinus secretions and bronchial mucosal tissue have concentrations comparable to those of serum.

Following 500 mg intravenously, concentrations up to 7 mg/l have been found in the aqueous humor. CSF penetration is poor, but increases with meningeal inflammation. It crosses the placenta readily to enter the fetal circulation, where it achieves 25–75% of the maternal plasma concentration. It is also present in breast milk.

Metabolism

A small amount is metabolized to 4-epitetracycline.

Excretion

Tetracycline is largely eliminated unchanged by glomerular filtration, with more than 50% excreted within 24 h after oral administration. This rises to approximately 70% following parenteral administration. Urinary concentrations of 300 mg/l occur within the first 2 h and persist for up to 12 h. Urinary excretion is enhanced in alkaline urine. Renal clearance is reduced in severe protein calorie malnutrition, possibly through reduced glomerular filtration. It accumulates in the presence of renal failure and is only slowly removed by hemodialysis and minimally by peritoneal dialysis.

The bile is an important route of excretion, accounting for about one-third of the dose. Biliary concentrations may be 10–25 times those found in serum. Impaired hepatic function or biliary obstruction lead to an increase in blood levels.

Toxicity and side effects

The gastrointestinal side effects common to the group (p. 395) are the most frequent cause of intolerance. Metallic taste and glossitis are less burdensome than diarrhea. Antibiotic-associated enterocolitis caused by *Clostridium difficile* toxin and staphylococcal enterocolitis have been reported. Steatorrhea and acute pancreatitis have been described. Irritation and ulceration of the esophagus has occurred with local impaction of the drug. *C. albicans* overgrowth is common and may result in symptomatic oral or vaginal candidiasis and occasionally candida diarrhea.

Hypersensitivity reactions include contact dermatitis, urticaria, facial edema and asthma. Anaphylaxis is rare. A lupus syndrome has been reported, but its cause is uncertain. Photosensitivity can be severe and cause vesiculation, desquamation and onycholysis. The Jarisch–Herxheimer reaction has been observed in the treatment of syphilis, louse-borne relapsing fever, leptospirosis, brucellosis and tularemia. Tetracycline deposition in deciduous teeth and bone (where it may temporarily inhibit growth) is of continuing concern. Between 3 and 44% of administered tetracycline is incorporated in the inorganic phase of bone, which may become visibly discolored and fluoresce. Concentrations as high as 290 mg/g have been recorded in bone in those on long-term tetracycline treatment for acne.

Existing renal insufficiency may be aggravated and is probably related to the antianabolic effect of this class of drugs; interference with protein synthesis places an additional burden on the kidney from amino acid metabolism. Acute renal failure may occur and can be aggravated by drug-induced diarrhea. Dehydration and salt loss from diuretic therapy may aggravate nephrotoxicity. Methoxyflurane and tetracycline in combination may be synergistically nephrotoxic.

An uncommon but serious adverse reaction is acute fatty liver, which may be complicated by renal insufficiency and electrolyte abnormalities. This is most likely to occur with high-dose intravenous administration, especially during pregnancy.

Hematological toxicity is uncommon. Leukopenia, thrombocytopenia and hemolytic anemia have been reported. Altered coagulation may also occur with high intravenous dosage. Phagocyte function may be impaired as a result of the increased excretion of vitamin C.

Neurological toxicity is uncommon but includes benign intracranial hypertension (p. 396). A transient myopathy has complicated long-term oral use for the treatment of acne, while intravenous administration has caused increased muscle weakness in those with myasthenia gravis and has also potentiated curare-induced neuromuscular blockade.

Metabolic effects include precipitation of lactic acidosis in diabetic patients receiving phenformin, a reduction in vitamins B_{12}, B_6 and pantothenic acid with long-term therapy, interference with laboratory tests of urinary catecholamines and urinary tests for glucose (Clinitest and Benedict's) and elevation of serum lithium concentrations. In addition, warfarin is potentiated and failures of oral contraceptives occur, justifying advice concerning the simultaneous use of a barrier contraceptive method in women of childbearing potential.

Clinical use

Uses are those listed in Table 33.2; p. 396. Along with doxycycline it is one of the most commonly used tetracyclines.

Preparations and dosage

Proprietary names: Achromycin, Sustamycin, Tetrabid-Organon, Tetrachel, Deteclo (in combination with chlortetracycline and demeclocycline), Mysteclin (in combination with nystatin).

Preparations: Tablets, capsules, i.v. infusion.

Dosage: Adults, oral, 250–500 mg every 6–8 h, depending on severity of infection; acne, 500 mg–1 g per day as a single or two divided doses; i.v. infusion, 500 mg every 12 h with a maximum of 2 g per day.

Widely available.

Further information

Anonymous 1999 Tetracycline (hydrochloride). In: Dollery C (ed.) *Therapeutic Drugs* 2nd edn. Churchill Livingstone, Edinburgh, pp. T66–T69.

Boer de WA, Driessen WM, Potters VP, Tytgat GN 1994 Randomized study comparing 1 with 2 weeks of quadruple therapy for eradicating *Helicobacter pylori*. *American Journal of Gastroenterology* 89: 1993–1997.

Enderlin G, Morales L, Jacobs RF, Cross JT 1994 Streptomycin and alternative agents for the treatment of tularemia: review of the literature. *Clinical Infectious Diseases* 19: 42–47.

Feurle GE, Marth T 1994 An evaluation of antimicrobial treatment for Whipple's disease. Tetracycline versus trimethoprim-sulfamethoxazole. *Digestive Diseases and Sciences* 39: 1642–1648.

Islam MR 1987 Single dose tetracycline in cholera. *Gut* 28: 1029–1032.

Labenz J, Ruhl GH, Bertrams J, Borsch G 1994 Effective treatment after failure of omeprazole plus amoxycillin to eradicate *Helicobacter pylori* infection in peptic ulcer disease. *Alimentary Pharmacology and Therapeutics* 8: 323–327.

Looareesuwan S, Vanijanota S, Viravan C et al 1994 Randomised trial of mefloquine-tetracycline and quinine-tetracycline for acute uncomplicated falciparum malaria. *Acta Tropica* 57: 47–53.

Murphy AA, Zacur HA, Charache P, Burkman RT 1991 The effect of tetracycline on levels of oral contraceptives. *American Journal of Obstetrics and Gynecology* 164: 28–33.

Nicolau DP, Mengedoht DE, Kline JJ 1991 Tetracycline-induced pancreatitis. *American Journal of Gastroenterology* 86: 1669–1671.

Oklund SA, Prolo DJ, Gutierrez RV 1981 The significance of yellow bone. Evidence for tetracycline in adult human bone. *Journal of the American Medical Association* 246: 761–763.

Pierog SH, Al-Salimi FL, Cinotti D 1986 Pseudotumor cerebri – a complication of tetracycline treatment of acne. *Journal of Adolescent Health Care* 7: 139–140.

Sinclair D, Phillips C 1982 Transient myopathy apparently due to tetracycline. *New England Journal of Medicine* 307: 821–822.

TIGECYCLINE

GAR-936; 9-t-butylglycylamido-minocycline. An investigational compound of the glycylcycline class.

Activity against common bacterial pathogens is shown in Table 33.3 (p. 397). It is as potent as, or more potent than, earlier tetracyclines and activity is retained against strains containing *tet* determinants (p. 394). The spectrum includes rapidly growing mycobacteria. *Ps. aeruginosa*, *Pr. mirabilis*, other *Proteus* spp. and some strains of *Corynebacterium jeikeium* are resistant.

Further information

Boucher HW, Wennersten CB, Eliopoulos GM 2000 In vitro activities of the glycylcycline GAR-936 against gram-positive bacteria. *Antimicrobial Agents and Chemotherapy* 44: 2225–2229.

Chopra I 2001 Glycylcyclines: third-generation tetracycline antibiotics. *Current Opinion in Pharmacology* 1: 464–469.

Gales AC, Jones RN 2000 Antimicrobial activity and spectrum of the new glycylcycline, GAR-936 tested against 1,203 recent clinical bacterial isolates. *Diagnostic Microbiology and Infectious Disease* 36: 19–36.

Johnson AP 2000 GAR-936. *Current Opinion in Anti-Infective Investigational Drugs* 2: 164–170.

Petersen PJ, Jacobus NV, Weiss WJ, Sum PE, Testa RT 1999 In vitro and in vivo antibacterial activities of a novel glycylcycline, the 9-*t*-butylglycylamido derivative of minocycline (GAR-936). *Antimicrobial Agents and Chemotherapy* 43: 738–744.

Sum P-E, Lee VJ, Testa RT, Hlavka JJ et al 1994 Glycylcyclines. 1. A new generation of potent antibacterial agents through modification of 9-aminotetracyclines. *Journal of Medicinal Chemistry* 37: 184–188.

Sum PE, Petersen P 1999 Synthesis and structure-activity relationship of novel glycylcycline derivatives leading to the discovery of GAR-936. *Bioorganic Medicinal Chemistry Letters* 9: 1459–1462.

34 Miscellaneous antibacterial agents

D. Greenwood

This chapter is concerned with various antimicrobial compounds that are structurally different from the major antimicrobial drug families and from each other. Most are of historical interest only and are not widely used in human medicine, except, in some cases, as topical agents.

PEPTIDE ANTIBIOTICS

Peptides of various kinds were among the earliest antibiotics isolated from natural sources. The recovery of tyrothricin from *Bacillus brevis* was reported in 1939 and its separation into gramicidin (a linear peptide) and tyrocidine (a cyclic peptide) in 1940. Gramicidin S (Soviet), which is also produced by a strain of *B. brevis*, is a cyclic peptide similar to tyrocidine. It was developed in the former Soviet Union and is not generally available.

Another cyclic peptide, bacitracin, was isolated from *Bacillus licheniformis* in 1945 and named after Margaret Tracy, the young girl from whom the organism was isolated. Polymyxin B, which was discovered almost simultaneously in the USA as a product of *Bacillus polymyxa* and in the UK as a product of *Bacillus aerosporus* followed in 1947. The disruptive activity of these peptides on cell membranes, to which they owe their mammalian toxicity, has limited their therapeutic use largely to topical application, but the polymyxins, notably as colistimethate sodium (colistin sulfomethate), are still occasionally used systemically against otherwise resistant organisms.

Antibacterial oligopeptides are virtually ubiquitous throughout the natural world and are thought to play a part in native defences against infection. Such peptides include, among many others, the cecropins (originally described in insects, but now known to be more widely distributed), magainins (from the skin of the toad *Xenopus laevis*), lantibiotics (lanthionine-containing peptides, like nisin, from bacteria) and the defensins (from mammalian phagocytes). Many of these compounds interfere with membrane integrity and exhibit differential activity against various species. Some of them, and related synthetic oligopeptides, are under investigation as possible therapeutic agents.

 Further information

Boman HG, Marsh J, Goode JA (eds) 1994 *Antimicrobial peptides* (Ciba Foundation Symposium 186). John Wiley, Chichester.
Evans ME, Feola DJ, Rapp RP 1999 Polymyxin B sulfate and colistin: old antibiotics for emerging gram-negative bacteria. *Annals of Pharmacotherapy* 33: 960–967.

 BACITRACIN

Molecular weight (bacitracin A): 1411.

A mixture of peptides produced by *Bacillus licheniformis*. Bacitracin A is the major constituent of commercial preparations. The more stable zinc salt is used in topical formulations. It has been widely used as a growth promoter in animals, but has been banned for that purpose in the European Union.

Antimicrobial activity

Bacitracin is highly active against many Gram-positive bacteria. Although strains of *Staphylococcus aureus* are usually susceptible, they are rather less so than most other Gram-positive bacteria. *Streptococcus pyogenes* is so much more susceptible than other hemolytic streptococci that bacitracin susceptibility is used as a screening test for identification. *Clostridium difficile* and *Actinomyces* spp. are susceptible, but *Nocardia* spp. are resistant. Among susceptible Gram-negative organisms are *Haemophilus influenzae*, *Neisseria* spp. and fusobacteria but enterobacteria and *Pseudomonas* spp. are resistant. *Entamoeba histolytica* is inhibited by 0.6–10 mg/l.

Acquired resistance

Resistance is uncommon, but has been detected in *Staph. aureus* following topical treatment.

Pharmacokinetics

Bacitracin is not absorbed by mouth. Absorption may occur from application to ulcerated areas.

Toxicity and side effects

Bacitracin is nephrotoxic when given parenterally and depression of renal function may persist for weeks. Although some absorption may occur, local applications do not appear to produce systemic toxicity, but occasional anaphylaxis has been described.

Clinical use

- Component of preparations for local application.
- Suppression of gut flora, including *Clostridium difficile* (oral).

 Preparations

Ointment and ophthalmic ointments.

Various preparations with polymyxin, neomycin and corticosteroids.

Widely available.

 Further information

Andrews BJ, Bjorvatn B 1994 Chemotherapy of *Entamoeba histolytica*: studies in vitro with bacitracin and its zinc salt. *Transactions of the Royal Society of Tropical Medicine and Hygiene* 88: 98–100.

Dudley MN, McLaughlin JC, Carrington G et al 1986 Oral bacitracin vs vancomycin therapy for *Clostridium difficile*-induced diarrhea. A randomized double-blind trial. *Archives of Internal Medicine* 146: 1101–1104.

Eedy DJ, McMillan JC, Bingham EA 1990 Anaphylactic reactions to topical antibiotic combinations. *Postgraduate Medical Journal* 66: 858–859.

Prescott JF, Baggot JD, Walker RD 2000 *Antimicrobial therapy in veterinary medicine* 3rd ed. Iowa State University Press, Ames.

Sprung J, Schedewie HK, Kampine JP 1990 Intraoperative anaphylactic shock after bacitracin irrigation. *Anesthesia and Analgesia* 71: 430–433.

 DAPTOMYCIN

A semisynthetic lipopeptide derived from a fermentation product of *Streptomyces roseosporus*.

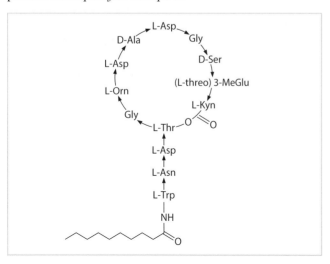

Daptomycin is a cyclic peptide with a lipophilic tail and thus resembles the polymyxins structurally. Its useful activity is restricted to Gram-positive cocci, and its chief attraction is that it retains activity against multiresistant strains. Its activity in vitro is greatly potentiated by the presence of calcium (but not magnesium) ions and in these conditions it is more potently bactericidal than the glycopeptides. Oral absorption is poor and it is administered intravenously. It is extensively protein bound (90–95%) and is eliminated by the kidneys with a half-life of around 8 h, rising to 30 h in patients with severe renal impairment. Various adverse reactions have been reported, including muscle toxicity, which may be irreversible at higher doses. Early development was halted because of side effects, but anxieties over antibiotic resistance in Gram-positive cocci have led to renewed clinical trials.

 Preparations and dosage

Preparation: Injection.

Dosage: Adults, i.v., 2–6 mg/kg once daily.

Very limited availability.

 Further information

Benson CA, Beaudette F, Trenholm G 1987 Comparative in vitro activity of LY 146032, a new peptolide with vancomycin and eight other agents against Gram-positive organisms. *Journal of Antimicrobial Chemotherapy* 20: 191–196.

de la Maza L, Ruoff KL, Ferraro MJ 1989 In vitro activity of daptomycin and other antimicrobial agents against vancomycin-resistant Gram-positive bacteria. *Antimicrobial Agents and Chemotherapy* 33: 1383–1384.

Snydman DR, Jacobus NV, McDermott LA, Lonks JR, Boyce JM 2000 Comparative activities of daptomycin and vancomycin against resistant gram-positive pathogens. *Antimicrobial Agents and Chemotherapy* 44: 3447–3450.

Tally FP, DeBruin MF 2000 Development of daptomycin for gram-positive infections. *Journal of Antimicrobial Chemotherapy* 46: 523–526.

 GRAMICIDIN

Molecular weight: gramicidin A 1883.3.

Gramicidin as used in topical formulations is a mixture of several closely related compounds, of which about 80% is in the form of gramicidin A. It is part of the tyrothricin complex originally isolated from *B. brevis* by Dubos.

Although gramicidin is a linear peptide antibiotic, it can adopt an open helical configuration, allowing it to act as a channel-forming molecule in cell membranes. It is active against most species of Gram-positive bacteria, including mycobacteria. Synergic activity with amphotericin B has been demonstrated against *Candida* spp. Gram-negative bacilli are completely insensitive, probably due to the presence of surface phospholipids that inhibit the activity. Gramicidin exhibits some activity against viruses, including HIV.

By intravenous injection, gramicidin is highly toxic to erythrocytes, liver and kidney, and it is not used therapeutically except for its inclusion in mixtures for local application. It has been used in the former Soviet Union as a spermicide.

Preparations

Topical applications with neomycin and other mixtures.
Widely available.

Further information

Bourinbaiar AS, Krasinski K, Borkowsky W 1994 Anti-HIV effect of gramicidin in vitro: potential for spermicide use. *Life Sciences* 54: PL5–9.

Bourinbaiar AS, Lee-Huang S 1994 Comparative in vitro study of contraceptive agents with anti-HIV activity: gramicidin, nonoxynol-9, and gossypol. *Contraception* 49: 131–137.

Franklin TJ, Snow GA 1998 *Biochemistry and Molecular Biology of Antimicrobial Drug Action.* Kluwer Academic Publishers, Dordrecht, pp. 46–55.

Pascal SM, Cross TA 1992 Structure of an isolated gramicidin A double helical species by high-resolution nuclear magnetic resonance. *Journal of Molecular Biology* 226: 1101–1109.

POLYMYXINS

Polymyxin B and colistin (polymyxin E); mixtures of sulfates of polypeptides produced by strains of *B. polymyxa* and *B. polymyxa* var *colistinus*. Colistimethate sodium (colistin sulfomethate sodium). Molecular weights: Polymyxin B_1 1203; polymyxin B_2 1189; colistimethate sodium 1748.

L-Leu → L-DAB

D-Leu ← L-DAB

L-DAB ← L-Thr

L-DAB

L-DAB

L-Thr

L-DAB—6—Me—octanoyl

DAB= diaminobutyric acid

A group of basic polypeptide antibiotics with a side chain terminated by characteristic fatty acids. Five polymyxins (A, B, C, D and E) were originally isolated and characterized and others have since been added. Polymyxin B and colistin (polymyxin E) sulfates have been commercially developed.

By treatment with formalin and sodium bisulfite, five of the six diaminobutyric acid groups of the polymyxins can be replaced by sulfomethyl groups to form undefined mixtures of the mono-, di-, tri-, tetra- and penta-substituted derivatives. Sulfomethyl polymyxins differ considerably in their properties

from the parent antibiotics: they are less active antibacterially, relatively painless on injection, more rapidly excreted by the kidney and less toxic. Only colistimethate sodium is now commercially available for systemic use, but polymyxin B and colistin sulfates are found as ingredients of several topical formulations.

Polymyxins bind specifically to the lipid A region of lipopolysaccharide with neutralization of its biological effects, notably endotoxin shock. In attempts to separate this desirable therapeutic property from the toxicity of the molecule, the lipid tail has been removed to leave the corresponding nonapeptide, which is 2–64 times less inhibitory than the parent compound, depending on the bacterial species, and about 100 times less toxic to cells in tissue culture. It is not available commercially.

Antimicrobial activity

All the polymyxins have a similar antibacterial spectrum, although there are slight quantitative differences in their activity in vitro (Table 34.1). They are inactive against Grampositive organisms, but nearly all enterobacteria, except *Proteus* spp., *Burkholderia cepacia* and *Serratia marcescens*, are highly susceptible, as are *H. influenzae*, *Bordetella pertussis* and *Pseudomonas aeruginosa*. *Bacteroides fragilis* is resistant, but other *Bacteroides* spp. and fusobacteria are susceptible. Resistance of *Vibrio cholerae* eltor to polymyxin B distinguishes it from the classical vibrio.

The sulfomethyl derivatives are generally 4–8 times less active than the sulfates, but their activity is difficult to measure precisely since on incubation they spontaneously decay to the parent compound, with a corresponding progressive increase in the antibacterial activity.

Through the disruptive effect on the cell membrane, polymyxins can admit hydrophilic compounds, including sulfonamides and trimethoprim, to the cell, producing significant synergy. Synergy with ciprofloxacin is also described. Calcium ions exert a strong pH-dependent competition for membrane

Table 34.1 Activity of polymyxins against common pathogenic bacteria: MIC (mg/l)

	Colistin sulfate	Colistimethate sodium	Polymyxin B sulfate
Staph. aureus	64–R	R	64–R
Str. pyogenes	32	32	16–R
E. faecalis	R	R	R
H. influenzae	0.5–1	No data	0.03
Neisseria spp.	R	R	R
Esch. coli	0.01–32	0.05–R	0.03
K. pneumoniae	0.01–1	0.01–4	0.03–0.5
Proteus spp.	R	R	R
Ps. aeruginosa	0.03–4	2–32	0.03–4
B. fragilis	R	R	R

R, resistant (MIC >64 mg/l).

binding sites, and the presence of calcium and magnesium ions in certain media adversely affects the bactericidal activity, notably against *Ps. aeruginosa*.

Acquired resistance

There is complete cross-resistance between the polymyxins, but stable acquired resistance in normally susceptible species is very rare. Adaptive resistance, probably due to changes in cell wall permeability, is readily achieved by passage of a variety of enterobacteria in the presence of the agents in vitro.

Pharmacokinetics

Oral absorption	Negligible
C_{max} (colistimethate sodium) 2 mega-units (c. 160 mg colistin base) i.m.	6–7 mg/l after 2–3 h
Plasma half-life (colistimethate sodium)	c. 4–6 h
Plasma protein binding	Very low

Absorption
Polymyxins are not absorbed from the alimentary tract or mucosal surfaces, but can be absorbed from denuded areas or large burns.

Distribution
After parenteral administration of the sulfates, blood levels are usually low (1–4 mg/l 2 h after a 500 000 unit intramuscular dose). Substantially higher plasma levels are obtained from intramuscular injections of sulfomethyl polymyxins. There is some accumulation in patients receiving 120 mg 8-hourly. In patients treated intravenously with a priming dose of 1.5–2.5 mg/kg followed by continuous infusion of 4.8–6.0 mg/h for 20–30 h, steady state levels were around 5–10 mg/l.

The volume of distribution is unknown, but polymyxins diffuse poorly into tissue fluids and penetration to cerebrospinal fluid is poor. As a result of binding to mammalian cell membranes (sulfomethates less so), they persist in the tissues, where they accumulate on repeated dosage, although they disappear from the serum. Polymyxin crosses the placenta, but the levels achieved are low. A small amount appears in the breast milk.

Metabolism and excretion
The sulfates are excreted almost entirely by the kidney, but after a considerable lag, with very little of the dose appearing in the first 12 h. The sulfomethyl derivatives are much more rapidly excreted, accounting for their shorter half-lives. Around 80% of a parenteral dose of colistimethate sodium is eventually found in the urine, with concentrations reaching around 100–300 mg/l at 2 h. The fate of the remainder is unknown, but no metabolic products have been described and none is excreted in the bile. Polymyxins accumulate in renal failure and are not removed by peritoneal dialysis.

Toxicity and side effects

Pain and tissue injury can occur at the site of injection of the sulfates, but this is less of a problem with the sulfomethyl derivatives. Neurological symptoms such as paresthesia with typical numbness and tingling around the mouth, dizziness and weakness are relatively common, and neuromuscular blockade, sometimes severe enough to impede respiration, occurs. Evidence of nephrotoxicity is observed in about 20% of patients, leading to acute tubular necrosis in about 2%. Damage is more likely in patients with pre-existing renal disease. The appearance of any evidence of deterioration of renal function or of neuromuscular blockade calls for immediate cessation of treatment. All the toxic manifestations appear to be reversible, but complete recovery may be slow.

Although less toxic than the sulfate, untoward effects have been observed in up to a quarter of those treated with colistimethate sodium. Evidence of nephrotoxicity is the most common (increase in urea and creatinine is almost invariable over the first few days of treatment) and potentially most serious, with acute tubular necrosis being heralded by the appearance of proteinuria, hematuria and casts, sometimes without prior evidence of functional impairment. Renal damage usually continues to progress for up to 2 weeks after withdrawal of therapy. Renal damage is likely to increase with the dose and with the simultaneous administration of other potentially nephrotoxic agents.

Manifestations of central and peripheral neurotoxicity occur particularly in patients with impaired renal function. Neuromuscular blockade is seen principally in patients also receiving anesthetics or other agents that impair neuromuscular transmission. Complete flaccid paralysis with respiratory arrest and subsequent complete recovery has been seen in a patient with myasthenia gravis. Allergy is occasionally seen, and nebulized colistin has caused bronchial hyperreactivity with tightness in the chest in adults with cystic fibrosis. Application of colistin or polymyxin B ear drops can lead to ototoxicity.

Clinical use

Colistimethate sodium
- Infections due to *Ps. aeruginosa* and other Gram-negative rods resistant to less toxic agents.
- Cystic fibrosis (inhalation therapy for pseudomonas infection).

Polymyxin B and colistin sulfate
- Component of preparations for local application.
- Superficial infections with *Ps. aeruginosa* and to prevent the colonization of burns.
- Selective decontamination of the gut (p. 569) and as a paste for control of upper respiratory tract colonization in patients on prolonged mechanical ventilation (in combination with other agents).

Preparations and dosage

Proprietary name: Aerosporin.

Preparations: Injection, ear and eye drops and ointment. Also in multi-ingredient topical preparations.

Dosage: Adults, i.v., 1.5–2.5 mg/kg per day.

Topical preparations widely available.

Proprietary name: Colomycin.

Preparations: Injection, tablets, syrup, multi-ingredient topical applications.

Dosage: Adults, oral, 1.5–3 million units every 8 h. Children, oral, 15–30 kg, 750 000 units–1.5 million units every 8 h; < 15 kg, 250 000–500 000 units every 8 h. Adults i.m., i.v., 2 million units every 8 h. Children, i.m., i.v., <60 kg, 50 000 units/kg/day in three divided doses; inhalation of nebulized solution, patients > 40 kg, 1 million units every 12 h, <40 kg, 500 000 units every 12 h.

Widely available.

 Further information

Anonymous 1999 Colistin (sulfate) and colistimethate (sodium). In: Dollery C (ed.). *Therapeutic Drugs* 2nd edn. Churchill Livingstone, Edinburgh, pp. C326–C329.

Anonymous 1999 Polymyxin B (sulfate). In: Dollery C (ed.). *Therapeutic Drugs* 2nd edn. Churchill Livingstone, Edinburgh, pp. P162–P164.

Duwe AK, Rupar CA, Horsman GB, Vas SI 1986 In vitro cytotoxicity and antibiotic activity of polymyxin B nonapeptide. *Antimicrobial Agents and Chemotherapy* 30: 340–341.

Evans ME, Feola DJ, Rapp RP 1999 Polymyxin B sulfate and colistin: old antibiotics for emerging gram-negative bacteria. *Annals of Pharmacotherapy* 33: 960–967.

Hartenauer U, Thülig B, Diemer W et al 1991 Effect of selective flora suppression on colonization, infection and mortality in critically ill patients: a one-year prospective consecutive study. *Critical Care Medicine* 19: 463–473.

Littlewood JM, Koch C, Lambert PA et al 2000 A ten year review of colomycin. *Respiratory Medicine* 94: 632–640.

Maddison J, Dodd M, Webb AK 1994 Nebulised colistin causes chest tightness in adults with cystic fibrosis. *Respiratory Medicine* 88: 145–147.

Rogers MJ, Cohen J 1986 Comparison of the binding of Gram-negative bacterial endotoxin by polymyxin B sulphate, colistin sulphate and colistin sulphomethate sodium. *Infection* 14: 79–81.

Warren HS, Kania SA, Siber GR 1985 Binding and neutralization of bacterial lipopolysaccharide by colistin nonapeptide. *Antimicrobial Agents and Chemotherapy* 28: 107–112.

Webb AK, Dodd ME 1997 Nebulized antibiotics for adults with cystic fibrosis. *Thorax* 52 (Suppl. 2): 69–71.

COUMARINS

This is a small group of naturally occurring antibiotics chemically related to the coumarin group of anticoagulants. The best known is novobiocin, but a few naturally occurring coumarins and some semisynthetic derivatives have been studied. They share a narrow range of antimicrobial activity largely directed against aerobic Gram-positive organisms. There has been some revived interest in coumarins as potentiating agents of antineoplastic drugs and as alternative agents for the treatment of infection with multiresistant Gram-positive cocci.

 Further information

Rappa G, Shyam K, Lorico A, Fodstad O, Sartorelli AC 2000 Structure-activity studies of novobiocin analogs as modulators of the cytotoxicity of etoposide (VP-16). *Oncology Research* 12: 113–119.

 NOVOBIOCIN

Cathomycin; streptonivicin. Molecular weight 612.6.

A fermentation product of *Streptomyces spheroides* and *Streptomyces niveus*, usually supplied as the calcium or the much more soluble monosodium salt.

Antimicrobial activity

The activity against common pathogenic bacteria is shown in Table 34.2. Novobiocin is active against β-lactamase-producing and methicillin-resistant strains of *Staph. aureus*. *Staph. saprophyticus* is resistant, and this property has been used to distinguish it from other coagulase-negative staphylococci, although the specificity of this has been questioned. Most enterobacteria are resistant, but some strains of *Pasteurella*, *Citrobacter* and *Proteus*, particularly *Proteus vulgaris*, are susceptible to moderate concentrations. *Corynebacterium diphtheriae* and *Listeria* spp. are susceptible.

Table 34.2 Activity of novobiocin against common pathogenic bacteria

	MIC (mg/l)
Staph. aureus	0.1–2
Str. pyogenes	0.5–4
Str. pneumoniae	0.2–2
E. faecalis	1–16
H. influenzae	0.5–1
N. meningitidis	0.5–4
N. gonorrhoeae	4
Esch. coli	R
K. pneumoniae	R
Ps. aeruginosa	R

R, resistant (MIC >64 mg/l).

Activity against *Staph. aureus* is bactericidal at, or close to, the minimum inhibitory concentration (MIC). The MIC is at least eight times higher at pH 8.0 than at pH 5.4, and is markedly increased by the presence of 10% or more serum, or by increase in the magnesium or nutrient content of the medium. Tetracyclines may enhance its effect by chelating magnesium ions, and this may be the basis of the bactericidal synergy claimed between them.

Novobiocin is a potent inhibitor of DNA gyrase and eliminates plasmids at concentrations 2–8-fold below the MIC. Cytokine-suppressing properties have been described in vitro.

Acquired resistance

Increase in the resistance of staphylococci may occur in vitro or during treatment. There is no cross-resistance with other common antibiotics.

Pharmacokinetics

Oral absorption	Good
C_{max} 250 mg oral	c. 11 mg/l after 1–4 h
Plasma half-life	1.7–4 h
Plasma protein binding	c. 90%

After repeated doses, serum levels of 50 to over 100 mg/l may be reached. Concentrations rather lower than those in the blood are found in serous effusions, but cerebrospinal fluid contains little or none. Less than 3% of the dose appears in the urine. It is excreted mainly in the bile, in which the concentration is high. There is extensive biliary recirculation and high concentrations are found in the feces.

Toxicity and side-effects

Nausea, abdominal pain and diarrhea are fairly common. Maculopapular, morbilliform or urticarial skin eruptions with or without fever are common, often developing about the ninth day. Stevens–Johnson syndrome and hemorrhagic rashes have been encountered. Rashes usually disappear on stopping the drug, but may promptly reappear on re-administration, together with a prompt and profound fall in circulating basophils indicative of sensitization. Allergic myocarditis and pneumonitis have been described. Novobiocin may displace other substances from protein binding sites and can lower the plasma-bound iodine by displacing thyroxine.

Eosinophilia and moderate transient leukopenia are occasionally seen. Thrombocytopenia, which may be severe, and hemolytic anemia have also been reported.

It gives rise to a yellow metabolite, which may give an indirect positive van den Bergh reaction, but in addition exerts a profound effect on hepatic excretory function by interfering with the uptake of various compounds by hepatic cells, inhibiting glucuronyl transferase and suppressing excretion of conjugates into the bile. Particularly severe effects may occur in the newborn, where glucuronide formation is imperfectly developed. It exerts a different depressant effect on the biliary excretion of different compounds and on the excretion of the same conjugate when this is produced endogenously or infused.

Clinical use

- Staphylococcal infections (especially infection due to methicillin-resistant strains).
- Elimination of methicillin-resistant staphylococci from the noses of carriers (in combination with rifampicin).

There has been considerable interest in the ability of novobiocin to inhibit various malignant cells and to potentiate the effects of anticancer agents.

 Preparations and dosage

Preparation: Capsules.

Dosage: Adults, oral, 250 mg every 6 h or 500 mg every 12 h. Children, oral, 15 mg/kg/day in 2–4 divided doses. Doses can be doubled in severe infections.

Very limited availability, not available in the UK.

 Further information

Ellis GK, Crowley J, Livingston RB, Goodwin JW, Hutchins L, Allen A 1991 Cisplatin and novobiocin in the treatment of non-small cell lung cancer. A Southwest Oncology Group Study. *Cancer* 67: 2969–2973.

French P, Venuti E, Fraimow HS 1993 In vitro activity of novobiocin against multi-resistant strains of *Enterococcus faecium*. *Antimicrobial Agents and Chemotherapy* 37: 2736–2739.

Murren JR, DiStasio SA Lorico A et al 2000 Phase I and pharmacokinetic study of novobiocin in combination with VP-16 in patients with refractory malignancies. *Cancer Journal* 6: 256–265.

Nordenberg J, Albukrek D, Hadar T et al 1992 Novobiocin-induced anti-proliferative and differentiating effects in melanoma. *British Journal of Cancer* 65: 183–188.

Rappa G, Lorico A, Sartorelli AC 1992 Potentiation by novobiocin of the cytotoxic activity of etoposide (VP-16) and teniposide (VM-26). *International Journal of Cancer* 51: 780–787.

Walsh TJ, Auger F, Tatem BA, Hansen SL, Standiford HC 1986 Novobiocin and rifampicin in combination against methicillin-resistant *Staphylococcus aureus*: an in-vitro comparison with vancomycin plus rifampicin. *Journal of Antimicrobial Chemotherapy* 17: 75–82.

 METHENAMINE

Methenamine (hexamine; hexamethylenetetraamine), under the name Urotropin, was successfully used in cystitis by the German physician Nicolaier in 1895. It has no intrinsic antibacterial activity and owes its effect to decomposition in acid conditions to formaldehyde, which is non-specifically microbicidal, and ammonia. It is often used in the form of organic acid salts, methenamine hippurate and methenamine mandelate, which have been claimed (unconvincingly) to keep the urinary pH low. Mandelic acid has some antibacterial activity in its own right and is sometimes given alone as a urinary antiseptic, usually as the calcium or ammonium salt. Infection with urea-splitting organisms such as *Proteus* spp. causes the urine to become alkaline and methenamine is unsuitable for these infections.

Methenamine is absorbed from the gut and mainly excreted unchanged in the urine, achieving concentrations of around 2–60 mg/l, sufficient to inhibit most bacteria and yeasts. Higher concentrations are achieved by the hippurate salt. It is given in enteric-coated tablets to prevent the liberation of formaldehyde by gastric acid. There is little breakdown in the blood and no systemic effect or toxicity.

Some patients complain of gastrointestinal upset or frequent and burning micturition. Attempts to control these side effects with alkali will abolish the antibacterial effect of the drug. Contact dermatitis and anterior uveitis have occasionally been encountered. Prolonged administration or high dosage may produce proteinuria, hematuria and bladder changes. Methenamine should not be given to patients with acidosis, gout or hepatic insufficiency. There have been fears about the potential carcinogenicity of formaldehyde.

Methenamine and its salts are unsuitable for the treatment of acute urinary tract infection. Their main use, now largely supplanted by other agents, has been in the long-term prophylaxis of recurrent cystitis.

Preparations and dosage

Preparation: Tablets.

Dosage: Adults, oral, 1 g 2–3 times daily. Children, oral, 6–12 years, 500 mg twice daily (maximum 2 g daily).

Widely available.

Further information

Dreyfors JM, Jones SB, Sayed Y 1989 Hexamethylenetetramine – a review. *American Industrial Hygiene Association Journal* 50: 579–585.

Gleckman R, Alvarez S, Joubert DW, Matthews SJ 1979 Drug therapy reviews: methenamine mandelate and methenamine hippurate. *American Journal of Hospital Pharmacy* 36: 1509–1512.

35 Antifungal agents

D. W. Warnock

Effective drugs are now available for a wide range of fungal infections, covering most of the major pathogens and providing a choice for many conditions. In the more common superficial infections it is now possible to cure many patients with topical treatment, and the details of administration are often more important than the choice of agent. There is less satisfactory provision for systemic fungal infections, and there are still conditions for which there is no effective treatment.

There are four main families of antifungal agents: the allylamines, the azoles, the echinocandins and the polyenes. In addition, there is a miscellaneous group of drugs that includes flucytosine, griseofulvin, amorolfine and various other agents that are used for topical treatment. New groups of compounds and new ways of using the older agents, such as liposomal formulations, are under constant development and review. Resistance, although not a major problem, has now been recorded with some azole antifungals and with flucytosine, usually in situations where the drugs have been given for long periods of time in the face of persistent infection.

 Further information

Arikan S, Rex JH 2000 New agents for treatment of systemic fungal infections. *Emerging Drugs* 5: 135–160.

Georgopapadakou NH 1998 Antifungals: mechanism of action and resistance, established and novel drugs. *Current Opinion in Microbiology* 1: 547–557.

Groll AH, Piscitelli SC, Walsh TJ 1999 Clinical pharmacology of systemic antifungal agents: a comprehensive review of agents in clinical use, current investigational compounds, and putative targets for antifungal drug development. *Advances in Pharmacology* 44: 343–500.

Pfaller MA, Rex JH, Rinaldi MG 1997 Antifungal susceptibility testing: technical advances and potential clinical applications. *Clinical Infectious Diseases* 24: 776–784.

Summers KK, Hardin TC, Gore SJ et al 1997 Therapeutic drug monitoring of systemic antifungal therapy. *Journal of Antimicrobial Chemotherapy* 40: 753–764.

White TC, Marr KA, Bowden RA 1998 Clinical, cellular and molecular factors that contribute to antifungal drug resistance. *Clinical Microbiology Reviews* 11: 382–402.

ALLYLAMINES

This group of synthetic agents contains compounds that are effective in the topical and oral treatment of dermatophytoses and superficial forms of candidosis. Two drugs, naftifine and terbinafine, have entered clinical use.

 ## NAFTIFINE

The original allylamine, synthesized in Switzerland in 1974. It is used as a 1% cream for the topical treatment of dermatophytoses, including tinea pedis, tinea corporis and tinea cruris.

 Preparation and dosage

Proprietary name: Naftin.

Preparation: Topical.

Dosage: Dosage and duration of treatment vary according to the condition being treated.

Available in a number of countries, including the USA. Not UK.

 Further information

Monk JP, Brogden RN 1991 Naftifine. A review of its antimicrobial activity and therapeutic use in superficial dermatomycoses. *Drugs* 42: 659–672.

TERBINAFINE

Molecular weight (free base): 291.4; (hydrochloride): 327.9.

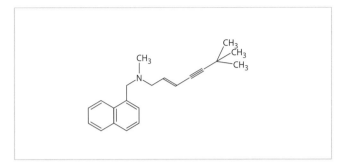

A synthetic allylamine available as the hydrochloride for oral and topical administration.

Antimicrobial activity

Terbinafine is active against a wide range of pathogenic fungi, including dermatophytes (*Epidermophyton*, *Microsporum* and *Trichophyton* spp.), dimorphic fungi (*Blastomyces dermatitidis*, *Histoplasma capsulatum* and *Sporothrix schenckii*), molds (including *Aspergillus* and *Fusarium* spp.), dematiaceous fungi, and some yeasts (including *Candida parapsilosis*).

Acquired resistance

This has not been reported.

Pharmacokinetics

Oral absorption	70–80%
C_{max} 250 mg oral	c. 1 mg/l after 2 h
Plasma half-life	c. 17 h
Volume of distribution	1000 l
Plasma protein binding	>95%

Blood concentrations of the drug increase in proportion to dosage. It is lipophilic and this results in accumulation in adipose tissue. It reaches the stratum corneum as a result of diffusion through the dermis and epidermis, and secretion in sebum. Diffusion from the nail bed is the major factor in its rapid penetration of nails. It is metabolized by the liver and the inactive metabolites are excreted in the urine. The elimination half-life is prolonged in patients with hepatic or renal impairment.

Interactions

Blood concentrations are reduced following concomitant administration with drugs, such as rifampicin, that induce cytochrome P_{450}-mediated metabolism. Conversely, levels are increased if it is given with drugs, such as cimetidine, which inhibit hepatic metabolism. Terbinafine does not affect the clearance of drugs that undergo cytochrome P_{450}-mediated hepatic metabolism, such as cyclosporin.

Toxicity and side effects

These include abdominal discomfort, loss of appetite, nausea, diarrhea, headache, impairment of taste, rash and urticaria. Serious skin reactions, including Stevens–Johnson syndrome, and rare hepatotoxic reactions, including jaundice, cholestasis and hepatitis, are occasionally encountered.

Clinical use

- tinea pedis, tinea corporis and tinea cruris.
- onychomycosis.

 Preparations and dosage

Proprietary name: Lamisil.

Preparations: Tablets, cream.

Dosage: Adults, oral, 250 mg/day for 2–6 weeks in tinea pedis, 2–4 weeks in tinea cruris, 2–4 weeks in tinea corporis, 6–12 weeks or longer in nail infections.

Widely available.

 Further information

Anonymous 1999 Terbinafine (hydrochloride). In: Dollery C (ed.) *Therapeutic Drugs* 2nd edn. Churchill Livingstone, Edinburgh, pp. T41–T45.

Evans EGV, Sigurgeirsson B 1999 Double blind, randomised study of continuous terbinafine compared with intermittent itraconazole in treatment of toenail onychomycosis. *British Medical Journal* 318: 1031–1035.

Faergemann J 1997 Pharmacokinetics of terbinafine. *Review of Contemporary Pharmacotherapy* 8: 289–297.

McClellan KJ, Wiseman LR, Markham A 1999 Terbinafine. An update of its use in superficial mycoses. *Drugs* 58: 179–202.

Ryder NS, Favre B 1997 Antifungal activity and mechanism of action of terbinafine. *Review of Contemporary Pharmacotherapy* 8: 275–287.

AZOLES

This large group of synthetic agents, which includes drugs used in bacterial and parasitic infections (5-nitroimidazoles, Ch. 27; benzimidazoles, Ch. 37), contains many compounds that are effective in the topical treatment of dermatophytoses and superficial forms of candidosis; a number are suitable for systemic administration.

Members of this group have in common an imidazole or triazole ring with *N*-carbon substitution. The activity is essentially fungistatic, but at high concentrations some azoles can exert fungicidal effects.

Interactions

Coadministration of systemic agents (fluconazole, itraconazole and ketoconazole) with cisapride, terfenadine or astemizole can lead to serious cardiac arrhythmias, due to inhibition of the metabolism of these drugs, and is therefore contraindicated. They can similarly precipitate the toxic side effects of phenytoin and may lead to increased serum concentrations of cyclosporin, warfarin, benzodiazepines, and hypoglycemic drugs such as chlorpropamide, glibenclamide, glipizide and tolbutamide. Concomitant administration with rifampicin leads to a marked reduction in blood levels, especially with itraconazole and ketoconazole.

 FLUCONAZOLE

Molecular weight 306.3.

A synthetic bis(triazole) available for oral or parenteral administration.

Antimicrobial activity

The spectrum of activity includes dermatophytes (*Epidermophyton*, *Microsporum* and *Trichophyton* species), dimorphic fungi (*Blast. dermatitidis*, *Coccidioides immitis*, *Hist. capsulatum* and *Paracoccidioides brasiliensis*), and some yeasts (including *Candida albicans*, *Candida parapsilosis*, *Candida tropicalis*, and *Cryptococcus neoformans*). Most strains of *Candida krusei* and *Candida glabrata* (formerly *Torulopsis glabrata*) appear to be insensitive.

Acquired resistance

Resistant strains of *Cand. albicans* have been isolated from acquired immune deficiency syndrome (AIDS) patients given long-term treatment for oral or esophageal candidosis. There are a few reports of fluconazole-resistant strains of *Cryp. neoformans* recovered from AIDS patients with relapsed meningitis. Most, but not all, *Cand. albicans* strains resistant to fluconazole are cross-resistant to other azoles.

Pharmacokinetics

Oral absorption	>90%
C_{max} 50 mg oral	c. 1 mg/l after 2 h
Plasma half-life	25–30 h
Volume of distribution	0.55–0.65 l/kg
Plasma protein binding	c. 12%

Absorption

Oral absorption is almost complete and is not affected by food or intragastric pH. Blood concentrations increase in proportion to dosage. Maximum serum concentrations increase to about 2–3 mg/l after repeated dosing with 50 mg.

Distribution

Fluconazole is widely distributed achieving therapeutic concentrations in most tissues and body fluids. Concentrations in cerebrospinal fluid (CSF) are 50–60% of the simultaneous serum concentration in normal individuals and even higher in patients with meningitis.

Metabolism and excretion

More than 90% of a dose is eliminated in the urine: about 80% as unchanged drug and 10% as inactive metabolites. The drug is cleared through glomerular filtration, but there is significant tubular reabsorption. The plasma half-life is prolonged in renal failure, necessitating adjustment of the dosage. Fluconazole is removed during hemodialysis and, to a lesser extent, during peritoneal dialysis. In children the volume of distribution and plasma clearance are increased, and the half-life is considerably shorter (16–20 h).

Toxicity and side effects

Untoward reactions include nausea, abdominal discomfort, diarrhea and headache. Transient abnormalities of liver enzymes and rare serious skin reactions, including Stevens–Johnson syndrome, have been reported.

Clinical use

- Mucosal, cutaneous and systemic candidosis.
- Coccidioidomycosis.
- Cryptococcosis.
- Dermatophytosis.
- Pityriasis versicolor.

Preparation and dosage

Proprietary name: Diflucan.

Preparations: Capsules, oral suspension, i.v. infusion.

Dosage: Adults, oral, vaginal candidosis or balanitis, 150 mg as a single dose; oropharyngeal candidosis, 50 mg/day for 7–14 days; atrophic candidosis, 50 mg/day for 14 days; esophageal and mucocutaneous candidosis, and candiduria, 50 mg/day for 14–30 days. Tinea pedis, corporis, cruris, pityriasis versicolor, 50 mg/day for 2–4 weeks. Systemic candidosis, cryptococcal meningitis and other forms of cryptococcosis, oral or i.v. infusion, 200–400 mg on first day, then 100–400 mg/day; treatment is continued according to response. For the prevention of relapse of cryptococcal meningitis in AIDS patients, 100–200 mg/day, indefinitely. Prevention of fungal infections in neutropenic patients, 50–400 mg/day.

Children >1 year, oral, i.v. infusion, superficial candidosis, 3 mg/kg daily; systemic candidosis and cryptococcosis, 6–12 mg/kg daily (maximum 400 mg/day).

Widely available.

Further information

Anonymous 1999 Fluconazole. In: Dollery C (ed.) *Therapeutic Drugs* 2nd edn. Churchill Livingstone, Edinburgh, pp. F62–F68.

Debruyne D 1997 Clinical pharmacokinetics of fluconazole in superficial and systemic mycoses. *Clinical Pharmacokinetics* 33: 52–77.

Goodman JL, Winston DJ, Greenfield RA et al 1992 A controlled trial of fluconazole to prevent fungal infections in patients undergoing bone marrow transplantation. *New England Journal of Medicine* 326: 845–851.

Lopez-Ribot JL, McAtee RK, Perea S et al 1999 Multiple resistant phenotypes of *Candida albicans* coexist during episodes of oropharyngeal candidiasis in human immunodeficiency virus-infected patients. *Antimicrobial Agents and Chemotherapy* 43: 1621–1630.

Powderly WG, Saag MS, Cloud GA et al 1992 A controlled trial of fluconazole or amphotericin B to prevent relapse of cryptococcal meningitis in patients with the acquired immunodeficiency syndrome. *New England Journal of Medicine* 326: 793–798.

Rex JH, Bennett JE, Sugar AM et al 1994 A randomized trial comparing fluconazole with amphotericin B for the treatment of candidemia in patients without neutropenia. *New England Journal of Medicine* 331: 1325–1330.

Saag MS, Cloud GA, Graybill JR 1999 A comparison of itraconazole versus fluconazole as maintenance therapy for AIDS-associated cryptococcal meningitis. *Clinical Infectious Diseases* 28: 291–296.

Saag MS, Powderly WG, Cloud GA, Robinson P, Grieco MH, Sharkey PK 1992 Comparison of amphotericin B with fluconazole in the treatment of acute AIDS-associated cryptococcal meningitis. *New England Journal of Medicine* 326: 83–89.

ITRACONAZOLE

Molecular weight: 705.6.

A synthetic dioxolane triazole available for oral or parenteral administration.

Antimicrobial activity

The spectrum of activity includes dermatophytes, dimorphic fungi (*Blast. dermatitidis*, *Cocc. immitis*, *Hist. capsulatum*, *Paracocc. brasiliensis* and *Spor. schenckii*), molds (including *Aspergillus* spp. and *Penicillium marneffei*), dematiaceous fungi, and yeasts (*Candida* spp. and *Cryp. neoformans*).

Acquired resistance

This is still rare, but ketoconazole-resistant and some fluconazole-resistant *Cand. albicans* are cross-resistant to itraconazole. There are several reports of itraconazole-resistant strains of *Asp. fumigatus*.

Pharmacokinetics

Oral absorption	55%
C_{max} 100 mg oral	0.1–0.2 mg/l after 2–4 h
Plasma half-life	20–30 h
Volume of distribution	10.7 l/kg
Plasma protein binding	>99%

Absorption

Itraconazole is a lipophilic compound. Absorption from the gastrointestinal tract is improved if the drug is given with food or an acidic beverage. In contrast, absorption is reduced if it is given together with compounds that reduce gastric acid secretion. Much higher concentrations are obtained with repeated dosing, but there is much variation among individuals. Incorporation of itraconazole into a solution of hydroxypropyl-β-cyclodextrin enhances bioavailability and leads to much higher blood levels in neutropenic individuals and persons with AIDS. This formulation is better absorbed if given without food.

Distribution

Levels in body fluids such as the CSF are low, but concentrations in tissues such as lung, liver and bone are 2–3 times higher than in serum, and concentrations in the genital tract are 3–10 times higher. High concentrations are also found in the stratum corneum, as a result of drug secretion in sebum.

Metabolism and excretion

It is degraded by the liver into a large number of metabolites, most of which are inactive, and these are excreted with the bile. It is not excreted as unchanged drug in the urine. No adjustment of dosage is required in hepatic or renal failure, or during hemodialysis or peritoneal dialysis.

Toxicity and side effects

Unwanted effects include nausea, abdominal pain, dyspepsia, diarrhea (with solution), headache, allergic reactions (pruritus and skin rash). Rare side effects include Stevens–Johnson syndrome, transient abnormalities of liver enzymes, reversible idiosyncratic hepatitis, and hypokalemia.

Clinical use

- Aspergillosis.
- Systemic mycoses with dimorphic fungi (blastomycosis, coccidioidomycosis, histoplasmosis, paracoccidioidomycosis, penicilliosis).
- Subcutaneous mycoses (chromoblastomycosis, sporotrichosis).
- Mucosal and cutaneous candidosis.
- Dermatophytosis.
- Phaeohyphomycosis.
- Pityriasis versicolor.

Preparations and dosage

Proprietary name: Sporanox.

Preparations: Capsules, oral solution, i.v. infusion.

Dosage: Adults, oral, oropharyngeal candidosis, 100 mg/day (200 mg/day in AIDS or neutropenia) for 15 days. Vaginal candidosis, 200 mg twice daily for 1 day. Pityriasis versicolor, 200 mg daily for 7 days; tinea corporis, tinea cruris, 100 mg/day for 15 days; tinea pedis, tinea manuum, 100 mg/day for 30 days or 200 mg twice daily for 7 days. Onychomycosis, 200 mg once daily for 3 months or 200 mg twice daily for 7 days repeated once after 21 days for fingernails and repeated twice at 21 day intervals for toenails. Aspergillosis and other systemic or subcutaneous fungal infections, oral or i.v. infusion, 200 mg once or twice daily; treatment is continued according to response. For the prevention of relapse of histoplasmosis or penicillosis in AIDS patients, 200 mg/day, indefinitely. Prevention of fungal infections in neutropenic patients, 200–400 mg/day.

Widely available.

Further information

Anonymous 1999 Itraconazole. In: Dollery C (ed.) *Therapeutic Drugs* 2nd edn. Churchill Livingstone, Edinburgh, pp. I120–I126.

Boogaerts MA, Maertens J, Van Der Geest R et al 2001 Pharmacokinetics and safety of a 7-day administration of intravenous itraconazole followed by a 14-day administration of itraconazole oral solution in patients with hematologic malignancy. *Antimicrobial Agents and Chemotherapy* 45: 981–985.

Denning DW, Lee JY, Hostetler JS et al 1994 NIAID mycoses study group multicenter trial of oral itraconazole therapy for invasive aspergillosis. *American Journal of Medicine* 97: 135–144.

Denning DW, Venkateswarlu K, Oakley KL et al 1997 Itraconazole resistance in *Aspergillus fumigatus. Antimicrobial Agents and Chemotherapy* 41: 1364–1368.

Haria M, Bryson HM, Goa KL 1996 Itraconazole. A reappraisal of its pharmacological properties and therapeutic use in the management of superficial fungal infections. *Drugs* 51: 585–620.

Morgenstern GR, Prentice AG, Prentice HG et al 1999 A randomised controlled trial of itraconazole versus fluconazole for the prevention of fungal infections in patients with haematological malignancies. *British Journal of Haematology* 105: 901–911.

Stevens DA 1999 Itraconazole in cyclodextrin solution. *Pharmacotherapy* 19: 603–611.

Wheat J, Hafner R, Korzun AH et al 1995 Itraconazole treatment of disseminated histoplasmosis in patients with the acquired immunodeficiency syndrome. *American Journal of Medicine* 98: 336–342.

 KETOCONAZOLE

Molecular weight: 531.4.

A synthetic dioxolane imidazole available for oral and topical use.

Antimicrobial activity

The spectrum of activity includes dermatophytes, dimorphic fungi (*Blast. dermatitidis, Cocc. immitis, Hist. capsulatum* and *Paracocc. brasiliensis*) and some yeasts (*Candida* spp.).

Acquired resistance

This is rare, but instances have been documented in patients treated for chronic mucocutaneous candidosis and AIDS patients with oropharyngeal or esophageal candidosis. Some fluconazole-resistant *Cand. albicans* are cross-resistant to ketoconazole.

Pharmacokinetics

Oral absorption	Variable
C_{max} 400 mg oral	*c.* 5–6 mg/l after 2 h
Plasma half-life	6–10 h
Volume of distribution	0.36 l/kg
Plasma protein binding	>95%

It is erratically absorbed after oral administration. Absorption is favored by an acid pH. Food delays absorption, but does not significantly reduce the peak serum concentration. Absorption is reduced if it is given together with compounds that reduce gastric acid secretion. Penetration into CSF is generally poor and unreliable, although effective concentrations have been recorded with high doses in some cases of active meningitis. It is metabolized by the liver, and the metabolites are excreted in the bile. Less than 1% of an oral dose is excreted unchanged in the urine.

Toxicity and side effects

Unwanted effects include nausea, vomiting, abdominal pain, headache, rashes, urticaria, pruritus. Transient abnormalities of liver enzymes, interference with testosterone synthesis (leading to gynecomastia, alopecia and oligospermia) and rare fatal hepatic damage have been reported.

Clinical use

- Mucosal candidosis.
- Pityriasis versicolor.
- Seborrheic dermatitis.
- Non-life-threatening forms of blastomycosis, coccidioidomycosis, histoplasmosis and paracoccidioidomycosis.

Preparations and dosage

Proprietary name: Nizoral.

Preparations: Tablets, suspension, topical cream, shampoo.

Dosage: Adult, oral, 200–400 mg/day for 14 days. Children, oral, 3 mg/kg daily.

Widely available.

Further information

Anonymous 1999 Ketoconazole. In: Dollery C (ed.) *Therapeutic Drugs* 2nd edn. Churchill Livingstone, Edinburgh, pp. K13–K17.

Daneshmend TK, Warnock DW 1988 Clinical pharmacokinetics of ketoconazole. *Clinical Pharmacokinetics* 14: 13–34.

Lake-Bakkar G, Scheuer PJ, Sherlock S 1987 Hepatic reactions associated with ketoconazole in the United Kingdom. *British Medical Journal* 294: 419–422.

National Institutes of Allergy and Infectious Disease Mycoses Study Group 1985 Treatment of blastomycosis and histoplasmosis with ketoconazole. *Annals of Internal Medicine* 103: 861–872.

Sugar AM, Alsip SG, Galgiani JN et al 1987 Pharmacology and toxicity of high-dose ketoconazole. *Antimicrobial Agents and Chemotherapy* 31: 1874–1878.

 # VORICONAZOLE

Molecular weight: 349.3.

A synthetic triazole formulated for oral and parenteral use.

Antimicrobial activity

The spectrum of activity includes most fungi that cause disease in humans: dimorphic fungi (*Blast. dermatitidis*, *Cocc. immitis*, *Hist. capsulatum*, *Paracocc. brasiliensis*, and *Pen. marneffei*), moulds (*Aspergillus* spp., *Fusarium* spp., and *Scedosporium* spp.), dematiaceous fungi, and yeasts (*Candida* spp., *Cryp. neoformans* and *Trichosporon* spp.).

Acquired resistance

This has not been reported, but some fluconazole-resistant *Cand. albicans* show reduced susceptibility to voriconazole.

Pharmacokinetics

Oral absorption	90%
C_{max} 250 mg oral	c. 2 mg/l after 1.5 h
Plasma half-life	c. 6 h
Volume of distribution	2 l/kg
Plasma protein binding	60%

Absorption
The human pharmacokinetics are non-linear, possibly as a result of partial saturation of first-pass metabolism and systemic clearance.

Distribution
Voriconazole is widely distributed into body tissues and fluids, including brain and cerebrospinal fluid.

Metabolism and excretion
It is extensively metabolized by the liver. About 78–88% of a single dose appears in the urine, but less than 5% is excreted in unchanged form.

Toxicity and side effects

Unwanted effects include mild to moderate visual disturbance, rashes, and transient abnormalities of liver enzymes.

Clinical use

- Acute and chronic invasive aspergillosis.
- Serious invasive *Candida* infections (fluconazole-resistant).
- Serious infections caused by *Scedosporium* and *Fusarium* spp.

 Preparations and dosage

Proprietary name: Vfend.

Preparations: Film-coated tablets (50 mg and 200 mg); lyophilised power (200 mg) for reconstitution for infusion.

Dosage: Adult, oral, 200–400 mg 12-hourly for 24 h, then 100–200 mg 12-hourly; i.v. 6 mg/kg 12-hourly for 24 h, then 4 mg/kg 12-hourly. Not recommended for children under 2 years.

Available in USA and Europe.

 Further information

European Commission: European Drug Regulatory Agency website: www.eudra.org/humandocs/PDFs/EPAR/vfend/404901en4.pdf.

Johnson EM, Szekely A, Warnock DW 1998 In-vitro activity of voriconazole, itraconazole and amphotericin B against filamentous fungi. *Journal of Antimicrobial Chemotherapy* 42: 741–745.

Li RK, Ciblak MA, Nordoff N et al 2000 In vitro activities of voriconazole, itraconazole, and amphotericin B against *Blastomyces dermatitidis*, *Coccidioides immitis*, and *Histoplasma capsulatum*. *Antimicrobial Agents and Chemotherapy* 44: 1734–1736.

Marco F, Pfaller MA, Messer S et al 1998 In vitro activities of voriconazole (UK-109,496) and four other antifungal agents against 394 clinical isolates of *Candida* spp. *Antimicrobial Agents and Chemotherapy* 42: 161–163.

Pfaller MA, Zhang J, Messer SA et al 1999 In vitro activities of voriconazole, fluconazole, and itraconazole against 566 clinical isolates of *Cryptococcus neoformans* from the United States and Africa. *Antimicrobial Agents and Chemotherapy* 43: 169–171.

Sheehan DJ, Hitchcock CA, Sibley CM 1999 Current and emerging azole antifungal agents. *Clinical Microbiology Reviews* 12: 40–79.

OTHER AZOLES

In addition to the systemic agents numerous imidazoles are presently available for topical use. They include:

- **Bifonazole.** Used for the topical treatment of dermatophytoses and pityriasis versicolor.
- **Butoconazole.** Used for the topical treatment of vaginal candidosis.
- **Clotrimazole.** Used for the topical treatment of dermatophytoses, and oral, cutaneous and vaginal candidosis.
- **Econazole nitrate.** Used for the topical treatment of dermatophytoses and cutaneous and vaginal candidosis.
- **Fenticonazole nitrate.** Used for the topical treatment of vaginal candidosis.
- **Isoconazole nitrate.** Used for the topical treatment of dermatophytoses and cutaneous and vaginal candidosis.
- **Miconazole nitrate.** Used for the topical treatment of dermatophytoses, pityriasis versicolor, and oral, cutaneous and

vaginal candidosis. (Formerly also available for intravenous use.)

- **Oxiconazole.** Used for the topical treatment of dermatophytoses and cutaneous candidosis.
- **Sulconazole nitrate.** Used for the topical treatment of dermatophytoses and cutaneous candidosis.
- **Terconazole.** Used for the topical treatment of dermatophytoses and cutaneous and vaginal candidosis.
- **Tioconazole.** Used for the topical treatment of dermatophytoses (including nail infections) and cutaneous and vaginal candidosis.

 Preparations and dosages

Bifonazole
Proprietary names: Amycor, Mycospor.

Preparation: Topical.

Dosage: For fungal skin infections dosage and duration of treatment varies according to condition.

Widely available.

Butoconazole
Proprietary names: Femstat.

Preparation: Pessaries, vaginal cream.

Dosage: Adults, pessaries, 100 mg/day for 3–6 consecutive days.

Widely available.

Clotrimazole
Proprietary names: Canesten, Gyne-Lotrimin, Lotrimin, Mycelex.

Preparations: Pessaries, vaginal cream, oral troche, topical.

Dosage: Adults, pessaries, 500 mg as a single dose, or 200 mg/day for three consecutive days, or 100 mg/day for 6 days. Oral troches, 10 mg five times daily for 2 weeks or longer. For fungal skin infections dosage and duration of treatment varies according to condition.

Widely available.

Econazole nitrate
Proprietary names: Ecostatin, Gyno-Pevaryl, Pevaryl, Spectazole.

Preparations: Pessaries, topical.

Dosage: Adults, pessaries, 150 mg/day for three consecutive days. For fungal skin infections dosage and duration of treatment varies according to condition.

Widely available.

Fenticonazole nitrate
Proprietary name: Lomexin.

Preparation: Pessaries.

Dosage: Adult, pessaries, 600 mg as a single dose or 200 mg/day for three consecutive days.

Widely available.

Isoconazole
Proprietary name: Fazol, Travogen, Travogyn.

Preparation: Pessaries, topical.

Dosage: Adult, pessaries, 600 mg as a single dose or 300 mg/day for three days. For fungal skin infections dosage and duration of treatment varies according to condition.

Widely available.

Miconazole nitrate

Proprietary names: Daktarin, Femeron, Gyno-Daktarin, Micatin, Micozole, Monistat.

Preparations: Pessaries, vaginal cream, oral gel, topical.

Dosage: Adults, pessaries, 200 mg/day for seven consecutive days, or 100 mg/day for 14 days; oral gel, 125 mg, four times daily. Children 2–6 years, 125 mg twice daily; infants <2 years, 62.5 mg twice daily. For fungal skin infections dosage and duration of treatment varies according to condition.

Widely available.

Oxiconazole

Proprietary name: Oxistat, Oxizole.

Preparation: Topical.

Dosage: For fungal skin infections dosage and duration of treatment varies according to the condition being treated.

Widely available.

Sulconazole nitrate

Proprietary name: Exelderm.

Preparation: Topical.

Dosage: For fungal skin infections dosage and duration of treatment varies according to the condition being treated.

Widely available.

Terconazole

Proprietary name: Terazol.

Preparation: Pessaries, vaginal cream.

Dosage: Adults, pessaries, 80 mg/day for three consecutive days.

Widely available.

Tioconazole

Proprietary name: Trosyd, Trosyl, Vagistat.

Preparation: Pessaries, nail solution, cream.

Dosage: Adults, pessaries, 300 mg as a single dose. For fungal skin and nail infections dosage and duration of treatment varies according to the condition being treated.

Widely available.

Further information

Anonymous 1999 Miconazole (nitrate). In: Dollery C (ed.) *Therapeutic Drugs* 2nd edn. Churchill Livingstone, Edinburgh, pp. M171–M174.

Anonymous 1999 Clotrimazole. In: Dollery C (ed.) *Therapeutic Drugs* 2nd edn. Churchill Livingstone, Edinburgh, pp. C305–C3308.

Anonymous 1999 Tioconazole. In: Dollery C (ed.) *Therapeutic Drugs* 2nd edn. Churchill Livingstone, Edinburgh, pp. T123–T126.

Como JA, Dismukes WE 1994 Oral azole drugs as systemic antifungal therapy. *New England Journal of Medicine* 330: 263–272.

Sanglard D, Ischer F, Calabrese D et al 1998 Multiple resistance mechanisms to azole antifungals in yeast clinical isolates. *Drug Resistance Updates* 1: 255–265.

Sheehan DJ, Hitchcock CA, Sibley CM 1999 Current and emerging azole antifungal agents. *Clinical Microbiology Reviews* 12: 40–79.

ECHINOCANDINS

A new class of semisynthetic cyclic lipopeptide antifungal agents that cause cell lysis of susceptible fungi by interfering with glucan formation (pp. 19–20). They are active against *Candida* spp. isolates that are resistant to azoles and amphotericin B.

Cilofungin, the first member of the group, reached clinical trials but was abandoned because of side effects associated with the carrier used for the parenteral formulation. A newer agent, caspofungin, has been licensed for use in systemic fungal infections in a number of countries, and several others (micafungin, anidulafungin) are in development.

Further information

Georgopapadakou NH 2001 Update on antifungals targeted to the cell wall: focus on beta-1,3-glucan synthase inhibitors. *Expert Opinion on Investigational Drugs* 10: 269–280.

CASPOFUNGIN

Molecular weight: 1213.42.

[chemical structure]

A semisynthetic derivative of pneumocandin Bo, a lipopeptide fermentation product derived from the fungus *Glarea lozoyensis*. Formulated as the acetate for intravenous infusion.

Antimicrobial activity

It is active against *Aspergillus* spp., *Candida* spp. and *Pneumocystis carinii*. Resistance has not been reported.

Pharmacokinetics

C_{max} 70 mg 1 h infusion	*c.* 10 mg/l end infusion
Plasma half-life	9–11 h
Plasma protein binding	*c.* 97%

Intravenous infusion of a 70 mg loading dose followed by 50 mg daily maintains the mean blood level above 1 mg/l throughout treatment.

The drug is widely distributed, the highest concentrations being found in the liver. It is metabolized by the liver and less than 5% of a dose is excreted unchanged in the urine. The terminal half-life is 40–50 h. No dosage adjustment is recommended in patients with renal impairment; however, a dose reduction to 35 mg following the 70 mg loading dose is recommended for patients with moderate hepatic impairment. Caspofungin is not cleared by hemodialysis.

Interactions

Coadministration with cyclosporin has resulted in transaminase elevations of two to three times the upper limit of normal, which resolved when both drugs were discontinued. In addition, caspofungin serum concentrations were increased, but there was no effect on cyclosporin pharmacokinetics. No other drug interactions have been reported.

Toxicity and side effects

Fever, rash, pruritus, nausea, vomiting, and transient abnormalities of liver enzymes have been reported.

Clinical use

- Invasive aspergillosis unresponsive to other antifungal drugs.

Preparations and dosage

Proprietary name: Cancidas.

Preparations: i.v. infusion.

Dosage: Adult, i.v., 70 mg on first day, then 50 mg/day; treatment is continued according to response.

Widely available.

Further information

Abruzzo GK, Gill CJ, Flattery AM et al 2000 Efficacy of the echinocandin caspofungin against disseminated aspergillosis and candidiasis in cyclophosphamide-induced immunosuppressed mice. *Antimicrobial Agents and Chemotherapy* 44: 2310–2318.

Bartizal K, Gill CJ, Abruzzo GK et al 1997 In vitro preclinical evaluation studies with the echinocandin antifungal MK-0991(L-743,872). *Antimicrobial Agents and Chemotherapy* 41: 2326–2332.

Groll AH, Gullick BM, Petraitiene R et al 2001 Compartmental pharmacokinetics of the antifungal echinocandin caspofungin (MK-0991) in rabbits. *Antimicrobial Agents and Chemotherapy* 45: 596–600.

POLYENES

Around 100 polyene antibiotics have been described, but few have been developed for clinical use. They are large amphipathic molecules: closed macrolide rings with a variable number of hydroxyl groups along the hydrophilic side, and along the hydrophobic side a variable number of conjugated double bonds to which they owe the name 'polyene'; e.g. tetraene (four double bonds), heptaene (seven double bonds). They bind to sterols of susceptible fungal cells (p. 19) but because they bind to host cell membranes as well they are toxic to both fungal and mammalian cells.

The most important member of the group is amphotericin B, a heptaene that is administered parenterally for the treatment of systemic fungal infections.

Further information

Sugar AM 1986 The polyene macrolide antifungal drugs. In: Peterson PK, Verhoef J (eds). *The antimicrobial agents annual.* Elsevier, Amsterdam, vol 1, p 229–244.

AMPHOTERICIN B

Molecular weight: 924.1.

A fermentation product of *Streptomyces nodosus* available for intravenous infusion or oral administration. The traditional micellar suspension formulation of this drug is often associated with serious toxic side effects, in particular renal damage, and this has stimulated efforts to develop chemical modifications and new formulations. Most of the chemical modifications that have been devised have been less toxic, but also less active than amphotericin B. None has achieved clinical importance. Three lipid-associated formulations have been licensed for use:

- Liposomal amphotericin B, in which the drug is encapsulated in phospholipid-containing liposomes.
- Amphotericin B colloidal dispersion, in which the drug is packaged into small lipid disks containing cholesterol sulfate.
- Amphotericin B lipid complex, in which the drug is complexed with phospholipids to produce ribbon-like structures.

These formulations appear to be less toxic than the micellar suspension because of their altered pharmacological distribution. They permit higher doses to be administered and encouraging results have been reported in patients with serious fungal infection.

Antimicrobial activity

The spectrum includes most fungi that cause human disease: *Aspergillus fumigatus*, *Blast. dermatitidis*, *Candida* spp., *Cocc. immitis*, *Cryp. neoformans*, *Hist. capsulatum*, *Paracocc. brasiliensis* and *Spor. schenckii*. Dermatophytes, *Fusarium* spp. and some other *Aspergillus* spp. may be less sensitive, while *Sced. apiospermum* (*Pseud. boydii*), *Sced. prolificans*, *Trichosporon beigelii* and some fungi that cause mucormycosis are resistant.

It also exhibits useful activity against *Prototheca* spp., some protozoa, including *Leishmania* spp., and the genera *Naegleria* and *Hartmanella*.

Acquired resistance

This is a rare problem. Resistant strains of *Cand. tropicalis*, *Cand. lusitaniae*, *Cand. krusei* and *Cand. guilliermondii*, with alterations in the cell membrane including reduced amounts of ergosterol, have occasionally been isolated after prolonged treatment, particularly of infections in partially protected sites, such as the vegetations of endocarditis. Significant resistance in yeasts, including *Cand. albicans* and *Cand.* (*Torulopsis*) *glabrata*, has also been reported in isolates from cancer patients with prolonged neutropenia. In some cases resistant strains have caused disseminated infection. There are a few reports of amphotericin-resistant strains of *Cryp. neoformans* recovered from AIDS patients with relapsed meningitis.

Pharmacokinetics

Oral absorption	Very poor
C_{max} 50 mg slow infusion (micellar suspension)	*c.* 2 mg/l
Plasma half-life	24–48 h
Volume of distribution	4 l/kg
Plasma protein binding	>90%

Less than 10% of a parenteral dose of the conventional micellar suspension formulation of amphotericin B remains in the blood 12 h after administration. The remainder is thought to bind to tissue cell membranes, the highest concentrations being found in the liver (up to 40% of the dose). Levels in the CSF are less than 5% of the simultaneous blood concentration. The conventional formulation has a third-phase half-life of about 2 weeks. About 2–5% of a given dose appears in the urine within 24 h, but the fate of the rest is unknown. No metabolites have been identified.

The pharmacokinetics of the different lipid-based formulations are quite diverse. Maximal serum concentrations of 25–60 mg/l have been obtained after parenteral administration of a 5 mg/kg dose of the liposomal formulation, and levels of 5–10 mg/l have been detected at 24 h. In contrast, the maximal serum concentrations attained with the colloidal dispersion and lipid complex formulations are lower than those attained after equivalent amounts of the conventional formulation due to more rapid distribution of the drug to tissue. Maximal blood levels have ranged from 1 to 2 mg/l for a 5 mg/kg dose of the lipid complex and a 1 mg/kg dose of the colloidal dispersion. Administration of lipid associated formulations of amphotericin B results in much higher drug concentrations in the liver and spleen than are achieved with the conventional formulation. Renal concentrations of the drug are much lower and its nephrotoxic side effects are greatly reduced.

Blood concentrations are unchanged in hepatic or renal failure. Likewise, hemodialysis does not influence serum concentrations unless the patient is hyperlipidemic, in which case there is some drug loss due to adherence to the dialysis membrane.

Interactions

Amphotericin B can augment the nephrotoxic effects of other drugs, such as aminoglycoside antibiotics, cyclosporin and certain antineoplastic agents. It can also augment corticosteroid-induced potassium loss.

Toxicity and side effects

Common side effects include fever, rigors, headache, backache, nausea, vomiting, anorexia, anemia, disturbances in renal function (including hypokalemia and hypomagnesemia), renal toxicity, abnormal liver function (discontinue treatment), rash, anaphylactoid reactions.

Infusion-related reactions are uncommon in patients receiving liposomal amphotericin B, but fever, rigors and hypotension have developed in up to 40% of patients given the colloidal dispersion. Patients who have developed renal impairment while receiving the conventional formulation of amphotericin B have improved or stabilized when lipid-associated amphotericin B was substituted, even when the dose was increased. Renal function should be measured at regular intervals, particularly in patients receiving other nephrotoxic drugs.

Clinical use

- Aspergillosis.
- Systemic mycoses with dimorphic fungi (blastomycosis, coccidioidomycosis, histoplasmosis, paracoccidioidomycosis, penicilliosis).
- Candidosis.
- Cryptococcosis.
- Hyalohyphomycosis, mucormycosis, phaeohyphomycosis.

Preparations and dosage

Proprietary names: Abelcet (lipid complex), AmBisome (liposomal), Amphocil (colloidal dispersion), Amphocin, Amphotec (colloidal dispersion), Fungilin, Fungizone.

Preparations: Tablets, lozenges, oral suspension, i.v. infusion.

Dosage: Adults, oral, 100–200 mg, four times daily. Lozenges, 1–2, four times daily. Infants and children, 1 ml of suspension four times daily. Intravenous infusion, adults and children, 0.25 mg/kg daily gradually increasing to 1 mg/kg daily. In severely ill patients the dose can be increased to 1.5 mg/kg daily. Lipid formulations, adults and children, i.v. infusion 1–5 mg/kg daily.

Widely available.

Further information

Anonymous 1999 Amphotericin B. In Dollery C (ed.) *Therapeutic Drugs* 2nd edn. Churchill Livingstone, Edinburgh, pp. A166–A171.

Ellis M, Spence D, de Pauw B et al 1998 An EORTC international multicenter randomized trial comparing two dosages of liposomal amphotericin B for treatment of invasive aspergillosis. *Clinical Infectious Diseases* 27: 1406–1412.

Gallis HA, Drew RH, Packard WW 1990 Amphotericin B: 30 years of clinical experience. *Reviews of Infectious Diseases* 12: 308–329.

Sterling TR, Merz WG 1998 Resistance to amphotericin B: emerging clinical and microbiological patterns. *Drug Resistance Updates* 1: 161–165.

Walsh TJ, Finberg RW, Arndt C et al 1999 Liposomal amphotericin B for empirical therapy in patients with persistent fever and neutropenia. *New England Journal of Medicine* 340: 764–771.

Walsh TJ, Hiemenz JW, Seibel NL et al 1998 Amphotericin B lipid complex for invasive fungal infections: analysis of safety and efficacy in 556 cases. *Clinical Infectious Diseases* 26: 1383–1396.

White MH, Bowden RA, Sandler ES et al 1998 Randomized, double-blind clinical trial of amphotericin B colloidal dispersion vs. amphotericin B in the empirical treatment of fever and neutropenia. *Clinical Infectious Diseases* 27: 296–302.

Wingard JR, Kubilis P, Lee L et al 1999 Clinical significance of nephrotoxicity in patients treated with amphotericin B for suspected or proven aspergillosis. *Clinical Infectious Diseases* 29: 1402–1407.

Wingard JR, White MH, Anaissie E et al 2000 A randomized, double-blind comparative trial evaluating the safety of liposomal amphotericin B versus amphotericin B lipid complex in the empirical treatment of febrile neutropenia. *Clinical Infectious Diseases* 31: 1155–1163.

Wong-Beringer A, Jacobs RA, Guglielmo BJ 1998 Lipid formulations of amphotericin B: clinical efficacy and toxicities. *Clinical Infectious Diseases* 27: 603–618.

OTHER POLYENES

Other clinically useful polyenes, which in general resemble amphotericin B in antifungal action and spectrum of activity, are mostly used only topically.

- **Mepartricin**; methyl partricin (heptaene). A product of *Streptomyces aureofaciens* used for intravenous treatment of deep candidosis and for the topical treatment of vaginal candidosis. It offers no conspicuous advantages over amphotericin B as a systemic antifungal.
- **Natamycin**; pimaricin (tetraene). A product of *Streptomyces chatanoogensis* or *Streptomyces natalensis* used for the topical treatment of ophthalmic and bronchopulmonary infections and vaginal candidosis.

- **Nystatin** (tetraene). A product of *Streptomyces albulus* or *Streptomyces noursei* used for the topical treatment of oral, esophageal, gastrointestinal and genital candidosis, and gastrointestinal prophylaxis. A liposomal formulation has entered clinical trials for intravenous treatment of systemic fungal infections.

Preparations and dosages

Mepartricin
Preparations: Tablets, vaginal preparations, topical cream, oral suspension. Not available in the UK. Available in continental Europe.

Natamycin
Preparations: Oral suspension, ophthalmic suspension, cream, vaginal preparations, lozenges.

Dosage: Adults, oral, 400 mg/day in divided doses.

Not available in the UK. Available in continental Europe.

Nystatin
Proprietary name: Mycostatin, Nystan.

Preparations: Tablets, pastilles, oral suspension, vaginal and topical preparations.

Dosage: Adults, oral, 500 000 units every 6 h, doubled in severe infections. Prophylaxis: adults, 1 million units daily; children, 100 000 units four times daily; neonates, 100 000 units daily as a single dose. Vaginal pessaries, 1–2 at night for at least 14 nights.

Widely available.

Further information

Anonymous 1999 Nystatin. In: Dollery C (ed.) *Therapeutic Drugs* 2nd edn. Churchill Livingstone, Edinburgh, pp. N149–N152.

Groll AH, Mickiene D, Werner K et al Compartmental pharmacokinetics and tissue distribution of multilamellar liposomal nystatin in rabbits. *Antimicrobial Agents and Chemotherapy* 44: 950–957.

Johnson EM, Ojwang JO, Szekely A et al 1998 Comparison of in vitro antifungal activities of free and liposome-encapsulated nystatin with those of four amphotericin B formulations. *Antimicrobial Agents and Chemotherapy* 42: 1412–1416.

OTHER SYSTEMIC AGENTS

FLUCYTOSINE

5-Fluorocytosine. Molecular weight: 129.1.

A synthetic fluorinated pyrimidine available for intravenous infusion or oral administration.

Antimicrobial activity

It has a restricted spectrum of activity including *Candida* spp., *Cryp. neoformans* and some fungi causing chromoblastomycosis.

Acquired resistance

About 10% of *Cand. albicans* isolates (more in some centers) are resistant before treatment starts, and resistance may develop during treatment. The most common cause of resistance appears to be loss of the enzyme uridine monophosphate pyrophosphorylase.

Pharmacokinetics

Oral absorption	Complete
C_{max} 25 mg/kg 6-hourly oral	70–80 mg/l after 1–2 h
Plasma half-life	3–6 h
Volume of distribution	0.7–1 l/kg
Plasma protein binding	*c.* 12%

Absorption is slower in persons with impaired renal function, but peak concentrations are higher. Levels in the CSF are around 75% of the simultaneous serum concentration. More than 90% of a dose of flucytosine is excreted in the urine in unchanged form. The serum half-life is much longer in renal failure, necessitating modification of the dosage regimen.

Toxicity and side effects

Nausea, vomiting, diarrhea are common. Rashes, headache, alteration in liver function tests (hepatitis and hepatic necrosis) and blood disorders (including thrombocytopenia, leukopenia and aplastic anemia) have been reported.

The nephrotoxic effects of amphotericin B can result in elevated blood concentrations of flucytosine, and levels of the latter drug should be monitored when these compounds are administered together.

Clinical use

- Candidosis (in combination with amphotericin B or fluconazole).
- Cryptococcosis (in combination with amphotericin B or fluconazole).

Monitoring of flucytosine concentrations is desirable in all patients, and mandatory in those with renal impairment, in whom the dosage must be modified (Table 35.1).

Preparations and dosage

Proprietary names: Alcobon, Ancobon, Ancotil.

Preparations: Tablets, capsules, i.v. infusion.

Dosage: Adults, oral, i.v., 200 mg/kg daily in four divided doses. For extremely sensitive organisms, 50–150 mg/kg daily in four divided doses may be sufficient.

Widely available.

Table 35.1 Regimens for administration of flucytosine in renal failure

Creatinine clearance (ml/min)	Individual dosage (mg/kg)	Dosage interval (h)
>40	25–37.5	6
40–20	25–37.5	12
20–10	25–37.5	24
<10		>24[a]

Renal function is considered to be normal when creatinine clearance is greater than 40–50 ml/min or the concentration of creatinine in serum is less than 180 mmol/l; concentration of creatinine in serum is not reliable unless renal function is stable.
[a] Dosage interval must be based on serum drug concentration measurement at frequent intervals. Maximum serum concentration should not exceed 80 mg/l.

 Further information

Anonymous 1999 Flucytosine. In: Dollery C (ed.) *Therapeutic Drugs* 2nd edn. Churchill Livingstone, Edinburgh, pp. F69–F70.

Francis P, Walsh TJ 1992 Evolving role of flucytosine in immunocompromised patients: new insights into safety, pharmacokinetics, and antifungal therapy. *Clinical Infectious Diseases* 15: 1003–1018.

Larsen RA, Bozette SA, Jones BE et al 1994 Fluconazole combined with flucytosine for treatment of cryptococcal meningitis in patients with AIDS. *Clinical Infectious Diseases* 19: 741–745.

Scholer HJ 1980 Flucytosine. In: Speller DCE (ed.) *Antifungal chemotherapy*. Wiley, Chichester, pp. 35–106.

 GRISEOFULVIN

Molecular weight: 352.8.

A fermentation product of various species of *Penicillium*, including *Penicillium griseofulvum*. Available as fine-particle or ultrafine-particle formulations for oral use.

Antimicrobial activity

The spectrum of useful activity is restricted to dermatophytes causing skin, nail and hair infections (*Epidermophyton*, *Microsporum* and *Trichophyton* spp.). Resistance has seldom been reported.

Pharmacokinetics

Absorption from the gastrointestinal tract is dependent on drug formulation. Administration with a high-fat meal will increase the rate and extent of absorption, but individuals tend to achieve consistently high or low blood concentrations. It appears in the stratum corneum within 4–8 h, as a result of secretion in perspiration. However, levels begin to fall soon after the drug is discontinued, and within 48–72 h it can no longer be detected. Griseofulvin is metabolized in the liver, the metabolites being excreted in the urine. The drug has an elimination half-life of 9–21 h.

Interactions

Griseofulvin can diminish the anticoagulant effect of warfarin. Its absorption is reduced in persons receiving concomitant treatment with phenobarbitone.

Toxicity and side effects

Adverse reactions occur in about 15% of patients and include headache, nausea, vomiting, rashes and photosensitivity.

Clinical use

- Dermatophyte infections of hair, skin and nail.

 Preparations and dosage

Proprietary names: Fulcin, Fulvicin, Grisactin, Grisovin.

Preparations: Tablets, capsules, oral suspension.

Dosage: Adults, oral, 500 mg/day as a single or divided dose. In severe infections the dose may be doubled, reducing when response occurs. Children, 10 mg/kg daily in divided doses, or as a single dose.

Widely available.

 Further information

Anonymous 1999 Griseofulvin. In: Dollery C (ed.) *Therapeutic Drugs* 2nd edn. Churchill Livingstone, Edinburgh, pp. G94–G96.

Bennett ML, Fleischer AB, Loveless JW et al 2000 Oral griseofulvin remains the treatment of choice for tinea capitis in children. *Pediatric Dermatology* 17: 304–309.

Davies RR 1980 Griseofulvin. In: Speller DCE (ed.) *Antifungal chemotherapy*. Wiley, Chichester, pp. 149–182.

OTHER TOPICAL AGENTS

There is also a large and miscellaneous group of topical antifungal agents, all of which are effective treatments for superficial mycoses. They include the following.

- **Amorolfine hydrochloride.** A synthetic morpholine derivative that inhibits ergosterol biosynthesis. It is used for the treatment of tinea corporis, tinea cruris, tinea pedis and onychomycosis.
- **Butenafine hydrochloride.** A synthetic benzylamine derivative which acts as an ergosterol biosynthesis inhibitor. It is used for the treatment of tinea corporis, tinea cruris and tinea pedis.
- **Ciclopirox.** A synthetic pyridinone used in onychomycosis and as the olamine salt in tinea corporis, tinea cruris, tinea pedis, cutaneous candidosis and pityriasis versicolor.
- **Haloprogin.** A halogenated phenolic which is effective in tinea corporis, tinea cruris, tinea pedis and pityriasis versicolor.
- **Tolnaftate.** A thiocarbamate used in tinea cruris and tinea pedis.

 Preparations and dosage

Amorolfine hydrochloride
Proprietary name: Loceryl.

Preparation: Nail solution, cream.

Dosage: For fungal skin infections, apply once daily for at least 2–3 weeks (up to 6 weeks for tinea pedis). For nail infections, apply solution 1–2 times weekly; treat fingernails for 6 months, toenails for 9–12 months.

Widely available.

Butenafine hydrochloride
Proprietary name: Mentax.

Preparation: Topical.

Dosage: For fungal skin infections dosage and duration of treatment varies according to condition.

Widely available.

Ciclopirox
Proprietary name: Loprox, Penlac.

Preparation: Nail solution, cream, powder.

Dosage: For fungal skin infections, apply twice daily for at least 2–4 weeks. For nail infections, apply solution once daily for at least 6 months.

Widely available.

Haloprogin
Proprietary name: Halotex.

Preparation: Topical.

Dosage: For fungal skin infections dosage and duration of treatment varies according to condition.

Widely available.

Tolnaftate
Proprietary name: Aftate, Tinactin.

Preparation: Topical.

Dosage: For fungal skin infections dosage and duration of treatment varies according to condition.

Widely available.

 Further information

Haria M, Bryson HM 1995 Amorolfine, a review of its pharmacological properties and therapeutic potential in the treatment of onychomycosis and other superficial fungal infections. *Drugs* 49: 103–120.

McNeely W, Spencer CM 1998 Butenafine. *Drugs* 55: 405–412.

36 Antimycobacterial agents

J. Grange

The mycobacteria causing human disease, and therefore requiring treatment by antibacterial agents, are divisible into three groups: the tuberculosis complex (*Mycobacterium tuberculosis*, *M. bovis* and *M. africanum*); the leprosy bacillus (*M. leprae*); and various environmental saprophytes that occasionally cause human disease. Patients with acquired immune deficiency syndrome (AIDS) are particularly likely to develop disease due to the latter species, notably the *Mycobacterium avium* complex (MAC), although the incidence of such infection has declined in developed nations since the introduction of highly active antiretroviral therapy (HAART).

Antimycobacterial agents include natural and semisynthetic antibiotics and synthetic agents. Some, such as rifampicin (rifampin; p. 376) and streptomycin (p. 179) are active against a wide range of bacteria, but their use is mostly restricted to the treatment of mycobacterial disease and some are active only against mycobacteria. In recent years, the increasing occurrence of tuberculosis resistant to the first-line drugs has led to the growing use of agents principally used for other infections. These include the newer macrolides (Ch. 24), fluoroquinolones (Ch. 29), minocycline (p. 401) and amoxicillin with clavulanic acid (p. 273).

The few species of rapidly growing mycobacteria that cause human disease, principally *M. abscessus*, *M. chelonae* and *M. fortuitum*, are resistant to the standard antituberculosis agents, but are often susceptible to agents used for other purposes, including macrolides, quinolones, imipenem, sulfonamides, trimethoprim, cephalosporins, gentamicin and amikacin.

The rifamycins (Ch. 30) are among the most important of the antimycobacterial agents. Rifampicin is included in drug regimens for the treatment of tuberculosis and leprosy and rifabutin is effective against MAC infection in AIDS patients. The aminoglycoside streptomycin is used in some antituberculosis regimens, particularly when resistance to other agents is suspected or known. Other aminoglycosides, notably amikacin (p. 171), are sometimes used in the treatment of disease due to environmental mycobacteria, particularly AIDS-related MAC infection.

Synthetic agents, which for practical purposes are active only against mycobacteria, are chemically diverse and were principally found as a result of extensive screening of compounds for activity against *M. tuberculosis*. Isoniazid and pyrazinamide are, with rifampicin,

the principal components of modern short-course antituberculosis regimens (Ch. 61). A fourth drug (usually ethambutol) is commonly included in short-course antituberculosis regimens on account of the increasing incidence of resistance to one or more of the other drugs. Thiacetazone has the advantage of cheapness, but because it has limited antibacterial activity and high incidence of serious side effects (including life-threatening exfoliative dermatitis, particularly in HIV-positive patients) it should be avoided whenever possible.

Second-line drugs include ethionamide and the closely related protionamide and *p*-aminosalicylic acid (PAS), and are principally used for treating cases of tuberculosis resistant to the first-line drugs. Dapsone has long been the key drug in the treatment of leprosy and is now used in combination with rifampicin and clofazimine. Clofazimine was also used for the treatment of disseminated MAC infection in HIV-positive patients, but is rarely used now on account of toxicity in such patients.

A number of new rifamycins and pyrazinamide analogs are being evaluated and the recent sequencing of the genome of *M. tuberculosis*, together with increasing understanding of mycobacterial metabolic pathways, has stimulated interest in the development of 'designer' drugs. Novel modes of drug delivery, including liposome encapsulation, are being investigated and there are indications that immunotherapeutic interventions may prove to be useful adjuncts to chemotherapy.

ANTIMICROBIAL ACTIVITY

The action of antimycobacterial agents in vivo depends on the population dynamics of the mycobacteria within the lesions. In the case of tuberculosis, some bacilli replicate freely in the walls of well-oxygenated cavities, some replicate more slowly in acidic and anoxic tissue and within macrophages and a few are in a near-dormant 'persister' state. Isoniazid exerts a powerful and rapid bactericidal activity against the freely replicating bacilli and thus kills up to 95%, with a substantial reduction of infectiousness, within a few days of commencing treatment; however, it has little or no effect against the near-dormant bacilli. These are killed by rifampicin, while the slowly replicating bacilli in acidic environments are killed by pyrazinamide, which is active only at low pH. Thus a distinction may be drawn between agents that are bactericidal in vitro and those that actually 'sterilize' lesions in vivo. Accordingly, the most widely used short-course antituberculosis regimen is based on a 2-month intensive phase of treatment with isoniazid, rifampicin, pyrazinamide and ethambutol, during which all except a few persisters are killed, and a 4-month continuation phase of rifampicin (which kills persisters during shorter bursts of metabolic activity) and isoniazid to kill any rifampicin-resistant mutants that might commence replication (Ch. 61). In both tuberculosis and leprosy, the great majority of bacilli are killed during the first few weeks of therapy; prolonged therapy, with its associated problems of cost, compliance and the need for supervision, is required to kill a few remaining metabolically inactive persisters and thus prevent relapse.

In the absence of acquired drug resistance, strains of *M. tuberculosis* and related members of the tuberculosis complex are remarkably constant in their susceptibility to the antituberculosis drugs. All strains of *M. bovis* and some strains of *M. africanum* are, however, naturally resistant to pyrazinamide. Environmental mycobacteria are often resistant to antituberculosis agents in vitro, although in patients with disease due to the slowly growing species (*M. kansasii*, *M. xenopi*, *M. avium*, *M. intracellulare* and *M. malmoense*) good clinical responses to regimens containing rifampicin, ethambutol and isoniazid are often seen. The rapidly growing pathogens, principally *M. chelonae* and *M. fortuitum*, are resistant to the antituberculosis drugs but susceptible to a range of other agents.

DRUG RESISTANCE

Mutation to drug resistance occurs at a low but constant rate in all mycobacterial populations and such mutants (Table 36.1) are readily selected if the patient is treated with a single drug. Successful therapy thus requires the use of at least two drugs to which the strain is susceptible. An exception is the use of a single drug, usually isoniazid, to prevent the emer-gence of active tuberculosis in infected but healthy persons who are assumed to have very small numbers of bacilli in their tissues. Emergence of drug resistance is uncommon in patients receiving a fully supervised course of modern short-course chemotherapy based on drugs of known quality.

Unfortunately, poor prescribing habits, unavailability of drugs, inadvertent use of time-expired or even counterfeit drugs, poor supervision of therapy and unregulated 'over-the-counter' sales of drugs have led to the emergence of drug-resistant tubercle bacilli in many countries. Even combination formulations occasionally lead to the development of single- or multiple-drug resistance if given intermittently. Tuberculosis resistant to rifampicin and isoniazid, with or without additional resistances, is termed multidrug resistant tuberculosis. Resistance may develop in an inadequately treated patient (acquired or secondary resistance), or a person may become infected with a resistant strain (initial or primary resistance). Likewise, primary and acquired drug resistance is encountered in leprosy, and the World Health Organization (WHO) has therefore advised that all cases of leprosy should be treated by combination therapy.

The WHO recommends that surveys of primary drug resistance should be undertaken as these give a good measure of the efficiency of control programs. The extent to which such surveys are carried out varies considerably from country to country: whereas in developed nations drug susceptibility tests are carried out on most clinical isolates of *M. tuberculosis*, such testing is often carried out only sporadically, and perhaps on unrepresentative isolates, in many developing countries.

Between 1994 and 1997 the WHO and the International Union Against Tuberculosis and Lung Disease undertook a global survey of resistance to the antituberculosis drugs. This revealed that the prevalence of initial and acquired resistance varied enormously from region to region, with particularly high levels of both forms of resistance in the Dominican Republic, Russia, the Baltic States and Sierra Leone (Figure 36.1). Certain 'hotspots' of resistance occur within countries, such as New York where, in 1991, 19% of all isolates were multi-drug resistant.

Table 36.1 Targets of antimycobacterial agents and genes determining resistance

Agent	Target	Gene(s) encoding target(s) or in which mutations conferring resistance occur
Isoniazid	Mycolic acid synthesis	*inhA*, *katG*, *oxyR-ahpC*
Pyrazinamide	? Fatty acid synthesis, requires enzymatic conversion to pyrazinoic acid	*pncA*
Ethambutol	Arabinosyl transferase (cell wall arabinogalactan synthesis)	*embA*, *embB* and *embC*
Thiacetazone	Mycolic acid synthesis	Unknown
p-Aminosalicylic acid	? Mycoside synthesis	Unknown
Ethionamide and protionamide	Mycolic acid synthesis	*inhA*
Capreomycin and viomycin	50S or 30S ribosomal subunit	*vicA* (50S) or *vicB* (30S)
Clofazimine	? RNA polymerase	Unknown
Cycloserine	Peptidoglycan	*alrA*
Dapsone	? folic acid synthesis	Unknown

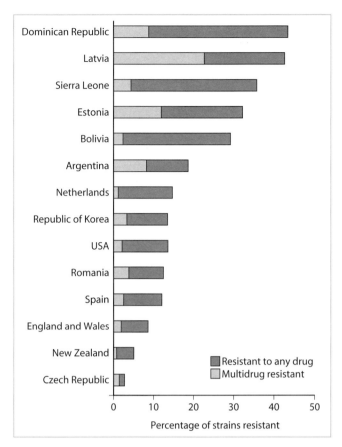

Fig. 36.1 Percentage of all isolates resistant to one or more of isoniazid, rifampicin, streptomycin and ethambutol, and strains resistant to rifampicin plus isoniazid (multidrug resistance). Data from the World Health Organization

PHARMACOKINETICS

With the exception of streptomycin (and other aminoglycosides) and the peptides, all the antimycobacterial agents currently in use are absorbed adequately when given orally. They are distributed to all tissues and organs and adequate amounts of the first-line antituberculosis agents cross the blood–brain barrier. Thus, in principle, standard regimens and doses are suitable for treatment of all forms of tuberculosis, although many clinicians prescribe more prolonged courses of therapy for extrapulmonary tuberculosis, particularly tuberculous meningitis, and for cases of HIV-related tuberculosis (Ch. 61). Rifampicin, isoniazid, pyrazinamide, ethionamide and protionamide are either eliminated in the bile or metabolized, and may therefore be given in standard doses to patients with impaired renal function. Ethambutol is eliminated predominantly by the kidney, and streptomycin and other aminoglycosides are excreted entirely by the kidney: these drugs should be avoided, if possible, in patients with impaired renal function.

Small amounts of isoniazid and even smaller amounts of the other antituberculosis drugs enter the milk, so breast feeding is not contraindicated.

TOXICITY AND SIDE EFFECTS

Unwanted side effects occur with all antituberculosis agents, but those caused by the first-line drugs (rifampicin, isoniazid, pyrazinamide) are less frequent and severe than those due to the older agents (streptomycin, *p*-aminosalicylic acid, thiacetazone). Side effects are particularly likely to occur in HIV-positive patients, who should never be given thiacetazone as fatal exfoliative dermatitis may occur (specific toxicities are discussed under the individual drugs). Transient and clinically insignificant rise in serum hepatic enzyme levels commonly occurs during the first few weeks of therapy and, unless the patient is known to have liver disease, routine assay of these enzymes is generally regarded as unnecessary. Clinically evident hepatitis occurs in about 1% of patients and the incidence increases with age, although it usually resolves rapidly when therapy ceases. In most cases therapy with the same drugs can be continued. More generalized reactions, with rashes, influenza-like symptoms and sometimes lymphadenopathy and hepatic enlargement with or without jaundice may occur in the first 2 months of therapy. Therapy must be stopped, the responsible drug identified by giving small challenge doses sequentially, and treatment resumed without that drug.

Interactions between the antimycobacterial drugs themselves have been described: pyrazinamide and ethionamide may increase serum concentrations of isoniazid while pyrazinamide may decrease that of rifampicin, but these effects are of no known clinical significance. More significant interactions occur between the antimycobacterial agents and drugs used for other purposes. Most recorded drug interactions involve rifampicin and quinolones but some interactions with isoniazid have been described, especially in slow acetylators (p. 437).

CLINICAL USE

Definite recommendations for the treatment of tuberculosis and leprosy have been made by the WHO (Chs. 60 and 61). These regimens are also used for treating human tuberculosis due to *M. bovis* and for the rare cases of disseminated disease due to the vaccine strain Bacille Calmette–Guérin (BCG), although both are naturally resistant to pyrazinamide.

Opinions differ as to the most suitable regimens for other mycobacterial infections. While standard regimens have been proposed, drug susceptibilities vary from species to species, and from strain to strain, so that some workers advocate individualized therapy.

The British and American Thoracic Societies recommend an 18-month course of rifampicin, ethambutol and isoniazid for treatment of pulmonary disease due to MAC, *M. kansasii*, *M. xenopi* and *M. malmoense*. The need for isoniazid has been questioned, but ethambutol is a key component and must be given throughout. A 9-month course appears adequate for *M. kansasii*. These recommendations are likely to be revised when the results of trials involving quinolones and the newer macrolides are available.

HIV-related disease, which is usually caused by MAC, has been treated with regimens containing rifabutin, clofazimine and ethambutol but the US Task Force on MAC now recommends that all patients should receive clarithromycin or azithromycin with companion drugs selected on the basis of in-vitro susceptibility tests.

No controlled clinical trials have been carried out on the therapy of disease due to the rapidly growing *M. chelonae* and *M. fortuitum*. Therapy is therefore empirical, but may be assisted by in-vitro susceptibility testing. Limited infections such as post-injection abscesses respond to co-trimoxazole together with erythromycin. More serious infections have responded to cefoxitin with amikacin. The outcome of therapy is, however, very unpredictable.

Johnson JL, Kamya RM, Okwera A et al 2000 Randomized controlled trial of *Mycobacterium vaccae* immunotherapy in non-human immunodeficiency virus-infected Ugandan adults with newly diagnosed pulmonary tuberculosis. *Journal of Infectious Diseases* 181: 1304–1312.

Mitchison DA 1998 How drug resistance emerges as a result of poor compliance during short course chemotherapy of tuberculosis. *International Journal of Tuberculosis and Lung Disease* 2: 10–15.

Mitchison DA 2000 Role of individual drugs in the chemotherapy of tuberculosis. *International Journal of Tuberculosis and Lung Disease* 4: 796–806.

Ramaswamy S, Musser JM 1998 Molecular genetic basis of antimicrobial agent resistance in *Mycobacterium tuberculosis*. *Tubercle and Lung Disease* 79: 3–29.

Rea TH 2000 Trials of daily, long term minocycline and rifampicin or clarithromycin and rifampicin in the treatment of borderline lepromatous and lepromatous leprosy. *International Journal of Leprosy* 68: 129–135.

Schraufnagel DE 1999 Tuberculosis treatment for the beginning of the next century. *International Journal of Tuberculosis and Lung Disease* 3: 651–662.

Winstanley PA 1998 Clinical pharmacology of antituberculosis drugs. In: Davies PDO (ed.) *Clinical tuberculosis* 2nd edn. Chapman & Hall Medical, London, pp. 225–242.

World Health Organization 1997 *Treatment of tuberculosis. Guidelines for national programmes*. WHO, Geneva.

FORMULATIONS

Compliance with antituberculosis therapy is aided by use of combination drug preparations and calendar blister-packs. Examples of combination preparations are:

- rifampicin + isoniazid (Rifinah, Rimactizid)
- rifampicin + isoniazid + pyrazinamide (Rifater)

It is essential that combination drugs are obtained from reputable manufacturers as the bioavailability of the component drugs may be seriously affected by the manufacturing process. Blister-packs are available for treatment of paucibacillary and multibacillary leprosy (PB-Combi, MB-Combi).

 Further information

Acocella G 1990 The use of fixed-dose combinations in antituberculosis chemotherapy. Rationale for their application in daily, intermittent and pediatric regimens. *Bulletin of the International Union Against Tuberculosis and Lung Disease* 65 (2–3): 77–83.

Baker RJ 1990 The need for new drugs in the treatment and control of leprosy. *International Journal of Leprosy* 58: 78–97.

Bartmann K (ed.) 1988 Antituberculosis drugs. In: *Handbook of experimental pharmacology*, vol 84. Springer, Berlin.

Crofton J, Chaulet P, Maher D 1997 *Guidelines for management of drug-resistant tuberculosis*. WHO, Geneva.

Farmer P, Kim JY 1998 Community based approaches to the control of multidrug resistant tuberculosis: introducing 'DOTS-plus'. *British Medical Journal* 317: 671–674.

Fox W 1990 Drug combinations and the bioavailability of rifampicin. *Tubercle* 71: 241–245.

Grange JM, Winstanley PA, Davies PDO 1994 Clinically significant drug interactions with antituberculosis agents. *Drug Safety* 11: 242–251.

Grosset JH 1992 Treatment of tuberculosis in HIV infection. *Tubercle and Lung Disease* 73: 378–383.

Grosset JH 1994 Progress in the chemotherapy of leprosy. *International Journal of Leprosy* 62: 268–277.

Heifets LB (ed.) 1991 *Drug susceptibility in the chemotherapy of mycobacterial infections*. CRC Press, Boca Raton, FL.

Israel HL 1993 Chemoprophylaxis for tuberculosis. *Respiratory Medicine* 87: 81–83.

 ***PARA*-AMINOSALICYLIC ACID**

PAS. Molecular weight (free acid): 153.1.

A salicylic acid derivative formulated as the dihydrate or sodium salt for oral administration.

Antimicrobial activity

The activity is bacteristatic. Inhibitory concentrations for *M. tuberculosis* are 0.5–10 mg/l, depending on the medium used and the inoculum size. Other mycobacterial species are resistant to 8 mg/l.

Acquired resistance

Resistance is very uncommon as the drug is rarely used.

Pharmacokinetics

Oral absorption	Good
C_{max} 4 g oral (free acid)	41–68 mg/l after 3–4 h
4 g oral (sodium salt)	76–104 mg/l after 0.5–1 h
Plasma half-life	0.75–1 h
Volume of distribution	0.24 l/kg
Plasma protein binding	50–73%

High tissue concentrations are achieved. The drug is rapidly acetylated in the liver and about 80% is excreted in the urine within 7 h, mostly in the acetylated form.

Toxicity and side effects

Adverse effects, leading to problems of compliance, occur in 10–30% of patients. Gastrointestinal effects, including abdominal pain, nausea and diarrhea are very common. It interferes with iodine metabolism in the thyroid, and prolonged therapy may lead to goitre, and less frequently to myxedema, which respond to thyroxine therapy. Allergic skin reactions are common. Other less common reactions include blood dyscrasias, crystalluria, a syndrome resembling infectious mononucleosis and, rarely, Löeffler's syndrome and encephalitis.

Clinical use

- Multidrug resistant tuberculosis (with other antituberculosis drugs).

Preparations and dosage

Preparations: Tablets, oral granules.

Dosage: Adults and children, oral, 150–300 mg/kg per day in 2–4 divided doses.

Limited availability; not available in the UK.

Further information

Anonymous 1999 Aminosalicylic acid. In: Dollery C (ed.) *Therapeutic Drugs* 2nd edn. Churchill Livingstone, Edinburgh, pp. A137–A140.

Peloquin CA, Berning SE, Huitt GA, Childs JM, Singleton MD, Jones GT 1999 Once-daily and twice daily doses of *p*-aminosalicylic acid granules. *American Journal of Respiratory and Critical Care Medicine* 159: 932–934.

Trnka L, Mison P 1988 *p*-Aminosalicylic acid (PAS). In: Bartmann K (ed.) *Antituberculosis drugs* (Handbook of experimental pharmacology, vol 84). Springer, Berlin, pp. 191–197.

CAPREOMYCIN

A mixture of four basic hexapeptides, capreomycin IA, IB, IIA and IIB, produced by *Streptomyces capreolus*. It is supplied as a water-soluble sulfate and at least 90% consists of capreomycin IA and IB. Like viomycin, to which it is related, part of the molecule is cyclized to form a 16-membered ring. It is thought to act by blocking protein synthesis.

Antimicrobial activity

Capreomycin inhibits *M. tuberculosis*, including strains resistant to most other antituberculosis agents, at a minimum inhibitory concentration (MIC) of 1.25–2.5 mg/l in liquid media. MICs are higher (8–16 mg/l) on egg media owing to protein binding. It has not been adequately determined whether the drug is bacteristatic or bactericidal.

Acquired resistance

Resistant strains are cross-resistant to viomycin and partly cross-resistant to aminoglycosides.

Pharmacokinetics

Capreomycin is not absorbed from the intestine and does not readily enter cells or the cerebrospinal fluid (CSF). Intramuscular injection of 1 g gives peak serum concentrations of 20–50 mg/l. It is mostly excreted unchanged in the urine. No metabolites have been described.

Toxicity and side effects

Pain, induration and excessive bleeding may occur at the injection site. Capreomycin is ototoxic, affecting both cochlear and vestibular functions, and nephrotoxic, causing loss of K^+, Ca^{2+} and Mg^{2+}, leading to neuromuscular blockade. Anorexia, thirst and polyuria occasionally occur. These toxic effects are uncommon if the drug is given two or three times weekly. Auditory and vestibular functions and serum potassium levels should be monitored before and regularly during therapy.

Clinical use

- Multidrug resistant tuberculosis (with other antituberculosis drugs).

Preparations and dosage

Proprietary name: Capastat.

Preparation: Injection.

Dosage: Adults, deep i.m. injection, 1 g/day (with a maximum of 20 mg/kg) for 2–4 months, then 1 g 2–3 times a week for the remainder of the therapy.

Limited availability, including the UK and the USA.

Further information

Black HR, Griffith RS, Peabody AM 1966 Absorption, excretion and metabolism of capreomycin in normal and diseased states. *Annals of the New York Academy of Sciences* 135: 974–982.

Heifets L, Lindholm-Levy P 1989 Comparison of bactericidal activities of streptomycin, amikacin, kanamycin and capreomycin against *Mycobacterium avium* and *Mycobacterium tuberculosis*. *Antimicrobial Agents and Chemotherapy* 33: 1298–1301.

Lehmann CR, Garrett LE, Winn RE et al 1988 Capreomycin kinetics in renal impairment and clearance by hemodialysis. *American Review of Respiratory Disease* 138: 1312–1313.

Otten H 1988 Capreomycin. In Bartmann K (ed.) *Antituberculosis drugs* (Handbook of experimental pharmacology, vol 84). Springer, Berlin, pp. 191–197.

CLOFAZIMINE

Molecular weight: 473.4.

One of a number of substituted iminophenazine dyes originally synthesized as potential antituberculosis agents. It is almost insoluble in water. It stimulates various phagocyte functions including release of free oxygen radicals, but it is not clear whether this contributes to its antimicrobial activity. It also has anti-inflammatory properties, probably due to its ability to stimulate prostaglandin E_2 synthesis and release, and this property makes it a useful drug for treating leprosy reactions.

Antimicrobial activity

There is some evidence that clofazimine binds preferentially to mycobacterial DNA on the guanine base, thereby preventing RNA transcription. It has bacteristatic and weak bactericidal activity against several species of mycobacteria and some species of *Actinomyces* and *Nocardia*. In-vitro MICs are: *M. tuberculosis* 0.5 mg/l; *M. scrofulaceum* 0.5 mg/l; *M. leprae* (assayed in a mouse model) 0.1–1 mg/l; *M. avium/intracellulare* 1–2 mg/l; *M. chelonae*, 0.2–4 mg/l, and *M. fortuitum* 0.5–8 mg/l. These MICs have limited clinical relevance as clofazimine shows marked differences in accumulation in various tissues. Activity against *M. leprae* is demonstrable in humans only after 50 days of therapy. Clofazimine-resistance, though reported, appears to be rare.

Pharmacokinetics

Clofazimine is well absorbed by the intestine and is taken up by adipose tissue and cells of the macrophage/monocyte series, including those in the wall of the small intestine. It has a very long half-life (variously estimated as 10–70 days) and is eliminated, mostly unchanged, in the urine and feces.

Toxicity and side effects

Clofazimine is usually well tolerated, but some patients develop nausea, abdominal pain and diarrhea, relieved to some extent by taking the drug with a meal or glass of milk. Dose-related, reversible, skin discoloration is very common and is unac-

ceptable to some patients. Discoloration of the hair, cornea, urine, sweat and tears also occurs. Infants born to mothers receiving clofazimine are reversibly pigmented at birth.

Edema of the wall of the small intestine leading to subacute obstruction is a rare but serious complication of prolonged high-dose therapy for leprosy reactions. Deposition of clofazimine in lymph nodes may interfere with lymphatic drainage, occasionally manifesting as edema of the feet.

Clinical use

- Multibacillary leprosy (in combination with dapsone and rifampicin).
- Erythema nodosum leprosum (anti-inflammatory activity).

Clofazimine has been suggested as a drug for treatment of multidrug resistant tuberculosis, although its efficacy is unproven. It has been used to treat *M. ulcerans* infection (Buruli ulcer) but with limited responses. It was included in regimens for AIDS-related MAC disease, but has largely been abandoned on account of toxicity.

Preparations and dosage

Proprietary name: Lamprene.

Preparation: Capsules.

Dosage: Multibacillary forms of leprosy: adults, oral, 300 mg once a month, supervised, and 50 mg/day or 100 mg on alternate days self-administered. Erythema nodosum leprosum: 300 mg once a day for no longer than 3 months.

Limited availability.

Further information

Anderson R, Zeis BM, Anderson IF 1988 Clofazimine-mediated enhancement of reactive oxidant production by human phagocytes as a possible therapeutic mechanism. *Dermatologia* 176: 234–242.

Anonymous 1999 Clofazimine. In: Dollery C (ed.) *Therapeutic Drugs* 2nd ed. Churchill Livingstone, Edinburgh, pp. C272–C275.

Grange JM 1991 Detection of drug resistance in *Mycobacterium leprae* and the design of treatment regimens for leprosy. In: Heifets L. (ed.) *Drug susceptibility in the chemotherapy of mycobacterial infections*. CRC Press, Boca Raton, FL, pp. 161–177.

Jamet P, Traore I, Husser JA, Ji B 1992 Short-term trial of clofazimine in previously untreated lepromatous leprosy. *International Journal of Leprosy* 60: 542–548.

Oommen ST, Natu MV, Mahajan MK, Kadyan RS 1994 Lymphangiographic evaluation of patients with clinical lepromatous leprosy on clofazimine. *International Journal of Leprosy* 62: 32–36.

Schaad-Lanyi Z, Dieterle W, Dubois JP, Theobold W, Vischer W 1987 Pharmacokinetics of clofazimine in healthy volunteers. *International Journal of Leprosy* 55: 9–15.

Zeis BM, Anderson R 1986 Clofazimine-mediated stimulation of prostaglandin synthesis and free oxygen radical production as novel mechanisms of drug-induced immunosuppression. *International Journal of Immunopharmacology* 8: 731–739.

CYCLOSERINE

Molecular weight: 102.1.

A fermentation product of *Streptomyces orchidaceus* and other organisms. Commercially produced synthetically. Aqueous solutions are stable at pH 7.8 but rapidly destroyed in acid conditions.

Antimicrobial activity

Cycloserine is active against a wide range of Gram-negative and Gram-positive bacteria, including *Staphylococcus aureus*, streptococci, including *Enterococcus faecalis*, a variety of enterobacteria, *Nocardia* and *Chlamydia* spp. *M. tuberculosis*, including streptomycin- and isoniazid-resistant strains, is inhibited by 8–16 mg/l. Environmental mycobacteria, including *M. avium*, are also susceptible. Its action is specifically antagonized by D-alanine, from which media for in-vitro tests should be free.

Acquired resistance

Primary resistance in *M. tuberculosis* is rare and develops only slowly in patients treated with cycloserine alone. Its inclusion in combinations deters the development of resistance to other drugs. There is no cross-resistance with other therapeutic antibiotics.

Pharmacokinetics

Oral absorption	>95%
C_{max} 250 mg oral	10 mg/l after 3–4 h
Plasma half-life	c. 10 h (mean)
Plasma protein binding	<20%

Doubling the dose approximately doubles the plasma level. Some accumulation occurs over the first 3 or 4 days of treatment. In children receiving 20 mg/kg orally, plasma levels of 20–35 mg/l have been found. It is widely distributed throughout the body fluids, including the CSF. About 50% is excreted unchanged in the glomerular filtrate over 24 h and 65–70% over the subsequent 2 days. The remainder is metabolized. There is no tubular secretion and no effect of probenecid. Cycloserine accumulates in renal failure, reaching toxic levels if dosage is uncontrolled. It can be removed by hemodialysis.

Toxicity and side effects

Rarely, rashes, drug fever and cardiac arrhythmia occur. Evidence of central nervous system (CNS) toxicity may develop over the first 2 weeks of treatment. Effects include headache, somnolence, vertigo, visual disturbances, confusion, depression, acute psychotic reactions and tremors. The effects may be exacerbated by alcohol. Treatment should be stopped promptly if any mental or neurological signs develop. Convulsions are said to occur in about 50% of patients when the plasma concentration exceeds 20–25 mg/l, but the relationship to dose is not particularly close. No permanent damage appears to be caused. Cycloserine inhibits mammalian transaminases and this and the convulsant effects of the drug have been attributed to a metabolite, amino-oxyalanine. The drug should be avoided in patients with previous fits or other neurological or psychiatric abnormalities. Peripheral neuritis has been rarely encountered.

Clinical use

- Multidrug resistant tuberculosis and other mycobacterioses (with other antituberculosis drugs).
- Formerly used for urinary tract infection.

 Preparations and dosage

Proprietary name: Cycloserine.

Preparation: Capsules.

Dosage: Adults, oral, 250 mg every 12 h for 2 weeks, with a maximum of 500 mg every 12 h. Children, initially 10 mg/kg per day, adjusted according to blood levels and response.

Limited availability; available in the UK.

Further information

Anonymous. Cycloserine. In: Dollery C (ed.) *Therapeutic Drugs* 2nd ed. Churchill Livingstone, Edinburgh, C355–C358.

DAPSONE

Diaminodiphenyl sulphone (DDS). Molecular weight 248.3.

The most effective of a number of sulfonamide derivatives to be tested against leprosy. The dry powder is very stable. It is only slightly soluble in water.

Antimicrobial activity

Dapsone is active against many bacteria and some protozoa. Fully susceptible strains of *M. leprae* are inhibited by a little as 0.003 mg/l. It is predominantly bacteristatic.

Acquired resistance

Resistance to high levels is acquired by several sequential mutations. As a result of prolonged use of dapsone monotherapy, acquired resistance emerged in patients with multibacillary leprosy in many countries. Initial resistance also occurs in patients with both paucibacillary and multibacillary leprosy. Thus, leprosy should always be treated with multidrug regimens.

Pharmacokinetics

Oral absorption	>90%
C_{max} 100 mg oral	c. 2 mg/l after 3–6 h
Plasma half-life	18–45 h
Plasma protein binding	c. 50%

Dapsone is slowly but almost completely absorbed from the intestine. It is widely distributed in the tissues but is selectively retained in skin, muscle, kidneys and liver. It is metabolized by *N*-oxidation and also by acetylation, which is subject to the same genetic polymorphism as isoniazid (p. 437). The elimination half-life is consequently very variable, but on standard therapy the trough levels are always well in excess of the inhibitory concentrations.

Dapsone is mostly excreted in the urine: in the unchanged form (20%), as *N*-oxidation products (30%), and as other metabolites.

Toxicity and side effects

Although dapsone is usually well tolerated at standard doses, gastrointestinal upsets, anorexia, headaches, dizziness and insomnia may occur. Less frequent reactions include skin rashes and photosensitivity, peripheral neuropathy, psychoses, hepatitis, nephrotic syndrome and generalized lymphadenopathy.

The term 'dapsone syndrome' is applied to a skin rash and fever occurring 2–8 weeks after starting therapy and sometimes accompanied by lymphadenopathy, hepatomegaly, jaundice and/or mononucleosis.

Blood disorders include anemia, methemoglobinemia, sulfhemoglobinemia, hemolysis (notably in patients with glucose-6-phosphate dehydrogenase deficiency), mononucleosis and, rarely, agranulocytosis. Severe anemia should be treated before patients receive dapsone.

There is some evidence that the incidence of adverse reactions declined in the 1960s but reappeared around 1982, the time when multidrug therapy was introduced, and may represent an unexplained drug interaction with rifampicin.

Clinical use

- Leprosy (multidrug regimens).
- Prophylaxis of malaria; treatment of chloroquine-resistant malaria (in combination with pyrimethamine).
- Prophylaxis of toxoplasmosis (in combination with pyrimethamine).
- Prophylaxis and therapy of *Pneumocystis carinii* pneumonia (in combination with trimethoprim).
- Dermatitis herpetiformis and related skin disorders.

Preparations and dosage

Preparation: Tablets.

Dosage: Paucibacillary leprosy (in combination with rifampicin): Adults, oral, 100 mg/day, children 1–2 mg/kg daily, for at least 6 months. Multibacillary leprosy (in combination with rifampicin and clofazimine), adults, 100 mg/day; children, 1–2 mg/kg daily, for at least 2 years.

Limited availability in Europe and the USA.

Further information

Ahrens EM, Meckler RJ, Callen JP 1986 Dapsone-induced peripheral neuropathy. *International Journal of Dermatology* 25: 314–316.

Anonymous 1999 Dapsone. In: Dollery C (ed.) *Therapeutic Drugs* 2nd edn. Churchill Livingstone, Edinburgh, pp. D13–D18.

Byrd SR, Gelber RH 1991 Effect of dapsone on haemoglobin concentration in patients with leprosy. *Leprosy Review* 62: 171–178.

Johnson DA, Cattau EL, Kuritsky JN, Zimmerman HJ 1986 Liver involvement in the sulphone syndrome. *Archives of Internal Medicine* 146: 875–877.

Kromann NP, Vihelmsen R, Stahl D 1982 The dapsone syndrome. *Archives of Dermatology* 118: 531–532.

Rai PP, Aschhoff M, Lilly L, Balakrishnan S 1988 Influence of acetylator phenotype of the leprosy patient on the emergence of dapsone resistant leprosy. *Indian Journal of Leprosy* 60: 400–406.

Rastogi N, Goh KS, Labrousse V 1993 Activity of subinhibitory concentrations of dapsone alone and in combination with cell wall inhibitors against *Mycobacterium avium* complex organisms. *European Journal of Clinical Microbiology* 12: 954–958.

Richardus JH, Smith TC 1989 Increased incidence in leprosy of hypersensitivity reactions to dapsone after introduction of multidrug therapy. *Leprosy Review* 60: 267–273.

Zuidema J, Hilbers-Modderman ES, Merkus FW 1986 Clinical pharmacokinetics of dapsone. *Clinical Pharmacokinetics* 11: 299–315.

ETHAMBUTOL

Hydroxymethylpropylethylene diamine. Molecular weight (dihydrochloride): 277.2.

$$CH_2OH \qquad\qquad C_2H_5$$
$$|\qquad\qquad\qquad\qquad |$$
$$HC - NH - CH_2 - CH_2 - NH - CH$$
$$|\qquad\qquad\qquad\qquad |$$
$$C_2H_5 \qquad\qquad CH_2OH$$

A synthetic ethylenediamine derivative formulated as the dihydrochloride for oral administration. The dry powder is very soluble and stable.

Antimicrobial activity

Ethambutol is active against several species of mycobacteria and nocardiae. MICs on solid media are: *M. tuberculosis* 0.5–2 mg/l; *M. kansasii* 1–4 mg/l; other slowly growing mycobacteria 2–8 mg/l; rapidly growing pathogens 2–16 mg/l; *Nocardia* spp. 8–32 mg/l. There is some evidence that ethambutol may enhance the activity of some of the other antimycobacterial drugs by affecting mycobacterial cell wall permeability. Resistance is uncommon.

Pharmacokinetics

Oral absorption	c. 80%
C_{max} 25 mg/kg oral	2.6–5 mg/l after 2 h
Plasma half-life	10–15 h
Volume of distribution	3.9 l/kg
Plasma protein binding	10–40%

Absorption is impeded by aluminum hydroxide and alcohol. It is concentrated in the phagolysosomes of alveolar macrophages. It does not enter the CSF in health but CSF levels of 25–40% of the plasma concentration, with considerable variation between patients, are achieved in cases of tuberculous meningitis.

Various metabolites are produced, including dialdehyde, dicarboxylic acid and glucuronide derivatives. About 90% is excreted in the urine, mostly unchanged, but 10–15% is excreted as metabolites.

Toxicity and side effects

The most important side effect is optic neuritis, which may be irreversible if treatment is not discontinued. This complication is rare if the higher dose (25 mg/kg) is given for no more than 2 months. National codes of practice for prevention of ocular toxicity should be adhered to; in particular, patients should be advised to stop therapy and seek medical advice if they notice any change in visual acuity, peripheral vision or color perception, and the drug should not be given to young children and others unable to comply with this advice.

Other side effects include peripheral neuritis, arthralgia, hyperuricemia, rashes and, rarely, thrombocytopenia and jaundice.

Clinical use

- Tuberculosis (initial intensive phase of short course therapy).
- Other mycobacterioses (*M. kansasii, M. xenopi, M. malmoense* and the *M. avium* complex) (with rifampicin and isoniazid).

Preparations and dosage

Proprietary names: Myambutol.

Preparations: Tablets (and syrup on special request).

Dosage: Adults and children, oral, 15–25 mg/kg daily for 2 months or 25–30 mg/kg three times a week or 45–50 mg/kg twice a week. If more prolonged therapy is indicated, the daily dose should not exceed 15 mg/kg; retreatment 25 mg/kg daily in first 60 days.

Widely available.

Further information

Anonymous. Ethambutol (hydrochloride). In: Dollery C (ed.) *Therapeutic Drugs* 2nd ed. Churchill Livingstone, Edinburgh, E68–E72.

Citron KM 1986 Ocular toxicity from ethambutol. *Thorax* 41: 737–739.

Hoffner SE, Kallenius G, Beezer AE, Svenson SB 1989 Studies on the mechanisms of the synergistic effects of ethambutol and other antibacterial drugs on *Mycobacterium avium* complex. *Acta Leprologica* 7 (Suppl. 1): 195–199.

Khanna BK, Gupta VP, Singh VP 1984 Ethambutol-induced hyperuricaemia. *Tubercle* 65: 215–217.

Prasad R, Mukerji PK 1989 Ethambutol-induced thrombocytopenia. *Tubercle* 70: 211–212.

Sarren M, Khuller GK 1990 Cell wall and membrane changes associated with ethambutol resistance in *Mycobacterium tuberculosis* H37Rv. *Antimicrobial Agents and Chemotherapy* 34: 1773–1776.

ETHIONAMIDE

Ethylthioisonicotinamide. Molecular weight: 166.2.

One of a number of synthetic nicotinamide analogs found to have antituberculosis activity, following the observation that nicotinamide inhibited the replication of *M. tuberculosis*. It is almost insoluble in water and is unstable on exposure to light

Antimicrobial activity

The MIC for *M. tuberculosis* on solid egg media is 0.8–1.6 mg/l; MICs for the *M. avium* complex, *M. kansasii* and *M. malmoense* are similar. Resistant strains show cross-resistance to protionamide and thiacetazone. Although resistance is associated with mutations in the *inhA* gene encoding for long-chain enoyl-ACP reductase, cross-resistance to isoniazid does not usually develop.

Pharmacokinetics

Oral absorption	>90%
C_max 250 mg oral (enteric coated)	1.8 mg/l after 2–3 h
Plasma half-life	1.8–2.4 h
Plasma protein binding	c. 30%

The uncoated drug is well absorbed from the intestine but not well tolerated. Enteric-coated tablets, though better tolerated, produce serum levels about half those found after ingestion of uncoated drug. CSF concentrations approach the unbound plasma levels. Ethionamide is degraded in the liver to up to seven metabolites, including a biologically active sulfoxide and various inert compounds including nicotinic acid. Less than 1% is excreted unchanged in the urine and about 1.2% is excreted as the sulfoxide metabolite.

Toxicity and side effects

The principal side effect is gastric irritation, which is more common in adults and women. This effect is reduced by commencing with a low dose and gradually increasing to the full dose, by the use of antacids and by taking the drug at bedtime. Hypersensitivity reactions and hepatitis also occur. Rare effects include hypothyroidism, menstrual irregularities, alopecia, convulsions, deafness, diplopia, peripheral neuropathy, mental disturbances (including depression) and, in male patients, impotence and gynecomastia.

Clinical use

- Multidrug resistant tuberculosis (with other antituberculosis drugs).
- Short-course (13 week) regimens for multibacillary leprosy, (with rifampicin and either dapsone or clofazimine).

Preparations and dosage

Proprietary name: Trecator.

Preparation: Tablets.

Dosage: Adult, oral, 500 mg/kg per day in divided doses, with meals. Children, 12–15 mg/kg per day to a maximum of 750 mg in divided doses, with meals.

Limited availability, not available in the UK.

Further information

Anonymous 1999 Ethionamide. In: Dollery C (ed.) *Therapeutic Drugs* 2nd edn. Churchill Livingstone, Edinburgh, pp. E81–E84.

Donald PR, Seifart HI 1989 Cerebrospinal fluid concentrations of ethionamide in children with tuberculous meningitis. *Journal of Pediatrics* 115: 483–486.

Jenner PJ, Ellard GA, Gruer PJK, Aber VR 1984 Plasma levels and urinary excretion of ethionamide and prothionamide in man. *Journal of Antimicrobial Chemotherapy* 13: 267–277.

Pattyn SR, Groenen G, Janssens L, Kuykens L, Mputu LB 1992 Treatment of multibacillary leprosy with a regimen of 13 weeks duration. *Leprosy Review* 63: 41–46.

ISONIAZID

Isonicotinic acid hydrazide; INH. Molecular weight: 137.1.

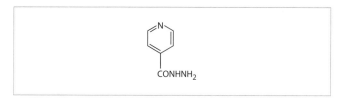

One of a number of nicotinamide analogs found to have antituberculosis activity, following the observation that nicotinamide inhibited the replication of *M. tuberculosis*. It is soluble in water. The dry powder is stable if protected from light.

Antimicrobial activity

Susceptibility to isoniazid is virtually restricted to the *M. tuberculosis* complex (MIC 0.01–0.2 mg/l). It is highly bactericidal against actively replicating *M. tuberculosis*. Other mycobacteria are resistant, except for some strains of *M. xenopi* (MIC 0.2 mg/l) and a minority of strains of *M. kansasii* (MIC 1 mg/l).

Acquired resistance

Several mutational changes induce isoniazid resistance (Table 36.1; p. 428) and the predominant mutation(s) show geographical variations in their distribution. Some resistant strains of *M. tuberculosis* lack catalase-peroxidase activity due to point mutations in, or deletion of, the *katG* gene encoding this enzyme. Conversely, many strains from south India have weak or no catalase-peroxidase activity, but are fully susceptible to isoniazid.

Worldwide, isoniazid resistance is one of the two most frequently encountered forms of drug resistance in *M. tuberculosis*; the other being streptomycin resistance. Almost all multiple resistant strains are resistant to isoniazid (*see* p. 428).

Pharmacokinetics

Oral absorption	>95%
C_max 300 mg oral	3–5 mg/l after 1–2 h
Plasma half-life	0.5–1.5 h (rapid acetylators)
	2–4 h (slow acetylators)
Volume of distribution	0.6–0.8 l/kg
Plasma protein binding	Very low

Absorption and distribution

Isoniazid is almost completely absorbed and is well distributed. Absorption is impaired by aluminum hydroxide. Therapeutic concentrations are achieved in sputum and CSF. It crosses the placenta and is found in breast milk.

Metabolism

Isoniazid is extensively metabolized to a variety of pharmacologically inactive derivatives, predominantly by acetylation. As a result of genetic polymorphism, patients are divisible into rapid and slow acetylators. About 50% of Caucasians and Blacks, but 80–90% of Chinese and Japanese, are rapid acetylators. Acetylation status does not affect the efficacy of daily-administered therapy. The rate of acetylation is reduced in chronic renal failure.

Excretion

Nearly all the dose is excreted into urine within 24 h, as unchanged drug and metabolic products.

Toxicity and side effects

Toxic effects are unusual on recommended doses and are more frequent in slow acetylators. Many side effects are neurological, including restlessness, insomnia, muscle twitching and difficulty in starting micturition. More serious but less common neurological side effects include peripheral neuropathy, optic neuritis, encephalopathy and a range of psychiatric disorders, including anxiety, depression and paranoia.

Neurotoxicity is usually preventable by giving pyridoxine (vitamin B_6) 10 mg/day. Pyridoxine should be given to patients with liver disease, pregnant women, alcoholics, renal dialysis patients, HIV-positive patients, the malnourished and the elderly. Encephalopathy, which has been reported in patients on renal dialysis, may not be prevented by, or respond to, pyridoxine, but usually resolves on withdrawal of isoniazid.

Isoniazid-related hepatitis occurs in about 1% of patients receiving standard short-course chemotherapy. The incidence is unaffected by acetylator status. It is more common in those aged over 35 years and isoniazid prophylaxis should be used with care in older people.

Other less common side effects include arthralgia, a 'flu'-like syndrome, hypersensitivity reactions with fever, rashes and, sometimes, eosinophilia, sideroblastic anemia, pellagra (which responds to treatment with nicotinic acid) and hemolysis in patients with glucose-6-phosphate dehydrogenase deficiency. It exacerbates acute porphyria and induces antinuclear antibodies, but overt systemic lupus erythematosus is rare.

Drug interactions

Isoniazid increases the plasma concentrations of the antiepileptics phenytoin and carbamazepine, sometimes enough to cause toxicity. It enhances the defluorination of the anesthetic enflurane. Drug interactions may be more pronounced in slow acetylators. Antiepileptic therapy requires monitoring and adjustment of dosage as necessary. Prednisolone reduces isoniazid levels in both slow and rapid acetylators, but the mechanism is unclear.

Clinical use

* Tuberculosis (intensive and continuation phases).
* Prevention of primary tuberculosis in close contacts and reactivation disease in infected but healthy persons (monotherapy).

Preparations and dosage

Proprietary name: Rimifon.

Preparations: Tablets, elixir and injectable form (Nydrazid).

Dosage: Unsupervised: adults, oral, 300 mg/day; children, 5–10 mg/kg daily with a maximum dose of 300 mg/day. Supervised: adults and children, 15–20 mg/kg 2–3 times a week. Adults, i.m., i.v., 200–300 mg as a single daily dose. Children, 10–20 mg/kg daily with a maximum of 300 mg/day. Neonates, 3–5 mg/kg daily, with a maximum of 10 mg/kg daily.

Widely available.

Further information

Anonymous 1999 Isoniazid. In: Dollery C (ed.) *Therapeutic Drugs* 2nd ed. Churchill Livingstone, Edinburgh, I92–I100.

Banerjee A, Dubnau E, Quemard A et al 1994 *InhA*, a gene encoding a target for isoniazid and ethionamide in *Mycobacterium tuberculosis*. *Science* 263: 227–230.

Cheung WC, Lo CY, Lo WK, Ip M, Cheng IKP 1993 Isoniazid induced encephalopathy in dialysis patients. *Tubercle and Lung Disease* 74: 136–139.

Ellard GA 1984 The potential clinical significance of the isoniazid acetylator phenotype in the treatment of pulmonary tuberculosis. *Tubercle* 65: 211–217.

Grosset J 1990/1991 New experimental regimens for preventive therapy of tuberculosis. *Bulletin of the International Union Against Tuberculosis and Lung Disease* 66 (Suppl. 1990/1991): 15–16.

Holdiness MR 1987 Neurological manifestations and toxicities of the antituberculosis drugs. *Medical Toxicology* 2: 33–51.

Israel HL 1993 Chemoprophylaxis for tuberculosis. *Respiratory Medicine* 87: 81–83.

Israel HL, Gottleib JE, Maddrey WC 1992 Perspective: preventive isoniazid therapy and the liver. *Chest* 101: 1298–1301.

Lee H, Cho SN, Bang HE, Lee JH, Bai GH, Kim SJ, Kim JD 2000 Exclusive mutations related to isoniazid and ethionamide resistance among *Mycobacterium tuberculosis* isolates from Korea. *International Journal of Tuberculosis and Lung Disease* 4: 441–447.

Snider DE, Tabas GJ 1992 Isoniazid associated hepatitis deaths: a review of available information. *American Review of Respiratory Disease* 145: 494–497.

Statement: International Union Against Tuberculosis and Lung Disease/World Health Organization 1994 Tuberculosis preventive therapy in HIV-infected individuals. *Tubercle and Lung Disease* 75: 96–98.

Tsukamura M 1990 In vitro bacteriostatic and bactericidal activity of isoniazid on the *Mycobacterium avium–Mycobacterium intracellulare* complex. *Tubercle* 71: 199–204.

Weber WW 1986 The molecular basis of hereditary acetylation polymorphism. *Drug Metabolism and Disposition* 14: 377–381.

PROTIONAMIDE

Prothionamide; propylthioisonicotinamide. Molecular weight: 180.29.

Structurally closely related to ethionamide, but with a propyl group replacing the ethyl substituent. The antibacterial activity and pharmacokinetics of the two drugs are almost identical, but protionamide is said to be better tolerated. It is seldom used in tuberculosis, but is used in place of clofazimine for the treatment of leprosy in patients who find skin pigmentation caused by that drug unacceptable. As gastric irritation often leads to non-compliance, supervised therapy is recommended. If given simultaneously with isoniazid, the blood level of protionamide may be raised, resulting in more side effects unless the dosage is adjusted.

Preparations and dosage

Proprietary names: Peteha.

Preparations: Tablets, injection, suppositories.

Dosage: Adults, oral, 500 mg/kg per day in divided doses, with meals. Children, 12–15 mg/kg per day to a maximum of 750 mg in divided doses, with meals.

Very limited availability; not available in the UK.

Further information

(*see also* ethionamide p. 435)

Anonymous 1999 Protionamide. In: Dollery C (ed.) *Therapeutic Drugs* 2nd edn. Churchill Livingstone, Edinburgh, pp. P270–P273.

Ellard GA, Kiran KU, Stanley JNA 1988 Long-term prothionamide compliance: a study carried out in India using a combined formulation containing prothionamide, dapsone and isoniazid. *Leprosy Review* 59: 163–175.

PYRAZINAMIDE

Pyrazinoic acid amide. Molecular weight 123.1.

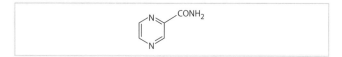

One of a number of synthetic nicotinamide analogs found to have antituberculosis activity, following the observation that nicotinamide inhibited the replication of *M. tuberculosis*.

Antimicrobial activity

Its activity against *M. tuberculosis* is highly pH dependent. At pH 5.6 the MIC is 8–16 mg/l, but it is almost inactive at neutral pH. Other mycobacterial species, including *M. bovis*, are resistant. Its activity requires its conversion to pyrazinoic acid by the mycobacterial enzyme pyrazinamidase, encoded for by the *pncA* gene, which is present in *M. tuberculosis* but not *M. bovis*. Pyrazinamide is principally active against actively metabolizing intracellular bacilli and those in acidic, anoxic inflammatory lesions.

Acquired resistance

Drug resistance is uncommon and cross-resistance to other antituberculosis agents does not occur. Susceptibility testing is technically demanding as it requires very careful control of the pH of the medium. As resistant mutants lose pyrazinamidase activity, tests for this activity offer an alternative to conventional susceptibility testing.

Pharmacokinetics

Oral absorption	>90%
C_{max} 20–22 mg/kg oral	10–50 mg/l after 2 h
Plasma half-life	c. 10 h
Plasma protein binding	c. 50%

Pyrazinamide readily crosses the blood–brain barrier, achieving CSF concentrations similar to plasma levels. It is metabolized to pyrazinoic acid in the liver and oxidized to inactive metabolites, which are excreted in the urine.

Toxicity and side effects

It is usually well tolerated. Moderate elevations of serum transaminases occur early in treatment. Severe hepatotoxicity is uncommon with standard dosage, except in patients with pre-existing liver disease.

Its principal metabolite, pyrazinoic acid, inhibits renal excretion of uric acid, occasionally causing gout requiring treatment with allopurinol. An unrelated arthralgia, notably of the shoulders and responsive to analgesics, also occurs.

Other side effects include anorexia, nausea, mild flushing of the skin and photosensitization.

Clinical use

- Tuberculosis (early, intensive, phase of therapy).

Preparations and dosage

Proprietary name: Zinamide.

Preparation: Tablets.

Dosage: Adult, oral, 2 g/day (over 50 kg), 1.5 g/day (under 50 kg); children, 35 mg/kg daily, in 3–4 divided doses. Alternatively, adults and children, oral, 50 mg/kg three times a week or up to 75 mg/kg twice a week.

Widely available.

Further information

Anonymous 1999 Pyrazinamide. In: Dollery C (ed.) *Therapeutic Drugs* 2nd edn. Churchill Livingstone, Edinburgh, pp. P287–P289.

Jain A, Mehta VL, Kulshrestha S 1993 Effect of pyrazinamide on rifampicin kinetics in patients with tuberculosis. *Tubercle and Lung Disease* 74: 87–90.

Lacroix C, Hoang TP, Nouveau J et al 1989 Pharmacokinetics of pyrazinamide and its metabolites in healthy subjects. *European Journal of Clinical Pharmacology* 36: 395–400.

Stamatakis G, Montes C, Trouvin JH et al 1988 Pyrazinamide and pyrazinoic acid pharmacokinetics in patients with chronic renal failure. *Clinical Nephrology* 30: 230–234.

Sun Z, Scorpio A, Zhang Y 1997 The *pycA* gene from naturally pyrazinamide-resistant *Mycobacterium avium* encodes pyrazinamidase and confers pyrazinamide susceptibility to resistant *M. tuberculosis* complex organisms. *Microbiology* 143: 3367–3373.

Trivedi S 1987 Pyrazinamidase activity of *Mycobacterium tuberculosis* – a test of sensitivity to pyrazinamide. *Tubercle* 68: 221–224.

 # THIACETAZONE

Thioacetazone; acetylaminobenzaldehyde thiosemicarbazone. Molecular weight: 236.3.

$$CH_3COHN-\bigcirc-CH=N_2HCSNH_2$$

A synthetic compound discovered during initial work on the sulfonamides, to which it is structurally related. It is only slightly soluble in water.

Antimicrobial activity

M. tuberculosis is inhibited by 0.5–1 mg/l in Dubos Tween–albumin liquid medium, but in-vitro MICs vary considerably according to the medium used and bear little relation to in-vivo efficacy. Many strains of *M. tuberculosis* isolated in East Africa, India and Hong Kong are naturally more resistant than strains from Europe. Acquired resistance, as a result of the use of monotherapy, is prevalent in the developing countries. Resistance develops rapidly in *M. leprae*.

Pharmacokinetics

Oral absorption	Good
C_{max} 100 mg oral	1–4 mg/l after 2–4 h
Plasma half-life	8–12 h
Plasma protein binding	c. 95%

Little information is available about the distribution of the drug. Several metabolites are described. About 20% is eliminated in the urine; the fate of the remainder is unknown.

Toxicity and side effects

Rashes are common, occurring in 2–4% of patients in Africa but much more frequently in those of Chinese ethnic origin. More severe skin reactions, exfoliative dermatitis and Stevens–Johnson syndrome occur in less than 0.5% of patients, but there is a 10-fold increase of these reactions in HIV-positive patients, proving fatal in up to 3% of such patients.

Other common side effects include gastrointestinal reactions, vertigo and conjunctivitis. Less common reactions include hepatitis, erythema multiforme, hemolytic anemia and, rarely, agranulocytosis. Prolonged therapy may rarely lead to hypertrichosis, gynecomastia and osteoporosis.

Clinical use

- Tuberculosis (with other antituberculosis drugs).

Thiacetazone has the single virtue of low cost. Owing to its low efficacy and frequent serious side effects, it should be avoided whenever possible and must never knowingly be given to an HIV-positive person. It has been evaluated in leprosy but abandoned because of the high incidence of side effects and rapid emergence of drug resistance.

 ### Preparations and dosage

Preparation: Tablets.

Dosage: Adults, oral, 150 mg/day. Children, 4 mg/kg to a maximum of 150 mg/day. Limited availability.

 ### Further information

Anonymous. Thiacetazone. In Dollery C (ed.) *Therapeutic Drugs* 2nd edn. Churchill Livingstone, Edinburgh, pp. T83–T86.

Heifets LB, Lindholm-Levy PJ, Flory M 1990 Thiacetazone in vitro activity against *Mycobacterium avium* and *M. tuberculosis*. *Tubercle* 71: 287–292.

Lawn SD, Griffin GE 2000 Further consequences of thiacetazone-induced cutaneous reactions. *International Journal of Tuberculosis and Lung Disease* 4: 92–93.

Okwera A, Johnson JL, Vjecha MJ et al 1997 Risk factors for adverse drug reactions during thiacetazone treatment of pulmonary tuberculosis in human immunodeficiency virus infected adults. *International Journal of Tuberculosis and Lung Disease* 1: 441–445.

 # VIOMYCIN

A basic hexapeptide with properties resembling those of capreomycin, to which it is structurally related. It is produced by several species of *Streptomyces* and is supplied as the sulfate.

Viomycin inhibits *M. tuberculosis* at concentrations of 2–12 mg/l. Although data are limited, other mycobacteria appear less susceptible. Resistance rapidly develops, with complete cross-resistance to capreomycin and one-way cross-resistance to streptomycin and kanamycin; strains resistant to streptomycin and kanamycin are usually susceptible to viomycin. It shows synergy with isoniazid against *M. tuberculosis*.

Low-level resistance, and cross-resistance to capreomycin, results from mutations in genes coding for the 50S (*vicA*) or 30S (*vicB*) ribosomal subunits. High-level resistance results from mutations in the *vicA* and *str* (streptomycin resistance) genes or in the *vicB* and both the *str* and *nek* (neomycin and kanamycin) genes. Thus cross-resistance with these aminoglycosides occurs.

It is not absorbed from the intestine. An intramuscular dose of 1 g produces peak plasma concentrations of around 42 mg/l at 2 h after injection. Viomycin is distributed in the extracellular space, does not pass the blood–brain barrier readily and is mostly excreted unchanged in the urine.

Side effects include ototoxicity, leading to deafness and giddiness, and nephrotoxicity. The incidence of these effects is greatly reduced by giving the drug on only two or three days each week.

It is now rarely used and is of very limited availability.

 Further information

McClatchy JK, Kanes W, Davidson PT, Moulding TS 1977 Cross resistance in *M. tuberculosis* to kanamycin, capreomycin and viomycin. *Tubercle* 58: 29–34.

37 Anthelmintics

G. A. Conder

The helminths, or parasitic worms, comprise the nematodes (roundworms), trematodes (flukes), cestodes (tapeworms) and acanthocephalans (thorny-headed worms). No new class of anthelmintic has come to the market in recent years and few companies are searching for new ones, particularly for use in human medicine. Most anthelmintics were discovered and developed for use in the veterinary field, where helminths significantly impact health and productivity. Commercial competition has produced a steady supply of new compounds for the veterinarian, although these generally have been from the same chemical class (same mode of action) as previously available compounds.

Despite the fact that no new class of anthelmintics has entered the market for many years, satisfactory results can be achieved with current products for nearly all helminth infections. Side effects usually include gastrointestinal upsets, but these are as likely to be related to the worm burden as to the drug. As helminths are often large and/or present in large numbers, their death and disintegration after chemotherapy can result in an obstruction or an allergic–anaphylactic type reaction, particularly given the superb activity of modern anthelmintics.

The biggest problems still remaining to be solved are treatment of infections with larval cestodes, especially *Echinococcus* spp., and macrofilarial stages in filarial infections. There is no satisfactory drug against larval cestodes; benzimidazole carbamates have useful activity but they are poorly absorbed from the gut when administered orally and painful injection-site reactions preclude parenteral use.

Another problem is the treatment of disseminated strongyloidiasis. This condition occurs when patients with a latent infection are immunosuppressed. The parasite, *Strongyloides stercoralis*, multiplies until the host is overwhelmed with worms in all tissues, as a result of autoinfection. The drug of choice is albendazole, and although tiabendazole (thiabendazole) is also useful, it has such unpleasant side effects that its use in patients who are already sick is a problem. No satisfactory chemotherapy is available to treat Guinea worm (*Dracunculus medinensis*) infection.

Although drug resistance is common in the veterinary field it has not been a problem in human medicine, except with regard to schistosomiasis where resistance is known for hycanthone and praziquantel. This discrepancy is because anthelmintics are very widely and frequently used in the veterinary world but much less so in human medicine, in part due to the poverty of most of the people who are infected. With increasing wealth in tropical countries where these infections are common, anthelmintics are being used much more widely and there is concern that drug resistance will develop.

 Further information

Campbell WC, Rew RS 1986 *Chemotherapy of parasitic diseases*. Plenum Press, New York.

Cioli D, Pica-Mattoccia L, Archer S 1995 Antischistosomal drugs: Past, present … and future? *Pharmacology and Therapeutics* 68: 35–85.

Conder GA 2001 Chemical control of animal-parasitic nematodes. In: Lee D (ed.) *The biology of nematodes*. Taylor & Francis, London, pp. 521–529.

Gustafsson LL, Beermann B, Abdi YA 1987 *Handbook of drugs for tropical parasitic infections*. Taylor & Francis, London.

James DM, Gilles HM 1985 *Human antiparasitic drugs. Pharmacology and usage*. Wiley, Chichester.

Vanden Bossche H, Thienpont D, Janssens PG 1985 *Chemotherapy of gastrointestinal helminths*. Springer-Verlag, Berlin.

World Health Organization 1995 *WHO model prescribing information. Drugs used in parasitic diseases*, 2nd edn. WHO, Geneva.

BENZIMIDAZOLES

These synthetic compounds exhibit useful activity against cestodes, trematodes and nematodes. They are widely used in veterinary medicine. The first compound of this class to be marketed for human use, tiabendazole (thiabendazole), has been largely superseded by the benzimidazole carbamates, especially albendazole and mebendazole.

ACQUIRED RESISTANCE

There are no published records of any human nematode developing resistance to benzimidazole derivatives. However, one patient with persistent and recurring *Enterobius vermicularis* (pinworm) infection failed to respond to a 5-day course of mebendazole but was subsequently cured with albendazole.

Since mebendazole is now available without prescription in some countries, there is a risk that resistance may develop in patients who do not complete the full course of treatment and such resistance may extend to related benzimidazoles. Experience in the veterinary world shows that if resistance to one benzimidazole occurs the parasite very rapidly becomes resistant to all members of the class.

 Further information

Various authors 1990 Benzimidazole anthelmintics. *Parasitology Today* 6: 106–136.

 ALBENDAZOLE

Molecular weight: 265.33.

$$CH_3CH_2CH_2S \quad \text{benzimidazole} \quad NHCOOCH_3$$

A benzimidazole carbamic acid methyl ester available for oral administration. Insoluble in water, soluble in dimethyl sulfoxide. Stable at room temperature.

Anthelmintic activity

Activity against the common intestinal nematodes is shown in Table 37.1. Albendazole is active against trichostrongyles and exhibits useful activity against tissue-dwelling larvae of *Trichinella spiralis*, larvae of animal hookworms (causing cutaneous larva migrans), and microfilariae of various filarial species. It also exhibits some activity against cysticercosis and hydatid stages of *Echinococcus granulosus* and *Echinococcus multilocularis*. It has been successfully used in infections with the protozoon *Giardia lamblia* and for microsporidiosis.

Pharmacokinetics

Albendazole is rather better absorbed after oral absorption than the other benzimidazole carbamates. It is extensively metabolized to the anthelmintically active albendazole sulfoxide, producing plasma concentrations of the metabolite of about 1.31 mg/l 2–5 h after a 400 mg oral dose. The half-life is about 8 h and the major route of excretion is via the bile. Plasma protein binding of the sulfoxide is around 70%.

Toxicity and side effects

Various intestinal and other upsets of a mild nature which resolved without treatment have been reported, but similar numbers were reported by patients who were given a placebo in double-blind trials. With extended use as for larval tapeworm infections, hepatic abnormalities or leukopenia may require discontinuation of treatment. In rare cases granulocytopenia, pancytopenia, agranulocytosis or thrombocytopenia may occur. It should not be given during pregnancy since it may cause fetal harm; women should be cautioned against becoming pregnant within a month of completing treatment.

Clinical use

- Intestinal worm infections.
- Trichinosis (including chronic stage).
- Cutaneous larva migrans.
- Hydatid disease (as an adjunct, or alternative, to surgery).
- Neurocysticercosis.
- Lymphatic filariasis (alone or in combination with ivermectin).
- Giardiasis.
- Microsporidiosis.

Table 37.1 Activity of currently used anthelmintics against common intestinal nematodes

Agent	*Enterobius vermicularis*	*Ascaris lumbricoides*	*Ancylostoma duodenale*	*Necator americanus*	*Strongyloides stercoralis*	*Trichuris trichiura*
Piperazine	++	+++	–	–	–	–
Levamisole	–	+++	+++	+++	–	–
Pyrantel	+++	+++	+++	++	–	–
Mebendazole	+++	+++	+++	+++	++	++
Albendazole	+++	+++	+++	+++	++	++
Ivermectin	+	+++	+	+	+++	+

+++, Highly effective; ++, moderately effective; +, poorly effective; –, no useful activity.

Preparations and dosage

Proprietary names: Albenza, Eskazole, Paranthil, Zentel.

Preparation: Tablets, 200 or 400 mg.

Dosage

Ascariasis, pinworm, hookworms, trichostrongyliasis: 400 mg as a single oral dose; for pinworm, a second dose may be needed after 2–3 weeks.

Strongyloidiasis, whipworm: 400 mg orally on each of three consecutive days.

Echinococcosis: therapy, presurgery, or postsurgery, 60 kg or greater, 400 mg twice daily orally with meals for 28 days followed by 14 tablet-free days; up to three cycles of treatment may be given; less than 60 kg, 15 mg/kg/day orally in divided doses twice daily with meals (800 mg/day maximum).

Neurocysticercosis: 60 kg or greater, 400 mg twice daily orally with meals for 8–30 days; less than 60 kg, 15 mg/kg/day orally in two divided doses with meals (800 mg/day maximum).

Widely available.

Further information

Anonymous 1999 Albendazole. In: Dollery C (ed.) *Therapeutic Drugs* 2nd edn. Churchill Livingstone, Edinburgh pp. A51–A56.

Firth M 1983 Albendazole in helminthiasis. Royal Society of Medicine, International Congress and Symposium Series, Number 57. Royal Society of Medicine, London.

Horton J 2000 Albendazole: a review of anthelmintic efficacy and safety in humans. *Parasitology* 121: S113–S132.

Teggi A, Lastilla MG, De Rosa F 1993 Therapy of hydatid disease with mebendazole and albendazole. *Antimicrobial Agents and Chemotherapy* 37: 1679–1684.

FLUBENDAZOLE

Molecular weight: 313.28.

A benzimidazole carbamate used in some countries in place of mebendazole for the treatment of ascariasis. It is even less well absorbed after oral administration than mebendazole.

Preparations and dosage

Dosage: Adults and children, oral, enterobiasis, 100 mg as a single dose, repeated if necessary after 2–3 weeks. Ascariasis, trichuriasis and hookworm, 100 mg twice daily on three consecutive days.

Limited availability.

MEBENDAZOLE

Molecular weight: 295.29.

A benzimidazole carbamic acid methyl ester available for oral administration. It is insoluble in water and stable at room temperature.

Anthelmintic activity

Activity against common intestinal nematodes is shown in Table 37.1.

Pharmacokinetics

Oral absorption is poor. Plasma concentrations achieved after oral administration of 100 mg twice daily for three consecutive days do not exceed 0.03 mg/l. All metabolites are inactive. Most of the dose, as unchanged drug or a primary metabolite, is retained in the intestinal tract and passed in the feces, with the remainder, approximately 2% of the dose, being excreted in the urine.

Toxicity and side effects

Diarrhea and gastrointestinal discomfort may occur, but adverse reactions are generally mild. Woman of childbearing age should be informed of a potential risk to the fetus if treated during pregnancy, particularly during the first trimester.

Clinical use

- Intestinal nematode infections.
- Trichinosis (larval stage).

Preparations and dosage

Proprietary name: Vermox (many others).

Preparations: Tablets, 100 mg; suspension 100 mg/5 ml

Dosage: Adults and children >2 years, not recommended for children <2 years of age.

Pinworm: 100 mg as a single dose; if reinfection occurs a second dose may be needed after 2–3 weeks.

Ascariasis, hookworms, and whipworm: 100 mg twice daily for three consecutive days.

Widely available.

Further information

Anonymous 1999 Mebendazole. In: Dollery C (ed.) *Therapeutic Drugs* 2nd edn. Churchill Livingstone, Edinburgh, pp. M12–M15.

TIABENDAZOLE

Thiabendazole. Molecular weight: 201.26.

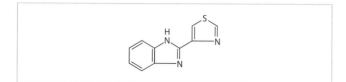

A thiazolyl benzimidazole available for oral administration. It is insoluble in water. The dry powder is stable at room temperature.

Anthelmintic activity

It is active against most common intestinal nematodes. As a result of its larvicidal and ovicidal activity, it is effective in strongyloidiasis, trichinosis, visceral larva migrans (caused predominantly by *Toxocara* spp. of canids and felids) and cutaneous larva migrans.

Pharmacokinetics

It is well absorbed from the small intestine. Peak plasma levels are reached about 1–2 h after a single oral dose of the suspension. It is extensively metabolized in the liver to the 5-hydroxy derivative, which is inactive. Most of the drug is excreted within 24 h. About 90% is excreted in the urine, chiefly as glucuronide or sulfate conjugates; the remainder is passed in the feces.

Toxicity and side effects

A wide range of unpleasant side effects occur, including nausea and other gastrointestinal upsets, fever and neurological effects.

Clinical use

- Infection with intestinal helminths.
- Disseminated strongyloidiasis.
- Cutaneous larva migrans (topical; emulsified in hand cream or petroleum jelly).

Tiabendazole has been largely replaced by the less toxic benzimidazole carbamates. Although active against *A. lumbricoides*, *E. vermicularis* and hookworms, it should not be used as primary therapy for these infections.

Preparations and dosage

Proprietary names: Mintezol, Triasox

Preparation: Tablets, 500 mg; oral suspension 500 mg/5 ml.

Dosage: Oral, based on patient's weight.

Strongyloidiasis: Two doses a day on two successive days or 50 mg/kg as a single dose.

Trichinosis: Two doses a day on 2–4 successive days, depending on response.

Cutaneous larva migrans: Two doses a day on two successive days, and repeat if active lesions are still present 2 days after completion of therapy.

Visceral larva migrans: Two doses a day on 5–7 successive days.

Widely available.

Further information

Anonymous 1999 Thiabendazole. In: Dollery C (ed). *Therapeutic Drugs* 2nd edn. Churchill Livingstone, Edinburgh, pp. T81–T83.

MISCELLANEOUS ANTHELMINTIC AGENTS

BEPHENIUM

Molecular weight: 443.53.

A quaternary ammonium compound formulated as the hydroxynaphthoate. It is almost insoluble in water.

Bephenium is effective as a single 5 g dose against several nematodes, including *A. lumbricoides* and *A. duodenale*, but not *N. americanus*. It is extremely bitter and may induce vomiting. It has been largely superseded by other drugs and no longer features in the World Health Organization (WHO) model prescribing information on drugs for use in parasitic diseases.

DIETHYLCARBAMAZINE

Molecular weight (free base): 199.29; (citrate): 391.42.

A carbamyl derivative of piperazine formulated as the citrate. It is readily soluble in water and slightly hygroscopic.

Anthelmintic activity

Useful activity is restricted to filarial worms. It is adulticidal and microfilaricidal against *Loa loa*. Against *Wuchereria bancrofti* and *Brugia malayi* it is predominantly microfilaricidal, but slowly kills adult worms. It kills microfilariae, but not adults, of *Onchocerca volvulus*.

Pharmacokinetics

Oral absorption	>90%
C_{max} 200 mg	1.5–2 mg/l after 2 h
Plasma half-life	c. 6–12 h
Volume of distribution	107–371 l
Plasma protein binding	Very low

Like piperazine (to which it is related), diethylcarbamazine is rapidly and completely absorbed. About half the dose is excreted unchanged in the urine; the rest is metabolized and eliminated by renal and extrarenal routes.

Toxicity and side effects

In uninfected people, diethylcarbamazine has virtually no side effects, but in people with various forms of filariasis it has unpleasant effects primarily due to the death of, often, millions of blood- or skin-dwelling microfilariae. In onchocerciasis the severe reactions, most frequently of the skin, that occur in treated patients have been named 'Mazzotti reactions'. Historically, these reactions were deliberately used as a diagnostic procedure, but now this is regarded as unethical. The Mazzotti reaction also may be systemic, including fever, headache, malaise to prostration, nausea, joint and muscle pain, vertigo, tachycardia, cough and respiratory distress, hypotension, and ocular signs. In patients with *L. loa* who harbor very large numbers of microfilariae in their blood, neurological problems may be very severe. Cardiological damage has also been reported. In patients with *W. bancrofti* and *B. malayi* high fever occurs in the first few days after treatment. Reversible proteinuria may occur.

Clinical use

- Filariasis.

It has also been used for visceral larva migrans, but experience is limited and there is little evidence of its efficacy.

Preparations and dosage

Proprietary names: Banocide, Filarcidan, Hetrazan, Loxuran.

Preparation: Tablets, 50 or 100 mg.

Dosage

Loiasis: Adults, oral, 1 mg/kg of body weight as a single dose, doubled on two successive days, and then adjusted to 2–3 mg/kg of body weight three times daily for a further 18 days.

Wuchereria bancrofti: Adults and children over 10 years of age, oral, 6 mg/kg of body weight daily for 12 days, preferably in divided doses after meals.

Brugia spp.: Adults and children over 10 years of age, oral, 3–6 mg/kg of body weight daily for 6–12 days, preferably as divided doses after meals.

Onchocerciasis: Adults, oral, a single 0.5 mg/kg of body weight dose initially, doubled on two successive days to 2 mg/kg, then 4–5 mg/kg divided into two doses daily for a further 5 days.

Limited availability.

Further information

Anonymous 1999 Diethylcarbamazine (citrate). In: Dollery C (ed.) *Therapeutic Drugs* 2nd edn. Churchill Livingstone, Edinburgh, pp. D103–D106.

Mackenzie CD, Kron MA 1985 Diethylcarbamazine: a review of its action in onchocerciasis, lymphatic filariasis and inflammation. *Tropical Diseases Bulletin* 82: R1–R37.

Maizels RM, Denham DA 1993 Diethylcarbamazine (DEC): immunopharmacological interactions of an anti-filarial drug. *Parasitology* 105: S49–S60.

IVERMECTIN

Molecular weight: (dihydroavermectin B_{1a}): 875.1; (dihydroavermectin B_{1b}): 861.07.

R
secbutyl (80%)
isopropyl (20%)

A mixture of two closely related semisynthetic derivatives of avermectins, a complex of macrocyclic lactone antibiotics produced by *Streptomyces avermitilis*. In commercial preparations the ratio of the two components, dihydroavermectin B_{1a} and dihydroavermectin B_{1b}, are present within the limits 80–90% and 10–20%, respectively.

Anthelmintic activity

Activity against intestinal nematodes is shown in Table 37.1 (p. 442). It is also active against *Onchocerca volvulus* and other filarial worms, but the effect is chiefly directed against the larval forms (microfilariae). Uniquely among anthelmintic agents it exhibits activity against some ectoparasites, including *Sarcoptes scabiei*.

Pharmacokinetics

Oral absorption	c. 60%
C_{max} 12 mg oral	c. 30–47 ng/ml after 4 h
Plasma half-life	c. 12 h
Volume of distribution	46.9 l
Plasma protein binding	93%

Ivermectin is rapidly metabolized in the liver and the metabolites are excreted in the feces over about 12 days with minimal (<1%) urinary excretion. Highest concentrations occur in the liver and fat. Extremely small amounts are found in the brain.

Toxicity and side effects

In the treatment of onchocerciasis mild Mazzotti-type reactions occur, with occasional neurological problems. Although ivermectin is highly effective against *L. loa*, care must be taken to avoid treating patients with high microfilarial counts: there is one report of a patient with a concomitant *L. loa* infection who died when treated for onchocerciasis. Mild gastrointestinal and nervous system signs may occur following treatment for strongyloidiasis.

Clinical use

- Onchocerciasis.
- Non-disseminated strongyloidiasis.
- Lymphatic filariasis (in combination with albendazole).
- Scabies.

If the patient is harboring *A. lumbricoides*, the worms will be passed in the feces. Head lice will also be killed, which is very much welcomed by the treated patients. Ivermectin has been widely used in the veterinary field, where use also is made of its effect on ectoparasites.

Preparations and dosage

Proprietary names: Mectizan, Stromectol.

Preparation: Tablets, 3 or 6 mg.

Dosage

Onchocerciasis: 15 kg or greater, oral, 150 µg/kg of body weight as a single dose. Re-treat at 6–12-month intervals.

Strongyloidiasis: 15 kg or greater, oral, 200 µg/kg of body weight as a single dose.

Ivermectin should not be used during pregnancy or in nursing mothers. Limited availability.

Further information

Anonymous 1999 Ivermectin. In: Dollery C (ed.) *Therapeutic Drugs* 2nd edn. Churchill Livingstone, Edinburgh, pp. 1127–1130.

Brown KR, Ricci FM, Ottesen EA 2000 Ivermectin: effectiveness in lymphatic filariasis. *Parasitology* 121: S133–S146.

Campbell WC 1989 Ivermectin and abamectin. Springer, New York.

Campbell WC 1991 Ivermectin as an antiparasitic agent for use in humans. *Annual Review of Microbiology* 45: 445–474.

Chodakewitz J 1995 Ivermectin and lymphatic filariasis: A clinical update. *Parasitology Today* 11: 233–235.

Goa KL, McTavish D, Clissold SP 1991 Ivermectin: A review of its antifilarial activity, pharmacokinetic properties and clinical efficacy in onchocerciasis. *Drugs* 42: 640–658.

Ottesen EA, Campbell WC 1994 Ivermectin in human medicine. *Journal of Antimicrobial Chemotherapy* 32: 195–203.

LEVAMISOLE

Molecular weight (free base): 204.29; (hydrochloride): 240.75.

C₆H₅ — N — S · HCl

The L isomer of tetramisole, available as the monohydrochloride. The D isomer has no anthelmintic activity. It is very soluble in water and is stable in the dry state.

Anthelmintic activity

Its principal activity is against *A. lumbricoides* and hookworms. Worms are paralyzed and passed out in the feces within a few hours.

Pharmacokinetics

Oral absorption	c. 90%
C_{max} 150 mg oral	0.5 mg/l after c. 2 h
Plasma half-life	c. 4 h
Volume of distribution	100–120 l

Levamisole is rapidly absorbed from the gut and extensively metabolized in the liver. It is excreted chiefly in the urine.

Toxicity and side effects

Nausea, gastrointestinal upsets, and very mild neurological problems have been reported.

Clinical use

- Ascariasis.
- Hookworm infection.

Levamisole has been used in rheumatoid arthritis and some other conditions that are said to respond to its immuno-modulatory activity. It has been reported to be effective against the rarely seen acanthocephalan parasite *Macracanthorhynchus hirudinaceus* in swine.

Preparations and dosage

Proprietary names: Ergamisol, Ketrax, Solaskil.

Preparation: Tablets, 40 or 50 mg.

Dosage

Ascariasis: Adults, oral, 120–150 mg as a single dose; children, 3 mg/kg as a single dose.

Hookworm: Oral, 2.5–5 mg/kg of bodyweight; in severe cases, a second dose may be given 7 days after the first dose.

Limited availability.

Further information

Anonymous 1999 Levamisole (hydrochloride). In: Dollery C (ed) *Therapeutic Drugs* 2nd edn. Churchill Livingstone, Edinburgh, pp. L26–L29.

METRIFONATE

Trichlorfon (USAN). Molecular weight: 257.44.

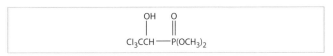

An organophosphorus compound. It is soluble in water and stable at room temperature. At higher temperatures it decomposes to the insecticide dichlorvos.

Anthelmintic activity

Useful activity is restricted to *Schistosoma haematobium*. It has little activity against other schistosomes (Table 37.2). Although it exhibits activity against several other helminths, it is not used for their treatment.

Pharmacokinetics

Metrifonate is rapidly absorbed after oral administration, achieving a peak concentration in plasma within 1–2 h. It undergoes chemical transformation to dichlorvos, which is the active molecule. Dichlorvos is rapidly and extensively metabolized and excreted mainly in the urine.

Toxicity and side effects

Various side effects such as abdominal pain, gastrointestinal upsets and vertigo occur in many patients. As the worms release their hold of the veins in the bladder they pass through the blood system to the lungs, where they disintegrate; this may cause some of the side effects. Cholinesterase levels in the blood and on erythrocytes are depressed, but the significance of this is unknown.

Clinical use

- Urinary schistosomiasis (especially mass chemotherapy control programs).

Preparations and dosage

Proprietary name: Bilarcil.

Preparation: Tablets, 100 mg.

Dosage: Adults and children, oral. *S. haematobium:* three doses of 7.5–10 mg/kg of body weight may be given at intervals of 14 days.

Limited availability.

Table 37.2 Activity of commonly used antischistosome agents

Agent	Schistosoma mansoni	Schistosoma haematobium	Schistosoma japonicum	Schistosoma intercalatum	Schistosoma mekongi
Praziquantel	+++	+++	+++	+++	+++
Metrifonate	–	+++	–	–	–
Oxamniquine	+++	–	–	–	–

+++, Highly effective; –, no useful activity.

Further information

Anonymous 1999 Trichlorfon. In: Dollery C (ed.) *Therapeutic Drugs* 2nd edn. Churchill Livingstone, Edinburgh, pp. T174–T179.

 NICLOSAMIDE

Molecular weight: 327.12.

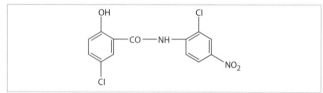

A synthetic chlorinated nitrosalicylanilide available for oral administration.

Anthelmintic activity

Useful activity is restricted to intestinal tapeworms, including *Taeniarhynchus saginatus* (Syn. *Taenia saginata*), *Taenia solium*, *Diphyllobothrium latum* and *Hymenolepis nana*. It is not effective against larval stages of tapeworms.

Pharmacokinetics

Conflicting data exist relative to the level of absorption of niclosamide from the gut. The metabolized drug is passed in the feces and urine, staining them yellow.

Toxicity and side effects

Very few side effects have been reported, but these include mild nausea, abdominal cramps, and dizziness.

Clinical use

- Intestinal tapeworm infections.

 Preparations and dosage

Proprietary names: Niclocide, Tredemine, Yomesan.

Preparation: Tablets, 500 mg.

Dosage

T. saginatus, *T. solium* (intestinal stage), and *D. latum:* Adults, 2 g as a single oral dose; children 10–35 kg, 1 g as a single oral dose; infants <10 kg, 0.5 g as a single oral dose. Chronically constipated patients should receive a purgative on the evening preceding treatment.

H. nana: A 7-day treatment is recommended; adults, 2 g on the first day and 1 g on each of the next 6 days; children 10–35 kg, 1 g on the first day and 0.5 g on each of the next 6 days; infants <10 kg, a total of 2 g should be given over 7 days.

Widely available.

 OXAMNIQUINE

Molecular weight: 279.33.

A synthetic quinolinemethanol, available for oral administration.

Anthelmintic activity

Activity against human schistosomes is shown in Table 37.2. Some strains of *Schistosoma mansoni*, particularly those in Egypt and Southern Africa, require higher doses for efficacy due to innate tolerance. There is no useful activity against other *Schistosoma* spp.

Pharmacokinetics

Oxamniquine is rapidly absorbed after oral administration, achieving a peak concentration of 0.3–2.5 mg/l 1–3 h after an oral dose of 15 mg/kg body weight. Peak levels following intramuscular treatment at 7.5 mg/kg generally do not exceed 0.15 mg/l. It is extensively metabolized to biologically inactive 6-carboxylic and 2-carboxylic acid derivatives, which are excreted in the urine, mostly within 12 h.

Toxicity and side effects

Dizziness, sleepiness, nausea, and headache occur frequently. Other side effects are probably due to the death and disintegration of the worms in the liver. Following treatment, urine may become red.

Clinical use

- Infection with *S. mansoni*.

Preparations and dosage

Proprietary name: Vansil.

Preparations: Capsule, 250 mg; syrup, 50 mg/ml.

Dosage

West Africa, South America, Caribbean Islands: Adults, a single oral dose of 15 mg/kg of body weight; children <30 kg, 10 mg/kg orally twice daily for 1 day.

East and Central Africa and Arabian Peninsula: Adults and children, 15 mg/kg orally twice daily for 1 day.

Egypt, Southern Africa, and Zimbabwe: Adults and children, 60 mg/kg administered orally over 2–3 days with no single dose to exceed 20 mg/kg.

Limited availability.

Further information

Anonymous 1999 Oxamniquine. In: Dollery C (ed.) *Therapeutic Drugs* 2nd edn. Churchill Livingstone, Edinburgh, pp. O35–O37.

Foster R 1987 A review of clinical experience with oxamniquine. *Transactions of the Royal Society for Tropical Medicine and Hygiene* 81: 55–59.

 # PIPERAZINE

Molecular weight: piperazine: 86.14; (edetate calcium): 416.44; (anhydrous citrate): 642.65.

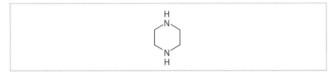

A synthetic chemical, most commonly formulated as the citrate, but also available as the adipate, edetate calcium and tartrate salts.

Anthelmintic activity

Activity against common intestinal nematodes is shown in Table 37.1 (p. 442). It has no other useful anthelmintic activity.

Pharmacokinetics

Activity against intestinal worms requires that a substantial amount remains in the gut. However, after oral administration a variable amount is rapidly absorbed from the small intestine and subsequently excreted in the urine. Its half-life is extremely variable.

Toxicity and side effects

Some people develop hypersensitivity, requiring cessation of treatment. Transient, mild gastrointestinal or neurological symptoms may occur.

Clinical use

- Ascariasis.
- Pinworm.

 ## Preparations and dosage

Proprietary names: Many (e.g. Pripsen, Antepar).

Preparations: Various oral presentations.

Dosage

The dosage of piperazine is generally expressed relative to piperazine hexahydrate.

Ascariasis: Adults and children over 12 years of age, the equivalent of 75 mg/kg body weight to a maximum of 3.5 g of piperazine hexahydrate as a single oral dose or divided over two consecutive days; children 2–12

years of age, as for adults but to a maximum of 2.5 g; children under 2 years of age, the equivalent of 50 mg/kg of bodyweight of piperazine hexahydrate administered under medical supervision. Alternative regimens exist.

Pinworm: Adults and children, the equivalent of 50 mg/kg of piperazine hexahydrate given orally on each of 7 consecutive days. Treatment should be repeated at an interval of 2 weeks and all family members should be treated. Alternative regimens exist.

Widely available without prescription in many countries under numerous trade names.

 Further information

Anonymous 1999 Piperazine. In: Dollery C (ed.) *Therapeutic Drugs* 2nd edn. Churchill Livingstone, Edinburgh, pp. P137–P139.

 # PRAZIQUANTEL

Molecular weight: 312.41.

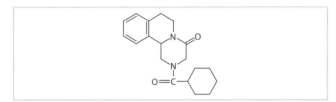

A synthetic pyrazinoquinoline formulated for oral administration. It is stable in the dry state, but hygroscopic.

Anthelmintic activity

All species of human schistosomes are susceptible (Table 37.2). Praziquantel is also effective against adult and tissue-dwelling larval tapeworms, against the intestinal flukes *Fasciolopsis buski*, *Metagonimus yokogawi*, *Heterophyes heterophyes* and *Nanophyetus salmincola*; against *Clonorchis* and *Opisthorchis* spp. in the bile ducts; and against *Paragonimus* spp. in the lungs. It has variable activity against zoonotic *Fasciola. hepatica* infections.

Acquired resistance

There is growing evidence that resistance to praziquantel is emerging in schistosomes, although there is debate as to whether treatment failures are due to resistance or innate tolerance.

Pharmacokinetics

Oral absorption	>80%
C_{max} 50 mg/kg oral	1 mg/l after 1–2 h
Plasma half-life: parent drug	1–1.5 h
metabolites	4–6 h
Plasma protein binding	80%

Praziquantel is rapidly absorbed when given orally, but it undergoes extensive first-pass biotransformation and the concentration of unchanged drug in plasma is low. The major metabolite, a 4-hydroxy derivative, retains little to no antiparasitic activity. About 80% of the oral dose, as parent drug and its metabolites, is excreted in the urine by the fourth day post-treatment, 90% of this in 24 h. A higher peak plasma concentration is achieved in infected people, but other pharmacokinetic values are unchanged.

Toxicity and side effects

Very few side effects have been reported. In the treatment of cerebral cysticercosis the death of cysts in the brain may cause local inflammation and edema, but this usually subsides quickly. Ocular cysticercosis should not be treated with this drug, because parasite destruction in the eye can lead to irreparable lesions. Adverse events seen in the treatment of schistosomiasis, including abdominal pain, nausea, anorexia, diarrhea, and mild neurological effects, are almost certainly due to the death and disintegration of the large adult worms.

Clinical use

- Schistosomiasis.
- Other trematode infections (except *F. hepatica*).
- Tapeworm infection, including cerebral cysticercosis.

Treatment may need to be prolonged in cerebral cysticercosis.

Preparations and dosage

Proprietary name: Biltricide

Preparation: Tablets, 600 mg

Dosage
Adults and children over 4 years of age.

Schistosomiasis: 20 mg/kg of body weight orally three times a day at 4–6 h intervals on one day or 40 mg/kg as a single dose.

Liver and lung flukes: 25 mg/kg of bodyweight orally three times a day at 4–6 h intervals on one day or two consecutive days.

Intestinal flukes: 25 mg/kg of bodyweight as a single oral dose.

Intestinal taeniasis: 5–10 mg/kg of body weight as a single oral dose.

Intestinal diphyllobothriasis: 10–25 mg/kg of bodyweight as a single oral dose.

Intestinal hymenolepiasis: 15–25 mg/kg of bodyweight as a single oral dose.

Cysticercosis: A total of 50 mg/kg of bodyweight daily in three divided doses for 14 consecutive days. A corticosteroid should be administered for 2–3 days before and throughout treatment.

Limited availability.

Further information

Anonymous 1999 Praziquantel. In: Dollery C (ed.) *Therapeutic Drugs* 2nd edn. Churchill Livingstone, Edinburgh, pp. P184–P189.

Davis A 1993 Antischistosomal drugs and clinical practice. In: Jordan P, Webbe G, Sturrock RF (eds) *Human schistosomiasis*. CAB international, Wallingford pp. 367–404.

Fritsche TR, Eastburn RL, Wiggins LH et al 1989 Praziquantel for treatment of human *Nanophyetus salmincola* (*Troglotrema salmincola*) infection. *Journal of Infectious Diseases* 160: 896–899.

Groll E 1984 Praziquantel. *Advances in Pharmacology and Chemotherapy* 20: 219–238.

King CH, Mahmoud AAF 1989 Drugs five years later: Praziquantel. *Annals of Internal Medicine*, 110: 290–296.

Ismail M, Botros S, Metwally A et al 1999 Resistance to praziquantel: Direct evidence from *Schistosoma mansoni* isolated from Egyptian villagers. *American Journal of Tropical Medicine and Hygiene* 60: 932–935.

Kumar V, Gryseels B 1994 Use of praziquantel against schistosomiasis: a review of current status. *International Journal of Antimicrobial Agents* 4: 313–320.

Pearson RD, Guerrant RL 1983 Praziquantel: A major advance in anthelmintic therapy. *Annals of Internal Medicine* 99: 195–198.

PYRANTEL

Molecular weight: (free base): 206.3; (pamoate): 594.68.

A tetrahydropyrimidine, formulated as the pamoate (embonate) in a 1:1 ratio and available as a suspension for oral administration. It is practically insoluble in water, but soluble in dimethyl sulfoxide. It is stable at room temperature.

Anthelmintic activity

Activity against the common intestinal nematodes is shown in Table 37.1 (p. 442). Pyrantel is less active against *N. americanus* than against *A. duodenale*.

Pharmacokinetics

By synthetic design most of the dose is passed unchanged in the feces. The portion that is absorbed (<5%) is metabolized and excreted in the urine.

Toxicity and side effects

Pyrantel should not be used at the same time as piperazine as their modes of action are antagonistic. Gastrointestinal upsets and, rarely, very mild neurological symptoms occur.

Clinical use

- Ascariasis.
- Pinworm.
- Hookworm (especially *A. duodenale*).
- Trichostrongyliasis.

Higher and more prolonged doses may be necessary in hookworm infection caused by *N. americanus*. Pyrantel has been used in combination with an analog (oxantel) where concurrent whipworm infection was likely.

 Preparations and dosage

Proprietary name: Antiminth, Combantrin.

Preparation: Tablets, 250 mg; oral suspension, 50 mg/ml.

Dosage: Adults and children >6 months of age, 10 mg/kg of body weight orally; treatment for pinworm should be repeated after 2 weeks; more severe infections of *N. americanus* require 20 mg/kg as a single dose on each of two consecutive days, or 10 mg/kg as a single dose on each of 3–4 consecutive days.

Widely available.

 Further information

Anonymous 1999 Pyrantel (pamoate). In: Dollery C (ed.) *Therapeutic Drugs* 2nd edn. Churchill Livingstone, Edinburgh, pp. P284–P286.

 SURAMIN

A complex symmetrical molecule originally developed in Germany in the early 1920s as a colorless derivative of the antitrypanosomal dye, trypan blue, for the treatment of African trypanosomiasis. Its useful anthelmintic activity is restricted to *O. volvulus* and it has been used to achieve a radical cure of onchocerciasis by killing the adult worms. However, it is an extremely toxic drug and its use has become increasingly uncommon since ivermectin became available. Its properties are described in Chapter 38 (p. 469).

OTHER ANTHELMINTIC AGENTS

Potassium antimony tartrate (tartar emetic), sodium antimony tartrate, the thioxanthone, hycanthone, and the 5-nitro-thiazole, niridazole, were formerly used in the treatment of schistosomiasis, but have been largely superseded by less toxic compounds. Niridazole has also been used in Guinea worm infection, but no drug interrupts transmission and metronidazole or benzimidazole carbamates are much safer and as useful in providing symptomatic relief. The chlorinated hydrocarbon tetrachloroethylene has been used since the 1920s in the treatment of hookworm infection. It is more effective in eliminating *N. americanus* than *A. duodenale* and has no useful effect against other intestinal worms. It has been replaced by safer and more effective agents. Pyrvinium, a cyanine dye formulated as the almost insoluble pamoate, was formerly used to treat pinworm infections. It is not absorbed from the gut, is very bright red in color, and stains the feces red.

38 Antiprotozoal agents

S. L. Croft

The treatment and prophylaxis of many protozoal diseases, such as malaria (which causes up to 250 million infections and 2 million deaths per annum) is inadequate. Malaria chemotherapy has been undermined by the development of resistance to chloroquine, pyrimethamine and other drugs (Ch. 64). Standard drugs for the treatment of human African trypanosomiasis (sleeping sickness), leishmaniasis and South American trypanosomiasis (Chagas' disease), caused by closely related flagellate parasites, remain arsenicals, antimonials or toxic nitroheterocyclic compounds respectively. During the past 20 years opportunistic protozoa, some previously unknown in humans, have emerged as important pathogens in immunocompromised patients. No drug has so far proved effective against cryptosporidiosis, and those for toxoplasmosis and microsporidiosis are limited.

Protozoa are unicellular, eukaryotic cells with an enormous diversity in morphology, life cycles, genomic and biochemical characteristics. This diversity is reflected in their very different sensitivity to antiprotozoal drugs.

Several antiprotozoal agents developed in the 1920s and 1930s, for example suramin, mepacrine, primaquine, chloroquine and sodium stibogluconate, are still widely used. Identification of new drugs has been hampered in part by lack of suitable in-vitro and in-vivo models; for example suitable in-vitro models for *Plasmodium falciparum* and *Trypanosoma brucei* were not discovered until the 1970s. Progress has also been hampered by the absence of economic incentive; the development of public–private partnerships is helping to address this problem. Several new antiprotozoal agents have been developed through therapeutic switching of antibacterial, antifungal or anticancer drugs.

Further information

Coombs G, North M (eds) 1991 *Biochemical protozoology.* Taylor & Francis, London.
Croft SL 1997 The current status of antiparasite chemotherapy. *Parasitology* 114: S3–S15.
Derouin F, Gangeux J-P 1998 Changing patterns of disease and treatment of opportunistic parasite infections in patients with AIDS. *Current Opinion in Infectious Diseases* 11: 711–716.
Khaw M, Panosian CB 1995 Human Antiprotozoal Therapy: past, present and future. *Clinical Microbiology Reviews* 8: 427–439.

ORGANOMETALS

The use of arsenic and antimony in the treatment of infectious diseases originates from traditional treatments: Fowler's solution, containing potassium arsenite, and tartar emetic (antimony potassium tartrate). Arsenical compounds were used for the treatment of African sleeping sickness and antimonial compounds for the treatment of leishmaniasis before 1920. The compounds presently used are considerably less toxic than their predecessors; they were developed in the 1930s (sodium stibogluconate) and 1940s (melarsoprol, meglumine antimonate). Tryparsamide was formerly used in sleeping sickness, but it is highly toxic and there is intrinsic resistance. A water-soluble compound, trimelarsen (Mel W) has also been used, but it is less effective and more toxic than melarsoprol.

MELARSOPROL

Molecular weight: 398.34.

Mel B. A derivative of trivalent melarsen oxide and dimercaprol (BAL), possessing a melaminyl moiety. Formulated for intravenous administration. It is almost insoluble in water, but soluble in propylene glycol.

Antimicrobial activity

Melarsoprol is highly and rapidly active against *T. brucei gambiense* and *T. brucei rhodesiense* in vitro at submicromolar concentrations. It is much less active against the animal trypanosomes *T. congolense* and *T. vivax*. Combinations with eflornithine and nitroimidazoles are highly active against central nervous system (CNS) infection with *T. brucei* in rodents.

Acquired resistance

About 3–11% of patients with *T. brucei gambiense* and *T. brucei rhodesiense* infections relapse. This rate remained constant for 40 years, but up to 25% cases of *T. brucei gambiense* in Central Africa now relapse. Patients infected with *T. brucei* normally respond to a second course of the drug, but those with *T. brucei gambiense* do not. Resistance is due to reduced uptake of the drug by trypanosomes. Laboratory-generated resistant trypomastigotes either lack an adenine/adenosine transporter or contain a transporter gene with point mutations.

Pharmacokinetics

Pharmacokinetic data are being re-examined. Serum levels of 2–4 mg/l at 24 h after administration of 3.6 mg/kg, falling to 0.1 mg/l at 120 h after the fourth daily injection, have been reported. Bioassay and atomic absorption spectroscopy indicated biphasic elimination with a half-life of 35 h and a volume of distribution of 100 l. It is rapidly metabolized by microsomal enzymes to melarsen oxide; the maximum plasma concentration of melarsen oxide was reached by 15 min with a half-life of 3.9 h. This metabolite can cross the blood–brain barrier and effect a CNS cure in mice. Levels of melarsoprol in the cerebrospinal fluid (CSF) reached around 300 µg/l, about 50 times lower than serum levels.

Toxicity and side effects

Melarsoprol is supplied in 3.6% propylene glycol, which can cause tissue trauma and long-term damage to veins. Reactions due to melarsoprol include fever on first administration, abdominal colic pain, dermatitis and arthralgia. Polyneuropathy has been reported in about 10% of patients. Reactive arsenical encephalopathy is a serious side effect that occurs in around 10% of those treated, with death in 1–3% of cases. The frequency of encephalopathy increases with a rise in the white cell count or the presence of trypanosomes in the CSF. The causes of the immunological responses involved in the encephalopathy and the possible existence of two forms (reactive and hemorrhagic) are subjects of debate. Concomitant administration of prednisolone has reduced the frequency of reactive encephalopathy in late stage *T. brucei gambiense* infection.

Clinical use

- Late-stage sleeping sickness caused by *T. brucei gambiense* and *T. brucei rhodesiense*.

It is not recommended for early-stage disease, in which alternatives with less serious side effects are available.

Preparations and dosage

Proprietary name: Arsobal.

Preparation: Injection.

Dosage: Adults, i.v., 3.6 mg/kg daily for 3–4 days and repeat 2–3 times with an interval of at least 7 days between courses. An alternative regimen of 10 daily doses, with no interval, of 2.2 mg/kg has similar efficacy.

Limited availability.

Further information

Barrett MP 2000 Problems for the chemotherapy of human African trypanosomiasis. *Current Opinion in Infectious Diseases* 13: 647–651.

Berger BJ, Fairlamb AH 1994 High-performance liquid chromatographic method for the separation and quantitative estimation of anti-parasitic melaminophenyl arsenical compounds. *Transactions of the Royal Society of Tropical Medicine and Hygiene* 88: 357–359.

Burri C, Nkunku S, Merolle A, Smith T, Blum J, Brun R 2000 Efficacy of new, concise schedule for melarsoprol in treatment of sleeping sickness caused by *Trypanosoma brucei gambiense*: a randomised trial. *Lancet* 355: 1419–1425.

Dumas M, Bouteille B 2000 Treatment of human African trypanosomiasis. *Bulletin of the World Health Organization* 78: 1474.

Kaminsky R, Maser P 2000 Drug resistance in African trypanosomes. *Current Opinion in Anti-infective Investigational Drugs* 2: 76–82.

Keiser J, Ericsson O, Burri C 2000 Investigations of the metabolites of the trypanocidal drug melarsoprol. *Clinical Pharmacology and Therapeutics* 67: 478–488.

Pepin J, Milord F 1994 The treatment of human African trypanosomiasis. *Advances in Parasitology* 33: 1–47.

SODIUM STIBOGLUCONATE

Pentavalent sodium antimony gluconate.

A pentavalent antimonial of uncertain chemical composition; probably a complex mixture of polymeric forms. There is batch-to-batch variation and solutions may contain 32–34% pentavalent antimony (Sb^V). The structural formula normally given is conjectural and based upon that of tartar emetic. It is freely soluble in water.

Antimicrobial activity

The drug has low activity against the extracellular promastigotes of *Leishmania* spp. in vitro, but is active against amastigotes in macrophages. There is higher level of metabolism of

Sb^V to toxic Sb^{III} in amastigotes than promastigotes. Variation in the sensitivity of different *Leishmania* species may contribute to differences in clinical response. It is more active against visceral than cutaneous leishmaniasis in animal models. Sodium stibogluconate cures CNS infections with *T. brucei* in rodents.

Acquired resistance

Increasing unresponsiveness and relapse of *L. donovani* infections in Bihar State, India (up to 30%) during the 1990s was assumed to be due to increasing acquired resistance. Lack of response is also reported in patients with mucosal leishmaniasis caused by *Leishmania braziliensis*. Relapse is common in patients with visceral leishmaniasis who are immunodepressed, for example by human immunodeficiency virus (HIV) infection, but this is due to the immune dependence of drug activity and not acquired resistance. In laboratory-generated resistant *Leishmania* promastigotes Sb^{III} is conjugated to intracellular thiols, for example trypanothione, and extruded by increased numbers of ABC transporters.

Pharmacokinetics

Peak concentrations of about 12–15 mg antimony/l are achieved in serum 1 h after a dose of 10 mg/kg. There is a slow accumulation in the central compartment, and tissue concentrations reach a maximum after several days. In contrast to trivalent derivatives, pentavalent antimonials are not accumulated by erythrocytes, but there is evidence of protein binding. Antimony is detected in the skin for at least 5 days after treatment. Some of the dose of Sb^V is converted to Sb^{III}, possibly by the liver or by macrophages. It is rapidly excreted into urine with a half-life of about 2 h; 60–80% of the dose appears in the urine within 6 h of parenteral administration. In a study on structurally related meglumine antimonate (*see below*) the pharmacokinetics of Sb^V and Sb^{III} were similar as measured by serum and urine levels.

Toxicity and side effects

The toxic effects are limited by the rapid excretion, but cumulative toxicity increases in proportion to dose. Myalgia, arthralgia, anorexia and electrocardiographic changes have been reported with high-dose regimens. Hepatocellular damage, hepatic and renal functional impairment and pancreatitis have also been reported. The changes are reversible on discontinuation of treatment.

Clinical use

- Visceral, cutaneous and mucocutaneous leishmaniasis.

The combination with allopurinol (visceral leishmaniasis) or with paromomycin (visceral and cutaneous leishmaniasis) has been used in unresponsive cases.

Preparations and dosage

Proprietary name: Pentostam.

Preparation: Injection.

Dosage: Adults, i.m., i.v., 10–20 mg/kg per day with a maximum of 850 mg for at least 20 days; the dose varies with different geographical regions.

Limited availability; not available in the USA.

Further information

Alvar J, Canavate C, Gutierrez-Solar B et al 1997 *Leishmania* and human immunodeficiency virus coinfection: the first 10 years. *Clinical Microbiology Reviews* 10: 298–319.

Anonymous 1999 Sodium stibogluconate. In: Dollery C (ed.) *Therapeutic Drugs* 2nd edn. Churchill Livingstone, Edinburgh, pp. S64–S67.

Berman JD 1997 Human leishmaniasis: clinical, diagnostic, and chemotherapeutic developments in the last 10 years. *Clinical Infectious Diseases* 24: 684–703.

Ephros M, Bitnun A, Shaked P, Waldan E, Zilberstein D 1999 Stage-specific activity of pentavalent antimony against *Leishmania donovani* axenic amastigotes. *Antimicrobial Agents and Chemotherapy* 43: 278–282.

Ouellette M, Legare D, Haimeur A et al 1998 ABC transporters in *Leishmania* and their role in drug resistance. *Drug Resistance Updates* 1: 43–48.

Sundar S, More DK, Singh MK et al 2000 Failure of pentavalent antimony in visceral leishmaniasis in India: report from the center of the Indian epidemic. *Clinical Infectious Diseases* 31: 1104–1107.

MEGLUMINE ANTIMONATE

N-Methylglucamine antimonate; methylaminoglucitol antimonate.

The Sb^V content varies around 28% between batches. The structures of this oligomeric drug have been re-examined and the major moiety identified as:

Activity, pharmacology and toxicology are similar to those of sodium stibogluconate, with which it is essentially interchangeable. The predominant use of sodium stibogluconate in the Middle East and Africa and meglumine antimoniate in South America is due to history and marketing policies.

Clinical use

- Treatment of visceral and cutaneous leishmaniasis.

Studies in Central and South America have indicated that the combination with interferon-γ is effective in the treatment of visceral and cutaneous leishmaniasis cases unresponsive to antimony alone.

Preparations and dosage

Proprietary name: Glucantime.

Preparation: Injection.

Dosage: Adults, i.m., i.v., 20 mg/kg/day for 20–28 days. The course can be repeated.

Limited availability, not available in the UK.

Further information

Roberts WL, McMurray WJ, Rainey PM 1998 Characterization of the antimonial agent meglumine antimonate (Glucantime). *Antimicrobial Agents and Chemotherapy* 42: 1076–1082.

QUINOLINES

Quinoline-containing drugs have been the mainstay of anti-malarial chemotherapy since the seventeenth century in the form of *Cinchona* bark, which contains quinine and related alkaloids. Synthetic quinolines were developed in the 1920s and 1930s. The most important of these, the 4-aminoquino-line chloroquine, has succumbed to global resistance in *P. fal-ciparum*. This has brought quinine and quinidine back into use for the therapy of severe malaria and prompted the search for new derivatives, a process that led to mefloquine. Amodiaquine is active against chloroquine-resistant strains of *P. falciparum*, but is not recommended for prophylaxis. Identification of the structure–function relationships for activity and resistance has enabled the development of quinolines active against chloro-quine-resistant *P. falciparum*; two bis(quinolines), piperaquine and hydroxypiperaquine, have been used in the treatment of drug-resistant malaria in China. The 8-aminoquinoline pri-maquine is used for the radical cure of benign tertian malaria, but the investigational derivative tafenoquine may have wider uses.

Further information

Egan TJ 2001 Quinoline antimalarials. *Expert Opinion in Therapeutic Patents* 11: 185–209.
Foley M, Tilley L 1998 Quinoline antimalarials: mechanisms of action and resistance and prospects for new agents. *Pharmacology and Therapeutics* 79: 55–87.
Lell B, Faucher JF, Missinou MA et al 2000 Malaria chemoprophylaxis with tafeno-quine: a randomised study. *Lancet* 355: 2041–2045.
Mungthin M, Bray PG, Ridley RG, Ward SA 1998 Central role of haemoglobin degra-dation in mechanisms of action of 4-aminoquinolines, quinoline methanols and phenanthrene methanols. *Antimicrobial Agents and Chemotherapy* 42: 2973–2977.
Olliaro PL, Yuthavong Y 1999 An overview of chemotherapeutic targets for anti-malarial drug discovery. *Pharmacology and Therapeutics* 81: 91–110.
Peters W 1999 The evolution of tafenoquine – antimalarial for a new millennium? *Journal of the Royal Society of Medicine* 92: 345–352.

CHLOROQUINE

Molecular weight 319.9.

A synthetic 4-aminoquinoline, formulated as the phosphate or sulfate for oral administration and as the hydrochloride or sulfate for parenteral use. The salts are soluble in water.

Antimicrobial activity

Chloroquine accumulates 300-fold in infected erythrocytes and acts against the early erythrocytic stages of all four species of *Plasmodium* that cause human malaria. It is also active against the gametocytes of *Plasmodium vivax*, *Plasmodium ovale* and *Plasmodium malariae*, but not against the hepatic stages or mature erythrocytic schizonts and merozoites.

Acquired resistance

Resistance of *P. falciparum* was first reported in South America and South-east Asia in 1959. It has since spread widely, including to Africa and has become a major problem in the control of malaria. The mechanism appears to be either decreased uptake of drug by the parasite or increased efflux from the parasite, or both. Changes in genes encoding a P-glycoprotein homolog, *Pfmdrl*, and another putative trans-porter, *Pfcrt*, are associated with resistance. Verapamil and desipramine reverse chloroquine resistance in experimental models, but human trials have been disappointing. Chloroquine-resistant *P. vivax* has been reported in South America and South-east Asia.

Pharmacokinetics

Oral absorption	80–90%
C_{max} 300 mg oral	0.25 mg/l after 1–6 h
Plasma half-life	c. 9 days (mean)
Volume of distribution	200 l/kg
Plasma protein binding	50–70%

There is extensive tissue binding and a high affinity for melanin-containing tissues. Chloroquine is extensively metab-olized to a biologically active monodesethyl derivative that forms about 20% of the plasma level of the drug. The mean elimination half-life results from an initial phase (3–6 days), slow phase (12–14 days) and terminal phase (40 days). Renal clearance is about 50% of the dose.

Toxicity and side effects

Minor side effects such as dizziness, headache, rashes, nausea and diarrhea are common. Pruritus occurs in up to 20% of Africans taking chloroquine. Long-term treatment can induce CNS effects and cumulative dosing over many years may cause retinopathy. Rarely, photosensitization, tinnitus and deafness have occurred.

Clinical use

- Prophylaxis and treatment of all types of malaria.
- Hepatic amebiasis (in sequential combination with dehydroemetine).

Activity against *P. falciparum* is seriously limited by the spread of resistance.

Preparations and dosage

Proprietary names: Avloclor, Nivaquine.

Preparations: Tablets, syrup, injection.

Dosage: Treatment of benign malarias: adult, oral, 600 mg chloroquine base as initial dose then a single dose of 300 mg after 6–8 h, then a single dose of 300 mg/day for 2 days. Children, oral, initial dose of 10 mg/kg of chloroquine base then a single dose of 5 mg/kg after 6–8 h, then a single dose of 5 mg/kg daily for 2 days. Malaria prophylaxis: consult specialist guidelines.

Widely available.

Further information

Anonymous 1999 Chloroquine. In: Dollery C (ed.) *Therapeutic Drugs* 2nd edn. Churchill Livingstone, Edinburgh, pp. C177–C182.

Babiker HA, Prongle SJ, Abdel-Muhsin A, et al 2001 High-level chloroquine resistance in Sudanese isolates of *Plasmodium falciparum* is associated with mutations in the chloroquine resistance transporter gene pfcrt and the multidrug resistance gene *pfmdr1. Journal of Infectious Diseases* 183: 1535–1538.

Krishna S, White NJ 1996 Pharmacokinetics of quinine, chloroquine and amodiaquine. Clinical implications. *Clinical Pharmacokinetics* 30: 263–299.

Pagola S, Stephens PW, Bohle DS et al 2000 The structure of malaria pigment β-haematin. *Nature* 404: 307–310.

Reed MB, Saliba KJ, Caruana SR 2000 Pgh1 modulates sensitivity and resistance to multiple antimalarials in *Plasmodium falciparum. Nature* 403: 906–909.

Sanchez CP, Lanzer M 2000 Changing ideas on chloroquine resistance in *Plasmodium falciparum. Current Opinion in Infectious Diseases* 13: 653–658.

 AMODIAQUINE

Molecular weight: 355.86.

A mono-Mannich-base 4-aminoquinoline, formulated as the dihydrochloride dihydrate or free base for oral administration.

Amodiaquine is active against *P. falciparum* and *P. vivax* and is more active than chloroquine for the treatment of uncomplicated *P. falciparum* malaria. Pharmacokinetic behavior is similar to that of chloroquine with a terminal elimination half-life of 1–3 weeks.

Clinical use

- Treatment of falciparum malaria.

Prophylactic use has been abandoned because of agranulocytosis and hepatotoxicity due to formation of a quinone–imine metabolite. There is renewed interest in its use in treatment owing to the spread of chloroquine resistance.

Preparations and dosage

Preparation: Tablets.

Dosage: Adults, oral, a total dose of 35 mg/kg has been given over 3 days. Limited availability.

Further information

Hawley SR, Bray PG, Ward SA 1996 Amodiaquine accumulation in *Plasmodium falciparum* as a possible explanation for its superior antimalarial activity over chloroquine. *Molecular and Biochemical Parasitology* 80: 15–25.

Krishna S, White NJ 1996 Pharmacokinetics of quinine, chloroquine and amodiaquine. Clinical implications. *Clinical Pharmacokinetics* 30: 263–299.

Olliaro P, Mussano P 2000 Amodiaquine for treating malaria. *Cochrane database Systematic Review* CD000016.

Olliaro P, Nevill C, Le Bras J et al 1996 Systematic review of amodiaquine treatment in uncomplicated malaria. *Lancet* 348: 1196–1201.

Ridley RG, Hudson AT 1998 Quinoline antimalarials. *Expert Opinions in Therapeutic Patents* 8: 121–136.

 IODOQUINOL

Molecular weight: 396.98.

Di-iodohydroxyquinoline. An 8-hydroxyquinoline derivative formulated for oral use.

Antimicrobial activity

Iodoquinol has direct, but feeble, activity against *Entamoeba histolytica* and *Dientamoeba fragilis* in vitro and in vivo. The mechanism of action is unknown.

Pharmacokinetics

Halogenated hydroxyquinolines are slowly and incompletely absorbed, with less than 10% of an oral dose reaching the circulation. Absorbed drug is metabolized to sulfate or glucuronide conjugates and excreted.

Toxicity and side effects

Side effects are normally mild, including nausea, diarrhea, rashes and cramps. Other halogenated hydroxyquinolines have been shown to cause subacute myelo-optic neuropathy from prolonged dosage and are banned in some countries.

Clinical use

- Asymptomatic or mild intestinal amebiasis.

Preparations and dosage

Preparations: Tablets, topical cream.

Dosage: Adults, oral, 500 mg three times daily for 10–20 days. Children, oral, 20–40 mg/kg daily in divided doses for 10–20 days.

Limited availability, not available in the UK.

Further information

Chan FT, Guan MX, Mackenzie AM, Diaz-Mitoma F 1994 Susceptibility testing of *Dientamoeba fragilis* ATCC30948 with iodoquinol, paromomycin, tetracycline, and metronidazole. *Antimicrobial Agents and Chemotherapy* 38: 1157–1160.

 MEFLOQUINE

Molecular weight (free base): 378.3; (hydrochloride): 414.8.

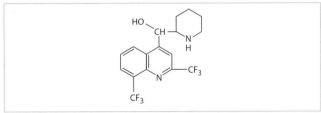

A synthetic 4-quinolinemethanol, formulated as the hydrochloride for oral administration. It is slightly soluble in water.

Antimicrobial activity

Mefloquine has rapid dose-related activity against erythrocytic stages of *Plasmodium* spp., with in-vitro activity at 10–40 nM. It is effective against strains of *P. falciparum* that are resistant to chloroquine, sulfonamides and pyrimethamine. The C-11 (hydroxy) enantiomers have equal antimalarial activity. Mefloquine also exhibits bactericidal activity (including methicillin-resistant *Staphylococcus aureus*), and is active against some fungi.

Acquired resistance

Resistance in *P. falciparum* is increasing; in South-east Asia high-grade resistance occurs in 15% of patients and low-grade resistance in about 50%. Use of lower initial doses could lead more rapidly to resistance. There is cross-resistance with quinine and halofantrine, and an inverse relationship with chloroquine resistance has been reported. The molecular basis of resistance remains unclear but polymorphisms of the *pfmdr1* gene, associated with chloroquine resistance, lead to increased sensitivity to mefloquine. Resistant strains of *P. falciparum* appeared in Africa before the drug was used in that continent, perhaps because of quinine abuse or intrinsic resistance.

Pharmacokinetics

Oral absorption	70–80%
C_{max} 1 g oral	1 mg/l after 2–12 h
Plasma half-life	20 days
Volume of distribution	16–25 l/kg
Plasma protein binding	98%

Mefloquine is concentrated 2- to 5-fold in erythrocytes. The major metabolites do not have antimalarial activity. Pregnant women require larger doses than non-pregnant women to achieve comparable blood levels. It is predominantly excreted in the bile. Less than 10% is excreted in urine.

Toxicity and side effects

At prophylactic doses risks of serious toxicity are about 1 in 10 000, similar to chloroquine. Doses used in therapy are more commonly associated with nausea, dizziness, fatigue, mental confusion and sleep loss. Psychosis, encephalopathy and convulsions are seen in about 1 in 1200–1700 patients.

Clinical use

- Antimalarial prophylaxis in areas of chloroquine resistance.
- Treatment of uncomplicated multidrug-resistant malaria (alone or in combination with artesunate).

Mefloquine has been used for the treatment of cutaneous leishmaniasis in South America.

Preparations and dosage

Proprietary names: Lariam, Mephaquine.

Preparation: Tablets.

Dosage: Malaria treatment, oral, 20–25 mg/kg as a single dose or in 2–3 divided doses 6–8 h apart. A lower dose of 15 mg/kg may suffice for partially immune individuals. Malaria prophylaxis, see specialist guidelines.

Widely available.

Further information

Anonymous 1999 Mefloquine (hydrochloride). In: Dollery C (ed.) *Therapeutic Drugs* 2nd edn. Churchill Livingstone, Edinburgh, pp. M24–M30.

Brockman A, Price RN, van Vugt M et al 2000 *Plasmodium falciparum* antimalarial drug susceptibility on the north-western border of Thailand during five years of extensive use of artesunate – mefloquine. *Transactions of the Royal Society of Tropical Medicine and Hygiene* 94: 537–544.

Duraisingh MT, Roper C, Walliker D, Warhurst DC 2000 Increased sensitivity to the antimalarials mefloquine and artemisinin is conferred by mutations in the *pfmdr1* gene of *Plasmodium falciparum*. *Molecular Microbiology* 36: 955–961.

Kunin CM, Ellis WY 2000 Antimicrobial activities of mefloquine and a series of related compounds. *Antimicrobial Agents and Chemotherapy* 44: 848–852.

Pukrittayakamee S, Chantra A, Simpson JA et al 2000 Therapeutic responses to different antimalarial drugs in Vivax malaria. *Antimicrobial Agents and Chemotherapy* 44: 1680–1685.

Simpson JA, Watkins ER, Price RN et al 2000 Mefloquine pharmacokinetic–pharmacodynamic models: implications for dosing and resistance. *Antimicrobial Agents and Chemotherapy* 44: 3414–3424.

Pennie RA, Koren G, Crevoisier C 1993 Steady state pharmacokinetics of mefloquine in long-term travellers. *Transactions of the Royal Society of Tropical Medicine and Hygiene* 87: 459–462.

PRIMAQUINE

Molecular weight (free compound): 259.3; (diphosphate): 455.3.

A synthetic 8-aminoquinoline, formulated as the diphosphate for oral administration.

Antimicrobial activity

Primaquine is highly active against the hepatic stages of the malaria life cycle, including the latent hypnozoite stage of *P. vivax*. It has poor activity against erythrocytic stages of malaria parasites, but kills gametocytes. The isomers have similar antiplasmodial activity but differ in toxicity. There is activity against *Pneumocystis carinii*. In experimental models primaquine has activity against *Babesia* spp. and the intracellular stages of *Leishmania* spp. and *T. cruzi*.

Acquired resistance

Failure rates of up to 35% have been reported in South-east Asia in patients treated with a standard course for *P. vivax* infections.

Pharmacokinetics

Oral absorption	>75%
C_{max} 45 mg oral	0.2 mg/l after 2–3 h
Plasma half-life	4–10 h
Volume of distribution	2 l/kg
Plasma protein binding	Extensive

Bioavailability is variable after oral administration. There is extensive tissue distribution. About 60% of the dose is metabolized to carboxyprimaquine, which can reach levels 50 times that of the parent drug; this metabolite has a half-life of 16 h, a low tissue distribution and is detectable at 120 h. Methoxy and hydroxy metabolites are also detectable. Less than 4% of the original dose is excreted unchanged in urine.

Toxicity and side effects

At standard doses side effects are mild: abdominal cramps, anemia, leukocytosis and methemoglobinemia. Patients with glucose-6-phosphate dehydrogenase deficiency, which occurs most frequently in Africans, are prone to intravascular hemolysis resulting from the oxidant stress induced by the drug.

Clinical use

- Radical cure of malaria caused by *P. vivax* or *P. ovale*.
- Mild or moderately severe infections with *Pneumocystis carinii* (in combination with clindamycin).

Because of its gametocytocidal properties primaquine has been used rarely in a single dose to prevent the spread of chloroquine resistant *P. falciparum*.

Preparations and dosage

Dosage: Malaria treatment, adults, oral, 15 mg per day for 14–21 days (after chloroquine). Children, oral, 250 microgram/kg per day as per adult. Malaria prophylaxis, see specialist guidelines.

Limited availability in the UK.

Further information

Anonymous 1999 Primaquine (phosphate). In: Dollery C (ed.) *Therapeutic Drugs* 2nd edn. Churchill Livingstone, Edinburgh, pp. P202–P205.

Bolchoz LJ, Budinsky RA, McMillan DC, Jollow DJ 2001 Primaquine-induced anemia: formation and hemotoxicity of the arylhydroxylamine metabolite 6-methoxy-8-hydroxyaminoquinoline. *Journal of Pharmacology and Experimental Therapeutics* 297: 509–515.

Kain KC, Shanks GD, Keystone JS 2001 Malaria chemoprophylaxis in the age of drug resistance. i. Currently recommended drug regimens. *Clinical Infectious Diseases* 33: 226–234.

Pukrittayakamee S, Chantra A, Simpson JA et al 2000 Therapeutic responses to different antimalarial drugs in vivax malaria. *Antimicrobial Agents and Chemotherapy* 44: 1680–1685.

Pukrittayakamee S, Vanijanonta S, Chantra A, Clemens R, White NJ 1994 Blood stage antimalarial efficacy of primaquine in *Plasmodium vivax* malaria. *Journal of Infectious Diseases* 169: 932–935.

Toma E, Thorne A, Singer J et al 1998 Clindamycin with primaquine vs. trimethoprim – sulfamethoxazole therapy for mild and moderately severe *Pneumocystis carinii* pneumonia in patients with AIDS: a multicentre, double blind, randomized trial (CTN 004). CTN-PCP Study Group. *Clinical Infectious Diseases* 27: 524–530.

Wernsdorfer H, Trigg PI (eds) 1987 *Primaquine: pharmacokinetics, metabolism, toxicity and activity.* WHO/Wiley, Chichester.

 # QUININE

Molecular weight (free base): 324.4.

A quinolinemethanol from the bark of the *Cinchona* tree; the laevorotatory stereoisomer of quinidine. Formulated as the sulfate, bisulfate or ethylcarbonate for oral use and as the dihydrochloride for parenteral administration. The salts are highly soluble in water.

Antimicrobial activity

Quinine inhibits the erythrocytic stages of human malaria parasites at <1 mg/l, but not the liver stages. It is also active against the gametocytes of *P. vivax*, *P. ovale* and *P. malariae*, but not *P. falciparum*. The dextrarotatory stereoisomer, quinidine, is more active than quinine, but epiquinine (cinchonine) and epiquinidine (cinchonidine) have much lower antimalarial activities.

Acquired resistance

Resistance in *P. falciparum* was first reported in Brazil in 1910. It is now widespread in South-east Asia, where some strains are also resistant to chloroquine, sulfadoxine-pyrimethamine and mefloquine. Cross-resistance with mefloquine has been demonstrated in *P. falciparum* in Central Africa and in laboratory studies.

Pharmacokinetics

Oral absorption	80–90%
C_{max} 600 mg oral	5 mg/l after 1–3 h
Plasma half-life	8.7 h
Volume of distribution	1.8 l/kg
Plasma protein binding	c. 70%

Quinine is well absorbed by the oral route. Intramuscular administration gives more predictable data than intravenous administration and may be more useful in children. Plasma protein binding rises to 90% in uncomplicated malaria and 92% in cerebral malaria due to high levels of acute-phase proteins. Similarly, the elimination half-life rises to 18.2 h in severe malaria. There is extensive hepatic metabolism to hydroxylated derivatives. Urinary clearance is <20% of total clearance.

Toxicity and side effects

Up to 25% of patients experience cardiac dysrhythmia, hypoglycemia, cinchonism (tinnitus, vomiting, diarrhea, headache). Severe effects, including hypotension and hypoglycemia, are of particular importance in children, pregnant women and the severely ill. Rarely, quinine can induce hemolytic anemia ('blackwater fever').

Clinical use

- Falciparum malaria (alone or in combination with tetracycline, doxycycline, clindamycin or pyrimethamine-sulfadoxine).
- Babesiosis (in combination with clindamycin).

Quinine is particularly used in cerebral malaria, if chloroquine resistance is suspected (Ch. 64). Quinidine, which is used as an antiarrhythmic drug and is more toxic, may be substituted in severe drug-resistant *P. falciparum* malaria if quinine is not available.

Preparations and dosage

Preparations: Tablets, injection.

Dosage: Treatment of falciparum malaria: Adults, oral, 600 mg of quinine salt every 8 h for 7 days; i.v., initial loading dose of 20 mg/kg quinine salt (up to a maximum of 1.4 g) infused over 4 h, then after 8–12 h a maintenance dose of 10 mg/kg (up to a maximum of 700 mg) infused over 4 h, every 8–12 h until oral therapy can be taken to complete the 7-day course. Children, oral, 10 mg/kg of quinine salt every 8 h for 7 days. Malaria prophylaxis: see specialist guidelines.

Widely available.

 ## Further information

Anonymous 1999 Quinine. In: Dollery C (ed.) *Therapeutic Drugs* 2nd edn. Churchill Livingstone, Edinburgh, pp. Q16–Q21.

Bjorkmann A, Willcox M, Marbiah N, Payne D 1991 Susceptibility of *Plasmodium falciparum* to different doses of quinine in vivo and to quinine and quinidine in vitro in relation to chloroquine in Liberia. *Bulletin of the World Health Organization* 69: 459–465.

Krishna S, Nagaraja NV, Planche T et al 2001 Population pharmacokinetics of intramuscular quinine in children with severe malaria. *Antimicrobial Agents and Chemotherapy* 45: 1803–1809.

Meshnick SR 1997 Why does quinine still work after 350 years of use? *Parasitology Today* 13: 89–90.

Meshnick SR 1998 From quinine to qinghaosu: historical perspectives. In: Sherman IW (ed.) *Malaria: Parasite Biology, Pathogenesis, and Protection*. ASM Press, Washington, USA, pp. 341–353.

Pukrittayakamee S, Supanaranond W, Looareesuwan S, Vanijanonta S, White NJ 1994 Quinine in severe falciparum malaria: evidence of declining efficacy in Thailand. *Transactions of the Royal Society of Tropical Medicine and Hygiene* 88: 324–327.

DIAMIDINES

Stilbamidine, propamidine, pentamidine and diminazene were initially developed for the treatment of African trypanosomiasis following the identification of the trypanocidal activity of structurally related biguanidines in 1937. Pentamidine has been used extensively for early stage infections with *T. brucei gambiense* and was formerly given half-yearly as part of a mass prophylaxis campaign in Central Africa. Pentamidine has acquired a new lease of life because of its efficacy in the prophylaxis and treatment of *P. carinii* infections. Another diamidine, diminazene aceturate (Berenil), is used for cattle trypanosomiasis, but is not registered for human use.

Propamidine and hexamidine have been used for the topical treatment of ocular amebiasis caused by *Acanthamoeba* spp.; therapeutic activity is also reported for the structurally related polyhexamethylene biguanide. Novel amidoxime derivatives have high activity against *T. brucei* and *P. carinii*.

 ## Further information

Loin L, Coster DJ, Badenoch PR 2000 Antimicrobial susceptibility of 19 Australian isolates of *Acanthamoeba*. *Clinical Experimental Ophthalmology* 28: 119–124.

Pepin J, Milord F 1994. The treatment of human African trypanosomiasis. *Advances in Parasitology* 33: 1–47.

Perrine D, Chenu JP, Georges P, Lancelot JC, Saturnino C, Robba M 1995 Amoebicidal efficiencies of various diamidines against two strains of *Acanthamoeba polyphaga*. *Antimicrobial Agents and Chemotherapy* 39: 339–342.

 ## PENTAMIDINE

Molecular weight (isethionate): 592.7.

A synthetic diamidine, available as the isethionate (2-hydroxymethane sulfonate) salt for parenteral use. It is also administered by instillation of a nebulized solution directly into the lungs.

Antimicrobial activity

Pentamidine has broad antiprotozoal activity in experimental models against *P. falciparum*, *Toxoplasma gondii*, *Leishmania* spp., *Trypanosoma* spp. and *Babesia* spp. It also has activity against *P. carinii*.

Acquired resistance

Relapse rates of 7–16% have been reported in the treatment of human African trypanosomiasis in West Africa. Patients usually respond to a subsequent course of treatment with melarsoprol. Arsenic-resistant *T. brucei* are cross-resistant to diamidines, but far more so to diminazene and stilbamidine than pentamidine.

Pharmacokinetics

Oral absorption	Negligible
C_{max} 4 mg/kg intramuscular	c. 0.5 mg/l after 1 h
Plasma half-life	c. 6.5 h
Volume of distribution	3 l/kg
Plasma protein binding	c. 70%

Pentamidine is rapidly and extensively metabolized by rat liver, and high concentrations are retained in renal and hepatic tissue for up to 6 months after administration. In humans distribution is mainly in the liver, kidney, adrenal glands and spleen, with lower accumulation in the lung. This tissue retention is the basis for its prophylactic use. Critically, for the treatment of African trypanosomiasis, the drug is unable to cross the blood–brain barrier in sufficient quantity to be trypanocidal: <1% of the plasma concentration has been measured in the CSF of sleeping-sickness patients. About 15–20% of the dose is excreted in the urine but because of retention in tissues there is an extremely long terminal half-life (>12 days).

Toxicity and side effects

Side effects range from local irritation and sterile abscess at the site of injection to transient effects (vomiting, abdominal discomfort) and serious systemic effects (hypotension, effects on heart, hypoglycemia and hyperglycemia, leukopenia, thrombocytopenia). In a study of the treatment of South American cutaneous leishmaniasis, 17% of patients prematurely terminated treatment due to toxicity and another 30% reported side effects.

Clinical use

- Human African trypanosomiasis (early stages before CNS involvement).
- Prophylaxis and therapy of *Pneumocystis carinii* pneumonia.
- Leishmaniasis unresponsive to pentavalent antimonials.

There is limited evidence for its use in the treatment of clinical babesiosis.

Preparations and dosage

Proprietary name: Pentacarinat.

Preparations: Injection, nebulizer solution.

Dosage

Visceral leishmaniasis: Adults, i.m., 3–4 mg/kg once or twice weekly until the condition resolves or i.v., 3–4 mg/kg on alternate days to a maximum of 10 injections.

Trypanosomiasis: Adults, i.m., 4 mg/kg daily or on alternate days to a total of 7–10 injections.

P. carinii pneumonia: i.v., 4 mg/kg/day for at least 14 days.

Widely available.

Further information

Anonymous 1999 Pentamidine. In: Dollery C (ed.) *Therapeutic Drugs* 2nd edn. Churchill Livingstone, Edinburgh, pp. P38–P43.

Barrett MP, Fairlamb AH 1999 The biochemical basis of arsenical-diamidine cross-resistance in African trypanosomes. *Parasitology Today* 15: 136–140.

Berger BJ, Henry L, Hall JE, Tidwell R 1992 Problems and pitfalls in the assay of pentamidine. *Clinical Pharmacokinetics* 22: 163–168.

Berman JD 1997 Human leishmaniasis: clinical, diagnostic, and chemotherapeutic developments in the last 10 years. *Clinical Infectious Diseases* 24: 684–703.

Bronner U, Doua F, Ericsson O et al 1991 Pentamidine concentrations in plasma, whole blood and cerebrospinal fluid during treatment of *Trypanosoma gambiense* infection in Côte d'Ivoire. *Transactions of the Royal Society of Tropical Medicine and Hygiene* 85: 608–611.

Pepin J, Milord F 1994 The treatment of human African trypanosomiasis. *Advances in Parasitology* 33: 1–47.

Stead AMW, Bray P, Edwards IG et al 2001 Diamidine compounds: selective uptake and targeting in *Plasmodium falciparum*. *Molecular Pharmacology* 59: 1298–1306.

Wei CC, Gardner S, Rachlis A, Pack LL, Chan CK 2001 Risk factors for prophylaxis failure in patients receiving aerosol pentamidine for *Pneumocystis carinii* pneumonia prophylaxis. *Chest* 119: 1427–1433.

Vöhringer HF, Arasteh K 1993 Pharmacokinetic optimisation in the treatment of *Pneumocystis carinii* pneumonia. *Clinical Pharmacokinetics* 24: 388–412.

PROPAMIDINE

A synthetic diamidine formulated as the isethionate or as dibromopropamidine isethionate for topical administration to the eye.

Its activity against bacterial pathogens is poor, but it exhibits specific activity against *Acanthamoeba* spp. Reduction in sensitivity of *Acanthamoeba* during encystation might reflect changes in drug uptake.

Clinical use

- Amebic keratitis (in combination with neomycin or other agents).

Further information

Turner NA, Russell AD, Furr JR, Lloyd D 2000 Emergence of resistance to biocides during differentiation of *Acanthamoeba castellanii*. *Journal of Antimicrobial Chemotherapy* 46: 27–34.

Varga JH, Wolf TC, Parmley VC, Rowsey JJ 1993 Combined treatment of *Acanthamoeba* keratitis with propamidine, neomycin and polyhexamethylene biguanide. *American Journal of Ophthalmology* 115: 466–470.

Preparations and dosage

Proprietary name: Brolene.

Preparation: Ophthalmic ointment and eye drops.

Widely available.

BIGUANIDES

The antimalarial activity of biguanides was discovered during the Second World War by Rose, Davey and Curd of the ICI pharmaceutical company. The most important compound, proguanil, is used widely as an antimalarial prophylactic. The closely related chlorproguanil is used in combination with dapsone. They are prodrugs, metabolized in vivo to the triazines cycloguanil and chlorcycloguanil, which have much enhanced activity. Along with the diaminopyrimidines (Ch. 19) these drugs are often referred to as antifolates due to their mechanism of action (p. 18).

PROGUANIL

Chlorguanide. Molecular weight (free base): 253.8; (hydrochloride): 290.2.

Cycloguanil

Proguanil

A synthetic arylbiguanide, formulated as the hydrochloride for oral use. It is slightly soluble in water.

Antimicrobial activity

Proguanil may have some direct antiplasmodial action, but most of the useful activity is attributable to its metabolite cycloguanil, which inhibits the early erythrocytic stages of all four *Plasmodium* spp. that cause human malaria and the primary hepatic stage of *P. falciparum*. Proguanil acts synergistically with atovaquone and probably enhances its effect on mitochondrial membrane charge.

Acquired resistance

Resistance of *P. falciparum* associated with point mutations of dihydrofolate reductase has been reported worldwide, although infrequently despite its use since the 1940s. Resistance in *P. vivax* and *P. malariae* has been reported in South-east Asia. Cross-resistance with pyrimethamine is not absolute, because differential resistance can arise from different point mutations on the dihydrofolate reductase gene. The chlorproguanil–dapsone combination is effective against *P. falciparum* strains with some mutations but not others.

Pharmacokinetics

Oral absorption	>90%
C_{max} 100 mg oral	0.4 mg/l after 2–4 h
Plasma half-life	10 h
Plasma protein binding	75%

Oral absorption is slow. It is 75% protein bound and is concentrated 10- to 15-fold by erythrocytes. About 20% of the drug is metabolized to dihydrotriazene derivatives, most importantly cycloguanil, by hepatic cytochrome P_{450} processes. Cycloguanil is detectable 2 h after administration of proguanil. High proportions of 'non-metabolizers' have been identified in Japan and Kenya, indicating another source of resistance. About 60% of the dose is excreted in urine.

A combination of chlorproguanil 1.2 mg/kg with dapsone 2.4 mg/kg achieved plasma levels of chlorproguanil of 0.1 mg/l with a half-life of 12 h.

Toxicity and side effects

Proguanil is well tolerated at recommended doses. Gastrointestinal and renal effects have been reported at doses exceeding 600 mg/day.

Clinical use

- Antimalarial prophylaxis (usually in combination with chloroquine).
- Treatment and prophylaxis for drug-resistant falciparum malaria (in combination with atovaquone).

The chlorproguanil–dapsone combination ('lapdap') has undergone extensive clinical trials and is under development.

 Preparations and dosage

Proprietary name: Paludrine.

Preparation: Tablets.

For malaria prophylaxis, see specialist guidelines.

Widely available.

 Further information

Anonymous 1999 Proguanil (hydrochloride). In: Dollery C (ed.) *Therapeutic Drugs* 2nd edn. Churchill Livingstone, Edinburgh, pp. P232–P236.

Amukoye E, Winstanley PA, Watkins PA et al 1997 Chlorproguanil–dapsone: effective treatment for uncomplicated malaria. *Antimicrobial Agents and Chemotherapy* 41: 2261–2264.

Bradley DJ, Warhurst DC 1995 Malaria prophylaxis: guidelines for travellers from the United Kingdom. *British Medical Journal* 341: 848–851.

Srivastava IK, Vaidya AB 1999 A mechanism for the synergistic antimalarial action of atovaquone and proguanil. *Antimicrobial Agents and Chemotherapy* 43: 1334–1339.

Watkins WN, Mberu EK, Winstanley PA, Plowe CV 1997 The efficacy of antifolate antimalarial combinations in Africa: a predictive model based on pharmacodynamic and pharmacokinetic analyses. *Parasitology Today* 13: 458–464.

Winstanley PA 2000 Chemotherapy for falciparum malaria: the armoury, the problems and the prospects. *Parasitology Today* 16: 146–153.

SESQUITERPENE LACTONES

In 1979, a research group in China described the use of a sesquiterpene peroxide, artemisinin (qinghaosu), in the treatment of malaria caused by *P. falciparum* and *P. vivax*. This compound, derived from a plant used in traditional Chinese medicine, *Artemisia annua*, has been used extensively in East Asia and Africa for the treatment of malaria. This drug, and derivatives that have higher intrinsic antimalarial activity and improved formulations (artesunate, artemether and arteether), have replaced quinine as a treatment of falciparum malaria in South-east Asia and are being used widely, alone and in combination with other antimalarials.

The novel structure, containing an endoperoxide bridge, has stimulated the development of semisynthetic and synthetic dioxane, trioxane and tetroxane compounds with activity against *Plasmodium* spp. and *Tox. gondii*.

 Further information

Meshnick SR 1998 From quinine to qinghaosu: historical perspectives. In: Sherman IW, (ed.) *Malaria: Parasite Biology, Pathogenesis, and Protection*, ASM Press, Washington, USA, pp. 341–353.

Meshnick SR, Taylor TE, Kamchonwongpaisan S 1996 Artemisinin and the antimalarial endoperoxides: from herbal remedy to targeted chemotherapy. *Microbiological Reviews* 60: 301–315.

Vroman JA, Alvim-Gaston M, Avery MA 1999 Current progress in the chemistry, medicinal chemistry and drug design of artemisinin-based antimalarials. *Current Pharmaceutical Design* 5: 101–138.

ARTEMISININ

Qinghaosu. Molecular weight (native compound): 282.3; (artemether): 298.4; (sodium artesunate): 407.4.

Artemisinin

R = CCH₂ CH₂ COOH: Artesunate

$R = CCH_2 CH_2 COOH$: Artesunate
‖
O

$R = CH_3$: Artemether

A sesquiterpene peroxide derived from *A. annua*, chiefly used in the form of artemether, the methyl ester synthesized from dihydroartemisinin, or artesunate, the water-soluble hemisuccinate. Formulated for administration by the oral, intramuscular or intrarectal routes; artesunate can also be given intravenously.

Antimicrobial activity

Artemisinin is active against the erythrocytic and gametocyte stages of chloroquine-sensitive and chloroquine-resistant strains of *P. falciparum* and other malaria parasites. Two anomers of artemether are produced on synthesis, α-artemether and β-artemether, of which the latter has higher antimalarial activity. Uptake into *Plasmodium*-infected erythrocytes is by a tubovesicular membrane network. Activities against the protozoa *Tox. gondii* and *Leishmania major* and the helminth *Schistosoma mansoni* have been demonstrated in experimental models.

Acquired resistance

Although artemisinin resistance has been developed in *Plasmodium* in experimental models, there have been no clinical reports of resistance.

Pharmacokinetics

Oral absorption	Incomplete
C_{max} 500 mg oral	0.4 mg/l after 1.8 h
Plasma half-life (dihydroartemisinin)	40–60 min
Volume of distribution	c. 0.25 l/kg
Plasma protein binding (artemether)	77%

Artemisinins are concentrated by erythrocytes and are rapidly hydrolyzed to dihydroartemisinin. They are hydroxylated by cytochromes 2B6, 2C19 and 3A4; the derivatives induce this metabolism. After injection peak plasma concen-

trations are reached within 1–3 h, when levels of dihydroartemisinin are included. The elimination half-life of intravenous artesunate is <30 min; artemether appears to have a much longer half-life (4–11 h).

Toxicity and side effects

Few toxic effects other than drug-induced fever and a reversible decrease in reticulocyte counts have been reported. High-dose studies in animal models show neurotoxicity and reproducible dose-related neuropathic lesions; dihydroartemisinin is a toxic metabolite but the precise causes of neurotoxicity are not clear.

Clinical use

- Malaria (including cerebral malaria).

Combinations of artesunate with mefloquine, or artemether with lumefantrine (benflumetol; an aryl-aminoalcohol) are also used in the treatment of uncomplicated falciparum malaria (Ch. 64). Prophylactic effects on *S. mansoni* infection have been shown in field trials.

Preparations and dosage

Preparations: Tablets, injection, suppositories.

Dosage: Adults, oral, 25 mg/kg on the first day, then 12.5 mg/kg on days two and three (plus mefloquine on day two to effect a radical cure). Other derivatives can also be given.

Limited availability.

Further information

Anonymous 1999 Artemisinin. In: Dollery C (ed.) *Therapeutic Drugs* 2nd edn. Churchill Livingstone, Edinburgh, pp. A208–A213.

Brewer TG, Peggins JO, Grate SJ et al 1994 Neurotoxicity in animals due to arteether and artemether. *Transactions of the Royal Society of Tropical Medicine and Hygiene* 88 (Suppl. 1): 33–36.

Davis TME, Phuong HL, Ilett KF et al 2001 Pharmacokinetics and pharmacodynamics of intravenous artesunate in severe falciparum malaria. *Antimicrobial Agents and Chemotherapy* 45: 181–186.

Giao PT, de Vries PJ 2001 Pharmacokinetic interactions of antimalarial drugs. *Clinical Pharmacokinetics* 40: 343–373.

Newton P, Suputtamongkol Y, Teja-Isavadharm P et al 2000 Antimalarial bioavailability and disposition of artesunate in acute falciparum malaria. *Antimicrobial Agents and Chemotherapy* 44: 972–977.

Olliaro P, Haynes RK, Meunier B, Yuthavong Y 2001 Possible modes of action of the artemisinin-type compounds. *Trends in Parasitology* 17: 122–125.

Smith SL, Sadler CJ, Dodd CC et al 2001 The role of glutathione in the neurotoxicity of artemisinin derivatives in vitro. *Biochemical Pharmacology* 61: 409–416.

Utzinger J, N'Goran EK, N'Dri A et al 2000 Oral artemether for prevention of *Schistosoma mansoni* infection: randomised controlled trial. *Lancet* 355: 1320–1325.

Wilairatna P, Krudsood S, Silachamroon U et al 2000 Clinical trial of sequential treatments of moderately severe and severe malaria with dihydroartemisinin suppository followed by mefloquine in Thailand. *American Journal of Tropical Medicine and Hygiene* 63: 290–294.

Winstanley PA 2000 Chemotherapy for falciparum malaria: the armoury, the problems and the prospects. *Parasitology Today* 16: 146–153.

MISCELLANEOUS ANTIPROTOZOAL AGENTS

 ## ATOVAQUONE

Molecular weight: 366.8.

A hydroxynaphthoquinone. Available as the *trans* isomer (which is more active than the *cis* form) for oral use. It is insoluble in water.

Antimicrobial activity

Atovaquone is more active than standard antimalarials in vitro against *P. falciparum*, with an IC_{50} value of about 1 nM. It is active against erythrocytic, liver and sexual stages of the malaria parasite. It is also active against *Babesia* spp. and both tachyzoites and cysts of *Tox. gondii* in vitro and in mice. *P. carinii* is sensitive in vitro at 0.1–3.0 mg/l and high doses are effective in the rat.

Acquired resistance

In clinical trials of the treatment of malaria there was up to 33% relapse rate following monotherapy. Recrudescent parasites were 1000 times more resistant to atovaquone than pretreatment parasites. Point mutations on parasite cytochrome b are associated with drug resistance. This rapid selection of parasites resistant to atovaquone led to the development of the synergistic combination with proguanil. Failure of *P. carinii* prophylaxis has also been associated with similar mutations.

Pharmacokinetics

Oral absorption	Poor
C_{max} 750 mg oral	27 mg/l (steady-state)
Plasma half-life	70 h
Plasma protein binding	>99%

Atovaquone is highly lipophilic and bioavailability is doubled when administered with meals. Steady-state plasma concentrations are up to 50% lower in AIDS patients than in asymptomatic HIV-positive cases and the elimination half-life is lower (55 h) in patients with AIDS. It penetrates the CSF, but the concentration is less than 1% of the plasma level. Unlike some other naphthoquinones it is not metabolized by human liver microsomes. Combinations with co-trimoxazole

(in HIV patients) and with proguanil plus artesunate in healthy adults did not produce any changes in atovaquone pharmacokinetics.

Toxicity and side effects

Most clinical trials have involved patients with AIDS in whom adverse effects are often difficult to detect; however, more than 20% reported fever, nausea, diarrhea and rashes. There were limited changes in hepatocellular function.

Clinical use

- *Pneumocystis carinii* pneumonia.
- Prophylaxis and treatment of malaria (in combination with proguanil).

The drug has been used in cerebral toxoplasmosis in AIDS patients and against human babesiosis but further studies are necessary.

 ## Preparations and dosage

Proprietary name: Malarone.

Preparations: Tablets, oral suspension.

Dosage

P. carinii pneumonia treatment: adults, oral, 750 mg twice daily for 21 days.

Malaria treatment: adults, oral, 1 g per day (plus proguanil 400 mg per day) for 3 days.

Malaria prophylaxis: see specialist guidelines.

Widely available.

Further information

Anonymous 1999 Atovaquone. In: Dollery C (ed.) *Therapeutic Drugs* 2nd edn. Churchill Livingstone, Edinburgh, pp. A233–A236.

Baggish AL, Hill DR 2002 Antiparasitic agent atovaquone. *Antimicrobial Agents and Chemotherapy* 46: 1163–1173.

Canfield CJ, Pudney M, Gutteridge WE 1995 Interactions of atovaquone with other antimalarials against *Plasmodium falciparum in vitro*. *Experimental Parasitology* 80: 373–381.

Hogh B, Clarke PD, Camus D et al 2000 Atovaquone-proguanil versus chloroquine-proguanil for malaria prophylaxis in non-immune travellers: a randomised, double-blind study. Malarone International Study Team. *Lancet* 356: 1864–1865.

Korsinczky M, Chen N, Kotecka B et al 2000 Mutations in *Plasmodium falciparum* cytochrome b that are associated with atovaquone resistance are located at a putative drug-binding site. *Antimicrobial Agents and Chemotherapy* 44: 2100–2108.

Krause PJ, Lepore T, Sikand VK et al 2000 Atovaquone and azithromycin for the treatment of babesiosis. *New England Journal of Medicine* 343: 1454–1458.

Lell B, Luckner D, Ndjave M, Scott T, Kremsner PG 1998 Randomised palcebo-controlled study of atovaquone plus proguanil for malaria prophylaxis in children. *Lancet* 351: 709–713.

Rosenberg DM, McCarthy W, Slavinsky J et al 2001 Atovaquone suspension for treatment of *Pneumocystis carinii* pneumonia in HIV-infected patients. *AIDS* 15: 211–214.

Srivastava IK, Vaidya AB 1999 A mechanism for the synergistic antimalarial action of atovaquone and proguanil. *Antimicrobial Agents and Chemotherapy* 43: 1334–1339.

Walter DJ, Wakefield AE, Dohn MN et al 1998 Sequence polymorphisms in the *Pneumocystis carinii* cytochrome b gene and their association with atovaquone prophylaxis failure. *Journal of Infectious Diseases* 178: 1767–1775.

 # DEHYDROEMETINE

Molecular weight (free compound): 478.61; (hydrochloride): 515.1.

The synthetic racemic derivative of the plant alkaloid emetine, which is no longer recommended for use. Formulated as the hydrochloride for intramuscular administration.

Antimicrobial activity

Like the parent compound, emetine, it inhibits *E. histolytica* at concentrations of 1–10 mg/l in vitro, but it is more active than the parent in animal models. It also has activity against *Leishmania* spp. in experimental models.

Acquired resistance

Drug-resistant *E. histolytica* is rare, but differences in sensitivity have been reported.

Pharmacokinetics

Dehydroemetine is administered parenterally. No human pharmacokinetic data are available. A half-life of 2 days, compared with 5 days for emetine, has been reported. There is selective tissue binding and accumulation in the liver, lung, spleen and kidney.

Toxicity and side effects

It is considerably less toxic than emetine, possibly because it is more rapidly eliminated. Nevertheless, nausea, vomiting, diarrhea and abdominal cramps frequently occur. Neuromuscular effects have also been reported. More serious cardiotoxic effects can lead to electrocardiogram (ECG) changes, tachycardia and a drop in blood pressure.

Clinical use

- Severe intestinal or hepatic amebiasis (second-line treatment).

 ### Preparations and dosage

Preparation: Injection.

Dosage: Adults, s.c., i.m., 1–1.5 mg/kg daily for 4–6 days with a maximum daily dose of 90 mg. Allow 6 weeks between courses.

Limited availability.

 ### Further information

Badalamenti S, Jameson JE, Reddy KR 1999 Amebiasis. *Current Treatment Options in Gastroenterology* 2: 97–103.

Ohnishi K, Murata M, Kojima H, Takemura N, Tsuchida T, Tachibana H 1994 Brain abscess due to infection with *Entamoeba histolytica*. *American Journal of Tropical Medicine and Hygiene* 51: 180–182.

DILOXANIDE

Molecular weight (furoate): 328.2.

Dichloro(hydroxyphenyl)methylacetamide. Available as the furoate, an insoluble ester, for oral administration.

Antimicrobial activity

Diloxanide inhibits *E. histolytica* with unusually high specificity at concentrations of 0.01–0.1 mg/l. It is more effective in mouse and rat models than in the hamster model of infection.

Acquired resistance

No resistance has been reported. Patients with dysentery have lower cure rates than cyst excreters.

Pharmacokinetics

Human pharmacokinetic data are limited. Animal data show that diloxanide furoate is rapidly absorbed from the intestine. The furoate is hydrolyzed in the gut, leaving high intraluminal concentrations of free diloxanide. About 75% is excreted via the kidney within 48 h, mostly as a glucuronide.

Toxicity and side effects

It is well tolerated, but flatulence is common, and nausea and vomiting may occur.

Clinical use

- Asymptomatic intestinal (luminal) amebiasis.

It is also used for the eradication of cysts after the treatment of acute amebiasis with nitroimidazoles.

Preparations and dosage

Proprietary names: Furamide, Entamizole.

Preparation: Tablets.

Dosage: Adults, oral, 500 mg every 8 h for 10 days. Children >25 kg, oral, 20 mg/kg daily in three divided doses for 10 days.

Limited availability. Available in the USA and UK.

Further information

Anonymous 1999 Diloxanide furoate. In: Dollery C (ed.) *Therapeutic Drugs* 2nd edn. Churchill Livingstone, Edinburgh, pp. D136–D138.

Badalamenti S, Jameson JE, Reddy KR 1999 Amebiasis. *Current Treatment Options in Gastroenterology* 2: 97–103.

Bhopale KK, Pradhan KS, Masani KB, Kaul CL 1995 A comparative study of experimental amoebiasis and the evaluation of amoebicides. *Annals of Tropical Medicine and Parasitology* 89: 253–259.

EFLORNITHINE

α-Difluoromethylornithine. Molecular weight (free base): 182.2; (hydrochloride monohydrate): 236.6.

$$H_2N(CH_2)_3 - \overset{\overset{\displaystyle NH_2}{|}}{\underset{\underset{\displaystyle CHF_2}{|}}{C}} - COOH$$

An analog of ornithine, formulated as the hydrochloride for intravenous infusion. It is freely soluble in water.

Antimicrobial activity

Cultured bloodstream trypomastigotes of *T. brucei* are relatively insensitive, but high doses are effective against bloodstream and CNS infections of *T. brucei brucei* and *T. brucei gambiense* in rodents, provided a strong antibody response is also present. *T. brucei rhodesiense* infections do not respond. Synergy with some arsenicals has been demonstrated. Eflornithine is also active against *P. falciparum* in experimental models and against *Leishmania* promastigotes and *Giardia lamblia* in culture.

Acquired resistance

Acquired resistance in *T. brucei gambiense* in West Africa has not been reported, but *T. brucei rhodesiense* strains from East Africa are innately less sensitive.

Pharmacokinetics

Oral absorption	55%
C_{max} 10 mg/kg oral	c. 7 mg/l after 4 h
200 mg/kg intravenously	15.9 mg/l (87.5 nmol/ml) (mean)
Plasma half-life	3.3 h
Volume of distribution	0.34 l/kg
Plasma protein binding	Very low

Renal clearance is 83%, with most eliminated unchanged. In a study in Zaire the mean serum concentration in children under 12 years old was half that of adults, probably due to more rapid renal clearance. CNS penetration is good in adults with a CSF:plasma ratio of 0.91 at the end of administration for 14 days. However, the CSF:plasma ratio in children under 12 years old was 0.58. Relapses have been recorded in patients in whom CSF levels dropped below 9 mg/l (50 nmol/ml) at the end of treatment.

Toxicity and side effects

Osmotic diarrhea and bone marrow suppression are common, and up to 50% of sleeping sickness patients develop leukopenia. Reversible anemia and thrombocytopenia have been observed. Convulsions and seizures, different from those observed in melarsoprol-induced encephalopathy, have been reported in 4–18% of treated sleeping sickness patients but not in patients treated for *P. carinii* pneumonia. This difference might be due to the CNS inflammation associated with sleeping sickness.

Clinical use

- Late-stage *T. brucei gambiense* infections (including arsenic-resistant cases).

It has been used speculatively for treatment of *P. carinii* infections in AIDS patients.

Preparations and dosage

Proprietary name: Ornidyl.

Preparation: Injection.

Dosage: Trypanosomiasis: adults, i.v., 400 mg/kg daily in divided doses for at least 14 days.

Limited availability. The manufacturers will donate it to the WHO and Médicines sans Frontières over a 5-year period.

Further information

Anonymous 1999 Eflornithine (hydrochloride). In: Dollery C (ed.) *Therapeutic Drugs* 2nd edn. Churchill Livingstone, Edinburgh, pp. E7–E10.

McCann PP, Pegg AE 1992 Ornithine decarboxylase as an enzyme target for therapy. *Pharmacology and Therapeutics* 54: 195–215.

Milord F, Loko L, Ethier L, Mpia B, Pepin J 1993 Eflornithine concentrations in serum and cerebrospinal fluid in 63 patients treated for *Trypanosoma brucei gambiense* sleeping sickness. *Transactions of the Royal Society of Tropical Medicine and Hygiene* 87: 473–477.

Pepin J, Khonde N, Maiso F et al 2000 Short-course eflornithine in Gambian trypanosomiasis: a multicentre randomized controlled trial. *Bulletin of the World Health Organization* 78: 1284–1295.

Vohringer HF, Arasteh K 1993 Pharmacokinetic optimisation in the treatment of *Pneumocystis carinii* pneumonia. *Clinical Pharmacokinetics* 24: 388–412.

HALOFANTRINE

Molecular weight (free base): 500.4; (hydrochloride): 536.9.

A phenanthrene methanol, formulated as the hydrochloride for oral administration. Parenteral formulations are not available. The enantiomers have equivalent activity in vitro. Aqueous solubility is extremely low.

Antimicrobial activity

Halofantrine inhibits erythrocytic stages of chloroquine-sensitive and chloroquine-resistant *P. falciparum* and other *Plasmodium* spp. in vitro at concentrations in the range of 0.4–4.0 mg/l. It is more active than mefloquine and the combination of proguanil and atovaquone against *P. falciparum*, but less effective than mefloquine or chloroquine against *P. vivax*.

Acquired resistance

Resistance in *P. falciparum* has been reported in Central and West Africa, where it has been used widely. Cross-resistance with mefloquine has been reported in Thailand, where it has not been used.

Pharmacokinetics

Absorption shows high intra- and inter-subject variability. Bioavailability is increased more than 6-fold after a fatty meal or by lipid-based formulations. In patients with malaria bioavailability is significantly lower than in healthy individuals. Peak plasma levels are variable and occur 6 h after administration. Unlike many other antimalarials, halofantrine is not concentrated by infected or uninfected erythrocytes. Distribution to lipoproteins is stereo-selective. About 20–30% of the dose is metabolized to an *N*-desbutyl derivative by cytochrome P_{450} 3A4 and 3A5. The elimination half-life of the parent drug is 1 day and that of the metabolite 3 days. Little unchanged drug is excreted in urine.

Toxicity and side effects

Abdominal pain, diarrhea and pruritus are the most frequent. High doses (24 mg/kg) have been reported to be cardiotoxic, inducing prolongation of the PR and QTc intervals; this is not stereo-selective. Mefloquine enhances these effects by increasing the circulating concentration of halofantrine; these drugs should not be used together.

Clinical use

- Treatment of multidrug-resistant falciparum malaria.

Preparations and dosage

Proprietary name: Halfan.

Preparation: Tablets.

Dosage: Treatment of falciparum malaria: Adults, oral, 1.5 g divided into three doses of 500 mg given at intervals of 6 h; repeat the course after an interval of 1 week. Children, oral, 24 mg/kg divided into three doses as adult.

Widely available.

Further information

Abernethy DR, Wesche DL, Barbey JT et al 2001 Steroselective halofantrine disposition and effect: concentration-related QTc prolongation. *British Journal of Clinical Pharmacology* 51: 231–237.

Anonymous 1999 Halofantrine (hydrochloride). In: Dollery C (ed.) *Therapeutic Drugs* 2nd edn. Churchill Livingstone, Edinburgh, pp. H1–H3.

Baune B, Flinois JP, Furlan V et al 1999 Halofantrine metabolism in microsomes in man: major role of CYP 3A4 and CYP 3A5. *Journal of Pharmacy and Pharmacology* 51: 419–426.

Bouchaud O, Monlun E, Muanza K et al 2000 Atovaquone plus proguanil versus halofantrine in the treatment of imported acute uncomplicated *Plasmodium falciparum* malaria in non-immune adults: a randomized comparative trial. *American Journal of Tropical Medicine and Hygiene* 63: 274–279.

Brasseur P, Bittsindou P, Moyou R et al 1993 Fast emergence of *Plasmodium falciparum* resistance to halofantrine. *Lancet* 341: 901–902.

Karbwang J, Bangchang KN 1994 Clinical pharmacokinetics of halofantrine. *Clinical Pharmacokinetics* 27: 104–119.

Khoo SM, Porter CJ, Charman WN 2000 The formulation of halofantrine as either non-solubilizing PEG6000 or solubilizing lipid based solid dispersions: physical stability and absolute bioavailability assessment. *International Journal of Pharmaceutics* 205: 65–78.

Mungthin M, Bray PG, Ridley RG, Ward SA 1998 Central role of hemoglobin degradation in mechanisms of action of 4-aminoquinolines, quinoline methanols, and phenanthrene methanols. *Antimicrobial Agents and Chemotherapy* 42: 2973–2977.

Pukrittayakamee S, Chantra A, Simpson JA et al 2000 Therapeutic responses to different antimalarial drugs in vivax malaria. *Antimicrobial Agents and Chemotherapy* 44: 1680–1685.

Wilson CM, Volkman SK, Thaithong S et al 1993 Amplification of *pfmdr I* associated with mefloquine and halofantrine resistance in *Plasmodium falciparum* from Thailand. *Molecular and Biochemical Parasitology* 57: 151–160.

Winstanley PA 2000 Chemotherapy for falciparum malaria: the armoury, the problems and the prospects. *Parasitology Today* 16: 146–153.

MEPACRINE

Quinacrine (USAN). Molecular weight (dihydrochloride): 472.88.

A synthetic acridine derivative, formulated as the hydrochloride for oral use.

Antimicrobial activity

Mepacrine is active against the asexual erythrocytic stage of all four *Plasmodium* spp. that infect humans and the gametocytes of *P. vivax* and *P. malariae*. The enantiomers have equal antimalarial activity. It exhibits broad antiprotozoal activity in experimental models against *T. cruzi*, *Leishmania* spp., *E. histolytica*, *Trichomonas vaginalis*, *G. lamblia* and *Blastocystis hominis*. It is also active against tapeworms.

Acquired resistance

The structural resemblance to chloroquine suggests the likelihood of cross-resistance with that drug, but evidence for this is equivocal.

Pharmacokinetics

Oral absorption	Good
C_{max} 100 mg oral	50 μg/l after 1–3 h
Plasma half-life	5 days
Plasma protein binding	85%

There is extensive tissue binding and a 6-fold concentration into leukocytes from plasma. About 10% of the daily dose is excreted in the urine.

Toxicity and side effects

Mepacrine causes dizziness, headache and gastric problems. Toxic psychoses, bone marrow depression, yellow skin and exfoliative dermatitis are described. Poor toleration is noted, especially in children. It should not be used in combination with 8-aminoquinolines.

Clinical use

- Giardiasis.
- Prophylaxis of malaria.
- Tapeworm infections.

It has been superseded by other drugs, but is useful in giardiasis if treatment with nitroimidazoles fails. Intralesional injections have been tried in cutaneous leishmaniasis. Its sclerosant effect has led to its use in the form of intravaginal pellets as a non-surgical method of female sterilization.

 Preparations and dosage

Preparation: Tablets.

Dosage: Adults, oral, 100 mg three times daily for 5–7 days. A second course of treatment after 2 weeks is sometimes required. Children, oral, 2 mg/kg three times daily.

Limited availability.

 Further information

Bonse S, Santelli-Rouvier C, Barbe J, Krauth-Siegel RL 1999 Inhibition of *Trypanosoma cruzi* trypanothione reductase by acridines: kinetic studies and structure-activity relationships. *Journal of Medicinal Chemistry* 42: 5448–5454.
Gardner TB, Hill DR 2001 Treatment of giardiasis. *Clinical Microbiological Reviews* 14: 114–128.
Vdovanko AA, Williams JE 2000 *Blastocystis hominis:* neutral red supravital staining and its application to in vitro drug sensitivity testing. *Parasitology Research* 86: 573–581.

MILTEFOSINE

Hexadecylphosphocholine. Molecular weight: 407.58.

$$H_3C\,(CH_2)_{14}-CH_2-O-\overset{\overset{\displaystyle O}{\|}}{\underset{\underset{\displaystyle O^-}{|}}{P}}-O-CH_2\,CH_2N^+\,(CH_3)_3$$

An alkyllysophospholipid, originally investigated as an anticancer compound, formulated for oral administration.

Antimicrobial activity

Concentrations of 1–5 μM inhibit the extracellular promastigotes and intracellular amastigotes of *Leishmania* spp. and the extracellular epimastigotes and intracellular amastigotes of *Trypanosoma cruzi*. Inhibitory concentrations against *Trypanosoma brucei* sspp. and *Entamoeba histolytica* are closer to 50 μM.

Acquired resistance

There have been no reports of experimental or clinical resistance in *Leishmania*.

Pharmacokinetics

In rodent models the drug is almost completely absorbed after oral administration. About 90% is bound to plasma proteins and the half-life is 48 h. Peak concentrations are achieved after 24 h with distribution to the liver, lung, spleen, heart and brain.

Toxicity and side effects

Mild to moderate gastrointestinal side effects are reported in 40–60% of patients in clinical trials.

Clinical use

- Visceral leishmaniasis.
- Cutaneous leishmaniasis.

Preparations and dosage

Dosage: Adults, oral, 100–150 mg per day for 28 days.

Under trial. Not generally available.

Further information

Croft SL, Snowdon D, Yardley V 1996 The activities of four anticancer alkyllysophospholipids against *Leishmania donovani, Trypanosoma cruzi* and *Trypanosoma brucei. Journal of Antimicrobial Chemotherapy* 38: 1041–1047.

Jha TK, Sundar S, Thakur CP et al 1999 Mitefosine, an oral agent, for the treatment of Indian visceral leishmaniasis. *New England Journal of Medicine* 341: 1795–1800.

PYRONARIDINE

Molecular weight: 518.06.

An aza-aminoacridine formulated for oral use.

Antimicrobial activity

Pyronaridine is active against the asexual erythrocytic stage of *P. falciparum* with little or no activity against gametocytes or the hepatic stage. In-vitro blood schizonticide activities are in the range of 0.001–0.03 mg/l, showing a moderate correlation to chloroquine resistance. It is also active against *P. vivax, P. ovale* and *P. malariae.*

Acquired resistance

No resistance has been reported.

Pharmacokinetics

Peak plasma concentrations are reached after 3–14 h depending upon the formulation; there is also considerable interindividual variation. Elimination half-lives of 63–190 h have been reported, again dependent upon the formulation.

Toxicity and side effects

It is well tolerated and no outstanding toxic effects have been reported.

Clinical use

- Treatment of uncomplicated *P. falciparum* and *P. vivax* malaria.

Preparations and dosage

Not widely available. Oral formulations have been used in China and in clinical trials in Thailand and Africa.

Further information

Fu S, Xiao S-H 1991 Pyronaridine: a new antimalarial drug. *Parasitology Today* 7: 310–313.

Olliaro P 2000 Pyronaridine development at a standstill: no one prepared to foot the bill? A review of Chinese development and more recent studies. *Current Opinion in Anti-Infective Investigational Drugs* 2: 71–75.

Ringwald P; Bickii J, Basco L 1996 Randomised trial of pyronardine versus chloroquine for acute uncomplicated falciparum malaria in Africa. *Lancet* 347: 24–28.

Ringwald P, Eboumbo ECM, Bickii J, Basco LK 1999 In vitro activities of pyronaridine, alone and in combination with other antimalarial drugs, against *Plasmodium falciparum. Antimicrobial Agents and Chemotherapy* 43: 1525–1527.

SURAMIN

Molecular weight (hexasodium salt): 1429.21.

A sulfated naphthylamine formulated for intravenous administration. It is freely soluble in water. The dry powder is stable, but it is hygroscopic and unstable in solution.

Antimicrobial activity

Suramin has no significant trypanocidal activity in vitro, but is effective in animals infected with *T. brucei*. Trypanosomes take up suramin bound to plasma protein by a combination of fluid phase and receptor-mediated endocytosis. It acts synergistically with nitroimidazoles and eflornithine in the elimination of trypanosomes from CSF of infected mice.

Acquired resistance

Relapse rates of 30–50% have been recorded in Kenya and Tanzania but there is no evidence of resistant parasites. Stable resistance has been described in the related camel parasite *Trypanosoma evansi*.

Pharmacokinetics

Oral absorption	Poor
C_{max} 1 g intravenous doses (6 doses at weekly intervals)	100 mg/l
Plasma half-life	44–54 days
Volume of distribution	20–80 l
Plasma protein binding	>99%

Suramin is normally administered by slow intravenous infusion. It can be detected in blood for 3 months; plasma levels >100 mg/l were observed for several weeks after a 6-week course of treatment. No metabolism was observed and 80% was removed by renal clearance. Tissue distribution is high to reticuloendothelial cells, especially liver macrophages, the adrenal glands and the kidney. Due to its large molecular size and anionic charge at physiological pH it does not enter erythrocytes and penetrates the blood–brain barrier poorly.

Toxicity and side effects

Suramin is a toxic drug, especially in malnourished patients. A test dose of 200 mg has been recommended. Immediate febrile reactions (nausea, vomiting, loss of consciousness) can be avoided by slow intravenous administration. Intramuscular or subcutaneous injections are painful and irritating. These reactions can be followed by fever and urticaria. Anaphylactic shock is rare (fewer than 1 in 2000 patients). Delayed reactions include renal damage, exfoliative dermatitis, anemia, leukopenia, agranulocytosis, jaundice and diarrhea.

Clinical use

- African sleeping sickness (early stage before CNS involvement).
- Onchocerciasis.

Preparations and dosage

Proprietary name: Suramin.

Preparation: Injection.

Dosage: The dose schedule varies depending on the stage of the disease. Available in South Africa.

Further information

Anonymous 1999 Suramin. In: Dollery C (ed.) *Therapeutic Drugs* 2nd edn. Churchill Livingstone, Edinburgh, pp. S154–S158.

Kaminsky R, Maser P 2000 Drug resistance in African trypanosomes. *Current Opinion in Anti-infective Investigational Drugs* 2: 76–82.

Pepin J, Milord F 1994 The treatment of human African trypanosomiasis. *Advances in Parasitology* 33: 1–47.

Voogd TE, Vansterkenburg ELM, Wilting J, Janssen LHM 1993 Recent research on the biological activity of suramin. *Pharmacological Reviews* 45: 177–203.

Willson M, Callens M, Kuntz DA, Perie J, Opperdoes F 1993 Synthesis and activity of inhibitors highly specific for the glycolytic enzymes from *Trypanosoma brucei*. *Molecular and Biochemical Parasitology* 59: 210.

ANTIBACTERIAL AND OTHER ANTIMICROBIAL AGENTS USED IN PROTOZOAL DISEASE

Properties of the diaminopyrimidines (Ch. 19), sulfonamides (Ch. 32) nitroimidazoles (Ch. 27) and nitrofurans (Ch. 26) that are used as antiprotozoal agents are described in the appropriate chapters. A broad-spectrum antiparasitic nitroheterocycle, nitazoxanide, was effective against *Cryptosporidium parvum* and *Enterocytozoon bieneusi* infections in limited trials. Among antibiotics, tetracyclines (Ch. 33), clindamycin (Ch. 23) and certain macrolides (Ch. 24) have a place in the treatment of some protozoal diseases, including malaria. The aminoglycoside paromomycin (Ch. 14) is sometimes used in amebiasis; it is also increasingly used in topical formulations for cutaneous leishmaniasis. A parenteral formulation has been shown to be effective in visceral leishmaniasis and paromomycin is one of the few drugs claimed to be useful in intractable cryptosporidiosis.

Antifungal polyene and azole derivatives (Ch. 35) are increasingly used in diseases caused by protozoa. Both extracellular and intracellular forms of *Leishmania* spp. and *T. cruzi* are highly sensitive to amphotericin B in vitro at concentrations below 1 mg/l. Lipid formulations, in particular liposomal amphotericin B (p. 422), have proved valuable in the treatment of visceral leishmaniasis, but immunocompromised patients often relapse after initial improvement. Amphotericin B is also used for the treatment of primarily amebic meningoencephalitis caused by *Naegleria fowleri*.

The imidazoles miconazole and ketoconazole (p. 418) and the triazole itraconazole (p. 417) are active against *Leishmania* spp. and *T. cruzi* in experimental models, but results have been equivocal in clinical trials. Investigational triazole derivatives, posaconazole and ravuconazole are effective against *T. cruzi* in experimental models and could be used in the treatment of Chagas' disease. The anthelmintic benzimidazole albendazole (p. 442) is effective in infections caused by *G. lamblia* and is on trial for the treatment of microsporidiosis in AIDS patients.

 ## Further information

Andrade ALS, Zicker F, Oliveira RM et al 1996 Randomised trial of efficacy of benznidazole in treatment of early *Trypanosoma cruzi* infection. *Lancet* 348: 1407–1412.

Berman JD, Badaro R, Thakur CP et al 1998 Efficacy and safety of liposomal amphotericin B (AmBisome) for visceral leishmaniasis in endemic developing countries. *Bulletin of the World Health Organization* 76: 25–32.

El-On J, Halevy S, Grunwald MH, Weinrauch L 1992 Topical treatment of Old World cutaneous leishmaniasis caused by *Leishmania major:* a double blind control study. *Journal of the American Academy of Dermatology* 27: 227–231.

Derouin F, Gangeux J-P 1998 Changing patterns of disease and treatment of opportunistic parasitic infections in patients with AIDS. *Current Opinion in Infectious Diseases* 11: 711–716.

Molina JM, Chastang C, Goguel J et al 1998 Albendazole for the treatment and prophylaxis of microsporidiosis due to *Encephalitozoon intestinalis* in patients with AIDS: a randomized double-blind controlled trial. *Journal of Infectious Diseases* 177: 1373–1377.

Navin TR, Arana BA, Arana FE, Berman J, Chajon JF 1992 Placebo-controlled clinical trial of sodium stibogluconate (Pentostam) versus ketoconazole for treating cutaneous leishmaniasis. *Journal of Infectious Diseases* 165: 528–534.

Pepin J, Milord F 1994 The treatment of human African trypanosomiasis. *Advances in Parasitology* 33: 1–47.

Pradines B, Spiegel A, Rogier C et al 2000 Antibiotics for prophylaxis of *Plasmodium falciparum* infections: *in vitro* activity of doxycycline against Senegalese isolates. *American Journal of Tropical Medicine and Hygiene* 62: 82–85.

Pukrittayakamee S, Chantra A, Vanijanonta S, Clemens R, Looareesuwan S, White NJ 2000 Therapeutic responses to quinine and clindamycin in multidrug-resistant falciparum malaria. *Antimicrobial Agents and Chemotherapy* 44: 2395–2398.

Reynoldson JA, Thompson RCA, Horton RJ 1992 Albendazole as a future antigiardial agent. *Parasitology Today* 8: 412–414.

Rossignol JF, Ayoub A, Ayers MS 2001 Treatment of diarrhea caused by *Cryptosporidium parvum:* a prospective double-blind, placebo-controlled study of nitazoxamide. *Journal of Infectious Diseases* 184: 103–106.

Thakur CP, Kanyok TP, Pandey AK, Sinha GP, Messick C, Olliaro P 2000 Treatment of visceral leishmaniasis with injectable paromomycin (aminosidine). An open-label randomized phase-II clinical study. *Transactions of the Royal Society of Tropical Medicine and Hygiene* 94: 432–433.

Thakur CP, Singh RK, Hassan SM, Kumar R, Narian S, Kumar A 1999 Amphotericin B deoxycholate treatment of visceral leishmaniasis with newer modes of administration and precautions: a study of 938 cases. *Transactions of the Royal Society of Tropical Medicine and Hygiene* 93: 319–323.

Upcroft JA, Campbell RW, Benakli K, Upcroft P, Vanelle P 1999 Efficacy of new 5-nitroimidazoles against metronidazole-susceptible and resistant *Giardia, Trichomonas* and *Entamoeba* spp. *Antimicrobial Agents and Chemotherapy* 43: 73–76.

Urbina JA 1999 Chemotherapy of Chagas disease: the how and the why. *Journal of Molecular Medicine* 77: 332–338.

39 Antiretroviral agents

Sean Emery and David A. Cooper

Some 35 million people around the world are presently infected with the human immunodeficiency virus (HIV). In untreated individuals this infection results almost uniformly in the progressive destruction of elements of the immune system and increasing immunodeficiency. Infected individuals are susceptible to life-threatening opportunistic infections and neoplasia.

Following the identification of HIV in 1983 and recognition of the significant threat this virus presents to global health there has been an enormous investment in the development of anti-HIV therapies. This has occurred in parallel with advances in understanding of HIV replication; in particular the identification of those steps in the replica-

tive cycle that are unique to the virus and thus potential targets for chemotherapy (Figure 39.1). HIV is a member of the lentivirus subfamily of human retroviruses with a double-stranded RNA genome encoding at least nine functional or regulatory proteins. There are several potential points at which the process of virus replication could be blocked:

- Attachment to host-cell membranes.
- Reverse-transcription of the virus genome.
- Integration of virus into the host genome.
- Virus assembly and maturation.

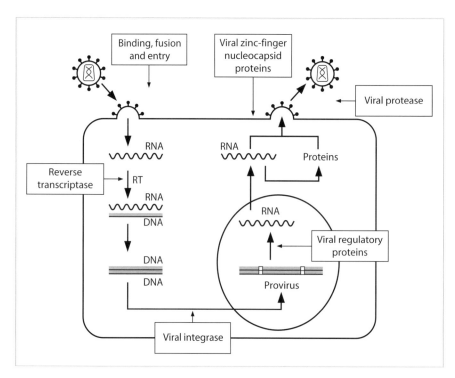

Fig. 39.1 Schematic representation of the HIV replicative cycle. Points at which antiretroviral therapies can inhibit virus replication are shown in boxed arrows.

None of the currently available therapies cure HIV infection. Once initiated, treatment is a lifelong commitment. Side effects and toxicities arise during long-term exposure (sometimes more troublesome than those revealed during the conduct of short-term clinical trials), but the causal relationship between individual drugs and specific side effects is often difficult to elucidate because these drugs are routinely administered in combination regimens.

The use of combination antiretroviral therapy has, thus far, resulted in significant and sustained reductions in morbidity and mortality in people with HIV infection. However, many challenges to dealing with this insidious virus remain:

- The increasing complexity of combination regimens.
- Interactions between the drugs themselves and those commonly used for the treatment of other illnesses in an HIV-infected patient.
- The difficulties associated with adherence to complex regimens.
- Drug resistance.
- Cumulative toxicities and side effects.

Antiretroviral drugs act intracellularly, where relative concentrations are virtually impossible to predict or measure. For this reason little reliable information is available that relates plasma concentrations to in-vivo effectiveness. Clinical studies are under way to determine the extent to which plasma drug level monitoring may be of clinical use in the treatment of HIV disease with antiretroviral therapy. Caution should also be employed in comparing in-vitro concentrations with in-vivo effectiveness.

 Further information

Beach JW 1998 Chemotherapeutic agents for human immunodeficiency virus infection: mechanism of action, pharmacokinetics, metabolism and adverse reactions. *Clinical Therapeutics* 20: 2–25.

Carpenter CCJ, Cooper DA, Fischl MA et al 2000 Antiretroviral therapy in adults. Updated recommendations of the International AIDS Society-USA panel. *Journal of the American Medical Association* 283: 381–390.

Carr A, Cooper DA 1996 Pathogenesis and management of HIV drug associated hypersensitivity. In: Volberding P, Jacobson MA (eds). *AIDS Clinical Review 1995/1996*. Marcel Dekker, New York.

Carr A, Cooper DA 2000 Adverse effects of antiretroviral therapy. *Lancet* 356: 1423–1430.

Flexner C, Hendrix CW 1997 Pharmacology of antiretroviral agents. In: De Vita VT, Hellman S, Rosenberg SA (eds). *AIDS: etiology, diagnosis, treatment and prevention*, 4th edn. Lippincott-Raven, Philadelphia, pp. 479–493.

Hirsch MS, Conway B, D'Aquila RT et al 2000 Antiretroviral drug resistance testing in adults with HIV infection: Implications for clinical management. *Journal of the American Medical Association* 283: 2417–2426.

Panel on Clinical Practices for Treatment of HIV infection 2001 Guidelines for the use of antiretroviral agents in HIV-1 infected adults and adolescents. Department of Health and Human Services and Henry J Kaiser Family Foundation. www.hivatis.org.

Panel on Clinical Practices for Treatment of HIV infection 2000 Guidelines for the use of antiretroviral agents in HIV-1 infected adults and adolescents. Department of Heath and Human Services and Henry J Kaiser Family Foundation January 28, 2000. *HIV Clinical Trials* 1: 60–110.

Piscitelli SC, Gallicano KD 2001 Interactions among drugs for HIV and opportunistic infections. *New England Journal of Medicine* 344: 984–996.

Schinazi RF, Larder BA, Mellors JW 1997 Resistance table: mutations in retroviral genes associated with drug resistance. *International Antiviral News* 5: 129–142.

CLASSIFICATION

Drugs that interfere with HIV replication, collectively known as antiretroviral agents, are categorized on the basis of where in the HIV replicative cycle they exert inhibitory effects.

HIV reverse transcriptase is an essential enzyme for virus replication. This RNA-dependent DNA polymerase is coded by the *pol* gene and permits the transcription of virus RNA into a DNA copy, which is then available for integration into the host cell genome. Nucleoside analog, non-nucleoside analog, and nucleotide analog inhibitors of HIV reverse transcriptase are presently used in treatment.

HIV protease inhibitors are structurally related molecules based on amino acid sequences that represent synthetic analogs of one of the HIV *gag–pol* target cleavage sites. Combination of HIV protease inhibitors with reverse transcriptase inhibitors yields regimens that inhibit the process of virus replication at two distinct enzymatic sites representing unrelated components of the virus life cycle.

NUCLEOSIDE ANALOGS

Nucleoside analog reverse transcriptase inhibitors are dideoxynucleosides. They undergo intracellular phosphorylation to yield dideoxynucleoside triphosphates that inhibit HIV-1 and HIV-2 replication (*see* pp. 21–22).

In addition to sharing a common mode of action these drugs have a number of overlapping toxicities that may arise through a common pathway. They are all able to inhibit some mammalian DNA polymerases, in particular those found exclusively within mitochondria, which are responsible for division of the organelle. Interference with mitochondrial replication and function is likely to be a mechanism through which several of the significant toxicities are mediated. Laboratory investigations indicate that the potency of this class of drugs for inhibition of cellular DNA polymerases is: zalcitabine >stavudine >didanosine >zidovudine >lamivudine and abacavir.

These drugs are all linked to fatal and non-fatal cases of lactic acidosis with hepatomegaly as a result of steatosis. Long-term use has been associated with significant changes in the deposition of body fat.

 Further information

Brinkmann K, ter Hofstede HJM, Burger DM et al 1998 Adverse effects of reverse transcriptase inhibitors: mitochondrial toxicity as a common pathway. *AIDS* 12: 1735–1744.

Brinkmann K, Smeitink JA, Romjin JA, Reiss P 1999 Mitochondrial toxicity induced by nucleoside analogue reverse transcriptase inhibitors is a key factor in the pathogenesis of antiretroviral therapy related lipodystrophy. *Lancet* 354: 1112–1115.

Lewis W, Dalakas MC 1995 Mitochondrial toxicity of antiviral drugs. *Nature Medicine* 1: 417–421.

Moyle GJ, Sadler M 1998 Peripheral neuropathy with nucleoside antiretrovirals: risk factors, incidence and management. *Drug Safety* 19: 481–494.

Shaer AS, Rastegar A 2000 Lactic acidosis in the setting of antiretroviral therapy for the acquired immunodeficiency syndrome. A case report and review of the literature. *American Journal of Nephrology* 20: 332–338.

Stein DS, Moore KH 2001 Phosphorylation of nucleoside analogue antiretrovirals: a review for clinicians. *Pharmacotherapy* 21: 11–34.

 # ABACAVIR

Molecular weight: 670.76.

An analog of guanidine formulated for oral administration. Aqueous solubility is approximately 77 g/l.

Antiviral activity

The in-vitro anti-HIV activity is additive in combination with didanosine, zalcitabine, lamivudine, stavudine, and amprenavir; it is synergistic with zidovudine and nevirapine.

Acquired resistance

In-vitro resistance is associated with specific changes in the HIV reverse transcriptase codon region (codons 184 with 65, 74 or 115). Sequential acquisition of multiple point mutations results in up to an 8-fold decline in susceptibility. Resistant isolates may also show reduced sensitivity to lamivudine, zalcitabine and/or didanosine, but may remain sensitive to zidovudine and stavudine.

Pharmacokinetics

Oral absorption	c. 83%
C_{max} 300 mg oral	3 mg/l after c. 1–1.5 h
Plasma half-life	c. 1.5 h
Volume of distribution	0.8 l/kg
Plasma protein binding	c. 49%

Absorption and distribution

There are no apparent differences between the tablet and liquid formulations for estimates of the area under the time–concentration curve (AUC). There is no significant accumulation after repeated oral administration. The overall pharmacokinetic characteristics in children are similar to those seen in adults with slightly greater variability in plasma concentrations. No studies have been performed in patients over 65 years old and no dosing recommendations have been made. The concentration in cerebrospinal fluid (CSF) is 30–44% of the simultaneous plasma level. Abacavir and its metabolites are secreted in milk and there are no data available on exposure in infants under 3 months old. Mothers should not breastfeed their infants while receiving treatment.

Metabolism and excretion

Abacavir is primarily metabolized in the liver, mainly by alcohol dehydrogenase and glucuronidation. Around 83% of the dose is eliminated in the urine, <2% as unchanged drug; the remainder is excreted in the feces.

No studies have been performed in individuals with established hepatic or renal impairment and no dosing recommendations have been made for this population. Concomitant ethanol consumption can result in an increase in the AUC by as much as 41% although the clinical significance of this remains unclear.

Toxicity and side effects

Life-threatening hypersensitivity reactions have been described in about 4% of all individuals to whom the drug has been administered in clinical trials. Typically patients present within the first 6 weeks of starting treatment (peak at 4 weeks after initiation) with fever and/or rash as part of a syndrome indicating multiorgan involvement. The mechanism has not been established and, since no diagnostic test is available to exclude other contributory causes, diagnosis is entirely clinical. Patients developing any symptoms and signs must be encouraged to contact their doctor immediately; treatment should be discontinued if hypersensitivity is suspected and other causes cannot be ruled out.

Symptoms in more than 10% of patients presenting with a hypersensitivity reaction include fatigue, malaise, headache, myalgia, nausea, vomiting, diarrhea, abdominal pain, dyspnea, sore throat and cough. Symptoms worsen with continued treatment and are life threatening. Patients may also complain of pruritus, chills and musculoskeletal symptoms.

If hypersensitivity is suspected therapy must *never* be restarted because accelerated hypersensitivity and deaths have been reported.

Other adverse events that occur in more than 10% of patients are nausea, vomiting, diarrhea, headache, fever, lethargy, fatigue, anorexia and rash. Most events are not treatment limiting.

Clinical use

- Treatment of HIV infection in adults and children (in combination with other antiretroviral drugs).

It should not be used in pregnant women unless the potential benefit to the mother outweighs the potential risk to the fetus.

Preparations and dosage

Proprietary name: Ziagen.

Preparations: Tablets (300 mg) and an oral solution (20 mg/ml). The oral solution contains sorbitol, which is metabolized to fructose and is unsuitable for patients with hereditary fructose intolerance.

Dosage: Adults, oral, 300 mg twice daily. Children >3 months, 8 mg/kg twice daily (maximum 300 mg twice daily).

Widely available alone and as a triple combination with zidovudine and lamivudine (Trizivir).

 Further information

Hervey PS, Perry CM 2000 Abacavir: a review of its clinical potential in patients with HIV infection. *Drugs* 60: 447–479.

 DIDANOSINE

2′, 3′-dideoxyinosine; ddI. Molecular weight 236.2.

An analog of deoxyadenosine, available for oral administration. The aqueous solubility is 27.3 g/l. It is rapidly degraded at acidic pH and tablets contain a buffering agent to increase the pH of the gastric environment. An enteric formulation has also been developed that avoids the need for the buffering agents. All formulations must be administered on an empty stomach.

Antiviral activity

Active against HIV-1 and HIV-2, and human T-cell lymphotrophic virus type 1.

Acquired resistance

Codon changes at positions 65 or 74 in HIV reverse transcriptase are associated with reduced sensitivity and reduced susceptibility to zalcitabine.

Virus with resistance to didanosine, stavudine, zalcitabine and zidovudine may arise by acquisition of specific point mutations at position 151 together with various combinations of changes at positions 62, 75, 77 and 116. Insertion or deletion mutations at position 68 in combination with a 215-point mutation also confer multidrug resistance.

Pharmacokinetics

Oral absorption	c. 40%
C_{max} 200 mg oral	c. 2 mg/l after 0.67–2.0 h
Plasma half-life	c. 1.4 h
Volume of distribution	c. 1 l/kg
Plasma protein binding	<5%

Absorption
Bioavailability is reduced by about half when taken with food and the drug should be given at least 30 min before a meal. In children absolute bioavailability is approximately 47%. The peak plasma concentration achieved by enteric-coated tablets is less than half that of buffered tablets.

Distribution
In adults penetration into the CSF relative to plasma concentrations is about 21%. In children up to 46% of the plasma concentration can be found in the CSF. The volume of distribution in children is 35.6 l/m². It is secreted in breast milk.

Metabolism
Based upon animal studies it is presumed that metabolism occurs by the pathways responsible for the elimination of endogenous purines.

Excretion
Renal clearance by glomerular filtration and active tubular secretion accounts for 50% of total body clearance after intravenous or oral administration. Urinary recovery accounts for about 20% of the oral dose in adults (17% in children). The elimination half-life after intravenous administration is 0.8 h in children. There is no evidence of accumulation after oral dosing up to 4 weeks in adults and 26 days in children. In patients with renal insufficiency doses must be reduced following assessment of creatinine clearance. There are no data on which to recommend specific dose modifications in patients with hepatic impairment.

Toxicity and side effects

Most serious are pancreatitis (fatal and non-fatal), lactic acidosis and severe hepatomegaly with steatosis (fatal and non-fatal), retinopathy, optical neuritis and dose-related peripheral neuropathy. Patients with low body weight or renal impairment may require dose modification.

In clinical trials pancreatitis occurred in around 6% of recipients. All recipients, particularly those with risk factors for pancreatitis, should be monitored regularly through assessment of serum amylase. Didanosine should not be given to patients who need to take other drugs known to cause pancreatic toxicity (e.g. intravenous pentamidine).

Most cases of lactic acidosis and hepatomegaly with steatosis have been in women. Obesity and prolonged exposure to nucleoside analogs are thought to be risk factors. The combination with stavudine should be used with caution in pregnant women because fatal cases of lactic acidosis have been reported. It is unclear whether pregnancy potentiates the development of the lactic acidosis. Caution should also be exercised when administering the drug to patients with known risk factors for liver disease. Therapy should be stopped in a patient who develops clinical or laboratory evidence of lactic acidosis or hepatotoxicity.

Caution should be exercised in coadministering other drugs with known neurotoxicity and in patients with a history of neuropathy. Treatment should stop once symptoms and signs of neuropathy are observed, but the condition is reversible and patients with resolved neuropathy may be retreated at a reduced dosage.

Retinal depigmentation has been observed in children and twice-yearly dilated retinal examination is recommended.

Other side effects reported during treatment include alopecia, anaphylaxis, asthenia, chills/fevers, pain, anorexia, dyspepsia, flatulence, sialoadenitis, parotid gland enlargement, dry mouth, dry eyes, anemia, granulocytopenia, leukopenia, thrombocytopenia, hepatitis, liver failure, diabetes mellitus, hypoglycemia, hyperglycemia, myalgia, rhabdomyolysis, arthralgia and myopathy. The buffered formulation contains phenylalanine, prompting caution in patients with phenylketonuria.

Clinical use

- Treatment of HIV infection (in combination with other antiretroviral drugs).

Preparations and dosages

Proprietary name: Videx.

Preparations: Chewable tablet containing either 25 mg or 100 mg. Also available as a powder for oral solution and in an enteric-coated formulation.

Dosage: Adults (weighing at least 60 kg with adequate renal function), oral, 200 mg twice daily. For adults weighing less than 60 kg the dose should be reduced to 125 mg twice daily. Dose reductions are also recommended for increasing severity of renal impairment. Children >3 months, 120 mg/m² twice daily (90 mg/m² twice daily with zidovudine).

Widely available.

Further information

Anonymous 1999 Didanosine. In: Dollery C (ed.) *Therapeutic Drugs* 2nd edn. Churchill Livingstone, Edinburgh, pp. D95–D100.
Perry CM, Noble S 1999 Didanosine: an updated review of its use in HIV infection. *Drugs* 58: 1099–1135.

 LAMIVUDINE

2′-3′-thiacytidine; 3TC. Molecular weight 229.3.

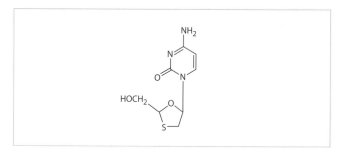

An analog of cytidine available for oral administration. It is highly soluble in water.

Antiviral activity

Lamivudine possesses potent anti-hepatitis B virus activity at doses below those used in the treatment of HIV disease.

In-vitro studies indicate that it interacts synergistically with zidovudine, didanosine and saquinavir. It competes with zalcitabine for the enzymes involved in intracellular phosphorylation.

Acquired resistance

A single codon change at position 184 in the HIV reverse transcriptase gene confers high-level resistance. Other changes at positions 44, 118, 215 or 41 are also associated with resistance. Resistant virus has been isolated from patients treated with the drug. In-vitro data indicate that lamivudine resistance may restore HIV sensitivity to zidovudine-resistant virus.

Pharmacokinetics

Oral absorption	80–85
C_{max} 150 mg oral	3.3 mg/l after c. 1 h
Plasma half-life	5–7 h
Volume of distribution	1.3 l/kg
Plasma protein binding	10–35%

Absorption

Ingestion with food reduces the peak plasma concentration by up to 47% and extends the time taken to reach the peak to 2.2 h. In children the oral bioavailability is about 65%, requiring the use of higher unit doses to attain effective plasma concentrations.

Distribution

Penetration into the CNS is poor. The CSF:serum concentration ratio is about 0.12 up to 4 h after oral administration. It is actively secreted in breast milk and mothers are advised not to breastfeed while taking the drug.

Metabolism

Less than 10% of the administered dose undergoes hepatic metabolism. Studies in patients with impaired hepatic function did not reveal any differences in the metabolic fate.

Excretion

Over 70% of the administered dose is subject to renal clearance via active tubular secretion. Impaired renal function assessed by creatinine clearance less than 50 ml/min requires dose reduction. An increase in systemic exposure by up to 40% occurs following coadministration with trimethoprim.

Toxicity and side effects

Lamivudine is relatively safe and non-toxic. Administration of very high doses in acute animal studies did not result in any organ toxicity. Use in children with a history of pancreatitis or risk factors for pancreatitis is cautioned. Fatal and non-fatal cases of lactic acidosis and hepatomegaly with steatosis have been reported in patients (mostly women) receiving combinations with other antiretroviral agents.

In patients coinfected with HIV and hepatitis B cessation of lamivudine therapy may result in clinical and/or laboratory evidence of recurrent hepatic disease that may be more severe in patients with hepatic decompensation. Liver function tests and markers of hepatitis B replication should be periodically monitored in such patients.

Other reported side effects are malaise, fever, fatigue, anemia, leukopenia, thrombocytopenia, headache, neuropathy, paresthesia, nausea, vomiting, diarrhea, abdominal discomfort, abnormal liver function tests, pancreatitis, alopecia and rash.

Clinical use

- Treatment of HIV infection (in combination with other antiretroviral drugs).
- Treatment of hepatitis B infection.

Safety in human pregnancy has not been established, but it appears to be a safe component of combination antiretroviral therapy in pregnancy.

 Preparations and dosage

Proprietary name: Epivir.

Preparations: Tablets containing 150 mg. Also available as an oral solution.

Dosage: Adults, oral, 150 mg twice daily. Children >3 months, 4 mg/kg twice daily to a maximum of 300 mg daily. Patients with impaired renal function require dose reduction.

Widely available alone, in combination with zidovudine (Combivir), and as a triple combination with zidovudine and abacavir (Trizivir).

 Further information

Perry CM, Faulds D 1997 Lamivudine: A review of its antiviral activity, pharmacokinetic properties and therapeutic efficacy in the management of HIV infection. *Drugs* 54: 657–680.

 STAVUDINE

2′, 3′-didehydro-3′-deoxythymidine; d4T. Molecular weight: 224.2.

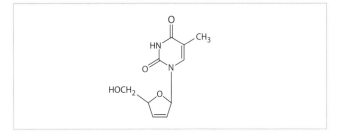

An analog of thymidine formulated for oral administration. It has an aqueous solubility of 83 g/l.

Antiviral activity

The anti-HIV activity in vitro is additive in combination with didanosine and synergistic with zalcitabine. It competes with zidovudine and ribavirin for the same intracellular phosphorylating enzymes and should not be used in combination with these drugs.

Acquired resistance

Reduced susceptibility arises with the acquisition of a single point mutation in the amino acid sequence of HIV reverse transcriptase at position 75. Specific point mutations associated with cross-resistance to other nucleoside analogs also occur (*see* didanosine).

Pharmacokinetics

Oral absorption	86%
C_{max} 40 mg oral	4 mg/l after 0.5–1 h
Plasma half-life	1.4 h
Volume of distribution	0.53 l/kg
Plasma protein binding	Very low

Absorption

The bioavailability after oral dosing is somewhat lower in children than in adults. Peak plasma concentrations after a high-fat meal are reduced by about half; the time taken to reach these levels is extended to 1.5 h, but concentrations are maintained for up to 6 h. Thereafter plasma levels are comparable between the two groups.

Distribution

The mean apparent volume of distribution following oral administration in children is 0.74 l/kg. Stavudine crosses the blood–brain barrier and attains levels in the range 31–45% (16–125% in children) of those measured in plasma. It is secreted in breast milk and nursing mothers should cease breastfeeding while taking the drug.

Metabolism and excretion

The metabolic fate in humans has not been elucidated. Renal elimination accounts for approximately 40% of overall clearance at a rate almost twice that of endogenous creatinine, indicating active tubular secretion in addition to glomerular filtration. In patients with renal impairment doses should be reduced on the basis of creatinine clearance rates. It is removed by hemodialysis.

Patients with stable hepatic insufficiency do not require dose modification, but patients with unstable hepatic insufficiency have not been studied. The mean terminal half-life in children is 1 h. No significant accumulation has been observed in adults or children following repeated dosing.

Toxicity and side effects

Side effects are similar to those of didanosine. They include peripheral neuropathy, lactic acidosis and hepatomegaly with steatosis and liver failure, and pancreatitis. Combination therapy with didanosine results in higher frequency of these toxicities, and fatalities have been reported in pregnant women.

Other side effects reported in more than 5% of patients include headache, fever, asthenia, abdominal pain, pain, malaise, allergic symptoms, neoplasm, chest pain, diarrhea, nausea/vomiting, anorexia, dyspepsia, constipation, lymphadenopathy, myalgia, arthralgia, insomnia, depression, anxiety, nervousness, dizziness, dyspnea, rash, sweating, pruritus and maculopapular rash.

Clinical use

- Treatment of HIV infection in adults and children.

Use in pregnant women is cautioned in the absence of clinical studies.

 Preparations and dosages

Proprietary name: Zerit.

Preparations: Capsules containing 15 mg, 20 mg, 30 mg and 40 mg. Also available as a powder for oral solution.

Dosage: Adults weighing at least 60 kg, oral, 40 mg every 12 h. Adults weighing <60 kg, 30 mg every 12 h. Children under 30 kg and >3 months, 1 mg/kg every 12 h.

Widely available.

 Further information

Anonymous 1999 Stavudine. In: Dollery C (ed.) *Therapeutic Drugs* 2nd edn. Churchill Livingstone, Edinburgh, pp. S94–S98.
Lea AP, Faulds D 1996 Stavudine: A review of its pharmacodynamic and pharmacokinetic properties and clinical potential in HIV infection. *Drugs* 51: 846–864.

 ZALCITABINE

2′, 3′-dideoxycytidine; ddC. Molecular weight: 211.2.

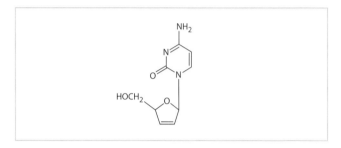

An analog of cytidine, formulated for oral administration. Aqueous solubility is 76.4 g/l.

Antiviral activity

Useful activity is restricted to HIV-1 and HIV-2. It interacts synergistically with zidovudine in tissue culture assays.

Acquired resistance

Clinically significant resistance in patients with HIV infection results from specific single changes in the reverse transcriptase at amino acid positions 65, 69, 74 or 75. Some of these changes are also associated with resistance to didanosine (65 or 74 or both) and stavudine (75). They may also contribute to resistance to abacavir. Specific point mutations associated with cross-resistance to other nucleoside analogs also occur (*see* didanosine).

Pharmacokinetics

Oral absorption	c. 80%
C_{max} 0.75 mg oral	c. 80 μg/l after 1–2 h
Plasma half-life	c. 2 h
Volume of distribution	0.53 l/kg
Plasma protein binding	<4%

Absorption and distribution

When taken with food the peak plasma concentration is significantly reduced. Concentrations in the CSF averaged 20% of those found concurrently in plasma.

Metabolism and excretion

The metabolic fate has not been fully evaluated. Renal elimination accounts for approximately 70% of orally administered drug. Less than 10% is excreted in feces.

Toxicity and side effects

The major clinically significant toxicity is peripheral neuropathy, which occurred in up to 31% of patients in clinical trials. The condition is characterized by numbness and burning dysesthesia involving distal extremities. It can progress to severe shooting and burning pains that may require narcotic analgesia unless therapy is stopped. In most patients symptoms slowly resolve on discontinuation of treatment. Clinical assessment and judgment is required to determine if the drug should be restarted at a reduced dose on resolution of neuropathy.

Fatal and non-fatal pancreatitis occurs with an incidence of about 1%. Careful monitoring of serum amylase levels is required and therapy discontinued if elevations are observed. Patients with known risk factors for pancreatitis should be treated cautiously.

Other serious side effects are esophageal ulcers, cardiomyopathy with congestive heart failure, anaphylactoid reactions, lactic acidosis and severe hepatomegaly with steatosis and oral ulceration.

Less serious adverse events include weight decrease, chest pain, fever, asthenia, pain, substernal chest pain, heart racing, abdominal pain, diarrhea, vomiting, dry mouth, dyspepsia, glossitis, constipation, rectal hemorrhage, hemorrhoids, enlarged abdomen, gum disorders, arthralgia, shoulder pain, hypertonia, hand tremor, twitching, confusion, impaired concentration, amnesia, insomnia, somnolence, depression, pharyngitis, coughing, dyspnea, cyanosis, dermatitis, rash, night sweats, alopecia, taste perversion, xerophthalmia, abnormal vision, eye pain, tinnitus, abnormal renal function, acute renal failure and renal cysts.

Clinical use

> • Treatment of HIV infection (alone or in combination with other antiretroviral agents).

Zalcitabine has teratogenic properties in rats and should not be used in pregnant women or those wishing to become pregnant. The safety and efficacy have not been demonstrated in children under 13 years of age.

 ## Preparations and dosage

Proprietary name: Hivid.

Preparations: Tablets containing 0.375 mg and 0.75 mg.

Dosage: Adults, oral, 0.75 mg three times daily (twice daily in patients with renal impairment).

Widely available.

 ## Further information

Anonymous 1999 Zalcitabine. In: Dollery C (ed.) *Therapeutic Drugs* 2nd edn. Churchill Livingstone, Edinburgh, pp. Z6–Z11.
Shelton MJ, O'Donnell AM, Morse GD 1993 Zalcitabine. *Annals of Pharmacotherapy* 27: 480–489.

 ## ZIDOVUDINE

3′-azido-3′-deoxythymidine; azidothymidine; AZT. Molecular weight 267.2.

An analog of thymidine, formulated for oral or intravenous use. Zidovudine was the first antiretroviral drug to be approved for the treatment of HIV infection in 1987. It is highly soluble in water.

Antiviral activity

Zidovudine is active against several human retroviruses in addition to HIV. It is also active against Epstein–Barr virus replication, although the clinical significance of this is unknown. In combination with all other antiretroviral drugs, except stavudine, the activity is additive or synergistic. Ribavirin appears to antagonize the antiretroviral activity through competition for intracellular phosphorylation and coadministration of these agents is not recommended.

Acquired resistance

High-level resistance develops in HIV strains with mutations at points 41, 67, 70, 215 or 219 within the reverse transcriptase amino acid sequence. Such mutants can be isolated during treatment. Specific point mutations associated with cross-resistance to other nucleoside analogs also occur (see didanosine).

Pharmacokinetics

Oral absorption	65%
C_{max} 250 mg oral	0.6 mg/l after 0.5–1.5 h
Plasma half-life	0.8–1.9 h
Volume of distribution	1.6 l/kg
Plasma protein binding	34–38%

Absorption

When taken with food absorption is slowed, with a consequent reduction in the peak concentration. The net effect is a variable reduction in the AUC with unclear clinical significance.

Distribution

Zidovudine crosses the blood–brain barrier and attains steady state CSF concentrations around 50% of those found simultaneously in plasma. It crosses the placenta and is found in amniotic fluid, fetal blood and semen. It is secreted in breast milk.

Metabolism

Zidovudine undergoes rapid first-pass metabolism in the liver to yield the glucuronide metabolite. A small proportion is metabolized to a 3'-amino-3'-deoxythymidine product that is implicated in myelosuppression.

Excretion

Following oral administration urinary recovery of zidovudine and its glucuronide metabolite accounted for 14 and 74% respectively of the dose, with a total urinary recovery of 90% of the administered dose. Elimination of unchanged drug and its principal metabolites occurs through glomerular filtration and active tubular secretion. There are limited data on the pharmacokinetic behavior in patients with renal or hepatic impairment.

Interactions

Coadministration with drugs known to cause nephrotoxicity, cytotoxicity or which interfere with red or white blood cell number and function may increase the risk of toxicity.

Probenecid and trimethoprim may reduce renal clearance of zidovudine and other drugs that are metabolized by glucuronidation may interfere with its metabolism.

Toxicity and side effects

In common with other drugs in this class, use has been associated with episodes of fatal and non-fatal lactic acidosis, hepatomegaly with steatosis. Careful clinical evaluation is needed in patients with evidence of hepatic abnormality.

Treatment is contraindicated in patients with neutrophil counts below 1×10^9/l and hemoglobin levels below 9 g/dl. Myelosuppression may occur within the first 4–6 weeks of therapy. Hematological parameters should be routinely monitored during this period with prompt dose modification if abnormalities are observed. Treatment with reduced doses may be reinstated in some patients once bone marrow recovery has been observed.

Other frequent side effects that may be dose limiting are asthenia, diaphoresis, fever, severe headache, malaise, nausea, vomiting, anorexia, diarrhea, dyspepsia, gastrointestinal pain, insomnia, dizziness, paresthesia, somnolence, dyspnea, rash, taste perversion, myopathy and myalgia.

Clinical use

- Treatment of HIV infection in adults and children (in combination with other antiretroviral drugs).
- Reduction of maternal transmission of HIV to the fetus.

Preparations and dosages

Proprietary names: Retrovir.

Preparations: Capsules (100 mg, 250 mg and 300 mg), tablets, syrup containing 10 mg/ml, oral solution, injection.

Dosage: Adults, oral, 500–600 mg per day in 2–3 divided doses. The optimal dose in children has not been established, although a dose of 360–480 mg/m²/day in 3–4 divided doses has been advocated by some investigators.

Widely available alone and in combination with lamivudine (Combivir) and lamivudine and abacavir (Trizivir).

Further information

Anonymous 1999 Zidovudine. In: Dollery C (ed.) *Therapeutic Drugs* 2nd edn. Churchill Livingstone, Edinburgh, pp. Z12–Z18.

NON-NUCLEOSIDE ANALOGS

The non-nucleoside reverse transcriptase inhibitors are a structurally unrelated group of compounds that selectively inhibit HIV-1 reverse transcriptase through allosteric inhibition following binding to the enzyme at regions remote from the active site. The unique mechanism of action results in a pattern of resistance distinct from other antiretroviral drug classes.

These drugs can inhibit or induce cytochrome P_{450} isozymes. As a consequence, use with several medications is contraindicated or cautioned. Importantly both nevirapine and efavirenz administration can reduce methadone concentrations by up to 50%. This may result in clinical features of opiate withdrawal, which requires careful management that may include increasing methadone dose.

Further information

Katlama C 1999 Review of NNRTIs: today and tomorrow. *International Journal of Clinical Practice (Supplement)* 103: 16–20.

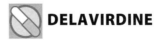
DELAVIRDINE

Molecular weight: 552.68.

A complex piperazine derivative, formulated for oral administration. Aqueous solubility is 2.9 g/l at pH 1; 0.30 g/l at pH 2.0 and 0.81 mg/l at pH 7.4.

Antiviral activity

Delavirdine is active against HIV-1 but not HIV-2. It exhibits synergy with zidovudine, didanosine, lamivudine, and zalcitabine in cell culture assays.

Acquired resistance

The predominant HIV amino acid substitution associated with resistance is at position 236 of the reverse transcriptase. This mutation may increase sensitivity of HIV to other non-nucleoside reverse transcriptase inhibitors. Resistance arising from changes at positions 103 and 181 has been implicated in resistance to other non-nucleoside reverse transcriptase inhibitors.

HIV strains exhibiting up to a 500-fold reduction in sensitivity have been isolated within 8 weeks in patients receiving delavirdine monotherapy.

Pharmacokinetics

Oral absorption	c. 50%
C_{max} 400 mg oral	30 μmol/l after c. 1 h
Plasma half-life	c. 5 h
Volume of distribution	1 l/kg
Plasma protein binding	98%

Absorption and distribution

Food has no significant affects on absorption. Concentrations in the CSF average 0.4% of the simultaneous plasma concentration, representing 20% of free drug in the plasma. It is secreted in breast milk.

Metabolism and excretion

Delavirdine is biotransformed to several metabolites by the CYP3A4 isoform of cytochrome P_{450} and is a potent inhibitor of this enzyme system. In radiolabel studies 44% of the drug was recovered in feces and 51% in urine. Renal excretion of unchanged drug accounts for about 5% of the dose.

Interactions

A large number of drugs that share cytochrome P_{450} CYP3A4 metabolism interact with delavirdine. It increases the plasma concentrations of saquinavir and indinavir, although the safety and efficacy of the combination has not been assessed. Ritonavir significantly increases the plasma concentration of delavirdine.

Specific drugs that are subject to clinically relevant interactions are summarized in Tables 39.1 and 39.2. As the biotransformation is identical to that of the HIV protease inhibitors it is not surprising that contraindications and cautions are the same.

Table 39.1 Drugs that should not be coadministered with delavirdine or HIV protease inhibitors because of demonstrated or predicted interactions with the potential for serious events or loss of efficacy

Drug class	Drug names
Antiarrhythmics	amiodarone, lignocaine (systemic), bepridil, quinidine
Antihistamines	astemizole (withdrawn), terfenadine (withdrawn)
Ergot derivatives	dihydroergotamine, ergotamine, ergonovine
Gastrointestinal motility agents	cisapride (withdrawn)
Neuroleptic	pimozide
Sedative/hypnotics	midazolam, triazolam
Antimycobacterial agents	rifampicin (rifampin)
Statins	lovastatin, simvastatin
Phosphodiesterase type 5 inhibitors	sildenafil
Herbal products	St John's wort

Table 39.2 Drugs that may require dose modification when administered with delavirdine or HIV protease inhibitors based upon demonstrated or predicted interactions with the potential for serious events or loss of efficacy

Drug class	Drug name
Anticoagulant	warfarin
Antimycobacterial	rifabutin
Antibacterial	erythromycin, dapsone
Antifungal	itraconazole, fluconazole
Immunosuppressants	cyclosporine, tacrolimus, rapamycin
Anticonvulsants	carbamazepine, phenobarbital, phenytoin
Narcotic analgesic	methadone

Toxicity and side effects

The principal dose-limiting side effect is skin rash. The overall frequency of rash was 18%, with treatment discontinuation being necessary in 4.3% of patients. Dose titration did not appear to reduce the incidence of this side effect. The rash is usually diffuse, maculopapular, erythematous and often pruritic. In most patients the rash first appears within 1 month of commencing therapy and resolves within 2 weeks, requiring no dose modification.

Delavirdine has been associated with fetal abnormalities in animal models.

Clinical use

- Treatment of HIV disease in adults and children over 12 years of age (in combination with other antiretroviral agents).

Preparations and dosages

Proprietary name: Rescriptor.

Preparations: Tablets (100 mg or 200 mg).

Dosage: Adults, oral, 400 mg three times daily.

Widely available.

Further information

Scott LJ, Perry CM 2000 Delavirdine: a review of its use in HIV infection. *Drugs* 60: 1411–1444.

EFAVIRENZ

Molecular weight: 315.68.

A synthetic heterocyclic compound formulated for oral administration. It is practically insoluble in water.

Antiviral activity

Efavirenz is active against HIV-1, but not HIV-2. Synergy against HIV-1 has been demonstrated in vitro in combination with zidovudine, didanosine and indinavir.

Acquired resistance

Single-codon substitutions in the HIV reverse transcriptase genome at positions 100 and 103 generate virus with up to 33-fold reduction in susceptibility. Further reduction in sensitiv-

ity arises when the 103 mutation occurs in addition to mutations at positions 100, 101, 108, 138, 188, 190 or 225. Many, but not all, of these point mutations confer reduced susceptibility to other non-nucleoside analog reverse transcriptase inhibitors.

Pharmacokinetics

Oral absorption	>65%
C_{max} 600 mg oral	4.5 mg/l
Plasma half-life	40–55 h
Plasma protein binding	>99%

Absorption and distribution

Absorption was dose related after single oral dosing in the range 100–1600 mg, but was non-proportional, indicating diminished absorption at higher doses. The mean peak and trough concentrations and AUC after single oral doses of 200 mg, 400 mg and 600 mg were linear. At the 600 mg dose, steady-state C_{max} was 12.9 µmol (14.2 µmol in children), steady state C_{min} was 5.6 µmol (same in children) and AUC was 184 µmol.h (214 µmol.h in children). Oral bioavailability following a standard high-fat meal was increased by an average of 50%, but was unaffected by a standard meal.

Concentrations in the CSF average 0.69% of the corresponding plasma concentration, representing a concentration of free drug three times higher than that found in plasma.

Metabolism

Efavirenz is metabolized by cytochrome P_{450} systems (predominantly CYP3A4 and CYP2B6 isozymes) to hydroxylated intermediates and excreted after subsequent glucuronidation. Metabolites are not active against HIV. It is thought to inhibit CYP3A4 isozyme at clinically relevant concentrations. Self-induction of P_{450} enzyme systems results in lower accumulation of drug than that predicted from modeling studies.

Formal studies of metabolism in patients with hepatic impairment have not been performed. Patients coinfected with hepatitis B or C and HIV experience more frequent elevations in serum transaminase concentrations after commencing treatment with efavirenz.

Excretion

Up to 34% of the administered dose can be recovered in urine, <1% as unchanged drug. The relatively low renal excretion indicates that the impact of renal impairment should be minimal.

Interactions

Use in patients treated concurrently with drugs that are metabolized through the same cytochrome P_{450} isozymes may alter the pharmacokinetic profiles of either drug and may therefore require caution or dose adjustment. Efavirenz should not be coadministered with astemizole, terfenadine, midazolam, triazolam, or cisapride and ergot derivatives. Indinavir dosage must be increased to 1000 mg every 8 h when coadministered with efavirenz.

There are potentially significant interactions with warfarin, saquinavir, clarithromycin, rifabutin, rifampicin (rifampin), ethinyl estradiol, methadone, phenobarbitone and phenytoin.

Toxicity and side effects

Rash occurs in up to 26% of patients, mostly in the first 2 weeks of therapy. Rash of more than grade 2 severity occurred in fewer than 1% of patients in clinical trials, but was sufficiently severe to limit treatment in 1.7% of patients. Rash may be more frequent (46%) and more frequently severe (5%) in children. In most patients the rash resolves within 1 month if treatment continues. Prophylactic use of antihistamines or corticosteroids is recommended if treatment is reinitiated in patients who interrupted therapy because of rash.

Disturbances of the central nervous system (CNS) with symptoms including, but not limited to, dizziness, insomnia, somnolence, impaired concentration and abnormal dreaming occurred in around 52% of clinical trial participants, with events of moderate to severe intensity occurring in about 3% of patients. Rare (0.2% of patients) episodes of severe delusional or inappropriate behavior and severe acute depression (including suicidal ideation) have also been reported. The symptoms commonly begin in the first 2 weeks of treatment.

Elevations in serum hepatic transaminase to levels more than five times the upper limit of normal are observed in about 3% of patients. This index increases to about 8% in patients who have hepatitis B or C and HIV coinfection.

An increase of up to 20% in non-fasting serum cholesterol concentrations has been observed. The effect on other serum lipid profiles has not been characterized.

Other side effects observed include alcohol intolerance, allergic reaction, asthenia, fever, hot flushes, malaise, influenza-like syndrome, pain, peripheral edema, syncope, ataxia, increased appetite, confusion, convulsions, impaired coordination, impotence, increased libido, migraine headaches, neuralgia, paresthesia, peripheral neuropathy, speech disorder, tremor, vertigo, gastritis, gastroenteritis, esophageal reflux, dry mouth, pancreatitis, tinnitus, flushing, palpitations, tachycardia, thrombophlebitis, hepatitis, weight gain, weight loss, arthralgia, myalgia, aggravated depression, agitation, amnesia, anxiety, apathy, emotional lability, euphoria, hallucination, psychosis, asthma, sinusitis, upper respiratory tract infection, acne, alopecia, eczema, folliculitis, seborrhea, skin exfoliation, urticaria, abnormal vision, diplopia, parosmia, and taste perversion.

Clinical use

- Treatment of HIV-1 infection in adults and children (in combination with other antiretroviral drugs).

Teratogenic effects have been noted in non-human primates. It should not be used in pregnant women or women attempting to conceive. The use in nursing mothers is also cautioned. It has not been evaluated in children below 3 years of age or who weigh less than 13 kg.

Preparations and dosages

Proprietary name: Sustiva; Stocrin.

Preparations: Capsules containing 50 mg, 100 mg, or 200 mg.

Dosage: Adults, oral, 600 mg once a day. Children, dosage determined by body weight. In order to alleviate some of the CNS side effects it is recommended the daily dose be taken at bedtime. It can be administered without food restrictions.

Widely available.

Further information

Adkins JC, Noble S, 1998 Efavirenz. *Drugs* 56: 1055–1064.

NEVIRAPINE

Molecular weight (anhydrous): 266.3; (hemihydrate): 275.3.

A synthetic heterocyclic compound, available in the anhydrous form in tablets and as the hemihydrate in a liquid oral preparation.

Antiviral activity

Nevirapine is active against HIV-1, but not HIV-2. It exhibits synergy with zidovudine, didanosine, stavudine, lamivudine, saquinavir and indinavir in cell culture assays.

Acquired resistance

Clinical isolates of HIV with reduced sensitivity have been described. One or more changes within the HIV reverse transcriptase at amino acid positions 103, 106, 108, 181, 188 and 190 have been implicated in the generation of resistance. These point mutations have also been implicated, either alone or in combination, in HIV resistance to other non-nucleoside reverse transcriptase inhibitors. Cross-resistance with other classes of antiretroviral drugs is unlikely and has not been described.

Pharmacokinetics

Oral absorption	93%
C_{max} 200 mg oral	1.5–2.5 mg/l after c. 4 h
Plasma half-life	25–30 h
Volume of distribution	1.21 l/kg
Plasma protein binding	c. 60%

Absorption

Peak plasma concentrations are linear for oral dosing at 200–400 mg. Absorption is unaffected by food, antacids or commonly used medicinal products.

Distribution

It is widely distributed. It crosses the placenta and blood–brain barrier readily and is found in breast milk. Concentrations in the CSF are around 45% of those found simultaneously in plasma.

Metabolism

It is extensively metabolized by cytochrome P_{450} enzymes into a number of hydroxylated intermediates that are subsequently biotransformed by conjugation with glucuronide. Oxidative metabolism of nevirapine is predominantly by the CYP3A isozymes of cytochrome P_{450}, although CYP2C9 and CYP2C19 isozymes may have a secondary role. As a result of autoinduction the drug has a shorter terminal half-life than that anticipated from single dosing models.

Excretion

Around 81% of the dose can be recovered in urine (80% as glucuronides) and 10% in feces. No more than 5% is excreted in urine as unchanged compound. The mean terminal half-life after multiple dosing in children is 18–24 h in young children and 31 h in older children

Interactions

Clinically significant interactions with other medications commonly used in patients with HIV infection are thought to be infrequent. Coadministration with indinavir requires a dose increase of indinavir to 1000 mg three times daily. Adjustment of methadone dose in patients experiencing narcotic withdrawal symptoms may be needed. The theoretical risk of interactions with drugs metabolized by the CYP3A and CYP2B6 cytochrome P_{450} enzyme systems remains.

Toxicity and side effects

Severe and life-threatening skin reactions, including hypersensitivity reactions characterized by rash, constitutional findings and visceral involvement, cases of toxic epidermal necrosis, and Stevens–Johnson syndrome occur mainly during the first 6 weeks of therapy. Patients should be monitored closely for isolated rash during the first 8 weeks of therapy. Treatment must be discontinued and not restarted in any patient presenting with symptoms and signs characteristic of a hypersensitivity reaction with mucosal or visceral involvement. About 16% of patients experience a rash, which is severe in around 7%. Use of lower doses for the first 2 weeks of treatment before escalating to recommended daily doses can reduce the frequency of this type of reaction.

Severe or life-threatening hepatotoxicity including fulminant hepatitis has occurred during the first 8 weeks of therapy and sometimes later. Treatment should stop, and not be restarted, in patients with evidence of clinical hepatitis. For an average 12-month period of follow-up the risk of such an event was 1.2% among 1121 patients.

Patients presenting with elevations in liver function tests to above five times the upper limit of normal should cease treatment immediately and only recommence at a reduced dose upon resolution of the abnormal findings.

Other side effects reported in patients treated with nevirapine as part of combination therapy are pruritus, abdominal pain, anorexia, constipation, diarrhea, dyspepsia, flatulence, gastroesophageal reflux, dry mouth, nausea, ulcerative stomatitis, vomiting, fatigue, fever, headache, malaise, pain, rigors, dizziness, insomnia, paresthesia, peripheral neuropathy, somnolence, flushing, increased sweating, depression, emotional lability, abnormal thinking, arthralgia, myalgia, frequent micturition, nocturia, granulocytopenia, lymphadenopathy, anemia, pancreatitis and thrombocytopenia

Clinical use

- Treatment of HIV-1 infection in adults and children over 2 months old (in combination with other antiretroviral therapies).

Use in pregnancy is cautioned, but perinatal transmission studies indicate that nevirapine monotherapy is effective in reducing mother-to-child transmission of HIV with no untoward fetal or maternal toxicity.

Preparations and dosages

Proprietary name: Viramune.

Preparations: 200 mg tablets and an oral suspension of nevirapine hemihydrate (10 mg/ml).

Dosage: Adults, oral, 200 mg once daily for the first 14 days followed by 200 mg twice daily, in combination with other antiretroviral therapies. Children (8–16 years), 4 mg/kg once daily for 2 weeks followed by 4 mg/kg twice daily. Children (2 months to 8 years), 4 mg/kg once daily for 2 weeks followed by 7 mg/kg twice daily. In children of all ages the total daily dose should not exceed 400 mg.

Widely available.

Further information

Bardsley-Elliot A, Perry CM 2000 Nevirapine: a review of its use in the prevention and treatment of paediatric infection. *Paediatric Drugs* 2: 373–407.

NUCLEOTIDE ANALOGS

Nucleotides are the monophosphorylated derivatives of nucleosides. Phosphorylation of nucleosides normally occurs within the cytoplasm of cells entering mitotic division and represents the rate-limiting step in the synthesis of bases for addition to growing nucleic acid chains. Nucleotides are actively taken up by most cells irrespective of the stage in the cell cycle. Several such drugs have been synthesized, including cidofovir (p. 506) and some have activity against HIV reverse transcriptase. They also inhibit mitochondrial DNA-polymerases.

 TENOFOVIR

Molecular weight 635.5.

A synthetic chemical formulated as the disproxil fumarate salt for oral administration. It has an aqueous solubility of 13.4 g/l.

Antiviral activity

In vitro the 50% inhibitory concentration for HIV is 0.04–8.5 μmol. Additive or synergic anti-HIV activity with nucleoside analog, non-nucleoside analog and protease inhibitors has been demonstrated in vitro.

Tenofovir also possesses antiviral activity against hepatitis B virus and is currently being evaluated as therapy for this infection.

Acquired resistance

In laboratory systems a point mutation at codon 65 of the HIV reverse transcriptase (a mutation associated with treatment with nucleoside reverse transcriptase inhibitors) was associated with 3–4 fold reduced sensitivity and may reduce the effec- tiveness of tenofovir in vivo. Isolates of HIV with multiple zidovudine-associated point mutations also showed reduced sensitivity to tenofovir. Multinucleoside-resistant HIV with an insertion mutation at codon 69 has shown reduced sensitivity.

Pharmacokinetics

Oral absorption	c.25%
C_{max}	296 ($\pm$ 90) ng/ml after 1 h
Plasma half-life	Not reported
Volume of distribution	1.3 ($\pm$ 0.6) l/kg
Plasma protein binding	<0.7%

Absorption

Tenofovir should be taken with food to increase bioavailability. High-fat food increases the oral bioavailability about 40% with an associated 14% increase in C_{max}.

Distribution

The extent of penetration into the CSF has not been reported. In animal studies the drug is secreted in breast milk.

Metabolism

Tenofovir is not a substrate for cytochrome P_{450} isozymes.

Excretion

Around 32% of an orally administered dose is recovered in urine as unchanged drug. It is eliminated by a combination of glomerular filtration and active tubular secretion. Treatment of patients with underlying renal disease is not recommended.

Interactions

Concomitant use with didanosine is associated with a 28% increase in the peak plasma concentration of that drug. Patients receiving the combination should be monitored for long-term adverse events associated with didanosine.

Coadministration with lopinavir/ritonavir results in approximately 30% increases in peak and trough concentrations of tenofovir.

There may be clinically relevant interactions with drugs that share the renal elimination pathway.

Toxicity and side effects

Lactic acidosis and severe hepatomegaly with steatosis occur and careful clinical evaluation is needed in patients with evidence of hepatic abnormality. Treatment should be stopped in any patient who develops clinical or laboratory findings indicative of hepatotoxicity or lactic acidosis.

The most frequent side effects associated with use in combination with other antiretroviral drugs were mild to moderate gastrointestinal events. Fewer than 1% of patients reporting such events required cessation of tenofovir therapy.

Clinical use

- Treatment of HIV infection in adults (in combination with other antiretroviral drugs).

Preparations and dosages

Proprietary name: Viread.

Preparations: Tablets (300 mg).

Dosage: Adults, oral, 75–300 mg once daily. The optimal dose in children has not been established.

Limited availability.

HIV PROTEASE INHIBITORS

Protease inhibitors are large molecules that are difficult to manufacture. As a class they possess complex pharmacokinetic properties including significant metabolic interactions, so that coadministration with many other drugs is either contraindicated or cautioned (Table 39.1 and 39.2; p. 481). They are active against HIV-1 and HIV-2.

The individual compounds possess signature toxicities, some of which are treatment limiting, in addition to class-specific side effects. All have been associated with significant abnormalities of body fat (lipodystrophy syndrome) that include central obesity, dorsocervical fat enlargement (buffalo hump), peripheral fat wasting and breast enlargement. The mechanism and long-term consequences of these changes are currently unknown. These drugs may also be associated with the development of glucose intolerance and diabetes mellitus (or worsening of previously stable diabetes). They cause significant changes in serum lipid profiles (including hypertriglyceridemia and hypercholesterolemia) and a range of glycemic effects in some patients. They have also been associated with spontaneous bleeding in patients with hemophilia A and B that required additional factor VIII treatment. There are rare reports of acute hemolytic anemia.

An important limitation of this drug class in patients experiencing treatment limiting side effects is the lack of recommended reductions in unit dose. For such patients alternate treatment regimens that may include an alternative protease inhibitor must be prescribed.

Virus isolates from patients with HIV who have been treated with these drugs but who are no longer responding to treatment are known to possess resistance mutations within the protease amino acid sequence. Some resistance mutations to one drug confer high-level resistance to all other protease inhibitors. In most cases increasing levels of virus resistance appears to be conferred by increasing numbers of primary mutations. This relationship appears to hold also in terms of conferring cross-resistance to other protease inhibitors.

Further information

Condra JH, Petropoulos CJ, Ziermann R, Scheif WA, Shivaprakash M, Emini EA 2000 Drug resistance and predicted virologic responses to human immunodeficiency virus type 1 protease inhibitor therapy. *Journal of Infectious Diseases* 182: 758–765.

Flexner C 1998 HIV protease inhibitors. *New England Journal of Medicine* 338: 1281–1292.

Flynn TE, Bricker LA 1999 Myocardial infarction in HIV infected men receiving protease inhibitors. *Annals of Internal Medicine* 131: 258–262.

Moyle G 2001 Use of HIV protease inhibitors as pharmacoenhancers. *AIDS Reader* 11: 87–98.

Ren S, Lien EJ 2001 Development of HIV protease inhibitors; a survey. *Progress in Drug Research* 1–34.

AMPRENAVIR

Molecular weight: 505.64.

A synthetic chemical formulated for oral use. The aqueous solubility is about 0.04 g/l.

Antiviral activity

In cell culture assays amprenavir exhibited synergic inhibition of HIV replication with abacavir, zidovudine, didanosine and saquinavir, and additive inhibition with indinavir, nelfinavir, and ritonavir.

Acquired resistance

Isolates of HIV with up to a 10-fold decrease in susceptibility have been selected in vitro and from patients. Genotypic analysis of these isolates has revealed mutations in the HIV protease at positions 46, 47, 50 54 and 84. Many of these mutations contribute to the reduced susceptibility of HIV to other protease inhibitors.

Pharmacokinetics

Oral absorption	Not known
C_{max}	5.36 mg/l after 1–2 h
Plasma half-life	7.1–10.6 h
Volume of distribution	430 l
Plasma protein binding	c. 90%

Absorption and distribution

The absolute oral bioavailability in humans has not been established, but it is rapidly absorbed. Fasting and high-fat meals did not significantly affect the relative bioavailability of single doses in HIV-negative volunteers. Patients with incremental levels of hepatic impairment have significantly higher systemic exposure and require dosage adjustment. In children the bioavailability of the oral solution is about 14% lower than that of the capsule formulation in adults. Levels in the CSF have not been evaluated.

Metabolism

Amprenavir is extensively metabolized by the cytochrome P_{450} CYP3A4 enzyme system. Two major metabolites have been identified that appear to result from the oxidation of the tetrahydrofuran and aniline moieties. Conjugation of these metabolites with glucuronide is not thought to be significant.

Excretion

Around 14% of a dose is eliminated in the urine and 75% in feces. Less than 3% is in the form of unchanged drug, and two metabolites account for >90% of administered drug found in fecal samples.

Interactions

Amprenavir is both metabolized by and inhibits CYP3A4 cytochrome P_{450}. Caution is therefore required when coadministering medications that are known to be substrates, inhibitors, or inducers of this enzyme (Tables 39.1 and 39.2; p. 481). Many other drugs are likely to interact with amprenavir but have not been studied.

Toxicity and side effects

The safety has been evaluated in adults and children who participated in single-or multiple-dose studies. There are no apparent differences in the types, severity or frequency of side effects.

About 15% of patients discontinued treatment because of side effects that included gastrointestinal events (11%), rash (3%) and paresthesias (1%). Most gastrointestinal events (nausea, vomiting, diarrhea and taste perversion) were of mild to moderate severity.

Skin rash occurs in around 28% of patients within 10 (range 7–73) days. The rash is usually maculopapular, of mild to moderate severity, and occasionally presents with pruritus. Treatment was often continued without interruption. If interrupted, rechallenge did not cause rash to recur. Severe or life-threatening rash, including Stevens–Johnson syndrome, occurred in 1% of patients (4% of all recipients who reported rash).

The principal laboratory abnormalities encountered are hyperglycemia, hypertriglyceridemia and hypercholesterolemia.

Clinical use

- Treatment of HIV infection (in combination with other antiretroviral drugs).

Preparations and dosage

Proprietary name: Agenerase.

Preparations: Capsules containing 50 mg and 150 mg and an oral solution containing 15 mg/ml.

Dosage: Adults, oral, 1200 mg twice daily. Children 4–12 years of age, 20 mg/kg twice daily or 15 mg/kg thrice daily to a maximum of 2400 mg per day in each instance. For pediatric patients treated with oral solution 22.5 mg/kg (1.5 ml/kg) twice daily or 17 mg/kg (1.1 ml/kg) thrice daily to a maximum of 2800 mg per day. Doses in the capsule and oral formulations are not interchangeable.

Limited availability.

Further information

Noble S, Goa KL 2000 Amprenavir: a review of its clinical potential in patients with HIV infection. *Drugs* 60: 1383–1410.

 INDINAVIR

Molecular weight (free base): 613.8; (sulfate): 711.88.

A synthetic chemical formulated as the sulfate for oral administration. The free base is poorly soluble in water, but the sulfate is freely soluble.

Antiviral activity

Indinavir exhibits synergistic antiretroviral activity in vitro when combined with zidovudine, didanosine or non-nucleoside reverse transcriptase inhibitors.

Acquired resistance

Loss of antiretroviral activity in patients is typically associated with the accumulation of mutations resulting in amino acids changes in the protease enzyme. At least eleven individual point mutations have been characterized. No single substitution appears able to cause measurable resistance, but resistance follows the expression of multiple and variable substitutions. Generally, the level of resistance rises with the number of point mutations.

Complete cross-resistance with all other HIV protease inhibitors has been described in clinical isolates of HIV, but the level of resistance is variable.

Pharmacokinetics

Oral absorption	60–65%
C_{max} 800 mg oral	7.7 mg/l after 0.8 h
Plasma half-life	1.8 h
Plasma protein binding	c. 39%

No pharmacokinetic data are available in children.

Absorption
Absorption is subject to significant variability. A standard high-fat meal reduces absorption by 80% and systemic exposure to the drug by 85%. Light meals have no impact on pharmacokinetic parameters. Grapefruit juice significantly reduces the systemic exposure and should be avoided.

An acid gastric pH is thought to be required for absorption. This contrasts with the alkaline buffering required for absorption of didanosine. When coadministered with didanosine the two drugs should be taken at least 1 h apart.

Distribution
The apparent volume of distribution is not known. Indinavir crosses the blood–brain barrier, but this is limited and yields mean plasma:CSF concentration ratios of around 0.18. It does not readily cross the placenta, but is secreted in milk.

Metabolism
Indinavir is metabolized in the liver by the CYP3A4 cytochrome P_{450} system. Seven major metabolites have been described, including one glucuronide conjugate and six oxidative metabolites.

Excretion
Around 83% of the dose is recovered in feces; 18% is excreted in urine, 10% as unchanged drug. Patients with mild to moderate hepatic impairment experience significantly increased systemic exposure with a mean terminal half-life of 2.8 h.

Interactions

Recommended contraindications and cautions are summarized in Tables 39.1 and 39.2 (p. 481). The dose must be reduced when coadministered with delavirdine and increased when coadministered with efavirenz.

Ritonavir inhibits the metabolism of indinavir and several novel regimens are showing some promise in terms of antiretroviral activity and safety.

Toxicity and side effects

The principal side effect is nephrolithiasis, including flank pain with or without hematuria. The low aqueous solubility can result in crystallization of unchanged drug in the kidneys within a few days of commencing treatment. The reported incidence is 3–15% in clinical studies. Patients should be encouraged to maintain an additional fluid intake of at least 1.5 l/day at all times.

Indirect hyperbilirubinemia (total bilirubin ≥ 43 µmol) has been reported in about 10% of patients. These rises are rarely associated with significant increases in other indices of liver function and most patients continue treatment without dose modification.

Increased serum triglycerides, hypercholesterolemia and hyperglycemia have been reported. Glucose intolerance, incident diabetes mellitus or worsening of previously stable diabetes have also been described.

Clinical use

- Treatment of adult HIV infection (in combination with other antiretroviral drugs).

There are no well-controlled studies to guide its use in pregnancy.

Preparations and dosage

Proprietary name: Crixivan.

Preparations: Capsules containing 200 mg or 400 mg.

Dosage: Adults, oral, 800 mg three times daily (2.4 g per day) taken without food 1 h before or 2 h after a meal. Children 4–17 years old, 500 mg/m² three times daily (maximum 800 mg three times daily).

Widely available.

Further information

Anonymous 1999 Indinavir (sulfate). In: Dollery C (ed.) *Therapeutic Drugs* 2nd edn. Churchill Livingstone, Edinburgh, pp. 136–140.
Plosker GL, Noble S 1999 Indinavir: a review of its use in the treatment of HIV infection. *Drugs* 58: 1165–1203.

LOPINAVIR

Molecular weight: 628.80.

A synthetic inhibitor of the HIV protease enzyme, coformulated with ritonavir for oral administration. In this formulation, ritonavir functions to inhibit the metabolic clearance of lopinavir, and does not contribute to the antiretroviral activity.

It is practically insoluble in water, freely soluble in methanol and ethanol, and soluble in isopropanol.

Antiviral activity

Lopinavir is active against HIV-1 and HIV-2.

Acquired resistance

Isolates of HIV with reduced susceptibility have been selected in vitro in the presence and absence of ritonavir. The genotypic characteristics have not been determined and it is not yet known whether such strains might arise during treatment. Virus from patients who have not responded to lopinavir/ritonavir has, in all cases, arisen in persons previously treated with other HIV protease inhibitors; such isolates exhibited preexisting protease resistance genotypes.

Further studies are needed to assess the issue of resistance to lopinavir/ritonavir. It is possible that plasma levels of lopinavir arising from coadministration with ritonavir may exceed the concentrations needed to inhibit replication of HIV with high resistance.

Pharmacokinetics

Oral absorption	Not known
C_{max} 400 mg (with 100 mg ritonavir)	9.6 mg/l after c. 4 h
Plasma half-life	5–6 h
Plasma protein binding	98–99%

Absorption and distribution

The absolute bioavailability of the coformulation with ritonavir has not been determined. The recommended dose in children achieves a peak concentration of c. 8.2 mg/l. The mean AUC for lopinavir in adults was 82.8 mg.h/l (72.6 mg.h/l in children). In individuals fed a moderate-fat meal at the time of dosing the peak plasma concentration increased by 23% and the AUC by 48%.

No information is available on the penetration into the CNS. It is secreted in breast milk.

Metabolism

Lopinavir is primarily metabolized by the CYP3A4 cytochrome P_{450} system. Ritonavir is a potent inhibitor of CYP3A4 isozymes and therefore the coformulation results in increased levels of plasma lopinavir. At least 13 oxidized metabolites of lopinavir have been identified in humans. Ritonavir also induces CYP3A4 isozymes and lopinavir concentrations stabilize after 10–16 days of multiple dosing.

Excretion

Over an 8-day period after single dosing with the combined formulation around 10.4% and 82.6% of the administered dose is recovered in urine and feces respectively. Less than 3% of the dose is recovered as unchanged drug in urine and 19.8% in feces.

Interactions

The coformulation is contraindicated with a large number of drugs that are biotransformed by the cytochrome P_{450} family of enzymes (Table 39.1; p. 481). Medications that should be coadministered judiciously are summarized in Table 39.2 (p. 481).

Preliminary studies of lopinavir/ritonavir in combination with amprenavir, indinavir or saquinavir suggest that the pharmacokinetic properties are not affected in ways that would require dose modification.

Toxicity and side effects

Clinical experience is presently limited to 612 patients who participated in clinical trials. The following side effects of moderate to severe intensity occurred in more than 2% of patients: abdominal pain, asthenia, headache, pain, abnormal stools, diarrhea, nausea, vomiting, insomnia and rash. The principal laboratory abnormalities were elevated serum triglycerides and cholesterol.

Episodes of pancreatitis have been reported and these may be related to the elevations in serum triglyceride levels. The toxicity in children is similar to that in adults.

Clinical use

- Treatment of HIV infection (in combination with ritonavir and other antiretroviral agents).

No well-controlled studies have been performed in pregnant women. Studies to determine the safety and efficacy in children are ongoing.

Preparations and dosages

Proprietary name: Kaletra.

Preparations: Capsules (133.3 mg lopinavir and 33.3 mg ritonavir); oral solution (400 mg lopinavir and 100 mg ritonavir per 5 ml).

Dosage: Adults, oral, 400 mg lopinavir plus 100 mg ritonavir twice daily with food. Children aged 6 months to 12 years, 12 mg lopinavir plus 3 mg ritonavir/kg twice-daily for those weighing 7–15 kg; 10 mg lopinavir plus 2.5 mg ritonavir/kg twice daily for those weighing 15–40 kg.

Widely available.

Further information

Hurst M, Faulds D 2000 Lopinavir. *Drugs* 60: 1380–1381.

NELFINAVIR

Molecular weight: 663.9.

A synthetic chemical formulated as the mesylate for oral administration. It is slightly soluble in water at low pH and freely soluble in methanol, ethanol, isopropanol and propylene glycol.

Antiviral activity

In cell culture assays of HIV replication combinations with didanosine or stavudine exhibited additive inhibition and combinations with zidovudine, lamivudine or zalcitabine exhibited synergy. Interactions ranging from antagonism to synergy were found with other HIV protease inhibitors.

Acquired resistance

Clinical isolates of HIV with 5- to 93-fold reduction in sensitivity have been identified. These isolates have combinations of mutations within the protease amino acid sequence at positions 30, 35, 36, 46, 71, 77, 88 or 90. The most common mutations are at positions 30 and 90. These mutations may play a role in the development of resistance to other HIV protease inhibitors.

Pharmacokinetics

Oral absorption	c. 78%
C_{max} 750 mg oral (with food)	3–4 mg/l after 2–4 h
Plasma half-life	c. 3.5–5 h
Volume of distribution	2–7 l/kg
Plasma protein binding	>98%

Absorption and distribution

Food improves the bioavailability and the drug should be administered with a light meal. If administered with didanosine, it should be given at least 1 h before or 2 h after. Penetration into the CNS has not been determined. It is secreted in breast milk.

Metabolism

Multiple cytochrome P_{450} isozymes, including CYP3A4, are responsible for the metabolism of the drug. One major and several minor oxidative metabolities have been found in plasma.

Excretion

Most of an oral dose is recovered in feces as unchanged drug (22%) and metabolites (78%). The remainder is recovered in urine, mainly unchanged.

Interactions

In addition to the drug interactions summarized in Tables 39.1 and 39.2 (p. 481), nelfinavir should not be coadministered with oral contraceptives containing ethinylestradiol on norethisterone.

Combinations with other protease inhibitors may provide prolonged exposure to one or both drugs (Table 39.3). The safety of these combinations has not been evaluated.

Table 39.3 Pharmacokinetic interactions between nelfinavir and other protease inhibitors

Combination	Increase in AUC (%)
Nelfinavir + indinavir	Nelfinavir 83; indinavir 51
Nelfinavir + ritonavir	Nelfinavir 152
Nelfinavir + saquinavir	Nelfinavir 18; saquinavir 392

Toxicity and side effects

The primary treatment-limiting side effect is diarrhea. This is generally of mild to moderate severity, but in clinical trials moderate to severe diarrhea was experienced by up to 32% of patients.

Adverse events that occurred in less than 2% of patients were fever, headache, malaise, pain, anorexia, dyspepsia, epigastric pain, gastrointestinal bleeding, hepatitis, mouth ulceration, pancreatitis, flatulence, nausea, vomiting, anemia, leukopenia, thrombocytopenia, increased liver function tests, increased serum amylase, hyperlipidemia, hyperuricemia, arthralgia, arthritis, cramps, myalgia, myasthenia, myopathy, anxiety, depression, dizziness, emotional lability, hyperkinesia, insomnia, migraine, paresthesia, seizures, sleep disorders, suicidal ideation, dyspnea, maculopapular rash, pruritus, sweating, urticaria, renal calculus and sexual dysfunction.

Clinical use

- Treatment of HIV infection (in combination with other antiretroviral drugs).

Preparations and dosages

Proprietary name: Viracept.

Preparations: Tables containing 250 mg; oral powder for solution containing 50 mg/g.

Dosage: Adults, oral, 750 mg three times daily. Children aged 2–13 years old, 20–30 mg/kg three times daily. Each dose in adults and children should be taken with a light snack.

Widely available.

Further information

Pai VB, Nahata MC 1999 Nelfinavir mesylate: a protease inhibitor. *Annals of Pharmacotherapy* 33: 325–339.

RITONAVIR

Molecular weight: 720.95.

A synthetic chemical formulated as capsules and as an alcoholic solution for oral administration. It is a white to light-tan powder that is practically insoluble in water but freely soluble in methanol and ethanol and soluble in isopropanol.

Antiviral activity

Ritonavir is active against HIV-1 and HIV-2.

Acquired resistance

Genotypic analysis of resistant isolates of HIV selected in vitro has revealed that resistance is attributable to specific amino acid substitutions in the HIV protease at positions 82 and 84. Virus from treated patients indicates that the development of resistance proceeds in an ordered and sequential manner leading to the accumulation of multiple mutations at codons 54, 71, 36 and 82.

Resistant strains are cross-resistant to indinavir, and nelfinavir. Studies to determine whether the cross-resistance extended to other protease inhibitors were inconclusive.

Pharmacokinetics

Oral absorption	c. 66–75%
C_{max} 600 mg oral	11.2 mg/l after 2–4 h
Plasma half-life	2–4 h
Volume of distribution	0.41 l/kg
Plasma protein binding	>98%

Absorption and distribution

Fasting and high-fat meals had no appreciable effect on the oral absorption. Penetration into the CNS is thought to be low because of the low free fraction in plasma.

Metabolism

Ritonavir is metabolized in the liver by the CYP3A4 and CYP2D6 isoforms of cytochrome P_{450}. Four oxidized metabolites have been identified, the major of which retains antiretroviral activity. As well as inhibiting cytochrome P_{450} isoforms, it is a potent inducer of this enzyme system. Consequently pharmacokinetic parameters may take up to 4 weeks to stabilize. Patients with hepatic impairment should be closely monitored.

Excretion

Around 11.3% of the dose can be recovered in the urine (only 4% as unchanged drug) and 86.4% in feces respectively. Metabolites are eliminated primarily via the feces.

Interactions

It is one of the most potent inhibitors of the CYP3A4 isoform of cytochrome P_{450} yet described and is contraindicated and cautioned with a greater number of medications than all other protease inhibitors. In addition to those listed in Table 39.1 (p. 481), it is contraindicated with bupropion, clozapine, encainide, flecainide, pethidine, propafenone and dextropropoxyphene, meperidine, clorazepate, estazolam and zolpidem.

Dose modification of either or both coadministered drugs should be considered when used with alfentanil, fentanyl, nefadozone, quinine, verapamil, tamoxifen, fenasteride, flutamide, prednisone, theophylline and clonazepam.

Effects on the pharmacokinetics of other protease inhibitors are exploited in the coformulation with lopinavir. Ritonavir boosts the AUC of saquinavir by approximately 20-fold and significantly increases indinavir concentrations.

It significantly reduces the AUC of ethinyloestradiol and alternative contraception should be sought. Since formulations contain ethanol it should not be administered in combination with disulfiram or metronidazole.

Toxicity and side effects

Adverse events of moderate to severe intensity that occurred in more than 2% of patients who participated in clinical trials included asthenia (27.6%), malaise (4.3%), vasodilation (2.6%), anorexia (7.8%), constipation (2.6%), diarrhea (21.6%), flatulence (2.6%), nausea (46.6%), vomiting (22.4%), circumoral paresthesia (5.2%), dizziness (5.2%), insomnia (3.4%), paresthesia (5.2%), somnolence (2.6%), abnormal thinking (2.6%), pharyngitis (2.6%), sweating (3.4%) and taste perversion (15.5%).

Changes in laboratory indices included hyperglycemia, hyperuricemia, elevated liver enzymes, hypertriglyceridemia, hypercholesterolemia, and elevated creatine phosphokinase.

Clinical use

- Treatment of HIV infection in adults and children aged 12 years and over (in combination with other antiretroviral agents).

The safety and efficacy have not been established in children less than 12 years of age.

 Preparations and dosage

Proprietary name: Norvir.

Preparations: Soft capsules containing 100 mg and an oral solution containing 80 mg/ml.

Dosage: Adults, oral, 600 mg twice daily. Children >12 years old, initially 250 mg/m² twice daily increasing by 50 mg/m² at intervals of 2–3 days to 350 mg/m² twice daily (maximum 600 mg twice daily).

Widely available.

 Further information

Hurst M, Faulds D 2000 Ritonavir. *Drugs* 60: 1371–1379.

 SAQUINAVIR

Molecular weight: 670.86

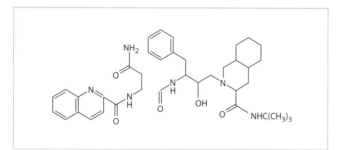

A synthetic chemical available for oral administration as the free base (soft gel capsule), which has superseded the former mesylate (hard gel capsule) formulation. It is insoluble in water.

Antiviral activity

In cell culture, saquinavir exhibits synergic antiretroviral effects in double and triple combinations with nucleoside analogs and nevirapine.

Acquired resistance

Isolates of HIV with reduced susceptibility selected in vitro have several mutations in the protease gene but only those at codons 48 and 90 were consistently associated with resistance. Similar mutations have been observed in HIV isolated from patients who have received saquinavir.

Mutations at positions 48 and 90 also confer resistance to at least one other HIV protease inhibitor, but the details of this cross-resistance have not been fully elucidated.

Pharmacokinetics

Oral absorption (soft gel capsule)	c. 13%
C_{max} 600 mg oral	c. 0.2 mg/l
Plasma half-life	c. 1–2 h
Volume of distribution	10 l/kg
Plasma protein binding	c. 97%

Absorption and distribution

The handling of oral doses is poorly characterized, though the soft gel formulation is better absorbed than the former hard gel capsule. The mean AUC at steady state is 7.25 mg.h/ml, although this figure is subject to considerable variability. Penetration into the CNS is less than 1% of simultaneous plasma concentrations.

Metabolism

Saquinavir is metabolized via the CYP3A4 isoenzyme of cytochrome P_{450} in the liver, principally to mono- and dihydroxylated derivatives. It may inhibit cytochrome P_{450} activity, but it is thought not to induce this enzyme system appreciably.

Excretion

Around 88% of the dose is excreted in the feces and 1% in urine. Data indicate that it undergoes extensive first-pass metabolism.

Interactions

The contraindications and precautions applicable to other HIV protease inhibitors remain valid despite the relatively low bioavailability and the absence in vivo of P_{450} induction.

The possibility of enhancing plasma levels by coadministering with other HIV protease inhibitors that inhibit cytochrome P_{450} metabolism has been investigated. Ritonavir increases the AUC c. 275%; nelfinavir increases the AUC c. 390%.

Plasma levels can also be significantly enhanced by co-administration with delavirdine (increase in AUC of c. 350%). Paradoxically, nevirapine and efavirenz reduce plasma exposure, and these two agents should not be used with saquinavir.

Toxicity and side effects

The most frequently observed side effects in 500 clinical trial participants were mild and principally involved gastrointestinal signs and symptoms: diarrhea (20%), nausea (18%), abdominal discomfort (13%), flatulence (12%) and dyspepsia (9%). Other events that were reported by more than 5% of patients were fatigue (6%), headaches (9%) and insomnia (6%).

Marked laboratory abnormalities include elevated liver function test, hypercalcemia, hypoglycemia, hyperglycemia, hyperkalemia, hyperamylasemia, hypophosphatemia and hyperbilirubinemia.

Clinical use

- Treatment of HIV infection (in combination with other antiretroviral drugs).

Safety and efficacy during pregnancy and in HIV-infected children have not been established.

Preparations and dosages

Proprietary names: Fortovase (soft gel capsules); Invirase (hard gel capsules).

Preparations: Fortovase capsules contain 200 mg

Dosage: Adults, oral, 1200 mg three times daily taken immediately after food (Fortovase).

Adults, oral, 600 mg three times daily (Invirase).

Widely available.

Further information

Anonymous 1999 Saquinavir. In: Dollery C (ed.) *Therapeutic Drugs* 2nd edn. Churchill Livingstone, Edinburgh, pp. S8–S12.

Figgitt DP, Plosker GL 2000 Saquinavir soft-gel capsules: an updated review of its use in the management of HIV infection. *Drugs* 60: 481–516.

EXPERIMENTAL THERAPIES

Despite the availability of 15 antiretroviral agents, investment in the development of new drugs to treat HIV infection continues. Many new drugs represent additional members of available classes that offer pharmacological improvements:

- **Nucleoside analog reverse transcriptase inhibitors:** diaminopurine dioxolane (DAPD) and emtracitabine (FTC).
- **Non-nucleoside reverse transcriptase inhibitors:** capravirine and DMP-083.
- **HIV protease inhibitors:** tipranavir, BMS-232632 (atazanavir) and DMP-450.

Agents directed against completely new targets in the virus replicative cycles are also entering clinical development. Inhibitors of the process by which HIV fuses with cell membranes during infection (fusion inhibitors) are currently being evaluated in phase III clinical trials, having shown antiretroviral activity in earlier phases of investigation. The fusion inhibitor pentafuside (T-20) requires twice daily subcutaneous administration.

Inhibitors of HIV integrase, nucleocapsid antagonists and chemokine/chemokine receptor antagonists are also under investigation.

CHAPTER

40 Other antiviral agents

R. J. Whitley

Numerous converging scientific events have led to an age of antiviral therapy: the achievements of the molecular virologist in defining the life cycle of many viral pathogens have contributed to the development of selective and specific inhibitors of viral replication, an example being aciclovir; the application of rapid viral diagnostic procedures, particularly the polymerase chain reaction (PCR), has paralleled the development of antiviral therapeutics; and the recognition of the medical impact of chronic viral infections, such as hepatitis B and C and HIV, has moved the field forward.

Inhibition of viral replication can be accomplished at several sites. These include:

- direct inactivation of the virus prior to cell attachment and entry
- blocking attachment of virus to host-cell membrane receptors and penetration
- prevention of viral uncoating
- impeding transcription or translation into viral messenger RNA and proteins
- interfering with glycosylation steps
- alteration of viral assembly and prevention of release.

Clearly, events of viral replication vary according to the genetic nature of the pathogen, i.e. single or double-stranded DNA or RNA virus. This chapter addresses compounds other than antiretroviral agents that are licensed for clinical use.

ADAMANTANES

The parent compound, amantadine, is a tricyclic primary amine that was discovered in the 1960s and was found to inhibit replication of strains of influenza A. Like its congener, rimantadine, amantadine prevents virus acidification required for fusion of the viral envelope to cells (p. 22).

 AMANTADINE

1-Aminoadamantane hydrochloride. Molecular weight (hydrochloride): 187.7.

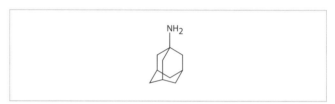

A symmetrical synthetic C-10 tricyclic amine with an unusual cage-like structure, supplied as the hydrochloride for oral administration.

Antiviral activity

Amantadine inhibits influenza A virus replication at concentrations of 0.2–0.6 mg/l. It has little activity against influenza B or C.

Acquired resistance

Resistance is the consequence of mutations in amino acid positions 27, 30 and 31 in the M2 transmembrane sequence. Cross-resistance between amantadine and rimantadine is universal. Resistant strains are recovered from nasopharyngeal secretions of approximately 30% of treated subjects. Resistant strains are transmissible. Postexposure family prophylaxis results in the prompt emergence of drug resistance after onset of treatment.

Pharmacokinetics

Oral absorption	>90%
C_{max} 200 mg oral daily	0.4–0.9 mg/l after c. 4–6 h
Plasma half-life	9.7–14.5 h
Volume of distribution	10.4 l/kg
Plasma protein binding	65%

Absorption and distribution

Amantadine is almost completely absorbed after oral administration. Levels in secretions approach plasma concentrations.

Metabolism and excretion

Drug is eliminated unchanged by the kidney. About 56% of a single oral dose is excreted within 24 h. Altogether 90% of an oral dose is excreted in the urine, with a mean elimination half-life of 11.8 h in subjects with normal renal function. In elderly men, the half-life is 28.9 h and in patients with renal insufficiency half-lives of 18.5 h to 33.8 days have been observed. The renal clearance is around 398 ml/min (range 112–772 ml/min), indicating active secretion as well as glomerular filtration. Less than 5% of a dose is removed during hemodialysis and average half-lives of 8.3 and 13 days have been reported in patients on chronic hemodialysis. Extreme care must be taken to ensure that drug does not accumulate to toxic levels.

Interactions

Central nervous system (CNS), gastrointestinal or other side effects provoked by anticholinergic drugs or L-dopa may be aggravated. Patients have developed visual hallucinations while concurrently taking amantadine and benzhexol; these respond to a reduction of the dose of benzhexol. Hemodialysis is not helpful because of the large volume of distribution.

Toxicity and side effects

Embryotoxicity and teratogenicity have been observed in rats receiving 50 mg/kg daily, about 15 times the usual human dose. Neurological side effects include drowsiness, insomnia, light-headedness, difficulty in concentration, nervousness, dizziness and headache in up to 20% of individuals. Other side effects include anorexia, nausea, vomiting, dry mouth, constipation and urinary retention. All develop during the first 3–4 days of therapy and are reversible by discontinuing the drug. An exception to rapid onset of adverse reactions is livedo reticularis. Convulsions, hallucinations and confusion are dose related, usually occurring at levels in excess of 1.5 mg/l; convulsions may occur at a lower threshold in patients with a history of epilepsy and the drug is best avoided in such patients.

Clinical use

- Prevention and treatment of influenza A.

Rational use requires laboratory and epidemiological evidence of influenza A in the community. Rimantadine is used preferentially over amantadine.

 Preparations and dosage

Proprietary name: Symmetrel.

Preparations: Capsules, syrup.

Dosage: Treatment or prophylaxis. Adults, oral, 100 mg once or twice daily for 5–7 days.

Children aged 1–9 years, 4–8 mg/kg per day; 10–15 years, 100 mg per day.

Widely available.

 Further information

Anonymous 1999 Amantadine (hydrochloride). In: Dollery C (ed.) *Therapeutic Drugs* 2nd edn. Churchill Livingstone, Edinburgh, pp. A116–A119.

Aoki FY, Stiver HG, et al 1985 Prophylactic amantadine dose and plasma concentration-effect relationships in healthy adults. *Clinical Pharmacology and Therapeutics* 37: 128–136.

Hayden FG, Belshe RM et al 1989 Emergence and apparent transmission of rimantadine resistant influenza A virus in families. *New England Journal of Medicine* 321: 1696–1702.

Hayden FG, Gwaltney Jr JM et al 1981 Comparative toxicity of amantadine hydrochloride and rimantadine hydrochloride in healthy adults. *Antimicrobial Agents and Chemotherapy* 19: 226–233.

 RIMANTADINE

Molecular weight (hydrochloride): 215.7.

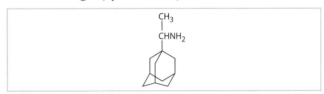

An analog of amantadine, supplied as the hydrochloride for oral administration.

Antiviral activity

In cell culture and animal models Rimantadine is more effective than amantadine on a weight-for-weight basis. There is complete cross-resistance with amantadine.

Pharmacokinetics

Oral absorption	>90%
C_{max} 100 mg oral (twice daily)	0.4–0.5 mg/l after 2–6 h
Plasma half-life	c. 35 h
Volume of distribution	Very large
Plasma protein binding	c. 40%

Absorption and distribution

Single- and multiple-dose pharmacokinetic studies in elderly patients and young adults are remarkably similar. The steady-state concentration in nasal mucus develops by day 5 at a concentration approximately 1.5-fold higher than plasma.

Metabolism

In contrast to amantadine, rimantadine is extensively metabolized by the liver by hydroxylation and glucuronidation.

Excretion

Less than 20% is excreted unchanged in the urine and most of the breakdown products are excreted by this route. Thus, the plasma half-life is much less affected by renal dysfunction than that of amantadine.

Toxicity and side effects

Rimantadine has significantly fewer side effects than amantadine at equivalent doses, perhaps because of differences in pharmacokinetics, since with equal doses the blood levels are considerably lower. Central nervous system (CNS) side effects are not significantly higher than placebo.

Clinical use

- Prophylaxis and treatment of influenza A infections.

Since prolonged administration is well tolerated by elderly patients, the drug is preferable to amantadine.

 Preparations and Dosage

Proprietary Name: Flumadine.

Preparations: Tablet and syrup.

Dosage: Adults, oral, 200 mg/day in single or divided doses, if >40 kg. Children, 5 mg/kg/day in 1–2 divided doses (maximum 150 mg/day).

Available in continental Europe and the USA.

 Further information

Tominack RL, Hayden FG 1987 Rimantadine hydrochloride and amantadine hydrochloride use in influenza A virus infections. *Infectious Disease Clinics of North America* 1: 459–478.

Tominack RL, Wills RJ et al 1988 Multiple dose pharmacokinetics of rimantadine in elderly adults. *Antimicrobial Agents and Chemotherapy* 32: 1813–1819.

INTERFERONS

Interferons are low molecular weight proteins that are produced by mammalian cells in vitro and in vivo in response to viral infection and certain other stimuli. There are three classes.

- Interferon-α, produced by lymphocytes.
- Interferon-β, produced by fibroblasts.
- Interferon-γ, produced by lymphoid cells in response to mitogens.

The interfereons are generally species specific and are now produced by recombinant genetic techniques. Only interferon-α is used in the context of viral disease, where its effectiveness may be due as much to immunomodulatory as antiviral properties.

 INTERFERON-α

Molecular weight: approximately 19 kDa.

A human protein produced by recombinant DNA technology in *Escherichia coli*, formulated for administration by intramuscular, subcutaneous or intralesional injection. A pegylated form, peginterferon, has been developed by attaching a 40-kDa branched chain polyethelene glycol moiety to interferon-α-2a, resulting in a prolonged half-life and better tolerability. Potency is expressed as international units (IU), defined as the amount needed to prevent lysis of 50% of cells by vesicular stomatitis virus in tissue culture assay.

Antiviral activity

Interferon-α renders cells resistant to infection by a wide range of viruses and mediates immunoregulation, inflammation, inhibition of cell multiplication, interaction with mixed histocompatability genes, and differentiation. It has no effect on extracellular virus and does not prevent virus from penetrating cells. It reversibly binds to specific cellular receptors, thereby activating cytoplasmic enzymes affecting messenger RNA translation and protein synthesis; the antiviral state takes several hours to develop but persists for days thereafter. Peginterferon has the same spectrum of activity as interferon-α.

Pharmacokinetics

Oral absorption	Poor
C_{max} 3 × 10⁶ IU intramuscularly	20 IU/ml after 2–4 h
9 × 10⁶ IU intramuscularly	50–100 IU/ml after 2–4 h
Plasma half-life	3–8 h
Peginterferon	36 h
Plasma protein binding	Not known

Interferon-α penetrates the cerebrospinal fluid (CSF) poorly and is not cleared by hemodialysis. Little or none is excreted in the urine, and its fate after release from the cell receptor is largely unknown. The extent of excretion in breast milk is unknown.

Interactions

Human hepatic cytochrome P_{450} systems and oxidative drug metabolism are inhibited, causing a modest prolongation in the half-life of drugs such as theophylline.

Toxicity and side effects

Toxicity has become increasingly apparent with the advent of purer preparations. 'Flu'-like symptoms (fever, arthralgia, myalgia, headache, malaise, chills) occur, which can usually be ameliorated by acetaminophen (paracetamol) administration. Lymphocytopenia is a common side effect, generally arising 2–4 h after administration of several million units. Liver function test values are frequently elevated at doses above 10^7 IU/day. These effects are rapidly reversible and tolerance may develop after several doses. Other toxic effects include gastrointestinal disturbances (anorexia, nausea, diarrhea, vomiting), weight loss, local pain, severe fatigue, alopecia, paresthesias, confusion, dizziness, drowsiness, nervousness and bone marrow suppression. The hematological toxicity is dose dependent (threshold around 3×10^6 IU/day) and reversible. Hypotension may develop during, or up to, 2 days after treatment, and arrhythmias and cardiac failure have been observed.

Administration of excessive doses to pregnant rhesus monkeys in the early to mid-trimester caused abortions. Its effect on human pregnancy is unknown. Neutralizing antibodies have been reported in around a quarter of treated patients but no clinical sequelae to their presence have been documented. Intralesional administration is generally well tolerated.

Peginterferon is associated with the same frequency of side effects as interferon for fatigue, headache, myalgia and fever; most other side effects occur less frequently.

Clinical use

- Chronic hepatitis B.
- Chronic hepatitis C (alone or in combination with ribavirin).
- Condyloma acuminata (intralesional).

It may also be of benefit in hairy cell and chronic myelogenous leukemias and Kaposi's sarcoma.

Preparations and dosage

Proprietary names: Interferon-α, Intron A, Roferon A, Wellferon, Viraferon, Interferon-γIb, Imukin; Pegasys (peginterferon).

Preparation: Injection.

Dosage: Dose varies according to the condition being treated.

Widely available.

Further information

Alexander GJM, Brahm J et al 1987 Loss of HBsAg with interferon therapy in chronic hepatitis B infection. *Lancet* ii: 66–69.

Anonymous 1999 Interferon alfa. In: Dollery C (ed.) *Therapeutic Drugs* 2nd edn. Churchill Livingstone, Edinburgh, pp. 146–152.

Heathcote JC, Shiffman ML, et al 2000 Peginterferon alfa-2a in patients with chronic hepatitis C and cirrhosis *New England Journal of Medicine* 343: 1673–1680.

Zeuzem S, Feinman SV et al 2000. Peginterferon alpha-2a in patients with chronic hepatitis C. *New England Journal of Medicine* 343: 1666–1672.

NEURAMINIDASE INHIBITORS

A new class of antiviral drugs that inhibit influenza A and B replication.

 OSELTAMIVIR

Molecular weight (ethyl ester): 312.

A selective neuraminidase inhibitor, formulated as the phosphate salt of the ethyl ester for oral administration.

Antiviral activity

Oseltamivir inhibits both influenza A and B virus replication by targeting the neuraminidase protein (p. 22). It has no activity against any other virus.

Acquired resistance

Mutations in the neuraminidase have been detected rarely in treated patients. In vitro the emergence of a resistant variant occurs with the substitution of a lysine for the conserved arginine at amino acid 292 of the neuraminidase. Cross-resistance with zanamivir has been described in vitro.

Pharmacokinetics

Oral absorption	c. 75%
C_{max} 75 mg oral	0.35–0.55 mg/l after 4 h
Plasma half-life	7–9 h
Plasma protein binding	Not known

The ethyl ester prodrug is hydrolyzed by hepatic esterases to release the active compound, oseltamivir carboxylate. Drug is excreted in the urine as the carboxylate derivative.

Toxicity and side effects

Adverse events relate to the gastrointestinal tract; the most common is nausea with or without vomiting in 10% of patients. Food alleviates side effects.

Clinical use

- Treatment and prevention of influenza A and B infections.

Preparations and Dosage

Proprietary Name: Tamiflu.

Preparations: 75 mg tablets, capsules.

Dosage: Adults, oral, 75–150 mg/day in 1–2 divided doses. Children >1 year old, 30–75 mg once or twice daily.

Widely available in North America and Europe.

Further information

Hayden FG, Atmar RL et al 1999 Use of the selective oral neuraminidase inhibitor oseltamivir to prevent influenza. *New England Journal of Medicine* 341: 1336–1343.

Treanor JJ, Hayden FG et al 2000 Efficacy and safety of the oral neuraminidase inhibitor oseltamivir in treating acute influenza. *Journal of the American Medical Association* 283: 1016–1024.

Nicholson KG, Aoki FY et al 2000 Treatment of acute influenza: efficacy and safety of the oral neuraminidase inhibitor oseltamivir. *Lancet* 355: 1845–1850.

Whitley RJ, Hayden FG et al 2001 Oral oseltamivir treatment of influenza in children. *Pediatric Infectious Diseases Journal* 20: 12–133.

Welliver R, Monto AS et al 2001 Effectiveness of oseltamivir in preventing influenza in household contacts. *Journal of the American Medical Association* 285: 748–754.

ZANAMIVIR

Molecular weight: 332.

A synthetic neuraminidase inhibitor formulated for administration by inhalation.

Antiviral activity

Zanamivir inhibits both influenza A and influenza B.

Acquired resistance

Resistance is presently uncommon. In clinical trials the frequency was no more than 1% of exposed patients.

Pharmacokinetics

Oral bioavailability is poor. After inhalation local respiratory mucosal concentrations greatly exceed those that are inhibitory for influenza A and B replication. The median concentrations in the sputum exceed 1 mg/l 6 h after inhalation and remain detectable for 24 h.

Toxicity

Most adverse effects are related to the respiratory tree. These include rhinorrhea and, rarely, bronchospasm. Nausea and vomiting have been reported at low incidence.

Clinical use

- Treatment and prevention of influenza A and B infections in patients over 7 years of age.

Preparation and dosage

Proprietary Name: Relenza.

Preparation: Powder for inhalation.

Dosage: Adults, by inhalation, 10 mg twice daily for 5 days.

Available in North America and Europe, including UK.

Further information

Hayden FG, Osterhaus ADME et al 1997 Efficacy and safety of the neuraminidase inhibitor zanamivir in the treatment of influenza virus infections. *New England Journal of Medicine* 337: 874–880.

Hayden, FG, Gubareva LV et al 2000 Inhaled zanamivir for the prevention of influenza in families. *New England Journal of Medicine* 282–1289.

NUCLEOSIDE ANALOGS

Derived from purines or pyrimidines, nucleoside analogs are the mainstay of antiviral chemotherapy. First-generation antiviral drugs such as vidarabine did not use unique virus-induced enzymes. Thus, while clinically effective, the therapeutic index was narrow because of host toxicity. Second-generation antiviral drugs, such as aciclovir, are selectively activated by viral enzymes (*see* p. 21).

ACICLOVIR

Acyclovir; acycloguanosine. Molecular weight (aciclovir): 225; (valaciclovir): 324.

Aciclovir   Valaciclovir

A synthetic acyclic purine nucleoside analog of the natural nucleoside 2′ deoxyguanosine, formulated for oral and topical use, and as the sodium salt for intravenous infusion. Valaciclovir (the L-valyl ester) is a prodrug formulation supplied as the hydrochloride for oral use.

Antiviral activity

Herpes simplex virus (HSV) types 1 and 2, simian herpes virus B and varicella zoster viruses (VZV), which encode thymidine kinase, are all susceptible to concentrations readily attainable in human plasma. The 50% inhibitory concentration (ID_{50}) for HSV-1 and HSV-2 is 0.1 µmol, in contrast to uninfected Vero cells (300 µmol). The concentration required to inhibit HSV-1 and HSV-2 replication by 90 and 99% is approximately 10- and 100-fold greater than that producing 50% inhibition. The ID_{50} for VZV is 3 µmol, while that for uninfected WI 38 cells is >3000 µmol. Valaciclovir is metabolized to aciclovir, and thus has the same antiviral profile.

Because thymidine-kinase-negative HSV mutants and cytomegalovirus (CMV) do not code for thymidine kinase, monophosphorylation of aciclovir cannot occur by this mechanism (see p. 21). Moreover, CMV DNA polymerase is not readily inhibited by aciclovir triphosphate. Although Epstein–Barr virus (EBV) may have reduced thymidine kinase activity, its DNA polymerase is susceptible to aciclovir triphosphate. Accordingly, EBV shows intermediate susceptibility, whereas CMV isolates are generally resistant. Human herpes viruses 6 and 7 are less susceptible than EBV.

There is little or no inhibitory activity against viruses other than those in the herpes group.

Acquired resistance

HSV may become resistant by several different mechanisms. Mutations that involve deficient thymidine kinase or an altered substrate are most common; alterations in the DNA polymerase gene also result in resistance. Resistant mutants may be found in wild virus populations; mutants lacking thymidine kinase activity may be readily induced by passage of HSV in the presence of the drug. Resistant strains have mostly been reported in immunocompromised patients, are generally thymidine-kinase negative, and have decreased virulence. Resistant mutants that retain thymidine kinase activity appear to retain virulence. Emergence of resistant HSV strains is less frequent in immunocompetent patients, occurring in about 2% of those receiving prolonged treatment.

Pharmacokinetics

Oral absorption, aciclovir	c. 20%
valaciclovir	c. 60%
C_{max} 200 mg oral 4-hourly	1.4–4 µmol after 1.5–1.75 h
5 mg/kg 8-hourly intravenous infusion	43.2 µmol steady state
10 mg/kg 8-hourly intravenous infusion	88.9 µmol steady state
Plasma half-life	3–3.3 h
Plasma protein binding	15%

Absorption

Therapeutic drug levels are readily attained after oral or intravenous administration, though concentrations achieved by an oral dose are over 90% lower than those after intravenous therapy. Accumulation of the drug is unlikely in patients without renal dysfunction.

Valaciclovir is readily absorbed and is converted rapidly and almost completely to aciclovir; absorption is unaffected by food. Peak plasma concentrations of 22 µmol are found in subjects after an oral dose of 1000 mg valaciclovir three times daily; systemic exposure is comparable to that of intravenous aciclovir 5 mg/kg every 8 h. The peak plasma concentration and AUC show a less than proportional increase with increasing doses of valaciclovir, presumably due to reduced absorption with increasing doses. The time to peak aciclovir concentration also displays dose dependency, ranging from 0.9 to 1.8 h after single oral doses of 100–1000 mg.

Distribution

Aciclovir is widely distributed in various tissues and body fluids. Delivery of the drug to the basal epidermis after topical administration is about 30–50% of that obtained by oral administration. Aciclovir ointment penetrates the corneal epithelium. CSF concentrations are about 50% of simultaneous plasma concentrations. Vesicular fluid concentrations approximate those in plasma. The drug is actively secreted into breast milk at a concentration several times than in plasma. Placental cord blood contains levels of 69–99% of maternal plasma and the drug is 3–6 times more concentrated in amniotic fluid.

Metabolism

About 15% of an intravenous dose is metabolized in persons with normal renal function. The only significant urinary metabolite is 9-carboxymethoxymethylguanine, which has no antiviral activity. Less than 0.2% of the dose is recovered as the 8-hydroxylation product, 8-hydroxy-9-(2-hydroxymethoxymethyl) guanine.

Excretion

The principal route of elimination is by the kidney; 45–79% of a dose is recovered unchanged, the percentage declining with decreasing creatinine clearance. In patients with renal failure, mean peak plasma concentrations nearly doubled and the elimination half-life increased to 19.5 h. Dosage reductions are advised for various stages of renal impairment. During hemodialysis the half-life is 5.7 h and after dialysis the plasma concentration is about 60% less than the predialysis concentration. Half-lives of 12–17 h have been reported for patients undergoing continuous peritoneal dialysis, with only 13% or less of administered drug being recovered in the 24-h dialysate. The half-life in a patient undergoing arteriovenous hemofiltration/dialysis is about 20 h.

Less than 1% of a dose of valaciclovir is recovered as unchanged drug in the urine. In multidose studies the amount of aciclovir recovered across dose levels ranged from about 40% to 50%. Between 7 and 12% of the dose is found as the 9-carboxymethoxymethylguanine metabolite. Overall, aciclovir accounts for 80–85% of total urinary recovery.

Interactions

Aciclovir does not significantly alter the pharmacokinetics of zidovudine, and high doses (3200 mg/day) do not affect trough cyclosporin levels in renal transplant recipients.

Toxicity and side effects

Few adverse reactions to topical, ocular, oral or intravenous formulations have been reported. Allergic contact dermatitis occasionally occurs with aciclovir cream. Superficial punctate keratopathy is the most common ophthalmic adverse event, occurring in 10% of patients; stinging or burning on application occurs in 4%. Less common complications of the ophthalmic preparation include conjunctivitis, blepharitis and pain.

During early trials, transient increases in blood urea nitrogen and creatinine occurred in 10% of patients given bolus injections. This is analogous to the renal dysfunction seen in experimental animals with deposition of aciclovir crystals in the renal tubules. It can be largely avoided by reducing the rate of infusion, adequate hydration and dosage adjustment in renal failure. Nausea, vomiting, diarrhea and abdominal pain occasionally occur, particularly in association with a raised creatinine concentration. Acute reversible renal failure has been reported. Reconstituted aciclovir has a pH of about 11; severe inflammation and ulceration have been reported after extravasation at the infusion site. Encephalopathy, tremors, confusion, hallucinations, convulsions, psychiatric disorders, bone-marrow depression and abnormal liver function have occasionally arisen. Skin rashes have been reported in a few patients but resolve on discontinuation of the drug.

Headache and nausea have been reported as side effects of valaciclovir, but occurred with similar frequency in subjects taking placebo.

Aciclovir is not embryotoxic or teratogenic to mice or rabbits, despite the presence of substantial concentrations of the drug in amniotic fluid and fetal tissue. However, teratogenicity in rats has been reported. Results of mutagenicity tests in vitro and in vivo indicate that it is unlikely to pose a genetic risk to humans, and the drug was not found to be carcinogenic in long-term studies in mice and rats. The Acyclovir in Pregnancy Registry has followed over 4000 aciclovir-exposed pregnancies with no detectable drug-related effects.

Clinical use

Aciclovir
- Herpes simplex keratitis and lesions of the skin and mucous membranes, including primary genital herpes.
- Varicella zoster infections.
- Herpes simplex encephalitis and neonatal herpes.
- Prophylaxis of HSV infections in the severely immunocompromised.

Valaciclovir
- Herpes zoster and genital HSV infections.

 Preparations and dosage

Proprietary name: Zovirax (aciclovir); Valtrex (valaciclovir).

Preparations: Tablets, suspension, i.v. infusion, cream, eye ointment (aciclovir); tablets (valaciclovir).

Dosage: Adults, children, oral, dose varies according to the condition being treated. I.v. infusion, adults, HSV or VZV, 5 mg/kg every 8 h, doubled in primary and VZV in the immunocompromised and in herpes simplex encephalitis. Children 3 months, 10 mg/kg every 8 h; 3 months to 12 years, 250 mg/m^2 every 8 h; dose doubled in the immunocompromised and HSV encephalitis; for neonatal HSV, 20 mg every 8 h × 21 days.

Valaciclovir: herpes zoster, 1000 mg three times a day for 7 days. Episodic therapy of genital herpes, 500 mg three times a day Suppressive treatment, 500 or 1000 mg/day in two divided doses.

Widely available.

 Further information

Anonymous 1999 Acyclovir. In: Dollery C (ed.) *Therapeutic Drugs* 2nd edn. Churchill Livingstone, Edinburgh, pp. A39–A44.
Balfour HH Jr 1999 Antiviral drugs. *New England Journal of Medicine* 340: 1255–1268.
Grant DM 1987 Acyclovir (Zovirax) ophthalmic ointment: a review of clinical tolerance. *Current Eye Research* 6: 231–235.
Wagstaff AJ, Faulds D, Goa KL 1994 Aciclovir: a reappraisal of its antiviral activity, pharmacokinetic properties and therapeutic efficacy. *Drugs* 47: 153–205.
Whitley R, Gnann J 1992 Acyclovir: A decade later. *New England Journal of Medicine* 327: 782–789.

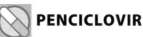 **PENCICLOVIR**

Molecular weight (penciclovir): 253.3; (famciclovir): 321.3.

Famciclovir   Penciclovir

A synthetic acyclic purine nucleoside analog, usually administered orally as the diacetyl ester, famciclovir, which acts as a prodrug undergoing rapid first-pass metabolism to release the active compound in vivo. The parent compound has virtually no oral bioavailability, but is supplied as a topical formulation.

Antiviral activity

Penciclovir is active against members of the herpes virus family, with greatest activity against HSV-1 (ID_{50} 1.6 µmol), somewhat lower activity against HSV-2 (ID_{50} 6.0 µmol), and less activity against VZV (ID_{50} 12 µmol). The ID_{50} values for aciclovir in the same cells were 0.9, 2.7 and 17 µmol, respectively. CMV is relatively resistant and EBV has intermediate susceptibility. The activity of hepatitis B virus is inhibited in vitro.

In cells infected with HSV-1, HSV-2 and VZV, it is monophosphorylated by virus-encoded thymidine kinase, phosphorylation proceeding more efficiently than that of aciclovir in herpes-infected cells. Conversion to the triphosphate is then accomplished by cellular enzymes. Although it has less affinity for viral DNA polymerases than aciclovir triphosphate, and does not act as a DNA chain terminator, it has a much longer half-life.

Acquired resistance

Penciclovir is inactive against thymidine kinase-deficient strains of HSV. Foscarnet-resistant HSV isolates appear to retain sensitivity to both penciclovir and aciclovir.

Pharmacokinetics

Oral absorption: penciclovir	5%
famciclovir	77%
C_{max} famciclovir 250 mg oral	1.6 mg/l after 0.5–1.5 h
famciclovir 500 mg oral	3.3 mg/l after 0.5–1.5 h
famciclovir 750 mg oral	5.1 mg/l after 0.5–1.5 h
Plasma half-life	2.1–2.7 h
Volume of distribution	c. 1.5 l/kg
Plasma protein binding	<20%

Following absorption famciclovir is converted rapidly by enzyme-mediated deacetylation and oxidation to the active antiviral metabolite, penciclovir, since little unchanged drug is detected in plasma. Food does not lead to any significant change in the availability or elimination.

The pharmacokinetics in elderly subjects are similar to those seen in younger subjects, although small increases in AUC and plasma half-lives were seen, consistent with slightly decreased renal clearance.

Renal excretion is the major route of elimination; 50.9, 56.5, 59.9 and 60.4% of oral doses of 125, 250, 500 and 750 mg, respectively, were recovered in the urine. Following intravenous infusion, approximately 70% is excreted unchanged in the urine. After oral administration of famciclovir, penciclovir accounts for 82% of urinary drug-related material. The remainder includes metabolites, of which the largest is the 6-deoxy precursor of penciclovir. Renal clearance exceeds glomerular filtration, indicating renal tubular secretion.

Interactions

Famciclovir has the potential for interactions with drugs that are metabolized by hepatic enzymes; no evidence exists for clinically significant pharmacokinetic interactions with allopurinol, cimetidine, theophylline, digoxin or zidovudine.

Toxicity and side effects

In clinical trials the incidence of adverse events after famciclovir, aciclovir and placebo were similar, the most common adverse events being headache and nausea.

Clinical use

- Herpes zoster and genital herpes.
- Orolabial herpes (topical).

Preparations and dosage

Proprietary name: Famvir, Denavir, Vectavir.

Preparations: Tablets and topical cream.

Dosage: Adults, oral, 125–500 mg three or four times daily for 7 days for HSV and VZV infections. Topical, four times a day.

Widely available.

Further information

Anonymous 1999 Famciclovir. In: Dollery C (ed.) *Therapeutic Drugs* 2nd edn. Churchill Livingstone, Edinburgh, pp. F9–F14.

Boyd MR, Bacon TH, Sutton D, Cole M 1987 Antiherpes activity of 9-(4-hydroxy-3-hydroxymethylbut-I-yl) guanine (BRL 39123) in cell culture. *Antimicrobial Agents and Chemotherapy* 31: 1238–1242.

Hodge RAV 1993 Famciclovir and penciclovir. The mode of action of famciclovir including its conversion to penciclovir. *Antiviral Chemistry and Chemotherapy* 4: 67–84.

Pue MA, Benet LZ 1993 Pharmacokinetics of famciclovir in man. *Antiviral Chemistry and Chemotherapy* 4(Suppl. 1): 47–55.

GANCICLOVIR

Molecular weight: (free acid): 255; (sodium salt): 277; (val-ganciclovir): 354.

A synthetic 2′-deoxyguanosine nucleoside analog, supplied for oral administration and as the sodium salt for parenteral use. A slow-release ocular implant device is also available. Valganciclovir is the L-valine ester and is rapidly converted to ganciclovir after oral administration.

Antiviral activity

Ganciclovir is phosphorylated to the monophosphate by a cellular deoxyguanosine kinase more rapidly in infected than uninfected cells. HSV and VZV thymidine kinases monophosphorylate ganciclovir, after which it is further metabolized to the active triphosphate by cellular enzymes. The UL97 open-reading frame of CMV encodes a phosphonotransferase, which can regulate phosphorylation. In CMV-infected cells the concentration of the triphosphate is approximately 10-fold higher than in uninfected cells.

HSV-1 and HSV-2 are inhibited by 0.2–8.0 μmol (0.05–2.0 mg/l). Its activity is similar to that of acyclovir against HSV-1 in vitro, but is slightly superior against HSV-2. The ID_{50} for CMV ranges from 0.5 to 11 μmol (0.125–2.75 mg/l). EBV is inhibited by 1–4 μmol and VZV by 4–40 μmol.

Acquired resistance

The use of prolonged repeated courses leads to the selection of resistant strains, occurring in 8% of patients receiving the drug for >3 months. Studies of laboratory-derived resistant strains indicate that drug resistance can result from alterations in the phosphonotransferase encoded by the gene region UL 27, the viral DNA polymerase (gene region UL 54), or both.

Pharmacokinetics

Oral absorption: ganciclovir	5.4–7.1%
valganciclovir	80%
C_{max} 5 mg/kg 1 h infusion	33.2 μmol end infusion
Plasma half-life (intravenous infusion)	2.9 h
Volume of distribution	c. 1.17 l/kg
Plasma protein binding	1–2%

Absorption

After an intravenous infusion of 5 mg/kg, the plasma level after 11 h was 2.2 μmol. After repeated 5 mg/kg doses every 8 h, the mean peak serum levels were 25 μmol and mean trough levels 3.6 μmol. Thus, when the drug is administered at a dose of 5 mg/kg, levels in plasma are in excess or in the same range as the CMV ID_{50}. In patients treated for 8–22 days with 1 or 2.5 mg/kg every 8 h, the mean steady-state plasma concentrations after a 1 h infusion of 1 mg/kg ranged from 7.2 μmol immediately after infusion to 0.8 μmol after 8 h. Corresponding values after a dose of 2.5 mg/kg were 19.6 and 3.2 μmol, respectively.

Multiple dosing with oral ganciclovir 1000 mg three times daily resulted in peak levels of 1.13 mg/l (4.3 μmol) and a trough of 0.52 mg/l (2.1 μmol). The poor oral bioavailability led to the development of valganciclovir, which is rapidly converted to ganciclovir in a fashion similar to valaciclovir. Resulting plasma levels are similar to those achieved with 5 mg/kg every 12 h.

Distribution

There are only limited data on distribution. The levels of the drug in CSF are estimated to be 24–67% of those in plasma. Mean intravitreal levels of 14 μmol were reported for samples taken a mean of 12 h after therapy with a mean dose of 6 mg/kg daily. However, no significant correlations are noted between time after the last dose and intravitreal concentration. The observed mean value in the eye is below the concentration required to achieve 50% or 90% inhibition of CMV plaque formation by clinical isolates, which may explain the difficulty in controlling CMV retinitis.

Metabolism and excretion

About 80% of the drug is eliminated unchanged in the urine within 24 h. Probenecid, as well as other drugs that impact renal tubular secretion or absorption, may reduce its renal clearance. In severe renal impairment, the mean plasma half-life is 28.3 h. Dosage must be reduced in patients with impaired renal function. Plasma levels of the drug can be reduced by approximately 50–90% with hemodialysis. The half-life on dialysis is about 4 h. Patients undergoing dialysis should be given 1.25 mg/kg daily; therapy should also be administered after dialysis.

No significant pharmacokinetic interaction occurs when ganciclovir and foscarnet are given as concomitant or daily alternate therapy.

Toxicity and side effects

The IC_{50} for human bone marrow colony-forming cells is 39 (± 73) μmol; for other cell lines it ranges from 110 to 2900 μmol. Toxicity frequently limits therapy. Marrow suppression may develop on as little as 5 mg/kg on alternate days and is exacerbated when the drug is given with zidovudine. Neutropenia of <1000/mm³ occurs in nearly 40% of recipients and <500/mm³ in upwards of 30% for those given induction therapy of 10 mg/kg daily for 14 days, followed by 5 mg/kg daily. Neutropenia is reversible and develops during the early treatment or maintenance phase, but may occur later. Thrombocytopenia of <20 000/mm³ and <50 000/mm³ develops in about 10% and 19% of patients, respectively. Frequent monitoring of the full blood count is recommended.

Adverse effects on the CNS, including confusion, convulsions, psychosis, hallucinations, tremor, ataxia, coma, dizziness, headaches and somnolence, occur in around 5% of patients. Liver function abnormalities, fever and rash occur in about 2%. Intraocular injection of ganciclovir is associated with intense pain, and occasionally amaurosis lasting for 1–10 min.

Animal studies indicate that inhibition of spermatogenesis and suppression of female fertility occurs. Ganciclovir is also potentially embryolethal, mutagenic and teratogenic and is contraindicated during pregnancy or lactation. It can cause local tissue damage and should not be administered intramuscularly or subcutaneously; patients should be adequately hydrated during treatment.

Clinical use

- Life- or sight-threatening CMV infections in immunocompromised individuals.
- Prevention of CMV disease in patients receiving immunosuppressive therapy for organ transplantation.

An ocular implant has been developed for the treatment of CMV retinitis.

Preparations and dosage

Proprietary name: Cytovene, Cymevene, Vitrasert (ocular implant), Valcyte (valganciclovir).

Preparations: Capsules, i.v. infusion, ophthalmic solution (ganciclovir); tablets (valganciclovir).

Dosage: Adults, i.v., treatment, 5 mg/kg every 12 h for 14–21 days. Maintenance dose, i.v., 6 mg/kg daily on 5 days per week *or* 5 mg/kg once every day. Oral, 1 g three times daily or 500 mg six times daily, following at least 3 weeks i.v. therapy.

Valganciclovir: 900 mg twice daily.

Widely available.

Further information

Anonymous 1999 Ganciclovir (sodium). In: Dollery C (ed.) *Therapeutic Drugs* 2nd edn. Churchill Livingstone, Edinburgh, pp. G16–G22.

Chow S, Erice A, Jordan MC et al 1995 Analysis of the UL97 phosphonotransferase coding sequence in clinical cytomegalovirus isolates and identification of mutations conferring ganciclovir resistance. *Journal of Infectious Diseases* 171: 576–583.

Crumpacker C 1996 Ganciclovir. *New England Journal of Medicine* 335: 721–728.

Cymeval RO 1999 Valganciclovir. *Drugs* 5: 318–319.

Drew WL, Miner RC et al 1991 Prevalence of resistance in patients receiving ganciclovir for serious cytomegalovirus infection. *Journal of Infectious Diseases* 163: 716–719.

Kupperman BD, Quiceno JI et al 1993 Intravitreal ganciclovir concentration after intravenous administration in AIDS patients with cytomegalovirus retinitis. *Journal of Infectious Diseases* 168: 1506–1509.

Lake KD, Fletcher CV et al 1988 Ganciclovir pharmacokinetics during renal impairment. *Antimicrobial Agents and Chemotherapy* 32: 1899–1900.

Littler E, Stuart E, Chee MS 1992 Human cytomegalovirus UL97 open reading frame encodes a protein that phosphorylates the antiviral analogue ganciclovir. *Nature* 358: 160–162.

Pescovitz MD, Rabkin J et al 2000 Valganciclovir results in improved oral absorption of ganciclovir in liver transplant recipients. *Antimicrobial Agents and Chemotherapy* 44: 2811–2815.

Sommadossi J-P, Bevan R et al 1988 Clinical pharmacokinetics of ganciclovir in patients with normal and impaired renal function. *Reviews in Infectious Diseases* 10: S507–S514.

RIBAVIRIN

Tribavirin. Molecular weight: 244.2.

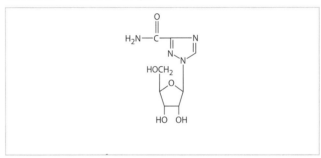

A synthetic nucleoside consisting of D-ribose attached to a 1,2,4-triazole carboxamide. It is neither a classic pyrimidine nor a purine, but stereochemical studies indicate that it is a guanosine analog. It is usually formulated for administration by inhalation, but oral and intravenous preparations are also used.

Antiviral activity

Ribavirin is phosphorylated in cells and inhibits inosine monophosphate dehydrogenase, which is involved in the synthesis of guanosine triphosphate. Decrease in intracellular thymidine triphosphate has also been noted. In most cell lines in which antiviral testing has been performed, the antiviral activity is distinct from the cytostatic dose, which ranges from 200 to 1000 mg/l.

In-vitro and in-vivo laboratory tests indicate that the herpes viruses are the most sensitive. Of the RNA viruses, activity has been noted with influenza types A and B; parainfluenza virus types 1, 2 and 3; mumps, measles and respiratory syncytial virus (RSV); Lassa fever and Machupo viruses; Rift Valley fever, sandfly fever, Hantaan and yellow fever viruses. RSV plaques are reduced 85–98% by 16 mg/l.

Ribavirin and interferon-α, particularly the pegylated forms, act synergistically in the treatment of chronic hepatitis C virus (HCV) infection, resulting in sustained reduction in alanine aminotransferase levels and loss of HCV RNA in 40% of patients who failed to respond to interferon previously.

Acquired resistance

In contrast to other antivirals, development of resistant virus strains has not been demonstrated with ribavirin.

Pharmacokinetics

Oral absorption	36–46%
C_{max} 3 mg/kg oral	4.1–8.2 µmol/l after 1–1.5 h
600 mg intravenous	43.6 µmol/l end infusion
Plasma half-life	c. 24 h
Volume of distribution	647 l
Plasma protein binding	<10%

Absorption

Drug is rapidly absorbed after oral administration. Mean peak concentrations after 1 week of oral doses of 200, 400 and 800 mg every 8 h were 5.0, 11.1 and 20.9 µmol/l, respectively. Trough levels 9–12 h after the final dose after 2 weeks' therapy were 5.1, 13.2 and 18.4 µmol/l, respectively, indicating continued accumulation of the drug. Drug was still detectable 4 weeks after discontinuation of oral dosing. Mean peak plasma concentrations after intravenous doses of 600, 1200 and 2400 mg were 43.6, 72.3 and 160.8 µmol/l, respectively; at 8 h the mean plasma concentrations were 2.1, 5.6 and 10.2 µmol/l.

Aerosolized ribavirin (6 g in 300 ml distilled water) has generally been administered at a rate of 12–15 ml/h using a Collison jet nebulizer, the estimated dosage being 1.8 mg/kg per h for infants and 0.9 mg/kg per h for adults. When administered by small particle aerosol for 2.5–8 h, plasma concentrations ranged from 0.44 to 8.7 µmol/l.

Metabolism and excretion

Ribavirin is rapidly degraded by deribosylation or amide hydrolysis, and together with its metabolites is slowly eliminated by the kidney. About 50% of the drug or its metabolites appears in the urine within 72 h and 15% excreted in the stools. The remainder seems to be retained in body tissues, principally in red blood cells, which concentrate the drug or metabolites to a peak at 4 days, the half-life in red cells being approximately 40 days. After intravenous administration 19.4% of the dose was eliminated during the first 24 h (compared with 7.3% after an oral dose), the difference reflecting the bioavailability.

Toxicity

Ribavirin is generally well tolerated, though adverse reactions appear to be related to dose and duration of therapy. Minor adverse reactions include metallic taste, dry mouth sensation and increased thirst, flatulence, fatigue and CNS complaints, including headache, irritability and insomnia. Daily doses of 1 g may cause unconjugated bilirubin levels to double and the reticulocyte count to increase. Hemoglobin concentrations may decrease with prolonged treatment or higher dosages; with doses of 3.9–12.6 g/day, a drop in hemoglobin was noted by day 7–13 of treatment, which was generally 'rapidly' reversible on withdrawal of the drug but in some instances necessitated blood transfusion.

Aerosol administration of about 2 g in 36 or 39 h during 3 days is well tolerated, does not affect results of pulmonary function tests, and seems non-toxic.

Ribavirin is both teratogenic and embryotoxic in laboratory animals, so precautions must be observed in women of child-bearing age.

Clinical use

- RSV infections in infants (by nebulizer).
- Lassa fever.
- Hepatitis C (in combination with interferon-α).

Use in treatment of RSV pneumonia in infants is no longer routine. Ribavirin has been shown to reduce mortality from Hantaan virus, the agent responsible for the hemorrhagic fever with renal syndrome.

 Preparations and dosage

Proprietary name: Virazid; Virazole.

Preparation: Inhalation, capsules or intravenous.

Dosage: By aerosol inhalation or nebulization (via small-particle aerosol generator) of solution containing 20 mg/ml for 12–18 h per day for at least 3 days and a maximum of 7 days. Adults, oral, <65 kg, 400 mg twice daily; 65–85 kg, 400 mg in the morning and 600 mg at night; >85 kg, 600 mg twice daily.

Widely available.

 Further information

Anonymous 1999 Ribavirin. In: Dollery C (ed.) *Therapeutic Drugs* 2nd edn. Churchill Livingstone, Edinburgh, pp. R20–R23.

Brillanti S, Garson J et al 1994 A pilot study of combination therapy with ribavirin plus interferon alpha for interferon alpha resistant chronic hepatitis C. *Gastroenterology* 107: 812–817.

Patterson JL, Fernandez-Larsson R 1990 Molecular mechanisms of action of ribavirin. *Reviews of Infectious Diseases* 12: 1139–1146.

Reichard O, Andersson J et al 1991 Ribavirin treatment for chronic hepatitis C. *Lancet* 337: 1058–1061.

OTHER NUCLEOSIDE ANALOGS

Idoxuridine

A synthetic halogenated pyrimidine analog originally synthesized as an anticancer agent. Formulated in dimethylsulfoxide for topical application and as a solution for ophthalmic use.

Activity is largely limited to DNA viruses, primarily HSV-1, HSV-2 and VZV. HSV-1 plaque formation in BHK 21 cells is sensitive to 6.25–25 mg/l; type 2 microplaques required 62.5–125 mg/l. RNA viruses are not affected, with the exception of oncogenic RNA viruses such as Rous sarcoma virus. Drug resistance is easily generated in vitro, and may be an obstacle to treatment. However, there is little or no cross-resistance with newer nucleoside analogs.

Idoxuridine is poorly soluble in water, and aqueous solutions are ineffective against infections other than those localized to the eye. In animals, therapeutic levels are achieved in the cornea within 30 min of ophthalmic application and persist for 4 h. Penetration is otherwise poor, with only the biologically inactive dehalogenated metabolite uracil entering the eye.

The drug is too toxic for systemic administration. Contact dermatitis, punctate epithelial keratopathy, follicular conjunctivitis, ptosis, stenosis and occlusion of the puncta and keratinization of the lid margins occur in up to 14% of those receiving ophthalmic preparations.

Clinical use

- Cutaneous herpes.
- Herpes keratitis.

It has largely been superseded by trifluridine or aciclovir.

Preparations and dosage

Proprietary names: Idoxene, Herpid, Iduridin, Virudox.

Preparations: Topical, ophthalmic.

Dosage: Apply to involved eye four times daily for 14 days. Paint on topical lesions four times daily for 4 days.

Widely available.

Further information

Anonymous 1999 Idoxuridine. In Dollery C (ed.) *Therapeutic Drugs* 2nd edn. Churchill Livingstone, Edinburgh, pp. I13–I15.

Lamivudine

An antiretroviral agent that also exhibits activity against hepatitis B virus and duck hepatitis B virus. Its properties are described in Ch. 39 (p. 476). A mutation at the MYDD locus of hepatitis B reverse transcriptase conveys resistance.

Clinical use

- Therapy of chronic hepatitis B.

Use is limited by the development of resistance within 1 year in up to 25% of treated patients. It is likely to be used with other drugs in the future.

Preparations and dosage

Proprietary name: Epivir.

Preparation: 100 mg tablets, oral solution.

Dosage: Adults, oral, 150 mg twice daily. Children 3 months to 12 years, 4 mg/kg twice daily (maximum 300 mg/day).

Widely available.

Further information

Lai CL, Chien RN, Leung NW et al 1998 A one-year trial of lamivudine for chronic hepatitis B. Asia hepatitis lamivudine study group. *New England Journal of Medicine* 339: 61–68.
Dusheiko G 1999 A pill a day, or two, for hepatitis B? *Lancet* 353: 1032–1023.
Grellier L, Mutimer D, Ahmed M et al 1996 Lamivudine prophylaxis against reinfection in liver transplantation for hepatitis B cirrhosis. *Lancet* 348: 1212–1215.

Trifluridine

Trifluorothymidine. A synthetic halogenated pyrimidine nucleoside, first synthesized in the early 1960s as an antitumor agent. It inhibits enzymes of the DNA pathway and is incorporated into both cellular and progeny viral DNA, causing faulty transcription of late messenger RNA and the production of incompetent virion protein. It does not require a viral thymidine kinase for phosphorylation to the monophosphate derivative and therefore is far less selective and more toxic than other analogs. It is active against HSV-1 and HSV-2, vaccinia virus, CMV and possibly adenovirus. When applied as a 1% ophthalmic solution, it rapidly enters the aqueous humor of HSV-infected rabbits' eyes but is cleared within 60–90 min.

Trifluridine causes sister chromatid exchange – an indicator of mutagenicity – at 0.5 mg/l in human lymphocytes and fibroblasts. It is teratogenic to chick embryos when injected directly into the yolk sac and its principal adverse effects in humans following systemic administration include leukopenia, anemia, fever and hypocalcemia. Accordingly, it is restricted to topical ophthalmic use. The ophthalmic 1% aqueous solution produces occasional punctate lesions; other side effects are similar to those of idoxuridine and vidarabine but arise less frequently.

Clinical use

- HSV ocular infections.

Preparations and dosage

Proprietary name: Viroptic.

Preparation: Ophthalmic drops.

Limited availability, including the USA.

Further information

Heidelberger C 1979 Trifluorothymidine. *Pharmacology and Therapeutics* 6: 427–442.

Weller S, Blum MR et al 1993 Pharmacokinetics of the acyclovir prodrug valaciclovir after escalating single- and multiple-dose administration to normal volunteers. *Clinical Pharmacology and Therapeutics* 54: 595–605.

Vidarabine

Adenine arabinoside; a purine nucleoside analog, originally synthesized in 1960 as an anti-cancer drug. Its antiviral spectrum includes all the herpesviruses and several poxviruses (vaccinia and myxoma). Polyoma and adenoviruses are only slightly sensitive. Among RNA viruses, it is active against Rous sarcoma virus, murine leukemia virus, rabies virus and vesicular stomatitis virus. It also inhibits hepatitis B DNA polymerase.

Vidarabine is rapidly metabolized to arabinosyl-hypoxanthine, a metabolite that posses antiviral activity. While originally licensed as both a topical ophthalmic and intravenous formulation, it is now available only in the ophthalmic form. When applied topically to the eye it does not penetrate; the metabolite can sometimes be found in the aqueous humor, but not at effective concentrations.

The ophthalmic preparation may cause lacrimation, foreign-body sensation, burning, irritation, superficial punctate keratitis, pain, photophobia, punctal occlusion and sensitivity.

Clinical use

- Herpes keratoconjunctivitis.

Preparations and dosage

Proprietary name: Vidarabine.

Preparations: Ophthalmic ointment.

Limited availability. Available in the USA.

Further information

Anonymous 1999 Vidarabine (monohydrate). In Dollery C (ed.) *Therapeutic Drugs* 2nd edn. Churchill Livingstone, Edinburgh, pp. V28–V31.

Whitley R, Alford C, Hess F, Buchanan R 1980 Vidarabine: a preliminary review of its pharmacological properties and therapeutic use. *Drugs* 20: 267–282.

NUCLEOTIDE ANALOGS

A new class of antiviral compounds that is receiving increased attention. The class includes cidofovir, adefovir, and tenofovir (which has antiretroviral activity and is described on p. 485). None of these drugs is metabolized by the host. They are phosphorylated intracellularly to the active metabolite, a diphosphate derivative that has antiviral activity. Because these drugs are non-specifically activated, the risk of toxicity is increased.

CIDOFOVIR

Molecular weight: 279.

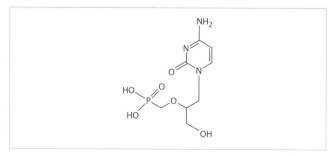

An acyclic cytosine analog containing a phosphonate group enabling it to mimic a nucleotide and bypass initial virus-dependent phosphorylation. Administered by intravenous infusion.

Antiviral activity

Cellular enzymes are responsible for serial conversion to the diphosphate and triphosphate, which is the active intracellular compound. Cidovir has in vitro and in vivo activity against CMV and other herpesviruses, including aciclovir-resistant HSV. Oral hairy leukoplakia resolved on therapy, suggesting that it has activity against EBV. It is also reported to have activity against adenovirus and papillomaviruses.

Resistance

Resistance can be generated in the laboratory but has not yet been encountered during treatment of patients.

Pharmacokinetics

Oral absorption	<5%
C_{max} 3 mg/kg intravenous infusion	7.7 mg/l end infusion
10 mg/kg intravenous infusion	23 mg/l end infusion
Plasma half-life	c. 3–4 h
Volume of distribution	c. 0.6 l/kg
Plasma protein binding	<6%

The intracellular half-life of the diphosphate is 17–65 h.

It is excreted unchanged by the kidney by glomerular filtration and tubular secretion.

Toxicity and side effects

Nephrotoxicity is the dose-limiting adverse effect; it was heralded by proteinuria and occurred at weekly doses of

≥3 mg/kg in two of five patients after 6 and 14 consecutive weeks of therapy. Two of five patients given 10 mg/kg developed nephrotoxicity after only two doses, which manifested as a Fanconi-like syndrome with proteinuria, glucosuria, bicarbonaturia, phosphaturia, polyuria and increased creatinine. Biopsy revealed proximal tubular effects. Prehydration and extended dosing intervals seems to be nephroprotective.

Clinical use

- Treatment of CMV retinitis.

Because of nephrotoxicity it is a drug of last resort. Cidofovir has been used experimentally in the treatment of adenovirus pneumonia and BK virus in transplant patients and juvenile laryngeal papillomatosis.

 Preparations and dosage

Proprietary Name: Vistide.

Preparation: Injection.

Dosage: Induction: adults, i.v., 5 mg/kg with hydration and probenecid once weekly for 2 weeks; then every other week.

Available in USA and Europe, including UK.

 Further information

Lalezari JP, Drew WL, Glutzer E et al 1995 (S)-1-[3-Hydroxy-2-(phosphonyl-methoxy)propyl]cytosine (Cidofir): results of a phase I/II study of a novel antiviral nucleotide analog. *Journal of Infectious Diseases* 171: 788–796.

OLIGONUCLEOTIDES

Short nucleotides with sequences of bases that mirror regions of mRNA and prevent translation of the RNA into protein.

 FOMIVIRSEN

Molecular weight: 6682.

An antisense oligonucleotide, 21 bases in length, representing the mirror image of a region of mRNA coding for a regulatory protein of CMV. It is administered as the sodium salt by intraocular injection. Experiments in monkeys suggest that it has a very long elimination half-life (c. 3 days). Because of its unique mode of action fomivirsen retains activity against strains of CMV resistant to other antiviral agents.

Side effects commonly include ocular inflammation, which is responsive to topical steroids, and raised intraocular pressure.

Clinical use

- CMV retinitis in AIDS patients intolerant of, or unresponsive to, other treatments.

 Preparations and dosage

Proprietary name: Vitravene.

Preparation: Injection.

Dosage: 0.33 mg intravitreal injection fortnightly for two doses, then every 4 weeks (half this dose for previously untreated patients).

Limited availability. Available in the USA and UK.

 Further information

Perry CM, Balfour JA 1999 Fomivirsen. *Drugs* 57: 375–380.

PHOSPHONIC ACIDS

This group includes the two aliphatic compounds phosphonoformic acid (foscarnet) and phosphonoacetic acid. Phosphonoacetate forms a six-ring chelate with metal ions and similar five-ring chelates would be expected for phosphonoformate. It is probable that this chelating activity is responsible for the effect of these agents on a wide range of polymerases and nucleases. Only phosphonoformic acid has been licensed for clinical use.

 FOSCARNET

Phosphonoformic acid; trisodium phosphonoformate. Molecular weight (anhydrous): 192; (trisodium salt): 300.1.

$$\begin{array}{c} \text{NaO} \\ \\ \text{NaO} \end{array} \!\! P \!\! \begin{array}{c} \text{O} \\ \| \\ \end{array} \!\! - \text{COONa}$$

A synthetic non-nucleoside pyrophosphate analog formulated as the trisodium hexahydrate for intravenous use. The solubility in water at pH 7 is only about 5% (w/w).

Antiviral activity

Foscarnet inhibits the RNA polymerase of influenza A virus, the DNA polymerases of HSV-1 and HSV-2, CMV, EBV, VZV and HBV more efficiently than host-cell DNA polymerases. Concentrations of 6–55 μmol are required to inhibit CMV plaque formation by 50%, but clinical isolates are generally 1.5–8 times less sensitive. In-vitro inhibition of CMV replication is reversed by withdrawal of the drug. Most strains of HSV that are resistant to aciclovir are susceptible. However, when treatment is discontinued, relapse is frequent. Foscarnet acts as a non-competitive inhibitor for substrates and templates of HIV reverse transcriptase in concentrations ranging from 0.1 to 5.0 µmol, but 680 µmol was required to block replication of the virus in H9 cell cultures.

Acquired resistance

Resistance has been generated in vitro, and CMV strains that are resistant to both ganciclovir and foscarnet have occasionally been recovered from humans.

Pharmacokinetics

Oral absorption	c. 17%
C_{max} 60 mg/kg intravenous 8-hourly	557 µmol/l
Plasma half-life	3.3–6.8 h
Volume of distribution	0.52–0.74 l/kg
Plasma protein binding	14–17%

Absorption and distribution

Oral bioavailability is poor. A wide range of plasma concentrations was noted (75–500 µmol/l) during 3–21 days of continuous intravenous infusion of 0.14–0.19 mg/kg per min. During continuous intravenous therapy the concentrations reached a plateau on day 3. Considerable differences in steady-state plasma concentrations exist between individuals. Drug penetrates the CSF; the mean concentration is about 40–60% of the mean plasma concentration, depending upon dose.

Metabolism and excretion

Elimination appears to be triphasic, with two initially short half-lives of 0.5–1.4 h and 3.3–6.8 h, followed by a long terminal phase of 88 h. About 88% of the cumulative intravenous dose is recovered unchanged in the urine within a week of stopping an infusion, indicating that the drug is not metabolized to any significant extent. Non-renal clearance accounts for 14–18% of total clearance and is believed to relate to uptake into bone. Plasma clearance decreases markedly with decreased renal function and the elimination half-life may be increased by up to 10-fold. Conventional dialysis will eliminate about 25% of a dose while high-flux dialysis can remove nearly 60%.

Interactions

Concomitant foscarnet and zidovudine therapy does not affect the pharmacokinetics of either drug. No significant pharmacokinetic interaction occurs when ganciclovir and foscarnet are given as concomitant or daily alternating therapy.

In view of its nephrotoxicity, coadministration with potentially nephrotoxic drugs (e.g. aminoglycosides, amphotericin B, pentamidine, and cyclosporin) should be avoided.

Toxicity and side effects

Treatment is more frequently limited by toxicity than with ganciclovir. Renal toxicity is the most common dose-limiting adverse event. A two- to three-fold increase in serum creatinine levels occurs in 20–60% (mean 45%) of patients given 130–230 mg/kg daily as a continuous intravenous infusion. Renal impairment usually develops within the first few weeks of treatment and is generally reversible within several weeks of discontinuing therapy. Foscarnet chelates metal ions, and serum electrolyte abnormalities, predominantly hypocalcemia, hypomagnesemia, hypokalemia and hypophosphatemia are common, occurring in about 30, 15, 16 and 8% of patients, respectively. Convulsions occur in 10–15%. Other side effects include anemia (25–50%), penile or vulval ulceration (3–9%), nausea and vomiting (20–30%), local irritation and thrombophlebitis at the infusion site, abdominal pain and occasional pancreatitis, headache (c. 25%), dizziness, involuntary muscle contractions, tremor, hypoesthesia, ataxia, neuropathy, anxiety, nervousness, depression and confusion, and skin rash. Nephrogenic diabetes insipidus has been reported.

Foscarnet is contraindicated in pregnancy. Topical application does not result in dermal toxicity similar to that produced by phosphonacetic acid.

Clinical use

- Treatment of CMV retinitis in patients for whom ganciclovir is contraindicated, inappropriate or ineffective.

It is also potentially of value in the treatment of aciclovir-resistant HSV infection.

Preparations and dosage

Proprietary name: Foscavir.

Preparation: Injection.

Dosage: Adults, i.v., 60 mg/kg every 8 h for 2–3 weeks, then 60 mg/kg/day increasing to 90–120 mg/kg/day if tolerated.

Widely available.

Further information

Anonymous 1999 Foscarnet (sodium). In: Dollery C (ed.) *Therapeutic Drugs* 2nd edn. Churchill Livingstone, Edinburgh, pp. F158–F161.

Aweeka F, Gambertoglio JG et al 1995 Foscarnet and ganciclovir pharmacokinetics during concomitant or alternating maintenance therapy for AIDS-related cytomegalovirus retinitis. *Clinical Pharmacology and Therapeutics* 57: 403–412.

Hengge UR, Brockmeyer NH et al 1993 Foscarnet penetrates the blood–brain barrier: rationale for therapy of cytomegalovirus encephalitis. *Antimicrobial Agents and Chemotherapy* 37: 1010–1014.

Jacobson MA, Causey D et al 1993 A dose ranging study of daily maintenance intravenous foscarnet therapy for cytomegalovirus retinitis in AIDS. *Journal of Infectious Diseases* 168: 444–448.

Safrin S, Crumpacker C et al 1991 A controlled trial comparing foscarnet with vidarabine for acyclovir-resistant mucocutaneous herpes simplex in the acquired immunodeficiency syndrome. *New England Journal of Medicine* 325: 551–555.

Sjövall J, Karlsson A et al 1988 Pharmacokinetics and absorption of foscarnet after intravenous and oral administration to patients with human immunodeficiency virus. *Clinical Pharmacology and Therapeutics* 44: 65–73.

Sjövall J, Bergdahl S et al 1989 Pharmacokinetics of foscarnet and distribution to cerebrospinal fluid after intravenous infusion in patients with human immunodeficiency virus infection. *Antimicrobial Agents and Chemotherapy* 33: 1023–1031.

Studies of Ocular Complications of AIDS Research Group, in collaboration with the AIDS Clinical Trials Group 1995 Morbidity and toxic effects associated with ganciclovir or foscarnet therapy in a randomised cytomegalovirus retinitis trial. *Archives of Internal Medicine* 155: 65–73.

Tatrowicz WA, Lurain NS, Thompson KD 1992 A ganciclovir resistant clinical isolate of human cytomegalovirus exhibiting cross-resistance to other DNA polymerase inhibitors. *Journal of Infectious Diseases* 166: 904–907.

Wagstaff AJ, Bryson HM 1994 Foscarnet. A reappraisal of its antiviral activity, pharmacokinetic properties and therapeutic use in immunocompromised patients with viral infections. *Drugs* 48: 199–226.

OTHER ANTIVIRAL COMPOUNDS

Several novel antiviral compounds that are approved for use or being considered for licensure in various countries of the world warrant brief note.

Docosanol

A 22-carbon straight chain alcohol licensed for over-the-counter sales for the topical treatment of herpes labialis. It is thought to act by blocking viral fusion with the host cell, although definitive studies are lacking. The clinical relevance of the antiviral activity has been debated and the place of this medication as a treatment of herpes labialis remains to be established.

Imiquimod

An imidazoquinoline used for the treatment of genital and perianal warts. While the mechanism of action is not precisely known, it is thought to induce interferon. It has no direct antiviral activity. The 5% cream applied three times a week for up to 16 weeks resulted in total wart clearance in 50% of patients, with a better response in women than in men. Local reactions are common and include erythema, erosion, excoriation and edema.

Pleconaril

An oxadiazole that is active against most enteroviruses and rhinoviruses. It binds to the hydrophobic pocket of the virus capsid protein VP1, inducing conformational changes that lead to altered receptor binding and viral uncoating. It is currently being assessed for the treatment of rhinovirus infections in Phase III trials. The regulatory applications demonstrate antiviral activity for rhinovirus colds and chronic enterovirus infections of the CNS in patients with agammaglobulinemia.

Adefovir dipivoxil

The orally bioavailable prodrug of the nucleotide analog adefovir. It is active against both herpes and hepadnaviruses. Treatment of chronic hepatitis B at 10 mg daily decreases HBV DNA polymerase (by 3.56 $\log_{10}$ steps compared with 0.55 in placebo recipients), improves hepatitic histopathology scores, and induces loss of hepatitis B e antigen.

Entecavir

A nucleoside analog that is orally bioavailable for the treatment of chronic hepatitis B. Phase III trials are in progress.

 Preparations and dosage

Docosanol
Proprietary name: Abreva.
Preparation: 10% cream.
Dosage: Topically, five times daily.
Limited availability. Available in USA.

Imiquimod
Proprietary name: Aldara.
Preparation: 5% cream.
Dosage: Topically three times a week at night.
Limited availability. Available in the USA and UK.

41 Sepsis

A. Norrby-Teglund and D. E. Low

In the last half of the twentieth century, the use of antibiotics for the treatment of bacterial infections resulted in sharp reductions in morbidity and mortality from infections. However, mortality has remained high when an acute bacterial infection induces sepsis with shock, metabolic acidosis, oliguria, or hypoxemia. In fact, in the United States alone, there are at least 500 000 episodes of sepsis annually, and the resultant mortality rate ranges from 30 to 50%, even with intensive medical care including antibiotics, intravenous fluids, nutrition, mechanical ventilation for respiratory failure, and surgery when indicated to eradicate the source of the infection.[1–3] However, our understanding of sepsis and sepsis syndrome has increased markedly over the last decade.[4] One of the major gains has been the identification of mediators or cytokines that appear to be responsible for the pathophysiologic changes associated with the systemic manifestations of infection. Both Gram-positive and Gram-negative bacterial infections trigger the macrophage to produce cytokines including tumor necrosis factor (TNF) and interleukin-1 (IL-1).[5] In addition, endotoxin produced by bacteria or other cell-wall components of the organism may elicit tissue damage directly by activating pathways such as the coagulation cascade,[6] the complement cascade,[7] vessel injury, or the release of arachidonic acid metabolites or nitric oxide.[8] Thus, the processes that result in the sepsis syndrome are the result of microbial products that profoundly dysregulate mediator release and the homeostasis of several important pathways.[9] Attempts to treat sepsis by blocking individual mediators or some of the common pathways have failed to reduce the overall mortality. This is probably due to the fact that in complex situations where multiple cellular activation processes are involved and many humoral cascades are triggered, merely blocking a single component may be insufficient to arrest the inflammatory process. However, it seems possible that the dysregulation that characterizes sepsis may be amenable to blockade of the bacterial components or to the intracellular pathways triggered by these products.[9]

EPIDEMIOLOGY

Recent publications using mortality and morbidity data from the US National Center for Health Statistics have reported a 58% increase in death rates due to infectious diseases between 1980 to 1992[10] and a rate of admission to hospital for infectious diseases that declined less steeply than for all admissions.[11] Among the 15 leading causes of death in the USA that have been reported since 1950, the greatest increase in death rates has been due to septicemia.

BACTEREMIA

Clinically significant bacteremia occurs with a frequency of 5–10 per 1000 hospital admissions, a figure that has been rising slowly during the last 10 years largely due to an increasing number of nosocomial infections. Mylotte et al[12] studied the epidemiology and outcome of community acquired bacteremia in a teaching hospital and a non-teaching hospital and found incidences of community-acquired bacteremia to be 12.6 and 11.9 episodes per 1000 admissions, respectively. The reported incidence of community-acquired bacteremia in recent studies has varied from 2.5 to 7.4 episodes per 1000 admissions in teaching hospitals and from 2.2 to 6.7 episodes in non-teaching hospitals. A number of sites are possible sources of bacteremia (Table 41.1). The type of pathogen and resistance pattern may vary according to site of infection, the type of

Table 41.1 Source of micro-organisms isolated from blood of patients with community and hospital-acquired bacteremia[12,77]

Source	Site of acquisition (%)		
	Community	Hospital	
		Teaching	Non-teaching
i.v. catheter	8	0	19
Respiratory tract	32	21	12
Urinary tract	29	40	18
Skin/soft tissue	9	3	6
Intra-abdominal	4	12	12
Other	6	5	7
Unknown	12	19	26

Table 41.2 Micro-organisms isolated from the blood of patients with community and hospital acquired bacteremia[12,77]

Organism	Prevalence of various organisms according to site (%)		
	Community		Hospital
	Teaching	Non-teaching	
Staphylococcus aureus			19
Methicillin-sensitive	25	9	
Methicillin-resistant	5	<1	
Coagulase-negative staphylococci	Not included in study		9
Streptococcus pneumoniae	10	15	4
Enterococci	10	5	7
Escherichia coli	14	41	15
Klebsiella pneumoniae	4	9	7
Pseudomonas aeruginosa	5	4	6
Proteus mirabilis	6	4	2
Others	20	12	20
% Gram-positives	59	38	34
% Gram-negatives	41	62	66

hospital and the location within the hospital in which the patient is being treated (Table 41.2). Such information may be of assistance in deciding the most likely pathogen and most appropriate antimicrobial therapy. Mylotte et al[12] found the proportion of episodes due to methicillin-sensitive *Staphylococcus aureus* was significantly higher at the teaching hospital, whereas the proportion of episodes due to *Escherichia coli* was significantly higher at the non-teaching hospital (Table 41.2). Except for these differences, the proportion of episodes due to other organisms was similar between the two groups. Community-acquired bacteremia caused by Gram-positive organisms (staphylococci, streptococci, and enterococci) occurred significantly more often at the teaching hospital, conversely, community-acquired bacteremia caused by Gram-negative bacilli occurred more often at the non-teaching hospital, reflecting the urinary tract as a more common source of bacteremia in this setting.

Edmond et al[13] carried out concurrent surveillance for nosocomial bloodstream infections at 49 hospitals over a 3-year period. Nearly two-thirds of the episodes (64.4%) were caused by Gram-positive organisms, 27% were due to Gram-negative bacteria, and fungi caused the remaining 8.4%. Coagulase-negative staphylococci accounted for nearly one-third of all nosocomial bacteremias (31.9%), followed by *Staph. aureus* (15.7%) and enterococci (11.1%). *Candida* species were the fourth most common cause (7.6%). The most common Gram-negative organisms were *Esch. coli* (5.7%), *Klebsiella* spp., (5.4%), and *Enterobacter* spp. (4.5%). Crude mortality rates ranged from 20.8% for coagulase-negative staphylococci to 39.9% for *Candida* spp. Of the ten major pathogens, *Enterobacter* spp., *Serratia* spp., coagulase-negative staphylococci, and *Candida* spp. were more likely to be isolated from patients in the critical care setting, whereas *Staph. aureus*, *Klebsiella* spp., *Esch. coli*, and viridans streptococci were more common in the ward setting.

The intensive care unit (ICU) is a center of development of nosocomial infections. In a 1-day point-prevalence infection surveillance performed in 1417 European ICUs, 45% of 10 038 patients were infected and 21% had ICU-acquired infections.[14] Richards et al[15] reported the epidemiology of nosocomial infections in adults in 112 medical ICUs in 97 hospitals in the USA that were part of the National Nosocomial Infections Surveillance (NNIS) system of the Centers for Disease Control and Prevention between January 1992 and July 1997. The most common pathogens reported were coagulase-negative staphylococci (36%), enterococci (16%), *Staph. aureus* (13%), and Gram-negative aerobes (17%). The most frequent Gram-negatives were *Klebsiella pneumoniae* and *Pseudomonas aeruginosa*. *Candida* species were found to be associated with urinary catheters, coagulase-negative staphylococci with central lines, and *Ps. aeruginosa* and *Acinetobacter* species with ventilators. In other reports from the NNIS, trends of increasing proportions of Gram-positive infections and decreasing proportions of Gram-negative infections during the last 15 years have become apparent.

SEPTICEMIA

There has been a major increase in the rates of admission to hospital due to septicemia: between 1980 and 1994, the annual change in the number of admissions due to septicemia was 10.5%, second only to that for HIV infection and/or AIDS.[11] Simonsen et al[11] found septicemia to be the fourth leading cause of hospital admission due to infectious diseases in the USA in 1994 (a total of 301 800, or 116 admissions per 100 000 persons). The age-adjusted death rate due to septicemia increased from 0.3 per 100 000 in 1950 to 4.2 per 100 000 in 1997, a 14-fold increase, which makes septicemia the thirteenth leading cause of death in 1997.[16] The unadjusted rate in 1997 was 8 per 100 000. Among elderly people, the mortality rate was 23 per 100 000 for persons 65–74 years old, 60 per 100 000 for 75–84 years old, and 178 per 100 000 for people of 85 years or more.

McBean and Rajamani[17] examined the rates of hospital admission of elderly people due to septicemia in the period 1986–1997. The sex- and race-adjusted annual rates in 1997 were more than double the rates in 1986 (Figure 41.1). For people between 65 and 74 years old, the rate in 1997 was 2.2 times the rate in 1986; for those of 75–84 years it was double and 2.3 times greater for patients ≥85. Rates of admission for septicemia were significantly higher for those of 85 years or older in all years ($p < 0.001$).

The overall 30-day postadmission mortality rate for persons admitted for treatment of septicemia in 1997 was 246.5 per 1000 patients admitted and was 6.9% greater among Black Americans (262 per 1000) than among White Americans (245 per 1000). The 30-day postadmission mortality rate for patients for whom the presumed source of infection was decubitus ulcer was 372 per 1000 admissions; for pneumonia it was 336 per 1000, for urinary tract infections and cystitis 193 per 1000, for cellulitis 177 per 1000 and 66 per 1000 for admissions due to kidney infections.

Reasons for the increase in septicemia over the 12 years of the study include the increased prevalence (due to both increased incidence and increased duration) of chronic diseases such as diabetes, cancer and end-stage renal disease in the elderly that put them at higher risk for infectious diseases. Medical devices, used either temporarily or permanently, may also increase the risk of septicemia.

PATHOPHYSIOLOGY

Severe sepsis develops as a consequence of microbial antigenemia inducing a generalized activation of numerous host defense systems, including the adaptive and the innate immune responses of which complement, coagulation, contact-phase, and fibrinolytic systems are prominent contributors.[6,18] Activation of these proinflammatory and procoagulatory cascades results in release of proinflammatory cytokines, nitric oxide, endothelins, tissue damaging proteinases, lipid mediators (platelet activating factor, arachidonic acid, and eicosanoids), and hypotensive molecules such as kinins.[6,18] These mediators regulate cellular and humoral immune responses and are essential for an adequate and efficient host defense against infecting micro-organisms. However, excessive and dysregulated release of these mediators is the key event leading to the clinical symptoms seen in sepsis and shock, i.e. circulatory collapse, organ failure and death (Figure 41.2). The initial proinflammatory phase of sepsis is followed by a second phase characterized by an anti-inflammatory state, commonly referred to as the compensatory anti-inflammatory response syndrome.[19] The compensatory anti-inflammatory response syndrome is believed to be a mechanism by which the host can minimize tissue damage caused by dysregulated inflammation. This may be achieved by release of anti-inflammatory cytokines as well as by downregulation and shedding of cytokine receptors; however, the exact actions of this anti-inflammatory system in the pathophysiology of sepsis have not yet been clearly established.

Gram-positive and Gram-negative bacteria produce numerous microbial factors, both cell-associated and secreted factors,

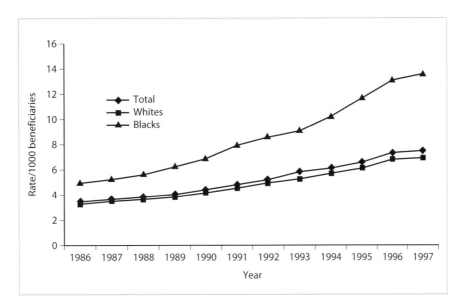

Fig. 41.1 Rates of admission to hospital for treatment of septicemia during the period 1986–1997. (◆, Total rate, ■, White patients; ▲, Black patients.) By 1997 the adjusted rate was 2.17 times the rate in 1986. The estimated annual percentage change for this period was 7.83%. (Reprinted from *Journal of Infectious Diseases* 183: 596–603, 2001.[17])

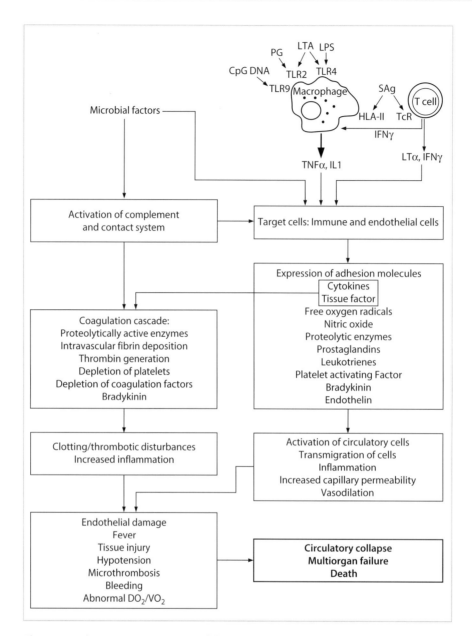

Fig. 41.2 Schematic representation of the pathophysiology of sepsis. Microbial factors such as lipopolysaccharide (LPS) produced by Gram-negative bacteria, or peptidoglycan (PG), lipoteichoic acid (LTA), and superantigens (SAg) produced by Gram-positive bacteria, as well as unmethylated oligonucleotides containing cytidine-phosphate-guanosine (CpG) motifs, interact with specific receptors such as HLA class II molecules (HLA-II) and Toll like receptors (TLR) on antigen-presenting cells and the T-cell receptor (TCR) on T cells. This triggers activation of the cells and release of the proinflammatory cytokines IL-1 and TNF, which results in activation of the cytokine cascade and the coagulation system. Activation of these host defense systems leads to excessive and dysregulated release of inflammatory mediators and consequently the clinical symptoms of sepsis.

capable of activating the host systems involved in sepsis. Lipopolysaccharide (LPS), which is a major constituent of the outer membrane of Gram-negative bacteria, has long been recognized as the principal mediator of sepsis, by virtue of its potent proinflammatory activities.[20] The cell wall of Gram-positive bacteria also contains several molecules capable of inducing potent proinflammatory responses, including peptidoglycan and lipoteichoic acid.[21] Interestingly, LPS, lipoteichoic acid and peptidoglycan all display pathogen-associated molecular patterns, which activate the innate immunity through interaction with pattern recognition receptors (i.e CD14) and activation of Toll-like receptors 2 and 4.[22] This results in activation of antigen-presenting cells, induction of proinflammatory cytokines (chemokines) and production of endogenous antimicrobial peptides.[22]

Streptococcus pyogenes and *Staph. aureus* also express and secrete exotoxins with superantigenic activity that induce very powerful immune responses.[23] Superantigens interact, without prior cellular processing, with the relatively invariable Vβ-region of the T-cell receptor and the MHC class II molecules on antigen-presenting cells (Figure 41.3). Cross-linking of T cells and antigen-presenting cells by superantigens results in potent activation of these cells and consequently excessive production of proinflammatory cytokines.[23]

Other virulence factors suggested to be involved in the pathogenesis of sepsis are hemolysins and unmethylated oligonucleotides containing cytidine-phosphate-guanosine (CpG) motifs that are present in both Gram-positive and Gram-negative bacteria.[24–27] Unmethylated CpG DNA is exclusively found in prokaryotes and triggers proinflammatory responses by interaction with Toll-like receptor 9.[28] Synergistic or additive effects have been shown for many of the above-mentioned virulence factors,[21,29] and sepsis is most likely to be caused by the interplay between multiple microbial factors and host cells.

One of the initial events in sepsis is induction of proinflammatory cytokines, which trigger activation of the cytokine cascade, complement and coagulation systems, injury to endothelium an vessels, and release of proteases, arachidonic acid metabolites and nitric oxide (Fig. 41.2).[18,30] The cytokines most commonly associated with sepsis are interleukins (IL) 1, 6, 8 and 12, tumor necrosis factor (TNF)-α, interferon (IFN)-γ, macrophage migration inhibitory factor (MIF), and high mobility group-1 (HMG-1).[30–33] However, several more

cytokines are being released during sepsis, and together with the above-mentioned they interact in a complex network involving several interaction points and feedback loops. The cytokine cascade is initiated by IL-1 and TNF-α, which are secreted by activated macrophages in response to proinflammatory microbial components, and these cytokines are therefore often referred to as 'early mediators of sepsis'. Activation of the cytokine cascade results in a rapid activation of different cell types, and further release of IL-1, TNF-α and several other important mediators.[30] IL-1 and TNF-α induce potent pyrogenic and hypotensive responses, and administration of either cytokine reproduces the clinical symptoms of sepsis.[30] One of the best markers for sepsis and outcome of sepsis is IL-6. However, IL-6 itself does not induce a proinflammatory response or hypotension, and does not cause shock in animal models. IL-8 is a highly powerful chemokine, which attracts and activates polymorphonuclear leukocytes, and has been postulated to have a central role in the pulmonary inflammation resulting in acute respiratory distress.[30] MIF, a pituitary- and macrophage-derived factor,[31] behaves as a proinflammatory cytokine, and was recently shown to be a critical mediator of septic shock.[34] One important attribute of MIF is that it is induced by glucocorticoid; it also counteracts the effect on glucocorticoids being released from the adrenals in order to inhibit the proinflammatory response by induction of anti-inflammatory cytokines, thus further promoting a proinflammatory response.[31] HMG-1 was recently shown to increase LPS-induced IL-1 and TNF-α and to be a critical mediator of septic shock in mice, which appears late in the cytokine cascade and is produced over a prolonged period.[33]

A positive correlation between development of shock in sepsis and activation of the coagulation response was reported as early as 30 years ago.[35] Microbial factors can activate the coagulation cascade either directly or indirectly via induction

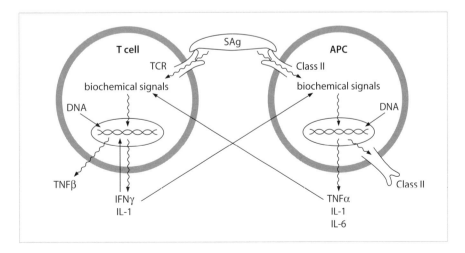

Fig. 41.3 Interplay between T-cell and antigen-presenting cell-derived cytokines and induction of an inflammatory cytokine cascade by superantigens. IFN, interferon; Sag, superantigens; TNF, tumor necrosis factor; IL, interleukin (Reprinted from *Clinical Microbiology Reviews*, 8: 411–426, 1995.[80])

of proinflammatory cytokines and subsequent expression of tissue factor on endothelial cells and monocytes, which is the main pathway of activation of coagulation activation in sepsis (Figure 41.2).[35] A drastic reduction in the levels of important endogenous coagulation inhibitors such as antithrombin III and activated protein C (APC) due to consumption, expression deficiency or proteolytic inactivation of these inhibitors further contributes to the procoagulatory state in sepsis.[35,36] Numerous studies have revealed that sepsis and disseminated intravascular coagulation are associated with decreased antithrombin III and protein C, and a disruption in the balance between coagulation and fibrinolysis.[35,36] Furthermore, a correlation between deficiency in these inhibitors and increased morbidity and mortality in sepsis has been reported.[35,36] Dysregulated expression of antithrombin III and activated protein C also affects the inflammatory processes due to increased thrombin production that promotes upregulation of expression of adhesion molecules and microvascular thrombosis, which subsequently increases the inflammatory response through tissue ischemia and neutrophil/endothelium activation.[35,36]

Activation of the complement and contact systems has also been postulated as contributing to the sepsis process, mainly by the release of hypotensive mediators, anaphylatoxins, and the consumption of coagulatory factors.[37] Herwald et al[38] recently demonstrated that the fibrous surface components of Gram-positive and Gram-negative bacteria bind to and trigger assembly of the components of the contact system, resulting in the release of hypotensive kinins, hypocoagulatory state, and dysregulated fibrin and clot formation.[38] Other virulence factors, such as the streptococcal M protein and the streptococcal proteinase, have also been shown to interact with components of the contact system.[38]

DIAGNOSTIC ISSUES

Sepsis is not a single disease but a syndrome that can result from diverse causes, and with a spectrum of severity that ranges from fever associated with transitory hypotension through to profound shock and high mortality (Box 41.1). The same clinical picture is seen in some non-infective conditions. Consequently, nomenclature may be confusing.

Identifying subgroups and giving them labels is worth while only if doing so aids design of better treatment or more accurate prediction of outcome.

Bacteremia, the presence of viable bacteria in the bloodstream, is a transient phenomenon (with the exception of

Box 41.1 Diagnostic criteria for conditions associated with bacteremia and sepsis.[78,79]

Bacteremia
The presence of viable bacteria in the bloodstream.

Septicemia
As bacteremia, but of greater severity.

Systemic inflammatory response syndrome (SIRS)
Two or more of the following criteria:

- Temperature >38°C or <36°C.
- Heart rate >90 beats/min.
- Respiratory rate >20 breaths/min *or* P_aCO_2 <32 mmHg.
- White blood cell count >12 × 10^9/l or <4 × 10^9/l.

Multiple organ dysfunction syndrome (MODS)
Presence of altered organ function in an acutely ill patient such that homeostasis cannot be maintained without intervention.

Sepsis
Two or more of the following criteria occurring as a result of infection:

- Temperature >38°C or <36°C.
- Heart rate >90 beats/min.
- Respiratory rate >20 breaths/min *or* P_aCO_2 <32 mmHg.
- White blood cell count >12 × 10^9/l or <4 × 10^9/l.

Sepsis syndrome
Sepsis plus evidence of altered organ perfusion with at least one of: hypoxemia, elevated lactate, oliguria, altered mentation.

Septic shock
Sepsis associated with hypotension despite adequate fluid resuscitation, and perfusion abnormalities that may include, but are not limited to, lactic acidosis, oliguria or an acute alteration in mental status.

endovascular infections such as endocarditis). *Septicemia* denotes a more severe form of bacteremia, whereas sepsis is a term used when there is clinical evidence of infection plus a systemic response as manifested by an elevated temperature, tachycardia, increased respirations, and leukocytosis or leukopenia. *Sepsis* is the inflammatory response to infection. This has been further modified by referring to the sepsis syndrome (sepsis with evidence of altered organ perfusion) or severe sepsis (sepsis associated with organ dysfunction, hypoperfusion abnormality or hypotension). *Septic shock* is a subset of severe sepsis, associated with a worse prognosis. The critical difference between systemic inflammatory response syndrome (SIRS) and sepsis is the requirement for clinical or laboratory evidence of infection.

The relationships between SIRS, sepsis, shock and death is well illustrated by a prospective study of nearly 4000 patients admitted to ICUs in the USA.[2] The incidence of SIRS on surgical ICUs was 857 episodes per 1000 patient-days, and the mortality of these patients was just 7%, emphasizing that SIRS is a very sensitive definition. However, in the small proportion (4%) that developed septic shock, mortality was 46%.

There are two major reasons why an infectious etiology is not identified in a patient presenting with sepsis:

- antibiotics are often used empirically in the outpatient and home care setting and the hospital before testing;
- bacteremia may be intermittent, except in the patient with an endovascular infection.

However, in patients with sepsis it is more important to initiate appropriate antimicrobial therapy in order to ensure optimal outcome than to wait for further blood culture sets.[39] Although 75–80% of neutropenic fevers are thought to be caused by infections, a causal organism can be confirmed in only 30–50% of episodes. In a prospective study of sepsis and septic shock, at least 15% of patients had no documented infection. Even among patients with presumed infection, less than half had bacteremia.[40] Ideally two or three blood cultures should be obtained several hours apart to increase the likelihood for detection.[41] The total volume of blood cultured is one of the most important factors in the recovery of bacterial pathogens: in one study, increasing the volume of blood cultured over a 24-hour period from 40 to 60 ml increased the recovery by 10%.[42]

TREATMENT

TRADITIONAL THERAPEUTIC STRATEGIES

Antimicrobial therapy

Antimicrobial therapy remains the mainstay of treatment of sepsis; Bryant et al[43] found that appropriate antimicrobial therapy for Gram-negative bacteremia significantly reduced

mortality. Such findings have supported empirical broad-spectrum therapy before results of culture are known. In addition, there is evidence that early therapy improves outcome. Pneumonia is the most frequent infectious cause of death among all patients of all ages.[44] In a study of the association between process and outcome of care for patients who were admitted to hospital with community-acquired pneumonia Meehan et al found a lower mortality associated with antibiotic administration within 8 h of hospital arrival (odds ratio, 0.85; 95% CI 0.75–0.96).[39]

The number of effective antimicrobial agents available is becoming limited because of the emergence of multidrug resistance in both Gram-negative and Gram-positive pathogens.[45] One of the consequences of infections due to resistant strains is the increased likelihood of inappropriate initial therapy. Leroy et al[46] found that ineffective initial antimicrobial therapy was the best predictor for a bad prognosis in community-acquired pneumonia.

The decision as to which antimicrobial or antimicrobial combination to use empirically depends on the source of the infection, whether it is community-acquired or nosocomial, whether or not the patient has an underlying illness that changes the predictability of the offending pathogen, and the local antimicrobial resistance rates. Another important aspect to consider in the choice of antimicrobial therapy is that the release of proinflammatory cell wall components and subsequent inflammatory responses varies with the antibiotic used.[47–49] This variation is a consequence of the mechanistic action of the antimicrobials. β-Lactam agents generally induce release of larger amounts of cell-wall components of Gram-negative and Gram-positive bacteria than do antimicrobials that act on protein synthesis.[47–49] It has recently been demonstrated that combination therapy significantly affects the amount of LPS released. For instance, tobramycin and cefuroxime in combination caused significantly lower levels of LPS to be released than each agent alone, despite increased bacterial killing.[50]

Volume replacement

The first goal of management of the patient with severe sepsis is adequate monitoring of vital signs so that any hemodynamic changes can be detected and treated. Insertion of a central venous pressure monitoring device, arterial catheter, and Swan-Ganz catheters to determine the left atrial end-diastolic pressure allows for optimal monitoring and fluid replacement.

A number of solutions are used to expand intravascular fluid volume and colloid oncotic pressure, including normal and hypertonic saline, fresh-frozen plasma, albumin, and various dextran preparations. However, the type of volume therapy used differs widely between ICUs and no standards exist for volume therapy in patients in such units.[51] Crystalloid solutions are the first choice to correct fluid and electrolyte deficits in non-hemorrhagic shock. In the case of major hypovolemia, particularly in situations of increased capillary permeability, colloid solutions have been thought to be indicated to achieve sufficient tissue perfusion. However, different colloids have different molecular weights and therefore vary in the length of time they remain in the circulatory system. Because of this and their other characteristics, colloids may differ in their safety and efficacy. Bunn et al[52] reviewed randomized and quasi-randomized trials comparing colloid solutions in critically ill and surgical patients thought to need volume replacement. The main outcomes measured were death, amount of whole blood transfused and incidence of adverse reactions. They found no evidence that one colloid solution was more effective or safe than any other, although the confidence intervals were wide and did not exclude clinically significant differences between colloids.

Colloids are widely used, having been recommended in a number of resuscitation guidelines and intensive care management algorithms.[53] However, a 1995 survey of American academic health centers found that the use of colloids far exceeded these recommendations.[54] In fact, the use of colloids for the treatment of septic shock has been recently challenged: they are more expensive than crystalloids, some colloid solutions may be associated with adverse outcomes and some clinical trials have found them to be no better than crystalloids. Roberts[55] carried out a systematic review of randomized controlled trials of resuscitation with colloids or crystalloids for volume replacement of critically ill patients. They found that the pooled relative risk of mortality for all patient groups was 1.19 (95% confidence interval 0.98–1.45). The risk of mortality with resuscitation using colloids was 24% (20% with resuscitation using crystalloids), giving an increase in absolute risk of mortality for resuscitation with colloids of 4% (95% CI 0–0.08). When only trials with adequate concealment of allocation were analyzed, the increase in absolute risk of mortality for resuscitation with colloids was 7% (95% CI– 1–0.15%), indicating no statistically significant increase in mortality for resuscitation with colloids, although the trend was in that direction. The overview concluded that the use of colloids for volume resuscitation in critically ill patients is not supported by the literature. Concern has been raised about the use of albumin, often the colloid of choice for replacement therapy.[56] The Cochrane Group carried out a review of randomized controlled trials comparing administration of albumin or plasma protein fraction with no administration, or with administration of crystalloid solution, in critically ill patients with hypovolemia, burns, or hypoalbuminemia. They found that for each patient category the risk of death in the albumin-treated group was higher than in the comparison group. For hypoalbuminemia the relative risk of death after albumin administration was 1.69 (1.07–2.67). They concluded that use of human albumin in critically ill patients should be urgently reviewed and that it should not be used outside the context of rigorously conducted, randomized controlled trials.

Vasopressor agents

If fluid therapy alone fails to restore adequate arterial pressure and organ perfusion, therapy with vasopressor agents should be initiated. For many years, norepinephrine and epinephrine were the principal agents available. However, because of their intense peripheral vasocontricting activity and increase in myocardial irritability, they have been replaced with alternative agents such as isoproterenol, dopamine, and dobutamine. These agents have an inotropic effect on myocardial function but because of β-adrenergic activity are capable of enhancing peripheral tissue perfusion. Norepinephrine was reserved only for those patients in whom it was not possible to support systemic blood pressure and vascular perfusion with dopamine or isoproterenol. However, the results from two studies have challenged this dogma.[57,58] Martin et al[58] carried out a study that was designed to identify factors associated with outcome in a cohort of septic shock patients. Special attention was paid to hemodynamic management and to the choice of vasopressor used, to determine whether the use of norepinephrine was associated with increased mortality. Five variables were significantly associated with outcome. One factor that was strongly associated with a favorable outcome was the use of norepinephrine as part of the hemodynamic support of the patients: the 57 patients who were treated with norepinephrine had significantly lower hospital mortality (62% vs. 82%, $p < 0.001$; relative risk = 0.68; 95% confidence interval 0.54–0.87) than the 40 patients treated with vasopressors other than norepinephrine (high-dose dopamine and/or epinephrine). Such studies have led to a re-evaluation of which sympathomimetic amines should be used and when. Dopamine and/or norepinephrine are now considered by some to be the first-line agents for shock. Epinephrine should be limited for use in patients unresponsive to other agents.

Low-dose dopamine is still commonly administered to critically ill patients in the belief that it reduces the risk of renal failure by increasing renal blood flow. However, Bellomo et al[59] carried out a multicenter, randomized, double-blind, placebo-controlled prospective study of low-dose dopamine in patients with at least two criteria for the SIRS and clinical evidence of early renal dysfunction and found no benefit for renal protection.

NOVEL THERAPEUTIC STRATEGIES

During the last two decades, significant advances have been made in the field of sepsis, revealing a complex interplay between several microbial factors and different host defense. This has allowed for novel therapeutic strategies, ranging from interventions with defined microbial factors to the various host systems (Table 41.3).

Neutralization of microbial factors

Anti-endotoxin therapies, including polyclonal and monoclonal antibodies and various lipid analogs, have been tested quite extensively in clinical trials, but have so far failed to reveal any significant effect on mortality rates.[20] Other anti-endotoxin approaches that are currently under investigation include bac-

Table 41.3 Novel therapeutic strategies in septic shock

Strategies*	Type of agent	References
Neutralization of microbial factors		
Anti-endotoxin	Polyclonal antiserum (J5, anti-Lipid A, IVIG)	20,66
	Monoclonal antibodies (HA-1A, E5, T88)	20,66
	Lipid A analogs (lipid X, monophosporyl lipid A, etc)	20,66
	Recombinant bactericidal/permeability-increasing protein	60
Anti-superantigen	IVIG	62,63
Modulation of pro-inflammatory mediators		
Anti-cytokines	Corticosteroids	65
Anti-TNF	Mononoclonal antibodies, receptor fusion proteins	65,66
Anti-interleukin 1	Interleukin-1 receptor antagonist	65,66
Anti-PAF	PAF antagonist	65
Anti-bradykinin	Bradykinin antagonist	65
Anti-prostaglandin	Ibuprofen (cyclooxygenase inhibitor)	66
Nitric oxide inhibitor	Nitric oxide synthase inhibitor	66
Modulation of coagulation		
Antithrombin III	Inhibitor of coagulation	72
Activated protein C	Inhibitor of coagulation	73

IVIG, intravenous polyclonal immunoglobulin; PAF, platelet-activating factor.
*Includes therapeutic agents that have been tested in controlled human sepsis trials.

tericidal-permeability-increasing protein[60] and inhibition of CD14 or LPS-binding proteins.[20]

Neutralization of Gram-positive microbial factors has mainly been achieved by intravenous polyspecific immunoglobulin G (IVIG), which has been demonstrated to contain neutralizing antibodies against streptococcal and staphylococcal superantigens, as well as opsonic antibodies against a variety of micro-organisms.[61,62] In addition to its direct toxin-neutralizing and opsonic activities, IVIG has a general immunomodulatory effect due to its interaction with Fc-receptors, complement, immune cell functions, cytokines and cytokine antagonists.[61,62] There have been several placebo-controlled trials of IVIG in sepsis, some of which (although not all) have shown clinical efficacy.[63] With the very potent neutralization of Gram-positive superantigens, IVIG may have the most pronounced effect in Gram-positive sepsis, in particular against invasive group A streptococcal infections. This notion was supported by a recent case-control study by Kaul et al,[64] which showed a significant reduction in mortality following IVIG therapy in patients with streptococcal toxic shock syndrome.

Inhibition of pro-inflammatory mediators

With all the knowledge implicating cytokines, especially TNF-α and IL-1, as principal mediators of sepsis and shock, these molecules were obvious therapeutic targets. However, despite animal experiments revealing drastic improvement in survival after anti-cytokine therapy, ranging from general cytokine inhibition by corticosteroids to agents targeting specific mediators,

none of these agents succeeded in lowering the mortality of sepsis in large phase III clinical trials (Table 41.3).[65–67] There are several potential reasons for why these therapies failed:

- blockage of one mediator may not suffice to arrest the whole process;[6]
- agents directed against early mediators have a narrow therapeutic window;
- the peak of production may have passed by the time of initiation of treatment, and downstream cascades may already be triggered.

There have been numerous studies of the use of corticosteroids in sepsis with highly varying results, ranging from beneficial to even harmful effect.[65] However, recent reports of a low-dose regimen have reported significant improvements in hemodynamics and survival in septic shock.[68–70]

Another therapeutic approach to attenuate the pathogenic proinflammatory response was recently described by Borovikova et al,[71] and involves a parasympathetic anti-inflammatory pathway by which the brain modulates systemic inflammatory responses. It was reported that an endotoxin-induced proinflammatory cytokine response could be inhibited in vitro by the principal vagal neurotransmitter acetylcholine. Furthermore, lethal endotoxic shock in rats could be prevented by direct electric stimulation of the peripheral vagus nerve, which decreased in-vivo levels of TNF.

Novel targets for intervention include among others MIF and HMG-1, which have been shown to be persistent mediators of severe sepsis; their neutralization results in protection against experimental septic shock.[33,34] In contrast to the early cytokines TNF-α and IL-1, HMG-1 and MIF are late mediators of sepsis and are produced over an extended period of time, which would facilitate intervention due to a wider therapeutic window.[32–34]

Modulators of coagulation

The important interplay between the inflammatory response and the coagulation system, in addition to the finding that patients with severe sepsis are deficient in important coagulation inhibitors, suggested that modulation of coagulation might be a potential therapeutic strategy.[72] Several anti-coagulant strategies have been proposed, among the most promising of which are the natural coagulation inhibitors antithrombin III and activated protein C.[72,73] Phase II clinical trials of antithrombin III replacement in sepsis indicated a possible clinical efficacy.[72] Promising results have also been presented for activated protein C replacement, where the reduction in morbidity and mortality noted in the phase II clinical trial[74] have been repeated in a phase III trial.[73] There are several reasons as to why activated protein C might be an effective therapy in patients with sepsis.

- Most patients with severe sepsis have diminished levels of activated protein C, because of the reduction in the components of the coagulation system that are necessary for the conversion of inactive protein C to activated protein C.[75]
- Activated protein C inhibits activated factors V and VIII, thereby decreasing the formation of thrombin, and stimulates fibrinolysis by reducing the concentration of plasminogen-activator inhibitor type 1.
- In addition to its central regulatory role in coagulation, protein C has been shown to have a strong anti-inflammatory effect, some of which may be mediated by its inhibition of the proinflammatory cytokines MIF and TNF-α.[76]

Bernard et al[73] conducted a randomized, double-blind, placebo-controlled, multicenter trial, assigning patients with systemic inflammation and organ failure due to acute infection to receive an intravenous infusion of either placebo or activated protein C. Patients receiving activated protein C demonstrated a dose-dependent reduction in the plasma levels of D-dimer and serum levels of IL-6, markers of coagulopathy and inflammation, respectively. The absolute reduction in the 28-day mortality rate was 6.1% (the rate in the placebo group was 30.8%, compared with a rate of 24.7% in the group assigned to receive activated protein C), and the relative risk of death in the treated group was reduced by nearly 20%. The treatment was effective regardless of age, severity of illness, the number of dysfunctional organs or systems, the site of infection, and the type of infecting organism. Treatment with activated protein C reduced mortality even though >70% of the patients were in shock and were already receiving mechanical ventilation. This provides evidence that mortality can be reduced among patients with severe sepsis through the use of a therapy that inhibits both the procoagulant and the inflammatory cascades.[3]

CONCLUSION

As the number of patients with chronic underlying disease and temporary or permanent foreign bodies increase so have the number of episodes of sepsis. The etiology of these episodes reflects the patient population and the geographic location of the healthcare facility they are treated in. Patients with severe underlying illness or chronic disease will always be at increased risk for endotoxin mediated Gram-negative sepsis, whereas those with intravascular catheters or prosthetic devices will be at greater risk for Gram-positive infections. Complicating the management of these infections has been the emergence of multidrug resistance in such pathogens, both in the hospital and the community setting. In some countries and regions, multidrug resistant strains are endemic and account for the large majority of infections. This often means that first-and second-line antimicrobials are ineffective, leaving few and often less acceptable alternatives. Infections caused by multiresistant organisms are associated with increased morbidity and mortality.

However, despite the advancements in medical treatment (including intensive medical care units, vasopressor agents, intravenous replacement fluids, nutrition, mechanical ventilation for respiratory failure, and surgery when indicated to eradicate the source of the infection), the outcome of patients with sepsis syndrome and septic shock has not greatly improved. This is because we treat only the cause and not the consequences of such infections. We now recognize that these conditions reflect stimulation of the process of innate immunity resulting in the excessive production of cytokines and chemokines and activation of the coagulation and complement cascades.

Blockage or antagonism of the actions of individual intermediary messenger molecules has proved unsuccessful. The most promising therapies today seem to be agents that target several different microbial factors and/or host systems involved in sepsis. Furthermore, several clinical trials have shown clinical efficacy in subgroups of patients, but not in the whole study material. This indicates that it is not the agents themselves that are wrong but rather the study design, and that targeting more defined patient populations based on specific clinical, immunological and/or microbiological parameters, will probably benefit the outcome of sepsis trials and provide a promising future for the therapy of these syndromes.

References

1. Hook EW; Horton CA, Schaberg DR 1983 Failure of intensive care unit support to influence mortality from pneumococcal bacteremia. *Journal of the American Medical Association* 249: 1055–1057
2. Rangel-Frausto MS, Pittet D, Costigan M, Hwang T, Davis CS, Wenzel RP 1995 The natural history of the systemic inflammatory response syndrome (SIRS). A prospective study. *Journal of the American Medical Association* 273: 117–123
3. Matthay MA 2001 Severe sepsis – a new treatment with both anticoagulant and antiinflammatory properties. *New England Journal of Medicine* 344: 759–762
4. Baumgartner JD, Calandra T 1999 Treatment of sepsis: past and future avenues. *Drugs* 57: 127–132

5. Van Der PT, Van Deventer SJ 1999 Cytokines and anticytokines in the pathogenesis of sepsis. *Infectious Disease Clinics of North America* 13: 413–426

6. Esmon CT, Fukudome K, Mather T et al 1999 Inflammation, sepsis, and coagulation. *Haematologica* 84: 254–259

7. Hoffmann JA, Kafatos FC, Janeway CA, Ezekowitz RA 1999 Phylogenetic perspectives in innate immunity. *Science* 284: 1313–1318

8. Murphy K, Haudek SB, Thompson M, Giroir BP 1998 Molecular biology of septic shock. *New Horizons* 6: 181–193

9. Glauser MP 2000 Pathophysiologic basis of sepsis: considerations for future strategies of intervention. *Critical Care Medicine* 28(Suppl. 9): S4–S8

10. Pinner RW, Teutsch SM, Simonsen L et al 1996 Trends in infectious diseases mortality in the United States. *Journal of the American Medical Association* 275: 189–193

11. Simonsen L, Conn LA, Pinner RW, Teutsch S 1998 Trends in infectious disease hospitalizations in the United States, 1980–1994. *Archives of Internal Medicine* 158: 1923–1928

12. Mylotte JM, Kahler L, McCann C 2001 Community-acquired bacteremia at a teaching versus a nonteaching hospital: Impact of acute severity of illness on 30-day mortality. *American Journal of Infection Control* 29: 13–19

13. Edmond MB, Wallace SE, McClish DK, Pfaller MA, Jones RN, Wenzel RP 1999 Nosocomial bloodstream infections in United States hospitals: a three-year analysis. *Clinical Infectious Diseases* 29: 239–244

14. Vincent JL, Bihari DJ, Suter PM et al 1995 The prevalence of nosocomial infection in intensive care units in Europe. Results of the European Prevalence of Infection in Intensive Care (EPIC) Study. EPIC International Advisory Committee. *Journal of the American Medical Association* 274: 639–644

15. Richards MJ, Edwards JR, Culver DH, Gaynes RP 1999 Nosocomial infections in medical intensive care units in the United States. National Nosocomial Infections Surveillance System. *Critical Care Medicine* 27: 887–892

16. Hoyert DL, Kochanek KD, Murphy SL 1999 Deaths: final data for 1997. *National Vital Statistics Report* 47: 1–104

17. McBean M, Rajamani S 2001 Increasing rates of hospitalization due to septicemia in the US elderly population, 1986–1997. *Journal of Infectious Diseases* 183: 596–603

18. Bone RC 1991 The pathogenesis of sepsis. *Annals of Internal Medicine* 115: 457–469

19. Vincent J 2000 The immune responses in critical illness: Excessive, inadequate or dysregulated. In: Marshall J, Cohen J (eds) *Update in intensive care and emergency medicine. Immune response in the critically ill.* Berlin, Heidelberg, New York: Springer-Verlag, pp. 12–22

20. Lynn WA. Anti-endotoxin therapeutic options for the treatment of sepsis 1998 *Journal of Antimicrobial Chemotherapy* 41(Suppl. A): 71–80

21. Sriskandan S, Cohen J 1999 Gram-positive sepsis. Mechanisms and differences from gram-negative sepsis. *Infectious Disease Clinics of North America* 13: 397–412

22. Medzhitov R, Janeway CJ Jr 2000 Innate Immunity. *New England Journal of Medicine* 5: 338–344

23. Kotb M 1998 Superantigens of gram-positive bacteria: structure-function analyses and their implications for biological activity. *Current Opinion in Microbiology* 1: 56–65

24. Ginsburg I, Ward PA, Varani J 1999 Can we learn from the pathogenetic strategies of group A hemolytic streptococci how tissues are injured and organs fail in post-infectious and inflammatory sequelae? FEMS *Immunology Medical Microbiology* 25: 325–338

25. Uhlen P, Laestadius A, Jahnukainen T et al 2000 Alpha-haemolysin of uropathogenic E. coli induces Ca2+ oscillations in renal epithelial cells. *Nature* 405: 694–697

26. Chatellier S, Kotb M 2000 Preferential stimulation of human lymphocytes by oligodeoxynucleotides that copy DNA CpG motifs present in virulent genes of group A streptococci. *European Journal of Immunology* 30: 993–1001

27. Wagner H, Lipford GB, Hacker H 2000 The role of immunostimulatory CpG-DNA in septic shock. *Springer Seminars in Immunopathology* 22: 167–171

28. Hemmi H, Takeuchi O, Kawai T et al 2000 A Toll-like receptor recognizes bacterial DNA. *Nature* 408: 740–745

29. Horn DL, Morrison DC, Opal SM, Silverstein R, Visvanathan K, Zabriskie JB 2000 What are the microbial components implicated in the pathogenesis of sepsis? Report on a symposium. *Clinical Infectious Diseases* 31: 851–858

30. Cavaillon J, Adib-Conquy M 2000 The pro-inflammatory cytokine cascade. In: Marshall J, Cohen J (eds) *Update in intensive care and emergency medicine. Immune responses in the critically ill.* New York, Springer-Verlag, pp. 37–66

31. Bernhagen J, Calandra T, Bucala R 1998 Regulation of the immune response by macrophage migration inhibitory factor: biological and structural features. *Journal of Molecular Medicine* 76: 151–161

32. Andersson U, Wang H, Palmblad K et al 2000 High mobility group 1 protein (HMG-1) stimulates proinflammatory cytokine synthesis in human monocytes. *Journal of Experimental Medicine* 192: 565–570

33. Wang H, Bloom O, Zhang M et al 1999 HMG-1 as a late mediator of endotoxin lethality in mice. *Science* 285: 248–251

34. Calandra T, Echtenacher B, Roy DL et al 2000 Protection from septic shock by neutralization of macrophage migration inhibitory factor. *Nature Medicine* 6: 164–170

35. Levi M, ten Cate H 1999 Disseminated intravascular coagulation. *New England Journal of Medicine* 341: 586–592

36. Fisher CJ, Yan SB 2000 Protein C levels as a prognostic indicator of outcome in sepsis and related diseases. *Critical Care Medicine* 28(Suppl. 9): S49–S56

37. Colman RW, Schmaier AH 1997 Contact system: a vascular biology modulator with anticoagulant, profibrinolytic, antiadhesive, and proinflammatory attributes. *Blood* 90: 3819–3843

38. Herwald H, Morgelin M, Olsen A et al 1998 Activation of the contact-phase system on bacterial surfaces – a clue to serious complications in infectious diseases. *Nature Medicine* 4: 298–302

39. Meehan TP, Fine MJ, Krumholz HM et al 1997 Quality of care, process, and outcomes in elderly patients with pneumonia. *Journal of the American Medical Association* 278: 2080–2084

40. Bone RC 1992 Toward an epidemiology and natural history of SIRS (systemic inflammatory response syndrome). *Journal of the American Medical Association* 268: 3452–3455

41. Weinstein MP, Murphy JR, Reller LB, Lichtenstein KA 1983 The clinical significance of positive blood cultures: a comprehensive analysis of 500 episodes of bacteremia and fungemia in adults. II. Clinical observations, with special reference to factors influencing prognosis. *Reviews of Infectious Diseases* 5: 54–70

42. Li J, Plorde JJ, Carlson LG 1994 Effects of volume and periodicity on blood cultures. *Journal of Clinical Microbiology* 32: 2829–2831

43. Bryant RE, Hood AF, Hood CE, Koenig MG 1971 Factors affecting mortality of gram-negative rod bacteremia. *Archives of Internal Medicine* 127: 120–128

44. Pneumonia and influenza death rates – United States, 1979–1994. *MMWR Morbidity and Mortality Weekly Report* 1995; 44: 535–537

45. Neu HC 1992 The crisis in antibiotic resistance. *Science* 257: 1064–1073

46. Leroy O, Georges H, Beuscart C et al 1996 Severe community-acquired pneumonia in ICUs: prospective validation of a prognostic score [see comments]. *Intensive Care Medicine* 22: 1307–1314

47. Periti P 2000 Current treatment of sepsis and endotoxaemia. *Expert Opinion in Pharmacotherapy* 1: 1203–1217

48. Mattsson E, Van Dijk H, Verhoef J, Norrby R, Roll of J 1996 Supernatants from *Staphylococcus epidermidis* grown in the presence of different antibiotics induce differential release of tumor necrosis factor alpha from human monocytes. *Infection and Immunity* 64: 4351–4355

49. Orman KL, English BK 2000 Effects of antibiotic class on the macrophage inflammatory response to *Streptococcus pneumoniae. Journal of Infectious Diseases* 182: 1561–1565

50. Sjolin J, Goscinski G, Lundholm M, Bring J, Odenholt I 2000 Endotoxin release from *Escherichia coli* after exposure to tobramycin: dose-dependency and reduction in cefuroxime-induced endotoxin release. *Clin Microbiol Infect* 6: 74–81

51. Boldt J, Lenz M, Kumle B, Papsdorf M 1998 Volume replacement strategies on intensive care units: results from a postal survey. *Intensive Care Medicine* 24: 147–151

52. Bunn F, Alderson P, Hawkins V 2000 Colloid solutions for fluid resuscitation. *Cochrane Database System Review* (2): CD001319

53. Vermeulen LC Jr, Ratko TA, Erstad BL, Brecher ME, Matuszewski KA 1995 A paradigm for consensus. The University Hospital Consortium guidelines for the use of albumin, nonprotein colloid, and crystalloid solutions. *Archives of Internal Medicine* 155: 373–379

54. Yim JM, Vermeulen LC, Erstad BL, Matuszewski KA, Burnett DA, Vlasses PH 1995 Albumin and nonprotein colloid solution use in US academic health centers. *Archives of Internal Medicine* 155: 2450–2455

55. Schierhout G, Roberts I 1998 Fluid resuscitation with colloid or crystalloid solutions in critically ill patients: a systematic review of randomised trials. *British Medical Journal* 316: 961–964

56. Cochrane Injuries Group Albumin Reviewers. Human albumin administration

in critically ill patients: systematic review of randomised controlled trials. *British Medical Journal* 1998; 317: 235–240

57. Martin C, Papazian L, Perrin G, Saux P, Gouin F 1993 Norepinephrine or dopamine for the treatment of hyperdynamic septic shock? *Chest* 103: 1826–1831

58. Martin C, Viviand X, Leone M, Thirion X 2000 Effect of norepinephrine on the outcome of septic shock. *Critical Care Medicine* 28: 2758–2765

59. Bellomo R, Chapman M, Finfer S, Hickling K, Myburgh J 2000 Low-dose dopamine in patients with early renal dysfunction: a placebo-controlled randomised trial. Australian and New Zealand Intensive Care Society (ANZICS) Clinical Trials Group. *Lancet* 356: 2139–2143

60. Levin M, Quint PA, Goldstein B et al 2000 Recombinant bactericidal/permeability-increasing protein (rBPI21) as adjunctive treatment for children with severe meningococcal sepsis: a randomised trial. rBPI21 Meningococcal Sepsis Study Group. *Lancet* 356: 961–967

61. Mouthon L, Kaveri SV, Spalter SH et al 1996 Mechanisms of action of intravenous immune globulin in immune-mediated diseases. *Clinical and Experimental Immunology* 104(Suppl. 1): 3–9

62. Norrby-Teglund A, Stevens DL 1998 Novel therapies in streptococcal toxic shock syndrome: attenuation of virulence factor expression and modulation of the host response. *Current Opinion in Infectious Diseases* 11: 285–291

63. Werdan K, Pilz G 1996 Supplemental immune globulins in sepsis: a critical appraisal. *Clinical and Experimental Immunology* 104(Suppl. 1): 83–90

64. Kaul R, McGeer A, Norrby-Teglund A et al 1999 Intravenous immunoglobulin therapy in streptococcal toxic shock syndrome – a comparative observational study. *Clinical Infectious Diseases* 28: 800–807

65. Abraham E 1999 Why immunomodulatory therapies have not worked in sepsis. *Intensive Care Medicine* 25: 556–566

66. Cohen J 1999 Adjunctive therapy in sepsis: a critical analysis of the clinical trial programme. *British Medical Bulletin* 55: 212–225

67. Lynn WA, Cohen J 1995 Adjunctive therapy for septic shock: a review of experimental approaches. *Clinical Infectious Diseases* 20: 143–158

68. Schneider AJ, Voerman HJ 1991 Abrupt hemodynamic improvement in late septic shock with physiological doses of glucocorticoids. *Intensive Care Medicine* 17: 436–437

69. Bollaert PE, Charpentier C, Levy B, Debouverie M, Audibert G, Larcan A 1998 Reversal of late septic shock with supraphysiologic doses of hydrocortisone. *Critical Care Medicine* 26: 645–650

70. Briegel J, Forst H, Haller M et al 1999 Stress doses of hydrocortisone reverse hyperdynamic septic shock: a prospective, randomized, double-blind, single-center study. *Critical Care Medicine* 27: 723–732

71. Borovikova LV, Ivanova S, Zhang M et al 2000 Vagus nerve stimulation attenuates the systemic inflammatory response to endotoxin. *Nature* 405: 458–462

72. Thijs LG 2000 Coagulation inhibitor replacement in sepsis is a potentially useful clinical approach. *Critical Care Medicine* 28(Suppl. 9): S68–S73

73. Bernard GR, Vincent JL, Laterre PF et al 2001 Efficacy and safety of recombinant human activated protein C for severe sepsis. *New England Journal of Medicine* 344: 699–709

74. Bernard G, Hartman D, Heltebrand J, Fisher C 1999 Recombinant human activated protein C (rhAPC) produces a trend toward improvement in morbidity and 28-day survival in patients with severe sepsis. *Critical Care Medicine* 27: A33

75. Esmon CT 2000 Regulation of blood coagulation. *Biochimica Biophysica Acta* 1477: 349–360

76. Schmidt-Supprian M, Murphy C, While B et al 2000 Activated protein C inhibits tumor necrosis factor and macrophage migration inhibitory factor production in monocytes. *European Cytokine Network* 11: 407–413

77. Kieft H, Hoepelman AI, Zhou W, Rozenberg-Arska M, Struyvenberg A, Verhoef J 1993 The sepsis syndrome in a Dutch university hospital. Clinical observations. *Archives of Internal Medicine* 153: 2241–2247

78. Hebert PC, Drummond AJ, Singer J, Bernard GR, Russell JA 1993 A simple multiple system organ failure scoring system predicts mortality of patients who have sepsis syndrome. *Chest* 104: 230–235

79. Bone RC 1992 Modulators of coagulation. A critical appraisal of their role in sepsis. *Archives of Internal Medicine* 152: 1381–1389

80. Kotb M 1995 Bacterial pyrogenic exotoxins as superantigens. *Clinical Microbiology Reviews* 8: 411–426

 Further information

Abraham E, Arcaroli J, Carmody A, Wang H, Tracey KJ 2000 HMG-1 as a mediator of acute lung inflammation. *Journal of Immunology* 165(6): 2950–2954

Abraham E, Matthay MA, Dinarello CA et al 2000 Consensus conference definitions for sepsis, septic shock, acute lung injury, and acute respiratory distress syndrome: time for a reevaluation. *Critical Care Medicine* 28(1): 232–235

Baue AE 2000 A debate on the subject 'Are SIRS and MODS important entities in the clinical evaluation of patients?' The con position. *Shock* 14(6): 590–593

Ben Nasr A, Herwald H, Sjobring U, Renne T, Muller-Esterl W, Bjorck L 1997 Absorption of kininogen from human plasma by Streptococcus pyogenes is followed by the release of bradykinin. *Biochemical Journal* 326(3): 657–660

Boman HG 2000 Innate immunity and the normal microflora. *Immunology Reviews* 173: 5–16

Calandra T, Spiegel LA, Metz CN, Bucala R 1998 Macrophage migration inhibitory factor is a critical mediator of the activation of immune cells by exotoxins of Gram-positive bacteria. *Proceedings of the National Academy of Science of the USA* 95(19): 11383–11388

Conner BD, Bernard GR 2000 Acute respiratory distress syndrome. Potential pharmacologic interventions. *Clinical Chest Medicine* 21(3): 563–587

Esmon C 2000 The protein C pathway. *Critical Care Medicine* 28(Suppl. 9): S44–S48

Esmon CT 2000 The endothelial cell protein C receptor. *Thrombosis and Haemostasis* 83(5): 639–643

Green J, Lynn WA 2000 Presentation and clinical features of severe sepsis. *Journal of the Royal College of Physicians of London* 34(5): 418–423

Herwald H, Collin M, Muller-Esterl W, Bjorck L 1996 Streptococcal cysteine proteinase releases kinins: a virulence mechanism. *Journal of Experimental Medicine* 184(2): 665–673

Heumann D, Glauser MP, Calandra T 1998 Molecular basis of host-pathogen interaction in septic shock. *Current Opinion in Microbiology* 1(1): 49–55

Hoffman JN, Faist E 2000 Coagulation inhibitor replacement during sepsis: useless? *Critical Care Medicine* 28(Suppl. 9): S74–S76

Kimbrell DA, Beutler B 2001 The evolution and genetics of innate immunity. *Nature Reviews in Genetics* 2(4): 256–267

Kotb M 1998 Superantigens of gram-positive bacteria: structure-function analyses and their implications for biological activity. *Current Opinion in Microbiology* 1(1): 56–65

Krutzik SR, Sieling PA, Modlin RL 2001 The role of Toll-like receptors in host defense against microbial infection. *Current Opinion in Immunology* 13(1): 104–108

Le Roy D, Di Padova F, Tees R et al 1999 Monoclonal antibodies to murine lipopolysaccharide (LPS)-binding protein (LBP) protect mice from lethal endotoxemia by blocking either the binding of LPS to LBP or the presentation of LPS/LBP complexes to CD14. *Journal of Immunology* 162(12): 7454–7460

Lee WL, Downey GP 2000 Coagulation inhibitors in sepsis and disseminated intravascular coagulation. *Intensive Care Medicine* 26(11): 1701–1706

Levi M 2000 Keep in contact: the role of the contact system in infection and sepsis. *Critical Care Medicine* 28(11): 3765–3766

Liaw PC, Neuenschwander PF, Smirnov MD, Esmon CT 2000 Mechanisms by which soluble endothelial cell protein C receptor modulates protein C and activated protein C function. *Journal of Biological Chemistry* 275(8): 5447–5452

Marshall JC 2000 SIRS and MODS: what is their relevance to the science and practice of intensive care? *Shock* 14(6): 586–589

Nasraway SA 2000 Norepinephrine: no more 'leave 'em dead'? *Critical Care Medicine* 28(8): 3096–3098

Norrby-Teglund A, Lustig R, Kotb M 1997 Differential induction of Th1 versus Th2 cytokines by group A streptococcal toxic shock syndrome isolates. *Infection and Immunity* 65(12): 5209–5215

Norrby-Teglund A, Basma H, Andersson J, McGeer A, Low DE, Kotb M 1998 Varying titers of neutralizing antibodies to streptococcal superantigens in different preparations of normal polyspecific immunoglobulin G: implications for therapeutic efficacy. *Clinical Infectious Diseases* 26(3): 631–638

Norrby-Teglund A, Chatellier S, Low DE, McGeer A, Green K, Kotb M 2000 Host variation in cytokine responses to superantigens determine the severity of invasive group A streptococcal infection. *European Journal of Immunology* 30(11): 3247–3255

Norrby-Teglund A, Ihendyane N, Kansal R et al 2000 Relative neutralizing activity in polyspecific IgM, IgA, and IgG preparations against group A streptococcal superantigens. *Clinical Infectious Diseases* 31(5): 1175–1182

Petros A, Schindler M, Pierce C, Jacobe S, Mok Q 1998 Human albumin administration in critically ill patients. Evidence needs to be shown in paediatrics. *British Medical Journal* 317(7162): 882

Shibata M, Kumar SR, Amar A et al 2001 Anti-inflammatory, antithrombotic, and neuroprotective effects of activated protein C in a murine model of focal ischemic stroke. *Circulation* 103(13): 1799–1805

Sieling PA, Modlin RL 2001 Activation of toll-like receptors by microbial lipoproteins. *Scandinavian Journal of Infectious Diseases* 33(2): 97–100

Sriskandan S, Cohen J 2000 Kallikrein-kinin system activation in streptococcal toxic shock syndrome. *Clinical Infectious Diseases* 30(6): 961–962

Sriskandan S, Kemball-Cook G, Moyes D, Canvin J, Tuddenham E, Cohen J 2000 Contact activation in shock caused by invasive group A Streptococcus pyogenes. *Critical Care Medicine* 28(11): 3684–3691

Taylor FB Jr, Chang A, Esmon CT, D'Angelo A, Vigano-D'Angelo S, Blick KE 1987 Protein C prevents the coagulopathic and lethal effects of *Escherichia coli* infusion in the baboon. *Journal of Clinical Investigation* 79(3): 918–925

Taylor FB Jr, Peer GT, Lockhart MS, Ferrell G, Esmon CT 2001 Endothelial cell protein C receptor plays an important role in protein C activation in vivo. *Blood* 97(6): 1685–1688

Totzke G, Smolny M, Seibel M, Czechowski M, Schobersberger W, Hoffmann G 2001 Antithrombin iii enhances inducible nitric oxide synthase gene expression in vascular smooth muscle cells. *Cellular Immunology* 208(1): 1–8

Vincent JL 2000 Update on sepsis: pathophysiology and treatment. *Acta Clinica Belgica* 55(2): 79–87

Vincent JL 2000 New therapeutic implications of anticoagulation mediator replacement in sepsis and acute respiratory distress syndrome. *Critical Care Medicine* 28(Suppl. 9): S83–S85

Vincent JL, Spapen H, Bakker J, Webster NR, Curtis L 2000 Phase II multicenter clinical study of the platelet-activating factor receptor antagonist BB-882 in the treatment of sepsis. *Critical Care Medicine* 28(3): 638–642

Vincent JL, Thijs L, Artigas A, Marshall J, Suter P 2000 Roundtable II: clinical implications of anticoagulation mediator replacement in sepsis and acute respiratory distress syndrome. *Critical Care Medicine* 28(Suppl. 9): S86–S87

Walport MJ 2001 Advances in immunology: Complement (First of two parts). *New England Journal of Medicine* 344(14): 1058–1066

White B, Livingstone W, Murphy C, Hodgson A, Rafferty M, Smith OP 2000 An open-label study of the role of adjuvant hemostatic support with protein C replacement therapy in purpura fulminans-associated meningococcemia. *Blood* 96(12): 3719–3724

Wray GM, Foster SJ, Hinds CJ, Thiemermann C 2001 A cell wall component from pathogenic and non-pathogenic gram-positive bacteria (peptidoglycan) synergises with endotoxin to cause the release of tumour necrosis factor-alpha, nitric oxide production, shock, and multiple organ injury/dysfunction in the rat. *Shock* 15(2): 135–142

42 Abdominal and other surgical infections

E. W. Taylor

Wound infection remains a common postoperative complication. These, and other infective complications such as intra-abdominal abscess, pneumonia, urinary tract infections and septicemia, may lead to the death of the patient. It has been estimated that over half of the patients who die in surgical intensive care units die of infective complications. Much work has been done to define the optimum prophylactic antibiotic regimen that will reduce the incidence of postoperative infection.

Many patients present with community-acquired infection or the infective complications of naturally occurring pathology such as osteomyelitis, perinephric abscess, pancreatitis, salpingitis and appendicitis. It is important to segregate these from subsequent, hospital-acquired infections when auditing the incidence of postoperative infections. Audit of surgical wound infection may become a hospital quality assurance indicator and has become an essential activity in many hospitals. But audit remains problematic, requiring agreed definitions of infection, analysis of risk factors and a validated method of surveillance after the patient has left hospital, post-discharge surveillance. Some published definitions have relied upon culture of the infecting organism, but this presupposes that a suitable specimen for culture is always sent, that laboratory facilities are available to confirm the infection, and that the isolation of an organism equates to clinical infection. This is clearly not so and most authorities feel that in most circumstances the diagnosis of superficial wound infection can be made on clinical grounds alone.[1] The definitions most commonly used are those published by the American Centers for Disease Control and Prevention (CDC).[2] The diagnosis of deep, cavity infection or infection around prosthetic implants can be more complex.

The CDC have shown that surveillance of patients for 30 days will identify 98% of superficial postoperative infections if there is no prosthetic implant, while up to 1 year's surveillance is required if there has been an implant. The increasing trend towards early discharge from hospital means that the signs and symptoms of an infection may develop only after the patient has left hospital, which accentuates the need for post-discharge surveillance. For example

Law et al found the rate of clean wound infection to be 1.3% in hospital,[3] but an additional 4% of patients developed infection after leaving hospital. Although there is a clear need for post-discharge surveillance if the true rate of postoperative infection is to be determined, the optimal method by which this is performed remains controversial.[2] Many methods have been assessed – special patient review clinics, review of patients at home by specially trained nurses, postal questionnaires, telephone calls with or without subsequent clinical review, review of general practitioners' notes, and review of antibiotic drug prescriptions.[3]

Each method has its advocates and its detractors. All methods are expensive and time consuming. Clearly, if results are to be comparable there must be a common definition of wound infection and the patient groups and category of operation must be comparable. Many patients have immunosuppressive diseases or are taking drugs that modify their body's immune status; risk factors for infection. Any audit of postoperative infection must take these risk factors into account.

While wound infection may be a primary event the discharge of a hematoma, seroma, collection of bile or gastrointestinal content, urine or cerebrospinal fluid (CSF) may leak through the wound, and bacteria will be isolated from this discharge. However these 'wound infections' represent an infection secondary to the underlying complication rather than a primary wound infection.

ETIOLOGY OF POSTOPERATIVE INFECTION

The risk of infection after an operation is a balance between

- the bacterial contamination of the operating field
- the extent to which tissue damage occurs or foreign bodies are implanted at the time of the operation and
- the ability of the patient's body to resist these threats.

BACTERIAL CONTAMINATION

Bacteria contaminating the wound or deep tissues of the body at operation may be either exogenous or endogenous in origin. *Exogenous* contamination may be airborne or transferred from the surgical team at operation. Many of the rituals and practices within the operating theatre have evolved in an attempt to prevent exogenous contamination. This preventative approach perhaps reached its peak with the development of the laminar air-flow systems with high efficiency particle air (HEPA) bacterial filters, total body exhaust systems and no-touch technique favored in some orthopedic units where ultra-clean prosthetic implant surgery is performed. However, there is little scientific evidence to show that the use of caps, masks, gloves or overshoes alters the infection rate after most non-implant operations. There is little doubt that most postoperative infections are caused by organisms *endogenous* to the patient.

The type of organism contaminating the wound also influences the incidence of infection. Some are more pathogenic and virulent than others. Endogenous bacteria rarely proliferate in normal tissue[4] but grow readily in the presence of damaged tissue or foreign bodies. In addition, bacteria may act synergistically to create abscesses; the presence of both aerobic and anaerobic bacteria promotes abscess formation, whereas each alone cause little morbidity.[5]

TISSUE DAMAGE

The proliferation of endogenous bacteria is dependent upon a degree of tissue damage, which will vary greatly from wound to wound, operation to operation and (perhaps more importantly) from surgeon to surgeon. The importance of delicate handling of the tissues and competent surgical technique cannot be overemphasized. A wound left with a seroma or hematoma provides an ideal culture medium for bacterial growth, as does tissue traumatized by overtight sutures, for example.

Many operations use prosthetic, non-absorbable materials which radically reduce the number of organisms necessary to create infection.[6] Suction or open drains inserted into the wound or into body cavities to drain fluids probably increase the risk of infection, both by providing a portal of entry for bacteria and by acting as foreign bodies.[7]

HOST RESISTANCE

The ability of the patient to resist the bacterial contamination that occurs at operation is the other major determinant of postoperative infection. Some of the many factors that influence host resistance are shown in Box 42.1. The role of blood transfusion in reducing immunocompetence has been well documented; it has long been known that blood transfusion reduces rejection after renal transplantation and there is evidence that transfusion increases the risk of recurrent tumor after cancer operations.[8–9] The influence on postoperative infection, however, was first highlighted by Tartter,[10] while Jensen et al[11] reported 28% incidence of infection after colorectal surgery if the patient received a perioperative blood transfusion, compared with 2% if no blood was transfused. This effect occurred when whole blood was transfused but not with red cell concentrates. Braga et al[12] found transfusion of more than 1000 ml of blood to be an independent risk factor for infection in 285 patients undergoing operations for gastrointestinal cancer.

Box 42.1 Factors reducing host resistance

- Extremes of age
- Obesity
- Malnutrition
- Cirrhosis
- Uremia
- Diabetes mellitus
- Malignancy
- Burns
- Splenectomy
- Corticosteroids
- Cytotoxic drugs
- AIDS
- Immunosuppressive diseases
- Acute infections
- Foreign bodies
- Blood transfusion

INCIDENCE OF INFECTION

The classification of operations into clean, clean-contaminated, contaminated and dirty has become internationally accepted, and the audit by Cruse and Foord[13] documents the influence this has on infection (Table 42.1). However, this classification takes into account only the presumed bacterial contamination and the distinction between clean-contaminated and contaminated can become arbitrary and subjective. Haley et al[14] assessed a number of risk factors in 59 352 patients and compared the results with the standard classification. They found only four significant risk factors: operations lasting more than 2 h, abdominal operations, operations classified as contaminated or dirty, and patients who had three or more recorded concomitant diagnoses. There was better correlation between the incidence of infection and the number of patient risk factors than with the standard classification of bacteriological contamination. Culver et al,[15] in a further assessment of risk factors in 84 961 patients, showed that the duration of

Table 42.1 Influence of bacterial contamination on postoperative infection[13]

Category	No. of patients	No. infected	%
Clean	73 589	1002	1.4
Clean-contaminated	14 018	879	6.3
Contaminated	9085	1211	13.3
Dirty	3038	1310	39.9
Total	100 000	4412	4.4

operation at which risk increased was dependent on the type of surgery performed, and showed that it was possible to replace the factor '3 or more concomitant diagnoses' with the American Society of Anesthesiology's (ASA) grading of fitness for operation. These analyses of risk, in such large cohorts of patients, suggest that some assessment of patient risk factors should be introduced into all future trials or audits of postoperative infection. The wound class, duration of operation and preoperative ASA status are now frequently used as risk factor indicators for audit. However, the data given by Culver[15] on the duration of operation is taken from the findings in the USA and has not been validated in other countries.

ANTIBIOTIC PROPHYLAXIS

The aim of antibiotic prophylaxis is to reduce the incidence of postoperative infection when bacterial contamination of the tissues at operation is inevitable or occurs unexpectedly.[16] The principal role of prophylaxis is to reduce the incidence of wound infection, but other forms of operation-related infection, particularly intra-abdominal abscess, septicemia and death, may also be reduced. The evidence that antibiotics reduce the incidence of respiratory and urinary tract infections is not so impressive.

Prophylaxis must be distinguished from *therapy*. Patients presenting with an infective problem for which an urgent operation is performed require antibiotic therapy to treat the established infection. Antibiotics may reduce the incidence of wound infection, but this is a secondary benefit. The type of antibiotic, the regimen and route of administration should all be chosen to treat the original infection and should be considered therapeutic, not prophylactic.

CHOICE OF ANTIBIOTIC

The prophylactic antibiotic should be active against those organisms most likely to contaminate the wound. While *Staphylococcus aureus* and other skin organisms represent the main contaminating organism from the environment, it is usually the organisms colonizing the body tract or cavity opened during the operation that cause postoperative infection, and it is these organisms that determine the prophylactic regimen. The choice of antibiotic regimen will depend upon the site of operation and the likely bacterial contaminants (Table 42.2).

Some authors have suggested that the prophylactic regimen should differ from that used for a subsequent postoperative infection.[17] Thus, in the USA cefalotin (cefalothin) and cefoxitin are widely used for prophylaxis, retaining cefotaxime, ceftazidine, piperacillin and the carbapenems for therapy. This is based on the assumption that postoperative infections are likely to be caused by organisms resistant to the antibiotic used for prophylaxis. However, there is little evidence to support this

view, which would be more credible if prolonged courses of antibiotic prophylaxis were adopted, thus selecting out resistant strains. Changes in susceptibility patterns of postoperative infections have not been documented where single-dose prophylaxis is used.

Cost

The cost of antibiotic prophylaxis is important, but must be seen in the context of cost versus benefit. If a cheaper antibiotic is less effective, the cost of consequent infections may far outweigh the cost of a more expensive but more effective agent. Lazorthes et al[18] randomized 162 patients undergoing groin hernia repair to receive a single dose of cefamandole and 162 patients to receive placebo. No patient receiving the antibiotic (which cost approximately US$500) developed infection, whereas seven of the patients receiving placebo developed wound infections, for which the treatment cost was approximately US$5000. However, if 10 doses (3–5 days') 'prophylaxis' had been given instead of single dose this cost benefit would have been lost.

Adverse reactions

The other major factor in the choice of the prophylactic antibiotic regimen is safety. Penicillin sensitivity and its cross-sensitivity with the cephalosporins, renal and ototoxicity with the aminoglycosides, and the development of pseudomembranous colitis with the expanded-spectrum cephalosporins (group 4; *see* Ch 15) are examples. Once again, the incidence of these complications is minimal with the use of single-dose prophylaxis.

TIME OF ADMINISTRATION

The antibiotic should be administered so that there is a high circulating blood level (and hence tissue concentrations) at the time of the operation. In practice this means the antibiotic should be given either intramuscularly with any premedication 1 h before surgery or intravenously on induction of anesthesia. Should contamination occur unexpectedly during the course of the operation, additional appropriate antibiotic(s) should be administered immediately. The importance of timing of administration of prophylaxis on the incidence of infection has been demonstrated by Classen et al.[19] Where the antibiotic was administered more than 2 h preoperatively or more than 3 h postoperatively, the infection rates were significantly higher than when the antibiotic was given perioperatively (3.8% and 3.3% compared with 0.4% infection).

DURATION OF PROPHYLAXIS

The duration of antibiotic prophylaxis has proved controversial. Increasing evidence suggests that single-dose prophylaxis is adequate for all operations, except where there is blood

Table 42.2 Antibiotic prophylaxis

Type of operation	Principal pathogens	Antibiotic regimens and doses recommended*	
Clean operations			
In hospitals without endemic MRSA			
Implanted prosthesis	*Staphylococcus* spp. including MRSA	Amoxicillin–clavulanic acid	1.2 g i.v.
Other clean operations for which prophylaxis is indicated		Flucloxacillin	2 g i.v.
		with gentamicin	2 mg/kg i.v.
		Cefazolin	1 g i.v.
		Cefuroxime	1.5 g i.v.
In hospitals with endemic MRSA		Glycopeptide e.g. vancomycin	1 g i.v. infusion over 60 min
For penicillin-allergic patients	(Clindamycin)	(600 mg i.v.)	
		(Clarithromycin	(500 mg i.v.)
		with gentamicin)	(2 mg/kg i.v.)
Clean-contaminated operations			
Head and neck			
(if sinus, nasal, oral or pharyngeal mucosa breached)	Staphylococci Streptococci Oral anaerobes	Amoxicillin–clavulanic acid	1.2 g i.v.
		Cefuroxime	1.5 g i.v.
		with metronidazole	500 mg i.v.
		Cefazolin	1 g i.v.
		with metronidazole	500 mg i.v.
		(Clindamycin)	(600 mg i.v.)
Thoracic			
Bronchial	Staphylococci	Amoxicillin–clavulanic acid	1.2 g i.v.
Esophageal	Streptococci GNAB Oral anaerobes	Cefuroxime	1.5 g i.v.
		with metronidazole	500 mg i.v.
		(Cefuroxime	(1.5 g i.v.)
		with metronidazole)	(500 mg i.v.)
Upper gastrointestinal			
Gastric	GNAB	Amoxicillin–clavulanic acid	1.2 g i.v.
		Gentamicin	5 mg/kg
		with metronidazole	500 mg i.v.
		Clarithromycin	500 mg i.v.
		Cefazolin	1 g i.v.
		(Cefuroxime)	(1.5 g i.v.)
Biliary	GNAB	Amoxicillin–clavulanic acid	1.2 g i.v.
ERCP	? Enterococci	Piperacillin	2 g i.v.
		with gentamicin	2 mg/kg i.v.
		Cefazolin	1 g i.v.
		(Cefuroxime)	(1.5 g i.v.)
		(Vancomycin)	(1 g i.v. infusion over 1 h)
Urology			
TURP	GNAB Enterococci	Amoxicillin–clavulanic acid	1.2 g i.v.
		Gentamicin	2 mg/kg i.v.
		(Ciprofloxacin)	(500 mg orally with premed)
Obstetrics and gynecology			
Hysterectomy	GNAB *Bacteroides* spp.	Amoxicillin–clavulanic acid	1 g i.v.
		Gentamicin	2 mg/kg i.v.
		with metronidazole	500 mg/kg i.v.
		Cefazolin	1 g i.v.
		with metronidazole	500 mg i.v.
		Cefotetan	1 g i.v.
		(Clindamycin)	(600 mg i.v.)

Table 42.2 Continued

Type of operation	Principal pathogens	Antibiotic regimens and doses recommended*	
Cesarean section	β-hemolytic streptococci *Bacteroides* spp Enterococci *Staph. aureus* *Chlamydia*[†]	Options as above	As above
Amputation	*Clostridium* spp.	Benzylpenicillin with gentamicin and metronidazole (Clarithromycin) (and metronidazole)	1.2 g i.v. 2 mg/kg i.v. 500 mg i.v. (500 mg i.v.) (500 mg i.v.)
Contaminated operations *Colorectal* Elective operations	GNAB *Bacteroides fragilis*	Amoxicillin–clavulanic acid	1.2 g i.v.
		Amoxicillin with Gentamicin and metronidazole Cefazolin with metronidazole Cefotetan (Cefuroxime) (with metronidazole)	1 g i.v. 2 mg/kg i.v. 500 mg i.v. 1 g i.v. 500 mg i.v. 1 g i.v. (1.5 g i.v.) (500 mg i.v.)
Intestinal obstruction	*Bacteroides* spp. GNAB	Options as above	As above
Compound trauma (within 4 h)	Other anaerobes *Staph. aureus* GNAB *Bacillus* spp.	Penicillin and gentamicin and metronidazole (Clarithromycin) with metronidazole	1.2–2.4 g 5 mg/kg i.v. 500 mg i.v. (500 mg i.v.) (500 mg i.v.)

*The evidence indicates, that single-dose prophylaxis is adequate, although some surgeons administer antibiotic prophylaxis for 24 hours.
[†]is not an acute surgical infection risk although it may be spread by surgery. If prophylaxis is considered appropriate azithromycin 1 g is recommended
ERCP, Endoscopic retrograde cholangiopancreatogram; GNAB, Gram-negative aerobic bacteria; MRSA, methicillin resistant *Staphylococcus aureus*; TURP, Transurethral prostatectomy.
Antibiotics shown in brackets are replacements for β-lactam antibiotics in the above regimen for patients allergic to penicillin.

loss in excess of 1.5 l for an adult patient, or the operation lasts for more than 2 h. Rowe-Jones et al[20] randomized 943 patients to receive cefotaxime (1 g intravenously) with metronidazole (0.5 g intravenously) on induction of anesthesia, or cefuroxime (1.5 g intravenously) with metronidazole 0.5 g intravenous preoperatively followed by two further doses at 8 and 16 h postoperatively. There was no statistically significant difference between the groups: mortality rates were 5.5 and 6.6% respectively, and incidence of wound infection 7.1 and 7.3%. Strachan et al[21] found no difference between one dose and 5 days' prophylaxis in biliary-tract surgery; Turano et al[22] no difference between one and three doses of cefotaxime in 273 patients having abdominal, gynecological and urological operations; Bates et al[23] no difference between one and three doses of amoxicillin–clavulanate in patients undergoing at-risk abdominal surgery; and Jensen et al[11] no difference between

one and three doses in colorectal surgery. A number of other studies have confirmed that a single dose is as effective as multidose prophylaxis, even in implant surgery.[24–27]

The effect of the duration of operation on the incidence of infection has been investigated extensively by Culver et al[15] and varies from operation to operation, but a procedure lasting longer than 2 h is a good general indicator of the need for a second dose of prophylactic antibiotic. This is governed by the half-life of many antibiotics or, where there is extensive blood loss, by falling drug concentrations. Even in the severely immunocompromised there is no evidence that more prolonged antibiotic prophylaxis is of benefit.[28] Prolonged prophylaxis is one of the major areas of antibiotic misuse and contributes to the development of drug resistance. Strict adherence to well constructed antibiotic policies is important for its control.

ROUTE OF ADMINISTRATION

Antibiotic prophylaxis is usually administered intravenously or occasionally intramuscularly, but has also been given subcutaneously in the area of the incision.[29,30] This route certainly provides a high level of the antibiotic in the region of the wound, but there is little evidence that this is more effective than giving the antibiotic parenterally. It has also been suggested that a suitable antibiotic can be given orally[31] for some operations. This may well be less expensive than the parenteral route, but presumes that the antibiotic is given on time, to a compliant patient, that there is satisfactory absorption of the drug, and that the operating list runs to time. A change may occur to any one of these factors, unknown to the surgeon. For this reason it is recommended that prophylaxis is administered intravenously on induction of anesthesia.

WHICH PATIENTS SHOULD RECEIVE ANTIBIOTIC PROPHYLAXIS?

It has been traditional teaching that patients should receive antibiotic prophylaxis only if a bacterially colonized tract or cavity will be opened at operation. In addition, those patients undergoing prosthetic implant procedures, neurosurgical or cardiothoracic operations often receive antibiotic prophylaxis because, although the incidence of infection is low, any resulting infection can be quite catastrophic. However, this teaching has been challenged by Platt et al,[32] who compared cefonicid and placebo in patients undergoing non-implant breast surgery and groin hernia repairs in a large multicenter study. Whilst the incidence of overall infection was low the outcome favored the group receiving the antibiotic (4.5% versus 8.1%); the study was sufficiently large (1218 patients) to render the difference in the overall incidence of infection statistically significant ($p < 0.01$). However, the incidence of wound infection alone (1.9% versus 1.3% in hernia and 8.6% versus 5.6% in breast operations) was not significantly different and other studies to assess the benefit of prophylactic antibiotics in clean, non-implant operations have not confirmed any benefit (Taylor et al[33] found no benefit in a study of 586 groin hernia repair operations and Gupta et al[34] found no benefit in 334 non-implant breast operations).

SELECTIVE DECONTAMINATION OF THE DIGESTIVE TRACT

Selective decontamination of the digestive tract (SDD) was developed as an attempt to reduce the incidence of morbidity and mortality resulting from nosocomial infection by Gram-negative aerobic bacilli (GNAB) in patients treated in intensive care units (ICU). The intention was to remove the GNAB and yeasts from the oropharynx and upper and lower gastrointestinal tract using non-absorbable antibiotics, thus reducing the colonization and infection of the lungs and other tissues

by these organisms (the topic is discussed in more detail in Ch. 44). Although the incidence of nosocomial pneumonia has been reduced by this regimen, a reduction in overall mortality has been less easy to demonstrate. The difficulty would appear to be related to the time it takes to eradicate the GNAB from the gastrointestinal tract: in these very sick patients it can take 5–10 days, by which time the organisms have already caused the infections from which the patients die. Two recently published meta-analyses of trials of SDD[35,36] have shown significant reduction in mortality in critically ill patients, but Webb[37] has expressed concern about the impact on antibiotic resistance of such use. He notes that other methods of preventing ventilator-associated pneumonia such as gastric nutrition, subglottic aspiration, semielevated positioning and continuous lateral rotation of the patient carry no such risks and have yet to be evaluated in comparison with SDD. Ebner et al[38] echo Webb's concern. However, SDD has been advocated for use prophylactically[39] with some persuasive literature, but failure to demonstrate clear evidence for a reduction in mortality has been the cause of much controversy.

Most organisms causing postoperative wound and other nosocomial infections arise from the gastrointestinal tract. Certainly the organisms responsible for the development of septicemia, multiple organ failure and overwhelming sepsis would appear to derive from the colon, which has been described as the 'motor' of multiple organ failure.[40] The colonic flora contains both aerobic and anaerobic organisms, which act synergistically to produce postoperative intra-abdominal infection. Preoperative eradication of the anaerobic bacteria from the colon would probably not be possible in view of the large number of organisms involved, and is not desirable because of the influence these organisms have on colonization resistance.[41] However, the smaller number of GNAB in the colon *can* be eradicated, or greatly suppressed, by standard SDD therapy or by use of fluoroquinolones,[42] and thus rendered unable to cause infection by direct contamination of the tissues, by synergy with anaerobic organisms or by bacterial translocation. This approach has been favorably assessed in cardiopulmonary bypass operations,[43] esophageal surgery,[44] liver transplantation,[45–46] small-bowel transplantation[48] and in colorectal surgery.[49]

ANTIBIOTIC THERAPY

Many emergency surgical procedures are undertaken in patients who present with primary infective pathology. In some situations surgical treatment of this infection is all that is required and, particularly in patients with superficial or deep abscesses, drainage of the abscess alone without antibiotic therapy may suffice. Antibiotics may be required when there is contamination of peritoneal or pleural cavities, cellulitis, lymphangitis or septicemia. In these situations an empirical, 'best-guess', antibiotic regimen is necessary[50] and can be modified subsequently in the light of laboratory information. The importance of bacteriological assessment of the infection and modification of the antibiotic therapy in light of the cultures is demonstrated by the audits reported by Mosdell et al[51] and Davey et al.[52] Patients receiving inappropriate empiric therapy have worse outcomes in terms of length of stay, need for reoperation, incidence of wound infection and mortality.

As with antibiotic prophylaxis, there is increasing evidence that short-course, high-dose therapy is at least as effective as the prolonged, 7–14 day therapy previously administered. This is particularly so where the focus of infection has been dealt with surgically as in patients with appendicitis, perforated colon, or penetrating or blunt abdominal trauma in whom the infecting lesion has been removed. In the case of abdominal trauma 12–24 h therapy is adequate; Oreskovich et al[53] compared 12 h with 5-day antibiotic therapy with penicillin G and doxycycline in 81 evaluable patients and found no difference in the average number of days with fever, the need for additional antibiotics or infective complications. Fabian et al[54] also compared 1-day with 5-day therapy in a randomized study of 285 patients who had sustained abdominal trauma. The colon had been injured in 15% of patients. There was no significant difference in the mortality (3% in each group) or in the incidence of abdominal infections (8% and 10%). Where the infective pathology cannot or has not been surgically eliminated, such as in patients with infected osteomyelitis, pancreatitis, salpingitis, cholangitis or diverticulitis, longer courses of therapy may be necessary.

HEAD AND NECK SURGERY

PROPHYLAXIS

Operations that breach the mucosa of the mouth or pharynx or which enter the antra or paranasal sinuses expose the tissues to the normal flora of these spaces. The most common pathogens are streptococci, staphylococci, GNAB and anaerobic bacteria. Head and neck operations have been classified according to the risk of postoperative wound infection (Box 42.2). GNAB have been reported in 29–82% of infected wounds[53] and probably contaminate the tissues via the nasogastric tube. Because of the wide range of infecting organisms, many different antibiotic prophylactic regimens have been adopted. A group 3 cephalosporin (Ch. 15) with metronidazole or amoxicillin–clavulanate would seem a reasonable option. Clearly, antibiotic prophylaxis would be indicated for clean-contaminated and contaminated operations, and antibiotic therapy may be necessary following the drainage of a neck abscess.

THERAPY

The neck structures are surrounded by fascial layers, between which lie a number of potential spaces infection of which may result in potentially serious or fatal complications such as

Box 42.2 Classification of head and neck operations[56]

Clean	Contaminated
Radical neck dissection	Total laryngectomy
Parotidectomy	Laryngo-pharyngectomy
Submandibular gland excision	Glossectomy
Thyroidectomy	Hemimandibulectomy
Excision of uninfected bronchial cyst	**Dirty**
	Drainage of neck abscess
Clean-contaminated	
Laryngeal fissure	
Excision laryngocele	

airway obstruction from soft tissue swelling, mediastinitis, septicemia, carotid artery hemorrhage, jugular vein thrombosis, meningitis or even cavernous sinus thrombosis.

Acute bacterial parotitis

Acute bacterial parotitis is uncommon, but may occur in elderly patients or with dehydration. *Staph. aureus* is the most common pathogen, but many organisms have been isolated and flucloxacillin, oxacillin, cefuroxime or amoxicillin–clavulanate would be appropriate choices of drug.

Peritonsillar abscess

Peritonsillar abscess or quinsy may form between the tonsil or capsule and the superior constrictor muscle of the pharynx. Again, a mixed bacterial flora is usual, which includes anaerobes. Incision and drainage is often required, although high-dose penicillin G, clindamycin or amoxicillin–clavulanate may be effective in reducing the risk of spread to fascial planes. Adequate drainage with appropriate antibiotic therapy has also reduced the need for subsequent tonsillectomy.

Parapharyngeal abscess

A parapharyngeal abscess may follow dental infection, tonsillitis or a quinsy. Such abscesses should be drained via a collar incision at the level of the hyoid bone and treated with an antibiotic regimen similar to that used to manage peritonsillar abscess.

Ludwig's angina

Ludwig's angina is a severe, acute cellulitis of the sublingual space and floor of the mouth and is frequently caused by poor dental hygiene. While the mortality has fallen from 50% to 10% since the advent of antibiotic therapy, the condition remains serious and life threatening.[57] Frequently there is little or no pus, but when organisms have been cultured these are streptococci, staphylococci or anaerobic organisms. The flora is frequently mixed and antibiotic therapy is essential. Parenteral broad-spectrum agent such as cefotaxime and metronidazole or clindamycin and gentamicin would be appropriate choices.

THORACIC AND VASCULAR SURGERY

The esophagus is normally colonized by organisms from the oropharynx and the upper respiratory tract. Esophageal operations are frequently combined with gastric surgery; in these operations, and where there is an esophageal stricture, overgrowth of both aerobic and anaerobic organisms with Enterobacteriaceae, enterococci and streptococci may occur.[58] Single-dose prophylaxis with cefuroxime, cefotaxime or piperacillin (possibly with the addition of metronidazole) or amoxicillin–clavulanate is recommended.

The lower respiratory tract is normally sterile. However, pulmonary pathology for which surgery is performed may well change this situation and antibiotic prophylaxis is standard in most thoracic units. The common infecting organisms are streptococci, staphylococci, GNAB and oral anaerobes. This is also true of empyema and lung abscesses.[59] The same antibiotics as used for esophageal surgery are recommended; a single dose is sufficient for prophylaxis, but prolonged therapy of up to 6–8 weeks may be necessary in the treatment of lung abscess (Ch. 48).

CARDIAC SURGERY

Before the advent of antibiotics, infective endocarditis (Ch. 49) had a mortality of 100%. This has been reduced to 30% by the introduction of antimicrobial agents and improved surgical techniques. The common organisms responsible are *Staph. aureus*, streptococci and coagulase-negative staphylococci, and occasionally yeasts. Surgery on the infected valve should always be covered by appropriate antimicrobial therapy (Ch. 49) and efforts made to eliminate any predisposing forms of infection such as dental disease.

Surgical technique is paramount in preventing early postoperative infection of prosthetic valves, although it is recognized that intravascular lines, pacing wires and urinary catheters provide other portals of infection. *Staph. aureus*, coagulase-negative staphylococci, streptococci and occasionally GNAB predominate (Ch. 49). Late infection of prosthetic valves may follow subsequent bacteremia, particularly from dental procedures. Methicillin-resistant *Staph. aureus* (MRSA) is becoming prevalent in many cardiac units and in the ICUs where these patients are nursed postoperatively. The influence of MRSA and prophylactic regimens are discussed in Ch. 49.

STERNOTOMY WOUND INFECTIONS AND MEDIASTINITIS

Minor wound infections may occur in up to 16% of patients following sternotomy,[60] and deep infections in 0.5–1.5% of patients.[61] The latter can produce mediastinitis, osteomyelitis, pericarditis, septicemia, disruption of coronary artery grafts, wound dehiscence, infection of prosthetic valves and possibly death. *Staph. aureus* is frequently isolated but coagulase-negative staphylococci can be important pathogens in the sternotomy site, which may contain bone debris, hematomata, bone wax and suture wires.

Superficial infections should be drained and treated with an antistaphylococcal agent such as flucloxacillin or oxacillin until microbiological information is available and MRSA excluded. Deeper infections may require aggressive surgical debridement and high-dose, long-term antibiotic therapy based on the bacterial cultures from the deep tissues and local sensitivity patterns. Where MRSA is isolated treatment with teicoplanin or vancomycin may be necessary.

Mediastinitis may complicate cardiac surgery, esophageal surgery, penetrating trauma and spontaneous or instrumental perforation. The surgical management depends upon the underlying cause and may involve thoracotomy with drainage of the mediastinum. The insertion of drains and irrigation with povidone iodine is favored by some,[62] but not others.[63] Whatever surgical management is instituted the use of broad-spectrum antibiotic therapy covering both aerobic and anaerobic organisms (e.g. cefotaxime and metronidazole, imipenem or amoxicillin–clavulanate) is mandatory, and evidence of MRSA infection should be sought.

CARDIAC PACEMAKERS

Approximately a quarter of a million cardiac pacemakers are implanted each year. Infection may occur in the pocket created to hold the pacemaker, the subcutaneous electrodes, or in the tissues surrounding the leads.[64] As might be expected the incidence of infection is higher for temporary, external pacemakers (1–5%) than for permanent pacemakers (1%).[65] *Staph. aureus* and *Staphylococcus epidermidis* are the predominant pathogens. *Staph. aureus* is more common within 2 weeks of operation, whereas *Staph. epidermidis* (coagulase-negative) is more commonly associated with late infection.[66] Fungal infections are rare but usually fatal.[67]

Pacemaker pocket abscess causes swelling, erythema and discharge of pus or extrusion of the prosthesis. Bacteria, usually *Staph. aureus*, can be isolated from the blood in some patients. Mural endocarditis may ensue. Management generally requires removal of both pacemaker and leads.[66] 32 of 75 patients with infected pacemakers were treated conservatively with antibiotics, debridement and irrigation or aspiration of infected sites but all but one patient failed such therapy and required pacemaker removal. In the remaining 43 patients the infected pacemaker was treated primarily by removal, with successful resolution of the infection in all cases. Removal of the pacemaker is not a minor surgical procedure and may necessitate open heart surgery with cardiopulmonary bypass or inflow occlusion.[64]

Although antibiotics are widely used prophylactically when

implanting a pacemaker, evidence for the efficacy is difficult to obtain. The infection rate is low (around 1%) and statistically valid trials are therefore virtually impossible to undertake. Bluhm et al[68] compared flucloxacillin with placebo in a prospective double-blind trial of 106 patients and found no infection in either group, with a follow-up of up to 35 months. Similarly, Ramsdale et al[69] found no difference between patients who did receive antibiotic prophylaxis and those who did not. However, like other implant procedures, although the incidence of infection is low the complications when they do occur can be life-threatening. Therefore it would seem wise to continue the normal practice of administering single-dose prophylaxis (flucoxacillin oxacillin or amoxicillin–clavulanate are suitable agents). In units where MRSA is endemic teicoplanin or vancomycin may be needed.

VASCULAR SURGERY

The number of patients presenting with arterial disease continues to increase. Consequently, the repertoire of vascular surgical procedures and range of materials from which the implanted grafts are made has increased. Graft infections are a major problem, with considerable cost implications. Grafts to or below the groin are most vulnerable, particularly when there is distal tissue necrosis or infection.

Graft infection can be difficult to diagnose and culture of perigraft fluid is often unrewarding. Coagulase-negative staphylococci and other organisms, when present within a biofilm bound to the prosthesis, are often protected from antibiotic inactivation. Culture of these organisms may be successful only after graft removal and ultrasonication, which releases the organism.

The serious consequences of graft infection have quite reasonably led to almost universal prescribing of perioperative antibiotic prophylaxis. Antibiotics active against both *Staph. aureus* and *Staph. epidermidis* and, if the operation extends to or below the groin, against the Enterobacteriaceae, are recommended. In units where MRSA is endemic teicoplanin or vancomycin may be needed. There is little evidence to indicate that more than single-dose prophylaxis is necessary.[70]

GASTROINTESTINAL SURGERY

PROPHYLAXIS

Although operations for benign peptic ulceration have become uncommon, those for gastric malignancy continue unabated. In normal health the stomach is essentially sterile because of the high acid secretion; however, with gastric carcinoma and situations where the acidity is inhibited by drug therapy or is neutralized, bacterial overgrowth readily occurs. The stomach becomes colonized with the oral bacteria and Enterobacteriaceae so that perioperative broad-spectrum antibiotic

prophylaxis with a group 3 or 4 cephalosporin (Ch. 15), ureidopenicillin or amoxicillin–clavulanate is indicated. This is also true for small-bowel surgery. Anaerobic organisms may also be found in all these sites, especially the distal small bowel, and so metronidazole is usually added to regimens that lack anaerobic activity.

SPLENECTOMY

The problems of overwhelming postsplenectomy sepsis are well recognized (Ch. 11). In addition to the long-term risk of infection there is increasing evidence that splenectomy increases the risk of immediate postoperative infection. In 1982, Standage and Goss[71] reported an incidence of 29% morbidity (mostly infective) and 9.4% mortality in a series of 277 patients who underwent splenectomy. The majority of the deaths were from infective complications. Operative mortality occurred in 15% of patients after incidental splenectomy, which was markedly higher than the incidence after splenectomy for other pathologies. The common surgical practice of placing a drain in the splenic bed at operation may have increased the incidence of infection.[72] Despite the findings of Standage and Goss,[71] the incidence of infective complications would appear to be higher in those patients undergoing splenectomy for malignant disease than splenectomy for trauma.

BILIARY TRACT OPERATIONS

Bacterial colonization of the bile occurs with increasing age, acute cholecystitis, gallstones and in the presence of strictures of the common bile duct, whether benign or malignant. The Enterobacteriaceae and fecal streptococci predominate; anaerobes are uncommon. Endoscopic retrograde choledochopancreatography is commonly performed in situations in which the bile may be colonized, and antibiotic prophylaxis is indicated to prevent septicemia occurring during the injection of contrast media. *Pseudomonas* septicemia has been reported,[73] occasionally from organisms contaminating the bridge of the endoscope.[74]

Patients with colonized bile are at a higher risk of postoperative infection and have been recommended to receive prophylactic antibiotics. This hypothesis was tested in 644 patients who received preoperative prophylaxis with sulbactam-ampicillin.[75] The bile was found to be colonized in 121 (19% of patients) and the incidence of infection in this group was 22% (compared with 2% in patients with sterile bile; $p < 0.001$). However, more than half of the patients who had colonized bile (65 of 121) had no high-risk factor. For this reason, the authors recommended that single-dose antibiotic prophylaxis be given to all patients undergoing open cholecystectomy.[76]

The advent of laparoscopic surgery has led to a reappraisal of the need for prophylaxis. In the early reports of large series of laparoscopic cholecystectomies, the incidence of infection was exceptionally low (0.5%), and is mainly infection of the umbilical port hole, through which the gall-bladder is removed.[77–79] The reason for this difference in the incidence of infection is not clear. There is considerable evidence that postoperative infection after open cholecystectomy is caused by organisms that colonize the bile,[80] and it could be anticipated that bile contamination would be at least as high during a laparoscopic operation. However, the degree of wound tissue damage is different. Because of the low incidence of infective complications the role of antibiotic prophylaxis for laparoscopic cholecystectomy remains uncertain but a number of reports are now suggesting that it is not necessary.[81,82]

APPENDECTOMY

Appendectomy remains a common abdominal operation, performed electively for acute appendicitis, 'en passant' to another intra-abdominal procedure, or at an interval after the resolution of an appendix abscess. When performed for acute appendicitis the state of the appendix ranges from normal to perforated and releasing fecoliths into the peritoneal cavity. Histological examination of the removed appendix often shows that surgical assessment of the state of the appendix at operation is unreliable – an apparently normal appendix may have mucosal appendicitis; an inflamed appendix may be histologically perforated and an apparently purulent, perforated appendix may not in fact show transmural perforation or infarction.

As would be expected wound infection is more common in patients with a perforated or gangrenous appendix, and antibiotic therapy rather than prophylaxis is indicated. In a retrospective series of more than 1000 appendectomies, Pieper et al[83] showed an overall incidence of infective complications of 11.5%, (ranging from 5% in patients with a normal appendix to 33.6% for those with a perforated appendix). Some researchers have contended that wound infection should be uncommon in low-risk patients such as children and those from whom a normal appendix is removed:[84] in a meta-analysis of antibiotic prophylaxis studies in appendectomy, Krukowski et al[85] showed a 10.4% incidence of infection in low-risk and 34.9% infection in high-risk patients in the control (no antibiotic) groups. Thus current opinion favors the use of antimicrobial prophylaxis in all operations for acute appendicitis.

Anaerobic organisms, particularly *Bacteroides* spp., are common in wound infections after appendectomy, which has led to the widespread use of metronidazole in Europe and similar antianaerobic agents in North America. However, the results with metronidazole are not always favorable: Krukowski's meta-analysis showed an incidence of 7.4% infection in low-risk and 31.9% in high-risk patients when metronidazole alone was used, either intravenously or rectally.[85] Many studies have been performed to assess metronidazole in combination with an antibiotic active against the

aerobic flora; Krukowski's meta-analysis suggests that an infection rate of 3.8% in low-risk and 15% in high-risk patients is then achieved.[85] Wilson et al[86] assessed the value of a single perioperative dose of cefotetan (2 g) to a 5-day regimen of metronidazole per rectum: 14 (9.5%) of 148 patients receiving the metronidazole alone developed postoperative infection, whereas only three of 141 patients (2.1%) who received the cefotetan did so ($p < 0.05$). The group 3 and 4 cephalosporins and the cefamycin antibiotics have become popular prophylaxis for appendicectomy; again, Krukowski's meta-analysis has shown an infection rate of 2.9% in low-risk and 21.2% in high-risk patients when these agents are used.[85]

Many studies do not separate high- and low-risk patients: al-Dhohayan et al[87] have shown amoxicillin–clavulanate to be at least as effective as metronidazole and gentamicin; Salam et al[88] have shown piperacillin to be as effective as cefoxitin; Pokorny et al[89] found ticarcillin–clavulanate to be as effective as triple therapy with ampicillin, gentamicin and clindamycin; while Uhari et al[90] showed that imipenem–cilastatin was as effective as tobramycin and metronidazole for appendicitis in children.

Coldham et al[91] have suggested that single-dose 'prophylaxis' is appropriate and cost-effective for appendectomy, and many surgeons would be happy to consider this for low-risk patients. The duration of therapy required for high-risk patients with perforated or gangrenous appendicitis remains to be determined. Provided the infected focus has been adequately extirpated, with or without peritoneal toilet, it is likely that 24 h or 48 h therapy will be as effective, although 5 days' treatment is usually administered.

It remains to be seen what effect minimally invasive techniques for appendicitis will have on postoperative infection.[92] To date, reports on the incidence of infection after laparoscopic appendectomy would suggest that, whilst the incidence of infection is lower the overall complication rate remains unchanged.[93,94]

If infection rates are significantly lower, as has become apparent following laparoscopic cholecystectomy, then current practice may need to be reassessed. However, it should be remembered that appendectomy is usually performed for an acute, infective episode, whereas cholecystectomy is performed in an elective, non-infected situation.

COLORECTAL SURGERY

The colon, particularly the descending colon and rectum, contain the largest number of bacteria; surgery to these sites is associated with the highest incidence of postoperative infection and mortality. However, with good surgical technique the contamination of the tissues during colorectal resection should be no greater than during procedures on other areas of the gastrointestinal tract, although the synergistic interaction between aerobes and anaerobes increases the risk of infection.

Bowel preparation

Most surgeons would accept that preoperative bowel preparation is a sensible if not essential part of the preparation of a patient for elective colorectal surgery. This view has been challenged[95,96] on the grounds that there is little evidence that adequate bowel preparation reduces the bacterial contamination of the tissues at the time of operation indeed, some forms of bowel preparation, such as the osmotic cathartic mannitol 10%, have been shown to increase the viable bacterial count of the residual flora in the mucus of the colon[97]. Nevertheless, it remains normal practice in most countries to attempt to remove the bulk of fecal material from the colon before surgery. The use of oral antibiotics has become an important part of this preparation in the USA (*see below*). When operating on the obstructed colon the fecal contents can be evacuated on the operating table by irrigation using a Foley catheter inserted through the appendix stump and disposable anesthetic trunking inserted into the cut distal end of the colon, which leads the fecally contaminated irrigation fluid away from the operative field.

Oral antibiotics

Attempts have been made to reduce the bacterial contamination that occurs when the colon is transected by reducing the viable bacterial load in the gut using preoperative antibiotics. The Nichols-Condon regimen of antibiotic prophylaxis favored in the USA is neomycin 1 g and erythromycin base 1 g given at 13.00, 14.00 and 23.00 h on the day before operation.[98] Erythromycin base is used because, like neomycin, it is poorly absorbed. However, this route of antibiotic administration has not found favor in Europe,[99,100] and in practice, most colorectal surgeons in the USA (and some in Europe) combine preoperative oral administration with perioperative parenteral prophylaxis.[101]

Selective decontamination to remove or suppress GNAB in the colon preoperatively has been advocated on the basis that any contamination that occurs would then be with anaerobes only, thus preventing the synergistic interaction necessary for postoperative wound and intra-abdominal infections. Oral ciprofloxacin selectively removes GNAB from the gastro-intestinal tract within 24 h using a cathartic agent in addition to the quinolone.[102] In a subsequent large multicenter study to investigate the efficacy of this form of bowel preparation after elective colorectal surgery, the incidence of wound infection was 11% in the antibiotic group and 23% in the controls ($p < 0.001$). All patients received the same parenteral antibiotic (piperacillin 4 g) intravenously on induction of anesthesia. When all operation-related infections were taken into account, the group receiving oral ciprofloxacin had a 14.5% incidence of infection, compared with 33% in the group that did not ($p < 0.0002$).[49]

Lazorthes et al,[103] in a small study of 90 patients undergoing elective colorectal operations, found similar benefit from a combined oral and parenteral approach. They gave 30 patients

kanamycin and metronidazole orally, a further 30 patients the same drugs parenterally on induction of anesthesia and a third group of 30 patients the same drugs preoperatively by mouth and parenterally at operation. Despite the small numbers, the difference in the incidence of infection in each of the groups (30%, 23%, 3.3%) was statistically significant ($p < 0.01$). However, Lau et al,[104] in a study of 194 patients undergoing elective colorectal surgery for carcinoma, randomized patients to receive oral neomycin and erythromycin base, systemic metronidazole and gentamicin or a combination of both regimens. Postoperative infective complications occurred in 27.4%, 11.9% and 12.3%, respectively. They concluded that systemic administration was preferable to oral prophylaxis, but that a combination added no special benefit. Stellato et al,[105] in a similar study, randomized 146 evaluable patients to receive oral neomycin and erythromycin or parenteral cefoxitin, or a combination of both: the incidence of infective complications was 11.4%, 11.7% and 7.8%. However, these differences were not statistically significant and they concluded that no advantage was gained by combining oral and parenteral antibiotic prophylaxis. Playforth et al[106] reported wound infection rates of 27.6% in patients who received no oral antibiotic and 13.9% in the group that did ($p < 0.04$). They concluded that it was important in colorectal operations not only to ensure adequate tissue levels of parenteral antimicrobials but also to reduce the risk of endogenous bacterial infection by partial decontamination of the bowel.

Although it is not normal practice in Europe, a combination of both preoperative oral and perioperative parenteral antibiotic prophylaxis is likely to reduce the incidence of infection to its lowest level in this form of surgery. In a systematic review of the literature published between 1984 and 1995 Song and Glenny[107] concluded that oral neomycin and erythromycin on the day before operation alone was an inadequate form of prophylaxis and that a single-dose regimen of a parenteral antibiotic was as effective as longer term prophylaxis.

Parenteral antibiotics

The work of Willis and others in the 1970s established the importance of activity against the anaerobes, particularly *Bacteroides* spp., of the antibiotic regimen used for prophylaxis in appendectomy and colorectal surgery.[108,109] Although a number of drugs such as clindamycin, cefoxitin and tinidazole have activity against anaerobes, metronidazole has been the mainstay of both therapy and prophylaxis in this area. Metronidazole can be given intravenously, orally or rectally, and all routes have been shown to be effective. Parenteral metronidazole is by far the most expensive formulation.

However, it is not only the anaerobes that cause infection after appendectomy or colorectal surgery, and hence it is common practice to add an agent active against the aerobic flora of the gastrointestinal tract, both Gram-positive and Gram-negative organisms. The incidence of staphylococcal infection should not be underestimated. In a study of infection after elective colorectal operations in which patients received either piperacillin or gentamicin and metronidazole, Walker et al[110] found 25% of the wound infections to be staphylococcal. Similarly, Morris et al[111] found a high incidence of Gram-positive organisms, in particular *Staph. aureus*, in infections after patients had received aztreonam with metronidazole. They concluded that the antibacterial combination chosen for prophylaxis in elective colorectal surgery must include adequate cover against Gram-positive organisms.

The literature is replete with clinical trials of the efficacy of various antibiotics for prophylaxis in elective colorectal surgery. Most studies have shown little or no difference between the agents used. Although it is no longer ethical to conduct placebo-controlled studies in colorectal surgery, it is of considerable interest to note the wide variation in the infection rates from different centers. They vary from approximately 5% infection in Scandinavia, where the use of doxycycline is popular,[112] to 26% in the UK.[113] Such differences cannot reflect the influence of the antibiotic chosen alone. There are many factors which determine the incidence of infection, of which the preoperative condition of the patient and the surgical expertise and degree of tissue damage are paramount. As has been emphasized previously,[107] there is no evidence that multiple-dose prophylaxis confers any benefit over a single-dose regimen. Broad-spectrum activity against anaerobes and aerobes, both Gram positive and Gram negative, is essential. Traditionally, a combination of gentamicin and metronidazole, with or without the addition of ampicillin to improve the activity against *Enterococcus faecalis*, has been considered to be the 'gold standard'. However, the possible toxic effect of gentamicin has encouraged the use of alternative regimens such as a group 3 or 4 cephalosporin or a ureidopenicillin plus metronidazole. Amoxicillin–clavulanate or imipenem are also used, without the addition of metronidazole. In their meta-analysis, Song and Glenny found no evidence that the later cephalosporins were more effective than the earlier (group 1 and 2) drugs.[107]

PERITONITIS

Peritonitis is a generalized or localized inflammation of the peritoneum leading to formation of a serous exudate, which rapidly becomes infected and purulent. Non-bacterial causes of peritonitis, usually chemical peritonitis, may be caused by the leakage of sterile gastric juices, bile, urine or pancreatic fluid into the peritoneal cavity. Meconium peritonitis may occur after intrauterine perforation of the gastrointestinal tract, while granulomatous peritonitis may result from sarcoidosis or tuberculosis. Occasionally, drugs, such as isoniazid, practolol and intraperitoneal cytolytics for malignant disease, may cause acute or chronic peritonitis. Starch peritonitis from talc on surgical gloves is a historical cause.

PRIMARY PERITONITIS

Primary or spontaneous bacterial peritonitis is unusual. It may occur in children who have undergone splenectomy or with the nephrotic syndrome, but is more commonly seen in adult patients with cirrhosis and ascites. In this latter group the prevalence has been estimated as 8–27% with a resultant mortality of 48–57%. The route by which bacteria gain access to the peritoneal cavity is not clear. Bacteria could gain access to the ascitic fluid by translocation from the colon, although bacteremia occurring in the presence of abnormal host resistance, intrahepatic shunting and impaired opsonic activity of ascitic fluid is probably more likely. Bacteremia is, in itself, more likely to occur in these patients because of compromised neutrophil and reticuloendothelial function in cirrhotic patients. The usual pathogens are *Escherichia coli*, streptococci, and *Klebsiella pneumoniae*. A single organism is usually cultured. In one-third of patients no organism is isolated (culture-negative neutrocytic ascites). Peritonitis is diagnosed by the presence of an ascitic fluid neutrophil count greater than $0.5 \times 10^9/l$, negative ascitic fluid culture, no other cause of intra-abdominal infection, no prior antibiotic treatment within 30 days and no alternative explanation for the elevated white cell count.

Antibiotic therapy should be guided by laboratory data. Because anaerobic organisms are unusual, cefotaxime, piperacillin or amoxicillin–clavulanate continued for 10–14 days are usually adequate.

Recurrence of spontaneous bacterial peritonitis is common, and has a high mortality rate. Prophylactic measures include reduction of ascitic fluid by diuretic therapy as well as more specific management of any precipitating disease. There is evidence that long-term prophylaxis is cost effective[114] and some have recommended prolonged use of antibiotics such as ciprofloxacin, which selectively removes the GNAB from the gastrointestinal tract, although long-term morbidity or the frequency of admission to hospital is unaltered.[115]

SECONDARY PERITONITIS

There are many causes of bacterial peritonitis, ranging from initially sterile collections of gastric fluid or bile, which subsequently become infected, to perforation of colonic diverticulae or carcinoma, leading to fecal peritonitis. The more distal the lesion is in the gastrointestinal tract the heavier the bacterial load. Wherever the lesion, the Enterobacteriaceae, acting either alone or in synergy with anaerobic bacteria, predominate. The role of enterococci and *Pseudomonas aeruginosa* as primary pathogens remains controversial. The former is frequently isolated from intra-abdominal infection but rarely as a single isolate, and pseudomonal infections are more common in repeat laparotomies than as a primary pathogen. Peritonitis following blunt or penetrating abdominal trauma may introduce exogenous infection, although the organisms from the injured viscus are most likely to be the pathogens.

The management of bacterial peritonitis involves adequate

preoperative resuscitation, laparotomy with repair or resection of the damaged viscera with or without fecal diversion, and appropriate antibiotic therapy such as cefotaxime and metronidazole or clindamycin and gentamicin. Since many of these patients will be seriously ill, the points discussed in Ch. 41 should also be considered. Saline or antibiotic peritoneal lavage is thought to have some merit, but the use of intraperitoneal drains should be minimized.

The antibiotic regimen should include activity against both aerobic and anaerobic organisms.[116] In most situation 5 days' high-dose therapy is sufficient. In future, other forms of supportive therapy, such as monoclonal antibodies against endotoxin, TNF and interleukin receptors, may prove helpful, but at present they are unproven.

PERITONEAL LAVAGE

The use of antibiotic solutions to lavage the infected peritoneal cavity has had some advocates who have used parenteral tetracycline together with a tetracycline solution (1 mg/ml saline) with impressive results.[117,118] However, the meticulous technical protocol used by these workers cannot be ignored, and whether the excellent results can be attributed to tetracycline lavage or to their expertise has been questioned.[119] Anxieties that the lavage will spread bacterial contamination to the remaining 'uncontaminated' peritoneal cavity, or that intraabdominal adhesions may result, seem unfounded. The lavage certainly removes debris from the peritoneal cavity that would otherwise function as foreign bodies. Silverman et al[120] reported infection in 25 of 74 patients (34%) who had saline lavage, compared with 15 (18%) of 85 patients whose peritoneal cavity was lavaged with tetracycline solution ($p < 0.05$), which counters the argument, suggesting that it is not purely the mechanical debridement which is of benefit.

INFLUENCE OF LAPAROSCOPIC SURGERY ON SURGICAL INFECTION

Elective laparoscopic operations have been associated with a lower incidence of postoperative infection and a lower metabolic response to injury. The development of this technology has encouraged surgeons to expand the range of operations undertaken. However, a number of anxieties have been expressed about the safety of inducing a pneumoperitoneum in the presence of infection such as appendicitis or a perforated duodenal ulcer or diverticulum. Does the pneumoperitoneum spread the contamination? Does the intra-abdominal pressure increase the risk of septicemia? Is the gas introduced sterile? Targarona et al[121] reviewed the published literature and concluded that laparoscopy is associated with greater preservation of the immune response and a lower incidence of infective complications in these situations. While CO_2 pneumoperitoneum influences the peritoneal response to infection this appears not to be harmful.

PANCREATITIS

Pancreatitis remains a common cause of acute peritonitis. The diagnosis is usually straightforward and, with appropriate resuscitation and analgesia, most patients recover. However, 5–10% die from the initial attack, and infection leading to septicemia and multiple organ failure is one of the more common causes. Acute pancreatitis causes necrosis of the peripancreatic parenchyma, while inflammation of the pancreas may lead to duct necrosis. There is considerable edema of the retroperitoneal and adjacent tissues (the retroperitoneal 'burn'), including the stomach, colon and upper small bowel.

Why, and by what route, the necrotic pancreas becomes infected is not clear. Pancreatitis frequently occurs in the presence of gallstones, and here the bile is frequently colonized. It is most probable that passage of bacteria from the bowel lumen or from the bile into the pancreatic duct is the route of infection, although bacterial translocation through the colonic wall into the lymphatics and retroperitioneal inflammatory edema is also possible. The value of antibiotics used from the onset of the attack remains debatable; many trials report too few patients and use possibly inappropriate antibiotics such as ampicillin or cefalotin. The incidence of infection has certainly not been altered by these antibiotics;[122,123] perhaps broader spectrum antibiotics may have resulted in a different outcome. In a study in which 74 patients with necrotizing pancreatitis were randomized to receive intravenous imipenem-cilastin 0.5 g for 2 weeks or no antibiotic, there was a significant benefit in favor of the antibiotic group (12.2% v 30.3% sepsis, $p < 0.01$).[124] A similarly beneficial result has been reported by Widdison et al[127] using cefotaxime in an experimental study of infected pancreatitis in cats. Recent review articles[126,127] conclude that the evidence is in favor of the use of antibiotic prophylaxis in this situation and a survey of clinicians in the UK has shown that 88% would administer antibiotics to such patients.[128]

The diagnosis of infection in acute pancreatitis can be very difficult. The onset of sepsis and multiple organ failure may occur despite the fact that no organism can be isolated from the necrotic pancreatic tissue. A sudden deterioration in a patient's condition may be associated with infection and ultrasound-guided or computed-tomography-guided fine-needle aspiration of the peripancreatic tissues may help to define whether the collection is infected or not. However, when deterioration occurs debridement and drainage of the pancreatic tissues may be indicated, whether or not the tissues are infected. Antibiotics are usually administered.

ABDOMINAL TRAUMA

Approximately 50% of deaths after major injuries occur within a few minutes of the accident and are caused by injuries to the brainstem, spinal cord, cardiac or major blood vessels. Other patients die within 2 h of respiratory failure or hemorrhage into body cavities or brain tissue, but approximately 20% of deaths after major injury occur over the next 20 weeks – and some 80% of these die of organ failure and infection. This infection might not be caused by the trauma but may be associated with endotracheal intubation, blood transfusion, catheterization, ICU management or nasogastric suction, all of which increase the risk of infection following trauma.[129] The risk of infection after abdominal trauma depends on the mechanism of injury and the organs involved. The interval between injury and treatment is an important factor, as is the occurrence of hypovolemic shock, particularly when associated with vascular injury.

Weigelt et al,[130] in a review of 949 patients, showed a higher incidence of infection after shotgun injuries (20–25%) than after gunshot wounds (3.6–16%) or stab injuries (4–4.7%). Similarly, Dellenger et al[131] showed that 42 (30%) of 140 patients sustaining gunshot wounds developed infection, compared with 31 (16%) of 190 patients who sustained stab wounds. The incidence of infection was higher when the colon was injured (35%) than when there was no colonic injury (18%). Weigelt et al[130] also showed that the incidence of infection increased when four or more intra-abdominal organs were injured.

In a review of injuries after vascular trauma Wilson et al[132] correlated the incidence of intra-abdominal infection with the blood pressure on admission to the accident and emergency department. Where the blood pressure was initially unrecordable, 40% of those surviving developed intra-abdominal infection; the incidence of intra-abdominal infection was 25% when the blood pressure was below 70 mmHg, 23% where the blood pressure was 70–90 mmHg and 11% where the blood pressure was in excess of 90 mmHg. It was initially postulated that bacterial translocation occurred more commonly in patients with hypovolemic shock. Bacterial translocation does occur after traumatic injury but may be independent of hemorrhagic shock and its clinical significance remains in some doubt.[133]

As might be expected, infection is more common after colonic injury. In a multicenter review of 54 361 patients, 2739 (5%) required laparotomy, and the colon was injured in 195 (11%) of these patients.[134] The colon was the organ most commonly injured, with small bowel injury occurring in 4%, liver injury in 3% and splenic injury in 3%. The factor most closely associated with the development of infection after trauma is peritoneal contamination by intestinal contents. The presence of a stoma is also a significant risk factor and this has led to re-evaluation of primary repair of the colon following such injuries. In the civilian context, most colon injuries can be managed by repair or resection with primary anastomosis. Ivatury et al,[135] in a multiple regression analysis of risk factors in 252 patients sustaining penetrating injuries of the colon, found the abdominal trauma index and the presence of a colostomy as the significant independent risk factors associated with the occurrence of intra-abdominal abscess. Demetriades et al[136] studied prospectively 100 patients with bullet injuries of the colon: 76% had primary repair of the colon, with 11.8% developing abdominal sepsis; the level of sepsis in the remaining 24 patients was 29.2%. In a review of 125 patients with intraperitoneal colonic injury, George et al[137]

reported an 18% complication rate in the 88 patients managed by primary closure and 42% in the 37 managed by end colostomy or ileostomy.

Nutrition is as important in the traumatized patient as in other patients requiring major surgery, particularly when the integrity of the gastrointestinal tract has been disturbed. Much has been written about the role played by individual elements of the diet, which is beyond the scope of this chapter. Nevertheless, there is increasing evidence to suggest that enteral nutrition is preferable to parenteral nutrition, and may reduce the incidence of postoperative septic complications. Kudsk et al[138] studied protein levels in 68 severely injured patients with abdominal trauma indexes of 15 or higher, randomized to enteral or parenteral feeding. Patients fed enterally showed lower levels of acute phase proteins, primarily caused by septic complications after severe trauma, and higher levels of constitutive proteins. Moore et al[139] conducted a meta-analysis of trials to compare enteral with parenteral feeding postoperatively and assess the incidence of septic complications: 118 patients receiving enteral and 112 patients receiving parenteral nutrition were evaluable. There were significantly ($p < 0.01$) fewer enteral patients (18%) with septic complications than those receiving parenteral nutrition (35%).

Clearly these patients require parenteral antibiotic therapy and it might be thought that selective decontamination of the digestive tract (SDD) (Ch. 44) might be of value in this situation. However, in 72 patients who had sustained multiple trauma with chest injuries requiring intermittent positive pressure ventilation, and who had a mean injury severity score of 29.5, Hammond et al[140] reported no difference in the number of patients infected (11 receiving SDD vs 11 receiving placebo), the number of infections (17 vs 16) or deaths (5 vs 3). The duration of stay both in the ICU and in the hospital were also similar.

Infection following abdominal trauma that involves the gastrointestinal tract is caused by both aerobic and anaerobic bacterial flora. Brook[141] has shown that infection is biphasic, with the Enterobacteriaceae as the major pathogens in the peritonitis stage and anaerobes, particularly *Bacteroides fragilis*, in the later abscess stage. For this reason, the antibiotic(s) must be active against both aerobic and anaerobic organisms.

The pharmacokinetics of antibiotics in trauma patients may be important. Reed et al[142] have shown a significant expansion in the apparent volume of distribution for amikacin, which correlated with fluid resuscitation. They previously noted failure to achieve adequate levels using standard regimens[143] and believed this was due to apparent underdosing. In their original study they found no significant difference between 72 and 24 h treatment with amikacin and clindamycin in 150 abdominal trauma patients requiring laparotomy (19% vs 21%). Their data suggested that higher doses of the antibiotic were more effective than longer courses in reducing infection in these patients.

There is increasing evidence that short-course, high-dose therapy is indicated in these patients, provided there has been adequate surgical elimination of the source of infection.

Oreskovich et al[53] showed no difference between 24 h and 5 days' antibiotic administration in patients with penetrating abdominal trauma; nor did Fabian et al[54] when they compared 24 h with 5 days in 500 traumatized patients. Nichols et al[144] suggested that patients can be stratified into those requiring short-term therapy and those who may benefit from longer term therapy, although this study showed no difference between short-term therapy of 2 days and a similar group of 145 historical control subjects who received 5 days of antibiotic therapy. The Surgical Infection Society of North America has published guidelines on the treatment of intra-abdominal infection, and recommend that prolonged antibiotic therapy is not required in patients sustaining traumatic enteric perforations if they are operated on within 12 h of injury.[116]

LIVER ABSCESS

Liver abscess is uncommon and tends to be diagnosed in the more elderly population.[145] However, it can occur in any age group and may be difficult to diagnose. Two types of abscess are well recognized – pyogenic and the occasional imported amebic abscess. Both need to be differentiated from other cystic conditions in the liver.

PYOGENIC ABSCESS

Pyogenic abscess used more commonly to follow portal pyemia associated with acute appendicitis. However, with the widespread use of antibiotics in managing appendicitis, pyogenic abscess is now more common in elderly people, where malignancy, biliary sepsis and diverticulitis disease are more common. A pyogenic abscess may be single or multiple, and is most often found in the right lobe of the liver. Patients with compromised host defences are more susceptible. For example, unusual pathogens such as the *Mycobacterium avium* complex in patients with acquired immune deficiency syndrome (AIDS)[146] and *Yersinia enterocolitica* associated with cirrhosis, diabetes mellitus, alcoholism or malnutrition have been reported.[147] In over half of patients no cause is found.

The organism responsible for pyogenic abscess often reflects the etiology. Abscesses are usually polybacterial. Anaerobes are particularly important.[148,149] Streptococci of the *anginosus* group (formerly *Streptococcus milleri*) are microaerophilic commensals of the gastrointestinal tract and have recently emerged as an important cause of hepatic abscesses.[150,151] *Klebsiella* spp. and *Esch. coli* (and occasionally *Proteus vulgaris* and *Pseudomonas* spp.) are responsible.

The diagnosis can be difficult. The classic features of abdominal pain, pyrexia, anorexia, malaise and weight loss are less common, particularly in older persons. A high white cell count, raised erythrocyte sedimentation rate and alkaline phosphatase are common. The chest radiograph may show a sympathetic pleural effusion or an air/fluid level within the liver; the latter carries a worse prognosis.[152] Ultrasound scans or a computed tomography (CT) scan are usually diagnostic. A CT scan with enhancement can detect an abscess of 1 cm diameter.[153]

Treatment of pyogenic liver abscess relies upon adequate drainage and appropriate antibiotic therapy.[154] Drainage may be either open or by percutaneous needle aspiration. The insertion of a catheter under ultrasonic or CT guidance is now widely practised.[155] Although antibiotics have been instilled via the needle or irrigated via the catheter they are not usually required. Where radiographic expertise is lacking, or when needle aspiration or catheter drainage fails, open transperitoneal drainage should be performed[152] (this is more likely in multiloculated or multiple abscesses). Moore et al[156] suggested that left lobe abscesses in children are best treated by elective early open surgical drainage.

Antibiotic therapy is essential and, until culture and sensitivity results are available, broad-spectrum therapy against both aerobes and anaerobes should be given. A combination of penicillin, gentamicin and metronidazole is appropriate, while vancomycin can be of use in the penicillin-allergic patient. Therapy should be guided by response and repeat ultrasound examination. Short-course therapy of 10–14 days may suffice for abscesses that drain adequately, while 4 weeks or more may be necessary for less rapidly responding infections. *Streptococcus anginosus* group infections are resistant to metronidazole, and penicillin is the drug of choice. Cefotaxime is a better choice than gentamicin in elderly patients with reduced renal function.

References

1. Peel ALG, Taylor EW 1991 Proposed definitions for the audit of post operative infection: a discussion paper. *Annals of the Royal College of Surgeons of England* 73: 385–388
2. Mangram AJ, Horan TC, Pearson ML, Silver LC, Jarvis WR 1999 Guideline for Prevention of Surgical Site Infection, 1999. Centers for Disease Control and Prevention (CDC) Hospital Infection Control Practices Advisory Committee. *American Journal of Infection Control* 27: 97–132
3. Law DJW, Mishriki SF, Jeffrey PJ 1990 The importance of surveillance after discharge from hospital in the diagnosis of post-operative wound infection. *Annals of the Royal College of Surgeons of England* 72: 207–209
4. Polk HC, Miles AA 1973 The decisive period in the primary infections of muscle by *Escherichia coli*. *British Journal of Experimental Pathology* 54: 99–101
5. Onderdonk AB, Bartlett JG, Louie T, Sullivan-Seigler N, Gorbach SL 1976 Microbial synergy in experimental intra-abdominal abscess. *Infection and Immunity* 13: 22–26
6. Elek SD, Conen PE 1957 The virulence of *Staphylococcus pyogenes* for man. A study of the problems of wound infection. *British Journal of Experimental Pathology* 38: 573–586
7. Simchen E, Rozin R, Wax Y 1990 The Israeli study of surgical infection of drains and the risk of wound infection in operations for hernia. *Surgery, Gynecology and Obstetrics* 170: 331–337
8. Burrows L, Tartter P 1982 Effect of blood transfusion on colonic malignancy rates. *Lancet* ii: 662
9. George CD, Marello PJ 1987 Immunological effect of blood transfusion upon renal transplantation tumor operation and bacterial infections. *American Journal of Surgery* 152: 329–337
10. Tarrter PI 1989 Blood transfusion and postoperative infection. *Transfusion* 29: 456–459
11. Jensen LS, Andersen A, Fristrup SC, Holme JB, Hvid HM, Kraglund K 1990

Comparison of one dose versus three doses of prophylactic antibiotics and the influence of blood transfusion on infectious complications after acute and elective colorectal surgery. *British Journal of Surgery* 77: 513–518

12. Braga M, Vignali A, Radaelli G, Gianotti L, Di Carlo V 1992 Association between perioperative blood transfusion and postoperative infection in patients having elective operations for gastrointestinal cancer. *European Journal of Surgery* 158: 531–536

13. Cruse PJE 1992 Classification of operations and audit of infection. In: Taylor EW (ed.) *Infection in surgical practice.* Oxford, Oxford University Press

14. Haley RW, Culver DH, Morgan WM et al 1985 Identifying patients at risk of surgical wound infection. A simple multi-variate index of patient susceptibility and wound contamination. *American Journal of Epidemiology* 121: 206–215

15. Culver DH, Horan TC, Gaines RP et al 1991 Surgical wound infection rates by wound class, operative procedure, and patient risk index. National Nosocomial Infections Surveillance System. *American Journal of Medicine* 91(Suppl. 3B): 152S–157S

16. Scottish Intercollegiate Guidelines Network 2000 Antibiotic prophylaxis in surgery. July Guideline no 45

17. Stuckey J, Gross RJ 1990 Infectious disease. In: Kammerer WS, Gross RJ (eds) *Medical consultation.* Baltimore, Williams & Wilkins

18. Lazorthes F, Chiotasso P, Massip P, Materre JP, Sarkissian M 1992 Local antibiotic prophylaxis in inguinal hernia repair. *Surgery, Gynecology and Obstetrics* 175: 569–570

19. Classen DC, Evans RS, Pestotnik SL, Horn SD, Menlove RL, Burke JP 1992 The timing of prophylactic administration of antibiotics and the risk of surgical wound infection. *New England Journal of Medicine* 326: 281–286

20. Rowe-Jones DC, Peel ALG, Shaw JFL, Teasdale C, Cole DS 1990 Single dose cefotaxime plus metronidazole versus three doses cefuroxime plus metronidazole as prophylaxis against wound infection in colorectal surgery: a multicentre prospective randomized study. *British Medical Journal* 300: 18–22

21. Strachan CJL, Black J, Powers SJA et al 1977 Prophylactic use of cephazolin against wound sepsis after cholecystectomy. *British Medical Journal* i: 1254–1256

22. Turano A 1992 Multicentre Study Group. New clinical data on the prophylaxis of infections in abdominal, gynecologic and urologic surgery. *American Journal of Surgery* 158(Suppl. 4a): 16S–20S

23. Bates T, Roberts JV, Smith K, German KA 1992 A randomized trial of one versus three doses of augmentin as wound prophylaxis in at-risk abdominal surgery. *Postgraduate Medical Journal* 68: 811–816.

24. Di Piro JT, Chung RPF, Bowden TA, Mannsburger JA 1986 Single dose antibiotic prophylaxis of surgical wound infections. *American Journal of Surgery* 152: 552–559

25. Scher KS, Wroczynski AF, Jones CW 1986 Duration of antibiotic prophylaxis. An experimental study. *American Journal of Surgery* 151: 209–212

26. Periti P, Mazzei T, Tonelli F 1989 Single dose cefotetan versus multi dose cefoxitin antimicrobial prophylaxis in colorectal surgery. *Diseases of the Colon and Rectum* 32: 121–127

27. University of Melbourne Colorectal Group 1989 A comparison of single dose systemic timetin with mezlocillin for prophylaxis of wound infection in colorectal surgery. *Diseases of the Colon and Rectum* 32: 940–943

28. Moesgaard F, Lukkegaard-Neilsen M 1989 Pre-operative cell mediated immunity and duration of antibiotic prophylaxis in relation to post-operative infective complications. A controlled trial in biliary gastroduodenal and colorectal surgery. *Acta Chirugica Scandinavica* 155: 281–286

29. Dixon JM, Armstrong CP, Duffy SW, Chetty U, Davies GC 1984 A randomized prospective trial comparing the value of intravenous and preincisional cefamandole in reducing postoperative sepsis after operations upon the gastrointestinal tract. *Surgery, Gynecology and Obstetrics* 158: 303–307

30. Taylor TV, Dawson DL, De Silva M, Shaw SJ, Durrans D, Makin D 1985 Preoperative intraincisional cefamandole reduces wound infection and postoperative inpatient stay in upper abdominal surgery. *Annals of the Royal College of Surgeons of England* 67: 235–237

31. McArdle CS, Morran CG, Pettit L, Gemmell CG, Sleigh JD, Tillotson GS 1991 The value of oral antibiotic prophylaxis in biliary tract surgery. *Journal of Hospital Infection* 19(Suppl. C): 59–64

32. Platt R, Zaleznik DF, Hopkins CC et al 1990 Perioperative antibiotic prophylaxis for hernia and breast surgery. *New England Journal of Medicine* 322: 153–160

33. Taylor EW, Byrne DJ, Leaper DJ, Karran SJ, Browne MK, Mitchell KJ 1997 Antibiotic prophylaxis and open groin hernia repair. *World Journal of Surgery* 21: 811–814

34. Gupta R, Sinnett D, Carpenter R, Preece PE, Royle GT 2000 Antibiotic prophylaxis for post-operative wound infection in clean elective breast surgery. *European Journal of Surgical Oncology* 26: 363–366

35. Nathens AB, Marshall JC 1999 Selective decontamination of the digestive tract in surgical patients: a systematic review of the evidence. *Archives of Surgery* 134: 170–176

36. Silvestri L, Mannucci F, van Saene HK 2000 Selective decontamination of the digestive tract: a life saver. *Journal of Hospital Infection* 45: 185–190

37. Webb CH 2000 Selective decontamination of the digestive tract, SDD: a commentary. *Journal of Hospital Infection* 46: 106–109

38. Ebner W, Kropec-Hubner A, Daschner FD 2000 Bacterial resistance and overgrowth due to selective decontamination of the digestive tract. *European Journal of Clinical Microbiology and Infectious Diseases* 19: 243–247

39. Donnelly JP 1993 Selective decontamination of the digestive tract and its role in antimicrobial prophylaxis. *Journal of Antimicrobial Chemotherapy* 31: 813–29

40. Carrico CJ, Meakins JL, Marshall JC, Fry D, Maier RV 1986 Multiple-organ-failure syndrome. *Archives of Surgery* 121: 196–208

41. Tetteroo GWM, Wagenvoort JHT, Bruining HA 1994 Bacteriology of selective decontamination: efficacy and rebound colonization. *Journal of Antimicrobial Chemotherapy* 34: 139–148

42. Maschmeyer G, Haralambie E, Gaus W et al 1988 Ciprofloxicin and norfloxicin for selective decontamination in patients with severe granulocytopenia. *Infection* 16: 98–104

43. Martinez-Pellus AE, Merino P, Bru M et al 1997 Endogenous endotoxemia of intestinal origin during cardiopulmonary bypass. Role of type of flow and protective effect of selective digestive decontamination. *Intensive Care Medicine* 23: 1251–1257

44. Tetteroo GWM, Wagenvoort JHT, Castelein A, Tilanus HW, Ince C, Bruining HA 1990 Selective decontamination to reduce Gram-negative colonization and infections after oesophageal resection. *Lancet* 335: 704–707

45. Weisner RH 1990 The incidence of Gram-negative bacterial and fungal infections in liver transplant patients treated with selective decontamination. *Infection* 18(Suppl. 1): 19–21

46. Bion JF, Badger I, Crosby HA et al 1994 Selective decontamination of the digestive tract reduces Gram-negative pulmonary colonization but not systemic endotoxemia in patients undergoing elective liver transplantation. *Critical Care Medicine* 22: 40–49

47. Emre S, Sebastian A, Chodoff L et al 1999 Selective decontamination of the digestive tract helps prevent bacterial infections in the early postoperative period after liver transplant. *Mount Sinai Journal of Medicine* 66: 310–313

48. Beath SV, Kelly DA, Booth IW, Freeman J, Buckels JAC, Mayer AD 1994 Postoperative care of children undergoing small bowel and liver transplantation. *British Journal of Intensive Care* 4: 302–308

49. Taylor EW, Lindsay G, West of Scotland Surgical Infection Study Group 1994 Selective decontamination of the colon before elective colorectal operations. *World Journal of Surgery* 18: 926–931

50. Evans RS, Classen DC, Pestotnik SL, Lundsgaarde HP, Burke JP 1994 Improving empiric antibiotic selection using computer decision support. *Archives of Internal Medicine* 154: 878–884

51. Mosdell DM, Morris DM, Voltura A et al 1991 Antibiotic treatment for surgical peritonitis. *Annals of Surgery* 214: 543–549

52. Davey P, Libby G, Hunter K et al 2001 How important is appropriate empirical antibiotic therapy for intra-abdominal infection. In Press

53. Oreskovich MR, Dellinger EP, Lennard ES, Wertz M, Carrico CJ, Minshew BH 1982 Duration of preventive antibiotic administration for penetrating abdominal trauma. *Archives of Surgery* 117: 200–205

54. Fabian TC, Croce MA, Payne EW, Minard G, Pritchard FE, Kudsk KA 1992 Duration of antibiotic therapy for penetrating abdominal trauma: a prospective trial. *Surgery* 112: 788–794

55. Swift AC, Bartzokas CA, Corkill JE 1984 The gastro-oral pathway of intestinal bacteria after head and neck cancer surgery. *Clinical Otolaryngology* 1: 263–269

56. Swift AC 1992 Infection in ENT surgery. In: Taylor EW (ed.) *Infection in surgical practice.* Oxford, Oxford University Press

57. Fritsch DE, Klein DG 1992 Ludwig's angina. *American Journal of Infection Control* 21: 39–46

58. Findlay IG, Wright PA, Menzies T, McCardle CS 1982 Microbial flora in carcinoma of oesophagus. *Thorax* 37: 181–184

59. Bartlett JG, Gorbach SL, Thadepalli H, Finegold SM 1974 Bacteriology of empyema. *Lancet* i: 338–340

60. Wilson AP, Gruneberg RN, Treasure T, Sturridge MF 1988 Staphylococcus epidermidis as a cause of postoperative wound infection after cardiac surgery: An assessment of pathogenicity and a wound scoring method. *British Journal of Surgery* 75: 168–170

61. Bor DH, Rose RM, Modlin JF, Weintraub R, Friedland GH 1983 Mediastinitis after cardiovascular surgery. *Reviews in Infectious Diseases* 5: 885–897

62. Angelini GD, Lamarra M, Azzu AA, Bryan AJ 1990 Wound infection following early repeat sternotomy for post-operative bleeding. An experience utilizing intraoperative irrigation with povidone iodine. *Journal of Cardiovascular Surgery (Torino)* 31: 793–795

63. Ko W, Lazenby WD, Zelano JA, Isom OW, Krieger KH 1992 The effects of shaving methods and intraoperative irrigation on suppurative mediastinitis after bypass operations. *Annals of Thoracic Surgery* 53: 301–305

64. Frame R, Brodman RF, Furman S, Andrews CA, Gross JN 1993 Surgical removal of infected transvenous pacemaker leads. *Pacing and Clinical Electrophysiology* 16: 2343–2348

65. Sugarman B, Young EJ 1989 Infections associated with prosthetic devices: magnitude of the problem. *Infectious Disease Clinics of North America* 3: 187–198

66. Lewis AB, Hayes DL, Holmes DR, Vlietstra RE, Pluth JR, Osborne MJ 1985 Update on infections involving permanent pacemakers. Characterisation and management. *Journal of Thoracic and Cardiovascular Surgery* 89: 758–763

67. Wilson HA, Downes TR, Julian JS, White WL, Haponik EF 1993 Candida endocarditis. A treatable form of pacemaker infection. *Chest* 103: 283–284

68. Bluhm G, Nordlander R, Ransjo U 1986 Antibiotic prophylaxis in pacemaker surgery: a prospective double blind trial with systemic administration of antibiotic versus placebo at implantation of cardiac pacemakers. *Pacing and Clinical Electrophysiology* 9: 720–726

69. Ramsdale DR, Charles RG, Roland DB, Singh SS, Gautam PC, Faragher EB 1984 Antibiotic prophylaxis for pace-maker implantation: a prospective randomized trial. *Pacing and Clinical Electrophysiology* 7: 844–849

70. Strachan CJL 1992 Infection in vascular surgery. In: Taylor EW (ed.) *Infection in surgical practice.* Oxford, Oxford University Press

71. Standage BA, Goss JC 1982 Outcome and sepsis after splenectomy in adults. *American Journal of Surgery* 143: 545–548

72. Rao GN 1988 Predictive factors in local sepsis after splenectomy for trauma in adults. *New England Journal of Medicine* 33: 68–70

73. Westphal JF, Brogard JM 1999 Biliary tract infections: a guide to drug treatment. *Drugs* 57: 81–91

74. Struelens MJ, Rost F, Deplano A et al 1993 *Pseudomonas aeruginosa* and Enterobacteriaceae bacteremia after biliary endoscopy: an outbreak investigation using DNA macrorestriction analysis. *American Journal of Medicine* 95: 489–498

75. Wells GR, Taylor EW, Lindsay G, Morton L, West of Scotland Surgical Infection Study Group 1989 The relationship between the colonization, high risk factors and postoperative sepsis in patients undergoing biliary tract operations while receiving a prophylactic antibiotic. *British Journal of Surgery* 76: 374–377

76. Cahill CJ, Payne JA 1988 Current practice in biliary surgery. *British Journal of Surgery* 75: 1169–1172

77. Southern Surgeons Club 1991 A prospective of analysis of 1518 laparoscopic cholecystectomies. *New England Journal of Medicine* 324: 1073–1078

78. Peters JH, Gibbons GD, Innes JT et al 1991 Complications of laparoscopic cholecystectomy. *Surgery* 110: 769–777

79. Litwin DE, Girotti MJ, Poulin EC, Mamazza J, Negy AG 1992 Laparoscopic cholecystectomy: trans Canada experience with 2201 cases. *Canadian Journal of Surgery* 35: 291–296

80. Edwards GFS, Lindsay G, Taylor EW, West of Scotland Surgical Infection Study Group 1990 Bacteriological assessment of ampicillin with sulbactam as antibiotic prophylaxis in patients undergoing biliary tract operations. *Journal of Hospital Infection* 16: 249–255

81. Higgins A, London J, Charland S et al 1999 Prophylactic antibiotics for elective laparoscopic cholecystectomy: are they necessary? *Archives of Surgery* 134: 611–613

82. Tocchi A, Lepre L, Costa G, Liotta G, Mazzoni G, Maggiolini F 2000 The need for antibiotic prophylaxis in elective laparoscopic cholecystectomy: a prospective randomized study. *Archives of Surgery* 135: 67–70

83. Pieper R, Kazer L, Nasman P 1982 Acute appendicitis. *Acta Chirugica Scandinavica* 148: 51–62

84. Kizilcan F, Tanyel FC, Buyukpamukcu N, Hicsonmez A 1992 The necessity of prophylactic antibiotics in uncomplicated appendicitis during childhood. *Journal of Pediatric Surgery* 27: 586–588

85. Krukowski ZH, Irwin ST, Denholm S, Matheson NA 1988 Preventing wound infection after appendicectomy: a review. *Archives of Surgery* 75: 1023–1023

86. Wilson RG, Taylor EW, Lindsay G et al 1987 A comparative study of cefotetan and metronidazole against metronidazole alone to prevent infection after appendectomy. *Surgery, Gynecology and Obstetrics* 164: 447–451

87. al-Dhohayan A, Alsebayl M, Shibl A, Al Eshalwy S, Kattan K, Al Saleh M 1993 Comparative study of augmentin versus metronidazole/gentamicin in the prevention of infections after appendicectomy. *European Surgical Research* 25: 60–64

88. Salam IM, Abu Galala KH, El Ashaal YI, Chandran VP, Asham NN, Sim AJ 1994 A randomized prospective study of cefoxitin versus pipericillin in appendicectomy. *Journal of Hospital Infection* 26: 133–136

89. Pokorny WJ, Kaplan SL, Mason EO 1991 A preliminary report of ticarcillin and clavulanate versus triple antibiotic therapy in children with ruptured appendicitis. *Surgery, Gynecology and Obstetrics* 172(Suppl.): 54–56

90. Uhari M, Seppanen J, Heikkinen E 1992 Imipenem-cilastatin versus tobramycin and metronidazole for appendicitis related infections. *Pediatric Infectious Disease Journal* 11: 445–450

91. Coldham GJ, Mickleson JC, Ali P-G 1993 Antibiotic protocol for appendicectomy – costs and benefits of single dose therapy. *New Zealand Medical Journal* 106: 13–14

92. Wilson APR 1995 Antibiotic prophylaxis and infection control measures in minimally invasive surgery. *Journal of Antimicrobial Chemotherapy* 36: 1–5

93. McCall JL, Sharples K, Jadallah F 1997 Systematic review of randomized controlled trials comparing laparoscopic with open appendicectomy. *Archives of Surgery* 84: 1045–1050

94. Fingerhut A, Millat B, Borrie F 1999 Laparoscopic versus open appendectomy: time to decide. *World Journal of Surgery* 23: 835–845

95. Irving AD, Scrimgeour D 1987 Mechanical bowel preparation for colonic resection and anastomosis. *Archives of Surgery* 74: 580–581

96. Santos JCM, Batista J, Sirimarco MT, Guimaraes AS, Levy CE 1994 Prospective randomized trial of mechanical bowel preparation in patients undergoing elective colorectal surgery. *Archives of Surgery* 81: 1673–1676

97. Keighley MRB, Taylor EW, Hares MM et al 1981 Influence of oral manitol bowel preparation on colonic microflora and the risk of explosion during endoscopic diathermy. *Archives of Surgery* 68: 554–556

98. Nichols RL, Condon RE, Gorbach SL, Nyhus LM 1972 Efficacy of preoperative antimicrobial preparation of the bowel. *Annals of Surgery* 176: 227–232

99. Keighley MRB, Arabi Y, Alexander-Williams J, Youngs D, Burden DW 1979 Comparison between systemic and oral antimicrobial prophylaxis in colorectal surgery. *Lancet* 28: 894–897

100. Weaver M, Burdon DW, Youngs DJ, Keighley MRB 1986 Oral neomycin and erythromycin compared with single dose systemic metronidazole and ceftriaxone prophylaxis in elective colorectal surgery. *American Journal of Surgery* 151: 437–442

101. Solla JA, Rothenberger DA 1990 Pre-operative bowel preparation. Surgery colon and rectal surgeons. *Diseases of the Colon and Rectum* 33: 154–159

102. Taylor EW, Lindsay G, Helyar AG 1990 Pre-operative selective decontamination of the colon by ciprofloxcin and mechanical catharsis in patients undergoing elective colorectal operations. *Surgical Research Communications* 7: 351–5

103. Lazorthes F, Legrand G, Monrozies X et al 1982 Comparison between oral and systemic antibiotics and their combined use for the prevention of complications in colorectal surgery. *Diseases of the Colon and Rectum* 25: 309–11

104. Lau WY, Chu KW, Poon GP, Ho KK 1988 Prophylactic antibiotics in elective colorectal surgery. *British Journal of Surgery* 75: 782–785

105. Stellato TA, Danzigger LH, Gordon N et al 1990 Antibiotics in elective colon surgery. A randomized trial of oral and oral/systemic antibiotics for prophylaxis. *American Surgeon* 56: 251–254

106. Playforth MJ, Smith GMR, Evans M, Pollock AV 1988 Antimicrobial bowel preparation – oral, parenteral or both? *Diseases of the Colon and Rectum* 31: 90–93

107. Song F, Glenny AM 1998 Antimicrobial prophylaxis in colorectal surgery: a systematic review of randomized controlled trials. *British Journal of Surgery* 85: 1232–1241

108. Willis AT, Ferguson IR, Jones PH et al 1976 Metronidazole in prevention and treatment of bacteroides infections after appendicectomy. *British Medical Journal* 1: 318–321

109. Willis AT, Ferguson IR, Jones PH et al 1977 Metronidazole in prevention and treatment of bacteroides infections in elective colonic surgery. *British Medical Journal* 1: 607–610

110. Walker AJ, Taylor EW, Lindsay G, Dewar EP 1988 A multicentre study to compare piperacillin with a combination of netilmycin and metronidazole in prophylaxis in elective colorectal surgery undertaken in district general hospitals. *Journal of Hospital Infection* 11: 340–348

111. Morris DL, Rodgers-Wilson S, Payne J et al 1990 A comparison of aztreonam/metronidazole and cefotaxime/metronidazole in elective colorectal surgery: antimicrobial prophylaxis must include Gram-positive cover. *Journal of Antimicrobial Chemotherapy* 95: 273–278

112. Bergman L, Solhaug JH 1987 Single dose chemoprophylaxis in elective colorectal surgery: comparison between doxycycline plus metronidazole and doxycycline. *Annals of Surgery* 205: 77–81

113. Karran SJ, Sutton G, Gartell P, Karran SE, Thinnes D, Blenkensopp J 1993 Imipenem prophylaxis in elective colorectal surgery. *British Journal of Surgery* 80: 1196–1198

114. Das AA 1998 Cost analysis of long term antibiotic prophylaxis for spontaneous bacterial peritonitis in cirrhosis. *American Journal of Gastroenterology* 93: 1895–1900

115. Bhuva M, Ganger D, Jensen D 1994 Spontaneous bacterial peritonitis: an update on evaluation management and prevention. *American Journal of Medicine* 97: 169–175

116. Bohnen JM, Solomkin JS, Dellinger EP, Bjornson HS, Page CP 1992 Guidelines for clinical care: anti-infective agents for intra-abdominal infection. A Surgical Infection Society policy statement. *Archives of Surgery* 127: 83–89

117. Stewart DJ 1978 Antibiotic lavage in the prevention of intraperitoneal sepsis. *Annals of the Royal College of Surgeons of England* 60: 240–243

118. Krukowski ZH, Koruth NM, Matheson NA 1986 Antibiotic lavage in emergency surgery for peritoneal sepsis. *Journal of the Royal College of Surgeons of Edinburgh* 31: 1–6

119. Sauven P, Playforth MJ, Smith GM, Evans M, Pollock AV 1986 Single dose antibiotic prophylaxis of abdominal surgical wound infection; a trial of pre-operative latamoxef against per-operative tetracycline lavage. *Journal of the Royal Society of Medicine* 79: 137–141

120. Silverman SH, Ambrose NS, Youngs DJ, Sheperd AF, Roberts AP, Keighley MR 1986 The effect of peritoneal lavage with tetracycline solution on postoperative infection. A prospective, randomized, clinical trial. *Diseases of the Colon and Rectum* 29: 165–169

121. Targarona EM, Balague C, Knook MM, Trias M 2000 Laparoscopic surgery and surgical infection. *British Journal of Surgery* 87: 536–544

122. Finch WT, Sawyers JL, Schenker S 1976 A prospective study to determine the efficacy of antibiotics in acute pancreatitis. *Annals of Surgery* 183: 667–670

123. Stone HM, Fabian TC 1980 Peritoneal analysis in the treatment of acute alcoholic pancreatitis. *Surgery, Gynecology and Obstetrics* 150: 878–882

124. Pederzoli P, Bassi C, Vesentini S, Campedelli A 1993 A randomized multi-centre clinical trial of antibiotic prophylaxis of septic complications in acute necrotizing pancreatitis with imipenem. *Surgery, Gynecology and Obstetrics* 176: 480–483

125. Widdison AL, Karanjia ND, Reber HA 1994 Antimicrobial treatment of pancreatic infection in cats. *British Journal of Surgery* 81: 886–889

126. Gumaste V 2000 Prophylactic antibiotic therapy in the management of acute pancreatitis. *Journal of Clinical Gastroenterology* 31: 6–10

127. Sharma VK, Howden CW 2001 Prophylactic antibiotic administration reduces sepsis and mortality in acute necrotizing pancreatitis: a meta-analysis. *Pancreas* 22: 28–31

128. Powell JJ, Campbell E, Johnson CD, Siriwardena AK 1999 Survey of antibiotic prophylaxis in acute pancreatitis in the UK and Ireland. *British Journal of Surgery* 86: 320–322

129. Oller DW 1990 Infection in victims of trauma. *Problems in Critical Care* 4: 3–20

130. Weigelt JL, Haley RW, Seibert B 1987 Factors which influence the risk of wound infection in trauma patients. *Trauma* 27: 774–781

131. Dellinger EP, Oreskovich MR, Wertz MJ, Hamasaki V, Lennard ES 1984 Risk of infection following laparotomy for penetrating abdominal injury. *Archives of Surgery* 119: 20–27

132. Wilson RF, Wiencek RG, Balog M 1989 Predicting and preventing infection after abdominal vascular injuries. *Trauma* 29: 1371–1375

133. Brathwaite CEM, Ross SE, Nagele R, Mure AJ, O'Malley KF, Garcia-Perez FA 1993 Bacterial translocation occurs in humans after traumatic injury: evidence using immunofluorescence. *Journal of Trauma* 34: 586–590

134. Ross SE, Cobean RA, Hoyt DB et al 1992 Blunt colonic injury – a multi-centre review. *Journal of Trauma* 33: 379–384

135. Ivatury RR, Gaudino J, Nallathambi MN, Simon RJ, Kazigo ZJ, Stahl WM 1993 Definitive treatment of colon injuries: a prospective study. *American Journal of Surgery* 59: 43–49

136. Demetriades D, Charalambides D, Pantanowitz D 1992 Gunshot wounds of the colon: role of primary repair. *Annals of the Royal College of Surgeons of England* 74: 381–384

137. George SM, Fabian TC, Mangiante EC 1988 Colon trauma: further support for primary repair. *American Journal of Surgery* 156: 16–20

138. Kudsk KA, Minard G, Wojtysiak SL, Croce MA, Fabian TC, Brown RO 1994 Visceral protein response to enteral versus parenteral nutrition and sepsis in patients with trauma. *Surgery* 116: 516–523

139. Moore FA, Feliciano DV, Andrassy RJ 1992 Early enteral feeding, compared with parenteral, reduces postoperative septic complications. The results of a meta-analysis. *Annals of Surgery* 216: 172–183

140. Hammond JMJ, Potgieter PD, Saunders GL 1994 Selective decontamination of the digestive tract in multiple trauma patients – Is there a role? Results of a prospective, double-blind, randomized trial. *Critical Care Medicine* 22: 33–39

141. Brook L 1988 Management of infection following intra-abdominal trauma. *Annals of Emergency Medicine* 17: 626–632

142. Reed RL, Ericsson CD, Wu A, Miller-Crotchett P, Fischer RP 1992 The pharmacokinetics of prophylactic antibiotics in trauma. *Journal of Trauma* 32: 21–27

143. Ericsson CD, Fischer RP, Rowlands BJ, Hunt C, Miller-Crotchett P, Reed L 1989 Prophylactic antibiotics in trauma: the hazards of underdosing. *Journal of Trauma* 29: 1356–1361

144. Nichols RL, Smith JW, Robertson GD et al 1993 Prospective alterations in therapy for penetrating abdominal trauma. *Archives of Surgery* 128: 55–64

145. Branum GD, Tyson GS, Branum MA, Meyers WC 1990 Hepatic abscess. Changes in etiology, diagnosis and management. *Annals of Surgery* 212: 655–662

146. Cappell MS 1991 Hepatobiliary manifestations of the acquired immune deficiency syndrome. *American Journal of Gastroenterology* 86: 1–15

147. Elliott TB, Partridge BW 1991 Multiple hepatic abscesses due to Yersinia enterocolitica. *Australia and New Zealand Journal of Surgery* 61: 708–10

148. Brook I, Fraizer EH 1993 Role of anaerobic bacteria and liver abscesses in children. *Pediatric Infectious Diseases* 12: 743–747

149. Chou FF, Sheen-Chen SM, Chen YS, Lee TY 1995 The comparison of clinical course and results of treatment between gas-forming and non gas-forming pyogenic liver abscess. *Archives of Surgery* 130: 401–405

150. Allison HF, Immelman EJ, Forder AA 1984 Pyogenic liver abscess caused by *Streptococcus milleri*. *South Africa Medical Journal* 65: 432–435

151. Molina JM, Leport C, Bure A, Wolff M, Michon C, Vilde JL 1991 Clinical and bacterial features of infections caused by *Streptococcus milleri*. *Scandinavian Journal of Infectious Diseases* 23: 659–666

152. Chou FF, Sheen-Chen SM, Chen YS, Chen MC, Chen FC, Tai DI 1994 Prognostic factors for pyogenic abscess of the liver. *Journal of the American College of Surgeons* 179: 727–732

153. Halvorsen RA, Korookin M, Foster WL, Silverman PM, Thomson WM 1984 The variable CT appearance of hepatic abscesses. *American Journal of Roentgenology* 142: 941–946.

154. Krige JEJ 1995 The changing pattern of pyogenic liver sepsis. *Current Opinion Surgery and Infection* 3: 25–32

155. Hashimoto L, Hermann R, Grundfest-Broniatowski S 1995 Pyogenic hepatic abscess; results of current management. *American Surgeon* 61: 407–411

156. Moore SW, Millar AJ, Cywes S 1994 Conservative initial treatment for liver abscesses in children. *British Journal of Surgery* 81: 872–874

43 Infections associated with neutropenia and transplantation

Chris Kibbler

Neutropenic patients and transplant recipients are at risk of a number of life-threatening opportunistic infections. Neither patient group suffers from a single specific immunological deficit, there being a subtle blend of physical and immunological defects which evolve with time. Judgments about management need to be based upon knowledge of the balance of these defects and the timing of the infection.

Since the 1970s large numbers of multicenter clinical trials of antimicrobial therapy or prophylaxis have been performed in neutropenic patients. However, until recently there have been few prospective, randomized studies of antimicrobial agents in organ-transplant recipients and most published work has reported experiences from single centers. The majority of hemato-oncology centers and transplant units base patient management (including that of infection) upon agreed protocols and the evidence base for these has become more robust in recent years. It is important that protocols are regularly updated and take account of local variations in risk, organisms and antimicrobial sensitivities.

INFECTIONS IN NEUTROPENIC PATIENTS

The inverse relationship between the numbers of circulating neutrophils and the risk of infection was established nearly four decades ago.[1] This effect becomes apparent when the absolute neutrophil count is less than $1.0 \times 10^9/l$. The risk increases considerably as the count falls below $0.5 \times 10^9/l$ and all patients with a count of less than $0.1 \times 10^9/l$ for more than 3 weeks have been found to develop an infective episode.[1] Criteria for enrollment in a febrile neutropenia trial usually include a neutrophil count less than $0.5 \times 10^9/l$.

CAUSES OF NEUTROPENIA

Most of these patients are neutropenic following chemotherapy for leukemia and some leukemic patients will present with neu-tropenia before chemotherapy. In addition, the neutrophils of patients with myelodysplasia or leukemia, particularly those with acute myeloid leukemia, may have impaired microbicidal activity.[2,3]

Patients receiving chemotherapy for high-risk or relapsed leukemia may be neutropenic for 2–3 weeks, especially if receiving regimens containing fludarabine. Those undergoing chemotherapy for lymphoma or for solid tumors may also suffer a reduction in circulating neutrophils, but this is rarely less than $0.1 \times 10^9/l$ and is often not below $0.5 \times 10^9/l$. Also, the duration of neutropenia is often less than 7 days. In patients with aplastic anemia, or bone marrow transplant (BMT) recipients who fail to engraft, neutropenia is often profound and prolonged. Normal engraftment in allogeneic BMT recipients takes place between 2 and 3 weeks after transplantation.

There has been a four-fold increase in the numbers of peripheral blood stem cell transplants (PBSCT) performed in Europe over the past 10 years,[4] and autologous PBSCT has virtually replaced autologous bone marrow transplantation. Autologous PBSCT recipients have a shorter duration of neutropenia.

Patients undergoing allogeneic bone marrow transplantation behave essentially like neutropenic patients during the early post-transplant phase, but remain immunosuppressed for up to 2 years, even without complications such as graft-versus-host disease.

Other causes of neutropenia are shown in Box 43.1.

FACTORS PREDISPOSING TO INFECTION

The pathogenesis of infection in these patients is multifactorial and is often the consequence of a breach in the skin or oral mucosa plus defects in cellular or humoral immunity.

Some defects are associated with specific infections (Table 43.1). Lymphopenia, as a consequence of lymphoid malig-

Box 43.1 Non-malignant causes of neutropenia

Congenital
- Cyclical neutropenia
- Chronic benign neutropenia
- Severe congenital neutropenia

Acquired
- Drug-induced
  - Cytotoxic chemotherapy (the most common cause of neutropenia)
  - Antimicrobial associated: chloramphenicol; β-lactams; sulfonamides; trimethoprim; nitrofurantoin; flucytosine; ganciclovir; zidovudine
  - Other drugs (e.g. phenothiazines, tolbutamide)
- Alcohol
- Radiation
- Megaloblastic anemia
- Autoimmune neutropenia

nancy or treatment, is associated with reactivation of intracellular organisms such as mycobacteria, the herpes viruses, *Toxoplasma gondii* and *Pneumocystis carinii*. Patients with chronic lymphoid malignancies and those receiving immunosuppressive chemotherapy, such as BMT recipients, have impaired antibody production which predisposes to infection with encapsulated organisms such as *Streptococcus pneumoniae*. The use of indwelling central venous catheters and mucosal damage caused by chemotherapy and herpes simplex virus (HSV) infection[5] allows penetration by commensal flora. In recent years changes in cytotoxic chemotherapy have rendered the oropharynx a major portal of entry for α-hemolytic streptococci. Likewise, splenectomy undertaken as treatment or for diagnosis renders the patient susceptible to infection with encapsulated organisms such as *Str. pneumoniae*. Others have pre-existing sites of chronic infection such as middle-ear disease or bronchiectasis, which may act as reservoirs of infection with organisms such as *Pseudomonas aeruginosa*. Ethnic origin and foreign travel may increase exposure to infections such as tuberculosis, malaria or strongyloidiasis.

CAUSATIVE ORGANISMS

Between 30 and 50% of febrile episodes in neutropenic patients can be confirmed microbiologically, and of these, most are due to bacteremia. Infections with Gram-positive bacteria, especially the coagulase-negative staphylococci and α-hemolytic streptococci, have increased in frequency over the past two decades. In the EORTC (European Organisation for Research and Treatment of Cancer) participatory centers the incidence of bacteremia due to Gram-positive organisms has increased from 29% in the first trial[6] to 67% in the ninth[7]. This increase correlates to some extent with the escalating use of central venous catheters, the development of alternative high-dose chemotherapy with attendant mucositis, and better prevention of Gram-negative infections. Of recent interest is the finding that cell-wall deficient (mostly Gram-positive) bacteria may be responsible for up to 25% of episodes of neutropenic fever in BMT recipients.[8]

Gram-negative bacteria continue to cause some of the most serious episodes of sepsis. Infections caused by the Enterobacteriaceae and *Ps. aeruginosa* carry a mortality of 40–60%.[9,10] Oropharyngeal candidosis is extremely common,

Table 43.1 Factors predisposing to infection in the neutropenic patient

Immune defect/risk factor	Example of opportunistic organisms
Neutropenia	*Streptococcus oralis*
	Pseudomonas aeruginosa
	Candida spp.
	Aspergillus spp.
Lymphoid cell defect	*Mycobacterium* spp.
	Toxoplasma gondii
	Herpes viruses
	Pneumocystis carinii
Humoral	*Streptococcus pneumoniae*
Mucosal barrier (e.g. HSV/chemotherapy-induced mucositis)	*Streptococcus oralis*
	Enterobacteriaceae
	Fungi
Vascular access	Coagulase-negative staphylococci
	Fungi
Foreign travel/ethnic origin	*Mycobacterium* spp.
	Strongyloides stercoralis
Anatomical defect/reservoir (e.g. chronic sinusitis)	*Pseudomonas* spp.
Splenectomy	*Streptococcus pneumoniae*

while invasive candidosis and aspergillosis account for 20–30% of fatal infections when treating acute leukemia.[11,12] Invasive aspergillosis is now the most important infective cause of death in childhood acute myeloid leukemia[13] and in our adult allogeneic bone marrow tranplant patients. Other important infectious agents are listed in Box 43.2.

CHEMOPROPHYLAXIS

Prevention of these serious infections, particularly those carrying a high mortality such as Gram-negative bacteremia or invasive aspergillosis, has been the goal of clinicians for many years. Strategies for preventing acquisition of organisms, such as the use of filtered room air, appear important in some profoundly neutropenic patients at risk from aspergillosis and has been increasingly emphasized in recent years.[14] However, detailed discussion is not possible here.

Box 43.2 Important infectious agents in neutropenic patients

Bacteria	Viruses
Staphylococci	Herpes simplex virus
Streptococci	Varicella zoster virus
Enterobacteriaceae	Cytomegalovirus
Pseudomonads	Epstein–Barr virus
Mycobacterium spp.	Hepatitis A, B, C viruses
Legionella spp.	Parvovirus
Clostridium septicum	Adenovirus
Clostridium difficile	Polyomavirus
Stomatococci	Measles virus
Fungi	**Protozoa/helminths**
Candida spp.	*Toxoplasma gondii*
Aspergillus spp.	*Strongyloides stercoralis*
Zygomycetes	
Cryptococcus neoformans	
Trichosporon beigelli	
Pneumocystis carinii	

Various trials have examined the efficacy of oral non-absorbable antibiotics. Although a number of these were flawed, several controlled trials showed a benefit only when they were combined with a protective environment.[15–23]

Trimethoprim–sulfamethoxazole was first used in patients with acute leukemia to prevent *Pneumocystis carinii* pneumonitis, but it also reduced the incidence of bacterial infection.[24] Further studies have shown variable results, although greatest benefit has been shown in patients with prolonged neutropenia, among whom a consistent reduction in Gram-negative bacterial infections has been found.[25–28] However, the incidence of side-effects (including bone marrow suppression) and the selection of multiresistant organisms has caused some concern.

Oral quinolones (ciprofloxacin, ofloxacin and norfloxacin) have been compared in a number of studies with placebo, trimethoprim–sulfamethoxazole and non-absorbable antibiotics. In the majority of these the 4-quinolone treated patients had significantly fewer Gram-negative bacterial infections, a delayed onset of fever and a reduction in the number of days of fever. Several meta-analyses have confirmed these effects, although a reduction in mortality has not been demonstrated.[29] There has been concern that quinolone resistance is increasing in some units[30] and, certainly, this has the potential to limit the use of quinolone prophylaxis. However, meta-analysis has not shown this to be a significant problem. A sequential study has recently shown that combining ciprofloxacin with colistin was associated with no significant change in quinolone resistance over a 12 year period.[31]

The problem of Gram-positive infections, particularly those due to α-hemolytic streptococci, has been addressed by a number of studies using different agents, including oral penicillins,[32] macrolides[33,34] and rifampicin (rifampin).[35] However, these have given mixed results and have been associated with the emergence of resistance. It is difficult, therefore, to make recommendations for prophylaxis of Gram-positive pathogens.

Attempts at antifungal prophylaxis have met with variable success. Initial studies examined oral polyenes. Nystatin, in doses up to 12×10^6 units/day had little effect on the incidence of invasive candidosis in neutropenic patients,[12] whereas amphotericin B, as suspension, tablets or lozenges, was superior to placebo in preventing the disease.[36]

While most invasive candidal infections are thought to gain entry via the gut,[36] non-absorbable antifungal agents do not protect against fungal infections at other sites, namely the skin, intravenous catheter sites and the respiratory tract. The oral, systemically active azoles have the potential to control colonization as well as prevent dissemination.

Ketoconazole, in daily doses of 200–600 mg, reduces yeast carriage and the incidence of both local and systemic candidosis compared with placebo or non-absorbable agents.[36] However, absorption is impaired in neutropenic patients, particularly in BMT recipients,[37] and breakthrough infections have occurred.[38] There is also the problem of elevated cyclosporin A levels as a result of activity on hepatic P_{450} enzymes and serious idiosyncratic hepatotoxicity.

Fluconazole, in daily doses of 50–400 mg reduces colonization and mucosal thrush as well as reducing the number of disseminated yeast infections.[39,40] Two placebo-controlled studies in bone marrow transplant recipients showed a significant reduction in invasive fungal infections,[41,42] and in one of these fluconazole was associated with a reduced mortality at 110 days.[42] Unfortunately, its use in some centers has been associated with an increase in colonization and infection with *Candida krusei*, which is intrinsically resistant to fluconazole.[43] Fluconazole is also inactive against the important invasive molds that which affect this population, especially *Aspergillus* spp. and the Zygomycetes.

In contrast, itraconazole has activity against the molds, particularly *Aspergillus* species (*see* Ch. 35). However, in its original capsule formulation it was poorly absorbed in these patients. This has been overcome by the introduction of an itraconazole–cyclodextrin complex in solution. Three large randomized controlled trials have shown this formulation to cause a lower overall incidence of fungal infection, a lower death rate from fungal infection and a reduction in the use of intravenous amphotericin B for suspected invasive fungal infection than fluconazole, oral amphotericin B and placebo.[44–46] However, although two of the studies showed a reduction in the incidence of invasive aspergillosis, this was not significant and the placebo-controlled study demonstrated an increase in association with itraconazole.

Amphotericin B administered as a nasal spray has produced conflicting results in preventing invasive aspergillosis,[47,48] although some studies have shown greater benefit when it is aerosolized.[49,50] A recent large prospective randomized study has shown no significant difference in proven, probable or possible invasive aspergillosis between aerosolized amphotericin B and no inhalation (4% vs 7%).[51]

Prophylaxis against *Pn. carinii* infection has proved remarkably effective in those undergoing treatment for acute lymphoblastic leukaemia[24] and for the first 6 months post-BMT. Trimethoprim–sulfamethoxazole three times weekly has been most studied, although some units are now using a 2-day regimen. Nebulized pentamidine is often used in adults during bone marrow engraftment to avoid the myelosuppressive effects of trimethoprim–sulfamethoxazole.

Most virus infections in the neutropenic patient are due to reactivation of the human herpes viruses. Aciclovir, 200 mg 8-hourly to 800 mg 12-hourly, is effective as prophylaxis against herpes simplex virus (HSV) infection in HSV-seropositive patients with leukaemia undergoing chemotherapy, or in BMT recipients.[52,53]

Chemoprophylaxis against cytomegalovirus (CMV) infection has been investigated in detail only in BMT recipients, although disease also occurs in patients with acute leukemia receiving chemotherapy. High-dose aciclovir has been shown to be partially effective in preventing CMV infection and disease post-BMT. A multicenter randomized trial compared 500 mg/m² intravenously 8-hourly for 1 month followed by 800 mg 6-hourly by mouth for 6 months with 200 or 400 mg 6-hourly orally for 1 month followed by placebo.[54] The incidence of CMV infection reduced and survival increased by day 210 post-BMT, although the rates of CMV pneumonia were similar in the two groups.

The use of ganciclovir as prophylaxis against CMV infection has shown some benefit in reducing the incidence of CMV disease but has no effect on survival during the first 4 months post-BMT.[39,55] When used as pre-emptive therapy following detection of CMV infection, survival was improved at 100 and 180 days post-transplant.[56] The difference in these two approaches may be due to the myelosuppressive effects of ganciclovir causing a higher number of deaths from non-viral infections when used as prophylaxis as well as failure to prevent CMV pneumonia. It would seem more appropriate to use ganciclovir as pre-emptive therapy, particularly now that tests for antigenemia and the CMV polymerase chain reaction (PCR) allow even earlier detection of infection.[57–59]

A summary of prophylactic regimens is shown in Table 43.2.

Table 43.2 Current antimicrobial prophylactic regimens for patients with prolonged neutropenia

Prophylaxis	Agent	Dosage	Duration
Antibacterial	Ciprofloxacin	500 mg 12-hourly	During period of neutropenia
Antifungal (high-risk patients)	Itraconazole suspension	400 mg once daily	During period of neutropenia 6 months post-BMT
	+ amphotericin B	500 mg 6-hourly	During period of neutropenia 6 months post-BMT
Anti-*Pn. carinii*	Trimethoprim–sulfamethoxazole	960 mg 12-hourly	1 week pre- and 6 months post-BMT 3 times/week throughout treatment in ALL
	(Nebulized pentamidine in adults)	(150 mg fortnightly)	During period of neutropenia
Antituberculosis*	Isoniazid	5 mg/kg daily	During period of neutropenia 6 months post-BMT
Herpes simplex virus†	Aciclovir	400–800 mg 4–5 times/day	During period of neutropenia
Cytomegalovirus‡	Seronegative blood products		
	Aciclovir	High dose	Not yet established
	Ganciclovir		Not yet established

*At-risk patients only.
† Seropositive patients only.
‡ BMT recipients only.

EMPIRICAL THERAPY

The use of empirical antibiotic therapy in febrile neutropenic patients is almost universally practised, because to await microbiological diagnosis is associated with a high mortality, particularly in patients with Gram-negative bacteremia. The trigger for this is usually a single oral temperature of 38.3°C or two separate temperatures of 38.0°C at least 1 h apart.

The regimen chosen should be active against the common organisms likely to result in overwhelming sepsis or death, and influenced by local antibiotic sensitivity patterns, the incidence of particular infections, the specific needs of the patient and the prophylactic regimen used. Traditionally the significant organisms have been the Enterobacteriaceae and *Ps. aeruginosa*, which carry a mortality of 40–60%.[9,10] Earlier regimens included an aminoglycoside in combination with a β-lactam antibiotic in an attempt to achieve broad-spectrum and synergistic activity against organisms such as *Ps. aeruginosa*. However, the potential renal, auditory and vestibular toxicity associated with prolonged and repeated courses of aminoglycosides has led investigators to study non-aminoglycoside containing regimens. These have consisted of combinations of two β-lactam agents (the 'double β-lactam combination') or a single broad-spectrum agent such as ceftazidime, cefoperazone, cefpirome, a quinolone or a carbapenem ('monotherapy'). The advantages and disadvantages of these different regimens are shown in Table 43.3.

The first studies of double β-lactam therapy gave results inferior to aminoglycoside-containing regimens,[6,60,61] but later studies using ceftazidime, latamoxef and cefoperazone in combination with a ureidopenicillin[62–64] concluded that such combinations were of equal efficacy and less nephrotoxic than aminoglycoside-containing regimens. However, it was unclear whether they were any better than β-lactam monotherapy.

Ceftazidime was the initial choice for monotherapy. A meta-analysis of carefully selected studies has shown that results of combination therapy are not significantly different from ceftazidime alone, even in bacteremic patients.[65] A number of other monotherapy regimens have been studied (Box 43.3). Imipenem, and more recently meropenem, has been compared with a number of regimens.[63,65–70] Outcome has been at least as good as with the comparator, although some failures, of Gram-positive infections, have occurred. There have also been reports that *Stenotrophomonas maltophilia* is selected out by the carbapenems, to which it is intrinsically resistant.[71] In addition, there have been concerns over central nervous system (CNS) toxicity with high-dose imipenem[64] or ciprofloxacin prophylaxis.[72]

One advantage of the carbapenems is their activity against the α-hemolytic streptococci,[74] allowing them to be used alone without the need for early glycopeptide therapy. Similar streptococcal activity can be provided by piperacillin–tazobactam.[75] The current excess of Gram-positive infections indicates that empirical therapy should contain a broad-spectrum anti-Gram-positive agent. Clinical trials of glycopeptides have provided conflicting evidence as to whether and when to add such an agent.

Early studies in centers in which there were significant numbers of Gram-positive infections showed initial vancomycin or teicoplanin increased response rates and reduced morbidity,[76,77] although no study has shown a reduction in mortality. In addition, vancomycin is associated with increased toxicity.[77,78] The large joint study conducted by the EORTC and the National Cancer Institute of Canada showed that

Table 43.3 Options for initial empirical therapy

Regimen	Advantages	Disadvantages
Aminoglycoside + β-lactam	Broad spectrum Proven efficacy Synergy vs Gram-negative bacteria and streptococci	Poor activity vs coagulase-negative staphylococci Nephrotoxic and ototoxic Serum assays required
Double β-lactam therapy	Broad spectrum Avoids aminoglycoside toxicity No monitoring required	No more effective than single-agent therapy Possible prolongation of neutropenia Electrolyte imbalance Possible antagonism
Monotherapy	Broad spectrum Avoids aminoglycoside toxicity Avoids antagonism No monitoring required Cheaper	Lack of synergy (? less effective vs *Ps. aeruginosa*) Less active versus Gram-positive bacteria (with ceftazidime) Risk of resistance Potential central nervous system toxicity (with imipenem)
Single agent + glycopeptide	Broad spectrum including coagulase-negative staphylococci and α-hemolytic streptococci No monitoring required (with teicoplanin)	Expensive Unnecessary in some units Nephro- and oto-toxicity (with vancomycin) Monitoring required (with vancomycin) Risk of glycopeptide resistance

Box 43.3 Representative antibiotic regimens that have been evaluated for empirical therapy in febrile neutropenic patients[73]

Penicillin and aminoglycoside combinations
Carbenicillin and gentamicin/amikacin/sisomicin

Ticarcillin and gentamicin/tobramycin/amikacin/netilmicin

Mezlocillin and tobramycin

Piperacillin and gentamicin/amikacin/netilmicin/tobramycin

Azlocillin and amikacin/netilmicin

Piperacillin–tazobactam and amikacin

Cephalosporin and aminoglycoside combinations
Cefalotin and gentamicin

Latamoxef and gentamicin/amikacin

Cefotaxime and amikacin

Ceftazidime and tobramycin/amikacin

Cefoperazone and amikacin

Ceftriaxone and amikacin/netilmicin

Double β-lactam combinations
Carbenicillin and cefalotin

Carbenicillin and cefamandole

Ceftazidime and flucloxacillin

Ticarcillin and latamoxef

Piperacillin and latamoxef

Ceftazidime and azlocillin

Ceftazidime and piperacillin

Triple agent combinations
Carbenicillin, cefalotin and gentamicin

Carbenicillin, cefazolin and amikacin

Cefotaxime, piperacillin and netilmicin

Monotherapy regimens
Latamoxef

Ceftazidime

Cefoperazone

Ceftriaxone

Imipenem

Meropenem

Ciprofloxacin

Cefpirome

Cefepime

Piperacillin–tazobactam

Other agents and combinations
Aztreonam and vancomycin

Imipenem and vancomycin

Trimethoprim–sulfamethoxazole and amikacin

Ticarcillin–clavulanate

including vancomycin in the initial therapy conferred no additional benefit.[79]

The increasing isolation of vancomycin-resistant enterococci[80,81] prompted the CDC (Centers for Disease Control and Prevention) to issue guidelines on the use of vancomycin that specifically exclude its use as empirical therapy in the neu-

tropenic patient.[82] This seems prudent, although the Infectious Diseases Society of America (IDSA) suggests that vancomycin may be used in initial regimens in institutions where fulminant Gram-positive infections are common and discontinued 3–4 days later if such an infection is not identified.[83]

There is also evidence that the choice of broad-spectrum agent for empirical therapy can influence the emergence of glycopeptide-resistant enterococci. A UK unit using ceftazidime and teicoplanin found colonization rates of up to 50%.[84] Changing the regimen to piperacillin–tazobactam monotherapy (whilst the total teicoplanin use remained the same) was followed by a fall in colonization with glycopeptide-resistant enterococci to 19%. A return to the previous regimen resulted in an increase to 36%.

The duration of treatment has not been studied independently, but since the first EORTC trial the evidence has suggested that prolonged treatment is associated with more superinfections, often fungal, but no improvement in outcome. Current EORTC trials are conducted on the basis of discontinuing antibiotics after 7 days minimum treatment and four consecutive afebrile days and this is similar to the IDSA guidelines where 5–7 days without fever is recommended.[83]

HOME THERAPY

Health services in general are moving towards earlier discharge of all groups of patients and attempts have been made to achieve this in the neutropenic population. Talcott and colleagues derived a risk assessment model in which patients were divided into four groups:[85] those with previous admissions, those having serious comorbidity, those with uncontrolled cancer and the remainder. The fourth group was found to be at low risk and was studied in subsequent trials, which showed that amoxicillin–clavulanate plus ciprofloxacin was as effective as intravenous ceftazidime or ceftriaxone plus amikacin in treating these patients.[86,87] This may allow patients to be discharged while still receiving treatment for resolving neutropenic fever, or even to be managed as outpatients. Such strategies are continuing to be explored.

MANAGEMENT OF THE PATIENT WITH PERSISTENT PYREXIA

Approximately 20–30% of febrile patients who remain persistently neutropenic fail to respond to apparently appropriate antibiotic therapy. Some remain febrile until recovery of their neutrophil counts, irrespective of the antimicrobial therapy administered. Many patients with persistent fever will have an occult fungal infection; autopsy studies have shown that up to 25% of those neutropenic patients who die have an undiagnosed fungal infection.[11] In view of the difficulties in diagnosis the use of empirical antifungal therapy has been advocated. The largest randomized study reported compared the effect of amphotericin B (0.6 mg/kg daily or equivalent) with no treatment in patients remaining febrile 4 days after empirical therapy.[88] Although more responded in the amphotericin B-treated group, the effect was only significant in patients not given antifungal prophylaxis (78% vs 45%; $p = 0.04$). Following this a number of other agents have been shown to be at least as effective as conventional amphotericin B. Liposomal amphotericin B (AmBisome) is less nephrotoxic than conventional amphotericin B, at least as effective in rendering patients afebrile and is associated with significantly fewer breakthrough fungal infections.[89,90] Intravenous itraconazole and voriconazole also appear likely to be useful for empirical antifungal therapy.

Patients who deteriorate during the first 48 h of empirical therapy pose a particularly difficult therapeutic challenge. It is important that there are no gaps in the spectrum of the selected regimen. Deterioration may be due to Gram-negative or Gram-positive organisms, such as α-hemolytic streptococci, which may cause features similar to those of sepsis syndrome

(including ARDS and septic shock), or enterococci. Gram-negative activity (including antipseudomonal activity) is essential. Consequently, the addition of an aminoglycoside to initial β-lactam monotherapy is recommended, and a glycopeptide should also be considered. The above approach is summarized in Figure 43.1.

ASPECTS OF THERAPY FOR SPECIFIC ORGANISMS AND INFECTIONS

Intravenous catheter-associated infections

Most neutropenic patients undergoing chemotherapy have an indwelling central line, which commonly becomes infected. The predominant pathogens are coagulase-negative staphylococci and *Staphylococcus aureus*.[91] Others include *Candida* spp.,

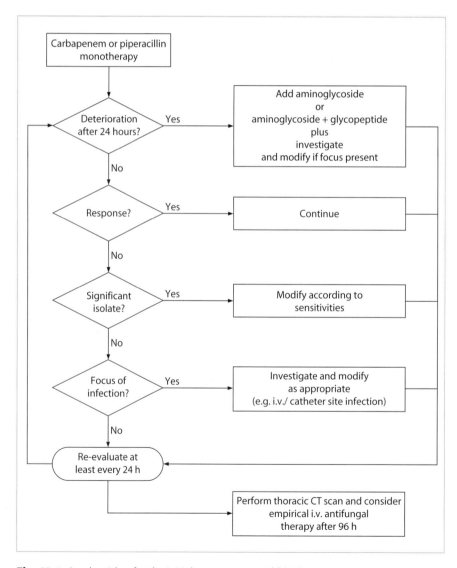

Fig. 43.1 An algorithm for the initial management of febrile neutropenic patients receiving prophylaxis.

coryneforms, *Acinetobacter*, *Stenotrophomonas* and *Pseudomonas* spp.[73] Ideally, infected catheters should be removed, but coagulase-negative staphylococcal infections may be effectively suppressed or eliminated by administering antibiotics via the catheter until neutropenia has resolved.[91] A high percentage of coagulase-negative staphylococci isolated on hematology units are resistant to methicillin and other β-lactams. A glycopeptide (most frequently vancomycin) is given for these, with the chance of success being more than 50%. Similar response rates can be obtained with coryneform infections but those due to *Candida* spp., Enterobacteriaceae, *Staph. aureus* and *Ps. aeruginosa*, and any form of tunnel infection, require the catheter to be removed and appropriate antimicrobial therapy administered.[92]

Pulmonary infections of unknown cause

Pulmonary infiltrates commonly occur in the febrile neutropenic patient and have a number of causes, especially in the BMT recipient. These include non-infective conditions such as pulmonary edema, alveolar hemorrhage, drug adverse effects and the idiopathic pneumonitis syndrome. Focal lesions are more indicative of fungal infection, and computed tomography (CT) or magnetic resonance imaging (MRI) scanning may reveal characteristic features of these.[93] However, in most cases treatment has to be given empirically.

Initial therapy should certainly include agents effective against common respiratory pathogens such as *Str. pneumoniae* and *Haemophilus influenzae* as well as Gram-negative organisms including *Ps. aeruginosa*, and hence a carbapenem, piperacillin–tazobactam or ceftazidime, with or without an aminoglycoside, is recommended.

Atypical pneumonias are extremely uncommon in this population and, unless there are particular clinical or epidemiological reasons to suggest Legionnaires' disease, erythromycin can be omitted from the initial therapy. Mycobacterial infections may occasionally complicate hematological malignancies. Patients with lymphoid malignancy and BMT recipients who have not been receiving trimethoprim–sulfamethoxazole prophylaxis are at risk of *P. carinii* pneumonitis; empirical high-dose trimethoprim–sulfamethoxazole therapy (120 mg/kg daily in divided doses) is warranted in such patients. BMT recipients are particularly at risk of CMV pneumonitis post-transplant. However, CMV or *Pn. carinii* pneumonitis usually present a month or so post-transplant, when the patient is no longer neutropenic, and the timing of the presentation should be taken into account when decisions are being made regarding empirical therapy. CMV pneumonitis is treated with ganciclovir (5 mg/kg intravenous, twice daily) plus intravenous immunoglobulin 200–400 mg/kg on alternate days for 14–21 days.[94–96] Despite this, mortality from CMV infection is still in excess of 50% in BMT recipients. Further, the myelosuppressive effect of ganciclovir can present a particular problem in these patients.

Patients discharged into the community are at risk of respiratory viral infections with agents such as respiratory syncytial virus, influenza and paramyxoviruses, which occasionally cause outbreaks on hematology units.[97]

Invasive aspergillosis

The mortality due to invasive aspergillosis remains high in neutropenic patients despite the use of high-dose (1.0–1.5 mg/kg daily) intravenous amphotericin B; the infection is now the most important cause of death in childhood AML and adult BMT recipients in BMT recipients case fatality rates have been 86.7% in the last 5 years.[98] Successful outcome is dependent upon early treatment and, to a considerable extent, on bone marrow recovery. High-dose conventional amphotericin B is also associated with a high incidence of nephrotoxicity. Lipid-associated formulations of the drug have been licensed for use in patients failing treatment or experiencing unacceptable toxicity with conventional amphotericin B. Liposomal amphotericin B (AmBisome) has been studied in a randomized prospective trial comparing two doses (1 mg/kg/day and 4 mg/kg/day) for the treatment of invasive aspergillosis in neutropenic patients:[99] 6-month mortality was approximately 60% with attributable mortality of around 20% in the two arms.

Itraconazole has been used with success in this population[100] and the drug is being increasingly used for completion therapy once a patient has responded to intravenous amphotericin B. Other alternatives becoming available include voriconazole, posaconazole (new triazoles) and the echinocandin caspofungin. The therapy of fungal infection is considered in detail in Ch. 62.

The development of mycotic lung sequestra (which have been mistakenly termed mycetomas) may require additional therapy. These lesions appear once the bone marrow is regenerating. Patients are at risk of life-threatening hemoptysis.[101] In addition, patients who require further chemotherapy or bone marrow transplantation are at considerable risk of relapse of the original infection. Resection of these lesions has been shown to be effective, preventing relapse following bone marrow transplantation, and is associated with a lower mortality than antifungal therapy alone.[102]

ADDITIONAL THERAPIES

Growth factors

Hematopoietic growth factors have been extensively used to treat neutropenic patients. Studies have consistently shown that granulocyte colony stimulating factor (G-CSF) reduces the duration of neutropenia. However, the reduction in infectious complications has been modest and most trials have been unable to demonstrate a reduction in infectious morbidity and mortality.[103–105] This is probably because the major effect of G-CSF is to accelerate the recovery of neutrophils, whereas it has no impact on the critical lag period of profound neutropenia.[106] The American Society of Oncology has published guidelines for the use of these agents in the setting of anti-cancer chemotherapy.[107]

Granulocyte–macrophage colony-stimulating factor and macrophage colony-stimulating factor may be beneficial in the treatment of invasive fungal infections,[108] although large-scale trials demonstrating this are regrettably still lacking.

Granulocyte transfusions

Transfusions of circulating white cells have been used to augment antimicrobial therapy in neutropenic patients with unresponsive infection. Their use was largely abandoned, although benefit had been demonstrated in children, in whom it is possible to achieve significant increases in neutrophil counts. Renewed interest is now being shown in this modality, coupled with improved methods of harvesting and increased yield following the use of growth factors.[109,110]

Immunoglobulin therapy

Passive immunotherapy has been used both for prevention of infection and for treatment. However, it has a significant benefit in a few conditions only. The addition of intravenous immunoglobulin to ganciclovir improves survival in CMV pneumonitis.

Routine prophylactic use of intravenous immunoglobulin in leukemia therapy does not reduce viral infections. Post-exposure immunoglobulin is indicated for the prevention of hepatitis A, measles and varicella-zoster infection (with hyper-immune immunoglobulin).

INFECTIONS IN TRANSPLANT RECIPIENTS

IMMUNOSUPPRESSIVE THERAPY

Between 1994 and 1998 the 1-year graft survival for cadaveric renal transplants in the USA was 87% (96% for living HLA-identical sibling renal allografts).[111] The results are similar for Europe. Developments in surgery and better control of rejection and infective complications have allowed a steady improvement in the survival of other organ grafts.

Most transplant units use a triple regimen of azathioprine, cyclosporin A and corticosteroids for immunosuppression. Azathioprine is a purine analog which inhibits both B and T cell proliferation and as a consequence both cell-mediated immunity (CMI) and humoral immunity are inhibited. The drug may take weeks or months to exert its full effect. Cyclosporin, a calcineurin inhibitor, arrests the lymphocyte cell cycle in the resting phase, having most effect on CD4-positive T cells and a minimal effect on B cells. This results in effective suppression of CMI, has little effect on humoral immunity and no effect on phagocytosis. The inflammatory response is preserved.

Corticosteroids in high dose have a very broad immunosuppressive action, producing a reduction in antigen-stimulated lymphocyte proliferation and a blunting of the primary antibody response. They also inhibit neutrophil chemotaxis and monocyte phagocytosis, dramatically reducing inflammatory responses at high dosage and disguising the presence of infection.

The aim of these regimens is to achieve a balance between graft rejection and risk of infection. Episodes of subsequent acute rejection require considerable immunosuppression and are accompanied by an increased risk of opportunistic infections. The phase of acute rejection varies in length for different transplants. Most episodes occur in the first 3 months of liver transplantation, whereas the phase of acute rejection lasts for 6 months for renal transplants.[112] Rejection episodes are usually treated with high-dose methylprednisolone or various antibody preparations such as polyclonal antithymocyte globulin (ATG), antilymphocyte globulin (ALG) or the pan-T-cell monoclonal antibody OKT3. Patients requiring a second or third graft are usually even more immunosuppressed and at increased risk of opportunistic infection.

Tacrolimus (FK506), another calcineurin antagonist, has been substituted for ciclosporin for certain indications; several studies have demonstrated it to have fewer infective complications,[113–116] which may be a consequence of the need for less episodic anti-rejection therapy. Mycophenolate mofetil, an inhibitor of inosine monophosphate dehydrogenase, which inhibits purine synthesis, has been used as a substitute for calcineurin inhibitors. Although it has no associated renal toxicity (and allows improvement in renal function) some studies have shown it to result in increased risk of rejection.[112] There is still considerable scope for refining immunosuppression with these and other new agents, hopefully enabling a further reduction in infective complications.

THE SEQUENCE OF INFECTIONS FOLLOWING TRANSPLANTATION

Infectious complications follow a relatively predictable chronological order after any transplantation procedure. Knowledge of this is helpful in guiding the use and duration of prophylaxis, establishing a diagnosis through appropriate investigations and administering empirical treatment if necessary.

In the first month after transplant, infections are largely associated with the transplant surgical procedure, particularly those complicating the anastomoses associated with the specific procedure (such as the biliary tract in liver transplantation). Some infections are transmitted with the allograft or are present in the recipient before transplantation.

Between the first and the sixth month following transplantation the most important infections are caused by the herpes group viruses (especially CMV), *Nocardia* species, *Listeria monocytogenes*, *Toxoplasma gondii*, *Pn. carinii* and other fungi. In addition, latent infections such as tuberculosis or histoplasmosis may reactivate at this time. The risk of infection correlates with the severity of immunosuppression required to treat rejection episodes.

Subsequent infections are usually the result of community-acquired organisms. A few patients will suffer chronic viral infections affecting the graft, while others who have been intensively immunosuppressed remain at risk of opportunistic infections.

Bacterial infections

Bacterial infections occur in approximately 50% of renal transplant recipients and in up to 70% of liver transplant patients. In some series patients have suffered at least one bacterial infection in the post-transplant period.[117] The common infections are intra-abdominal abscess, cholangitis, bacteremia, wound infection, lower respiratory tract infection and urinary tract infection, with intra-abdominal infection responsible for approximately 30% in liver transplantation.[117–120] The overall mortality is less than 5%, but varies according to site and organ.

In recent years resistant organisms have become established as endemic pathogens in many transplant units. MRSA was found to be the leading cause of bacteremia in liver transplant recipients in one center, responsible for 37% of all episodes.[121] Vancomycin-resistant enterococci and extended-spectrum β-lactamase-producing Gram-negative organisms are also increasingly causing infections in these patients.

Representative organisms isolated from infected patients in the postoperative period are shown in Box 43.4. Bacteria isolated from the graft perfusion fluid differ in their propensity to cause post-transplantation infection. Positive cultures have been found in up to 40% of cases in renal transplantation, but most of these have been due to Gram-positive skin bacteria and do not seem to have serious consequences. However, the isolation of the Enterobacteriaceae and *Ps. aeruginosa* correlate with vascular infection and postoperative sepsis[122–124] and warrant systemic antibiotic therapy following transplantation.

Infections due to *Nocardia* spp. are important late complications following transplantation, usually occurring after the first month, and which correlate with the degree of immunosuppression. Outbreaks in renal transplant units have been described[125] and the incidence is up to 4% in this group.

Tuberculosis tends to occur several months after transplantation. The onset is significantly later in renal transplants than in other groups of organ transplant recipients (median time 11.5 months post-transplant versus 4, 4 and 3.5 months in liver, heart, and lung transplants respectively).[126] Approximately one-third have disseminated infection and the overall mortality is 29%. The overall incidence of mycobacterial infection in the transplant population is 1%, more than 50-fold greater than the incidence in the general population.[127]

Transplant recipients are at increased risk of Legionnaires' disease by virtue of their immunosuppression. In addition, a UK study demonstrated that *Legionella* spp. could be isolated from the water in approximately 50% of transplant units.[128]

Fungal infections

Colonization with yeasts is common in this population, although the incidence varies according to the number and frequency of sites sampled and the use of antifungal prophylaxis. Infection rates vary with the type of transplant, being least for renal transplant recipients (approximately 5%).[129] There is evidence that the incidence of fungal infections is falling, possibly as a consequence of reduced immunosuppression and improvement in surgical technique.[130] Most infections are caused by *Candida* spp. (approximately 80%), with *Aspergillus* spp. accounting for the majority of invasive mold infections.[129,131] *Pn. carinii* pneumonitis occurred in 4–10% of kidney, 10–11% of liver, 5–41% of heart, and 16–43% of heart–lung and lung transplant recipients before routine prophylaxis was implemented.[132] It is closely linked with CMV disease.

Severe fungal infections carry a high mortality rate. Candidal infections are associated with death in more than 50% and invasive aspergillosis is almost universally fatal in this group.[129] The site of infection is transplant dependent. Thus urinary tract candidosis is mostly confined to the renal transplant group and lung transplant recipients have a much increased risk of pulmonary infections. Although occurring very infrequently, focal brain infection in solid organ transplant patients is almost exclusively due to fungi, usually *Aspergillus* spp.;[133–135] *Cryptococcus neoformans* is the most frequent cause of meningitis.

Most fungal infections occur in the first 2 months after transplant,[129] although *Pn. carinii* infection tends to be delayed and cryptococcosis usually affects patients in the late trans-

Box 43.4 Organisms causing post-transplant infections

Gram-positive bacteria	Fungi
Coagulase-negative staphylococci	*Candida* spp.
Staphylococcus aureus	*Aspergillus* spp.
Enterococci	*Pneumocystis carinii*
Streptococci	*Cryptococcus neoformans*
Listeria monocytogenes	
Nocardia spp.	**Viruses**
	Herpes simplex virus
Gram-negative bacteria	Cytomegalovirus
Enterobacteriaceae	Hepatitis B virus
Pseudomonas spp.	Hepatitis C virus
Stenotrophomonas maltophilia	Varicella zoster virus
Legionella spp.	Polyoma viruses
	Adenovirus
	Human herpesvirus-6
Anaerobic bacteria	Human herpesvirus-8
Bacteroides spp.	
Clostridium spp.	**Others**
	Mycobacterium spp.
	Toxoplasma gondii

plant period. The management of these infections is discussed further in Ch. 62.

Viral infections

Cytomegalovirus is responsible for the greatest number of all types of infection in these patients. The incidence varies from 45%[136] to 100%,[136] reflecting the incidence of seropositivity among the recipient population and the numbers of seropositive to seronegative transplantations. However, incidence is transplant dependent, being lowest in renal transplants, in whom it is symptomatic in less than 10%.[137]

Overall, 25–30% of infected patients develop disease,[136–138] although of those at highest risk (seropositive to seronegative transplants) 50–60% will develop clinical disease.[127] The site of disease is transplant dependent, being focused on the graft. About 3% of all transplant recipients affected will develop CMV pneumonitis.[138]

Post-transplant hepatitis occurs in more than 10% of solid organ transplant recipients overall. The most common cause is hepatitis C virus (HCV). In liver transplant patients most of these infections occur as a result of reinfection in patients who have been transplanted for HCV-related cirrhosis. Polymerase chain reaction techniques have shown that virtually all infected patients suffer reinfection post-transplant. Before universal screening of blood donors and awareness of donor status, primary HCV infections occurred in more than 35%;[139] the incidence is now much lower. In one study, 95% of patients with pretransplant infection developed post-transplant hepatitis, mostly due to HCV.

Reinfection with hepatitis B virus (HBV) following liver transplantation is almost inevitable unless long-term prophylaxis is used. The highest recurrence is seen in those who are HBV-DNA positive before transplant.[140]

Epstein–Barr virus (EBV) infection following transplant is probably underdiagnosed. Most clinical disease is due to reactivation although primary infection does occur, usually after the patient is discharged, and is responsible for more severe disease. The most important complication of EBV infection is post-transplant lymphoproliferative disorder (PTLD). The overall incidence of this condition is approximately 1%.[141] In a large series of various solid organ graft recipients, viremia was found in 3.9%, and 75% of those with primary viremia developed PTLD compared with 11% of secondary viremia cases.[141] The risk of this disease is also increased by the use of anti-rejection therapy such as OKT3 anti-T cell antibodies.

Before the advent of aciclovir, HSV infections (almost exclusively the consequence of reactivation) were responsible for clinical disease in approximately 50% of seropositive patients.[127] HSV infections are now much less clinically significant than other herpes group infections.

Human herpesvirus-6 (HHV-6) may be responsible for central nervous system disease post transplantation. CNS symptoms occurred in 25% of liver transplant recipients with HHV-6 viremia, compared with 12% of those without.[142]

Infection with HHV-6 may also have an immunomodulatory role, being associated with an increased risk of CMV infection and fungal infection.[143]

Human herpesvirus-8 (HHV-8) is transmitted from donor to recipient, resulting in Kaposi's sarcoma in up to 8% of cases who seroconvert.[144]

Polyomavirus causes latent infection in the kidney in the immunocompetent subject and in renal transplant recipients may be responsible for tubulointerstitial nephritis and graft dysfunction.[145]

Infections due to other organisms

The incidence of toxoplasmosis varies according to the type of transplant and is most common in heart transplant recipients, of whom more than 50% of seronegative patients receiving a heart from a seropositive donor will seroconvert.[146] In addition, toxoplasmosis is governed by the seroprevalence of the infection (20% in the UK, higher in other countries such as France) and the serological status of donor and recipient: the highest rate and most severe infections occur when transplanting a seropositive donor to a seronegative recipient. In renal transplant recipients less than 1% develop primary toxoplasmosis. Most such cases occur within 2 months of transplant and are characterized by encephalitis, brain abscess, retinitis, pneumonitis, cardiac involvement and hepatitis.[147–149]

CHEMOPROPHYLAXIS

Until recently, most prophylactic regimens used in transplant recipients have been based on the risk of infection and likely organisms. Regimens shown to be effective in the neutropenic patient or in surgical prophylaxis have been adopted, yet few have been subject to randomized comparative trials. A short course of prophylactic antibiotics is probably appropriate to prevent wound infection related to the procedure itself. Selective decontamination of the digestive tract may be of benefit in some transplant groups, although there is conflicting evidence. Gram-negative infections are reduced in liver transplant recipients[150] but an increase in Gram-positive infections, including MRSA and vancomycin-resistant enterococci, has been seen in several heart transplant centres.[151]

A number of studies have demonstrated the benefit of long-term prophylaxis for urinary tract infections in renal transplant recipients. Both trimethoprim–sulfamethoxazole (960 mg nightly) and ciprofloxacin have been effective, although the former has the additional benefit of preventing *Pn. carinii* infection.[152,153]

The issue of mycobacterial prophylaxis remains controversial and policies vary internationally. There is a significant risk of isoniazid hepatic toxicity and so this drug should be used selectively. However, this risk varies according to the transplant, from 2.5% in renal transplant recipients to 41% in liver transplant.[126] Patients in whom such treatment is justified are those of Asian or other high-risk ethnic origin, those with a history of tuberculosis and those with radiographic changes suggesting past chest infection. In the USA the tuberculin skin test is often used as a determinant for prophylaxis.

The high risk of fungal infection in liver transplant recipients has led to the administration of antifungal agents in the post-transplant period. Non-absorbable agents such as amphotericin B or nystatin, sometimes in combination with oral antibiotics such as gentamicin and polymyxin B, are widely used. Fluconazole and itraconazole have been studied in randomized comparative trials in liver transplantation and both are better than placebo in preventing superficial and invasive candidosis.[154,155]

Prophylaxis against *Pn. carinii* pneumonia with trimethoprim–sulfamethoxazole is probably only necessary during the first year post-transplant, except in lung transplant recipients, when there is a significant persisting risk of the disease.[156]

Several randomized comparative studies have demonstrated that early (first 14 days or until discharge) post-transplant ganciclovir, with[157] or without[158] gammaglobulin is more effective that aciclovir (various doses) in preventing CMV symptomatic infection in liver transplants. Symptomatic infection was reduced to 5–9%.

Pre-emptive prophylaxis targets patients at highest risk of disease and limits duration of drug administration, reducing toxicity and cost. Hence, kidney–pancreas transplant patients receiving OKT3 pan-T-cell monoclonal antibody therapy and CMV-shedding liver transplant recipients both appear to benefit from pre-emptive prophylaxis with ganciclovir.[159,160] CMV antigenemia-guided pre-emptive therapy is as effective as, but less expensive than, universal oral ganciclovir prophylaxis for 90 days or intravenous ganciclovir for 14 days.[161]

Trials of prophylaxis with lamivudine to prevent recurrence of HBV following liver transplantation have shown that, although HBV-DNA levels become undetectable in virtually all patients, this effect is not sustained because of the emergence of resistant mutants.[162]

TREATMENT

Although transplant recipients are severely immunocompromised, they do not have the same paucity of signs as neutropenic patients in the face of serious sepsis and, in the immediate postoperative period behave more like non-transplant patients with surgical sepsis.[163] Consequently, the concept of early empirical therapy in response to fever alone has not been applied to these patients.

All attempts should be made to identify a focus of sepsis or the non-infective cause for fever in a transplant patient. Antimicrobial therapy may reasonably be withheld if the patient is otherwise well and there is no identifiable infective cause, but this should be kept under review. If empirical treatment is considered necessary the choice of antimicrobials should be governed by the timing of the infection (and hence the probable organisms), the type of transplant, the site of sepsis, knowledge of colonization with resistant organisms (such as MRSA and VRE), and local antimicrobial resistance patterns, as discussed previously.

ASPECTS OF THERAPY FOR SPECIFIC INFECTIONS

Fungal infections

Fungal infections should be managed using the same agents as used in the neutropenic patient (p. 551). No antifungal is contraindicated but care is a required in their use because of toxicity (especially in renal and liver transplant recipients) and drug interaction (especially flucytosine with antimetabolites and itraconazole with cyclosporin and tacrolimus – *see below*).

It is probably appropriate to reduce immunosuppression in the face of a progressive life-threatening fungal infection such as invasive aspergillosis, especially in the setting of a non-essential organ graft such as a kidney transplant, although the evidence for benefit is anecdotal. Other attempts at immunomodulation have included the use of colony-stimulating factors. Granulocyte colony-stimulating factor antagonizes the effect of triazoles in an immunocompromised mouse model of invasive aspergillosis.[164] Granulocyte macrophage colony-stimulating factor has been used with some success in the neutropenic patient and might prove of more use than G-CSF in the transplant setting.

Pulmonary infections of unknown cause

Patients presenting with pulmonary infiltrates and fever 1 month or more post-transplant are most likely to have CMV or *Pn. carinii* infection (unless they are receiving trimethoprim–sulfamethoxazole prophylaxis). These infections should be managed as in the BMT recipient (*see* p. 551). The possibility of other community-acquired respiratory tract infections, including those due to influenza and respiratory syncytial viruses, should always be borne in mind.

Post-transplant lymphoproliferative disorder

The incidence of this occurring in renal transplant recipients is 1–2%,[165,166] is related to the degree of immunosuppression (it is seen particularly in patients receiving OKT3) and is more likely in primary EBV infection.[167] At present, the mainstay of therapy is the reduction of immunosuppression together with intravenous aciclovir (10 mg/kg 8-hourly). However, many patients will require local resection or radiotherapy of affected tissue and/or antilymphoma chemotherapy. Developments in this field include the possibility of immunotherapy by means of donor leukocyte infusions.[168]

DRUG INTERACTIONS DURING TREATMENT OF INFECTION

Cyclosporin and tacrolimus are metabolized by the cytochrome P_{450} enzyme system and therefore interact with a number of important antimicrobial agents likely to be prescribed in transplant recipients (Table 43.4). Levels of these drugs may be altered by the induction or inhibition of this system and it is essential that these are measured to prevent toxicity, as well as to avoid inadequate or excessive immunosuppression with the consequences of rejection or infection. Rifampicin is a potent inducer of the CYP 3A4 isoenzyme and causes increased metabolism of cyclosporin and tacrolimus. Erythromycin, some of the newer macrolides, and the azole antifungal agents, particularly ketoconazole and itraconazole (and fluconazole at high doses), competitively inhibit this pathway, thus increasing levels of cyclosporin and tacrolimus. The levels of corticosteroids may be reduced by rifampicin and doses should be increased during treatment of tuberculosis in the transplant patient.

Renal function is often impaired in the transplantation setting and there may be a complex interaction between cyclosporin (itself potentially nephrotoxic, particularly during initial therapy) and nephrotoxic antimicrobial agents such as the aminoglycosides, high-dose trimethoprim–sulfamethoxazole, vancomycin and amphotericin B. Therapeutic drug monitoring is mandatory (with the exception of amphotericin B) to prevent additional toxicity and alternative agents be chosen whenever possible.

CONCLUSION

Prevention should always be the goal in the management of infective complications in neutropenia and organ transplantation. This has become increasingly important over the past decade with the advent of MRSA, vancomycin-resistant enterococci and other resistant organisms. Despite the development of antimicrobials with good activity against the infecting agents, the mortality from many of these infections remains high. The spectrum of immunocompromised patients is changing with the evolution of chemotherapy, stem-cell transplantation, immunosuppression regimens and tissue and organ transplantation techniques – and we can expect to see the pattern of opportunistic infections also shifting.

References

1. Bodey GP, Buckley M, Sathe YS, Freireich EJ 1966 Quantitative relationships between circulating leucocytes and infection in patients with acute leukaemia. *Annals of Internal Medicine* 64: 328–340
2. Cline MJ 1973 A new white cell test which measures individual phagocyte function in a mixed leukocyte population. I. A neutrophil defect in acute myelocytic leukemia. *Journal of Laboratory and Clinical Medicine* 81: 311–316
3. Cline MJ 1973 Defective mononuclear phagocytic function in patients with myelomonocytic leukemia and in some patients with lymphomas. *Journal of Clinical Investigation* 52: 2815–2190
4. Gratwohl A, Passweg J, Baldomero H, Hermans J 1999 Blood and marrow transplantation activity in Europe 1997. *BMT* 24: 231–245
5. Hann I, Prentice HG, Blacklock HA et al 1983 Acyclovir prophylaxis against herpes virus infections in severely immunocompromised patients: randomised double blind trial. *British Medical Journal* 287: 384–388

Table 43.4 Potential drug interactions during management of infections in organ transplant recipients

Antimicrobial agent	Immunosuppressive agent	Effect
Aminoglycosides	Cyclosporin	Exacerbation of nephrotoxicity
Amphotericin B	Cyclosporin	Exacerbation of nephrotoxicity
Trimethoprim–sulfamethoxazole	Cyclosporin	Possible exacerbation of nephrotoxicity
Trimethoprim–sulfamethoxazole (i.v.)	Cyclosporin	Reduced levels of cyclosporin
Doxycycline	Cyclosporin	Increased cyclosporin levels
Erythromycin*	Cyclosporin	Increased cyclosporin levels
Fluconazole	Cyclosporin	Increased cyclosporin levels
Flucytosine	Azathioprine	Possible exacerbation of myelosuppression
Ganciclovir	Azathioprine	Possible exacerbation of myelosuppression
Itraconazole	Cyclosporin	Increased cyclosporin levels
Ketoconazole	Cyclosporin	Increased cyclosporin levels
Pentamidine (i.v.)	Cyclosporin	Possible exacerbation of nephrotoxicity
Rifampicin	Cyclosporin	Reduced levels of cyclosporin
	Prednisone	Reduced levels of prednisone
Sulfonamides	Azathioprine	Possible exacerbation of myelosuppression
Trimethoprim	Azathioprine	Possible exacerbation of myelosuppression
Vancomycin	Cyclosporin	Exacerbation of nephrotoxicity

*And other macrolides

6. The EORTC International Antimicrobial Therapy Project Group 1978 Three antibiotic regimens in the treatment of infection in febrile granulocytopenic patients with cancer. *Journal of Infectious Diseases* 137: 14–29

7. Cometta A, Zinner S, De Bock R et al 1995 Piperacillin–tazobactam plus amikacin as empiric therapy for fever in granulocytopenic patients with cancer. *Antimicrobial Agents and Chemotherapy* 39: 445–452

8. Woo PCY, Wong SSY, Lum PNL, Hui W-T, Yuen K-Y 2001 Cell-wall-deficient bacteria and culture-negative febrile episodes in bone-marrow-transplant recipients. *Lancet* 357: 675–679

9. Schimpff SC, Greene WH, Young VW, Wiernik PH 1974 Significance of *Pseudomonas aeruginosa* in the patient with leukemia or lymphoma. *Journal of Infectious Diseases* 130: S24–S31

10. Bodey GP, Jadeja J, Elting L 1985 Pseudomonas bacteremia. Retrospective analysis of 410 episodes. *Archives of Internal Medicine* 145: 1621–1629

11. Bodey GP, Bueltmann B, Duguid W et al 1992 Fungal infections in cancer patients – an international autopsy survey. *European Journal of Clinical Microbiology* 11: 99–109

12. DeGregorio MW, Lee WMF, Linker CA et al 1982 Fungal infections in patients with acute leukemia. *American Journal of Medicine* 73: 543–548

13. Riley LC, Hann IM, Wheatley K, Stevens RF 1999 Treatment-related deaths during induction and first remission of acute myeloid leukaemia in children treated on the Tenth Medical Research Council Acute Myeloid Leukaemia Trial (MRC AML 10). *British Journal of Haematology* 106: 436–444

14. Manuel RJ, Kibbler CC 1998 The epidemiology and prevention of invasive aspergillosis. *Journal of Hospital Infection* 39: 95–109

15. Jameson B, Gamble DR, Lynch J, Kay HEM 1971 Five-year analysis of protective isolation. *Lancet* i: 1034–1040

16. Levine AS, Siegal SE, Schreiber AD et al 1973 Protected environments and prophylactic antibiotics. A prospective controlled study of their utility in the therapy of acute leukemia. *New England Journal of Medicine* 288: 477–483

17. Yates JW, Holland JF 1973 A controlled study of isolation and endogenous microbial suppression in acute myelocytic leukemia patients. *Cancer* 32: 1490–1498

18. Schimpff SC, Greene WH, Young VW et al 1975 Infection prevention in acute nonlymphocytic leukemia. Laminar air flow room reverse isolation with oral nonabsorbable antibiotic prophylaxis. *Annals of Internal Medicine* 82: 351–358

19. Dietrich M, Gaus W, Vossen J et al 1977 Protective isolation and antimicrobial decontamination in patients with high susceptibility to infection. A prospective co-operative study of gnotobiotic care in acute leukemia patients. I. Clinical results. *Infection* 5: 107–114

20. Storring RA, Jameson B, McElwain TJ, Wiltshire E 1977 Oral nonabsorbed antibiotics prevent infection in acute non-lymphoblastic leukaemia. *Lancet* ii: 837–840

21. Rodriguez V, Bodey GP, Freireich EJ et al 1978 Randomized trial of protected environment prophylactic antibiotics in 145 adults with acute leukemia. *Medicine* 57: 253–266

22. Buckner CD, Clift RA, Sanders JE et al 1978 Protective environment for marrow transplant recipients. *Annals of Internal Medicine* 89: 893–901

23. Bodey GP 1979 Treatment of acute leukemia in protected environment units. *Cancer* 44: 431–436

24. Hughes WT, Price RA, Kim HK et al 1973 *Pneumocystis carinii* pneumonia in children with malignancies. *Journal of Pediatrics* 82: 404–415

25. Gurwith MJ, Brunton JL, Lank BL et al 1979 A prospective controlled investigation of prophylactic trimethoprim-sulfamethoxazole in hospitalized granulocytopenic patients. *American Journal of Medicine* 66: 248–256

26. Dekker AW, Rozenberg-Arska M, Sixma JJ et al 1981 Prevention of infection by trimethoprim-sulfamethoxazole plus amphotericin B in patients with acute nonlymphocytic leukemia. *Annals of Internal Medicine* 95: 555–559

27. Wade JC, Schimpff SC, Hargadon MT et al 1981 A comparison of trimethoprim–sulfamethoxazole plus nystatin with gentamicin plus nystatin in the prevention of infections in acute leukemia. *New England Journal of Medicine* 304: 1057–1062

28. EORTC International Antimicrobial Therapy Project Group 1984 Trimethoprim–sulfamethoxazole in the prevention of infection in neutropenic patients. *Journal of Infectious Diseases* 150: 372–379

29. Cruciani M, Rampazzo R, Malena M et al 1996 Prophylaxis with fluoroquinolones for bacterial infections in neutropenic patients: a meta-analysis. *Clinical Infectious Diseases* 23: 795–805

30. Krcmery V Jr, Spanik S, Krupova I, Trupl J, Kunova A, Smid MPE 1998 Bacteremia due to multiresistant gram-negative bacilli in neutropenic cancer patients: a case controlled study. *Journal of Chemotherapy* 10: 320–325

31. Prentice HG, Kibbler CC, Prentice AG 2000 Towards a targeted, risk-based, antifungal strategy in neutropenic patients. *British Journal of Haematology* 110: 273–284

32. Fanci R, Leoni F, Bosi A et al 1993 Chemoprophylaxis of bacterial infections in granulocytopenic patients with ciprofloxacin vs ciprofloxacin plus amoxicillin. *Journal of Chemotherapy* 5: 119–123

33. Kern WV, Hay B, Kern P, Marre R, Arnold R 1994 A randomized trial of roxithromycin in patients with acute leukemia and bone marrow transplant recipients receiving fluoroquinolone prophylaxis. *Antimicrobial Agents and Chemotherapy* 38: 465–472

34. Wimperis JZ, Baglin TP, Marcus RE, Warren RE 1991 An assessment of the efficacy of antimicrobial prophylaxis in bone marrow autografts. *Bone Marrow Transplantation* 8: 363–367

35. Bow EJ, Mandell LA, Louie TJ, Feld R, Palmer M, Zee B, Pater J 1996 Quinolone-based antibacterial chemoprophylaxis in neutropenic patients: effect of augmented gram-positive activity on infectious morbidity. National Cancer Institute of Canada Clinical Trials Group. *Annals of Internal Medicine* 125: 183–190

36. Odds FC 1988 *Candida and candidosis,* 2nd ed. London, Baillière Tindall

37. Hann IM, Corringham R, Keaney M et al 1982 Ketoconazole versus nystatin plus amphotericin B for fungal prophylaxis in severely immunocompromised patients. *Lancet* i: 826–829

38. Hansen RM, Reinerio N, Sohnle PG et al 1987 Ketoconazole in the prevention of candidiasis in patients with cancer. A prospective, randomized, controlled, double-blind study. *Archives of Internal Medicine* 147: 710–712

39. Winston DJ, Ho WG, Bartoni et al 1993 Ganciclovir prophylaxis of cytomegalovirus infection and disease in allogeneic bone marrow transplant recipients. Results of a placebo-controlled, double-blind trial. *Annals of Internal Medicine* 118: 179–184

40. Philpott-Howard JN, Wade JJ, Mufti GJ, Brammer KW, Ehninger G 1993 Randomized comparison of oral fluconazole versus oral polyenes for the prevention of fungal infection in patients at risk of neutropenia. Multicentre Study Group. *Journal of Antimicrobial Chemotherapy* 31: 973–984

41. Goodman JL, Winston DJ, Greenfield RA et al 1992 A controlled trial of fluconazole to prevent fungal infections in patients undergoing bone marrow transplantation. *New England Journal of Medicine* 326: 845–851

42. Slavin MA, Osborne B, Adams R et al 1995 Efficacy and safety of fluconazole prophylaxis for fungal infections after marrow transplantation – A prospective, randomised, double-blind study. *Journal of Infectious Diseases* 171: 1545–1552

43. Wingard JR, Merz WG, Rinaldi MG et al 1991 Increase in *Candida krusei* infection among patients with bone marrow transplantation and neutropenia treated prophylactically with fluconazole. *New England Journal of Medicine* 325: 1274–1277

44. Morgenstern GR, Prentice AG, Prentice HG, Ropner JE, Schey SA, Warnock DW 1999 A randomized controlled trial of itraconazole versus fluconazole for the prevention of fungal infections in patients with haematological malignancies. *British Journal of Haematology* 105: 901–911

45. Harousseau JL, Dekker A, Stamatoullas A, Bassaris H, Linkesch W, Fassas A 2000 Prophylaxis of fungal infections in haematological malignancies: a double blind trial comparing itraconazole oral solution to amphotericin B capsules. *Antimicrobial Agents and Chemotherapy* 44: 1887–1893

46. Menichetti F, Del Favero A, Martino P et al 1999 Itraconazole oral solution as prophylaxis for fungal infections in neutropenic patients with hematologic malignancies: a randomised, placebo-controlled, double blind, multicentre trial. GIMEMA infection programme. Groupo Italiano Malattie Ematologiche del Adulto. *Clinical Infectious Diseases* 28: 250–255

47. Meunier F 1987 Prevention of mycoses in immunocompromised patients. *Reviews in Infectious Diseases* 9: 408–416

48. Jorgensen CJ, Dreyfus F, Vaixeler J et al 1989 Failure of amphotericin B spray to prevent aspergillosis in granulocytopenic patients. *Nouvelle Revue Française d'Hématologie* 31: 327–328

49. Conneally E, Cafferkey MT, Daly PA et al 1990 Nebulized amphotericin B as prophylaxis against invasive aspergillosis in granulocytopenic patients. *Bone Marrow Transplantation* 5: 403–406

50. Myers SE, Devine SM, Topper RL et al 1992 A pilot study of prophylactic aerosolized amphotericin B in patients at risk for prolonged neutropenia. *Leukemia and Lymphoma* 8: 229–233

51. Schwartz S, Behre G, Heinemann V et al 1999 Aerosolized amphotericin B inhalations as a prophylaxis of invasive aspergillus infections during prolonged neutropenia: results of a prospective randomized multicenter trial. *Blood* 93: 3654–3661

52. Zaia JA 1990 Viral infections associated with bone marrow transplantation. *Hematology/Oncology Clinics of North America* 4: 603–623

53. Wade JC 1993 Management of infection in patients with acute leukemia. *Hematology/Oncology Clinics of North America* 7: 293–315

54. Prentice HG, Gluckman E, Powles RL et al 1994 Impact of long-term acyclovir on cytomegalovirus infection and survival after allogeneic bone marrow transplantation. European Acyclovir for CMV Prophylaxis Study Group. *Lancet* 343: 749–753

55. Goodrich JM, Bowden RA, Fisher L et al 1993 Ganciclovir prophylaxis to prevent cytomegalovirus disease after allogeneic marrow transplant. *Annals of Internal Medicine* 118: 173–178

56. Goodrich JM, Mori M, Gleaves CA et al 1991 Prevention of cytomegalovirus disease after allogeneic marrow transplantation by early treatment with ganciclovir. *New England Journal of Medicine* 325: 1601–1607

57. Einsele H, Steidle M, Vallbracht A et al 1991 Early occurrence of human cytomegalovirus infection after bone marrow transplantation as demonstrated by polymerase chain reaction technique. *Blood* 77: 1104–1110

58. Boeckh M, Bowden RA, Goodrich JM et al 1992 Cytomegalovirus antigen detection in peripheral blood leukocytes after allogeneic marrow transplantation. *Blood* 80: 1358–1364

59. Kidd M, Fox JC, Pillay D et al 1993 Provision of prognostic information in immunocompromised patients by routine application of the polymerase chain reaction for cytomegalovirus. *Transplantation* 56: 867–871

60. Bodey GP, Buckley Valdivieso M, Feld R, Rodriguez V, McCredie K 1977 Carbenicillin plus cephalothin or cefazolin as therapy for infections in neutropenic patients. *American Journal of Medical Sciences* 273: 309–318

61. Gurwith M, Brunton JL, Lank B et al 1978 Granulocytopenia in hospitalised patients. II. A prospective comparison of two antibiotic regimens in the empiric therapy of febrile patients. *American Journal of Medicine* 64: 127–132

62. Winston DJ, Barnes RC, Ho WG et al 1984 Moxalactam plus piperacillin versus moxalactam plus amikacin in febrile granulocytopenic patients. *American Journal of Medicine* 77: 442–450

63. Winston DJ, Ho WG, Bruckner DA, Gale RP, Champlin RE 1988 Controlled trials of double beta-lactam therapy with cefoperazone plus piperacillin in febrile granulocytopenic patients. *American Journal of Medicine* 85(Suppl. IA): 21–30

64. Kibbler CC, Prentice HG, Sage RJ et al 1989 Do double beta-lactam combinations prolong neutropenia in patients undergoing chemotherapy or bone marrow transplantation for haematological disease? *Antimicrobial Agents and Chemotherapy* 33(4): 503–507

65. Sanders JW, Powe NR, Moore RD 1991 Ceftazidime monotherapy for empiric treatment of febrile neutropenic patients: a meta-analysis. *Journal of Infectious Diseases* 164: 907–916

66. Liang R, Yung R, Chiu E et al 1990 Ceftazidime versus imipenem–cilastatin as initial monotherapy for febrile neutropenic patients. *Antimicrobial Agents and Chemotherapy* 34: 1336–1341

67. Rikonen P 1991 Imipenem compared with ceftazidime plus vancomycin as initial therapy for fever in neutropenic children with cancer. *Pediatric Infectious Disease Journal* 10: 918–923

68. Cornelissen JJ, De Graeff A, Verdonck LF et al 1992 Imipenem versus gentamicin combined with either cefuroxime or cephalothin as initial therapy for febrile neutropenic patients. *Antimicrobial Agents and Chemotherapy* 36: 801–807

69. Rolston KVI, Berkey P, Bodey GP et al 1992 A comparison of imipenem ceftazimide with or without amikacin as empiric therapy in febrile neutropenic patients. *Archives of Internal Medicine* 152: 283–291

70. Cometta A, Calandra T, Gaya H et al 1996 Monotherapy with meropenem versus combination therapy with ceftazidime plus amikacin as empiric therapy for fever in granulocytopenic patients with cancer. *Antimicrobial Agents and Chemotherapy* 40: 1108–1115

71. Kerr KG, Hawkey PM, Child JA, Norfolk DR, Anderson AW 1990 *Pseudomonas maltophilia* infections in neutropenic patients and the use of imipenem. *Postgraduate Medical Journal* 66: 1090

72. McWhinney PHM, Kibbler CC, Prentice HG et al 1991 A prospective trial of imipenem versus ceftazidime/ vancomycin as empirical therapy for fever in neutropenic patients. Proceedings of the 17th International Congress of Chemotherapy, Berlin, abstract 1276

73. Bodey GP 1986 Infection in cancer patients. A continuing association. *American Journal of Medicine* 81(Suppl. 1A): 11–26

74. McWhinney PH, Patel S, Whiley RA et al 1993 Activities of potential therapeutic and prophylactic antibiotics against blood culture isolates of viridans group streptococci from neutropenic patients receiving ciprofloxacin. *Antimicrobial Agents and Chemotherapy* 37: 2493–2495

75. Klastersky J 1998 Science and pragmatism in the treatment and prevention of neutropenic infection. *Journal of Antimicrobial Chemotherapy* 41(Suppl. D): 13–24

76. Karp JE, Merz WG, Dick JD, Saral R 1991 Strategies to prevent or control infections after bone marrow transplants. *Bone Marrow Transplantation* 8: 1–6

77. Chow AW, Jewesson PJ, Kureishi A, Phillips GL 1993 Teicoplanin versus vancomycin in the empirical treatment of febrile neutropenic patients. *European Journal of Haematology* 51: 18–24

78. Ramphal R, Bolger M, Oblon DJ et al 1992 Vancomycin is not an essential component of the initial empiric treatment regimen for febrile neutropenic patients receiving ceftazidime: a prospective randomized study. *Antimicrobial Agents and Chemotherapy* 36: 1062–1067

79. EORTC International Antimicrobial Therapy Cooperative Group and the National Cancer Institute of Canada – Clinical Trials Group 1991 Vancomycin added to empirical combination antibiotic therapy for fever in granulocytopenic cancer patients. *Journal of Infectious Diseases* 163: 951–958

80. Shlaes DM, Binczewski B, Rice LB 1993 Emerging antibiotic resistance and the immunocompromised host. *Clinical Infectious Diseases* 17(Suppl. 2): S527–S536

81. Handwerger S, Rancher B, Alterac D et al 1993 Outbreak due to *Enterococcus faecium* highly resistant to vancomycin, penicillin, and gentamicin. *Clinical Infectious Diseases* 16: 750–755

82. Centers for Disease Control and Prevention 1994 Preventing the spread of vancomycin resistance: report from the hospital infection control practices advisory committee. *Federal Register* 59: 25 757

83. Hughes WT, Armstrong D, Bodey GP et al 1997 guidelines for the use of antimicrobial agents in neutropenic patients with unexplained fever. *Clinical Infectious Diseases* 25: 551–573

84. Bradley SJ, Wilson ALT, Allen MC, Sher HA, Goldstone AH, Scott GM 1999 The control of hyperendemic glycopeptide-resistant *Enterococcus* spp. on a haematology unit by changing antibiotic usage. *Journal of Antimicrobial Chemotherapy* 43: 261–266

85. Talcott JA, Siegel RD, Finberg R, Goldman L 1992 Risk assessment in cancer patients with fever and neutropenia: a prospective, two-center validation of a prediction rule. *Journal of Clinical Oncology* 10: 316–322

86. Freifeld A, Marchigiani D, Walsh T et al 1999 A double-blind comparison of empirical oral and intravenous antibiotic therapy for low-risk febrile patients with neutropenia during cancer chemotherapy. *New England Journal of Medicine* 341: 305–311

87. Kern WV, Cometta A, De Bock R et al for the International Antimicrobial Therapy Cooperative Group of the European Organization for Research and Treatment of Cancer 1999 Oral versus intravenous empirical therapy for fever in patients with granulocytopenia who are receiving cancer chemotherapy. *New England Journal of Medicine* 341: 312–318

88. Anonymous 1989 Empiric antifungal therapy in febrile granulocytopenic patients. EORTC International Antimicrobial Therapy Cooperative Group. *American Journal of Medicine* 86: 668–672

89. Prentice HG, Hann IM, Herbrecht R et al 1997 A randomized comparison of liposomal versus conventional amphotericin B for the treatment of pyrexia of unknown origin in neutropenic patients. *British Journal of Haematology* 98: 711–718

90. Walsh TJ, Finberg RW, Arndt C et al 1999 Liposomal amphotericin B for empirical therapy in patients with persistent fever and neutropenia. *New England Journal of Medicine* 340: 764–771

91. Winston DJ, Dudnick DV, Chapin M et al 1983 Coagulase-negative staphylococcal bacteremia in patients receiving immunosuppressive therapy. *Archives of Internal Medicine* 143: 32–36.

92. Smith JG, Summerfield GP, Adam A et al 1997 BCSH guidelines on the insertion and management of central venous lines. *British Journal of Haematology* 98: 1041–1047

93. Berger LA 1998 Imaging in the diagnosis of infections in immunocompromised patients. *Current Opinion in Infectious Diseases* 11: 431–436

94. Emanuel D, Cunningham I, Jules-Elysee K et al 1988 Cytomegalovirus pneumonia after bone marrow transplantation successfully treated with the com-

bination of ganciclovir and high-dose intravenous immune globulin. *Annals of Internal Medicine* 109: 777–782

95. Reed EC, Bowden RA, Dandliker PS, Lilleby KE, Meyers JD 1988 Treatment of cytomegalovirus pneumonia with ganciclovir and intravenous cytomegalovirus immunoglobulin in patients with bone marrow transplants. *Annals of Internal Medicine* 109: 783–788

96. Ljungman P, Engelhard D, Link H et al 1992 Treatment of interstitial pneumonitis due to cytomegalovirus with ganciclovir and intravenous immune globulin: experience of European Bone Marrow Transplant Group. *Clinical Infectious Diseases* 14(4): 831–835

97. Harrington RD, Hooton TM, Hackman RC et al 1992 An outbreak of respiratory syncytial virus in a bone marrow transplant center. *Journal of Infectious Diseases* 165: 987–993

98. Lin S-J, Schranz J, Teutsch SM 2001 Aspergillus case-fatality rate: systematic review of the literature. *Clinical Infectious Diseases* 32: 358–366

99. Ellis M, Spence D, De Pauw B et al 1998 An EORTC international multicenter randomized trial (EORTC number 19923) comparing two dosages of liposomal amphotericin B for treatment of invasive aspergillosis. *Clinical Infectious Diseases* 27: 1406–1412

100. Denning DW, Tucker RM, Hanson LH, Stevens DA 1989 Treatment of invasive aspergillosis with itraconazole. *American Journal of Medicine* 86: 791–800

101. Kibbler CC, Milkins SR, Bhamra A et al 1988 Apparent pulmonary mycetoma following invasive aspergillosis in neutropenic patients. *Thorax* 43: 108–112

102. Yeghen T, Kibbler CC, Prentice HG et al 2000 Management of invasive pulmonary aspergillosis in hematology patients: a review of 87 consecutive cases at a single institution. *Clinical Infectious Diseases* 31: 859–868

103. Demetri GD, Antman KHS 1992 Granulocyte–macrophage colony-stimulating factor (GMCSF): preclinical and clinical investigations. *Seminars in Oncology* 19: 362–385

104. Glaspy JA, Golde DW 1992 Granulocyte colony-stimulating factor (GCSF): preclinical and clinical investigations. *Seminars in Oncology* 19: 386–394

105. Pettengell R, Gurney H, Radford JA et al 1992 Granulocyte colony-stimulating factor to prevent dose-limited neutropenia in non-Hodgkin's lymphoma: a randomized controlled trial. *Blood* 80: 1430–1436

106. Singer JW 1992 Role of colony-stimulating factors in bone marrow transplantation. *Seminars in Oncology* 19: 27–31

107. American Society of Clinical Oncology Committee 1996 Update of recommendations for the use of hematopoietic colony-stimulating factors. Evidence-based clinical practice guidelines. *Journal of Clinical Oncology* 14: 1957–1960

108. Bodey GP, Anaissie E, Gutterman J, Vadhan-Raj S 1993 Role of granulocyte–macrophage colony-stimulating factor as adjuvant therapy for fungal infection in patients with cancer. *Clinical Infectious Diseases* 17: 705–707

109. Hubel K, Dale DC, Engbert A, Liles WC 2001 Current status of granulocyte (neutrophil) transfusion therapy for infectious diseases. *Journal of Infectious Diseases* 183(2): 321–328

110. Price TH, Bowden RA, Boeckh M et al 2000 Phase I/II trial of neutrophil transfusions from donors stimulated with G-CSF and dexamethasone for treatment of patients with infections in hematopoietic stem cell transplantation. *Blood* 95(11): 3302–3309

111. Cecka JM 1999 The UNOS Scientific Renal Transplant Registry

112. Ascher NL 2001 Immunosuppressant substitutes in liver transplantation. *Lancet* 357: 571–572

113. Torre-Cisneros J, Manez R, Kusne S, Alessiani M, Martin M, Starzl TE 1991 The spectrum of aspergillosis in liver transplant patients: comparison of FK506 and cyclosporin immunosuppression. *Transplantation Proceedings* 23: 3040–3041

114. Sakr M, Hassanein T, Gaveler J et al 1992 Cytomegalovirus infection of the upper gastrointestinal tract following liver transplantation: incidence, location and severity in cyclosporin and FK506 treated patients. *Transplantation* 53: 786–791

115. Kusne S, Fung J, Alessiani M et al 1992 Infections during a randomized trial comparing cyclosporine to FK506 immunosuppression in liver transplantation. *Transplantation Proceedings* 24: 429–430

116. European FK506 Multicentre Liver Study Group 1994 Randomised trial comparing tacrolimus (FK506) and cyclosporin in prevention of liver allograft rejection. *Lancet* 344: 423–428

117. George DL, Arnow PM, Fox AS et al 1991 Bacterial infection as a complication of liver transplantation: epidemiology and risk factors. *Reviews of Infectious Diseases* 13: 387–396

118. Kusne S, Dummer JS, Singh N et al 1988 Infections after liver transplantation. An analysis of 101 consecutive cases. *Medicine Baltimore* 67: 132–143

119. Colonna JO, Winston DJ, Brill JE et al 1988 Infectious complications in liver transplantation. *Archives of Surgery* 123: 360–364

120. Paya CV, Hermans PE, Washington JA et al 1989 Incidence, distribution and outcome of episodes of infection in 100 orthotopic liver transplantations. *Mayo Clinic Proceedings* 64: 555–564

121. Chang FY, Singh N, Gayowski T, Drenning SD, Wagener MM, Mariono R 1998 Staphylococcus aureus nasal colonisation and association with infections in liver transplant recipients. *Transplantation* 65: 1169–1

122. Fernando ON, Higgins AF, Moorhead JF 1976 Secondary haemorrhage after renal transplantation. *Lancet* ii: 368

123. Weber TR, Freier DT, Turcotte JF 1979 Transplantation of infected kidneys. *Transplantation* 27: 63–65

124. Nelson PW, Delmonicao FL, Tolkoff-Rubin NE et al 1984 Unsuspected donor *Pseudomonas* infection causing arterial disruption after renal transplantation. *Transplantation* 37: 313–314

125. Leaker B, Hellyar A, Neild GH et al 1989 Nocardia infection in a renal transplant unit. *Transplantation Proceedings* 21: 2103–2104

126. Singh N, Paterson DL 1998 *M. tuberculosis* infection in solid organ transplant recipients: impact and implications for management. *Clinical Infectious Diseases* 27: 1266–1277

127. Rubin RH 1994 Infection in the organ transplant recipient. In: Rubin RH, Young LS (eds). *Clinical approach to infection in the compromised host*, 3rd edn. New York, Plenum, pp. 629–705

128. Patterson WJ, Hay J, Seal DV, McLuckie JC 1997 Colonization of transplant unit water supplies with *Legionella* and protozoa: precautions required to reduce the risk of legionellosis. *Journal of Hospital Infection* 37: 7–17

129. Paya CV 1993 Fungal infections in solid-organ transplantation. *Clinical Infectious Diseases* 16: 677–688

130. Singh N 1998 Infectious diseases in the liver transplant patient. *Seminars in Gastrointestinal Disease* 9: 136–146

131. Wajszczuk CP, Dummer JS, Ho M et al 1985 Fungal infections in liver transplant recipients. *Transplantation* 40: 347–353

132. Sepkowitz KA, Brown AE, Armstrong D 1995 Pneumocystis carinii pneumonia without acquired immunodeficiency syndrome: more patients, same risk. *Archives of Internal Medicine* 155: 1125–1128

133. Martinez AJ, Ahdab-Barmada M 1993 The neuropathology of liver transplantation: comparison of main complications in children and adults. *Modern Pathology* 6: 25–32

134. Singh N, Yu VL, Gayowski T 1994 Central nervous system lesions in adult liver transplant recipients – clinical review with implications for management. *Medicine* 73: 110

135. Bonham CA, Dominguez EA, Fukui MB, Paterson DL, Pankey GA, Wagener MM 1998 Central nervous system lesions in liver transplant recipients: prospective assessment of indications for biopsy and implications for management. *Transplantation* 66: 1596–1604

136. Umana JP, Mutimer DJ, Shaw JC et al 1992 Cytomegalovirus surveillance following liver transplantation: does it allow presymptomatic diagnosis of CMV disease? *Transplantation Proceedings* 24: 2643

137. Ho M 1994 Advances in understanding cytomegalovirus infection after transplantation. *Transplantation Proceedings* 26: 7–11

138. Mustafa MM 1994 Cytomegalovirus infection and disease in the immunocompromised host. *Pediatric Infectious Disease Journal* 13: 249–259

139. Wright TL, Donegan E, Hsu HH et al 1992 Recurrent and acquired hepatitis C viral infection in liver transplant recipients. *Gastroenterology* 103: 317–322

140. Samuel D, Muller R, Alexander G 1993 Liver transplantation in European patients with the hepatitis B surface antigen. *New England Journal of Medicine* 329: 1842–1847

141. Rostaing L, Icart J, Durand D et al 1993 Clinical outcome of Epstein–Barr viraemia in transplant patients. *Transplant Proceedings* 25: 2286–2287

142. Rogers J, Singh N, Carrigan DR et al 1999 Clinical relevance of human herpesvirus-6 infection in liver transplant recipients: role in pathogenesis of fungal infections, neurologic complications and impact on outcome. In: Program and abstracts of the 39th Interscience Conference on Antimicrobial Agents and Chemotherapy, San Francisco, USA, pp. 457–472

143. Dockrell DH, Mendez JC, Jones M et al 1999 Human herpesvirus 6 seronegativity before transplantation predicts the occurrence of fungal infection in liver transplant recipients. *Transplantation* 67: 399–403

144. Ragamey N, Tamm M, Wernli M et al 1998 Transmission of human her-

pesvirus 8 infection from renal-transplant donors to recipients. *New England Journal of Medicine* 339: 358–1363

145. Nickeleit V, Hirsch HH, Binet IF et al 1999 Polyomavirus infection of renal allograft recipients: from latent infection to manifest disease. *Journal of the American Society of Nephrology* 10: 1080–1089

146. Gallino A, Maggioroni M, Kiowski W 1996 Toxoplasmosis in heart transplant recipients. *European Journal of Clinical Microbiology and Infectious Diseases* 15: 389–393

147. Speirs GE, Hakim M, Wreghitt TG 1998 Relative risk of donor transmitted *Toxoplasma gondii* infection in heart, liver and kidney transplant recipients. *Clinical Transplants* 2: 257–269

148. Michaels MG, Wald ER, Fricker FJ, del Nido PJ, Armitage J 1992 Toxoplasmosis in pediatric recipients of heart transplant. *Clinical Infectious Diseases* 14: 847–851

149. Singer MA, Hagler WS, Grossniklaus HE 1993 *Toxoplasma gondii* retinochoroiditis after liver transplantation. *Retina* 13: 40–45

150. Smith SD, Jackson RJ, Hannaken CJ, Wadowsky RM, Tzakis AG, Rowe MI 1993 Selective decontamination in paediatric liver transplantation. A randomised prospective study. *Transplantation* 55: 1306–1309

151. Murphy OM, Gould FK 1999 Prevention of nosocomial infection in solid organ transplantation. *Journal of Hospital Infection* 42: 177–183

152. Tolkoff-Rubin NE, Cosimi AB, Russell PS et al 1982 A controlled study of trimethoprim–sulfamethoxazole prophylaxis of urinary tract infections in renal transplant recipients. *Reviews of Infectious Diseases* 4: 614–618

153. Fox BC, Sollinger HW, Belzer FO et al 1990 A prospective, randomized, double-blind study of trimethoprim–sulfamethoxazole for prophylaxis of infections in renal transplantation: clinical efficacy, absorption of trimethoprim–sulfamethoxazole, effects on the microflora, and the cost benefit of prophylaxis. *American Journal of Medicine* 89: 255

154. Winston DJ, Pakrasi A, Busuttil RW 1999 Prophylactic fluconazole in liver transplant recipients. A randomised, double-blind, placebo-controlled trial. *Annals of Internal Medicine* 131: 729–737

155. Colby WD, Sharpe MD, Ghent CN et al 1999 Efficacy of itraconazole prophylaxis against systemic fungal infection in liver transplant recipients. Program and abstracts of the 39th Interscience Conference on Antimicrobial Agents and Chemotherapy, San Francisco, USA, Washington

156. Gordon SM, LaRossa SP, Kalmadi S et al 1999 Should prophylaxis for Pneumocystis carinii pneumonia in solid organ transplant recipients ever be discontinued? *Clinical Infectious Diseases* 28: 240–246

157. Kakazato PZ, Burns W, Moore P, Garcia-Kennedy R, Cox K, Esquivel C 1993 Viral prophylaxis in hepatic transplantation: preliminary report of a randomized trial of acyclovir and ganciclovir. *Transplantation Proceedings* 25: 1935–1937

158. Martin M 1993 Antiviral prophylaxis for CMV infection in liver transplantation. *Transplantation Proceedings* 25(Suppl. 4): 10–14

159. Hopt UT, Pfeffer F, Schareck W, Busing M, Ming C 1994 Ganciclovir for prophylaxis of CMV disease after pancrease/kidney transplantation. *Transplantation Proceedings* 26: 434–435

160. Singh N, Yu VL, Mieles L et al 1994 High-dose acyclovir compared with short-course preemptive ganciclovir therapy to prevent cytomegalovirus disease in liver transplant recipients: a randomized trial. *Annals of Internal Medicine* 120: 375–381

161. Kusne S, Grossi P, Irish W et al 1999 Cytomegalovirus PP65 antigenaemia monitoring as a guide for preemptive therapy: a cost effective strategy for prevention of cytomegalovirus disease in adult liver transplant recipients. *Transplantation* 68: 1125–1131

162. Dodson SF, Balart LA, Shakil O et al 1998 Lack of efficacy of lamivudine for HBV infection after liver transplantation. *Hepatology* 28: 262A

163. Sawyer RG, Crabtree TD, Gleason TD et al 1999 Impact of solid organ transplantation and immunosuppression on fever, leukocytosis and physiologic response during bacterial and fungal infections. *Clinical Transplants* 13: 260–265

164. Graybill J, Loebenberg R, Bocanegra R, Najvar L 1998 Granulocyte colony stimulating factor (G-CSF) and azole antifungal therapy in murine aspergillosis: surprises. Program and abstracts of the 38th International Conference on Antimicrobial Agents and Chemotherapy, San Diego, USA

165. Cockfield SM, Preiksatis JK, Jewell LD, Parfrey NA 1993 Post-transplant lymphoproliferative disorder in renal allograft recipients. *Transplantation* 56: 88–96

166. Strauss SE, Cohen JI, Tosato G et al 1993 Epstein–Barr virus infection: biology, pathogenesis, and management. *Annals of Internal Medicine* 118: 45–58

167. Nalesnik MA, Starzl TE 1994 Epstein–Barr virus, infectious mononucleosis, and posttransplant lymphoproliferative disorders. *Transplantation Science* 4: 61–79

168. Papadopoulos EB, Ladanyi M, Emanuel D et al 1994 Infusions of donor leukocytes to treat Epstein-Barr virus-associated lymphoproliferative disorders after allogeneic bone marrow transplantation. *New England Journal of Medicine* 330: 1185–1191

169. Winston DJ, Chandrasekar PH, Lazarus HM et al 1993 Fluconazole prophylaxis of fungal infections in patients with acute leukemia. Results of a randomized placebo-controlled, double-blind, multicenter trial. *Annals of Internal Medicine* 118: 495–503

 Further information

Brammer KW 1990 Management of fungal infection in neutropenic patients with fluconazole. *Haematologie und Bluttransfusion* 33: 546–550.

Calandra T, Zinner SH, Viscoli C et al 1993 Efficacy and toxicity of single daily doses of amikacin and ceftriaxone versus multiple daily doses of amikacin and ceftazidime for infection in patients with cancer and granulocytopenia. *Annals of Internal Medicine* 119: 584–593.

Castaldo P, Stratta RJ, Wood RP et al 1991 Clinical spectrum of fungal infections after orthotopic liver transplantation. *Archives of Surgery* 126: 149–156.

Castaldo P, Stratta RJ, Wood RP et al 1991 Fungal infections in liver allograft recipients. *Transplantation Proceedings* 23: 1967.

De Pauw BE, Deresinski SC, Feld R et al 1994 Ceftazidime compared with piperacillin and tobramycin for the empiric treatment of fever in neutropenic patients with cancer – a multicenter randomized trial. *Annals of Internal Medicine* 120: 834–844.

Donnelly JP, Maschmeyer G, Daenen S 1992 Selective oral antimicrobial prophylaxis for the prevention of infection in acute leukaemia – ciprofloxacin versus co-trimoxazole plus colistin. *European Journal of Cancer* 28A: 873–878.

Eickhoff TC, Olin DB, Anderson RJ et al 1972 Current problems and approaches to diagnosis of infection in renal transplant recipients. *Transplantation Proceedings* 4: 693–697.

EORTC International Antimicrobial Therapy Group 1987 Ceftazidime combined with a short or long course of amikacin for empirical therapy of Gram-negative bacteraemia in cancer patients with granulocytopenia. *New England Journal of Medicine* 317: 1692–1628.

Fisher BD, Armstrong D, Yu B, Gold JW 1981 Invasive aspergillosis: progress in early diagnosis and treatment. *American Journal of Medicine* 71: 571–577.

GIMENA Infection Program 1991 Prevention of bacterial infection in neutropenic patients with hematologic malignancies. A randomized multicenter trial comparing norfloxacin with ciprofloxacin. *Annals of Internal Medicine* 115: 7–12.

Hawkins C, Armstrong D 1984 Fungal infections in the immunocompromised host. *Clinics in Haematology* 13: 599–630.

Kern WV 1998 Epidemiology of fluoroquinolone-resistant *Escherichia coli* among neutropenic patients. *Clinical Infectious Diseases* 27: 235–237.

Kibbler CC, Prentice HG, Sage RJ et al 1989 A comparison of double beta-lactam combinations with netilmicin/ureidopenicillin regimens in the empirical therapy of febrile neutropenic patients. *Journal of Antimicrobial Chemotherapy* 23: 759–771.

Kirby RM, McMaster P, Clements D et al 1987 Orthotopic liver transplantation: postoperative complications and their management. *British Journal of Surgery* 74: 3–11.

Klastersky J, Glauser MP, Schimpff SC, Gaya H 1986 Antimicrobial Therapy Project Group for Research on Treatment of Cancer. Prospective randomised comparison of three antibiotic regimens for empirical therapy of suspected bacteremic infection in febrile granulocytopenic patients. *Antimicrobial Agents and Chemotherapy* 29: 263–270.

Majeski JA, Alexander JW, First MR et al 1982 Transplantation of microbially contaminated cadaver kidneys. *Archives of Surgery* 117: 221–224.

McCoy GC, Loening S, Braun WE et al 1975 The fate of cadaver renal allografts contaminated before transplantation. *Transplantation* 20: 467–472.

McWhinney PH, Kibbler CC, Hamon MD et al 1993 Progress in the diagnosis and management of aspergillosis in bone marrow transplantation: 13 years' experience. *Clinical Infectious Diseases* 17: 397–404.

Mills W, Chopra R, Linch DC, Goldstone AH 1994 Liposomal amphotericin B in the treatment of fungal infections in neutropenic patients: a single-centre experience of 133 episodes in 116 patients. *British Journal of Haematology* 86: 754–760.

Montgomery JR, Barrett FF, Williams TW Jr 1973 Infectious complications in cardiac transplant patients. *Transplantation Proceedings* 5: 1239–1243.

Pizzo PA, Commers J, Cotton D et al 1984 Approaching the controversies in the antibacterial management of cancer patients. *American Journal of Medicine* 76: 436–449.

Pizzo PA, Hathorn JW, Hiemenz J et al 1986 A randomised trial comparing ceftazidime alone with combination antibiotic therapy in cancer patients with fever and neutropenia. *New England Journal of Medicine* 315: 552–558.

Pizzo PA, Rubin M, Freifeld A, Walsh TJ 1991 The child with cancer and infection. I. Empiric therapy for fever and neutropenia, and preventive strategies. *Journal of Pediatrics* 119: 679–694.

Schroter GPJ, Hoelscher M, Putnam CW, Porter KA, Starzl TE 1977 Fungus infections after liver transplantation. *Annals of Surgery* 186: 115–122.

Shenep JL, Hughes WT, Roberson PK et al 1988 Vancomycin, ticarcillin, and amikacin compared with ticarcillin–clvulanate and amikacin in the empirical treatment of febrile, neutropenic children with cancer. *New England Journal of Medicine* 319: 1053–1058.

The International Antimicrobial Therapy Project Cooperative Group of the European Organization for Research and Treatment of Cancer 1993 Efficacy and toxicity of single daily doses of amikacin and ceftriaxone versus multiple daily doses of amikacin and ceftazidime for infection in patients with cancer and granulocytopenia. *Annals of Internal Medicine* 119: 584–593.

Viviani MA, Tortorano AM, Malaspina C et al 1992 Surveillance and treatment of liver transplant recipients for candidiasis and aspergillosis. *European Journal of Epidemiology* 8: 433–436.

Working Party of the British Society for Antimicrobial Chemotherapy 1993 Chemoprophylaxis for candidosis and aspergillosis in neutropenia and transplantation: a review and recommendation. *Journal of Antimicrobial Chemotherapy* 32: 5–21.

44 Infections in intensive care patients

M. G. Thomas and S. J. Streat

Infection is a common reason for admission to an intensive care unit (ICU) and a common complication of stay in an ICU. Approximately one in three patients in the ICU will have an infection. Approximately half the infections in ICU patients are acquired before admission to the ICU, usually before admission to hospital.[1,2] Community-acquired infection is common in pediatric and adult medical and surgical ICUs but infrequent in neonatal and cardiac surgical ICUs.[1] Between 1984 and 2000, 1624 patients with sepsis were admitted to the adult ICU in our hospital in Auckland, New Zealand. These patients comprised 10.3% of ICU admissions but used 17.3% of ICU days and accounted for 17.3% of all ICU deaths over the 17-year period. Most required ventilatory (81%) and inotropic (87%) support. Renal replacement therapy was given to 8.4%. Their overall mortality within the ICU was 26%. Table 44.1 shows the number of ICU admissions for all septic sites together with the mean age, length of ICU stay and ICU survival for each site.

The most common sites of infection were intraperitoneal from a gastrointestinal source (35.5% of admissions); respiratory tract 20.4%; urinary tract 10.5%; meninges 8.4%; bacteremia with an unknown source 6.8% and soft tissue infections 5.4%. ICU survival varied strikingly with septic site, being relatively good for meningitis (91%) and urinary tract infection (81%) poorer for respiratory infection (68%) or bacteremia (61%) and worst for mediastinitis (55%) and septic arthritis (51%). ICU admissions for sepsis continue to rise steadily (at around 5% per year) while survival is improving very slowly (at c. 0.8% per year). Currently, the total cost of treating all patients with sepsis per ICU survivor is approximately $NZD19 934 (£5885).

Approximately half the infections present in patients in an ICU are acquired following admission to the unit. Richards et al[3] found six nosocomial infections per 100 patients in medical-surgical ICUs in the USA; while 21% of patients in European ICUs had nosocomial infec-

Table 44.1 Admissions with infection to the Auckland Hospital ICU of during the period 1984–2000

Septic site/source	Number of admissions	Mean age (years)	Mean length of stay (days)	ICU survival (%)
Gastrointestinal	577	61	6.8	75
Respiratory	331	53	6.9	68
Urinary tract	170	55	4.2	81
Meninges	137	35	3.3	91
Bacteremia (unknown source)	111	45	5.1	61
Soft tissues	88	45	6.8	78
Joints	51	62	5.3	51
Genital	30	37	3.5	87
Unknown	29	50	8.5	66
Endovascular and endocarditis	26	48	5.2	65
Prosthetic device/graft	20	54	1.7	80
Brain (abscess, ventriculitis)	19	39	5.5	89
Mediastinum	11	56	4.4	55
Epidural abscess	10	62	6.9	90
Osteomyelitis	8	57	10.9	75
CAPD peritonitis	6	39	6.7	67
Total	**1624**	**53**	**6**	**74**

CAPD, continuous ambulatory peritoneal dialysis.

Table 44.2 Site of nosocomial infection in intensive care units*

	Study	
	Vincent et al[2]	Richards et al[3]
Total no. of infections	2485	29041
Site of infection (%)		
Respiratory tract	54	37
Genitourinary tract	15	23
Wound	6	8
Gastrointestinal	4	4
Bacteremia	10	14
Skin	4	3
Other	8	11

*Infection at each site as a proportion of total infection rate.

Table 44.3 Etiology of community-acquired pneumonia in intensive care units

	BTS[13]	Moine[126]	Leroy[127]	Oleacha[128]
Total No. of patients	60	132	299	262
Organism (%)				
Str. pneumoniae	18	33	27	11
Staph. aureus	5	4	19	4
H. influenzae	12	11	8	4
Enteric Gram-negative bacilli	3	11	18	3
L. pneumophila	12	3	0	8
Unknown	42	28	34	41

tions. The most important sites of nosocomial infection in these patients are the respiratory tract, the urinary tract and the bloodstream (Table 44.2). The spectrum of organisms responsible for infections acquired in the ICU differs from that causing community-acquired infections: *Neisseria meningitidis* and *Streptococcus pneumoniae* are important causes of community-acquired infection in adults[4] but are unusual causes of ICU acquired infection; enteric Gram-negative bacilli, *Staphylococcus aureus* and *Staphylococcus epidermidis* are responsible for most nosocomial ICU infections.[2,5]

The presence of infection in patients in the ICU is an important risk factor for increased mortality and morbidity.[6] Infection on admission to the ICU and nosocomial intra-abdominal infection have been shown to be independently predictive of fatality, after allowing for other variables such as acute physiology (APACHE score) or the use of steroids or chemotherapy.[8] Commonly death is due to inadequate treatment of a nosocomial infection (often caused by an unusually resistant organism) following successful treatment of a community-acquired infection.[5] All ICUs need to have in place effective strategies to minimize the nosocomial transmission of infection and the selection of pathogens with increased resistance to antimicrobials.

PNEUMONIA

Pneumonia (Ch. 48) is a common reason for admission to the ICU and among the most common nosocomial infections in patients in these units. Both community-acquired and nosocomial pneumonia have a high mortality in such patients, and management is complicated by the need to cover a wide range of pathogens.

COMMUNITY-ACQUIRED PNEUMONIA

The presence of clinical features such as tachypnea (>30/min), hypotension (systolic BP<90 and/or diastolic BP<60 mmHg), confusion, multilobar involvement, hypoxemia ($P_aO_2/F_iO_2<250$) and renal impairment (serum creatinine >1.8 mmol/l) can help identify patients with severe community-acquired pneumonia.[9,10] *Str. pneumoniae, Staph. aureus, Haemophilus influenzae*, enteric Gram-negative bacilli and *Legionella pneumophila*

are the most commonly identified bacterial causes of community-acquired pneumonia in patients admitted to the ICU (Table 44.3). It seems likely that *Str. pneumoniae* is the etiological agent for many patients in whom no microbial cause can be proven. Enteric Gram-negative bacilli, particularly *Pseudomonas aeruginosa* and *Klebsiella pneumoniae*, are uncommon causes of community-acquired pneumonia in patients admitted to the ICU, but are associated with a mortality of 50–75%, in contrast to an overall mortality of 20–50%.[11-14]

The clinical presentation is usually an unreliable guide to the etiology of community-acquired pneumonia,[12,14,15] and initial treatment will often need to cover the most common pathogens. Occasionally the clinical features on admission may provide useful clues to the etiology. For example, a history of chronic respiratory disease, alcoholism, immunosuppression or bronchiectasis should alert the doctor to the possibility that the pneumonia is due to an enteric Gram-negative bacillus. Other clues to a specific diagnosis include admission during an epidemic due to mycoplasma or influenza. During an influenza epidemic secondary infection with *Staph. aureus* should be suspected. The admission radiographic findings in patients admitted with pneumonia usually do not allow a reliable discrimination between the various possible etiologies. Sputum Gram stain suggests the etiology in approximately 10% of patients, while sputum culture and blood culture are diagnostic in 12–44% and 10–35% respectively.[11,13,14] A variety of methods (including fiberoptic bronchoscopy with protected brush sampling or bronchoalveolar lavage; percutaneous lung aspiration with ultrathin needles) have been proposed to increase the rate of microbiological diagnosis, however none has entered routine clinical practice. Bronchoscopy with bronchoalveolar lavage should at present be reserved for selected patients, such as those in whom infection with *Mycobacterium tuberculosis, Pneumocystis carinii* or cytomegalovirus is thought likely.

Treatment

An essential goal of treatment of severe community-acquired pneumonia is to ensure adequate activity against *Str. pneumoniae*, the most common cause of death in such patients. The rapid dissemination of penicillin-non-susceptible *Str. pneumoniae* has raised concern about the role of penicillins and cephalosporins in the treatment of disease due to this organism. However, high-dose intravenous therapy with many β-lactams provides serum levels well in excess of the minimum inhibitory concentrations (MICs) of non-susceptible strains of *Str. pneumoniae*, and (with the exception of rare strains for which the MIC of penicillin is greater than 4 mg/l) cure rates for non-susceptible strains are comparable to those seen with susceptible strains. At present, therefore, it does not appear necessary to include vancomycin in empiric regimens for the treatment of severe community-acquired pneumonia.

Because *L. pneumophila* may cause severe community-acquired pneumonia, treatment with a macrolide (e.g. erythromycin, clarithromycin or azithromycin) or a 'respiratory' fluoroquinolone (e.g. levofloxacin, gatifloxacin or moxifloxacin) is widely considered an essential component of the initial antimicrobial regimen.[15,16] Both of these classes of antimicrobial agents possess the advantages of providing activity against other common respiratory pathogens. Macrolides have useful activity against *Str. pneumoniae*, *Mycoplasma pneumoniae*, *Chlamydophila* (*Chlamydia*) *pneumoniae* and, to a variable degree, *Haemophilus influenzae*, while the 'respiratory' quinolones are active against *Str. pneumoniae* (including penicillin non-susceptible strains), *M. pneumoniae*, *C. pneumoniae* and enteric Gram-negative bacilli. Two recent North American guidelines have recommended a combination of a group 4 cephalosporin (e.g. ceftriaxone or cefotaxime) or a penicillin with a penicillinase inhibitor (e.g. amoxicillin–clavulanate, or ampicillin–sulbactam) together with a macrolide or a 'respiratory' quinolone for most patients in the ICU with community-acquired pneumonia.[15,16] It seems likely that a group 3 cephalosporin (such as cefuroxime), given in high doses, would provide comparable efficacy for pneumococcal pneumonia and only marginally less efficacy against enteric Gram-negative bacilli. Units that wish to limit their use of group 4 cephalosporins may consider replacing this component of the regimen with high-dose cefuroxime. Patients whose initial sputum (or tracheal aspirate) Gram stain suggests infection due to enteric Gram-negative bacilli should be treated with a regimen with enhanced antipseudomonal activity (e.g. ceftazidime or gentamicin, combined with a fluoroquinolone). Patients with suspected or proven anaerobic infection should be treated with clindamycin, or a penicillin with a penicillinase inhibitor.

NOSOCOMIAL PNEUMONIA

Ventilator-associated pneumonia is a common nosocomial infection in the ICU:[1–3] in patients ventilated for more than 48 h the incidence of pneumonia is approximately 20% with an associated mortality of 40–60%.[17,18] Ventilator-associated pneumonia remains a diagnostic and therapeutic dilemma, pneumonia can be diagnosed with certainty in a minority of patients in whom it is suspected, the pathogen(s) responsible for pneumonia are often uncertain, and the outcome is poor despite aggressive investigation and antibiotic treatment.[19] Furthermore, ventilator-associated pneumonia is frequently a marker of terminal illness rather than an independently important cause of death, and most of the deaths associated with this condition cannot be attributed to it.[20,21]

Aspiration of oropharyngeal secretions is the usual route of acquiring lung infection. Impaired consciousness, immobility, the presence of endotracheal and nasogastric tubes, and tracheostomies all increase the risk of aspiration and the incidence of pneumonia. The organisms aspirated into the lungs reflect those present in the oropharynx and stomach. Following admission to the ICU, the oropharynx and stomach become increasingly colonized with enteric Gram-negative bacilli. Thus, aspiration of oropharyngeal secretions at the onset of the illness or injury which leads to ICU admission commonly will result in pneumonia due to methicillin-sensitive *Staph. aureus*, *Str. pneumoniae* or *H. influenzae*, while aspiration occurring 3 or more days after admission to the unit is more likely to be due to enteric Gram-negative bacilli or methicillin-resistant *Staph aureus*.[22,23]

Diagnosis

Diagnosis of pneumonia in patients in the ICU, particularly those who are being ventilated, may be difficult. Although fever, leukocytosis, hypoxemia, purulent sputum and the presence of pathogenic bacteria in the tracheobronchial secretions will raise concerns about the possibility of pneumonia, these clinical features are more commonly present in the absence of pneumonia. A simple assessment based on these clinical features can effectively identify patients with a low risk of pneumonia who do not require intensive or prolonged antimicrobial therapy.[24]

Because the organisms responsible for causing nosocomial pneumonia in ICU patients are commonly derived from those colonizing the oropharynx, the use of sputum or tracheal aspirates to identify the causative organism(s) is hampered by the problem of distinguishing between contaminants and true pathogens. A variety of techniques, including transthoracic aspiration and bronchoscopy with sampling by bronchoalveolar lavage or protected specimen brush, have been evaluated, but none has been shown consistently to lower mortality rates.[19,22,25]

Gram-negative enteric bacilli, *Staph. aureus*, *Str. pneumoniae* and *H. influenzae* are the pathogens most commonly responsible for ventilator-associated pneumonia. In one study of 168 patients with bacteremic nosocomial pneumonia the organisms isolated from blood cultures were members of the *Klebsiella-Enterobacter-Serratia* family (26%), *Ps. aeruginosa* (13%), *Escherichia coli* (8%), other aerobic Gram-negative organisms (8%), *Staph. aureus* (23%), *Str. pneumoniae* (11%) and other Gram-positive organisms (10%).[26] Polymicrobial bacteremia, most commonly with *Staph. aureus*, *K. pneumoniae* or *Ps. aeruginosa*, occurred in 10% of episodes.

Treatment

Nosocomial pneumonia should be treated with an agent or combination of agents that covers this spectrum of pathogens.

Occasionally, previous consistent isolation of a pathogen from surveillance cultures of the patient's sputum will assist with selection of an antibiotic regimen. Similarly, the knowledge that *H. influenzae* and *Staph. aureus* are much more likely to cause pneumonia in a patient who has not recently received antibiotic therapy, and that *Ps. aeruginosa* is a particularly common cause in patients who have received prior antibiotic therapy,[27] can assist with antibiotic selection. Finally, the occurrence of endemic or epidemic transmission of a nosocomial pathogen within the ICU may need to be considered.

The combination of an aminoglycoside plus a third-generation cephalosporin or a broad-spectrum penicillin have been most commonly recommended for initial treatment of nosocomial pneumonia in the ICU.[28,29] These regimens have been selected on the basis of having adequate activity against the usual spectrum of pathogens plus *Ps. aeruginosa*, because of the especially high mortality associated with pneumonia due to this organism. In ICUs where *Ps. aeruginosa* and other multiresistant organisms are unusual causes of ventilator-associated pneumonia, a less broad-spectrum regimen may be used (e.g. a combination of an aminoglycoside with cefuroxime or amoxicillin–clavulanic acid). Concern about the nephrotoxicity and ototoxicity associated with aminoglycoside therapy has led to the use of regimens in which ciprofloxacin or aztreonam is substituted for the aminoglycoside. However, aztreonam lacks activity against Gram-positive organisms and generally should be used in combination with another agent with Gram-positive activity such as clindamycin, vancomycin or flucloxacillin.

Ceftazidime, imipenem–cilastatin, ciprofloxacin and a number of other agents have been evaluated as monotherapy for nosocomial pneumonia. Ceftazidime, imipenem–cilastatin and ticarcillin–clavulanic acid have all given high cure rates in patients with ventilator-associated pneumonia.[30–34] In contrast monotherapy with ciprofloxacin or pefloxacin has been associated with unacceptably high failure rates.[35,36] None of the monotherapy regimens evaluated was adequate treatment for pneumonia due to *Pseudomonas* spp. Persistent infection during treatment, development of resistance to the agent used, and clinical failure of monotherapy, occasionally with an improved response when a second agent was added to the regimen, were common problems when *Pseudomonas* pneumonia was treated with any of the monotherapy regimens. Although the overall outcome of monotherapy is similar to that of combination therapy,[37] pneumonia known or suspected to be caused by *Ps. aeruginosa* (or by *Enterobacter* or *Serratia* spp.) should be treated with a combination regimen.

The patient in the ICU with a nosocomial pneumonia should usually be treated initially with a broad-spectrum cephalosporin (e.g. cefuroxime, ceftriaxone or cefotaxime) or penicillin (e.g. amoxicillin–clavulanate) plus an aminoglycoside. In patients in whom infection with *Pseudomonas* is more likely (e.g. those who have had a prolonged ICU stay plus prior antibiotic therapy) an aminoglycoside plus a β-lactam with activity against pseudomonas (e.g. ceftazidime) should be used. A macrolide or quinolone should be a component of the regimen in hospitals experiencing epidemic or endemic infection with *Legionella*. Treatment should be modified on the basis of the microbiology results, for example to flucloxacillin or vancomycin in patients with staphylococcal infection, or to amoxicillin or cefuroxime alone in patients with infection due to a sensitive *Esch. coli*. Treatment can often be discontinued after 5–7 days but ventilator-associated pneumonia due to *Ps. aeruginosa* should be treated for at least 14 days.

INTRA-ABDOMINAL INFECTION

Intra-abdominal infection (Ch. 42) is a common important cause of sepsis in the ICU, especially in those units with surgical patients. The overall mortality of patients with severe generalized peritonitis or abdominal abscess(es), the most common intra-abdominal infections in the ICU, is 30–60%,[38,39] but varies greatly dependent on the degree of multiorgan dysfunction.

Microbiology

The organisms responsible for intra-abdominal sepsis vary with the source of infection. Peritonitis secondary to contamination by intestinal contents usually results in a polymicrobial mixed aerobic and anaerobic infection, with *Bacteroides fragilis* and *Esch. coli* the most commonly isolated species.[40] Spontaneous bacterial peritonitis is usually a monomicrobial infection. *Esch. coli*, *K. pneumoniae* and Gram-positive cocci are the usual pathogens. Anaerobes are rarely present.[41] Tertiary peritonitis, which occurs in severely ill patients following laparotomy, and which is not usually associated with peritoneal contamination by intestinal contents, is often monomicrobial and commonly due to *Staph. epidermidis*, *Enterococcus* spp., *Enterobacter* spp., *Pseudomonas* spp. or *Candida albicans*.[42]

Treatment

Antimicrobial therapy, other than brief perioperative prophylaxis, is not necessary either in patients with peritoneal contamination without infection (e.g. gastroduodenal ulcer perforation operated on within 24 h of onset) or in patients in whom a localized infectious process is treated by excision (e.g. acute suppurative appendicitis, simple acute cholecystitis and ischemic bowel without perforation). Peritonitis following contamination of the peritoneal cavity usually should be treated with a regimen active against enteric Gram-negative bacilli and anaerobes. An agent active against *Staph aureus* should be used in patients with peritonitis following gastric perforation. A combination of an aminoglycoside (e.g. gentamicin or tobramycin) with an anti-anaerobic agent (e.g. metronidazole or clindamycin) are established regimens for patients with intra-abdominal sepsis. Aztreonam is widely used as an alternative to an aminoglycoside for those patients at significant risk from the nephrotoxicity of aminoglycosides. Aztreonam plus clindamycin was found to have similar efficacy to tobramycin (or gentamicin) plus clindamycin in five clinical trials reviewed by Di Piro and Fortson.[43] Monotherapy with imipenem–cilastatin, piperacillin–tazobactam, cefotetan or cefoxitin is as effective as combination treatment with an aminoglycoside plus an anti-anaerobic drug,[44–46] and is associated with significantly less nephrotoxicity. These data have led Gorbach to suggest that aminoglycoside-containing regimens should not be used routinely for the initial treatment of uncomplicated intra-abdominal infection.[40] Enterococci are frequently present in polymicrobial intra-abdominal infections but are seldom found alone. Treatment with an agent active against enterococci (e.g. amoxicillin) is not routinely required.[40,47] Monotherapy with cefoxitin, combination therapy with cefuroxime plus metronidazole or gentamicin plus metronidazole (or clindamycin) are cheap, widely used alternatives for treatment of intra-abdominal infection. More expensive alternatives such as imipenem–cilastatin or piperacillin–tazobactam should be reserved for patients with complicated infections. Patients with generalized peritonitis or localized abdominal abscess should ordinarily be treated for 5–7 days.[48] Runyon et al (1991)[49] treated spontaneous bacterial peritonitis with cefotaxime 2 g 8-hourly for 5 days, with no deaths due to infection and a 93% microbiologic cure rate. As spontaneous bacterial peritonitis is usually due to community-acquired infection with relatively sensitive organisms it seems likely that very similar results could be achieved with cefuroxime or amoxicillin–clavulanate.

Tertiary peritonitis should initially be treated with amoxicillin, gentamicin and metronidazole, but treatment should be modified when appropriate microbiology results are available. When infection is due to *Candida* spp. other antimicrobial agents should be discontinued, foreign bodies removed if possible, and treatment with amphotericin B given for at least 4 weeks.[50]

Infection is a common complication of severe acute pancreatic necrosis. It usually occurs 2 or 3 weeks after the onset of acute pancreatitis and is commonly due to enteric Gram-negative bacilli, *Staph. aureus*, streptococci or *Bacteroides fragilis*. Antimicrobial prophylaxis (e.g. monotherapy with imipenem–cilastatin or cefuroxime, or combination therapy with ceftazidime, metronidazole and amikacin) appears to be useful in preventing infection in high-risk patients, those with necrosis of more than one-third of the pancreas. However, no trial has shown a significant benefit in mortality. It seems reasonable to treat patients with severe acute pancreatic necrosis with cefuroxime for 14 days in the expectation that preventing infection will reduce morbidity, if not mortality.[51]

URINARY TRACT INFECTION

Urinary tract infections are the third most common cause of admissions to ICUs for sepsis and are present in approximately 10% of such patients.[52,53] Although mortality from urinary tract sepsis is slightly lower than for the two more common sources (intra-abdominal infections and pneumonia), it is nevertheless still approximately 30%.[54,55] Most patients with urinary tract sepsis who require admission to an ICU have infections that are complicated; that is, they are associated with structural abnormalities of the urinary tract (e.g. congenital abnormalities, urolithiasis, malignancy). Rarely, and most often in patients with diabetes, there may be an associated perinephric abscess[56] or emphysematous pyelonephritis.[57]

Microbiology

The organisms most commonly responsible for complicated urinary infections are *Esch. coli*, *Proteus* and *Klebsiella*, other enteric Gram-negative bacilli, and less commonly enterococci. *Staph. aureus*, *Candida* and other fungi are sometimes responsible, particularly in patients with a renal abscess. Azotemia should not be assumed to be acute as underlying chronic renal impairment is often present. Initial empiric antibiotic therapy should include amoxicillin and either an aminoglycoside or aztreonam. Immediate investigation should include imaging of the urinary tract with ultrasonography or computed tomography (CT) to define the site and nature of any obstruction and detect the presence of an abscess or free gas in the tissues. Initial diagnostic radiology should be combined with either percutaneous nephrostomy or uteretic stenting (performed following the first dose of antibiotics). Treatment of perinephric abscess(es) should include an anti-staphyloccocal antibiotic (e.g. flucloxacillin or vancomycin)[58] and consideration of operative drainage. Nephrectomy is usually recommended in emphysematous pyelonephritis.[57]

Colonization and infection of the urinary tract occur in 6–18% of ICU patients.[1,2] In most of these patients urinary tract infection is a relatively insignificant complication of urinary catheterization, which resolves on removal of the catheter but in a minority it is the cause of systemic illness and in a few it may contribute to mortality. Antimicrobial treatment is not indicated in the majority of patients and should be reserved for those with evidence of systemic sepsis.

Treatment

A variety of different antimicrobials have been evaluated in the treatment of hospital patients with serious urinary tract infection. The most important requirement of a regimen is adequate activity against aerobic Gram-negative bacilli, including *Pseudomonas*. Gentamicin, or another aminoglycoside, has long been considered the standard parenteral treatment for pyelonephritis, but concerns about nephrotoxicity and ototoxicity have prompted the assessment of other agents.

Aztreonam, ceftazidime, imipenem–cilastatin, ciprofloxacin and a host of other agents have demonstrated generally similar efficacy to the aminoglycosides.[59–61] The selection of initial empiric therapy is influenced more by the relative costs of these agents than by any differences in clinical efficacy. Once the urinary pathogen has been identified treatment can often be modified to use a cheaper narrow-spectrum agent. Pyelonephritis should be treated for 7–10 days but colonized patients can usually be managed by observation until removal of the catheter. The management of urinary tract infection is discussed in Ch. 57.

INTRAVASCULAR CATHETER-ASSOCIATED INFECTIONS

Infections of intravascular cannulas may range in severity from asymptomatic colonization of the cannula hub or skin insertion site to suppurative thrombophlebitis. Bacteremia is a common complication of severe catheter-associated infection, and in ICU patients is associated with a significantly increased mortality.[62] The incidence of intravascular catheter-associated sepsis is particularly affected by the spectrum and density of bacterial colonization of the skin at the insertion site, the duration of catheterization and the type of catheter used. The rate of cannula-related bacteremia is approximately 0.2% for peripheral intravenous cannulas, 1% for arterial catheters used for hemodynamic monitoring and 3–5% for short-term non-cuffed central venous catheters.[63] Infection rates in patients with burns are commonly much higher.[64] The organisms most commonly responsible for cannula-related sepsis in ICU patients are *Staph. epidermidis*, enteric Gram-negative bacilli, *Staph. aureus*, *Enterococcus faecalis* and *C. albicans*[65–67] (Table 44.4).

Catheter-associated infection should be suspected in all febrile patients who lack an identified source of sepsis. Infection of central venous catheters is not usually associated with any signs of sepsis at the insertion site. In contrast, insertion-site inflammation may be a useful sign of infection associated with peripheral venous and arterial catheters. However, most patients with peripheral catheter insertion-site inflammation do not have significant infection. Furthermore, sepsis may occur in the absence of local inflammation. In one study of 130 arterial catheters, bacteremia occurred in 3 of 14 patients with inflammation at the site of catheter insertion and 2 of 116 patients without local inflammation.[68]

The management of catheter-associated infection is discussed in detail in Ch. 45.

All patients with intravascular catheter-associated sepsis, especially those with infection due to *Staph. aureus*, should be carefully evaluated for the development of distant foci of

infection (e.g. endocarditis, epidural abscess, septic arthritis). While these complications most commonly occur during the first 14 days after onset of the catheter-associated infection[69] they may present as late as 2 months after the completion of antibiotic treatment.[70] Patients who have clinical evidence of suppurative thrombophlebitis or perivascular abscess may need adjunctive treatment with heparin, surgical removal of the infected vein, or drainage of a perivascular abscess.[71]

The optimal duration of treatment for apparently uncomplicated intravascular catheter-associated sepsis is uncertain. Jernigan and Farr[70] reviewed 11 studies of short-course therapy of catheter-related *Staph. aureus* bacteremia and concluded that treatment should be for more than 2 weeks. Fowler et al[72] have suggested that patients with cannula-related *Staph. aureus* bacteremia who have no indwelling prosthetic devices, clinical resolution within 3 days of removal of the infected cannula, sterile blood cultures at 2–4 days after starting appropriate therapy and a normal trans-esophageal echocardiogram after 5–7 days of therapy should be treated for only 7 days. The duration of treatment for patients with cannula-related bacteremia due to other organisms is even less certain. Use of central venous cannulas, coated with either chlorhexidine and silver sulfadiazine or rifampicin and minocycline has a significant benefit in the prevention of cannula-associated bacteremia.[73]

SINUSITIS

Sinusitis (Ch. 47), particularly affecting the maxillary sinuses, is an occasional cause of fever in ICU patients.[74,75] Complications of sinusitis include bronchopneumonia, septicemia and subdural empyema.

Sinusitis should be suspected in febrile patients who have endotracheal and gastric tubes inserted through the nares. Purulent rhinorrhea and middle ear effusion(s) (detected by pneumatic otoscopy) are useful clinical associations with sinusitis.[76] Partial or complete opacification of the sinuses has been demonstrated in 30–60% of patients admitted to an ICU for at least 7 days.[74,75] However, in approximately half of these patients the maxillary sinus fluid does not grow significant numbers (>10^3 cfu/ml) of organisms. The demonstration of fluid in the sinuses (by computed tomography, radiography or ultrasonography) should not therefore be regarded as proof of the presence of purulent sinusitis. In patients who do have purulent sinusitis the infection is commonly polymicrobial, with Gram-negative bacilli present in most. *Candida* and anaerobes are occasional causes of sinusitis.

The initial treatment of sinusitis should include removal of any nasal tubes and treatment with a broad-spectrum antibiotic such as cefoxitin. In patients with persistent fever, radiological evidence of significant sinus opacification and no other focus of infection, the affected sinuses should be surgically drained and lavaged and treatment modified on the basis of culture results.

Table 44.4 Etiology of primary bacteremia in patients in intensive care units

	Richards et al[3]	Richards et al[5]
Total no. of isolates	2971	4394
Organisms (%)		
Staph. aureus	13	12
Staph. epidermidis	36	39
Enterococci	16	11
Enteric Gram-negative bacilli	17	20
Candida spp.	11	12

SOLID ORGAN TRANSPLANTATION

Solid organ transplant recipients are admitted to an ICU under two circumstances – immediately postoperatively or at some later time following transplantation. Infection is the most common reason for such admission.

Prophylactic perioperative antimicrobial therapy in solid organ transplant recipients should be effective against the common bacterial and fungal pathogens responsible for infection during this period of maximal immunosuppression. The regimen should represent the consensus views of transplant clinicians, intensivists and infectious disease physicians and should be in the form of a written protocol. Prophylaxis should begin immediately preoperatively so as to provide high blood levels during surgery. The agents used should be appropriate to the (site and organ-specific) infective risks and should be given for short periods only (less than 24 h). Finally, account should be taken of co-morbidity such as renal impairment so as to minimize iatrogenic complications. These recommendations are consistent with the general principles for the prevention of surgical site infections.[77]

Common regimens in abdominal organ transplantation include either a group 3 cephalosporin (cefuroxime or cefoxitin) or a combination of an antistaphylococcal penicillin (or vancomycin) and either an aminoglycoside or aztreonam. A short course of prophylactic systemic antifungal therapy is recommended in high-risk patients undergoing liver transplantation.[78]

Perioperative regimens in heart transplantation should be similar to those used in non-transplant cardiac surgery (e.g. cefazolin). Lung transplant recipients with cystic fibrosis or bronchiectasis are frequently colonized with multiresistant enteric Gram-negative bacilli and should receive prophylaxis with a dual antipseudomonal regimen (e.g. ceftazidime and an aminoglycoside). Other lung transplant patients, for example those with pulmonary hypertension, should have similar prophylaxis to heart transplant recipients.

Bacterial infections in critically ill transplant recipients early after transplantation should be treated according to protocols designed for other critically ill patients, bearing in mind the local microbial flora, the nature of the putative septic site and the state of immunosuppression. Empiric treatment may consist of a group 3 cephalosporin (perhaps in combination with an aminoglycoside) in pneumonia or urinary tract infection; an anti-staphylococcal penicillin (or vancomycin) with an aminoglycoside and perhaps amphotericin B[79,80] in clinical sepsis without an identified site; and either triple combination therapy (aminoglycoside, metronidazole and amoxicillin or vancomycin) or monotherapy with a carbapenem in intra-abdominal infection. *Enterococcus faecium*, including vancomycin-resistant strains, is a particular problem in biliary and intra-abdominal infection after liver transplantation, as are multiresistant organisms after lung transplantation.[81]

Serious fungal infections are particularly problematic[82–84] and constitute the most common unsuspected finding at autopsy in transplant recipients who die in the ICU.[85] Early recourse to liposomal amphotericin B is recommended in life-threatening fungal infections in transplant recipients, although successful use of caspofungin or voriconazole has been reported for invasive aspergillosis.[86,87]

Infections occurring more than a month after transplantation are more likely to be due to opportunistic organisms[88] and invasive means should be used if necessary to establish the nature of the causative organisms.

The prophylaxis and therapy of viral and other opportunistic infections in transplant patients is covered in Ch. 43.

SEPSIS MODULATORS

Sepsis (that is, the clinical syndrome usually associated with severe life-threatening infections) has a complex pathophysiology that has proved difficult to elucidate.[89] Although understanding of many of the underlying mediators and mechanisms of disease (e.g. the inflammatory and coagulation cascades) is increasing[90,91] attempts to convert this understanding into effective therapeutic strategies have so far been largely unsuccessful.[52,92,93] In large part this is because of the extreme heterogeneity of clinical sepsis with respect to patient factors (e.g. co-morbidity), quality of clinical care (e.g. the appropriateness of surgical and antimicrobial therapy),[94,95] the nature of the septic process (e.g. abscess or bacteremia), the timing of intervention with respect to the stage of evolution of the underlying pathophysiology, and the redundancy of disease mechanisms which limit the possible efficacy of a 'single magic bullet' intervention strategy.

The lack of specific clinical correlates of underlying disease mechanisms has prompted calls for a reappraisal of the utility of the clinical definition of sepsis and for a classification of septic patients in ways that ensure more homogeneity with respect to these mechanisms.[96] However, despite these formidable methodological difficulties, a meta-analysis[97] of 18 trials of a variety of anti-inflammatory therapies showed a small but statistically significant reduction in absolute mortality (from around 39% to 36%) in the 'active' arm. This suggests that such therapies may indeed have therapeutic benefit. It seems likely that some of these agents may be less effective than others and that the size of the 'benefit' in the meta-analysis may be an underestimate of the efficacy of a few 'strong performers'. Nevertheless, very large trial sizes (*c.* 6000 patients) would be required to detect such small (3%) benefits, unless trial design improved. After a number of small trials of anti-thrombin-III suggested that this agent might be beneficial,[98] a large multi-center study (*c.* 2300 patients) was recently completed, but the results were unfortunately confounded by the adverse effects in the anti-thrombin-III arm of simultaneous heparin administration and the future of this agent is unclear.[99] Another agent with both anti-inflammatory and anti-thrombotic activity, recombinant human activated protein C or drotrecogin-alfa, has recently been shown to reduce all-cause 28-day mortality from 30.8% to 24.7% in yet another large trial.[53] However, the cost-effectiveness and clinical applicability of the results of this trial have yet to be established.

PREVENTION OF INFECTION IN THE ICU

SELECTIVE DECONTAMINATION OF THE DIGESTIVE TRACT

The use of selective decontamination of the digestive tract (SDD) to reduce the incidence of infection in multiple trauma patients was first reported by Stoutenbeek et al.[100] The regimen used for SDD is commonly a mixture of polymyxin, tobramycin (or gentamicin) and amphotericin B. This mixture is applied as a paste to the oral mucosa, and a liquid suspension is swallowed or administered via a nasogastric tube four times daily. The regimen is intended to eliminate fungi and aerobic Gram-negative bacteria from the gastrointestinal tract but to have little effect on the predominant anaerobic flora and thus maintain 'colonization resistance' due to their continued growth. The purpose of SDD is to reduce the rate of pneumonia and other serious infections caused by pathogenic organisms originating from the gastrointestinal tract. In a modification of SDD the topical oral and enteric regimen used throughout a patients stay in the ICU has been supplemented by the addition of a systemic broad-spectrum antibiotic (usually cefotaxime) for the first 4 days of the stay. This selective parenteral and enteral anti-sepsis regimen (SPEAR) is intended to improve upon the efficacy of SDD by treating occult or incubating infections present at admission to ICU. Whether or not regimens have included an initial period of systemic antimicrobial therapy the acronym SDD is most frequently used to describe this form of chemoprophylaxis.

Colonization of the oropharynx, stomach and rectum is dramatically affected by SDD regimens. Aerobic Gram-negative bacilli are eliminated from the oropharynx and stomach within 3–4 days of starting SDD. In contrast, they continue to be isolated from these sites in 20–50% of control patients not given SDD. The proportion of patients with aerobic Gram-negative bacilli present in rectal swabs also declines from approximately 60–90% to 10–20% over a period of 10–14 days.[101–103]

The reduction in colonization of the upper gastrointestinal tract by aerobic Gram-negative bacilli is associated in most studies with a marked reduction in the incidence of nosocomial infection, especially pneumonia. Thus, analysis of the results from 16 randomized controlled trials (including 3361 patients) of SDD regimens that included a systemic antimicrobial demonstrated a strong protective effect (odds ratio = 0.35, 95% CI = 0.29–0.41) against respiratory tract infections.[104]

SDD regimens that include a systemic antimicrobial have shown a positive but less dramatic effect (odds ratio 0.79, 95% CI = 0.65–0.97) on overall mortality, which was approximately 30% in control patients and 24% in the patients given SDD. This suggests that approximately 23 patients would need to be treated to prevent one death. The adverse effects of SDD reg-

imens include the significantly increased expenditure on antibiotics, the potential for increased antibiotic resistance in the endemic bacterial flora of the ICU due to the selective pressure exerted by the SDD regimen, and the toxicity of the agents used. Opinion is divided between those who consider SDD of proven benefit[104] and those who consider that further study is required to determine whether it is cost-effective in selected subgroups (e.g. trauma and burn patients).[22,23]

OTHER STRATEGIES TO PREVENT VENTILATOR-ASSOCIATED PNEUMONIA

Semi-recumbent positioning, enteral rather than gastric feeding, use of sucralfate rather than antacids or H_2 antagonists as prophylaxis against stress-induced gastric ulceration, continuous subglottic aspiration and removal of nasogastric and endotracheal tubes at the earliest opportunity have all been shown to reduce the incidence of ventilator-associated pneumonia.[23]

HAND HYGIENE

Despite clear evidence that micro-organisms are disseminated within the ICU on the hands of staff,[105] and increasing concern about nosocomial infection with ever more resistant organisms, ICU staff wash their hands on approximately only one-third of the occasions when they should do so. The level of compliance with handwashing guidelines in ICUs tends to be lower than it is in other parts of the hospital, perhaps because of heavier staff workloads in the ICU. Placing labels on ICU equipment that remind staff to wash their hands, provision of easily accessible handbasins and dispensers, and use of an antiseptic handrub rather than handwashing, have all been found to improve hand hygiene in the ICU.[106] Maintaining high levels of hand hygiene requires adequate staffing and continuous education and motivation of staff. While these actions may appear mundane, improvements in hand hygiene are likely to dramatically reduce nososcomial infection.

POLICIES TO MAXIMIZE THE EFFECTIVENESS OF ANTIMICROBIAL USE IN THE ICU

The prevalence of infection with antibiotic-resistant organisms is rising in ICUs,[107] as it is in hospitals generally. Such infections are difficult and costly to treat.[108] Intensive care units are often accused of indiscriminate use of antibiotics and of creating antibiotic-resistant organisms, which then spread to the rest of the hospital. While it is evident that the patients with the most severe infections in the hospital are often admitted to the ICU as a result of their infection, there is much that can be done in the ICU to limit the inappropriate use of antibiotics and the selection of resistant microbial strains.[109]

Crucial to the success of these endeavors, however, is the creation of a conservative culture with respect to the use of antibiotics, both prophylactically and therapeutically. This requires the cooperation of all clinicians practising within the ICU. This culture should be expressed in an antibiotic management program. Infectious disease physicians have a detailed knowledge of the local microbiological flora, both in hospital and in the surrounding community and can provide evidence-based advice and facilitate consensus among other clinicians on appropriate antibiotic use.[109]

Antibiotic management programs should be specific and applicable to the clinical situation, where decisions often need to be made without supporting microbiological information. They should specifically cover 'surgical prophylaxis' and should specify the indications, agent, dose and duration of therapy.[110] They should also explicitly prohibit the use of antibiotic prophylaxis in situations where it is not indicated and should specify initial empiric therapy based on presenting clinical syndromes (i.e. before microbiological information comes to hand). Once again, the agents, dose and duration should be specified. Certain agents (e.g. perhaps expanded-spectrum cephalosporins, amphotericin B, carbapenems, amikacin, streptogramins, linezolid) could be designated as mandating either prior approval or early review by an infectious disease physician specializing in infectious diseases. A policy commitment by the treating clinicians to reserve empiric antibiotic therapy for 'clinical sepsis' and not to treat 'colonization' is crucial to the success of an antibiotic management program in reducing unnecessary and probably harmful antibiotic use. Finally, these policies should also stipulate a commitment to rationalize antibiotics (narrower spectrum, less 'reserved', cheaper) in the light of appropriate definitive microbiological information.

Specifying the most appropriate investigation strategy for common syndromes of clinical infection[19] may reduce mortality, improve the quality of microbiological information and reduce unnecessary investigation, antibiotic use and cost.

INFECTIONS DUE TO UNUSUALLY RESISTANT BACTERIA

Colonization and infection with bacteria resistant to commonly used antibiotics is a rapidly growing problem in ICUs. Recent reports have described resistance to methicillin in 65% of infections due to *Staph. aureus*, gentamicin resistance in 46% of infection due to *Ps. aeruginosa* in European ICUs,[111] resistance to cefotaxime, ceftriaxone and aztreonam in 20–30% of isolates of *K. pneumoniae* from ICUs in France,[112] and resistance to vancomycin in 17% of enterococcal isolates from ICUs in the USA.[113] Potential adverse consequences of colonization or infection with multiresistant strains include failure of antimicrobial therapy, increased expense of antimicrobial therapy, spread of infection to other patients, and transfer of resistance to other bacterial species. Epidemics of multiresistant bacteria in ICU patients are often followed by spread to patients in other parts of the hospital and then to the community, or back to the ICU. When formulating policies for antibiotic use in the ICU, doctors should be influenced by the distant effects of their antibiotic choices and avoid unnecessary prescription of those agents most likely to facilitate the selection of multiresistant strains (Ch. 3).

Colonization and infection with multiresistant bacteria is usually the result of acquisition of endemic or epidemic strains following admission to the ICU.[114] A variety of factors (including greater severity of the underlying illness, prolonged stay in the ICU, the use of invasive devices and prolonged use of broad-spectrum antimicrobial therapy) increase the rate of infection with these organisms.[115] Resistance of a bacterial isolate to commonly tested antibiotics (e.g. methicillin resistance in *Staph. aureus*, vancomycin resistance in enterococci, aminoglycoside and group 4 cephalosporin resistance in Gram-negative bacilli) frequently serves as a marker of an epidemic of nosocomial infection, which might otherwise remain unsuspected. Such epidemics are of importance in themselves, but should also be regarded as the visible tip of an iceberg of undetected nosocomially transmitted infection.

Pseudomonas, Klebsiella, Enterobacter, Serratia and *Acinetobacter* spp., methicillin-resistant *Staph. aureus* and enterococci are the most commonly reported causes of epidemics of nosocomial bacteremia in ICU patients.[116] Such epidemics usually last less than 3 months, affect an average of 10 patients per outbreak, commonly arise from contaminated medical equipment, and often depend on transmission of infection by the hands of ICU staff. Similar factors no doubt contribute to the much larger problem of endemic nosocomial infection, but are less easily identified because the organisms responsible often lack unusual antibiotic resistance patterns.

Methicillin-resistant *Staph. aureus*

Methicillin-resistant *Staph. aureus* (MRSA) is a common cause of epidemics of infection in ICUs. Burns, surgical wounds, prolonged stay in the unit, and prolonged courses of multiple antibiotics all increase the risk of MRSA infection. Although persistent colonization of hospital staff has been suspected as the source of infection in some MRSA outbreaks, this is not found in most outbreaks. However, transient contamination of the hands is common in staff directly involved in the care of patients with MRSA infection, and is presumed to be the most common mode of transmission of infection between patients. Control and, not infrequently, termination of epidemics of MRSA can be achieved by surveillance of patients for MRSA colonization or infection, strict isolation of colonized or infected patients, consistent use of hand hygiene between each patient contact and appropriate treatment to minimize colonization or eradicate infection in affected patients and staff.

MRSA colonization may be reduced or eliminated by stopping antibiotic treatment whenever possible, effective treatment of underlying skin disorders, application of mupirocin ointment to colonized sites, and washing with an antiseptic.[117] Infection with MRSA is usually treated with intravenous vancomycin or linezolid, or oral clindamycin or fusidic acid supplemented by oral rifampicin.

Resistant enterococci

Enterococci (especially *E. faecalis* and *Enterococcus faecium*) resistant to gentamicin, ampicillin or vancomycin have emerged as an important cause of nosocomial infection in ICUs. Prolonged stay in the unit, persistent intra-abdominal infection, and prolonged broad-spectrum antimicrobial therapy with agents inactive against enterococci are common features in patients with enterococcal infection. Feces and urine of colonized patients are the usual sources of infection, and transmission on the hands of hospital staff is presumed to be the major route of cross-infection. The urinary tract, bloodstream and surgical wounds are the most common sites of infection.[5]

Bacteremia due to enterococci highly resistant to gentamicin (MIC >1000 mg/l) but susceptible to ampicillin or vancomycin may be successfully treated with amoxicillin (or ampicillin) or vancomycin monotherapy.[118,119] This is in contrast to enterococcal endocarditis, which requires combination treatment with amoxicillin or vancomycin plus an aminoglycoside for cure. Optimal treatment of infection with enterococci resistant to ampicillin, vancomycin and aminoglycosides is at present unclear, but linezolid and quinupristin–dalfopristin show some promise.

The rapid emergence of multiresistant enterococci, the difficulties posed by treatment of these infections, and the spectre of transfer of resistance to *Staph. aureus* are important reasons to limit the use of vancomycin as much as possible. Vancomycin should not ordinarily be used for perioperative prophylaxis, initial treatment of antibiotic-associated colitis, initial empirical treatment of febrile neutropenic patients, selective decontamination of the digestive tract, or eradication of MRSA colonization.[120]

Extended-spectrum β-lactamase-positive *K. pneumoniae*

Since its first appearance in 1983, *K. pneumoniae* resistant to broad-spectrum cephalosporins and aminoglycosides has caused epidemics of infection in ICUs worldwide.[121] Resistance is due to readily transmissible plasmids which encode for extended spectrum β-lactamases and for aminoglycoside and quinolone resistance. The β-lactamases are usually susceptible to inhibitors such as clavulanic acid and sulbactam, which may assist with identification of these strains in the laboratory.[112] Outbreaks of infection may involve multiple strains of *K. pneumoniae* and may spread to involve other bacteria such as *Esch. coli*, *Citrobacter freundii*, *Serratia marcescens* and *Enterobacter aerogenes*.

Infection with multiresistant *K. pneumoniae* usually involves the urinary tract, the respiratory tract or wounds.[121] Enteric colonization and transmission on the hands of hospital staff appear to contribute to epidemic spread. Treatment with cefotaxime or related cephalosporins may be effective against urinary tract infections due to multiresistant *K. pneumoniae*, but these agents will not be adequate for the treatment of major infections at other sites.[121] Imipenem–cilastatin, cephamycins such as cefoxitin, and piperacillin–tazobactam or ticarcillin–clavulanate, are active against most broad-spectrum β-lactamase-producing *K. pneumoniae*. Despite resistance to many other aminoglycosides, sensitivity to gentamicin is often retained.

Gram-negative bacilli with inducible β-lactamases

Another important source of infection due to multiresistant Gram-negative bacilli is the selection of organisms with chromosomally encoded class I β-lactamase production. *Pseudomonas*, *Enterobacter*, *Citrobacter* and *Serratia* spp. are the organisms that most frequently produce class I β-lactamase (*see* Ch. 17). Induction of enzyme production or selection of stably depressed mutant cells which constitutively manufacture class I β-lactamase at a high level may lead to development of resistance to β-lactams during treatment.[122,123] Enzyme production is strongly induced when organisms are exposed to cephalosporins of groups 1 and 2 (*see* Ch. 15), cefoxitin or imipenem–cilastatin, but is only weakly induced by exposure to groups 3 and 4 cephalosporins, ureidopenicillins and monobactams. Induced enzyme production ceases promptly when treatment with the inducing antibiotic is stopped. Selection of stably depressed mutants constitutively producing large amounts of β-lactamase occurs when inducible strains (especially *Ps. aeruginosa* and *Enterobacter cloacae*) are exposed to broad-spectrum cephalosporins, ureidopenicillins or monobactams. Resistance persists even when treatment with the antibiotic responsible for selecting the mutant strain is stopped. Development of resistance during treatment occurs in approximately 10–20% of patients,[123] and spread within the ICU may result in multiresistance in 30% of ICU isolates of *Ent. cloacae*.[122]

Imipenem–cilastatin, despite being a strong inducer of class I β-lactamase, is not susceptible to the enzyme's action. Alternative regimens include imipenem–cilastatin monotherapy or combination therapy using imipenem–cilastatin plus an aminoglycoside or a fluoroquinolone selected on the basis of careful susceptibility testing.[124] Patients treated with a broad-spectrum cephalosporin, ureidopenicillin or monobactam for an infection due to an initially sensitive strain should be carefully observed for the emergence of resistant mutants during treatment.

Multiresistant *Acinetobacter calcoaceticus*

Multiresistant *A. calcoaceticus* is an occasional cause of epidemics of infection in ICU patients. Epidemic strains are resistant to many broad-spectrum cephalosporins, and have variable susceptibility to aminoglycosides. Colonization and infection of the respiratory tract in artificially ventilated patients is a common feature of epidemics, and improvements in the methods used to sterilize ventilator equipment has led to termination of epidemics.[125] In most patients *A. calcoaceticus* merely colonizes the respiratory tract; however, it may be responsible for pneumonia and other serious infections. Imipenem–cilastatin alone, or in combination with an aminoglycoside, is often appropriate treatment.

A frequent theme for many epidemics caused by multiresistant bacteria has been the widespread use of antibiotics in response to increased resistance in other commonly isolated bacterial species. For example, vancomycin resistance in enterococci has emerged following increased use of vancomycin to treat suspected or proven MRSA (or methicillin-resistant *Staph. epidermidis* infections. Similarly, epidemics of infection due to multiresistant *K. pneumoniae* and *A. calcoaceticus* have followed increased use of group 4 cephalosporins and imipenem–cilastatin.[124] Thus the increased use of potent antibiotics with ever broader spectra of activity acts as a stimulus to the evolution of new epidemics of ever more resistant pathogens. The effect is to mortgage the future of antibiotic treatment to pay for our present practices. While there is no one solution to this problem that can be applied to all ICUs, the use of prescribing guidelines which encourage the use of older narrow-spectrum antibiotics and limit the use of new broad-spectrum antibiotic agents should prolong the utility of new drugs, delay the emergence of resistant strains and set a better example for prescribing patterns in the rest of the hospital[126] (Ch. 11).

References

1. Brown RB, Hosmer D, Chen HC et al 1985 A comparison of infections in different ICUs within the same hospital. *Critical Care Medicine* 13: 472–476

2. Vincent J-L, Bihari DJ, Suter PM et al 1995 The prevalence of nosocomial infection in intensive care units in Europe – the results of the EPIC study. *Journal of the American Medical Association* 274: 639–644

3. Richards MJ, Edwards JR, Culver DH, Gaynes RP and the National Nosocomial Infections Surveillance System 1999 Nosocomial infections in medical intensive care units in the United States. *Critical Care Medicine* 27: 887–892

4. Khoo SH, Creagh-Barry P, Wilkins EGL, Pasvol G 1992 Fulminant community acquired infections admitted to an intensive care unit. *Quarterly Journal of Medicine* NS83: 381–388

5. Richards MJ, Edwards JR, Culver DH, Gaynes RP and the National Nosocomial Infections Surveillance System 2000 Nosocomial infections in combined medical-surgical intensive care units in the United States. *Infection Control and Hospital Epidemiology* 21: 510–515

6. Chandrasekar PH, Kruse JA, Mathews MF 1986 Nosocomial infection among patients in different types of intensive care units at a city hospital. *Critical Care Medicine* 14: 508–510

7. Craven DE, Kunches LM, Lichtenberg DA et al 1988 Nosocomial infection and fatality in medical and surgical intensive care unit patients. *Archives of Internal Medicine* 148: 1161–1168

8. Kollef MH, Sherman G, Ward S, Fraser VJ 1999 Inadequate antimicrobial treatment of infections. A risk factor for hospital mortality among critically ill patients. *Chest* 115: 462–474

9. British Thoracic Society and the Public Health Laboratory Service 1987 Community-acquired pneumonia in adults in British hospitals in 1982–1983: a survey of aetiology, mortality, prognostic factors and outcome. *Quarterly Journal of Medicine* NS62: 195–220

10. American Thoracic Society 1993 Guidelines for the initial management of adults with community-acquired pneumonia; diagnosis, assessment of severity, and initial antimicrobial therapy. *American Review of Respiratory Disease* 148: 1418–1426

11. Ortqvist A, Sterner G, Nilsson JA 1985 Severe community-acquired pneumonia: factors influencing need of intensive care treatment and prognosis. *Scandinavian Journal of Infectious Diseases* 17: 377–386

12. Torres A, Serra-Batlles J, Ferrer A et al 1991 Severe community-acquired pneumonia. *American Review of Respiratory Disease* 144: 312–318

13. British Thoracic Society Research Committee and the Public Health Laboratory Service 1992 The aetiology, management and outcome of severe community-acquired pneumonia on the intensive care unit. *Respiratory Medicine* 86: 7–13

14. Potgieter PD, Hammond JMJ 1992 Etiology and diagnosis of pneumonia requiring ICU admission. *Chest* 101: 199–203

15. Bartlett JG, Dowell SF, Mandell LA, File TM, Musher DM, Fine MJ 2000 Practice guidelines for the management of community-acquired pneumonia in adults. *Clinical Infectious Diseases* 31: 347–382

16. Mandell LA, Marrie TJ, Grossman RF, Chow AW, Hyland RH and the Canadian Community. Acquired Pneumonia Working Group 2000 Canadian guidelines for the initial management of community-acquired pneumonia: an evidence-based update by the Canadian Infectious Diseases Society and the Canadian Thoracic Society. *Clinical Infectious Diseases* 31: 383–421

17. Craven DE, Kunches LM, Kilinsky V, Lichtenberg DA, Make BJ, McCabe WR 1986 Risk factors for pneumonia and fatality in patients receiving continuous mechanical ventilation. *American Review of Respiratory Disease* 133: 792–796

18. Rello J, Quintana E, Ausina V et al 1991 Incidence, etiology and outcome of nosocomial pneumonia in mechanically ventilated patients. *Chest* 100: 439–444

19. Fagon JY, Chastre J, Wolff M et al 2000 Invasive and noninvasive strategies for management of suspected ventilator-associated pneumonia. A randomized trial. *Annals of Internal Medicine* 132: 621–630

20. Fagon J-Y, Chaistre J, Hance AJ, Montravers P, Novara A, Gibert C 1993 Nosocomial pneumonia in ventilated patients: a cohort study evaluating attributable mortality and hospital stay. *American Journal of Medicine* 94: 281–288

21. Kollef MH, Silver P, Murphy DM, Trovillion E 1995 The effect of late-onset ventilator-associated pneumonia in determining patient mortality. *Chest* 108: 1655–1662

22. American Thoracic Society 1995 Hospital-acquired pneumonia in adults: diagnosis, assessment of severity, initial antimicrobial therapy, and preventative strategies. *American Journal of Respiratory and Critical Care Medicine* 153: 1711–1725

23. Kollef MH 1999 The prevention of ventilator-associated pneumonia. *New England Journal of Medicine* 340: 627–634

24. Singh N, Rogers P, Atwood CW, Wagener MM, Yu VL 2000 Short-course empiric antibiotic therapy for patients with pulmonary infiltrates in the intensive care unit. A proposed solution for indiscriminate antibiotic prescription. *American Journal of Respiratory and Critical Care Medicine* 162: 505–511

25. Grossman RF 2000 Evidence-based assessment of diagnostic tests for ventilator-associated pneumonia. *Chest* 117: 77S–181S

26. Bryan CS, Reynolds KL 1984 Bacteremic nosocomial pneumonia. Analysis of 172 episodes from a single metropolitan area. *American Review of Respiratory Disease* 129: 668–671

27. Rello J, Ausina V, Ricart M, Castella J, Prats G 1993 Impact of previous antimicrobial therapy on the etiology and outcome of ventilator-associated pneumonia. *Chest* 104: 1230–1235

28. Scheld WM, Mandell GL 1991 Nosocomial pneumonia: pathogenesis and recent advances in diagnosis and therapy. *Reviews of Infectious Diseases* 13 (Suppl. 9): S743–S751

29. La Force FM 1992 Lower respiratory tract infections. In: Bennett JV, Brachman PS (eds) *Hospital infections*, 3rd edn. Little, Brown and Co., Boston, pp. 611–639

30. Cone LA, Woodard DR, Stoltzman DS, Byrd RG 1985 Ceftazidime versus tobramycin-ticarcillin in the treatment of pneumonia and bacteremia. *Antimicrobial Agents and Chemotherapy* 28: 33–36

31. Salata RA, Gebhart RL, Palmer et al 1985 Pneumonia treated with imipenem/cilastatin. *American Journal of Medicine* 78 (Suppl. 6A): 104–109

32. Schwigon CD, Hulla FW, Schulze B, Maslak A 1986 Timentin in the treatment of nosocomial bronchopulmonary infections in intensive care units. *Journal of Antimicrobial Chemotherapy* 17 (Suppl. C): 115–122

33. Mandell LA, Nicolle LE, Ronald AR et al 1987 A prospective randomized trial of ceftazidime versus cefazolin/tobramycin in the treatment of hospitalized patients with pneumonia. *Journal of Antimicrobial Chemotherapy* 20: 95–107

34. Norrby SR, Finch RG, Glauser M, European Study Group 1993 Monotherapy in serious hospital-acquired infections: a clinical trial of ceftazidime versus imipenem/cilastatin. *Journal of Antimicrobial Chemotherapy* 31: 927–937

35. Martin C, Gouin F, Fourrier F, Junginger W, Prieur BL 1988 Pefloxacin in the treatment of nosocomial lower respiratory tract infections in intensive care patients. *Journal of Antimicrobial Chemotherapy* 21: 795–799

36. Peloquin CA, Cumbo TJ, Nix DE, Sands MF, Schentag JJ 1989 Evaluation of intravenous ciprofloxacin in patients with nosocomial lower respiratory tract infections. *Archives of Internal Medicine* 149: 2269–2273

37. La Force FM 1989 Systemic antimicrobial therapy of nosocomial pneumonia: monotherapy versus combination therapy. *European Journal of Clinical Microbiology and Infectious Diseases* 8: 61–68

38. Bohnen J, Boulanger M, Meakins JL, McLean APH 1983 Prognosis in generalized peritonitis. Relation to cause and risk factors. *Archives of Surgery* 118: 285–290

39. Bohnen JMA, Mustard RA, Oxholm SE, Schouten BD 1988 APACHE II score and abdominal sepsis. A prospective study. *Archives of Surgery* 123: 225–229

40. Gorbach SL 1993 Treatment of intra-abdominal infections. *Journal of Antimicrobial Chemotherapy* 31 (Suppl. A): 67–78

41. Mbopi Keou F-X, Bloch F, Buu Hoi A et al 1992 Spontaneous peritonitis in cirrhotic hospital in-patients: retrospective analysis of 101 cases. *Quarterly Journal of Medicine* NS 83: 401–407

42. McClean KL, Sheehan GJ, Harding GKM 1994 Intra-abdominal infection: a review. *Clinical Infectious Diseases* 19: 100–116

43. DiPiro JT, Fortson NS 1993 Combination antibiotic therapy in the management of intra-abdominal infection. *American Journal of Surgery* 165 (Suppl. 2A): 82S–88S

44. Ho JL, Barza M 1987 Role of aminoglycoside antibiotics in the treatment of intra-abdominal infection. *Antimicrobial Agents and Chemotherapy* 31: 485–491

45. Solomkin JS, Dellinger EP, Christou NV, Busutti RW 1990 Results of a multicenter trial comparing imipenem/cilastatin to tobramycin/clindamycin for intra-abdominal infections. *Annals of Surgery* 212: 581–591

46. Eklund A-E, Nord CE, Swedish Study Group 1993 A randomized multicenter trial of piperacillin/tazobactam versus imipenem/cilastatin in the treatment of severe intraabdominal infections. *Journal of Antimicrobial Chemotherapy* 31 (Suppl. A): 79–85

47. Nichols RL, Muzik AC 1992 Enterococcal infections in surgical patients: the mystery continues. *Clinical Infectious Diseases* 15: 72–76

48. Bohnen JMA, Solomkin JS, Dellinger EP, Bjornson HS, Page CP 1992 Guidelines for clinical care: anti-infective agents for intra-abdominal infection. *Archives of Surgery* 127: 83–89

49. Runyon BA, McHutchison JG, Antillon MR, Akriviadis EA, Montano AA 1991 Short-course versus long-course antibiotic treatment of spontaneous bacterial peritonitis. *Gastroenterology* 100: 1737–1742

50. British Society for Antimicrobial Chemotherapy Working Party 1994 Management of deep *Candida* infection in surgical and intensive care unit patients. *Intensive Care Medicine* 20: 522–528

51. Kramer KM, Levy H 1999 Prophylactic antibiotics for severe acute pancreatitis: the beginning of an era. *Pharmacotherapy* 19: 592–602

52. Opal SM, Fisher CJ Jr, Dhainaut JF et al 1997 Confirmatory interleukin-1 receptor antagonist trial in severe sepsis: a phase III, randomized, double-blind, placebo-controlled, multicenter trial. The Interleukin-1 Receptor Antagonist Sepsis Investigator Group. *Critical Care Medicine* 25: 1115–1124

53. Bernard GR, Vincent JL, Laterre PF et al 2001 Recombinant human protein C Worldwide Evaluation in Severe Sepsis (PROWESS) study group. Efficacy and safety of recombinant human activated protein C for severe sepsis. *New England Journal of Medicine* 344: 699–709

54. Knaus WA, Sun X, Nystrom O, Wagner DP 1992 Evaluation of definitions for sepsis. *Chest* 101: 1656–1662

55. Buisson C, Doyon F, Carlet J 1996 Bacteremia and severe sepsis in adults: a multicenter prospective survey in ICUs and wards of 24 hospitals. French Bacteremia-Sepsis Study Group. *American Journal of Respiratory and Critical Care Medicine* 154: 617–624

56. Hutchison FN, Kaysen GA 1988 Perinephric abscess:the missed diagnosis. *Medical Clinics of North America* 72: 993–1014

57. Huang JJ, Tseng CC 2000 Emphysematous pyelonephritis: clinicoradiological classification, management, prognosis, and pathogenesis. *Archives of Internal Medicine* 160: 797–805

58. Dembry LM, Andriole VT 1997 Renal and perirenal abscesses. *Infectious Disease Clinics of North America* 11: 663–680

59. Sattler FR, Moyer JE, Schramm M, Lombard JS, Appelbaum PC 1984 Aztreonam compared with gentamicin for treatment of serious urinary tract infections. *Lancet* i: 1315–1318

60. Fang G, Brennen C, Wagener M et al 1991 Use of ciprofloxacin versus use of aminoglycosides for therapy of complicated urinary tract infection: prospective, randomized, clinical and pharmacokinetic study. *Antimicrobial Agents and Chemotherapy* 35: 1849–1855

61. Cox CE 1993 Comparison of intravenous fleroxacin with ceftazidime for treatment of complicated urinary tract infections. *American Journal of Medicine* 94 (Suppl. 3A): 118S–125S

62. Renaud B, Brun-Buisson C 2001 Outcomes of primary and catheter-related bacteremia. A cohort and case-controlled study in critically ill patients. *American Journal of Respiratory and Critical Care Medicine* 163: 1584–1590

63. Maki DG 1992 Infections due to infusion therapy. In: Bennett JV, Brachman PS (eds) *Hospital infections*, 3rd edn. Little, Brown and Co., Boston, pp. 849–898

64. Pruitt BA, McManus WF, Kim SH, Treat RC 1980 Diagnosis and treatment of cannula-related intravenous sepsis in burn patients. *Annals of Surgery* 191: 546–554

65. Collignon P, Soni N, Pearson I, Sorrell T, Woods P 1988 Sepsis associated with central vein catheters in critically ill patients. *Intensive Care Medicine* 14: 227–231

66. Richet H, Hubert B, Nitemberg G et al 1990 Prospective multicenter study of vascular-catheter-related complications and risk factors for positive central-catheter cultures in intensive care unit patients. *Journal of Clinical Microbiology* 28: 2520–2525

67. Pittet D, Tarara D, Wenzel RP 1994 Nosocomial bloodstream infection in critically ill patients. *Journal of the American Medical Association* 271: 1598–1601

68. Band JD, Maki DG 1979 Infections caused by arterial catheters used for hemodynamic monitoring. *American Journal of Medicine* 67: 735–741

69. Arnow PM, Quimosing EM, Beach M 1993 Consequences of intravascular catheter sepsis. *Clinical Infectious Diseases* 16: 778–784

70. Jernigan JA, Farr BM 1993 Short-course therapy of catheter-related *Staphylococcus aureus* bacteremia: a meta-analysis. *Annals of Internal Medicine* 119: 304–311

71. Verghese A, Widrich WC, Arbeit RD 1985 Central venous septic thrombophlebitis – the role of medical therapy. *Medicine* 64: 394–400

72. Fowler VG Jr, Sanders LL, Sexton DJ et al 1998 Outcome of *Staphylococcus aureus* bacteremia according to compliance with recommendations of infectious diseases specialists: experience with 244 patients. *Clinical Infectious Diseases* 27: 478–486

73. Darouiche RO, Raad II, Heard So et al 1999 A comparison of two antimicrobial-impregnated central venous catheters. *New England Journal of Medicine* 340: 1–8

74. Holzapfel L, Chevret S, Madinier G et al 1993 Influence of long-term oro- or nasotracheal intubation on nosocomial maxillary sinusitis and pneumonia: results of a prospective, randomized, clinical trial. *Critical Care Medicine* 21: 1132–1138

75. Rouby J-J, Laurent P, Gosnach M et al 1994 Risk factors and clinical relevance of nosocomial maxillary sinusitis in the critically ill. *American Journal of Respiratory and Critical Care Medicine* 150: 776–783

76. Borman KR, Brown PM, Mezera KK, Jhaveri H 1992 Occult fever in surgical intensive care unit patients is seldom caused by sinusitis. *American Journal of Surgery* 164: 412–416

77. Mangram AJ, Horan TC, Pearson ML, Silver LC, Jarvis WR 1999 Guideline for prevention of surgical site infection, 1999. Hospital Infection Control Practices Advisory Committee. *Infection Control and Hospital Epidemiology* 20: 250–278

78. Singhal S, Ellis RW, Jones SG et al 2000 Targeted prophylaxis with amphotericin B lipid complex in liver transplantation. *Liver Transplantation* 6: 588–595

79. Wagener MM, Yu VL 1992 Bacteremia in transplant recipients: a prospective study of demographics, etiologic agents, risk factors, and outcomes. *American Journal of Infection Control* 20: 239–247

80. Palmer SM, Alexander BD, Sanders LL et al 2000 Significance of blood stream infection after lung transplantation: analysis in 176 consecutive patients. *Transplantation* 69: 2360–2366

81. Metras D, Viard L, Kreitmann B et al 1999 Lung infections in pediatric lung transplantation: experience in 49 cases. *European Journal of Cardiothoracic Surgery* 15: 490–494

82. Paradowski LJ 1997 Saprophytic fungal infections and lung transplantation-revisited. *Journal of Heart and Lung Transplantation* 16: 524–531

83. Mehrad B, Paciocco G, Martinez FJ, Ojo TC, Iannettoni MD, Lynch JP 2001 Spectrum of *Aspergillus* infection in lung transplant recipients: case series and review of the literature. *Chest* 119: 169–175

84. Grossi P, Farina C, Fiocchi R, Dalla Gasperina D 2000 Prevalence and outcome of invasive fungal infections in 1,963 thoracic organ transplant recipients: a multicenter retrospective study. Italian Study Group of Fungal Infections in Thoracic Organ Transplant Recipients. *Transplantation* 70: 112–116

85. Mort TC, Yeston NS 1999 The relationship of pre mortem diagnoses and post mortem findings in a surgical intensive care unit. *Critical Care Medicine* 27: 299–303

86. Linden P, Williams P, Chan KM 2000 Efficacy and safety of amphotericin B lipid complex injection (ABLC) in solid-organ transplant recipients with invasive fungal infections. *Clinical Transplantation* 14: 329–339

87. Denning DW, Ribaud P, Milpied N et al 2002 Efficacy and safety of voriconazole in the treatment of acute invasive aspergillosis. *Clinical Infectious Diseases* 34: 563–571

88. Fishman JA, Rubin RH 1998 Infection in organ-transplant recipients. *New England Journal of Medicine* 338: 1741–1751

89. Bone RC, Balk RA, Cerra FB et al 1992 Definitions for sepsis and organ failure and guidelines for the use of innovative therapies in sepsis. The ACCP/SCCM Consensus Conference Committee. American College of Chest Physicians/Society of Critical Care Medicine. *Chest* 101: 1644–1655

90. Glauser MP 2000 Pathophysiologic basis of sepsis: considerations for future strategies of intervention. *Critical Care Medicine* 28: S4–S8

91. Wanecek M, Weitzberg E, Rudehill A, Oldner A 2000 The endothelin system in septic and endotoxin shock. *European Journal of Pharmacology* 407: 1–15

92. Angus DC, Birmingham MC, Balk RA et al 2000 E5 murine monoclonal antiendotoxin antibody in gram-negative sepsis: a randomized controlled trial. E5 Study Investigators. *Journal of the American Medical Association* 283: 1723–1730

93. Abraham E, Anzueto A, Gutierrez G et al 1998 Double-blind randomised controlled trial of monoclonal antibody to human tumour necrosis factor in treatment of septic shock. NORASEPT II Study Group. *Lancet* 351: 929–933

94. Clark MA, Plank LD, Connolly AB et al 1998 Effect of a chimeric antibody to tumor necrosis factor-alpha on cytokine and physiologic responses in patients with severe sepsis – a randomized, clinical trial. *Critical Care Medicine* 26: 1650–1659

95. Streat SJ, Plank LD, Hill GL 2000 An overview of Modern management of patients with critical injury and severe sepsis. *World Journal of Surgery* 24: 655–663

96. Abraham E, Matthay MA, Dinarello CA et al 2000 Consensus conference definitions for sepsis, septic shock, acute lung injury, and acute respiratory distress syndrome: Time for a reevaluation. *Critical Care Medicine* 28: 232–235

97. Natanson C 1997 Anti-inflammatory therapies to treat sepsis and septic shock: a reassessment. *Critical Care Medicine* 25: 1095–1100

98. Eisele B, Lamy M, Thijs LG et al 1998 Antithrombin III in patients with severe sepsis. A randomized, placebo-controlled, double-blind multicenter trial plus a meta-analysis on all randomized, placebo-controlled, double-blind trials with antithrombin III in severe sepsis. *Intensive Care Medicine* 24: 663–672

99. Warren BL, Eid A, Singer P et al 2001 High-dose antithrombin III in severe sepsis. A randomized controlled trial. *Journal of the American Medical Association* 286: 1869–1878

100. Stoutenbeek CP, van Saene HKF, Miranda DR, Zandstra DF 1984 The effect of selective decontamination of the digestive tract on colonisation and infection rate in multiple trauma patients. *Intensive Care Medicine* 10: 185–192

101. Ledingham IM, Alcock SR, Eastaway AT, McDonald JC, McKay IC, Ramsay G 1988 Triple regimen of selective decontamination of the digestive tract, systemic cefotaxime, and microbiological surveillance for prevention of acquired infection in intensive care. *Lancet* i: 785–790

102. Hammond JMJ, Potgieter PD, Saunders GL, Forder AA 1992 Double-blind study of selective decontamination of the digestive tract in intensive care. *Lancet* 340: 5–9

103. Hamer DH, Barza M 1993 Prevention of hospital-acquired pneumonia in critically ill patients. *Antimicrobial Agents and Chemotherapy* 37: 931–938

104. Liberati A, D'Amico R, Pifferi S, Telaro E 2000 Antibiotic prophylaxis in intensive care units: meta-analyses versus clinical practice. *Intensive Care Medicine* 26: S38–S44

105. Paterson DL, Yu VL 1999 Extended-spectrum beta-lactamases: a call for improved detection and control. *Clinical Infectious Diseases* 29: 1419–1422

106. Boyce JM 1999 It is time for action: improving hand hygiene in hospitals. *Annals of Internal Medicine* 130: 153–155

107. Fridkin SK 2001 Increasing prevalence of antimicrobial resistance in intensive care units. *Critical Care Medicine* 29: N64–N68

108. Niederman MS 2001 Impact of antibiotic resistance on clinical outcomes and the cost of care. *Critical Care Medicine* 29: N114–N120

109. DeLisle S, Perl TM 2001 Antimicrobial management measures to limit resistance: A process-based conceptual framework. *Critical Care Medicine* 29: N121–N127

110. Namias N, Harvill S, Ball S, McKenney MG, Salomone JP, Civetta JM 1999 Cost and morbidity associated with antibiotic prophylaxis in the ICU. *Journal of the American College of Surgeons* 188: 225–230

111. Vincent J-L 2000 Microbial resistance: lessons from the EPIC study. *Intensive Care Medicine* 26: S3–S8

112. Sirot DL, Goldstein FW, Soussy CJ et al 1992 Resistance to cefotaxime and seven other β-lactams in members of the family Enterobacteriaceae: a 3-year survey in France. *Antimicrobial Agents and Chemotherapy* 36: 1677–1681

113. National Nosocomial Infections Surveillance System 2000 National Nosocomial Infections Surveillance (NNIS) System report, data summary from January 1992 – April 2000, issued June 2000. *American Journal of Infection Control* 28: 429–448

114. Warren DK, Fraser VJ 2001 Infection control measures to limit antimicrobial resistance. *Critical Care Medicine* 29: N128–N134

115. Pittet D, Herwaldt LA, Massanari RM 1992 The intensive care unit. In: Bennett JV, Brachman PS (eds) *Hospital infections*, 3rd edn. Little, Brown and Co., Boston, pp. 405–439

116. Pittet D 1993 Nosocomial bloodstream infections. In: Wenzel RP (ed.) *Prevention and control of nosocomial infections*, 2nd edn. Williams & Wilkins, Baltimore, pp. 512–555

117. Duckworth G 1990 Revised guidelines for the control of epidemic methicillin-resistant *Staphylococcus aureus*. *Journal of Hospital Infection* 16: 351–377

118. Watanakunakorn C, Patel R 1993 Comparison of patients with enterococcal bacteremia due to strains with and without high-level resistance to gentamicin. *Clinical Infectious Diseases* 17: 74–78

119. Graninger W, Ragette R 1992 Nosocomial bacteraemia due to *Enterococcus faecalis* without endocarditis. *Clinical Infectious Diseases* 15: 49–57

120. Hospital Infection Control Practices Advisory Committee 1995 Recommendations for preventing the spread of vancomycin resistance. *Infection Control and Hospital Epidemiology* 16: 105–113

121. Brun-Buisson C, Legrand P, Philippon A, Montravers F, Ansquer M, Duval J 1987 Transferable enzymatic resistance to third-generation cephalosporins during nosocomial outbreak of multi-resistant *Klebsiella pneumoniae*. *Lancet* ii: 302–306

122. Livermore DM 1991 Mechanisms of resistance to β-lactam antibiotics. *Scandinavian Journal of Infectious Diseases* (Suppl. 78): 7–16

123. Snydman DR 1991 Clinical implications of multi-drug resistance in the intensive care unit. *Scandinavian Journal of Infectious Diseases* (Suppl. 78): 54–63

124. Meyer KS, Urban C, Eagan JA, Berger BJ, Rahal JJ 1993 Nosocomial outbreak of *Klebsiella* infection resistant to late-generation cephalosporins. *Annals of Internal Medicine* 119: 353–358

125. Hartstein AI, Rashad AL, Liebler JM et al 1988 Multiple intensive care unit outbreak of *Acinetobacter calcoaceticus* subspecies *anitratus* respiratory infection and colonization associated with contaminated, reusable ventilator circuits and resuscitation bags. *American Journal of Medicine* 85: 624–631

126. Neu HC 1993 Antimicrobial agents: role in the prevention and control of nosocomial infections. In: Wenzel RP (ed.) *Prevention and control of nosocomial infections*, 2nd edn. Williams & Wilkins, Baltimore, pp. 406–419

127. Moine P, Vercken JB, Chevret S, Gajdos P and The French Study Group of Community-Acquired Pneumonia in ICU 1995 Severe community-acquired pneumococcal pneumonia. *Scandinavian Journal of Infectious Diseases* 27: 201–206

128. Leroy O, Santre C, Beuscart C et al 1995 A five-year study of severe community-acquired pneumonia with emphasis on prognosis in patients admitted to an intensive care unit. *Intensive Care Medicine* 21: 24–31

129. Oleacha PM, Quintana JM, Gallardo MS, Insausti J, Maravi E, Alvarez B 1996 A predictive model for the treatment approach to community-acquired pneumonia in patients needing ICU admission. *Intensive Care Medicine* 22: 1294–1300

45 Infections associated with implanted medical devices

Christopher J. Crnich, Nasia Safdar and Dennis G. Maki

This chapter provides an overview of the risk of infection associated with the use of the most important implanted medical devices (*see* Table 45.1), their clinical features, pathogenesis, epidemiology, diagnosis and treatment and, perhaps most importantly, strategies for their prevention.

GENERAL ASPECTS OF PATHOGENESIS

Implantation of prosthetic material evokes a host response, which intrinsically increases the risk of infection. Animal models have shown that the inoculum needed to establish infection is greatly reduced in the presence of a foreign body.[1] The characteristics of the implanted device and the material from which it is manufactured, the likelihood that the device might be exposed to micro-organisms, the intrinsic virulence of the involving organisms and the capacity of the host to resist infection all contribute to the overall risk of device related infection.

'Biomaterial' is a generic term for the material from which a medical device, manufactured for the distinct purpose of implantation in the human body, is constructed. Most devices are constructed of hydrocarbon polymers, which can now be engineered with predictable mechanical properties. Biomaterial in contact with deep tissues can have one or more physiologic effects:[2]

- the biomaterial releases chemicals toxic to contiguous tissue;
- the biomaterial is non-toxic, but unable to resist the inflammatory response its presence elicits, and the material is absorbed over time (e.g. chromic gut sutures);
- the biomaterial is non-toxic and unaffected by the inflammatory response, avoiding absorption by the body, but elicits chronic inflammation, resulting in encapsulation of the device (e.g. hip arthroplasty) or local thrombosis (e.g. vascular catheters);[3,4]
- the biomaterial is both non-toxic and biocompatible, and well tolerated by tissue, resulting in adhesive bonds that

stabilize the device and attenuate the inflammatory reaction (e.g. bioactive glass-ceramics and bioactive composites[5]).

Almost all implanted medical devices in use today fall into the third category. Development of a biologically totally inert material that does not induce a host response and is non-thrombogenic remains the 'holy grail' of biomaterials research.

The ensuing host–foreign body reaction plays an integral role in promotion of implant infection by distorting the local immune response and coating ('processing') of the surface by matrix proteins.[6] Animal models show striking derangement of the immune response in the peri-implant environment, most notably in phagocytosis.[1,7] Neutrophils recovered from the surface of foreign bodies show greatly reduced levels of granule-associated bactericidal enzymes and oxidative burst-dependent bactericidal activity.[1,7,8]

The presence of a foreign body not only perturbs local immune dysfunction but also provides an altered surface to which bacteria can more readily adhere and form a complex microenvironment, or biofilm. While non-specific physio-chemical forces, such as surface tension, electrostatic forces, hydrophobic interactions and van der Waal's forces mediate the initial microbial adherence to a foreign body,[9] durable adherence is also influenced by specific host–protein–microbial interactions.

After placement, vascular catheters are rapidly coated by host proteins, including albumin, fibrinogen, fibrin, fibronectin and platelets;[10–12] a similar process probably occurs with other implanted devices. Studies with *Staphylococcus aureus* have identified specific microbial fibronectin-[13–16] and fibrinogen-binding surface proteins,[15,17,18] and other proteins with broader specificity that can bind fibronectin as well as fibrinogen, vitronectin, thrombospondin and bone sialoprotein.[19,20] Direct support for the importance of these bacterial surface proteins comes from both in-vitro and animal models:[21,22] knockout strains of *Staph. aureus* that are deficient in fibronectin-binding surface proteins show a markedly reduced capacity to bind to polymethylmethacrylate (PMMA) coated slides in vitro[22] or to traumatized heart valves in a rat model.[21] Moreover, strains of

Staph. aureus deficient in the gene for production of the fibrinogen-binding surface protein lack the ability to adhere to PMMA-coated slides that are covered with fibrinogen.[18] The capacity to adhere is regained when the gene is restored to the knockout strain.

Coagulase-negative staphylococci also have the ability to bind fibronectin, although with less avidity than *Staph. aureus*.[15,16] In contrast, fibrinogen does not appear to be a major receptor for binding of coagulase-negative staphylococci to implant surfaces,[16] although other surface binding proteins unique to this micro-organisms have been reported.[23] A polysaccharide capsular adhesin that mediates the attachment to uncoated polysterene catheters has been identified, and antibodies to this epitope have been shown to inhibit binding to silicone catheters and prevent catheter-related infection in a rabbit model.[24]

Once bound to an implanted device, most micro-organisms that cause device-related infection are able to produce an extracellular polysaccharide matrix.[25] The combination of host proteins in intimate association with microcolonies of the infecting organism, embedded in massive quantities of exoglycocalyx, comprises a unique microecosystem, the biofilm.[26,27] Biofilms can be found almost universally on infected implanted materials of all types,[26] and have been best characterized with:

- Gram-positive bacteria, especially *Staph. aureus*,[28] *Staphylococcus epidermidis*,[29] and *Enterococcus faecalis*;[30]
- Gram-negative bacilli, such as *Escherichia coli*,[31] *Pseudomonas aeruginosa*[26] and *Burkholderia cepacia*;[32]
- yeasts, such as *Candida albicans*.[33]

Organisms within a biofilm are uniquely adapted to extreme environments and form a nidus of chronic infection on the surface of the implanted device from which planktonic phase organisms are released, producing signs and symptoms of infection.

Biofilms greatly facilitate surface adherence, protect the micro-organism and allow its survival, even under intense attack from the immune system and high concentrations of antimicrobial drugs. Several mechanisms appear to be responsible.

1. Micro-organisms encased in a biofilm are resistant to phagocytosis,[34] and there is evidence that antimicrobial oxidants produced by phagocytic cells are inactivated in the superficial layers of a biofilm.[26]
2. Antimicrobial drugs penetrate biofilms poorly[35,36] and lose activity in the acidic and anaerobic environment of the deepest layers of a biofilm.[27]
3. Micro-organisms in a biofilm are in a sessile, or slow-growing phase of growth that further enhances resistance to antimicrobials, most of which are most effective against rapidly multiplying organisms.[37]
4. Micro-organisms in a biofilm exhibit unique phenotypic features,[27] expressing genes that are not expressed in the plank-tonic, rapidly growing phase encountered in infections unrelated to implanted devices.

The extraordinary capacity of the biofilm to produce refractory infection can be seen in in-vitro experiments: studies have shown that concentrations of a bactericidal antibiotic 100 to 1000 times those effective against the planktonic phase of the organism (the minimal inhibitory concentration or MIC) do not kill the micro-organisms within a biofilm.[38] Thus, while antimicrobial therapy is often effective in resolving the acute features of device-associated infection, such as local inflammation and fever, antimicrobial therapy alone rarely kills the indolent sessile organisms within the deepest layers of an implant-associated biofilm. For these reasons, the management of most implanted device-related infections requires removal of the infected device as well as appropriate antimicrobial therapy.

INFECTIONS ASSOCIATED WITH ORTHOPEDIC DEVICES

EPIDEMIOLOGY

Over seven million orthopedic procedures were performed in the USA in 1996, including 500 000 total knee arthroplasties and total hip arthroplasties.[39] The site of prosthetic joint implantation, characteristics of the implant, and events surrounding the operation have a profound impact on the risk of infection.

Rates of deep infection after total hip arthroplasty range from *c.* 0.5 to 1.5% at most centers;[40,41] rates of infection with total knee arthroplasty appear to be somewhat higher, in the range of 0.8–2.5% (Table 45.1).[41–43] The risk of infection appears to be highest in the first 2–3 years after surgery: combined rates of hip and knee prosthetic infection are 6.5 per 1000 joint years in the first year after surgery, 3.2 per 1000 during the second postoperative year and 1.4 per 1000 in the total years thereafter.[44] Rates of infection with other prosthetic joint implants have been less well characterized but average 1% for shoulders,[45] 2.4–6.0% for ankles and wrists[46,47] and as high as 7–9% for elbows.[46]

The characteristics of the artificial joint clearly influence the risk of infection. Use of metal-on-metal hinged knee prostheses have been shown to be associated with a risk of infection 20 times higher than encountered with the modular metal-on-polyethylene prosthetic joints most widely used today.[48] Host factors associated with an increased risk of postoperative infection of the prosthesis include rheumatoid arthritis,[41,48–50] diabetes mellitus,[51] malignancy,[52] concurrent corticosteroid use,[53] hemophilia[54] and revision arthroplasty. Other factors that may increase the risk of infection, such as obesity[55] and active urinary tract infection at the time of surgery, have been less rigorously evaluated.

Table 45.1 Risk of infection with the implanted medical devices in widest clinical use

Device	Approximate risk of infection over the lifetime of the device (%)
Orthopedic devices	
Total joint prostheses	
Hip	0.5–1.5
Knee	0.8–2.5
Elbow, ankle, and wrist	1–9
Cardiovascular devices	
Prosthetic heart valves	
Mechanical	~5
Bioprosthetic	~6
Coronary stents	<0.01
Pacemakers and implantable cardiac defibrillators	1–7
Left ventricular assist devices	15–70
Implanted artificial heart	Unknown
Intravascular devices	
Short-term vascular catheters	
Peripheral venous catheters and needles	0.2–0.4
Arterial catheters	1–2
Central venous catheters	3–4
Temporary hemodialysis catheters	13–18
Long-term devices	
Cuffed and tunneled central venous (Hickman and Broviac) catheters	18–22
Peripheral inserted central catheters	0.5–2
Subcutaneous central ports	4–6
Tunneled and cuffed hemodialysis catheters	4–9
Vascular Gore-tex and Dacron arterial grafts	1–5
Neurosurgical devices	
Ventriculoperitoneal, ventriculoatrial and lumboperitoneal shunts	2–9
Ventriculostomy catheters	~10
Intra-arterial coils	<0.01
Urological/renal devices	
Urethral catheters	10–50
Ureteral stents	~7
Peritoneal dialysis catheters	20–50
Penile implants	1–3
Miscellaneous	
Breast implants	~3
Intra-abdominal mesh	2–8

PATHOGENESIS

Several staging systems have been proposed for prosthetic joint sepsis but consensus is lacking. The most widely accepted system is that formulated originally by Coventry[56] and modified by Gillespie.[57]

Stage 1 infections are defined as those occurring within 1 month of surgery; patients with stage 1 infections typically present with signs of sepsis as well as local signs of infection, with local erythema and wound discharge. The organisms most commonly recovered from stage 1 infections derive from the patient's skin, bacteria in operating room air, or the skin of members of the surgical team.[58,59]

Stage 2 infections are defined as those that occur after 1 month but within 2 years of surgery. These infections are also thought to derive from the introduction of organisms of low pathogenicity, such as coagulase-negative staphylococci and *Propionibacterium* sp., at the time of surgery. Patients typically exhibit gradual impairment of prosthetic function, (i.e. early loosening of the prosthesis and increasing joint pain).

Stage 3 infections are arbitrarily defined as infections that occur more than 2 years after surgery and are assumed to derive from hematogenous seeding of the joint.

There are limitations with the above classification. The Coventry system fails to take into account the possibility of hematogenous seeding of the newly placed joint that might occur from intravascular device-related bloodstream infections as well as from intercurrent urinary tract or other remote infections.[60–62] Furthermore, the capacity of certain micro-organisms, such as coagulase-negative staphylococci to be present in the joint for prolonged periods before manifesting signs of overt infection is well known,[63] and an arbitrary cutoff of 2 years to define local versus hematogenous infection fails to take this into account. Nevertheless, most stage 3 infections behave differently than stage 2 infections in that patients typically have completely normal joint function then abruptly develop acute pain and inflammation of the joint, in contrast to the gradual decline in function seen with most stage 2 infections.

While definitively identifying the source of a prosthetic joint infection may be difficult, several lines of evidence suggest that the vast majority derive from contamination of the wound at the time of surgery.

1. The risk of prosthetic joint infection is highest in the perioperative period.[44]
2. Most late infections are caused by *Staph. aureus* and coagulase-negative staphylococci,[44] which are acquired from skin of the patient or members of the operating team at the time of surgery.
3. Operating theaters that provide ultrafiltered air, to reduce airborne microbial counts to <5 colony forming units (cfu)/m^3, have 10–60% lower rates of infection than operating rooms that do not employ such systems.[64,65]
4. Studies of perioperative antibiotic prophylaxis have shown a 64–85% reduction in rates of prosthetic joint infection,[57,63,64,66] with the benefit of prophylaxis becoming ever greater the longer the period after surgery.[63]
5. Studies that have rigorously attempted to identify the source

of prosthetic joint infections have found that hematogenous seeding appears to account for only 7–11% of all cases.[67–69]

MICROBIOLOGY

Staph. aureus and coagulase-negative staphylococci predominate in prosthetic joint infections (Figure 45.1); infections with other Gram-positive organisms, such as streptococci and enterococci, are less common.[44] Infections caused by aerobic Gram-negative bacilli usually occur in association with Gram-positive organisms (mixed infections),[44] and in this situation probably reflect gross intraoperative contamination of the surgical wound or, perhaps, postoperative invasion of micro-organisms through surgical drains. Hematogenous seeding is more likely when organisms are isolated in pure culture, although direct inoculation is still possible. The microbial profile of prosthetic joint infections has been remarkably stable over time,[44] which suggests that the pathogenesis of infection in both early and late infection is similar (i.e. most originate in the operating theater, even most late-onset infections).

DIAGNOSIS

Patients with early postoperative prosthetic joint infection usually show impressive signs and symptoms of joint inflammation: severe pain and limited range of motion, usually in association with erythema of the surgical wound, with or without discharge. Signs of systemic sepsis, with fever, tachycardia and even shock, may be present, depending on the virulence of the infecting organism(s) (e.g. *Staph. aureus* or Gram-negative bacilli). Patients with late hematogenous infection often show a similarly fulminant course complicating recent skin or respiratory tract infection, or dental manipulation. This

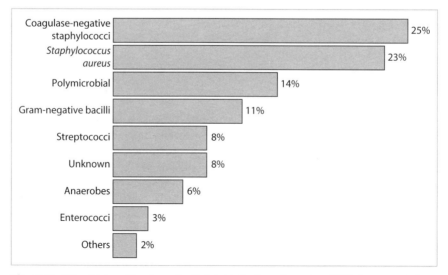

Fig. 45.1 Microbial profile of prosthetic joint infections, based on 1033 documented cases seen at the Mayo Clinic from 1969 to 1991.[549]

pattern was highlighted in a recent report where 16 of 59 patients with orthopedic devices and documented nosocomial *Staph. aureus* bacteremia developed prosthetic device infection 0–65 days (median 3 days) after the onset of bacteremia.[70]

Patients with stage 2 infections often follow an indolent course, characterized by increasing pain and slowly deteriorating joint function that may or may not be associated with loosening of the prosthesis radiographically. Most are afebrile. No single test or clinical finding is pathognomonic of infection, thus it is necessary to interpret the results of multiple tests and, especially, to obtain joint aspirates or deep operative cultures off antibiotics.

Routine laboratory studies usually, but not always, show leukocytosis.[71] The erythrocyte sedimentation rate (ESR) is elevated in most cases but is a non-specific finding, with a sensitivity ranging from 54 to 82% and specificity 65–85%.[71–73] C-reactive protein (CRP) appears to be a better dagnostic test, with reported sensitivities of 80–96% and specificities ranging from 93 to 100%, respectively.[73,74] CRP is particularly useful in the early postoperative period as the level should normalize within 2–3 weeks after surgery;[75–77] persistent elevation should prompt suspicion of indolent infection. Finally, the combined use of the ESR and CRP, when both are normal, virtually rules out prosthetic joint infection.[74]

Plain radiographs are usually normal in early postoperative and hematogenously derived infections. Loosening of the joint prosthesis may be seen with chronic infection but this finding is not specific.[78] Periosteal reaction or scalloping of the bone is more specific for infection but is often absent in chronic infections,[78,79] especially those caused by coagulase-negative staphylococci. Ultrasound may be useful for identifying hematomas in the early postoperative period as well as guiding needle aspiration of a joint suspicious for infection.

Numerous studies have evaluated nuclear imaging modalities for the diagnosis of prosthetic joint infection. Unfortunately, most studies were limited by bias introduced through patient selection, lack of randomization, the use of multiple sequential scans,[80] and, especially, lack of a rigorous definition infection. Published studies have reported sensitivities of 38–68% for technetium/gallium radionuclear scanning,[81–83] 72–83% for technetium/indium [111]-labelled granulocyte scanning,[81,84] and 64–100% for indium [111]-labeled IgG scanning.[84–86] Specificity is not much better, ranging from 40 to 100% for the above three tests.[81–86]

Microbiologic confirmation of infection remains the gold standard for the diagnosis of prosthetic joint infection and should always be sought. Blood cultures are positive in only 20% of prosthetic joint infections and are rarely positive in the absence of systemic signs of sepsis. Superficial swabs of surgical wounds or draining sinuses are unreliable for identifying the specific organism(s) infecting the prosthetic joint.[87] The failure of non-invasive tests to be able to reliably confirm the presence of infection requires imaging guided aspiration of the suspect joint or intraoperative sampling. The sensitivity of preoperative joint aspiration is >80% (range 50–100%)[73,83,88,89] and recovery of an organism usually is indicative of infection

(specificity, 92 to 100%).[73,83,88,89] Concurrent antimicrobial therapy clearly reduces the yield of joint aspiration culture and its use should be deferred until all appropriate microbiological studies have been completed.

Intraoperative Gram stain has been advocated by some as a method for rapidly identifying or ruling out the presence of prosthetic joint infection. Unfortunately, the Gram stain is positive in less than one-third of prosthetic joint infections and is almost certainly less accurate with intercurrent antibiotic therapy.[73,83,90,91] Intraoperative cultures have the highest yield, provided that antibiotic therapy is withheld until immediately after obtaining specimens for culture. Tissue samples, rather than swabs, are preferable and obtaining multiple samples (three or more) improves the specificity.[90] Sampling from the sonicated removed implant may further increase yield by the release of biofilm organisms.[92] It is imperative that multiple samples be inoculated on solid media in the microbiology lab rather than cultured solely in liquid media: multiple colonies growing on solid media almost always represent true infection, whereas microbial growth only in broth is most often indicative of contamination.

TREATMENT

Management of a patient with confirmed prosthetic joint infection requires careful consideration of the stage of the infection (early postoperative, chronic or acute hematogenous infection), the characteristics of the infecting organism, the patient's co-morbidities and life expectancy.

Surgical management

Historically, infection of a prosthetic joint has been most effectively managed with two-stage exchange arthroplasty:[93–95] surgical debridement with removal of the infected prosthetic device and all cement, followed by a prolonged period of parenteral antimicrobial therapy—6–12 weeks or longer—during which time the joint is immobilized, increasingly with the use of an antibiotic-impregnated spacer;[96,97] when all clinical signs of infection have resolved and, ideally, the ESR and CRP have normalized, a new prosthetic device is implanted, often with the use of antibiotic-impregnated cement[98] or a cementless prosthesis.[99] Multiple intraoperative specimens are cultured and if persistent infection is found parenteral antibiotic therapy is continued postoperatively, guided by resolution of the clinical features of infection and laboratory measures of inflammation (ESR and CRP). With this approach, long-term eradication of a prosthetic joint infection can be achieved in 87–96% of infected total hip arthroplasties[100–103] and in 83–96% of infected total knee arthroplasties.[96,97,102,104]

Obviously, this approach is costly, both for the healthcare system and the patient, who must endure prolonged immobilization, deconditioning and not one but two major operations. This has led to three alternative approaches to management: initial irrigation and debridement with retention of the prosthetic device, followed by prolonged antimicrobial therapy; one-stage exchange arthroplasty followed by antimicrobial therapy; and the use of indefinite antimicrobial suppression.

Irrigation and debridement with retention of the prosthetic device has been best evaluated with early postoperative infections and has shown encouraging results.[105,106] In contrast, attempts to salvage the prosthesis in patients who have late infections or evidence of ongoing infection for more than 5 days have shown failure rates ranging from 62% to 86%.[104,107–110] Debridement with retention of the prosthesis may achieve rates of success of about 70% in carefully selected patients who are in the early postoperative period (< one month):[107,111–113] (1) patients must have a hyperacute presentation (< 2–5 days),[105,108,110] as shown in one study where the failure with debridement and retention greatly increased if symptoms of infection had been present for more than two days (RR = 4.2, 95% confidence interval = 1.6–10.3);[108] (2) the prosthesis must be stable without radiologic evidence of loosening; (3) the patient must be willing to comply with prolonged antimicrobial therapy for 3–6 months or longer; and (4) most importantly, the infecting micro-organism must be highly susceptible to both parenteral and oral antibiotics, such as α-hemolytic or group A streptococci.

Published studies of one-step exchange arthroplasty have reported success rates that exceed 80%,[114–118] which approaches the rate seen with the traditional two-step exchange arthroplasty. However, almost all of the published experiences are case series of highly selected patients (i.e. prosthetic infections caused by Gram-negative bacilli or methicillin-resistant *Staph. aureus* (MRSA) were excluded). Notably, Hanssen et al found that only 11% of patients presenting with prosthetic joint infection at their institution met criteria for one-step exchange arthroplasty.[119] Moreover, a study of 118 unselected infected total knee arthroplasties found that one-step exchange arthroplasty was successful in only 63% of cases,[120] and a retrospective analysis from the UK revealed that the rate of recurrent infection after one-stage exchange was three times higher than two stage exchange arthroplasty.[121] The lack of randomized trials, the lack of proven benefit with resistant Gram-positive and Gram-negative infections, and concerns over the emergence of resistance with the use of antimicrobial-impregnated cement during refractory infection[116] limit the utility of this surgical approach.

Despite its proven benefit in the treatment of late prosthetic joint infection, there are situations where exchange arthroplasty is not feasible and where the quality of life associated with prolonged immobilization is unacceptable to the patient. In these situations, debridement with retention of the infected prosthesis, followed by indefinite suppressive antibimicrobial therapy, has been proposed.[122,123] In contrast to prosthesis retention in the early postoperative period, the goal of therapy in this situation is not cure but rather indefinite suppression of infection. Segreti et al reported the utility of this approach in 18 patients with both early and late prosthetic joint infections;[123] eight were infected with *Staph. aureus*, two with MRSA, and seven with coagulase-negative staphylococci.

Eleven of the 18 patients (61%) remained successfully suppressed at the end of the study period (median 49 months); seven discontinued antibiotic therapy, three because of breakthrough infection and four chose voluntarily to stop – relapse of infection occurred in only one of the four. Other studies have met with lesser rates of success, ranging from 23 to 63%.[122,124]

Antimicrobial therapy

Staphylococci are the most common infecting organisms and treatment of these infections is often most challenging. For strains susceptible to methicillin, nafcillin (oxacillin or flucloxacillin) is the agent of choice; for patients with well-documented allergy to penicillin, vancomycin or clindamycin is recommended. For staphylococci resistant to methicillin vancomycin is always the drug of choice and should be combined with rifampicin (rifampin).

Animal models have demonstrated the beneficial impact of rifampicin-containing antimicrobial regimens in implant-associated infections.[125,126] Growing clinical data confirm these findings;[105,127] a randomized study conducted by Zimmerli et al found that administration of a rifampicin-containing regimen to patients with prosthetic joint infections, who underwent irrigation and debridement with retention of their prosthesis, resulted in long-term cure in all of the 12 patients who completed at least 3–6 months of therapy.[105] Unless the infecting organism demonstrates in-vitro resistance or the patient has known allergy to rifampicin, based on these data we believe rifampicin should be routinely included in the regimen for all staphylococcal prosthetic joint infections, especially if vancomycin is used.

Newer fluoroquinolones (other than ciprofloxacin), such as levofloxacin and gatifloxacin, exhibit excellent in-vitro activity against staphylococci (although they are often inactive against MRSA), are highly bioavailable orally, and attain high joint fluid concentrations in experimental animal models of staphylococcal prosthetic joint infection.[128] Moreover, clinical trials of oral therapy in chronic osteomyelitis have demonstrated their equivalency to parenteral regimens,[129,130] although the studies were underpowered. Fluoroquinolone-containing regimens for treatment of staphylococcal prosthetic joint infection have shown benefit in a limited number of clinical studies.[105,127] However, in our opinion the role of fluoroquinolones in the initial antimicrobial regimen for treatment of prosthetic joint infections caused by staphylococci remains undefined. Rather, their utility at this time appears to be in the consolidation phase of therapy, after a patient has completed a prescribed period of intravenous nafcillin (oxacillin or flucloxacillin) or vancomycin in conjunction with rifampicin; or for the patient where chronic suppression, rather than cure is the goal. In-vitro confirmation of susceptibility is necessary before their use can be considered, and any fluoroquinolone-containing regimen should also include another effective antimicrobial, usually rifampicin, as at least one prospective study has described the emergence of fluoroquinolone resistance during prolonged monotherapy.[105]

For prosthetic joint infections caused by Gram-negative bacilli, the initial regimen must be guided by the in-vitro susceptibilities of the infecting organism. In general, a fluoroquinolone with excellent Gram-negative activity – such as ciprofloxacin – or a carbapenem (such as imipenem or meropenem) are most likely to be effective. For *Ps. aeruginosa* infections, two antipseudomonal drugs of different classes, such as ciprofloxacin and cefepime (or ceftazidime), are recommended. Aminoglycosides, which achieve bone and joint levels similar to the β-lactams, are associated with a high risk of toxicity with long-term use, and their use in prosthetic joint infections is generally discouraged.[131]

Rare fungal prosthetic joint infections are best treated with amphotericin B, with consideration for one of the lipid-based formulations (e.g., amphotericin B lipid complex or liposomal amphotericin B), which exhibit better marrow penetration than the standard formulation and are associated with greatly reduced toxicity.[132] In general, azoles, such as fluconazole, are not as effective in bone and joint infections.[133,134]

PREVENTION

Interventions to reduce the number of micro-organisms in operating room air were among the first novel approaches to reduce rates of postoperative prosthetic joint infection.[49,58,64,135] Modern ventilation systems that utilize ultrafiltration and directional airflow can reduce concentrations of airborne micro-organisms from 10^4 cfu/m^3 to less than 5 cfu/m^3.[65] Despite wide use of ultrafiltration by hospitals in the early 1980s, convincing evidence of its benefit was lacking.[49] A European multi-center trial, published in 1982, showed unequivocally that providing ultrafiltered air in operating rooms was beneficial: rates of prosthetic joint infection were reduced 55% (RR = 0.45, 95% CI = 0.21–0.93).[64] Unfortunately, the study did not strictly control for perioperative antibiotic prophylaxis, although ultrafiltered air and antimicrobial prophylaxis appeared to be synergistic in a post-hoc analysis; prosthetic joint infection occurred in 1.2% of patients randomized to ultrafiltered air alone (compared with a rate of 3.4% in the control group), while only 0.3% of patients randomized to ultrafiltered air but also receiving antibiotic prophylaxis developed infection (4.2% in the control group).[64] A later trial enrolled over 6000 patients, all of whom received antibiotic prophylaxis, and showed that ultraclean operating room air reduced rates of prosthetic joint infections by 10% but this result did not reach statistical significance (RR 0.90; 95% CI 0.36–2.3).[135] These studies confirm the benefit of both ultraclean air and perioperative antibiotic prophylaxis in total joint arthroplasty and show that if antimicrobial prophylaxis is used the impact of ultrafiltered air is minimal; however, if antibiotic prophylaxis is not employed, ultraclean air assumes a much greater role in the prevention of infection.

The use of ultraviolet light to sterilize operating room air has also been shown to be effective and compares favorably to ultraclean air systems.[136] The use of impermeable clothing and ventilation suits can reduce operating counts of airborne micro-organisms even further;[137] however, their utility in reducing rates of infection remains unproven, and their cost-effectiveness is questionable.

The simplest and perhaps most important advance for the prevention of prosthetic joint infection has been the adoption of routine perioperative antimicrobial prophylaxis, in which the first dose is always given immediately before the incision. Pooled analysis of four randomized placebo-controlled trials of antibiotic prophylaxis in prosthetic joint surgery demonstrates a 76% reduction in infection (odds ratio, 0.24; 95% CI, 0.15–0.37).[57] The classic study by Hill et al[63] shows that the cumulative benefit of prophylaxis increases the further out the patient is from surgery; 99.5%, 99.3% and 99% of patients randomized to antibiotic prophylaxis remained free of prosthetic joint infection at 12, 24 and 36 months, respectively, compared with 97.5%, 97%, and 96% in the control group during the same periods. The duration of perioperative prophylaxis in these trials ranged from 24 h to 2 weeks; subsequent studies of antibiotic prophylaxis in orthopedic and other types of surgery have shown unequivocally that no added benefit is gained by extending prophylaxis beyond 24 h.[138,139]

Giving prophylactic antibiotics by other routes, such as incorporation into the PMMA cement, has been examined in several studies. A randomized trial in 1688 primary total hip arthroplasties demonstrated that the use of antibiotic-impregnated cement was equivalent to systemic antibiotic therapy alone; 13 late infections occurred in the systemic antibiotic prophylaxis group and nine in the antibiotic-impregnated cement group.[140] An analysis of 10 905 cemented primary hip arthroplasties in the Norwegian Arthroplasty Register suggests that combined use of systemic prophylactic antibiotics and antibiotic-impregnated cement is associated with a lower rate of infection than either intervention alone (5-year incidence of infection 0.2% in the combined prophylaxis group vs. 0.8% with systemic prophylaxis alone, $P = 0.001$),[141] however, a randomized trial comparing systemic prophylactic antibiotics alone with combined systemic antibiotic/antibiotic impregnated cement regimens is lacking.

The use of late antibiotic prophylaxis after successful joint implantation to prevent hematogenous prosthetic joint infection, particularly with invasive dental procedures, is a routine practice of most orthopedic surgeons[142] but has come under scrutiny, given the very low rates of late hematogenous infection seen in large series (7–11% of all prosthetic joint infections[67–69]) and the absence of studies demonstrating efficacy or cost benefit.[66,143] Administration of a single dose of semisynthetic penicillin poses a risk of anaphylaxis of approximately 0.04%, of skin rash of 5% and of *Clostridium difficile* antibiotic-associated colitis of 0.01%.[65] A decision analysis study of antibiotic prophylaxis for dental procedures to prevent prosthetic joint infections concluded that US $480 000 would need to be spent to prevent a single case of late prosthetic joint infection and that adoption of routine penicillin prophylaxis would actually result in more deaths than not using prophylaxis because of adverse effects from the prophylactic drugs.[144] A retrospective study of 3490 patients with prosthetic joints found that only seven developed prosthetic joint infection temporally related to a dental procedure.[69] Five of these seven had underlying co-morbidity that predisposed them to infection, such as diabetes mellitus or rheumatoid arthritis. Based on these data, recent recommendations for the use of antibiotic prophylaxis in patients with prosthetic joints undergoing invasive procedures include patients with rheumatoid arthritis with a prosthesis implanted within the past year, an overt oral infection, a prolonged dental procedure (>115 minutes) and, possibly, diabetes mellitus or chronic corticosteroid therapy.[145]

INFECTIONS ASSOCIATED WITH PROSTHETIC HEART VALVES

EPIDEMIOLOGY

Of all complications seen with implanted devices used in modern medicine, infection of a prosthetic valve is perhaps the most feared. It is estimated that 60 000 prosthetic valve replacements are performed in the USA each year.[146] Prosthetic valve endocarditis (PVE) accounts for 10–20% of all cases of endocarditis,[147–149] and the 5-year risk of developing infection of a prosthetic valve after surgery has remained in the range of 3–6% since the 1960s.[150–154] The risk of PVE is highest within the first 2–3 months after surgery then falls to approximately 0.1–0.7% per patient-year thereafter.[150,152,154,155]

The risk of infection of mitral and aortic valves appears to be similar.[150–152,156] However, the risk of infection with mechanical and bioprosthetic valves differs with the proximity to surgery: mechanical prosthetic valves have a higher incidence of infection in the first 12 months after implantation[150,151] whereas the incidence of infection after 12 months is higher with bioprosthetic valves.[150,151] This results in an overall 5-year risk of infection that is similar for the two types of valves – 5.0% for mechanical and 6.3% for bioprosthetic valves.[150,151,156–158]

Outcome with PVE has improved greatly over the past two decades but mortality remains high and is estimated to range from 32 to 64%.[150,156,159–161] The highest mortality is seen with early PVE (≤60 days): 92 deaths occurred in a pooled analysis of 180 cases of early PVE (51%).[156,160,162–165] Mortality in late PVE (>60 days) is lower: 97 deaths occurred in the pooled analysis of 298 cases of late PVE (32%).[156,160–163]

PATHOGENESIS AND MICROBIAL ETIOLOGY

Infection of newly implanted mechanical and bioprosthetic valves may begin at the annular sewing line or on the valve itself. Early studies showed that mechanical valves are relatively resistant to infection of the prosthetic valvular component and that most infections begin at the interface between the endocardium of the annulus and the cloth sewing ring. In contrast, infection of bioprosthetic valves is more likely to begin on the valve structure itself. These observations are supported by older studies showing a much higher rate of perivalvular abscess with infection of mechanical valves.[150,166] More recent studies have failed to show such a difference.[151,167,168]

As with orthopedic devices, most prosthetic valve infections are thought to derive from contamination of the valve at the time of surgery or in the early postoperative period. Similar to the definitions for early and late infection with orthopedic devices, infection of a prosthetic valve is arbitrarily defined as early or late based on whether it manifests within 60 days or later or, as now promoted by Karchmer, within 12 months of surgery or later.[168] These arbitrary cutoffs are relevant pathophysiologically because the risk of infection and the organisms encountered in early and late PVE differ significantly (Table 45.2). Most infecting organisms within the first 12 months after surgery are common nosocomial pathogens, most notably *Staph. aureus* and coagulase-negative staphylococci (Table 45.2);[151] the coagulase-negative staphylococci recovered from PVE during the first year after surgery are far more likely to be resistant to methicillin than those recovered more than one year after surgery (87% versus 22%),[168] strongly suggesting that the former were acquired intraoperatively or in the immediate postoperative period. Furthermore, infections classically associated with native-valve endocarditis, such as streptococci and the 'HACEK' organisms are rarely (if ever) encountered in PVE until 12 months or longer after valve implantation (Table 45.2).

Although intraoperative contamination of the valve during surgery almost certainly accounts for most early postoperative prosthetic valve infections,[169,170] the contribution of hemato-

Table 45.2 Micro-organisms involved in early and late prosthetic valve endocarditis[a]

Organism	Early PVE[b] (≤ 12 months) (n = 262) No. (%)	Late PVE[b] (> 12 months) (n = 219) No. (%)
Coagulase-negative staphylococci	98 (37.4)	23 (10.5)
Staphylococcus aureus	49 (18.7)	41 (18.7)
Fungi	25 (9.5)	3 (1.4)
Gram-negative bacilli	24 (9.1)	11 (5.0)
Enterococci	23 (8.8)	25 (11.4)
Streptococci	12 (4.6)	74 (33.8)
Diphtheroids	10 (3.8)	5 (2.2)
HACEK[c]	0 (0)	11 (5.0)
Culture-negative	15 (5.7)	17 (7.8)
Miscellaneous	6 (2.3)	9 (4.1)

[a] Pooled data from eight studies of early and late prosthetic valve endocarditis.[151,161–165,172,547]
[b] PVE = Prosthetic valve endocarditis.
[c] HACEK: *Haemophilus parainfluenzae*, *Haemophilus aphrophilus*, *Actinobacillus actinomycetemcomitans*, *Cardiobacterium hominis*, *Eikenella corrodens*, and *Kingella kingae*.

genous seeding cannot be overlooked. Heavy use of invasive devices, especially intravascular and urinary catheters, in the early postoperative period and the risk of nosocomial bloodstream infection related to their use is very high (*see below*).[171,172] Studies suggest that 31–92% of cases of early postoperative PVE stem from another nosocomial infection.[166,168,172] A study by Fang et al further highlights the risk of PVE in the setting of nosocomial bacteremia: 24% and 10% of patients with a prosthetic valve exposed to nosocomial bloodstream infection with *Staph. aureus* or Gram-negative bacilli developed secondary PVE, respectively.[173]

The organisms causing PVE greatly influence the outcome. PVE with *Staph. aureus* and coagulase-negative staphylococci is associated with a mortality ranging from 28% to 100%[156,159–161,163,174–178] and, although data are limited, infections with aerobic Gram-negative bacilli and fungi appear to be associated with worse outcomes.[173,179] In contrast, mortality from PVE caused by streptococci appears to be much lower, ranging from 5% to 35%.[161,163,165]

PVE is not only associated with a higher mortality than that seen with native valve endocarditis but is also associated with a higher rate of complications.[151,166–168,180] Infection involving the suture line results in invasive infection of the annulus and underlying myocardium, with development of ring abscess, conduction abnormalities, and dehiscence of the prosthesis (with valvular incompetence). Moreover, the vegetations on a mechanical valve can interfere with normal closure, producing regurgitation or, alternatively, functional stenosis. Both complications are associated with a worse outcome and help define 'complicated PVE':

- a new or worsening murmur due to valve dysfunction;
- new or worsening congestive heart failure due to valvular dysfunction or abscess;
- new electrocardiographic conduction abnormalities; or
- an intracardiac abscess detected by echocardiogram, surgery, or autopsy.[159,168,178,181]

Each of these complications is regarded as a clear-cut indication for surgical replacement of the infected prosthetic valve.

DIAGNOSIS

The clinical presentation of PVE does not differ greatly from that seen with native valve endocarditis. Signs and symptoms include fever (>90%),[182] a new or changing murmur (40–70%),[182] congestive heart failure (30–100%),[182] petechiae (30–60%),[182] splenomegaly (15–40%),[182] embolic phenomenona, including strokes or transient ischemic attacks (5–40%),[182] shock (0–30%),[182] and conduction abnormalities (5–20%).[182] Osler's nodes, Janeway lesions and Roth's spots are relatively infrequent (5–15%).[182] The likelihood that a patient will present with one or more clinical signs or symptoms is influenced in greatest measure by the virulence of the infecting organism. For example, in recent studies, PVE caused by *Staph. aureus* was associated with a necrologic event in

25–67% of cases, septic shock in 30% of cases and an overall mortality of 33–75%.[161,163,178]

Leukocytosis, anemia and elevations in the ESR and CRP are common in PVE but are non specific, especially in the early postoperative period.[182] Isolation of a micro-organism from blood cultures is usually the first and best clue to PVE, and obtaining at least two – preferably three – blood cultures before beginning empiric antimicrobial therapy, is mandatory when evaluating unexplained fever in a patient with a prosthetic heart valve. If at least 20–30 ml of blood is obtained from each of three separate venepuncture sites, 99% of detectable bacteremias should be identified *if* the patient has not received recent antimicrobial therapy.[183,184] In rare situations where blood cultures remain negative despite strong clinical suspicion of PVE, the use of special cultures or serologic tests to detect fastidious organisms, such as the 'HACEK' species, *Legionella* spp., rapid growing mycobacteria, *Coxiella burnetii*, *Mycoplasma hominis* and fungi other than *Candida*, should be employed.[185] The presence of a sustained, high-grade bacteremia or fungemia strongly suggests PVE and must prompt further evaluation of the prosthetic valve.[186,187]

The availability of transesophageal echocardiography (TEE) has greatly improved the capacity of clinicians to make a definitive diagnosis of PVE. For a variety of reasons, but most importantly because of the distance between the transducer and the heart, transthoracic echocardiography (TTE) can detect only the largest vegetations on a prosthetic valve in any location (>10 mm):[188] compared with sensitivity of 17–40% for TTE[189–191] the sensitivity of TEE for the diagnosis of PVE ranges from 77 to 100%.[165,189,191] Moreover, TEE is greatly superior to TTE for detection of perivalvular abscess (up to 100% for TEE, 0–40% for TTE)[192,193] and valvular dysfunction (86% for TEE, 43% for TTE). TEE visualizes the mitral valve extremely well but may have difficulty visualizing the entire aortic valve as well as portions of the left ventricular outflow track, and thus an approach that utilizes both TEE and TTE is recommended.[194]

The combination of clinical signs and symptoms, the results of blood cultures and echocardiography has been used to formulate criteria for the diagnosis of native valve endocarditis.[195] Application of the Duke criteria to PVE has been evaluated in several studies;[161,165,178] in confirmed cases of PVE, Duke criteria for definite PVE were met in 76–79% and criteria for possible PVE in an additional 20–24% cases.[161,165] Perez-Vasquez et al have recommended amending these criteria for the diagnosis of PVE, adding heart failure and conduction disturbances to the minor criteria;[165] adding these two additional criteria increased the percentage of definite cases of PVE from 79 to 90%, although the effect on specificity was not addressed.

TREATMENT

The best management of patients with PVE often requires a combined medical and surgical approach. A careful analysis of the nature of the infection and the infecting micro-organism is imperative to determine the best approach. Unfortunately, even when armed with this information, many aspects of the care of the patient with PVE remain unclear. For example, the findings that mandate surgical intervention and the timing of that intervention are still areas of dispute. Moreover, whether to continue or discontinue anticoagulation in a patient with an infected mechanical PVE is also unclear.

Antimicrobial therapy

Antimicrobial therapy must always be withheld until appropriate cultures can be obtained. The decision to then begin empiric antimicrobial therapy, before the results of cultures are available, is influenced by the perceived clinical urgency. With patients who are hemodynamically stable and without signs of complicated PVE, antimicrobial therapy can generally be safely withheld until bloodstream infection is confirmed.

With the patient who warrants immediate therapy because of fulminant sepsis or signs of dehiscence or other complications, therapy should be based on whether he or she has early PVE (<12 months after surgery) or late PVE (>12 months after surgery) and whether there is infection at a distant focus, such as urosepsis, surgical site infection, or an infected intravascular device, that points to a specific organism. Empiric therapy of patients with PVE should include vancomycin and gentamicin to cover resistant staphylococci, especially MRSA, enterococci and enteric Gram-negative bacilli. Antipseudomonal drugs may be indicated for early PVE in certain clinical settings, such as ventilator-associated pneumonia with suspected PVE. It is important to recognize that whereas the use of either vancomycin or gentamicin alone has a low risk of nephrotoxicity or ototoxicity (1–2%), when these drugs are used in combination for longer than 3–5 days, especially in elderly patients, the risk of toxicity rises sharply, to 25% or higher.[196] Most importantly, the definitive regimen must be based on the identification and susceptibilities of the infecting organism.

Guidelines for antimicrobial therapy of native and prosthetic valve endocarditis caused by various organisms are summarized in Table 45.3. In general a bactericidal agent to which the micro-organism is susceptible should be used; for staphylococci, streptococci and enterococci in combination with gentamicin for at least 2 weeks to enhance the bactericidal activity of the regimen.[197,198] The duration of therapy for PVE is longer than for native valve endocarditis, and antibiotic therapy should generally be continued for a minimum of 6 weeks, often longer, regardless of whether surgical intervention has occurred or is planned. Rifampicin may be added to the regimen with staphylococcal infections, based on its adjunctive value in osteomyelitis and prosthetic joint infections.[105,125–127] Resistance to rifampicin develops rapidly when it is used as a single agent or when the microbial burden is high,[126] and it may be desirable to delay adding rifampicin to the regimen until after 3–5 days of therapy with other agents.[168] In the presence of high-level aminoglycoside resistance, therapy for enterococcal PVE should be prolonged to 8–12 weeks. The best

therapy for vancomycin-resistant *Enterococcus faecium* PVE remains uncertain at this point, although there have been reports of successful outcomes, both with linezolid[199] and with quinupristin–dalfopristin.[200]

Fungal PVE has been associated with a very poor outcome and current management mandates surgical replacement of the infected valve followed by prolonged antifungal therapy.[179,187] Amphotericin B, with or without 5-fluorocytosine, is recommended for *Candida* PVE, and some have recommended follow-up long-term suppressive therapy with an azole, based on reports of recurrent infection after parenteral therapy has been completed.[179]

Surgical therapy

The onset of PVE within 2 months of valve replacement, new or worsening congestive heart failure due to valve dysfunction, new high-grade electrocardiographic conduction abnormalities, an intracardiac abscess detected echocardiographically, infection with staphylococci, *Ps. aeruginosa* or fungi, uncontrolled infection with persistent bloodstream infection despite appropriate antimicrobial therapy, relapse of endocarditis after a full course of appropriate antimicrobial therapy, and fever that persists beyond 10 days despite appropriate antimicrobial therapy are all associated with a poor outcome,[198] and are regarded as indications for surgical intervention, with removal of the infected prosthetic valve, debridement of the annulus (and any abscesses found), and implantation of a new prosthetic valve. The decision to intervene surgically must take into account all of these factors as well as host factors predictive of poor surgical outcome such as stage IV heart failure, acute renal failure or, especially, multiorgan failure.

PVE presenting with severe heart failure, while associated with high operative mortality, is almost universally fatal within 6 months without surgery.[181] Studies have shown that patients with paravalvular abscesses, which occur in 45–60% of patients with PVE,[150,166] have survival rates approaching 80% when a combined medical–surgical approach is employed.[201,202] In a recent study, *Staph. aureus* PVE treated medically was associated with a mortality of 83% whereas treatment with a combined medical–surgical approach was associated with a 20% mortality,[178] a difference that remained highly significant, even after correcting for age, severity of illness and medical comorbidities.

Ideally, patients with clear indications for surgery but risk factors for a poor outcome should be taken immediately to the operating room before their heart failure worsens or their renal function is compromised – but, understandably, surgeons may be hesitant to perform valve replacement, which is associated with a mortality of 10–30% in experienced hands,[201,202] when patients appear to be clinically stable and seem to be responding to antimicrobial therapy. Moreover, there is obviously theoretical concern about reimplanting a new prosthetic valve in an infected surgical site; however, the data indicate that the rate of recurrent PVE is low, 6–15%.[159,202,203] Finally, delaying surgery to provide a longer duration of antimicrobial therapy

Table 45.3 Recommended antimicrobial regimens for specific micro-organisms causing prosthetic valve endocarditis[a]

Organism	Antibiotic	Dose	Duration (weeks)
Penicillin-susceptible streptococci (MIC ≤ 0.1 µg/ml	Penicillin G plus	18–24 million units i.v. daily by continuous infusion or divided doses every 4 h	≥ 6
	gentamicin *or*	1 mg/kg i.m. or i.v. every 8 h	2
	Ceftriaxone plus	2 g i.v. or i.m. daily as a single dose	≥ 6
	gentamicin *or*	1 mg/kg i.m. or i.v. every 8 h	2
	Vancomycin[b] plus	15 mg/kg i.v. every 12 h	≥ 6
	gentamicin	1 mg/kg i.m. or i.v. every 8 h	2
Penicillin-intermediate streptococci (> 0.1 µg/ml to < 0.5 µg/ml)	Penicillin G plus	24–30 million units i.v. daily by continuous infusion or divided doses every 4 h	≥ 6
	gentamicin	1 mg/kg i.m. or i.v. every 8 h	4
Enterococci and streptococci with MIC ≥ 0.5 µg/ml[c]	Penicillin G plus	24–30 million units i.v. daily by continuous infusion or divided doses every 4 h	≥ 6
	gentamicin *or*	1 mg/kg i.m. or i.v. every 8 h	6
	Ampicillin plus	2 g i.v. every 4 h	≥ 6
	gentamicin *or*	1 mg/kg i.m. or i.v. every 8 h	6
	Vancomycin[b] plus	15 mg/kg i.v. every 12 h	≥ 6
	gentamicin	1 mg/kg i.m. or i.v. every 8 h	6
Methicillin-sensitive staphylococci	Nafcillin plus	2 g i.v. every 4 h or 12 g by continuous infusion	≥ 6–8
	gentamicin plus	1 mg/kg i.m. or i.v. every 8 h	2
	rifampicin	600 mg orally once daily	≥ 6–8
Methicillin-resistant staphylococci[d]	Vancomycin[b] plus	15 mg/kg i.v. every 12 h	≥ 6–8
	gentamicin plus	1 mg/kg i.m. or i.v. every 8 h	2
	rifampicin	600 mg orally once daily	≥ 6–8
HACEK group	Ceftriaxone *or*	2 g i.v. or i.m. as a single dose	≥ 6
	Ampicillin plus	2 g i.m. every 4 h	≥ 6
	gentamicin	1 mg/kg i.m. or i.v. every 8 h	4
Diphtheroids	Penicillin G plus	18–24 million units i.v. by continuous infusion or divided doses every 4 h	≥ 6
	gentamicin *or*	1 mg/kg i.m. or i.v. every 8 h	6
	Vancomycin	15 mg/kg i.v. every 12 h	≥ 6
Fungi	Amphotericin B +/–	0.7–1.0 mg/kg i.v. once daily	≥ 6
	5-fluorocytosine	150 mg/kg divided into four doses daily	≥ 6

[a] Adapted in part from Wilson et al 1995.[198]
[b] Should be used only in patients with immediate or severe penicillin or cephalosporin allergy.
[c] In-vitro evaluation of MIC of penicillin and vancomycin, β-lactamase production, and high level resistance to gentamicin and streptomycin considered mandatory.
[d] Regimen can also be used for patients with methicillin-sensitive staphylococcal PVE who have a severe penicillin allergy.

in the hopes of sterilizing the surgical bed has not been shown to improve outcome.[202] Thus, the data indicate that a patient presenting with one or more indications listed in Table 45.6 will benefit from early cardiac surgery.

Anticoagulation

A final controversial aspect of the care of patients with PVE is the decision whether to continue anticoagulation. Currently, most patients with bioprosthetic heart valves are anticoagulated for the first 3 months after valve replacement;[204] however, in the setting of bioprosthetic valve endocarditis, the risk of anticoagulation outweighs the benefit and oral anticoagulants should be discontinued.

In contrast, patients with mechanical prosthetic heart valves have an annual risk of embolic stroke that approaches 4% without anticoagulation,[205] and discontinuing anticoagulation in these patients is more problematic. Anticoagulation of patients with infected mechanical valves appears to offer protection against embolic stroke: in a large cohort study, patients with mechanical PVE who were anticoagulated had a much lower risk of stroke than patients who were not receiving anticoagulants (12% versus 42%).[206]

Unfortunately, when stroke occurs in anticoagulated patients there is a higher risk of hemorrhagic extension,[161,178,207] especially if *Staph. aureus* is the infecting pathogen. Studies suggest that the risk of neurologic deterioration is increased when patients with an embolic stroke undergo cardiac surgery within 2–3 weeks of the event, presumably because of the need for heparinization during cardiopulmonary bypass.[208] Thus, it is generally considered desirable to continue anticoagulants in patients with mechanical valves and PVE, but every effort must be made to avert excessive anticoagulation; using intravenous heparin may provide a safer alternative during the early phase of therapy. Finally, if cerebral embolism does occur, anticoagulation should be withheld for several days to reduce the risk of hemorrhagic complications, and surgical intervention should be delayed, if possible, for at least 2–3 weeks to allow stabilization of the cerebral vasculature.[208]

PREVENTION

Prosthetic heart valves, whether bioprosthetic or mechanical, are considered at high risk for endocarditis in the latest American Heart Association guideline,[209] and the use of prophylactic antibiotics before procedures that are likely to produce bacteremia is recommended to prevent late PVE. Interventions that reduce the risk of intraoperative contamination at the time of surgery will have the greatest impact on prevention of early PVE.[210,211] Therefore, scrupulous asepsis and meticulous surgical technique combined with perioperative antimicrobial prophylaxis with drugs exhibiting antistaphylococcal activity – cefazolin, cefuroxime or cefamandole – forms the cornerstone of prevention of PVE. Vancomycin should not be routinely used for prophylaxis unless the hospi-

tal has a high rate of MRSA infection or the patient is a known MRSA carrier.[210,212]

A novel silver-coated St. Jude valve (Silzone®, St. Jude Medical Inc.) has been advocated to prevent recurrent PVE, with anecdotal success. The large, multicenter, Artificial Valve Endocarditis Reduction Trial (AVERT) trial was undertaken in 1999[213] with the goal of assessing the efficacy of the novel medicated valve; however, there have been reports of recurrent PVE despite its use.[214] Most importantly, enrollment in the AVERT trial was suspended in January 2001 because of evidence of increased paravalvular incompetence in patients who received the silver-coated valve.

PACEMAKER INFECTIONS

EPIDEMIOLOGY

Approximately 370 000 pacemakers were implanted in the USA in 1996.[39] Pacemaker infection manifests clinically in one of three ways depending on the type of pacing leads used:

- localized infection of the pulse generator pocket;
- pericarditis and/or mediastinitis due to infection of epicardial pacing leads; or
- primary bloodstream infection in association with rightsided endocarditis due to infection of transvenous endocardial pacing leads.

Overall rates of infection following implantation of a permanent pacemaker range from 1 to 7%.[215–219]

Pacemaker endocarditis, a complication seen almost exclusively with endocardial pacing leads and caused mainly by *Staph. aureus*, occurs least commonly (0.5–1% of implantations).[217,220,221] However, mortality is high, approaching 40% without removal of the infected leads.[217,220]

Infection of the pulse-generator pocket is far more common in the early post-implant period, but can occur years later when the pacemaker battery is replaced.[216] Invasive infection of the pacing leads typically manifests late, although infection may develop early if the leads become contaminated at the time of implantation.

The risk of pacemaker infection is increased in patients with diabetes mellitus or underlying malignancy,[217,222] with operator inexperience,[222,223] with manipulation of the pacemaker such as replacement of the battery,[216] and if the patient requires a temporary transvenous pacemaker before implantation of the permanent pacemaker.[222]

PATHOGENESIS

Infection occurs early (< 2 weeks), intermediate (2 weeks to 6 months), or late in the post-implantation period (> 6 months). Infections of the pulse-generator pocket constitute the majority of early and intermediate pacemaker infections, deriving from contamination of the pulse generator pocket by cutaneous organisms at the time of implantation.[224] Seeding of epicardial leads also occurs most frequently at the time of implantation, less often later, by migration of infection from the pulse-generator pocket, and thus also tends to present in the early and intermediate post-implantation period. Infection of transvenous pacemaker leads may occur at implantation,[217] with migration of micro-organisms from an infected pulse-generator pocket, or derive from hematogenous seeding during a late bloodstream infection,[225,226] and these infections tend to present in the intermediate or late post-implantation period, few presenting early.

MICROBIOLOGY

Predictably, most pacemaker infections are caused by Gram-positive organisms, especially *Staph. aureus* or coagulase-negative staphylococci.[222,226,227] *Propionibacterium acnes*, Gram-negative bacilli and *Candida albicans* account for most of the rest. Rare cases of late pacemaker endocarditis caused by viridans streptococci or enterococci have been reported.[221] Finally, rare organisms implicated in pacemaker infection have included *Brucella melitensis*,[228] non-tuberculosis mycobacteria,[229] *Aspergillus* spp.[230] and *Petriellidium boydii*.[231]

DIAGNOSIS

The clinical presentation of pacemaker infection depends on whether it involves the pulse-generator pocket or the pacing leads. Infection of the pulse-generator pocket typically occurs shortly following implantation or battery exchange, and manifests with localized erythema, pain, and fluctuance, occasionally with erosion of the overlying skin. Rarely, migration of infection from the pocket produces pericardial involvement (when epicardial leads are used) or bloodstream infection, with endocardial leads. Infection of endocardial pacing leads typically presents as a primary bloodstream infection that varies in severity, depending on the causative organism: indolent febrile illness with coagulase-negative streptococci as contrasted with fulminant sepsis with *Staph. aureus*. In either case, signs and symptoms of right-sided endocarditis are often present, including fever and chills (> 80%),[225,226] septic pulmonary emboli (20–45%),[225,226] and tricuspid regurgitation (25%).[225,226]

A presumptive diagnosis of a pulse-generator pocket infection can usually be made on clinical grounds alone and is confirmed by a percutaneous aspirate from the pocket that shows micro-organisms on Gram stain or in culture. Diagnosing infection of an epicardial pacing lead can be more challenging unless bloodstream infection is present. Cryptogenic pericarditis or mediastinitis are usually identifiable by computed tomography (CT) or magnetic resonance imaging (MRI) of the chest but microbiologic confirmation is mandatory if blood cultures are non-diagnostic. As seen with PVE, foreign body-related endovascular infections are associated with high-grade bloodstream infection that typically does not quickly clear after starting antimicrobial therapy. Therefore, patients with endocardial pacing lead infection, in addition to manifesting signs of right-sided endocarditis, usually show high-grade bloodstream infection, despite days of appropriate antimicrobial therapy.[195,225] Echocardiography shows vegetations on the endocardial leads and/or the tricuspid valve, and is valuable for confirming infection. TEE, with a sensitivity that ranges from 91 to 96% (compared with a 22–43% sensitivity seen with TTE) is preferred.[217,225,226,232]

TREATMENT

Successful treatment of pacemaker-related infection usually requires a combined medical and surgical approach. While isolated reports have claimed successful eradication of pacemaker infections with limited debridement followed by prolonged antimicrobial therapy, most of the published series report an unacceptably high failure rate unless the entire pacing system, including the battery pack and pacing wires, is removed.[218,225–227,233,234] Lewis et al found that 31 of 32 patients with pacemaker infection treated at their center with medical therapy alone recurred and ultimately required removal of the entire pacing system to achieve cure.[227] Similar experiences were reported by Molina et al, who found that 12 of 12 patients treated medically suffered recurrence.[233] Most importantly, the mortality with infected endocardial leads is greatly increased in patients treated medically, as shown in an analysis of 182 cases by Cacoub et al, who found a 41% mortality in medically treated patients, compared with 18% in patients whose entire pacemaker was removed.[226]

Traditional management mandates removal of the entire infected pacing system, placement of a temporary pacemaker, if indicated (not indicated in 13–52% of patients[235]), followed by several weeks of parenteral antibiotic therapy, after which a new battery and endocardial pacing system are implanted. Recent studies have shown low recurrence rates with removal of the entire infected pacemaker followed by immediate placement of a new permanent epicardial pacing system, obviating the need for temporary pacing.[236]

Transcutaneous extraction of infected endocardial leads that have been in place for prolonged periods is often difficult, as the lead is incorporated into a fibrous sheath in the right atrium and traction fails to dislodge the infected lead in 14–36% of cases.[235,237] In this situation, open-heart surgical extraction is usually necessary. Recently, a transvenous excimer laser sheath[237,238] has permitted successful lead extraction in 94% of cases, as contrasted with only 64% in a group where simple traction and a telescoping sheath were utilized.[237]

Removal of an infected lead with large vegetations by transcutaneous extraction engenders concern over potential embolization. A study by Klug et al demonstrated that 30% of patients with endocardial lead vegetations had scintigraphic evidence of pulmonary emboli following removal of the lead,[225] although none of these patients developed clinical symptoms.

Several series have reported successful transcutaneous extraction of infected leads with vegetations >10 mm in size;[232,239] however, concerns remain with vegetations this size and some authorities recommend proceeding directly to surgical removal.[240]

PREVENTION

Strict aseptic technique and well-trained, experienced operators are be associated with reduced rates of pacemaker-related infection.[223] Antibiotic prophylaxis has traditionally been discouraged, except in high-risk patients,[241] however, a recent meta-analysis that encompassed 2023 patients found that routine antibiotic prophylaxis with anti-staphylococcal drugs was associated with a 75% reduction in pacemaker-related infections (CI 0.10–0.66, $p = 0.005$).[242] Unfortunately, heterogeneity of the studies and inclusion of only a single, double-blinded, randomized trial limits application of this analysis. If prophylaxis is to be used, an antistaphylococcal drug, such as cefuroxime or cefazolin, is recommended (vancomycin if the patient has been colonized by or has had previous infection with MRSA).

INFECTIONS RELATED TO INTRAVASCULAR DEVICES

EPIDEMIOLOGY

Reliable vascular access for administration of fluids and electrolytes, blood products, drugs, nutritional support and for hemodynamic monitoring has become one of the most essential features of modern medical care. Unfortunately, vascular access is associated with substantial and generally under-appreciated potential for producing iatrogenic disease, particularly bloodstream infection originating from infection of the percutaneous device used for vascular access or from contamination of the infusate administered through the device.[243] More than one-half of all epidemics of nosocomial bacteremia or candidemia derive from vascular access in some form.[244,245]

More than 250 000 intravascular device (IVD) related bloodstream infections occur in the USA each year,[246] each associated with 12–25% attributable mortality,[243,247–249] prolongation of hospital stay,[243,248–251] and an added cost to healthcare of $33 000–$35 000.[243,248,250,251]

Prospective studies in which every IVD was cultured at the time of removal show that every device carries some risk of causing bloodstream infection, but the magnitude of risk varies greatly (Table 45.4).[252]

PATHOGENESIS

There are two major sources of IVD-related bloodstream infection:

1. Colonization of the IVD; catheter-related infection.
2. Contamination of the fluid administered through the device; infusate-related infection.[253]

Contaminated infusate is the cause of most epidemic IVD-related infections and has been reviewed elsewhere.[246] In contrast, catheter-related infections are responsible for most endemic infections and comprise the focus of this review.

In order for micro-organisms to cause IVD-related infection they must first gain access to the extraluminal or intraluminal surface of the device, where they can adhere and become incorporated into a biofilm that allows sustained infection and hematogenous dissemination.[254] Micro-organisms gain access by one of three mechanisms (Figure 45.2): (1) skin organisms invade the percutaneous tract, probably facilitated

Table 45.4 Rates of intravascular device-related bloodstream infection associated with the major types of devices used in clinical practice[a]

Type of intravascular device (no. studies)	Rates of infection			
	per 100 devices		per 1000 device days	
	Pooled mean	95% CI	Pooled mean	95% CI
Peripheral venous catheters (13)	0.2	0.1–0.3	0.6	0.3–1.2
Arterial catheters used for hemodynamic monitoring (6)	1.5	0.9–2.4	2.9	1.8–4.5
Short-term, non-cuffed, non-medicated central venous catheters (61)	3.3	3.3–4.0	2.3	2.0–2.4
Pulmonary artery catheters (12)	1.9	1.1–2.5	5.5	3.2–12.4
Hemodialysis catheters				
Non-cuffed (15)	16.2	13.5–18.3	2.8	2.3–3.1
Cuffed (5)	6.3	4.2–9.2	1.1	0.7–1.6
Peripherally inserted central catheters (8)	1.2	0.5–2.2	0.4	0.2–0.7
Long-term tunneled and cuffed central venous catheters (18)	20.9	18.2–21.9	1.2	1.0–1.3
Subcutaneous central venous ports (13)	5.1	4.0–6.3	0.2	0.1–0.2

[a] Based on 206 published prospective studies in which every device was evaluated for infection; Kluger and Maki, 2001.[252]

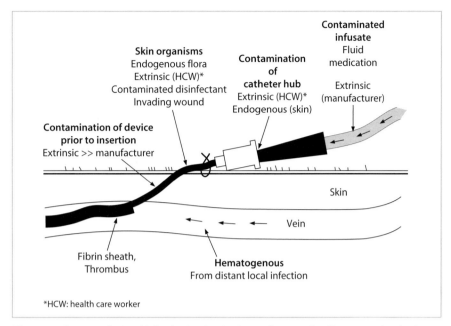

*HCW: health care worker

Fig. 45.2 Routes of microbial colonization in the pathogenesis of intravascular device-related bloodstream infection (adapted from Maki and Mermel, 1998[246]).

by capillary action[255] at the time of insertion or in the days following; (2) micro-organisms contaminate the catheter hub (and lumen) when the catheter is inserted over a percutaneous guidewire or later manipulated;[256] or (3) organisms are carried hematogenously to the implanted IVD from remote sources of local infection, such as a pneumonia.[244,257]

With short-term IVDs (in place <10 days) – peripheral intravenous catheters, arterial catheters and non-cuffed, non-tunneled central venous catheters – most device-related bloodstream infections are of cutaneous origin, from the insertion site, and gain access extraluminally, occasionally intraluminally.[258,259]

In contrast, contamination of the catheter hub and lumen appears to be the predominant mode of infection with long-term, permanent IVDs (in place >10 days), such as cuffed

Hickman- and Broviac-type catheters, cuffed hemodialysis central venous catheters (CVCs), subcutaneous central ports and peripherally inserted central catheters.[260–262]

MICROBIOLOGY

Micro-organisms found on patients' skin and which gain access to the IVD extraluminally, occasionally intraluminally – coagulase-negative staphylococci (39%), *Staph. aureus* (26%), and *Candida* species (11%) – account for 76% of IVD-related infections with short-term, non-cuffed devices of all types; only 14% are caused by Gram-negative bacilli (Figure 45.3).[263] In contrast, with long-term surgically implanted devices such as cuffed and tunneled catheters, peripherally inserted central

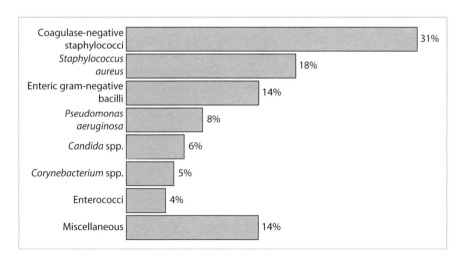

Fig. 45.3 Microbial profile of intravascular device-related bloodstream infection based on an analysis 159 published prospective studies.[263]

catheters and subcutaneous central venous ports, coagulase-negative staphylococci (25%) and Gram-negative bacilli (45%) (which most commonly gain access intraluminally and contaminate infusate in the device) account for 76% of IVD-related bloodstream infections; only 2% are caused by *Candida* species (Figure 45.3).[263]

DIAGNOSIS

Despite the challenge in identifying the source of a patient's signs of sepsis,[264] several clinical, epidemiological, and microbiologic findings point strongly towards an IVD as the source of a septic episode.[246] Patients with the abrupt onset of signs and symptoms of sepsis without any other identifiable source should prompt suspicion of infection of an IVD.[246] The presence of inflammation, with or without purulence, at the IVD insertion site, while present in the minority of cases, when combined with signs and symptoms of sepsis has been shown to be predictive of IVD-related bacteremia and should prompt removal of the IVD.[246] Finally, recovery of certain microorganisms in multiple blood cultures, such as staphylococci, *Corynebacterium* or *Bacillus* spp., or *Candida* or *Malassezia* spp., strongly suggests infection of the IVD.

Removal and culture of the IVD has historically been the gold standard for the diagnosis of IVD-related infections, particularly with short-term catheters. Numerous studies have demonstrated the superiority of semiquantitative or quantitative culture methods over qualitative broth culture for the diagnosis of such infections.[265,266] Growth of ≥ 15 cfu from an IVD segment by semiquantitative culture or growth of $\geq 10^3$ cfu from a catheter segment cultured after sonication, when accompanied by local signs of infection or the systemic inflammatory response syndrome (SIRS) usually indicates infection of the IVD. The diagnosis of IVD-related bloodstream infection is completed when a heavily colonized IVD is associated with concurrent infection, with no other plausible source (i.e. primary bloodstream infection); the linkage becomes virtually certain when the strains recovered from the colonized IVD and from blood cultures are shown to be identical by phenotypic or, better, genotypic subtyping.[267–269]

Semiquantitative and quantitative cultures of IVDs obviously require their removal. As noted, this can be a major problem in patients with long-term, surgically implanted IVDs such as Hickman and Broviac catheters, cuffed and tunneled hemodialysis catheters and subcutaneous central venous ports. Prospective studies of patients with long-term IVDs have shown that only 25–45% of episodes of sepsis represent true IVD-related bloodstream infection.[270,271] Thus, it would seem that development of in-situ methods of detecting such infections that do not require removal of the IVD would be of great utility to clinicians and patients, and in research studies.

If a laboratory is prepared to do pour-plate blood cultures or has available an automated quantitative system for culturing blood, such as the Isolator® lysis centrifugation system (Wampole Laboratories, Cranbury, NJ), quantitative blood cultures drawn through the IVD and concomitantly by venepuncture from a peripheral vein (or another IVD) can permit the diagnosis of IVD-related bacteremia or fungemia to be made with sensitivity and specificity in the range of 80–95%,[266] without removal of the catheter, if empiric antimicrobial therapy has not yet been initiated. With infected IVDs, the blood culture drawn through the device usually shows a five- to ten-fold rise in the concentration of organisms compared to the quantitative blood culture drawn percutaneously from a peripheral site. High grade peripheral candidemia (≥ 25 cfu/ml) reflects an infected IVD 90% of the time.[186] Quantitative IVD-drawn blood cultures are most useful for the diagnosis of infection with long-term devices but, because of their expense, have had limited utility for the diagnosis of infections associated with short-term devices.[272] There is evidence that a single quantitative culture drawn from a long-term device, even without an accompanying quantitative culture drawn from the periphery, can accurately identify IVD-related infection if there is >100 cfu/ml of growth.[266]

Quantitative blood cultures are labor intensive and cost almost twice as much as standard blood cultures.[266] The wide availability of radiometric blood culture systems (e.g. BACTEC system®, Becton Dickenson), in which blood cultures are continuously monitored for microbial growth (approximately every 20 min), has led to a clever application of this system for the detection of IVD-related bloodstream infection. The differential-time-to-positivity of blood cultures drawn through the IVD and concomitantly from a peripheral site has been evaluated as a surrogate for paired quantitative blood cultures. Detection of positivity in a blood culture drawn from the IVD more than 2 h before positivity of the culture drawn from a peripheral site has been shown to be highly predictive of IVD-related infection, in one study correctly identifying 16 of 17 such infections with long-term catheters, yielding an overall sensitivity of 94% and specificity of 91%.[273] Subsequent studies with short-term catheters, used mainly in the intensive care unit (ICU), have generally found lower predictive values,[274] probably related to the extraluminal pathogenesis of infection with most of these devices.

Another simple but rapid and potentially cost-effective method of detecting IVD-related infection is acridine-orange leukocyte cytospin (AOLC) staining, combined with Gram staining, of a sample of lysed and centrifuged blood drawn from the suspected IVD. In a recent prospective study of 124 adult surgical patients, this method was found to be 96% sensitive and 92% specific.[275] In contrast, AOLC with Gram staining was found in a recent prospective study to be of limited utility in diagnosing infection with short-term IVDs (mean duration of catheterization 6 days): AOLC failed to diagnose all 12 confirmed IVD-related infections. Therefore, AOLC with Gram stain will probably remain useful primarily for diagnosing infections associated with long-term IVDs.[270]

In-situ testing using a novel culture-brush, which can be passed down the lumen and out the end of a long-term IVD to pick up luminal biofilm and colonized fibrin and thrombus around the tip, has also been proposed as an alternative to removal and culture of the IVD. A prospective study that compared use of the endoluminal brush with semiquantitative culture of removed IVDs found the brush to be 95% sensitive and 84% specific.[276] However, a subsequent study failed to demonstrate this level of efficacy: van Heerdan et al found that use of the endoluminal brush was associated with a sensitivity of 21% although the specificity was 100%.[277] The predominance of organisms on the extraluminal surface of infected short-term catheters may limit the utility of the brush-culture in the ICU.

TREATMENT

If a short-term vascular catheter is suspected of being infected because the patient has no obvious other source of infection to explain fever, there is inflammation at the insertion site, or cryptogenic staphylococcal bacteremia or candidemia has been documented, blood cultures should be obtained and the catheter should be removed and cultured. Failure to remove an infected catheter puts the patient at risk of developing septic thrombophlebitis with peripheral intravenous catheters, septic thrombosis of a great central vein with central venous catheters,[278] or even endocarditis. Continued access, if necessary, can be established with a new catheter inserted in a new site. A new catheter should never be placed in an old site over a guidewire if the first catheter is suspected of being infected, especially if there is purulence at the site.

Bloodstream infection that might have originated from a cuffed and tunneled central venous catheter does not automatically mandate removal of the device, unless:

- there has been persistent exit site infection,
- the tunnel is obviously infected,
- there is evidence of complicating endocarditis, septic thrombosis, or septic pulmonary emboli, the infecting pathogen is *Staph. aureus*,[279] *Corynebacterium jeikeium*,[280] a *Bacillus* species,[281] *Stenotrophomonas* spp., *Burkholderia cepacia* and all pseudomonal species,[282] a filamentous fungus or *Malassezia* species,[283] or a mycobacterial species;[284]
- bacteremia or candidemia persists for more than 3 days despite adequate therapy.

Studies of 7–21 days of antibiotics infused through the infected line have shown success rates of 60–91% without catheter removal,[285–287] although there was significant variability in the response rates depending on the infecting microorganism; with infections due to coagulase-negative staphylococci, the risk of recurrent bacteremia has been approximately 20%.[288] Several studies have reported successful treatment of IVD-related infections due to *Candida* spp. without removing the device by administering prolonged courses of amphotericin B administered through the catheter;[289,290] however, this is in contrast to the results of other prospective studies that found an increased duration of candidemia and mortality in patients who retained their infected IVD.[291,292]

In addition to infusion of systemic antibiotics through the infected line, which is mandatory for any patient with documented IVD-related infection, instillation of a highly concentrated solution of the antibiotic or antibiotic combination, 'locked' into the infected tunneled catheter, may be of adjunctive value to 'cure' an infected long-term IVD. In-vitro testing has proven the long-term stability of solutions of most antimicrobial agents over periods of time as long as 10 days.[293]

In small, uncontrolled clinical trials, 'antibiotic lock therapy', usually in conjunction with systemic antibiotic therapy, has shown 'cure' rates with infected IVDs in excess of 90%[294,295] but the vast majority of IVDs reported in these studies were infected with Gram-positive organisms other than *Staph. aureus* or *Bacillus* spp. (primarily coagulase-negative staphylococci or Gram-negative bacilli other than *Ps. aeruginosa*). Data are lacking on the value of lock therapy for IVD-related fungemia, and therefore at this time it cannot be recommended for the management of long term IVDs infected by *Staph. aureus*, *Bacillus* spp., *Corynebacterium jeikeium*, *Stenotrophomonas* spp., *Burk. cepacia*, all pseudomonas species, fungi or mycobacterial species.

Historically, central ports are rarely curable with medical therapy alone if the device is clearly infected (e.g. an aspirate from the port shows heavy growth).[296,297] In-vitro studies of antibiotic lock solutions in simulated models of infected central ports raise the possibility of using antibiotic lock therapy to preserve these long-term devices when they become infected. A recent study of patients with AIDS with central ports who developed IVD-related bloodstream infection found that lock therapy combined with systemic antibiotic therapy resulted in 70% of the ports being salvaged (although long-term follow-up was not reported). A recent larger clinical trial of antibiotic lock therapy for central port infections achieved salvage rates less than 50%.[298] Based on the marginal efficacy of the technique in these two studies and the historically poor cure rate achieved with systemic antibiotics alone, we believe that definitive treatment of infected central ports mandates their removal.

The decision to treat a suspected IVD-related infection before microbiologic confirmation (i.e. empirically) comes down to clinical judgment, weighing the evidence suggesting bloodstream infection and the risks of delaying treatment. In general, fever or other signs of sepsis in a granulocytopenic patient must be regarded as infection until proven otherwise.

If IVD-related bloodstream infection is suspected after cultures have been obtained, the combination of intravenous vancomycin (for staphylococci resistant to methicillin) with a fluoroquinolone (preferably ciprofloxacin) or with cefepime or a carbapenem (for aerobic Gram-negative bacilli) should prove effective against the bacterial pathogens most likely to be encountered. Initial therapy can then be modified based on the microbiologic identity and susceptibility of the infecting organisms.

While there are no prospective data to guide the duration of antimicrobial therapy for IVD-related infections, most coagulase-negative staphylococci infections can be cured with 5–7 days of therapy[246,288,299,300] whereas most infections caused by other micro-organisms can be adequately treated with 10–14 days of antimicrobial therapy.[299–301] These recommendations hold only as long as there are no complications related to the infection – endocarditis, septic thrombophlebitis, septic thrombosis, or metastatic infection such as osteomyelitis – and the infection clears within 72 h of initiating therapy. Nosocomial enterococcal bacteremia deriving from an IVD is rarely associated with persistent endovascular infection, and unless there is clinical or echocardiographic evidence of endocarditis, treatment with intravenous ampicillin or vancomycin alone for 7–14 days should suffice.[302]

The management of *Staph. aureus* device-related infection deserves special mention, as there have been no prospective studies to evaluate the optimal duration of therapy for such infection. Historically, high rates of associated infectious endocarditis and late complications led to a universal policy of 4–6 weeks of antimicrobial therapy for all patients with *Staph. aureus* bacteremia. Earlier diagnosis and initiation of bactericidal therapy of nosocomial *Staph. aureus* bacteremias in recent years have been associated with lower rates of infectious endocarditis and metastatic complications, prompting suggestions that short-course therapy (14 days) is effective and safe for most cases of IVD-related *Staph. aureus* bacteremia if the patient defervesces within 72 h and there is no evidence of metastatic infection.[303,304] In a study where TEE was routinely performed in 103 hospital patients with *Staph. aureus* bacteremia, 69 related to an IVD, Fowler et al found a surprisingly high rate of late complications, 23% with IVD-related *Staph. aureus* bacteremia.[305] More recently, these authors reported that TEE is a cost-effective way to stratify patients with IVD-related *Staph. aureus* infection into short-course or long-course regimens. However, at this time there are no prospective studies to confirm this approach. Until more data are available, short-course antimicrobial therapy for IVD-related *Staph. aureus* bacteremia therapy should be used only when TEE is unequivocally negative, the patient has defervesced within 72 h of starting therapy, and there is no evidence of distant metastatic infection.

All patients with IVD-related candidemia should be treated, even if the patient becomes afebrile and blood cultures spontaneously revert to negative following removal of the IVD without antifungal therapy.[306,307] IVD-related candidemia that responds rapidly to removal of the catheter and institution of intravenous amphotericin B can be reliably treated with a daily dose of 0.3–0.5 mg/kg and a total dose of 3–5 mg/kg.[306,307] Fluconazole (400 mg/day) has been shown to be as effective as amphotericin B in randomized trials in non-neutropenic patients,[308] and has further been shown to be comparable to amphotericin B in observational studies of neutropenic patients with *Candida* IVD-related infection[309] but should not be used with infections associated with septic thrombosis and high-grade candidemia or, obviously, with infections caused by fluconazole-resistant organisms such as *Candida krusei* or *Candida glabrata*.

All patients with an IVD-related bloodstream infection must be monitored closely, for at least 6 weeks after completing therapy, especially if they have had high-grade bacteremia or candidemia, to detect late-appearing endocarditis,[278,306] retinitis[306] or other metastatic infections, such as vertebral osteomyelitis.[310]

PREVENTION

Over the past decade many investigators have evaluated strategies for the prevention of IVD-related infections, with greater success than with any other form of nosocomial infection.[246,311,312] Guidelines for the prevention of such infections were last issued by the Hospital Infection Control Practices Advisory Committee in 1996 and have recently been revised.[313] Wide adoption of these measures has resulted in a substantial decline in hospital-acquired primary bloodstream infections in centers in the USA.[314] More consistent application of control measures and wider acceptance of novel technologies shown to be effective (and cost-effective) will be needed to reduce this rate further.

Aseptic technique

Although there has been considerable controversy as to the level of barrier precautions necessary during insertion of a CVC, recent studies[259,315] have shown that the use of maximal barriers – a long-sleeved, sterile surgical gown, mask, cap and large sterile drape, sterile gloves – significantly reduces the risk of CVC-related infection. The use of maximal barriers has further been shown to be highly cost-effective.[315] Such measures are not necessary, however, for peripheral venous or arterial catheters used for hemodynamic monitoring, where sterile gloves and a small sterile fenestrated drape will suffice.

Given the evidence for the importance of cutaneous micro-organisms in the genesis of IVD-related infection, the choice of the chemical antiseptic for disinfection of the insertion site would seem of high priority. In the USA, iodophors such as 10% povidone-iodine are widely used. Eight randomized, prospective trials have compared a chlorhexidine-containing antiseptic with povidone-iodine for disinfection of the skin before insertion of IVDs: both agents were well tolerated in every trial, seven of eight found lower rates of catheter colonization, and three showed a significant reduction in CVC-related infections in the chlorhexidine-containing antiseptic group.[316–318] These studies indicate that chlorhexidine is superior to iodophors and should be the antiseptic of first choice for vascular access.[313]

Novel dressings

IVDRs can be dressed with sterile gauze and tape or with a sterile transparent, semipermeable, polyurethane film dressing. The available data suggest that the two types of dressings are equivalent in terms of their impact on IVD-related infections.[267,319–321]

Based on the superiority of chlorhexidine for cutaneous disinfection of vascular access sites, a novel chlorhexidine-impregnated sponge dressing has been developed (Biopatch®, Johnson and Johnson Medical Inc.) and evaluated in three trials to date.[322–324] A large prospective, randomized trial comparing the use of the chlorhexidine dressing to a standard polyurethane dressing with short-term central venous and arterial catheters in adults admitted to two teaching hospital ICUs showed a 60% reduction in catheter-related bloodstream infections with use of the chlorhexidine sponge dressing (adjusted RR 0.38, $p = 0.01$), with no adverse reactions associated with its use.[324] Moreover, testing of the in-vitro susceptibility of isolates from infected catheters in both groups showed no evidence that the antiseptic dressing promoted resistance to chlorhexidine.

Innovative IVD design

Hickman and Broviac catheters incorporate a subcutaneous Dacron® cuff which becomes ingrown by host tissue, creating a mechanical barrier against invasion of the tract by skin organisms. Rates of bloodstream infection per 1000 days with these catheters are far lower than with short-term percutaneously inserted, non-cuffed CVCs inserted in the ICU (Table 45.4).[246,252] and can be considered a quantum advance for safer long-term vascular access.

Surgically implanted subcutaneous central venous ports, which can be accessed intermittently with a steel needle, have been associated with the lowest rates of bloodstream infection (Table 45.4; p. 588). A prospective observational study of Hickman catheters and central ports in oncology patients showed that for patients needing intermittent central access, ports appear to carry lower risk of IVD-related infection.[290]

Studies also suggest that peripherally inserted central catheters pose substantially lower risks of infection than standard non-tunneled, non-cuffed CVCs (Table 45.4),[252] perhaps because bacterial colonization on the arm is lower than the neck or upper chest.[262]

A novel CVC made of polyurethane that is impregnated with minute quantities of silver sulfadiazine and chlorhexidine (ArrowGard®, Arrow International) became available approximately 10 years ago. There have now been 15 randomized trials of this catheter for prevention of related infection. Most have demonstrated a reduction in colonization of the catheter but only two studies were able to show a significant reduction in CVC related bloodstream infections.[268,325] In the most rigorous study to date,[268] which used molecular subtyping to conclusively identify CVC-related infections, the antiseptic catheter was associated with a two-fold reduction in catheter colonization and a five-fold reduction in catheter-related bloodstream infection (RR 0.21, $p = 0.03$). In-vitro analysis of 58 isolates from infected catheters in the two groups showed no evidence that use of the antiseptic catheter induced resistance to chlorhexidine and silver sulfadiazine. Use of the antiseptic catheter was shown to be highly cost effective if baseline rates of catheter-related blood infection exceeded 2% (3.3 per 1000 IVD-days).

Recent meta-analyses by Veenstra et al[326] and Mermel[311] have shown that chlorhexidine–silver sulfadiazine-impregnated CVCs reduce rates of catheter related infection by at least 40% (OR 0.40–0.56). Veenstra et al have also published analyses suggesting that use of the antiseptic catheter is cost-effective if the baseline incidence of CVC-related infection is greater than 0.4 per 1000 IVD-days,[327,328] they project that $59 000 will be saved, seven cases of bloodstream infection avoided and one death prevented for every 300 antiseptic catheters used.

Raad et al proposed the use of a minocycline-rifampicin-coated catheter, based on in-vitro and animal data demonstrating potent activity of this novel combination against Gram-positive, and Gram-negative organisms and *Candida albicans*.[329,330] A randomized clinical trial with nearly 300 short-term CVCs found that the coated catheters were associated with greatly reduced catheter colonization (8% versus 26%; $p = < 0.001$) and CVC-related infection (0% versus 5%; $p = <0.01$).[269] No resistance to the minocycline–rifampicin combination was detected.

A multicenter trial comparing minocycline-rifampicin-coated and chlorhexidine–silver sulfadiazine-impregnated CVCs found that antibiotic-coated catheters were far less likely to be colonized at removal (RR 0.34, $p < 0.001$).[331] While Kaplan–Meier analysis showed the two catheters to be equivalent with regard to the risk of catheter-related blood infection until day 7, overall rates of such infection were much lower among patients with the minocycline–rifampicin-coated catheter (0.3 versus 4.1 per 1000 IVD-days $p = <0.001$).

The major theoretical deterrents to using antibiotics for coating percutaneous intravascular catheters are the ineffectiveness of antibiotics against antibiotic-resistant nosocomial bacteria and yeasts, the risk of promoting bacterial resistance with long-term topical use[332,333] and potential for hypersensitization.[334] Although no induction of resistance to minocycline–rifampicin has been identified in the three clinical trials to date,[269,331,335] an in-vitro study has shown that resistance can develop.[336] It would seem of high priority that future studies carefully evaluate the long-term impact of anti-infective-coated catheters on nosocomial microbial resistance.

Two second-generation silver-impregnated catheters have been studied clinically. The Erlanger® catheter uses a microdispersed silver technology to greatly increase the quantity of available ionized silver and has been evaluated in two trials.[337,338] Adult patients randomized to the Erlanger® catheter had lower rates of catheter colonization and rates of 'catheter-associated sepsis' than those in the control catheter arm (5.3 versus 18.3 per 1000 IVD-days, $p = <0.05$).

A novel silver-impregnated CVC utilizing oligodynamic iontophoretic technology has also been developed and evaluated in two clinical trials. This novel catheter incorporates both silver and platinum in the polyurethane, putatively increasing the surface release of silver ions. A single randomized clinical trial, while underpowered, found a trend towards reduced catheter-related bloodstream infection with the use of this catheter (4% versus 12%; $p = 0.09$).[339] A larger trial that used historical controls, demonstrated rates of CVC-related infections in the year after the silver-platinum catheter was introduced markedly lower than rates seen in the years when standard polyurethane CVCs were in use (0% versus 4%; $p = <0.001$).[340]

Anti-infective hubs

A novel hub developed by Segura et al (Segur-Lock®, Inibsa Laboratories) contains a connecting chamber filled with iodinated alcohol and was shown in a randomized clinical trial to be associated with greatly reduced rates of catheter colonization and CVC-related bloodstream infection (4% versus 16%; $p = <0.01$),[341] although a subsequent trial failed to show benefit with the use of this hub.[342] Another model, using a povidone-iodine saturated sponge to encase the hub, also showed significant reductions in CVC-related infection, compared to a control hub (0% versus 24%, $P = <0.05$).[343]

Antibiotic lock therapy

Prophylactic use of systemic antibiotics at the time of IVD implantation has not proven effective in reducing the incidence of IVD-related bloodstream infections and is strongly discouraged.[313] However, studies of continuous infusion of vancomycin, incorporated into total parenteral nutrition admixtures, have shown reduced rates of coagulase-negative staphylococcal bacteremia in low-birth-weight infants.[344] Unfortunately, this form of prophylaxis results in prolonged low blood levels of vancomycin, which may be conducive to promoting resistance.

The 'antibiotic lock' is a novel technique of local prophylaxis: an antibiotic solution is instilled into the catheter lumen and allowed to dwell for a defined period of time, usually 6–12 hours, after which it is removed. There have been six prospective randomized trials of antibiotic lock solutions for the prevention of bloodstream infections with long-term IVDs. The largest trial and most recent trial by Henrickson et al[345] randomized 126 pediatric oncology patients (36 944 IVD-days) who had recently had a tunneled CVC implanted to three prophylactic lock regimens: heparin (10 U/ml) (control); heparin and vancomycin (25 µg/ml); and heparin, vancomycin and ciprofloxacin (2 µg/ml). Use of the vancomycin-ciprofloxacin containing lock solution was associated with a markedly lower rate of IVD-related infection, than that with heparin alone (0.55 versus 1.72 per 1000 IVD-days; $p = 0.005$). Similarly, the rate of infection with vancomycin-containing lock solution was significantly reduced (0.37 per 1000 IVD-days; $p = 0.004$). The two antimicrobial lock solutions showed comparable protection against Gram-positive and Gram-negative IVD-related infection. Unfortunately, failure to separate local infections from bloodstream infections in the final data limits analysis of the results of this study. While rates of nosocomial colonization or infection with vancomycin-resistant enterococci, as detected by clinical cultures ordered by patients' physicians, were comparable in the three groups, no effort was made to proactively assess the impact of antibiotic-containing lock solu-

tions on nosocomial colonization by vancomycin-resistant enterococci, MRSA and fluoroquinolone-resistant Gram-negative bacilli.

Most studies used a lock solution containing vancomycin. It seems unlikely that micro-organisms in the exposed patient's flora could develop resistance to vancomycin from the minute quantities of drug in a catheter lumen (<15 µg), yet there is just concern over the possible effect of wide prophylactic use of vancomycin lock solutions, and more data are needed before their routine use can be recommended, specifically, randomized studies that prospectively assess the impact on nosocomial colonization by resistant micro-organisms. However, because antibiotic lock solutions clearly reduce the risk of implant-related infections with long-term IVDs, the new HICPAC Guideline considers their use acceptable in individual cases in which a patient who requires indefinite vascular access continues to experience such infections despite maximal compliance with infection control guidelines.[313]

INFECTION OF CEREBROSPINAL FLUID SHUNTS

EPIDEMIOLOGY

Cerebrospinal fluid (CSF) shunts are widely used for surgical decompression and diversion of excess CSF in the management of hydrocephalus. Approximately 25 000 shunt procedures are performed in the USA annually, making it the most commonly performed neurosurgical operation.[346] While considerable success in the treatment of hydrocephalus has been achieved, the most serious complication remains infection. Early studies reported rates of CSF shunt infection ranging from 1.5 to 39% (mean 10–15%);[347,348] however, during the past two decades infection rates have dropped to 2–9%.[349–352] Most reported series are from infant and pediatric populations, as most shunts are placed for treatment of congenital hydrocephalus. Ventricular shunt infection rates range from 3.9 to 5.2%[353] in the most recent US national nosocomial infection surveillance report, with the highest risk in children, particularly premature infants,[354] and elderly people.[349] CSF shunt infections are associated with a mortality of 20–50%,[355,356] prolonged stay in hospital, and an increased risk of seizure disorder[357] and decreased intellectual performance in survivors.[358]

A CSF shunt system consists of a catheter placed either in the ventricle or the lumbar subarachnoid space which is connected to a subcutaneous silastic tube through which CSF drains into the central great veins, the pleural space or, most commonly, the peritoneum. A reservoir to allow percutaneous access for CSF sampling and intraventricular administration of antibiotics or chemotherapy may be incorporated (e.g., Hakim system) or may be independent (Rickham or Ommaya reservoir). Pressure-regulating valves are also usually integrated into the system.

A variety of different shunt systems have been evaluated but ventriculoatrial (VA) and ventriculoperitoneal (VP) shunts have been employed most widely in clinical practice (Figure 45.4). VP shunting has become the diversion procedure of choice because of its shorter operative time and the need for fewer revisions than VA shunts.[359] The rate of infection does not appear to differ greatly between VA and VP shunts.[360]

A number of studies have identified risk factors that predispose to the occurrence of shunt-related ventriculitis or meningitis. One large, recent prospective study of 299 patients using multivariable techniques of data analysis found the presence of a CSF leak (odds ratio 19.2), infant prematurity (odds ratio 4.7) and a breach in surgical asepsis (odds ratio 1.07) to be the most important risk factors for shunt infection.[363] Other risk factors include younger age (10–20% rates of infection in infants <6 months of age)[354,364] and high cutaneous floral density.[365]

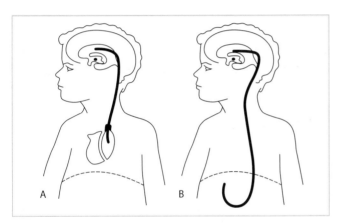

Fig. 45.4 Schematic of (A) ventriculoatrial (VA) and (B) ventriculoperitoneal (VP) cerebrospinal fluid shunts.

PATHOGENESIS

Micro-organisms gain access to the shunt by three routes: (1) intraoperative colonization; (2) hematogenous seeding of the shunt; or (3) retrograde spread of infection from the distal portion of the catheter, such as the peritoneal cavity or bloodstream. Intraoperative contamination of the shunt is widely considered to be most important, since 80% of infections occur within 6 months of surgery.[347–349] Bayston et al compared organisms cultured from the surgical wound at the time of shunt insertion or revision with those cultured from the patient's nose, ear or skin before operation:[366] 58% of wounds were colonized, and in one-half the colonizing organism originated from the patient's own flora. The level of contamination of the wound was directly proportional to the duration of the surgical procedure. More recently, airborne bacteria in the operating room have been identified as an important source of shunt infection.[367]

Three factors play a central role in the development of shunt infection: the microbial inoculum; microbial virulence, and the patient's host defenses. CSF shunt implantation is a clean neu-

rosurgical procedure; hence, the inoculum should be small. Coagulase-negative staphylococci cause most infections and are of low intrinsic virulence. Host defenses are severely impaired, however, because of the foreign body nature of the shunt.[368] The pressure valves have been found to be the most heavily colonized portion of an infected shunt.[368]

Bacteremia from a remote source can also cause secondary infection of CSF shunts. The frequency of VP shunt infection by this route is unclear but is thought to be low. VA shunts, however, are continuously and directly exposed to potential infection by silent transient bacteremias. Reports of late *Haemophilus influenzae* with VA shunts infections in children affirm the potential for hematogenous infection of these devices.[369]

Infection of the distal portion of a VP shunt may derive from perforation of an intra-abdominal viscus or pelvic inflammatory disease in women, with retrograde extension of infection throughout the drainage tubing and valve apparatus.[370] Although lumbo-ureteral shunts are now rarely used, retrograde infection by Gram-negative bacilli derive from silent bacteriuria.[371]

MICROBIOLOGY

Staphylococcus epidermidis and other coagulase-negative staphylococci are responsible for the vast majority of CSF shunt infections,[347,355,372,373] and *Staph. aureus* causes about 25% of cases (Table 45.5). Gram-negative enteric bacteria and *Pseudomonas* spp. account for about 5–10% of infections and are associated with greater morbidity and mortality.[374]

Anaerobic organisms, particularly *Propionibacterium* species, account for 3–20% of infections in various series.[375] Polymicrobial infection must prompt suspicion of bowel perforation as the source.[376] Fungal infections, fortunately, are rare, accounting for less than 1% of infections; *C. albicans* is the leading pathogen,[377] although infections with *Coccidioides immitis*,[378] *Cryptococcus neoformans*[379] and *Histoplasma capsulatum*[380] have been reported.

Table 45.5 Microbiologic profile of CSF shunt infections[a]

Organism	Incidence (%)
Staphylococcus epidermidis	60–70
Staphylococcus aureus	12–25
Streptococcal species	8–10
Enteric Gram-negative bacilli	6–20
Anaerobes	6
Diphtheroids	1–14
Organisms of traditional meningitis[b]	2–8

[a] Pooled data.[347,355,372,373]
[b] *H. influenzae*, *Str. pneumoniae* and *N. meningitidis*

DIAGNOSIS

The clinical manifestations and diagnostic approach to shunt infections vary, depending in part on the type and location of the shunt. Fever is the most common manifestation of infection with all types of shunts but is not universally present, especially if the infecting organism is CNS.[347,381] With proximal infection (ventriculitis), headache may be absent and non-specific symptoms such as lethargy and malaise may be the only clinical clues to infection; meningismus is present in less than one-third of cases.[382]

Complications of VA shunt infections include septic pulmonary emboli,[383] perforation of the myocardium leading to tamponade,[384] perforation of the interatrial septum, superior or inferior vena caval obstruction,[385] atrial thrombus[386] and right-sided endocarditis.[387] A rare manifestation of chronic VA shunt infection is shunt nephritis,[388] caused by deposition of antigen–antibody complexes onto the glomerular basement membrane, similar to the immune complex nephritis of bacterial endocarditis. The nephritis characteristically resolves when the underlying shunt infection is eradicated.[388]

Up to one-third of patients with VP shunts present with abdominal symptoms. A loculated CSF collection often develops; however, if encystation by the peritoneum is unsuccessful, frank peritonitis may occur.[389] The presence of a peritoneal pseudocyst in a patient with a VP shunt almost always indicates shunt infection.[390] VP shunts are also well known to spontaneously perforate the bowel. In the early postoperative period, local signs of inflammation with wound infection or infection of the subcutaneous course of the drainage tubing may be present. The first indication of occult infection is often shunt malfunction.[391] Occult infection must be ruled out in every case of shunt malfunction.

The diagnosis of shunt infection requires a high index of suspicion because of its insidious and frequently nonspecific presentation. Fever in a shunted patient should always prompt suspicion of shunt infection. Blood cultures reliably identify the causative organism in 95% of VA shunt infections;[392] in contrast only 20% of VP infected shunts produce bacteremia.[348]

The peripheral white blood cell count (WBC) is of limited value in diagnosing shunt infection; up to 25% of patients have a normal WBC count.[393] CSF leukocytosis is also usually modest: one study reported a median CSF WBC count of 79 cells/mm^3.[348] Gram-stained smears of CSF were positive in the majority of cases of infection with *Staph. aureus* and Gram-negative bacilli (82% and 91% respectively) but in only a minute fraction of cases (4%) caused by coagulase-negative staphylococci.[372] Other CSF changes are rarely helpful in the diagnosis: hypoglycorrachia is infrequent and slight, when present;[394] protein elevation is often present but is non-specific.[372]

Cultures of CSF obtained from the shunt are essential to establish the diagnosis and are positive in 90% of patients when pleocytosis is > 100 white cells/mm^3, but only 50% of patients when pleocytosis is <20 white cells/mm^3.[347] The highest yield is when the CSF is aspirated directly from the shunt (92%).[394]

Radiologic imaging is useful if the patient has abdominal symptoms or a palpable mass, to evaluate for the presence of a peritoneal pseudocyst, which almost always signifies infection. If the shunt is malfunctioning, brain imaging may show hydrocephalus.

TREATMENT

Management of the shunt

Once CSF shunt infection is diagnosed, usually by a positive CSF culture, options for treatment include;

- complete removal of the shunt apparatus, delaying replacement until the infection has been eradicated with parenteral antibiotics;
- surgical removal of the shunt, temporary external CSF drainage, parenteral antimicrobial therapy, with shunt replacement after the infection has been eradicated;
- externalization of distal portion of shunt (for VP shunts), followed by delayed replacement, in conjunction with systemic antimicrobial therapy;
- retention of shunt, attempting to eradicate the infection with antibiotic therapy alone.

All of these approaches, except the last, subject the patient to one or more surgical procedures, with attendant risks. The most widely accepted approach has been complete removal of the entire shunt apparatus, followed by prolonged antimicrobial therapy, with later implantation of a new shunt on the contralateral side.[356,372,381,395] If CSF drainage is necessary during the interim period temporary external CSF drainage can be provided with a ventriculostomy catheter.

In a prospective randomized study, James et al compared three groups of patients with VP shunt infections who were treated by three different approaches:[355] one group underwent shunt removal, systemic antibiotic therapy and external ventricular drainage; the second, shunt removal with immediate shunt replacement, followed by intrashunt antibiotic therapy; and the third, systemic and intraventricular antibiotic therapy alone without shunt removal. The cure rates were 100%, 90% and 30%, respectively. The group that received antimicrobial therapy alone had a much longer hospital course and two of the ten patients died. Larger retrospective series have corroborated these results (Table 45.6), and removal of an infected shunt is considered mandatory to achieve reliable cure of shunt infections.[347,392]

McLaurin et al have suggested that some VP shunt infections may be cured without removing the ventricular portion of the apparatus, by externalizing the peritoneal catheter and closed system drainage, combined with intraventricular and systemic antimicrobial therapy;[396] of 11 patients with VP shunts (age range three weeks to 14 years), 10 were reportedly cured of infection with this approach. Follow-up periods ranged from 4 months to 5 years. However, in a more recent study, externalization of distal tubing with retention of the

Table 45.6 Cure rates with different approaches to management of CSF shunt infection: an analysis of 20 series published between 1975 and 1987[a]

	Antibiotics alone	Antibiotics + shunt removal + immediate shunt replacement	Antibiotics + shunt removal + external ventriculostomy + delayed shunt replacement
No. treated	254	161	227
No. cured	95 (37%)	114 (71%)	213 (94%)

[a] Adapted from Bisno and Sturnau, 1994.[548]

shunt and systemic antimicrobial therapy in patients with VP shunt infections showed persistently positive CSF cultures in 10 of 21 patients.[397] The most common infecting organisms were coagulase-negative staphylococci.

Meningitis due to fastidious, highly sensitive organisms that reach the CSF from the primary bloodstream infections (e.g. *H. influenzae*, *Str. pneumoniae* and *Neisseria meningitidis*) has been treated successfully without shunt removal.[369]

Antimicrobial therapy

Several factors must be taken into consideration when choosing systemic antimicrobial therapy, including: CSF penetration of the agent; susceptibility of the infecting organism; and the potential for neurotoxicity. Nearly 90% of coagulase-negative staphylococcal infections acquired in the hospital implicated in shunt infections are now resistant to methicillin,[353] and vancomycin is thus the drug of choice for most Gram-positive infections. Although its CSF penetration is modest, with meningeal inflammation it is usually possible to achieve therapeutic CSF levels.[398] Rifampicin is often added for enhanced bactericidal activity, high CSF penetration, in-vitro synergism with vancomycin and β-lactams, and its adjunctive value in other device-related infections.[105,125–127] For Gram-negative infections, group 4 cephalosporins or carbapenems, such as imipenem, provide effective treatment if the infecting organism is susceptible, however, with imipenem use in the setting of meningitis or ventriculitis, the risk of seizures is considerable (33% in some series);[399] meropenem appears to pose a lower risk.[400]

Intraventricular antimicrobial therapy has been extensively used in the past, with or without systemically administered antibiotics for treatment of CSF shunt infections, although the indications for intraventricular therapy are uncertain.[401] The most commonly used intraventricular antimicrobials have been the aminoglycosides and vancomycin.

Intrathecal aminoglycosides have been widely used for the treatment of shunt infections,[402] however, ototoxicity has been encountered,[402,403] and no randomized trials have confirmed their benefit. The only prospective randomized trial to compare systemic to intrathecal administration of gentamicin, a study of neonates with Gram-negative meningitis, showed that mortality was higher in infants given intrathecal gentamicin (43%) than in those given systemic gentamicin (13%).[404] Some authors have recommended routine measurement of CSF aminoglycoside levels to reduce the risk of toxicity; however, accurate measurement of CSF drug levels is fraught with difficulty[401] and studies have failed to show a correlation between toxicity and CSF aminoglycoside levels,[405] even with peak levels as high as 450 mg/l[406] and trough levels as high as 76 mg/l.[407]

No prospective studies have compared the efficacy of intrathecal vancomycin with systemic vancomycin, although anecdotal reports suggest that intrathecal vancomycin therapy is beneficial.[408,409] Vancomycin penetrates the CSF poorly in the absence of inflammation,[410] and even in the presence of inflammation attains CSF levels only one-fifth of those it reaches in serum.[411] Vancomycin typically is administered intrathecally in doses of 5–20 mg per 24 h. There have been no reports of neurotoxicity, even with CSF levels as high as 100 mg/l.[364]

Intraventricular β-lactams and cephalosporins cause seizures and neurological deficits and their use is strongly discouraged.[412]

Antimicrobials given intrathecally should be constituted in a preservative-free medium to reduce the risk of arachnoiditis. In general, removal of the infected shunt and intravenous antibiotic therapy will prove effective in the vast majority of cases, and intraventricular antibiotic therapy should be used only if there is reason to believe that therapeutic CSF concentrations cannot be achieved with systemically administered antibiotics, such as in patients with severe scarring of the choroid plexus or if the antimicrobial of choice is known to have poor CSF penetration, such as an aminoglycoside.

There is a paucity of clinical data regarding the duration of therapy for CSF shunt infections; a minimum of 7 days has been suggested, with the final duration influenced by the rapidity of clinical improvement and results of serial CSF cultures.[364]

PREVENTION

As it appears that intraoperative contamination by skin flora or airborne skin organisms is the most important mechanism of infection of CSF shunts, efforts have been directed at improving intraoperative asepsis and reducing contamination of the operative field. Novel measures that have been evaluated include adhesive plastic drapes,[413] use of ultraviolet lights in the operating room,[414] soaking shunts in an antimicrobial solution[415] and irrigating the wound with an antibiotic solution.[416] None has been evaluated in a randomized trial, and thus most cannot be routinely recommended.

Faillace et al reported a meticulous 'no-touch' protocol for CSF shunt implantation,[417] which involved minimal handling of shunt components during implantation through use of special instruments, placing the shunt on a separate table away from skin dissection instruments, limiting the number of personnel in the operating room, and intensive education of surgical assistants and nurses: a threefold decrease in the rate of shunt infection was observed, from 9.1% before implementation of the new protocol to 2.9% (odds ratio 0.30; $P = 0.05$).

Choux et al employed an even more intensive perioperative protocol, including not shaving the operative site, using chlorhexidine or povidone-iodine for site disinfection, implantation early in the morning before other operations, single-dose perioperative prophylaxis, meticulous surgical technique and limiting the implantation procedure to 40 minutes.[418] With adoption of these measures, the authors observed a decreased infection rate from 7% to 0.2%. However, because so many modifications of the surgical procedure were made, it is difficult to draw conclusions about the independent role of each measure. While most neurosurgeons shave their patients preoperatively, randomized trials have shown that shaving may increase the risk of CSF shunt infection.[419]

The use of perioperative prophylactic antibiotics for shunt implantation procedures has been controversial.[420] Most studies have suffered from methodologic problems: most were uncontrolled, retrospective comparisons. Few of the randomized trials done were adequately powered to detect a clear-cut benefit from use of preoperative prophylactic antibiotic therapy. In one prospective trial of 243 patients undergoing 300 CSF shunt implantations, oral trimethoprim and rifampicin were administered 2 h before surgery and for 48 h postoperatively.[421] A lower infection rate (12%) was found in the treatment group than the placebo group (19%); however, the results did not achieve statistical significance. In another randomized trial, Blomstedt reported significantly fewer infections among patients receiving perioperative trimethoprim–sulfamethoxazole than those receiving placebo;[422] however, children less than 12 years of age were excluded from the study, and the 29% baseline rate of infection is very high.

Bayston et al determined that a randomized trial with power to detect a statistically significant difference, if one exists, would require 712 patients.[423] Their multicenter trial was not able to achieve this goal and was terminated after 2.5 years.[423] Several meta-analyses have attempted to resolve this issue.[350,424,425] Two suggest benefit;[424,425] one early and smaller meta-analysis did not:[350] Haines et al found a 50% risk reduction from prophylactic antibiotic use with a baseline infection rate above 5%;[425] Langley et al in a meta-analysis of 12 randomized trials came to a similar conclusion.[424] It thus appears that short-term perioperative antimicrobial prophylaxis may be of benefit in preventing shunt infections: anti-staphylococcal antibiotics, such as cefuroxime or trimethoprim–sulfamethoxazole, are recommended.

Novel technology

Incorporation of antibiotics into the shunt material has been attempted to decrease the incidence of shunt infection. Bayston et al demonstrated that impregnation of silicone rubber with clindamycin hydrochloride was effective in preventing in-vitro bacterial colonization by *Staph. epidermidis* for as long as 9 days.[426] The same authors also showed that catheters impregnated with clindamycin and rifampicin resisted three successive challenge doses of *Staph. epidermidis* over a 28-day period[427] as well as biweekly challenges with strains of *Staph. aureus* and *Staph. epidermidis* over periods as long as 56 days.[428] While these in-vitro studies are promising, the efficacy, thrombogenic and epileptogenic potential of medicated shunts must be evaluated by randomized clinical trials before they can be recommended.

An ineffective immune response against infection in infants is thought to contribute to the higher infections rates of CSF shunts in patients less than one year of age. A prospective randomized trial of administering a single dose of intravenous immunoglobulin prior to shunt implantation in infants showed a lower rate of infection in the group given immunoglobulin (0 versus 5.1%), however, the study was underpowered (60 patients), and the results did not achieve statistical significance.[429]

VENTRICULOSTOMY-RELATED INFECTIONS

EPIDEMIOLOGY

Intracranial pressure monitoring has become essential for the management of patients with closed head injuries or who have undergone major neurosurgical operations.[430,431] Techniques used to measure intracranial pressure include use of ventriculostomy catheters (72%), intraparenchymal catheters (47%), subarachnoid bolts (25%), epidural catheters (15%) and subdural catheters (5%).[432] The most accurate and widely used method to continuously measure intracranial pressure is by placement of an intraventricular catheter through a burr hole into the lateral ventricle. Unfortunately, ventriculostomy catheters are associated with a substantial risk of ventriculitis and meningitis, which has significant morbidity.[431,433]

Infection is the primary complication associated with the use of ventriculostomies, ranging from 0 to 40%.[433–440] Most studies average 10%[431] and a large meta-analysis, which included more than 6000 patients, found an overall rate of infection of 5.8%.[441] Prospective studies indicate that the greatest risk factor for development of ventriculostomy-related infection is the duration of ventricular catheterization.[433,437] Mayhall et al, in the largest prospective study, found that the risk of infection rose to 9% after 5 days of catheterization (RR, 7.0).[433] Paramore et al found that the rate of infection rose to 10.3% by the sixth day.[430] Irrigation of the system,[433] intracerebral or intraventricular hemorrhage (RR 3.5)[433,437] and high intracranial pressures[433] have also been found to increase the risk of nosocomial ventriculitis.

PATHOGENESIS AND MICROBIOLOGY

The pathogenesis of ventriculostomy-related infection is poorly understood: infecting organisms can be introduced at the time of catheter insertion, but probably more often gain access during later manipulation of the system for CSF drainage or calibration.[440]

Ventriculostomy-related infection is very similar to post-operative neurosurgical wound infection. The most common infecting micro-organisms have been coagulase-negative staphylococci and *Staph. aureus*, which cause 60–80% of all cases;[433,442] however, a significant number of cases of nosocomial meningitis are caused by Gram-negative bacilli, ranging from 16 to 33%.[443,444]

TREATMENT

Similar to the treatment of CSF shunt infections, the treatment of ventriculostomy-related infection should be guided by the results of the CSF Gram-stain and culture. If feasible, the catheter should be removed unless intrathecal therapy is considered essential (e.g. for *Ps. aeruginosa* ventriculitis). For most nosocomial staphylococcal infections, intravenous vancomycin and oral rifampicin are required, unless in-vitro susceptibility testing shows susceptibility to β-lactams.

For ventriculitis caused by Gram-negative bacilli, a cephalosporin such as cefepime or cefotaxime or a carbapenem (meropenem, rather than imipenem, given the higher risk of seizures with the latter[400]), with or without ciprofloxacin, should prove effective in most cases.

As noted, the role of intraventricular antimicrobial therapy in the treatment of CSF infections related to neurosurgery is undefined, but its use should be considered in patients who fail to improve despite the use of appropriate systemic antimicrobial therapy.

PREVENTION

Prevention of catheter-related ventriculitis begins with limiting the duration of catheterization to the fewest days necessary and maintaining a stringently closed system. Mayhall et al have recommended relocating the ventricular catheter to a new site if monitoring exceeds 5 days;[433] however, the risks associated with placement of a new ventriculostomy catheter, especially intracranial hemorrhage, have been estimated to be as high as 6%.[430]

Data on the prophylactic use of antibiotics at the time of catheter insertion and/or throughout the duration of ventricular catheterization are also conflicting. Of five retrospective[431,434–436,438] and two prospective trials,[433,437] only two retrospective studies found the use of antimicrobial prophylaxis to be beneficial.[434,435]

One randomized trial in 228 patients receiving ventriculostomy catheters compared brief perioperative administration of prophylactic antibiotics with prolonged prophylaxis, in which the patients received therapy for the entire period of catheterization, and showed a lower infection rate in patients receiving prolonged prophylaxis with ampicillin–sulbactam and aztreonam (3% versus 11%, $P = 0.01$).[445] However, the pathogens causing infection in patients receiving prolonged prophylaxis showed greater antimicrobial resistance. Two other randomized trials, one in 52 patients and the other in 95 patients, did not demonstrate any benefit from prophylactic antibiotic use, but the studies were severely underpowered.[422,446] Prophylactic antibiotics to prevent monitoring-related ventriculitis with ventriculostomy catheters are probably not effective, are likely to promote infection by multiresistant pathogens, and based on current data, are not recommended.

CATHETER-ASSOCIATED URINARY TRACT INFECTIONS

EPIDEMIOLOGY

Catheter-associated urinary tract infections (CAUTIs) account for 40% of all nosocomial infections in the USA, affecting an estimated 800 000 patients per year.[447] In the 25% of patients that have a urinary catheter inserted at some time during their hospital stay the incidence of nosocomial UTI is approximately 5% per day, with virtually all patients developing bacteriuria by 30 days of catheterization.[448] Even though the vast majority of these infections are asymptomatic,[449] silent CAUTIs comprise the largest pool of antibiotic-resistant pathogens in the hospital[353] and drive a great deal of generally unnecessary antibiotic therapy.

Large, prospective studies in which catheterized patients were cultured daily and which used multivariable techniques of statistical analysis have identified risk factors independently predictive of an increased risk for CAUTI:[450–453] females have a higher risk than males (RR, 2.5–3.7), and patients with other active sites of infection (RR, 2.3–2.4) or a major pre-existing chronic condition such as diabetes (RR, 2.2–2.3), malnutrition (RR, 2.4), or renal insufficiency (RR, 2.1–2.6), are also at higher risk; inserting the catheter outside the operating room (RR, 2.0–5.3) or late in hospitalization (RR, 2.6–8.6), the presence of a ureteral stent (RR, 2.5) or using the catheter to measure urine output (RR, 2.0) further increase risk. The most important modifiable risk factor, identified in every study, is prolonged catheterization – beyond six days. Antimicrobial therapy is protective against CAUTI for short-term catheterizations (RR, 0.1–0.4) but clearly selects for infection caused by multiresistant micro-organisms such as *Ps. aeruginosa* and other resistant Gram-negative bacilli, enterococci and yeasts.

A recent large, prospective study monitored compliance on a daily basis with seven recommended precepts for catheter care, including closed drainage, proper position of the drainage tubing and collection bag, and protection of the drainage port.[453] The only violation predictive of an increased risk of CAUTI was improper position of the drainage tube, above the level of the bladder or sagging below the level of the collection bag. This study suggests we may be at the point of diminishing returns in terms of behavioral modification for further reduction in CAUTI, and that technologic innovations will be needed to further reduce risk.

PATHOGENESIS

Excluding rare hematogenous pyelonephritis, most CAUTIs derive from micro-organisms in the patient's own colonic and perineal flora or transmitted from the hands of healthcare personnel during catheter insertion or manipulation of the collection system.[447,448] Organisms gain access extraluminally – by direct inoculation when the catheter is inserted or later, by organisms ascending from the perineum by capillary action in the thin mucous film contiguous to the external catheter surface – or intraluminally, by reflux of micro-organisms gaining access to the catheter lumen from failure of closed drainage or contamination of collection bag urine (Figure 45.5). Recent studies suggest that CAUTIs most frequently are extraluminally-acquired, but both routes are important.[454]

Infected urinary catheters are covered by a thick biofilm, which forms intraluminally, extraluminally or both, usually advancing in a retrograde fashion. Anti-infective-impregnated and silver-hydrogel catheters, which inhibit adherence of micro-organisms to the catheter surface, significantly reduce the risk of CAUTI,[455–458] particularly infections caused by Gram-positive organisms or yeasts, which are most likely to be acquired extraluminally from the periurethral flora. These data suggest that microbial adherence to the catheter surface is important in the pathogenesis of many, but not all, CAUTIs.

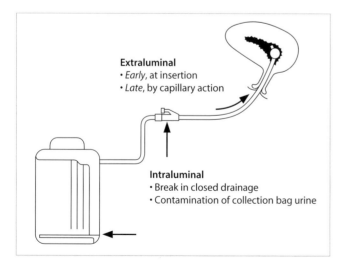

Fig. 45.5 Routes of microbial colonization in the pathogenesis of catheter-associated urinary tract infections (adapted from Maki and Tambyah, 2001[447]).

Infections in which the biofilm does not play a pathogenic role are probably caused by mass transport of intraluminal contaminants into the bladder by reflux of microbe-laden urine when a catheter or collection system is moved or manipulated.

MICROBIOLOGY

As noted, CAUTIs comprise the largest institutional reservoir of nosocomial antibiotic-resistant pathogens,[353,447] the most important of which are multidrug-resistant Enterobacteriaceae other than *Escherichia coli* (such as *Klebsiella*, *Enterobacter*, *Proteus*, and *Citrobacter* spp.) *Ps. aeruginosa*, enterococci and staphylococci, and *Candida* spp. (Figure 45.6).

DIAGNOSIS

Clinical presentation

Classically, urinary tract infections (UTIs) in non-catheterized patients present with dysuria and frequency, often associated with lower abdominal pain or even flank pain. The irritating effects of a urinary catheter can mimic some of these symptoms in the absence of infection, and thus corroborating evidence of CAUTI is needed before initiation of antimicrobial therapy.

Although there have been recommendations to treat CAUTIs only when they are symptomatic,[264] until recently the symptoms associated with CAUTI had not been clearly defined. In a recent prospective study of 1497 newly catheterized patients, over half of whom were in an ICU, undertaken to determine the prevalence of signs and symptoms attributable to CAUTI and the relative contribution of CAUTI to nosocomial bloodstream infections, quantitative urine cultures and urine leukocyte counts were taken daily and each patient was questioned by a research nurse regarding symptoms.[449] In this study, there were no significant differences between patients with and without CAUTI in subjective symptoms commonly associated with urinary tract infection; most were afebrile. There were also no significant differences between the two groups in mean peripheral leukocyte counts, although the urine WBCs in patients with CAUTI were significantly higher than in uninfected catheterized patients. Of 79 nosocomial bloodstream infections identified in the study population, there was only one that appeared unequivocally to have derived from a CAUTI; interestingly, this patient had no symptoms referable to the urinary tract.

This study shows that, although a large proportion of patients with indwelling urinary catheters develop bacteriuria, fewer than 10% with microbiologically documented CAUTI (most with active infection and pyuria for many days) report any symptoms commonly associated with community-acquired UTI unrelated to a urinary catheter, such as dysuria, urgency, fever or chills. Symptoms referable to the urinary tract not only are infrequent in patients with UTI but also have little pre-

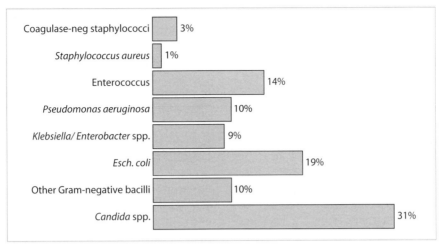

Fig. 45.6 Microbiologic profile of catheter-associated urinary tract infection, based on data from the National Nosocomial Infection Surveillance system report.[353]

dictive value for the diagnosis of infection. Moreover, despite their ubiquity, CAUTIs only rarely cause secondary bloodstream infection.

An association between fever and CAUTI has not been convincingly demonstrated in other studies. In a prospective study of elderly patients in nursing homes, Kunin et al found that, although 74% of catheterized patients ultimately developed CAUTI, fewer than 2% had temperatures higher than 38 °C.[459] More recently, in a study of the contribution of CAUTI to febrile morbidity in a long-term care facility, CAUTI was found to be the cause of fewer than 10% of episodes of fever, despite the high prevalence of bacteriuria.[460] Warren et al evaluated 47 women in a nursing home with long-term urinary catheters, all of whom had chronic bacteriuria, and reported a very low incidence of febrile episodes of urinary tract origin.[461]

All of these data show clearly that although CAUTI is common in catheterized patients, including in the ICU, fever and symptoms referable to the urinary tract are very infrequent in patients with UTI and have little predictive value for the diagnosis of infection.

Laboratory tests

Pyuria has become universally regarded as an essential criterion for the diagnosis and management of urinary tract infection in the non-catheterized patient.[462] However, studies that have examined the utility of quantitative pyuria in catheterized patients have found conflicting results on its prognostic value.[463,464] In a study of 761 hospital patients with newly inserted indwelling urinary catheters,[465] Tambyah et al found that 82 (10.8%) patients studied developed CAUTI while catheterized, and the mean urine WBC in patients with CAUTI was significantly higher than in patients without infection (71 vs. 4 per mm^3; $P = 0.006$). However, using a urine WBC count greater than 10 per mm^3 (>5 per high-powered field in a conventional urinalysis) as the cutoff for defining its

presence, pyuria had a specificity of 90% for predicting CAUTI with >10^5 cfu/ml but a sensitivity of only 37%.

The clinical relevance of this study seems clear: pyuria cannot and should not be used as the sole criterion for obtaining a urine culture in the catheterized patient. This is especially true in the case of infections caused by yeasts or Gram-positive cocci,[466,467] which account for nearly one-half of nosocomial CAUTIs in the ICU. It is clear that most patients with CAUTI are asymptomatic and do not have fever.[449] If a catheterized patient develops fever or signs of sepsis that cannot be linked to another source such as nosocomial pneumonia, surgical site infection or vascular catheter-related infection,[264] urine cultures should be obtained even if the patient does not have demonstrable pyuria.

In the outpatient setting, particularly in clinics that may not have rapid access to laboratory testing, non-cultural rapid diagnostic tests are widely used, most commonly the leukocyte esterase and bacterial nitrite rapid dipstick tests. These tests have shown excellent sensitivity in non-catheterized patients with a high pre-test probability of UTI because of characteristic symptoms; however, in a non-selected patient population sensitivity of the tests has been poor, in the range of 50%.[468] In a recent prospective study of the leukocyte esterase and nitrite urinary dipstick in catheterized ICU patients, the sensitivity (50 and 79%), specificity (48 and 55%), and predictive value (60 and 81%) of both tests were poor.[469]

Gram stains of urine, of either unspun or centrifuged specimens, have high sensitivity and specificity for detection of high-level quantitative bacteriuria (>10^5 CFU/per ml), with specificity and positive and negative predictive values all greater than 90%.[470] However, inexplicably, clinicians encountering patients with symptomatic UTI or even frank urosepsis rarely use Gram stains. A Gram stain of urine is simple, can be done rapidly, and is highly reliable (>90%) for detecting bacteriuria or candiduria; moreover, it permits immediate determination of whether the infection is caused by Gram-negative bacilli,

Gram-positive cocci such as enterococci or staphylococci, or yeasts, such as *Candida* Spp.

Microbiologic studies

In clinical practice, a quantitative culture of a spontaneously voided, clean-catch urine specimen showing >10^5 cfu/ml is widely considered to represent infection.[462] Studies have shown that a count >10^2 cfu/ml of enteric Gram-negative bacilli recovered in culture of a clean catch specimen from a woman with pyuria and symptoms of UTI correlates highly with recovery of the same organism from bladder urine obtained by urethral catheterization or suprapubic aspiration, and can reliably be considered to represent true lower urinary tract infection, i.e. cystourethritis.[471]

Because urine cultures obtained by aspiration from an indwelling urethral catheter bypass potentially contaminating periurethral flora, it seemed likely that microbiologic concentrations considerably below 10^5 cfu/ml in a culture of urine taken from a catheterized patient might well be relevant pathogenetically, epidemiologically, and clinically. In a prospective study of 110 newly catheterized patients, low-level bacteriuria or candiduria (<10^5 cfu/ml), which developed in 41 patients, progressed to concentrations >10^5 cfu/ml 96% of the time (*P*<0.001), usually within 3 days of the first culture showing growth, unless the patient received intercurrent, suppressive antimicrobial therapy.[472] Even with very low-level bacteriuria or candiduria (1–99 organisms per ml), 90% of the cases progressed to high-level bacteria within 48–72 h, demonstrating that in the catheterized patient a considerably lower level of bacteriuria than 10^5 cfu/ml, (probably ≥ 10^2 cfu/ml) is valid as an index of infection; 10^2 cfu/ml is a concentration that can be easily and reproducibly detected in a clinical laboratory.

In sum, a quantitative urine culture showing growth but less than 10^5 cfu/ml should not reflexly be disregarded, especially if the patient is immunologically compromised or has clinical signs of UTI. In this circumstance, the culture result may reasonably form the basis for antimicrobial therapy if symptomatic CAUTI or, especially, urosepsis is suspected clinically.

TREATMENT

Only patients with symptomatic CAUTI should receive antimicrobial therapy; however, two clinical exceptions to this dictum exist: asymptomatic CAUTI in patients who are profoundly granulocytopenic[473] and patients who have silent CAUTI in association with urinary tract obstruction.[473] Urosepsis in the presence of obstruction rapidly converts silent bacteriuria to symptomatic urosepsis, which if unrelieved, culminates in bacteremia and septic shock. Harding et al reported that of 27 catheterized patients with asymptomatic catheter-associated bacteriuria seven (26%) developed symptoms referable to the urinary tract, but only *after* the catheter had been removed.[474]

In the absence of the above exceptions, empiric therapy may be initiated, in the symptomatic patient, based on the results of Gram stain and culture and then modified based on the results of in-vitro sensitivity testing. The optimal duration of therapy in patients with symptomatic CAUTI remains undefined, but in general, antimicrobials should be continued for 7–14 days.[475]

PREVENTION

Catheter-care practices universally recommended to prevent or at least delay the onset of CAUTI include[447,448] avoiding unnecessary catheterizations, using a condom or suprapubic catheter, having trained professionals insert catheters aseptically, removing the catheter as soon as it is no longer needed, maintaining uncompromising closed drainage, ensuring dependent drainage, minimizing manipulations of the system and geographically separating catheterized patients. While entirely defensible, few of these practices have been proven to be effective by randomized controlled trials.

Systemic antimicrobial prophylaxis with trimethoprim–sulfamethoxazole, methenamine mandelate, or especially, a fluoroquinolone[476] can reduce the risk of CAUTI for short-term catheterizations. Although use of antimicrobials in this way may reduce the rate of CAUTI, infections that do occur are far more likely to be caused by antibiotic-resistant bacteria and yeasts. Since most CAUTIs are asymptomatic and do not result in urosepsis,[449] it is difficult to justify antimicrobial prophylaxis to prevent asymptomatic bacteriuria.

Novel technology

Many technologic innovations proposed and evaluated during the past 25 years have not proven beneficial,[447,448] including the use of anti-infective lubricants when inserting the catheter, soaking the catheter in an antimicrobial solution before insertion, regular meatal cleansing or periodically applying anti-infective creams or ointments to the meatus, continuously irrigating the catheterized bladder with an anti-infective solution through a triple-lumen catheter or periodically instilling an anti-infective solution into the collection bag. Bladder irrigation with antimicrobial solution has not only shown no benefit for prevention but has also been associated with a strikingly increased proportion of CAUTIs caused by micro-organisms resistant to the drugs in the irrigating solution.[332]

Given the widely accepted importance of closed catheter drainage, efforts have been made to seal the connection between the catheter and collection tubing. An initial trial with a sealed junction showed modest benefit and suggested a reduction in hospital deaths; however, follow up studies have not demonstrated a reduction in CAUTI with a sealed catheter–collecting tube junction.[477]

Medicated catheters, which reduce adherence of micro-organisms to the catheter surface, may confer the greatest benefit for preventing CAUTI. Two catheters impregnated with anti-infectives have been evaluated clinically, one with the urinary antiseptic nitrofurazone[455] and the other with minocycline and rifampicin.[457] Both catheters showed a significant reduction in bacterial CAUTIs; however the studies were small and the impact of the coating on selection of antimicrobial-resistant uropathogens was not satisfactorily resolved. Coating the catheter surface with an antiseptic, such as a silver compound, offers another alternative to reduce the risk of CAUTI. Silver oxide-coated catheters, however, did not show efficacy in large, well-controlled trials.[451,452] In one trial, male patients receiving a coated catheter had a paradoxical and inexplicably increased risk of CAUTI.[452]

A silver-hydrogel catheter has been developed that inhibits adherence of micro-organisms to the catheter surface in vitro and has also been evaluated clinically.[456,458,478] In a recent, large, double-blind trial in 850 patients, the silver-hydrogel catheter reduced the incidence of CAUTI by 26%,[456] and was most effective in preventing infections caused by Gram-positive organisms, enterococci, staphylococci and *Candida*, microorganisms that appeared to gain access to the bladder extraluminally; the catheter conferred no protection against CAUTIs with Gram-negative bacilli, which most often gain access intraluminally. Use of the silver-hydrogel catheter was not associated with an increased incidence of infections caused by antibiotic-resistant organisms or *Candida*, and in-vitro susceptibility testing of isolates from both treatment groups showed no infections caused by silver-resistant micro-organisms. Cost-utility analysis indicates that use of this catheter could bring substantial cost savings to healthcare institutions.[447] In a large crossover trial of a silver-hydrogel catheter in 27 878 patients, Karchmer et al also found a lower risk of CAUTI with the novel catheter (RR 0.70; $p = 0.04$).[458]

INFECTIONS ASSOCIATED WITH PERITONEAL DIALYSIS CATHETERS

EPIDEMIOLOGY

It is estimated that 115 000 patients worldwide were maintained on peritoneal dialysis (PD) in 1997.[479] Nearly two-thirds of patients maintained on peritoneal dialysis in the United States receive continuous ambulatory PD (CAPD) while the remainder receive their dialysis by other mechanisms, such as continuous cycler PD (CCPD).[479]

Infection is the most common complication of PD, occurring at the catheter exit site; the catheter tunnel; or the peritoneum. Infection of the catheter exit site and the tunnel are relatively unusual but infection of the peritoneum is very common and remains the leading indication for conversion to hemodialysis in this population.[480] Between 63 and 90% of patients undergoing CAPD retain their catheters for 3 years,[481–483] although at least 60% will experience an episode of peritonitis within the first 12 months of initiating dialysis,

and 80% will have experienced at least one episode by 30 months.[484]

PATHOGENESIS

Infection of the peritoneum occurs by one of several routes:[485] intraluminal contamination of the catheter during dialysate exchange, migration of skin micro-organisms in the space contiguous to the external surface of the catheter, transmural migration of intestinal organisms, hematogenous seeding, extrinsic contamination of dialysate (mainly in association with CCPD) and transvaginal spread.

Considerable evidence suggests that most infections derive from contamination of the PD catheter, either extraluminally or, more often, intraluminally by the patient's endogenous skin flora: surveillance cultures from the patients' skin and peritoneal fluid have shown concordance,[486] use of Y systems, which reduce the number of times that patients are required to open their drainage system, has resulted in a significant decline in the incidence of CAPD.[487–490] Use of CCPD, which requires patients to access their PD catheters only once a day, has similarly been associated with reduced rates of peritonitis.[482,491] Finally, nasal carriers of *Staph. aureus* are more likely to develop concurrent *Staph. aureus* exit-site infections and peritonitis.[492,493]

The presence of a foreign body that is exposed to the external environment is the primary reason for the high rates of infection with PD; however, the presence of a large volume of non-physiologic fluid in the peritoneum impairs local host defenses, further increasing the risk of infection. Intraperitoneal activated macrophages and opsonins – immunoglobulin G and complement (C3) – are found in greatly reduced concentrations with repeated dialysate exchanges.[494,495] The high osmolarity and low pH of the dialysate, which has been shown to reduce granulocytic function in vitro,[496] may also contribute to susceptibility to infection.

MICROBIOLOGY

Table 45.7 summarizes the range and frequencies of pathogens causing PD-related peritonitis. Gram-positive organisms account for 60–80% of culture-proven cases. Unusual organisms include *Alcaligenes xylosidans, Stenotrophomonas maltophilia, Burkholderia cepacia, Agrobacterium* spp., *Mycobacterium* spp., and *Fusarium* spp.

In approximately 20% of cases, cultures of the peritoneal fluid fail to grow any organisms despite the presence of a large number of inflammatory cells. These patients usually respond to empiric antimicrobial therapy.

Staph. aureus accounts for approximately 50% of PD catheter exit site and tunnel infections, and coagulase-negative staphylococci are implicated in 30%.[479] In contrast to surgical peritonitis, Gram-negative bacilli are less commonly involved with PD catheter exit site and tunnel infections, with *Ps. aerug-*

Table 45.7 Distribution of micro-organisms causing peritoneal dialysis-related peritonitis.[a]

Organisms	%
Coagulase-negative staphylococci	30–40
Staphylococcus aureus	10–20
Streptococcus spp.	10–15
Enterococci	3–6
Escherichia coli	5–10
Pseudomonas spp.	5–10
Other Gram-negative bacilli	7–16
Anaerobic organisms	2–5
Fungi	2–10
Other	3–7
Culture negative	0–30

[a] Adapted from Vas, 1994.[486]

inosa and *Esch. coli* being isolated in 8% and 4% of cases, respectively.[479]

DIAGNOSIS

Patients with PD-related peritonitis present clinically with cloudy dialysate (98%), abdominal pain (79%)[479] and abdominal tenderness (70%), although frank rebound tenderness is infrequent (50%).[486] In contrast to surgical peritonitis, PD-related peritonitis is associated with fever only 53% of the time.[479] Nausea and vomiting are common (25% of cases); however, septic shock is unusual unless the infecting organism is *Staph. aureus*.

Exit-site infection usually manifests with erythema and crusting around the exit site. Frank purulence with fluctuance over the subcutaneous portion of the catheter suggests tunnel infection and is often associated with extrusion of the cuff.

The normal WBC in returned dialysate from uninfected patients is <8 white cells/mm^3; in contrast, 90% of patients with PD-related peritonitis will show a dialysate WBC >100/mm^3,[497] many >500/mm^3,[498] associated with a neutrophilic predominance. However, up to 15% present with monocytosis.[497] Delay in the rise of the dialysate WBC has been reported[499] and therefore abdominal pain in a patient with a PD catheter should be assessed with serial dialysate cell counts and cultures to rule out PD-related peritonitis. Lymphocytic pleocytosis may be the first clue to the presence of an usual organism, such as *Mycobacterium tuberculosis* or anomalous mycobacteria. Peritoneal eosinophilia has been described with fungal infections[500] and hypersensitivity to intraperitoneal antibiotics.[501]

Gram-stain of centrifuged dialysate is positive in only 9–28% of cases[497,502] but when positive is useful for guiding empiric antimicrobial therapy. Peripheral blood cultures are usually negative and in the absence of signs of sepsis their value is dubious. Whereas dialysate cultures are usually positive they remain sterile in up to 30% of cases. Negative cultures are thought to most often represent a failure of culture methods rather than infection with an unusual organism.[503] The most common mistakes are obtaining cultures too early in the course of peritonitis, before microbial counts rise to detectable levels; culturing inappropriately small volumes of dialysate (<10 ml);[504] and administration of antibiotics before obtaining cultures.[505] Persistently elevated cell counts despite appropriate empiric antibiotic therapy should raise suspicion of an unusual pathogen, such as *M. tuberculosis* or fungi, especially if monocytosis or eosinophilia is present, or a non-infectious cause, such as renal cell carcinoma, leukemia or peritoneal lymphoma.[479]

Plain films and CT scans of the abdomen are generally not useful or recommended, and often reveal a small volume of pneumoperitoneum that does not represent bowel perforation. However, if the patient presents with signs of sepsis or multiple organisms are seen on the Gram stain or recovered in culture, or if a large volume of free air is seen radiographically, a perforated viscus must be suspected, and appropriate combination antibiotic therapy and surgical consultation are indicated.

TREATMENT

Initial anti-infective therapy of PD-related peritonitis is based on the most likely infecting organisms, namely Gram-positive bacteria, unless the initial Gram-stain indicates to the contrary. Since PD-related peritonitis is a local infection, treatment with intraperitoneal antibiotics is preferred as very high levels are achieved quickly, as are therapeutic blood levels, with most antimicrobials.

Historically, concerns over infection caused by methicillin-resistant organisms led to the use of vancomycin in empiric regimens; however, the appearance of vancomycin resistance among enterococci[506] (and, even more alarmingly, among *Staph. aureus*[507]) has prompted recommendations to limit the empiric use of this critical antibiotic.[508] Empiric regimens that include a group 1 cephalosporin, either cephalotin or cefazolin, or cefepime combined with an aminoglycoside have been shown to be equivalent to vancomycin containing regimens,[509] and vancomycin can be withheld unless a patient has infection caused by MRSA or has life-threatening allergy to β-lactam drugs (Table 45.8). Studies of once-daily intraperitoneal cephalosporin regimens have shown blood and intraperitoneal drug levels far above the MIC of most infecting Gram-positive organisms for the entire 24-h period, with therapeutic success rates comparable to continuous administration of intraperitoneal cephalosporins.[510,511]

Combined use of an aminoglycoside must take into account the patient's residual renal function: patients with a urine output >100 ml/day should not receive an aminoglycoside, based on studies showing accelerated decline in renal function,[512] but should receive a higher dose of the β-lactam in monotherapy; in contrast, patients with a urine output <100 ml/day may safely receive a combined β-lactam/amino-

Table 45.8 Empiric antibiotic regimens for suspected peritoneal dialysis related peritonitis[a]

Antibiotic	Daily dose	
	Residual urine output	
	<100 ml/day	>100 ml/day
Cefazolin or cephalotin	1 g/bag *or* 15 mg/kg/bag[b]	20 mg/kg/bag
Ceftazidime or cefepime	1 g/bag[b]	20 mg/kg/bag
Gentamicin, tobramycin, or netilmicin	0.6 mg/kg/bag	Not recommended
Amikacin	2 mg/kg/bag	Not recommended

[a] Adapted from Keane et al, 2000.[508]
[b] Coadministered with an aminoglycoside: gentamicin, tobramycin, netilmicin, or amikacin.

glycoside regimen (Table 45.8). Clindamycin, vancomycin, and ciprofloxacin are acceptable alternatives in patients with β-lactam allergies.[508]

When the Gram stain or culture confirms the presence of a specific organism, therapy should be adapted to reflect the sensitivities of that organism (Table 45.9). *Staph. aureus* usually responds to 21 days of therapy with an intraperitoneal group 1 cephalosporin; however, in 20–51% of cases this results in catheter loss,[479,513] especially when there is a concurrent exit site or tunnel infection (which results in loss of the catheter in 70–80% of episodes[514,515]). If symptoms of infection persist for more than 72 h or a patient has experienced a recurrent bout of peritonitis, rifampicin should be added.[508]

Ps. aeruginosa infections are very difficult to treat and even with combination antimicrobial therapy have been associated with failure rates and catheter loss ranging from 20% to 80%.[516,517] Initial therapy requires two drugs, such as ceftazidime, cefepime or an antpseudomonal penicillin, in combination with an aminoglycoside or ciprofloxacin (Table 45.9). If peritonitis fails to clear or recurs within 4 weeks of discontinuing therapy, removal of the PD catheter is usually necessary.

Management of fungal peritonitis also represents a formidable challenge to the clinician, and is associated with failure rates approaching 35%,[518,519] despite therapy that includes early removal of the PD catheter and prolonged antifungal therapy. Fungal peritonitis has been associated with a mortality ranging from 17% to 32%.[520,521] A single retrospective study reported a catheter salvage rate of 64% with the use of prolonged antifungal therapy,[515] although the number of cases was small. Other, larger, case series have reported high rates of catheter loss, in the range of 66–86%.[518,519,521] Fluconazole combined with flucytosine is the anti-infective combination of choice for peritonitis caused by *C. albicans*,[479] which has been implicated in >75% of cases of fungal peritonitis,[520] and is generally continued for 4–6 weeks. Amphotericin B exhibits broader antifungal activity than the currently available azoles,

but does not penetrate the peritoneum well when given intravenously[522] and is irritating when given by intraperitoneal route.[523] However, its use is recommended in critically ill patients, when definitive identification of the fungus is pending, and in known infections with filamentous fungi, such as *Aspergillus*, which are intrinsically resistant to fluconazole.[508]

Patients with PD-related peritonitis should be instructed to increase their dialysate dwell times as this is associated with increased peritoneal levels of IgG and activated macrophages.[524] Some authors have recommended discontinuing PD altogether for at least 48 h in an attempt to allow recovery of a local inflammatory response to help control the infection.[525] Anecdotally, the use of thrombolytics has been reported to be beneficial[526] but at this time neither intervention can be routinely recommended.

The decision to remove the PD catheter must take into account the patient's dialysis requirements, the availability of vascular access if transitioning to hemodialysis, the type of infection and, obviously, the patient's wishes. Fungal peritonitis, as noted, is associated with high mortality,[520,521] as is peritonitis caused by *Staph. aureus*.[527] In seriously ill patients with peritonitis caused by these two organisms, a low threshold for early PD catheter removal is advisable. Additional indications for PD catheter removal include *Ps. aeruginosa* peritonitis not responding to therapy, obvious tunnel or refractory exit site infection, fecal peritonitis, relapsing bouts of peritonitis with the same organism or recurrent bouts of culture-negative peritonitis.[479] Several studies have demonstrated the utility of one-stage removal of the infected catheter with simultaneous placement of a new PD catheter,[528,529] with success rates as high as 83%.[529]

PREVENTION

Given the dominance of catheter contamination in the pathogenesis of PD-related peritonitis, interventions aimed at reducing microbial colonization of the extraluminal and intraluminal surfaces of the PD catheter would seem most likely to impact favorably on the risk of infection. The first effective technologic innovation was the Y-set connector system, which reduces the number of times that patients must access their PD catheter by allowing simultaneous connection of the drainage and infusion bag.[530] This initial single bag system, which only comes with an attached drainage bag, to which the patient must connect a fresh dialysate bag, also allows for a 'flush before fill' technique whereby micro-organisms that may have gained intraluminal access during the initial connection of the dialysate bag to the connector are flushed from the catheter into the drainage bag, after which the peritoneum is emptied, then refilled with fresh dialysate. Randomized trials have shown a reduction in the rate of PD-related peritonitis from one episode per 7.5–11 patient-months with standard delivery systems to 1 episode per 15–43 patient-months with Y-delivery systems.[487–489,531]

Newer twin-bag systems that come pre-attached with both

Table 45.9 Recommended regimens for specific organisms causing peritoneal dialysis-related peritonitis[a]

Infecting organism	Initial antibiotics	At 48–96 h	Duration of therapy
Enterococci	Ampicillin 125 mg/l/bag combined with an aminoglycoside[b] or Vancomycin[c] 15–30 mg/kg i.v. every 5–7d	If no improvement, reculture and evaluate for a concurrent exit site or tunnel infection	14 days
Staphylococcus aureus	Group 1 cephalosporin or Vancomycin[c] 15–30 mg/kg i.v. every 5–7d	Start rifampicin 600 mg/day orally. If no improvement, reculture and evaluate for a concurrent exit site or tunnel infection	21 days
Coagulase-negative staphylococci	Continue cephalosporin	Consider vancomycin if methicillin resistance documented. If no improvement, reculture and evaluate for a concurrent exit site or tunnel infection	14 days
Pseudomonas spp.	Ceftazidime or cefepime 1 g/bag daily plus an aminoglycoside[b] if UO<100 ml/day Ciprofloxacin 500 mg p.o. twice daily if UO>100 ml/day or Piperacillin 4 g i.v. every 12 h plus an aminoglycoside[b] if UO<100 ml/day. Ciprofloxacin 500 mg p.o. twice daily if UO>100 ml/day or Aztreonam 1 g/l load followed by 250 mg/l/bag plus an aminoglycoside[b] if UO<100 ml/day. Ciprofloxacin 500 mg p.o. twice daily if UO>100 ml/day	If no improvement, reculture and evaluate for a concurrent exit site or tunnel infection. Consider removal of peritoneal dialysis catheter	21 days
Stenotrophomonas spp.	Trimethroprim–sulfamethoxasole 1–2 DS tabs/day ± ciprofloxacin 500 mg p.o. twice daily (confirm sensitivities)	Consider removal of dialysis catheter	21 days
Other Gram-negative bacilli	Aminoglycoside[b] if UO<100 ml/day Ceftazidime 1 g/bag daily if UO>100 ml/day	If no improvement, reculture and evaluate for a concurrent exit site or tunnel infection	14 days
Fungi	Remove PD catheter and start fluconazole 200 mg p.o. or i.p. qd plus flucytosine 1 g p.o. qd Amphotericin B if resistant yeast or filamentous fungi are present or the patient is severely ill	If dialysis catheter retained it should be removed at 48 hours if infection not clearing	4–6 weeks
Culture-negative	Continue cepahlosporin and stop aminoglycoside, if given with empiric regimen	Reculture fluid if patient not improving and adjust based on results. Consider infection with fungi and mycobacteria	14 days

UO, urine output; i.p., intraperitoneally; p.o., by mouth; DS, double strength.
[a] Adapted from Keane et al, 2000.[508]
[b] Refer to Table 45.13 for dosing.
[c] Use only with confirmed ampicillin or methicillin resistance or in patients with major penicillin allergy.

a drainage and new infusion bag have demonstrated even lower rates of infection than single bag systems, with rates of PD-related peritonitis ranging from one episode per 12–14 patient-months for the single bag system to one episode per 25–46 patient-months for the dual bag system.[532,533] Use of these systems has resulted in a reduction in cases of coagulase-negative staphylococcal peritonitis but has had little impact on rates of *Staph. aureus* infection.[534] Given the predominance of coagulase-negative staphylococci in PD-related peritonitis, wider use of Y-systems should result in significant declines in rates of PD-related infection.

The use of CCPD, which requires only a single night-time connection, also reduces the number of times a PD catheter must be handled, and several studies have reported lower rates of infection than in CAPD, which requires the PD catheter to be accessed 3–4 times a day (one episode per 8–14 patient-months in CAPD patients; one per 20–25 patient-months in patients using CCPD[482,491]).

Reducing rates of PD catheter exit site infections should, in theory, also reduce the rate of PD-related peritonitis. Patients with nasal colonization by *Staph. aureus* are much more likely to develop PD catheter exit site infections[492,493,513,535,536] and at least two studies have demonstrated that these patients are also at increased risk of peritonitis.[535,536] A randomized clinical trial of oral rifampicin, 600 mg/day for 5 days every 3 months, regardless of *Staph. aureus* colonization, demonstrated a significant reduction in the rate of *Staph. aureus* exit-site infection.[537] Studies of the application of 2% nasal mupirocin ointment to the anterior nares, 2–3 times daily for 5 days each month, have also shown reduced rates of PD catheter exit site infection but no effect on rates of peritonitis;[538–540] moreover, re-colonization by *Staph. aureus* occurred in the majority of patients after 1 year.[540] Direct application of 2% mupirocin ointment to intravascular catheter access sites has been shown to reduce rates of IVD-related bloodstream infections in patients undergoing hemodialysis,[541] and studies of direct application to PD catheter exit-sites has similarly shown a reduction in CAPD exit-site infections.[542] However, these studies did not show any favorable cost-benefit with mupirocin use,[543] and sharply rising mupirocin resistance in *Staph. epidermidis*[333] and *Staph. aureus*[544] clinical isolates have been seen with routine use. We believe further studies are needed before prophylactic mupirocin can be routinely recommended in PD or hemodialysis.

Use of perioperative antibiotics for placement of permanent PD catheters has recently been studied.[545,546] Rates of peritonitis occurring within 10 days of catheter placement were lower in patients given perioperative cefuroxime compared to placebo in one randomized trial;[545] another study demonstrated a reduced rate of PD-related peritonitis within 2 weeks of the procedure with prophylactic use of either vancomycin or cefazolin.[546]

References

1. Zimmerli W, Waldvogel FA, Vaudaux P, Nydegger UE 1982 Pathogenesis of foreign body infection: description and characteristics of an animal model. *Journal of Infectious Diseases* 146: 487–497
2. Hench LL, Wilson J 1984 Surface-active biomaterials. *Science* 226: 630–636
3. Fuller RA, Rosen JJ 1986 Materials for medicine. *Scientific American* 255: 118–125
4. Murabayashi S, Nose Y 1986 Biocompatibility: bioengineering aspects. *Artificial Organs* 10: 114–121
5. Hench LL 1998 Biomaterials: a forecast for the future. *Biomaterials* 19: 1419–1423
6. Vaudaux P, Francois P, Lew DP, Waldvogel FA 2001 Host responses to implanted biomaterials. In: Waldvogel FA, Bisno AL (eds) *Infections Associated with Indwelling Medical Devices*, 3rd edn. Washington, DC; ASM Press, pp. 1–26
7. Hermann M, Jaconi ME, Dahlgren C, Waldvogel FA, Stendahl O, Lew DP 1990 Neutrophil bactericidal activity against Staphylococcus aureus adherent on biological surfaces. Surface-bound extracellular matrix proteins activate intracellular killing by oxygen-dependent and -independent mechanisms. *Journal of Clinical Investigations* 86: 942–951
8. Zimmerli W, Lew PD, Waldvogel FA 1984 Pathogenesis of foreign body infection. Evidence for a local granulocyte defect. *Journal of Clinical Investigations* 73: 1191–1200
9. Dickinson GM, Bisno AL 1989 Infections associated with indwelling devices: infections related to extravascular devices. *Antimicrobial Agents and Chemotherapy* 33: 602–607
10. Hoshal VL, Ause RG, Hoskins PA 1971 Fibrin sleeve formation on indwelling subclavian central venous catheters. *Archives of Surgery* 102: 253–258
11. Grasel TG, Wilson RS, Lelah MD, Bielich HW, Cooper SL 1986 Blood flow and surface-induced thrombosis. *ASAIO Transactions* 32: 515–520
12. Park K, Mosher DF, Cooper SL 1986 Acute surface-induced thrombosis in the canine ex vivo model: importance of protein composition of the initial monolayer and platelet activation. *Journal of Biomedical Materials Research* 20: 589–612
13. Vaudaux P, Suzuki R, Waldvogel FA, Morgenthaler JJ, Nydegger UE 1984 Foreign body infection: role of fibronectin as a ligand for the adherence of *Staphylococcus aureus*. *Journal of Infectious Diseases* 150: 546–553
14. Vaudaux PE, Waldvogel FA, Morgenthaler JJ, Nydegger UE 1984 Adsorption of fibronectin onto polymethylmethacrylate and promotion of *Staphylococcus aureus* adherence. *Infection and Immunity* 45: 768–774
15. Hermann M, Vaudaux PE, Pittet D et al 1988 Fibronectin, fibrinogen, and laminin act as mediators of adherence of clinical staphylococcal isolates to foreign material. *Journal of Infectious Diseases* 158: 693–701
16. Vaudaux P, Pittet D, Haeberli A et al 1989 Host factors selectively increase staphylococcal adherence on inserted catheters: a role for fibronectin and fibrinogen or fibrin. *Journal of Infectious Diseases* 160: 865–875
17. Hermann M, Lai QJ, Albrecht RM, Mosher DF, Proctor RA 1993 Adhesion of *Staphylococcus aureus* to surface-bound platelets: role of fibrinogen/fibrin and platelet integrins. *Journal of Infectious Diseases* 167: 312–322
18. McDevitt D, Francois P, Vaudaux P, Foster TJ 1994 Molecular characterization of the clumping factor (fibrinogen receptor) of *Staphylococcus aureus*. *Molecular Microbiology* 11: 237–248
19. McGavin MH, Krajewska-Pietrasik D, Ryden C, Hook M 1993 Identification of a *Staphylococcus aureus* extracellular matrix-binding protein with broad specificity. *Infection and Immunity* 61: 2479–2485
20. Jonsson K, McDevitt D, McGavin MH, Patti JM, Hook M 1995 *Staphylococcus aureus* expresses a major histocompatibility complex class II analog. *Journal of Biological Chemistry* 270: 21457–21460
21. Kuypers JM, Proctor RA 1989 Reduced adherence to traumatized rat heart valves by a low-fibronectin-binding mutant of *Staphylococcus aureus*. *Infection and Immunity* 57: 2306–2312
22. Greene C, McDevitt D, Francois P, Vaudaux PE, Lew DP, Foster TJ 1995 Adhesion properties of mutants of *Staphylococcus aureus* defective in fibronectin-binding proteins and studies on the expression of fnb genes. *Molecular Microbiology* 17: 1143–1152
23. Tojo M, Yamashita N, Goldmann DA, Pier GB 1988 Isolation and characterization of a capsular polysaccharide adhesin from *Staphylococcus epidermidis*. *Journal of Infectious Diseases* 157: 713–722
24. Kojima Y, Tojo M, Goldmann DA, Tosteson TD, Pier GB 1990 Antibody to the capsular polysaccharide/adhesin protects rabbits against catheter-related bacteremia due to coagulase-negative staphylococci. *Journal of Infectious Diseases* 162: 435–441
25. Donlan RM 2001 Biofilms and device-associated infections. *Emergency Infectious Diseases* 7: 277–281
26. Costerton JW, Stewart PS, Greenberg EP 1999 Bacterial biofilms: a common cause of persistent infections. *Science* 284: 1318–1322
27. Stewart PS, Costerton JW 2001 Antibiotic resistance of bacteria in biofilms. *Lancet* 358: 135–138
28. Williams I, Paul F, Lloyd D et al, 1999 Flow cytometry and other techniques show that *Staphylococcus aureus* undergoes significant physiological changes in the early stages of surface-attached culture. *Microbiology* 145: 1325–1333
29. Gallimore B, Gagnon RF, Subang R, Richards GK 1991 Natural history of chronic Staphylococcus epidermidis foreign body infection in a mouse model. *Journal of Infectious Diseases* 164: 1220–1223
30. Stickler D, Hewett P 1991 Activity of antiseptics against biofilms of mixed bacterial species growing on silicone surfaces. *European Journal of Clinical Microbiology and Infectious Diseases* 10: 416–421
31. Ganderton L, Chawla J, Winters C, Wimpenny J, Stickler D 1992 Scanning electron microscopy of bacterial biofilms on indwelling bladder catheters. *European Journal of Clinical Microbiology and Infectious Diseases* 11: 789–796
32. Kaitwatcharachai C, Silpapojakul K, Jitsurong S, Kalnauwakul S 2000 An outbreak of *Burkholderia cepacia* bacteremia in hemodialysis patients: an epidemiologic and molecular study. *American Journal of Kidney Diseases* 36: 199–204
33. Chandra J, Kuhn DM, Mukherjee PK, Hoyer LL, McCormick T, Ghannoum MA 2001 Biofilm formation by the fungal pathogen *Candida albicans*: development, architecture, and drug resistance. *Journal of Bacteriology* 183: 5385–5394
34. Shiau AL, Wu CL 1998 The inhibitory effect of *Staphylococcus epidermidis* slime on the phagocytosis of murine peritoneal macrophages is interferon-independent. *Microbiology and Immunology* 43: 33–40
35. Shigeta M, Tanaka G, Komatsuzawa H, Sugai M, Suginaka H, Usui T 1997 Permeation of antimicrobial agents through *Pseudomonas aeruginosa* biofilms: a simple method. *Chemotherapy* 43: 340–345

36. Anderl JN, Franklin MJ, Stewart PS 2000 Role of antibiotic penetration limitation in *Klebsiella pneumoniae* biofilm resistance to ampicillin and ciprofloxacin. *Antimicrobial Agents and Chemotherapy* 44: 1818–1824

37. Xu KD, McFeters GA, Stewart PS 2000 Biofilm resistance to antimicrobial agents. *Microbiology* 146: 547–549

38. Ceri H, Olson ME, Strernick C, Read RR, Morck D, Buret A 1999 The Calgary Biofilm Device: new technology for rapid determination of antibiotic susceptibilities of bacterial biofilms. *Journal of Clinical Microbiology* 37: 1771–1776

39. Graves E, Kozak L 1998 Detailed diagnosis and proceedures. National Hospital Discharge Survey, 1996. *Vital Health Statistics 13* 138: 1–151

40. Schmalzried TP, Amstutz HC, Au MK, Dorey FJ 1992 Etiology of deep sepsis in total hip arthroplasty. The significance of hematogenous and recurrent infections. *Clinical Orthopaedics and Related Research* 280: 200–207

41. Wymenga AB, van Horn JR, Theeuwes A, Muytjens HL, Slooff TJ 1992 Perioperative factors associated with septic arthritis after arthroplasty. Prospective multicenter study of 362 knee and 2,651 hip operations. *Acta Orthopaedica Scandinavica* 63: 665–671

42. Lazzarini L, Pellizzer G, Stecca C, Viola R, de Lalla F 2001 Postoperative infectious following total knee replacement: an epidemiological study. *Journal of Chemotherapy* 13: 182–187

43. Meding JB, Ritter MA, Faris PM 2001 Total knee arthroplasty with 4.4 mm of tibial polyethylene: 10-year followup. *Clinical Orthopaedics and Related Research* 388: 112–117

44. Steckelberg JM, Osmon DR 2001 Prosthetic joint infections. In: Bisno AL, Waldvogel FA (eds). *Infections Associated with Indwelling Medical Devices*, 3rd ed. Washington, D.C, ASM Press pp. 173–209

45. Sperling JW, Kozak TK, Hanssen AD, Cofield RH 2001 Infection after shoulder arthroplasty. *Clinical Orthopaedics and Related Research* 382: 206–216

46. Rand JA, Morrey BF, Bryan RS 1984 Management of the infected total joint arthroplasty. *Orthopedic Clinics of North America* 15: 491–504

47. Wynn AH, Wilde AH 1992 Long-term follow-up of the Conaxial (Beck-Steffee) total ankle arthroplasty. *Foot and Ankle* 13: 303–306

48. Poss R, Thornhill TS, Ewald FC, Thomas WH, Batte NJ, Sledge CB 1984 Factors influencing the incidence and outcome of infection following total joint arthroplasty. *Clinical Orthopaedics and Related Research* 182: 117–126

49. Salvati EA, Robinson RP, Zeno SM, Koslin BL, Brause BD, Wilson PD Jr 1982 Infection rates after 3175 total hip and total knee replacements performed with and without a horizontal unidirectional filtered air-flow system. *Journal of Bone and Joint Surgery – American Volume* 64: 525–535

50. Luessenhop CP, Higgins LD, Brause BD, Ranawat CS 1996 Multiple prosthetic infections after total joint arthroplasty. Risk factor analysis. *Journal of Arthroplasty* 11: 862–868

51. Yang K, Yeo SJ, Lee BP, Lo NN 2001 Total knee arthroplasty in diabetic patients: a study of 109 consecutive cases. *Journal of Arthroplasty* 16: 102–106

52. Berbari EF, Hanssen AD, Duffy MC et al 1998 Risk factors for prosthetic joint infection: case-control study. *Clinical Infectious Diseases* 27: 1247–1254

53. Espehaug B, Havelin LI, Engesaeter LB, Langeland N, Vollset SE 1997 Patient-related risk factors for early revision of total hip replacements. A population register-based case-control study of 674 revised hips. *Acta Orthopaedica Scandinavica* 68: 207–215

54. Beeton K, Rodriguez-Merchan EC, Alltree J 2000 Total joint arthroplasty in haemophilia. *Haemophilia* 6: 474–481

55. Perka C, Labs K, Muschik M, Buttgereit F 2000 The influence of obesity on perioperative morbidity and mortality in revision total hip arthroplasty. *Archives of Orthopedic Trauma Surgery* 120: 267–271

56. Coventry MB 1975 Treatment of infections occurring in total hip surgery. *Orthopedic Clinics of North America* 6: 991–1003

57. Gillespie WJ 1997 Prevention and management of infection after total joint replacement. *Clinical Infectious Diseases* 25: 1310–1317

58. Charnley J 1972 Postoperative infection after total hip replacement with special reference to air contamination in the operating room. *Clinical Orthopaedics and Related Research* 87: 167–187

59. Lidwell OM, Lowbury EJ, Whyte W, Blowers R, Stanley SJ, Lowe D 1983 Bacteria isolated from deep joint sepsis after operation for total hip or knee replacement and the sources of the infections with *Staphylococcus aureus*. *Journal of Hospital Infections* 4: 19–29

60. Wroblewski BM, del Sel HJ 1980 Urethral instrumentation and deep sepsis in total hip replacement. *Clinical Orthopaedics and Related Research* 146: 209–212

61. Friedman RJ 1988 Infection in total joint arthroplasty from distal intravenous lines. A case report. *Journal of Arthroplasty* 3(Suppl): S69–71

62. Wilkins J, Patzakis MJ 1990 Peripheral teflon catheters. Potential source for bacterial contamination of orthopedic implants? *Clinical Orthopaedics and Related Research* 254: 251–254

63. Hill C, Flamant R, Mazas F, Evrard J 1981 Prophylactic cefazolin versus placebo in total hip replacement. Report of a multicentre double-blind randomised trial. *Lancet*. 1: 795–796

64. Lidwell OM, Lowbury EJ, Whyte W, Blowers R, Stanley SJ, Lowe D 1982 Effect of ultraclean air in operating rooms on deep sepsis in the joint after total hip or knee replacement: a randomised study. *British Medical Journal (Clinical Research Edition)* 285: 10–14

65. Norden C, Gillespie WJ, Nade S 1994 Infections in total joint replacement. *Infections in Bones and Joints.* Boston, Blackwell Scientific Publications: pp. 291–319

66. Norden CW 1991 Antibiotic prophylaxis in orthopedic surgery. *Reviews of Infections Diseases* 13(Suppl. 10): S842–846

67. Glynn MK, Sheehan JM 1983 An analysis of the causes of deep infection after hip and knee arthroplasties. *Clinical Orthopaedics and Related Research* 178: 202–206

68. Ainscow DA, Denham RA 1984 The risk of haematogenous infection in total joint replacements. *Journal of Bone and Joint Surgery – British Volume* 66: 580–582

69. Waldman BJ, Mont MA, Hungerford DS 1997 Total knee arthroplasty infectious associated with dental procedures. *Clinical Orthopaedics and Related Research* 343: 164–172

70. Murdoch DR, Roberts SA, Fowler Jr, VG Jr et al 2001 Infection of orthopedic prostheses after *Staphylococcus aureus* bacteremia. *Clinical Infectious Diseases*. 32: 647–649

71. Cuckler JM, Star AM, Alavi A, Noto RB 1991 Diagnosis and management of the infected total joint arthroplasty. *Orthopedic Clinics of North America* 22: 523–530

72. Canner GC, Steinberg ME, Heppenstall RB, Balderston R 1984 The infected hip after total hip arthroplasty. *Journal of Bone and Joint Surgery – American Volume* 66: 1393–1399

73. Spangehl MJ, Masri BA, O'Connell JX, Duncan CP 1999 Prospective analysis of preoperative and intraoperative investigations for the diagnosis of infection at the sites of two hundred and two revision total hip arthroplasties. *Journal of Bone and Joint Surgery – American Volume* 81: 672–683

74. Sanzen L, Carlsson AS 1989 The diagnostic value of C-reactive protein in infected total hip arthroplasties. *Journal of Bone and Joint Surgery – British Volume* 71: 638–641

75. Aalto K, Osterman K, Peltola H, Rasanen J 1984 Changes in erythrocyte sedimentation rate and C-reactive protein after total hip arthroplasty. *Clinical Orthopaedics and Related Research* 184: 118–120

76. Shih LY, Wu JJ, Yang DJ 1987 Erythrocyte sedimentation rate and C-reactive protein values in patients with total hip arthroplasty. *Clinical Orthopaedics and Related Research* 225: 238–246

77. Bilgen O, Atici T, Durak K, Karaeminogullari, Bilgen MS 2001 C-reactive protein values and erythrocyte sedimentation rates after total hip and total knee arthroplasty. *Journal of International Medical Research* 29: 7–12

78. Thoren B, Hallin G 1989 Loosening of the Charnley hip. Radiographic analysis of 102 revisions. *Acta Orthopaedica Scandinavica* 60: 533–539

79. Tigges S, Stiles RG, Roberson JR 1994 Appearance of septic hip prostheses on plain radiographs. *AJR. American Journal of Roentgenology* 163: 377–380

80. Owen RJ, Harper WM, Finlay DB, Belton IP 1995 Isotope bone scans in patients with painful knee replacements: do they alter management? *British Journal of Radiology* 68: 1204–1207

81. Merkel KD, Brown ML, Dewanjee MK, Fitzgerald RH Jr 1985 Comparison of indium-labeled-leukocyte imaging with sequential technetium-gallium scanning in the diagnosis of low-grade musculoskeletal sepsis. A prospective study. *Journal of Bone and Joint Surgery – American Volume* 67: 465–476

82. Merkel KD, Brown ML, Fitzgerald RH 1986 Sequential technetium-99m HMDP-gallium-67 citrate imaging for the evaluation of infection in the painful prosthesis. *Journal of Nuclear Medicine* 27: 1413–1417

83. Kraemer WJ, Saplys R, Waddell JP, Morton J 1993 Bone scan, gallium scan, and hip aspiration in the diagnosis of infected total hip arthroplasty. *Journal of Arthroplasty* 8: 611–616

84. de Lima Ramos PA, Martin-Comin J, Bajen MT et al 1996 Simultaneous administration of 99Tcm-HMPAO-labelled autologous leukocytes and 111In-labelled non-specific polyclonal human immunoglobulin G in bone and joint infections. *Nuclear Medicine Communications* 17: 749–757

85. Oyen WJ, van Horn JR, Claessens RA, Slooff TJ, van der Meer JW, Corstens FH 1992 Diagnosis of bone, joint, and joint prosthesis infections with In-111-labeled nonspecific human immunoglobulin G scintigraphy. *Radiology* 182: 195–199

86. Nijhof MW, Oyen WJ, van Kampen A, Claessens RA, van der Meer JW, Corstens FH 1997 Hip and knee arthroplasty infection. In-111-IgG scintigraphy in 102 cases. *Acta Orthopaedica Scandinavica* 68: 332–336

87. Mackowiak PA, Jones SR, Smith JW 1978 Diagnostic value of sinus-tract cultures in chronic osteomyelitis. *Journal of the American Medical Association* 239: 2772–2775

88. Roberts P, Walters AJ, McMinn DJ 1992 Diagnosing infection in hip replacements. The use of fine-needle aspiration and radiometric culture. *Journal of Bone and Joint Surgery – British Volume* 74: 265–269

89. Lachiewicz PF, Rogers GD, Thomason HC 1996 Aspiration of the hip joint before revision total hip arthroplasty. Clinical and laboratory factors influencing attainment of a positive culture. *Journal of Bone and Joint Surgery – American Volume* 78: 749–754

90. Atkins BL, Athanasou N, Deeks JJ et al 1998 Prospective evaluation of criteria for microbiological diagnosis of prosthetic-joint infection at revision arthroplasty. The OSIRIS Collaborative Study Group. *Journal of Clinical Microbiology* 36: 2932–2939

91. Spangehl MJ, Masterson E, Masri BA, O'Connell JX, Duncan CP 1999 The role of intraoperative gram stain in the diagnosis of infection during revision total hip arthroplasty. *Journal of Arthroplasty* 14: 952–956

92. Tunney MM, Patrick S, Gorman SP et al 1998 Improved detection of infection in hip replacements. A currently underestimated problem. *Journal of Bone and Joint Surgery – British Volume* 80: 568–572

93. Colyer RA, Capello WN 1994 Surgical treatment of the infected hip implant. Two-stage reimplantation with a one-month interval. *Clinical Orthopaedics and Related Research* 298: 75–79

94. Garvin KL, Hanssen AD 1995 Infection after total hip arthroplasty. Past, present, and future. *Journal of Bone and Joint Surgery – American Volume* 77: 1576–1588

95. Garvin KL, Mormino MA, McKillip TM 2001 Management of infected implants. In: Szabo RM, Marder R, Vince KG, et al (eds). *Chapman's Orthopaedic Surgery*. Vol Four. 3rd edn. Philadelphia, Lippincott Williams & Wilkins; pp. 1: 3577–3594

96. Henderson MH, Booth RE 1991 The use of an antibiotic-impregnated spacer block for revision of the septic total knee arthroplasty. *Seminars in Arthroplasty* 2: 34–39

97. Haddad FS, Masri BA, Campbell D, McGraw RW, Beauchamp CP, Duncan CP 2000 The PROSTALAC functional spacer in two-stage revision for infected knee replacements. Prosthesis of antibiotic-loaded acrylic cement. *Journal of Bone and Joint Surgery – British Volume* 82: 807–812

98. Hanssen AD, Rand JA, Osmon DR 1994 Treatment of the infected total knee arthroplasty with insertion of another prosthesis. The effect of antibiotic-impregnated bone cement. *Clinical Orthopaedics and Related Research* 309: 44–55

99. Haddad FS, Muirhead-Allwood SK, Manktelow AR, Bacarese-Hamilton I 2000 Two-stage uncemented revision hip arthroplasty for infection. *Journal of Bone and Joint Surgery – British Volume* 82: 689–694

100. McDonald DJ, Fitzgerald RH Jr, Ilstrup DM 1989 Two-stage reconstruction of a total hip arthroplasty because of infection. *Journal of Bone and Joint Surgery – American Volume* 71: 828–834

101. Garvin KL 1994 Two-stage reimplantation of the infected hip. *Seminars in Arthroplasty* 5: 142–146

102. Brandt CM, Duffy MC, Berbari EF, Hanssen AD, Steckelberg JM, Osmon DR 1999 Staphylococcus aureus prosthetic joint infection treated with prosthesis removal and delayed reimplantation arthroplasty. *Mayo Clinic Proceedings* 74: 553–558

103. Haddad FS, Masri BA, Garbuz DS, Duncan CP 1999 The treatment of the infected hip replacement. The complex case. *Clinical Orthopaedics and Related Research* 369: 144–156

104. Segawa H, Tsukayama DT, Kyle RF, Becker DA, Gustilo RB 1999 Infection after total knee arthroplasty. A retrospective study of the treatment of eighty-one infections. *Journal of Bone and Joint Surgery – American Volume* 81: 1434–1445

105. Zimmerli W, Widmer AF, Blatter M, Frei R, Ochsner PE 1998 Role of rifampin for treatment of orthopedic implant-related staphylococcal infections: a randomized controlled trial. Foreign-Body Infection (FBI) Study Group. *Journal of the American Medical Association* 279: 1537–1541

106. Krasin E, Goldwirth M, Hemo Y, Gold A, Herling G, Otremski I 2001 Could irrigation, debridement and antibiotic therapy cure an infection of a total hip arthroplasty? *Journal of Hospital Infection* 47: 235–238

107. Burger RR, Basch T, Hopson CN 1991 Implant salvage in infected total knee arthroplasty. *Clinical Orthopaedics and Related Research* 273: 105–112

108. Brandt CM, Sistrunk WW, Duffy MC, et al 1997 *Staphylococcus aureus* prosthetic joint infection treated with debridement and prosthesis retention. *Clinical Infectious Diseases* 24: 914–919

109. Crockarell JR, Hanssen AD, Osmon DR, Morrey BF 1998 Treatment of infection with debridement and retention of the components following hip arthroplasty. *Journal of Bone and Joint Surgery – American Volume* 80: 1306–1313

110. Tattevin P, Cremieux AC, Pottier P, Huten D, Carbon C 1999 Prosthetic joint infection: when can prosthesis salvage be considered? *Clinical Infectious Diseases* 29: 292–295

111. Borden LS, Gearen PF 1987 Infected total knee arthroplasty. A protocol for management. *Journal of Arthroplasty* 2: 27–36

112. Schoifet SD, Morrey BF 1990 Treatment of infection after total knee arthroplasty by debridement with retention of the components. *Journal of Bone and Joint Surgery – American Volume* 72: 1383–1390

113. Tsukayama DT, Estrada R, Gustilo RB 1996 Infection after total hip arthroplasty. A study of the treatment of one hundred and six infections. *Journal of Bone and Joint Surgery – American Volume* 78: 512–523

114. Miley GB, Scheller AD Jr, Turner RH 1982 Medical and surgical treatment of the septic hip with one-stage revision arthroplasty. *Clinical Orthopaedics and Related Research* 170: 76–82

115. Wroblewski BM 1986 One-stage revision of infected cemented total hip arthroplasty. *Clinical Orthopaedics and Related Research* 211: 103–107

116. Hope PG, Kristinsson KG, Norman P, Elson RA 1989 Deep infection of cemented total hip arthroplasties caused by coagulase-negative staphylococci. *Journal of Bone and Joint Surgery – British Volume* 71: 851–855

117. Goksan SB, Freeman MA 1992 One-stage reimplantation for infected total knee arthroplasty. *Journal of Bone and Joint Surgery – British Volume* 74: 78–82

118. Raut VV, Siney PD, Wroblewski BM 1995 One-stage revision of total hip arthroplasty for deep infection. Long-term followup. *Clinical Orthopaedics and Related Research* 321: 202–207

119. Hanssen AD, Osmon DR 2000 Assessment of patient selection criteria for treatment of the infected hip arthroplasty. *Clinical Orthopaedics and Related Research* 381: 91–100

120. von Foerster G, Kluber D, Kabler U 1991 Mid- to long-term results after treatment of 118 cases of periprosthetic infections after knee joint replacement using one-stage exchange surgery. *Orthopade* 20: 244–252

121. Elson RA 1993 Exchange arthroplasty for infection. Perspectives from the United Kingdom. *Orthopedic Clinics of North America* 24: 761–767

122. Goulet JA, Pellicci PM, Brause BD, Salvati EM 1988 Prolonged suppression of infection in total hip arthroplasty. *Journal of Arthroplasty* 3: 109–116

123. Segreti J, Nelson JA, Trenholme GM 1998 Prolonged suppressive antibiotic therapy for infected orthopedic prostheses. *Clinical Infectious Diseases* 27: 711–713

124. Tsukayama DT, Wicklund B, Gustilo RB 1991 Suppressive antibiotic therapy in chronic prosthetic joint infections. *Orthopedics (Thorofare, NJ)* 14: 841–844

125. Widmer AF, Frei R, Rajacic Z, Zimmerli W 1990 Correlation between in vivo and in vitro efficacy of antimicrobial agents against foreign body infections. *Journal of Infectious Diseases* 162: 96–102

126. Chuard C, Herrmann M, Vaudaux P, Waldvogel FA, Lew DP 1991 Successful therapy of experimental chronic foreign-body infection due to methicillin-resistant *Staphylococcus aureus* by antimicrobial combinations. *Antimicrobial Agents and Chemotherapy* 35: 2611–2616

127. Drancourt M, Stein A, Argenson JN, Zannier A, Curvale G, Raoult D 1993 Oral rifampin plus ofloxacin for treatment of *Staphylococcus*-infected orthopedic implants. *Antimicrobial Agents and Chemotherapy* 37: 1214–1218

128. Cremieux AC, Mghir AS, Bleton R et al 1996 Efficacy of sparfloxacin and autoradiographic diffusion pattern of [14C]Sparfloxacin in experimental *Staphylococcus aureus* joint prosthesis infection. *Antimicrobial Agents and Chemotherapy* 40: 2111–2116

129. Gentry LO, Rodriguez GG 1990 Oral ciprofloxacin compared with parenteral antibiotics in the treatment of osteomyelitis. *Antimicrobial Agents and Chemotherapy* 34: 40–43

130. Gentry LO, Rodriguez-Gomez G 1991 Ofloxacin versus parenteral therapy for chronic osteomyelitis. *Antimicrobial Agents and Chemotherapy* 35: 538–541

131. Esterhai JL Jr, Bednar J, Kimmelman CP 1986 Gentamicin-induced ototoxicity

complicating treatment of chronic osteomyelitis. *Clinical Orthopaedics and Related Research* 209: 185–188

132. Hiemenz JW, Walsh TJ 1996 Lipid formulations of amphotericin B: recent progress and future directions. *Clinical Infectious Diseases* 22(Suppl. 2): S133–144

133. Dan M, Priel I 1994 Failure of fluconazole therapy for sternal osteomyelitis due to *Candida albicans*. *Clinical Infectious Diseases* 18: 126–127

134. Flanagan PG, Barnes RA 1997 Hazards of inadequate fluconazole dosage to treat deep-seated or systemic *Candida albicans* infection. *Journal of Infection* 35: 295–297

135. Fitzgerald RH, Ilstrup DM 1990 A prospective study of unidirectional airflow in operating rooms (Abstract). Paper presented at 57th Annual Meeting of the Academy of Orthopedic Surgeons, 1990, New Orleans

136. Lidwell OM 1994 Ultraviolet radiation and the control of airborne contamination in the operating room. *Journal of Hospital Infection* 28: 245–248

137. Shaw JA, Bordner MA, Hamory BH 1996 Efficacy of the Steri-Shield filtered exhaust helmet in limiting bacterial counts in the operating room during total joint arthroplasty. *Journal of Arthroplasty* 11: 469–473

138. Conte JE, Cohen SN, Roe BB, Elashoff RM 1972 Antibiotic prophylaxis and cardiac surgery. A prospective double-blind comparison of single-dose versus multiple-dose regimens. *Annals of Internal Medicine* 76: 943–949

139. Nelson CL, Green TG, Porter RA, Warren RD 1983 One day versus seven days of preventive antibiotic therapy in orthopedic surgery. *Clinical Orthopaedics and Related Research* 176: 258–263

140. Josefsson G, Kolmert L 1993 Prophylaxis with systematic antibiotics versus gentamicin bone cement in total hip arthroplasty. A ten-year survey of 1,688 hips. *Clinical Orthopaedics and Related Research* 292: 210–214

141. Espehaug B, Engesaeter LB, Vollset SE, Havelin LI, Langeland N 1997 Antibiotic prophylaxis in total hip arthroplasty. Review of 10,905 primary cemented total hip replacements reported to the Norwegian arthroplasty register, 1987 to 1995. *Journal of Bone and Joint Surgery – British Volume* 79: 590–595

142. Shrout MK, Scarbrough F, Powell BJ 1994 Dental care and the prosthetic joint patient: a survey of orthopedic surgeons and general dentists. *Journal of the American Dental Association* 125: 429–436

143. Deacon JM, Pagliaro AJ, Zelicof SB, Horowitz HW 1996 Prophylactic use of antibiotics for procedures after total joint replacement. *Journal of Bone and Joint Surgery – American Volume* 78: 1755–1770

144. Jacobson JJ, Schweitzer S, DePorter DJ, Lee JJ 1990 Antibiotic prophylaxis for dental patients with joint prostheses? A decision analysis. *International Journal of Technology Assessment in Health Care* 6: 569–587

145. Segreti J, Levin S 1989 The role of prophylactic antibiotics in the prevention of prosthetic device infections. *Infectious Disease Clinics of North America* 3: 357–370

146. Vongpatanasin W, Hillis LD, Lange RA 1996 Prosthetic heart valves. *New England Journal of Medicine* 335: 407–416

147. Wilson WR, Danielson GK, Giuliani ER, Geraci JE 1982 Prosthetic valve endocarditis. *Mayo Clinic Proceedings* 57: 155–161

148. van der Meer JT, Thompson J, Valkenburg HA, Michel MF 1992 Epidemiology of bacterial endocarditis in The Netherlands. I. Patient characteristics. *Archives of Internal Medicine* 152: 1863–1868

149. Berlin JA, Abrutyn E, Strom BL et al 1995 Incidence of infective endocarditis in the Delaware Valley, 1988–1990. *American Journal of Cardiology* 76: 933–936

150. Ivert TS, Dismukes WE, Cobbs CG, Blackstone EH, Kirklin JW, Bergdahl LA 1984 Prosthetic valve endocarditis. *Circulation* 69: 223–232

151. Calderwood SB, Swinski LA, Waternaux CM, Karchmer AW, Buckley MJ 1985 Risk factors for the development of prosthetic valve endocarditis. *Circulation* 72: 31–37

152. Rutledge R, Kim BJ, Applebaum RE 1985 Actuarial analysis of the risk of prosthetic valve endocarditis in 1,598 patients with mechanical and bioprosthetic valves. *Archives of Surgery* 120: 469–472

153. Arvay A, Lengyel M 1988 Incidence and risk factors of prosthetic valve endocarditis. *European Journal of Cardio-Thoracic Surgery* 2: 340–346

154. Agnihotri AK, McGiffin DC, Galbraith AJ, O'Brien MF 1995 The prevalence of infective endocarditis after aortic valve replacement. *Journal of Thoracic and Cardiovascular Surgery* 110: 1708–1720; discussion 1720–1704

155. Puvimanasinghe JP, Steyerberg EW, Takkenberg JJ et al 2001 Prognosis after aortic valve replacement with a bioprosthesis: predictions based on meta-analysis and microsimulation. *Circulation* 103: 1535–1541

156. Grover FL, Cohen DJ, Oprian C, Henderson WG, Sethi G, Hammermeister KE 1994 Determinants of the occurrence of and survival from prosthetic valve endocarditis. Experience of the Veterans Affairs Cooperative Study on Valvular Heart Disease. *Journal of Thoracic and Cardiovascular Surgery* 108: 207–214

157. Bloomfield P, Wheatley DJ, Prescott RJ, Miller HC 1991 Twelve-year comparison of a Bjork-Shiley mechanical heart valve with porcine bioprostheses. *New England Journal of Medicine* 324: 573–579

158. Hammermeister KE, Sethi GK, Henderson WG, Oprian C, Kim T, Rahimtoola S 1993 A comparison of outcomes in men 11 years after heart-valve replacement with a mechanical valve or bioprosthesis. Veterans Affairs Cooperative Study on Valvular Heart Disease. *New England Journal of Medicine* 328: 1289–1296

159. Calderwood SB, Swinski LA, Karchmer AW, Waternaux CM, Buckley MJ 1986 Prosthetic valve endocarditis. Analysis of factors affecting outcome of therapy. *Journal of Thoracic and Cardiovascular Surgery* 92: 776–783

160. Yu VL, Fang GD, Keys TF et al 1994 Prosthetic valve endocarditis: superiority of surgical valve replacement versus medical therapy only. *Annals of Thoracic Surgery* 58: 1073–1077

161. Tornos P, Almirante B, Olona M, et al 1997 Clinical outcome and long-term prognosis of late prosthetic valve endocarditis: a 20-year experience. *Clinical Infectious Diseases* 24: 381–386

162. Sett SS, Hudon MP, Jamieson WR, Chow AW 1993 Prosthetic valve endocarditis. Experience with porcine bioprostheses. *Journal of Thoracic and Cardiovascular Surgery* 105: 428–434

163. Wolff M, Witchitz S, Chastang C, Regnier B, Vachon F 1995 Prosthetic valve endocarditis in the ICU. Prognostic factors of overall survival in a series of 122 cases and consequences for treatment decision. *Chest* 108: 688–694

164. Gordon SM, Serkey JM, Longworth DL, Lytle BW, Cosgrove DM 3rd 2000 Early onset prosthetic valve endocarditis: the Cleveland Clinic experience 1992–1997. *Annals of Thoracic Surgery* 69: 1388–1392

165. Perez-Vazquez A, Farinas MC, Garcia-Palomo JD, Bernal JM, Revuelta JM, Gonzalez-Macias J 2000 Evaluation of the Duke criteria in 93 episodes of prosthetic valve endocarditis: could sensitivity be improved? *Archives of Internal Medicine* 160: 1185–1191

166. Dismukes WE, Karchmer AW, Buckley MJ, Austen WG Swartz MN 1973 Prosthetic valve endocarditis. Analysis of 38 cases. *Circulation* 48: 365–377

167. San Roman JA, Vilacosta I, Sarria C et al 1999 Clinical course, microbiologic profile, and diagnosis of periannular complications in prosthetic valve endocarditis. *American Journal of Cardiology* 83: 1075–1079

168. Karchmer AW 2000 Infections of prosthetic heart valves. In: Bisno AL, Waldvogel FA (eds) *Infections Associated with Indwelling Devices*, 3rd edn. Washington, DC, ASM press, pp. 145–172

169. Blakemore WS, McGarrity GJ, Thurer RJ, Wallace HW, MacVaugh H 3rd, Coriell LL 1971 Infection by air-borne bacteria with cardiopulmonary bypass. *Surgery* 70: 830–838

170. Kluge RM, Calia FM, McLaughlin JS, Hornick RB 1974 Sources of contamination in open heart surgery. *Journal of The American Medical Association* 230: 1415–1418

171. Freeman R, Hjersing N, Burridge A 1981 Catheter tip cultures on open-heart surgery patients: associations with site of catheter and age of patients. *Thorax* 36: 355–359

172. Keys TF 1993 Early-onset prosthetic valve endocarditis. *Cleveland Clinical Journal of Medicine* 60: 455–459

173. Fang G, Keys TF, Gentry LO et al 1993 Prosthetic valve endocarditis resulting from nosocomial bacteremia. A prospective, multicenter study. *Annals of Internal Medicine* 119: 560–567

174. Richardson JV, Karp RB, Kirklin JW, Dismukes WE 1978 Treatment of infective endocarditis: a 10-year comparative analysis. *Circulation* 58: 589–597

175. Karchmer AW, Archer GL, Dismukes WE 1983 *Staphylococcus epidermidis* causing prosthetic valve endocarditis: microbiologic and clinical observations as guides to therapy. *Annals of Internal Medicine* 98: 447–455

176. Kuyvenhoven JP, van Rijk-Zwikker GL, Hermans J, Thompson J, Huysmans HA 1994 Prosthetic valve endocarditis: analysis of risk factors for mortality. *European Journal of Cardio-Thoracic Surgery* 8: 420–424

177. Roder BL, Wandall DA, Espersen F, Frimodt-Moller N, Skinhoj P, Rosdahl VT 1997 A study of 47 bacteremic *Staphylococcus aureus* endocarditis cases: 23 with native valves treated surgically and 24 with prosthetic valves. *Scandinavian Cardiovascular Journal* 31: 305–309

178. John MD, Hibberd PL, Karchmer AW, Sleeper LA, Calderwood SB 1998 *Staphylococcus aureus* prosthetic valve endocarditis: optimal management and risk factors for death. *Annals of Thoracic Surgery* 26: 1302–1309

179. Nguyen MH, Nguyen ML, Yu VL, McMahon D, Keys TF, Amidi M 1996 *Candida*

prosthetic valve endocarditis: prospective study of six cases and review of the literature. *Clinical Infectious Diseases* 22: 262–267

180. Rocchiccioli C, Chastre J, Lecompte Y, Gandjbakhch I, Gibert C 1986 Prosthetic valve endocarditis. The case for prompt surgical management. *Journal of Thoracic and Cardiovascular Surgery* 92: 784–789

181. Karchmer AW, Dismukes WE, Buckley MJ, Austen WG 1978 Late prosthetic valve endocarditis: clinical features influencing therapy. *American Journal of Medicine* 64: 199–206

182. Douglas JL, Cobbs CG 1992 Prosthetic valve endocarditis. In: Kaye D (ed.) *Infective Endocarditis*. 2nd edn. New York, Raven Press, pp. 375–396

183. Weinstein MP, Murphy JR, Reller LB, Lichtenstein KA 1983 The clinical significance of positive blood cultures: a comprehensive analysis of 500 episodes of bacteremia and fungemia in adults. II. Clinical observations, with special reference to factors influencing prognosis. *Reviews of Infectious Diseases* 5: 54–70

184. Mermel LA, Maki DG 1994 Detection of bacteremia in adults: consequences of culturing an inadequate volume of blood. *Annals of Internal Medicine* 119: 270–272

185. Berbari EF, Cockerill FR, 3rd, Steckelberg JM 1997 Infective endocarditis due to unusual or fastidious microorganisms. *Mayo Clinic Proceedings* 72: 532–542

186. Telenti A, Steckelberg JM, Stockman L, Edson RS, Roberts GD 1991 Quantitative blood cultures in candidemia. *Mayo Clinic Proceedings* 66: 1120–1123

187. Melgar GR, Nasser RM, Gordon SM, Lytle BW, Keys TF, Longworth DL 1997 Fungal prosthetic valve endocarditis in 16 patients. An 11-year experience in a tertiary care hospital. *Medicine* 76: 94–103

188. Krivokapich J, Child JS 1996 Role of transthoracic and transesophageal echocardiography in diagnosis and management of infective endocarditis. *Cardiology Clinics* 14: 363–382

189. Daniel WG, Mugge A, Grote J et al 1993 Comparison of transthoracic and transesophageal echocardiography for detection of abnormalities of prosthetic and bioprosthetic valves in the mitral and aortic positions. *American Journal of Cardiology* 71: 210–215

190. Lowry RW, Zoghbi WA, Baker WB, Wray RA, Quinones MA 1994 Clinical impact of transesophageal echocardiography in the diagnosis and management of infective endocarditis. *American Journal of Cardiology* 73: 1089–1091

191. Morguet AJ, Werner GS, Andreas S, Kreuzer H 1995 Diagnostic value of transesophageal compared with transthoracic echocardiography in suspected prosthetic valve endocarditis. *Herz* 20: 390–398

192. Taams MA, Gussenhoven EJ, Bos E et al 1990 Enhanced morphological diagnosis in infective endocarditis by transoesophageal echocardiography. *British Heart Journal* 63: 109–113

193. Daniel WG, Mugge A, Martin RP et al 1991 Improvement in the diagnosis of abscesses associated with endocarditis by transesophageal echocardiography. *New England Journal of Medicine* 324: 795–800

194. Ryan EW, Bolger AF 2000 Transesophageal echocardiography (TEE) in the evaluation of infective endocarditis. *Cardiology Clinics* 18: 773–787

195. Durack DT, Lukes AS, Bright DK 1994 New criteria for diagnosis of infective endocarditis: utilization of specific echocardiographic findings. Duke Endocarditis Service. *American Journal of Medicine* 96: 200–209

196. Rybak MJ, Albrecht LM, Boike SC, Chandrasekar PH 1990 Nephrotoxicity of vancomycin, alone and with an aminoglycoside. *Journal of Antimicrobial Chemotherapy* 25: 679–687

197. Rice LB, Calderwood SB, Eliopoulos GM, Farber BF, Karchmer AW 1991 Enterococcal endocarditis: a comparison of prosthetic and native valve disease. *Reviews of Infectious Diseases* 13: 1–7

198. Wilson WR, Karchmer AW, Dajani AS et al 1995 Antibiotic treatment of adults with infective endocarditis due to streptococci, enterococci, staphylococci, and HACEK microorganisms. American Heart Association [see comments]. *Journal of the American Medical Association* 274: 1706–1713

199. Babcock HM, Ritchie DJ, Christiansen E, Starlin R, Little R, Stanley S 2001 Successful treatment of vancomycin-resistant Enterococcus endocarditis with oral linezolid. *Clinical Infectious Diseases* 32: 1373–1375

200. Furlong WB, Rakowski TA 1997 Therapy with RP 59500 (quinupristin/dalfopristin) for prosthetic valve endocarditis due to enterococci with VanA/VanB resistance patterns. *Clinical Infectious Diseases* 25: 163–164

201. Glazier JJ, Verwilghen J, Donaldson RM, Ross DN 1991 Treatment of complicated prosthetic aortic valve endocarditis with annular abscess formation by homograft aortic root replacement. *Journal of the American College of Cardiology* 17: 1177–1182

202. Jault F, Gandjbakhch I, Chastre JC et al 1993 Prosthetic valve endocarditis with ring abscesses. Surgical management and long-term results. *Journal of Thoracic and Cardiovascular Surgery* 105: 1106–1113

203. Baumgartner WA, Miller DC, Reitz BA et al 1983 Surgical treatment of prosthetic valve endocarditis. *Annals of Thoracic Surgery* 35: 87–104

204. Stein PD, Alpert JS, Bussey HI, Dalen JE, Turpie AG 2001 Antithrombotic therapy in patients with mechanical and biological prosthetic heart valves. *Chest* 119(1 Suppl): 220S–227S

205. Cannegieter SC, Rosendaal FR, Briet E 1994 Thromboembolic and bleeding complications in patients with mechanical heart valve prostheses. *Circulation* 89: 635–641

206. Davenport J, Hart RG 1990 Prosthetic valve endocarditis 1976–1987. Antibiotics, anticoagulation, and stroke. *Stroke* 21: 993–999

207. Tornos P, Almirante B, Mirabet S, Permanyer G, Pahissa A, Soler-Soler J 1999 Infective endocarditis due to *Staphylococcus aureus*: deleterious effect of anticoagulant therapy. *Archives of Internal Medicine* 159: 473–475

208. Gillinov AM, Shah RV, Curtis WE et al 1996 Valve replacement in patients with endocarditis and acute neurologic deficit. *Annals of Thoracic Surgery* 61: 1125–1129; discussion 1130

209. Dajani AS, Taubert KA, Wilson W et al 1997 Prevention of bacterial endocarditis: recommendations by the American Heart Association. *Clinical Infectious Diseases* 25: 1448–1458

210. Maki DG, Bohn MJ, Stolz SM, Kroncke GM, Acher CW, Myerowitz PD 1992 Comparative study of cefazolin, cefamandole, and vancomycin for surgical prophylaxis in cardiac and vascular operations. A double-blind randomized trial. *Journal of Thoracic and Cardiovascular Surgery* 104: 1423–1434

211. Vuorisalo S, Pokela R, Syrjala H 1998 Comparison of vancomycin and cefuroxime for infection prophylaxis in coronary artery bypass surgery. *Infection Control and Hospital Epidemiology* 19: 234–239

212. Anonymous 1994 Recommendations for preventing the spread of vancomycin resistance. Recommendations of the Hospital Infection Control Practices Advisory Committee (HICPAC). *Morbidity and Mortality Weekly Reports* 44: 1–13

213. Schaff H, Carrel T, Steckelberg JM, Grunkemeier GL, Holubkov R 1999 Artificial Valve Endocarditis Reduction Trial (AVERT): protocol of a multicenter randomized trial. *Journal of Heart Valve Disease* 8: 131–139

214. Kjaergard HK, Tingleff J, Abildgaard U, Pettersson G 1999 Recurrent endocarditis in silver-coated heart valve prosthesis. *Journal of Heart Valve Disease* 8: 140–142

215. Phibbs B, Marriott HJ 1985 Complications of permanent transvenous pacing. *New England Journal of Medicine* 312: 1428–1432

216. Wade JS, Cobbs CG 1998 Infections in cardiac pacemakers. *Current Clinical Topics in Infectious Diseases* 9: 44–61

217. Arber N, Pras E, Copperman Y et al 1994 Pacemaker endocarditis. Report of 44 cases and review of the literature. *Medicine* 73: 299–305

218. Trappe HJ, Pfitzner P, Klein H, Wenzlaff P 1995 Infections after cardioverter-defibrillator implantation: observations in 335 patients over 10 years. *British Heart Journal* 73: 20–24

219. Lai KK, Fontecchio SA 1998 Infections associated with implantable cardioverter defibrillators placed transvenously and via thoracotomies: epidemiology, infection control, and management. *Clinical Infectious Diseases* 27: 265–269

220. Morgan G, Ginks W, Siddons H, Leatham A 1979 Septicemia in patients with an endocardial pacemaker. *American Journal of Cardiology* 44: 221–224

221. Bluhm G, Julander I, Levander-Lindgren M, Olin C 1982 Septicaemia and endocarditis – uncommon but serious complications in connection with permanent cardiac pacing. *Scandinavian Journal of Thoracic and Cardiovascular Surgery* 16: 65–70

222. Eggimann P, Waldvogel F 2000 Pacemaker and defibrillator infections. *Infections Associated with Indwelling Medical Devices*. Washington, DC American Society for Microbiology Press, pp. 247–257

223. Harcombe AA, Newell SA, Ludman PF et al 1998 Late complications following permanent pacemaker implantation or elective unit replacement. *Heart* 80: 240–244

224. Da Costa A, Lelievre H, Kirkorian G et al 1998 Role of the preaxillary flora in pacemaker infections: a prospective study. *Circulation* 97: 1791–1795

225. Klug D, Lacroix D, Savoye C et al 1997 Systemic infection related to endocarditis on pacemaker leads: clinical presentation and management. *Circulation* 95: 2098–2107

226. Cacoub P, Leprince P, Nataf P et al 1998 Pacemaker infective endocarditis. *American Journal of Cardiology* 82: 480–484

227. Lewis AB, Hayes DL, Holmes DR, Vlietstra RE, Pluth JR, Osborn MJ 1985 Update

on infections involving permanent pacemakers. Characterization and management. *Journal of Thoracic and Cardiovascular Surgery* 89: 758–763

228. de la Fuente A, Sanchez JR, Uriz J, Reparaz J, Lopez-Coronado JL, Moriones I 1997 Infection of a pacemaker by *Brucella melitensis*. *Texas Heart Institute Journal* 24: 129–130

229. Verghese S, Mullaseri A, Padmaja P, Subhadra AC, Cherian KM 1998 Pacemaker implant site infection caused by atypical mycobacteria. *Indian Heart Journal* 50: 201–202

230. Acquati F, Semeraro F, Respighi E, Gallotti R, Repetto S, Binaghi G 1987 *Aspergillus flavus*-infection of a pacemaker wire: continuing evidence for active management of infected pacemakers. *Giornale Italiano di Cardiologia* 17: 467–468

231. Davis WA, Isner JM, Bracey AW, Roberts WC, Garagusi VF 1980 Disseminated *Petriellidium boydii* and pacemaker endocarditis. *American Journal of Medicine* 69: 929–932

232. Victor F, De Place C, Camus C et al 1999 Pacemaker lead infection: echocardiographic features, management, and outcome. *Heart* 81: 82–87

233. Molina JE 1997 Undertreatment and overtreatment of patients with infected antiarrhythmic implantable devices. *Annals of Thoracic Surgery* 63: 504–509

234. Chua JD, Wilkoff BL, Lee I, Juratli N, Longworth DL, Gordon SM 2000 Diagnosis and management of infections involving implantable electrophysiologic cardiac devices. *Annals of Internal Medicine* 133: 604–608

235. Bracke FA, Meijer A, van Gelder LM 2001 Pacemaker lead complications: when is extraction appropriate and what can we learn from published data? *Heart* 85: 254–259

236. Abad C, Manzano JJ, Quintana J, Bolanos J, Manzano JL 1995 Removal of infected dual chambered transvenous pacemaker and implantation of a new epicardial dual chambered device with cardiopulmonary bypass: experience with seven cases. *Pacing and Clinical Electrophysiology* 18: 1272–1275

237. Wilkoff BL, Byrd CL, Love CJ et al 1993 Pacemaker lead extraction with the laser sheath: results of the pacing lead extraction with the excimer sheath (PLEXES) trial. *Journal of the American College of Cardiology* 33: 1671–1676

238. Kennergren C 1999 Excimer laser assisted extraction of permanent pacemaker and ICD leads: present experiences of a European multi-centre study. *European Journal of Cardio-Thoracic Surgery* 15: 856–860

239. Nguyen KT, Neese P, Kessler DJ 2000 Successful laser-assisted percutaneous extraction of four pacemaker leads associated with large vegetations. *Pacing and Clinical Electrophysiology* 23: 1260–1262

240. Voet JG, Vandekerckhove YR, Muyldermans LL, Missault LH, Matthys LJ 1999 Pacemaker lead infection: report of three cases and review of the literature. *Heart* 81: 88–91

241. Kusumoto FM, Goldschlager N 1996 Cardiac pacing. *New England Journal of Medicine* 334: 89–97

242. Da Costa A, Kirkorian G, Cucherat M et al 1998 Antibiotic prophylaxis for permanent pacemaker implantation: a meta-analysis. *Circulation* 97: 1796–1801

243. Arnow PM, Quimosing EM, Beach M 1993 Consequences of intravascular catheter sepsis. *Clinical Infectious Diseases* 16: 778–784

244. Maki DG 1981 Nosocomial bacteremia. An epidemiologic overview. *American Journal of Medicine* 70: 719–732

245. Maki D 1990 The epidemiology and prevention of nosocomial bloodstream infections (Abstract). Programs and Abstracts of the Third International Conference on Nosocomial Infections, Atlanta, GA

246. Maki D, Mermel L 1998 Infections due to infusion therapy. In: Bennett JV, Brachman PS, (eds). *Hospital Infections*, 4th edn. Philadelphia, Lippincott-Raven, pp. 689–724

247. Smith RL, Meixler SM, Simberkoff MS 1991 Excess mortality in critically ill patients with nosocomial bloodstream infections. *Chest* 100: 164–167

248. Pittet D, Tarara D, Wenzel R 1994 Nosocomial bloodstream infection in critically ill patients. Excess length of stay, extra costs, and attributable mortality. *Journal of the American Medical Association* 271: 1598–1601

249. Collignon PJ 1994 Intravascular catheter associated sepsis: a common problem. The Australian Study on Intravascular Catheter Associated Sepsis. *Medical Journal of Australia* 161: 374–378

250. Digiovine B, Chenoweth C, Watts C, Higgins M 1999 The attributable mortality and costs of primary nosocomial bloodstream infections in the intensive care unit. *American Journal of Respiratory Critical Care Medicine* 160: 976–981

251. Rello J, Ochagavia A, Sabanes E et al 2000 Evaluation of outcome of intravenous catheter-related infections in critically ill patients. *American Journal of Respiratory Critical Care Medicine* 162: 1027–1030

252. Kluger D, Maki D 2001 The relative risk of intravascular device-related bloodstream infections with different types of intravascular devices in adults. A meta-analysis of 206 published studies. *Presented in abstract form at the Fourth Decennial International Conference on Nosocomial and Healthcare-Associated Infections, Atlanta, GA, 2000. Submitted for publication*

253. Maki DG, Goldman DA, Rhame FS 1973 Infection control in intravenous therapy. *Annals of Internal Medicine* 79: 867–887

254. Marrie TJ, Costerton JW 1984 Scanning and transmission electron microscopy of in situ bacterial colonization of intravenous and intraarterial catheters. *Journal of Clinical Microbiology* 19: 687–693

255. Cooper GL, Schiller AL, Hopkins CC 1988 Possible role of capillary action in pathogenesis of experimental catheter-associated dermal tunnel infections. *Journal of Clinical Microbiology* 26: 8–12

256. Sitges-Serra A, Linares J, Garau J 1985 Catheter sepsis: the clue is the hub. *Surgery* 97: 355–357

257. Maki DG, Jarrett F, Sarafin HW 1977 A semiquantitative culture method for identification of catheter-related infection in the burn patient. *Journal of Surgical Research* 22: 513–520

258. Cooper GL, Hopkins CC 1988 Rapid diagnosis of intravascular catheter-associated infection by direct Gram staining of catheter segments. *New England Journal of Medicine* 312: 1142–1147

259. Mermel LA, McCormick RD, Springman SR, Maki DG 1991 The pathogenesis and epidemiology of catheter-related infection with pulmonary artery Swan-Ganz catheters: a prospective study utilizing molecular subtyping. *American Journal of Medicine* 91: 197S–205S

260. Cheesbrough JS, Finch RG, Burden RP 1986 A prospective study of the mechanisms of infection associated with hemodialysis catheters. *Journal of Infectious Diseases* 154: 579–589

261. Flynn PM, Shenep JL, Stokes DC, Barrett FF 1987 In situ management of confirmed central venous catheter-related bacteremia. *Pediatric Infectious Diseases Journal* 6: 729–734

262. Maki DG, Narans LL, Banton J 1998 A prospective study of the pathogenesis of picc-related bsi (Abstract). Proceedings and Abstracts of the 38th Interscience Conference of Antimicrobial Agents and Chemotherapy; September 24–27, 1998; San Diego, CA

263. Maki DG, Kluger DM, Crnich CJ 2001 The microbiology of intravascular device-related infection in adults: an analysis of 159 prospective studies and implications for prevention and treatment. *Submitted for publication*

264. O'Grady NP, Barie PS, Bartlett J et al 1998 Practice parameters for evaluating new fever in critically ill adult patients. Task Force of the American College of Critical Care Medicine of the Society of Critical Care Medicine in collaboration with the Infectious Disease Society of America. *Crtical Care Medicine* 26: 392–408

265. Sherertz RJ, Heard SO, Raad II 1997 Diagnosis of triple-lumen catheter infection: comparison of roll plate, sonication, and flushing methodologies. *Journal of Clinical Microbiology* 35: 641–646

266. Siegman-Igra Y, Anglim AM, Shapiro DE, Adal KA, Strain BA, Farr BM 1997 Diagnosis of vascular catheter-related bloodstream infection: a meta-analysis. *Journal of Clinical Microbiology* 35: 928–936

267. Maki DG, Stolz SS, Wheeler S, Mermel LA 1994 A prospective, randomized trial of gauze and two polyurethane dressings for site care of pulmonary artery catheters: implications for catheter management. *Crtical Care Medicine* 22: 1729–1737

268. Maki DG, Stolz SM, Wheeler S, Mermel LA 1997 Prevention of central venous catheter-related bloodstream infection by use of an antiseptic-impregnated catheter. A randomized, controlled trial. *Annals of Internal Medicine* 127: 257–266

269. Raad I, Darouiche R, Dupuis J et al 1997 Central venous catheters coated with minocycline and rifampin for the prevention of catheter-related colonization and bloodstream infections. A randomized, double-blind trial. The Texas Medical Center Catheter Study Group. *Annals of Internal Medicine* 127: 267–274

270. Gowardman JR, Montgomery C, Thirlwell S et al 1998 Central venous catheter-related bloodstream infections: an analysis of incidence and risk factors in a cohort of 400 patients. *Intensive Care Medicine* 24: 1034–1039

271. Tacconelli E, Tumbarello M, Pittiruti M et al 1997 Central venous catheter-related sepsis in a cohort of 366 hospitalised patients. *European Journal of Clinical Microbiology and Infectious Diseases* 16: 203–209

272. Sherertz RJ, Raad, II, Belani A et al 1990 Three-year experience with sonicated vascular catheter cultures in a clinical microbiology laboratory. *Journal of Clinical Microbiology* 28: 76–82

273. Blot F, Nitenberg G, Chachaty E et al 1999 Diagnosis of catheter-related bacteraemia: a prospective comparison of the time to positivity of hub-blood versus peripheral-blood cultures. *Lancet* 354: 1071–1077

274. Rijnders BJ, Verwaest C, Peetermans WE et al 2001 Difference in time to positivity of hub-blood versus nonhub-blood cultures is not useful for the diagnosis of catheter-related bloodstream infection in critically ill patients. *Critical Care Medicine* 29: 1399–1403

275. Kite P, Dobbins BM, Wilcox MH, McMahon MJ 1999 Rapid diagnosis of central-venous-catheter-related bloodstream infection without catheter removal. *Lancet* 354: 1504–1507

276. Kite P, Dobbins BM, Wilcox MH et al 1997 Evaluation of a novel endoluminal brush method for in situ diagnosis of catheter related sepsis. *Journal of Clinical Pathology* 50: 278–282

277. van Heerden PV, Webb SA, Fong S, Golledge CL, Roberts BL, Thompson WR 1996 Central venous catheters revisited – infection rates and an assessment of the new Fibrin Analysing System brush. *Anaesthesia and Intensive Care* 24: 330–333

278. Verghese A, Widrich WC, Arbeit RD 1985 Central venous septic thrombophlebitis – the role of medical therapy. *Medicine* 64: 394–400

279. Dugdale DC, Ramsey PG 1990 *Staphylococcus aureus* bacteremia in patients with Hickman catheters. *American Journal of Medicine* 89: 137–141

280. Riebel W, Frantz N, Adelstein D, Spagnuolo PJ 1986 *Corynebacterium JK*: a cause of nosocomial device-related infection. *Reviews of Infectious Diseases* 8: 42–49

281. Banerjee C, Bustamante CI, Wharton R, Talley E, Wade JC 1988 *Bacillus* infections in patients with cancer. *Archives of Internal Medicine* 148: 1769–1774

282. Elting LS, Bodey GP 1990 Septicemia due to *Xanthomonas* species and non-aeruginosa *Pseudomonas* species: increasing incidence of catheter-related infections. *Medicine* 69: 296–306

283. Marcon MJ, Powell DA 1992 Human infections due to *Malassezia* spp. *Clinical Microbiology Reviews* 5: 101–119

284. Raad, II, Vartivarian S, Khan A, Bodey GP 1991 Catheter-related infections caused by the Mycobacterium fortuitum complex: 15 cases and review. *Reviews of Infectious Diseases* 13: 1120–1125

285. Hartman GE, Shochat SJ 1987 Management of septic complications associated with Silastic catheters in childhood malignancy. *Pediatric Infectious Diseases Journal* 6: 1042–1047

286. Benezra D, Kiehn TE, Gold JW, Brown AE, Turnbull AD, Armstrong D 1988 Prospective study of infections in indwelling central venous catheters using quantitative blood cultures. *American Journal of Medicine* 85: 495–498

287. Marr KA, Sexton DJ, Conlon PJ, Corey GR, Schwab SJ, Kirkland KB 1997 Catheter-related bacteremia and outcome of attempted catheter salvage in patients undergoing hemodialysis. *Annals of Internal Medicine* 127: 275–280

288. Raad I, Davis S, Khan A, Tarrand J, Elting L, Bodey GP 1992 Impact of central venous catheter removal on the recurrence of catheter-related coagulase-negative staphylococcal bacteremia. *Infection Control and Hospital Epidemiology* 13: 215–221

289. Kulak K, Maki DG 1992 Treatment of hickman catheter-related candidemia without removing the catheter. Programs and Abstracts of the 32nd Interscience Conference on Antimicrobial Agents and Chemotherapy, Anaheim, CA

290. Groeger JS, Lucas AB, Thaler HT et al 1993 Infectious morbidity associated with long-term use of venous access devices in patients with cancer. *Annals of Internal Medicine* 119: 1168–1174

291. Dato VM, Dajani AS 1990 Candidemia in children with central venous catheters: role of catheter removal and amphotericin B therapy. *Pediatric Infectious Diseases Journal* 9: 309–314

292. Rex JH, Bennett JE, Sugar AM et al 1995 Intravascular catheter exchange and duration of candidemia. NIAID Mycoses Study Group and the Candidemia Study Group. *Clinical Infectious Diseases* 21: 994–996

293. Anthony TU, Rubin LG 1999 Stability of antibiotics used for antibiotic-lock treatment of infections of implantable venous devices (ports). *Antimicrobial Agents and Chemotherapy* 43: 2074–2076

294. Messing B, Man F, Colimon R, Thuillier F, Beliah M 1990 Antibiotic lock technique is an effective treatment of bacterial catheter-related sepsis during parenteral nutrition. *Clinical Nutrition* 19: 220–224

295. Krzywda EA, Andris DA, Edmiston CE Jr, Quebbeman EJ 1995 Treatment of Hickman catheter sepsis using antibiotic lock technique. *Infection Control and Hospital Epidemiology* 16: 596–598

296. Champault G 1986 Totally implantable catheters for cancer chemotherapy: French experience on 325 cases. *Cancer Drug Delivery* 3: 131–137

297. Brothers TE, Von Moll LK, Niederhuber JE, Roberts JA, Walker-Andrews S, Ensminger WD 1988 Experience with subcutaneous infusion ports in three hundred patients. *Surgery, Gynecology and Obstetrics* 166: 295–301

298. Longuet P, Douard MC, Maslo C, Benoit C, Arlet G, Leport C 1995 Limited efficacy of antibiotic lock techniques (ALT) in catheter related bacteremia of totally implanted ports (TIP) in HIV infected oncologic patients (Abstract). Programs and Abstracts of the 35th Interscience Conference of Antimicrobial Agents and Chemotherapy, San Francisco

299. Raad I 2000 Management of intravascular catheter-related infections. *Journal of Antimicrobial Chemotherapy* 45: 267–270

300. Mermel LA, Farr BM, Sherertz RJ et al 2001 Guidelines for the management of intravascular catheter-related infections. *Clinical Infectious Diseases* 32: 1249–1272

301. Raad, II, Sabbagh MF 1992 Optimal duration of therapy for catheter-related *Staphylococcus aureus* bacteremia: a study of 55 cases and review. *Cleveland Clinical Journal of Medicine* 14: 75–82

302. Maki DG, Agger WA 1988 Enterococcal bacteremia: clinical features, the risk of endocarditis, and management. *Medicine* 67: 248–269

303. Bowler I, Conlon C, Crook D, Peto K 1992 Optimum duration of therapy for catheter related Staphylococcus aureus bacteremia: A cohort study of 75 patients (Abstract). Programs and Abstracts of the Thirty-Second Interscience Conference on Antimicrobial Agents and Chemotherapy, 1992; Anaheim, CA

304. Raad, II, Luna M, Khalil SA, Costerton JW, Lam C, Bodey GP 1994 The relationship between the thrombotic and infectious complications of central venous catheters. *Journal of the American Medical Association* 271: 1014–1016

305. Fowler VG, Li J, Corey GR et al 1997 Role of echocardiography in evaluation of patients with *Staphylococcus aureus* bacteremia: experience in 103 patients. *Journal of the American College of Cardiology* 30: 1072–1078

306. Rose HD 1978 Venous catheter-associated candidemia. *American Journal of Medical Science* 275: 265–269

307. Lecciones JA, Lee JW, Navarro EE et al 1992 Vascular catheter-associated fungemia in patients with cancer: analysis of 155 episodes. *Clinical Infectious Diseases* 14: 875–883

308. Phillips P, Shafran S, Garber G et al 1997 Multicenter randomized trial of fluconazole versus amphotericin B for treatment of candidemia in non-neutropenic patients. Canadian Candidemia Study Group. *European Journal of Clinical Microbiology and Infectious Diseases* 16: 337–345

309. Nguyen MH, Peacock JE Jr, Tanner DC et al 1995 Therapeutic approaches in patients with candidemia. Evaluation in a multicenter, prospective, observational study. *Archives of Internal Medicine* 155: 2429–2435

310. Lee YH, Kerstein MD 1971 Osteomyelitis and septic arthritis. A complication of subclavian venous catheterization. *New England Journal of Medicine* 285: 1179–1180

311. Mermel LA 2000 Prevention of intravascular catheter-related infections. *Annals of Internal Medicine* 132: 391–402

312. Crnich CJ, Maki DG 2001 The promise of novel technology for prevention of intravascular device-related bloodstream infection, part I: short-term devices. *Clinical Infectious Diseases* in press

313. O'Grady NP, Alexander M, Dellinger EP et al 2001 HICPAC Guideline (Draft) for the prevention of intravascular catheter-related infection. *Federal Register* in Press

314. CDC 2000 Monitoring hospital-acquired infections to promote patient safety – United States, 1990–1999. *MMWR Morbidity and Mortality Weekly Reports* 49: 149–153

315. Raad, II, Hohn DC, Gilbreath BJ et al 1994 Prevention of central venous catheter-related infections by using maximal sterile barrier precautions during insertion. *Infection Control and Hospital Epidemiology* 15: 231–238

316. Maki DG, Ringer M, Alvarado CJ 1991 Prospective randomized trial of povidone-iodine, alcohol, and chlorhexidine for prevention of infection associated with central venous and arterial catheters. *Lancet* 338: 339–343

317. Mimoz O, Pieroni L, Lawrence C et al 1996 Prospective, randomized trial of two antiseptic solutions for prevention of central venous or arterial catheter colonization and infection in intensive care unit patients. *Critical Care Medicine* 24: 1818–1823

318. Maki DG, Knasinski V, Narans LL, Gordon BJ 2001 A randomized trial of a novel 1% chlorhexidine-75% alcohol tincture versus 10% povidone-iodine for cutaneous disinfection with vascular catheters (Abstract). Paper presented at: 31st Annual Society for Hospital Epidemiology of America Meeting, Toronto

319. Conly JM, Grieves K, Peters B 1989 A prospective, randomized study comparing transparent and dry gauze dressings for central venous catheters. *Journal of Infectious Diseases* 159: 310–319

320. Maki D, Will L 1984 Colonization and infection associated with transparent dressings for central venous, arterial, and Hickman catheters: A comparative trial (Abstract). Programs and Abstracts of the 24th Interscience Conference on Antimicrobial Agents and Chemotherapy, Washington, DC

321. Maki D, Mermel LA, Martin M, Knasinski V, Berry D 1996 A highly semipermeable polyurethane dressing does not increase the risk of CVC-related BSI: a prospective, multicenter, investigator-blinded trial (Abstract). Programs and Abstracts of the 36th Interscience Conference on Antimicrobial Agents and Chemotherapy; September 15–18, New Orleans, LA

322. Hanazaki K, Shingu K, Adachi W, Miyazaki T, Amano J 1999 Chlorhexidine dressing for reduction in microbial colonization of the skin with central venous catheters: a prospective randomized controlled trial. *Journal of Hospital Infections* 42: 165–168

323. Garland JS, Harris MC, Alex CP et al 2001 A randomized trial comparing povidone-iodine to chlorhexidine gluconate impregnated dressing for prevention of central venous catheter infections in neonates. *Pediatrics* 107: 1431–1437

324. Maki DG, Mermel LA, Kluger DM et al 2000 The efficacy of a chlorhexidine-impregnated sponge (biopatch) for the prevention of intravascular catheter-related infection – a prospective, randomized, controlled, multicenter trial. Programs and Abstracts of the 40th Interscience Conference on Antimicrobial Agents and Chemotherapy, Toronto, Ontario, Canada

325. Hanley EM, Veeder A, Smith T, Drusano G, Currie E, Venezia RA 2000 Evaluation of an antiseptic triple-lumen catheter in an intensive care unit. *Critical Care Medicine* 28: 366–370

326. Veenstra DL, Saint S, Saha S, Lumley T, Sullivan SD 1999 Efficacy of antiseptic-impregnated central venous catheters in preventing catheter-related bloodstream infection: a meta-analysis. *Journal of the American Medical Association* 281: 261–267

327. Veenstra DL, Saint S, Sullivan SD 1999 Cost-effectiveness of antiseptic-impregnated central venous catheters for the prevention of catheter-related bloodstream infection. *Journal of the American Medical Association* 282: 554–560

328. Saint S, Veenstra DL, Lipsky BA 2000 The clinical and economic consequences of nosocomial central venous catheter-related infection: are antimicrobial catheters useful? *Infection Control and Hospital Epidemiology* 21: 375–380

329. Raad I, Darouiche R, Hachem R, Sacilowski M, Bodey GP 1995 Antibiotics and prevention of microbial colonization of catheters. *Antimicrobial Agents and Chemotherapy* 39: 2397–2400

330. Raad I, Darouiche R, Hachem R, Mansouri M, Bodey GP 1996 The broad-spectrum activity and efficacy of catheters coated with minocycline and rifampin. *Journal of Infectious Diseases* 173: 418–424

331. Darouiche RO, Raad, II, Heard SO et al 1999 A comparison of two antimicrobial-impregnated central venous catheters. Catheter Study Group. *New England Journal of Medicine* 340: 1–8

332. Warren JW, Platt R, Thomas RJ, Rosner B, Kass EH 1978 Antibiotic irrigation and catheter-associated urinary-tract infections. *New England Journal of Medicine* 299: 570–573

333. Zakrzewska-Bode A, Muytjens HL, Liem KD, Hoogkamp-Korstanje JA 1995 Mupirocin resistance in coagulase-negative staphylococci, after topical prophylaxis for the reduction of colonization of central venous catheters. *Journal of Hospital Infection* 31: 189–193

334. Martinez E, Collazos J, Mayo J 1999 Hypersensitivity reactions to rifampin. Pathogenetic mechanisms, clinical manifestations, management strategies, and review of the anaphylactic-like reactions. *Medicine* 78: 361–369

335. Marik PE, Abraham G, Careau P, Varon J, Fromm RE Jr 1999 The ex vivo antimicrobial activity and colonization rate of two antimicrobial-bonded central venous catheters. *Critical Care Medicine* 27: 1128–1131

336. Sampath L, Tambe S, Modak S 1999 Comparison of the efficacy of antiseptic and antibiotic catheters impregnated on both their luminal and outer surfaces (Abstract). Programs and Abstracts of the 39th Interscience Conference on Antimicrobial Agents and Chemotherapy; September 26–29, San Francisco, CA

337. Boswald M, Lugauer S, Regenfus A et al 1999 Reduced rates of catheter-associated infection by use of a new silver-impregnated central venous catheter. *Infection* 27 (Suppl. 1): S56–60

338. Carbon RT, Lugauer S, Geitner U et al 1999 Reducing catheter-associated infections with silver-impregnated catheters in long-term therapy of children. *Infection* 27 (Suppl. 1): S69–73

339. Bong JJ, Kite P, Wilcox MH et al 1998 Reduction of the incidence of catheter-related sepsis (CRS) in high-risk patients by silver iontophoretic central venous catheters (CVCs) (Abstract). 38th Interscience Conference on Antimicrobial Agents and Chemotherapy, San Diego, CA

340. Shaikh LS 2001 Catheter-related infection rates in intensive care patients after changing to silver and platinum impregnated central venous catheters (Abstract). Society of Critical Care Meeting, San Fransisco, CA

341. Segura M, Alvarez-Lerma F, Tellado JM et al 1996 A clinical trial on the prevention of catheter-related sepsis using a new hub model. *Annals of Surgery* 223: 363–369

342. Luna J, Masdeu G, Perez M et al 2000 Clinical trial evaluating a new hub device designed to prevent catheter-related sepsis. *European Journal of Clinical Microbiology and Infectious Diseases* 19: 655–662

343. Halpin DP, O'Byrne P, McEntee G, Hennessy TP, Stephens RB 1991 Effect of a betadine connection shield on central venous catheter sepsis. *Nutrition* 7: 33–34

344. Spafford PS, Sinkin RA, Cox C, Reubens L, Powell KR 1994 Prevention of central venous catheter-related coagulase-negative staphylococcal sepsis in neonates. *Journal of Pediatrics* 125: 259–263

345. Henrickson KJ, Axtell RA, Hoover SM et al 2000 Prevention of central venous catheter-related infections and thrombotic events in immunocompromised children by the use of vancomycin/ciprofloxacin/heparin flush solution: A randomized, multicenter, double-blind trial. *Journal of Clinical Oncology* 18: 1269–1278

346. Guertin SR 1987 Cerebrospinal fluid shunts. Evaluation, complications, and crisis management. *Pediatric Clinics of North America* 34: 203–217

347. Schoenbaum SC, Gardner P, Shillito J 1975 Infections of cerebrospinal fluid shunts: epidemiology, clinical manifestations, and therapy. *Journal of Infectious Diseases* 131: 543–552

348. Forward KR, Fewer HD, Stiver HG 1983 Cerebrospinal fluid shunt infections. A review of 35 infections in 32 patients. *Journal of Neurosurgery* 59: 389–394

349. George R, Leibrock L, Epstein M 1979 Long-term analysis of cerebrospinal fluid shunt infections. A 25-year experience. *Journal of Neurosurgery* 51: 804–811

350. Rieder MJ, Frewen TC, Del Maestro RF, Coyle A, Lovell S 1987 The effect of cephalothin prophylaxis on postoperative ventriculoperitoneal shunt infections. *Canadian Medical Association Journal.* 136: 935–938

351. Rotim K, Miklic P, Paladino J, Melada A, Marcikic M, Scap M 1997 Reducing the incidence of infection in pediatric cerebrospinal fluid shunt operations. *Childs Nervous System* 13: 584–587

352. Davis SE, Levy ML, McComb JG, Masri-Lavine L 1999 Does age or other factors influence the incidence of ventriculoperitoneal shunt infections? *Pediatric Neurosurgery* 30: 253–257

353. Anonymous 2000 National Nosocomial Infections Surveillance (NNIS) system report, data summary from January 1992–April 2000, issued June 2000. *American Journal of Infection Control* 28: 429–448

354. James HE, Bejar R, Gluck L et al 1984 Ventriculoperitoneal shunts in high risk newborns weighing under 2000 grams: a clinical report. *Neurosurgery* 15: 198–202

355. James HE, Walsh JW, Wilson HD, Connor JD, Bean JR, Tibbs PA 1980 Prospective randomized study of therapy in cerebrospinal fluid shunt infection. *Neurosurgery* 7: 459–463

356. Walters BC, Hoffman HJ, Hendrick EB, Humphreys RP 1984 Cerebrospinal fluid shunt infection. Influences on initial management and subsequent outcome. *Journal of Neurosurgery* 60: 1014–1021

357. Chadduck W, Adametz J 1988 Incidence of seizures in patients with myelomeningocele: a multifactorial analysis. *Surgical Neurology* 30: 281–285

358. Mapstone TB, Rekate HL, Nulsen FE, Dixon MS, Glaser N, Jaffe M 1984 Relationship of CSF shunting and IQ in children with myelomeningocele: a retrospective analysis. *Childs Brain* 11: 112–118

359. Little JR, Rhoton AL, Mellinger JF 1972 Comparison of ventriculoperitoneal and ventriculoatrial shunts for hydrocephalus in children. *Mayo Clinic Proceedings* 47: 396–401

360. Lam CH, Villemure JG 1997 Comparison between ventriculoatrial and ventriculoperitoneal shunting in the adult population. *British Journal of Neurosurgery* 11: 43–48

361. Renier D, Lacombe J, Pierre-Kahn A, Sainte-Rose C, Hirsch JF 1984 Factors causing acute shunt infection. Computer analysis of 1174 operations. *Journal of Neurosurgery* 61: 1072–1078

362. Spanu G, Karussos G, Adinolfi D, Bonfanti N 1986 An analysis of cerebrospinal fluid shunt infections in adults. A clinical experience of twelve years. *Acta Neurochirurgica* 1986 80: 79–82

363. Kulkarni AV, Drake JM, Lamberti-Pasculli M 2001 Cerebrospinal fluid shunt

infection: a prospective study of risk factors. *Journal of Neurosurgery* 94: 195–201

364. Bayston R 2001 Epidemiology, diagnosis, treatment, and prevention of cerebrospinal fluid shunt infections. *Neurosurgery Clinics of North America* 36: 703–708

365. Pople IK, Quinn MW, Bayston R 1990 Morbidity and outcome of shunted hydrocephalus. *Zeitschrift fur Kinderchirurgie* 45(Suppl 1): 29–31

366. Bayston R 1975 Antibiotic prophylaxis in shunt surgery. *Developmental Medicine and Child Neurology – Supplement* 35: 99–103

367. Duhaime AC, Bonner K, McGowan KL, Schut L, Sutton LN, Plotkin S 1991 Distribution of bacteria in the operating room environment and its relation to ventricular shunt infections: a prospective study. *Childs Nervous System* 7: 211–214

368. Borges LF 1982 Cerebrospinal fluid shunts interfere with host defenses. *Neurosurgery* 10: 55–60

369. Stern S, Bayston R, Hayward RJ 1988 *Haemophillus influenzae* meningitis in the presence of cerebrospinal fluid shunts. *Childs Nervous System* 4: 164–165

370. Sathyanarayana S, Wylen EL, Baskaya MK, Nanda A 2000 Spontaneous bowel perforation after ventriculoperitoneal shunt surgery: case report and a review of 45 cases. *Surgical Neurology* 54: 388–396

371. Ferrera PC, Thibodeau L, Shillito J 1994 Long-term lumboureteral shunt removed secondary to iatrogenic meningitis. *Surgical Neurology* 42: 231–233

372. Odio C, McCracken GH Jr, Nelson JD 1984 CSF shunt infections in pediatrics. A seven-year experience. *American Journal of Diseases of Children* 138: 1103–1108

373. Shapiro S, Boaz J, Kleiman M, Kalsbeck J, Mealey J 1988 Origin of organisms infecting ventricular shunts. *Neurosurgery* 22: 868–872

374. Sells CJ, Shurtleff DB, Loeser JD 1977 Gram-negative cerebrospinal fluid shunt-associated infections. *Pediatrics* 59: 614–618

375. Greene KA, Clark RJ, Zabramski JM 1993 Ventricular CSF shunt infections associated with Corynebacterium jeikeium: report of three cases and review. *Clinical Infectious Diseases* 16: 139–141

376. Snow RB, Lavyne MH, Fraser RA 1986 Colonic perforation by ventriculoperitoneal shunts. *Surgical Neurology* 25: 173–177

377. Chiou CC, Wong TT, Lin HH et al 1994 Fungal infection of ventriculoperitoneal shunts in children. *Clinical Infectious Diseases* 19: 1049–1053

378. Wages DS, Helfend L, Finkle H 1995 Coccidioides immitis presenting as a hyphal form in a ventriculoperitoneal shunt. *Archives of Pathology and Laboratory Medicine* 119: 91–93

379. Ingram CW, Haywood HB 3rd, Morris VM, Allen RL, Perfect JR 1993 Cryptococcal ventricular-peritoneal shunt infection: clinical and epidemiological evaluation of two closely associated cases. *Infection Control and Hospital Epidemiology* 1993 14: 719–722

380. Schwartz JG, Tio FO, Fetchick RJ 1986 Filamentous *Histoplasma capsulatum* involving a ventriculoatrial shunt. *Neurosurgery* 18: 487–490

381. Yogev R 1985 Cerebrospinal fluid shunt infections: a personal view. *Pediatric Infectious Diseases Journal* 4: 113–118

382. Ronan A, Hogg GG, Klug GL 1995 Cerebrospinal fluid shunt infections in children. *Pediatric Infectious Diseases Journal* 14: 782–786

383. Valk PE, Morris JG, McRae J 1970 Pulmonary embolism as a complication of ventriculoatrial shunt. *Australasian Radiology* 14: 272–274

384. Dzenitis AJ, Mealey J Jr, Waddell JR 1965 Myocardial perforation by ventriculoatrial-shunt tubing. *Journal of The American Medical Association* 194: 1251–1253

385. Parizek J, Nytra T, Zemankova M, et al 1994 Catheterobronchial fistula due to vena cava superior thrombosis as a late complication of ventriculoatrial shunt. *Childs Nervous System* 10: 468–471

386. Yavuzgil O, Ozerkan F, Erturk U, Islekel S, Atay Y, Buket S 1999 A rare cause of right atrial mass: thrombus formation and infection complicating a ventriculoatrial shunt for hydrocephalus. *Surgical Neurology* 52: 54–60; discussion 60–51

387. Bellamy CM, Roberts DH, Ramsdale DR 1990 Ventriculo-atrial shunt causing tricuspid endocarditis: its percutaneous removal. *International Journal of Cardiology* 28: 260–262

388. Bayston R, Rodgers J, Tabara ZB 1991 Ventriculoatrial shunt colonisation and immune complex nephritis. *European Journal of Pediatric Surgery* 1(Suppl. 1): 46–47

389. Salomao JF, Leibinger RD 1999 Abdominal pseudocysts complicating CSF shunting in infants and children. Report of 18 cases. *Pediatric Neurosurgery* 31: 274–278

390. Egelhoff J, Babcock DS, McLaurin R 1985 Cerebrospinal fluid pseudocysts:

sonographic appearance and clinical management. *Pediatric Neuroscience* 12: 80–86

391. Haines SJ, Taylor F 1982 Prophylactic methicillin for shunt operations: effects on incidence of shunt malfunction and infection. *Childs Brain* 9: 10–22

392. Morissette I, Gourdeau M, Francoeur J 1993 CSF shunt infections: a fifteen-year experience with emphasis on management and outcome. *Canadian Journal of Neurological Sciences* 20: 118–122

393. Hubschmann OR, Countee RW 1980 Acute abdomen in children with infected ventriculoperitoneal shunts. *Archives of Surgery* 115: 305–307

394. Noetzel MJ, Baker RP 1984 Shunt fluid examination: risks and benefits in the evaluation of shunt malfunction and infection. *Journal of Neurosurgery* 61: 328–332

395. Walters BC 1992 Cerebrospinal fluid shunt infection. *Neurosurgery Clinics of North America* 3: 387–401

396. McLaurin RL, Frame PT 1987 Treatment of infections of cerebrospinal fluid shunts. *Reviews of Infectious Diseases* 9: 595–603

397. Wang KC, Lee HJ, Sung JN, Cho BK 1999 Cerebrospinal fluid shunt infection in children: efficiency of management protocol, rate of persistent shunt colonization, and significance of 'off-antibiotics' trial. *Childs Nervous System* 15: 38–43; discussion 43–34

398. Odio C, Mohs E, Sklar FH, Nelson JD, McCracken GH Jr 1984 Adverse reactions to vancomycin used as prophylaxis for CSF shunt procedures. *American Journal of Diseases of Children* 138: 17–19

399. Wong VK, Wright HT Jr, Ross LA, Mason WH, Inderlied CB, Kim KS 1991 Imipenem/cilastatin treatment of bacterial meningitis in children. *Pediatric Infectious Diseases Journal* 10: 122–125

400. Klugman KP, Dagan R 1995 Carbapenem treatment of meningitis. *Scandinavian Journal of Infectious Diseases – Supplementum* 96: 45–48

401. Wen DY, Bottini AG, Hall WA, Haines SJ 1992 Infections in neurologic surgery. The intraventricular use of antibiotics. *Neurosurgery Clinics of North America* 3: 343–354

402. Mangi RJ, Holstein LL, Andriole VT 1977 Treatment of Gram-negative bacillary meningitis with intrathecal gentamicin. *Yale Journal of Biology and Medicine* 50: 31–41

403. Hodges GR, Watanable IS, Singer P et al 1985 Ototoxicity of intraventricularly administered gentamicin in adult rabbits. *Research Communications in Chemical Pathology and Pharmacology* 50: 337–347

404. McCracken GH, Mize SG, Threlkeld N 1980 Intraventricular gentamicin therapy in gram-negative bacillary meningitis of infancy. Report of the Second Neonatal Meningitis Cooperative Study Group. *Lancet* 1: 787–791

405. Rahal JJ, Simberkoff MS 1982 Host defense and antimicrobial therapy in adult gram-negative bacillary meningitis. *Annals of Internal Medicine* 96: 468–474

406. Kourtopoulos H, Holm SE 1976 Intraventricular treatment of *Serratia marcescens* meningitis with gentamicin. Pharmacokinetic studies of gentamicin concentration in one case. *Scandinavian Journal of Infectious Diseases* 8: 57–60

407. Olsen L, Grotte G, Nordbring F 1977 Successful treatment of *pseudomonas aeruginosa*-ventriculitis with intraventricular gentamicin in a child with hydrocephalus. *Scandinavian Journal of Infectious Diseases* 9: 243–245

408. Bayston R 1987 Intraventricular vancomycin for treatment of shunt-associated ventriculitis. *Journal of Antimicrobial Chemotherapy* 20: 283

409. Swayne R, Rampling A, Newsom SW 1987 Intraventricular vancomycin for treatment of shunt-associated ventriculitis. *Journal of Antimicrobial Chemotherapy* 19: 249–253

410. Krontz DP, Strausbaugh LJ 1980 Effect of meningitis and probenecid on the penetration of vancomycin into cerebrospinal fluid in rabbits. *Antimicrobial Agents and Chemotherapy* 18: 882–886

411. Andes DR, Craig WA 1999 Pharmacokinetics and pharmacodynamics of antibiotics in meningitis. *Infectious Disease Clinics of North America* 13: 595–618

412. Manzella JP, Paul RL, Butler IL 1988 CNS toxicity associated with intraventricular injection of cefazolin. Report of three cases. *Journal of Neurosurgery* 68: 970–971

413. Venes JL 1976 Control of shunt infection. Report of 150 consecutive cases. *Journal of Neurosurgery* 45: 311–314

414. Taylor GJ, Bannister GC, Leeming JP 1995 Wound disinfection with ultraviolet radiation. *Journal of Hospital Infections* 30: 85–93

415. Gower DJ, Gower VC, Richardson SH, Kelly DL 1985 Reduced bacterial adherence to silicone plastic neurosurgical prosthesis. *Pediatric Neuroscience* 12: 127–133

416. Maurice-Williams RS, Pollock J 1999 Topical antibiotics in neurosurgery: a re-

evaluation of the Malis technique. *British Journal of Neurosurgery* 13: 312–315

417. Faillace WJ 1995 A no-touch technique protocol to diminish cerebrospinal fluid shunt infection. *Surgical Neurology* 43: 344–350

418. Choux M, Genitori L, Lang D, Lena G 1992 Shunt implantation: reducing the incidence of shunt infection. *Journal of Neurosurgery* 77: 875–880

419. Horgan MA, Piatt JH Jr 1997 Shaving of the scalp may increase the rate of infection in CSF shunt surgery. *Pediatric Neurosurgery* 26: 180–184

420. Haines SJ 1992 Antibiotic prophylaxis in neurosurgery. The controlled trials. *Neurosurgery Clinics of North America* 3: 355–358

421. Walters BC, Goumnerova L, Hoffman HJ, Hendrick EB, Humphreys RP, Levinton C 1992 A randomized controlled trial of perioperative rifampin/trimethoprim in cerebrospinal fluid shunt surgery. *Childs Nervous System* 8: 253–257

422. Blomstedt GC 1985 Results of trimethoprim-sulfamethoxazole prophylaxis in ventriculostomy and shunting procedures. A double-blind randomized trial. *Journal of Neurosurgery* 62: 694–697

423. Bayston R, Bannister C, Boston V et al 1990 A prospective randomised controlled trial of antimicrobial prophylaxis in hydrocephalus shunt surgery. *Zeitschrift für Kinderchirurgie* 45(Suppl. 1): 5–7

424. Langley JM, LeBlanc JC, Drake J, Milner R 1993 Efficacy of antimicrobial prophylaxis in placement of cerebrospinal fluid shunts: meta-analysis. *Clinical Infectious Diseases* 17: 98–103

425. Haines SJ, Walters BC 1994 Antibiotic prophylaxis for cerebrospinal fluid shunts: a metanalysis. *Neurosurgery* 34: 87–92

426. Bayston R, Milner RD 1981 Antimicrobial activity of silicone rubber used in hydrocephalus shunts, after impregnation with antimicrobial substances. *Journal of Clinical Pathology* 34: 1057–1062

427. Bayston R, Grove N, Siegel J, Lawellin D, Barsham S 1989 Prevention of hydrocephalus shunt catheter colonisation in vitro by impregnation with antimicrobials. *Journal of Neurology, Neurosurgery and Psychiatry* 52: 605–609

428. Bayston R, Lambert E 1997 Duration of protective activity of cerebrospinal fluid shunt catheters impregnated with antimicrobial agents to prevent bacterial catheter-related infection. *Journal of Neurosurgery* 87: 247–251

429. Ersahin Y, Mutluer S, Kocaman S 1997 Immunoglobulin prophylaxis in shunt infections: a prospective randomized study. *Childs Nervous System* 13: 546–549

430. Paramore CG, Turner DA 1994 Relative risks of ventriculostomy infection and morbidity. *Acta Neurochirurgica* 127: 79–84

431. Rebuck JA, Murry KR, Rhoney DH, Michael DB, Coplin WM 2000 Infection related to intracranial pressure monitors in adults: analysis of risk factors and antibiotic prophylaxis. *Journal of Neurology, Neurosurgery and Psychiatry* 69: 381–384

432. Mollman HD, Rockswold GL, Ford SE 1988 A clinical comparison of subarachnoid catheters to ventriculostomy and subarachnoid bolts: a prospective study. *Journal of Neurosurgery* 68: 737–741

433. Mayhall CG, Archer NH, Lamb VA et al 1984 Ventriculostomy-related infections. A prospective epidemiologic study. *New England Journal of Medicine* 310: 553–559

434. Wyler AR, Kelly WA 1972 Use of antibiotics with external ventriculostomies. *Journal of Neurosurgery* 37: 185–187

435. Smith RW, Alksne JF 1976 Infections complicating the use of external ventriculostomy. *Journal of Neurosurgery* 44: 567–570

436. Kanter RK, Weiner LB, Patti AM, Robson LK 1985 Infectious complications and duration of intracranial pressure monitoring. *Critical Care Medicine* 13: 837–839

437. Aucoin PJ, Kotilainen HR, Gantz NM, Davidson R, Kellogg P, Stone B 1986 Intracranial pressure monitors. Epidemiologic study of risk factors and infections. *American Journal of Medicine* 80: 369–376

438. Clark WC, Muhlbauer MS, Lowrey R, Hartman M, Ray MW, Watridge CB 1989 Complications of intracranial pressure monitoring in trauma patients. *Neurosurgery* 25: 20–24

439. Bader MK, Littlejohns L, Palmer S 1995 Ventriculostomy and intracranial pressure monitoring: in search of a 0% infection rate. *Heart and Lung* 24: 166–172

440. Holloway KL, Barnes T, Choi S et al 1996 Ventriculostomy infections: the effect of monitoring duration and catheter exchange in 584 patients. *Journal of Neurosurgery* 85: 419–424

441. Aschoff A, Annecke A, Kockro R, Maywald N, Scheihing M, Tronnier V 1996 Complications of external CSF drainage: fatal or avoidable? A meta-analysis of 6000 literature and 485 own cases (Abstract). *European Journal of Pediatric Surgery* 6(Suppl. 1): 48

442. Ohrstrom JK, Skou JK, Ejlertsen T, Kosteljanetz M 1989 Infected ventriculostomy: bacteriology and treatment. *Acta Neurochirurgica* 100: 67–69

443. Durand ML, Calderwood SB, Weber DJ et al 1993 Acute bacterial meningitis in adults. A review of 493 episodes. *New England Journal of Medicine* 328: 21–28

444. Korinek AM 1997 Risk factors for neurosurgical site infections after craniotomy: a prospective multicenter study of 2944 patients. The French Study Group of Neurosurgical infections, the SEHP, and the C-CLIN Paris-Nord. Service Epidémiologie Hygiène et Prévention. *Neurosurgery* 41: 1073–1079; discussion 1079–1081

445. Poon WS, Ng S, Wai S 1998 CSF antibiotic prophylaxis for neurosurgical patients with ventriculostomy: a randomised study. *Acta Neurochirurgica – Supplementum* 71: 146–148

446. Flanagan PP, Riley DK, Bost JW, Wilson J, Whiting D 1996 Prophylactic antibiotics in ventriculostomies: a randomized double-blind pilot study. Programs and Proceedings of the American Association of Neurosurgical Surgeons Annual Meeting, Minneapolis, MN

447. Maki DG, Tambyah PA 2001 Engineering out the risk for infection with urinary catheters. *Emergency Infectious Diseases* 7: 342–347

448. Warren JW 1997 Catheter-associated urinary tract infections. *Infectious Disease Clinics of North America* 11: 609–622

449. Tambyah PA, Maki DG 2000 Catheter-associated urinary tract infection is rarely symptomatic: a prospective study of 1,497 catheterized patients. *Archives of Internal Medicine* 160: 678–682

450. Platt R, Polk BF, Murdock B, Rosner B 1986 Risk factors for nosocomial urinary tract infection. *American Journal of Epidemiology* 124: 977–985

451. Johnson JR, Roberts PL, Olsen RJ, Moyer KA, Stamm WE 1990 Prevention of catheter-associated urinary tract infection with a silver oxide-coated urinary catheter: clinical and microbiologic correlates. *Journal of Infectious Diseases* 162: 1145–1150

452. Riley DK, Classen DC, Stevens LE, Burke JP 1995 A large randomized clinical trial of a silver-impregnated urinary catheter: lack of efficacy and staphylococcal superinfection. *American Journal of Medicine* 98: 349–356

453. Maki DG, Knasinski V, Tambyah PA 2000 Risk factors for catheter-associated urinary tract infection: a prospective study showing the minimal effects of catheter care violation on the risk of CAUTI (Abstract). *Infection Control and Hospital Epidemiology* 21: 165

454. Tambyah PA, Halvorson KT, Maki DG 1999 A prospective study of pathogenesis of catheter-associated urinary tract infections. *Mayo Clinic Proceedings* 74: 131–136

455. Maki DG, Knasinski V, Halvorson KT, Tambyah PA, Holcomb RG 1997 A prospective, randomized, investigator-blinded trial of a novel nitrofurazone-impregnated urinary catheter (Abstract). *Infection Control and Hospital Epidemiology* 18(Suppl) 50

456. Maki DG, Knasinski V, Halvorson KT, Tambyah PA 1998 A novel silver-hydrogel-impregnated indwelling urinary catheter reduces CAUTI (Abstract). Proceedings and Abstracts of the Eighth International Meeting of the Society for Healthcare Epidemiology in America, 1998; Orlando, FL

457. Darouiche RO, Smith JA Jr, Hanna H et al 1999 Efficacy of antimicrobial-impregnated bladder catheters in reducing catheter-associated bacteriuria: a prospective, randomized, multicenter clinical trial. *Urology* 54: 976–981

458. Karchmer TB, Giannetta ET, Muto CA, Strain BA, Farr BM 2000 A randomized crossover study of silver-coated urinary catheters in hospitalized patients *Archives of Internal Medicine* 160: 3294–3298

459. Kunin CM, Chin QF, Chambers S 1987 Morbidity and mortality associated with indwelling urinary catheters in elderly patients in a nursing home – confounding due to the presence of associated diseases. *Journal of the American Geriatrics Society* 35: 1001–1006

460. Orr PH, Nicolle LE, Duckworth H, et al 1996 Febrile urinary infection in the institutionalized elderly. *American Journal of Medicine* 100: 71–77

461. Warren JW, Damron D, Tenney JH, Hoopes JM, Deforge B, Muncie HL 1987 Fever, bacteremia, and death as complications of bacteriuria in women with long-term urethral catheters. *Journal of Infectious Diseases* 155: 1151–1158

462. Stamm WE 1992 Criteria for the diagnosis of urinary tract infection and for the assessment of therapeutic effectiveness. *Infection* 20(Suppl. 3): S151–154; discussion S160–151

463. Gribble MJ, Puterman ML, McCallum NM 1989 Pyuria: its relationship to bacteriuria in spinal cord injured patients on intermittent catheterization. *Archives of Physical Medicine and Rehabilitation* 70: 376–379

464. Peterson JR, Roth EJ 1989 Fever, bacteriuria, and pyuria in spinal cord injured

patients with indwelling urethral catheters. *Archives of Physical Medicine and Rehabilitation* 70: 839–841

465. Tambyah PA, Maki DG 2000 The relationship between pyuria and infection in patients with indwelling urinary catheters: a prospective study of 761 patients. *Archives of Internal Medicine* 160: 673–677

466. Rimland D, Alexander W 1989 Absence of factors associated with significant urinary tract infections caused by coagulase-negative staphylococci. *Diagnostic Microbiology and Infectious Disease* 12: 123–127

467. Huang CT, Leu HS, Ko WC 1995 Pyuria and funguria. *Lancet* 346: 582–583

468. Lachs MS, Nachamkin I, Edelstein PH, Goldman J, Feinstein AR, Schwartz JS 1992 Spectrum bias in the evaluation of diagnostic tests: lessons from the rapid dipstick test for urinary tract infection. *Archives of Internal Medicine* 117: 135–140

469. Mimoz O, Bouchet E, Edouard A, Costa Y, Samii K 1995 Limited usefulness of urinary dipsticks to screen out catheter-associated bacteriuria in ICU patients. *Anaesthesia and Intensive Care* 23: 706–707

470. Kunin CM 1961 The quantitative significance of bacteria visualized in the urinary sediment. *New England Journal of Medicine* 265: 589

471. Stamm WE, Counts GW, Running KR, Fihn S, Turck M, Holmes KK 1982 Diagnosis of coliform infection in acutely dysuric women. *New England Journal of Medicine* 307: 463–468

472. Stark RP, Maki DG 1984 Bacteriuria in the catheterized patient. What quantitative level of bacteriuria is relevant? *New England Journal of Medicine* 311: 560–564

473. Quintiliani R, Klimek J, Cunha BA, Maderazo EG 1978 Bacteraemia after manipulation of the urinary tract. The importance of pre-existing urinary tract disease and compromised host defences. *Postgraduate Medical Journal* 54: 668–671

474. Harding GK, Nicolle LE, Ronald AR et al 1991 How long should catheter-acquired urinary tract infection in women be treated? A randomized controlled study. *Archives of Internal Medicine* 114: 713–719

475. Stamm WE, Hooton TM 1993 Management of urinary tract infections in adults. *New England Journal of Medicine* 329: 1328–1334

476. van der Wall E, Verkooyen RP, Mintjes-de Groot J et al 1992 Prophylactic ciprofloxacin for catheter-associated urinary-tract infection. *Lancet* 339: 946–951

477. Huth TS, Burke JP, Larsen RA, Classen DC, Stevens LE 1992 Clinical trial of junction seals for the prevention of urinary catheter-associated bacteriuria. *Archives of Internal Medicine* 152: 807–812

478. Saint S, Veenstra DL, Sullivan SD, Chenoweth C, Fendrick AM 2000 The potential clinical and economic benefits of silver alloy urinary catheters in preventing urinary tract infection. *Archives of Internal Medicine* 160: 2670–2675

479. Burkart JM 2000 Peritoneal dialysis. In: Brenner BM (ed.) *Brenner & Rector's The Kidney*, 6th edn. Philadelphia, W. B. Saunders; pp. 2454–2517

480. Gokal R, Alexander S, Ash S, et al 1998 Peritoneal catheters and exit-site practices toward optimum peritoneal access: 1998 update. (Official report from the International Society for Peritoneal Dialysis). *Peritoneal Dialysis International* 18: 11–33

481. Weber J, Mettang T, Hubel E, Kiefer T, Kuhlmann U 1993 Survival of 138 surgically placed straight double-cuff Tenckhoff catheters in patients on continuous ambulatory peritoneal dialysis. *Peritoneal Dialysis International* 13: 224–227

482. Burkart JM, Jordan JR, Durnell TA, Case LD 1992 Comparison of exit-site infections in disconnect versus nondisconnect systems for peritoneal dialysis. *Peritoneal Dialysis International* 12: 317–320

483. Eklund BH, Honkanen EO, Kala AR, Kyllonen LE 1995 Peritoneal dialysis access: prospective randomized comparison of the Swan neck and Tenckhoff catheters. *Peritoneal Dialysis International* 15: 353–356

484. Peterson PK, Matzke G, Keane WF 1987 Current concepts in the management of peritonitis in patients undergoing continuous ambulatory peritoneal dialysis. *Reviews of Infectious Diseases* 9: 604–612

485. Oliver MJ, Schwab SJ 2000 Infections related to hemodialysis and peritoneal dialysis. In: Waldvogel FA, Bisno AL (eds) *Infections Associated with Indwelling Medical Devices*, 3rd edn. Washington, DC, ASM Press, pp. 345–372

486. Vas SL 1994 Infections associated with the peritoneum and hemodialysis. In: Bisno AL, Waldvogel FA (eds). *Infections Associated with Indwelling Medical Devices*, 2nd edn. Washington, DC, ASM Press; pp. 309–346

487. Burkart JM, Hylander B, Durnell-Figel T, Roberts D 1990 Comparison of peritonitis rates during long-term use of standard spike versus Ultraset in continuous ambulatory peritoneal dialysis (CAPD). *Peritoneal Dialysis International* 10: 41–43

488. Scalamogna A, De Vecchi A, Castelnovo C, Guerra L, Ponticelli C 1990 Long-term incidence of peritonitis in CAPD patients treated by the Y set technique: experience in a single center. *Nephron* 55: 24–27

489. Port FK, Held PJ, Nolph KD, Turenne MN, Wolfe RA 1992 Risk of peritonitis and technique failure by CAPD connection technique: a national study. *Kidney International* 42: 967–974

490. Bonnardeaux A, Ouimet D, Galarneau A et al 1992 Peritonitis in continuous ambulatory peritoneal dialysis: impact of a compulsory switch from a standard to a Y-connector system in a single North American Center. *American Journal of Kidney Diseases* 19: 364–370

491. Holley JL, Bernardini J, Piraino B 1990 Continuous cycling peritoneal dialysis is associated with lower rates of catheter infections than continuous ambulatory peritoneal dialysis. *American Journal of Kidney Diseases* 16: 133–136

492. Sewell CM, Clarridge J, Lacke C, Weinman EJ, Young EJ 1982 Staphylococcal nasal carriage and subsequent infection in peritoneal dialysis patients. *Journal of The American Medical Association* 248: 1493–1495

493. Luzar MA, Coles GA, Faller B et al 1990 *Staphylococcus aureus* nasal carriage and infection in patients on continuous ambulatory peritoneal dialysis. *New England Journal of Medicine* 322: 505–509

494. Verbrugh HA, Keane WF, Conroy WF, Peterson PK 1984 Bacterial growth and killing in chronic ambulatory peritoneal dialysis fluids. *Journal of Clinical Microbiology* 20: 199–203

495. Brulez HF, Verbrugh HA 1995 First-line defense mechanisms in the peritoneal cavity during peritoneal dialysis. *Peritoneal Dialysis International* 15(7 Suppl): S24–33; discussion S33–24

496. Duwe AK, Vas SI, Weatherhead JW 1981 Effects of the composition of peritoneal dialysis fluid on chemiluminescence, phagocytosis, and bactericidal activity in vitro. *Infection and Immunity* 33: 130–135

497. Tranaeus A, Heimburger O, Lindholm B 1989 Peritonitis in continuous ambulatory peritoneal dialysis (CAPD): diagnostic findings, therapeutic outcome and complications. *Peritoneal Dialysis International* 9: 179–190

498. Kraus ES, Spector DA 1983 Characteristics and sequelae of peritonitis in diabetics and non-diabetics receiving chronic intermittent peritoneal dialysis. *Medicine* 62: 52–57

499. Koopmans JG, Boeschoten EW, Pannekeet MM, et al 1996 Impaired initial cell reaction in CAPD-related peritonitis. *Peritoneal Dialysis International* 16(Suppl. 1): S362–367

500. Nankivell BJ, Pacey D, Gordon DL 1991 Peritoneal eosinophillia associated with Paecilomyces variotii infection in continuous ambulatory peritoneal dialysis. *American Journal of Kidney Diseases* 18: 603–605

501. Piraino B, Bernardini J, Johnston J, Sorkin M 1987 Chemical peritonitis due to intraperitoneal vancomycin. *Peritoneal Dialysis Bulletin* 7: 156–159

502. Rubin J, Rogers WA, Taylor HM et al 1980 Peritonitis during continuous ambulatory peritoneal dialysis. *Annals of Internal Medicine* 92: 7–13

503. Bunke M, Brier ME, Golper TA 1994 Culture-negative CAPD peritonitis: the Network 9 Study. *Advances in Peritoneal Dialysis* 10: 174–178

504. Sewell DL, Golper TA, Hulman PB et al 1990 Comparison of large volume culture to other methods for isolation of microorganisms from dialysate. *Peritoneal Dialysis International* 10: 49–52

505. Eisele G, Adewunni C, Bailie GR, Yocum D, Venezia R 1993 Surreptitious use of antimicrobial agents by CAPD patients. *Peritoneal Dialysis International* 13: 313–315

506. Low DE, Keller N, Barth A, Jones RN 2001 Clinical prevalence, antimicrobial susceptibility, and geographic resistance patterns of enterococci: results from the SENTRY Antimicrobial Surveillance Program, 1997–1999. *Clinical Infectious Diseases* 32(Suppl 2): S133–145

507. Tenover FC, Biddle JW, Lancaster MV 2001 Increasing resistance to vancomycin and other glycopeptides in *Staphylococcus aureus*. *Emergency Infectious Diseases* 7: 327–332

508. Keane WF, Bailie GR, Boeschoten E et al 2000 Adult peritoneal dialysis-related peritonitis treatment recommendations: 2000 update. *Peritoneal Dialysis International* 20: 396–411

509. Gucek A, Bren AF, Hergouth V, Lindic J 1997 Cefazolin and netilmycin versus vancomycin and ceftazidime in the treatment of CAPD peritonitis. *Advances in Peritoneal Dialysis* 13: 218–220

510. Goldberg L, Clemenger M, Azadian B, Brown EA 2001 Initial treatment of peritoneal dialysis peritonitis without vancomycin with a once-daily cefazolin-based regimen. *American Journal of Kidney Diseases* 37: 49–55

511. Lai MN, Kao MT, Chen CC, Cheung SY, Chung WK 1997 Intraperitoneal once-daily dose of cefazolin and gentamicin for treating CAPD peritonitis. *Peritoneal Dialysis International* 17: 87–89

512. Shemin D, Maaz D, St Pierre D, Kahn SI, Chazan JA 1999 Effect of aminoglycoside use on residual renal function in peritoneal dialysis patients. *American Journal of Kidney Diseases* 34: 14–20

513. Davies SJ, Ogg CS, Cameron JS, Poston S, Noble WC 1989 *Staphylococcus aureus* nasal carriage, exit-site infection and catheter loss in patients treated with continuous ambulatory peritoneal dialysis (CAPD). *Peritoneal Dialysis International* 9: 61–64

514. Holley JL, Bernardini J, Piraino B 1991 Risk factors for tunnel infections in continuous peritoneal dialysis. *American Journal of Kidney Diseases* 18: 344–348

515. Millikin SP, Matzke GR, Keane WF 1991 Antimicrobial treatment of peritonitis associated with continuous ambulatory peritoneal dialysis. *Peritoneal Dialysis International* 11: 252–260

516. Bunke M, Brier ME, Golper TA 1995 *Pseudomonas* peritonitis in peritoneal dialysis patients: the Network #9 Peritonitis Study. *American Journal of Kidney Diseases* 25: 769–774

517. Szeto CC, Chow KM, Leung CB et al 2001 Clinical course of peritonitis due to Pseudomonas species complicating peritoneal dialysis: a review of 104 cases. *Kidney International* 59: 2309–2315

518. Nagappan R, Collins JF, Lee WT 1992 Fungal peritonitis in continuous ambulatory peritoneal dialysis–the Auckland experience. *American Journal of Kidney Diseases* 20: 492–496

519. Chan TM, Chan CY, Cheng SW, Lo WK, Lo CY, Cheng IK 1994 Treatment of fungal peritonitis complicating continuous ambulatory peritoneal dialysis with oral fluconazole: a series of 21 patients. *Nephrology. Dialysis, Transplantation* 9: 539–542

520. Michel C, Courdavault L, al Khayat R, Viron B, Roux P, Mignon F, 1994 Fungal peritonitis in patients on peritoneal dialysis. *American Journal of Nephrology* 14: 113–120

521. Goldie SJ, Kiernan-Tridle L, Torres C et al 1996 Fungal peritonitis in a large chronic peritoneal dialysis population: a report of 55 episodes. *American Journal of Kidney Diseases* 28: 86–91

522. Kerr CM, Perfect JR, Craven PC et al 1983 Fungal peritonitis in patients on continuous ambulatory peritoneal dialysis. *Annals of Internal Medicine* 99: 334–336

523. Arfania D, Everett ED, Nolph KD, Rubin J 1981 Uncommon causes of peritonitis in patients undergoing peritoneal dialysis. *Archives of Internal Medicine* 141: 61–64

524. Vlaanderen K, Bos HJ, de Fijter CW, et al 1991 Short dwell times reduce the local defence mechanism of chronic peritoneal dialysis patients. *Nephron* 57: 29–35

525. Cairns HS, Beckett J, Rudge CJ, Thompson FD, Mansell MA 1989 Treatment of resistant CAPD peritonitis by temporary discontinuation of peritoneal dialysis. *Clinical Nephrology* 1989; 32: 27–30

526. Murphy G, Tzamaloukas AH, Eisenberg B, Gibel LJ, Avasthi PS 1991 Intraperitoneal thrombolytic agents in relapsing or persistent peritonitis of patients on continuous ambulatory peritoneal dialysis. *Internal Journal of Artificial Organs* 14: 87–91

527. Digenis GE, Abraham G, Savin E et al 1990 Peritonitis-related deaths in continuous ambulatory peritoneal dialysis (CAPD) patients. *Peritoneal Dialysis International* 10: 45–47

528. Majkowski NL, Mendley SR 1997 Simultaneous removal and replacement of infected peritoneal dialysis catheters. *American Journal of Kidney Diseases* 29: 706–711

529. Swartz RD, Messana JM 1999 Simultaneous catheter removal and replacement in peritoneal dialysis infections: update and current recommendations. *Advances in Peritoneal Dialysis* 15: 205–208

530. Buoncristiani U, Cozzari M, Quintaliani G et al 1983 Abatement of exogenous peritonitis risk using the Perugia CAPD system. *Dialysis and Transplantation* 12: 14

531. Anonymous 1989 Peritonitis in continuous ambulatory peritoneal dialysis (CAPD): a multicentre randomized clinical trial comparing the Y connector disinfectant system to standard systems. Canadian CAPD Clinical Trials Group. *Peritoneal Dialysis International* 9: 159–163

532. Harris DC, Yuill EJ, Byth K, Chapman JR, Hunt C 1996 Twin- versus single-bag disconnect systems: infection rates and cost of continuous ambulatory peritoneal dialysis. *Journal of the American Society of Nephrology* 7: 2392–2398

533. Monteon F, Correa-Rotter R, Paniagua R et al 1988 Prevention of peritonitis with disconnect systems in CAPD: a randomized controlled trial. The Mexican Nephrology Collaborative Study Group. *Kidney International* 54: 2123–2128

534. Holley JL, Bernardini J, Piraino B 1994 Infecting organisms in continuous ambulatory peritoneal dialysis patients on the Y-set. *American Journal of Kidney Diseases* 23: 569–573

535. Piraino B, Perlmutter JA, Holley JL, Bernardini J, 1993 *Staphylococcus aureus* peritonitis is associated with *Staphylococcus aureus* nasal carriage in peritoneal dialysis patients. *Peritoneal Dialysis International* 13(Suppl. 2): S332–334

536. Oxton LL, Zimmerman SW, Roecker EB, Wakeen M 1994 Risk factors for peritoneal dialysis-related infections. *Peritoneal Dialysis International* 14: 137–144

537. Zimmerman SW, Ahrens E, Johnson CA et al 1991 Randomized controlled trial of prophylactic rifampin for peritoneal dialysis-related infections. *American Journal of Kidney Diseases* 18: 225–231

538. Perez-Fontan M, Garcia-Falcon T, Rosales M, et al 1993 Treatment of *Staphylococcus aureus* nasal carriers in continuous ambulatory peritoneal dialysis with mupirocin: long-term results. *American Journal of Kidney Diseases* 22: 708–712

539. Mylotte JM, Kahler L, Jackson E 1999 'Pulse' nasal mupirocin maintenance regimen in patients undergoing continuous ambulatory peritoneal dialysis. *Infection Control and Hospital Epidemiology* 20: 741–745

540. Crabtree JH, Hadnott LL, Burchette RJ, Siddiqi RA 2000 Outcome and clinical implications of a surveillance and treatment program for *Staphylococcus aureus* nasal carriage in peritoneal dialysis patients. *Advances in Peritoneal Dialysis* 16: 271–275

541. Sesso R, Barbosa D, Leme IL et al 1998 *Staphylococcus aureus* prophylaxis in hemodyalysis patients using central venous catheter: effect of mupirocin ointment. *Journal of the American Society of Nephrology* 9: 1085–1092

542. Bernardini J, Piraino B, Holley J, Johnston JR, Lutes R 1996 A randomized trial of Staphylococcus aureus prophylaxis in peritoneal dialysis patients: mupirocin calcium ointment 2% applied to the exit site versus cyclic oral rifampin. *American Journal of Kidney Diseases* 27: 695–700

543. Davey P, Craig AM, Hau C, Malek M 1999 Cost-effectiveness of prophylactic nasal mupirocin in patients undergoing peritoneal dialysis based on a randomized, placebo-controlled trial. *Journal of Antimicrobial Chemotherapy* 43: 105–112

544. Miller MA, Dascal A, Portnoy J, Mendelson J 1996 Development of mupirocin resistance among methicillin-resistant *Staphylococcus aureus* after widespread use of nasal mupirocin ointment. *Infection Control and Hospital Epidemiology* 17: 811–813

545. Wikdahl AM, Engman U, Stegmayr BG, Sorenssen JG 1997 One-dose cefuroxime i.v. and i.p. reduces microbial growth in PD patients after catheter insertion. *Nephrology. Dialysis, Transplantation* 12: 157–160

546. Gadallah MF, Ramdeen G, Mignone J, Patel D, Mitchell L, Tatro S 2000 Role of preoperative antibiotic prophylaxis in preventing postoperative peritonitis in newly placed peritoneal dialysis catheters. *American Journal of Kidney Diseases* 36: 1014–1019

547. Chen SC, Sorrell TC, Dwyer DE, Collignon PJ, Wright EJ 1990 Endocarditis associated with prosthetic cardiac valves. *Medical Journal of Australia* 152: 458, 461–453

548. Bisno AL, Sternau LL 1994 Infections of central nervous system shunts. In: Bisno AL, Waldvogel FA (eds). *Infections Associated with Indwelling Medical Devices*, 2nd edn. Washington DC. ASM Press; pp. 91–109

549. Steckelberg JM, Osmon DR 1994 Prosthetic joint infections. In: Bisno AL, Waldvogel FA (eds). *Infections Associated with Indwelling Medical Devices*, 2nd edn. Washington DC. ASM Press, pp. 259–290

46 Antiretroviral therapy for HIV

Anton Pozniak

Before 1988 the treatment of human immunodeficiency virus (HIV) and aquired immune deficiency syndrome (AIDS) was primarily the treatment and prevention of opportunistic infections. When zidovudine became available on compassionate grounds to those patients with AIDS, the era of antiviral therapy for HIV began. Early studies with zidovudine monotherapy showed short-term benefits in symptomatic patients in delaying disease progression[1] and the results of one of the first AIDS treatment trials, ACTG 019, suggested that even asymptomatic patients with a CD4 count of less than 500 cells/mm^3 should be treated.[2] However, by 1993, the usefulness of HIV treatment was questioned. The results of the Concorde trial indicated little benefit in early intervention[3] and ACTG 155[4] showed no advantage of dual therapy with zidovudine and ddC over zidovudine or zalcitabine monotherapy, generating a mood of therapeutic pessimism.

All that changed by mid-1995, when the results of several large-scale prospective studies proved that dual nucleoside analog regimens, especially zidovudine–didanosine, effectively delayed disease progression and prolonged life. Both the Delta and ACTG 175 trials[5,6] established the superiority of dual therapy over monotherapy and paved the way for the understanding of the importance of use of surrogate markers, particularly viral load and CD4 enumerations, in measuring the efficacy of a regimen as well as the role of resistance in virological failure. At the same time, phase II studies of another dual nucleoside regimen with zidovudine and lamivudine demonstrated impressive CD4+ and viral load benefits up to 1 year of follow-up.[7] Dual nucleoside-reverse transcriptase inhibitor (NRTI)-based regimens became commonplace, and AIDS-related mortality began to decrease.

In 1996, treatment of HIV changed dramatically for several reasons.

- First, there was an improved understanding of the pathogenesis of HIV infection.
- Second, tests became available to measure plasma HIV RNA levels down to below 1000 copies/ml.
- Third, a new and powerful class of drugs, the protease inhibitors, was introduced which, when added to the two nucleoside 'backbone' analogs, were capable of almost completely suppressing plasma HIV RNA levels. At the 10th International Conference on

AIDS in 1996, the optimism surrounding the results of these triple drug regimens led to a belief that eradication of the virus and a cure was possible.

As a result of increasing use of this highly active antiretroviral therapy (HAART), hospital admission rates for HIV-related complications and mortality rates decreased dramatically, AIDS hospice units closed and patients returned to work. Opportunistic infections, such as those caused by cytomegalovirus (CMV), *Mycobacterium avium* complex (MAC), and toxoplasmosis became exceedingly rare.[8] Published data in the late 1990s estimated the mortality rate in patients with CD4 counts of less than 100×10^6/l had fallen by nearly two-thirds to less than 8 per 100 patient-years.

However, further pathogenesis studies documented reservoirs of HIV in latently infected resting T lymphocytes and other long-lived cell populations, making it unlikely that HIV could be eradicated by antiretroviral therapy alone.[9] Strategies to sustain suppression of viral replication in the long term were required. Drug development concentrated on therapy that was potent, simple to adhere to, and could be used against resistant strains. The non-nucleoside analogs with their low pill burden, lack of food requirements and a perceived lack of long-term toxicity, as emerged for the protease inhibitors, made them an increasingly common first line treatment option. New classes of drugs are in development. Fusion inhibitors, which block the activity of the GP41 viral transmembrane protein, are in Phase III clinical trials and are likely to be the first new class of drug to reach the bedside[10] (*see* Ch. 39).

In addition to drugs that inhibit targets in the viral replication cycle, immunotherapeutic approaches are being assessed. Treatment with cycles of the cytokine interleukin (IL)-2 results in substantial increase in CD4 counts but has little effect on plasma viral load levels.[11] IL-2 may also improve immune responses to HIV and a large randomized international trial is under way to assess its efficacy in combination with effective antiretroviral regimens. Therapeutic vaccines are also under evaluation, which might improve specific immune responses and assist immunological control of HIV replication. Their clinical effectiveness remains unknown.

The long-term efficacy of current antiretroviral regimens remains uncertain; in clinical practice 40–50% of patients do not have sustained falls in plasma viral load after one year of therapy. However, the biological rationale for maintaining a clinical response has been established as sustained inhibition of viral replication results in partial reconstitution of the immune system in most patients, substantially reducing the risk of clinical progression and death. Although enthusiasm for antiretroviral therapy persists, problems are emerging, such as long-term metabolic complications of therapy.[12,13] Failure rates on HAART in clinic-based cohorts are about 50% or more[14,15] and, even among patients whose HIV RNA levels are undetectable for years, evidence of continuing viral replication can be detected.[16,17] Adherence to current regimens has to be 95% or more to ensure virological success and limit the risk of resistance emerging.

INITIATING ANTIRETROVIRAL THERAPY

AIMS OF TREATMENT

With currently available antiretroviral agents, eradication of HIV infection is not likely to be possible;[18] thus, the aim of treatment is to prolong and improve quality of life by maintaining suppression of virus replication for as long as possible.

Where possible, the objective of antiretroviral therapy is to reduce and sustain plasma viral load levels to below the level of detectability of the current ultrasensitive viral load assays (<50 copies/ml). If patients are adherent to therapy, the likelihood of a viral load rebound and drug resistance is minimal. However, in spite of inhibition of viral replication in plasma, lymph nodes, and other sites, reservoirs of HIV infection in latently infected resting macrophages and T lymphocytes remain. New cells probably continue to be infected as a result of either bursts of viral replication from these reservoirs or loss of the antiretroviral effect of the treatment regimen. Even in patients who have sustained, undetectable levels of plasma viral load for several years, discontinuation of antiretroviral therapy results in rapid rebound of plasma viral load to pre-treatment levels.[19]

The three groups of treatment-naïve patients for whom treatment might be considered are patients with primary HIV infection, patients with asymptomatic HIV infection and patients with symptomatic HIV disease or AIDS.

Primary HIV infection

There is no definitive evidence of clinical benefit from treatment of primary infection, apart from early data from a placebo-controlled study of zidovudine monotherapy.[20] The rationale for starting treatment during or shortly after infection is to attempt to maintain specific and robust CD4 helper HIV responses,[21–24] which are generally lost with the exception of long-term non-progressors[23] in chronic HIV infection.[25] Such immune responses appear to be maintained in people treated with potent antiretroviral therapy shortly after primary HIV infection. Recent data suggest that there is more rapid

and complete immune reconstitution in patients starting therapy during primary infection than in those starting treatment later.[26] There is, however, no evidence to date that any of these immunological benefits persist indefinitely with continuing treatment or after treatment is withdrawn.

Control of viral replication with no return of viremia for several weeks after withdrawal of antiretroviral therapy has been reported in a few patients treated very soon after primary infection.[27] Data suggest that stopping and starting therapy in a controlled way, so called 'strategic treatment interruptions', allows virus to intermittently rebound, which then stimulates the host immune responses.[28] This leads to a lowering of the viral load set point. In contrast, others have found that discontinuing therapy initiated during primary infection had no apparent effect upon the set point that would have been expected in the absence of any treatment.[29]

The possible benefits of treatment during primary infection with HIV should be considered against the known risks of toxicity,[30,31] the associated risk of development of drug resistance and the difficulties of long-term adherence. This remains an area of intense research.

Chronic HIV infection

Symptomatic disease

Any patient with a CD4 lymphocyte count consistently less than 200 cells/mm^3 or who has been diagnosed with AIDS or severe/recurrent HIV-related illnesses should start therapy. There is a high risk that further opportunistic infections may cause irreversible damage or be life threatening.

Asymptomatic disease

There are no controlled clinical trials to specifically address when to begin therapy in asymptomatic patients. CD4 count and plasma viral load are predictors of the estimated risk of progression to AIDS but in asymptomatic patients whether CD4 count alone or a combination of CD4 count and viral load should be used to decide when to initiate treatment has not been resolved.[32] Although clinical practice across Europe and North America varies, most clinicians would consider initiating therapy at some point when the CD4 count is 200–350 × 10^6 cells/l.

One of the strongest arguments for starting treatment early[14] comes from observational studies and controlled trials[33–35] suggesting that patients who delay therapy until the CD4 lymphocyte count is <200 cells/µl have a poorer virological and immunological response. Similar data exist from prospective clinical studies,[36] although the effect of baseline CD4 on response to therapy may not be the same for all drug regimens,[37] which may vary in potency and efficacy.

Another reason for starting early is that toxicity appears to occur less frequently at higher baseline CD4 counts. In addition, patients with a rapidly falling CD4 count (e.g. falling by more than 80 cells/ml per year on repeated testing) should be considered for initiation of therapy relatively earlier within the CD4 count range 200–350 cells/µl.

Box 46.1 Recommendations for starting antiretroviral therapy in adults: 2001

Disease stage	British HIV Association	US Department of Health and Human Services
Symptomatic	Treat	Treat
Asymptomatic		
CD4 <200 × 10⁶/l	Treat	Treat
CD4 200-350 × 10⁶/l	Consider therapy depending on rate of CD4 count decline, symptoms, and patient's wishes	Therapy should generally be offered
CD4 >350 × 10⁶/l	Defer	Defer or consider therapy if high viral load

Historically, therapy was started relatively early in patients with a high plasma viral load.[38,39] A viral load >55 000 copies/ml predicts a faster rate of decline in CD4 cells and is an independent risk factor for subsequent disease progression and death. These data are from an era before the introduction of HAART; recent cohort studies[40,41] suggest that baseline viral load does not predict subsequent mortality independently of the baseline CD4 count after starting therapy.

The arguments against starting early include growing concerns over the long-term complications of therapy. In addition, as adherence is a critical determinant of the long-term virologic response to therapy[42] clinical guidelines suggest that therapy can (and should) be deferred until patients are committed to long-term strict adherence. Unfortunately for a few patients, the motivation to start therapy may not develop until symptomatic disease is present or until the CD4+ count drops to low levels. Another reason to delay therapy is the concern that starting early may lead to virological failure, with drug-resistant variants being generated, thus limiting future options. For patients for whom there are concerns about toxicity or adherence, delayed therapy may be more prudent until better therapeutic options and/or strategies have been developed. Pill burden, dosing schedules and concomitant medication may effect both the timing of treatment and the choice of regimen (Box 46.2).

Box 46.2 Factors determining when to start and choice of therapy

- Risk of clinical disease progression (CD4 count, viral load)
- Willingness of patient to start therapy
- Clinical effectiveness of combination regimen
- Ability and motivation of patient to adhere to therapy
- Drug toxicity profile
- Pill burden and dosing schedule
- Transmitted drug resistance
- Future therapy options
- Likelihood of drug resistance
- Drug–drug interactions

In asymptomatic patients with chronic HIV infection and CD4 cell counts consistently above 350 cells/ml, few data support starting therapy. Indeed, there are good reasons to consider delaying therapy in order to minimize the long-term drug toxicity and the development of drug-resistant virus. As therapy-naïve patients consistently achieve the best results from any given combination, delaying therapy may enable patients to take simpler, less toxic and possibly more potent therapies when they eventually do start.

THERAPEUTIC STRATEGIES IN THE TREATMENT-NAÏVE PATIENT

The very dramatic fall in AIDS-related mortality and frequency of AIDS events in the developed world coincide with the introduction of HAART.[43] Any HAART regimen should be individualized in order to achieve the best potency, adherence and tolerability, to minimize potential toxicity, and to avoid any likely drug–drug interactions. A measurement of a regimen's success is achieving a viral load of <50 HIV-1 RNA copies/ml within 6–9 months of starting treatment. Although complete viral suppression may be the ultimate goal of therapy, whether this aim can be achieved is unclear with current regimens. Various observations suggest that ongoing viral replication occurs among patients in whom HIV appears to be completely suppressed.[44–46] This is particularly true among patients who have occasional bouts of viremia.[47]

No definitive clinical controlled trials demonstrate the long-term superiority of one HAART regimen over another. The advantages and disadvantages in terms of potency, adherence, toxicity, salvageability and potential drug–drug interactions should be considered for each patient and therapy individualized accordingly. For patients with very high viral loads, more than three active drugs may result in a more rapid decline in viral load.[48] Studies are in progress to determine whether this will lead to better long term outcomes as compared with standard HAART.

The most common categories of drug regimens that might be considered for a patient initiating antiretroviral therapy, are listed below.

- A single protease inhibitor: nelfinavir or saquinavir soft gel formulation.
- Two protease inhibitors, usually low-dose ritonavir and lopinavir or saquinavir or indinavir.
- One non-nucleoside reverse transcriptase inhibitor (NNRTI) such as nevirapine or efavirenz.
- Three nucleoside reverse transcriptase inhibitors (NRTIs), usually zidovudine + lamivudine + abacavir.

Two NRTIs plus one or two protease inhibitors

Protease inhibitors have clinical and surrogate marker efficacy in clinical practice. The AIDS Clinical Trials Group protocol 320 was a landmark clinical endpoint study which demonstrated long-term virological suppression and improved clinical outcome in patients taking zidovudine/lamivudine with the protease inhibitor indinavir.[49] Sustained suppression of plasma HIV-1 RNA levels for more than 4 years occurs in most patients in the Merck 035 study taking indinavir and two NRTIs.[50] Similar results occur with nelfinavir.

The hard gel formulation of saquinavir has also shown clinical benefit when used in combination,[51] but is not recommended as the sole protease inhibitor in a HAART regimen because of its poor bioavailability (*see* Ch. 39).

Many clinicians use protease inhibitors in combination to provide a pharmacokinetic boosting effect when they start patients on a protease inhibitor-based regimen. The rationale for dual protease inhibitor combinations is that these drugs are extensively metabolized by the cytochrome P_{450} system, resulting in short half-lives and low trough concentrations. Ritonavir, a potent inhibitor of the hepatic enzyme responsible for much of the drug metabolism (cytochrome P_{450} CYP3A) enhances plasma concentrations of saquinavir, indinavir, amprenavir, and lopinavir, raising trough levels and extending the half-life. This may improve potency and could be associated with a reduced risk of resistance development. In addition, a boosted protease inhibitor regimen may improve convenience by reducing dosage frequency and pill burden, facilitating adherence. However, some toxicities, such as nephrotoxicity, dry skin and nail dystrophy with indinavir–ritonavir, gastrointestinal toxicity with other boosted protease inhibitors, and lipid abnormalities, may be more common with combination protease inhibitor regimens.[52]

NNRTI-based regimens

A number of studies using NNRTI combinations have shown impressive surrogate marker results but they have not been as well evaluated as protease inhibitor combinations in controlled clinical endpoint trials.[53] Direct data comparing the two currently available NNRTIs efavirenz and nevirapine, in terms of their effects on surrogate markers and safety, are awaited.

Impressive results have been obtained using efavirenz with the nucleosides zidovudine and lamivudine. In a randomized open-label study, this combination was compared with indi-

navir together with these two drugs and showed superior surrogate marker endpoints up to 104 weeks of follow up when analyzed by 'intention to treat' and 'on treatment' analyses.[54] The major drawback of this study was the high discontinuation rate in both arms and at 48 weeks as 35% of the indinavir group and 25% of the efavirenz group withdrew from the study. Efavirenz has a long plasma half-life and one major advantage of a regimen containing this drug is a once-daily dose, which may improve adherence. Nevirapine plus the nucleosides didanosine and zidovudine have been compared with these two agents alone in antiretroviral-naïve patients;[55] superior HIV-1 RNA suppression at 48 weeks was seen in the triple therapy arm.

NNRTIs have limitations. There is less long-term experience with these drugs. They have significant side effects in the short term and the long-term safety has not been fully determined. Unfortunately, there is virtually complete cross-resistance among the NNRTIs and only one mutation confers high-level drug resistance to all the compounds in the class.

Triple NRTI regimens

The data supporting the use of triple NRTI-based regimens are more limited than with other regimens. The 48-week data from the Atlantic study showed no significant difference in viral load suppression (to below the 50 copies/ml threshold) for the triple NRTI arm (stavudine–didanosine–lamivudine) compared with the other two arms (which included a non-nucleoside, nevirapine or a protease inhibitor, indinavir) by intention to treat or on treatment analysis.[56] However triple NRTI-based regimens may be less effective in patients with high baseline HIV RNA levels (> 100 000 copies/ml).[57] When a similar study was performed in an open fashion, in spite of much higher adherence for the triple nucleoside arm, no significant differences were seen in the high viral load strata,[58] suggesting that adherence and potency are both important.

Some triple NRTI regimens have easy dosing schedules and limited drug–drug interactions. The combination of zidovudine/lamivudine into a single tablet taken twice daily simplifies dosing still further. In addition, patients who fail zidovudine, lamivudine and abacavir will usually have a virus with a mutation only at codon 184, allowing potential re-use of zidovudine and abacavir.

Triple NRTI regimens may be attractive starting regimens for patients with low viral loads or who are reluctant or unable to commit themselves to taking more complex HAART regimens.

Protease inhibitor/NNRTI combinations

The interest in protease inhibitor/NNRTI-based ('nucleoside-sparing') regimens has arisen out of concern over the long-term toxicities of NRTIs (such as lipodystrophy, pancreatitis and lactic acidosis) Although these combinations should be highly effective, dosing schedules tend to be complicated as both

NNRTIs and protease inhibitors are substrates of the cytochrome P_{450} system and have complex drug interactions (*see* Ch. 39). Additonally, failure of this regimen would leave limited options for salvage therapy.

MONITORING TREATMENT

Patients on HAART should have their CD4 count and plasma viral load levels monitored at regular intervals. Laboratory evaluations are performed usually at 2–4 week intervals initially and then eventually about 3 monthly, unless specifically needed. On effective therapy, plasma viral load falls rapidly as viral replication is inhibited. By 4 weeks a fall of greater than 1 log, and by 3–6 months a fall to <50 copies/ml, in viral load should be expected.

Even in patients who initiate therapy with CD4 counts below $100 \times 10^6/l$ substantial increases in CD4 count and clinical benefit can be achieved.

TREATMENT FAILURE AND SALVAGE THERAPY

FIRST TREATMENT FAILURE

One measure of treatment success is whether complete viral suppression is achieved and therefore any evidence of consistant ongoing viral replication indicates treatment failure. Once treatment failure is suspected, a repeat confirmatory viral load needs to be performed. There are several reasons why the viral load may increase on therapy and not all are the result of the development of viral resistance.

The major causes of treatment failure include:

- insufficient drug exposure due to poor adherence;
- drug–drug interactions leading to poor pharmacokinetics;
- drug toxicity leading to cessation of the regimen.

Less common causes are:

- lack of potency;
- inadequate drug absorption;
- inability of the agents to penetrate viral reservoirs.

Starting treatment at a late stage of HIV disease (high HIV RNA levels[59] and/or CD4+ count less than 100 cells/mm[3]) was strongly associated with early virologic failure.[14] Recently, primary drug resistance acquisition at time of infection has been associated with treatment failure.

Although many patients may fail therapy in the long term, predictors of the durability of the virologic response to therapy include the viral load nadir achieved within the first few months on treatment. In one cohort study, the risk of virological failure was four times greater in those achieving a viral load <400 but >50 HIV-1 RNA copies/ml than in those achieving undetectable (<50 copies/ml) viral loads.[60]

Transient increase in viral load

If a patient's viral load rises to just above detectable (50–500 copies/ml), the viral load count should be repeated as soon as possible, preferably within 2 weeks. The patient should be clinically assessed to determine any contributing factors such as drug–drug interactions, poor adherence, coexisting infections and/or vaccinations, which can all increase the viral load transiently. Rises in viral load to just above detectable levels occur in a significant proportion of patients on treatment.[61,62] Those whose viral load is transiently detectable because of laboratory assay-related problems or other factors will show no further rise or revert to undetectable, and are called 'blips'. Patients who develop virological failure show further increases in viral load. Whether viral 'blips' are associated with an increased future risk of virological failure is unclear for those who have already achieved viral suppression. One study showed no such association,[61] but another suggested that, although a low-level viral 'blip' was not a predictor of failure, those with repeated episodes or sustained low-level viral rebound were more likely to experience future virological failure.[62] Patients with frequent 'blips' should be monitored more regularly than others.

Sustained viral load rebound

Falls in CD4 count and clinical disease progression is the usual outcome in patients whose viral load continues to rise towards pretreatment levels.[63] Although resistance to all drugs in a treatment regimen may not be detected in patients experiencing virological failure, a persistently high viral load will lead to the accumulation of resistance mutations. For some drugs, such as lamivudine and NNRTIs, mutations at one position in the reverse transcriptase gene usually emerge at low levels of viral load rebound and result in significant phenotypic resistance. Reduced susceptibility to other drugs usually requires the accumulation of two or more mutations, as can occur with ongoing viral replication. Thus, changing therapy should be considered if viral replication persists and other available options exist to completely suppress it. However, a decision to switch to a second regimen is complicated, and depends on several factors, including addressing the etiology of virologic failure. A change of therapy should be considered if HIV load has never become undetectable or after being undetectable on antiviral therapy has subsequently becomes consistently detectable.

Some patients who are receiving non-HAART therapy, usually single or double NRTI may or may not want to change such therapy – especially if their viral load is stable and CD4 count is at a relatively high level. There is a risk that ongoing viral replication will lead to an increasing number of mutations in the viral genome, making subsequent therapy more difficult. Falls in CD4 count, however, should result in switching to a more effective regimen.

CHOICE OF SUBSEQUENT REGIMEN

Protease inhibitor failure

Optimal virological responses to a second or subsequent regimen will be obtained only when adherence is maximized and ineffective drugs eliminated from the regimen. Resistance testing may help guide choices of drugs in all classes. Patients failing protease inhibitor therapy are often difficult to treat because of broad cross-resistance within this class.[14,64,65] Use of a low-dose ritonavir-based dual protease inhibitor regimen should be strongly considered if treatment failure is due to poor adherence or suboptimal pharmacokinetics. In these cases resistance to protease inhibitors will often not be found on testing. Subsequent use of dual protease inhibitors may be more successful if nelfinavir was the initial protease inhibitor.[66-68]

Initial studies with low-dose ritonavir-boosted protease inhibitor plus an NNRTI and one or two NRTIs (a triple class regimen) provide good therapeutic results[69] but subsequent choices are severely limited. A resistance test with expert interpretation is recommended.

NNRTI failure

Patients who begin therapy with a combination of two NRTIs and an NNRTI retain susceptibility to protease inhibitors. Unfortunately, there is broad cross-resistance among the currently available licensed NNRTIs. Thus, they cannot be used reliably after failure of other drugs in the same class. There are a number of second-generation agents in development which may have some activity against NNRTI-resistant strains but activity depends on the level of phenotypic resistance that has developed to the existing agents.

Triple nucleoside failure

Both protease inhibitor and NNRTI regimens can be used. The limiting factor is the number of nucleosides available that do not show cross resistance to the initial failed regimen.

SALVAGE

For those who have experienced virologic failure on two or more HAART regimens (often referred to as 'salvage therapy') the therapeutic approach and goal of therapy is usually very different. In heavily pretreated patients there is difficulty in optimizing treatment as complete viral suppression may no longer be achievable. Partial viral suppression becomes the goal of therapy and CD4+ count guides clinical decision making. Even viral load reductions of greater than $0.5 \log_{10}$ copies/ml may result in clinical improvement and imply that a new salvage regimen is worth pursuing.[70] However, continuing viral replication on antiretroviral therapy will probably select for further resistance, limiting future options. Unfortunately, many patients have exhausted all options as cross-resistance frequently extends even to investigational agents.

The definition of salvage therapy varies. Here, it is defined as treatment following exposure to multiple drugs and, usually, all classes of antiretroviral agents. However, many so-called 'salvage studies' have been carried out in patients who are naïve with respect to one class of drugs. Unfortunately, the definition of salvage becomes a moving target as more classes of drugs (e.g. nucleotides, fusion inhibitors) enter the market place. The reasons for drug failure are complex. Most studies of salvage therapy have not distinguished between virological failure due to poor adherence and failure due to other causes (e.g. poor pharmacokinetics). Individuals who have been poorly adherent to therapy but have not developed resistant virus may be effectively treated if adherence is improved. Adherence counselling and directly observed, rather than self-administered, therapy results in significantly better surrogate marker responses, demonstrating the importance of adherence.[71,72] Low blood levels of protease inhibitors because of either poor absorption or unforeseen pharmacokinetic interactions, may also lead to failure without the development of resistance to this class of drugs.

Measuring the success of salvage regimens

Many salvage studies have been of short duration with little follow-up data and viral suppression is not often achievable.

Box 46.3 What to change to after first virological failure

Initial regimen	Options to consider		
two NRTIs + PI	Two NRTIs + NNRTI	*or* Two NRTIs + two PIs	*or* Two NRTIs + NNRTI + PI *or* two PIs
two NRTIs + NNRTI	Two NRTIs + PI	*or* Two PIs	
Three NRTIs	Two NRTIs + NNRTI	*or* Two NRTIs + PI or two PIs	*or* Two NRTIs + NNRTI + PI or 2 PIs

NRTI, Nucleoside reverse transcriptase inhibitor; PI, protease inhibitor; NNRTI, non-nucleoside reverse transcriptase inhibitor.

In late disease, the immediate risk of death is much more closely associated with the CD4 count than with the viral load. Perhaps a more important criterion is the degree to which the CD4 count rises. There are some general principles to consider when deciding upon a salvage regimen. Salvage will have the greatest likelihood of success if individuals are naïve to one class of drugs. If this is the NNRTI class, they should be prescribed whenever possible as part of a fully suppressive regimen to avoid the rapid emergence of resistance. This is often not possible without also adding other drugs such as the recently licensed class of nucleotides (e.g. tenofovir)[73] or the investigational fusion inhibitors.[74] Improved outcome is also more likely with the use of drugs within classes to which the patient has not been exposed and to which resistance is unlikely or proven to be absent. Salvage therapy is more successful at reducing the viral load to undetectable levels in those who commence at a lower viral load (e.g. <5000–10 000 copies/ml) as the potency of new regimens (although suboptimal) may be enough to suppress low viral loads. Resistance testing should be performed in cases where there are difficult choices to make concerning the most beneficial treatment. A result suggesting that the virus remains sensitive to a particular drug does not guarantee a long-term response, as drug exposure history is also an important factor. Although resistance tests are useful at first failure,[75–77] results for subsequent failure are conflicting.[78,79] Finally, plasma drug concentrates may influence therapy outcome. The Viradapt study[80] demonstrated that the best virological response occurred in patients who had optimal plasma drug concentrations as well as resistance genotyping to guide future choices.

Both cohort data and clinical controlled trials suggest that 60–70% of subjects who are experiencing failure of single-agent protease inhibitor-based therapy and who are NNRTI naïve will achieve viral load reductions to below 400 copies/ml at 16 weeks by switching to new NRTIs plus two protease inhibitors and an NNRTI. In a number of cohort studies lopinavir, enhanced with low-dose ritonavir, in combination with either efavirenz or nevirapine, reduced viral loads to below detectable limits in NNRTI-naïve, protease inhibitor-experienced patients.[81,82]

Amprenavir may retain activity after failure of other protease inhibitors. From one study of 108 patients, amprenavir maintained viral sensitivity in patients failing the other four licensed protease inhibitors in half to three-quarters of isolates.[83]

In patients with multiple class resistance being NNRTI naïve and receiving two protease inhibitors improves the chance of virological success (ACTG 398). However, less than half the study population remained on therapy at 6 months: 33% stopped because of toxicity and 20% stopped because of virological failure. As cross-resistance between NNRTIs and protease inhibitors is unlikely, a good choice of salvage therapy in patients who are NNRTI-experienced would be to use a dual protease inhibitor combination in those previously naïve to this class of drug or who have only been exposed to a single protease inhibitor previously. Other approaches have been tried

and some success has been reported by combining five or more drugs,[84] so-called mega-HAART, even though resistance to many of the individual components is present. Unfortunately, these small studies are difficult to analyse and, in the long term, toxicity is likely to outweigh benefit. Although the regimens contain multiple drugs and many pills, drug adherence was often relatively good, partly because the drugs were taken only twice a day.

ANTIRETROVIRAL RESISTANCE

Therapeutic failure is often associated with the emergence of resistance mutations and the pattern of mutations that emerges affects not only drug susceptibility but also the fitness of viral replication. For some antiretrovirals, such as lamividine or NNRTIs, the development of high-level resistance may require only a single mutation and probably has little effect on viral fitness. For others, such as the protease inhibitors or abacavir, the development of high-level resistance requires the accumulation of multiple mutations because single or a few mutations result in an unfit virus that replicates slowly, if at all. This may explain why prolonged virologic failure exists before resistance occurs to many of the protease inhibitors. Two multidrug-resistant genotypes for all NRTIs have been identified: the '151 complex' and the '69-S-S-S' insertion mutation. While uncommon, these mutations may account for some of the drug failures observed in patients whose treatment history would not suggest cross-resistance. Many randomized studies demonstrate the clinical value of HIV drug resistance tests in improving short-term virological outcome following a change of therapy.[75–78,85–88] A number of factors enhance the usefulness of the information provided by resistance testing.

- Ensuring that resistance tests are performed on samples taken while the patient is receiving therapy, because wild-type virus emerges rapidly after treatment is stopped.[89] The current assays are unable to consistently detect minority quasi-species, and resistant strains that represent a small proportion of the total viral pool may not be identified.
- At present the success of the resistance test procedure is significantly enhanced with a viral load of over 1000 HIV-1 RNA copies/ml. For those with low level viremia, it may not be possible to amplify enough material for sequencing.
- The virus subtype (clade) may determine the significance of certain mutations that are polymorphisms.[90,91] The genotypic patterns and phenotypic cut-offs for resistance of some drugs (e.g. abacavir and stavudine)[92] are evolving and novel mutations can confer resistance to some drugs. Complex mutational patterns emerge after prolonged virologic failure, especially to protease inhibitors, making interpretation difficult.

The overall benefit of a resistance test for any individual patient is dependent on other factors, including adherence, drug levels and experience of the physician interpreting the resistance test.

PRIMARY DRUG RESISTANCE

Sexual transmission of multidrug-resistant HIV was first reported in 1998.[93] Since then, a number of reports have demonstrated transmission of drug-resistant HIV. Some strains are resistant to more than one class of antiretroviral agents. Little and colleagues performed a similar analysis on 141 recently infected individuals from five urban centers. A 2.5- to 10-fold reduction in sensitivity to at least one class was noted in 26% of isolates, although only 2% of isolates exhibited 10-fold or higher reductions in drug susceptibility.[94] Primary resistance also exists among chronically infected treatment-naïve patients.[95]

USE OF ANTIVIRAL THERAPY TO REDUCE PERINATAL TRANSMISSION OF HIV

Preventing transmission of HIV to the fetus or neonate is a complex and multifactorial problem. Before the use of antiviral drugs in pregnancy, methods of preventing perinatal transmission included cesarian section and withholding breast feeding. Although withholding breast feeding is still recommended in developed countries, antiretroviral therapy that successfully reduces HIV-1 RNA to levels <1000 copies/ml substantially lowers the risk of perinatal HIV-1 transmission and limits consideration of elective cesarean delivery as an intervention.

The first study to quantify the reduction in transmission by antiretroviral drugs was the ACTG 076 study.[96] When zidovudine is administered alone before, during and after birth, perinatal transmission is reduced by approximately 70%. Based on these data, zidovudine should be included as a component of combination antiretroviral therapy in pregnancy. Interestingly, the development of resistance to this drug was unusual among the healthy population of women who participated in ACTG 076.[97] If a woman has not received zidovudine as a component of her antenatal antiretroviral regimen, some believe that it should be given during the birth and to the newborn. However, if an infected mother has adequate viral suppression, this is probably not necessary. Antiretroviral prophylaxis should be offered to all pregnant women with HIV infection as its use has been shown to provide benefit in preventing perinatal transmission even for infected pregnant women with low HIV-1 RNA levels (<1000 copies/ml). In a meta-analysis of factors associated with perinatal transmission despite having HIV-1 RNA <1000 copies/ml at or near delivery, transmission was only 1.0% among women receiving antenatal antiretroviral therapy (primarily zidovudine alone), compared with 9.8% among those receiving no antenatal therapy.[98]

The three-part zidovudine chemoprophylaxis regimen, started after the first trimester, should be recommended for all pregnant women with HIV infection, regardless of antenatal HIV viral load. The drug is usually given as part of a HAART combination for all HIV-infected women who have symptomatic disease, a low CD4 count or an HIV RNA over 1000 copies/ml. The use of antiretrovirals is associated with risks and benefits during pregnancy, both known and hypothetical. Because of the possibility of drug-induced teratogenesis, women who are in the first trimester of pregnancy may consider delaying therapy until after 12 weeks' gestation. Treatment with efavirenz should be avoided during the first trimester because significant teratogenic effects in monkeys were seen at drug exposures similar to those of humans. Combinations of stavadine and didanosine have been associated with lactic acidosis and are also best avoided.[99]

Some women on therapy who plan to become pregnant discontinue treatment before conception, risking immunological deterioration and potential for transmission because of rising viral loads. HIV-1 infected women receiving antiretroviral therapy in whom pregnancy is identified after the first trimester should continue therapy, although the benefits and potential risks of antiretroviral administration during this period should be discussed and discontinuation of therapy considered. If therapy is discontinued, all drugs should be stopped and reintroduced simultaneously to avoid the development of drug resistance.

If an HIV-infected woman presents in labor and has had no prior antiviral therapy, one of several effective regimens should be offered.

1. Single-dose nevirapine at the onset of labor followed by a single dose of nevirapine for the newborn at 48 h. This recommendation is based in part on a study of a breastfeeding population in Uganda that demonstrated that a single 200 mg oral dose of nevirapine given to the mother at onset of labor combined with a single 2 mg/kg oral dose given to her infant at 48–72 h of age reduced transmission by nearly 50% compared with a very short regimen of zidovudine given orally during labor and to the infant for one week.[100] Transmission at 6 weeks of age was 12% in the nevirapine group and 21% in the group receiving zidovudine.
2. Oral zidovadine and lamivudine during labor, followed by one week of oral zidovudine/lamivudine for the newborn. The PETRA African trial in breastfeeding HIV-infected women showed that an intrapartum/postpartum regimen, started during labor and continued for one week postpartum in the woman and infant, reduced transmission at 6 weeks from 17% in the placebo group to 11% with the two-part regimen, a reduction of 38%).[95] Oral zidovudine–lamivudine administered solely during the intrapartum period was not effective in lowering transmission.
3. Intrapartum intravenous zidovudine followed by 6 weeks of zidovudine for the newborn.

4. A two-dose nevirapine regimen combined with intrapartum intravenous zidovudine and 6 week zidovudine for the newborn.

If breastfeeding is continued the benefits fo these therapies can be lost in the long term. If an infant is born to an HIV-infected mother who has received no antiretroviral therapy during pregnancy or the birth, a 6-week course of therapy should be started for the infant as soon as possible after delivery – preferably within 6–12 hours of birth. In the immediate postpartum period, the woman should have appropriate surrogate marker assessments (e.g. CD4+ count and HIV-1 RNA copy number) to determine whether she should commence long term antiretroviral therapy.

FOLLOW-UP

Infants born to HIV-infected women should undergo early diagnostic testing so that if they are HIV-infected, long-term treatment can be started. The care and follow-up of the neonate is briefly outlined below.

TREATMENT OF HIV-INFECTED CHILDREN

Although many of the principles of treatment for HIV-infected adults apply to children, important differences are noted. Importantly, the clinical trial treatment data are more limited for children and there are often situations for which definitive data concerning efficacy are not available. Participation by the parents, caregivers and child in any decision-making process is absolutely crucial. A family clinic where children and parents can be seen together and individually is one successful model of care.

Viral loads are often much higher in infected children. Furthermore, the normal range for CD4 cells is different in adults and children and changes throughout childhood. In addition, children present with a different clinical disease pattern. Thus, a different clinical and immunologic categorization has been developed to guide initiation of therapy.

HIV-INFECTED CHILDREN WITH IMMUNE SUPPRESSION OR CLINICAL SYMPTOMS OF INFECTION

As in adults, antiretroviral therapy is associated with clinical benefit in infected children with either evidence of disease or immunosuppression. Initial clinical trials of monotherapy with zidovudine, didanosine, lamivudine or stavudine demonstrated substantial improvements in neurodevelopment, growth, and immunologic and/or virologic status.[102–107] Subsequent pediatric clinical trials in symptomatic, antiretroviral-naïve children demonstrate that combination therapy with either zidovudine and lamivudine or zidovudine and didanosine is clinically superior to monotherapy as initial therapy. Antiretroviral therapy in symptomatic patients slows clinical and immunologic disease progression and reduces mortality.[102,108]

For antiretroviral-experienced children, combination therapy that includes a protease inhibitor is virologically and immunologically superior to dual nucleoside combination therapy.[109] The use of protease inhibitor-containing HAART (from 0% before 1996 to over 70% by 1998) is accompanied by a substantial decrease in mortality (1% in 1997/1998; 5% in 1995/1996).[110] Consequently, antiretroviral therapy is recommended for all HIV-infected children in CDC (Centers for Disease Control and Prevention) categories A, B, or C (Table 46.1) or with evidence of immune suppression (i.e. those in CDC immune categories 2 or 3; Table 46.2) regardless of the age of the child or viral load.

ASYMPTOMATIC HIV-INFECTED CHILDREN

The effectiveness of antiretroviral therapy in infants and older children who have normal immune function and are asymptomatic is under investigation. The very high levels of HIV RNA seen during the first 1–2 years of life following perinatal transmission reflects the poor control of viral replication in infected infants. The situation can be likened to that found in adult acute seroconverters. Starting HAART early in this period might preserve immune function, diminish viral dissemination, lower the steady state viral load, and result in improved clinical outcome. (there are some clinical trial data to suggest this is true in some children).[112,113] However, because virologic response is partly related to viral load at the time of starting therapy,[108,114] and as infants have substantially higher viral loads, complete virologic response may not be attained in all children. Some studies have suggested that immunologic and clinical benefit may be observed in children who partially respond to therapy.[115] The risks of short- and long-term toxicity have to be taken into account, especially as there are only limited data on pharmacokinetics, dosing, and safety. Treatment may be lifelong and, if viral replication is not fully suppressed, viral mutations will arise and result in the development of resistance, potentially limiting future treatment options.

Treating asymptomatic children in the first year of life

Although HIV-infected infants under 12 months old are at high risk for disease progression, the predictive value of CD4 counts and viral load is not as useful in infants as in older children. Prospective cohort studies indicate that most HIV-infected infants will have clinical symptoms by 1 year of age.[116,117] In spite of the lack of definitive clinical trial data, antiretroviral therapy should be started in this age group as soon as the diagnosis is established, regardless of immune status or viral load.

Table 46.1 Human immunodeficiency virus pediatric classification system: clinical categories*

Category N: not symptomatic

Children who have no signs or symptoms considered to be the result of HIV infection or who have only *one* of the conditions listed in category A.

Category A: mildly symptomatic

Children with *two* or more of the following conditions but none of the conditions listed in categories B and C:

    Lymphadenopathy (>0.5 cm at more than two sites; bilateral = one site)

    Hepatomegaly

    Splenomegaly

    Dermatitis

    Parotitis

    Recurrent or persistent upper respiratory infection, sinusitis or otitis media

Category B: moderately symptomatic

Children who have symptomatic conditions, other than those listed for category A or category C, that are attributed to HIV infection. Examples of conditions in clinical category B include but are not limited to the following:

    Anemia (< 8 g/dl), neutropenia (<1000/mm³), or thrombocytopenia (<100 000/mm³) persisting >30 days

    Bacterial meningitis, pneumonia, or sepsis (single episode)

    Candidiasis, oropharyngeal (i.e. thrush) persisting for >2 months in children aged >6 months

    Cardiomyopathy

    Cytomegalovirus infection with onset before age 1 month

    Diarrhea, recurrent or chronic

    Hepatitis

    Herpes simplex virus (HSV) stomatitis, recurrent (i.e. more than two episodes within 1 year)

    HSV bronchitis, pneumonitis, or esophagitis with onset before age 1 month

    Herpes zoster (i.e. shingles) involving at least two distinct episodes or more than one dermatome

    Leiomyosarcoma

    Lymphoid interstitial pneumonia (LIP) or pulmonary lymphoid hyperplasia complex

    Nephropathy

    Nocardiosis

    Fever lasting >1 month

    Toxoplasmosis with onset before age 1 month

    Varicella, disseminated (i.e. complicated chickenpox)

Category C: severely symptomatic

Children who have any condition listed in the 1987 surveillance case definition for acquired immunodeficiency syndrome, with the exception of LIP (which is a category B condition).

---

*Centers for Disease Control and Prevention.[111]

Asymptomatic HIV-infected children older than 1 year

Most asymptomatic infected children older than 1 year have low CD4 + T cell percentages (i.e. <25%), indicating immunosuppression. Such children should start antiretroviral therapy. In asymptomatic children over 1 year of age with a normal immune status treatment can be delayed if the risk for clinical disease progression is low (i.e. a low viral load) or there are concerns about adherence and safety. The virologic, immunologic, and clinical status should be regularly monitored and therapy started if any deterioration occurs.

There are some caveats to these guidelines. Regardless of age, any child with HIV RNA levels >100 000 copies/ml is at high risk for death and should be started on antiretroviral therapy, as should those whose viral load consistently increases by than 0.5–0.7 $\log_{10}$.

CHOICE OF INITIAL ANTIRETROVIRAL THERAPY

Use of zidovudine as a single agent is only appropriate when used in infants of indeterminate HIV status during the first 6 weeks of life to prevent perinatal HIV transmission. Infants who are confirmed as being HIV-infected should be given a standard combination regimen. As the ACTG 076 study showed that zidovudine resistance did not occur in most infants who became infected despite maternal treatment with the drug,[118,119] the antiretroviral regimen for infected infants does not have to be chosen on the basis of maternal antiretroviral use. However, this may not always be the case because as more mothers may have been on more than one antiviral drug it is possible that those with detectable viral loads might transmit resistant virus to their children. When resistance is known or suspected in the mother resistance testing of the infant's viral isolate should be considered to assist in the choice of initial antiretroviral therapy.

Clinical trial data suggests that in initial therapy a protease inhibitor based regimen should be given,[112,113,120–122] which is more effective than therapy with two NRTIs, reducing viral load to undetectable levels. An alternative regimen for initial therapy includes efavirenz in combination with one or two NRTIs and nelfinavir. This regimen reduced viral load to below 50 copies/ml in 63% of children at 48 weeks and was well tolerated.[123]

Other regimens used include the combination of nevirapine with two NRTIs and the triple nucleoside analog regimen of abacavir, zidovudine and lamivudine. However, while each of these regimens result in virologic suppression in some children, experience is limited and the durability of viral suppression is not well defined.

Antiretroviral therapy will need to be taken for many years and will start at various stages of maturation of liver metabolism. Therefore, the choice of an initial regimen is complex and should consider barriers to adherence, the complexity of the regimen, food requirements, formulation and dosing.

VIROLOGIC CONSIDERATIONS FOR CHANGING THERAPY

The indications for changing therapy include similar virological critera as in adults but also may be considered if there is a reproducible CD4+ decline of 5% or more, especially in those

Table 46.2 Human immunodeficiency virus pediatric classification system: immune categories based on age-specific CD4 + T cell and percentage*

Immune category	<12 months No./mm³		1–5 years No./mm³		6–12 years No./mm³	
Category 1: no suppression	>1500	(>25%)	>1000	(>25%)	>500	(>25%)
Category 2: moderate suppression	750–1499	(15–24%)	500–999	(15–24%)	200–499	(15–24%)
Category 3: severe suppression	<750	(<15%)	<500	(<15%)	<200	(<15%)

*Modified from CDC 1994[114]

with CD4 counts less than 15%. Progressive neurodevelopmental and growth failure are clinical reasons to change treatment. However, disease progression may not necessarily reflect a failure of antiretroviral therapy but persistent immunologic dysfunction despite adequate antiviral response.

References

1. Fischl MA, Richman DD, Hansen N, et al 1990 The safety and efficacy of zidovudine (AZT) in the treatment of subjects with mildly symptomatic human immunodeficiency virus type 1 (HIV) infection. A double-blind, placebo-controlled trial. *Annals of Internal Medicine* 112: 727–737.

2. Volberding PA 1990 Zidovudine in asymptomatic HIV infection: a controlled trial in persons with fewer than 500 CD4-positive cells per cubic millimetre. *New England Journal of Medicine* 322: 941–949.

3. Concorde Coordinating Committee 1994 Concorde: MRC/ANRS randomised double-blind controlled trial of immediate and deferred zidovudine in symptom-free HIV infection. *Lancet* 343: 871–881.

4. Fischl MA, Stanley K, Collier AC et al 1995 Combination and monotherapy with zidovudine and zalcitabine in patients with advanced HIV disease. *Annals of Internal Medicine* 122: 24–32.

5. Delta Coordinating Committee 1996 Delta: a randomized double-blind controlled trial comparing combinations of zidovudine plus didanosine or zalcitabine with zidovudine alone in HIV-infected individuals. *Lancet* 348: 283–291.

6. Hammer SM, Katzenstein DA, Hughes MD et al 1996 A trial comparing nucleoside monotherapy with combination therapy in HIV-infected adults with CD4 cell counts from 200 to 500 per cubic millimeter. *New England Journal of Medicine* 335: 1081–1090.

7. CAESAR Coordinating Committee 1997 Randomized trial of addition of lamivudine plus loviride to zidovudine-containing regimens for patients with HIV-1 infection: the CAESAR trial. *Lancet* 349: 1413–1421.

8. Kovacs JA, Masur H 2000 Prophylaxis against opportunistic infections in patients with human immunodeficiency virus infection. *New England Journal of Medicine* 342: 1416–1429.

9. Finzi D, Blankson J, Siliciano JD et al 1999 Latent infection of CD4+ T cells provides a mechanism for lifelong persistence of HIV-1, even in patients on effective combination therapy. *Nature Medicine* 5: 512–525.

10. Kilby JM, Hopkins S, Venetta TM et al 1998 Potent suppression of HIV-1 replication in humans by T-20, a peptide inhibitor of gp41-mediated virus entry. *Nature Medicine* 4: 1302–1307.

11. David D, Nait-Ighil L, Dupont B, Maral J, Gachot B, Theze J 2001 Rapid effect of interleukin-2 therapy in human immunodeficiency virus-infected patients whose CD4 cell counts increase only slightly in response to combined antiretroviral treatment. *Journal of Infectious Diseases,* 183: 730–735.

12. Brinkman K, Smeitink JA, Romijn J, Reiss P 1999 Mitochondrial toxicity induced by nucleoside-analogue reverse transcriptase inhibitors is a key factor in the pathogenesis of antiretroviral-therapy-related lipodystrophy. *Lancet* 354: 1112–1115.

13. Carr A, Samaras K, Thorisdottir A et al 1999 Diagnosis, prediction, and natural course of HIV-1 protease-inhibitor-associated lipodystrophy, hyperlipidemia, and diabetes mellitus: a cohort study. *Lancet* 353: 2093–2099.

14. Deeks SG, Hecht FM, Swanson M et al 1999 Virologic outcomes with protease inhibitor therapy in an urban AIDS clinic: relationship between baseline characteristics and response to both initial and salvage therapy. *AIDS* 13: F35–F44.

15. Lucas GM, Chaisson RE, Moore RD 1999 Highly active antiretroviral therapy in a large urban clinic: risk factors for virologic failure and adverse drug reactions. *Annals of Internal Medicine* 131: 81–87.

16. Zhang L, Ramratnam B, Tenner-Racz K et al 1999 Quantifying residual HIV-1 replication in patients receiving combination antiretroviral therapy. *New England Journal of Medicine* 21: 1605–1613.

17. Gunthard HF, Frost SD, Leigh-Brown AJ et al 1999 Evolution of envelope sequences of human immunodeficiency virus type 1 in cellular reservoirs in the setting of potent antiviral therapy. *Journal of Virology* 73: 9404–9412.

18. Gazzard B, Hill A, Gartland M, for the AVANTI Study Group 1998 Different analyses give highly variable estimates of HIV-1 RNA undetectability and $\log_{10}$ reduction in clinical trials. *AIDS* 12(Suppl. 4): S36 [Abstract P77].

19. Ruiz L, Martinez-Picada J, Romeu J et al 2000 Structured treatment interruption in chronically HIV-1 infected patients after long-term viral suppression. *AIDS* 14: 397–403.

20. Kinloch de Loes S, Hirschel BJ, Hoen B et al 1995 A controlled trial of zidovudine in primary human immunodeficiency virus infection. *New England Journal of Medicine* 333: 408–413.

21. Koup RA, Safrit JT, Cao Y et al 1994 Temporal association of cellular immune responses with the initial control of viremia in primary human immunodeficiency virus type 1 syndrome. *Journal of Virology* 68: 4650–4655.

22. Borrow P, Lewicki H, Hahn BH, Shaw GM, Oldstone MB 1994 Virus-specific CD8+ cytotoxic T-lymphocyte activity associated with control of viremia in primary human immunodeficiency virus type 1 infection. *Journal of Virology* 68: 6103–6110.

23. Rosenberg ES, Billingsley JM, Caliendo AM et al 1997 Vigorous HIV-1-specific CD4+ T cell responses associated with control of viremia. *Science* 278: 1447–1450.

24. Rosenberg ES, Altfeld M, Poon SH et al 2000 Immune control of HIV-1 after early treatment of acute infection. *Nature* 407: 523–526.

25. Walker BD, Rosenberg ES, Hay CM, Basgoz N, Yang OO 1998 Immune control of HIV-1 replication. *Advances in Experimental Medicine and Biology* 452: 159–167.

26. Kaufmann GR, Bloch M, Zaunders JJ, Smith D, Cooper DA 2000 Long-term immunological response in HIV-1-infected subjects receiving potent antiretroviral therapy. *AIDS* 14: 959–969.

27. Lisziewicz J, Rosenberg E, Lieberman J et al 1999 Control of HIV despite the discontinuation of antiretroviral therapy. *New England Journal of Medicine* 340: 1683–1684.

28. Walker B 2001 Structured treatment interruption: state-of-the-art lecture. 8th Conference on Retroviruses and Opportunistic Infections. Chicago, IL, February 2001 [Session 37].

29. Markowitz M, Jin X, Ramratnam B et al 2001 Prolonged HAART initiated within 120 days of infection does not result in sustained control of HIV-1 after cessation of therapy. 8th Conference on Retroviruses and Opportunistic Infections. Chicago, February 2001 [Abstract 288].

30. Miller J, Finlayson R, Smith D et al 1999 The occurrence of lipodystrophic phenomena in patients with primary HIV infection (HIV) treated with anti-retroviral therapy (ARV). 7th European Conference on Clinical Aspects and Treatment of HIV Infection. Lisbon, Portugal, October, 1999 [Abstract 519].

31. Goujard C, Boufassa F, Deveau C, Laskri D, Meyer L 2001 Incidence of clinical lipodystrophy in HIV-infected patients treated during primary infection. AIDS 15: 282–284.

32. Ho DD 1995 Time to hit HIV, early and hard. New England Journal of Medicine 333: 450–451.

33. Kaplan J, Hanson D, Karon J et al 2001 Late initiation of antiretroviral therapy (at CD4+ lymphocyte count <200 cells/mL) is associated with increased risk of death. 8th Conference on Retroviruses and Opportunistic Infections. Chicago, IL, February 2001 [Abstract 520].

34. Hogg RS, Yip B, Wood E et al 2001 Diminished effectiveness of antiretroviral therapy among patients initiating therapy with CD4+ cell counts below 200/mm^3. 8th Conference on Retroviruses and Opportunistic Infections. Chicago, IL, February 2001 [Abstract 342].

35. Sterling TR, Chaisson RE, Bartlett JG, Moore RD 2001 CD4+ lymphocyte level is better than HIV-1 plasma viral load in determining when to initiate HAART. 8th Conference on Retroviruses and Opportunistic Infections. Chicago, IL, February 2001 [Abstract 519].

36. Wood R, Team TS 2000 Sustained efficacy of nevirapine (NVP) in combination with two nucleosides in advanced treatment-naive HIV infected patients with high viral loads: a B1090 substudy. 13th International AIDS Conference. Durban, South Africa, July 2000 [Abstract WeOrB604].

37. Nelson M, Staszewski S, Morales-Ramirez JO et al 2000 Successful virologic suppression with efavirenz in HIV-infected patients with low baseline CD4 cell counts: post hoc results from Study 006. 10th European Conference of Clinical Microbiology and Infectious Diseases. Stockholm, Sweden, May 2000 [Abstract 3–349].

38. Mellors JW, Munoz A, Giorgi JV et al 1997 Plasma viral load and CD4 lympho-cytes as prognostic markers of HIV-1 infection. Annals of Internal Medicine 126: 946–954.

39. Phillips AN, Staszewski S, Weber R et al 2000 Viral load changes in response to antiretroviral therapy according to the baseline CD4 lymphocyte count and viral load. 5th International Congress on Drug Therapy in HIV Infection. Glasgow, UK, October 2000 [Abstract PL3.4].

40. Cozzi-Lepri A, Phillips AN, d'Arminio Monforte A et al 2000 When to start HAART in chronically HIV-infected patients? A collection of pieces of evidence from the ICONA study. 5th International Congress on Drug Therapy in HIV Infection. Glasgow, UK, October 2000 [Abstract PL3.5].

41. Hogg RS, Yip B, Chan KJ et al 2001 Rates of disease progression by baseline CD4 cell count and viral load after initiating triple-drug therapy. JAMA 286: 2568–2577.

42. Haubrich RH, Little SJ, Currier JS et al 1999 The value of patient-reported adherence to antiretroviral therapy in predicting virologic and immunologic response. AIDS 130: 1099–1107.

43. Palella FJ, Delaney KM, Moorman AC et al 1998 Declining morbidity and mor-tality among patients with advanced human immunodeficiency virus infec-tion. New England Journal of Medicine 338: 853–860.

44. Gunthard H, Frost SDW, Leigh-Brown AJ et al 1999 Evolution of envelope sequences of human immunodeficiency virus type 1 in cellular reservoirs in the setting of potent antiretroviral therapy. Journal of Virology 73: 9404–9412.

45. Dornadula G, Zhang J, VanUitert B et al 1999 Residual HIV-1 RNA in blood plasma of patients taking suppressive highly active antiretroviral therapy. Journal of the American Medical Association 282: 1627–1632.

46. Zhang L, Ramratnam B, Tenner-Racz K et al 1999 Quantifying residual HIV-1 replication in patients receiving combination antiretroviral therapy. New England Journal of Medicine 21: 1605–1613.

47. Ramratnam B, Mittler JE, Zhang L et al 2000 The decay of the latent reservoir of replication competent HIV-1 is inversely correlated with the extent of residual viral replication during prolonged anti-retroviral therapy. Nature Medicine 6: 82–85.

48. Hoetelmans RMW, Reijers MHE, Weverling GJ et al 1998 The effect of plasma drug concentrations on HIV-1 clearance rate during quadruple drug therapy. AIDS 12: F111–F115.

49. Gulick RM, Mellors JW, Havlir D et al 1997 Treatment with indinavir, zidovu-dine, and lamivudine in adults with human immunodeficiency virus infection and prior antiretroviral therapy. New England Journal of Medicine 337: 734–739.

50. Hammer SM, Squires KM, Hughes MD et al 1997 A controlled trial of two nucleoside analogs plus indinavir in persons with human immunodeficiency virus infection and CD4 cell counts of 200 per cubic millimeter or less. New England Journal of Medicine 337: 725–733.

51. Haubrich R, Lalezari J, Follansbee SE et al 1998 Improved survival and reduced clinical progression in HIV-infected patients with advanced disease treated with saquinavir plus zalcitabine. Antiviral Therapy 3: 33–42.

52. Gatell JM, Lange J, Arnaiz JA et al 2000 A randomized study comparing continued indinavir (800 mg tid) vs switching to indinavir/ritonavir (800/100 mg bid) in HIV patients having achieved viral load suppression with indinavir plus 2 nucleoside analogues: the BID Efficacy and Safety Trial (BEST). 12th World AIDS Conference. Durban, South Africa, July 2000 [Abstract WeOrB484].

53. D'Aquila RT, Hughes MD, Johnson VA et al 1996 Nevirapine, zidovudine, and didanosine compared with zidovudine and didanosine in patients with HIV-1 infection. A randomized, double-blind, placebo-controlled trial. National Institute of Allergy and Infectious Diseases AIDS Clinical Trials Group Protocol 241 Investigators. Annals of Internal Medicine 124: 1019–1030.

54. Staszewski S, Morales-Ramirez J, Tashima KT et al 1999 Efavirenz plus zidovu-dine and lamivudine, efavirenz plus indinavir, and indinavir plus zidovudine and lamivudine in the treatment of HIV-1 infection in adults. Study 006 Team. New England Journal of Medicine 341: 1865–1873.

55. Montaner JSG, Reiss P, Cooper D et al 1998 A randomized, double-blind trial comparing combinations of nevirapine, didanosine, and zidovudine for HIV-infected patients. The INCAS Trial. Journal of the American Medical Association 279: 930–937.

56. Murphy RL, Katlama C, Johnson V et al 1999 The Atlantic Study: a randomized, open-label trial comparing two protease inhibitor (PI)-sparing antiretroviral strategies versus a standard PI-containing regimen, 48 week data. Programs and Abstracts of the 39th Interscience Conference on Antimicrobial Agents and Chemotherapy. San Francisco, CA, October 1999 [Abstract LB-22]

57. Staszewski S, Keiser P, Gathe J et al 1999 Comparison of antiviral response with abacavir/Combivir to indinavir/Combivir in therapy-naive adults at 48 weeks (CNA3005). Program and abstracts of the 39th Interscience Conference on Antimicrobial Agents and Chemotherapy; September 26–29, 1999; San Francisco, CA [Abstract 505]

58. Vibhagool A, Cahn P, Schechter M et al 2001 Abacavir/Combivir (ABC/COM) is comparable to indinavir/Combivir in HIV-1-infected antiretroviral therapy-naive adults: preliminary results of a 48-week open label study (CNA3014). I IAS Conference on HIV Pathogenesis and Treatment, Buenos Aires, Argentina, 8–11 July, 2001 [Abstract 63]

59. Deeks SG, Barbour J, Martin J, Swanson M, Grant RM 2000 Sustained CD4+ T cell response after virologic failure of protease inhibitor-based regimens in patients with human immunodeficiency virus infection. Journal of Infectious Diseases 181(3): 946–953

60. Pilcher CD, Miller WC, Beatty ZA, Eron JJ 1999 Detectable HIV-1 RNA at levels below quantifiable limits by Amplicor HIV-1 Monitor is associated with viro-logical relapse on antiretroviral therapy. AIDS 13: 1337–1342

61. Greub G, Cozzi Lepri A, Ledergerber B et al 2001 Lower level HIV viral rebound and blips in patients receiving potent antiretroviral therapy. 8th Conference on Retroviruses and Opportunistic Infections. Chicago, IL, 4–8 February 2001 [Abstract 522]

62. Havlir D, Levitan D, Bassett R, Gilbert P, Richman D, Wong J 2000 Prevalence and predictive value of intermittent viraemia in patients with viral suppres-sion. Antiviral Therapy, 5 (Suppl. 3): 89 [Abstract 112a]

63. Deeks SG, Barbor JD, Martin JN, Grant RM 2000 Delayed immunological dete-rioration among patients who virologically fail protease inhibitor therapy. 7th Conference on Retroviruses and Opportunistic Infections. San Francisco, CA, 30 January–2 February 2000 [Abstract 236]

64. Gallant JE, Hall C, Barnett S, Raines C 1998 Ritonavir/saquinavir (RTV/SQV) as salvage therapy after failure of initial protease inhibitor (PI) regimen. 5th Conference on Retroviruses and Opportunistic Infections; 1998; Chicago, II [Abstract 427]

65. Deeks SG, Grant RM, Beatty G, Horton C, Detmer J, Eastman S, 1998 Activity of a ritonavir plus saquinavir-containing regimen in patients with virologic evidence of indinavir or ritonavir failure. *AIDS* 12: F97–F102

66. Patick AK, Duran M, Cao Y et al 1994 Genotypic and phenotypic characterization of human immunodeficiency virus type 1 variants isolated from patients treated with the protease inhibitor nelfinavir. *Antimicrobial Agents and Chemotherapy* 42: 2637–2644

67. Tebas P, Patick AK, Kane E et al 1999 Virologic responses to a ritonavir-saquinavir-containing regimen in patients who had previously failed nelfinavir. *AIDS* 13: F23–28

68. Zolopa AR, Hertogs K, Shafer R et al 1999 A comparison of phenotypic, genotypic and clinical/treatment history predictors of virological response to saquinavir/ritonavir salvage therapy in a clinic based cohort. *Antiviral Therapy*, 4(Suppl. 1): 47 [Abstract 68]

69. Deeks SG, Hellmann N, Grant RM et al 1999 Novel four drug salvage treatment regimens after failure of a protease inhibitor-containing regimen: antiviral activity and correlation of baseline phenotypic drug susceptibility with virologic outcome. *Journal of Infectious Diseases* 179: 1379–1381

70. Deeks S, Bargour J, Grant R et al 2001 Incidence and predictors of clinical progression among HIV-infected patients experiencing virologic failure of protease inhibitor-based regimens. 8th Conference on Retroviruses and Opportunistic Infections. Chicago, IL, February 2001 [Abstract 428].

71. Tuldrà A, Fumaz CR, Ferrer MF et al 2000 Prospective randomized two-arm controlled study to determine the efficacy of a specific intervention to improve long-term adherence to highly active antiretroviral therapy. *Journal of AIDS* 25: 221–228.

72. Fischl M, Castro J, Monroig R et al 2001 Impact of directly observed therapy on long-term outcomes in HIV clinical trials. 8th Conference on Retroviruses and Opportunistic Infections. Chicago, IL, 4–8 February, 2001 [Abstract 528].

73. Miller MD, Margot NA, Schooley R, McGowan I 2001 Baseline and week 48 final phenotypic analysis of HIV-1 from patients adding tenofovir disoproxil fumarate (TDF) therapy to background ART. 8th Conference on Retroviruses and Opportunistic Infections. Chicago, IL, February 2001 [Abstract 441].

74. Lalezari J, Eron J, Carlson M et al 1999 Sixteen week analysis of heavily pretreated patients receiving T-20 as a component of multi-drug salvage therapy. Program and Abstracts of the 39th Interscience Conference on Antimicrobial Agents and Chemotherapy; September 26–29, 1999; San Francisco, CA [Abstract LB-18].

75. Durant J, Clevenbergh P, Halfon P et al 1999 Drug-resistance genotyping in HIV-1 therapy: the Viradapt randomised controlled trial. *Lancet* 353: 2195–2199.

76. Baxter JD, Mayers DL, Wentworth DN et al 2000 A randomised study of antiretroviral management based on plasma genotypic antiretroviral resistance testing in patients failing therapy. CPCRA 046 Study team for the Terry Beirn Community Programs for Clinical Research on AIDS. *AIDS* 14: F83–F93.

77. Cohen C, Kessler H, Hunt S et al 2000 Phenotypic resistance testing significantly improves response to therapy: final analysis of a randomised trial (VIRA3001). *Antiviral Therapy* 5 (Suppl. 3): 67.

78. Meynard JL, Vray M, Morand-Joubert L et al 2000 Impact of treatment guided by phenotypic or genotypic resistance tests on the response to antiretroviral therapy: a randomised trial (NARVAL, ANRS 088). *Antiviral Therapy* 5 (Suppl. 3): 67–68.

79. De Luca A, Antinor A, Cingolani A et al 2001 A prospective, randomised study on the usefulness of genotypic resistance testing and the assessment of patient-reported adherence in unselected patients failing potent HIV therapy (ARGENTA): final 6 month results. 8th Conference on Retroviruses and Opportunistic Infections. Chicago, IL, February 2001 [Abstract 433].

80. Clevenbergh P, Durant J, Verbiest W et al 2000 Phenotypic analysis of the Viradapt study: correlation with genotypic resistance and PI plasma levels. *Antiviral Therapy* 5 (Suppl. 3): 71–72.

81. Rockstroh, Brun SC, Sylte J et al 2000 ABT-378/ritonavir (ABT-378/r) and efavirenz: one year safety/efficacy evaluation in multiple PI-experienced patients. *AIDS* 14 (Suppl. 4): S29 [Abstract P43].

82. Day JN, Uriel AJ, Daintith R et al 2000 Evaluation of ABT-378/ritonavir (ABT-378/r) based salvage regimens in a cohort of HIV-infected patients. *AIDS* 14 (Suppl. 4): S29 [Abstract P44].

83. Race E, Dam E, Obry V et al 1999 Analysis of HIV phenotypic cross resistance to protease inhibitors in patients failing on combination therapies. 6th Conference on Retroviruses and Opportunistic Infections. Chicago, IL, January–February 1999 [Abstract 119].

84. Workman C, Mussen R, Sullivan J Salvage therapy using six drugs in heavily pretreated patients. 5th Conference on Retroviruses and Opportunistic Infections. Chicago, IL, February 1998 [Abstract 426]. Conference on Retroviruses and Opportunistic Infections. Chicago, IL, February 2001 [Abstract 357].

85. Lorenzi P, Opravil M, Hirschel B et al 1999 Impact of drug resistance on virologic response to salvage therapy. Swiss HIV Cohort Study. *AIDS*; 13: F17–F21.

86. Clevenbergh F, Durant J, Halfon F et al 2000 Persisting long-term benefit of genotype-guided treatment for HIV-infected patients failing HAART. The Viradapt study: week 48 follow-up. *Antiviral Therapy* 5: 65–70.

87. Vandamme A-M, Houyez F, Bànhegyi D et al 2001 Laboratory guidelines for the practical use of HIV drug resistance tests in patient follow-up. *Antiviral Therapy* 6: 21–39.

88. Tural C, Ruiz L, Holtzer C et al 2001 Utility of HIV genotyping and clinical expert advice: the Havana trial. 8th Conference on Retroviruses and Opportunistic Infections. Chicago, IL, February 2001 [Abstract 434].

89. Devereux HL, Youle M, Johnson MA et al 1999 Rapid decline in detectability of HIV-1 drug resistance mutations after stopping therapy. *AIDS* 13: F123–F127.

90. Cane PA, de Ruiter A, Rice P, Wiselka M, Fox R, Pillay D 2001 Resistance associated mutations in subtype C HIV-1 protease gene from treated and untreated patients in the United Kingdom. *Journal of Clinical Microbiology* 39: 2652–2654.

91. Grossman Z, Alkan M, Bentwich Z et al 2001 Patterns of drug resistance: do we need to adjust treatment to clade? 8th Conference on Retroviruses and Opportunistic Infections. Chicago, IL, February 2001 [Abstract 456].

92. Pellegrin I, Izopet J, Reynes J et al 1999 Emergence of zidovudine and multi-drug-resistance mutations in the HIV-1 reverse transcriptase gene in therapy-naïve patients receiving stavudine plus didanosine combination therapy. *AIDS* 13: 1705–1709.

93. Hecht FM, Grant RM, Petropoulos CJ et al 1998 Sexual transmission of an HIV-1 variant resistant to multiple reverse-transcriptase and protease inhibitors. *New England Journal of Medicine* 339: 307–311.

94. Little SJ, Daar ES, D'Aquila RT et al 1999 Reduced antiretroviral drug susceptibility among patients with primary infection. *Journal of the American Medical Association* 282 1142–1149.

95. UK Collaborative Group on Monitoring the Transmission of HIV Drug Resistance 2001 Analysis of prevalence of HIV-1 drug resistance in primary infections with the UK. *British Medical Journal* 322: 1087–1088.

96. Connor EM, Sperling RS, Gelber R et al 1994 Reduction of maternal-infant transmission of human immunodeficiency virus type 1 with zidovudine treatment. *New England Journal of Medicine* 331: 1173–1180.

97. Eastman PS, Shapiro DE, Coombs RW et al 1998 Maternal viral genotypic zidovudine resistance and infrequent failure of zidovudine therapy to prevent perinatal transmission of human immunodeficiency virus type 1 in Pediatric AIDS Clinical Trial Group Protocol 076. *Journal of Infectious Diseases* 177: 557–564.

98. Ioannidis JPA, Abrams EJ, Ammann A et al 2001 Perinatal transmission of human immunodeficiency virus type 1 by pregnant women with RNA virus loads <1000 copies/ml. *Journal of Infectious Diseases* 183: 539–545.

99. Bristol-Myers Squibb Company 2001 Healthcare Provider Important Drug Warning Letter. January 5, 2001.

100. Guay LA, Musoke P, Fleming T et al 1999 Intrapartum and neonatal single-dose nevirapine compared with zidovudine for prevention of mother-to-child transmission of HIV-1 in Kampala, Uganda: HIVNET 012 randomised trial. *Lancet* 354: 795–802.

101. Saba J on behalf of the PETRA Trial Study Team 1999 Interim analysis of early efficacy of three short ZDV/3TC combination regimens to prevent mother-to-child transmission of HIV-1: the PETRA trial. 6th Conference on Retroviruses and Opportunistic Infections. Chicago, IL, January 1999 [Abstract S-7].

102. Pizzo PA, Eddy J, Falloon J et al 1988 Effect of continuous intravenous infusion of zidovudine (AZT) in children with symptomatic HIV infection. *New England Journal of Medicine* 319: 889–896.

103. McKinney RE, Maha MA, Connor EM et al 1991 A multicenter trial for oral zidovudine in children with advanced human immunodeficiency virus disease. *New England Journal of Medicine* 324: 1018–1025.

104. Butler KM, Husson RN, Balis FM et al 1991 Dideoxyinosine in children with symptomatic human immunodeficiency virus infection. *New England Journal of Medicine* 324: 137–144.

105. Lewis LL, Venzon D, Church J et al 1996 Lamivudine in children with human

immunodeficiency virus infection: a phase I/II study. *Journal of Infectious Diseases* 174: 16–25.

106. Kline MW, Dunkle LM, Church JA et al 1995 A phase I/II evaluation of stavudine (d4T) in children with human immunodeficiency virus infection. *Journal of Pediatrics* 96: 247–252.

107. Kline MW, Culnane M, Van Dyke RB et al 1998 A randomized comparative trial of zidovudine (ZDV) versus stavudine (d4T) in children with HIV infection. *Pediatrics* 101: 214–220.

108. Englund J, Baker C, Raskino C et al 1997 Zidovudine, didanosine, or both as the initial treatment for symptomatic HIV-infected children. *New England Journal of Medicine* 336: 1704–1712.

109. Nachman S, Stanley K, Yogev R et al 2000 Nucleoside analogs plus ritonavir in stable antiretroviral therapy-experienced HIV-infected children – a randomized controlled trial. *Journal of the American Medical Association* 283: 492–498.

110. Gortmaker S, Hughes M, Oyompito R et al 2000 Impact of introduction of protease inhibitor therapy on reductions in mortality among children and youth infected with HIV-1. 7th Conference on Retroviruses and Opportunistic Infections. San Francisco, CA, 2000 [Abstract 691].

111. Centers for Disease Control 1994 Revised classification system for human immunodeficiency virus infection in children less than 13 years of age. *Morbidity and Mortality* weekly Reports 43: 1–10.

112. Luzuriaga K, McManus M, Catalina M et al 2000 Early therapy of vertical human immunodeficiency virus type 1 (HIV-1) infection: control of viral replication and absence of persistent HIV-1-specific immune responses. *Journal of Virology* 74: 6984–6991.

113. Chadwick EG, Palumbo P, Rodman J et al 2001 Early therapy with ritonavir (RTV), ZDV and 3TC in HIV-1-infected children 1–24 months of age. 8th Conference on Retroviruses and Opportunistic Infections. Chicago, IL, 2001 [Abstract 677].

114. Powderly WG, Saag MS, Chapman S et al 1999 Predictors of optimal virological response to potent antiretroviral therapy. *AIDS* 13: 1873–1880.

115. Fessel WJ, Krowka JF, Sheppard HW et al 2000 Dissociation of immunologic and virologic responses to highly active antiretroviral therapy. *Journal of AIDS* 23: 314–320.

116. Barnhart HX, Caldwell MB, Thomas P et al 1996 Natural history of human immunodeficiency virus disease in perinatally infected children: an analysis from the Pediatric Spectrum of Disease Project. *Pediatrics* 97: 710–716.

117. Blanche S, Newell ML, Mayaux MJ et al 1997 Morbidity and mortality in European children vertically infected by HIV-1: the French Pediatric HIV Infection Study Group and European Collaborative Study. *Journal of Acquired Immune Deficiency Syndromes and Human Retrovirology* 14: 442–450.

118. Eastman PS, Shapiro DE, Coombs RW et al 1998 Maternal viral genotypic zidovudine resistance and infrequent failure of zidovudine therapy to prevent perinatal transmission of human immunodeficiency virus type 1 in pediatric AIDS Clinical Trials Group Protocol 076. *Journal of Infectious Diseases* 177: 557–564.

119. McSherry GD, Shapiro DE, Coombs RW et al 1999 The effects of zidovudine in the subset of infants infected with human immunodeficiency virus type 1 (Pediatric AIDS Clinical Trials Group Protocol 076). *Journal of Pediatrics* 134: 717–724.

120. Mueller BU, Nelson RP Jr, Sleasman J et al 1998 A phase I/II study of the protease inhibitor ritonavir in children with human immunodeficiency virus infection. *Pediatrics* 101: 335–343.

121. Krogstad P, Wiznia A, Luzuriaga K et al 1999 Treatment of human immunodeficiency virus 1-infected infants and children with the protease inhibitor nelfinavir mesylate. *Clinical Infectious Diseases* 28: 1109–1118.

122. Van Rossum AMC, Niesters HGM, Geelen SPM et al 2000 Clinical and virologic response to combination treatment with indinavir, zidovudine and lamivudine in children with human immunodeficiency virus type-1 infection: a multicenter study in the Netherlands. *Journal of Pediatrics* 136: 780–788.

123. Starr SE, Fletcher CV, Spector SA et al 1999 Combination therapy with efavirenz, nelfinavir, and nucleoside reverse-transcriptase inhibitors in children infected with human immunodeficiency virus type I. *New England Journal of Medicine* 341: 1874–1881.

47 Infections of the upper respiratory tract

R. G. Finch and C. Carbon

The vulnerability of the upper respiratory tract to infections needs no emphasis. Despite a complex array of defense mechanisms, which include particle filtration, humidification, mucous entrapment, ciliary clearance augmented by a rich supply of lymphoid tissue and local antibody production, it is subject to repeated attacks by a plethora of viruses and bacteria and, to a lesser extent, yeasts. Factors such as age, transmissibility, crowding, immunological naïvety and immunosuppression and (in the case of the middle ear and paranasal sinuses) anatomical features and permanently damaged mucosa, contribute to this state of affairs.

Infections of the upper respiratory tract (URTIs) account for a large number of physician visits and represent the leading cause of antibiotic prescriptions in the community, both in children and adults. Although they are usually not life-threatening, serious complications can arise following late or improper antibiotic prescription.

The main problems raised by these infections are as follows:

- The vast majority of such infections have a viral origin.
- Currently, millions of courses of antibiotic therapy are prescribed for viral URTIs, which account for one in six physician visits in the USA or Canada.[1] In France, the frequency of URTIs with a presumed viral etiology that were diagnosed and treated with an antibiotic, increased by 86% in adults and 115% in children, in the period from 1980 to 1991.[2]
- Several factors may lead physicians to overtreat URTIs: parental pressure, physician workload, fear of litigation for possible delayed diagnosis of a true bacterial episode, promotional activities of industry, concerns over excessive return visits for persistent illness and poor ratings on patient satisfaction surveys.[3]
- Over-diagnosis of infections requiring antibiotics due to inadequate assessment and non-specificity of clinical features.[4]
- The three major bacterial pathogens responsible for URTIs (*Streptococcus pneumoniae*, *Haemophilus influenzae*, and group A streptococci, have exhibited decreasing susceptibility or true resistance to a variety of antibiotics during the past decades.[5] Susceptibility patterns differ widely between countries. *Str. pneumoniae* strains with decreased susceptibility to β-lactams continue to increase worldwide and are often associated with resistance to macrolides, trimethoprim–sulfamethoxazole, tetracyclines and fluoroquinolones.[6–8]

- Resistance among *H. influenzae* caused by β-lactamase production ranges from 0 to more than 40% in some places. Macrolide susceptibility among *H. influenzae* varies widely, with many strains beyond the in-vitro breakpoints for these drugs.[5] The main problem of group A streptococci is that resistance to macrolides can exceed 40% and exhibits a close relationship with macrolide usage in the community.[9]
- Amoxicillin remains a drug of choice for the treatment of pneumococcal infections, provided that a sufficient dose is given three times a day for pneumococci with MICs less than 4 mg/l (most isolates from the community).[10] Oral cephalosporins do not exhibit equivalent anti-pneumococcal activity, and some dosage regimens will obviously under-dose against such isolates. The long-acting parenteral cephalosporin ceftriaxone exhibits a high level of activity against both *Str. pneumoniae* and *H. influenzae*, and may be required for severe or unresponsive infections. Macrolides are no longer considered first-line agents for the treatment of infections involving *Str. pneumoniae* or *H. influenzae*, and their use in treating group A streptococci may be limited by high prevalence of resistance in some areas. Trimethoprim–sulfamethoxazole and tetracyclines have similar limitations to macrolides against *Str. pneumoniae* and *H. influenzae*. Where it is available, pristinamycin is considered a satisfactory alternative to β-lactams.
- The recently licensed respiratory fluoroquinolones are contraindicated in children. It is recommended that their use in the treatment of URTIs in adults should be limited and highly selective.
- The huge cost of antibiotics for treating URTIs, and the relationship between duration of treatment and risk of selection of resistance[2] should encourage shortened antibiotic courses. Short courses (less than 5 days) have the added advantage of improving compliance and reducing the rate of side effects[11]

THE COMMON COLD

Most colds are of viral origin (predominantly rhinoviruses and adenoviruses) and, although, some experimental methods of preventing and treating them are beginning to emerge, no specific treatment is available for most of these common illness. A variety of symptomatic treatments, such as simple analgesics, anti-inflammatory and anti-histamine-containing preparations have a role in disease management and are widely used. The presumed, but seldom established, role of secondary bacterial infection prompted the unacceptable widespread use of antibacterial chemotherapy in these conditions.

Antibiotics are especially widely used in respiratory infections in children who receive, on average, one course of antibiotics a year in the first 6 years of life. This reflects the difficulties in establishing a clinical and microbiological diagnosis of many URTIs in childhood, and the recognition that coryzal symptoms may precede a number of more serious bacterial infections. However, it has to be noted that acute otitis media may occur in 7–30% of cases, mainly in children aged from 6 months to 2 years. Acute sinusitis is observed in 0.5–10% of cases. Acute ethmoiditis may occur in infants and should be treated with antibiotics. Maxillary sinusitis usually occurs from 3 years of age.[12–14] It is recognized that patients with chronic ill health, especially those with chronic bronchitis, are more at risk of secondary bacterial complications (*see* Ch. 48). The general tendency for these infections to recover rapidly without specific treatment emphasizes the importance of a restrictive antibiotic policy.

The use of antibiotics for new episodes of respiratory illness varies greatly between practitioners. Five randomized, double-blind studies[15–19], concluded that the benefits of antimicrobial treatment were marginal and that routine prescribing for this type of illness was not indicated.[20,21] The common belief that prescribing antibiotics saves the general practitioner from extra work has been disproved by Howie and Hutchison.[22] Immunosupression and a past history of more than three episodes of acute otitis media within 6 months are risk factors for complications of rhinopharyngitis.[23] Persistence of fever for more than 3 days, may indicate failure but should be used selectively. Purulent conjunctivitis or a persistent cough, or rhinorrhea of more than 10 days are indications for antibiotic therapy. Early purulent nasal discharge is not associated with the presence of bacteria and per se is no indication for antibiotic treatment.[24]

Several trials have shown that interferon, given intranasally for 4–5 days, is protective against rhinovirus colds.[25,26] This effect has been achieved with partially purified leukocyte interferon and with, interferon purified by monoclonal antibody or by recombinant DNA methods. Intranasal administration of interferon for a few days was well tolerated, but attempts at longer term prophylaxis for 2 weeks often led to local symptoms of nasal irritation. Another approach that has shown some benefit has been to treat family contacts prophylactically.[27,28] However, at present, widespread use of interferon for treatment of the common cold is unlikely and remains investigative. The logistics and costs of treatment would be prohibitive for a largely self-limiting condition.

ACUTE SORE THROAT

Although most acute sore throats are caused by virus infections *Streptococcus pyogenes* (Lancefield group A, β hemolytic streptococci) accounts for 25–33% of acute sore throats seen in many studies in general practice. In some countries diphtheria remains important and has re-emerged in the former USSR as a result of failures in immunization policy. *Corynebacterium haemolyticum* is an established cause of sore throat and scarlatiniform rash in children and young adults.[29] Other less common bacterial causes include *Neisseria gonorrhoeae*, *Neisseria meningitidis*, *Yersinia enterocolitica* and *Mycoplasma pneumoniae*. The role of group C and G streptococci remains unclear, although they can be isolated from symptomatic patients. Vincent's angina is found especially, but not exclusively, in association with gingival sepsis. Clinical signs are often unreliable as a guide to etiology. Hemolytic streptococci are more likely to be found in association with high fever, follicular tonsillitis, tender anterior cervical glands and neutrophilia in the peripheral blood, but may be grown from patients with mild severe throat – or, indeed, from symptomless carriers. Conversely, bad sore throat, even with pharyngeal exudate, may be caused by Epstein–Barr virus, Herpes simplex virus and, occasionally, enteroviruses or adenoviruses. For these reasons, antibiotic treatment is most satisfactory if based on examination of a throat swab. The use of tests for rapid detection of group A streptococcal antigen has a sensitivity of >90% and is cost-effective in the selection of patients to be treated with an antibiotic.

The conventional treatment for streptococcal sore throat is penicillin, given orally as phenoxymethylpenicillin (250 mg four times daily in adults). In order to ensure eradication of streptococci in a high proportion of patients it is necessary to continue penicillin for 10 days.[30] This is uncommonly achieved in practice, because patients feel well again in a few days and do not complete the course. A 3-day course of penicillin is not effective and tends towards an increased recurrence rate in the following 6 months. A 7-day course seems to be acceptable.[31] Failure rates of penicillin therapy are 10–25%, depending on the populations studied. Shorter treatment, 5 days of various oral cephalosporins, various oral aminopenicillins (6 days of amoxicillin), and macrolides (5 days azithromycin) are reasonable alternatives, with faster resolution of symptoms, better compliance, and lower recurrence rates.[11,32] There is no need to routinely monitor the bacteriological efficacy of treatment. The rate of recolonization at day 30 is around 20%, similar to the carriage rate in family contacts.[33]

Recent trials have shown that antibiotic therapy does have a role in alleviating the illness caused by streptococcal pharyngitis, and treatment within 1 week of the onset of symptoms will prevent the now rare complication of acute rheumatic fever. Krober et al[34] showed significant differences in resolution of fever and other markers of clinical activity between patients given penicillin and those given placebo. In a larger trial involving 260 children, Randolph et al[35] showed that significantly fewer children given oral penicillin or cefadroxil showed persistence of fever or local signs of infection 18–24 h after treatment was started than those given placebo.

The possibility that treatment failures with penicillin may be caused by the presence of β-lactamase-producing bacteria in the pharynx has attracted attention. Brook[36] reviewed the evidence that β-lactamase-resistant aerobic and anaerobic flora frequently emerge during penicillin treatment and may spread to household contacts. Clindamycin can be considered such but should be used selectively.

When managing patients with acute sore throat, in the absence of microbiological support, it is useful to have a policy for the use of penicillin that includes patients most likely to have streptococcal infection but avoids its widespread use in viral syndromes. Such circumstances, include:

- scarlet fever, because its exact etiology is implicit and *Str. pyogenes* remains penicillin sensitive
- follicular tonsillitis with fever and tender anterior cervical glands
- bacterial complications of acute pharyngitis, such as peritonsillar abscess, acute otitis media, sinusitis, mastoiditis and suppurative cervical lymphadenitis
- acute sore throat in a family or community in which streptococcal infections are prevalent.

STREPTOCOCCAL CARRIAGE

Although it is now an uncommon requirement in most developed countries, the prevention of streptococcal throat infections in patients with a history of acute rheumatic fever is best achieved with penicillin. The most successful method is a monthly intramuscular injection of benzathine penicillin. The disadvantages of this method are the need for repeated injections (albeit infrequently) and the possibility that any allergic reaction will be prolonged in its effects.

DIPHTHERIA

Antibiotics are an essential but adjunctive part of treatment, and do not obviate the need for antitoxin.

Corynebacterium diphtheriae is moderately susceptible to penicillin, and is susceptible to amoxicillin, erythromycin and clindamycin. Erythromycin remains active, apart from a few strains of the *mitis* biotype, and is preferred for the treatment of the index case as well as household contacts or known carriers.[37]

ACUTE EPIGLOTTITIS

This rapidly progressive and life-threatening illness is encountered mainly in children, but is increasingly being recognized in adults. It is caused by infections with *H. influenzae* type b, which may often be cultured from the blood as well as from the local lesion. The favorable impact of conjugate vaccines on

H. influenzae meningitis has also fortunately reduced the incidence of acute epiglottitis in childhood. Treatment is as much concerned with maintaining the airway as with control of the infection. Ampicillin has been widely used in the past but the relative rarity of the condition does not allow objective judgment of its continued benefit. Ampicillin resistance is now widespread in *H. influenzae*, and a cephalosporin, such as cefotaxime of ceftriaxone, is now preferred on account of β-lactamase stability, high potency and excellent safety records.

The differential diagnosis of acute croup includes not only laryngotracheobronchitis, which is largely viral in etiology (RSV, parainfluenza), but may also occasionally be bacterial in nature (*M. pneumoniae*); but also acute epiglottitis, diphtheria, and many non-infectious conditions. Pseudomembranous croup is a severe bacterial tracheitis.[38] *Staphylococcus aureus* is most commonly involved, although sometimes with other organisms,[39] and treatment should include a β-lactamase-resistant penicillin.

ACUTE SINUSITIS

Acute sinusitis is an acute infection of the mucosal lining of the maxillary, frontal, sphenoidal or ethmoidal sinuses, characterized by facial pain, swelling, purulent nasal discharge, headhache, and sometimes fever. It is the fifth most common reason for primary care physicians to prescribe an antibiotic. More than 90% of acute cases are maxillary sinusitis. In young children, signs and symptoms are difficult to differentiate from those of a common cold. The duration of symptoms, location of pain and some specific signs (such as edema of the internal angle of the eye) are important for an accurate clinical diagnosis. Orbital and nervous system complications are rare.

Most episodes of acute bacterial sinusitis complicate viral URTIs. *H. influenzae* is the most common isolate in acute sinusitis, but detailed studies have shown a great variety of pathogens. A detailed quantitative study of 65 needle punctures in 81 adults with acute infections of the antrum[40] showed *H. influenzae* and *Str. pneumoniae* as the most frequent isolates with occasional high counts of staphylococci, *Moraxella catarrhalis*, α-hemolytic streptococci, anaerobes and viruses. Anaerobic isolates are common in chronic sinus infections; heavy pure cultures of anaerobes were found in 23 of 83 specimens removed aseptically at operation.[41] As with acute otitis media, results of treatment have generally correlated well with antibiotic concentrations in the sinus secretions; but even with high concentrations eradication of bacteria is not easily achieved, perhaps because the low pO_2 and high pCO_2 tension of purulent sinus secretions can increase bacterial resistance to some antibiotics.

In the vast majority of cases of acute sinusitis no specific investigation is required. Radiographic examination of the sinuses is appropriate in patients with bilateral pain or failure of a first course of treatment. Bacteriological examination of material provided by sinus puncture or sampling at the middle meatus is also desirable.

Whether antibiotic therapy should be given to all patients with acute sinusitis remains controversial. Clinical trials have largely included patients with acute maxillary sinusitis, so their conclusions should be extended to other conditions with caution. Lindbaek et al[42] showed that amoxicillin had a moderate benefit (86% cured vs 57% cured with placebo). Other studies[43] and meta-analyses[44] have shown amoxicillin to have no clear-cut benefit in terms of cure rate, control of symptoms or relapse rate. Other antibiotics did not appear superior to amoxicillin in the meta-analyses. It is important to note that the placebo response rate was greater than 50%, indicating that acute maxillary sinusitis is frequently a self-limiting illness. The problem for physicians is to distinguish the 50% of patients who will respond to decongestants alone from those who need antibiotics. In adults without underlying disease, a decongestant alone can be prescribed because of the benefit of antibiotics in such cases is low compared with the risk of side effects. Sinusitis in younger children is difficult to distinguish from the common cold, and the criterion for the use of an antibiotic should be the duration of symptoms.[45]

Persistence or progression of symptoms should be considered as an indication for antibiotic therapy. In the most severe cases, with intense pain and high fever, an antibiotic should be started quickly. A short-term course (less than 7 days) of corticosteroids has been demonstrated to be more effective than analgesics in controlling pain and speeding recovery, but corticosteroids should be used selectively.

In other conditions, such as frontal, sphenoidal or ethmoidal sinusitis, or infection occurring in immunosuppressed patients, antibiotic therapy should be considered. Use of amoxicillin or a macrolide (including the most recent compounds) may not be optimal in areas with a high prevalence of β-lactamase-producing *H. influenzae* or *Mor. catarrhalis* or high rates of multiresistant *Str. pneumoniae*: amoxicillin–clavulanate or group 3 cephalosporins would be more suitable in such situations. Antipneumococcal fluoroquinolones should be restricted to failures of first-line therapy. Several studies have shown the efficacy of shortening courses of antibiotic therapy down to 4–5 days.[11] In recalcitrant cases, sinus puncture with drainage should be considered, together with bacteriological examination of the fluid.

Acute sinusitis occurring in patients admitted to intensive care units is now increasingly recognized. Such patients are predisposed to this by impaired sinus drainage, nasogastric intubation and repeat aspirations used in airways toilet, but especially nasotracheal intubation. This will predispose patients to lower respiratory tract infections, and in particular pneumonia, which may have serious consequences.

ACUTE OTITIS MEDIA

Acute otitis media is the second most common infectious disease encountered in children in industrialized countries: 80% of children under 1 year of age develop the condition, one-third having at least three episodes, with a maximum incidence between 6 months and 1 year. The etiology of acute otitis media can be reliably established only by myringotomy or tympanocentesis but these procedures are rarely performed, and indeed are not indicated in the great majority of patients. The correlation between nasopharyngeal and middle-ear fluid cultures in children with otitis media is too weak for nasopharyngeal cultures to be a marker for the bacteriological documentation of otitis media.[46] The predominant organisms are *Str. pneumoniae* and *H. influenzae*; the latter was formerly thought to affect mainly children under 5 years old, but it is now known to can cause otitis at all ages. *Mor. catarrhalis* has been isolated in pure culture in a small but significant proportion of exudates. *Str. pyogenes*, formerly important, is now rarely found, and *Staph aureus*, enterobacteria and *Pseudomonas* spp. are frequent contaminants arising from the external meatus. Some authors have questioned the need for routine antibiotic treatment of acute otitis media. Van Buchem et al[47] studied 239 infections in 171 children, all of whom were given analgesics and decongestants. Groups were then given either no additional treatment, amoxicillin alone, amoxicillin with myringotomy or myringotomy alone. No difference was found between any of the groups in the rates of resolution of pain, temperature, ear discharge, otoscopic appearance or recurrence. Van Buchem et al suggest that initial treatment should be symptomatic only and other measures reserved for those with persistent symptoms. In a later study, Van Buchem et al[48] showed that more than 90% of 4860 children diagnosed as having acute otitis media recovered uneventfully with symptomatic treatment only. A severe course (defined as persistent illness, high temperature and/or severe pain after 3–4 days) was experienced by only 126 (2.7%), 30 of whom had *Str. pyogenes* infections. In the same study, a trial of 100 severe cases showed that amoxicillin alone or with myringotomy was more effective than myringotomy alone. Considering that the question of myringotomy remained unsolved, Engelhard et al[49] conducted a trial in 105 infants, in which the recovery rate in patients treated with antibiotic, with or without myringotomy, was 60% (compared with 23% in those receiving myringotomy with placebo). Full recovery at follow-up was judged by otoscopic findings. The meta-analysis published by Del Mar et al[50] from seven studies in children showed that the use of antibiotics decreases pain at 2–7 days after presentation, and reduces contralateral otitis and deafness at 3 months. Antibiotics did not reduce pain within 24 h or prevent recurrent otitis. An interesting study included in this meta-analysis was that of Kaleida et al[51], in which children were divided into two groups: those with mild symptoms (little pain and no, or low-grade fever), and those with more severe symptoms (substantial pain and fever). In the first group the failure rate in the patients treated with placebo was twice that of those receiving amoxicillin; in the second group, which included children under 2 years of age, placebo treatment failed six times more frequently than amoxicillin.

According to a report from the drug-resistant *Str. pneumoniae* therapeutic working group in the USA[52] oral amoxicillin should remain the first-line agent for treating acute otitis media. However, in order to achieve effective concentrations against *Str. pneumoniae* strains with decreased susceptibility to penicillin, an increase in the dosage used, from 40–45 mg/kg/day up to 80–90 mg/kg/day (divided into three doses) is recommended. For patients with clinically defined treatment failure after 3 days of therapy, useful alternatives include oral amoxicillin–clavulanate, cefuroxime axetil, and intramuscular ceftriaxone. Many other approved drugs for treatment of otitis media lack good evidence for efficacy against *Str. pneumoniae* with decreased susceptibility to penicillin.

The French recommendations[53] include high-dose (80–90 mg/kg/day) amoxicillin–clavulanate as the first-line choice, especially in children below 2 years or with more than three previous episodes of acute otitis media, which takes into account both the consequences of decreased susceptibility to penicillin of *Str. pneumoniae* and the high rate of β-lactamase production by *H. influenzae*. Intramuscular ceftriaxone may be a good alternative in cases of treatment failure.

The study by Dagan et al,[54] using bacteriological evaluation of otitis media at days 0 and 3–4 of therapy, suggests that persistence of bacteria at day 3–4 is highly predictive of clinical failure. The susceptibility breakpoints for *H. influenzae* should be considerably lower for both cefaclor and azithromycin than those currently in use for otitis media caused by *H. influenzae*.

The meta-analysis performed by Kozyrskyj et al[55] suggests that 5 days of short-acting antibiotics is effective treatment for uncomplicated otitis media in children.

Recurrent otitis media in childhood presents a difficult problem. Adenoidectomy is often the treatment of choice, but in some children recurrent attacks justify a trial of prolonged antibiotic prophylaxis, usually with ampicillin or amoxicillin. Limited trial evidence supports this strategy.[56] For example, Maynard et al[57] showed that ampicillin (125 or 250 mg/day) reduced attacks of otitis media by 47% (67% in good compliers) of Eskimo children with a high incidence of the problem. However, development of drug resistance is the price paid by this approach. Conjugate pneumococcal vaccines could not only substantially reduce the occurrence of pneumococcal otitis media but also lower complication rates.[58]

CONCLUSIONS

The treatment of URTIs is a major area for the development of policies promoting the judicious use of antibiotics. Several targets for intervention can be envisaged:

- public education campaigns to counter the prevailing culture of expectations of routine prescription of antibiotics;
- education of prescribers in management of prescribing demand (a willingness to explain the nature of the illness, to deal directly with specific concerns, and to discuss the reasons for arriving at a therapeutic decision correlates more closely with patient satisfaction than does prescribing an antimicrobial);

- reduction of uncertainty by helping clinicians recognize those situations that do not require an antibiotic by providing evidence-based guidance to patients that focuses on the major diagnostic and treatment decisions.

It is hoped that the development of rapid diagnostic tests, such as those already available for group A streptococcal infections, will be available and widely used in the future.

References

1. Gonzales R, Steiner JF, Sande MA 1997 Antibiotic prescribing for adults with colds, URTIs and bronchitis by ambulatory care physicians. *Journal of the American Medical Association* 278: 901–904.
2. Guillemot D, Maison P, Carbon C et al 1998 Trends in antimicrobial use in the community. France 1981–1992. *Journal of Infectious Diseases* 177: 492–497.
3. Schwartz B, Mainous AG, Marey SM 1995 Why do physicians prescribe antibiotics for children with URTIs? *Journal of the American Medical Association* 279: 881–882.
4. Gerber MA, Marey SM 1999 Editorial response: judicious use of antimicrobial agents for RTIs in children-why are the pediatricians in Toronto area doing so well? *Clinical Infectious Diseases* 29: 318–320.
5. Felmingham D 2000 Alexander Project. *Journal of Antimicrobial Chemotherapy*.
6. Arason VA, Kristinsson KG, Sigurdsson JA et al 1996 Do antimicrobial increase the carriage rate of penicillin-resistant pneumococci in children? Cross sectional prevalence study. *British Medical Journal* 313: 387–391.
7. Baquero F, Garcia-Rodriguez JA, Garcia de Lomas J, Aguilar L 1999 Antimicrobial resistance of 1113 *Streptococcus pneumoniae* isolates from patients with RTIs in Spain. *Antimicrobial Agents and Chemotherapy* 43: 357–359.
8. Chen DK, McGeer A, de Azavedo JC et al 1999 Decreased susceptibility of *Streptococcus pneumoniae* to fluoroquinolones in Canada. *New England Journal of Medicine* 341: 233–239.
9. Seppala H, Klaukka T, Vuopio-Verkien J et al 1997 The effects of changes in the consumption of macrolide antibiotics on erythromycin-resistance in group A streptococci in Finland. *New England Journal of Medicine* 337: 441–446.
10. Andes D, Craig WA 1998 In vivo activities of amoxicillin and amoxicillin-clavulanate *against Streptococcus pneumoniae*: application to breakpoint determination. *Antmicrobial Agents and Chemotherapy* 42: 2375–2379.
11. Pichichero ME, Cohen R 1997 Shortened course of antibiotic therapy for acute otitis media, sinusitis and tonsillopharyngitis. *Pediatric Infectious Disease Journal* 16: 680–695.
12. Heikkinen T, Ruuskanen O 1994 Temporal development of acute otitis media during upper respiratory tract infections. *Pediatric Infectious Disease Journal* 13: 659–661.
13. Ueda D, Yoto Y 1996 The ten-day mark as a practical diagnostic approach for acute paranasal sinusitis in children. *Pediatric Infectious Disease Journal* 15: 576–579.
14. Wald ER. Sinusitis in children. *New England Journal of Medicine* 326: 319–323.
15. Heikkinen T, Ruuskanen O, Ziegler T, Waris M, Puhakka H 1995 Shortened use of amoxicillin-clavulanate during upper respiratory tract infections for prevention of acute otitis media. *Journal of Pediatrics* 126: 313–316.
16. Howie JGR, Clark GA 1970 Double-blind trial of early demethyl-chlortetracycline in minor respiratory illness in general practice. *Lancet* 1099–1102.
17. Kaiser L, Lew D, Hirschel B et al 1996 Effects of antibiotic treatment in the subset of common cold patients who have bacteria in naso-pharyngeal secretions. *Lancet* 347: 1507–1510.
18. Taylor B, Abbot GD, Kerr MM, Ferguson DM 1977 Amoxycillin and cotrimoxazole in presumed viral respiratory infections in childhood; a placebo-controlled trial. *British Medical Journal* 2: 552–554.
19. Todd JK, Todd M, Dammato J, Todd W 1984 Bacteriology and treatment of purulent naso-pharyngitis: a double-blind, placebo-controlled evaluation. *Pediatric Infectious Disease Journal* 3: 226–232.
20. Arrol B, Kenealy T 1998 Antibiotics vs placebo in the common cold. Cochrane latest version 8 April 1998. Cochrane Library Oxford, Update Software.

21. Dowell SF, Schwartz B, Phillips WR 1998 Appropriate use of antibiotics for URTIs in children. Part II: cough, pharyngitis and the common cold. The Pediatric URI Consensus Team. *American Family Physician* 58: 1335–1345.

22. Howie JGR, Hutchinson KR 1978 Antibiotics and respiratory illness in general practice: prescribing policy and work load. *British Medical Journal* 2: 1342.

23. Berman S. Otitis media in children. *New England Journal of Medicine* 332: 1560–1565.

24. Mainous AG, Huston WJ, Eberlin C 1997 Color of respiratory discharge and antibiotic use. *Lancet* 350(9084): 1077–1079.

25. Scott GM, Phillpotts RJ, Wallace J et al 1982 Purified interferon as protection against rhinovirus infection. *British Medical Journal* 284: 1822–1825.

26. Hayden FJ, Gwaltney JM 1983 Intranasal interferon for prevention of rhinovirus infection and illness. *Journal of Infectious Diseases* 148: 543–547.

27. Hayden FG, Gwaltney JM, Johnson ME 1985 Prophylactic efficacy and tolerance of low dose, intranasal interferon-alpha 2 in natural respiratory viral infections. *Antiviral Research* 5: 11–15.

28. Douglas RM, Moore BW, Miles HB et al 1986 Prophylactic efficacy of intransal alpha-2-interferon against rhinovirus infections in the family setting. *New England Journal of Medicine* 314: 65–70.

29. Editorial 1978 Bacterial pharyngitis. *Lancet* I: 1241–1242.

30. Peter G 1992 Streptococcal pharyngitis: current therapy and criteria for evaluation of new agents. *Clinical Infectious Diseases* 14 (Suppl.) S218–S223.

31. Swart S, Sachs AP, Ruijs G et al 2000 Penicillin for sore throat: randomized, double-blind trial of seven day vs three d treatment or placebo in adults. *British Medical Journal* 320: 150–154.

32. Adam D, Scholz H, Helmerking M 2000 Short-course antibiotic treatment of 4782 of culture-proven cases of group A streptococcal tonsillopharyngitis and incidence of post-streptococcal sequelae. *Journal of Infectious Diseases* 182: 509–516.

33. Nguyen L, Levy D, Ferroni A, Gehanno P, Berche P 1997 Molecular epidemiology of *Streptococcus pyogenes* in an area where acute pharyngotonsillitis is endemic. *Journal of Clinical Microbiology* 35: 211–2114.

34. Krober MS, Bass JW, Michels GN 1985 Streptococcal pharyngitis. Placebo-controlled, double-blind evaluation of clinical response to penicillin therapy. *Journal of the American Medical Association* 253: 1271–1274.

35. Randolph MF, Gerber MA, de Meo KK, Wright L 1985 Effects of antibiotic therapy on the clinical course of streptococcal pharyngitis. *Journal of Pediatrics* 106: 870–875.

36. Brook I 1984 The role of beta-lactamase producing bacteria in the persistence of streptococcal tonsillar infection. *Reviews of Infectious Diseases* 6: 601–607.

37. Wilson APR 1995 Treatment of infection caused by toxigenic and non-toxigenic strains of *Corynebacterium diphtheriae*. *Journal of Antimicrobial Chemotherapy* 35: 717–720.

38. Donnelly BW, Mc Millan JA, Weiner LB 1990 Bacterial tracheitis: report of eight new cases and review. *Reviews of Infectious Diseases* 12: 729–735.

39. Henry RL, Mellis CM, Benjamin B 1983 Pseudomembranous croup. *Archives of Diseases in Childhood* 58: 180–183.

40. Hamory BH, Sande MA, Sydnor A, Seale DL, Gwaltney JM 1979 Etiology and antimicrobial therapy of acute maxillary sinusitis. *Journal of Infectious Diseases* 139: 197–202.

41. Frederick J, Braude AI 1974 Anaerobic infection of the paranasal sinuses. *New England Journal of Medicine* 290: 135–137.

42. Lindbaek M, Hjortdahl P, Johnasen UL 1996 Amoxycillin compared to placebo in the treatment of acute maxillary sinusitis in adults. *British Medical Journal* 313: 325–329.

43. Van Buchem FL, Knotterus JA, Schrijnemaekens VJ, Peeters MF 1997 Primary-care-based randomized, placebo-controlled trial of antibiotic treatment in acute maxillary sinusitis. *Lancet* 349: 683–687.

44. Williams JW, Aguilar C, Makela M et al 1999 Antimicrobial therapy for acute maxillary sinusitis. The Cochrane Data Base of Systematic Reviews, The Cochrane Library, Oxford.

45. Dowell SF, Schwartz B, Phillips WR 1998 Appropriate use of antibiotics in URIs in children. Part I: otitis media and sinusitis, The Pediatric URI Consensus Team. *American Family Physician* 58: 1113–1118.

46. Gehanno P, Lenoir G, Barry B et al 1996 Evaluation of naso-pharyngeal cultures for bacteriologic assessment of acute otitis media in children. *Pediatric Infectious Disease Journal* 15: 329–332.

47. Van Buchem F, Birk JHM, Van't Hof MA 1981 Therapy of acute otitis media: myringotomy, antibiotics or neither? *Lancet* ii: 883–887.

48. Van Buchem FL, Peeters MF, Van't Hof MA 1985 Acute otitis media: a new treatment strategy. *British Medical Journal* 290: 1033–1037.

49. Engelhard D, Cohen D, Strauss N et al 1989 Randomized study of myringotomy, amoxicillin-clavulanate or both for acute otitis media in infants. *Lancet* ii: 141–143.

50. Del Mar C, Glasziou P, Hayenm M 1997 Are antibiotics indicated as initial treatment for children with acute otitis media? A meta-analysis. *British Medical Journal* 314: 1526–1529.

51. Kaleida PH, Casselbrandt ML, Rockette HE et al 1991 Amoxicillin or myringotomy or both for acute otitis media: results of a randomized clinical trial. *Pediatrics* 87: 466–474.

52. Dowell SF, Butler JC, Giebink GS et al 1999 AOM: management and surveillance in an era of pneumococcal resistance: a report from the Drug-Resistant *Streptococcus pneumoniae* Therapeutic Working Group. *Pediatric Infectious Disease Journal* 18: 1–9.

53. 4e Conference de Consensus en therapeutique anti-infectieuse de la SPILF. Les infections des voies respiratoires. Lille 18 Octobre 1991. *Med Mal Infect* 1992: 22.

54. Dagan R, Leibovitz E, Fliss DM et al 2000 Bacteriologic efficacies of oral azithromycin and oral cefaclor in treatment of acute otitis media in infants and young children. *Antmicrobial Agents and Chemotherapy* 44: 43–50

55. Korzyrskyj AL, Hildes-Rostein E, Longstaffe E et al 1998 Treatment of acute otitis media with a shortened course of antibiotic. *Journal of the American Medical Association* 279: 1736–1742.

56. Bonati M, Marchetti F, Pistotti V et al 1992 Meta-analysis of antimicrobial prophylaxis for recurrent acute otitis media. *Clinical Trials Meta-analysis* 28: 39–50.

57. Maynard JE, Fleshman JK, Tshopp CF 1972 Otitis media in Alaskan Eskimo children; prospective evaluation of chemoprophylaxis. *Journal of the American Medical Association* 219: 597–599.

58. Dagan R, Givan-Lavi N, Shkolnik L et al 2000 Acute otitis media caused by antibiotic-resistant *S. pneumoniae* in Southern Israel; implications for immunizing with conjugate vaccines. *Journal of Infectious Diseases* 181: 1322–1329.

 ## Further information

Adam D 2000 The management of bacterial infections of the upper respiratory tract in children: pharyngitis and otitis media. 13: 83–88.

Aronovitz GH 2000 Antimicrobial therapy of acute otitis media: review of treatment recommendations. *Clinical Therapeutics* 22: 29–39.

Arroll B, Kenealy T 2000 Antibiotics for the common cold. Cochrane Database Systematic Review CD000247.

Bisno AL, Gerber MA, Gwaltney JM et al 1997 Diagnosis and management of group A streptococcal pharyngitis: a practice guideline. *Clinical Infectious Diseases* 25: 574–583.

Block SL 1999 Management of acute otitis media in the 1990s: the decade of resistant penumococcus. *Pediatric Drugs* 1: 31–50.

Braun BL, Fowels JB 2000 Characteristics and experiences of parents and adults who want antibiotics for cold symptoms. *Archives of Family Medicine* 9: 589–595.

Brooks I, Gooch WM, Jenkins SG et al 2000 Medical management of acute bacterial sinusitis. Recommendations of a clinical advisory committee on pediatric and adults sinusitis. *Annals of Otology: Rhinology and Laryngology Supplement* 182: 2–20.

Cohen R, de Gouvello A, Levy C et al 1998 Utilization of rapid diagnostic tests for group A streptococcus and bacteriologic and clinical correlations with acute angina in general medicine. *Presse Médicale* 27: 1131–1134.

Damm M, Eckel HE, Jungehulsing M et al 1999 Management of acute inflammatory childhood stridor. *Otolaryngology – Head and Neck Surgery* 121: 633–638.

Del Mar CB, Galsziou PP, Spinks AB 2000 Antibiotics for sore throat. Cochrane Database Systematic Review 4: CD000023.

Dippel DW, Touw-Otten F, Habbema JD 1992 Management of children with acute pharyngitis: a decision analysis. *Journal of Family Practice* 34: 149–159.

Engels EA, Terrin N, Barza M et al 2000 Meta-analysis of diagnostic tests for acute sinusitis. *Journal of Clinical Epidemiology* 53: 852–862.

English JA, Bauman KA 1997 Evidence-based management of upper respiratory infection in a family practice teaching clinic. *Family Medicine* 29: 38–41.

Gooch WM 1999 Antibacterial management of acute and chronic sinusitis. *Manag Care Interface* 12: 92–94.

Guay DR 2000 Short-course antimicrobial therapy for upper respiratory tract infections. *Clinical Therapeutics* 22: 673–684.

Harley EH, Sdralis T, Berkowitz RG 1997 Acute mastoiditis in children: a 12 year retrospective study. *Otolaryngology – Head and Neck Surgery* 116: 26–30.

Hedges JR, Singal BM, Estep JL 1991 The impact of a rapid screen for streptococcal pharyngitis on clinical decision making in the emergency department. *Medical Decision Making* 11: 119–124.

Hoberman A, Paradise JL 2000 Acute otitis media: diagnosis and management in the year 2000. *Pediatric Annual* 29: 609–620.

Jacobs RF 2000 Judicious use of antibiotics for common pediatric respiratory infections. *Pediatric Infectious Disease Journal* 19: 938–943.

Jiang CB, Chiu NC, Hsu CH et al 2000 Clinical presentation of acute mastoiditis in children. *Journal Microbiol Immunol Infect* 33: 187–190.

Kaaerner KJ, Nafsrad P, Jaakkola JJ 2000 Upper respiratory morbidity in preschool children: a cross-sectional study. *Archives of Otolaryngology and Head and Neck Surgery* 126: 1201–1206.

Kaplan SL, Mason EO, Wald ER et al 2000 Pneumococcal mastoidis in children. *Pediatrics* 106: 695–699.

Klein JO 2000 Clinical implications of antibiotic resistance for management of acute otitis media. *Journal of Laboratory and Clinical Medicine* 135: 220–224.

Klein JO 2000 Management of otitis media: 2000 and beyond. *Pediatric Infectious Disease Journal* 19: 383–387.

Klein JO 1999 Review of consensus reports on management of acute otitis media. *Pediatric Infectious Disease Journal* 18: 1152–1155.

Little DR, Mann BL, Godbout CJ 2000 How family physicians distinguish acute sinusitis from upper respiratory infections: a retrospective analysis. *Journal of the American Board of Family Practice* 13: 101–106.

Low DE, Desrosiers M, McSherry J et al 1997 A practical guide for the diagnosis and treatment of acute sinusitis. *CMAJ* 156: S1–14.

Mehra P, Caiazzo A, Bestgen S 1999 Odontogenic sinusitis causing orbital cellulitis. *Journal of the American Dental Association* 130: 1086–1092.

Mortimore S, Wormald PJ 1999 Management of acute complicated sinusitis: a 5-year review. *Otolaryngology – Head and Neck Surgery* 121: 639–642.

Murphy TF 2000 Bacterial otitis media: pathogenetic considerations. *Pediatric Infectious Disease Journal* 19: S9–15.

Pichichero ME, Reiner SA, Brook I et al 2000 Controversies in the medical management of persistent and recurrent acute otitis media. Recommendations of a clinical advisory committee. *Annals of Otology: Rhinology and Laryngology Supplement* 183: 1–12.

Pichichero ME 2000 Recurrent and persistent otitis media. *Pediatric Infectious Disease Journal* 19: 911–916.

Poole MD 1999 A focus on acute sinusitis in adults: changes in disease management. *American Journal of Medicine.* 106: 38S–47S.

Ramilo O 1999 Role of respiratory viruses in acute otitis media: implications for management. *Pediatric Infectious Disease Journal* 18: 1125–1129.

Shackley F, Knox K, Morris JB et al 2000 Outcome of invasive pneumococcal disease: a UK based study. Oxford Pneumococcal Surveillance Group. *Archives of Diseases in Childhood* 83: 231–233.

Sivertsen LM, Pattemore PK, Abbot GD 1998 The changing face of epiglottitis in Canterbury 1970–1996. *New Zealand Medical Journal* 111: 208–210.

Solomon P, Weisbrod M, Irish JC et al 1998 Adult epiglottitis: the Toronto hospital experience. *Journal of Otolargngology* 27: 332–336.

Stone S, Gonzales R, Maselli J et al 2000 Antibiotic prescribing for patients with colds, upper respiratory tract infections, and bronchitis: a national study of hospital-based emergency departments. *Annals of Emergency Medicine* 36: 320–327.

Trinh N, Ngo HH 2000 Practice variations in the management of sinusitis. *Journal of Otolaryngology* 29: 211–217.

Van Balen FA, de Melker RA 2000 Persistent otitis media with effusion: can it be predicted? A family practice follow-up study in children aged 6 months to 6 years. *Journal of Family Practice* 49: 605–611.

Van Cauwenberge PB, Van Kempen MJ, Bachert C 2000 The common cold at the turn of the millennium. *American Journal of Rhinology* 14: 339–343.

48 Infections of the lower respiratory tract

Lionel A. Mandell

Respiratory infections are usually divided into those involving the upper and those involving the lower respiratory tract. The former typically include infections of the sinuses, the tonsillopharyngeal area and the middle ear. Lower respiratory tract infections include acute bronchitis, acute exacerbations of chronic bronchitis and pneumonia. Pneumonia is further subdivided into community-, nursing home- and hospital-acquired infections.

Acute lower respiratory tract infections are a significant cause of morbidity and mortality worldwide and most occur in developing countries where poverty and inadequate medical care contribute to the high mortality rates. Pneumonia continues to be the most common cause of death from infectious diseases worldwide. Although our understanding of the various etiologic agents and the pathogenic mechanisms involved in various respiratory infections has increased, our ability to accurately diagnose the causative agent(s) has not kept pace. This means that often the physician initiates treatment on an empirical basis and in far too many situations antibiotics are used when the infection is viral in nature.

ACUTE BRONCHITIS

Lower respiratory tract infections are typically divided into either bronchitis or pneumonia. These can also be thought of as infections involving the airways and the pulmonary parenchyma, respectively. Acute bronchitis is very common and can be viewed as one end of a continuum that extends from bronchitis to pneumonia. While it is generally not a particularly serious infection, it still has a considerable economic impact because of the frequency of physician visits and the fact that despite the lack of any compelling evidence supporting antimicrobial therapy, physicians who diagnose acute bronchitis prescribe antibiotics for 66% of such patients.[1]

In the USA it is estimated that acute bronchitis results in approximately 12 000 000 visits to physicians per year at a cost of $200–300 million.[2]

ETIOLOGY AND EPIDEMIOLOGY

Acute bronchitis can occur as the result of infection or inhalation of substances that are toxic and irritating to the airways. For the purposes of this chapter the focus is on the infectious causes but the reader should be aware of possible environmental or occupational pollutants such as ammonia, sulfur dioxide and chlorine (among others), which may cause acute inflammation of the airways.

The most common infectious agents are viruses, and typically respiratory viruses such as, rhinovirus, corona virus, adenovirus and, at times, influenza virus, are implicated. Other viral agents include respiratory syncytial virus (RSV), parainfluenza virus, measles virus and herpes simplex virus.[3–5]

While the term 'atypical respiratory pathogens' can include a large and diverse number of etiologic agents, by convention they usually refer to *Mycoplasma pneumoniae*, *Chlamydophila* (formerly *Chlamydia*) *pneumoniae* and *Legionella* species. *Mycoplasma* and *C. pneumoniae* and the etiologic agent of whooping cough, *Bordetella pertussis*, are the most commonly encountered non-viral causes of acute bronchitis.[6]

Like many other respiratory infections, acute bronchitis is most common during the winter months. The mean attack rate in the USA is 87 cases per 100 000 persons per week, reaching a peak of 150 cases per 100 000 during the winter season.[7]

PATHOGENESIS

In cases of acute bronchitis the disease process is limited to the mucous membrane lining the tracheobronchial tree. The mucous membrane becomes edematous and hyperemic and increased bronchial secretion is typically seen. Epithelial injury is usually mild to moderate but in cases of influenza virus infection there may be fairly significant epithelial damage.

Studies of pulmonary function during attacks of acute bronchitis have demonstrated abnormal findings in both airway resistance and reactivity. Such results are in keeping with the association that has been described between an increased incidence of mild asthma and patients with a history of recurrent episodes of acute bronchitis.[8]

The increased airway reactivity and resistance may manifest themselves clinically as a persistent cough lasting up to several weeks following the initial infection.

CLINICAL MANIFESTATIONS

The predominant symptom is cough. This may last up to several weeks and, depending upon the etiologic agent, may be non-productive or productive of either mucoid or purulent sputum. In some cases the sputum may be mucoid initially, but if secondary bacterial infection results it may become purulent.

Patients may also experience a burning retrosternal sensation on inspiration.

Physical examination may reveal the presence of rhonchi or coarse rales but bronchial breath sounds should not be heard.

The patient may be febrile but usually does not appear particularly ill. The exceptions to this are herpes simplex infection or bronchitis complicating influenza, which can produce marked malaise.

DIAGNOSIS

The diagnosis of acute bronchitis in an otherwise well adult is usually not difficult from the clinical features. If there is any question of pneumonia, a chest radiograph will exclude the presence of a pulmonary infiltrate.

In general, it is not worth obtaining blood samples for serology or sputum for Gram stain and culture.

TREATMENT

Acute bronchitis is a common condition and most patients are managed at home. The treatment of acute bronchitis can be symptomatic or specific. Symptomatic treatment relies primarily upon maintenance of adequate hydration and cough suppression in those unable to sleep. If bronchospasm is a problem, then inhaled β_2-adrenergic bronchodilators may be used. At present there is insufficient evidence for the routine use of oral or inhaled steroids. Smokers should be encouraged to stop.

In patients with underlying cardiopulmonary disease, an episode of acute bronchitis may precipitate cardiac failure and the patient may need to be admitted to hospital for appropriate ventilatory and cardiac support.

Antimicrobial chemotherapy is generally not recommended: a number of placebo-controlled trials have evaluated the role of antibiotics in acute bronchitis and there is minimal benefit at best. Antibiotics might be considered in the following circumstances:

- a patient with a particularly severe attack on initial presentation;
- a patient whose symptoms have persisted for longer than 1 week and who shows no evidence of resolving or is obviously worsening;
- a patient with known cardiopulmonary disease whose underlying condition is worsened by an attack of acute bronchitis.

In such situations, doxycycline, or a macrolide (erythromycin, azithromycin or clarithromycin) should be considered. Influenza treatment is discussed on page 650.

ACUTE EXACERBATION OF CHRONIC BRONCHITIS

Chronic bronchitis is defined as the presence of a productive cough for at least 3 months of the year for 2 consecutive years. Chronic bronchitis itself constitutes a common component of chronic obstructive pulmonary disease (COPD), a clinical entity characterized by reduced expiratory air flow that is relatively stable over several months of observation. The prognosis for COPD correlates best with the forced expiratory volume in one second (FEV_1), and when this falls below 50% of predicted value the prognosis worsens.

Most physicians do not differentiate among COPD, acute bronchitis, and acute exacerbation of chronic bronchitis (AECB). In fact, even pneumonia is often simply included as part of the designation 'lower respiratory tract infections'. It is difficult to obtain accurate data on the exact economic impact of such entities, although COPD has been estimated to afflict one-fifth of the population of the USA.[9] In the UK 28 million working days are lost every year because of bronchitis, and the disease accounts for 5% of deaths annually.[10]

ETIOLOGY AND EPIDEMIOLOGY

Chronic bronchitis is the result of a variety of insults to the lung over time. These include predominantly cigarette smoke, infection, and environmental pollutants and irritants. Once chronic bronchitis is established the episodic worsening referred to as acute exacerbations of chronic bronchitis can be triggered by similar causes. For the purposes of this chapter, however, we will focus on infectious triggers.

Viruses account for up to 50% of acute exacerbations of chronic bronchitis and a variety of agents have been implicated; RSV, rhinovirus, influenza virus and parainfluenza virus. The remaining 50% of acute exacerbations are bacterial in nature, with the most common pathogens being *Haemophilus influenzae*, *Streptococcus pneumoniae*, and *Moraxella catarrhalis*. The role of atypical pathogens such as *M. pneumoniae* and *C. pneumoniae* is unclear but it is thought that they may account for a small percentage of infections.

Infection results in the release of inflammatory mediators

and further impairment of mucociliary clearance. This in turn alters the local milieu, making it easier for pathogens to further colonize the airways. Progressive airway damage is thought to occur as the result of injury caused either by the pathogens themselves or by the host response to the various infective agents.

CLINICAL MANIFESTATIONS

The clinical manifestations of patients with AECB represent a common pathway of underlying pulmonary disease in the form of chronic bronchitis or emphysema and the acute exacerbation triggered by infection or environmental pollutants. Patients may present with any or all of the following: increase in dyspnea, sputum volume or sputum purulence. In 1987, Anthonisen demonstrated that patients with at least two of these three findings experienced better clinical outcomes when treated with antibiotics than with placebo.[11] The Anthonisen classification refers to patients with one of these findings as type 3, two of the findings as type 2 and three of the findings as type 1. Other symptoms that may be noted during an exacerbation include wheezing, elevated temperature, and a feeling of malaise.

The duration of an exacerbation can vary from a few days to several weeks. On average, most patients experience approximately three exacerbations annually although significant variation has been described.

DIAGNOSIS

The diagnosis of AECB is usually clinical. Patients with a known history of chronic bronchitis who suffer periodic flare-ups are usually well aware of the signs and symptoms heralding the onset of an exacerbation. Increasing dyspnea, sputum volume, and purulence are the main clues that an exacerbation has occurred.

One of the difficulties in defining etiology is that many, if not most, individuals with chronic bronchitis normally have bacteria in their respiratory secretions. These bacteria colonize the airways but during an exacerbation are present in higher numbers. *H. influenzae*, *Str. pneumoniae*, and *Mor. catarrhalis* are the predominant pathogens. However, among those with severe exacerbations requiring admission to an intensive care unit (ICU) and mechanical ventilation these pathogens seem to be present less frequently and organisms such as *H. parainfluenzae* and *Pseudomonas aeruginosa* are more frequently found.[12,13]

In most patients treatment is begun empirically. In those with more severe underlying disease or in whom the exacerbations appear to be more serious, it may be worth while obtaining sputum samples for culture and susceptibility testing in order to rule out the presence of a resistant pathogen. Data are available suggesting that as severity of the illness increases (as indicated by markers such as illness lasting longer than 10

years, more than four exacerbations per year, steroid therapy, recent antibiotics, and severe airway obstruction (FEV$_1$ <35% predicted)) the microbiology becomes more complex.[14,15]

On the basis of a clinical examination, it may be impossible to differentiate between an acute exacerbation of chronic bronchitis and pneumonia. In such cases, a chest radiograph is necessary.

TREATMENT

Anthonisen was the first to assess response to treatment based upon stratification of patients according to their symptoms.[11] A meta-analysis of nine randomized placebo-controlled trials of patients treated for AECB demonstrated a statistically significant improvement in outcomes in those treated with antibiotics.[16] The effect size favored antibiotics in seven of the nine studies.

Despite such data, however, it is clear that routine antibiotic treatment fails in 13–25% of exacerbations.[17] Such failures carry an economic burden because they require additional visits to physicians, additional treatment regimens and more days lost from work.

A number of risk factors have been defined for treatment failure. These include the presence of cardiopulmonary disease and increased frequency of pulmonary infections during the previous year (>4).[17] A subgroup of patients is at risk, not only of treatment failure but also of respiratory failure. Mortality rates in hospital inpatients of 10–30% have been described, typically in patients older than 65 years, those with co-morbid respiratory and extrapulmonary organ dysfunction, and those residing in hospital before transfer to the ICU.[18,19]

It has been suggested that stratification of patients according to risk factors will allow physicians to treat more appropriately. No single stratification scheme has been agreed upon but those that do exist attempt to rank patients according to increased risk factors for treatment failure and possibly admission to hospital. Three schema have been published to date: Lode – Germany (1991), Balter – Canada (1994), and Wilson – UK (1995).[20–22] The most recent of these publications is summarized in Table 48.1. Niroumand and Grossman have published an excellent review of this topic.[6]

Patients with AECB should be considered as being possibly infected with a 'core' group of pathogens such as *H. influenzae*, *Str. pneumoniae* and *Mor. catarrhalis*; those who are more complicated (such as elderly patients, patients with more frequent exacerbations, and those with reduced lung function) may be infected not only by the core pathogens but also by Gram-negative bacilli such as the Enterobacteriaceae and *Ps. aeruginosa* or possibly resistant core pathogens.

The advantage of such an approach lies in the fact that they identify patients at increased risk of failure so that treatment may be initiated with antibiotic regimens most likely to be effective against all of the potential etiologic pathogens.

A variety of adjunctive or supportive measures including the use of bronchodilators, steroids (oral and/or inhaled) and

Table 48.1 Stratification and treatment[20]

Category	Characteristics	Suggested treatment
Group 1	Postviral tracheobronchitis; previously healthy person	None
Group 2	Simple chronic bronchitis; young person; mild–moderate impairment of lung function ($FEV_1 > 50\%$ predicted); Less than 4 exacerbations/year	β-Lactam antibiotic
Group 3	'Chronic bronchitis plus risk factors' older person; FEV_1 50% predicted or FEV_1 50–60% predicted but concurrent medical illnesses; CHF, diabetes mellitus, chronic renal disease, chronic liver disease, more than 4 exacerbations/year	Fluoroquinolone, amoxicillin–clavulanic acid, group 3 or 4 cephalosporin* azithromycin or clarithromycin
Group 4	'Chronic bronchial sepsis,' bronchiectasis, chronic airway colonization	Tailor antimicrobial treatment to airway pathogens

FEV_1, forced expiratory volume 1 second; CHF, congestive heart failure.
*See Ch 15 for classifications of cephalosporin.

oxygen therapy may be necessary. Preventive measures such as cessation of smoking, annual influenza vaccination, and administration of the pneumococcal vaccine should be emphasized.

COMMUNITY-ACQUIRED PNEUMONIA

Community-acquired pneumonia (CAP) has a significant impact on both individual patients and society, and pneumonia is currently the sixth leading cause of death in the USA with an estimated 3–4 million cases annually, accounting for more than 600 000 hospital admissions and 64 million days of restricted activity.[23]

CAP is not a reportable disease so exact figures are not available. It is clear, however, that it has a significant impact on the individual patient and society as a whole. Most (80%) patients are treated as outpatients while 20% are admitted to hospital; it is these 20% who generate most of the costs. The annual costs of treatment, are US $4.8 billion (patients older than 65 years) and $3.6 billion (patients under 65 years).[24]

ETIOLOGY AND EPIDEMIOLOGY

As with many other infections, the incidence rates of CAP are greatest at the extremes of age. Although the overall annual rate of pneumonia in the USA is 12 cases per 1000 the rate is 12–18 cases per 1000 in children below 4 years of age and 20

cases per 1000 in people over 60 years age.[25,26] Between the ages of 5 and 60 years, the annual rate ranges from one to five cases per 1000 and the incidence of CAP requiring admission to hospital in adult patients is 2.6 cases per 1000.[27]

Risk factors for pneumonia have been defined particularly for people over 60 years. A Finnish study lists the following risk factors: alcoholism, asthma, immunosuppression, institutionalization, and age greater than or equal to 70 years versus age 60–69 years.[28] Specific risk factors for pneumococcal infection include dementia, seizure disorders, congestive heart failure, cerebrovascular disease, COPD and HIV infection.[29]

Numerous microbial pathogens are potential etiologic agents. Determining the cause of infection in any particular patient is made difficult by the fact that CAP is not a single homogeneous entity and is further complicated by the recent realization that more than one pathogen may be responsible for disease in any patient. Such mixed infections are well known in hospital-acquired pneumonia, from a study which showed that multiple pathogens are present in more than half of the nosocomial pneumonia patients studied.[30] In CAP, the incidence of mixed infections is lower, ranging from 2.7% to 10% in three well defined studies of inpatients with CAP.[31–33]

The single most important etiologic agent is undoubtedly *Str. pneumoniae*. In a meta-analysis covering a 30-year period and including 7000 cases of pneumonia in which an etiologic diagnosis was made, *Str. pneumoniae* accounted for two-thirds of all cases and for two-thirds of fatalities.[34]

At one time it was thought that atypical pathogens such as

M. pneumoniae, C. pneumoniae and *Legionella* species were not important causes of pneumonia and that if they did cause infection they were usually mild and affected primarily the young. A study in 1997 of more than 2700 patients admitted to hospital with CAP ranked these pathogens second, third, and fourth of all etiologic agents meeting the criteria for a 'definite' diagnosis.[35] Another recent study described three outbreaks of *C. pneumoniae* in nursing homes with high attack and mortality rates.[36] These two studies have helped to dispel the earlier misconceptions surrounding infection with the atypical pathogens.

Gram-negative rods such as *Escherichia coli* and *Klebsiella* sp. are not particularly common causes of CAP but are nevertheless important to consider, particularly in elderly people or in those with co-morbid illness, especially if they are ill enough to require hospital treatment.[31,37] There has been considerable debate about whether or not *Ps. aeruginosa* is a significant pathogen requiring treatment. The consensus is that, while it is certainly not common, it can occur in selected patients if risk factors such as a recent course of antibiotics or steroids or a prolonged stay in hospital are present.

PATHOGENESIS

The lung has a formidable and effective array of defenses, which may be classified in a number of ways although a functional classification is probably best (e.g. resident or surveillance mechanisms versus augmenting mechanisms). The resident or surveillance mechanisms are primarily mechanical or anatomic and are operative from the point of air entry to the respiratory bronchioles. Beyond this point, the mechanical defenses are ineffective and resident or surveillance mechanisms that rely on immunoglobulin and phagocytic cells take over. In response to invasion by potential pathogens, the augmenting mechanisms are recruited.

Surveillance mechanisms include ciliated and squamous epithelium in the nasopharynx, mechanical barriers such as the larynx and airway angulation, mucociliary clearance, cough, and secretory IgA. In the alveolar milieu, surveillance mechanisms include opsonic IgG, the alternate complement pathway, surfactant and phagocytic cells. The augmenting mechanisms include the initiation of immune responses and generation of an inflammatory response.

The occurrence of pulmonary infection depends not only on the integrity of the host's defenses but also on the type of microbial challenge. A particularly virulent organism or a large inoculum of a less virulent pathogen may overwhelm even normal defenses. Once defense mechanisms are impaired or bypassed, infection even by usually non-pathogenic organisms may occur.

The various etiologic pathogens can gain access to the lower respiratory tract by a number of possible routes. These include inhalation, aspiration, and hematogenous spread. For bacterial pneumonia, aspiration of organisms colonizing the oropharynx appears to be the most important route.[38]

CLINICAL MANIFESTATIONS

Until relatively recently, physicians tended to divide cases of CAP into typical or atypical pneumonia based upon their clinical presentation. Typical or classic pneumonia refers to infection caused by bacterial pathogens such as *Str. pneumoniae* or *H. influenzae*, whereas atypical pneumonia refers to infection caused by the atypical pathogens (*M. pneumoniae, C. pneumoniae*, and *Legionella* spp.). It was thought that those with classic bacterial pneumonia presented with fairly sudden onset of signs and symptoms with cough productive of purulent sputum, pleuritic chest pain, and rigors. In contrast, those with atypical infection presented with an illness of undefined duration, a non-productive cough and often a frontal headache. It has become clear, however, that it is not possible to determine the etiologic agent from a careful history, physical examination, and non-specific laboratory tests and chest radiographs.

The symptoms of CAP may be constitutional and non-specific or they may be localized to the respiratory tract and be fairly specific for respiratory infection. The former category includes such findings as malaise, anorexia, myalgias and arthralgias, chills and rigors; the latter includes shortness of breath, pleuritic chest pain, cough, and sputum production.

In elderly patients the findings may be imprecise because constitutional symptoms such as confusion may predominate and there may be fewer findings related to the respiratory tract.

DIAGNOSIS

The problem of the diagnosis of CAP has generated much debate among physicians. Unfortunately, despite extensive testing even in university medical centers, no specific etiologic agent may be found in up to one-half of the cases. In routine clinical practice, the etiologic agent is determined in approximately 25% of cases but results in a change in antimicrobial therapy in less than 10% of cases.[39] Furthermore, an improvement in clinical outcome does not always result from identification of the etiologic agent.

Generally, diagnostic tests fall into two categories: clinical and invasive/quantitative. Clinical testing relies on information obtained from the patient history, physical examination, and selected tests or procedures such as chest radiography, sputum Gram stain, and blood and sputum cultures. Invasive/quantitative methods include bronchoscopic techniques, pleural fluid aspiration, and (in selected cases) lung biopsy. As a rule, the clinical method is too sensitive and lacks specificity while the invasive/quantitative methods require special expertise and laboratory support, and are more costly.

Clinical evaluation

The first step is to determine whether the patient has pneumonia rather than some other infective process such as bronchitis, or whether a non-infectious etiology (e.g. congestive heart failure, pulmonary embolism is the cause of the patient's problem. If a diagnosis of pneumonia is made, the next step is to determine the etiologic agent if possible. Unfortunately, it is impossible to accurately identify the pathogen based on clinical findings even when multiple clinical variables are used.[31,40] There is significant intra-observer variation in the ability to elicit abnormal physical findings and the sensitivity and specificity of the history and physical examination are currently undetermined.[41]

Chest radiograph

The presence of an infiltrate on the chest radiograph can help to establish the diagnosis of pneumonia but does not determine the causative pathogen. However, the radiograph is important in defining the presence of a lobar or multilobar infiltrate and in assessing the severity of illness and prognosis.

Laboratory assessment

Routine laboratory assessment is unnecessary for ambulatory patients with CAP, who are likely to be managed as outpatients. However, for those ill enough to require admission to hospital (or even for those considered for admission), a complete blood and differential count, serum electrolytes, liver function tests, serum creatinine, and an oxygen saturation assessment should be obtained. Significant abnormalities have been identified as risk factors for a complicated course or increased mortality. These abnormalities constitute the basis for assigning points to patients based upon Fine's rule used to assess mortality risk and to help in the site of care decision (*see* page 646).[42]

Microbiologic assessment

Sputum Gram stain and culture

Of the two tests, the sputum Gram stain is more reliable, but it is neither sensitive nor specific.[43] Many patients are unable to produce a sputum sample, and of those samples produced a significant percentage may not be adequate. Although current data suggest that atypical pathogens are responsible for 20–25% of all CAP cases, none is detectable by the sputum Gram stain. There is also considerable inter- and intra-observer variation in Gram stain interpretation.[44] The sputum culture also lacks sensitivity and specificity. Even in patients with confirmed pneumococcal pneumonia based upon positive blood cultures, a simultaneously obtained sputum culture tested positive in only one-half of patients.[45]

Blood cultures

The incidence of positive blood cultures in ambulatory patients with CAP is less than 1%.[46] In hospital inpatients it ranges from 6.6% to 17.6% but may reach 27% in patients in ICUs.[32] The most common pathogen is *Str. pneumoniae*, and pneumococcal pneumonia is complicated by bacteremia more frequently than pneumonia caused by other pathogens. It is generally recommended that blood cultures be obtained from all patients who are admitted with CAP but not from those treated in the community.

Serology

To determine the role of a specific micro-organism as a pathogen, serologic assessments should be based on the results of paired (acute and convalescent) serum samples. Unfortunately, such results are never available at the time the initial treatment decision is being made. Therefore, other than helping to define the epidemiologic role of selected pathogens, serologic testing is not helpful and is not recommended for routine use.

Legionella urinary antigen

This test is easy to perform and yields rapid results with a sensitivity of 70% and specificity of 100%. It is limited by the fact that it identifies only *Legionella pneumophila* serogroup 1. However, this serogroup accounts for most *Legionella* infections.

DNA probes and amplification

Unfortunately, rapid diagnostic techniques are not generally available and simply identifying the presence of a particular micro-organism does not confirm infection, the micro-organism may only be colonizing and not invading the patient. There are, however, a few micro-organisms whose mere presence indicates infection. These include *Mycobacterium tuberculosis*, *Coxiella burnetii*, and *Pneumocystis carinii*.

Invasive procedures

For most patients with CAP, invasive tests such as bronchoscopy, bronchoalveolar lavage, protected specimen brush, and percutaneous lung needle aspiration are not required. However, they may be appropriate in certain situations (e.g. patients with fulminant pneumonia or those unresponsive to a standard course of antimicrobials), when it may be necessary to identify a resistant or fastidious pathogen or to rule out a non-infectious cause.

Thoracocentesis should be performed in CAP patients, with a significant pleural effusion defined as a collection greater than 10 mm thickness on the lateral decubitus view.[47] The incidence of pleural effusion with pneumonia varies from 36% to 57% and is most common in patients with pneumococcal infection.[48]

TREATMENT

Therapy can be directed or empirical. Directed therapy implies that the etiologic agent is known and that therapy is aimed specifically at that pathogen. Empirical therapy is the more usual; it is, in effect, an educated guess and the physician institutes a course of treatment aimed at the most likely causes. Of these two options, directed therapy is clearly more desirable because it limits the breadth of spectrum required of the treatment agent(s), it may limit the number of drugs, reduces the adverse reactions associated with antibiotics, reduces antibiotic selection pressure and may result in less antimicrobial resistance.

Before discussing the various regimens, it is important to consider how the decision is made in terms of outpatient versus inpatient therapy and the problem of antimicrobial resistance.

SITE OF CARE DECISION

This decision is an important one, with considerable economic implications. The cost of inpatient care exceeds that of outpatient treatment by a factor of 15–20, and the cost of hospital management accounts for most of the money spent annually on CAP in the USA.[49]

In some cases it is immediately obvious that a patient can be treated outside the hospital; in other situations it is equally apparent that a patient requires hospital treatment and possibly admission to an ICU.

Effective prognostic scoring and outcome assessment tools are necessary to help physicians make the site of care decision. Such tools provide objective methods to assess the risk of adverse outcomes, including death.

Studies by Fine and others have attempted to identify patients at increased risk for adverse outcomes and to define independent predictors of mortality or poor outcome.[34,42,50] However, weaknesses or design flaws were found in each of them.[49]

The use of prediction rules may minimize unnecessary hospital admissions and help to identify patients who will benefit from care and intervention in the hospital and the ICU. The best known and most widely used prognostic tool is that of Fine.[42] This is a two-step rule designed to identify patients at low risk for mortality. Points are given based on age, coexisting disease, and abnormal physical and laboratory findings and patients are assigned to classes 1–5 based on the total number of points assigned.

Fine's rule has been adopted into recommendations published by the Infectious Diseases Society of America (IDSA) and the joint guidelines prepared by the Canadian Infectious Disease Society and the Canadian Thoracic Society.[51,52] The rule's main strengths are its accuracy as a mortality prediction model and its systematic approach, which provides a rational basis for decisions about admitting patients. However, it was neither designed nor validated as a triage rule and relies on an inordinately large number of prognostic variables. The rule also fails to consider other variables that may affect patient outcomes, such as cognitive impairment and substance abuse, and may oversimplify the interpretation of important predictor variables.

Finally, Fine's rule does not deal with severe CAP and does not help the physician to decide whether to admit a patient to the ICU. Criteria for severe CAP were presented in the American Thoracic Society guidelines and are given in Table 48.2.[53,54]

Table 48.2 Criteria for Severe Community-acquired Pneumonia[53,54]

- Respiratory rate > 30 min
- Severe respiratory failure: PaO_2/FiO_2 <250
- Need for mechanical ventilation
- Chest radiograph
  - presence of bilateral infiltrates, or
  - multilobar infiltrates, or
  - increase in infiltrate size by 50% within 48 h of admission
- Blood pressure <90 systolic or <60 diastolic
- Need for pressors > 4 h
- Urine output <20 ml/h

ANTIMICROBIAL RESISTANCE

Antimicrobial resistance among respiratory pathogens has become a major concern and it is important that clinicians understand and appreciate the general mechanisms and implications of this phenomenon. The emergence of resistance to penicillin among *Str. pneumoniae* isolates represents a gradual reduction in-vitro susceptibility. The National Committee for Clinical Laboratory Standards defines strains for which the minimum inhibitory concentration (MIC) of penicillin is <0.06 mg/l as sensitive, 0.1–1.0 mg/l as intermediate and ≥2 mg/l as resistant.[55] With *Str. pneumoniae*, the DNA incorporation and remodelling that results in resistance is from the DNA of closely related oral commensal bacteria (*see* Ch. 3). By such a process, our own flora can develop resistance when we are treated with antibiotics and pathogens such as *Str. pneumoniae* can subsequently acquire resistance coding DNA from our own colonizing microflora.[56] Pneumococcal resistance to β-lactams is due solely to the presence of low-affinity penicillin-binding proteins. Macrolide resistance, however, can occur either by target site modification or by an efflux pump (*see* Chapters 3 and 24). The relative frequencies of the two mechanisms vary internationally but in North America account for approximately 45% and 55%, respectively, of resistant isolates. Recent reports of breakthrough pneumococcal bacteremia in patients treated with macrolides have highlighted concerns about resistance to this class of agents.[58]

Resistance to ciprofloxacin and to newer fluoroquinolones among pneumococcal isolates has been reported.[59] Pneumococcal resistance to fluoroquinolones may be mediated by changes in one or both target sites (topoisomerase II and IV), usually resulting from mutations in the *gyrA* and *parC* genes, respectively, and possibly also by an efflux pump (*see* Ch. 3).[60] Of greatest concern, however, are the multidrug resistant isolates; those that are resistant to two or more antibiotics having different mechanisms of action. Recent data on more than 1500 pneumococcal isolates from across the USA indicate that 10% are macrolide resistant and 9.1% are multidrug resistant.[61]

Pathogens such as *H. influenzae* and the Enterobacteriaceae are also important to consider. *H. influenzae* is the third most common cause of CAP requiring admission to hospital and, while the Enterobacteriaceae are not particularly common, they are important because of the high mortality rates associated with them. Among such pathogens resistance is usually mediated by β-lactamases, and the highest prevalence of β-lactamase genes is found on plasmids rather than chromosomes. Members of the TEM and SHV families are the most successful of the plasmid-encoded β-lactamases, and the TEM-1 β-lactamase accounts for almost 80% of all plasmid-encoded β-lactamases.[62] The extended-spectrum β-lactamases include oxyimino enzymes that are TEM and SHV mutants and cephalosporinases unrelated to TEM and SHV enzymes (*see* Ch. 17).

THERAPEUTIC REGIMENS

Once the diagnosis of pneumonia has been made the physician must decide whether to treat the patient outside or inside the hospital and this in turn will help to determine the appropriate therapeutic regimen. The correct choice of antimicrobial(s) has generated considerable discussion, and a number of societies have produced guidelines to help physicians with the initial management of patients with CAP.[51–54,64–68] Some are from the UK and Europe, a number are from North America. The fact that there are four sets of recent guidelines from North America highlights the degree of controversy associated with this topic.[51,52,54,68]

Some have argued that physicians should not rely upon guidelines and that they should make their own decisions based on the circumstances of a particular case. An interesting paper reviewing the use of antibiotics for CAP at several prominent US medical centers before the development of the guidelines revealed a disturbing range in the number and types of antibiotics used.[69] It demonstrated quite clearly that before the guidelines were produced, the treatment of CAP was far from ideal. In fact, the guidelines have served a number of useful functions. They have codified our management of patients with CAP and (at the very least) they have highlighted the gaps in our knowledge and have helped to direct future studies and research. It is also quite clear that following the guidelines lowered the amount of money spent on antibiotics, lowered mortality rates and shortened hospital stay.[70,71]

The original guidelines published in North America in 1993 suggested that macrolides should be used for the management of outpatients.[53,67] This had nothing to do with concerns about pneumococcal resistance to penicillin but was because of concerns about the atypical pathogens. Penicillin would be the agent of choice for *Str. pneumoniae* but it would be ineffective against any of the atypicals. However, a macrolide would provide good-to-excellent coverage for all these likely pathogens.

Recently in North America the fluoroquinolones have assumed an important role in the management of CAP coinciding with rising resistance to β-lactams and macrolides, the appreciation of the potential importance of Gram-negative rods in selected CAP patients and the availability of the 'respiratory' fluoroquinolones which offer once-daily monotherapy, compared with the multiple dosing required if a β-lactam and macrolide regimen is used.[51,52,54]

One of the fundamental differences between the Centers for Disease Control and Prevention (CDC) document and the other North American guidelines is that it assumes that the physician knows that he or she is dealing with a pneumococcal infection.[51,52,54,68] The basis for the CDC recommendation lies in the fact that it feels that there are no treatment failures for infection with *Str. pneumoniae* for which the MIC of penicillin is up to 1 mg/l. For strains for which the MIC of penicillin is 2–4 mg/l, some data suggest that there is no increase in treatment failure, while other data suggest increased mortality or complications.[72–75]

Many experts feel that penicillin still has a role to play in the treatment of pneumococcal pneumonia and that it is effective against infections caused by susceptible organisms. For strains of *Str. pneumoniae* with intermediate levels of resistance to penicillin, higher doses may be used. Unfortunately, the identity or susceptibility of the etiologic agent is unknown in most cases at the time of initial antibiotic treatment.

Efflux resistance to macrolides results in low-level resistance while the target change mechanism results in high-level resistance. Low-level resistance predominates in North America, while the latter is more frequent in Europe. In the USA and Canada, therefore, macrolides are still seen as having a significant role to play in the management of many patients with CAP.

Approaches to the initial empiric treatment of patients with CAP based upon the Canadian and British guidelines are given in Tables 48.3 and 48.4.

The IDSA, American Thoracic Society and Canadian documents are in fact quite similar.[51,54,52] While the IDSA statement lists outpatients as a single group, specific considerations are provided in their main treatment table and are addressed in the body of the IDSA document.[51] For example, the IDSA indicates that some clinicians may prefer to use macrolides or doxycycline for patients under 50 years of age without co-morbidity, and fluoroquinolones in those over 50 years of age or with co-morbidity. In the Canadian guidelines outpatients are divided into those without modifying factors in whom a macrolide may be used, and those with modifying factors (such as COPD) who have or have not received antibiotics or steroids within 3 months.[52] A final grouping is patients with suspected gross aspiration.

Fluoroquinolones are reserved for those with COPD who have recently taken antibiotics, i.e. those at increased risk of infection with penicillin-resistant *Str. pneumoniae*, or even possibly Gram-negative rods. The American Thoracic Society guidelines are very similar to the Canadian guidelines in terms of how the outpatient groups are stratified and the regimens suggested.[54]

Table 48.3 Empirical antimicrobial selection for adults with community-acquired pneumonia (Canadian guidelines)

Type of patient, factor(s) involved	Treatment regimen	
	First choice	**Second choice**
Outpatient without modifying factors	Macrolide[a]	Doxycycline
Outpatient with modifying factors;		
COPD (no recent antibiotics or oral steroids within past 3 months)	Newer macrolide[b]	Doxycycline
COPD (recent antibiotics or oral steroids within past 3 months)	'Respiratory' fluoroquinolone[c]	Amoxicillin–clavulanate + macrolide or group 3 cephalosporin + macrolide*
Suspected macroaspiration	Amoxicillin–clavulanate ± macrolide	'Respiratory' fluoroquinolone + clindamycin or metronidazole
Nursing home resident	'Respiratory' fluoroquinolone alone *or* amoxicillin–clavulanate + macrolide	Group 3 cephalosporin + macrolide*
Nursing home – hospitalized	Identical to treatment for other inpatients	
Hospital patient on medical ward	'Respiratory' fluoroquinolone	Group 3–6 cephalosporin + macrolide*
Patient in ICU:		
a. *Ps. aeruginosa* not suspected	i.v. respiratory fluoroquinolone + cefotaxime, ceftriaxone, or β-lactam β-lactamase inhibitor	i.v macrolide + cefotaxime, ceftriaxone, or β-lactam–β-lactamase inhibitor
b. *Ps. aeruginosa* suspected	Antipseudomonal fluoroquinolone (e.g. ciprofloxacin) + antipseudomonal β-lactam or aminoglycoside	Triple therapy with anti-pseudomonal β-lactam (e.g. ceftazidime, piperacillin–tazobactam, imipenem, or meropenem) + aminoglycoside (e.g. gentamicin, tobramycin or amikacin) + macrolide

COPD, chronic obstructive pulmonary disease; p.o., by mouth.
[a] Erythromycin, azithromycin, or clarithromycin
[b] Azithromycin or clarithromycin
[c] Levofloxacin, gatifloxacin, or moxifloxacin; trovafloxacin is restricted because of severe hepatotoxicity.
*See Ch 15 for classifications of cephalosporin.

For those treated in hospital, all three guidelines divide patients into those treated on a medical ward and those treated in the ICU, and use the risk of infection with *Ps. aeruginosa* as a means of further subdividing ICU patients. In previous guidelines, the first choice for ward patients was a β-lactam with or without a macrolide.[51,52,54] In the most recent guidelines the Canadian document recommends a fluoroquinolone alone as the first choice and a β-lactam plus a macrolide as second choice for ward patients. The IDSA suggests that either regimen may be used. For patients treated in the ICU, a fluoroquinolone or macrolide in combination with a β-lactam is suggested if *Ps. aeruginosa* is not a concern. If it is, then an antipseudomonal β-lactam plus ciprofloxacin is recommended. The American Thoracic Society differs from the IDSA and Canadian guidelines in the management of ward patients in one sense: it suggests that azithromycin alone may be used in patients without cardiopulmonary disease and with no modifying factors. Neither the IDSA nor the Canadian guidelines

have such a category and neither group suggests monotherapy with azithromycin.

The recent British Thoracic Society guidelines provide an exhaustive evidence-based approach to the management of CAP patients.[65] They differ from the IDSA, American Thoracic Society and Canadian statements in a number of significant aspects and in some ways are closer to the CDC guidelines. For outpatients, the British Thoracic Society does not feel that atypical pathogens such as *M. pneumoniae* or *C. pneumoniae* are important enough to warrant routine coverage, and therefore treatment is aimed primarily at *Str. pneumoniae* and the drug of choice is amoxicillin.[65] This differs substantially from the three aforementioned guidelines, which all recommend routine coverage of *Str. pneumoniae* and the atypicals with either a macrolide or a fluoroquinolone. Of the North American guidelines, only the CDC offers a regimen without atypical coverage as an option for outpatients with CAP (i.e. macrolide, doxycycline or a β-lactam).

Table 48.4 British Thoracic Society recommendations for initial empirical treatment of CAP

Type of patient	First choice	Second choice
Home treated, not severe	Amoxicillin 0.5–1 g p.o. every 8 h	Erythromycin 500 mg p.o. every 6 h or clarithromycin 500 mg p.o. twice daily
Hospital treated, not severe[a]	Amoxicillin 0.5–1 g p.o. every 8 h	Erythromycin 500 mg p.o. every 6 h or clarithromycin 500 mg p.o. twice daily
Hospital treated, not severe	1. Amoxicillin 0.5–1 g p.o. every 8 h + erythromycin 500 mg p.o. every 6 h or clarithromycin 500 mg p.o. twice daily 2. Ampicillin 500 mg every 6 h i.v. or benzylpenicillin 1.2 g every 6 h i.v. + erythromycin 500 mg every 6 h i.v. or clarithromycin 500 mg twice daily i.v.	Fluoroquinolone with enhanced *Str. pneumoniae* activity[b]
Hospital treated, severe	Amoxicillin–clavulanate 1.2 g every 8 h i.v. or cefuroxime 1.5 g every 8 h i.v. cefotaxime 1 g every 8 h i.v. *or* ceftriaxone 2 g once daily i.v. + erythromycin 500 mg every 6 h i.v. *or* clarithromycin 500 mg twice daily i.v.	Fluoroquinolone with enhanced *Str. pneumoniae* activity[b] + benzylpenicillin 1.2 g every 6 h i.v.

[a] Admitted for non-clinical reasons or previously untreated in community.
[b] At time of writing levofloxacin 500 mg p.o. once daily or 500 mg i.v. once daily is only licensed agent.
p.o., by mouth.

For hospital inpatients the North American documents divide patients into those managed on a ward or in the ICU while the British guidelines consider hospital-treated patients under three categories: (1) not severe and admitted for non-clinical reasons or previously treated in the community; (2) not severe; (3) severe. The first group is treated with amoxicillin, the second is given amoxicillin plus a macrolide (erythromycin or clarithromycin) and the third group is given a β-lactam (amoxicillin–clavulanate, cefuroxime, ceftriaxone or cefotaxime) plus intravenous erythromycin or clarithromycin. The only fluoroquinolone available in the UK is levofloxacin; this is recommended as an alternative only for the second and third categories. The CDC and British guidelines are alike in that neither sees a first-line role for fluoroquinolones, both are prepared to treat outpatients with a β-lactam only and neither feels that *Ps. aeruginosa* is important in severe cases.

Initiation of treatment should not be delayed, particularly when dealing with patients over 65 years of age. A study of elderly patients presenting to emergency departments with CAP showed that those who received antibiotics within 8 h of presentation had a significantly lower 30-day mortality rate than those who waited longer for initiation of treatment.[76]

Intravenous to oral sequential treatment is strongly recommended because it reduces costs, encourages patient mobility and allows earlier discharge from hospital. Ancillary measures such as supplemental oxygen, drainage of significant pleural effusions and hydration are also important.

The patient should be followed and objective parameters monitored. These include the resolution of cough, shortness of breath and elevated temperature and (for those in hospital) improvement in the oxygen saturation and white blood cell count.

NURSING HOME PNEUMONIA

Nursing home pneumonia or pneumonia in elderly residents of long-term care facilities is an important entity and is only now becoming the subject of serious clinical investigation. Pneumonia is the main cause of death among residents of such facilities, with acute mortality rates ranging from 5% to 40% per infection. It is the most common reason for transfer of nursing home residents to an acute care hospital, with approximately one-third of pneumonia patients requiring hospital admission.[77]

ETIOLOGY AND EPIDEMIOLOGY

The incidence of pneumonia among residents of nursing homes is considerably higher than among persons living in the community, ranging from 1.2 to 2.5 episodes per 1000 resident days with a median incidence of 1 per 1000 resident days.[77] One of the difficulties in establishing the etiology of nursing home pneumonia is the fact that studies in this area have depended almost exclusively on results of sputum cultures. Such studies are compromised from the outset because over half the elderly patients do not produce any sputum. The likely pathogens are somewhat different from those in patients with CAP. In cases of CAP, the predominant etiologic agents are *Str. pneumoniae* and the atypicals (in selected cases Gram-negative rods may be encountered). In nursing home pneumonia, *Str. pneumoniae* is still a significant pathogen, but (it is important to note that age >65 years and residence in a nursing home have been identified as risk factors for penicillin-resistant *Str. pneumoniae* infection) there is a greater proportion of cases caused by *Staphylococcus aureus*, *H. influenzae* and Gram-negative rods in this population than in a younger cohort and a disconcertingly high percentage of the *Staph. aureus* isolates are methicillin resistant.[78] Atypicals are more common in younger patients.

The role of anaerobes is still not definitely settled and appropriately designed studies to substantiate their role as pathogens in the elderly do not appear to have been undertaken.

In addition to aerobic and possibly anaerobic bacterial pathogens, viruses and *Mycobacterium tuberculosis* must also be considered. Epidemics of influenza, respiratory syncytial virus and parainfluenza have been described in such populations, and must always be considered if an institutional outbreak is encountered. The incidence of tuberculosis is substantially higher in the institutionalized elderly and must be included in the assessment of such patients.

PATHOGENESIS

A number of risk factors have been defined in a prospective cohort study of respiratory tract infections in nursing home residents.[77] Older age, male sex, inability to take oral medications and swallowing difficulties were identified as independent risk factors for the development of pneumonia. Swallowing difficulty, confusion and altered levels of consciousness have often been evoked as surrogate markers for aspiration and by inference as indicators of infection with anaerobes.

Nasogastric tube feeding and tracheostomy have also been identified as potential risk factors for pneumonia, presumably because of the increased risk of aspiration.

CLINICAL MANIFESTATIONS AND DIAGNOSIS

The physician must be aware that in an elderly patient with pneumonia rather than a history of elevated temperature, chills and cough with purulent sputum, the story may be that of confusion, weakness, anorexia and falls. The difficulty in making a diagnosis of pneumonia in a nursing home population is enhanced by the fact that nursing homes lack laboratory and radiographic facilities and many often do not have a physician in attendance on a full-time basis.

Ideally, if a patient presents with findings suggestive of pneumonia, he or she should be evaluated by a physician and a chest radiograph should be obtained. If feasible, an expectorated sputum sample should be sent for Gram stain and culture, and for people with more serious illness in whom par-

enteral therapy or transfer to a hospital is contemplated, the following additional tests should be done: blood samples for culture and susceptibility testing, complete blood count and differential, serum creatinine, urine for *Legionella* antigen.

If pneumonia occurs in the setting of an influenza outbreak or if a particular case is suggestive of influenza infection, a nasopharyngeal swab should be obtained for rapid detection of viral antigen by immunofluorescence. Similarly, if tuberculosis is a possibility, sputum samples for acid-fast staining should be obtained. In both of these circumstances respiratory precautions must be instituted and the patient should be isolated to prevent spread of the disease.

TREATMENT

As with any patient, the use of an antimicrobial directed at a known pathogen is the ideal; however, at the time that the treatment decision is made it is unlikely that a definitive etiologic agent will have been identified. As with most cases of pneumonia, an empirical regimen is usually selected, based upon local epidemiology and susceptibility patterns and risk stratification of the patient.

The site of care decision is an important one and nursing home residents with pneumonia can be evaluated using the same prediction rules for hospital admission as are used for other patients with CAP.[42] For patients who can be treated in the nursing home setting, a 'respiratory fluoroquinolone' such as moxifloxacin, gatifloxacin or levofloxacin (according to availability), or a combination regimen consisting of amoxicillin-clavulanate plus a macrolide is recommended as first choice.[52] The potential disadvantage of the amoxicillin–clavulanate plus macrolide regimen is that it requires two drugs (three counting clavulanate) rather than one, and is associated with a higher incidence of diarrhea. A group 3 cephalosporin such as cefuroxime plus a macrolide is an alternative.

Patients who are transferred to the hospital would be treated according to the regimens outlined in Table 48.3.

Influenza outbreaks in an institutional setting can be associated with high attack rates and mortality rates. Annual immunoprophylaxis using vaccines offers protection and is recommended for all residents. Four drugs are currently available for use in prevention and/or treatment of influenza. Amantidine and rimantidine may be used for chemoprophylaxis and treatment of influenza A infection only. Zanamivir and oseltamivir are two newer neuraminidase inhibitors with activity against both influenza A and influenza B. Both of these agents are approved for treatment of uncomplicated influenza and if given within 48 h of onset of symptoms may decrease severity and duration of symptoms.

HOSPITAL-ACQUIRED PNEUMONIA

Hospital-acquired or nosocomial pneumonia is by definition infection that occurs 48 h or more after admission to hospital.

Although it is the second most common nosocomial infection in the USA, accounting for 13–18% of all hospital-acquired infections, it is the one most frequently associated with a fatal outcome, and is associated with significant morbidity and mortality.[79]

Current figures are based on estimates from hospital records because nosocomial pneumonia is not a reportable disease. It is felt, however, that currently more than 300 000 cases occur annually in the USA, resulting in an average increase in length of hospital stay of 8 days.[79]

Mortality figures range from 15 to 70%; however, the more relevant attributable mortality figures are estimated at 33–50%.

ETIOLOGY AND EPIDEMIOLOGY

The estimated rate of occurrence is 4–8 episodes per 1000 hospital admissions in non-teaching hospitals and 8 per 1000 in teaching hospitals.[79] In patients who are intubated, the rate is up to twenty times higher than in non-intubated patients. Rates of ventilator-associated pneumonia are reported to be approximately 15 per 1000 ventilator days.[80]

Risk factors for nosocomial pneumonia include increasing age, COPD, neuromuscular disease, decreased consciousness, aspiration, endotracheal intubation, thoracic and upper abdominal surgery, and nasogastric intubation.[81] Of the various pathogens, perhaps the most important with defined risk factors are *Staph. aureus* (head injury, coma longer than 24 h, and intravenous drug use) and *Ps. aeruginosa* (prior antibiotics, structural lung disease, and steroid treatment).[82]

The most common pathogens encountered in nosocomial pneumonia are the Gram-negative bacilli, which have been reported in up to 60% of cases, and *Staph. aureus*, which has been reported in up to 40% of patients. In infections occurring during the first 4 days of hospital stay, bacteria typically associated with CAP, such as *Str. pneumoniae* and *H. influenzae*, have also been reported.

The Gram-negative rods of interest are *Esch. coli*, *Klebsiella* spp., *Enterobacter* spp., *Proteus* sp. and *Serratia marcescens*. *Esch. coli* is the third most common coliform isolated from patients with nosocomial pneumonia and appears to affect predisposed hosts such as the critically ill. *K. pneumoniae* is the most commonly isolated of the *Klebsiella* species and may cause severe necrotizing lobar pneumonia in the elderly, in alcoholics and in diabetics. *K. pneumoniae* and *Esch. coli* are the bacteria that most commonly carry the extended-spectrum β-lactamases rendering them resistant to oxyimino-β-lactams such as cefotaxime, ceftazidime and aztreonam.

Among *Enterobacter* spp., *E. cloacae* and *E. aerogenes* are the primary cause of nosocomial pneumonia and frequently colonize patients who have received a course of antibiotics. Resistance to group 4 cephalosporins among these pathogens may develop within days of treatment.

Proteus mirabilis and *Proteus vulgaris* can act as opportunistic respiratory pathogens in a manner similar to that of the *Enterobacter* spp. Indole-positive species such as *Pr. vulgaris*

may undergo a single-step mutation to become constitutive high-level producers of β-lactamase enzymes, which is manifested as resistance to group 4 cephalosporins. *Ser. marcescens* preferentially colonizes the respiratory and urinary tracts and has been associated with common source outbreaks of pneumonia in the setting of inhalation therapy and contaminated bronchoscopes. Like all Enterobacteriaceae, this organism may spread to patients by hand transfer from healthcare personnel.

The non-fermentative Gram-negative bacilli of importance are *Ps. aeruginosa* and *Acinetobacter* spp. *Ps. aeruginosa* is one of the leading causes of Gram-negative pneumonia. The most common mechanism of infection is direct contact with environmental reservoirs, including respiratory devices such as contaminated nebulizers or humidifiers. *Acinetobacter* spp. can also result in serious nosocomial infection and has been shown to be an important cause of ventilator-associated pneumonia.

H. influenzae frequently colonizes the upper respiratory tract of individuals with predisposing conditions such as COPD. Most adult infections are caused by non-typeable strains and *H. influenzae* (along with *Str. pneumoniae*) can often be isolated from tracheal secretions following intubation. *Str. pneumoniae*, like *H. influenzae*, colonizes the oropharynx and, although it is predominantly a pathogen associated with CAP, *Str. pneumoniae* is being recognized with increasing frequency as a cause of hospital-acquired infection.[83]

Anaerobes may be found as pathogens in patients predisposed to aspiration. The anaerobes that have been implicated in nosocomial pneumonia are those that colonize the oropharynx such as *Fusobacterium* spp., *Prevotella melaninogenica*, and *Bacteroides ureolyticus*.

Legionella pneumophila serogroup 1 is the most common of the *Legionella* spp. to be associated with both CAP and hospital-acquired pneumonia. The exact mode of transmission is controversial and there is evidence for both aspiration and inhalation. Contaminated potable water, and contaminated aerosols have been reported as sources of infection in hospitals.

It is important to realize that nosocomial pneumonia may be caused by multiple pathogens in any one patient, emphasizing the need for broad coverage when empirical treatment is initiated. Bartlett demonstrated that more than one pathogen could be documented in over half of the cases studied.[30]

PATHOGENESIS

The pathogenesis of nosocomial pneumonia is complex. Pathogens may gain access to the lower respiratory tract by inhalation, microaspiration or silent aspiration of oropharyngeal secretions, gross aspiration of gastric contents, hematogenous spread, translocation from the gastrointestinal tract, spread from a contiguous focus (e.g. pleural space), and direct inoculation during surgery.

For certain pathogens, such as *Mycobacteria*, and *Aspergillus* sp., inhalation of aerosols is important. In patients being mechanically ventilated, contamination of a humidification reservoir may result in aspiration of potential pathogens directly into the airways. The most important mechanism, however, particularly for Gram-negative rods, is the microaspiration of bacteria colonizing the oropharynx.

Studies have shown that while oropharyngeal colonization by Gram-negative rods is unusual in healthy people it occurs with increasing frequency in those with underlying disease.[84,85] Once oropharyngeal colonization is established, the silent aspiration of these potentially virulent bacteria eventually results in the overwhelming of host defenses in the lung and the development of pneumonia.

In addition to the oropharyngeal-pulmonary route, the gastro-pulmonary route has also been suggested as a means of introducing pathogens to the distal airways. Normally, the acidic pH of the stomach provides a hostile environment to bacteria, rendering the stomach contents virtually sterile, but above pH 4 bacterial overgrowth may occur. However, studies of stress ulcer prophylaxis have failed to demonstrate a definitive correlation between colonization of the stomach by bacteria and pneumonia.[86,87] A recent review of the literature concluded that the stomach should be regarded as an amplifier but not as the primary source of pathogens causing pneumonia and that the oropharyngeal-pulmonary route is more important than the gastro-pulmonary route.[88]

In patients who are being mechanically ventilated, the endotracheal tube plays an important role in the pathogenesis of ventilator-associated pneumonia. The tube itself breaches the upper airway defenses, and the inflated cuff allows the oropharyngeal secretions containing various pathogens to collect until they eventually pass the inflated cuff to the distal airways. In addition, the tube acts as a template upon which a layer of biofilm is deposited.[89] Pieces of this biofilm containing millions of bacteria may subsequently break off and reach the distal airways, thereby seeding remote sites of the lung.

CLINICAL MANIFESTATIONS

Much of what has been said in the discussion of the clinical manifestations of CAP and nursing home-acquired pneumonia applies to nosocomial pneumonia. The findings will vary, depending upon the age of the patient and the severity of the illness. As with CAP and nursing home-acquired infection, the symptoms may be constitutional and non-specific or localized to the respiratory tract.

DIAGNOSIS

As with CAP, two approaches may be used: clinical and invasive/quantitative.

With the clinical approach, pneumonia is defined as the presence of a new pulmonary infiltrate unexplained by other obvious causes plus one of a number of additional features, such as elevated temperature, production of purulent sputum, or leukocytosis. While the clinical approach is relatively easy and straightforward and is not associated with significant costs, it is overly sensitive and does not reliably discriminate among the various causes. The invasive/quantitative approach, on the other hand, generally has greater precision but requires special training and laboratory support, is associated with significant costs, and has the potential for serious adverse effects.

Whichever approach is used, every patient with nosocomial pneumonia requires a careful history, including risk factors for specific pathogens, a physical examination, posteroanterior and lateral chest radiographs, complete blood count, blood chemistry, blood cultures, and either oximetry or arterial blood gases.

Chest radiography is useful in helping to determine the extent of the pneumonia and the presence of a pleural effusion. Multilobar involvement, cavitation, or rapid radiographic progression indicates the presence of a severe infection.

Routine blood counts and chemistry may indicate evidence of end-organ dysfunction and can be helpful in adjusting treatment regimens. Blood cultures may be useful in identifying the pathogen in up to 20% of patients with nosocomial pneumonia. The presence of a pathogen in blood indicates not only that it is the etiologic agent but also that the patient is at increased risk for a complicated course.

Serology is not normally useful in the management of individual patients with nosocomial pneumonia. It may, however, be helpful for epidemiologic purposes, although this is more likely to be the case in patients with CAP.

The value of sputum Gram stain and culture is controversial as there are significant problems with both the sensitivity and specificity of these tests. Most studies have been carried out in patients with CAP; however, the results can be extrapolated to patients with nosocomial pneumonia. In selected cases direct staining of sputum samples for fungi or mycobacteria, or direct fluorescent antibody staining for *Legionella pneumophila* may help in directing therapy.

Invasive techniques are not performed routinely in patients with nosocomial pneumonia. However, invasive techniques should be considered in selected cases, such as:

- patients receiving appropriate empirical antimicrobial coverage but who are failing to respond;
- certain immunocompromised patients;
- patients in whom an alternative diagnosis (e.g. carcinoma) is suspected.

A number of methods have been developed to obtain samples of lower respiratory tract secretions that are not contaminated by oropharyngeal micro-organisms. They are endotracheal aspirate, protected catheter aspirate, protected specimen brush, and bronchoalveolar lavage. The studies that claim to support these techniques suffer from a lack of standardization, which makes comparison difficult at best. The discordant findings among the investigators studying these techniques make it difficult for practitioners to determine the most effective method.

Other invasive tests include transthoracic needle aspiration, transbronchial biopsy, thoracoscopy, and open lung biopsy. One study comparing invasive and non-invasive strategies for management of suspected ventilator-associated pneumonia showed that there was a statistically significant reduction in mortality, sepsis-related organ failure and antibiotic free days in the cohort managed with invasive diagnostic tests.[90]

TREATMENT

When devising an antimicrobial regimen, the patient, the pathogen, and the drug should all be considered individually and the interactions among them taken into account.

Patient-related factors

These include any previous history of adverse reactions (and, in particular, anything suggesting type 1 hypersensitivity to any antimicrobial), and increasing age (since adverse drug effects are more common in elderly people). The macrolides, lincosamides, chloramphenicol, and metronidazole are eliminated via the liver, while most other antibiotics are eliminated by the kidney. When treating women of child-bearing age it is important to determine if the patient is pregnant because teratogenicity and fetotoxicity must be considered.

Pathogen-related factors

Ideally, the narrowest spectrum agent associated with the least toxicity and lowest cost should be administered if the pathogen is known. Unfortunately, empirical therapy is usually the norm, and one must consider the likely pathogens based upon the local epidemiology, the risk factors for pneumonia and for specific pathogens, and the severity of illness. The prevalence of resistance among pathogens to various antimicrobials must also be considered.

Drug-related factors

When selecting any antibiotic, the first step is to select an agent to which the pathogen is known or likely to be susceptible. Other considerations include pharmacokinetic and pharmacodynamic properties, toxicity, drug interactions, and cost. Pharmacokinetics refers to the absorption, distribution and elimination of drugs, while pharmacodynamics is the relationship between the concentration of the drug in serum and its pharmacologic and toxicologic effects (*see* Ch. 4). Depending upon the class of antibiotic being used, different pharmacokinetic/pharmacodynamic parameters correlate more or less closely with clinical or therapeutic efficacy. For β-lactam drugs, macrolides, and clindamycin, the time during which the antibiotic concentration at the site of action in the tissues is above the minimum inhibitory concentration (MIC) for the organism correlates best with efficacy. However, for aminoglycosides, fluoroquinolones, and vancomycin, the 24 h area-under-the-

curve/MIC ratio correlates best. Higher ratios of peak serum concentrations to MIC (C_{max}/MIC) have been shown to prevent the emergence of resistance during treatment with fluoroquinolones and aminoglycosides. Furthermore, aminoglycosides do not achieve high levels in lung tissue, and this problem is compounded by the fact that they are also relatively inactivated by the acidic pH present at the site of infection in the lung.

In North America two sets of guidelines have been developed that provide a structured approach to the management of patients with nosocomial pneumonia, and which take into account the risk factors, severity of illness and time of onset of the illness.[91,92] The risk factors are for infection with specific pathogens; severity of illness is either mild to moderate or severe; time of onset refers to early versus late (i.e. less than 5 or 5 or more days, respectively). Based upon these variables, a hierarchical approach to the patient with nosocomial pneumonia has been developed. While it is recognized that a large number of bacteria are potential pathogens, there is a 'core' group of organisms that must be considered for each patient for which antimicrobial coverage must be provided. This group consists of Gram-negative bacilli (such as *Enterobacter* spp., *Esch. coli*, *Klebsiella* and *Proteus* spp., *Ser. marcescens*), *H. influenzae*, *Staph. aureus*, and *Str. pneumoniae*. Depending upon the risk factors present and the severity of illness, anaerobes, methicillin-resistant *Staph. aureus*, *Legionella* spp., *Ps. aeruginosa* and *Acinetobacter* spp. should also be considered.

The American Thoracic Society regimens are presented in Tables 48.5, 48.6, and 48.7.[91] Other countries have produced guidelines for local use which reflect variation in the target pathogens and choice of therapy. Until the evidence base surrounding nosocomial pneumonia improves, variations in practice are likely to continue. The decision to select an agent should be based upon the host, pathogen, and drug-related issues outlined earlier. A few specific issues, however, deserve comment. Single-agent therapy is recommended in many situations. Two drugs should be used to achieve synergistic or additive activity against *Ps. aeruginosa* but there are no data to support the routine use of combination therapy for other bacterial pathogens in non-neutropenic patients.[93]

In patients who are either severely ill with risk factors and early onset or severely ill without risk factors but with late onset, combination therapy should be instituted. If the patient was not receiving any prior antibiotics and deep suction aspirates or bronchoscopy samples fail to yield *Ps. aeruginosa* or other often-resistant pathogens such as *Acinetobacter* spp., treatment may be modified to a single-drug regimen.

Enterobacter spp. are among the most common causes of Gram-negative bacillary hospital-acquired pneumonia. A major concern with infection caused by this organism is that in the presence of a group 4 cephalosporin it can become a hyperproducer of β-lactamase.[94]

The final issue is that of duration of therapy. Unfortunately, there are no appropriately designed randomized controlled trials that specifically address this issue. The general consensus, however, is that patients with severe infec-

Table 48.5 Initial empirical treatment of patients with mild-to-moderate hospital-acquired pneumonia, no unusual risk factors and onset at any time; or with severe, early onset hospital-acquired pneumonia. (Adapted from American Thoracic Society guidelines)

Core organisms	Core antibiotics

Enteric Gram-negative bacilli
  Enterobacter spp.
  Escherichia coli
  Klebsiella spp.
  Proteus spp.
  Serratia marcescens
  Haemophilus influenzae
Methicillin-sensitive *Staphylococcus aureus*
Streptococcus pneumoniae
	Cephalosporin (group 3 or 4)*
	
	β-lactam–β-lactamase inhibitor combination, (e.g. piperacillin–tazobactam)
	If allergic to penicillin: fluoroquinolone or clindamycin + aztreonam

*See Ch 15 for classifications of cephalosporin.

Table 48.6 Initial empirical treatment of patients with mild-to-moderate, hospital-acquired pneumonia with risk factors; onset any time (adapted from American Thoracic Society guidelines)

Core organisms	Core antibiotics plus

Anaerobes
  (recent abdominal surgery, witnessed aspiration)
	Clindamycin
	  or β-lactam–β-lactamase inhibitor (alone)
	  e.g. piperacillin–tazobactam

Staphylococcus aureus
  (coma, head trauma, diabetes mellitus, renal failure)
	+/– Vancomycin
	  (until methicillin-resistant *Staph. aureus* is ruled out)

Legionella spp. (high-dose steroids)	Erythromycin +/– rifampicin
Pseudomonas aeruginosa (prolonged ICU stay, steroids, antibiotics, structural lung disease)	Treat as severe hospital-acquired pneumonia

Table 48.7 Initial empirical treatment of patients with severe early onset hospital-acquired pneumonia with risk factors or with severe late onset hospital-acquired pneumonia (adapted from American Thoracic Society guidelines)

Core organisms plus	Therapy		
Pseudomonas aeruginosa	Antipseudomonal penicillin *or* piperacillin–tazobactam *or* ceftazidime *or* carbapenem[a]	+	aminoglycoside *or* ciprofloxacin
Acinetobacter sp.	Piperacillin–tazobactam *or* carbapenem	+	aminoglycoside *or* ciprofloxacin

[a] Imipenem or meropenem.

tion caused by pathogens such as *Ps. aeruginosa* or *Acinetobacter* spp. should be treated for a minimum of 14 days, whereas patients with less severe infection may only require 7–10 days of treatment.

References

1. Gonzales R, Steiner JF, Sande MA 1997 Antibiotic prescribing for adults with colds, upper respiratory tract infections, and bronchitis by ambulatory care physicians. *Journal of The American Medical Association* 278: 901–904.
2. Rodnick JE, Gude JK 1988 The use of antibiotics in acute bronchitis and acute exacerbations of chronic bronchitis. *Western Journal of Medicine* 149: 347–351.
3. Boldy DAR, Skidmore SJ, Ayres JG 1990 Acute bronchitis in the community: Clinical features, infective factors, changes in pulmonary function and bronchial reactivity to histamine. *Respiratory Medicine* 84: 377–385.
4. Sherry, MK, Klainer AD, Wolff M et al 1988 Herpetic febrile tracheobronchitis. *Annals of Internal Medicine* 1: 229–233.
5. Smith CB, Golden CA, Kanner RE et al 1980 Association of viral and *Mycoplasma pneumoniae* infections with acute respiratory illness in patients with chronic obstructive pulmonary diseases. *American Reviews of Respiratory Diseases* 121: 225–232.
6. Niroumand M, Grossman RF 1998 Airway Infection (eds). *Infectious Disease Clinics of North America* 12: 671–687.
7. Ayres JG 1986 Seasonal pattern of acute bronchitis in general practice in the United Kingdom. *Thorax* 41: 106–110.
8. Reynolds HY 1995 Chronic bronchitis and acute infectious exacerbations. In: Mandell, Douglas, Bennett, (eds). *Principles and Practice of Infectious Diseases*, 4th edn. New York, Churchill Livingstone Inc, p. 608.
9. US Bureau of the Census 1994 *Statistical Abstract of the United States*, 14th edn. Washington, DC, US Bureau of the Census, p. 95.

10. Turner-Warwick M, Hodson ME, Corrin B et al 1990 *Clinical Atlas of Respiratory Diseases.* London, Gower Medical Publishing.

11. Anthonisen NR, Manfreda J, Warren CPW et al 1987 Antibiotic therapy in exacerbations of chronic obstructive lung disease. *Annals of Internal Medicine* 106: 196–204.

12. Monso E, Ruiz J, Rosell A et al 1995 Bacterial infection in chronic obstructive pulmonary disease: A study of stable and exacerbated outpatients using the protected specimen brush. *American Journal of Respiratory Critical Care Medicine* 152: 1316–1320.

13. Soler N, Torres A, Ewig S et al 1998 Bronchial microbial patterns in severe exacerbations of chronic obstructive pulmonary disease (COPD) requiring mechanical ventilation. *American Journal of Respiratory Critical Care Medicine* 157: 1498–1505.

14. Eller J, Ede A, Schaberg T et al 1998 Infective exacerbations of chronic bronchitis: Relation between bacteriologic etiology and lung function. *Chest* 113: 1542–1548.

15. Miravitlles M, Espinosa C, Fernandez-Laso E et al 1999 Relationship between bacterial flora in sputum and functional impairment in patients with acute exacerbations of COPD. *Chest* 116: 40–46.

16. Saint S, Vittinghoff E, Grady D 1995 Antibiotics in chronic obstructive pulmonary disease exacerbations. A meta-analysis. *Journal of The American Medical Association* 273: 957–960.

17. Ball P, Harris JM, Lowson D et al 1995 Acute infective exacerbations of chronic bronchitis. *Quarterly Journal of Medicine* 88: 61–68.

18. Derenne JP, Fleury B, Parienta R 1998 Acute respiratory failure of chronic obstructive lung disease. *American Reviews of Respiratory Diseases* 138: 1006–1033.

19. Seneff MG, Wagner DP, Wagner RP et al 1999 Hospital and 1-year survival of patients admitted to intensive care units with acute exacerbation of chronic obstructive lung disease. *Journal of The American Medical Association* 274: 1852–1857.

20. Lode H 1991 Respiratory tract infections: When is antibiotic therapy indicated? *Clinical Therapeutics* 13: 149–156.

21. Balter NS, Hyland RH, Low DE et al 1994 Recommendations on the management of chronic bronchitis. *Canadian Medical Association Journal* 151(Suppl.): 7–23.

22. Wilson R 1995 Outcome predictors in bronchitis. *Chest* 108(Suppl.): 53–57.

23. National Center for Health Statistics 1998 National hospital discharge survey: Annual summary 1990. *Vital Health Statistics*, 13: 1–225.

24. Niederman MS, McCombs JS, Unger AN et al 1998 The cost of treating community-acquired pneumonia. *Clinical Therapeutics* 20: 820–837.

25. Foy HM, Cooney MK, Allan I et al 1979 Rates of pneumonia during influenza epidemics in Seattle, 1964 to 1975. *Journal of The American Medical Association* 241: 253–258.

26. Jokinen C, Heiskanen L, Juvonen H et al 1993 Incidence of community-acquired pneumonia in the population of four municipalities in eastern Finland. *American Journal of Epidemiology* 137: 977–988.

27. Koivula I, Sten M, Makela PH 1994 Risk factors for pneumonia in the elderly. *American Journal of Medicine* 96: 313–320.

28. Sankilampi U, Herva E, Haikala R et al 1997 Epidemiology of invasive *Streptococcus pneumoniae* infections in adults in Finland. *Epidemiology and Infection* 118: 7–15.

29. Nielsen SV, Henrichsen J 1996 Incidence of invasive pneumococcal disease and distribution of capsular types of pneumococci in Denmark, 1989–94. *Epidemiology and Infection* 117: 411–416.

30. Bartlett JG, O'Keefe P, Tally FP et al 1986 Bacteriology of hospital-acquired pneumonia. *Archives of Internal Medicine* 146: 868–871.

31. Fang GD, Fine M, Orloff J et al 1990 New and emerging etiologies for community-acquired pneumonia with implications for therapy: A prospective multicenter study of 359 cases. *Medicine* 69: 307–316.

32. Marrie TJ 1994 Community-acquired pneumonia. *Clinical Infectious Diseases* 18: 501–515.

33. Moine P, Vercken J-B, Chevret S et al 1994 Severe community-acquired pneumonia: Etiology, epidemiology and prognostic factors. *Chest* 105: 1487–1495.

34. Fine MJ, Smith MA, Carson CA et al 1996 Prognosis and outcomes of patients with community-acquired pneumonia. *Journal of the American Medical Association* 275: 134–141.

35. Marston BJ, Plouffe JF, File TM et al 1997 Incidence of community-acquired pneumonia requiring hospitalization. *Archives of Internal Medicine* 157: 1709–1718.

36. Troy CJ, Peeling RW, Ellis AG et al 1997 *Chlamydia pneumoniae* as a new source of infectious outbreaks in nursing homes. *Journal of the American Medical Association* 277: 1214–1218.

37. Pachon J, Prados MD, Capote F et al 1990 A. Severe community-acquired pneumonia: Etiology, prognosis and treatment. *American Reviews of Respiratory Diseases* 142: 369–373.

38. Johanson WG Jr, Pierce AK, Sanford JP, Thomas GD 1972 Nosocomial respiratory infections with gram-negative bacilli. *Annals of Internal Medicine* 77: 701–706.

39. Woodhead MA, Arrowsmith J, Chamberlain-Webber R et al 1991 The value of routine microbial investigation in community-acquired pneumonia. *Respiratory Medicine* 85: 313–317.

40. Farr BM, Kaiser DL, Harrison BDW et al 1989 Prediction of microbial aetiology at admission to hospital for pneumonia from the presenting clinical features. *Thorax* 44: 1031–1035.

41. Spiteri MA, Cook DG, Clarke SW 1988 Reliability of eliciting physical signs in examination of the chest. *Lancet* 1: 873–875.

42. Fine MJ, Auble TE, Yealy DM et al 1997 A prediction rule to identify low-risk patients will community-acquired pneumonia. *New England Journal of Medicine* 336: 243–250.

43. Reed WW, Byrd GS, Gates RH Jr et al 1996 Sputum Gram's stain in community-acquired pneumococcal pneumonia. A meta-analysis. *Western Journal of Medicine* 165: 197–204.

44. Geckler RW, McAllister K, Gremillion DH et al 1985 Clinical value of paired sputum and transtracheal aspirates in the initial management of pneumonia. *Chest* 87: 631–635.

45. Barrett-Connor E 1971 The nonvalue of sputum culture in the diagnosis of pneumococcal pneumonia. *American Reviews of Respiratory Diseases* 103: 845–848.

46. Woodhead 1987 Prospective study of the aetiology and outcome of pneumonia in the community. *Lancet* 1(8534): 671–674.

47. Light RW, Girard WM, Jenkinson SG et al 1980 Parapneumonic effusions. *American Journal of Medicine* 69: 507–512.

48. Sahn SA 1993 Management of complicated parapneumonic effusions. *American Reviews of Respiratory Diseases* 148: 813–817.

49. Auble TE, Yealy DM, Fine MJ 1998 Assessing prognosis and selecting an initial site of care for adults with community-acquired pneumonia. *Infectious Disease Clinics of North America* 12: 741–759.

50. Fine MJ, Hanusa BH, Lave JR et al 1995 Comparison of a disease-specific and a generic severity of illness measure for patients with community-acquired pneumonia. *Journal of General Internal Medicine* 10: 359–368.

51. Bartlett JG, Dowell SF, Mandell LA et al 2000 Practice guidelines for the management of community-acquired pneumonia in adults. *Clinical Infectious Diseases* 31: 347–382.

52. Mandell LA, Marrie TH, Grossman RF et al and the Canadian Community-Acquired Pneumonia Working Group 2000 Canadian guidelines for the initial management of community-acquired pneumonia: an evidence-based update by the Canadian Infectious Disease Society and the Canadian Thoracic Society. *Clinical Infectious Diseases* 31: 383–421.

53. Niederman MS, Bass JB Jr, Campbell GD et al 1993 American Thoracic Society guidelines for the initial management of adults with community-acquired pneumonia: diagnosis, assessment of severity, and initial antimicrobial therapy. American Thoracic Society. Medical Section of the American Lung Association. *American Reviews of Respiratory Diseases* 1418–1426.

54. American Thoracic Society 2001 Guidelines for the Management of Adults with Community-acquired Pneumonia: Diagnosis, Assessment of Severity, Antimicrobial Therapy and Prevention. *American Journal of Respiratory Critical Care Medicine* 163: 1730–1754.

55. National Committee for Clinical Laboratory Standards 1994 Performance Standards for Antimicrobial Susceptibility Testing. Villanova, PA, National Committee for Laboratory Standards. NCCLS document M100-S5 supplement, vol 24, no 16.

56. Ferrándiz MJ, Fernoll A, Li n ares J, de La Campa AG 2000 Horizontal transfer of *parC* and *parA* in fluoroquinolone-resistant clinical isolates of *Streptococcus pneumoniae*. *Antimicrobial Agents and Chemotherapy* 44: 840–847.

57. Johnston NJ, deAzavedo JC, Kellner JD et al 1997 Prevalence and characterization of the mechanisms of macrolide, lincosamide, and streptogramin resistance in *Streptococcus pneumoniae* from across Canada. Program and abstracts of the 37th Interscience Conference on Antimicrobial Agents and Chemotherapy, Toronto, Ontario, Canada, Sept. 28–Oct. 1, 1997. Abstract C-77a.

58. Kelley MA, Weber DJ, Gilligan P et al 2000 Breakthrough pneumococcal bacteremia in patients being treated with azithromycin and clarithromycin. *Clinical Infectious Diseases* 31: 1008–1011.

59. Wise R, Brenwald N, Gill M et al 1996 *Streptococcus pneumoniae* resistance to fluoroquinolones [letter]. *Lancet* 348: 1660.

60. Kohler T, Pechere JC 1998 Bacterial resistance to quinolones. In: Andriole VT (ed.) *The Quinolones*. Academic Press, San Diego, pp. 117–142.

61. Doern GV, Brueggemann A, Holley HP Jr et al 1996 Antimicrobial resistance of *Streptococcus pneumoniae* recovered from outpatients in the United States during the winter months of 1994 to 1995: Results of a 30-center national surveillance study. *Antimicrobial Agents and Chemotherapy* 40: 1208–1213.

62. Livermore DM 1995 Beta-lactamses in laboratory and clinical resistance. *Clinical Microbiology Reviews* 8: 557–584.

63. Henquell C, Chanal C, Sirot D et al 1995 Molecular characterization of nine different types of mutants among 107 inhibitor-resistant TEM beta-lactamases from clinical isolates of *Escherichia coli. Antimicrobial Agents and Chemotherapy* 39: 427–430.

64. Bartlett JG, Breiman RF, Mandell LA et al 1998 Community-acquired pneumonia in adults: guidelines for management. *Clinical Infectious Diseases* 26: 811–838.

65. Macfarlane J, Boswell T, Douglas G et al 2002 The British Thoracic Society Guidelines for the Management of Community Acquired Pneumonia in Adults. *Thorax* (in press).

66. ERS 1998 Guidelines for management of adult community-acquired lower respiratory tract infections. ERS Task Force Report. *European Respiratory Journal* 11: 986–991.

67. Mandell LA, Niederman M and the Canadian Community Acquired Pneumonia Consensus Conference Group 1993 Antimicrobial treatment of community acquired pneumonia in adults: A conference report. *Canadian Journal of Infectious Diseases* 4: 25–28.

68. Heffelfinger JD, Dowell SF, Jorgensen JH et al 2000 Management of community-acquired pneumonia in the era of pneumococcal resistance: a report from the Drug-Resistant *Streptococcus pneumoniae* Therapeutic Working Group. *Archives of Internal Medicine* 160: 1399–1408.

69. Gilbert K, Gleason PP, Singer DE et al 1998 Variations in antimicrobial use and cost in more than 2,000 patients with community-acquired pneumonia. *American Journal of Medicine* 104: 17–27.

70. Gleason PP, Meehan TP, Fine JM et al 1999 Associations between initial antimicrobial therapy and medical outcomes for elderly patients with pneumonia. *Archives of Internal Medicine* 159: 2562–2572.

71. Stahl JE, Barza M, DesJardin J et al 1999 Effect of macrolides as part of initial empiric therapy on length of stay in patients with community-acquired pneumonia. *Archives of Internal Medicine* 159: 2576–2580.

72. Choi E, Lee H 1998 Clinical outcome of invasive infections by penicillin-resistant *Streptococcus pneumoniae* in Korean children. *Clinical Infectious Diseases* 26: 1346–1354.

73. Deeks SL, Palacio R, Ruinsky R et al 1999 Risk factors and course of illness among children with invasive penicillin-resistant *Streptococcus pneumoniae. Pediatrics* 103: 409–413.

74. Feikin D, Schuchat A, Kolczak M et al 2000 Mortality from invasive pneumococcal pneumonia in the era of antibiotic resistance, 1995–1997. *American Journal of Public Health* 90: 223–229.

75. Dowell SF, Smith T, Leversedge K, Snitzer J 1999 Pneumonia treatment failure associated with highly resistant pneumococci. *Clinical Infectious Diseases* 29: 462–463.

76. Meehan TP, Fine MJ, Krumholz HM et al 1997 Quality of care, process and outcomes in elderly patients with pneumonia. *Journal of The American Medical Association* 278: 2080–2084.

77. Loeb M, McGeer A, McArthur M, Walter S et al 1999 Risk factors for pneumonia and other lower respiratory tract infections in elderly residents of long-term care facilities. *Archives of Internal Medicine* 159: 2058–2064.

78. Woodhead M 1994 Pneumonia in the elderly. *Journal of Antimicrobial Chemotherapy* 34(Suppl. 34): 85–92.

79. American Thoracic Society 1995 Hospital-acquired pneumonia in adults: Diagnosis, assessment of severity, initial antimicrobial therapy, and preventative strategies: A consensus statement. *American Journal of Respiratory Critical Care Medicine* 153: 1711–1725.

80. Craven DE, Steger KA, LaForce FM 1998 Pneumonia. In: Bennett JV, Brachman PS (eds). *Hospital Infections*, 4th edn. Lippincott-Raven Press, Philadelphia.

81. Wiblin RT, Wenzel RP 1996 Hospital-acquired pneumonia. *Current Clinical Topics in Infectious Diseases* 16: 194–214

82. Loeb M, Mandell LA, 1997 Microbiology of hospital-acquired pneumonia. *Seminars in Respiratory Critical Care Medicine* 18: 111–120.

83. Schleupner CJ, Cobb DK 1992 A study of the etiologies and treatment of nosocomial pneumonia in a community-based teaching hospital. *Infection Control and Hospital Epidemiology* 13: 515–525.

84. Valenti WM, Trudell RG, Bentley DW 1978 Factors predisposing to oropharyngeal colonization with gram-negative bacilli in the aged. *New England Journal of Medicine* 298: 1108–1111.

85. Johanson WG, Pierce AK, Sanford JP 1969 Changing pharyngeal bacterial flora of hospitalized patients: emergence of gram-negative bacilli. *New England Journal of Medicine* 281: 1137–1140.

86. Reusser P, Zimmerli W, Scheidegger D et al 1989 Role of gastric colonization in nosocomial infections and endotoxemia: A prospective study in neurosurgical patients on mechanical ventilation. *Journal of Infectious Diseases* 160: 414–421

87. Bonten MJM, Gaillard CA, van der Geest S et al 1997 The role of intragastric acidity and stress ulcus prophylaxis on colonization and infection in mechanically ventilated ICU patients: A stratified, randomized double-blind study of sucralfate versus antacids. *American Journal of Respiratory Critical Care Medicine* 152: 1825–1834

88. Stoutenbeek CP, van Saene HKF 1997 Nonantibiotic measures in the prevention of ventilator-associated pneumonia. *Seminars in Respiratory Infection* 12: 294–299

89. Inglis TJJ, Millar MR, Jones JG et al 1989 Tracheal tube biofilm as a source of bacterial colonization of the lung. *Journal of Clinical Microbiology* 27: 2014–2018

90. Fagen J 2000 Invasive and noninvasive strategies for management of suspected VAP. *Annals of Internal Medicine* 132: 621–630.

91. American Thoracic Society 1996 Hospital-acquired pneumonia in adults: diagnosis, assessment of severity, initial antimicrobial therapy, and preventative strategies. *American Journal of Respiratory Critical Care Medicine* 153: 1711–1725.

92. Mandell LA, Marrie TJ, Niederman MS and the Canadian Hospital Acquired Pneumonia Consensus Conference Group 1993 Initial antimicrobial treatment of hospital-acquired pneumonia in adults: a conference report. *Canadian Journal of Infectious Diseases* 4: 317–321.

93. Hilf M, Yu VL, Sharp J et al 1989 Antibiotic therapy for *Pseudomonas aeruginosa* bacteremia: Outcome correlations in a prospective study of 200 patients. *American Journal of Medicine* 87: 540–546.

94. Chow JW, Fine MJ, Shlaes DM et al 1991 *Enterobacter* bacteremia: Clinical features and emergence of antibiotic resistance during therapy. *Annals of Internal Medicine* 115: 585–590.

49 Endocarditis

David T. Durack

The diagnosis 'infective endocarditis' (IE) refers to microbial infection of the heart valves or endocardium. This is not a single disease, but a diverse group of diseases. Many different species of micro-organisms can infect the interior of the heart, the primary lesions can occur in a variety of locations; the pathology is variable, and the time course of the illness can range from chronic to fulminant (Box 49.1). These features present in a variety of combinations, requiring many different antimicrobial treatment regimens. Treatment for each individual patient should be selected after careful assessment of all available clinical and microbiological information.

Box 49.1 Infective endocarditis and endarteritis: a variety of diseases

Location	Native heart valves; prosthetic heart valves; endocardium or endothelium; intracardiac devices (e.g. catheters, pacemakers, patches, implants); ventricular assist devices; intravascular grafts and devices
Organisms	Bacteria; yeasts; molds; rickettsiae; chlamydiae
Pathologies	Vegetations on valves; vegetations at other sites; abscess; perforation of valves; pseudoaneurysms; mycotic aneurysms; infected thrombi
Rate of progression	Acute; subacute; chronic

PRINCIPLES OF TREATMENT

These include accurate diagnosis of IE, assessment of the patient's cardiac status, assessment of complications arising from IE, choice of initial empirical or specific antibiotic treatment, identification of the etiological organism, reliable antibiotic susceptibility information, modification of the antibiotic regimen to achieve total eradication of the etiological organisms, correct timing of surgical intervention, (when indicated), adequate follow-up after treatment, and consideration of prophylaxis against future episodes.

ACCURATE DIAGNOSIS

Because IE is not one but many different diseases, it is not surprising that its clinical manifestations can be numerous and confusing. The differential diagnosis is wide, and confirmation of a presumptive diagnosis of IE can be difficult. Older diagnostic criteria required evidence from either surgery or autopsy before the diagnosis of 'definite IE' could be accepted; modern criteria allow reasonably sensitive and highly specific diagnosis of definite IE based on clinical evidence. Alternative diagnoses such as bacteremia without IE and other infective and non-infective conditions should be carefully considered and excluded before a secure diagnosis of IE is made.

ASSESSMENT OF CARDIAC STATUS

Many patients with IE have new intracardiac pathology due to IE itself in addition to pre-existing heart disease. Both of these should be accurately assessed by echocardiography and, if necessary, other investigations.

ASSESSMENT OF COMPLICATIONS

There may be systemic complications such as arterial emboli, infarcts, hemorrhages, abscesses or mycotic aneurysms. To guide optimal management, all such lesions should be identified and assessed by means of appropriate imaging techniques. At a minimum, this requires echocardiography, preferably using transesophageal imaging. Other imaging techniques that may provide useful information include cardiac catheterization, radiography, computed tomography (CT) and magnetic resonance imaging (MRI).

CHOICE OF INITIAL ANTIBIOTIC TREATMENT

In the early stages of the illness, IE may be suspected or considered, but a definitive diagnosis cannot be made. Under these circumstances, the question arises of whether to give empirical antimicrobial therapy immediately, or to wait for the results of blood cultures and other tests. This can best be decided by determining whether the patient has acute or subacute endocarditis.

IDENTIFICATION OF THE ETIOLOGICAL ORGANISM

Because the natural history, treatment and prognosis are highly dependent upon the infecting organism, correct speciation is desirable. For example, group D streptococcal endocarditis could be caused by *Streptococcus bovis*, *Enterococcus faecalis* or *Enterococcus faecium*, but the treatment for each of these often differs.

RELIABLE ANTIBIOTIC SUSCEPTIBILITY INFORMATION

Dependable information on susceptibility must be available to choose the best treatment. The advent of widespread antibiotic resistance among common species of Gram-positive cocci over the past 20 years makes identification of methicillin-resistant *Staphylococcus aureus* and vancomycin-resistant enterococci especially important.

TOTAL ERADICATION OF THE ETIOLOGICAL ORGANISMS

In most bacterial and fungal infections of humans, cure can be achieved by antimicrobial treatment without necessarily killing all of the etiological organisms. In IE, however, host defences are partially or completely excluded from the vegetations, so that a total bactericidal effect is desirable to prevent possible relapse. Bacteristatic antimicrobials are inappropriate. When the results of susceptibility testing are available, the antibiotic regimen should be chosen to ensure the most effective and least toxic regimen that will eradicate all the infecting organisms. Achievement of this goal represents *microbiological cure*, which is necessary but not always sufficient for *clinical cure*. For example, patients with IE may die of stroke or heart failure, or suffer other serious complications, despite being microbiologically 'cured'.

CORRECT TIMING OF SURGICAL INTERVENTION, WHEN INDICATED

Surgery is indicated in up to one-third of cases of IE to achieve the best possible outcome. Selection of cases for surgery, and choice of the optimal time at which to intervene, are critically important aspects of management. This is a complex subject, the details of which are outside the scope of this chapter.

ADEQUATE FOLLOW-UP AFTER TREATMENT

Recurrent endocarditis includes relapses (with the same organism) and re-infections (with a new organism). Relapse after correct treatment of IE is uncommon. The observed frequency of relapse varies according to the infecting organism and the site of the infection. For example, less than 2% of patients relapse after treatment of native valve IE due to penicillin-sensitive streptococci so that recurrent IE after treatment is more likely to be due to reinfection than to relapse. Higher rates of relapse (5–15%) follow treatment of staphylococcal, Gram-negative and prosthetic valve IE, especially if a valve-ring abscess has developed. In all cases, appropriate follow-up is needed to identify possible relapses. In the asymptomatic patient whose blood count, C-reactive protein and erythrocyte sedimentation rate are normal or returning toward normal after treatment, follow-up blood cultures are unnecessary. However, the possibility of relapse should be kept in mind; any indication (especially recurrent fever) that cure has not been achieved should lead to immediate re-evaluation, including follow-up blood cultures.

CONSIDERATION OF PROPHYLAXIS AGAINST FUTURE EPISODES

After microbiological cure of an episode of IE, the patient is in double jeopardy of another episode. The original predisposition remains, and the cured IE itself is an additional risk factor for IE. Therefore, prophylaxis is indicated for selected future medical and dental procedures which might cause bacteremias, possibly leading to IE. Most important of these is dental extraction, but other dental manipulations and certain medical procedures such as urinary tract instrumentation also constitute relative indications for administration of prophylactic antibiotics.

LABORATORY SUPPORT FOR TREATMENT OF ENDOCARDITIS

Laboratory information is essential for optimal management of IE because the choice of treatment depends primarily upon the identity and antibiotic sensitivities of the infecting organism. For each case, tests should be chosen which give the necessary information in a cost-effective manner.

IDENTIFICATION

The minimum information required is the type of bacteria and the relevant antibiotic sensitivity. For example, subacute IE caused by a fully penicillin-sensitive streptococcus can usually be cured without any further information. However, such a minimalist approach would yield little understanding of the pathogenesis or the portal of entry for the organism. To illustrate, a patient with IE due to a penicillin-sensitive streptococcus could be infected by either a viridans group organism originating from the mouth, or by a strain of *Str. bovis* originating from the bowel. The implications are quite different: one patient needs dental treatment, the other investigation for a possible colonic tumor. Therefore, proper speciation of the etiological organism is generally advisable. Selective use of molecular typing techniques offer reliable means to distinguish between epidemic strains, and between relapse and reinfection in patients with recurrent IE caused by similar organisms. Biochemical profiles and antibiograms are no longer considered specific enough to establish that two isolates are the same or different.

ANTIMICROBIAL SUSCEPTIBILITY TESTS

Accurate determination of susceptibility to relevant antimicrobials is needed to choose the best therapeutic regimens for IE. Standard methods such as manual disk diffusion tests or automated systems using liquid media are acceptable for most organisms that cause IE. Measurement of both minimum inhibitory concentration (MIC) and minimum bactericidal concentration (MBC) for organisms causing IE has been recommended in the past. This arose from the well-documented observation that bactericidal antibiotics are more likely to cure IE than bacteristatic agents. However, convincing evidence has now accumulated showing that IE due to 'tolerant' organisms (which are inhibited but not killed by antibiotics that are normally bactericidal) can usually be cured by these same antibiotics. This observation indicates that measurement of the MBC does not provide essential information, so it is no longer routinely recommended.

Other relevant tests include detection or measurement of methicillin resistance among *Staph. aureus* and *Staph. epidermidis*, low- and high-level aminoglycoside resistance among enterococci, vancomycin resistance among enterococci, penicillinase production and serum antibiotic concentrations. Penicillinase production by enterococci can be missed by standard sensitivity assays because the results are inoculum dependent; the nitrocefin assay should be used.

Measurement of serum antibiotic concentrations at appropriate intervals is needed for most patients receiving aminoglycosides or vancomycin, whether or not they have endocarditis. However, these tests are frequently ordered more often than is necessary, thus wasting resources. Patients with normal renal function who are receiving once-daily doses of aminoglycosides at standard dosage (*see* Table 49.3) are unlikely to develop toxicity unless the duration of treatment is longer than 2–4 weeks. Except in patients of advanced age, or with any degree of renal insufficiency, or with other special factors which might raise the likelihood of aminoglycoside toxicity, measuring serum creatinine three times weekly and aminoglycoside trough concentrations once or twice weekly is generally sufficient.

To monitor the activity of antimicrobials during treatment, serum inhibitory and bactericidal titres (SIT and SBT) may be determined. This entails measuring that dilution of serum obtained from a patient receiving antimicrobial treatment which will inhibit (SIT) and kill (SBT) the patient's own infecting organism. In the past, this test was popular, even routine, for monitoring of treatment of IE. However, these tests are difficult to standardize, difficult to interpret, neither necessary nor helpful in most cases of IE and are not routinely recommended. If an unusual or unproven regimen is chosen, especially if treatment seems to be failing, it may occasionally be informative to measure SIT and SBT which is best performed by a specialized reference or research laboratory.

TREATMENT

The standard approach for treatment of IE is to administer one or more antimicrobials that meet two simple criteria: they can fully inhibit growth of the etiological organism, and have a history of proven effectiveness in treatment of IE due to the same or similar species. It is not always possible to meet these criteria. In the early stages of management of acute IE, it is usually necessary to choose empirical treatment before susceptibility results are available. This can be done by determining the most likely organisms on the basis of clinical evidence, then choosing antimicrobials which have a track record of efficacy against them. Initial tests may reveal that the organism is not fully susceptible to any of the standard antimicrobials. This is especially likely to occur in the case of enterococci such as *E. faecium*. Finally, the etiological organism may cause IE so rarely that there is little or no published experience available to guide treatment.

In general, the treatment regimen chosen for bacterial pathogens should include a cell-wall-active agent, (i.e. a β-lactam (preferably) or a glycopeptide, either alone or in combination). Drug toxicity is common because most recommended regimens utilize full dosages for several weeks. Therefore, side effects should be anticipated, and minimized by appropriate monitoring of kidney function and serum concentrations of drugs with timely dose adjustments as needed. IE is less common in children than in adults, but poses similar therapeutic problems. Continuous intravenous infusion of antibiotics can be substituted for divided intravenous doses in any of the regimens recommended below. Antimicrobial efficacy is probably similar for both methods, but continuous infusion by means of a pump may be more convenient, especially if the patient receives part of the course of treatment as an outpatient.

EMPIRICAL THERAPY FOR IE

The decision to commence empiric therapy depends mainly upon whether the patient has an acute or subacute endocarditis syndrome. Acute endocarditis is a rapidly progressive disease caused by pathogens such as *Staph. aureus* or *Streptococcus pneumoniae*. These organisms can destroy cardiac valves rapidly, the associated septicemia can cause severe symptoms, and they may give rise to 'metastatic' foci of infection by seeding tissues elsewhere in the body. Therefore, immediate antimicrobial therapy is indicated, allowing time only for urgently obtaining three sets of blood cultures (separate venepunctures) and a transthoracic echocardiogram. Patients with suspected acute endocarditis should be treated as if they had staphylococcal infection, because this is one of the most likely causes of acute IE.

Subacute IE is usually caused by organisms of low virulence such as the viridans streptococci, and is more slowly progressive. This does not necessarily imply that the symptoms will be mild; a stroke or other serious complication can occur at any time. Subacute infection has usually been present for at least several weeks before the diagnosis is suspected, and antibiotics cannot immediately reverse the risk of progressive valvular damage or emboli; this requires 1–2 weeks. Therefore, in most subacute cases antibiotic therapy may be withheld for 1–2 days, awaiting the initial results of blood cultures and other diagnostic tests, and the detailed interpretation of echocardiographs. This approach is advisable because, if antibiotics are given too early, the opportunity to recover the pathogen from further blood cultures may be lost. After 18–48 h initial blood culture results will often be available to confirm the diagnosis and to guide optimal choice of therapy. If after 24–48 h blood cultures remain negative but the diagnosis of subacute IE still seems likely, antibiotic treatment should not be further delayed; two additional sets of blood cultures should be taken (separate venepunctures) and empirical therapy should be started. The antibiotic regimen chosen should cover most species of streptococci, which are the organisms most likely to cause subacute endocarditis. The recommended regimens for empirical therapy are listed in Table 49.1.

STREPTOCOCCAL ENDOCARDITIS

Streptococci are the most common cause of subacute IE. Many different species fall under this classification, with a variety of antibiotic sensitivity patterns (Table 49.2).

Table 49.1 Empirical regimens for treatment of IE when the pathogen is unknown[1]

Indication	Drug/dose	Route	Frequency	Duration	Notes
Acute endocarditis syndrome					
First-line regimen	Flucloxacillin or nafcillin 2 g +	i.v.	Every 4 h	Until pathogen is identified, or 4 weeks, whichever is longer	Serum concentrations of gentamicin and vancomycin should be monitored, and doses adjusted accordingly
	gentamicin 1 mg/kg +	i.v.	Every 8 h		
	vancomycin 15 mg/kg not to exceed 2 g/day	i.v.	Every 12 h		
Alternative regimen	Ceftazidime 2.0 g +	i.v.	Every 8 h	Until pathogen is identified, or 4 weeks, whichever is longer	For patients allergic to penicillins but not cephalosporin. Serum concentrations of gentamicin and vancomycin should be monitored, and doses adjusted accordingly
	gentamicin 1 mg/kg +	i.v.	Every 8 h		
	vancomycin 15 mg/kg not to exceed 2 g/day	i.v.	Every 12 h		
Subacute endocarditis syndrome					
First-line regimen	Ampicillin 2.0 g +	i.v.	Every 4 h	Until pathogen is identified, or 4 weeks, whichever is longer	
	gentamicin 1.5 mg/kg or	i.v.	Every 12 h		
	Vancomycin 15 mg/kg not to exceed 2 g/day +	i.v.	Every 12 h		
	gentamicin 1.5 mg/kg	i.v.	Every 12 h		

Table 49.2 Summary of treatment options for various species and strains of streptococci that may cause infective endocarditis

Group or genus	Selected species	Sensitivity	Main options for treatment
Viridans streptococci	*Str. sanguis, Str. mutans, Str. mitior, Str. oralis*	Majority fully sensitive to penicillin; some intermediate; a few resistant	1. Penicillin or cephalosporin alone 2. Penicillin or cephalosporin + aminoglycoside 3. Vancomycin
Nutritionally variant strains of viridans streptococci	*Abiotrophia (Str.) adjacens*	More likely to be tolerant or partially resistant to penicillin	β-Lactam + aminoglycoside
Group D Enterococci	*E. faecalis* *E. faecium* *E. durans* *E. gallinarum* *E. casseliflavus*	Usually resistant to penicillin; high and increasing rate of resistance to aminoglycosides and vancomycin	1. Penicillin + aminoglycoside 2. Vancomycin 3. Vancomycin + aminoglycoside
Non-enterococci	*Str. bovis* *Str. equinus*	Fully sensitive to penicillin	As for viridans group
Group B streptococci	*Str. agalactiae*	Fully sensitive to penicillin	
Group A, C, G streptococci	*Str. pyogenes*	Fully sensitive to penicillin	
Pneumococci	*Str. pneumoniae*	Majority fully sensitive to penicillin; some intermediate, a few resistant	

Penicillin-sensitive streptococci

Most strains of non-enterococcal streptococci are still fully penicillin sensitive, defined by an MIC of penicillin of <0.1 mg/l, (this includes the common non-enterococcal group D species, *Str. bovis*). Several reliable regimens are available for treatment of uncomplicated IE caused by the sensitive streptococci (Table 49.2). The microbiological cure rate achieved by these regimens against such organisms is approximately 98%, a rate so high that clinical trials have been unable to demonstrate significant differences between the regimens. The choice of regimen should be made on grounds of convenience and cost, for each case. Intravenous once-daily ceftriaxone for 4 weeks has the advantage of allowing many patients without complications or other contraindications to be discharged from hospital on outpatient parenteral therapy well before the end of treatment. If patients are properly selected, outpatient therapy is safe, popular with patients and economical.

A minority of strains of viridans streptococci are partially resistant to penicillin, with MICs between 0.1 and 1.0 mg/l. This is usually termed 'intermediate penicillin sensitivity'. IE due to these strains should be treated with a regimen that includes an aminoglycoside to ensure high cure rates (Table 49.4). Alternatively, vancomycin alone could be used. The frequency of penicillin-resistant viridans streptococci, defined as strains for which the MIC is 1.0 mg/l or more, has risen significantly in recent years. These strains should be treated as if they were enterococci (Table 49.3).

Enterococci

These important species (Table 49.2) cause 5–15% of cases of subacute IE. Because enterococci show high rates of both intrinsic and acquired resistance to antibiotics, some cases of enterococcal IE are very difficult to treat. This problem has recently worsened because of the appearance of strains that are

Table 49.3 Regimens for infectious endocarditis due to enterococci and penicillin-resistant streptococci (MIC ≥ 1 mg/l), including prosthetic valve endocarditis caused by these species[1]

Indication	Drug/dose	Route	Frequency	Duration (weeks)	Notes
First-line regimen	Penicillin 4 million units (2–3 g) *or* ampicillin 2 g + gentamicin 1 mg/kg	i.v.	Every 4 h	4–6	For strains that do not have high-level resistance to gentamicin
Alternative regimen	Vancomycin 15 mg/kg not to exceed 2 g/day total dose +	i.v.	Every 12 h	4–6	For highly penicillin- resistant strains; monitoring for toxicity essential
	gentamicin 1 mg/kg	i.v.	Every 8 h	4–6	

Table 49.4 Recommended regimens for treatment of streptococcal (non-enterococcal) infective endocarditis

Indication	Drug/dose	Route	Frequency	Duration (weeks)	Notes
Penicillin-sensitive strains	Penicillin 2–4 million units (1.2–2.4 g)	i.v.	Every 6 h	4	Suitable for most patients who are not hypersensitive to penicillin
First-line regimens	Ceftriaxone 1–2 g	i.v. or i.m.	Once daily	4	Suitable for most patients; convenient for outpatient therapy
	Penicillin 3–4 million units (1.8–2.4 g) +	i.v.	Every 4 h	2	For patients <60 years old with no major complications
	gentamicin 3 mg/kg	i.v. or i.m.	Once daily	2	
	Ceftriaxone 1–2 g +	i.v. or i.m.	Once daily	2	For patients <60 years old with no major complications
	gentamicin 3 mg/kg	i.v. or i.m.	Once daily	2	
Alternative regimens	Ceftriaxone 2 g *followed by*	i.v. or i.m.	Once daily	2	Economical regimen; convenient for outpatient therapy
	amoxicillin 1 g	Orally	4 times daily	2	
	Vancomycin 15 mg/kg, not to exceed total dose of 2 g/day	i.v.	Every 12 h	4	For patients who cannot tolerate any β-lactam antibiotics
Partially resistant strains (MIC 0.1–1.0 mg/l)					
First-line regimen	Penicillin 3–4 million units (1.8–2.4 g) +	i.v.	Every 4 h	4	
	gentamicin 1 mg/kg	i.v. or i.m.	Every 8 h	4	
Alternative regimen	Vancomycin 15 mg/kg, not to exceed total dose of 4 g/day +	i.v.	Every 12 h	4	For patients hypersensitive to penicillin; needs careful monitoring of serum creatinine and antibiotic concentrations to manage toxicity
	gentamicin 1 mg/kg	i.v. or i.m.	Every 8 h	4	

vancomycin resistant (mostly *E. faecium*) or β-lactamase producing (mostly *E. faecalis*).

Each isolate should be tested for antibiotic sensitivity to guide choice of treatment. Standard strains of *E. faecalis* are killed synergistically by penicillin plus an aminoglycoside, even if standard tests show that they are partially resistant to both drugs. The combination has long been proven effective for treatment of enterococcal IE, and therefore is recommended as the first-line regimen (Tables 49.3 and 49.5). However, synergistic killing is unlikely if the strain has one or more of the following properties: high-level resistance to gentamicin and/or streptomycin (MIC >500 mg/l or >2000 mg/l, respectively), high-level intrinsic resistance to penicillin (MIC >64 mg/l), or β-lactamase production (MIC >64 mg/l). For these strains, a regimen including vancomycin (Table 49.3 and 49.5) should be used, unless the strain is resistant to it. Unfortunately, multiple-drug resistance is common among enterococci. For example, vancomycin-resistant strains frequently have high-level intrinsic resistance to penicillins.

Because published experience with treatment of IE caused

Table 49.5 Potential drugs for treatment of infectious endocarditis caused by highly resistant or multiresistant enterococci. In each case, the choice will be affected by the sensitivity pattern of the individual strain isolated (M. E. Levison, personal communication)

Resistance profile	Potential therapeutic options
High-level gentamicin resistance, MIC >500 mg/l	Cell wall active drug plus streptomycin
High-level streptomycin resistance, MIC >2000 mg/l	Cell wall active agent plus gentamicin
High-level resistance to both gentamicin and streptomycin	Cell wall active drug for 12 weeks or more, plus surgery as indicated
β-Lactamase-producing organism with high-level aminoglycoside resistance	Ampicillin–sulbactam, imipenem or glycopeptide
High-level penicillin resistance, MIC >64 mg/l	Glycopeptide plus aminoglycoside
Vancomycin A resistance, penicillin sensitive	β-Lactam plus aminoglycoside
Vancomycin A resistance, high-level penicillin resistance	Fluoroquinolone, doxycycline, teicoplanin, novobiocin, streptogramins (two or more, according to sensitivity test results)
Vancomycin B resistance, penicillin sensitive	β-Lactam or teicoplanin plus aminoglycoside
Vancomycin B resistance, high-level penicillin resistance	Teicoplanin plus aminoglycoside

by the most resistant strains of enterococci is limited, validated treatment regimens are not available. Some potentially useful alternative antimicrobials are listed in Table 49.5. For strains resistant to both vancomycin and aminoglycosides but partially sensitive to ampicillin, treatment can be attempted with an extended course of high-dose ampicillin alone: 16–20 g/day intravenously for 12 weeks or more. For vancomycin-resistant strains that also produce penicillinase, treatment can be attempted with ampicillin–sulbactam or amoxicillin–clavulanate. Other antibiotics may be chosen on the basis of sensitivity testing. Potentially active drugs include linezolid, teicoplanin, daptomycin, quinupristin–dalfopristin, fluoroquinolones, doxycycline and novobiocin. When non-standard regimens are used to treat these resistant strains treatment should be prolonged (8–12 weeks or more, if toxicity allows) and valve replacement surgery should be considered early to improve the chance of microbiological cure.

STAPHYLOCOCCI

Staphylococci are the second most common group of bacteria causing IE, after the streptococci. They cause a variety of IE syndromes, the two most important being acute IE due to *Staph. aureus* and prosthetic valve infection by *Staph. epidermidis*. The outcome of staphylococcal IE is generally less favorable than for streptococcal infections, and surgical intervention for complications, especially abscesses, is more likely to be needed. Because most strains are penicillin-resistant due to β-lactamase production, the first-line treatment is a penicillinase-resistant β-lactam agent (Table 49.6). Patients who are hypersensitive to β-lactam drugs should be treated with vancomycin. Methicillin-resistant strains of *Staph. aureus* and *Staph. epidermidis* have become common (15–50% of isolates);

these also require treatment with vancomycin. Because there are few satisfactory alternatives, the emergence of partial or full vancomycin resistance among staphylococci poses a serious threat to the effective treatment of IE. Currently linezolid appears to be an effective alternative to vancomycin, but experience with this new antibiotic is limited and resistance may emerge in the future, as it has for all other major antibiotics. Daptomycin, under clinical trial at the time of writing, is also likely to be effective.

Prosthetic valve infection with *Staph. epidermidis* is difficult to cure. Therefore, treatment with two or three antibiotics for at least 6 weeks is usually recommended, with surgical intervention as needed. Recommended regimens for the treatment of staphylococcal IE are listed in Table 49.6.

FASTIDIOUS GRAM-NEGATIVE ('HACEK') ORGANISMS

The acronym HACEK derives from the initials of the following species: *Haemophilus* spp., *Actinobacillus actinomycetemcomitans*, *Cardiobacterium hominis*, *Eikenella* spp. and *Kingella kingae*. These are small Gram-negative bacilli, which cause 3–5% of cases of IE. They usually cause subacute infection, sometimes with larger-than-usual vegetations, they are often nutritionally fastidious and slow-growing in blood culture, and they are usually sensitive to ampicillin and cephalosporins. Ceftriaxone 2 g (intravenous or intramuscular) plus gentamicin 3 mg/kg (intravenous or intramuscular), both given once daily, is a convenient first-line regimen that can be completed as outpatient therapy in selected patients. Microbiological cure is usually achieved in 3–4 weeks and the overall prognosis is fairly good, although not as favorable as for subacute endocarditis due to penicillin-sensitive streptococci.

Table 49.6 Regimens for treatment of infective endocarditis caused by staphylococci, on native or prosthetic valves[1,4]

Indication	Drug/dose	Route	Frequency	Duration (weeks)	Notes
Staph. aureus Methicillin sensitive	Flucloxacillin or nafcillin 2 g	i.v.	Every 4 h	4–6	Neutropenia may occur. Gentamicin 3 mg/kg daily may be added for the first 3 days to achieve rapid killing by synergy, but is not of proven value
Methicillin resistant	Vancomycin 15 mg/kg, not to exceed 2 g/day	i.v.	Every 12 h	4–6	
Staph. epidermidis	Vancomycin 15 mg/kg, not to exceed 2 g/day +	i.v.	Every 12 h	4–6	
	gentamicin 1.5 mg/kg +	i.v.	Every 12 h	4–6	
	rifampicin 300 mg	i.v.	Twice daily	4–6	

GRAM-NEGATIVE BACILLI

Although the aerobic Gram-negative bacilli are common human pathogens that often cause bacteremias, they seldom cause endocarditis. For example, IE caused by *Escherichia coli* or *Klebsiella* spp. is rare, even when bacteremia occurs in a patient with pre-existing valvular disease. The most important genus with respect to IE is *Pseudomonas*, which occasionally causes IE in parenteral drug addicts or in patients with prosthetic valves. IE caused by *Brucella* species is important in some geographic regions, especially Spain and other countries bordering the Mediterranean.

Gram-negative bacilli tend to cause acute endocarditis, which is more difficult to cure and carries high morbidity and mortality. Treatment for each case should be chosen on the basis of antibiotic sensitivity testing of the etiological organism. The preferred regimens combine a β-lactam antibiotic with an aminoglycoside, to be given parenterally for 6 weeks. Toxicity or drug hypersensitivity may occur during this long period of treatment, requiring either dose adjustment or change to another regimen. The rate of relapse after treatment is notably higher than for antibiotic-sensitive Gram-positive bacteria.

ENDOCARDITIS DUE TO UNUSUAL PATHOGENS

The list of other organisms known to cause IE is long, but most are uncommon or rare. Strict anaerobes only rarely infect the heart, causing less than 1% of cases of IE. *Coxiella burnetii* causes a subacute systemic infection that may involve native or prosthetic heart valves. Microbiological cure is difficult to achieve with antimicrobials alone, so relapse is common. The highest chance of cure requires prolonged treatment with a tetracycline plus hydroxychloroquine, for 12 months, plus valve replacement. If surgery cannot be undertaken, treatment for at least 18 months is recommended; some experts suggest continuing suppressive therapy for life in these cases. *Chlamydia* spp. can cause IE, but are even more rare than infection by *Coxiella* spp. About 50 cases of IE caused by *Bartonella* spp. have been reported, often in homeless men, alcoholics, or occasionally in patients with AIDS. The optimal treatment for IE caused by *Bartonella* appears to be parenteral aminoglycoside plus either rifampicin or a macrolide for 6 weeks.

IE caused by two or more organisms (polymicrobial infection) occurs occasionally, especially in parenteral drug addicts, but even in these patients accounts for less than 3% of cases.

FUNGAL ENDOCARDITIS

The most common form of fungal endocarditis is caused by yeasts, usually *Candida* spp. Most at risk are parenteral drug addicts, patients in hospital, (especially neonates and those on prolonged parenteral nutrition), and patients with prosthetic valves. Blood cultures are less likely to be positive than in untreated bacterial endocarditis; repeated sampling will increase the chance of isolating yeasts. The best chance of cure requires valve replacement plus antifungal therapy. The disease is too rare to allow clinical trials comparing regimens such as amphotericin B and imidazoles, and the optimal duration of therapy is unknown. A few cases have been cured with antifungal therapy alone when surgery could not be performed. In this situation, an imidazole such as fluconazole should be administered for 6–24 months, and possibly even longer. If the yeast is resistant to imidazoles, amphotericin B can be given until toxicity prevents its continuation. The prognosis for IE due to yeasts is worse than for bacterial endocarditis, but much better than for IE due to molds.

Either native or prosthetic valves may become infected with a mold. The most common pathogen is an *Aspergillus* species,

---

Box 49.2 Estimates of risk for infective endocarditis related to pre-existing cardiac disorders[3,4]

Relatively high risk	Intermediate risk	Low or negligible risk
Prosthetic heart valves	Mitral valve prolapse with regurgitation	Mitral valve prolapse without regurgitation
Previous infective endocarditis	Pure mitral stenosis	Trivial valvular regurgitation by echocardiography
Cyanotic congenital heart disease	Tricuspid valve disease	without structural abnormality
Patent ductus arteriosus	Pulmonary stenosis	Isolated atrial septal defect
Aortic regurgitation*	Asymmetric septal hypertrophy	Arteriosclerotic plaques
Aortic stenosis*	Bicuspid aortic valve or calcific aortic sclerosis	Coronary artery disease
Mitral regurgitation	with minimal hemodynamic abnormality	Cardiac pacemaker
Mitral stenosis and regurgitation	Degenerative valvular disease in elderly patients	Surgically repaired intracardiac lesions with minimal
Ventricular septal defect	Surgically repaired intracardiac lesions, with	or no hemodynamic abnormality, less than 6
Coarctation of the aorta	minimal or no hemodynamic abnormality, more	months after operation
Surgically repaired intracardiac lesions	than 6 months after operation	
with residual hemodynamic abnormality		

* Includes tricuspid, bicuspid and unicuspid valves.

but many other molds have been reported as rare causes of IE. This distinct form of fungal IE is characterized by a high rate of negative blood cultures, and a very poor prognosis. Surgery is the mainstay of treatment, but amphotericin B or another antifungal drug should be given according to the sensitivity of the etiological species. Valve replacement should be performed whenever feasible, because cure without surgery is rare.

PREVENTION OF INFECTIVE ENDOCARDITIS

Although IE is an uncommon disease, prevention is desirable because of its high morbidity and significant mortality. Most cases cannot be prevented, because the time of onset and the portal of entry for causative organisms cannot precisely be predicted. However, up to 5–7% of cases could be due to bacteria introduced during dental, surgical and diagnostic procedures. Tooth extraction appears to present a significant risk for viridans streptococcal IE in patients with predisposing cardiac conditions. For this reason, antibiotics are recommended before such procedures in an attempt to prevent some cases of IE.

Antibiotics can prevent experimental endocarditis in rabbits and rats, but have not been proven effective in humans. Therefore, this remains an empiric practice, which may have been overused in the past. Unnecessary use of antibiotics could promote emergence of resistant bacteria. Prophylaxis for IE is probably not cost-effective as a general strategy, but it may be worth while in selected situations. The recommended approach is to give antibiotic to selected patients with higher risk cardiac conditions such as prosthetic valves or previous endocarditis (Box 49.2) before higher risk procedures such as tooth extraction or urinary tract surgery (Box 49.3). Prophylaxis should be considered optional for intermediate risk and unnecessary for low-risk situations.

Each patient should be given clear instruction on the procedure for notifying healthcare providers of his or her condition and for obtaining antibiotic premedication. Preferably this information should be communicated in writing, in the form of a letter or printed wallet card kept by the patient. The regimen should be chosen according to standard recommendations such as those provided by the British Society for Antimicrobial Chemotherapy[6] and the American Heart Association[5] (Table 49.7).

Box 49.3 Recommendations for use of prophylaxis for endocarditis with various procedures which may cause bacteremia[3,5]

Prophylaxis recommended	Prophylaxis not recommended
Dental extractions, and intra-oral procedures that cause bleeding, including professional cleaning and scaling	Minor dental procedures not likely to cause bleeding, such as adjustment of orthodontic appliances, simple fillings above the gum line, root canal
Tonsillectomy, adenoidectomy and other operations that involve upper respiratory mucosa	Injection of intraoral local anesthetic
Sclerotherapy for esophageal varices and esophageal dilatation	Shedding of primary teeth
Cystoscopy, urethral dilatation	Tympanostomy tube insertion
Urethral catheterization if urinary infection present	Endotracheal tube insertion
Urinary tract surgery, including prostatic surgery	Bronchoscopy with flexible bronchoscope, with or without biopsy
Incision and drainage of infected tissue	Cardiac catheterization
Vaginal delivery complicated by infection	Gastrointestinal endoscopy with or without biopsy
Vaginal hysterectomy	Cesarian section and hysterectomy
	In the absence of infection: urethral catheterization, dilatation and curettage, uncomplicated vaginal delivery, therapeutic abortion, insertion or removal of intra-uterine device, sterilization procedures, laparoscopy

Table 49.7 Current recommendations for prophylaxis of endocarditis[a]

Indication	Regimen
Standard regimen	
For dental procedures; oral or upper respiratory tract surgery; minor gastrointestinal (GI) or genitourinary (GU) tract procedure	Amoxicillin 3.0 g orally 1 h before, then 1.5 g 6 h later
Special regimens	
Oral regimen for penicillin-allergic patients (oral and respiratory tract only)	Clindamycin 600 mg orally 1 h before, then 300 mg 6 h later
Parenteral regimen for high-risk patients; also for GI or GU tract procedures	Ampicillin 2 g i.v. or i.m. plus gentamicin 1.5 mg/kg i.v. or i.m. 0.5 h before
Parenteral regimen for penicillin-allergic patients	Vancomycin 1 g i.v. slowly over 1 h, starting 1 h before; add gentamicin 1.5 mg/kg i.v. or i.m. 0.5 h before
Parenteral regimen for penicillin-allergic patients	Vancomycin 1 g i.v. slowly over 1 h, starting 1 h before; add gentamicin 1.5 mg/kg i.m. or i.v. if gastrointestinal or genitourinary tract involved
Cardiac surgery including implantation of prosthetic valves	Cefazolin 2 g i.v. at induction of anesthesia, repeated 8 and 16 h later *or* Vancomycin 1 g i.v. slowly over 1 h starting at induction, then 1 g i.v. 12 h later

[a] Note that occasional prevention failures may occur with any regimen. These are recommendations only; clinical judgment as to safety and cost-benefit of prophylaxis should guide the decision in individual cases. One or two additional doses may be given if the period of risk for bacteremia is prolonged. Gentamicin, 1.5 mg/kg i.v., may be given with each dose to increase activity against Gram-negative bacteria. Adapted from Dajani et al[5], Durack[3] and Working Party of the British Society for Antimicrobial Chemotherapy[6]

References

1. Wilson WR, Karchmer AW, Dajani AS et al 1995 Antibiotic treatment of adults with infective endocarditis due to viridans streptococci, enterococci, other streptococci, staphylococci, and HACEK microorganisms. *Journal of the American Medical Association* 274: 1706–1713

2. Durack DT, Lukes AS, Bright DK, Duke Endocarditis Service 1994 New criteria for diagnosis of infective endocarditis: utilization of specific echocardiographic findings. *American Journal of Medicine* 96: 200–209

3. Durack DT 1995 Prevention of infective endocarditis. *New England Journal of Medicine* 332: 38–44

4. Durack DT 1997 Infective and noninfective endocarditis. In: Schlant RC (ed.) *The heart*, 9th edn. McGraw Hill, New York

5. Dajani AS, Bisno AL, Chung KJ et al 1990 Prevention of bacterial endocarditis. Recommendations by the American Heart Association. *Journal of the American Medical Association* 264: 2919–2922

6. Working Party of the British Society for Antimicrobial Chemotherapy 1985 Antibiotic treatment of streptococcal and staphylococcal endocarditis. *Lancet* 2: 815–817

Further information

Fowler VG, Durack DT 1994 Infective endocarditis. *Current Opinion in Cardiology* 9: 389–400

Francioli P, Etienne J, Hoigne R, Thys JP, Gerber A 1992 Treatment of streptococcal endocarditis with a single daily dose of ceftriaxone sodium for 4 weeks: efficacy and outpatient treatment feasibility. *Journal of the American Medical Association* 267: 264–267

Stamboulian D, Bonvehi P, Arevalo C 1991 Antibiotic management of outpatients with endocarditis due to penicillin-susceptible streptococci. *Reviews of Infectious Diseases* 13 (Suppl. 2): S160–S163

50 Infections of the gastrointestinal tract

Peter Moss

Infectious diseases may affect any part of the gastrointestinal tract from the mouth to the anus. Most infections of the mouth, oropharynx, and esophagus are caused either by commensal organisms or by opportunist pathogens. These infections are usually secondary to underlying problems, either local (such as poor oral hygiene, or malignancy) or systemic (particularly immunosuppression). Infections of the stomach are relatively unusual, with the exception of *Helicobacter pylori*, which is associated with peptic ulceration and gastric neoplasms. It is infections of the lower gastrointestinal tract, the small and large bowel, which are of the greatest clinical significance.

Intestinal infections usually present with diarrhea, sometimes accompanied by vomiting, abdominal pain, and fever. In severe cases there may be dehydration, hypovolemic shock, and renal failure. Persistent infection may cause anorexia and weight loss. Gastroenteritis may be caused by viruses, bacteria, protozoa, or (rarely) by helminths. Symptoms and signs may be produced by one or more of a number of different pathologic mechanisms. The clinical presentation of gastroenteritis rarely allows a specific diagnosis, and it is not usually possible to identify the causative organism, at least in the early stages of illness. Management is therefore usually empirical, and is based on the recognition of common clinical syndromes. These include acute watery diarrhea, dysentery, persistent diarrhea with or without malabsorption, and enteric fever. Identification of these patterns, along with a knowledge of the likely pathogens in a particular location and patient population, will guide treatment in most cases.

EPIDEMIOLOGY

Gastroenteritis causing diarrhea with or without vomiting is the third most common infectious cause of death (behind HIV/AIDS and lower respiratory tract infection). Although oral rehydration programs have cut the death toll significantly, at least 2.25 million people die every year as a direct result of diarrheal disease.[1] Gastroenteritis is a major cause of morbidity as well as mortality, with a disease burden of 100 million disability-adjusted life years (DALY) in the developing world.[2] The main burden falls on the poorest countries, where children can expect on average 3–6 bouts of infective diarrhea every year, and 15–30% of deaths under the age of 5 are due to diarrheal disease. In the Western world gastroenteritis is both less common and less likely to cause death, but it remains an important cause of mortality and morbidity. In Europe diarrheal disease is responsible for 30 000 deaths per year, and results in a burden of over one million DALY annually.[1]

Viral gastroenteritis is a common cause of diarrhea and vomiting in young children in both developed and developing countries, but is less often seen in adults. The viruses responsible (principally rotavirus and enteric adenoviruses) are spread from person to person, mainly by the feco-oral route, but also as an aerosol. Seasonal outbreaks are seen in developed countries, and in comparison with other diarrheal diseases there is less association with poverty and poor hygiene.

The main cause of adult gastroenteritis is bacterial infection. In developed countries this is often related to food poisoning, a problem exacerbated by modern methods of food production and the globalization of food supply. In less developed areas transmission is frequently by the direct feco-oral route, or from a contaminated water supply. Massive water-borne outbreaks may occur, especially in association with natural disasters or war. Protozoal and helminthic gut infections are rare in the West but are widespread in developing countries.

In all parts of the world it is children who are at most risk of catching diarrheal disease, and at most risk of dying from it. Mortality is mainly related to dehydration, although other factors such as malnutrition are important in developing countries. Elderly people are also at increased risk of complications from gastroenteritis. In the developed world certain other groups have a higher incidence of diarrheal disease: these include travellers to developing countries, gay men, and infants in daycare facilities.

PATHOGENESIS OF ENTERIC INFECTION

Micro-organisms with the potential to cause enteric infection are ubiquitous, and the development of disease depends on a number of host and microbial factors.

- Host factors include age and general health, personal hygiene, specific and non-specific immunity, and composition of normal intestinal microflora.
- Microbial factors include a number of virulence traits which determine the pathogenic mechanisms responsible for causing gastrointestinal infection.

Bacteria can cause diarrhea in three different ways: mucosal adherence, toxin production, and mucosal invasion (Table 50.1). Many species employ more than one of these methods. In most cases the first step in the pathogenic process is adherence to the intestinal mucosa; the exception being those bacteria which secrete toxin in food before consumption. A number of different molecular adhesion mechanisms have been elaborated, typically involving microbial cell surface proteins (often located on pili or fimbriae) which bind to specific host glycoproteins.[3] Expression of many of these adhesion proteins is encoded by transmissable plasmids. Usually attachment to the mucosa is merely the prelude to invasion or toxin production, but a few organisms such as enteropathogenic *Escherichia coli* can produce mucosal damage and secretory diarrhea directly as a result of adherence.

Some bacteria, having attached to the intestinal mucosa, simply colonize the surface epithelium. Others, such as *Shigella* species and the invasive strains of *Esch. coli*, penetrate and destroy the cells of the intestinal mucosa. Many different mechanisms may be involved in the invasive process, including attachment to transmembrane glycoproteins, production of cytotoxic exotoxins, and deliberate induction of host inflammatory response.[4] Invasion leads to destruction of the epithelial cells, and produces the typical symptoms of dysentery: low volume bloody diarrhea with abdominal pain.

Many bacterial enteric pathogens produce symptoms by means of toxin production. Gastroenteritis can be caused by three different types of bacterial toxins.

- Enterotoxins induce excessive fluid secretion into the bowel lumen without physically damaging the mucosa.
- Neurotoxins affect the autonomic nervous system, causing diarrhea and vomiting.

- Cytotoxins damage the intestinal mucosa and, in some cases, vascular endothelium as well.

Usually these toxins are produced by bacteria adhering to the intestinal epithelium, but neurotoxins (often stable to heat and gastric acid) may be elaborated exogenously by pathogens in poorly prepared food.

The pathogenic mechanisms underlying viral gastroenteritis are less well understood. The initial event is again adhesion, a viral capsid protein binding to specific glycolipid receptors in the mucosal cell membrane. This is followed by invasion, mainly of mature villus epithelial cells in the small intestine. A direct cytopathic effect leads to cell death, causing villus shortening, relative loss of absorptive epithelial cells relative to secretory crypt cells, and decreased production of intestinal disaccharidases.[5,6] In some cases (such as infection with Norwalk virus) there is significant mucosal inflammation, while in others (including rotavirus infection) there is little host inflammatory response. Diarrhea is probably produced by a combination of secretory/resorptive imbalance and disaccharide/fat malabsorption (which may persist for some time following acute infection).

Protozoa can cause diarrhea by both invasive and non-invasive mechanisms. *Entamoeba histolytica* (and probably *Balantidium coli*) attaches to the colonic mucosa by specific binding proteins. It then causes local destruction of the epithelium by a combination of lytic enzyme release and phagocytosis, leading to the clinical symptoms of dysentery. *Giardia lamblia (intestinalis)*, by contrast, is very rarely invasive. The parasite attaches to the duodenal and jejunal mucosa using a combination of mechanical and molecular bonds. Local disruption of the brush border ensues, with disaccharidase deficiency. There may also be more extensive damage to the epithelium with partial villous atrophy and inflammatory infiltrates: this is probably due to a cellular immune response to infection.[7] Several different pathogenic mechanisms may be important in the production of diarrhea by *Cryptosporidium parvum* (depending in part on the integrity of the host immune system), while the role of other parasites such as *Dientamoeba*

Table 50.1 Pathogenic mechanisms of bacterial gastroenteritis

Mechanism	Mode of action	Clinical presentation	Examples
Mucosal adherence	Effacement of intestinal mucosa	Moderate watery diarrhea	Enteropathogenic *Escherichia coli*
Toxin production			
Neurotoxin	Paralysis of autonomic nervous system	Short-lived, profuse watery diarrhea and vomiting	*Bacillus cereus*
Enterotoxin	Fluid secretion without mucosal damage	Variable diarrhea +/− vomiting	*Vibrio cholerae*
Cytotoxin	Damage to mucosa	Bloody diarrhea	Enterohaemorrhagic *Escherichia coli*
Mucosal invasion	Penetration and destruction of mucosa	Dysentery	*Shigella* spp.

fragilis and *Blastocystis hominis* in causing gastroenteritis remains unclear.

Although helminthic infection of the gut is very common, it rarely causes significant enteric symptoms. Schistosomal colitis can result from the inflammatory response to parasite eggs lodged in the bowel wall, and some nematodes (notably *Trichuris trichuria*) may cause symptoms due to superficial invasion of the colonic mucosa. Heavy worm infestations may cause mechanical problems such as obstruction or prolapse.

SYNDROMIC MANAGEMENT OF GASTROENTERITIS

SYNDROMES

Acute watery diarrhea

Acute, self-limiting, watery diarrhea is the most common form of gastroenteritis. It is produced by direct or toxin-mediated damage to the secretory and absorptive gut mucosal cells, and may be caused by a number of different pathogens (Table 50.2). Specific microbiological diagnosis is rarely necessary, as antimicrobial therapy is not usually required. The morbidity and mortality of acute watery diarrhea is largely related to dehydration (especially in children), and by far the most important component of management is adequate rehydration. In most cases this can be achieved by oral rehydration solutions (ORS), although intravenous fluids may occasionally be needed.

Dehydration is assessed clinically (Table 50.3), and treatment depends on the degree of fluid loss. Mildly dehydrated individuals should be given increased fluids; infants and children should continue feeding normally if possible. For moderate dehydration, ORS 75–100 ml/kg is given within the first 4 h, followed by further fluids to replace loss. Children should continue feeding once initial rehydration is completed. Intravenous rehydration is required only for severely dehydrated individuals with features of collapse. Several liters of intravenous fluid are usually required to overcome the features of shock: adults and older children should be given 30 ml/kg in the first 30 minutes, then 70 ml/kg over the next 2½ h; the rates should be halved for infants under 12 months.[8] Maintenance of hydration can usually be achieved with ORS. In moderate and severe dehydration the patient must be reassessed regularly to ensure that adequate fluid is being given. Attention should also be paid to nutrition, acid–base status and electrolytes, especially if the diarrhea is prolonged.

Antimicrobial therapy is rarely indicated in the empirical management of acute watery diarrhea. Antibiotics may lead to a decrease in the duration and severity of symptoms in some cases, but the improvement is small, and the condition is usually mild and self-limiting anyway.[9,10] The use of antibiotics depends on individual circumstances, the benefits of treatment being balanced against cost, risk of drug side effects, and the

Table 50.2 Clinical syndromes of gastroenteritis, and typical causative organisms

	Acute watery diarrhea	**Bloody diarrhea**	**Persistent diarrhea**
Viruses	Rotavirus Enteric adenoviruses Caliciviruses Astroviruses		Recurrent infections with rotavirus
Bacteria	*Salmonella enterica* serotypes *Campylobacter jejuni* Enteropathogenic *Escherichia coli* Enterotoxigenic *Escherichia coli* Enteroaggregative *Escherichia coli* *Vibrio cholerae* *Vibrio parahaemolyticus* *Clostridium difficile* *Staphylococcus aureus* (toxin b) *Bacillus cereus*	*Salmonella enterica* serotypes *Campylobacter jejuni* *Shigella* spp. Enteroinvasive *Escherichia coli* Enterohemorrhagic *Escherichia coli* *Yersinia enterocolitica* *Clostridium difficile*	*Mycobacterium tuberculosis* Recurrent or relapsing infections with other bacterial pathogens
Protozoa	*Giardia lamblia* *Cryptosporidium parvum* *Isospora belli* *Cyclospora cayetanensis* *Dientamoeba fragilis*	*Entamoeba histolytica* *Balantidium coli*	*Giardia lamblia* *Entamoeba histolytica* *Cryptosporidium parvum* *Isospora belli* *Cyclospora cayetanensis*
Miscellaneous		*Schistosoma mansoni* *Trichuris trichiura*	Postinfectious irritable bowel syndrome Disaccharidase deficiency

Table 50.3 Assessment of dehydration in acute diarrhea

Symptom/sign	No/minimal dehydration	Moderate dehydration	Severe dehydration
Mental state	Alert	Restless, irritable	Lethargic or unconscious; floppy infant
Eyes	Normal	Sunken	Very sunken, dry
Tears	Present	Absent	Absent
Tongue	Moist	Dry	Very dry
Thirst	Drinks normally	Drinks very eagerly	Unable to drink
Skin pinch	Goes back rapidly	Goes back slowly	Goes back very slowly
Probable fluid deficit	<2.5% body weight	2.5–10% body weight	>10% body weight
Management	Increased fluids	Oral rehydration	Intravenous fluids

likelihood of promoting antibiotic resistance. In cases in which there is strong clinical suspicion of cholera or other infection that requires specific treatment antibiotics should be started empirically while awaiting confirmation. Occasionally acute watery diarrhea may be the presenting symptom of an enteric infection which develops into persistent diarrhea (for example giardiasis) or dysentery (shigellosis or *Campylobacter* infection). In these cases antibiotic therapy may be necessary when the diagnosis becomes clear.

Dysentery

Dysentery is a clinical syndrome of bloody, usually low volume, diarrhea, often associated with abdominal pain and fever. It is caused by infection with invasive enteropathogens (Table 50.2). Fluid and electrolyte loss is not as great as in watery diarrhea, although ORS may still be important, especially in children. Morbidity and mortality are often due to complications other than dehydration, including perforation, sepsis, and hemolytic uremic syndrome (HUS). In most cases of bacillary dysentery antibiotics significantly reduce the severity and duration of illness, and in some instances decrease mortality.[8] Antimicrobials should always be used in shigellosis and amebic dysentery, and may be helpful in other forms of bacillary dysentery. However, in dysentery caused by verotoxigenic *Esch. coli* antibiotic treatment increases the risk of toxin-mediated HUS, and antibiotics should be used with caution if this is suspected.[11]

Persistent diarrhea

Infective diarrhea that continues for more than 14 days is defined as persistent, and may occur with or without malabsorption. It may be continuous, but is frequently intermittent, varying from day to day. Persistent diarrhea is often associated with weight loss and malnutrition, and accounts for most diarrheal deaths in children. It may be due to recurrent or relapsing infection with common and usually self-limiting

bacterial or viral pathogens, especially in malnourished individuals. In other cases, such as giardiasis, Whipple's disease, and intestinal tuberculosis, chronic diarrhea is the normal presentation in the absence of specific treatment (Table 50.2). Immunocompromised patients, especially those infected with HIV, are susceptible to a variety of pathogens causing persistent diarrhea.

It is important to identify the infecting organism as specific treatment is often required. If this is not possible, empirical treatment based on local patterns of infection in relevant patients should be used. This is particularly important in people with HIV/AIDS. If malnutrition is either contributing to or resulting from infection, nutritional supplements should be given. Antimotility agents may give symptomatic relief when the underlying cause cannot be diagnosed or treated.

In some cases persistent diarrhea may be triggered by an acute and self-limiting infection. A number of pathogens, including rotavirus, can cause villus damage and disaccharidase deficiency, leading to malabsorption. This is managed by temporary withdrawal of the malabsorbed nutrient. Postinfectious irritable bowel may follow infection with some gastrointestinal pathogens.

Enteric fever

Enteric fever is primarily a systemic illness, although the spread is feco-oral and the portal of entry gastrointestinal. The diagnosis is based on typical features, confirmed by isolation of the organism from blood or bone marrow. Treatment is with specific antimicrobial therapy.

Travellers' diarrhea

Travellers' diarrhea is defined as the passage of three or more unformed stools per day in a resident of an industrialized country travelling in or recently returned from a developing nation. Infection is usually food- or water-borne, and younger travellers are most often affected (probably reflecting behavior patterns). Reported attack rates vary from country to country, but approach 50% for a 2-week stay in many tropical countries. It may be caused by a wide variety of pathogens, the most common being enterotoxigenic *Esch. coli*.[12,13] The severity and duration of symptoms can be reduced by antibiotic treatment,[12–14] but the illness is usually relatively mild and self-limiting. ORS should be used to prevent dehydration. The decision to treat with antibiotics should be based on individual circumstances, bearing in mind the cost, potential side effects, and the possible effects on antimicrobial resistance.

SOLUTIONS FOR ORAL AND INTRAVENOUS REHYDRATION

The use of oral rehydration solutions (ORS) is based on the observation that glucose (and other carbohydrates) enhance sodium absorption in the small intestine, even in the presence of secretory loss due to toxins. The recognition of this principle, and the widespread promotion of the use of ORS by the World Health Organization (WHO) and other organizations, has saved millions of lives over the past 20 years. The composition of standard WHO/UNICEF and other ORS is shown in Table 50.4. Because of concerns about hypernatremia, a lower sodium formulation of ORS than that recommended by the WHO and UNICEF is generally used in industrialized countries.

Although standard ORS is effective in replacing fluid loss it does not have any impact on the duration and severity of diarrhea. Other forms of ORS have been developed in an attempt to address this. ORS based on cereal carbohydrate (usually rice) rather than glucose has been shown significantly to decrease stool volume and length of illness in cholera, both in adults and in children.[15] In other forms of acute diarrhea it is at least as good as glucose ORS in replacing fluid loss (even in infants under 6 months), but does not have such a marked impact on the course of the illness.[15–17] Hypo-osmolar ORS has been shown to decrease stool fluid loss in children,[18] although this effect has not been demonstrated in adults, and may be affected by other factors such as concurrent breast feeding.[19,20] Short-chain fatty acids (which are produced in the colon from non-absorbed carbohydrates) enhance sodium absorption, and the addition of amylase-resistant starch to ORS has a significant effect on fluid loss in adults with cholera.[21] Further research is needed to assess the effect of this type of ORS in other types of diarrhea.

Several other supplements have been added to ORS in an attempt to improve its efficacy. The addition of lactobacilli has been shown to improve outcomes in children with rotavirus and non-rotavirus diarrhea, although this has not become standard practice.[22,23] Supplementation of ORS with zinc significantly decreases fluid requirements in malnourished children with persistent diarrhea,[24] but other nutritional supplements such as folic acid have not been shown to help.[25] It is impor-

Table 50.4 Solutions for oral and intravenous rehydration

Solution	Components (mmol/l)		Substance added (grams/l of water)	
Oral				
WHO/UNICEF	Na	90	NaCl	3.5
	Cl	80	Trisodium citrate	2.9
	K	20	KCl	1.5
	Citrate	10	Glucose	20.0
	Glucose	111		
Household (salt based)	Na	85	NaCl	5
	K	80	Glucose	20
	Glucose	111		
Household (rice based)	Na	85	NaCl	5
	K	80	Cooked rice	80
UK/Europe	Na	35–60	Commercial	
	K	20–40	preparations	
	Glucose	90–200		
Intravenous				
Ringer's lactate	Na	130	Commercial	
	Cl	109	preparation	
	K	4		
	Lactate	28		
Dacca solution	Na	134	NaCl	5
	Cl	99	NaHCO$_3$	4
	K	13	KCl	1

tant to keep the preparation and administration of ORS simple: community-based studies have shown that despite instruction a high proportion of mothers are unable to prepare even standard ORS correctly.[26]

In severely dehydrated patients intravenous fluids may be needed for initial resuscitation. The fluid used should contain electrolytes to replace those lost, and bicarbonate or lactate to correct any acid–base imbalance. Examples of suitable commercial and generic solutions are shown in Table 50.4.

DRUGS IN SYNDROMIC MANAGEMENT

Antibiotics

Antibiotics are often prescribed for acute watery diarrhea in developed countries, even though the disease is usually mild and self-limiting (Table 50.5). Quinolones have been shown slightly to decrease the duration and severity of symptoms in adults in industrialized countries;[9,10] there is little information on children (in whom viral diarrhea is much more common), or from the developing world. By decreasing fluid loss antibiotic therapy should help to prevent dehydration, but there is no good evidence that the use of antimicrobials decreases mortality from dehydration or other complications of acute watery diarrhea. It may occasionally be justified on symptomatic grounds in adults with particularly severe or prolonged symp-

toms: in these cases ciprofloxacin 500 mg twice daily for 3–5 days is the best choice. Any benefit from antibiotic therapy has to be balanced against cost, the risk of side effects, and the possibility of inducing resistance.

Treatment with antibiotics is definitely indicated in shigellosis, which is the most common cause of dysentery in the developing world. The benefits are less marked in dysentery due to other organisms such as *Salmonella* and *Campylobacter*, which account for a large proportion of bloody diarrhea in industrialized countries. In general, in countries where shigellosis is relatively rare, antibiotic therapy should be reserved for those with more serious or prolonged symptoms of bloody diarrhea: ciprofloxacin is again the drug of choice. In developing countries adults and children should receive antibiotics: the choice of drug is guided by local patterns of resistance in *Shigella* spp. (*see below*).

Enteric fever should always be treated with antibiotics, and if clinical suspicion is high treatment should be started empirically while results are awaited.

A variety of different antibiotics have been shown to decrease the severity and duration of symptoms in travellers' diarrhea, including trimethoprim–sulfamethoxazole, erythromycin, and quinolones.[14] Ciprofloxacin is effective in a single dose of 500 mg,[27] and is the best choice if antimicrobial therapy is needed. Antibiotic prophylaxis has been recommended in certain cases, but for most travellers the adverse effects (both personal and environmental) are likely to outweigh the benefits.

Table 50.5 Antibiotics in the empirical treatment of acute gastroenteritis

Condition	Drug of choice	Alternatives	Indications	Benefits
Acute watery diarrhea	Ciprofloxacin 500 mg twice daily (15 mg/kg twice daily)	Nalidixic acid 1 g every 6 h (15 mg/kg every 6 h) Erythromycin 500 mg every 6 h (12.5 mg/kg every 6 h) Trimethoprim–sulfamethoxazole 960 mg twice daily (30 mg/kg twice daily)	Severe symptoms, prolonged illness, immunosuppressed patient	Relieves symptoms, shortens illness
Dysentery[a]	Ciprofloxacin 500 mg twice daily (15 mg/kg twice daily)	Ofloxacin 200 mg twice daily (15 mg/kg in two divided doses) Nalidixic acid 1 g every 6 h (15 mg/kg every 6 h) Trimethoprim–sulfamethoxazole 960 mg twice daily (30 mg/kg twice daily)	Most patients	Relieves symptoms, shortens illness. Decreases mortality in children
Travellers' diarrhea	Ciprofloxacin 1 g single dose	Trimethoprim–sulfamethoxazole 960 mg twice daily (30 mg/kg twice daily)	Rarely needed	Relieves symptoms, shortens illness

Treatment is for 5 days unless otherwise stated.
Doses for children are given in parentheses (not to exceed adult dose).
Fluoroquinolones are not licensed for children under 12 years old.
[a]Antibiotics should be used with caution if enterohemorrhagic *Esch. coli* is suspected.

Antimotility and antisecretory agents

A number of antimotility agents are available for the symptomatic relief of diarrhea. The most widely used are codeine phosphate, loperamide, diphenoxylate, and kaolin/opiate preparations: proprietary formulations of these are available over the counter in many countries. None is recommended for use in infants or young children with acute diarrhea because of the risk of precipitating respiratory depression or paralytic ileus. In adults antimotility agents may be useful for short-term relief of the symptoms of acute watery diarrhea (for example during a journey), although they can cause abdominal bloating. The use of these agents in dysentery is controversial. There is some evidence that they do provide symptomatic relief, but concerns exist about both increased risk of toxic dilation and prolonged excretion of pathogens. In general the use of opiates is not recommended in dysentery. Loperamide and codeine have a role in the management of chronic infective diarrhea, particularly in HIV-associated diarrhea where definitive treatment of the infection may be impossible.

Due to the problems associated with antimotility drugs, attention has focused on the development of new antisecretory agents to relieve symptoms and decrease fluid loss. Racecadotril, an enkephalinase inhibitor, increases the levels of the antisecretory neurotransmitter enkephalin. It has been shown to cause a 50% reduction in stool volume in infants with acute watery diarrhea of viral and other origin without significant side effects.[29,30] It is also effective in adults, and may become an important adjunct to ORS in the management of acute diarrhea.

MANAGEMENT OF SPECIFIC INFECTIONS

BACTERIAL INFECTIONS (TABLE 50.6)

Cholera

Cholera is characterized by watery diarrhea that is often profuse and may be life-threatening. It is caused by secretory enterotoxins (principally cholera toxin) produced by *Vibrio cholerae*. There are two main pathogenic strains of *V. cholerae*: O1 (seen in two biotypes, El Tor and classical), and O139. The mainstay of treatment for cholera is rehydration, and with appropriate and effective rehydration therapy mortality can be reduced to less than 1%. Oral rehydration with ORS is usually adequate, but severely dehydrated individuals may need intravenous fluids. Several liters of intravenous fluid may be required initially, and fluids must be continued to keep up with ongoing loss.

Antibiotics reduce the duration and volume of diarrhea, and may limit transmission by reducing the infectivity of the stools.[31,32] Treatment should be started as soon as possible in order to decrease the fluid requirement. Tetracycline (250–500 mg four times daily for 3 days) remains the most widely used antibiotic, but resistance is becoming a major problem. Resistance patterns vary greatly from place to place, and can change rapidly even in the same area.[33] Doxycycline, ampicillin, chloramphenicol, furazolidone, or trimethoprim–sulfamethoxazole may be effective, although resistance to all of these agents has been reported.[34–36] *V. cholerae* is generally sensitive to fluoroquinolones and a single dose of ciprofloxacin has been shown to be as effective as tetracycline or doxycycline in treating cholera.[37,38] Recently, however, some resistance to these drugs has been reported.[34,36] Because of these problems antibiotic treatment should ideally be based on local antibiotic sensitivity testing, although in some cases this may not be available.

Effective surveillance and improvements in hygiene and sanitation are the main factors in limiting the spread of cholera. Antibiotic prophylaxis (with the same drugs that are used for treatment) may decrease the attack rates in contacts of the disease, although widespread use of antibiotics may help to promote resistance.

Enteric fever

The enteric fever syndrome is an acute systemic illness characterized by fever, headache, and abdominal discomfort. Typhoid, the typical form of enteric fever, is caused by *Salmonella enterica* serotype Typhi. A similar but generally less severe illness known as paratyphoid is due to infection with *Salmonella enterica* serotypes Paratyphi A, B, or C. Untreated typhoid carries a mortality of up to 30%, but this can be reduced dramatically with appropriate therapy. After clinical recovery 5–10% of patients will continue to excrete *S.* Typhi for several months: these are termed convalescent carriers. Between 1 and 4% will continue to carry the organism for more than a year: this is chronic carriage.

Until recently the drug of choice for enteric fever was chloramphenicol, preferably given orally (2 g daily in divided doses for adults, 50 mg/kg for children). The past 10 years have seen the rapid spread of chloramphenicol resistance and, although the presence of in-vitro resistance does not necessarily mean that treatment will fail, it can no longer be considered adequate treatment in many parts of the world. Chloramphenicol resistance is usually plasmid mediated, and is frequently associated with amoxicillin and trimethoprim–sulfamethoxazole resistance. Such multiresistant organisms account for 80% of *S.* Typhi isolates in parts of Asia[39,40] and are becoming increasingly common in other parts of the world. Of cases detected in the USA in 1996–1997, 17% were resistant to five or more antibiotics.[41] Most of these were imported from the Indian subcontinent, and endemic cases of typhoid in the USA and southern Europe have a relatively low rate of antibiotic resistance.[41,42] Nalidixic acid, fluoroquinolones and group 4 cephalosporins are being used with increasing frequency but, although recent studies from India and Nigeria did not find any evidence of quinolone resistance,[43,44] ciprofloxacin and cef-

Table 50.6 Antibiotic treatment of specific bacterial causes of acute gastroenteritis

Condition	Drug of choice	Alternatives	Indications	Benefits
Cholera	Ciprofloxacin 1 g single dose	Tetracycline 500 mg every 6 h (12.5 mg/kg every 6 hª); 3 days Erythromycin 250 mg every 6 h (10 mg/kg every 8 h); 3 days	All patients	Relieves symptoms, shortens illness Reduces transmission
Enteric fever	Ciprofloxacin 500 mg twice daily (15 mg/kg twice daily); 7 days	Ofloxacin 200 mg twice daily (15 mg/kg in two divided doses only); 7 days Nalidixic acid 1 g every 6 h (15 mg/kg every 6 h); 7 days Azithromycin 500 mg once daily (10 mg/kg once daily); 5–7 days Chloramphenicol 500 mg every 6 h (12.5 mg/kg every 6 h); 7 days	All patients	Reduces morbidity and mortality
Non-typhoidal salmonellosis	Ciprofloxacin 500 mg twice daily (15 mg/kg twice daily)	Nalidixic acid 1 g every 6 h (15 mg/kg every 6 h) Trimethoprim–sulfamethoxazole 960 mg twice daily (30 mg/kg twice daily)	Prolonged illness; severe symptoms; immunosuppressed	Relieves symptoms, shortens illness. *May* decrease complications in selected groups
Shigellosis	Ciprofloxacin 500 mg twice daily (15 mg/kg twice daily)	Ofloxacin 200 mg twice daily (15 mg/kg in two divided doses only) Nalidixic acid 1 g every 6 h (15 mg/kg every 6 h) Trimethoprim–sulfamethoxazole 960 mg twice daily (30 mg/kg twice daily) Ampicillin 1 g every 6 h (25 mg/kg every 6 h)ᵇ	All patients	Relieves symptoms, shortens illness Decreases morbidity and mortality
Campylobacter	Erythromycin 500 mg every 6 h (12.5 mg/kg every 6 h)	Ciprofloxacin 500 mg twice daily (15 mg/kg twice daily)	Immunosuppressed; severe symptoms (rarely needed)	

Treatment is for 5 days unless otherwise stated.
Doses for children are given in parentheses (not to exceed adult dose).
Fluoroquinolones are not licensed for children under 12 years old.
Therapy should be guided by local antimicrobial sensitivities where known.
ᵃ Not recommended for children under 8 years old.
ᵇ Resistance common in many areas.

triaxone-resistant isolates have been reported from a number of areas.[45–47]

Wherever possible the treatment of enteric fever should be based on individual or local antibiotic susceptibility patterns. Chloramphenicol (and to a lesser extent trimethoprim–sulfamethoxazole and ampicillin) remain useful drugs in some places, and may be the only agents affordable or available (Table 50.7). Quinolones have been shown to be effective in both fully sensitive and multiresistant typhoid, and should now be used as the drug of choice in areas where multiresistance is encountered. No one drug of this class has been shown to be better than others: ciprofloxacin is the most widely used, and short courses of both ofloxacin and fleroxacin have proved

Table 50.7 Approximate drug costs and availability in developing countries

Antibiotic	Cost	Availability
Ampicillin	Medium	Widespread
Trimethoprim–sulfamethoxazole	Low	Widespread
Chloramphenicol	Low	Widespread
Nalidixic acid	Medium	Moderate
Ciprofloxacin	High	Rare
Ofloxacin	High	Rare

Low, <US$1; medium, US$ 1–4; high, US$ 5–30, each for 5 days adult treatment in conventional dose. Costs vary considerably; these are based on the cheapest bulk purchase.[129]

effective in children.[49–51] Despite concerns about the use of these agents in children (because of the risk of damage to developing cartilage) there is now considerable evidence to suggest that ciprofloxacin is sufficiently safe to be used in the treatment of childhood typhoid.[52,53] Studies using group 4 cephalosporins have produced variable results; some have shown good cure rates[54] but others have demonstrated less efficacy with cephalosporins than with other drugs, especially in short course regimens.[45,50,55] In general, comparative trials have shown better results using quinolones than cephalosporins. Several recent studies in both adults and children have shown excellent results using a 5- or 7-day oral course of azithromycin.[56–58] This drug, which is given once daily, is well tolerated and may have an important role in the treatment of typhoid in the future.

Most of these studies have been carried out in patients with mild or moderate typhoid. Patients with hypotension, impaired mental function, or evidence of decreased organ perfusion have a worse prognosis, and the impact of newer antibiotics in this group has not been assessed. The role of steroids in severe typhoid remains controversial: one trial (with relatively small numbers) demonstrated increased survival in patients treated with high-dose dexamethasone,[59] but there is little corroborating evidence for this. Complications such as intestinal perforation and renal failure should be managed aggressively, with surgical intervention and intensive care support where necessary.

Chronic carriage of *S.* Typhi may be difficult to eradicate, especially in the presence of gall bladder disease or urinary schistosomiasis. Prolonged courses of amoxicillin or trimethoprim–sulfamethoxazole are sometimes effective, and quinolones appear to have a higher success rate.[60,61] Treating underlying gall bladder or parasitic disease may help, but cholecystectomy is not justified on public health grounds alone.

Shigellosis

Infection with *Shigella* species can cause either watery diarrhea (clinically indistinguishable from other causes of acute watery diarrhea) or, more typically, dysentery. Four species can cause enteritis in humans: *Shigella dysenteriae* produces the most severe dysentery, and may also secrete a toxin which can induce hemolytic uremic syndrome. Antibiotic treatment of *Shigella* dysentery leads to a reduction in the severity and duration of symptoms, as well as a decrease in mortality in children.[8] In theory the use of antibiotics in toxigenic *S. dysenteriae* could lead to an increased risk of hemolytic uremic syndrome (as has been demonstrated in infections with verotoxigenic *Esch. coli*), but this remains to be confirmed.

Shigella spp. can rapidly develop resistance to antimicrobials, due to their ability to acquire plasmid-borne resistance genes from other species such as *Esch. coli*.[62] Following the introduction of nalidixic acid during an epidemic in Burundi, resistance to this drug rose from 0% to 57% in just 10 months.[63] Multiresistance is common, and some of the older and cheaper antibiotics such as ampicillin and trimetho-

prim–sulfamethoxazole are now ineffective in many developing and developed countries.[64,65] Most isolates remain sensitive to quinolones,[65] and a number of studies have demonstrated the clinical efficacy of ciprofloxacin, norfloxacin, and ofloxacin.[64,66] The use of these drugs in children is now becoming more widely accepted. Short courses of quinolones (e.g. ofloxacin 15 mg/kg in two divided doses in children) appear to be effective in many cases, making their use more economically viable.[64] Ceftibuten, cefixime and ceftriaxone have all been shown to be effective in various regimens,[67,68] as has azithromycin (500 mg, followed by 250 mg daily for 4 days).[69] Ideally the choice of antibiotic for shigellosis should be guided by current local resistance patterns. In the absence of these, a fluoroquinolone is the drug of choice in most areas, while nalidixic acid is probably the best of the cheaper drugs.

Although dehydration is not usually a major feature of shigella dysentery ORS should be given, especially to children.

Non-typhoidal salmonellosis

Salmonella serotypes other than Typhi and Paratyphi most commonly cause self-limiting gastroenteritis, which is usually watery but may be dysenteric. Bacteremia is documented in about 5% of cases: this may be transient and benign, but can lead to serious complications such as metastatic infection. Clinical trials suggest that fluoroquinolones may reduce the duration and severity of gastrointestinal symptoms in *Salmonella* infection, but the effect is small (1–2 days reduction).[9] In general, antibiotics are not recommended for people with mild or moderate *Salmonella* enteritis: even the presence of bacteremia in an otherwise healthy person is not a definite indication. Treatment is justified in patients with severe or prolonged symptoms, neonates, and for those at increased risk of invasive disease (in particular the immunocompromised, and patients with significant underlying disease).[10] Some authorities recommend a short (48–72 h) 'pre-emptive' course of antibiotics in those who have other risk factors for metastatic disease (e.g. elderly people, and people with known atherosclerotic lesions or aortic aneurysm),[70] while others suggest a 10–14 day course in the same group:[71] the clinical efficacy of either approach is unproven.

If antibiotic treatment is indicated then fluoroquinolones are the best choice. Group 4 cephalosporins, azithromycin and aztreonam are also effective; trimethoprim–sulfamethoxazole may be used although resistance is increasing. A number of studies have looked at the effect of quinolone treatment on fecal excretion of *Salmonella*, which typically persists for several weeks after infection. Treated patients usually have negative stool cultures immediately after treatment, but overall antibiotics have little effect on the time taken to clear the organism.[72] Even this limited response may be effective in interrupting spread of the disease in institutional outbreaks.[73] The management of symptomatic *Salmonella* bacteremia (which is common in HIV-positive patients in developing countries) is difficult: antibiotics may help, but eradication often proves impossible. Metastatic *Salmonella* infection, which typically affects atheromatous endothelium, also requires prolonged antibiotic therapy, often in conjunction with surgery.[74]

Escherichia coli infection

Esch. coli infection of the gut with enterotoxigenic (ETEC), enteropathogenic (EPEC), enteroinvasive (EIEC), enterohemorrhagic (EHEC) or enteroaggregative (EAggEC) strains can cause human disease, but these pathogens are not routinely identified in most microbiological laboratories. Consequently information about these infections is limited, and there are few therapeutic trials.

Verotoxin-secreting strains of EHEC (principally O157:H7) can cause hemolytic uremic syndrome (HUS) and thrombotic thrombocytopenic purpura (TTP), especially in children, and have therefore been the focus of much attention in industrialized countries. Several large food-borne outbreaks of *Esch. coli* O157 have been reported: most patients had a mild self-limiting bloody diarrhea, but 2.5–14% of children (and occasional adults) developed HUS.[11,75] Antibiotic treatment appears to increase the risk of HUS, presumably by increasing toxin release from dying bacteria.[11] Some antibiotics seem to have a greater effect than others,[76] but antibiotics should be avoided in *Esch. coli* O157 enteritis. EHEC has also been reported as a cause of gastroenteritis in adults and children in Africa.[77]

ETEC, which can produce both heat-stable and heat-labile toxins, is an important cause of acute watery diarrhea in children and adults throughout the world.[77–79] It has been responsible for large food-and water-borne outbreaks, and is the most commonly confirmed cause of travellers' diarrhea.[12,13,78] Widespread antibiotic resistance has been reported, with isolates from many parts of the world showing resistance to multiple drugs, including trimethoprim–sulfamethoxazole and amoxicillin.[80,81] The majority of ETEC remain sensitive to fluoroquinolones, but a survey in Thailand showed 1% of isolates to be ciprofloxacin resistant;[82] 15% of isolates in the same study were azithromycin resistant. The illness caused by ETEC is usually mild and self-limiting, but if treatment is deemed necessary then a fluoroquinolone should be used if available.

EIEC causes bacillary dysentery indistinguishable from shigellosis. It is rarely isolated, and most cases are probably treated empirically as shigellosis. If EIEC is cultured treatment should be guided by sensitivities.

EPEC is now recognized as a cause of acute watery diarrhea in infants and children worldwide, although it appears to be more common in developing countries.[77,83,84] Relatively little is known about antibiotic sensitivities of EPEC: resistance to trimethoprim–sulfamethoxazole has been reported,[80] but it is generally sensitive to quinolones.[80,84] Antibiotic treatment is rarely indicated.

EAggEC can be isolated from healthy people, but it also appears to be responsible for episodes of travellers' diarrhea,[85] persistent diarrhea in children,[86] and HIV-associated diarrhea.[87] The symptoms of both travellers' diarrhea and HIV-related chronic diarrhea can be alleviated by ciprofloxacin,[85,87] although in the former case this is not usually necessary. The epidemiology and treatment of EAggEC diarrhea in developing countries remains unclear.

Campylobacter infection

Infection with *Campylobacter jejuni* can cause acute watery diarrhea or, less commonly, dysentery. The illness is usually relatively mild and self-limiting, although there may occasionally be more severe dysenteric or systemic features. *Campylobacter coli* causes a similar but generally less severe illness. *Campylobacter* spp., which are widespread in livestock animals, have considerable potential to develop antibiotic resistance. This is usually plasmid mediated, and has been associated with the use of antibiotics in both humans and animals. Resistance to fluoroquinolones has become a major problem in many European countries, with up to 50% of human isolates in Spain showing quinolone resistance.[88,89] Some studies have linked this directly to the veterinary use of these drugs,[90] but resistance has also been shown to develop in humans during a course of treatment.[91] Most human *C. jejuni* isolates remain sensitive to macrolides,[89,92] although there is no good evidence that these drugs routinely improve the clinical course of illness. There is little information available on the antibiotic sensitivity of *Campylobacter* spp. in developing countries.

Most cases of *Campylobacter* enteritis resolve without specific treatment. More severe cases are likely to be treated empirically, often with a fluoroquinolone. If a *Campylobacter* species is grown and significant symptoms persist (especially in patients with HIV/AIDS) then antibiotic treatment should be guided by in-vitro sensitivities.

Yersinia infection

Yersinia enterocolitica is a relatively unusual cause of enteric infection in all ages. The spectrum of illness is very variable, and includes severe dysentery, septicemia, and extraintestinal manifestations such as lymphadenopathy and reactive arthritis. More severe cases should be treated with antibiotics: fluoroquinolones appear to be the most effective agents, although data are limited.[93] The effect of antibiotic treatment on *Yersinia*-triggered reactive arthritis has been assessed in small trials, without definite evidence of benefit.[94,95]

Non-cholera *Vibrio, Aeromonas* and *Plesiomonas* species

These organisms are being isolated with increasing frequency from patients with gastroenteritis, although whether this represents a genuine increase in prevalence or simply better laboratory techniques is unclear. *Vibrio parahaemolyticus* has caused major food- and waterborne outbreaks in Asia,[96] while *Aeromonas* and *Plesiomonas* species are common causes of diarrhea in children and travellers in some parts of the world.[71,97,98] All three usually cause self-limiting watery diarrhea. Almost all of these organisms are sensitive to fluoroquinolones in vitro;

there is widespread and variable resistance to other antibiotics.[98,99] Clinical data are very limited: one small retrospective study in Thailand showed no benefit from the use of antibiotics in *Plesiomonas* enteritis.[98]

Toxin-secreting bacteria

Some bacteria, notably *Clostridium perfringens*, *Bacillus cereus* and strains of *Staphylococcus aureus*, can produce heat-stable neurotoxins that affect the autonomic nervous system to cause diarrhea and vomiting. If toxin is ingested in contaminated food symptoms start within a few hours. Although diarrhea may be profuse the illness is usually short lived (24–48 h) and no specific treatment is required. Bacterial toxins are a common cause of food poisoning in Europe and the USA; the prevalence in developing countries is unknown. Ingestion of preformed toxins of *Clostridium botulinum* (especially from inadequately processed canned food) is a rarer but potentially fatal form of food poisoning.

Clostridium difficile

C. difficile, a spore-forming bacterium, is widespread in the environment.[100] However, it is usually prevented from colonizing the human gut by the presence of normal intestinal microflora. If the normal bowel commensals are eradicated by antibiotic treatment, *C. difficile* is able to move into the vacant niche: this is especially likely in elderly people. Once established, it produces cytopathic toxins (principally *C. difficile* toxins A and B). These are responsible for the symptoms, which can range from mild watery diarrhea to potentially fatal pseudomembranous colitis. All antibiotics except for parenteral aminoglycosides have been associated with *C. difficile* infection: the most common triggers are cephalosporins, aminopenicillins, and clindamycin.[101] Clinical infection is occasionally seen in the absence of antibiotic treatment, and asymptomatic carriage does occur. *C. difficile* diarrhea is well described as a hospital-acquired infection in the UK and the USA, but there is a paucity of information on the epidemiology of the disease in many countries, especially in the developing world.

The first approach in *C. difficile* diarhea is to stop antibiotic therapy if possible. This alone may lead to resolution in 15–25% of patients, but in most cases specific antimicrobial treatment is also given.[102] Both metronidazole (400 mg three times daily) and vancomycin (125 mg four times daily) for 7 days by mouth have a clinical response rate of >80%; bowel concentrations of either drug following intravenous administration are unpredictable.[103] No significant differences in overall response have been found between the two drugs, although resolution of symptoms appears to be more rapid with vancomycin.[103] Relapse rates are also similar at 15–25%: these are usually due to reinfection with the same or different strains of *C. difficile* rather than failure to clear the original infection.[104] It is common to treat relapses with the antibiotic that was not used initially, although there are no data to support this prac-

tice. Some patients suffer multiple relapses: prolonged courses of vancomycin, and combinations of vancomycin and rifampicin, have occasionally been reported to be effective in such cases.[103] Careful attention to infection control procedures and avoidance of 'high-risk' antibiotics will decrease the risk of recurrent infection. Attempts have been made to restore normal bowel flora following *C. difficile* infection using a variety of probiotic agents: no clear evidence of benefit has been published.[105]

Whipple's disease

Whipple's disease (caused by infection with *Tropheryma whippelii*) is a multisystem disorder, but the most commonly affected site is the small intestine. It is extremely rare, with less than 1000 confirmed cases reported worldwide. Antibiotic treatment may be curative, but relapse after treatment is common, especially in the central nervous system. There have been no randomized prospective trials comparing different drug therapy. A reasonable regimen is to give 2 weeks of intravenous therapy with benzylpenicillin (2.4 g daily) and streptomycin (15 mg/kg daily), followed by 1 year of trimethoprim–sulfamethoxazole 960 mg twice daily.[106] Central nervous system relapse may respond to chloramphenicol or ceftriaxone.

Intestinal mycobacterial infection

Intestinal tuberculosis should be treated with standard antituberculosis chemotherapy (Ch. 61). Symptomatic intestinal infection with mycobacteria other than tuberculosis (such as the *Mycobacterium avium* complex and *Mycobacterium genevense*) is only seen in patients with AIDS and related conditions.

Small bowel overgrowth

Colonization of the small intestine with exogenous bacteria may occur in patients with structural abnormalities of the small bowel (such as strictures or diverticula), bypassed surgical loops, or in conditions associated with hypomotility such as scleroderma. Bacterial overgrowth may lead to diarrhea and malabsorption. Clinical improvement is usually seen after treatment with metronidazole, tetracycline, or a fluoroquinolone, but repeated courses are often required if the underlying abnormality remains.

Helicobacter pylori

Infection with *H. pylori* is common throughout the world. It is characterized by a mild chronic active gastritis, but this is usually asymptomatic. However, *H. pylori* gastritis is implicated in the pathogenesis of duodenal and gastric ulcers, MALT lymphomas, and some gastric adenocarcinomas.[107] Eradication of *H. pylori* virtually abolishes duodenal ulcer relapse, and all patients with peptic ulcer disease in association with *H. pylori* infection should receive antibiotics. Eradication therapy should also be used in the treatment of gastric lymphomas. The effect of treatment on the progression of adenocarcinoma is less clear, but patients with high-grade gastric dysplasia or frank adenocarcinoma in association with *H. pylori* should be given eradication therapy.[107] Non-ulcer dyspepsia is commonly associated with *H. pylori* infection, but there is no evidence of a causal connection. Some patients do get symptomatic improvement after clearance of *H. pylori*, but expert opinion is divided on who should be treated.[107,108]

Several different therapeutic regimens have been used for treating *H. pylori* infection, including various combinations of antibiotics, proton pump inhibitors, H_2-receptor antagonists and bismuth compounds. Evidence suggests that the most effective combination is a 1-week course of omeprazole, combined with any two of amoxicillin, clarithromycin, or a nitroimidazole (metronidazole 500 mg twice daily or tinidazole 1 g daily). These all give an eradication rate of >90%, with few side effects, at a relatively modest cost.[109,110] The European *Helicobacter pylori* Study Group recommends a proton pump inhibitor (standard dose twice daily), clarithromycin 500 mg twice daily, and amoxicillin 500 mg twice daily for 1 week as first-line therapy.[108] Treatment success can be evaluated with endoscopy or urea breath test. Patients with persistent infection should receive a further week of treatment with a proton pump inhibitor, bismuth subsalicylate (120 mg four times daily), metronidazole (500 mg three times daily), and tetracycline (500 mg four times daily).[108] In children, *H. pylori* is associated with gastric and duodenal ulcer disease, as well as chronic gastritis. Eradication of the infection leads to long-term resolution of these conditions. However, there is a lack of data on treatment regimens, and no clear consensus on optimal management.[111]

VIRAL INFECTIONS

Viral gastroenteritis is extremely common throughout the world, especially in children. It can be caused by several different organisms, notably rotavirus, enteric adenovirus (types 40 and 41), Caliciviridae and Astroviridae. The last two families were formerly known as 'small round-structured viruses', and many members are named after the geographical location at which they were first isolated, e.g. Norwalk virus. All these viruses cause self-limiting watery diarrhea, and require only supportive treatment and rehydration. Occasionally mucosal damage or disaccharidase deficiency caused by the infection may result in more prolonged diarrhea. Viral gastroenteritis, often in association with malnutrition, is a major cause of morbidity and mortality in children in the developing world.

Some viruses, notably cytomegalovirus and herpes simplex, can cause severe ulcerating infection of the gastrointestinal tract in patients with HIV/AIDS or other immunosuppressing conditions.

PROTOZOAL INFECTIONS

Giardiasis

Infection with *Giardia lamblia* can produce a variety of responses including acute watery diarrhea, persistent diarrhea (often associated with nausea, anorexia, and belching), and asymptomatic colonization. Most people recover spontaneously, and treatment is often unnecessary. Treatment of symptomatic patients probably accelerates parasitological and clinical cure, and is definitely indicated in patients with a more protracted illness. There is little point in treating people with asymptomatic infection in endemic areas, as reinfection rates are high, but those living in non-endemic areas should be treated. The most commonly used drugs are metronidazole and tinidazole: furazolidone and mepacrine (quinacrine) are also effective.[112] Various regimens of nitroimidazoles have been used: there is some evidence that single-dose treatment may be as effective as longer courses,[113] although good-quality data are scarce.[114] Mepacrine, an acridine dye, is reasonably effective, but it has a high incidence of side effects (including toxic psychosis) and is poorly tolerated. Furazolidone, by contrast, is well tolerated but is less effective.[115] Albendazole has antigiardial activity, and has been used in courses ranging from 1 to 5 days. The results have been varied, but overall the cure rate with albendazole does not appear to be as good as with metronidazole.[114,116,117] Treatment regimens are described in Chapter 65.

Amebiasis

Infection with *Entamoeba histolytica* can be divided into three clinical pictures: asymptomatic cyst passage, dysentery, and liver abscess. The management of asymptomatic carriage has been complicated by the recognition that there are two species of ameba, *E. histolytica* and *Entamoeba dispar*, which are indistinguishable by microscopy of the cysts. Only the former is potentially pathogenic. In endemic areas attempts to eradicate cyst carriage are of limited value due to the high rate of reinfection. In non-endemic areas people with *E. histolytica* in the gut should certainly be treated, because of the potential pathogenicity and the risk of transmission. Until tests to distinguish *E. histolytica* from *E. dispar* are widely available, all cyst carriers should be treated. The drug of choice is diloxanide furoate, a non-absorbed luminal amebicide: paromomycin is also effective.

Proven amebic dysentery and amebic liver abscess should always be treated. The best agents are nitroimidazoles, either metronidazole or tinidazole. Appropriate regimens are described in Chapter 65.

Other protozoal infections

The treatment of cryptosporidiosis, microsporidiosis, isosporiasis and infection with *Cyclospora cayetanensis* is described in Chapter 65.

Carriage of *Balantidium coli* is usually asymptomatic,[118] but it can cause a syndrome similar to amebic dysentery. Tetracycline and metronidazole are effective,[119] although there are no good clinical trials to guide therapy. *Dientamoeba fragilis* is often found in association with other gut parasites, but there is evidence that isolated *D. fragilis* infection can cause gastrointestinal symptoms.[120] Treatment with tetracycline or metronidazole may be effective. The role of *Blastocystis hominis* in human disease remains uncertain, and presence of this organism should not be accepted as a cause of symptoms.

Intestinal helminths

See Ch. 66.

References

1. World Health Organization 1999 The World Health Report 1999. Online. Available: www.who.int/whosis/statistics/.
2. The Global Burden of Disease Project 1999 *The Global Burden of Disease*. Cambridge, Harvard University Press Vol 1, pp 247–294 (Executive summary online. Available: www.hsph.harvard-edu/organisations/bdu/summary.html)
3. Hultgren SJ, Abraham S, Caparon M, Falk P, St Geme JW, Normark S 1993 Pilus and non-pilus bacterial adhesins: assembly and function in cell recognition. *Cell* 73: 887–901.
4. Parsot C, Sansonetti PJ 1996 Invasion and pathogenesis of *Shigella* infections. *Current Topics in Microbiology and Immunology* 209: 25–42.
5. Haffejee IE 1995 The epidemiology of rotavirus infections: a global perspective. *Journal of Pediatric Gastroenterology and Nutrition* 20: 275–286.
6. Burke B, Desselburger U 1996 Rotavirus pathogenicity. *Virology* 218: 299–305.
7. Farthing MJ 1993 Diarrhoeal diseases: current concepts and future challenges. Pathogenesis of giardia. *Transactions of the Royal Society of Tropical Medicine and Hygiene* 87S3: 17–21.
8. World Health Organization 1995 *The treatment of diarrhoea. A manual for physicians and other senior health workers*. Geneva; WHO/CDR/95.3.
9. Dryden MS, Gabb RJ, Wright SK 1996 Empirical treatment of severe community acquired gastroenteritis with ciprofloxacin. *Clinical Infectious Diseases* 22: 1019–1025.
10. Moss PJ, Read RC 1995 Empiric antibiotic therapy for acute diarrhoea in the developed world. *Journal of Antimicrobial Chemotherapy* 35: 903–913.
11. Wong CS, Jelacic S, Habeeb RL, Watkins SL, Tarr PI 2000 The risk of the hemolytic-uremic syndrome after antibiotic treatment of *Escherichia coli* O157:H7 infections. *New England Journal of Medicine* 342: 1930–1936.
12. Jiang ZD, Mathewson JJ, Ericsson CD, Svennerholm AM, Pulido C, DuPont HL 2000 Characterisation of enterotoxigenic *Escherichia coli* strains in patients with travellers' diarrhea acquired in Guadalajara, Mexico, 1992–7. *Journal of Infectious Diseases* 181: 797–782.
13. Schultsz C, van den Ende J, Cobelens F et al 2000 Diarrheagenic *Escherichia coli* and acute and persistent diarrhea in returned travellers. *Journal of Clinical Microbiology* 38: 3550–3554.
14. De Bruyn G, Hahn S, Borwick A 2001 Antibiotic treatment for travellers' diarrhoea. Cochrane Database of Systematic Reviews, Issue 1.
15. Fontaine O, Gore SM, Pierce NF 2000 Rice-based oral rehydration solution for treating diarrhoea. Cochrane Database of Systematic Reviews, CD001264.
16. Cohen MB, Metzoff AG, Laney DW et al 1995 Use of a single solution for oral rehydration and maintenance therapy of infants with diarrhoea and mild to moderate dehydration. *Pediatrics* 95: 639–645.
17. Iynkaran N, Yadav M 1998 Rice-starch oral rehydration therapy in neonates and young infants. *Journal of Tropical Pediatrics* 44: 199–203.
18. Dutta P, Mitra U, Dutta S 2000 Hypo-osmolar oral rehydration salts (ORS) solution in dehydrating persistent diarrhoea in children: double-blind, randomised, controlled, clinical trial. *Acta Paediatrica* 89: 411–416.
19. Valentiner-Branth P, Steinsland H, Gjessing HK et al 1999 Community-based randomised controlled trial of reduced osmolarity oral rehydration solution in acute childhood diarrhoea. *Pediatric Infectious Disease Journal* 18: 789–795.
20. Alam NH, Majumder RN, Fuchs GJ 1999 Efficacy and safety of oral rehydration solution with reduced osmolarity in adults with cholera: a randomised double-blind clinical trial. *Lancet* 354: 296–299.
21. Ramakrishna BS, Venkataraman S, Srinivasan P et al 2000 Amylase resistant starch plus oral rehydration solution for cholera. *New England Journal of Medicine* 342: 308–313.
22. Simakachorn N, Pichaipat V, Rithipornpaisarn P 2000 Clinical evaluation of the addition of lyophilised heat-killed *Lactobacillus acidophilus* LB to oral rehydration therapy in the treatment of acute diarrhea in children. *Journal of Pediatric Gastroenterology and Nutrition* 30: 68–72.
23. Guandalini S, Pensebene L, Zikri MA et al 2000 *Lactobacillus* GG administered in oral rehydration solution to children with acute diarrhea: a multicenter European trial. *Journal of Pediatric Gastroenterology and Nutrition* 30: 54–60.
24. Dutta P, Mitra U, Datta A et al 2000 Impact of zinc supplementation in malnourished children with acute watery diarrhea. *Journal of Tropical Pediatrics* 46: 259–263.
25. Ashref H, Rahman MM, Fuchs GJ et al 1998 Folic acid in the treatment of acute watery diarrhoea in children: a double-blind, randomised controlled trial. *Acta Paediatrica* 87: 1113–1115.
26. Ahmed FU, Rahman ME, Mahmood CB 2000 Mothers' skill in preparing oral rehydration salt solution. *Indian Journal of Pediatrics* 67: 99–102.
27. Salam I, Katelaris P, Leigh-Smith S, Farthing MJ 1994 Randomised trial of single-dose ciprofloxacin for travellers' diarrhoea. *Lancet* 334: 1537–1539.
28. Murphy GS, Bodhidatta L, Echeverria P 1993 Ciprofloxacin and loperamide in the treatment of bacillary dysentery. *Annals of Internal Medicine* 118: 582–586.
29. Cezard JP, Duhamel JF, Meye M et al 2001 Efficacy and tolerability of racecadotril in acute diarrhea in children. *Gastroenterology* 120: 799–805.
30. Salazar Lindo E, Santisteban-Ponce J, Chea-Woo E, Gutierrez M 2000 Racecadotril in the treatment of acute watery diarrhea in children. *New England Journal of Medicine* 343: 463–467.
31. World Health Organization Programme for Control of Diarrhoeal Diseases 1992 Management of the patient with cholera. Geneva: World Health Organization: WHO/CDD/SER91.15 Rev 1.
32. Roy SK, Islam A, Ali R et al 1998 A randomised clinical trial to compare the efficacy of erythromycin, ampicillin and tetracycline for the treatment of cholera in children. *Transactions of the Royal Society for Tropical Medicine and Hygiene* 92: 460–462.
33. Mukhopadhyay AK, Garg S, Nair GB et al 1995 Biotype traits and antibiotic susceptibility of *Vibrio cholerae* serogroup O1 before during and after the emergence of the O139 serogroup. *Epidemiology and Infection* 115: 427–434.
34. Bhattacharya MK, Deb A et al 2000 Outbreak of cholera caused by *Vibrio cholerae* O1 intermediately resistant to norfloxacin at Malda, West Bengal. *Journal of the Indian Medical Association* 98: 389–390.
35. Ranjit K, Nurahan M 2000 Tetracycline resistant cholera in Kelantan. *Medical Journal of Malaysia* 55: 143–145.
36. Garg P, Chakraborty S, Basu I et al 2000 Expanding multiple antibiotic resistance among clinical strains of *Vibrio cholerae* isolated from 1992–7 in Calcutta, India. *Epidemiology and Infection* 124: 393–399.
37. Gotuzzo E, Seas C, Echeverria J et al 1995 Ciprofloxacin for the treatment of cholera: a randomised double-blind controlled clinical trial of a single daily dose in Peruvian adults. *Clinical Infectious Diseases* 20: 1485–1490.
38. Khan WA, Bennish M, Seas C et al 1996 Randomised controlled trial of single-dose ciprofloxacin and doxycycline for cholera caused by *Vibrio cholera*, O1 or O139. *Lancet* 348: 296–300.
39. Arora RK, Gupta A, Joshi NM et al 1992 Multidrug resistant typhoid fever: study of an outbreak in Calcutta. *Indian Journal of Paediatrics* 29: 61–66.
40. Kabra SK, Madhulika, Talati A, Soni N, Patel S, Modi RR 2000 Multidrug resistant typhoid fever. *Tropical Doctor* 30: 195–199.
41. Ackers ML, Puhr ND, Tauxe RV, Mintz ED 2000 Laboratory based surveillance of *Salmonella* serotype typhi infections in the United States: antimicrobial resistance on the rise. *Journal of the American Medical Association* 283: 2668–2673.
42. Scuderi G, Fantasia M, Niglio T 2000 The antibiotic resistance patterns of *Salmonella typhi* isolates in Italy 1980–96. *Epidemiology and Infection* 124: 17–23.
43. Ciraj AM, Seetha KS, Gopalkrishna BK, Shivananda PG 1999 Drug resistance patterns and phage types of *Salmonella typhi* isolates in Manipal, South Karnataka. *Indian Journal of Medical Sciences* 53: 486–499.

44. Akinyemi KO, Coker AO, Olukoya DK et al 2000 Prevalence of multidrug resistant *Salmonella typhi* among clinically diagnosed typhoid fever patients in Lagos, Nigeria. *Zeitschrift für Naturforschung* 55: 489–493.

45. Bhutta ZA, Khan IA, Shadmani M 2000 Failure of short course ceftriaxone chemotherapy for multidrug resistant typhoid fever in children: a randomised controlled trial in Pakistan. *Antimicrobial Agents and Chemotherapy* 44: 450–452.

46. Saha SK, Talukder SY, Islam M, Saha S 1999 A highly ceftriaxone-resistant *Salmonella typhi* in Bangladesh. *Pediatric Infectious Disease Journal* 18: 387.

47. Rowe B, Ward LR, Threlfall EJ 1995 Ciprofloxacin resistant *Salmonella typhi* in the UK. *Lancet* 346: 302.

48. Wallace MR, Yousuf AA, Mahroos GA 1993 Ciprofloxacin versus ceftriaxone in the treatment of multiresistant typhoid fever. *European Journal of Clinical Microbiology and Infectious Diseases* 12: 907–910.

49. Duong NM, Vinh Chau NV, Van Anh DC et al 1995 Short course fleroxacin in the treatment of typhoid fever. *Journal of the American Medical Association (Southeast Asia)* 11: 6–11.

50. Cao XT, Kneen R, Nguyen TA, Truong DL, White NJ, Parry CM 1999 A comparative study of ofloxacin and cefixime for the study of typhoid fever in children. *Pediatric Infectious Disease Journal* 18: 245–248.

51. Hien TT, Bethell DB, Hoa NT et al 1995 Short course of ofloxacin for treatment of multidrug resistant typhoid. *Clinical Infectious Diseases* 20: 917–923.

52. Bethell DB, Hien TT, Phi LT et al 1996 The effects on growth of single short courses of fluoroquinolones. *Archives of Diseases in Childhood* 74: 44–64.

53. Doherty CP, Saha SK, Cutting WA 2000 Typhoid fever, ciprofloxacin, and growth in young children. *Annals of Tropical Paediatrics* 20: 297–303.

54. Girgis NJ, Kilpatrick ME, Farid Z, Mikhail IA, Bishay E 1990 Ceftriaxone versus chloramphenicol in the treatment of typhoid fever. *Drugs Under Experimental and Clinical Research* 16: 607–609.

55. Smith MD, Doung NM, Hoa NT et al 1994 Comparison of ofloxacin and ceftriaxone for short-course treatment of enteric fever. *Antimicrobial Agents and Chemotherapy* 38: 1716–1720.

56. Frenck RW, Nakhla I, Sultar Y et al 2000 Azithromycin versus ceftriaxone for the treatment of uncomplicated typhoid fever in children. *Clinical Infectious Diseases* 31: 1134–1138.

57. Chinh N, Parry CM, Ly NT et al 2000 A randomised controlled comparison of azithromycin and ofloxacin for the treatment of multidrug resistant or nalidixic acid resistant enteric fever. *Antimicrobial Agents and Chemotherapy* 44: 1855–1859.

58. Butler T, Sridhar CB, Daga MK et al 1999 Treatment of typhoid fever with azithromycin versus chloramphenicol in a randomised multicentre trial in India. *Antimicrobial Agents and Chemotherapy* 44: 243–250.

59. Hoffman SL, Punjabi NH, Kumala S 1984 Reduction of mortality of chloramphenicol-treated severe typhoid fever by high dose dexamethasone. *New England Journal of Medicine* 310: 82–88.

60. Ferrecio C, Morris JG, Valdirieso C et al 1988 Efficacy of ciprofloxacin in the treatment of chronic typhoid carriers. *Journal of Infectious Diseases* 157: 1235–1239.

61. Gotuzzo E, Guerro JG, Benavente L et al 1998 Use of norfloxacin to treat chronic typhoid carriage. *Journal of Infectious Diseases* 157: 1221–1225.

62. Bratoeva MP, John JF 1994 In vivo R plasmid transfer in a patient with a mixed infection of shigella dysentery. *Epidemiology and Infection* 112: 247–252.

63. Engels D, Madaras T, Nyandwi S, Murray J 1995 Epidemic dysentery caused by *Shigella dysenteriae* type 1: a sentinel site surveillance of antimicrobial resistance patterns in Burundi. *Bulletin of the World Health Organization* 73: 787–791.

64. Vinh H, Wain J, Chinh MT et al 2000 Treatment of bacillary dysentery in Vietnamese children: two doses of ofloxacin versus 5 days nalidixic acid. *Transactions of the Royal Society of Tropical Medicine and Hygiene* 94: 323–326.

65. Jamal WY, Rotimi VO, Chugh TD, Pal T 1998 Prevalence and susceptibility of *Shigella* species to 11 antibiotics in a Kuwait teaching hospital. *Journal of Chemotherapy* 10: 285–290.

66. Salam MA, Dhar U, Khan WA, Bennish ML 1998 Randomised comparison of ciprofloxacin suspension and pivmecillinam for childhood shigellosis. *Lancet* 352: 522–527.

67. Martin JM, Pitetti R, Maffei F, Tritt J, Smail K, Wald ER 2000 Treatment of shigellosis with cefixime: two days versus five days. *Pediatric Infectious Disease Journal* 19: 522–526.

68. Moolasart P, Eampokalap B, Ratanasrithong M 1999 Comparison of the efficacy of ceftibuten and norfloxacin in the treatment of acute gastrointestinal infection in children. *Southeast Asian Journal of Tropical Medicine and Public Health* 30: 764–769.

69. Khan WA, Seas C, Dhar U, Salam MA, Bennish ML 1997 Treatment of shigellosis: comparison of azithromycin and ciprofloxacin. A double-blind, radomised, controlled trial. *Annals of Internal Medicine* 26: 697–703.

70. Hohmann EL 2001 Nontyphoidal salmonellosis. *Clinical Infectious Diseases* 32: 263–269.

71. Arduino RC, DuPont HL 1999 In Cohen J, Armstrong D (eds) *Infectious Diseases*. Mosby, London, 2.35.9.

72. Barbara G, Stanghellini V, Berti-Ceroni C et al 2000 Role of antibiotic therapy on long term germ excretion in faeces and digestive symptoms in *Salmonella* infection. *Alimentary Pharmacology and Therapeutics* 14: 1127–1131.

73. Dyson C, Ribeiro CD, Westmoreland D 1995 Large scale use of ciprofloxacin in the control of a *Salmonella* outbreak in a hospital for the mentally handicapped. *Journal of Hospital Infection* 29: 287–296.

74. Moss PJ, Read RC, Channer KC, McKendrick MW 1996 Persistent fever following gastroenteritis. *Lancet* 347: 1662.

75. Fukushima H, Hashizume T, Morita T et al 1999 Clinical experiences in Sakai City Hospital during the massive outbreak of enterohemorrhagic *Escherichia coli* O157 infections in Sakai City 1996. *Pediatrics International* 41: 213–217.

76. Ikeda A, Ida O, Kimoto K et al 1999 Effect of early fosfomycin treatment on prevention of hemolytic uremic syndrome accompanying *Escherichia coli* O157:H7 infection. *Clinical Nephrology* 52: 357–362.

77. Akinyemi KO, Oyefolu AO, Opere B, Otunba-Payne VA, Oworu AO 1998 *Escherichia coli* in patients with acute gastroenteritis in Lagos, Nigeria. *East African Medical Journal* 75: 512–515.

78. Clemens JD, Rao MR, Chakraborty J et al 1997 Breastfeeding and the risk of life threatening enterotoxicenic *Escherichia coli* diarrhea in Bangladeshi infants and children. *Pediatrics* 100: E2.

79. Roels TH, Proctor ME, Robinson LC, Hulbert K, Bopp CA, Davis JP 1998 Clinical features of infections due to *Escherichia coli* producing heat stable toxin during an outbreak in Wisconsin: a rarely suspected cause of diarrhea in the United States. *Clinical Infectious Diseases* 26: 898–892.

80. Mikhail IA, Fox E, Haberberger RL, Ahmed EH, Abbatte EA 1990 Epidemiology of bacterial pathogens associated with infectious diarrhea in Djibouti. *Journal of Clinical Microbiology* 28: 956–961.

81. Ghosh AR, Koley H, De D, Paul M, Nair GB, Sen D 1996 Enterotoxigenic *Escherichia coli* associated diarrhoea among infants aged less than six months in Calcutta, India. *European Journal of Epidemiology* 12: 81–84.

82. Hoge CW, Gambel JM, Srijan A, Pitarangsi C, Echeverria P 1998 Trends in antibiotic resistance among diarrheal pathogens isolated in Thailand over 15 years. *Clinical Infectious Disease* 26: 341–345.

83. Asrat D 2001 Screening for enteropathogenic *Escherichia coli* in paediatric patients with diarrhoea and controls using pooled antisera. *Ethiopian Medical Journal* 39: 23–28.

84. Obi CL, Coker AO, Epoke J, Ndip RN 1998 Distributional patterns of bacterial diarrhoeagenic agents and antibiograms of isolates from diarrhoeaic and non-diarrhoeaic patients in urban and rural areas of Nigeria. *Central African Journal of Medicine* 44: 223–229.

85. Glandt M, Adachi JA, Mathewson JJ et al 1999 Enteroaggregative *Escherichia coli* as a cause of travellers' diarrhoea: clinical response to ciprofloxacin. *Clinical Infectious Diseases* 29: 335–338.

86. Sang WK, Oundo JO, Mwituria JK et al 1997 Multidrug resistant enteroaggregative *Escherichia coli* associated with persistent diarrhoea in Kenyan children. *Emerging Infectious Diseases* 3: 373–374.

87. Wanke CA, Gerrior J, Blais V, Mayer H, Acheson D 1998 Succesful treatment of diarrheal disease associated with enteroaggregative *Escherichia coli* in adults infected with human immunodeficiency virus. *Journal of Infectious Diseases* 178: 1369–1372.

88. Navarro F, Miro E, Fuentes I, Mirelis B 1993 *Campylobacter* species: identification and resistance to quinolones. *Clinical Infectious Diseases* 17: 825–826.

89. Gomez-Garces JL, Cogollos R, Alos JL 1995 Susceptibility of fluoroquinolone resistent strains of *Campylobacter jejuni* to 11 oral antimicrobial agents. *Antimicrobial Agents and Chemotherapy* 39: 542–542.

90. Endtz HP, Ruijs GJ, van Klingeren B, Jansen WH, van der Ryden T, Moulton RP 1991 Quinolone resistance in campylobacter isolated from man and poultry following the introduction of fluoroquinolones in vetinary medicine. *Journal of Antimicrobial Chemotherapy* 27: 199–208.

91. Adler-Mosca H, Luthy-Hottehstein J, Martinetti Lucchini G, Burnens A, Altwegg M 1991 Development of resistance to quinolones in five patients with campylobacteriosis treated with ciprofloxacin or norfloxacin. *European Journal of Clinical Microbiology and Infectious Diseases* 10: 953–959.

92. Varga J, Fodor L 1998 Biochemical characteristics, sero group distribution, antibiotic susceptibility and age related significance of campylobacter strains causing diarrhoea in humans in Hungary. *Zentralblatt für Bakteriologie* 288: 67–73.

93. Gatraud M, Scavizzi MR, Mollaret HH, Guillevin L, Hornstein MJ 1993 Antibiotic treatment of *Yersinia enterocolitica* septicaemia. *Clinics in Infectious Diseases* 17: 402–410.

94. Hoogkamp-Korstanje JA, Moesker H, Bruyn GA 2000 Ciprofloxacin versus placebo for the treatment of *Yersinia enterocolitica* triggered reactive arthritis. *Annals of Rheumatic Diseases* 59: 914–917.

95. Sieper J, Fendler C, Laitko S et al 1999 No benefit of long-term ciprofloxacin treatment in patients with reactive arthritis and undifferentiated oligoarthritis: a three month, multicenter, double-blind, randomised, placebo-controlled study. *Arthritis and Rheumatism* 42: 1386–1396.

96. Wong HC, Liu SH, Wang TK et al 2000 Characteristics of *Vibrio parahaemolyticus* O3:K6 from Asia. *Applied and Environmental Microbiology* 66: 3981–3986.

97. Gomez Campdera J, Munoz P, Lopez Prieto F et al 1996 Gastroenteritis due to *Aeromonas* in pediatrics. *Anales Españoles de Pediatria* 44: 548–552.

98. Visitsunthorn N, Komolpis P 19XX Antimicrobial therapy in *Plesiomonas shigelloides*-associated diarrhea in Thai children. *Southeast Asian Journal of Tropical Medicine and Public Health* 26: 86–90.

99. Ahmed A, Hafiz S, Ahmed QT et al 1998 Sensitivity pattern and beta-lactamase production in clinical isolates of *Aeromonas* strains. *Journal of the Pakistan Medical Association* 48: 158–161.

100. Al Saif N, Brazier JS 1996 The distribution of *Clostridium difficile* in the environment of South Wales. *Journal of Medical Microbiology* 45: 133–137.

101. Spencer RC 1998 Clinical impact and associated costs of *Clostridium difficile*-associated disease. *Journal of Antimicrobial Chemotherapy* 41(Suppl. C): 5–12.

102. Olson MM, Shanholtzer CJ, Lee JT, Gerding DN 1994 Ten years of *Clostridium difficile*-associated disease surveillance and treatment at the Minneapolis VA Medical Center 1982–1991. *Infection Control and Hospital Epidemiology* 15: 371–381.

103. Wilcox MH 1998 Treatment of *Clostridium difficile* infection. *Journal of Antimicrobial Chemotherapy* 41 (Suppl. C): 41–46.

104. Wilcox MH, Fawley NN, Settle CD, Davidson A 1998 Recurrence of symptoms in *Clostridium difficile* infection – relapse or reinfection? *Journal of Hospital Infection* 38: 93–100.

105. Rolfe C 1996 Biotherapy for antibiotic-associated and other diarrhoeas. *Journal of Infection* 32: 1–10.

106. Veitch AM, Farthing MJG 1999 Whipple's disease. In: Cohen J, Armstrong D (eds). *Infectious Diseases*. Mosby, London, 2.36.1–4.

107. Goddard AF, Atherton JC 1999 Gastritis, peptic ulceration and related conditions. In: Cohen J, Armstrong D (eds). *Infectious Diseases*. Mosby, London, 2.34.1–6.

108. European *Helicobacter pylori* Study Group 2000 The Maastricht 2–2000 consensus report. Online. Available: www.helicobacter.org/ehpsg_guidelines_patients_2000.htm

109. Penstone JG, McColl KE 1997 Eradication of *Helicobacter pylori*: an objective assessment of current therapies. *British Journal of Clinical Pharmacology* 43: 223–243.

110. Goddard AF, Spiller RC 1996 *Helicobacter pylori* eradication in clinical practice: one week low dose therapy is preferable to bismuth triple therapy. *Alimentary Pharmacology and Therapeutics* 10: 1009–1013.

111. EHPSG guidelines for children.

112. Davidson RA 1984 Issues in clinical parasitology: the treatment of giardiasis. *American Journal of Gastroenterology* 79: 256–261.

113. Bulut BU, Gulnat SB, Aysev D 1996 Alternative treatment protocols in giardiasis: a pilot study. *Scandinavian Journal of Infectious Diseases* 28: 493–495.

114. Zaat JOM, Mank TG, Assendelft WJJ 2001 Drugs for treating giardiasis. Cochrane database of Systematic Reviews. Issue 1.

115. Quiros-Buelna E 1984 Furazolidone and metronidazole for treatment of giardiasis in children. *Scandinavian Journal of Gastroenterology* 24(Suppl. 159): 65–69.

116. Misra PK, Kumar A, Agarwal V, Jagota SC 1995 A comparative clinical trial of albendazole versus metronidazole in children with giardiasis. *Indian Pediatrics* 32: 291–294.

117. Pengsaa K, Sirivichayakul C, Pojjaroen-anant C, Nimnual S, Wisetsing P 1999 Albendazole treatment for *Giardia intestinalis* in school children. *Southeast Asian Journal of Tropical Medicine and Public Health* 30: 78–83.

118. Esteban JG, Aguirre C, Angle R, Ash LR, Mas-Coma S 1998 Balantidiasis in Aymara children from the northern Bolivian Altiplano. *American Journal of Tropical Medicine and Hygiene* 59: 922–927.

119. Garcia-Laverde A, De Bonilla L 1975 Clinical trials with metronidazole in human balantidiasis. *American Journal of Tropical Medicine and Hygiene* 24: 781–783.

120. Ayadi A, Bahri I 1999 *Dientamoeba fragilis*: pathogenic flagellate? *Bulletin de la Société de Pathologie Exotique* 92: 299–301.

121. World Health Organization 1995 Guidelines for the control of epidemics due to *Shigella dysenteriae* type 1. Online. Available: www.who.int/emc-documents/cholera/whocdr954c.html.

51 Hepatitis

J. Main and H. C. Thomas

Acute and chronic viral hepatitis continue to cause significant morbidity and mortality worldwide. While many viral infections can cause hepatitis this chapter concentrates on the hepatotropic viruses, particularly those associated with chronic hepatitis.

HEPATITIS A VIRUS INFECTION

Hepatitis A virus (HAV) is a member of the Picornaviridae family and a major cause of acute hepatitis. HAV is transmitted via the fecal–oral route. Most cases of acute HAV infection are subclinical but life-threatening fulminant infection can occur and is particularly seen in older patients, especially those with a background of significant alcohol consumption or pre-existing chronic liver disease such as chronic hepatitis B or C. There are anecdotal reports of interferon-β being used in severe cases[1] but this is an experimental approach and referral to a transplant center is recommended for patients with life-threatening disease.

PREVENTION

A major advance in the prevention of HAV infection has been the development of a safe and effective vaccine.[2] Before this the only strategy available was the administration of normal human immunoglobulin as passive prophylaxis. The efficacy of this depended on the presence of anti-HAV antibodies in the pool of blood donors but the seroprevalence of markers of previous HAV infection has declined with improved sanitation in many countries and failures have occurred. The vaccine has also been combined with hepatitis B vaccine and in another preparation with typhoid vaccine. There is considerable country-to-country variation in vaccine strategies, and in some countries hepatitis A vaccine is limited to travellers or to those in occupations where HAV infection could be a personal risk or a risk to others (e.g. food handlers). Some countries are employing HAV vaccine as part of the routine childhood immunization program however, there are concerns that if immunity wanes there will be susceptible adults potentially at risk of more severe disease.

HEPATITIS B VIRUS INFECTION

EPIDEMIOLOGY

Hepatitis B virus (HBV) can be transmitted sexually, by blood, blood products or vertically (mother to child). There are an estimated 350 million carriers of HBV worldwide. In some areas of South-east Asia approximately 20% of the population are HBV carriers, with many infected by the vertical route. Although vaccine programs have already made an impact it will be many years before the disease can be eradicated. In the Western world HBV infection is mainly seen in high-risk individuals such as homosexual men or intravenous drug users.

NATURAL HISTORY

HBV is a small (3.2 kB) partially double-stranded DNA virus and a member of the hepadnavirus group.

The incubation period of HBV infection is 2–6 months and, although many cases are subclinical, fulminant disease can occur.

It is thought that much of the liver damage that occurs with both acute and chronic HBV infection is secondary to the host immune response.

Chronic carriage is defined by ongoing viral replication 6 months or more after infection. Only 5% of healthy adults fail to clear the initial infection and develop chronic viral carriage but if infection occurs perinatally then the risk of chronic infection is 95%. The prognosis is better in infected women but it is estimated that 40% of infected men will, if not treated, die because of the subsequent complications which include cirrhosis, liver failure and the development of hepatocellular carcinoma.[3,4] The high risk of chronicity with perinatal infection is thought to relate to the immaturity of the neonatal immune system and possible viral factors, which include the circulating hepatitis B e antigen (HBeAg) inducing immune tolerance. Host immune factors are also thought to be important in adult-acquired infection and higher rates of chronic carriage are seen in those with underlying immunodeficiency such as advanced HIV infection. Certain major histocompatibility complex (MHC) subtypes may also determine outcome following infection.[5]

Wild-type virus and viral variants

Most patients with acute and chronic HBV infection are infected with the wild-type HBV and HBeAg is found in the blood. It was recognized for many years that a subgroup of patients, particularly around the Mediterranean, were HBeAg negative and yet had evidence of ongoing liver damage with abnormal liver biochemistry and histology and ongoing viral replication with the presence of HBV DNA in the blood. Viral isolates were sequenced from these patients and a mutation was found in the precore gene of the virus which resulted in a stop codon and prevented viral synthesis of HBeAg.[6]

These viral variants are known as pre-core variants or anti-HBe variants and can arise following infection with wild-type virus, following antiviral therapy; alternatively, patients can be infected de novo by these variants.

Animal models

Hepadnavirus infections with similar outcomes are seen in several animal species including woodchucks, Beechey ground squirrels and Pekin ducks. Antiviral agents have been tried as therapy for infection in these animals, and they are sources of hepatocyte cell lines for assessing future antiviral agents.

ACUTE HEPATITIS

The development of the acute hepatitic illness appears to coincide with the host immune response and the detection of anti-hepatitis B core antigen (HBc) IgM antibodies. Fatigue is not uncommon for some months after infection but does not seem to relate to ongoing viral replication. Large multicenter trials would be required to determine whether immunomodulatory or antiviral therapy could limit disease and reduce the risk of chronicity. Small trials have shown no significant toxicity with interferon-α in this setting,[7] and there are reports that lamivudine may be helpful in severe cases.[8]

CHRONIC HBV

The aims of antiviral therapy are to clear the infection and to reduce the risks of developing life-threatening liver disease. Viral clearance also reduces the risks of viral transmission to others.

Candidates for therapy

A chronic carrier is defined as the presence of ongoing viral replication for at least 6 months and will be HBeAg, hepatitis B surface antigen (HBsAg) and HBV DNA-positive (wild-type infection) or HBsAg, anti-HBe and HBV DNA-positive (anti-HBe variant).

Assessing the response to antiviral therapy

A complete response to antiviral therapy is defined as the complete clearance of infection.

In wild-type infection:

1. Sustained clearance of HBeAg and the appearance of anti-HBe antibodies (known as the HBeAg/anti-HBe 'seroconversion').
2. Sustained clearance of HBsAg and the appearance of anti-HBs antibodies (this can occur many years after (1)).
3. Sustained clearance of HBV DNA.

In chronically infected patients with anti-HBe antibodies only (2) and (3) are applicable.

In a successfully treated patient the clearance of virus should be associated with a biochemical response and normalization of the elevation in the transaminase values and a histological response with decreased inflammation and fibrosis. In a patient with advanced cirrhosis the aims of therapy may be to improve survival by maintaining liver function or by reducing the risk of eventual hepatocellular carcinoma.

Treatment

Interferons

Interferon-α has been administered for chronic HBV infection since 1976 and is now a licensed therapy in many countries.

It is thought that the combination of antiviral and immunomodulatory effects of interferon are important in this setting.

Interferon-α induces intracellular enzymes, that inhibit viral protein synthesis. Interferons stimulate the production of about 30 host proteins including 2′,5′-oligoadenylate synthetase, which leads to activation of ribonuclease enzymes that cleave viral mRNA. Protein kinases are also induced, these can further inhibit viral protein synthesis.

Hepatocytes have very little MHC Class I display and it is thought that this can facilitate chronic infection within the liver. Interferons can enhance the MHC Class I display and aid immune recognition and lysis of infected cells. Natural killer activity is also enhanced by interferons.

In successfully treated patients a sustained decline is observed in the HBV DNA levels and 6–8 weeks into therapy there is a surge in the transaminase value, which is thought to coincide with immune lysis of infected cells. In patients with HIV and HBV infection a similar phenomenon is seen following CD4 increases with antiretroviral therapy.[9] This 'transaminitis' is generally asymptomatic and detected on bio-

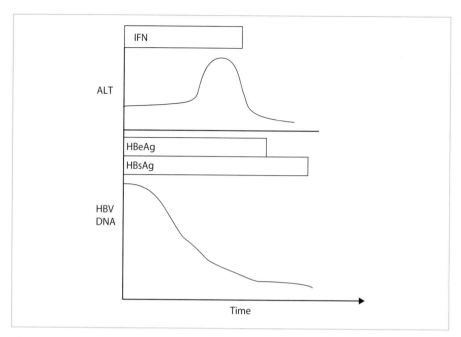

Fig 51.1 Chronic hepatitis B; successful response to interferon. IFN, interferon; ALT, alanine transaminase.

chemical testing. Hepatic decompensation is a risk, however, in patients with advanced disease (Figure 51.1).

In the successfully treated case the patient clears HBeAg and develops anti-HBe antibodies. Patients may continue to be HBsAg positive for some years but eventually this is also generally cleared and the patients become anti-HBs antibody positive.[10] Follow-up studies have also shown an improvement in the inflammatory activity in the liver but it will be many years before we can determine whether the risk of hepatocellular carcinoma is reduced in these patients.

Interferon-α is administered by intramuscular or subcutaneous injection and the usual dose is 5–10 megaunits (MU) three times weekly for 3–6 months. Most patients can be taught to self-administer the drug. The response rate is 20–40% in those with adult acquired disease.[11–14]

In one of the larger multicenter studies[15] 238 patients were randomized to receive no treatment, 2.5, 5 or 10 MU/m² of interferon-α three times weekly for 12–24 weeks. The clearance rate of HBeAg was 37% in the treatment group versus a spontaneous clearance rate of 13% in the no-treatment arm. There was no significant difference in the responses with the different doses although there was a trend towards higher response rates with the higher doses.

The response rate is very low in patients with vertically acquired disease, HIV infection or other immunodeficiency. Patients with low baseline HBV DNA levels and high transaminase levels or active inflammation on the liver biopsy are more likely to respond to therapy.

The main adverse effect of interferon-α is myelotoxicity, and careful monitoring of the blood count and dose adjustment is required (Box 50.1). Patients with advanced disease and baseline leukopenia or thrombocytopenia require particularly careful monitoring. Influenza-like symptoms with

Box 51.1 Side effects of interferon-α

Fever and chills (less with subsequent doses)

Myalgia

Fatigue

Myelotoxicity (regular monitoring of full blood count required)

Impaired concentration

Altered mood (particularly depression – can be severe)

Exacerbation or development of underlying autoimmune disease (e.g. hyperthyroidism or hypothyroidism)

Alopecia

Arthralgia

Hypersensitivity reactions (rare)

Pulmonary infiltrates (very rare)

malaise, fever and myalgia are particularly troublesome with the first doses of treatment. These can be minimized by administration of the interferon at bedtime and adjunctive paracetamol (acetaminophen).

Depression is another major side effect and interferon therapy is contraindicated in people with a background of severe depressive symptomatology. Patients can usually persevere with treatment if they develop mild depression and can find antidepressants helpful. For more major psychiatric side effects the interferon should be discontinued and expert help sought.

Most of the interferons in clinical use today are manufactured by recombinant technology using cultures of *Escherichia coli* with DNA insertions for human interferon-α. Interferon-α-2a (Roferon, Roche) and interferon-α-2b (Viraferon, Schering Plough) are two examples; there is only one amino acid difference between these two products.

A recent advance has been the development of pegylated interferon (peginterferon)-α, which has a longer half-life and can be given weekly. The experience with interferon-β has been more limited but results appear similar to those with interferon-α.

Interferon-γ as monotherapy or in combination with interferon-α has been tried in small studies and found to confer no advantage to interferon-α monotherapy.

Other immunomodulatory approaches

Corticosteroid therapy

It had been observed that the administration and subsequent withdrawal of corticosteroid therapy to patients with chronic HBV for other indications is, on occasion, associated with an 'immune rebound' hepatitis similar to the pattern observed with the administration of interferon-α and associated with viral clearance.[16] Generally, when this approach was evaluated formally in trials as monotherapy or in combination with interferon there appeared to be no significant benefit[13] and concerns were raised about treating patients with advanced disease and at risk of hepatic decompensation.[17]

However, early studies of nucleoside analogs with adenine arabinoside in combination with corticosteroid therapy suggested that this approach may be helpful for some patients,[18] and similar studies are in progress with corticosteroids and lamivudine, suggesting that further study of this approach is warranted.[19]

Thymic hormones

A number of naturally occurring and synthetic thymic peptides have been evaluated with no convincing benefit.[20]

Levamisole and inosine pranobex

Levamisole and inosine pranobex have also been evaluated, with disappointing results.

Vaccines as therapy

Patients with chronic HBV infection generally have very high levels of circulating HBsAg and the parenteral administration of exogenous HBsAg in the form of vaccine seems unlikely to be of benefit. In one study,[21] 32 patients were given three doses of HBV vaccine (GenHevacB, 20 mg of HBsAg and pre-S2 protein) with aluminum hydroxide as adjuvant. Interferon therapy was offered to all the patients in the study 6–9 months after the vaccine course and overall it was felt that the vaccination alone inhibited viral replication in 44% of the patients in the study.

Other immune approaches

Chronic HBV carriers given bone marrow transplants for life-threatening hematological malignancies have cleared HBV infection if the donor had immunity following HBV infection or vaccine administration. Lymphocyte transfer or modulation of the host immune response by ex-vivo stimulation of host lymphocytes are approaches under further study.

Nucleoside and nucleotide analogs

Nucleoside analogs have been assessed as potential therapy for chronic HBV for many years and there has been considerable renewed interest in this, with the development of agents for HIV infection that also have activity against HBV.

Adenine arabinoside and adenine arabinoside monophosophate

Adenine arabinoside (ara-A) and the water-soluble derivative adenine arabinoside monophosphate (ara-AMP) were among the first antiviral agents found to have activity against HBV.[22,23] Studies showed a decrease in the HBV DNA levels and some patients cleared HBeAg. The agents were administered as monotherapy or in combination with interferon-α[24] or corticosteroids. Prolonged treatment courses, however, were complicated by peripheral neuropathy.

Ribavirin

Ribavirin has broad-spectrum antiviral activity but has only modest activity against HBV.[23]

Aciclovir

Aciclovir at high serum levels has inhibitory activity against HBV replication. Unlike herpes viruses, HBV does not possess thymidine kinase activity and it is presumed that the first phosphorylation step towards the active triphosphate form required host intracellular enzymes. However, the use of aciclovir has been limited by the need to use intravenous dosing to achieve the necessary drug levels.[26]

Famciclovir

Famciclovir has greater oral bioavailability, and a pilot study demonstrated activity against HBV.[27] A 4-month study with famciclovir confirmed this activity,[28] however, famciclovir is not as potent as agents such as lamivudine and its role as monotherapy is limited, although it may have a role in combination therapy.

Lamivudine

Although hepadnaviruses are DNA viruses, the polymerase has reverse transcriptase acitivity and several nucleoside analogs developed as anti-HIV agents have activity against HBV. Mostly this is at a modest level, but lamivudine (3′-thiacytidine) was found to have potent activity against HBV replication and now has a major role in the therapy of chronic HBV. The initial pilot study was with 1 month of therapy,[29] and larger trials with longer duration of therapy followed.[30–36] Many patients have now been safely treated for several years. It is thought that the low toxicity of lamivudine is in part related to its minus enantiomer configuration.

After 1 year of therapy 17% of patients have a successful response; this increases to 27% after a second year.[34] An incremental increase is seen with longer treatment periods and a success rate of up to 66% has been reported with 4 years of therapy.[35]

A sustained response is generally seen following loss of HBeAg;[36] however, there have been concerns about the durability of this[37] and it is now recommended that lamivudine is continued for 3–6 months following HBeAg seroconversion.

Inevitably with monotherapy in a chronic viral infection, resistance is seen and was first reported in the setting of liver transplantation.[38,39] The main mutations are reported to involve the YMDD motif (the equivalent of the 184 mutation in the HIV reverse transcriptase gene).

The emergence of viral resistance has led to several controversies in the management of chronic HBV. It is thought that the YMDD variant is less replication competent[40] and, certainly, although an increase in the transaminase value may follow the emergence of such variants, the value often remains below pretreatment levels.[41,42] There have been reports of patients clearing HBV infection despite their emergence.[43] However acute 'flares' have been reported, with the emergence of resistant variants, and life-threatening disease can occur, particularly in those with end-stage disease or in the setting of transplantation.[44,45]

Lamivudine has revolutionized the outcome for patients with end-stage hepatitis HBV.[42,46–48] Pre-lamivudine the only option for the transplant patient was the suppression of infection with the administration of HBV immune globulin in the form of immune serum or monoclonal antibody. However, this is an expensive approach and merely temporarily suppresses infection. Potential candidates for liver transplantation were given lamivudine as suppressive therapy before transplantation and some patients had a dramatic clinical response and significantly improved liver function. Various regimens with the administration of lamivudine pre-, peri- and post-transplant have been tried;[43] however, currently there are limited options for the emergence of lamivudine-resistant mutants for patients undergoing liver transplantation.

For the patient with moderate disease activity who has failed on previous interferon therapy or where interferon is contraindicated lamivudine appears a reasonable approach. For the patient with more advanced disease who may be a candidate for liver transplantation it is important to liaise with the transplant unit regarding local protocols for antiviral therapy. For asymptomatic patients with only mild disease the emergence of lamivudine-resistant variants may limit future options with combination therapy and an expectant approach may be the preferred option.[49] One study has monitored the initial virologic response to lamivudine in an attempt to recognize which patients are likely to benefit most from therapy,[50] and it has been shown that reduced response may be seen in patients infected with certain viral subtypes.[51]

Lamivudine has also been tried in combination with interferon-α, which increased the success rate only marginally.[52] Lamivudine has also been used in combination with corticosteroid therapy in a small study.[18]

Adefovir

Adefovir is a nucleotide analog with broad-spectrum activity. There have been concerns about renal toxicities when used as therapy for HIV infection.[53,54] The drug nevertheless has potent activity against HBV,[55] and it is hoped that lower doses than those used in HIV studies will be effective and less toxic. Lamivudine-resistant strains have been shown to be sensitive to adefovir.[56]

Other agents

Other nucleoside analogs such as entecavir demonstrate promising activity against HBV.[57]

Anti-HBe variants

A high relapse rate is evident with interferon therapy for patients infected with the anti-HBe variant,[58,59] but those who have a sustained response achieve improved long-term outcome.[60]

Lamivudine has inhibitory effects against the antiHBe variant but the sustained response rate with prolonged therapy has yet to be determined.[61,62]

PREVENTION

Safe and effective vaccines have now been developed against HBV.[63] Passive prophylaxis with immune globulin continues to be used to limit vertical transmission and in patients undergoing liver transplantation.

HEPATITIS C VIRUS INFECTION

The existence of hepatitis C virus (HCV) infection had been suspected for many years as some patients who have been exposed to blood products developed acute and chronic hepatitis but were negative for HAV or HBV infection. The terms 'post-transfusion' or 'parenterally transmitted' non-A, non-B hepatitis evolved. HCV was discovered in 1989,[64] and appears to explain most of these cases. The virus is a member of the Flaviviridae family.

EPIDEMIOLOGY

Before the screening of blood products HCV accounted for more than 90% of cases of post-transfusion hepatitis, and it remains a common pathogen in intravenous drug users and in those exposed to pooled blood products. Contaminated needles and blood products are the main sources of infection but vertical transmission can occur; some patients may have been infected sexually. In many patients, however, there is no clear source of infection.

There is very little detailed information on the seroprevalence of HCV. There are thought to be 170 million carriers in the world.[65] The seroprevalence in UK blood donors is 0.07%,[66] but is thought to be 0.7% in the general population.[67]

In the USA there are thought to be 2.7 million people with HCV infection.[68] Seroprevalence rates as high as 25% have been recorded in areas of Egypt[69] and have led to theories regarding mass immunization programs or schistosomiasis treatment programs with contaminated needles.[70]

There appear to be six major genotypes of HCV:[71] in Europe and the USA the predominant genotypes are 1, 2 and 3;[68] in north Africa, for example, genotype 4 predominates.[72]

NATURAL HISTORY

The incubation period of HCV infection is 6–12 weeks, although shorter periods have been described following blood transfusion.[73] The primary infection is generally subclinical and HCV is not a major cause of fulminant hepatitis. Between 60 and 80% of those infected develop chronic infection and most carriers are asymptomatic, but chronic liver disease can insidiously develop over decades, leading to cirrhosis with risks of hepatocellular carcinoma.[74,75] In patients with established cirrhosis the risk of developing hepatocellular carcinoma is 2–5% per year.[76,77]

The varying rates of disease progression are not understood, but host factors[78] such as male gender, older age at time of infection, heavy alcohol consumption and immunosuppression such as HIV infection[79] are also associated with more rapid progression. It is also recognized that some patients complain of fatigue,[80] which is not explained by the degree of liver damage and may be related to involvement of the central nervous system.[81]

TREATMENT

Acute HCV

Despite the difficulty with the diagnosis of primary HCV infection, a number of small studies suggest that early intervention with antiviral therapy may reduce the chance of chronic infection.[82–86] This is an important strategy when dealing with patients and healthcare workers who have sustained a needlestick infection from an infected patient, but there are controversies regarding the regimens used and the timing and duration of the treatment courses.

Chronic HCV

Just as with chronic HBV infection the aims of treatment are to clear the infection and to reduce the chance of the fatal liver disease. There is no vaccine for HCV and successful treatment of the infection is important for limiting spread of infection.

The main treatments used for HCV infection are interferon-α and ribavirin. A sustained virological response is indicated when the HCV RNA level remains negative 6 months after therapy (Figure 51.2) and this is usually associated with a biochemical response and improvement in the liver histology.

Interferon-α

Interferon-α has been used in trials since 1986,[87] and is licensed as therapy in many countries. With successful therapy a reduction is seen in the HCV RNA levels (Figure 51.2) and, in contrast to the biochemical response seen with treatment

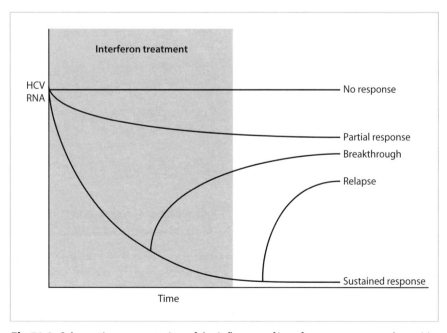

Fig 51.2 Schematic representation of the influence of interferon treatment on hepatitis C virus RNA levels.

for HBV infection, this is paralleled with a reduction in the transaminase levels. Although 50% of patients may show an initial viral or biochemical response, for many patients this is only partial – and even in those who achieve negative HCV RNA levels at the end of the treatment period about a half relapse.[88–93] A sustained response to interferon-α monotherapy is seen in only 10–20%, and those patients with genotype 1, genotype 4 HCV or high viral loads are less likely to respond.[94–96]

Ribavirin

Ribavirin, a guanosine analog, is a broad-spectrum antiviral agent (*see* Ch. 40). In initial monotherapy studies a reduction was seen in the transaminase values during therapy.[97] Studies with the availability of HCV RNA analysis demonstrated that this reduction was associated with, at most, a modest reduction in the HCV RNA levels.[98–101] It is thought that ribavirin's other properties such as immunomodulation may therefore be of more importance in this setting. The main side effect of ribavirin is hemolysis, and regular hemoglobin checks are therefore required throughout therapy (Box 51.2). Concerns have been expressed about the potential for fetal teratogenecity and prospective patients and their partners should be carefully counseled about this issue. It is recommended that both men and women avoid conception while on therapy and for several months afterwards.

Box 51.2 Side effects of ribavirin

Hemolysis – caution in patients with cardiac problems
Risk of teratogenicity – avoid conception
Rash – continue therapy if transient or mild
Pruritus – may limit continuation of therapy
Acute hypersensitivity – rare

Combination therapy

Combination studies have shown an improved sustained response rate (30–45%) with interferon and ribavirin;[102–105] this is now standard treatment in many countries. This combination is also an option for patients who have relapsed after interferon monotherapy.[106,107]

These trials confirmed that patients infected with the type 1 viral genotype had a lower response rate and that there was no extra benefit in treating patients with type 2 or 3 genotype for more than 6 months.[104] These studies have been used to develop national and international treatment guidelines.

Pegylated interferons

A further advance has been the development of peginterferon, which has more sustained absorption and decreased clearance than the standard interferons.[108,109] Measurement of 2′,5′-oligoadonylate synthetase activity confirms that biological activity is increased in level and duration with peginterferon and the side effects appear similar, although more local skin reactions are noted with the pegylated products. Peginterferons given as monotherapy have sustained response rates (39%), which are comparable to the combination of ribavirin and standard thrice-weekly interferon.[110,111]

Patients with HCV-associated cirrhosis have a very low response rate to standard thrice-weekly interferon but improved response rates with peginterferon.[112] Even if no sustained virological response is achieved with interferon therapy incidence of hepatocellular carcinoma development is reduced.[113–115] It is unclear whether this relates to the antiviral, immunomodulatory or antifibrotic effects of interferon.

For patients with end-stage disease liver transplantation should be considered; HCV infection is an increasing indication for this. However, graft reinfection is a major concern.

Combination of peginterferon and ribavirin

Sustained response rates of 82% in patients with genotypes 2 or 3 and 42% in patients with genotype 1 have been reported with a combination of peginterferon and ribavirin.[116] Tailored regimens based on the viral genotype and load, patient weight and initial response to therapy are being developed.

Amantadine

A pilot study has suggested that amantadine may have some activity against HCV,[117] but later studies including combination trials with interferon and ribavirin in treatment-naïve and previously treated patients have produced variable results.[118–121] In one study of 200 patients[118] a sustained response was reported in 29% of patients who received a combination of interferon and amantadine, compared with 17% in those who received interferon monotherapy. In a similar study,[83] only 10% of those who received combination therapy cleared the virus. However, those who received amantadine reported improved wellbeing compared with the interferon monotherapy arm, and it has been suggested that this may relate to the central nervous system stimulatory effects of amantadine[122] rather than any antiviral effect.

Future agents

HCV has serine protease and helicase activity. It is hoped that specific inhibitors can be developed as future treatment strategies.

HEPATITIS D VIRUS INFECTION

Hepatitis D virus (HDV) infection requires the presence of HBV to replicate. It is a major cause of rapidly progressive liver disease. Interferon-α is helpful for only a minority of patients,[123,124] and transplantation should be considered for those with advanced disease.[125] Lamivudine, despite its inhibitory effect on HBV replication, has little effect in on HDV infection.[126]

CONCLUSION

Significant advances have been made in the treatment of chronic HBV and HCV and it is now possible to offer virological cure for many patients.

References

1. Yoshiba M, Inoue K, Sekiyama K et al 1994 Interferon for hepatitis A. *Lancet* 343: 288–289.

2. Lemon SD, Thomas D 1997 Vaccines to prevent viral hepatitis. *New England Journal of Medicine* 336: 196.

3. De Jongh FE, Jamssea HL, De Man RA, Hopw WC, Schalm SW, Blankenstein MV 1992 Survival and prognostic indicators in hepatitis B surface antigen-positive cirrhosis of the liver. *Gastroenterology* 103: 1630–1635.

4. Liaw YF, Tai DI, Chu CM, Chen TJ 1988 The development of cirrhosis in patients with chronic type B hepatitis: a prospective study. *Hepatology* 8: 493–496.

5. Thursz MR, Thomas HC, Greenwood BM, Hill AV 1997 Heterozygote advantage for HLA class-II type in hepatitis B virus infection. *Nature Genetics* 17: 11–12.

6. Carman WF, Jacyna MR, Hadziyannis S et al 1989 Mutation preventing formation of hepatitis HB e antigen in chronic hepatitis B virus infection. *Lancet* ii: 588–591.

7. Kundu SS, Kundu AK, Pal NK 2000 Interferon-alpha in the treatment of acute prolonged hepatitis B virus infection. *Journal of the Association of Physicians of India* 48: 671–673.

8. Reshef R, Sbeit W, Tur-Kaspa R 2000 Lamivudine in the treatment of acute hepatitis. *New England Journal of Medicine* 343: 1123–1124.

9. Carr A, Cooper DA 1997 Restoration of immunity to chronic hepatitis B infection in HIV-infected patient on protease inhibitor. *Lancet* 349: 995–996.

10. Korenman J, Baker B, Waggoner J et al 1991 Long term remissions of chronic hepatitis B after alpha interferon. *Annals of Internal Medicine* 114: 629–634.

11. Anderson MG, Harrison TJ, Alexander GJM et al 1986 Randomised controlled trial of lymphoblastoid interferon for chronic active hepatitis B. *Journal of Hepatology* 3 (Suppl.): S225–S227.

12. Brook MG, Chan G, Yap I et al 1989 Randomised controlled trial of lymphoblastoid interferon alfa in Europid men with chronic hepatitis B virus infection. *British Medical Journal* 299: 652–656.

13. Perrillo RP, Schiff ER, Davis GL et al 1990 A randomised controlled trial of interferon alfa 2-b alone and after prednisone withdrawal for the treatment of chronic hepatitis B. *New England Journal of Medicine* 323: 295–301.

14. Wong DK, Cheung AM, O'Rourke K, Naylor CD, Detsky AS, Heathcote J 1993 Effect of alpha interferon treatment in patients with hepatitis B e antigen positive chronic hepatitis B. A meta analysis. *Annals of Internal Medicine* 119: 312–323.

15. Thomas HC, Lok ASF, Carreno V et al 1994 Comparative study of three doses of interferon-a$_{2a}$ in chronic active hepatitis B. *Journal of Viral Hepatology* 1: 139–148.

16. Nair PV, Tong M, Stevenson D et al 1985 Effects of short term high dose prednisone treatment of patients with HBsAg positive chronic active hepatitis. *Liver* 5: 8–12.

17. Krogsgaard K, Marcellin P, Trepo C et al 1996 Prednisolone withdrawal therapy enhances the effect of human lymphoblastoid therapy in chronic hepatitis B. *Journal of Hepatology* 25: 803–813.

18. Perrillo R, Regenstein F, Bodicky C et al 1985 Comparative efficacy of adenine arabinoside 5'-monophosphate and prednisone withdrawal followed by adenine arabinoside 5'-monophosphate in the treatment of chronic active hepatitis type B. *Gastroenterology* 88: 780–786.

19. Liaw YF, Tsai SL, Chien RN, Yeh CT, Chu CM 2000 Prednisolone priming enhances Th1 response and efficacy of subsequent lamivudine therapy in patients with chronic hepatitis B. *Hepatology* 32: 604–609.

20. Fattovich G, Giustina G, Alberti A et al 1994 A randomised controlled trial of thymopentin therapy in patients with chronic hepatitis B. *Journal of Hepatology* 21: 361–366.

21. Pol S, Driss F, Michel M-L et al 1994 Specific vaccine therapy in chronic hepatitis B infection. *Lancet* 344: 342.

22. Bassendine MF, Chadwick RG, Salmeron J et al 1981 Adenine arabinoside therapy in HBsAg-positive chronic liver disease: a controlled study. *Gastroenterology* 80: 1016–1021.

23. Hoofnagle JH, Hanson RG, Minuk GY et al 1984 Randomised controlled trial of adenine arabinoside monophosphate for chronic type B hepatitis. *Gastroenterology* 86: 150–157.

24. Garcia G, Smith CI, Weissberg JI et al 1987 Adenine arabinoside monophosphate (vidarabine phosphate) in combination with human leukocyte interferon in the treatment of chronic hepatitis B. *Annals of Internal Medicine* 107: 278–285.

25. Fried MW, Fong T-L, Swain MG et al 1994 Therapy of chronic hepatitis B with a 6 month course of ribavirin. *Journal of Hepatology* 21: 145–150.

26. Weller IVD, Carreno V, Fowler MJF et al 1983 Acyclovir in hepatitis B antigen positive chronic liver disease; inhibition of viral replication and transient renal impairment with IV bolus administration. *Journal of Antimicrobial Chemotherapy* 12: 223–231.

27. Main J, Brown JL, Howells C et al 1996 A double blind placebo controlled study to assess the effect of famciclovir on virus replication in patients with chronic hepatitis B virus infection. *Journal of Viral Hepatitis* 3: 211–215.

28. Trepo C, Jezek P, Atkinson G, Boon R, Young C 2000 Famciclovir in chronic hepatitis B: results of a dose-finding study. *Journal of Hepatology* 32: 1011–1018.

29. Tyrrell DLJ, Mitchell MC, De Man RA et al 1993 Phase II trial of lamivudine for chronic hepatitis B. *Hepatology* 18 (Suppl.): 112A.

30. Dienstag JL, Perrillo RP, Schiff ER, Bartholomew M, Vicary C, Rubin M 1995 A preliminary trial of lamivudine for chronic hepatitis B infection. *New England Journal of Medicine* 333: 1657–1661.

31. Dienstag JL, Schiff ER, Wright TL et al 1999 Lamivudine as initial treatment for chronic hepatitis B in the United States. *New England Journal of Medicine* 341: 1256–1263.

32. Nevens F, Main J, Honkoop P et al 1997 Lamivudine therapy for chronic hepatitis B: a six-month randomized dose-ranging study. *Gastroenterology* 113: 1258–1263.

33. Lai CL, Chien RN, Leung NW et al 1998 A one-year trial of lamivudine for chronic hepatitis B. Asia Hepatitis Lamivudine Study Group. *New England Journal of Medicine* 339: 61–68.

34. Liaw YF, Leung NW, Chang TT et al 2000 Effects of extended lamivudine therapy in Asian patients with chronic hepatitis B. Asia Hepatitis Lamivudine Study Group. *Gastroenterology* 119: 172–180.

35. Chang TT, Lai CL, Liaw YF et al 2000 Incremental increases in HBeAg seroconversion and continued ALT normalization in Asian chronic HBV patients treated with lamivudine for four years. *Antiviral Therapeutics* 5 (Suppl. 1): 44.

36. Dienstag JL, Schiff ER, Mitchell M et al 1999 Extended lamivudine retreatment for chronic hepatitis B: maintenance of viral suppression after discontinuation of therapy. *Hepatology* 30: 1082–1087.

37. Song BC, Suh DJ, Lee HC, Chung YH, Lee YS 2000 Hepatitis B e antigen seroconversion after lamivudine therapy is not durable in patients with chronic hepatitis B in Korea. *Hepatology* 32: 803–806.

38. Ling R, Mutimer D, Ahmed M et al 1996 Selection of mutations in the hepatitis B virus polymerase during therapy of transplant recipients with lamivudine. *Hepatology* 24: 711–713.

39. Bartholomew MM, Jansen RW, Jeffers LJ et al 1997 Hepatitis B virus resistance to lamivudine given for recurrent infection after orthotopic liver transplantation *Lancet* 349: 20–22.

40. Melegari M, Scaglioni PP, Wands JR 1998 Hepatitis B mutants associated with 3TC and famciclovir administration are replication defective. *Hepatology* 27: 628–633.

41. Hunt CM, McGill JM, Allen MI, Condreay LD 2000 Clinical relevance of hepatitis B viral mutations. *Hepatology* 31: 1037–1044.

42. Perrillo RP, Wright T, Rakela J et al 2001 A multicenter United States-Canadian trial to assess lamivudine monotherapy before and after liver transplantation for chronic hepatitis B. *Hepatology* 33: 424–432.

43. Liaw YF, Chien RN, Yeh CT, Tsai SL, Chu CM 1999 Acute exacerbation and hepatitis B virus clearance after emergence of YMDD motif mutation during lamivudine therapy. *Hepatology* 30: 567–572.

44. Mutimer D, Pillay D, Shields P et al 2000 Outcome of lamivudine resistant hepatitis B virus infection in the liver transplant recipient. *Gut* 46: 107–113.

45. Peters MG, Singer G, Howard T et al 1999 Fulminant hepatic failure resulting from lamivudine-resistant hepatitis B virus in a renal transplant recipient: durable response after orthotopic liver transplantation on adefovir dipivoxil and hepatitis B immune globulin. *Transplantation* 68: 1912–1914.

46. Yao FY, Bass NM 2000 Lamivudine treatment in patients with severely decompensated cirrhosis due to replicating hepatitis B infection. *Journal of Hepatology* 33: 301–307.

47. Kapoor D, Guptan RC, Wakil SM et al 2000 Beneficial effects of lamivudine in hepatitis B virus-related decompensated cirrhosis. *Journal of Hepatology* 33: 329–342.

48. Villeneuve J-P, Condreay LD, Willems B, et al. 2000 Lamivudine treatment for decompensated cirrhosis resulting from chronic hepatitis B. *Hepatology* 31: 207–210.

49. Lok ASF 2000 Lamivudine therapy for chronic hepatitis B; is longer duration of treatment better? *Gastroenterology* 119: 263–266.

50. Buti M, Sanchez F, Cotrina M et al 2001 Quantitative hepatitis B virus DNA testing for the early prediction of the maintenance of response during lamivudine therapy in patients with chronic hepatitis B. *Journal of Infectious Diseases* 183: 1277–1280.

51. Zollner B, Petersen J, Schroter M, Laufs R, Schoder V, Feucht H-H 2001 20-fold increase in risk of lamivudine resistance in hepatitis B virus subtype adw. *Lancet* 357: 934–935.

52. Schalm SW, Heathcote J, Cianciara J et al 2000 Lamivudine and alpha interferon combination treatment of patients with chronic hepatitis B infection: a randomised trial. *Gut* 46: 562–528.

53. Noble S, Goa KL 1999 Adefovir dipivoxil. *Drugs* 58: 479–487.

54. Ho ES, Lin DC, Mendel DB, Cihlar T 2000 Cytotoxicity of antiviral nucleotides adefovir and cidofovir is induced by the expression of human renal organic anion transporter 1. *Journal of the American Society of Nephrology* 11: 383–393.

55. Gilson RJ, Chopra KB, Newell AM et al 1999 A placebo-controlled phase I/II study of adefovir dipivoxil in patients with chronic hepatitis B virus infection. *Journal of Viral Hepatitis* 6: 387–395.

56. Perrillo R, Schiff E, Yoshida E et al 2000 Adefovir dipivoxil for the treatment of lamivudine-resistant hepatitis B mutants. *Hepatology* 32: 129–134.

57. Farrell GC 2000 Clinical potential of emerging new agents in hepatitis B. *Drugs* 60: 701–710.

58. Hadziyannis S, Bramou T, Makris A et al 1990 Interferon alfa-2b treatment of HBeAg negative/serum HBV DNA positive chronic active hepatitis type B. *Journal of Hepatology* 11: S133–S136.

59. Brunetto MR, Oliveri F, Demartini A et al 1991 Treatment with interferon of chronic hepatitis B associated with antibody to hepatitis B e antigen. *Journal of Hepatology* 13 (Suppl. 1): S8–S11.

60. Papatheodoridis GV, Manesis E, Hadziyannis SJ 2001 The long term outcome of interferon-α treated and untreated patients with HBeAg-negative chronic hepatitis B. *Journal of Hepatology* 34: 306–313.

61. Tassopoulos NC, Volpes R, Pastore G et al 1999 Efficacy of lamivudine in patients with hepatitis B e antigen-negative/hepatitis B virus DNA-positive (precore mutant) chronic hepatitis B Lamivudine Precore Mutant Study Group. *Hepatology* 29: 889–896.

62. Hadziyannis SJ, Papatheodoridis GV, Dimou E et al 2000 Efficacy of long-term lamivudine monotherapy in patients with hepatitis B e antigen-negative chronic hepatitis B. *Hepatology* 32: 847–851.

63. Zuckerman JN, Zuckerman AJ 2000 Current topics in hepatitis B. *Journal of Antimicrobial Chemotherapy* 41: 130–136.

64. Choo QI, Kuo G, Weiner AJ et al 1989 Isolation of a cDNA clone derived from blood-borne non-A, non-B viral hepatitis genome. *Science* 244: 359–362.

65. WHO 1997 Hepatitis C global prevalence. *Weekly Epidemiological Record* 72: 341–344.

66. Ryan KW, McLennan S, Barbara JA, Hewitt PE 1994 Follow-up of blood donors positive for antibiodies to hepatitis C. *British Medical Journal* 308: 696–697.

67. Sallie R, King R, Silva E, Tibbs C, Johnson P, Williams R 1994 Community prevalence of hepatitis C viraemia: a polymerase chain reaction study. *Journal of Medical Virology* 43: 111–114.

68. Alter MJ, Kruszon-Moran D, Nainan OV et al 1999 The prevalence of hepatitis C virus infection in the United States, 1988 through 1994. *New England Journal of Medicine* 341: 556–562.

69. Abdel-Aziz F, Habib M, Mohamed MK et al 2000 Hepatitis C virus (HCV) infection in a community in the Nile Delta: population description and HCV prevalence. *Hepatology* 32: 111–115.

70. Frank C, Mohamed MK, Strickland GT et al 2000 The role of parenteral antischistosomal therapy in the spread of hepatitis C virus in Egypt. *Lancet* 355: 887–889.

71. Simmonds P 1999 Viral heterogeneity of the hepatitis C virus. *Journal of Hepatology* 31 (Suppl. 1): 54–60.

72. Ray SC, Arthur RR, Carella A, Bukh J, Thomas DL 2000 Genetic epidemiology of hepatitis C virus throughout Egypt. *Journal of Infectious Diseases* 182: 698–707.

73. Alter HJ, Purcell RH, Shih JW et al 1989 Detection of antibody to hepatitis C virus in prospectively followed transfusion recipients with acute and chronic non-A, non-B hepatitis. *New England Journal of Medicine* 321: 1494–1500.

74. Seeff LB, Buskell-Bales Z, Wright EC et al 1992 Long term mortality after transfusion-associated non-A, non-B hepatitis. *New England Journal of Medicine* 327: 1906–1911.

75. Tong MJ, El-Farra NS, Reikes AR et al 1995 Clinical outcomes after transfusion associated hepatitis C. *New England Journal of Medicine* 332: 1463–1466.

76. Poynard T, Ratziu V, Benhamou Y, Opolon P, Cacoub P 2000 Natural history of HCV infection. *Baillière's Clinical Gastroenterology* 14: 211–218.

77. Bruno S, Silini E, Crosignani A et al 1997 Hepatitis C virus genotypes and risk of hepatocellular carcinoma in cirrhosis: a prospective study. *Hepatology* 25: 754–758.

78. Poynard T, Redossa P, Opolon P 1997 Natural history of liver fibrosis progression in patients with chronic hepatitis C. *Lancet* 349: 825–832.

79. Benhamou Y, Bochet M, Di Martino V et al 1999 Liver fibrosis progression in human immunodeficiency virus and hepatitis C virus coinfected patients. *Hepatology* 30: 1054–1058.

80. Foster GR, Goldin RD, Thomas HC 1998 Chronic hepatitis C virus infection causes a significant reduction in quality of life in the absence of cirrhosis. *Hepatology* 27: 209–212.

81. Forton DM, Allsop JM, Main J, Foster GR, Thomas HC, Taylor-Robinson SD 2001 Evidence for a cerebral effect of hepatitis C virus. *Lancet* 358: 38–39.

82. Omata M, Yokosuka O, Takano S et al 1991 Resolution of acute hepatitis C after therapy with natural beta interferon. *Lancet* 338: 914–915.

83. Viladomiu L, Genesca J, Estaban JI et al 1992 Interferon alpha in acute post-transfusion hepatitis C; a randomised controlled trial. *Hepatology* 16: 767–769.

84. Hwang SJ, Lee SD, Chan CY et al 1994 A randomized controlled trial of recombinant interferon alpha-2b in the treatment of Chinese patients with acute post-transfusion hepatitis C. *Journal of Hepatology* 19: 19–22.

85. Lampertico P, Rumi MG, Romeo R et al 1994 A multicenter randomized controlled trial of recombinant interferon alpha 2b in patients with acute transfusion associated hepatitis C. *Hepatology* 19: 19–22.

86. Poynard T, Leroy V, Cohard M et al 1996 Meta-analysis of interferon randomized trials in the treatment of viral hepatitis C; effects of dose and duration. *Hepatology* 24: 778–789.

87. Hoofnagle JH, Mullen KD, Jones DB et al 1986 Treatment of chronic non-A, non-B hepatitis with recombinant human alpha interferon. A preliminary report. *New England Journal of Medicine* 315: 1575–1578.

88. Davis GL, Balart LA, Schiff ER et al 1989 Treatment of chronic hepatitis C with recombinant interferon alpha. *New England Journal of Medicine* 321: 1501–1506.

89. Di Bisceglie AM, Martin P, Kassianides C et al 1989 Recombinant interferon alfa therapy for chronic hepatitis C: a randomized double blind placebo-controlled trial. *New England Journal of Medicine* 321: 1506–1510.

90. Saracco G, Rosina F, Torrani et al 1990 Randomised controlled trial of interferon alfa 2b as therapy for chronic non-A, non-B hepatitis. *Journal of Hepatology* 11: S34–S49.

91. Causse X, Godinot H, Chevallier M et al 1991 Comparison of 1 or 3 MU of interferon alfa-2b and placebo in patients with chronic non-A, non-B hepatitis. *Gastroenterology* 101: 497–502.

92. Cimino L, Nardone G, Citarella C et al 1991 Treatment of chronic hepatitis C with recombinant interferon alfa. *Italian Journal of Gastroenterology* 23: 399–342.

93. Marcellin P, Boyer N, Giostra E et al 1991 Recombinant human alpha-interferon in patients with chronic non-A, non-B hepatitis. A multi-centre randomised controlled trial from France. *Hepatology* 13: 393–397.

94. Martinot-Peignoux M, Marcellin P, Pouteau M et al 1995 Pretreatment serum HCV RNA levels and HCV genotype are the main and independent prognostic factors of sustained response to alfa interferon therapy in chronic hepatitis C. *Hepatology* 22: 1050–1056.

95. Yamada G, Takatani M, Kishi F et al 1995 Efficacy of interferon alfa therapy in chronic hepatitis C patients depends primarily on hepatitis C virus RNA level. *Hepatology* 22: 1351–1354.

96. el-Zayadi A, Selim O, Haddad S et al 1999 Combination treatment of interferon alpha-2b and ribavirin in comparison to interferon monotherapy in treatment of chronic hepatitis C genotype 4 patients. *Italian Journal of Gastroenterology and Hepatology* 31: 472–475.

97. Reichard O, Andersson J, Schvarcz R et al 1991 Ribavirin treatment for chronic hepatitis C. *Lancet* 337: 1058–1061.

98. Reichard O, Yun Z-B, Sonnersborg A et al 1993 Hepatitis C viral RNA titers in serum prior to, during and after oral treatment with ribavirin for chronic hepatitis C. *Journal of Medical Virology* 41: 99–102.

99. Di Bisceglie AM, Conjeevaram HS, Fried MW et al 1995 Ribavirin as therapy for chronic hepatitis C. A randomized, double-blind, placebo-controlled trial. *Annals of Internal Medicine* 123: 897–903.

100. Dusheiko G, Main J, Thomas HC et al 1996 Ribavirin treatment for patients with chronic hepatitis C: results of a placebo controlled study. *Journal of Hepatology* 25: 591–598.

101. Bodenheimer HC, Lindsay KL, Davis GL et al 1997 Tolerance and efficacy of oral ribavirin treatment of chronic hepatitis C; a multicenter trial. *Hepatology* 26: 1493–1497.

102. Chemello L, Cavalletto L, Bernardinello E et al 1995 The effect of interferon alfa and ribavirin combination therapy in naive patients with chronic hepatitis C. *Journal of Hepatology* 23 (Suppl. 2): 8–12.

103. McHutchison JG, Gordon S, Schiff ER et al 1998 Interferon alfa-2b plus ribavirin as initial treatment for chronic hepatitis C; results of a US multicenter randomized controlled trial. *New England Journal of Medicine* 339: 1485–1492.

104. Poynard T, Marcellin P, Lee SS et al 1998 Randomised trial of interferon alpha2b plus ribavirin for 48 weeks or for 24 weeks versus interferon alpha 2b plus placebo for 48 weeks for treatment of chronic infection with hepatitis C. *Lancet* 352: 1426–1432.

105. Lai MY, Kao JH, Yang PM et al 1996 Long term efficacy of ribavirin plus interferon alfa in the treatment of chronic hepatitis C. *Gastroenterology* 111: 1307–1312.

106. Brillanti S, Garson J, Foli M et al 1994 A pilot study of combination therapy with ribavirin plus interferon alfa for interferon resistant chronic hepatitis C. *Gastroenterology* 107: 812–817.

107. Davis GL, Esteban-Mur R, Rustgi V et al 1998 Interferon alfa-2b alone or in combination with ribavirin for the treatment of relapse of chronic hepatitis C. *New England Journal of Medicine* 339: 1493–1499.

108. Glue P, Fang JW, Rouzier-Panis R et al 2000 Pegylated interferon-alpha 2b: pharmacokinetics, pharmacodynamic, safety and preliminary efficacy data. Hepatitis C Intervention Therapy Group. *Clinical Pharmacology and Therapeutics* 68: 556–567.

109. Wang YS, Youngster S, Bausch J et al 2000 Identification of the major positional isomer of pegylated interferonalpha-2b. *Biochemistry* 39: 10634–10640.

110. Zeuzem S, Feinman SV, Rasenack J et al 2000 Peginterferon alfa-2a in patients with chronic hepatitis C. *New England Journal of Medicine* 343: 1666–1672.

111. Reddy KR, Wright TL, Pockros PJ et al 2001 Efficacy and safety of pegylated interferon alpha-2a compared with interferon alpha-2a in non-cirrhotic patients with chronic hepatitis C. *Hepatology* 33: 433–438.

112. Heathcote EJ, Shiffman ML, Cooksley WG et al 2000 Peginterferon alfa-2a in patients with chronic hepatitis C and cirrhosis. *New England Journal of Medicine* 343: 1673–1680.

113. Manns MP, McHutchison JG, Gordon S et al 2000 Peginterferon alfa-2b plus ribavirin compared to interferon alfa-2b plus ribavirin for the treatment of chronic hepatitis C: 24 week treatment analysis of a multicenter, multinational, phase III randomized controlled trial. *Hepatology* 32: 297.

114. International Interferon-alpha hepatocellular carcinoma study group. Effect of interferon alpha on progression of cirrhosis to hepatocellular carcinoma: a retrospective cohort study. *Lancet* 351: 1535–1539.

115. Nishiguchi S, Kuroki T, Nakatani S et al 1995 Randomised trial of effects of interferon alpha on incidence of hepatocellular carcinoma in chronic active hepatitis C with cirrhosis. *Lancet* 346: 1051–1055.

116. Benvegnu L, Chemello L, Noventa F, Fattovich G, Pontisso P, Alberti A 1998 Retrospective analysis of the effect of interferon monotherapy on the clinical outcome of patients with viral cirrhosis. *Cancer* 83: 901–909.

117. Smith JP 1997 Treatment of chronic hepatitis C with amantadine. *Digestive Disease and Sciences* 42: 1681–1687.

118. Mangia A, Minerva N, Annese M et al 2001 A randomized trial of amantadine and interferon versus interferon alone as initial treatment for chronic hepatitis C. *Hepatology* 33: 989–993.

119. Zeuzem S, Teuber G, Naumann U et al 2000 Randomized, double-blind, placebo-controlled trial of interferon alfa2a with and without amantadine as initial treatment for chronic hepatitis C. *Hepatology* 32: 835–841.

120. Younossi ZM, Mullen KD, Zakko W et al 2001 A randomized, double-blind controlled trial of interferon alpha-2b and ribavirin vs. interferon alpha-2b and amantadine for treatment of chronic hepatitis C non-responder to interferon monotherapy. *Journal of Hepatology* 34: 128–133.

121. Di Martino V, Boudjema H, Delacour T et al 2001 Treatment of chronic Hepatitis C with amantadine hydrochloride in patients who had not responded to previous treatment with interferon-alpha and/or ribavirin. *Clinical Infectious Diseases* 32: 830–831.

122. Lieb K, Hufert FT, Bechter K, Bauer J, Kornhuber J 1997 Depression, Borna disease, and amantadine. *Lancet* 349: 958.

123. Farci P, Mandas A, Coiana A et al 1994 Treatment of chronic hepatitis D with interferon alfa-2a. *New England Journal of Medicine* 330: 88–94.

124. Rosina F, Pintus C, Meschievitz C et al 1991 A randomised controlled trial of a 12 month course of recombinant human interferon alpha in chronic delta (type D) hepatitis: a multicenter Italian study. *Hepatology* 13: 1052–1056.

125. Samuel D, Muller R, Alexander G et al 1993 Liver transplantation in European patients with the hepatitis B surface antigen. *New England Journal of Medicine* 329: 842–1847.

126. Wolters LM, van Nunen AB, Honkoop P et al 2000 Lamivudine-high dose interferon combination therapy for chronic hepatitis B patients co-infected with the hepatitis D virus. *Journal of Viral Hepatitis* 7: 428–434.

52 Skin and soft tissue infections

Daniel A. Carrasco and Stephen K. Tyring

The skin and underlying soft tissues form a usually formidable defensive barrier against infection despite the fact that the skin's surface is normally colonized by a variety of organisms. Disruption of the integrity of the integument, immunocompromised conditions, or spread of an organism via the circulation can lead to a variety of skin and soft tissue infections. Diagnosis may rely solely upon the appearance of the skin lesions or on simple diagnostic tests such as cultures or skin biopsies. Isolation of the causative organism may be difficult, in many cases due to contamination by normal commensal skin flora. Treatment with systemic antiviral or antibacterial agents offers excellent tissue penetration and rapid recovery. Topical antimicrobial therapy is limited by lack of adequate tissue penetration and skin hypersensitivity; however, the advantage of topical therapy is its lack of systemic toxicity and ease of application.

CHILDHOOD EXANTHEMS

Viral exanthems are common in children. In some cases the morphology of the rash and associated findings may allow for a specific diagnosis and treatment although many cases are non-specific and not pathognomonic for a specific virus. There are now more than 50 specific agents known to cause viral exanthems. The classic six childhood exanthems are not all viruses (Table 52.1).

Table 52.1 Classic childhood exanthems

First disease	Rubeola (measles)
Second disease	Scarlet fever
Third disease	Rubella
Fourth disease	Filatov–Duke's disease
Fifth disease	Erythema infectiosum
Sixth disease	Exanthem subitum (roseola infantum)

All childhood exanthems cause a rather non-specific generalized rash that occurs in a predictable pattern. Most are benign and self-limiting viral diseases with no specific treat-

ment except for supportive care. For example, rubella is a benign disease but the effects of congenital rubella can be very serious. If a pregnant woman is afflicted with German measles (rubella) in the first trimester, the incidence of fetal damage approaches 50%.[1] Likewise, if erythema infectiosum (fifth disease; caused by parvovirus B19 infection) is acquired during pregnancy the risk of spontaneous abortion or hydrops fetalis in a surviving offspring is increased. Some viral exanthems are known for the unique skin lesions they produce; measles (rubeola) causes the characteristic Koplik's spots; erythema infectiosum is known for the erythematous 'slapped cheek' appearance.

Treatment for viral exanthems is supportive, although childhood vaccination remains the most effective means of prevention in the case of measles and rubella.

ENTEROVIRAL INFECTIONS

Enterovirus infections such as hand, foot and mouth disease, herpangina and echovirus 9 infection are the leading cause of childhood exanthems in the summer and fall. Enteroviruses enter through the gastrointestinal tract, and are said to account for two-thirds of all exanthems in August, September, and October in the USA. More than 30 have been identified to cause exanthems. Enteroviral infections are spread by the oral-oral or fecal-oral route, and the typical incubation period is 3–5 days. The cutaneous manifestations are quite pleomorphic and include rubelliform, morbilliform, roseola-like, scarlatiniform, urticarial, pustular, petechial, purpuric, and hemangioma-like eruptions. A specific enteroviral diagnosis is not possible for most exanthems. Hand, foot and mouth disease is characterized by vesicular lesions in the mouth and on the extremities associated with a mild fever. Herpangina is a specific infectious disease characterized by sudden onset of fever, headache and neck pain, and gray–white papulovesicular lesions on the anterior pillars, soft palate, uvula, and tonsils. No specific treatment is available; only supportive care is recommended for enteroviral infections.

HERPESVIRUSES

HERPES SIMPLEX (HSV)

HSV-1 and HSV-2 are double-stranded DNA viruses. Both types are characterized by a primary infection, which may or may not be symptomatic, followed by the establishment of a latent infection in the spinal ganglion.

HSV-1 commonly causes herpes labialis, also known as cold sores. Primary infection is more severe than recurrences, and may be associated with fever and lymphadenopathy. Infection usually recurs on or near the vermilion border of the lip due to sunlight, emotional stress, trauma to the lips, fatigue, or fever. The onset of recurrence is heralded by a typical prodrome of itching or burning at the site, followed by the classic appearance of an erythematous macule, followed by a papule, vesicle and finally a crust.

Genital herpes is commonly caused by HSV-2, generally acquired through sexual contact. More than 50% of persons with asymptomatic HSV-2 actively shed the virus; 70–80% of cases of genital herpes are thought to be spread by asymptomatic viral shedding.[2] As with herpes labialis a prodrome occurs in 40–50% of episodes.

Both oral and genital herpes infection appear as vesicles on an inflamed base. The vesicles erode quickly or become pustular before crusting over. Healing usually occurs in about 9 days for recurrent lesions, and up to 3 weeks for primary infections.

Herpetic lesions such as herpetic whitlow are caused by primary or recurrent HSV infection on the fingers, most commonly due to digital to genital contact.

Herpes gladiatorum, caused by direct skin-to-skin contact, is seen among wrestlers and rugby players and may affect the head, trunk, and extremities.

Eczema herpeticum is a widespread cutaneous infection with HSV, which occurs in patients with skin disorders such as atopic dermatitis, Darier's disease, and pemphigus. It is frequently superinfected with bacteria and is associated with fever, lymphadenopathy, and malaise.

Diagnosis

Diagnosis of herpes can be made by identifying multinucleated balloon keratinocytes on a Tzanck smear taken from the floor of an early vesicle stained with Wright or Giemsa stain. Culture is the gold standard for diagnosis and Western blot is used to distinguish between HSV-1 and HSV-2.

Treatment

Primary and recurrent genital herpes may be treated with oral aciclovir, famciclovir or valaciclovir: aciclovir 200 mg 5 times per day for 10 days for primary HSV and for 5 days with recurrent HSV is the recommended regimen. Aciclovir 200–400 mg twice daily for suppressive therapy remains a cost-effective means of treating genital herpes.

Primary genital HSV infection is treated with famciclovir, 250 mg three times daily for 10 days, 125 mg twice daily for 5 days for recurrences and 250 mg twice daily for suppressive therapy.

Recommended treatment for a primary genital infection is valaciclovir, 1000 mg twice daily for 10 days; recurrences 500 mg twice daily for 5 days. For suppressive therapy a dose of 500–1000 mg a day is required. Both famciclovir and valaciclovir are equally effective, more conveniently dosed and better absorbed than the prototype aciclovir. However, they are more expensive.

Penciclovir and aciclovir creams are approved for herpes labialis; however, their effectiveness is limited by poor tissue penetration and by the frequent inconvenient dosing regimen. Oral antivirals such as famciclovir, valaciclovir and aciclovir, although not approved for use for herpes labialis in the USA are effective in healing fever blister lesions more quickly.

VARICELLA ZOSTER VIRUS (HHV-3)

Varicella (chickenpox) and herpes zoster (shingles) are both caused by a single member of the herpesvirus family (human herpesvirus-3; HHV-3). Varicella results from a primary infection in a susceptible person, whereas zoster is a reactivation in persons who have had varicella. Varicella is highly contagious and usually transmitted via the respiratory route or by direct contact. The clinical manifestations of primary varicella include an occasional prodrome and, in children, low-grade fever and malaise may proceed or occur simultaneously with the onset of the rash. In adults, a headache, myalgia, nausea, vomiting and anorexia can precede the rash. The rash is characterized by small erythematous macules appearing initially on the face and trunk, spreading to the proximal upper limbs and somewhat sparing of the distal lower limbs. The skin lesions rapidly evolve in crops over 12–14 h. The rash progresses in a predictable manner: first papules, next vesicles and finally crust. Vesicles may have slightly hemorrhagic bases and are called 'dewdrops on a rose petal'. Infection tends to be more severe in older children and adults.

For primary varicella in healthy children treatment has traditionally been symptomatic, using only calamine lotion, cool compresses, tepid baths and non-aspirin antipyretics. Healthy children with primary varicella virus infection should be treated with oral aciclovir.

Treatment of primary varicella in older children, adults and immunocompromised patients is mandatory. If the patient is an adult or of adult size, the dosage of aciclovir is 800 mg 5 times a day for 7 days; in smaller children the recommendation is 20 mg/kg four times a day for 5 days. The use of famciclovir and valaciclovir have not been studied for treatment in primary varicella; however, zoster equivalent doses are effective.

Herpes zoster is an acute inflammatory unilateral dermatosis having both dermatological and neurological manifestations. It is estimated to afflict 15–20% of the population, with incidence increasing with rising age.[3] Immune senescence, resulting in a decline in T-cell-mediated immunity, is suspected to contribute to the reactivation of the varicella zoster virus lying dormant in the spinal cord dorsal root ganglia.[4] The patient may experience prodromal symptoms of low-grade fever, pain, numbness, pruritus, and paresthesia several days before cutaneous involvement. These signs foreshadow the appearance of the classical rash, most often described as unilateral grouped vesicles on an erythematous and edematous base along a dermatomal distribution. Frequently there are a few scattered non-dermatomal lesions, and rarely a generalized eruption may occur. Complete cutaneous healing is expected in 3–4 weeks and patients are considered contagious until the lesions are crusted.

Varicella and zoster are usually diagnosed clinically. The Tzanck smear is positive in 80–100% of zoster cases. Traditionally treatment for herpes zoster has included oral aciclovir 800 mg five times daily. However, famciclovir (500 mg three times daily or valaciclovir (1000 mg three times daily) are more conveniently dosed and achieve higher plasma concentrations than oral aciclovir.

EPSTEIN–BARR VIRUS (HHV-4)

Epstein–Barr Virus (EBV) is a double-stranded DNA virus with an envelope and is a member of the herpesvirus family (HHV-4). Humans become infected through oral secretions. EBV persists for life as a latent infection in B cells. It is the etiologic agent of infectious mononucleosis, and is associated with oral hairy leukoplakia and B-cell lymphoma in patients with AIDS, Burkitt's lymphoma, nasopharyngeal carcinoma, Hodgkin's disease, and some T-cell lymphomas,

The triad of fever, sore throat, and lymphadenopathy characterizes infectious mononucleosis.[5] Infection is acquired by contact with salivary secretions. Mononucleosis is usually self-limiting and patients need only rest and antipyretics.

Oral hairy leukoplakia is a non-malignant hyperplasia of the epithelial cells due to active replication of EBV, commonly seen in HIV-positive individuals.[6,7] Lesions are usually present on the lateral tongue and appear slightly raised and white with a corrugated or hairy appearance. Oral hairy leukoplakia will resolve with oral aciclovir, but it will recur 2 weeks to 2 months after stopping therapy.

The monospot test is used to diagnose EBV.

CYTOMEGALOVIRUS (HHV-5)

Cytomegalovirus (CMV) is an enveloped double-stranded DNA virus of the herpes family, also known as HHV-5. By old age nearly everyone has been infected with CMV. After primary infection, which is usually asymptomatic and sub-

clinical, the virus is present for life in a latent stage. The main danger of CMV is to immunocompromised patients and neonates. Transmission occurs via intimate contact with body fluids such as saliva, vaginal secretions, semen, breast milk, feces, or blood. Cutaneous lesions associated with CMV are rare and non-specific, and usually occur only in immunocompromised states. The most specific manifestation of cutaneous CMV is ulceration of the perianal area.

Treatment is usually with ganciclovir, foscarnet, or cidofovir. Fomivirsen is also approved.

HUMAN HERPESVIRUS 6 (ROSEOLA)

Roseola (also known as exanthem subitum) is a very common childhood exanthem in which HHV-6 has been shown to play a causal role. Roseola is characterized by a prodrome of high fever (102–105°F) for 3–5 days, followed by an abrupt decrease in fever and sudden appearance of an exanthem (hence 'subitum') that occurs almost exclusively in children under 2 years old. Ganciclovir and foscarnet may be helpful in cases with severe complications, but are not approved for this purpose in the USA. Primary infections confer lasting immunity.

HUMAN HERPESVIRUS 7

This is also known to cause roseola, but much less commonly than HHV-6. it is susceptible to ganciclovir and foscarnet, and shows minimal susceptibility to aciclovir, but these agents are not routinely used.

HUMAN HERPESVIRUS 8 (KAPOSI'S SARCOMA)

Kaposi's sarcoma is a malignancy associated with HHV-8 infection.[8] It presents as violaceous, red–dark-brown firm macules or papules, irregularly oval-shaped and parallel to skin tension lines. Systemic therapy should be restricted to patients with disseminated disease or with massive involvement of visceral organs. In HIV-positive patients therapy should be postponed until the patient has had time to respond to highly active antiretroviral therapy (HAART). Therapies for Kaposi's sarcoma include radiotherapy, interferon-α, cidofovir, conventional chemotherapy, and topical and systemic retinoids.[9]

POXVIRUSES

SMALLPOX

Smallpox is caused by a DNA-containing virus known as variola. The last known case occurred in October 1977 and worldwide eradication was announced in 1979. Smallpox was 25% fatal and no treatment was ever found.

CONTAGIOUS ECTHYMA (CONTAGIOUS PUSTULAR DERMATITIS) (ORF)

Contagious ecthyma is a member of the parapox genus. It is acquired from infected sheep or goats with crusted lesions on the lips. The lesions appear as flat or dome-shaped bullae with minimal fluid and a central umbilicated crust. They bleed easily and heal without scarring. During a period of approximately 35 days the lesions pass through six clinical stages, each lasting about 6 days.[10] The diagnosis is based on history and physical examination, viral culture on sheep cells, fluorescent antibody tests, electron microscopy and complement fixation test.[11] No treatment is usually necessary as the lesions resolve in 4–6 weeks. Liquid nitrogen or shave excision may be used to speed recovery; antibiotics are indicated for superinfection.

MILKER'S NODULE

Milker's nodule (caused by paravaccinia virus) is similar to orf, the virus is endemic in cattle.[12] It is transmitted by direct contact with cattle. Lesions have been described as passing through six clinical stages similar to the orf virus. Milker's nodule resolves without therapy.

MOLLUSCUM CONTAGIOSUM

Molluscum contagiosum is caused by a double-stranded DNA virus of the poxvirus group. It affects mainly children, sexually active adults, and immunocompromised individuals, and is spread by direct inoculation between humans. The lesions are small, discrete waxy, flesh-colored, dome-shaped papules with central umbilication, 3–6 mm in size. In patients with AIDS several systemic fungal infections commonly mimic molluscum contagiosum, including cryptococcosis, histoplasmosis, and *Penicillium marneffei* infection.

Histologically, molluscum bodies are present. The stratum corneum disintegrates in the center of the lesion, releasing the molluscum bodies and creating a central crater.

Treatment consist of cryosurgery, curettage, incision and expression of the molluscum body; cantharidin, topical podophyllotoxin cream, salicylic acid preparations, imiquimod, and topical cidofovir are also successful.

HUMAN PAPILLOMAVIRUSES

Warts are caused by papillomaviruses, members of the papovavirus group. Papillomaviruses are double-stranded DNA viruses that do not have an envelope and thus can remain infectious for long periods of time after drying. More than 80 different types of human papillomavirus (HPV) have been identified by their separate DNA genotypes as detected by polymerase chain reaction.[13] Incubation period is 2–9 months (average 3 months). Table 52.2 lists the various HPV types and their common lesions.

Palmoplantar warts usually occur on the palms, soles and the lateral aspects of the fingers and toes. They can be painful on pressure and look similar to a callus, but are differentiated by their loss of skin lines, and multiple black dots (which represent punctate hemorrhages from thrombosed dermal capillaries). Common warts (verruca vulgaris) can occur on any skin surface and are described as scaly, rough spiny papules. Flat warts (verruca plana) are most common on the face, lower legs and dorsal hands.

Epidermodysplasia verruciformis represents a unique susceptibility to cutaneous HPV infection.[14,15] About 50% of cases are inherited, usually with an autosomal recessive pattern. The warts resemble those of verruca plana.

Table 52.2 Human papillomaviruses and their common lesions

Human papillomavirus type	Wart type
HPV-1, HPV-2, HPV-4	Palmoplantar warts
HPV-2, HPV-4, HPV-27, HPV-29	Common warts
HPV-3, HPV-10, HPV-28, HPV-49	Flat warts
HPV-6, HPV-11	Condyloma (low risk of carcinoma)
HPV-16, HPV-18, HPV-31, HPV-33–35, HPV-40, HPV-51–60	Squamous cell carcinoma (high risk of carcinoma)
HPV-6, HPV-11	Laryngeal papillomas
HPV-30	Laryngeal carcinoma
HPV-13, HPV-32	Oral focal epithelial hyperplasia (Heck's disease)
HPV-16, HPV-18, HPV-31, HPV-33–35, HPV-39, HPV-40, HPV-51–60	Bowenoid papulosis
HPV-7	Butcher's warts
HPV-5, HPV-8, HPV-9, HPV-12, HPV-14, HPV-15, HPV-17, HPV-19–26, HPV-36, HPV-47, HPV-50	Epidermodysplasia verruciformis
HPV-6, HPV-11	Giant condyloma of Buschke and Loewenstein

Condyloma acuminatum commonly occurs on the penis, vulva, and anal region. The lesions appear as soft verrucous papules that coalesce into cauliflower-like masses.

Giant condyloma acuminata of Buschke and Loewenstein has been associated with HPV-6 and HPV-11 DNA, and is regarded as a low-grade verrucous carcinoma that resembles a large aggregate of condyloma acuminata. It is most common on the glans penis, vulva and anal region.

Bowenoid papulosis is described as multiple, small, reddish-brown flat-topped papules of the genitalia of men and women. Squamous cell carcinoma may arise in a Bowenoid papule, and is most commonly associated with HPV-16.

Oral focal epithelial hyperplasia (Heck's disease) is a rare condition described in Native Americans and Eskimos. Heck's disease is a chronic disease associated with HPV-13 and HPV-32. Lesions commonly present on the oral mucosa of the lower lip, buccal and gingival mucosa.

Therapy depends on the type of HPV.

- For common and palmoplantar warts, daily topical salicylic acid preparations, cryotherapy, curettage, electrodesiccation, cantharidin, intralesional bleomycin and CO_2 laser ablation are routine therapies.
- Genital warts respond to imiquimod, cryotherapy, trichloroacetic acid 50–80%, electrosurgery, excision, laser ablation, and interferon-α intralesionally. Imiquimod induces interferon-α and is the most effective with the lowest recurrence rate. Podophyllin is contraindicated because it contains mutagens, which are potential carcinogens.
- Flat warts may respond to topical treatment with the vitamin A derivative tretinoin or 5-fluorouracil, cryotherapy, and imiquimod.
- Epidermodysplasia verruciformis may also respond to systemic retinoids.
- Radiation of verrucas is contraindicated due to its association with the development of malignancy.

GRAM-POSITIVE ORGANISMS

STAPHYLOCOCCAL INFECTIONS

Impetigo

Both bullous and non-bullous forms of impetigo exist; however, non-bullous impetigo caused by *Staphylococcus aureus* accounts for the majority of cases.

A prodrome of itching and pain heralds the appearance of a vesicle or pustule, after which the classic honey-colored crusted plaque with surrounding erythema appears.

Treatment with topical mupirocin is sufficient for localized involvement, although a course of oral antibiotics with a penicillinase-resistant semisynthetic penicillin may be needed (Table 52.3). Oral dicloxacillin 125–500 mg 6-hourly, flu-

cloxacillin 250–500 mg 6-hourly or oxacillin 500–1000 mg 4–6-hourly (Table 52.3) are recommended. A group 2 cephalosporin such as oral cefalexin 250–500 mg 6-hourly (Table 52.4) may also be used. Alternatives include ampicillin plus clindamycin and either azithromycin or clarithromycin (Tables 52.3 and 52.5).

Table 52.3 Common penicillin doses (for adults) used in skin and soft-tissue infections

Penicillin	Route	Dose
Natural penicillins		
Aqueous penicillin G	i.v.	8–24 MU* every 2–6 h
Procaine penicillin G	i.m.	0.6–1.2 MU once
Benzathine penicillin G	i.m.	1.2–2.4 MU once
Procaine+benzathine penicillin	i.m.	2.4 MU once
Penicillin V	oral	250–500 mg four times daily
Penicillin-resistant penicillins		
Dicloxacillin	oral	125–500 mg every 6 h before meals
Cloxacillin	oral	250–500 mg every 6 h
Flucloxacillin	oral	250–500 mg every 6 h before meals
	i.m.	250–500 mg every 6 h
	i.v.	250–1 g every 6 h
Nafcillin	i.m.	500 mg every 4 h
	i.v.	500–2000 mg every 4–6 h
Oxacillin	oral	500–1000 mg every 6 h
	i.m. i.v.	250–2000 mg every 4–6 h
Aminopenicillins		
Amoxicillin	oral	250–500 mg every 8 h
	i.m.	500–1000 mg every 6 h
	i.v.	1–2 g every 4–6 h
Ampicillin	oral	250–1000 mg every 6 h
	i.m.	500–1000 mg every 6 h
	i.v.	1–2 g every 4 h
Ampicillin–sulbactam	i.v.	1.5–3 g every 6 h
Amoxicillin–clavulanate	oral	250/125 mg every 8 h
		500/125 mg every 12 h
		875/125 mg every 12 h
Antipseudomonal penicillins		
Piperacillin–tazobactam	i.v.	3.375 g every 6 h
		4.5 g every 8 h
Ticarcillin–clavulanate	i.v.	3.1 g every 4–6 h
Ticarcillin	i.v.	3 g every 4 h or 4 g every 6 h
Mezlocillin	i.v./i.m.	3 g every 4 h or 4 g every 6 h
Piperacillin	i.m./i.v.	6–24 g/day in divided doses

*1 megaunit (MU) = 600 mg.

Ecthyma

Impetigo can evolve into ecthyma if left untreated. Either *Staphylococcus aureus* or *Streptococcus pyogenes* causes ecthyma (Table 52.6). The lesions of ecthyma penetrate the epidermis,

Table 52.4 Common cephalosporin doses (for adults) used in skin and soft-tissue infections

Cephalosporin	Route	Dose
Cefalexin	oral	250–500 mg every 6 h
Cefadroxil	oral	1–2 g daily
Cefamandole	i.v./i.m.	500–1000 mg every 4–8 h
Cefazolin	i.m., i.v.	500–2000 mg every 8 h
Cefaclor	oral	250–1000 mg every 8 h
Cefuroxime	i.m. i.v.	750–1500 mg every 8 h
Loracarbef	oral	200 mg every 12 h
Cefotaxime	i.v./i.m.	1–2 g every 6–12 h
Ceftriaxone	i.m. i.v.	1–2 g daily
Cefixime	oral	400 daily or 200 twice daily
Ceftazidime	i.m., i.v.	1–2 g every 8–12 h
Cefoperazone	i.v./i.m.	2–4 g every 12 h
Cefepime	i.v.	500–2000 mg every 12 h

Table 52.5 Common macrolide doses (for adults) used in skin and soft-tissue infections

Macrolide	Route	Dose
Erythromycin base	oral	250–500 mg four times daily
Erythromycin ethyl succinate	oral	400 mg four times daily
Erythromycin estolate	oral	250 mg four times daily
Erythromycin lactobionate	i.v.	15–20 mg/kg/days (max 4 g), every 6 h
Azithromycin	oral	500 mg for one day followed by 250 mg per day for 4 days or 1–2 g single dose
	i.v.	500 mg daily
Clarithromycin	oral	250–500 mg twice daily

creating a yellow–gray crusted ulcer up to 3 cm in diameter. The lesions most commonly affect the lower extremities in neglected debilitated patients with poor hygiene. Healing can take several weeks, despite antibiotic therapy. Topical mupirocin, and the same oral antibiotic regimen as used in impetigo, are recommended.

Folliculitis

Folliculitis is most commonly caused by *Staph. aureus* (Table 52.6). There are two common types of folliculitis, superficial and deep. The superficial types are referred to as follicular or Bockhart's impetigo and commonly are located on the beard area, axilla, buttocks and extremities. The deep form of folliculitis typically occurs in the beard areas and involves perifollicular inflammation. Treatment with topical mupirocin is usually sufficient; systemic treatment with antibiotics is reserved for deep extensive cases. Folliculitis left untreated can evolve into a furuncle or carbuncle.

Furuncles and carbuncles

A furuncle, also known as a boil, is a deep, firm, erythematous painful inflammatory nodule, which occurs around hair follicles and gradually enlarges to form a fluctuant abscess. *Staph. aureus* is the etiologic agent (Table 52.6). Following rupture of a furuncle, pus is expressed along with a core of necrotic material and the lesion begins to heal. Several furuncles can coalesce into a deeper network of more extensive lesions and form a carbuncle.

Carbuncles are usually more erythematous and indurated than furuncles. Carbuncles and furuncles can evolve into more serious diseases such as cellulitis and bacteremic spread.

Treatment is aimed at incision and drainage of the pus. If a carbuncle or furuncle is complicated by fever or cellulitis, treatment with a semisynthetic penicillin is indicated: either oral dicloxacillin or flucloxacillin 250–500 mg 6-hourly or intravenous nafcillin/oxacillin 2 g 6-hourly (Table 52.3). Alternatively, intravenous cefazolin 1–2 g 8-hourly or vancomycin 1 g 12-hourly may be used.

Paronychia

Paronychia are infections caused predominately by *Staph. aureus* entering a break in the skin around the fingernails in persons exposed to hand trauma or chronic moisture[16] (Table 52.6). Other organisms causing paronychia include *Streptococcus, Candida, Pseudomonas* spp., and dermatophytes. Paronychia usually presents as red-hot, tender, proximal and lateral nail-fold inflammation.

Treatment of *Staph. aureus* paronychia includes both topical and oral antibiotic therapy plus incision and drainage of any abscess formation. Oral clindamycin (300 mg four times daily) or erythromycin-base (500 mg four times daily) are the suggested regimens (Table 52.5).

Staphylococcal scalded skin syndrome

Staphylococcal scalded skin syndrome is a severe skin exfoliation caused by a staphylococcal exotoxin (Table 52.6). Children under the age of 5 years are most commonly affected because their immune systems have not fully evolved; however, immunocompromised adults can also be afflicted.

The generalized syndrome can begin with an upper respiratory tract, eye, or ear infection[17]. Areas around the mouth and axilla initially become tender and slightly erythematous; this heralds the appearance of the generalized blisters that evolve into large flaccid bullae. Next, large sheets of epidermis are shed, leaving an erythematous denuded base exposed. Uniquely, the mucous membranes are spared. Healing of the lesions can be expected in 5–7 days. Culture and biopsy confirm diagnosis.

Treatment with an intravenous penicillinase-resistant antibiotic and subsequent substitution with an oral agent within a few days is appropriate (Table 52.3). Diligent management of

Table 52.6 Skin and soft tissue infections, causative organisms and primary and secondary treatment regimens

Disease	Causative organism	Primary treatment	Secondary treatment
Acne	*Propionibacterium acnes*	Doxycycline Minocycline Tetracycline	Erythromycin base Clindamycin
Actinomycosis	*Actinomyces israelii* *Actinomyces gerencseriae*	Penicillin V	Clindamycin
Anthrax	*Bacillus anthracis*	Penicillin G (aqueous) Ciprofloxacin	Erythromycin base Doxycycline
Bacillary angiomatosis	*Bartonella henselae,* *Bartonella quintana*	Erythromycin base	Doxycycline
Blistering distal dactylitis	*Staphylococcus aureus,* *Streptococcus pyogenes*	Dicloxacillin Penicillin V	Cephalosporin (group 2) Erythromycin base Clindamycin
Boils (carbuncles, furuncles)	*Staphylococcus aureus*	Dicloxacillin	Cephalosporin (group 2) Erythromycin base Clindamycin Levofloxacin
Cat bite	*Pasteurella multocida,* *Staphylococcal aureus*	Amoxicillin–clavulanate	Doxycycline Cefuroxime Penicillin G (aqueous) Penicillin V
Cat-scratch disease	*Bartonella henselae*	Ciprofloxacin	Trimethoprim–sulfamethoxazole
Cellulitis	*Streptococcus pyogenes,* *Staphylococcus aureus*	Nafcillin Oxacillin Dicloxacillin Cefazolin	Cephalosporin (group 2) Erythromycin base Azithromycin or clarithromycin Clindamycin Levofloxacin Linezolid
Clostridium cellulitis	*Clostridium perfringens*	Penicillin G (aqueous)	Clindamycin Metronidazole Tetracycline Chloramphenicol Imipenem
Diphtheria	*Corynebacterium diphtheriae*	Erythromycin base	Penicillin V Benzylpenicillin
Dog bites	*Pasteurella multocida,* Viridans group streptococci *Staphylococcus aureus*	Amoxicillin–clavulanate	Clindamycin plus: 1. fluoroquinolone (adults) 2. Trimethoprim–sulfamethoxazole (children)
Ecthyma	*Staphylococcus aureus*	Dicloxacillin	Cephalosporin (group 2) Erythromycin Clindamycin
Ehrlichiosis	*Ehrlichia* spp.	Doxycycline	Chloramphenicol
Erysipelas	*Streptococcus pyogenes*	Penicillin G (benzathine) Nafcillin Oxacillin Dicloxacillin	Erythromycin base Azithromycin Clarithromycin Cephalosporin (group 2)
Erysipeloid	*Erysipelothrix rhusiopathiae*	Penicillin G (aqueous) Ampicillin	Erythromycin base Fluoroquinolones Cephalosporin (group 4) Clindamycin
Erythema gangrenosum	*Pseudomonas aeruginosa*	Ceftazidime Amikacin	Piperacillin Tobramycin Ciprofloxacin

Table 52.6 *Continued*

Disease	Causative organism	Primary treatment	Secondary treatment
Erythrasma	*Corynebacterium minutissimum*	Erythromycin base	Topical benzoyl peroxide Topical Clindamycin
Folliculitis	*Staphylococcus aureus*	Topical mupirocin	Dicloxacillin Penicillin V Oxacillin Penicillin G (benzathine) Erythromycin base
Gangrenous cellulitis (necrotizing fasciitis)	*Peptostreptococcus* spp. *Bacteroides* spp. *Enterobacter* spp. *Proteus* spp.	Ampicillin–sulbactam Imipenem–cilastatin Ticarcillin–clavulanate	Cephalosporin (group 3) Clindamycin Metronidazole + aminoglycoside
Gangrenous cellulitis (streptococcal gangrene)	*Streptococcus* group A/B/C/G	Penicillin G (aqueous) Penicillin V	Erythromycin base Cephalosporin Vancomycin Clarithromycin Azithromycin Clindamycin
Gas gangrene	*Clostridium perfringens*	Penicillin G (aqueous) Clindamycin	Doxycycline Erythromycin base Chloramphenicol Cefazolin Cefoxitin
Human bites	Viridans group streptococci *Staphylococcus epidermidis* *Bacteroides* spp. *Corynebacterium* spp. *Eikenella corrodens*	Amoxicillin–clavulanate	Amoxicillin–sulbactam Cefoxitin Ticarcillin–clavulanate Piperacillin–tazobactam Clindamycin + ciprofloxacin or trimethoprim–sulfamethoxazole
Impetigo	*Staphylococcus aureus,* *Streptococcus pyogenes*	Dicloxacillin Penicillin V Oxacillin Penicillin G (benzathine)	Cephalosporin (group 2 or 3) Erythromycin base Clindamycin Azithromycin Clarithromycin Mupirocin
Kawasaki syndrome	*Staphylococcus aureus* superantigens	Intravenous immunoglobulin + aspirin	none
Listeriosis	*Listeria monocytogenes*	Ampicillin Penicillin G (aqueous)	Trimethoprim–sulfamethoxazole
Lyme disease (erythema migrans)	*Borrelia burgdorferi*	Ceftriaxone Cefuroxime Doxycycline Amoxicillin	Penicillin G (aqueous) Azithromycin Clarithromycin
Meningococcemia	*Neisseria meningitidis*	Penicillin G (aqueous)	Ceftriaxone Chloramphenicol Minocycline
Nocardiosis	*Nocardia asteroides*	Trimethoprim–sulfamethoxazole	Minocycline
Paronychia	*Staphylococcus aureus*	Clindamycin	Erythromycin
Plague	*Yersinia pestis*	Gentamicin Streptomycin	Doxycycline Chloramphenicol
Pseudomonal infection	*Pseudomonas aeruginosa*	Gentamicin Tobramycin Amikacin	Ciprofloxacin Ofloxacin *plus* an antipseudomonal penicillin or ceftazidime

Table 52.6 *Continued*

Disease	Causative organism	Primary treatment	Secondary treatment
Rat bite fever	*Streptobacillus moniliformis*	Ampicillin Clindamycin Penicillin G (aqueous)	Doxycycline Erythromycin base Clindamycin
Rocky Mountain spotted fever	*Rickettsia rickettsii*	Doxycycline	Chloramphenicol
Rosacea	*Unknown*	Minocycline Doxycycline Tetracycline Erythromycin Metronidazole (topical 1%) Ampicillin	Trimethoprim–sulfamethoxazole Metronidazole (oral) Dapsone
Saltwater contaminated wound	*Vibrio vulnificus* *Vibrio damsela*	Ceftazidime + doxycycline	Cefotaxime Ciprofloxacin
Scarlet fever	*Streptococcus pyogenes*	Penicillin (all)	Cephalosporins (all) Macrolides (all)
Staphylococcal scalded skin syndrome	*Staphylococcus aureus* exotoxin	Nafcillin	Oxacillin
Toxic shock syndrome	*Staphylococcus aureus* exotoxin	Nafcillin or Oxacillin + Intravenous immunoglobulins	Cephalosporin (group 1)
Tularemia	*Francisella tularensis*	Streptomycin	Gentamicin Doxycycline Chloramphenicol
Wound infection postoperative	*Staphylococcus aureus* *Streptococcus* Enterobacteriaceae	Cephalosporin (group 2) Amoxicillin–clavulanate	Doxycycline Cephalosporin (groups 3 and 4) Levofloxacin Linezolid

Note: Flucloxacillin can be substituted for nafcillin, oxacillin or dicloxacillin in countries in which it is available.

electrolytes and supportive skin care will speed recovery; however, despite all efforts approximately 2–3% of patients die (mortality rates are higher in adults than in children). Care must be taken to avoid epidemics in neonatal care units by eradicating *Staph. aureus* from healthcare workers who are nasal carriers and by implementing strict handwashing policies.

The recommended penicillinase-resistant antibiotic is intravenous nafcillin, oxacillin or flucloxacillin (2 g 4-hourly in adults; 150 mg/kg/6-hourly in children). Treatment should last 5–7 days (Table 52.3).

Staphylococcal toxic-shock syndrome

Staphylococcal toxic-shock syndrome, like staphylococcal scalded skin syndrome, is an illness that results from an exotoxin produced by *Staph. aureus* (Table 52.6). In addition, it is a multisystem disease involving at least three organ systems, with hypotension, fever, and a rash resembling that of scarlet fever followed by skin desquamation.

Menstruating women using tampons for a prolonged period of time account for up to 90% of cases. The conjunctiva may become injected; the oral mucosa and vagina may appear intensely erythematous. Between 1 and 2 weeks later palmar and plantar desquamation follows.

Initial treatment is aimed at controlling the hypotension and shock with fluid replacement. The tampon must be removed and intravenous penicillinase-resistant antibiotics started. If therapy is instituted early, intravenous γ-globulins and fresh-frozen plasma containing immunoglobins will expedite recovery.[16] Treatment with intravenous nafcillin, oxacillin or flucloxacillin 2 g 4-hourly or a group 1 cephalosporin such as cefazolin 1–2 g 8-hourly is recommended (Table 52.3 and 52.4).

Kawasaki syndrome

Kawasaki syndrome is an acute multisystem vasculitis of infancy and childhood associated with high fever, mucocutaneous inflammation, and the development of coronary artery abnormalities.[18] The etiology of Kawasaki syndrome is unknown; however, it is suspected that *Staph. aureus* superantigens may trigger the disease (Table 52.6). Treatment with intravenous immunoglobulin 2 g/kg over 12 h plus oral aspirin 80–100 mg/kg daily in four divided doses, followed by aspirin

3–5 mg/kg daily for 6–8 weeks. If the patient remains febrile after the first dose of immunoglobulin a second dose may be administered.

STREPTOCOCCAL INFECTIONS

Impetigo

Streptococcal impetigo is often indistinguishable from the staphylococcal variant (Table 52.6). Patients may be infected with both staphylococcal and streptococcal impetigo. Treatment of the streptococcal form with mupirocin ointment is effective, but more severe forms of group A streptococcal impetigo should be treated with oral or intramuscular penicillin. Oral penicillin V 250–500 mg daily is the recommended regimen (Table 52.3). If an intramuscular dose of penicillin is preferred, then benzathine penicillin G (0.6–1.2 million units) is advocated (Table 52.3). An alternative oral antibiotic is a group 2 cephalosporin (Table 52.4). Second-line treatment consists of a macrolide antibiotic or a group 3 cephalosporin (Table 52.4 and 52.5).

Blistering distal dactylitis

Blistering distal dactylitis is caused most commonly by *Streptococcus pyogenes* (Table 52.6). Mostly children and adolescents are affected.[19] The lesion is described as a seropurulent blister on an erythematous base that develops on the distal palmar or plantar aspect of the fingers and toes. Treatment with oral penicillin or erythromycin base is appropriate (Table 52.3 and 52.5).

Erysipelas

Erysipelas is a form of superficial cellulitis with lymphatic vessel involvement, caused mainly by group A β-hemolytic streptococci (Table 52.6). The lesions may be precursors to a more invasive cellulitis. The painful lesions are well demarcated and the plaques appear very erythematous and edematous, with an advancing raised border.[20] The diagnosis is usually clinical; however, Gram stain and culture will confirm the organism. It is important to differentiate between the more superficial erysipelas and the deeper cellulitis so that appropriate treatment can be instituted.

Treatment is with either oral or intramuscular penicillin; erythromycin base can be used in the penicillin-allergic patient (Table 52.3 and 52.5). A penicillin-resistant semisynthetic penicillin such as oral dicloxacillin or flucloxacillin 500 mg 6-hourly or, for a more severe infection, intravenous nafcillin, oxacillin or flucloxacillin 2 g every 4 hours is preferred. Second-line agents include macrolide antibiotics, group 1 cephalosporins or ampicillin and clindamycin (Tables 52.4 and 52.5). Improvement can be expected in 24–28 h with antibiotic therapy.

Cellulitis

Cellulitis is caused by most commonly by *Staph. aureus* and group A streptococci (Table 52.6). Other pathogens involved include group B streptococci, cryptococci, pneumococci, and Gram-negative bacilli. Unlike erysipelas, the deep dermis and subcutaneous soft tissues are affected, the margins are indistinct, not raised and are indurated. However, like erysipelas cellulitis is very painful. Diagnosis is clinical and confirmed with Gram stain and culture.

Treatment must be implemented rapidly to avoid any complications such as superinfections, bacteremia, necrotizing fasciitis, and amputations. Treatment can be customized depending on the offending pathogen (if cultures are available). Realistically, when patients present with cellulitis, cultures are not immediately available, therefore, empiric treatment with an intravenous penicillinase-resistant penicillin should be initiated to treat both staphylococcal and streptococcal infections intravenous nafcillin and oxacillin 2 g 4-hourly are appropriate (Table 52.3). Subsequent culture results can help guide specific therapy. For moderately complicated infections oral levofloxacin 500–750 mg twice daily is acceptable (Table 52.7). Treatment with vancomycin is the drug of choice for methicillin-resistant cases of cellulitis. Linezolid is an alternative to vancomycin with a similar spectrum of activity, including coverage for methicillin-resistant *Staphylococcus aureus*.[21] Linezolid is available in intravenous and oral preparations and is 100% orally bioavailable so patients may be switched from intravenous preparations to oral preparations without dose changes. Linezolid is available in 600 mg tablets, an oral suspension containing 100 mg/ml and an intravenous solution. The recommended oral dose for uncomplicated skin infections is 400 mg every 12 hours.[21] Immobilization and elevation of the affected limb will aid in reducing edema and pain. Frequent dressing changes with sterile saline will keep the lesion clean. Oral analgesics may be necessary for pain management.

Table 52.7 Common fluoroquinolones doses (for adults) used in skin and soft-tissue infections

Fluoroquinolone	Route	Dose
Nalidixic acid	oral	1 g four times daily
Ciprofloxacin	oral	250–750 mg twice daily
	i.v.	200–400 mg every 12 h
Ofloxacin	oral, i.v.	200–400 mg every 12 h
Levofloxacin	oral, i.v.	200–750 mg daily or twice daily
Trovafloxin/alatrofloxacin	oral	100–200 mg once daily
	i.v.	300 mg once daily
Sparfloxacin	oral	400 mg first day, followed by 200 mg once daily
Gatifloxacin	i.v./oral	400 mg once daily
Moxifloxacin	oral	400 mg once daily

Gangrenous cellulitis

Necrotizing fasciitis is a type of gangrenous cellulitis. The various forms of necrotizing fasciitis include a non-streptococcal gangrene, streptococcal gangrene, synergistic necrotizing cellulitis and Fournier's gangrene. Gangrenous cellulitis begins usually on an extremity, the perineum, or postoperative wound or trauma site and initially appears as a cellulitis infection. As the infection evolves gangrenous changes become apparent within 36–72 h. The area becomes purple followed by formation of vesicles and bullae that quickly rupture, producing sharply demarcated areas of necrotic eschar and crepitus that destroy all soft tissues, including vessels and nerves. A foul-smelling discharge and palpable gas in the tissues can sometimes be detected.

Streptococcal gangrene is caused principally by group A streptococci.

Non-streptococcal gangrene is a type of necrotizing fasciitis caused by pathogens other than group A streptococci such as anaerobes plus at least one facultative species.[20] These same pathogens can also cause Fournier's gangrene, which involves the scrotum and penis.

Another type of highly lethal necrotizing fasciitis is the polymicrobial synergistic necrotizing cellulitis, which involves necrosis of all layers of soft tissues and commonly involves the perineum. The diagnosis is based on Gram stain, culture, and clinical findings. Treatment with broad-spectrum antibiotics plus wide surgical debridement of the gangrenous tissue is recommended. For groups A, B, C and G streptococcus, penicillin G or V remain first-line agents (Table 52.3). Despite therapy morality remains high.

Scarlet fever

Scarlet fever is usually caused by a pharyngeal infection with group A streptococci and subsequent elaboration of a pyrogenic exotoxin occurring in children under 10 years of age (Table 52.6). Between 24 and 48 h after the appearance of the fever and pharyngitis the unique cutaneous manifestations of scarlet fever, including the characteristic diffuse erythematous 'sandpaper' like rash, and 'strawberry' red tongue appear. Diagnosis is confirmed by the presence of a positive group A streptococcal throat culture.

Following treatment with penicillin the symptoms improve quickly; however, a desquamation may persist for a few weeks. If untreated, uncomplicated infection may last 4–5 days.

CORYNEBACTERIUM MINUTISSIMUM

Erythrasma

Erythrasma caused by *Corynebacterium minutissimum* is a common tropical disease, occurring more often in men and with a predilection for the intertriginous areas (Table 52.6). The organism possesses keratolytic properties and lesions cause thick lamellated plaques on affected areas. The toe web spaces are commonly affected; a Wood's lamp examination revealing a striking bright coral red-pink fluorescence will confirm the diagnosis, as will a culture. Recommended treatment for widespread involvement is oral erythromycin (250 mg every six hours for 14 days) and, for more localized involvement, benzoyl peroxide (Table 52.5).

BACILLUS ANTHRACIS (ANTHRAX)

Anthrax is caused by infection with *Bacillus anthracis*, an aerobic, encapsulated, square rod (Table 52.6). Although primarily a disease of animals, humans can be infected by contact with infected carcases, during animal product handling. Other means of infection include aerosolized spores, which may cause pulmonary infection. A painless malignant pustule occurring on an exposed surface of the body is the hallmark of cutaneous anthrax.

Treatment of choice is aqueous penicillin G 20 million units a day intravenously in four divided doses (Table 52.3). For aerosolized anthrax, ciprofloxacin would be an effective alternative (Table 52.7).

ERYSIPELOTHRIX RHUSIOPATHIAE (ERYSIPELOID)

E. rhusiopathiae is a rod-shaped Gram-positive organism (Table 52.6), which occurs most commonly in people handling raw fish, poultry, or other meat products. The organism is inoculated through a break in the skin.

The macular and plaque-like lesions appear violaceous with sharply defined borders. A culture may confirm the presence of E. rhusiopathiae; however, the clinical history is usually enough to suggest the diagnosis.

Treatment with oral or intramuscular penicillin 2–3 million units (1.2–1.8 g) daily for 7–10 days is recommended (Table 52.3). In the penicillin-allergic patient a group 4 cephalosporin, imipenem, or ciprofloxacin would be adequate; however, most isolates are resistant to vancomycin[24] (Tables 52.4 and 52.7).

BARTONELLA HENSELAE (CAT SCRATCH DISEASE)

Cat scratch disease caused by *B. henselae* is the most common cause of localized chronic lymphadenopathy in children and young adults (Table 52.6).[25] Infection is typically benign and is caused by a bite or scratch from a cat. The initial inoculation may start as a papule and evolve into a vesicle and subsequent crust within 5 days.[26] The gold standard for diagnosis is the cat scratch disease skin test.

Treatment with antibiotics remains controversial, because most cases of this disease spontaneously resolve. *B. henselae* is sensitive to fluoroquinolones, macrolides, tetracyclines, and

Table 52.8 Common tetracycline doses (for adults) used in skin and soft-tissue infections

Tetracycline	Route	Dose
Short-acting tetracyclines		
Tetracycline	oral	250–500 mg 4 times daily
Long-acting tetracyclines		
Doxycycline	oral, i.v.	200 mg initially then 50–100 mg every 12 h
Minocycline	oral, i.v.	200 mg initially then 100 mg every 12–24 h

group 3 and 4 cephalosporins (Tables 52.5, 52.7, 52.8). A recommended regimen would be oral azithromycin 500 mg for one day followed by 250 mg for 4 additional days (Table 52.5); oral ciprofloxacin 500–750 mg twice daily is also effective (Table 52.7).

BARTONELLA QUINTANA (BACILLARY ANGIOMATOSIS)

Either *B. henselae* or *B. quintana* may cause bacillary angiomatosis (Table 52.6). Bacillary angiomatosis typically affects severely immunocompromised patients, such as advanced cases of HIV with CD4+ lymphocytes <50 cells/mm³.[27] Symptoms of bacillary angiomatosis include fever, lymphadenopathy, abdominal pain, and the classic grouped dark red and violaceous papules and nodules that are friable and painful. The lesions of bacillary angiomatosis appear similar to Kaposi's sarcoma and pyogenic granulomas, and should be distinguished from these conditions.

Treatment is with either oral macrolide antibiotic (clarithromycin 500 mg twice daily or azithromycin 250 mg daily) or erythromycin (500 mg four times daily) (Table 52.5). Ciprofloxacin (oral 500–750 mg twice daily) is also a first-line agent (Table 52.7); oral doxycycline (100 mg twice daily) is also recommended (Table 52.8). Treatment must continue for up to 6 months.

PROPIONIBACTERIUM ACNES (ACNE)

Acne is an inflammatory condition caused by the accumulation of free fatty acids in the follicles of the skin, produced by the action of bacterial lipolytic enzymes on triglycerides (Table 52.6). Acne begins with the formation of a comedome, sometimes papules, pustules, and nodules. The ensuing inflammation is a result of the presence of *P. acnes* which is the target of the inflammatory response. The accumulation of sebum in the follicles of the face, chest, shoulders and back produces nutrients on which *P. acnes* thrives.

The disruption in keratinization is a fundamental component of acne at for which therapy is directed. Topical agents include use of products containing benzoyl peroxide, salicylic acid, vitamin A derivatives, and synthetic retinoids adapalene and tazarotene. Topical antibacterial agents such as clindamycin, and erythromycin are effective (Table 52.9). Another cream intended to effect the keratinization process is azelaic acid. Cleansing is of limited value because soaps will not remove bacteria or lipids from inside the follicle. Intralesional steroid injection of larger nodular lesions will decrease inflammation and avoid potential scar formation. Daily oral tetracycline, erythromycin, clindamycin, doxycycline, and minocycline decrease the concentration of free fatty acids and suppress *P. acnes* (Table 52.5 and 52.8). Oral contraceptives containing estrogen will decrease sebum production and therefore, decrease acne lesions. Isotretinoin, a synthetic oral retinoid that produces profound decreases in sebum production has several side effects, including pronounced dryness of the skin and mucous membranes. A dose of 0.5–1.0 mg daily is recommended for a 20-week treatment. Baseline complete blood cell counts, liver function test, and triglyceride levels should be checked and repeated at 3–4 weeks and 6–8 weeks of therapy. Women of childbearing age should start contraception 1 month before therapy because isotretinoin is teratogenic.

CLOSTRIDIUM PERFRINGENS (CLOSTRIDIUM CELLULITIS)

Clostridium perfringens infection can cause a crepitant cellulitis of the subcutaneous tissue, possibly muscle, following traumatic tissue injury associated with soil contamination (Table 52.6). The crepitus present is caused by gas in the underlying tissues (gas gangrene). Pure clostridial infections do not emit foul odors; however, mixed and non-clostridial infections will produce foul-smelling hydrogen through incomplete oxidation produced by anaerobic organisms.[28]

The pain of a clostridium cellulitis is often mild and infection appears superficial, although tissue damage may be extensive. Treatment requires surgery and adjunct penicillin G, with possibly clindamycin and hyperbaric oxygen therapy (Table 52.3).

LISTERIA MONOCYTOGENES (LISTERIOSIS)

Listeria monocytogenes is found in the feces of wild animals, birds and soil, although, infection can not usually be associated with exposure to any of the common sources (Table 52.6). Treatment is with either ampicillin or penicillin (Table 52.3). For adults the dosage of aqueous penicillin G is 12–24 million units (7.2–14.4 g) intravenously daily in divided doses every 2–4 h; the dose of ampicillin is 12 g intravenously in divided doses every 3–4 hours (Table 52.3). In non-pregnant adults allergic to penicillin, trimethoprim–sulfamethoxazole is an alternative.[29]

Table 52.9 Topical antimicrobial agents

Antibiotic/strength	Indications	Bacterial coverage	Available forms
Azelaic acid 20%	Acne	Gram-positive	Cream
Bacitracin	Impetigo, furunculosis	Gram-positive	Ointment
Chloramphenicol 1%	Minor skin infections	Gram-positive and negative	Cream
Clindamycin 1%	Acne	Gram-positive	Solution, gel, pledget, lotion
Clioquinol	Tinea pedis	Broad spectrum	Cream, ointment
Demeclocycline	Skin infections	Gram-positive	Cream
Erythromycin 1.5–2%	Acne	Gram-positive and negative	Solution, gel, pledget, ointment solution
Fusidic acid	Skin infections	Gram-positive	Cream, ointment, impregnated gauze
Gentamicin 0.01%	Prophylaxis of malignant otitis externa	Gram-negative	Cream, ointment
Gramicidin	Skin infections	Gram-positive	Ointment
Metronidazole 0.75%	Rosacea	Anaerobes	Gel, cream
Mupirocin 2%	Impetigo, antimicrobial prophylaxis, and eliminating *Staph. aureus* nasal carriage	Gram-positive	Ointment
Neomycin	Abrasions, burns	Gram-negative	Ointment
Neomycin + polymyxin	Abrasions	Gram-negative	Cream
Neomycin + polymyxin + bacitracin	Abrasions	Gram-positive and negative	Ointment
Nitrofurazone 0.2%	Burns	Gram-positive and negative	Cream, solution
Paromomycin	Cutaneous leishmaniasis	Broad spectrum antibacterial and antiparasitic	
Polymyxin B	Infected atopic, nummular, stasis dermatitis, and swimmer's ear	Gram-negative	Ointment
Silver sulfadiazine	Burns	Broad spectrum	Cream
Tetracycline	Acne	Gram-positive and negative	Ointment, solution

ACTINOMYCES (ACTINOMYCOSIS)

Either *Actinomyces israelii* or *Actinomyces gerencseriae* cause actinomycosis (Table 52.6). Infection typically involves the cervicofacial anatomy following a traumatic procedure such as a dental extraction. Infection can result in a painful indurated soft tissue swelling around the oral mucosa known as 'woody fibrosis'. As the lesion enlarges at the angle of the jaw it is referred to as 'lumpy jaw'. Direct extension to adjacent thoracic structures may occur.

Diagnosis is based on clinical suspicion and detection of the organism on Gram stain, culture, exudates or biopsy.

Treatment is with intravenous aqueous penicillin G 10–20 million units (6–12 g)/day for 4–6 weeks (Table 52.3) or ampicillin 50 mg/kg daily intravenously for 4–6 weeks, followed by amoxicillin 500 mg/day for 6–12 additional months to prevent relapse (Table 52.3).

GRAM-NEGATIVE ORGANISMS

NEISSERIA MENINGITIDIS (MENINGOCOCCEMIA)

Neisseria meningitidis is an obligate aerobic, encapsulated Gram-negative coccus (Table 52.6). Humans are the only known host. Asymptomatic exposure to *N. meningitidis* can elicit protective bactericidal antibodies and so immunity increases with age.[30] A brief upper respiratory tract infection and subsequent nausea, vomiting, myalgia, fever, meningismus, stupor, hypotension, and hemorrhagic rash can precede acute meningococcemia. The hemorrhagic rash is a result of the pathogen damaging the small dermal blood vessels. The rash may transiently appear macular and papular with an erythematous hue with evolving purpura, and sometimes there are large red–black geographic-appearing areas of tissue infarction with a gray center.

Polymorphonuclear leukocytosis will be noted in the peripheral blood and cerebrospinal fluid. The organism may be seen on Gram stain, and is easily cultured in cases of meningococcemia.

Untreated infection with *N. meningitidis* is fatal. Adults should be given aqueous penicillin G, 4 million units (2.4 g) intravenously 4-hourly for 7 days after the temperature has returned to normal (Table 52.3); in the penicillin-allergic patient, chloramphenicol 1 g intravenously every 6 hours is the recommended regimen. In parts of the world where meningococcal resistance to penicillin has been isolated (e.g. Spain or the UK), a group 4 cephalosporin should be used[31] (Table 52.4). The recommended prophylactic dose of rifampicin (rifampin) is 600 mg orally twice daily for 2 days.[32] In cases of rifampicin resistance a fluoroquinolone is an effective oral single dose substitute (Table 52.7). Ceftriaxone is an alternative parenteral single dose for children and adults[31,33] (Table 52.4). Immunization with polysaccharide vaccines is safe and effective in preventing disease in adults and children over the age of 2 years.[32, 34]

PSEUDOMONAS AERUGINOSA

Pseudomonas aeruginosa is an obligate aerobic Gram-negative bacillus (Table 52.6). Some strains produce the characteristic blue pigment pyocyanin or the yellow–green pigment fluorescein, which will fluoresce under Wood's ultraviolet lamp. An odor of grapes, characteristic of trimethylamine, is typical of pseudomonal infection.[35] Healthy people infected with pseudomonas will typically be affected in areas exposed to increased humidity and moisture: such as the toe webs, fingernails (green nail syndrome), and the ear canal (swimmer's ear). People in public swimming pools or hot tubs (hot tub folliculitis) can also be affected.[36] Local infections will improve with topical therapy and drying of the affected area. Superficial skin infections such as toe web infections respond to acetic acid, silver nitrate and gentian violet each applied 2–3 times per day. Paronychia best responds to 4% thymol in chloroform, surgical drainage and nail trimming. For external ear infection acetic acid in 50% alcohol, 0.1% polymyxin in acetic acid or glucocorticoids with neomycin are effective. Systemic infection is rare in the immunocompetent host.

Patients with *Pseudomonas* infections are typically immunocompromised and may be afflicted with gangrenous cellulitis, or possibly ecthyma gangrenosum. Ecthyma gangrenosum lesions are painless and begin with an area of erythema surrounding a gray region of infarcted tissue. The lesions evolve to become black necrotic eschars. Treatment for systemic infections requires intravenous antibiotic therapy. Aminoglycosides, gentamicin, tobramycin and amikacin are recommended intravenous agents (Table 52.10). In patients that are acutely ill a second agent such as an anti-pseudomonal penicillin or ceftazidime should be added to the regimen.

BORRELIA BURGDORFERI (LYME BORRELIOSIS)

Lyme disease is caused by a tick vector that transmits the offending Gram-negative bacterial spirochete *Borrelia burgdorferi* to humans (Table 52.6). Lyme borreliosis is common throughout the northern hemisphere. Lyme disease can be classified into three stages: the first stage is called the early localized stage, the second the early disseminated and the last stage the late or chronic stage of lyme disease.

The hallmark cutaneous manifestation of Lyme disease, erythema migrans, begins at the site of a tick bite. Initially, the lesion appears as a confluent erythematous macule or patch, however, as the lesion spreads centrifugally the center of the lesion fades, leaving an annular area of erythema. The rash may be asymptomatic; however, systemic symptoms such as lymphadenopathy, headache, fever, malaise, myalgia, arthralgia, and gastrointestinal symptoms may be present.

Diagnosis is based on the history of exposure to a tick bite plus the appearance and evolution of the characteristic rash and serology.

Doxycycline, amoxicillin, penicillin, cefuroxime, clarithromycin, or azithromycin for 14–21 days have all been suggested for treatment (Tables 52.3–52.5 and 52.8). A vaccine is available for persons seeking prevention.

YERSINIA PESTIS (PLAGUE)

The plague is an infection in humans caused by *Yersinia pestis*, which is endemic in wild rodents and spread to humans via flea bites (*see* Ch. 63). Bubonic plague is the most common in the USA. Treatment is with intravenous gentamicin 2 mg/kg loading dose then 1.7 mg/kg 8-hourly, or intramuscular streptomycin 1 g 12-hourly for 10 days[37] (Table 52.10) Chloramphenicol, doxycycline or tetracycline are alternatives if infection with strains resistant to streptomycin are present (Table 52.8).

Table 52.10 Adult doses of aminoglycosides for treatment of skin and soft tissue infections

Aminoglycoside	Route	Dose
Amikacin	i.m./i.v.	15 mg/kg daily every 8–12 h
Gentamicin	i.m./i.v.	1.7–5.0 mg/kg daily every 8 h
Spectinomycin	i.m.	2 g once
Tobramycin	i.m./i.v.	3–5 mg/kg daily every 8 h
Streptomycin	i.m./i.v.	15 mg/kg daily or 25–30 mg/kg 2–3 times per week

FRANCISELLA TULARENSIS (TULAREMIA)

Tularemia is an infection of humans that typically follows direct inoculation by animals or by insect vectors with *Francisella tularensis* (*see* Ch. 63). Treatment is with streptomycin 1–2 g per day for 7–10 afebrile days. Gentamicin, tetracycline, and chloramphenicol are alternatives (Tables 52.8 and 52.10).

STREPTOBACILLUS MONILIFORMIS (RAT BITE FEVER)

Rat bite fever is acquired from rodents and is characterized by fever, polyarthralgia, and a rash[38] (Ch. 63). Treatment is with penicillin G 600 000 units (360 mg) intramuscularly every 6 hours for 10–12 days (Table 52.3). Doxycycline, erythromycin or clindamycin are alternatives in the penicillin-allergic patient[37] (Tables 52.5 and 52.8).

PASTEURELLA MULTOCIDA

Pasteurella multocida infection typically follows an animal bite (Ch. 63). (*P. multocida* can be isolated from the upper respiratory tract of healthy dogs, cats, rats and mice). Treatment of choice is oral penicillin V 500–750 mg 4 times daily (Table 52.3). For the penicillin-allergic patient doxycycline, chloramphenicol or trimethoprim–sulfamethoxazole (Table 52.8) are alternatives. Group 4 cephalosporins are also effective (Table 52.4); alternatively oral clindamycin 150–300 mg 4-times daily plus a fluoroquinolone may be effective (Table 52.7).

VIBRIO VULNIFICUS

Vibrio vulnificus is the most pathogenic of the *Vibrio* species. The soft-tissue infection and septicemia caused by *V. vulnificus* is deadly 50% of the time (Table 52.6). *V. vulnificus* produces a toxin and lytic enzymes that contribute to its pathogenicity. Gastroenteritis and saltwater wound injuries are common clinical findings. Septicemia following consumption of raw oysters can develop within 24 h.

Treatment of septicemia initially involves fluid replacement for shock followed by treatment with ceftazidime 2 g intravenously every 8 h plus doxycycline 100 mg (intravenously or orally) twice daily (Tables 52.4 and 52.8). Alternative regimens include cefotaxime 2 g intravenously 8-hourly or ciprofloxacin (oral 750 mg twice daily or intravenous 400 mg twice daily) (Table 52.4 and 52.7). Surgical debridement of necrotic lesions is indicated.[37]

RICKETTSIA RICKETTSII

Rickettsiae are obligate intracellular parasites transmitted to humans by arthropod vectors. The most common rickettsial disease in the USA is Rocky Mountain spotted fever. Others include typhus, trench fever, and Q fever. Rocky Mountain spotted fever can range from virtually asymptomatic disease to fulminate fatal disease.[39] The disease begins with abrupt fever, chills headache, myalgias, arthralgias, followed by a characteristic rash. The rash is a result of diffuse vasculitis that often begins first on the wrist, ankles and forearms, progresses to involve the palms and soles and then spreads centrally to involve the trunk, arms thighs, and face. The lesions initially appear as blanchable macules and papules, which become hemorrhagic with time. Treatment is with oral or intravenous doxycycline 100 mg for 7 days or for 2 days after the temperature returns to normal (Table 52.8). An alternative is oral or intravenous chloramphenicol 500 mg 4 times daily for 7 days or 2 days after the temperature reaches normal.

PARASITES

SCABIES

Scabies is caused by the itch mite *Sarcoptes scabiei* var *humanus*. The scabies mite is transmitted by skin-to-skin contact between sexual partners or family members. Infestation is usually bilateral and commonly involves the finger web spaces, wrist, elbows, genital and axillary folds. Diagnosis is made by identifying the mite, eggs, or fecal pellets.

Treatment is permethrin 5% cream, applied to the entire body from the neck down, paying special attention to the commonly infested areas. The cream must be washed off approximately 10 h after application. A second application may be used a week later it necessary. Lindane 1% (discontinued in the UK) is equally effective, and since low systemic absorption may occur, central nervous system toxicity has been reported. Permethrin and lindane must not be used on children under 2 years of age but sulfur 6% in petrolatum (petroleum jelly), applied each night for three nights and washed off is safe and effective for infants (and pregnant mothers). Symptomatic therapy of pruritus that may persist for weeks after effective therapy should include oral and topical antihistamines, and low to mid-potency topical steroids.

In serious cases, systemic treatment with ivermectin (p. 445) may be effective.

PEDICULOSIS (LICE)

Lice are blood-sucking insects. Their bites are painless and a person would be unaware of infestation if it were not for the body's immune system recognizing the foreign saliva, and anticoagulant produced by the bite of the insect feeding on the underlying dermis. Head lice (*Pediculus humanus* var. *capitis*) are typically isolated to the scalp. Crab lice or pubic lice (*Phthirus pubis*) are typically sexually transmitted. Body lice (*Pediculus humanus*) are found on people with poor hygiene.

Head lice are treated with synthetic pyrethroids: permethrin 1% cream rinse applied to a previously shampooed and rinsed hair and scalp, allowed to set for 10 minutes and then rinsed off with water. Alternatives include synergized pyrethrins applied in a similar manner. A second application of the medication 7–10 days later will kill any surviving eggs or nymphs that were not killed with the first treatment.

Crab lice are treated similarly with either synergized pyrethrins or lindane shampoo. The pubic area and the surrounding abdomen and thighs should be treated, especially if the patient is hairy. All undergarments and linens should be washed in hot water and dried on a high heat dryer cycle.

Body lice should be treated with a single application of permethrin 5% cream, exactly as one would treat scabies. Clothing and bed linens should be discarded or washed thoroughly in hot water.

OTHER INFECTIONS

- **Fungal infections** are discussed in detail in Ch. 62.
- **Mycobacterial infections** are discussed in detail in Ch. 61.
- **Sexually transmitted diseases** are discussed in detail in Ch. 59.
- **Protozoal infections** are discussed in detail in Ch. 65.
- **Helminthic infections** are discussed in detail in Ch. 66.
- **Hepatitis infection** is discussed in detail in Ch. 51.
- **HIV infection** is discussed in detail in Ch. 46.
- **Leprosy** is discussed in detail in Ch. 60.

References

1. Chapter 210. In: Freedberg IM, Eisen AZ, Wolff K et al (eds). *Fitzpatrick's Dermatology in General Medicine* 5th edn. McGraw-Hill, New York.
2. Wald A, Zeh J, Selke S et al 2000 Reactivation of genital herpes simplex virus type 2 infection in asymptomatic HSV-2 seropositive persons. *New England Journal of Medicine* 342: 844–850.
3. Hope Simpson RE 1965 The nature of herpes zoster: a long term study and new hypothesis. *Proceedings of the Royal Society of London, Series B* 58: 9–20.
4. Weksler ME 1994 Immune senescence. *Annals of Neurology* 35: S35–37.
5. Straus SE 1993 Epstein Barr virus infections: Biology, pathogenesis, and management. *Annals of Internal Medicine* 118: 45.
6. Epstein JB 1998 Hairy leukoplakia-like lesions in immunosuppressed patients following bone marrow transplatation. *Transplantation* 46: 462
7. Schmidt-Westhausen A 1990 Oral hairy leukoplakia in an HIV seronegative heart transplant patient. *Journal of Oral Pathology and Medicine* 19: 192.
8. Chang Y, Cesarman E, Pessin MS et al 1994 Identification of herpes-like DNA sequences in AIDS-associated Kaposi's sarcoma. *Science* 266: 1865–1869
9. Vander Straten MR, Carrasco DA, Tyring SK 2000 Treatment of human herpesvirus 8 infections. *Dermatological Therapy* 13: 2277–284.
10. Leavell UW Jr 1965 Ecthyma contagiosum (Orf). *Southern Medical Journal* 58: 238.
11. Nagington J 1964 The structure of the orf virus. *Virology* 23: 461.
12. Moscovici C 1963 Isolation of a viral agent from pseudocowpox disease. *Science* 141: 915.
13. Zur Hausen H 1996 Papillomavirus infections–a major cause of human cancers. *Biochimica Biophysica Acta Reviews of Cancer* 1288: F55.
14. Majewski S 1997 Epidermodysplasia verruciformis. Immunological and nonimmunological surveillance mechanisms: Role in tumor progression. *Clinical Dermatology* 15: 321.
15. Orth G 1986 Epidermodysplasia verruciformis: A model for understanding the oncogenicity of human papillomaviruses. *Ciba Foundation Symposium* 120: 157.
16. In: Freedberg IM, Eisen AZ, Wolff K et al (eds). *Fitzpatrick's Dermatology in General Medicine* 5th edn. McGraw-Hill, New York.
17. Chapter 196 In: Freedberg IM, Eisen AZ, Wolff K et al (eds). *Fitzpatrick's Dermatology in General Medicine* 5th edn. McGraw-Hill, New York.
18. Leung DY 1995 The potential role of bacterial superantigens in the pathogenesis of Kawasaki syndrome. *Journal of Clinical Immunology* 15: 11S.
19. Mc Cray MK, Esterly NB 1981 Blistering distal dactylitis. *Journal of the American Academy of Dermatology* 5: 592.
20. Chapter 197. In: Freedberg IM, Eisen AZ, Wolff K et al (eds). *Fitzpatrick's Dermatology in General Medicine* 5th edn. McGraw-Hill, New York.
21. Abramowicz M 2000 Linezolid (Zyvox). *The Medical Letter* 14: 45–46.
22. Laucks SS 1994 Fournier's gangrene. *Surgical Clinics of North America* 74: 1339.
23. Reboli AC, Farrar WE 1989 *Erysipelothrix rhusiopathiae*: An occupational pathogen. *Clinical Microbiology Reviews* 2: 354.
24. Venditti M 1990 Antimicrobial susceptibles of *Erysipelothrix rhusiopathiae*, *Antimicrobial Agents and Chemotherapy* 34: 2038.
25. Midani S 1996 Cat Scratch disease. *Advances in Pediatrics* 43: 387.
26. Carithers HA 1985 Cat scratch disease: and overview based on a study of 1200 patients. *American Journal of Diseases of Childhood* 139: 1124.
27. Maurin M. Raoult D 1996 *Bartonella* (*Rochalimaea*) *quintana* infections. *Clinical Microbiology Reviews* 9: 273.
28. Feingold DS 1982 Gangrenous and crepitant cellulitis. *Journal of the American Academy of Dermatology* 6: 289
29. Lorber B 1997 Listeriosis. *Clinical Infectious Diseases* 24: 1.
30. Goldschneider I 1969 Human immunity to the meningococcus: Development of natural immunity. *Journal of Experimental Medicine* 129: 1327.
31. Oppenheim BA 1997 Antibiotic resistance in *Neisseria meningitidis*. *Clinical Infectious Diseases* 24: 598.
32. Centers for Disease Control 1997: Control and prevention of meningococcal disease. *Morbidity and Mortality Weekly Reports* 46: RR-5, 1
33. Gilja OH 1993 Use of single dose of ofloxacin to eradicate tonsillopharyngeal carriage of neisseria meningitidis. *Antimicrobial Agents and Chemotherapy* 37: 2024.
34. Fass RJ, Saslaw S 1972 chronic meningococcemia: possible pathogenic role of IgM deficiency. *Archives of Internal Medicine* 130: 943
35. Chapter 198. In: Freedberg IM, Eisen AZ, Wolff K et al (eds). *Fitzpatrick's Dermatology in General Medicine* 5th edn. McGraw-Hill, New York.
35. Sharma PK, Yadav TP, Gautam RK, Taneja N, Satyanarayana L 2000 Erythromycin in pityriasis rosea: A double blind, placebo-controlled clinical trial. *Journal of the American Academy of Dermatology* 42: 241–244.
36. Agger WA, Mardan A 1995 *Pseudomonas aeruginosa* infection of intact skin. *Clinical Infectious Diseases* 20: 302
37. Chapter 200. In: Freedberg IM, Eisen AZ, Wolff K et al (eds). *Fitzpatrick's Dermatology in General Medicine* 5th edn. McGraw-Hill, New York.
38. Brown TMP, Nunemaker JC 1942 Ratbite fever. A review of the American cases with reevaluation of etiology. *Bulletin of the Johns Hopkins Hospital* 70: 210
39. Chapter 227. In: Freedberg IM, Eisen AZ, Wolff K et al (eds). *Fitzpatrick's Dermatology in General Medicine* 5th edn. McGraw-Hill, New York.

53 Bacterial infections of the central nervous system

Hisham M. Ziglam and Roger G. Finch

Bacterial meningitis remains an important cause of mortality and morbidity despite the widespread availability of effective antibiotics.[1] In the pre-antibiotic era, bacterial meningitis was a fatal disease. Following the introduction of penicillin, mortality fell to 15–30%. Today, despite the availability of potent antibacterials, the overall mortality from bacterial meningitis in adults has not decreased, averaging approximately 25% over the past three decades.[2] In children, major progress was achieved in the 1990s following the successful implementation of immunization against *Haemophilus influenzae* type b. However, in the neonate bacterial meningitis remains a serious disease; while the incidence has changed little in the past 30 years, the mortality rate has declined in industrialized countries from almost 50% in the 1970s to less than 10% in 1997. Nevertheless, neurological sequelae remain problematic is spite of improvements in treatment.

BACTERIAL MENINGITIS

Epidemiological data are largely derived from developed countries, in which the most common infecting organisms are *Streptococcus pneumoniae*, *Neisseria meningitidis*, Group B streptococci, *Escherichia coli* and *Listeria monocytogenes*. In contrast, Gram-negative bacilli such as *Klebsiella pneumoniae* and *Pseudomonas aeruginosa* are important but occasional pathogens, both in the context of nosocomial meningitis and community-acquired meningitis. In the latter, elderly and individuals with chronic debilitating diseases such as diabetes mellitus, cirrhosis, and malignancy are at risk from Gram-negative meningitis. *Str. pneumoniae* is numerically now the most important cause of community-acquired meningitis; strains resistant to penicillin and cephalosporins are increasingly recognized worldwide and have led to significant changes in management.

The etiology of bacterial meningitis varies by age and region of the world. One million cases of bacterial meningitis are estimated to occur worldwide, and of these 200 000 people die annually. Case-fatality rates vary by age and the causative organism, ranging from 3 to 19% in developed countries, and rates of 37–60% have been reported from developing

countries.[3] Up to 54% of survivors are left with disability due to bacterial meningitis, especially following pneumococcal meningitis. These include deafness, mental retardation, and other neurological sequelae.[4]

The etiology of bacterial meningitis has changed substantially since the introduction of conjugate *Haemophilus influenzae* (Hib) vaccine in the early 1990s. In addition, the frequency of neonatal group B streptococcal meningitis has declined in some countries because of the implementation of screening and treatment protocols in obstetric patients.[5] *Str. pneumoniae* is a well recognized cause of meningitis following fracture of the skull. Nosocomial cases of bacterial meningitis are almost invariably associated with neurosurgery and are caused by Gram-negative and other antibiotic-resistant strains including *Staphylococcus aureus*. Mixed infections, sometimes involving anaerobic organisms, are also found (Table 53.1).

Bacterial meningitis exhibits seasonal variation. The lowest incidence is in the summer months while pneumococcal infections are most common in the winter and meningococcal infections in the spring. Epidemic meningococcal infections are uncommon in developed countries but still occur in parts of Africa, India, and other emerging nations.

PRINCIPLES OF DIAGNOSIS AND TREATMENT

Early diagnosis of bacterial meningitis is essential for successful treatment. The age of the patient is of some value in indicating which of the common bacteria might be responsible. However, the only helpful physical sign is the characteristic rash found in some patients with severe meningococcal infection. Because of this paucity of clinical evidence, early bacteriological diagnosis is of the utmost importance, and an expert opinion on a Gram-stained film of a specimen of cerebrospinal fluid (CSF) should be regarded as one of the few bacteriological emergencies. One of the most important factors contributing to delayed diagnosis and therapy is the decision to perform a head computed tomography (CT) scan prior to

Table 53.1 Recommended empirical antibiotics for patients with meningitis according to age

Empirical therapy	Frequent pathogens	Recommended antibiotics
Patients <3 months	Group B streptococci *Escherichia coli* *Listeria monocytogenes*	Cefotaxime 50 mg/kg every 12 h in <1 month age ⎤ plus ampicillin 50 mg/kg every 6 h in >1 month age ⎦ 200 mg/kg daily
Patients 3 months to 50 years	*Streptococcus pneumoniae* *Neisseria meningitidis* *Listeria monocytogenes*	Ceftriaxone 80 mg/kg daily (children) 2 g every 12 h (adult) *or* cefotaxime 200 mg/kg daily (children) 2 g every 6 h (adult) ± vancomycin 60 mg/kg daily (children) or 1 g every 12 h (adult)
Adults over 50 years	*Streptococcus pneumoniae* *Listeria monocytogenes* Gram-negative bacilli	Ceftriaxone 2 g every 12 h *or* cefotaxime 2 g every 6 h *plus* ampicillin 2 g every 4 h *plus or minus* vancomycin 1 g every 12 h
Immunocompromised patients	*Listeria monocytogenes* *Streptococcus pneumoniae* Gram-negative bacilli (*Pseudomonas aeruginosa*)	Ceftazidime 1–2 g every 8–12 h *plus* ampicillin 2 g every 4 h
Head trauma, postneurosurgery patient	Enteric Gram-negative bacilli, Staphylococci, including *Staphylococcus aureus* and coagulase-negative staphylococci; *Pseudomonas aeruruginosa*	Ceftazidime 1–2 g every 8–12 h *plus* vancomycin 1 g every 12 h

lumbar puncture and therapy (Table 53.2). In patients with papilledma, focal neurological symptoms or a seizure, a CT scan should be obtained: a lumbar puncture should not be performed for fear of coning. If cranial imaging is deemed necessary, patients should have blood cultures drawn and empiric antibiotics administered before CT evaluation. One or two hours of antibiotic therapy before lumbar puncture does not decrease diagnostic sensitivity as long as CSF culture is perfomed in conjunction with CSF antigens and blood culture.[6]

Other methods to supplement the Gram stain and culture are now becoming more widely available. Rapid methods can be used to detect microbial antigen in CSF, blood or urine, using specific sera against the common causal pathogens.

These methods enable a rapid causal diagnosis to be made in some patients, (especially those who have received antibiotic treatment before lumbar puncture, in whom no bacteria can be seen in the Gram-stained CSF deposit). Countercurrent immunoelectrophoresis and other methods such as enzyme-linked immunosorbent assay have been supplanted by commercially prepared latex agglutination kits which are easy to use and give a result in a few minutes, although they vary in their sensitivity and specificity.[7] Obtaining a CSF sample for polymerase chain reaction assay between 24 and 72 h after admission is now standard practice in many centers and is reported to have increased the diagnostic rate and led to improved management.[8]

Table 53.2 Guidelines for the role of computed tomography (CT) scans and lumbar puncture in suspected intracranial infection

Urgent CT scan indicated, lumbar puncture contraindicated	Urgent CT scan indicated, followed by lumbar puncture if CT satisfactory	Lumbar puncture contraindicated, urgent CT scan may not alter management, antibiotics should not be delayed

1. Raised intracranial pressure
  (a) focal neurological signs
  (b) definite papilledema
2. Computed tomography findings
  (c) lateral shift of midline structures
  (d) loss of suprachiamsic or context of suspected basilar cisterns
  (e) obliteration of fourth ventricle
  (f) obliteration of superior cerebellar/quadrigeminal plate cisterns with sparing of ambient cisterns.
	(a) Altered level of consciousness, confusion, Glasgow Coma Scale <13
	(b) Convulsions (obviously convulsions in the intracranial infection)
	(c) When abscess suspected in view of ear/sinus or other focus of infection ± a subacute onset.
	(d) Immunocompromised patient
		Fulminant presentation ± purpuric rash ± coagulopathy ± low blood pressure

Lumbar puncture must be performed without preceding CT scan in the absence of all of the above.

No organism can be isolated from the CSF in some cases of purulent meningitis; the proportion varies between 12% and 25% in different series. The major reason for this is the preadmission administration of antibiotic, which reduces the number of positive CSF Gram-stained films and cultures. The low CSF glucose concentration normally found in pyogenic meningitis tends to persist and in the presence of a predominantly lymphocytic reaction strongly suggests tuberculous meningitis. Recently, a variety of studies have investigated the use of various CSF biochemical markers as a means of differentiating between bacterial and viral meningitis; elevated CSF lysozyme, procalcitonine, complement C3 and factor B levels have all been advocated as useful diagnostically.[9–11]

PHARMACOKINETIC FACTORS

Factors affecting antibiotic penetration into CSF

The factors affecting penetration of antibiotics into CSF include molecular size and configuration, lipophilicity, binding to plasma protein, the presence of an active transport system and the degree of meningeal inflammation, molecular charge and active efflux from the CSF.[12] Numerous studies have focused on the penetration of antibacterials into CSF, brain tissues and the pus of brain abscesses. Most concentration measurements were performed with lumbar CSF. The majority of the studies consist of a single determination in several individuals either after a single dose or repeated bolus dose. The available data on CSF levels varies greatly from drug to drug (Table 53.3), but it is possible to make a clinical classification (Box 53.1) into four groups:

1. Therapeutic CSF concentrations may be reached by standard dosage and route of administration.
2. A high therapeutic ratio allows an adequate CSF concentrations to be achieved by high intravenous or intramuscular doses; the CSF concentration is usually higher when the meninges are inflamed.

Box 53.1 Penetration of antimicrobial agents into CSF

1. Therapeutic CSF concentrations achieved by standard doses and routes of administration
Chloramphenicol
Sulfonamides
Trimethoprim
Fluroquinolones
Metronidazole
Doxycycline
Isoniazid
Rifampicin
Pyrazinamide
Ethionamide

2. Therapeutic CSF concentrations achieved by high intravenous or intramuscular doses, especially in meningitis
Penicillins
Cephalosporins

3. Therapeutic CSF concentrations may be achieved by standard doses and routes in meningitis
Clindamycin
Vancomycin
Tetracycline
Erythromycin
Ethambutol

4. Therapeutic CSF concentrations cannot be reliably achieved except where intrathecal route is possible
Aminoglycosides
Polymyxin
Fusidic acid

Table 53.3 Penetration of some agents into human CSF in relation to MIC_{90} for selected meningeal pathogens

Agent	Dose (g) (route/frequency)	Concentration in CSF (mg/l) meninges	CSF:serum ratio (%)	MIC_{90} against common meningeal pathogen					
				NM	HI	PSSP	PRSP	EC	PA
Pencillin G	1.5×10^5 i.v./M	0.8/I	8	0.03	1–256	≤0.06	4	NA	NA
Ampicillin	15 mg/kg i.v./S	0–0.9/I	3.4	0.004–32	0.5–256	0.06	4	≥8	NA
Ceftriaxone	100 mg/kg i.v./M	2–42/I	8.6	≤0.06	≤0.125	≤0.06	16	≤0.06	≥16
Cefotaxime	40 mg/kg i.v./M	3.7±5.5/I	18	≤0.06	≤0.06	≤0.05	0.5	0.125	≥32
Ceftazidime	2.0 g i.v./M	2–56/I	23.5	≤0.125	0.125–0.5	≤0.125	4	0.25–4	≥8
Meropenem	40 mg/kg i.v./S	0.3–6.5/I	21	≤0.06	0.015–0.25	≤0.06	16	0.015–4	0.015–16
Gentamicin	1.5 mg/kg i.m./S	0–0.10/I	2.5	NA	1–4	32	32	≥0.5	≥4
Ciprofloxacin	500 mg oral/S	0.3–0.5/U	25	≤0.06	≤0.06	1–2	12	0.03–0.125	0.5–4
Chloramphenicol	100 mg/kg i.v./M	2.0–15.6/I	38	0.06–8	0.5–8	1	16	4	NA

M, multiple; S, single; I, inflamed; U, non-inflamed; NA, not available; NM, *Neisseria meningitidis*; HI, *Haemophilus influenzae*; PSSP, Penicillin-sensitive pneumococci; PRSP, penicillin-resistant pneumococci; EC, *Escherichia coli*; PA, *Pseudomonas aeruginosa*.

3. Drug toxicity disallows an increase in dose, and the CSF concentration may reach therapeutic levels only when meninges are inflamed.
4. Little or no drug is found in the CSF with or without meningitis; intrathecal administration may be needed.

Logical decisions regarding antibiotic dosing depend not only on knowledge of drug penetration but also on knowledge of the pharmacokinetic and pharmacodynamic properties of the antibiotic.

Because of the general limitation in antibiotic penetration into the CSF, the use of oral antibiotics is discouraged since the dose and tissue levels tend to be considerably lower than with parenteral agents. An exception can be made for rifampicin (rifampin), given either as a synergistic drug or for eradication of mucosal carriage of *H. influenzae* or *N. meningitidis*.

Because of erratic distribution within the CSF, and failure of antibiotics injected into lumbar theca to become distributed throughout the ventricular system, intrathecal therapy is discouraged by many physicians as risks outweigh the doubtful therapeutic advantage. There are, nevertheless, a few situations in which intrathecal treatment is indicated, when the ventricular route must be used. In some patients a ventricular reservoir may be needed when injections at this site are easily made. Doses and preparations for intrathecal injection should be very carefully checked.

Contribution of experimental studies

Although much information has been gathered about antibiotic concentrations in serum and CSF in humans with meningitis, ethical and practical limitations make it difficult to achieve a full picture of the conditions necessary for successful treatment. Many factors certainly contribute to the poor results of treatment in neonatal meningitis, and in Gram-negative bacillary meningitis in older age groups, but recent studies indicate that failure to achieve appropriate concentration of the correct antibiotic at relevant sites correlates with poor results. As elsewhere in the body, local foci of infection remain important and, in neonatal meningitis especially, persistent ventriculitis results in treatment failure. General principles apply here as elsewhere: the antibiotic regimen used must be active and, in this situation, bactericidal against the causal organism at concentrations regularly achieved in body fluids. Additional factors related to success or failure have been clarified by work on experimental animals, especially in a rabbit model of experimental meningitis, in which repeated estimations of bacterial counts and of antibiotic concentrations can be made. McCracken has shown that, for some agents, the pharmacokinetic factors can be quite similar in the rabbit and the human infant.[13] McCracken concludes that measurement of the ratio of CSF area under curve to serum area under curve (CSF AUC/serum AUC × 100) after single doses and the mean relative concentrations after 9 h infusions give good predictors for CSF penetration in infants

and children. Both in rabbits and children, best results are achieved if the bactericidal titer of the CSF for the relevant organism is at least 1:8, but the rate of decline in the bacterial population of the CSF is no greater even if this titer is much exceeded. Measurements of this type, both in experimental animals and in humans, are helpful in the initial evaluation of new putative agents for treating meningitis, but are usually unnecessary in clinical practice once pharmacokinetic features of the drug have been well established.

SPECIFIC FEATURES OF ANTIBIOTICS COMMONLY USED IN THE TREATMENT OF MENINGITIS

Benzylpenicillin and ampicillin

In common with other β-lactam agents, these compounds penetrate the CSF poorly. Their low toxicity, however, enables this disadvantage to be overcome by high systemic dosage, which normally necessitates intravenous therapy. Where conditions make this impracticable or hazardous, intramuscular injections can be used but the large injection volumes are painful. CSF concentrations appropriate for the treatment of penicillin-susceptible meningococcal or pneumococcal meningitis can be achieved with dosage of 150 mg/kg (250 000 units/kg) daily divided into 4-hourly intravenous doses.[14] The same general points apply to ampicillin and its congeners. The range of doses in controlled trials has varied from 150 to 400 mg/kg daily. The highest doses are unnecessary, and a standard dose regimen of 200 mg/kg daily is recommended. Notably, none of the oral forms of penicillin or ampicillin is suitable for treating meningitis. Thus, the whole treatment course must be given by injection – CSF penetration diminishing even further as meningeal inflammation begins to resolve. The short half-lives of these compounds make it unwise to prolong the dose interval beyond 4–6 h.

Two specific unwanted effects have also to be considered. Neurological toxicity from penicillin presents a danger only when excessively high blood or CSF concentrations are reached. This sometimes occurs when very large doses are given intravenously in the presence of renal failure, but was especially associated with incorrectly high intrathecal dosage at a time when this form of administration was commonly used.

Cephalosporins

The extended-spectrum group 4 cephalosporins (cefotaxime and ceftriaxone) are characterized by excellent antibacterial activity against common meningitis-causing bacteria, and are currently recommended as the drugs of choice for the empirical therapy of bacterial meningitis. Cephalosporins, like other antibacterials, are not known to be metabolized in the CSF; thus, their concentrations in CSF depend on the balance between penetration and elimination. In most clinical trials, the penetration of cephalosporins through the blood–brain barrier is expressed as the ratio of CSF to blood concentration at particular time-point (Table 53.3). Because of the slow entry of cephalosporins secondary to low lipophilicity, their concentration–time curves in CSF lag behind those in blood.[15] Furthermore, the most important determinant predicting efficacy in meningitis is the relationship between the actual antibacterial concentration in CSF and the minimum bactericidal concentration (MBC) of the common organisms causing meningitis. The wide variability and occasional low CSF concentrations are worth noting because higher dosages are well tolerated and therapeutic concentrations in the CSF still be achieved. During the 1980s many controlled trials (reviewed in the previous editions of this book) were made of different cephalosporins in treating meningitis. The largest groups studied were children with *H. influenzae* meningitis. In most trials the compound under trial was compared with ampicillin and chloramphenicol in combination, the prevailing standard of treatment for community-acquired childhood meningitis at the time. These trials gave results generally similar to, but not better than, the standard regimen. Of the many compounds available, cefotaxime and ceftriaxone have been especially well studied.

In addition to clinical comparisons with the standard regimens, many trials included measurements of the rate of decline of bacterial counts in the CSF, and time to negative CSF cultures, which were again generally comparable in the two groups. In one trial comparing twice-daily ceftriaxone with chloramphenicol and ampicillin, repeat lumbar puncture 10–18 h after the start of treatment showed similar reductions of bacterial counts, but the median bactericidal titer in the CSF was 1:1024 in the ceftriaxone group, compared with 1:4 in the conventional therapy group.[16] Ceftriaxone concentrations in the CSF were 3–24% (mean 11.8%) of the serum concentration. These generally good results emboldened workers to study once-daily ceftriaxone dosage, allowing the possibility of largely outpatient treatment in patients who were well enough after the initial diagnostic assessment and initiation of treatment. Again, results were satisfactory:[17] diarrhea, the main unwanted effect, was not severe enough to necessitate a change of treatment. Duration of treatment has also been reduced, Lin et al[18] showing that the results with 7 days' treatment with ceftriaxone were as good as those after 10 days although, recently Roine *et al* found that 4 days of ceftriaxone therapy proved to be almost as safe as a 7-day course, especially in patients with rapid initial recovery from bacterial meningitis.[19]

Ceftriaxone, like the other cephalosporins used in meningitis, is normally given intravenously, but sometimes this route is difficult to maintain through the entire course of therapy. A study involving CSF examination 4–6 h after intramuscular injection on the third, sixth or ninth day of treatment (the normal intravenous route being used on the other days) showed satisfactory serum concentrations of ceftriaxone, and all CSF specimens showed bactericidal titers of a least 1:64 against the three common organisms.[20]

Cefotaxime has also been extensively studied and shown effective in the common forms of bacterial meningitis, often used mostly in a dose of 50 mg/kg four times daily, especially in treating sensitive organisms (include sensitive pneumococci). However, cefotaxime may be administered at a dose of 300 mg/kg daily, with a maximum daily dose of 24 g in treating resistant pneumococci.[21] A large study of 285 children prospectively randomized to receive cefotaxime or meropenem showed similar progress in the two groups.[22]

The increasing importance of drug resistance in *H. influenzae* infection, and the possible antagonism between ampicillin and chloramphenicol, led Finnish workers to conduct an important multicenter comparison in 220 children with meningitis (in 146 caused by *H. influenzae*) of chloramphenicol, ampicillin (initially with chloramphenicol), cefotaxime and ceftriaxone.[23] Results were similar in the four treatment groups, but all four bacteriological failures were with chloramphenicol and treatment had to be changed more frequently in this group. Use of ampicillin was limited by the problem of resistance. These workers were unable to rank the other two agents. Cefotaxime has fewer adverse effects, but the cost of both drugs limits their potential in developing countries.

Although cefotaxime and ceftriaxone are perhaps the most widely used cephalosporins in the treatment of meningitis, other β-lactam compounds have also been studied in *Haemophilus* meningitis, including ceftazidime, ceftizoxime and aztreonam – again, usually in comparison with ampicillin and chloramphenicol.

Cefuroxime, once used fairly widely in meningitis, proved inferior to ceftriaxone in a comparative trial of 106 children with the common forms of bacterial meningitis. Cultures in CSF remained positive at 18–36 h in 1 of 52 in the ceftriaxone group, compared with 6 of 52 receiving cefuroxime, and substantial hearing loss was present at follow-up in two of the ceftriaxone and nine of the cefuroxime group.[24] Although undoubtedly effective, this agent does appear as inferior to many later compounds and is not recommended for the treatment of meningitis. Lebel et al,[25] reviewing the results of four trials, noted positive CSF cultures 24 h into therapy in 9% of 174 patients given cefuroxime (compared with none in 159 treated with ceftriaxone), and subsequent hearing impairment in 18% (compared with 11%).

Other cephalosporins that are currently available or under development for clinical use are cefpirome, cefepime, cefoselis, cefclidin, cefozopran and cefluprenam (*see* Ch. 15). Cefepime is active against a broader spectrum of bacteria than earlier cephalosporins. This cephalosporin penetrates inflamed meninges to produce CSF concentrations ±20% of the serum concentrations.[26] This concentration is two to fourfold greater than that achieved by ceftriaxone and cefotaxime. In 1995, Saez-Llorens et al compared the use of cefepime and cefotaxime in 90 children with bacterial meningitis aged between 2 months and 15 years, randomized to receive cefepime 50 mg/kg every 8 h or cefotaxime 50 mg/kg every 6 h.[27] Concentrations of cefepime in CSF varied from 55 to 95 times greater than the maximal MIC required to inhibit the causative pathogens. Clinical response, cerebrospinal fluid sterilization, development of complications, and hospital stay were similar for the two treatment regimens, leading the authors to conclude that cefepime is safe and therapeutically equivalent.[27] This study has recently been confirmed by the same group in 345 pediatric patients recruited to two randomized trials that compared cefepime with either ceftriaxone or cefotaxime.[28] However, non-convulsive status epilepticus and reversible severe encephalopathy have been observed as unwanted side effects, especially if given in higher dose than required or in patients with renal failure.[29]

Carbapenems

Carbapenems (meropenem and imipenem) have a broad spectrum of antimicrobial activity that exceeds that of most other antimicrobial classes. Their potency extends to organisms resistant to many other types of antibiotics, including other β-lactam agents. The mean CSF concentration of meropenem following a single dose of 40 mg/kg in patients with inflamed meninges who had received dexamethasone (which markedly reduces the CSF concentrations of β-lactam antibiotics) has been reported to be 3.28 mg/l 2.5–3.5 h after administration.[30]

Meropenem has been extensively evaluated in treating bacterial meningitis in children but few studies have been comparative. Worldwide over 1200 children with different serious infections, including meningitis, have been treated and satisfactory responses have been seen in 90–100% of cases. The drug was well tolerated even at high doses.[31] Schmutzhard et al randomized 56 adults to meropenem ($n = 28$), cefotaxime ($n = 17$) or ceftriaxone ($n = 11$).[32] The dose of meropenem was 40 mg/kg, up to a maximum of 2 g, every 8 h. In the meropenem group, the causative pathogens included meningococci, pneumococci, *Ps. aeruginosa and H. influenzae*. All bacterial isolates were eliminated, regardless of the drug used. Among evaluable patients at the end of treatment, all patients on meropenem, 9 of 12 on cefotaxime and 8 of 10 on ceftriaxone were classified as cured.[32] Klugman *et al* randomized 98 children with bacterial meningitis to meropenem 40 mg/kg every 8 h and 98 children to cefotaxime 75–100 mg/kg every 8 h.[33] Two cefotaxime-treated patients died while receiving therapy and one meropenem-treated patient died of trauma 26 days after therapy. None of the deaths was judged to be related to the study drug. In evaluable patients, cure without sequelae was reported in 54 of 75 (72%) patients on meropenem and 52 of 64 (81%) randomized to cefotaxime; 21 patients (28%) on meropenem and 10 on cefotaxime (16%) had neurological and/or audiological sequelae. Seizures after the start of therapy were seen in five patients randomized to meropenem and three who were given cefotaxime.[33] Meropenem would appear to be as effective as cefotaxime for this indication.

Glycopeptides

Vancomycin is approximately 55% bound to serum proteins. It does not diffuse well into CSF, especially in the absence of inflamed meninges, although therapeutic concentrations can be achieved when higher dosages (15 mg/kg) are administered 6-hourly or by continuous infusion.[34] However, as dosages above 2 g/day are not recommended in adults because of nephrotoxicity, intraventricular administration has been used to treat staphylococcal infections of the CNS. The elimination half-life is 6–11 h and increases 20 h in case of intraventricular injection thus permitting once daily dosing.[35] Whether the bactericidal activity of vancomycin in CSF is time dependent, as it is in serum, has yet to be confirmed. However, animal studies reveal that maximal bacterial killing rate is achieved with C_{max}:MBC ratios of 5:1 to 10:1; any further increases in vancomycin CSF concentration does not result in a greater bacterial killing rate.[36] It has been suggested that vancomycin should be used in penicillin-resistant pneumococcal meningitis only when high-dose cephalosporin therapy has failed.[37] However, vancomycin in combination with a cephalosporin has been recommended to treat pneumococcal meningitis caused by strains with diminished susceptibility to the cephalosporin, especially in children older than 1 month.[38,39]

CHOICES OF EMPIRICAL ANTIBIOTICS

All adults in whom a diagnosis of bacterial meningitis is suspected should receive antibiotics in the community. There is little published evidence to indicate that the diagnosis is obscured by preadmission antibiotics. In view of the serious nature of this disease, it is strongly recommended that primary care physicians should give benzylpenicillin 1.2 g intravenously without delay. Cefotaxime or ceftriaxone 1 g should be given as an alternative in patients who have experienced an allergic reaction to penicillin other than anaphylaxis.

For patients admitted to hospital with suspected bacterial meningitis empirical antibiotic therapy is indicated if the lumbar puncture is to be delayed or if the CSF findings are compatible with bacterial meningitis with or without a diagnostic Gram stain. Antibiotic therapy should be started as soon as possible. Early antibiotic administration does not hinder microbiological diagnosis when polymerase chain reaction testing is used. The concern that early antibiotic administration may aggravate the clinical condition by causing antibiotic-induced endotoxin release[40,41] has not been confirmed clinically.[42] In contrast, delayed antibiotic therapy will simply result in an increase in bacterial biomass and the damaging effects of a more severe inflammatory response.

Because the CNS is an immunologically defective site, optimal therapy for bacterial meningitis depends on using antibiotics with bactericidal activity in vitro and in vivo. Empirical treatment must cover the full spectrum of possible causative pathogen(s), based on the patient's age, co-morbidity and whether infection is community or hospital acquired (Table 53.1). It is also important to note any history of drug allergy, recent travel, recent exposure to someone with meningitis, recent infections (especially respiratory and otic), recent use of antibiotics, injection drug use, and the presence of a progressive petechial or ecchymotic rash.

Presently a cephalosporin (usually cefotaxime or ceftriaxone) is recommended for the empirical treatment of community-acquired meningitis in adults and children older than 3 months. Empiric therapy for children younger than 3 months of age, consists of ampicillin and cefotaxime (in preference to ceftriaxone, which can bind albumin and alter bilirubin metabolism). Group 4 cephalosporins such as cefotaxime and ceftriaxone have emerged as the β-lactams of choice in the empiric treatment of meningitis in all other age groups. These drugs have potent activity against the major pathogens, with the notable exception of *Listeria*. They are clinically equivalent to, or better than, penicillin and ampicillin owing to their consistent CSF penetration. Their activity also includes most strains of penicillin-resistant *Str. pneumoniae*. Furthermore, synergistic activity has been reported between ceftriaxone and vancomycin in vitro and in experimental meningitis with strains for which the MIC of ceftriaxone was >4 mg/l. These findings have led most authorities to recommend vancomycin and ceftriaxone as empiric therapy for patients with meningitis in areas with a high incidence of pneumococcal resistance.

ROLE OF CORTICOSTEROIDS IN MANAGING (NON-TUBERCULOUS) BACTERIAL MENINGITIS

Since 1990 several studies have identified a wide variety of host inflammatory factors involved in the complex pathophysiology of bacterial meningitis that may serve as targets for adjunctive therapy. Adjunctive therapy with dexamethasone has been the most widely evaluated since a beneficial effect was observed in experimental bacterial meningitis. Early administration of corticosteroids such as dexamethasone in childhood meningitis, although showing no survival advantage, reduced the incidence of severe neurologic complications and deafness in *H. influenzae* infection.[43] A meta-analysis of five studies in children showed a relative risk of bilateral deafness of 4.1 and of late neurological sequelae of 3.9 in controls compared with children treated with steroids.[44] Several concerns have been raised over the adjunctive use of steroids: these include gastrointestinal bleeding, secondary fever, and difficulties in the clinical assessment of bacteriological cure due to quicker defervescence and penetration of antimicrobials through the blood–brain barrier, particularly in penicillin-resistant pneumococcal meningitis.[45] From Denmark a failure rate of 4% was reported in penicillin-sensitive cases receiving dexamethasone,[46] and from San Diego three failures in children were reported: one who relapsed, one with tuberculous meningitis and one with a brain abscess. Children with bacterial meningitis may be in septic shock and the role of steroids in septic shock and viral infections is unclear.[47] Sterilization of CSF by ampicillin and gentamicin in the presence of steroids also needs clarification. Not much is known about the use of dexamethasone in malnourished patients or those with HIV infection or other serious illness. Another major problem was that 65–70% of the children in studies from developed countries

had *H. influenzae* bacterial meningitis (excluding one retrospective study of pneumococcal infections from Dallas),[43,48] whereas in developing countries the causative organisms for bacterial meningitis are different.[48,49] In adults with bacterial meningitis (largely caused by *Str. pneumoniae*), the benefit of dexamethasone as an adjunctive therapy is still unclear.

Although many recommend that dexamethasone is considered for children with pneumococcal meningitis, the evidence from recent meta-analyses confirms benefit from dexamethasone in *H. influenzae* type b meningitis and efficacy in pneumococcal meningitis only if given early (before or during initial parenteral antibiotics). However, steroid therapy has not had any apparent effect on the mortality rates of pneumococcal meningitis. The American Academy of Pediatrics recommends that adjunctive therapy with dexamethasone should be considered for infants and children 6 weeks of age and older; the potential benefits and risks must be carefully weighed.[38] A potentially important concern is that the administration of steroids in combination with vancomycin may be disadvantageous. Vancomycin does not penetrate into non-inflamed CSF and the addition of steroids has been shown to decrease CSF vancomycin concentrations in adults.[50] This effect has not been observed in children.[51] In the context of antibiotic-resistant pneumococci, the clinician is forced to make a difficult decision: give steroids, as is appropriate for most patients who will respond to β-lactams, or withhold steroids, as is appropriate for those few who may have non-susceptible pneumococci requiring vancomycin. This decision can be made only on an individual basis with knowledge of the prevalence of antibiotic-resistant strains in a given community. In adults, rifampicin can substitute for vancomycin in patients receiving steroids.

Agents other than dexamethasone that are capable of intervening with inflammatory mediators such as nitric oxide synthase inhibitors, peroxynitrite scavenger, endothelin antagonist and matrix metaloproteinase inhibitor are beneficial in experimental bacterial meningitis and await clinical trials in humans.

DURATION OF THERAPY

The duration of antimicrobial therapy in patients with bacterial meningitis has traditionally been 10–14 days for non-meningococcal isolates (Table 53.4). Further information is presented later when each pathogen is discussed.

PATHOGEN-DIRECTED THERAPY

Meningococcal meningitis

Although meningococcal meningitis is a serious illness and meningococcal shock syndrome one of the most rapidly fatal of all infections, the organism itself is easily eliminated by appropriate chemotherapy. The success of sulfonamides in meningococcal disease was an outstanding triumph of chemotherapy, but the rapid spread of resistant strains since the first

Table 53.4 Recommended antibiotic regimens for patients with culture proven meningitis

Organism	Antibiotic therapy	Dosage in children	Dosage in adults	Duration of treatment (days)
Streptococcus pneumoniae				10–14
Penicillin MIC <0.1 mg/l	Penicillin G	300 000–400 000 U[a] every 4–6 h	2.4 g every 4 h	
Penicillin MIC 0.1–1.0 mg/l	Cefotaxime or	200–225 mg every 6–8 h	2 g every 6 h	
	ceftriaxone ±	100 mg every 12–24 h	2 g every 12 h	
	vancomycin	60 mg/every 6 h	1 g every 12 h	
Penicillin MIC >1.0 mg/l	Cefotaxime or	300 mg/every 6–8 h	2 g every 6 h (up to 24 g)	
	ceftriaxone ±	100 mg every 12–24 h	2 g/every 12 h	
	vancomycin	60 mg every 6 h	1 g every 12 h	
Ceftriaxone	Cefotaxime or	300 mg every 6–8 h	2 g every 6 h (up to 24 g)	
MIC >0.5 mg/l	ceftriaxone ±	100 mg every 12–24 h	2 g every 12 h	
	vancomycin plus	60 mg every 6 h	1 g every 12 h	
	rifampicin	20 mg every 12 h	300–600 mg every 12 h	
Haemophilus influenzae				7
β-lactamase negative	Ampicillin	Half adult dose	2 g every 4 h	
β-lactamase positive	Cefotaxime or	200–225 mg every 6–8 h	2 g every 4 h	
	ceftriaxone	100 mg every 12–24 h	2 g every 4 h	
Neisseria meningitidis	Penicillin G	300 000–400 000 U[a] every 4–6 h	2.4 g every 4 h	7
Listeria monocytogenes	Ampicillin plus	Half adult dose	2.4 g every 4 h	14–21
	aminoglycoside	Depends on aminoglycoside	Depends on aminoglycoside	
Streptococcus agalactiae	Ampicillin ±	Half adult dose	2.4 g every 4 h	14–21
	aminoglycoside	Depends on aminoglycoside	Depends on aminoglycoside	
Enterobacteriaceae	Ceftriaxone or	300 mg every 6–8 h	2 g every 4 h	21
	cefotaxime ±	100 mg every 12–24 h	2 g every 4 h	
	aminoglycoside	Depends on aminoglycoside	Depends on aminoglycoside	
Pseudomonas aeruginosa	Ceftazidime +	25–100 mg/kg every 8–12 h depending on age	1–2 g every 8–12 h	21
	aminoglycoside	Depends on aminoglycoside	Depends on aminoglycoside	

[a]300 000–400 000 U penicillin G = 180–240 mg

use of the drugs in 1963 rendered these agents unsuitable for first-choice treatment within a few years. The mainstay of treatment is benzylpenicillin, administered as described earlier (page 711). Susceptibility testing is necessary, because of the appearance of strains of reduced susceptibility to penicillin, described especially from Spain and now internationally. In the UK, the MIC of penicillin for most strains is less than 0.1 mg/l, but in 1993 6% showed MICs of 0.16–1.28 mg/l. These levels of reduced susceptibility are not clinically important if the correct dosage is used.

Ampicillin is as suitable as benzylpenicillin for meningococcal disease. When the microbial diagnosis of pyogenic meningitis is uncertain, the cephalosporins (discussed above) are fully active also against meningococci; a cephalosporin is the preferred agent in patients allergic to the penicillin or whose illness is caused by a penicillin-resistant meningococcus. Ceftriaxone has the added advantage of eradicating nasopharyngeal carriage (see below) in the index case, which is not true of benzylpenicillin.

In sharp contrast to the situation with many other forms of meningitis, eradication of the organism can be achieved readily and unduly prolonged treatment is unnecessary. Treatment is

often continued for 7 days, but 5 days suffices to eradicate infection and even shorter treatments have been effective. Viladrich et al[52] treated 50 patients with meningococcal meningitis with intravenous penicillin for 4 days. Even shorter regimens, such as 2 days of ceftriaxone[53] or single-dose therapy with a parenteral preparation of long-acting chloramphenicol have been successful.[54]

If meningococcal disease is suspected the patient should be given parenteral penicillin and admitted to hospital immediately. All suspected cases should be notified to the relevant public health authority. Although formerly widely used, nasal or throat swabs are no longer routine practice. Chemoprophylaxis should be offered promptly to all household and mouth-kissing contacts, to patients before discharge and anyone who has had contact with a patient's nasopharyngeal secretion (healthcare workers whose mouth or nose has been directly and heavily exposed to respiratory droplets/secretions from a case of meningococcal disease around the time of hospital admission).[55] Contacts should be carefully advised about possible early symptoms and of the persisting risk, even if they have received prophylaxis. In epidemic situations the use of vaccine should be considered if a group C (or A) strain is responsible, although prevention of epidemics of meningococcal disease in developing countries will be difficult until long-lasting conjugate vaccines capable of interrupting transmission of *N. meningitidis* can be incorporated into routine infant immunization schedules. Until then, the strategy of surveillance and response advocated by the World Health Organization is as effective as, and more practical than, a strategy of routine childhood and adult vaccination with currently available polysaccharide vaccines.[56]

Prophylaxis of meningococcal meningitis

Outbreaks of meningococcal meningitis in closed communities, especially military recruits, are well recognized, but spread within family groups may also occur, especially in conditions of overcrowding. Sulfadiazine has been very effective for chemoprophylaxis, but the emergence of sulfonamide-resistant strains has posed a problem. Rifampicin (rifampin) is much more effective than penicillin, ampicillin, tetracycline or erythromycin in controlling the carriage of sulfonamide-resistant strains and has therefore become the drug of first choice for chemoprophylaxis. A number of trials in the early 1970s established the degree of efficacy of rifampicin (85–90%) in immediate reduction of meningococcal carrier rate, but a substantial proportion of the residual strains isolated in the post-treatment period were rifampicin resistant; it is therefore possible that widespread use of rifampicin will be accompanied by an increase in strains resistant to this drug. The dosage of rifampicin is 600 mg twice daily for four doses (10 mg/kg body weight 12-hourly for four doses for children). Moderate success in controlling meningococcal carriage has also been achieved with minocycline 200 mg followed by 100 mg twice daily for 5 days. Total clearance of carriers was achieved using a combination of rifampicin and minocycline, but a third of the patients given both drugs experienced unpleasant side effects. Sequential use of minocycline followed by rifampicin has also been employed. Single-dose oral ciprofloxacin, in a dose of either 500 or 750 mg, has proved notably effective, and is now the preferred agent for adult contacts. For example, Cuevas *et al* conducted randomized comparative study of rifampicin and ciprofloxacin for eradicating nasopharyngeal carriage of meningococci.[57] Ciprofloxacin proved a safe and effective alternative to rifampicin for eradication of meningococcal carriage in adults but remains contraindicated in children. Similarly, 46 persistent carriers were treated with 750 mg in a single oral dose in a placebo-controlled double-blind trial:[58] 20 of the 22 placebo recipients remained positive, whereas 20 of 23 recipients of active drug showed negative results on swabbing 7 and 21 days later. Adverse drug reactions occur rarely following a single dose of ciprofloxacin but have included hypersensitivity reactions. Single-dose injection treatment with ceftriaxone has also been successful in clearing nasopharyngeal carriage[59] and this is the agent of choice in pregnant contacts. The adult dose is 250 mg as a single intramuscular injection; children under 12 years should receive half this dose. Furthermore, single doses of ofloxacin or azithromycin were found to be 97.2%[60] and 95%, respectively,[61] effective in eradicating carriage of *N. meningitidis*.

Chemoprophylaxis may fail because it is given too late or given to the wrong person, or because of non-compliance. Rifampicin resistance, although fortunately rare, is another cause of failure.[62] The effect of chemoprophylaxis is further limited because it does not prevent reintroduction of the pathogenic strain from a carrier outside the group, and therefore late secondary cases may occur.

Based on the observation that approximately half of the secondary cases in families develop within 24 h in children under 15 years, the Norwegian health authorities have advised treating these possible co-primary cases with phenoxymethylpenicillin for 1 week. Although this strategy has substantially reduced the number of co-primary fatalities in families, no controlled studies are available and this strategy has not been widely adopted elsewhere.

Pneumococcal meningitis

Initially, all *Str. pneumoniae* isolates were exquisitely susceptible to penicillin (MIC ≤0.06 mg/l), and this antibiotic served as the drug of choice. Beginning in the 1960s, however, clinical resistance to penicillin and other agents began to be reported. Today, drug-resistant *Str. pneumoniae* is recognized worldwide. Several reports of treatment failures related to pneumococcal isolates with decreased susceptibility to penicillin were published in the 1970s. In these cases, pneumococci for which the MIC of penicillin was between 0.1 and 1.0 mg/l were associated with microbiologic and/or clinical treatment failures in patients with bacterial meningitis being administered penicillin. These cases led to the conclusion that penicillin at routine doses did not result in high enough levels in the CSF (peak, about 1.0 mg/l) to reliably treat meningitis caused by intermediately susceptible pneumococcal strains (penicillin MIC 0.1–1.0 mg/l). At that time, ampicillin and chloramphenicol were the standard empiric agents for suspected bacterial meningitis in children. Chloramphenicol was considered an acceptable alternative to complete therapy if a penicillin-resistant *Str. pneumoniae* isolate was recovered, which at that time was still an infrequent occurrence. However, by the early 1990s, as penicillin-resistant pneumococcal isolates became more common throughout the world, treatment failures associated with cefotaxime or ceftriaxone administration for pneumococcal meningitis were reported. Vancomycin has also been used, but the correct drug concentration is difficult to achieve and a number of failures have been recorded. It is suggested that vancomycin be used (in penicillin and chloramphenicol-resistant pneumococcal meningitis) only when high-dose cephalosporins have failed.[37] Vancomycin may also have a place in combination with cephalosporins when diminished susceptibility to the cephalosporin has been demonstrated.[63] Although optimal therapy for infections caused by drug-resistant pneumococci is not known at the present, several options are available to the clinician facing this challenge. This should reflect the local epidemiology of resistance.

Where the majority of isolates remain sensitive to penicillin this drug can continue to be used, although for empirical therapy ceftriaxone would be a more reliable choice. Where resistance rates are high, it seems prudent to treat all patients with purulent meningitis empirically with vancomycin combined with either cefotaxime or ceftriaxone while awaiting CSF culture and antimicrobial susceptibility test results. The recommended dose of vancomycin in cases resistant to other drugs is 60 mg/kg/day. Alternative combination regimens for penicillin- and cephalosporin-resistant pneumococcal meningitis include rifampicin with either ceftriaxone or cefotaxime, rifampicin and vancomycin and vancomycin and chloramphenicol. Both cefepime, a broad-spectrum cephalosporin, and meropenem, a carbapenem antibiotic, have been evaluated in clinical trials for the treatment of bacterial meningitis. Randomized comparative studies assessed the efficacy of cefepime as empiric monotherapy in the treatment of bacterial meningitis. This drug represents an important therapeutic option for the empiric treatment of bacterial meningitis in children based on the good clinical response and bacteriologic eradication rates observed in this study.[28] However, no penicillin-resistant pneumococci were identified in the study; the effectiveness of cefepime for treating pneumococcal meningitis due to resistant strains could not be assessed and thus remains unknown.

Although meropenem is an alternative to extended-spectrum cephalosporins, much more experience with the drug is required before it can be reliably recommended as an effective antibiotic for the treatment of antibiotic-resistant pneumococcal meningitis.

In summary, the initial treatment of suspected pneumococcal meningitis should be altered especially in areas where resistant pneumococci have been encountered. Initial therapy with cefotaxime or ceftriaxone combined with vancomycin is recommended (Table 53.4). Once the results of culture and susceptibility testing are available, modifications of therapy should be made. If the strain is susceptible to penicillin, cefotaxime or ceftriaxone, vancomycin should be discontinued. Vancomycin plus cefotaxime or ceftriaxone should be used only if the organism is either intermediately or highly resistant to both penicillin and the cephalosporins. The addition of rifampicin or substitution of rifampicin for vancomycin after 24–48 h could be considered if the organism is susceptible to rifampicin, if there is evidence to suggest an inadequate clinical or bacteriologic response, or dexamethasone is used initially. It is prudent to perform a repeat CSF examination and culture at 24–48 h, until more experience is gained in treating meningitis caused by penicillin-resistant pneumococci.

Haemophilus meningitis

With the widespread addition of conjugate *H. influenzae* b vaccine in developed countries, very few cases of meningitis now occur in childhood. *H. influenzae* meningitis, although very much less common overall, is now encountered more frequently in adults.

The treatment for *Haemophilus* meningitis over the years illustrates the progressive limitation of therapeutic choice that results from the spread of antibiotic resistance. For many years chloramphenicol was unquestionably the drug of choice: it is bactericidal at concentrations that can readily be achieved in the CSF and is, indeed, superior to ampicillin in that respect. Ampicillin appeared to be equally effective, and being free from the possible hematologic toxicity, it became the preferred drug, especially in the USA.

In 1974, the situation changed when resistant strains of *H. influenzae* type b emerged. Resistance of *H. influenzae* is most commonly due to the plasmid-mediated β-lactamase production. Ampicillin resistance in *H. influenzae* has increased globally and ranges from 0% to 94%, depending on the geographic area. Resistance to chloramphenicol, though reported in the early 1970s, has remained rare, the incidence being about 0.5%. These changing resistance patterns have led to the widespread use of cephalosporins as initial treatment of *Haemophilus* meningitis. It is important to note that there is no evidence that cephalosporins give better results; the sole reason for their use is the presence of antibiotic resistance. Treatment with chloramphenicol or ampicillin is entirely appropriate when isolates are susceptible, an especially important consideration in the many parts of the world with financial limitations on antibiotic budgets. Practice in the USA, before ampicillin resistance became common, favored the initial use of chloramphenicol together with high-dose ampicillin. The antagonism between ampicillin (or penicillin) and chloramphenicol makes it likely that this form of combined treatment effectively relies on the chloramphenicol component,[64] and equivalent results are obtained whether chloramphenicol is used alone or in combination with penicillin.[65]

A number of choices are available when cephalosporins are indicated for the treatment of *Haemophilus* meningitis, and the agent used will depend on availability and the prevalent antibiotic policy of the country or institution. After disappointing results with the earliest cephalosporins, the first notable success was achieved with cefuroxime, but the possible limitations of this particular cephalosporin have already been discussed (page 712). In many countries cefotaxime or ceftriaxone are chiefly used but, as indicated, many other extended-spectrum cephalosporins are equally suitable for *Haemophilus* meningitis. The generally low toxicity of β-lactam agents permits high parenteral dosage and this, together with the high intrinsic activity which these compounds show against common bacterial causes of meningitis, overcomes their other relevant general property of poor CSF penetration. CSF concentrations and CSF:serum ratios for these compounds are summarized in Table 53.3; p. 710. The wide variability and occasional low concentrations in CSF are worth noting.

Protection of contacts

The risk of child contacts of patients with *Haemophilus* meningitis (and possibly other systemic *Haemophilus* infections) is of a similar order to that experienced by contacts of meningococcal disease. The overall risk is about 0.5% but nearer 2% in household contacts under 5 years of age. The high rate of nasopharyngeal carriage of the organism in contacts suggests the need for chemoprophylaxis. As with meningococcal infections, many agents that are effective in vitro, or even in the treatment of established infection, are ineffective in reducing nasopharyngeal carriage. Rifampicin, given in a dose of 20 mg/kg once-daily for 4 days, has been shown to reduce carriage rates by 90% and the effect persists, to a lessening extent, for several weeks. Resistance to rifampicin has been documented, although most re-isolates are still susceptible. These findings provided the basis for a number of trials, which showed a significant reduction of risk in contacts given rifampicin. The importance of correct dosage emerged clearly; in one study, carriage was reduced by 97% in children given 20 mg/kg of rifampicin but only by 63% in those given half that dose (and by 28% in the placebo group). Current recommendations have been influenced by the success of vaccination against invasive *Haemophilus* disease. Rifampicin chemoprophylaxis is now offered to all contacts in households in which there are any unvaccinated or incompletely vaccinated children less than 4 years old. The index case should also be given rifampicin, because persistent nasopharyngeal carriage may re-emerge after the acute infection has been treated. Chemoprophylaxis is also given to adult and child contacts in pre-school-age groups if two or more cases of disease have occurred within 120 days.

Chemoprophylaxis does not obviate the need for careful observation of all contacts, because a workable policy for chemoprophylaxis cannot include all those at risk. Rifampicin does sometimes fail to eradicate carriage, and the risk of rifampicin resistance is as yet uncertain. Moreover, although the recolonization rate is reduced, it does still occur. Failure of rifampicin prophylaxis has been reported a number of times. Rifampicin chemoprophylaxis, although marginally effective, will have negligible effect on the total number of patients with invasive *H. influenzae* disease and is much less important than vaccination as a control measure.

Staphylococcal meningitis

Staphylococcus aureus meningitis is usually encountered as a component of a generalized hematogenous infection, commonly in the elderly or in patients with serious underlying disease[66] such as postneurosurgical or post-trauma patients and those with CSF shunts; other underlying conditions include diabetes mellitus, alcoholism, chronic renal failure requiring hemodialysis, injection drug use, and malignancies. Other sources of community-acquired *Staph. aureus* meningitis include patients with sinusitis, osteomyelitis, and pneumonia. Mortality rates have ranged from 14 to 77% in various series. The course of the illness is difficult to modify, even with appropriate therapy. Flucloxacillin or oxacillin or equivalent compounds are suitable choices pending information from susceptibility tests. Results in the series quoted gave a suggestion that prognosis might be improved by the use of fusidic acid in conjunction with the penicillin. In countries where this drug is not available or in the presence of antibiotic resistance other choices include vancomycin and rifampicin. *Staphylococcus epi-*

dermidis is the most common cause of meningitis in patients with CSF shunts (discussed in detail in Ch. 45).

Streptococcus suis meningitis

Streptococcus suis meningitis has a strong occupational association with pigs or pork. Arthritis, endocarditis and other septicemic manifestations have been reported, and deafness is a common sequel. Kay, in a review that included 25 of their own cases,[67] indicated that *Str. suis* is susceptible to penicillin, ampicillin, cephalosporins, trimethoprim–sulfamethoxazole and vancomycin. Although 2–3 weeks' treatment with penicillin or ampicillin is usually satisfactory, relapses sometimes occur and require further treatment.

Gram-negative bacillary meningitis

Meningitis caused by organisms such as *Esch. coli*, *Klebsiella* and *Proteus* spp. is mainly encountered in neonates. It has become less unusual in older patients and those with immunosuppression or other conditions such as chronic renal failure. Group 4 cephalosporins (notably ceftriaxone and cefotaxime) have revolutionized the approach to their management, with reported recovery rates of 78–94%. Ceftazidime is active in vitro against *Pseudomonas aeruginosa* and has demonstrated clinical efficacy in infected patients. It is recommended that ceftazidime be combined with a parenteral aminoglycoside for the treatment of *Ps. aeruginosa* meningitis. Concomitant intraventricular aminoglycoside therapy should be considered in patients who fail to respond.[68] Other cephalosporins such as cefepime have been successful in the treatment of patients with Gram-negative enteric bacillary meningitis. However, although the MICs of these drugs for many Gram-negative bacilli found in meningitis are low and greatly exceeded by attainable serum and CSF concentrations, MICs for some organisms such as *Enterobacter cloacae* and *Acinetobacter baumannii* may be relatively high and treatment may fail for this reason.

The fluoroquinolones (e.g., ciprofloxacin) have also been used to treat these infections but are contraindicated in infants and children because of concerns about cartilage damage. Fluoroquinolones are most useful against multiresistant Gram-negative organisms or when the response to conventional β-lactam therapy is slow.[69]

Gram-negative organisms are also especially associated with nosocomial meningitis, especially complicating neurosurgery, CSF fistulas or ventriculostomies. A variety of organisms may be involved and the serious potential of such episodes is illustrated by the report of 25 cases of *Acinetobacter* meningitis in a neurosurgical unit over a 5-year period.[70] Initial empiric antibiotic therapy was with a ureidopenicillin plus an aminoglycoside. Intrathecal administration of amikacin was given on a number of occasions. Reflecting the desperate nature of these infections, intravenous colistin has also been used with success against a multiresistant strain of *Acinetobacter baumannii*.[71]

The fluoroquinolones penetrate well into the CSF, producing CSF:serum ratios of 20–30% for ciprofloxacin and ofloxacin.[72] Hence, they find occasional utility in the treatment of Gram-negative bacillary meningitis, especially for organisms resistant to standard regimens.[73]

NEONATAL MENINGITIS

Meningitis is a frequent accompaniment of neonatal septicemia, and carries both a high mortality and risk of residual neurological damage. The organisms responsible are summarized in Table 53.1 (p. 709). Among these, *Esch. coli* and *Str. agalactiae* (group B. streptococcus) predominate. Factors predisposing to neonatal meningitis are low birthweight, a complicated labor and maternal puerperal infection. Other causes include meningomyelocele or other neurologic defects. Gram-negative bacilli causing meningitis often demonstrate a varied antibiotic susceptibility pattern, and prompt laboratory guidance on positive CSF and blood cultures is essential.

Historically neonatal meningitis was often treated empirically with penicillin, usually ampicillin, and an aminoglycoside, usually gentamicin, as initial treatment. The poor penetration of aminoglycosides into CSF led to frequent supplementary administration of daily intrathecal injections of gentamicin. The erratic distribution of drug into the ventricular system following administration led to the introduction of ventricular reservoirs, allowing repeated CSF sampling and drug administration. The achievement of adequate ventricular concentrations of antibiotic is not merely a theoretical requirement. However, successive trials have also shown that addition of gentamicin by the lumbar intrathecal route to a parenteral regimen of ampicillin and gentamicin does not improve the outlook, and that intraventricular administration carries a substantial risk.

The most appropriate initial regimen, if no organism is seen on the Gram stain of the CSF deposit, is a combination of ampicillin and an appropriate cephalosporin, usually cefotaxime or ceftriaxone. If Gram-negative bacilli are seen, the cephalosporin can be used as sole initial agent. The former regimen of ampicillin and gentamicin (or other aminoglycoside) is still widely employed, especially when health budgets are low. However, failure to achieve adequate concentrations in the CSF and increasing resistance among Gram-negative bacilli accounts for some treatment failures with persistent meningitis.

Listeria monocytogenes

L. monocytogenes meningitis is less uncommon than previously thought. When it occurs in the newborn, it appears to result from maternal genital tract infection. It is also encountered in adults and is especially associated with lymphoreticular disease, immune suppression (as in transplant patients), pregnancy, diabetes mellitus and alcoholism.[74] Some patients have no underlying disease.

Ampicillin or penicillin G should be used as therapy for meningitis caused by *L. monocytogenes*. Many add an aminoglycoside for proven infection due to documented in-vitro synergy, even though a controlled trial comparing ampicillin with ampicillin plus gentamicin has never been performed in humans. Group 4 cephalosporins are inactive against *L. monocytogenes* and should not be used alone as an empiric regimen in neonates or when this organism is considered a likely pathogen.

Trimethoprim-sulfamethoxazole is increasingly used in patients who are allergic to penicillin, despite the in-vitro activity of chloramphenicol against *Listeria*, because the latter drug has an unacceptably high failure rate. Intraventricular vancomycin has been successful in one patient with recurrent *L. monocytogenes* meningitis. Meropenem, which is active in vitro and in experimental animal models of *Listeria* meningitis, may be a further useful alternative.[75]

Streptococcus agalactiae

Neonatal infections caused by *Str. agalactiae* (group B streptococcus) have come to prominence in recent years, especially in the USA. Much is now known of their epidemiology and pathogenesis. Two syndromes are seen: an early septicemic variety of rapid course and high mortality (50%) closely simulating the respiratory distress syndrome, and a meningitic syndrome developing somewhat later in the neonatal period. Group B streptococcal meningitis carries a high mortality (20%), as do other forms of neonatal meningitis. The median MICs of benzylpenicillin and ampicillin are 0.02 and 0.04 mg/l, respectively, with conventional inocula (10^5 colony forming units, but rises appreciably with larger inocula. Since the CSF may contain 10^6–10^8 bacteria/ml, treatment with high doses of penicillin, in excess of 150 mg/kg daily by intravenous injection, is recommended.

In most patients treated with high-dose penicillin or ampicillin alone, the CSF rapidly becomes and remains sterile. In some patients, however, poor response or relapse has been noted. One reason may be failure to eradicate the organisms from focal sites such as the ventricles or cardiac valves; another possibility is infection by a penicillin-tolerant strain, showing a high MBC:MIC ratio. These difficulties, together with the demonstration of synergy in vitro and in animal models between penicillin and aminoglycosides against group B streptococci, suggest the initial use of benzylpenicillin in high dosage with an aminoglycoside. The latter drug may be withdrawn if clinical progress and further laboratory data on the causal organism are satisfactory. Some units, following the recommendation of the American Academy of Pediatrics,[76] use penicillin or ampicillin as single agents.

Prophylaxis

Acquisition of these organisms by neonates is highly correlated with maternal carriage, although nosocomial transmission acts as an additional source. Attempts to reduce the risk of neonatal group B streptococcal disease are discussed elsewhere in this book (p. 778).

BRAIN ABSCESS

The mortality from brain abscess is high and has changed little in the antibiotic era. The reasons for this are certainly complex, but particularly important among them is the dangerously rapid rise of intracranial pressure which so often accompanies the development of brain abscess during the early stage of cerebritis. Discussion here is confined to antimicrobial aspects of treatment, but other aspects of management are of crucial importance, notably the control of raised intracranial pressure, and drainage (using stereotactic CT scanning) or excision of the abscess, as important in the brain as elsewhere. As in other forms of abscess, bacteria may be found in the abscess contents after many days of systemic chemotherapy. Surgical intervention may not be possible with multiple abscesses, and the advent of modern scanning has increased the frequency of non-surgical treatment if the condition can be recognized early and treatment closely monitored.

The causal organisms differ to some extent in their order of frequency with the origins of the abscess, but several studies have amply confirmed the importance of anaerobic Gram-negative bacteria, especially *Bacteroides* and *Fusobacterium* spp., and of aerobic and anaerobic streptococci. Enterobacteria of various genera are also commonly found, and staphylococci are important in infection associated with trauma and in spinal epidural abscess. Several species are often isolated from a single specimen when suitable selective techniques are used, especially in abscesses of middle ear origin. De Louvois et al stressed the strong association of *Bacteroides* spp. with temporal lobe abscess and the general importance of streptococci,[77] especially streptococci of the *anginosus* group (formerly *Streptococcus milleri*). Streptococci were the most prominent single pathogen in non-temporal lobe abscesses but, as Grace and Drake-Lee point out,[78] *Bacteroides* spp. may also be found in abscesses of sinus origin. A similar distribution of causal organisms is found in cerebral abscess in childhood, common associations of which are cyanotic congenital heart disease, otitis, sinusitis, head injuries and cystic fibrosis. It has to be remembered that, although the dominant organism in cerebral abscesses are well documented, other less common agents are sometimes encountered, including species of *Actinomyces* and *Nocardia* and fungi.

An appropriate first-choice antimicrobial drug regimen must take into account not only this diverse flora, but also the characteristics of potentially effective drugs in penetrating brain tissue, CSF and abscess cavities. Data on these aspects may be found in the work of Black et al,[79] Picardi et al,[80] De Louvois et al,[77,81] and a report by the British Society for Antimicrobial Chemotherapy.[82] Microbiological data are occasionally available at the time chemotherapy is started, for example, when brain abscess is diagnosed during the course of a septicemia of known etiology. Generally, however, no such information is available and initial antibiotic policy must be based on the organisms known to be dominant in the etiology of cerebral abscess (Table 53.5), as described above, bearing in mind especially that the common forms of brain abscess are often polymicrobial. Some authors recommend variations of regimen based on the different frequency of various species found in cerebral abscess associated with different parameningeal or pulmonary sources. These differences are not big enough to allow this sort of fine tuning; a single-unit policy for brain abscess associated with parameningeal or pulmonary sepsis is preferable.

These data indicate the basis of modern antibiotic treatment. High-dose ampicillin or penicillin retain an important role as effective against streptococci, including the microaerophilic species not susceptible to metronidazole, and against most of the relevant anaerobes. The recognition of anaerobes as an important component of the flora of many brain abscesses led to the use of metronidazole, especially relevant

Table 53.5 Initial empirical antibiotic therapy for patients with brain abscess

Infective source	Intracerebral location	Antimicrobial regimen[a]
Paranasal sinuses	Frontal lobe	Cefuroxime 1.5 g three times daily or cefotaxime 2 g four times daily or ceftriaxone 3–4 g once daily and metronidazole 500 mg three times daily
Teeth	Frontal lobe	Cefuroxime 1.5 g three times daily and metronidazole 500 mg three times daily
Middle ear (less often, sphenoidal sinuses)	Temporal lobe	Ampicillin 2–3 g three times daily and metronidazole 500 mg three times daily together with ceftazidime 2 g three times daily or gentamicin 5 mg/kg once daily[b]
Middle ear (less often, sphenoidal sinuses)	Cerebellum	Ampicillin 2–3 g three times daily and metronidazole 500 mg three times daily together with ceftazidime 2 g three times daily or gentamicin 5 mg/kg once daily[b]
Penetrating trauma	Depends on site of wound	Flucloxacillin 2–3 g four times daily or cefuroxime 1.5 g three times daily/ cefotaxime 2 g four times daily/ceftriaxone 3–4 g once daily
Metastatic and cryptogenic	Multiple lesions (usually in area supplied by middle cerebral artery)	Depends on source: benzylpenicillin 8–2.4 g every 6 h if endocarditis or cyanotic congenital heart disease; alternatively cefuroxime 1.5 g three times daily or cefotaxime 2 g four times daily or ceftriaxone 3–4 g once daily with or without metronidazole 500 mg three times daily

[a] Adult daily dosages.
[b] Gentamicin serum concentrations must be monitored.

as *Bacteroides fragilis* and perhaps some strains of *Prevotella melaninogenica*[83] are penicillin resistant but susceptible to metronidazole. This has led to the widespread use of metronidazole, together with ampicillin or penicillin, as agents of first choice. Good results in otogenic abscess were reported by Ingham et al,[84] who found that metronidazole, given orally or intravenously, achieved high concentrations in pus or ventricular fluid. In addition to high-dose ampicillin or penicillin and metronidazole, it is now customary to include a group 4 cephalosporin such as cefotaxime, ceftriaxone or ceftazidime in the treatment of patients with intracranial infections. Sjölin et al successfully treated 15 patients with a combination of cefotaxime (3 g thrice daily) and metronidazole (500 mg thrice daily) for a minimum of 3 weeks.[85] There are also a number of other reports of the successful use of cefotaxime to treat patients with brain abscess. Both ceftriaxone and ceftazidime achieve therapeutic concentrations in intracranial pus. However, to date, the numbers of patients treated with group 4 cephalosporins are small.[86] Cerebral abscesses in neonates caused by *Proteus mirabilis*, *Esch. coli* or *Serratia marcescens* have been successfully treated with combinations of cefotaxime and gentamicin or, with an even higher success rate, ceftriaxone and amikacin.[87] Formerly, chloramphenicol was widely used but now remains a reserve agent because of its toxicity concerns. There is very little information on the efficacy of more recently introduced antibiotics, such as the carbapenems, in the treatment of brain abscess.

Causal organisms in subdural empyema are generally similar to those in brain abscess and a similar antibiotic policy may be used. For staphylococcal brain abscess, pending detailed microbiological information a combination of flucloxacillin (or a similar isoxazolyl penicillin) and fusidic acid is suggested. Other abscesses of hematogenous origin may require specific chemotherapy different from those recommended for the common types associated with parameningeal sources in the ear or sinuses; these must be tailored to the particular organism.

EPIDURAL ABSCESS

SPINAL EPIDURAL ABSCESS

Spinal epidural abscess is a rare but potentially devastating condition. Many abscesses begin as a focal pyogenic infection involving the vertebral disk or the junction between the disk and the vertebral body (pyogenic infectious diskitis); in such cases the abscesses are often located in the anterior aspect of the spinal canal. However, hematogenous spread was identified in 26% of cases, primarily located in the posterior aspect of the spinal canal. The dominant organism is *Staph. aureus*, which accounts for about two-thirds of all cases. In a review of five studies between 1930 and 1982, Danner and Hartman found that *Staph. aureus* was isolated in 62%, other Gram-positive cocci cultured in 10%, Gram-negative organisms in

18%, and anaerobes in 2%.[88,89] In children, Auletta et al reviewed the literature over 15 years and confirmed that *Staph. aureus* is the predominant pathogen in spinal epidural abscess and community-acquired MRSA has been recognized in pediatric populations.[90] For this reason, initial antibiotic choice should be broad-spectrum, including a combination of drugs with bactericidal activity against staphylococci, anaerobes, and Gram-negative organisms. If a methicillin-sensitive *Staph. aureus* is isolated, successful treatment is possible with a group 1 or 2 cephalosporin, a penicillinase-resistant penicillin, a combination of vancomycin plus aminoglycoside, or trimethoprim-sulfamethoxazole. Parenteral treatment should be continued for at least 4 weeks and may be prolonged for 8 weeks or longer if vertebral osteomyelitis is suspected. When no pathogen is isolated, broad 'best-guess' bactericidal cover is safest and best. Instillation of penicillin into the abscess cavity is best avoided because the procedure has potential dangers and failure to sterilize the abscess contents is not usually attributable to deficiency of antibiotic in the pus.

INTRACRANIAL EPIDURAL ABSCESS

Intracranial epidural abscesses are less common than spinal epidural abscesses, and less acute in their evolution. They are usually associated with frontal sinusitis, prior craniotomy or mastoiditis. The morbidity and mortality of intracranial epidural abscesses in isolation are low. However, the great majority of patients have an associated brain abscess (up to 17%), subdural empyema (up to 81%) or meningitis (up to 38%). Treatment usually consists of surgical drainage of the abscess and associated infected sinus in addition to intravenous antimicrobial therapy. Empiric antibiotic therapy should be chosen based upon the probable infection. The regimens listed above for the treatment of spinal epidural abscesses when the etiology is unknown are also appropriate here.

References

1. Quagliarello V, Scheld WM 1992 Bacterial meningitis: pathogenesis, pathophysiology, and progress. *New England Journal of Medicine* 327: 864–872.
2. Durand ML, Calderwood SB, Weber DJ et al 1993 Acute bacterial meningitis in adults. A review of 493 episodes. *New England Journal of Medicine* 328: 21–28.
3. Salih MA, Khaleefa OH, Bushara M et al 1991 Long term sequelae of childhood acute bacterial meningitis in a developing country. A study from the Sudan. *Scandinavian Journal of Infectious Diseases* 23: 175–182.
4. Ciana G, Parmar N, Antonio C, Pivetta S, Tamburlini G, Cuttini M 1995 Effectiveness of adjunctive treatment with steroids in reducing short-term mortality in a high-risk population of children with bacterial meningitis. *Journal of Tropical Pediatrics* 41: 164–168.
5. Centers for Disease Control 1996 Prevention of perinatal group B streptococcal disease: a public health perspective. *Morbidity and Mortality Weekly Report* 45: 1–24.
6. Coant PN, Kornberg AE, Duffy LC, Dryja DM, Hassan SM 1992 Blood culture results as determinants in the organism identification of bacterial meningitis. *Pediatric Emergency Care* 8: 200–205.
7. Landgraf IM, Alkmin M, Vieira M 1995 Bacterial antigen detection in cerebrospinal fluid by the latex agglutination test. *Revista di Instituto de Medicina Tropical de São Paolo* 37(3): 257–260.

8. Carrol ED, Thomson AP, Shears P, Gray SJ, Kaczmarski EB, Hart CA 2000 Performance characteristics of the polymerase chain reaction assay to confirm clinical meningococcal disease. *Archives of Diseases in Childhood* 83: 271–273.

9. Bohuon C, Assicot M, Raymond J, Gendrel D 1998 Procalcitonin, a marker of bacterial meningitis in children. *Bulletin of the National Academy of Medicine* 182: 1469–1475.

10. Gendrel D, Raymond J, Assicot M et al 1997 Measurement of procalcitonin levels in children with bacterial or viral meningitis. *Clinical Infectious Diseases* 24: 1240–1242.

11. Stahel PF, Nadal D, Pfister HW, Paradisis PM, Barnum SR 1997 Complement C3 and factor B cerebrospinal fluid concentrations in bacterial and aseptic meningitis. *Lancet* 349: 1886–1887.

12. Nau R, Sorgel F, Prange HW 1998 Pharmacokinetic optimisation of the treatment of bacterial central nervous system infections. *Clinical Pharmacokinetics* 35: 223–246.

13. McCracken GH Jr 1983 Pharmacokinetic and bacteriological correlations between antimicrobial therapy of experimental meningitis in rabbits and meningitis in humans: a review. *Journal of Antimicrobial Chemotherapy* 12(Suppl. D): 97–108.

14. Hieber JP, Nelson JD 1977 A pharmacologic evaluation of penicillin in children with purulent meningitis. *New England Journal of Medicine* 297: 410–413.

15. Trang JM, Jacobs RF, Kearns GL et al 1985 Cefotaxime and desacetylcefotaxime pharmacokinetics in infants and children with meningitis. *Antimicrobial Agents and Chemotherapy* 28: 791–795.

16. Barson WJ, Miller MA, Brady MT, Powell DA 1985 Prospective comparative trial of ceftriaxone vs. conventional therapy for treatment of bacterial meningitis in children. *Pediatric Infectious Disease Journal* 4: 362–368.

17. Scholz H, Hofmann T, Noack R, Edwards DJ, Stoeckel K 1998 Prospective comparison of ceftriaxone and cefotaxime for the short-term treatment of bacterial meningitis in children. *Chemotherapy* 44: 142–147.

18. Lin TY, Chrane DF, Nelson JD, McCracken GH Jr 1983 Seven days of ceftriaxone therapy is as effective as ten days' treatment for bacterial meningitis. *Journal of the American Medical Association* 253: 3559–3563.

19. Roine I, Ledermann W, Foncea LM, Banfi A, Cohen J, Peltola H 2000 Randomized trial of four vs. seven days of ceftriaxone treatment for bacterial meningitis in children with rapid initial recovery. *Pediatric Infectious Disease Journal* 19: 219–222.

20. Bradley JS, Farhat C, Stamboulian D, Branchini OG, Debbag R, Compogiannis LS 1994 Ceftriaxone therapy of bacterial meningitis: cerebrospinal fluid concentrations and bactericidal activity after intramuscular injection in children treated with dexamethasone. *Pediatric Infectious Disease Journal* 13: 724–728.

21. Viladrich PF, Cabellos C, Pallares R et al 1996 High doses of cefotaxime in treatment of adult meningitis due to *Streptococcus pneumoniae* with decreased susceptibilities to broad-spectrum cephalosporins. *Antimicrobial Agents and Chemotherapy* 40: 218–220.

22. Odio CM, Puig JR, Feris JM et al 1999 Prospective, randomized, investigator-blinded study of the efficacy and safety of meropenem vs. cefotaxime therapy in bacterial meningitis in children. Meropenem Meningitis Study Group. *Pediatric Infectious Disease Journal* 18: 581–590.

23. Peltola H, Anttila M, Renkonen OV 1989 Randomised comparison of chloramphenicol, ampicillin, cefotaxime, and ceftriaxone for childhood bacterial meningitis. Finnish Study Group. *Lancet* 1: 1281–1287.

24. Schaad UB, Suter S, Gianella-Borradori A et al 1990 A comparison of ceftriaxone and cefuroxime for the treatment of bacterial meningitis in children. *New England Journal of Medicine* 322: 141–147.

25. Lebel MH, Hoyt MJ, McCracken GH Jr 1989 Comparative efficacy of ceftriaxone and cefuroxime for treatment of bacterial meningitis. *Journal of Pediatrics* 114: 1049–1054.

26. Blumer JL, Reed MD, Knupp C 2001 Review of the pharmacokinetics of cefepime in children. *Pediatric Infectious Disease Journal* 20: 337–342.

27. Saez-Llorens X, Castano E, Garcia R et al 1995 Prospective randomized comparison of cefepime and cefotaxime for treatment of bacterial meningitis in infants and children. *Antimicrobial Agents and Chemotherapy* 39: 937–940.

28. Saez-Llorens X, O'Ryan M 2001 Cefepime in the empiric treatment of meningitis in children. *Pediatric Infectious Disease Journal* 20: 356–361.

29. Martinez-Rodriguez JE, Barriga FJ, Santamaria J et al 2001 Nonconvulsive status epilepticus associated with cephalosporins in patients with renal failure. *Journal of Neurosurgery* 111: 115–119.

30. Dagan R, Velghe L, Rodda JL, Klugman KP 1994 Penetration of meropenem into the cerebrospinal fluid of patients with inflamed meninges. *Journal of Antimicrobial Chemotherapy* 34: 175–179.

31. Bradley JS 1998 Selecting therapy for serious infections in children: maximizing safety and efficacy. *Diagnostic Microbiology and Infectious Diseases* 31: 405–410.

32. Schmutzhard E, Williams KJ, Vukmirovits G, Chmelik V, Pfausler B, Featherstone A 1995 A randomised comparison of meropenem with cefotaxime or ceftriaxone for the treatment of bacterial meningitis in adults. Meropenem Meningitis Study Group. *Journal of Antimicrobial Chemotherapy* 36(Suppl. A): 85–97.

33. Klugman KP, Dagan R 1995 Randomized comparison of meropenem with cefotaxime for treatment of bacterial meningitis. Meropenem Meningitis Study Group. *Antimicrobial Agents and Chemotherapy* 39: 1140–1146.

34. Albanese J, Leone M, Bruguerolle B, Ayem ML, Lacarelle B, Martin C 2000 Cerebrospinal fluid penetration and pharmacokinetics of vancomycin administered by continuous infusion to mechanically ventilated patients in an intensive care unit. *Antimicrobial Agents and Chemotherapy* 44: 1356–1358.

35. Reesor C, Chow AW, Kureishi A, Jewesson PJ 1988 Kinetics of intraventricular vancomycin in infections of cerebrospinal fluid shunts. *Journal of Infectious Diseases* 158: 1142–1143.

36. Ahmed A, Jafri H, Lutsar I et al 1999 Pharmacodynamics of vancomycin for the treatment of experimental penicillin- and cephalosporin-resistant pneumococcal meningitis. *Antimicrobial Agents and Chemotherapy* 43: 876–881.

37. Viladrich PF, Gudiol F, Linares J et al 1991 Evaluation of vancomycin for therapy of adult pneumococcal meningitis. *Antimicrobial Agents and Chemotherapy* 35: 2467–2472.

38. American Academy of Pediatrics 1997 Pneumococcal Infection. In: Peter G. (ed.) *Red Book*.

39. Klugman KP, Feldman C 1999 Penicillin- and cephalosporin-resistant. *Streptococcus pneumoniae.* Emerging treatment for an emerging problem. *Drugs* 58: 1–4.

40. Kirikae T, Nakano M, Morrison DC 1997 Antibiotic-induced endotoxin release from bacteria and its clinical significance. *Microbiology and Immunology* 41: 285–294.

41. Morrison DC 1998 Antibiotic-mediated release of endotoxin and the pathogenesis of gram-negative sepsis. *Progress in Clinical Biological Research* 397: 199–207.

42. Horn DL, Opal SM, Lomastro E 1996 Antibiotics, cytokines, and endotoxin: a complex and evolving relationship in gram-negative sepsis. *Scandinavian Journal of Infectious Diseases Supplement* 101: 9–13.

43. Schaad UB, Lips U, Gnehm HE, Blumberg A, Heinzer I, Wedgwood J 1993 Dexamethasone therapy for bacterial meningitis in children. Swiss Meningitis Study Group. *Lancet* 342: 457–461.

44. Prasad K, Haines T 1995 Dexamethasone treatment for acute bacterial meningitis: how strong is the evidence for routine use? *Journal of Neurology, Neurosurgery and Psychiatry* 59: 31–37.

45. Paris MM, Hickey SM, Uscher MI, Sholton S, Olsen KD, McCracken GH Jr 1994 Effect of dexamethasone on therapy of experimental penicillin and cephalosporin resistant pneumococcal meningitis. *Antimicrobial Agents and Chemotherapy* 38: 1320–1324.

46. Nielsen PE, Thelle T, Tvede M 1995 Recrudescence and relapse of meningococcal meningitis and septicaemia. *Acta Paediatrica* 84: 342–345.

47. Warrell DA, Looareesuwan S, Warrell MJ et al 1982 Dexamethasone proves deleterious in cerebral malaria. A double-blind trial in 100 comatose patients. *New England Journal of Medicine* 306: 313–319.

48. Kennedy WA, Hoyt MJ, McCracken GH Jr 1991 The role of corticosteroid therapy in children with pneumococcal meningitis. *American Journal of Diseases in Childhood* 145: 1374–1378.

49. Macaluso A, Pivetta S, Maggi RS, Tamburlini G, Cattaneo A 1996 Dexamethasone adjunctive therapy for bacterial meningitis in children: a retrospective study in Brazil. *Annals of Tropical Paediatrics* 16: 193–198.

50. Quagliarello VJ, Scheld WM 1997 Treatment of bacterial meningitis. *New England Journal of Medicine* 336: 708–716.

51. Klugman KP, Friedland IR, Bradley JS 1995 Bactericidal activity against cephalosporin-resistant *Streptococcus pneumoniae* in cerebrospinal fluid of children with acute bacterial meningitis. *Antimicrobial Agents and Chemotherapy* 39: 1988–1992.

52. Viladrich PF, Pallares R, Ariza J, Rufi G, Gudiol F 1986 Four days of penicillin therapy for meningococcal meningitis. *Archives of Internal Medicine* 146: 2380–2382.

53. Marhoum eF, Noun M, Chakib A, Zahraoui M, Himmich H 1993 Ceftriaxone versus penicillin G in the short-term treatment of meningococcal meningitis in adults. *European Journal of Clinical Microbiology and Infectious Diseases* 12: 766–768.

54. Pecoul B, Varaine F, Keita M et al 1991 Long-acting chloramphenicol versus intravenous ampicillin for treatment of bacterial meningitis. *Lancet* 338: 862–866.

55. Stuart JM, Gilmore AB, Ross A et al 2001 Preventing secondary meningococcal disease in health care workers: recommendations of a working group of the PHLS meningococcus forum. *Community Disease and Public Health* 4: 102–105.

56. Woods CW, Armstrong G, Sackey SO et al 2000 Emergency vaccination against epidemic meningitis in Ghana: implications for the control of meningococcal disease in West Africa. *Lancet* 355: 30–33.

57. Cuevas LE, Kazembe P, Mughogho GK, Tillotson GS, Hart CA 1995 Eradication of nasopharyngeal carriage of *Neisseria meningitidis* in children and adults in rural Africa: a comparison of ciprofloxacin and rifampicin. *Journal of Infectious Diseases* 171: 728–731.

58. Dworzack DL, Sanders CC, Horowitz EA et al 1998 Evaluation of single-dose ciprofloxacin in the eradication of Neisseria meningitidis from nasopharyngeal carriers. *Antimicrobial Agents and Chemotherapy* 32: 1740–1741.

59. Schwartz B, Al Tobaiqi A, Al Ruwais A et al 1988 Comparative efficacy of ceftriaxone and rifampicin in eradicating pharyngeal carriage of group A *Neisseria meningitidis*. *Lancet* 1: 1239–1242.

60. Halstensen A, Gilja OH, Digranes A et al 1995 Single dose ofloxacin in the eradication of pharyngeal carriage of *Neisseria meningitidis*. *Drugs* 49(Suppl. 2): 399–400.

61. Girgis N, Sultan Y, Frenck RW Jr, El Gendy A, Farid Z, Mateczun A 1998 Azithromycin compared with rifampin for eradication of nasopharyngeal colonization by *Neisseria meningitidis*. *Pediatric Infectious Disease Journal* 17: 816–819.

62. Yagupsky P, Ashkenazi S, Block C 1993 Rifampicin-resistant meningococci causing invasive disease and failure of chemoprophylaxis. *Lancet* 341: 1152–1153.

63. Klugman KP 1994 Management of antibiotic-resistant pneumococcal infections. *Journal of Antimicrobial Chemotherapy* 34: 191–193.

64. Asmar BI, Dajani AS 1983 Ampicillin-chloramphenicol interaction against enteric Gram-negative organisms. *Pediatric Infectious Disease Journal* 2: 39–42.

65. Kumar P, Verma IC 1993 Antibiotic therapy for bacterial meningitis in children in developing countries. *Bulletin of the World Health Organization* 71: 183–188.

66. Jensen AG, Espersen F, Skinhoj P, Rosdahl VT, Frimodt-Moller N 1993 *Staphylococcus aureus* meningitis. A review of 104 nationwide, consecutive cases. *Archives of Internal Medicine* 153: 1902–1908.

67. Kay R, Cheng AF, Tse CY 1995 *Streptococcus suis* infection in Hong Kong. *Quarterly Journal of Medicine* 88: 39–47.

68. Saha V, Stansfield R, Masterton R, Eden T 1993 The treatment of *Pseudomonas aeruginosa* meningitis – old regime or newer drugs? *Scandinavian Journal of Infectious Diseases* 25: 81–83.

69. Modai J 1991 Potential role of fluoroquinolones in the treatment of bacterial meningitis. *European Journal of Clinical Microbiology and Infectious Diseases* 10: 291–295.

70. Siegman-Igra Y, Bar-Yosef S, Gorea A, Avram J 1993 Nosocomial acinetobacter meningitis secondary to invasive procedures: report of 25 cases and review. *Clinical Infectious Diseases* 17: 843–849.

71. Jimenez-Mejias ME, Becerril B, Marquez-Rivas FJ, Pichardo C, Cuberos L, Pachon J 2000 Successful treatment of multidrug-resistant *Acinetobacter baumannii* meningitis with intravenous colistin sulfomethate sodium. *European Journal of Clinical Microbiology and Infectious Diseases* 19: 970–971.

72. Scheld WM 1989 Quinolone therapy for infections of the central nervous system. *Reviews in Infectious Diseases* 11(Suppl. 5): S1194–S1202.

73. Wolfson JS, Hooper DC 1991 Pharmacokinetics of quinolones: newer aspects. *European Journal of Clinical Microbiology and Infectious Diseases* 10: 267–274.

74. Mylonakis E, Hohmann EL, Calderwood SB 1998 Central nervous system infection with *Listeria monocytogenes* 33 years' experience at a general hospital and review of 776 episodes from the literature. *Medicine (Baltimore)* 77: 313–336.

75. Nairn K, Shepherd GL, Edwards JR 1995 Efficacy of meropenem in experi-

mental meningitis. *Journal of Antimicrobial Chemotherapy* 136(Suppl. A): 73–84.

76. American Academy of Pediatrics Committee on Infectious Diseases 1988 Treatment of bacterial meningitis. *Pediatrics* 81: 904–907.

77. De Louvois J, Gortavai P, Hurley R 1997 Bacteriology of abscesses of the central nervous system: a multicentre prospective study. *British Medical Journal* 2: 981–984.

78. Grace A, Drake-Lee A 1984 Role of anaerobes in cerebral abscesses of sinus origin. *British Medical Journal (Clinical Research Edition)* 288: 758–759.

79. Black P, Graybill JR, Charache P 1973 Penetration of brain abscess by systemically administered antibiotics. *Journal of Neurosurgery* 38: 705–709.

80. Picardi JL, Lewis HP, Tan JS, Phair JP 1975 Clindamycin concentrations in the central nervous system of primates before and after head trauma. *Journal of Neurosurgery* 43: 717–720.

81. De Louvois J 1983 Antimicrobial chemotherapy in the treatment of brain abscess. *Journal of Antimicrobial Chemotherapy* 12: 205–207.

82. Report 2000 The rational use of antibiotics in the treatment of brain abscess. *British Journal of Neurosurgery* 14: 525–530.

83. Nau R, Behnke-Mursch J 1999 Diagnosis and treatment of brain abscesses. *Therapeutische Umschau* 56: 659–663.

84. Ingham HR, Slekon JB, Roxby CM 1977 Bacteriological study of otogenic cerebral abscesses: chemotherapeutic role of metronidazole. *British Medical Journal* 2: 991–993.

85. Sjölin J, Lilja A, Eriksson N, Arneborn P, Cars O, 1993 Treatment of brain abscess with cefotaxime and metronidazole: prospective study on 15 consecutive patients. *Clinical Infectious Diseases* 17: 857–863.

86. Mathisen GE, Johnson JP 1997 Brain abscess. *Clinical Infectious Diseases* 25: 763–779.

87. Renier D, Flandin C, Hirsch E, Hirsch JF 1988 Brain abscesses in neonates. A study of 30 cases. *Journal of Neurosurgery* 69: 877–882.

88. Danner RL, Hartman BJ 1987 Update on spinal epidural abscess: 35 cases and review of the literature. *Reviews of Infectious Diseases* 9: 265–274.

89. Hlavin ML, Kaminski HJ, Ross JS, Ganz E 1990 Spinal epidural abscess: a ten-year perspective. *Neurosurgery* 27: 177–184.

90. Auletta JJ, John CC 2001 Spinal epidural abscesses in children: a 15-year experience and review of the literature. *Clinical Infectious Diseases* 32: 9–16.

 ## Further information

The rational use of antibiotics in the treatment of brain abscess. *British Journal of Neurosurgery* 2000; 14: 525–530.

Blazer S, Berant M, Alon U 1983 Bacterial meningitis. Effect of antibiotic treatment on cerebrospinal fluid. *American Journal of Clinical Pathology* 80: 386–387.

Chaudhry R, Dhawan B, Laxmi BV, Mehta VS 1998 The microbial spectrum of brain abscess with special reference to anaerobic bacteria. *British Journal of Neurosurgery* 12: 127–130.

Coyle PK 1999 Glucocorticoids in central nervous system bacterial infection. *Archives of Neurology* 56: 796–801.

Darouiche RO, Hamill RJ, Greenberg SB, Weathers SW, Musher DM 1992 Bacterial spinal epidural abscess. Review of 43 cases and literature survey. *Medicine (Baltimore)* 71: 369–385.

Kaiser AB, McGee ZA 1975 Aminoglycoside therapy of gram-negative bacillary meningitis. *New England Journal of Medicine* 293: 1215–1220.

Kanra GY, Ozen H, Secmeer G, Ceyhan M, Ecevit Z, Belgin E 1995 Beneficial effects of dexamethasone in children with pneumococcal meningitis. *Pediatric Infectious Disease Journal* 14: 490–494.

Lebel MH, Freij BJ, Syrogiannopoulos GA et al 1988 Dexamethasone therapy for bacterial meningitis. Results of two double-blind, placebo-controlled trials. *New England Journal of Medicine* 319: 964–971.

McIntyre PB, Berkey CS, King SM et al 1997 Dexamethasone as adjunctive therapy in bacterial meningitis. A meta-analysis of randomized clinical trials since 1988. *Journal of the American Medical Association* 278: 925–931.

54 Viral infections of the central nervous system

Kevin A. Cassady

Viral infections of the central nervous system (CNS) occur infrequently and most often result in relatively benign, self-limiting disease. Nevertheless, these infections have tremendous importance because of the potential for death and neurologic damage. Neural tissues are exquisitely sensitive to metabolic derangements and injured brain tissue recovers slowly and often incompletely. The diseases discussed in this chapter include viral meningitis, encephalitis, and transmissible spongiform encephalopathies (TSEs). The definitions of viral CNS disease are often based on both virus tropism and disease duration. Inflammation occurs at multiple sites within the CNS and accounts for the myriad of clinical descriptors of viral neurological disease. *Aseptic meningitis* is a misnomer frequently used to refer to a benign, self-limiting, viral infection causing inflammation of the leptomeninges. *Encephalitis* refers to inflammation of parenchymal brain tissue and is usually accompanied by depressed level of consciousness, altered cognition, and frequently focal neurological signs. Slow progressive neurological deterioration, gliosis, abnormal accumulation of prion proteins in the brain, and the lack of CNS inflammation characterize the TSEs. Meningitis and encephalitis represent separate clinical entities; however, a continuum exists between these distinct forms of disease. A change in a patient's clinical condition can reflect disease progression with involvement of different regions in the CNS. Therefore, in many cases it is difficult to accurately and prospectively predict the etiology and extent of CNS infection. To provide organization for this chapter, viral meningitis and encephalitis will be discussed as discrete entities.

EPIDEMIOLOGY

Acute viral meningitis and meningoencephalitis represent most viral CNS infections and frequently occur in epidemics or in seasonal distribution.[1,2] The etiology and frequency differs based on geography and immunization practices. Enteroviruses cause an estimated 90% of cases (in countries that immunize against mumps), while arboviruses constitute the majority of the remaining reported cases in the USA.[3–6] Mumps virus is also an important cause of viral CNS disease in countries that do not immunize against it. In a recent study performed in Japan, mumps infection was the second leading cause of aseptic meningitis, accounting for approximately 30% of the cases.[7] A retrospective survey performed in the 1980s found that the annual incidence of 'aseptic meningitis' was approximately 10.9 per 100 000 persons or at least four times the incidence passively reported to the Centers for Disease Control (CDC) during the period.[2] Virus was identified in only 11% of patients in this study. This low viral isolation rate likely reflects the technological limits of the period, the infrequency with which viral cultures were performed, and the decreased incidence of viral CNS disease resulting from widespread vaccination against mumps and polio viruses.[2] With the advent of more rapid molecular based diagnostic techniques the isolation rates now approach 50–86% and will provide more reliable epidemiologic estimates.[5,7]

Similar to viral meningitis, passive reporting systems underestimate the incidence of viral encephalitis.[2] For example, an estimated 20 000 cases of encephalitis occur each year in the USA; however, the CDC received only between 740 (0.3 per 100 000) and 1340 (0.54 per 100 000) annual reports of cases from 1990 to 1994.[8,9] A recent prospective multicenter study in Finland, a region with a low incidence of arboviral encephalitis, found the incidence of encephalitis to be 10.5 per 100 000.[10] Herpes simplex virus CNS infections occur without seasonal variation, affect all ages, and cause most fatal cases of endemic encephalitis in the USA.[1] The arboviruses, a group of over 500 arthropod-transmitted RNA viruses, are the leading cause of encephalitis worldwide.[11] Arboviral infections occur in epidemics and show a seasonal predilection, reflecting the prevalence of the transmitting vector.[12] Encephalitis occurs in a minority of persons with arboviral infections, but the case fatality rate varies extremely, from 5% to 70%, depending upon viral etiology and age of the patient. LaCrosse encephalitis is the most commonly reported arboviral disease; St. Louis encephalitis is the most frequent cause of epidemic encephalitis in the USA.[12] Japanese B encephalitis and rabies cause most cases of encephalitis outside of North America. Japanese encephalitis virus, a member of the flavivirus genus, occurs throughout Asia and causes epidemics in China despite routine immunization.[1] The disease typically affects children, although adults with no history of exposure to the virus are also susceptible.[9] The disease has a high case-fatality rate and leaves half of the survivors with a significant degree of neurologic morbidity.[1] Rabies virus remains endemic around much of the world. Human infections in the USA have decreased over the last decades to 1–3 cases per year due to the immunization of domesticated animals. Bat exposure is increasingly recognized as the source of infection: 15% (685 of 4470) of bats tested carried the rabies virus in one study.[13] Since 1990, bat-associated variants of the virus have accounted for 24 of the 32 cases reported. In most cases (22 of 24) there was no evidence of a bite; however, in half of the cases direct contact (handling of bats) was documented.[14] In areas outside the USA, human cases of rabies encephalitis number in the thousands and are caused by bites from unvaccinated domestic animals that have had contact with infected wild animals.

Postinfectious encephalitis, an acute demyelinating process, has also been referred to as acute disseminated encephalomyelitis or autoimmune encephalitis. It accounts for approximately 100–200 additional cases of encephalitis annually in the USA, and is associated with antecedent upper respiratory virus (notably influenza virus) and varicella infections.[1,8,9] In locations that do not immunize measles and mumps, acute disseminated encephalomyelitis causes about one-third of the encephalitis cases and remains associated with the exanthematous viruses.[1,15] Measles continues to be the leading cause of postinfectious encephalitis worldwide and complicates one of every 1000 measles infections.[9]

The slow infections of the brain or transmissible spongiform encephalopathies (TSEs) occur sporadically worldwide. Creutzfeldt–Jakob disease (CJD) is a prototypical TSE with high rates of familial occurrence and an estimated incidence of 0.5–1.5 cases per million population.[16] In 1986, cases of a TSE in cattle, bovine spongiform encephalopathy (BSE), were reported in the UK. Concomitant with the increase in cases of BSE in Europe, an increase in atypical CJD also occurred, suggesting animal-to-human transmission. The report of atypical CJD (unique clinical and histopathologic findings) affecting young adults (an age at which CJD rarely has been diagnosed) led to the designation of a new disease: variant Creutzfeldt–Jakob disease. The epidemiology of this disease is currently being defined.

PATHOGENESIS

Viruses use two basic pathways to gain access to the CNS: hematogenous and neuronal. Most cases of viral meningitis occur following a high-titer secondary viremia. A combination of host and viral factors combined with seasonal, geographic, and epidemiologic probabilities influence the proclivity to develop viral CNS infection. Enteroviral meningitis occurs more often during the summer and early autumn months, reflecting the seasonal increase in enteroviral infections. Such

infections also exemplify the difference host physiology plays in determining the extent of viral disease. In children less than 2 weeks of age, enterovirus infections can produce a severe systemic infection, including meningitis or meningoencephalitis:[6] 10% of neonates with systemic enteroviral infections die, while as many as 76% are left with permanent sequelae. In children over 2 weeks of age, however, enteroviral infections are rarely associated with severe disease or significant morbidity.[6]

Viral hematogenous dissemination to the CNS involves initial inoculation, local spread and replication, often in regional lymph nodes (e.g. measles, influenza). Next, the virus enters the circulatory system (primary viremia), enabling virus to seed distant locations of the body. In rare circumstances such as disseminated neonatal herpes simplex infection, viruses infect the CNS during primary viremia; however, most viruses infect an intermediate tissue such as the liver and spleen, replicate and then infect the CNS during a prolonged high-titer secondary viremia.[17,18] The pathophysiology of viral transport from blood to brain, and viral endothelial cell tropism, is poorly understood. Virus infects endothelial cells, leaks across damaged endothelia, passively channels through endothelium (pinocytosis or colloidal transport) or bridges the endothelium within migrating leukocytes.[1,19]

Historically, the peripheral neural pathway was considered the only pathway of viral neurologic infection.[20] Contemporary data, however, demonstrate that the circulatory system provides the principal pathway for most CNS infections in humans.[1] Herpes simplex virus and rabies infect the CNS by neuronal spread. Rabies classically infects by the myoneural route and provides a prototype for peripheral neuronal spread.[21] Rabies virus replicates locally in the soft tissue following a bite from a rabid animal. After primary replication, the virus enters the peripheral nerve by acetylcholine receptor binding. Once in the muscle the virus buds from the plasma membrane, crosses myoneural spindles or enters across the motor end plate.[21,22] The virus travels by anterograde and retrograde axonal transport to infect neurons in the brainstem and limbic system. Eventually it spreads from the diencephalic and hippocampal structure to the remainder of the brain, killing the animal.[21]

In patients with acute encephalitis, the parenchyma exhibits neuronophagia and cells containing viral nucleic acids or antigens.[9] The pathologic findings are unique for each virus and reflect differences in pathogenesis and virulence. For example, in cases of typical herpes simplex encephalitis, a hemorrhagic necrosis occurs in the inferomedial temporal lobe with evidence of perivascular cuffing, lymphocytic infiltration and neuronophagia.[23] Pathological specimens in animals with rabies encephalitis demonstrate microglial proliferation, perivascular infiltrates, and neuronal destruction.

Some viruses do not directly infect the CNS but produce immune system changes that result in parenchymal damage. Patients with postinfectious encephalitis exhibit focal neurologic deficits and altered consciousness associated temporally with a recent (1–2 week) viral infection or immunization.[15] Pathologic specimens, while they show evidence of demyelination by histologic or radiographic analysis, do not demonstrate evidence of viral infection in the CNS by culture or antigen tests. Patients with postinfectious encephalitis have subtle differences in their immune system and some authors have proposed an autoimmune reaction as the pathogenic mechanism of disease.[9] Postinfectious encephalitis occurs most commonly following measles, varicella zoster infection, mumps, influenza, or parainfluenza infections.

The TSEs are non-inflammatory CNS diseases involving the accumulation of an abnormal form of a normal glycoprotein, the prion protein (PrP).[24] These encephalopathies differ in mode of transmission. While most TSEs are experimentally transmissible by direct inoculation in the CNS, this mode rarely occurs except for iatrogenic transmissions.[16] The scrapie agent of sheep spreads by contact and lateral transmission. There is no evidence for lateral transmission in the case of BSE or variant CJD, and all cases appear to have occurred following parenteral inoculation or ingestion of affected materials. The transmissible agents remain infectious after treatments that would normally inactivate viruses or nucleic acids (detergent, formalin, ionizing radiation, nucleases).[24] Most of the experimental work on TSEs has involved analysis of the scrapie agent. The current working model is that post-translational alteration of the normally α-helical form of the PrP protein results in a protease-resistant β-pleated sheet structure that accumulates in neurons, leading to progressive dysfunction, cell death and subsequent astrocytosis. In studies on the scrapie agent, gastrointestinal tract involvement with infection of abdominal lymph nodes occurs first, followed by brain involvement a year or more later.[16] Experimental subcutaneous inoculation in mice and goats also lead to local lymph node involvement followed by splenic spread and then CNS involvement. The mode of transmission to the CNS (direct versus hematogenous) and the infectivity of body fluids at different stages of infection are not known at this time.

DIAGNOSIS

Historically, investigators identified an agent in only 25–67% of presumed CNS infections.[25,26] The techniques for identifying viral CNS infection were invasive and often insensitive, as they relied on viral culture.[27] With the advent of the polymerase chain reaction (PCR), reliable diagnosis has improved the timely management of patients of viral CNS infections. The demonstration of viral nucleic acid in the cerebrospinal fluid of patients with symptoms of meningitis or encephalitis has replaced viral culture and serologic diagnosis.[28,29]

In the case of herpes simplex encephalitis, cerebrospinal fluid PCR has a sensitivity of >95% and a specificity approaching 100%.[30] Investigators are increasingly using these sensitive PCR-based diagnostic techniques to correlate treatment response and predict clinical outcomes.[31] As with any PCR-based technique, nucleic acid contamination of the laboratory area is a concern and results must always be interpreted within a clinical context. While PCR-based assays exist for many

viruses, there are still some (notably the arthropod-borne viral infections) for which universal primers are still being developed.[32] In other cases (cytomegalovirus, human herpesvirus-6) the presence of latent virus or a virus associated with inflammatory cells can produce positive results of unknown significance.

Molecular diagnostic techniques have greatly improved the speed, sensitivity, and specificity for the diagnosis of enterovirus infections.[26,33] The polymerase chain reaction (PCR) and other molecular biologic assays provide a rapid and reliable test for verifying the etiology of certain types of meningitis and can detect low copy numbers of viral RNA in patients with agammaglobulinemia or hyper IGM syndrome. Enterovirus is the cause of ~90% of aseptic meningitis cases for which a pathogen is detected.[6] These techniques provide results within 24–36 hours and therefore may limit the duration of hospitalization, antibiotic use, and excessive diagnostic procedures.[28]

The TSEs are currently only diagnosed by histologic examination, characteristic Electroencephalographic (EEG) changes, and the clinical context. Most laboratory tests are of little value in the diagnosis. Cerebrospinal fluid examination shows normal values or slighlty elevated protein levels. The EEG in classic CJD reveals generalized slowing early in the disease, punctuated by biphasic or triphasic peaks late in the disease with the onset of myoclonus. MRI changes late in the illness reveal global atrophy with hyperintense signal from the basal ganglia.[16] Histopathologic examination of the brain using a specific antibody to the PrP-res protein confirms the disease. In addition evidence of gliosis, neuronal loss, and spongiform changes support the diagnosis. In cases of vCJD characteristic amyloid plaques (so called florid plaques) microscopically define the disease. The florid plaques are not seen in other TSEs and consist of flower-like amyloid deposits surrounded by vacuolor halos. The detection of PrP-res in the tonsillar tissue by immunohistochemical staining is also diagnostic of vCJD.[16]

GENERAL THERAPY

The approach to a patient with a presumed CNS viral infection must be tailored to the severity and distribution of neurologic involvement. After establishing the degree of CNS disease by history and physical exam and stabilizing the patient (airway, breathing, circulation), the clinician next must ascertain a diagnosis. With the advent of highly sensitive and less invasive diagnostic techniques (CSF-PCR) identification of treatable forms of viral CNS disease (notably HSE) is essential in preventing further CNS damage. Potentially treatable diseases (fungal CNS infections, partially treated bacterial meningitis, tuberculous meningitis, parameningeal infection, mycoplasma, and fastidious bacterial infections) can mimic viral CNS disease and should be vigorously investigated before attributing the illness to an untreatable viral etiology. The same logic applies to treatable viral infections and non-infectious etiologies. In the normal host, viral meningitis is a relatively benign self-limiting disease and does not usually warrant specific antiviral treatment.[35] In certain cases, for example neonates or patients with immunoglobulin deficiency, patients can develop life-threatening infections and may benefit from therapy. After establishing a presumptive diagnosis and instituting therapy, the clinician must anticipate and treat complications (seizures, syndrome of inappropriate antidiuretic hormone secretion, cerebral edema, cardiac arrhythmias or respiratory arrest from brainstem inflammation). Patients in coma from encephalitis can recover after long periods of unconsciousness. The physician should limit the amount of iatrogenic damage and vigorously support the patient during the acute phase of the illness.

CHEMOTHERAPY

A limited number of antiviral medications are available to treat CNS infections, and prevention remains the mainstay of therapy. Historically the most common cause of viral CNS disease, mumps, has largely been eliminated through vaccination. Live attenuated vaccines against measles, mumps, and rubella have resulted in a dramatic decrease in the incidence of encephalitis in industrialized countries. Measles continues to be the leading cause of postinfectious encephalitis in developing countries, however, and complicates 1 of every 1000 measles infections.[9] Vaccination has also changed the character of previously common viral CNS disease. For instance, in 1952, poliomyelitis affected 57 879 Americans, but widespread vaccination has eradicated the disease from the Western hemisphere.[36] Vaccines exist for some arboviral infections. Vaccination against Japanese encephalitis virus has reduced the incidence of encephalitis in Asia; however, in China where 70 million children are vaccinated against this virus, 10 000 cases still occur annually.[37]

The US Food and Drug Administration (FDA), to reduce the potential exposure to TSE agents in the blood supply, has implemented guidelines eliminating whole blood or blood components prepared from individuals who later developed CJD or variant CJD. Changes in the agricultural practices in Europe and bans on infected cattle have been associated with a decline in cases of variant CJD. In North America no cases of this disease have been reported, and the Department of Agriculture has programs in place to monitor for TSE in livestock. Further discussion will be limited to those infections for which therapies exists (herpes simplex virus-1 and -3, varicella zoster, cytomegalovirus, HIV, B-virus, and enterovirus infection).

HSV ENCEPHALITIS

The introduction of aciclovir has resulted in a sharp decline in mortality and morbidity from herpes infections. For example,

neonatal mortality from disseminated herpes simplex (HSV) disease and herpes simplex encephalitis has declined from 70% to 40% since the development of aciclovir and vidarabine.[1] The Clinical Antiviral Study Group randomized controlled trials in the 1980s established that 81% of adults with biopsy-proven herpes simplex encephalitis who received aciclovir at 10 mg/kg every 8 h for 10–14 days survived and 38% of the recipients regained normal neurologic function.[38] The early initiation of antiviral therapy is essential for optimal recovery. Patients with encephalitis lasting longer than 4 days had a worse outcome. For herpes encephalitis intravenous administration of aciclovir is the treatment of choice and oral antivirals should not be used.

In cases of neonatal HSV infection, dosage of aciclovir, treatment duration, and toxicities differ from adult therapy. Encephalitis occurs in 33% of neonates perinatally infected with HSV. Neonates with evidence of CNS dysfunction or cutaneous manifestations of HSV infection should be empirically started on high-dose aciclovir until HSV neurologic infection can be excluded. In neonates with localized cutaneous or mucocutaneous disease, aciclovir administered intravenously 20 mg/kg every 8 h (60 mg/kg daily) for a minimum of 14–21 days is the treatment of choice. Neonates demonstrate a much lower rate of viral clearance than do immunocompromised adults, thus justifying the longer duration of treatment.[39] Prolonged therapy of 20 mg/kg intravenously every 8 h (60 mg/kg daily) for a minimum of 21 days is used for neonates with disseminated disease or evidence of neurologic involvement. In patients with evidence of viral DNA in the cerebrospinal fluid following 21 days of aciclovir treatment, antiviral therapy is extended until virus is no longer detectable. Studies are currently ongoing evaluating the utility of aciclovir therapy for reactivations and suppressive therapy during the first 6 months of life.

Aciclovir is associated with few adverse effects. In patients receiving large doses by rapid infusion, a dose-related nephrotoxicity from crystal deposition has been reported, but this is readily reversible with slower infusion times and improved hydration.[40] CNS disturbances (hallucinations, disorientation, tremors) have also been reported with aciclovir therapy. Neutropenia is well documented in children receiving prolonged therapy.

HSV MENINGITIS

Although no definitive clinical trials have been conducted, most authors recommend the use of intravenous aciclovir (10 mg/kg every 8 h) for HSV meningitis associated with primary HSV-2 infection, as it decreases the duration of primary herpes disease and may limit meningeal involvement.[41] Recurrent HSV-2 meningitis occurs rarely and recently a single case of meningitis associated with HSV-1 reactivation has been reported. At this time there are no data on benefit of antiviral treatment or on suppressive therapy for recurrent HSV CNS disease.[42,43]

VARICELLA ZOSTER VIRUS

Varicella immunoglobulin and aciclovir have reduced the complications from primary varicella infection and herpes zoster in the neonate and immunocompromised patient. Although controlled trials have not evaluated the efficacy of aciclovir in varicella CNS infections, the medication is routinely used to treat this complication.[44,45] Varicella can produce cerebral vasculitis, postinfectious encephalitis, ventriculitis, meningitis, and, historically, encephalopathy (Reye's syndrome). Other than postinfectious encephalitis, most of the varicella CNS manifestations are rare and occur most frequently in immunocompromised patients. Empiric therapy with intravenous aciclovir 10–15 mg/kg every 8 h for 10 days combined with prednisone 60–80 mg for 3–5 days is recommended for patients with large-vessel cerebral vasculitis. Small-vessel encephalitis should also be treated with aciclovir, 5–10 mg/kg every 8 hours for a minimum of 10 days.[46] Myelitis can complicate acute varicella zoster or zosteriform reactivation, especially in immunocompromised patients, and presents as paraparesis 1–2 weeks after development of a rash. MRI studies demonstrate significant spinal cord involvement, while the cerebrospinal fluid from patients frequently demonstrates an inflammatory infiltrate or increased protein levels. The demonstration of varicella zoster in the cerebrospinal fluid by PCR, or the demonstration of specific antibodies in the cerebrospinal fluid, confirms the diagnosis. Aggressive treatment with intravenous aciclovir, as described above for small-vessel encephalitis, can produce clinical improvements.[47]

CONGENITAL CYTOMEGALOVIRUS INFECTION

Ganciclovir and foscarnet are used for the treatment of cytomegalovirus encephalitis, although controlled clinical trials have not confirmed the efficacy of treatment. A recent multi-center study has demonstrated that there is a slight protection against hearing deterioration in congenitally infected neonates with severe CNS disease who received 6 weeks of intravenous ganciclovir.[48] Therapy was initiated within the first month of life and all of the children receiving ganciclovir required central venous lines. Drug toxicities were monitored routinely and severe neutropenia occurred in 63% of the treated, versus 20% of the untreated, patients.[48] One of the limitations of the study was that a large percentage of the children were lost to follow up and only about 50% of the enrolled children were evaluable. The children receiving intravenous ganciclovir maintained their level of hearing or demonstrated improvements at the 6-month follow up whereas in 44% of the no-treatment group hearing worsened. At one year or more after therapy 20% of ganciclovir-treated patients had worsening of hearing, compared with 70% of the no-treatment group.[48] A second study is currently in progress to evaluate the effect of ganciclovir on CNS disease aside from hearing loss. It should be emphasized that this study evaluates severely affected congenitally infected children (microcephaly, CNS calcifications). At this time there are no data on ganciclovir therapy in congenitally infected children without severe CNS disease.

CERCOPITHECINE HERPES INFECTION (B VIRUS)

B virus is indigenous in Old World monkeys (rhesus, cynologous, and Asian species of the *Macaca* genus) and causes a frequently fatal disease in humans if not treated. Infection has been documented in most cases following direct inoculation (bites), although cases exist following exposure to infected materials (animal bedding) or human-to-human spread. In humans bitten by an infected animal the risk of transmission is low, as the frequency of virus excretion is only 2–3% in infected animals at any given time.[49] Nevertheless, because of the severity of infection, therapy should be immediately instituted. B virus infection in humans produces a rapid infection, with evidence of a vesicular rash and an ascending myelitis in most cases within 3–7 days. Ultimately 90% of the documented infected persons progressed to develop encephalomyelitis and 70% died.

Management of potential B virus exposure is controversial but guidelines set up by a Centers for Disease Control and Prevention panel provides a framework for postexposure management.[50] Similar to rabies postexposure treatments, rapid wound decontamination minutes after the injury is the only way of preventing infection. Thorough irrigation for 15 minutes with water or sterile saline and washing with detergent is critical in preventing infection. If someone is bitten by a known infected or seropositive animal, cultures should be obtained from the animal (buccal mucosa of the biting monkey, urogenital area for urine exposure, swab from the cage for infected bedding). Some authors recommend culturing the patient after thorough cleansing and irrigation have been completed. Even more controversial are the recommendations for instituting prophylactic aciclovir. For high-risk exposures (infected shedding monkeys, monkeys of unknown B virus serology, ill macaques, or a high titer fluid source) prophylaxis is indicated, especially if the wound was not immediately cleansed/irrigated for 15 minutes, or if the wound is a deep laceration or puncture.

Because the inhibitory concentration of aciclovir for B virus is about ten times that for HSV-1, high-dose prophylaxis should be administered, consisting of oral aciclovir (800 mg per dose, five times daily) or intravenous aciclovir (10 mg/kg every 8 h) started immediately and continued pending culture results.[50] These recommendations were made before the improved accessibility of the highly bioavailable prodrugs valaciclovir and famciclovir, which provide higher serum levels of aciclovir or penciclovir and provide better prophylaxis than oral aciclovir. Again, the higher dosage used for varicella infections (valaciclovir 1 g per dose orally three times daily; famciclovir 500 mg per dose orally three times daily) should be used for B virus prophylaxis. If B virus is cultured from the wound, from the monkey, or if the bitten worker develops signs or symptoms of B virus infection, the patient must be immediately admitted to hospital (with body fluid precautions) and intravenous aciclovir instituted until symptoms resolve and three consecutive culture sets are negative.[49] Patients with cutaneous or peripheral neurologic signs of B virus infection should receive aciclovir 10 mg/kg intravenously every 8 h; patients with CNS dysfunction should receive 15 mg/kg every 8 h.[50]

It is equally important in the management of these patients to obtain acute and convalescent serologic studies. In patients with B virus infection (seroconversion or clinical disease) longterm management is essential. Experts at the Centers for Disease Control and Prevention in the USA or national reference facilities in other countries should be consulted for more detailed information on this subject. In general, long-term management requires monitoring the patient for evidence of virus shedding and in most instances long-term oral antiviral prophylaxis (minimum of 6 months, although some authors recommend lifelong suppression).

ENTEROVIRUS INFECTION

Currently antibody preparations and an antiviral agent, pleconaril, have shown activity against enterovirus in case reports and animal studies. Randomized controlled trials, however, have not supported their use in routine enterovirus meningitis. In case reports immunoglobulin preparations, given systemically or intrathecally, retarded mortality and morbidity in agammaglobulinemic patients with enteroviral meningitis. Despite the administration of immunoglobulin, these patients did not eliminate the virus from the cerebrospinal fluid and in turn developed chronic enteroviral meningitis.[51,52] Enteroviral infections in neonates frequently produce overwhelming viremia and CNS disease: 10% of neonates with systemic enteroviral infections die, while as many as 76% are left with permanent sequelae. A blinded randomized control trial did not demonstrate clinical benefit for neonates with severe life-threatening enteroviral infection who received intravenous immunoglobulin.[53] While the role of antibody in immuno-compromised patients with life-threatening infections remains unproven but debatable, there are currently no data supporting the use of immunoglobulin preparations for non-life-threatening infections in the normal host.

A recently developed antiviral agent, pleconaril (ViroPharma Inc.: Exton, Pa), is a bioavailable small-molecule inhibitor of picornavirus that binds the capsid and prevents receptor uncoating of viral RNA. Because of homology between the picornavirus, enterovirus, and rhinovirus capsid structure, the drug has activity against these viruses as well. Initial cell culture and animal studies using pleconaril demonstrated that the drug had potent anti-enteroviral activity.[54] Randomized controlled, double-blind clinical trials, while demonstrating slight improvements in adults with enteroviral meningitis, have not demonstrated the dramatic efficacy initially anticipated and have not been published in peer-reviewed

literature. In the 32 adults with aseptic meningitis studied, duration of headache was the most dramatic improvement, with the pleconaril group experiencing on average 6.5 days of headache versus 18.3 days of headache for the placebo-control population.[55] The duration of headache in the placebo-control group is much greater than previously published for enteroviral meningitis. Similarly, if one uses an objective measurement such as the duration of analgesic use (historical average control = 5 days) versus that reported in the pleconaril study (placebo group = 11.5 days), the statistically significant 5.3 days of analgesic use by the pleconaril group is less dramatic.[55,56]

While pleconaril does not have the dramatic effect previously predicted in cases of uncomplicated enterovirus meningitis, it may still prove beneficial in the treatment of severe life-threatening disease (neonatal sepsis, disease in the immunocompromised patient, encephalomyelitis). A non-randomized study of life-threatening cases of enteroviral infection demonstrated a clinical, laboratory, or virologic response in 78–92% of the patients available for follow up. The adults in the study received either 200 or 400 mg while children were treated with 5 mg/kg three times per day for a total of 7–10 days.[57] A multicenter randomized controlled trial is ongoing evaluating pleconaril in severe neonatal infection but preliminary information is unavailable at this time (David Kimberlin, personal communication).

RABIES VIRUS INFECTION

Pre- and immediate postexposure prophylaxis are the only ways known to prevent death in rabies-exposed individuals.[21] Case reports exist of patients surviving symptomatic rabies, but all of these patients had some prior immunity or received postexposure prophylaxis before developing symptoms. Individuals exposed to rabies require vigorous cleansing of the wound, passive immunization with direct administration of rabies hyper-immunoglobulin at the site of the animal bite, and postexposure intramuscular vaccination with human diploid cell vaccine or rhesus diploid cell vaccine on the first day of treatment and repeat doses on days 3, 7, 14, and 28 after the initial dose. Individuals with frequent contact with potentially rabid animals (veterinarians, animal control staff, workers in rabies laboratories, and travellers to rabies-endemic areas) should receive pre-exposure vaccination.

POSTINFECTIOUS ENCEPHALITIS

In cases of postinfectious encephalitis or acute disseminated encephalomyelitis, no randomized controlled trial has confirmed the benefit of immunomodulatory drugs. In practice the condition is often treated with different immunomodulators (corticosteroids, intravenous immunoglobulin preparations, plasmapheresis) in an attempt to limit immune mediated destruction of the CNS.[58–60] It must be emphasized, however, that no placebo-controlled studies have been performed and immunomodualtory therapy is based simply on isolated case reports. As with most case reports, clinical failures and iatrogenic morbidity from a therapeutic modality are rarely ever reported.

CONCLUSIONS

The pathogenic mechanism of a viral disease provides clues toward the development of antiviral medications and strategies for the prevention of viral CNS infections. The CNS is extremely sensitive to infection or secondary metabolic damage. Recovery is often prolonged and incomplete. Rapid diagnosis and prompt therapeutic intervention are critical for recovery. Application of viral PCR and other molecular diagnostic techniques have changed some of the fundamental concepts of viral infection. Improved diagnostic techniques are essential for advancing both research and therapy of viral neurologic infections. Basic research in neurosciences and infectious diseases will result in a better understanding of the host–virus interaction in the central nervous system. These advances have the potential for improving the care of patients with neurologic diseases.

References

1. Cassady KA, Whitley RJ 1977 Pathogenesis and pathophysiology of viral central nervous system infections. In: Scheld WM, Whitley RJ, Durack DT (eds). *Infections of The Central Nervous System*. Philadelphia, Lippincott-Raven, pp. 7–22.
2. Nicolosi A, Hauser WA, Beghi E, Kurland LT 1986 Epidemiology of central nervous system infections in Olmstead County, Minnesota, 1950–1981. *Journal of Infectious Diseases* 154–399.
3. Nigrovic LE, Chiang VW 2000 Cost analysis of enteroviral polymerase chain reaction in infants with fever and cerebrospinal fluid pleocytosis [see comments]. *Archives of Pediatrics and Adolescent Medicine* 154: 817–821.
4. Hammer SM, Connolly KJ 1992 Viral aseptic meningitis in the United States: clinical features, viral etiologies, and differential diagnosis. *Current Clinical Topics in Infectious Disease* 12: 1–25.
5. Pozo F, Casas I, Tenorio A, Trallero G, Echevarria JM 1998 Evaluation of a commercially available reverse transcription-PCR assay for diagnosis of enteroviral infection in archival and prospectively collected cerebrospinal fluid specimens. *Journal of Clinical Microbiology* 36: 1741–1745.
6. Sawyer MH 1999 Enterovirus infections: diagnosis and treatment. *Pediatric Infectious Disease Journal* 18: 1033–1039.
7. Hosoya M, Honzumi K, Sato M, Katayose M, Kato K, Suzuki H 1998 Application of PCR for various neurotropic viruses on the diagnosis of viral meningitis. *Journal of Clinical Virology* 11: 117–124.
8. Anonymous 1999 Summary of Notifiable Diseases, United States, 1998. *Morbidity and Mortality Weekly Report* 47. 53: 1–116.
9. Johnson RT 1987 The pathogenesis of acute viral encephalitis and postinfectious encephalomyelitis. *Journal of Infectious Diseases* 155: 359–364.
10. Koskiniemi M, Korppi M, Mustonen K et al 1997 Epidemiology of encephalitis in children. A prospective multicentre study. *European Journal of Pediatrics* 156: 541–545.
11. Ho DD, Hirsch MS 1985 Acute viral encephalitis. *Medical Clinics of North America* 69: 415.
12. Anonymous 1998 Arboviral infections of the central nervous system – United States, 1996–1997. *Morbidity and Mortality Weekly Report* 47: 517–522.
13. Pape WJ, Fitzsimmons TD, Hoffman RE 1999 Risk for rabies transmission from encounters with bats, Colorado, 1977–1996. *Emerging Infectious Diseases* 5: 433–437.
14. Anonymous 2000 Human Rabies – California, Georgia, Minnesota, New York, and Wisconsin, 2000. *Morbidity and Mortality Weekly Report* 49: 1111–1115.
15. Stuve O, Zamvil SS 1999 Pathogenesis, diagnosis, and treatment of acute disseminated encephalomyelitis. *Current Opinion in Neurology* 12: 395–401.
16. Whitley RJ, Macdonald N, Ascher DM 2000 Technical Report: transmissible spongiform encephalopathies: A review for pediatricians. *Pediatrics* 106: 1160–1165.
17. Kimura H, Futamura M, Kito H 1991 Detection of viral DNA in neonatal herpes simplex virus infections: frequent and prolonged presence in the serum and cerebrospinal fluid. *Journal of Infectious Diseases* 164: 289.
18. Stanberry LR, Floyd-Reising SA, Connelly BL 1994 Herpes simplex viremia: report of eight pediatric cases and review of the literature. *Clinical Infectious Diseases* 18: 401.
19. Wiestler OD, Leib SL, Brustle O, Spiegel H, Kleihues P 1992 Neuropathology and pathogenesis of HIV encephalopathies. *Acta Histochemica Supplementum* 42: 107–114.
20. Friedemann U 1943 Permeability of the blood–brain barrier to neurotropic viruses. *Archives of Pathology* 35: 912.
21. Mrak RE, Young L 1994 Rabies encephalitis in humans: pathology, pathogenesis and pathophysiology. *Journal of Neuropathology and Experimental Neurology* 53: 1–10.
22. Lentz TL 1990 The recognition event between virus and host cell receptor: a target for antiviral agents? *Journal of General Virology* 71: 751.
23. Nahmias AJ, Whitley RJ, Visintine AN, Takei Y, Alford CA Jr 1982 Herpes simplex encephalitis: laboratory evaluations and their diagnostic significance. *Journal of Infectious Diseases* 145: 829–836.
24. Pruisner SB 1982 Novel proteinaceous infectious particles cause scrapie. *Science* 216: 136–144.
25. Whitley RJ, Cobbs CG, Alford CA Jr. et al 1989 Diseases that mimic herpes simplex encephalitis. Diagnosis, presentation, and outcome. NIAD Collaborative Antiviral Study Group. *Journal of the American Medical Association* 262: 234–239.
26. Ahmed A, Brito F, Goto C et al 1997 Clinical utility of the polymerase chain reaction for diagnosis of enteroviral meningitis in infancy. *Journal of Pediatrics* 131: 393–397.
27. Wilfert CM, Lehrman SN, Katz SL 1983 Enterovirus and meningitis. *Pediatric Infectious Disease Journal* 2: 333.
28. Ramers C, Billman G, Hartin M, Ho S, Sawyer MH 2000 Impact of a diagnostic cerebrospinal fluid enterovirus polymerase chain reaction test on patient management. *Journal of the American Medical Association* 283: 2680–2685.
29. Sawyer MH 1999 Enterovirus infections: diagnosis and treatment. *Pediatric Infectious Disease Journal* 18: 1033–1039.
30. Lakeman AD, Whitley RJ 1995 Diagnosis of herpes simplex encephalitis: application of polymerase chain reaction to the cerebrospinal fluid from brain-biopsied patients and correlation with disease. *Journal of Infectious Disease* 171: 857.
31. Domingues RB, Lakeman FD, Pannuti CS, Fink MC, Tsanaclis AM 1997 Advantage of polymerase chain reaction in the diagnosis of herpes simplex encephalitis: presentation of 5 atypical cases. *Scandinavian Journal of Infectious Diseases* 29: 229–231.
32. Kuno G 1998 Universal diagnostic RT-PCR protocol for arboviruses. *Journal of Virological Methods* 72: 27–41.
33. van Vliet KE, Glimaker M, Lebon P et al 1998 Multicenter evaluation of the Amplicor Enterovirus PCR test with cerebrospinal fluid from patients with aseptic meningitis. The European Union Concerted Action on Viral Meningitis and Encephalitis. *Journal of Clinical Microbiology* 36: 2652–2657.
34. Ramers C, Billman G, Hartin M, Ho S, Sawyer MH 2000 Impact of a diagnostic cerebrospinal fluid enterovirus polymerase chain reaction test on patient management. *Journal of the American Medical Association* 283: 2680–2685.
35. Rorabaugh ML, Berlin LE, Heldrich F et al 1993 Aseptic meningitis in infants younger than 2 years of age: acute illness and neurologic complications. *Pediatrics* 92: 206.
36. Anonymous 1994 Expanded program on immunization: Certification of poliomyelitis eradication – the Americas. *Morbidity and Mortality Weekly Report* 43: 720.
37. Rosen L 1986 The natural history of Japanese encephalitis virus. *Annual Reviews in Microbiology* 40: 395–414.
38. Whitley RJ, Alford CA, Hirsch MS et al 1986 Vidarabine versus acyclovir therapy in herpes simplex encephalitis. *New England Journal of Medicine* 31:144–149.

39. Whitley RJ, Roizman B 1997 Herpes simplex viruses. In: Richman DD, Whitley RJ, Hayden FG (eds) *Clinical Virology.* New York, Churchill Livingstone Inc, pp. 375–410.

40. Bianchetti MG, Roduit C, Oetliker OH 1991 Acyclovir induced renal failure: course and risk factors. *Pediatric Nephrology* 5: 238–239.

41. Whitley RJ, Gnann JW Jr 1992 Acyclovir: a decade later. *New England Journal of Medicine* 327: 782.

42. Jensenius M, Myrvang B, Storvold G, Bucher A, Hellum KB, Bruu AL 1998 Herpes simplex virus type 2 DNA detected in cerebrospinal fluid of 9 patients with Mollaret's meningitis. *Acta Neurologica Scandinavica* 98: 209–212.

43. Conway JH, Weinberg A, Ashley RL, Amer J, Levin MJ 1997 Viral meningitis in a preadolescent child caused by reactivation of latent herpes simplex (type 1). *Pediatric Infectious Disease Journal* 16: 627–629.

44. Balfour HH Jr 1993 Current management of varicella zoster virus infections. *Journal of Medical Virology Supplemental* 1: 74.

45. Cinque P, Bossolasco S, Vago L et al 1997 Varicella-zoster virus (VZV) DNA in cerebrospinal fluid of patients infected with human immunodeficiency virus: VZV disease of the central nervous system or subclinical reactivation of VZV infection? *Clinical Infectious Diseases* 25: 634–639.

46. Gilden DH, Kleinschmidt-DeMasters BK, LaGuardia JJ, Mahalingam R, Cohrs RJ 2000 Neurologic complications of the reactivation of varicella-zoster virus. *New England Journal of Medicine* 342: 635–645.

47. de Silva SM, Mark AS, Gilden DH et al 1996 Zoster myelitis: improvement with antiviral therapy in two cases. *Neurology* 47: 929–931.

48. Kimberlin DW, Lin CY, Sanchez P et al 2000 Ganciclovir (GCVLin) Treatment of Symptomatic Congenital Cytomegalovirus (CMV) Infections: Results of a Phase III Randomized Trial. Program and abstracts of the 40th Interscience Conference on Antimicrobial Agents and Chemotherapy, Toronto, Ontario, Canada. Abstract #1942.

49. Keeble SA, Christofinis GJ, Wood W 1958 Natural virus B infection in rhesus monkeys. *Journal of Pathology and Bacteriology* 76: 189–199.

50. Holmes GP, Chapman LE, Stewart JA et al 1995 Guidelines for the prevention and treatment of B-virus infections in exposed persons. *Clinical Infectious Diseases* 20: 421–439.

51. McKinney RE Jr, Katz SL, Wilfert CM 1987 Chronic enteroviral meningoencephalitis in agammaglobulinemic patients. *Reviews of Infectious Disease* 9: 334–356.

52. Dwyer JM, Erlendsson K 1988 Intraventricular gamma-globulin for the management of enterovirus encephalitis. *Pediatric Infectious Disease Journal* 7: S30–S33.

53. Abzug M, Keyserling HL, Lee ML, Levin MJ, Rotbart HA 1995 Neonatal enterovirus infection: virology, serology, and effects of intravenous immunoglobulin. *Clinical Infectious Diseases* 20: 1201–1206.

54. Pevear DC, Tull TM, Seipel ME, Groarke JM 1999 Activity of pleconaril against enteroviruses. *Antimicrobial Agents and Chemotherapy* 43: 2109–2115.

55. Rotbart HA 1999 Antiviral therapy for enteroviral infections. *Pediatric Infectious Disease Journal* 18: 632–633.

56. Rotbart HA, Brennan PJ, Fife KH et al 1998 Enterovirus meningitis in adults. *Clinical Infectious Diseases* 27: 896–898.

57. Rotbart HA, Webster AD, Pleconrail Registry Group 2001 Treatment of potentially life-threatening enterovirus infections with pleconaril. *Clinical Infectious Diseases* 32: 228–235.

58. Pradhan S, Gupta RP, Shashank S, Pandey N 1999 Intravenous immunoglobulin therapy in acute disseminated encephalomyelitis. *Journal of the Neurological Sciences* 165: 56–61.

59. Stuve O, Zamvil SS 1999 Pathogenesis, diagnosis, and treatment of acute disseminated encephalomyelitis. *Current Opinion in Neurology* 12: 395–401.

60. Balestri P, Grosso S, Acquaviva A, Bernini M 2000 Plasmapheresis in a child affected by acute disseminated encephalomyelitis. *Brain and Development* 22: 123–126.

55 Bone and joint infections

D. A. Wininger and R. J. Fass

Acute hematogenous osteomyelitis and septic arthritis are most common in infants, children and elderly people.[1,2] Skeletal involvement may be obvious during the acute bacteremic phase or 1–2 weeks after a course of treatment for *Staphylococcus aureus* bacteremia, when the patient presents with osteomyelitis of the femur, a spinal disk space infection or a septic hip. Occasionally, the bacteremic episode is transient or inapparent.

In adults, osteomyelitis is usually a consequence of contiguous spread of infection from infected wounds, teeth, sinuses, ulcers, open fractures or after surgery.[2] Host defenses and early, vigorous antimicrobial treatment of these infections frequently prevents spread to bone or aborts progression of early bone involvement. Joint involvement due to soft-tissue infection is uncommon unless there is penetrating trauma, an overlying ulcer or spread from contiguous bone.[3–5]

Early, aggressive treatment of acute bone and joint infections is important to achieve cure and prevent chronic infection, for which cure is more difficult to achieve.[1–5] Suboptimal or delayed treatment of skin or soft-tissue infections when there is devitalized tissue due to trauma or vascular disease, as occurs with diabetic feet and pressure sores, are particularly common problems.[2,6,7]

Nosocomial skeletal infections complicating total joint replacement or internal fixation of fractures present unique challenges.[4,8,9] They may occur early, due to contamination at the time of injury or surgery, from infection in the postoperative period, or later, as a recrudescence of chronic, indolent infection or following bacteremic seeding.[9–11]

DIAGNOSIS

The diagnoses of osteomyelitis and septic arthritis require clinical suspicion and reliable microbiological data.[1–6,12] Imaging techniques can help confirm diagnoses in many settings.

To establish the diagnosis of osteomyelitis, imaging the involved bone or bones with X-rays, magnetic resonance imaging (MRI) and/or computed tomography (CT) are important diagnostic tools.[13–15] Both enhanced and unenhanced images should be obtained. Bone scans and radio-labelled white cell scans, while used extensively in the past, are less useful in adults today. However, bone scans are still commonly used in the evaluation of children with suspect osteomyelitis.

In acute disease, initial radiographs are typically normal because radiographic abnormalities require time to evolve. They are still useful, however, to establish a baseline for subsequent comparisons. MRI and CT scans are more sensitive for early disease and are often indicated for the diagnosis of acute hematogenous infection. They are not uniformly necessary, however, for suspected acute contiguous infection. Vigorous antimicrobial therapy of high-risk skin and soft-tissue infections, which assumes that bone involvement is present, may abort the development of established bone involvement. Clinical healing and normal plain radiographs at the time of follow-up may obviate the need for these expensive pretreatment evaluations.

Chronic osteomyelitis evolves over months or years. The resultant inflammatory bone destruction with sequestration of devascularized bone and reactive new bone formation cause obvious radiographic abnormalities. MRI and CT scans are helpful for defining the anatomical extent of disease, primarily for planning surgery.[14–16] Performing these tests routinely in all such patients, however, such as those with diabetic foot ulcers, is not always essential for effective patient management.[17] Palpating bone when probing a pedal ulcer has reasonable specificity (85%) and positive predictive value (89%) for osteomyelitis.[18]

The interpretation of imaging studies may be confounded by neighboring soft-tissue infection, fractures, underlying skeletal, vascular or neuropathic disease, previous surgery or the presence of prostheses.[6,7,14,15] The combination of indium-111 white blood cell scans and technetium-99m sulfur colloid marrow scans may help differentiate infected from uninfected neuropathic bone disease,[19–21] but is not yet in wide use at most centers.

Blood cultures should be performed in patients with osteomyelitis if bacteremia is a reasonable consideration. Gram stains and cultures of material obtained from the site of infection are also essential elements for establishing etiology: open debridement provides reliable material. Specimens obtained by aspiration or biopsy through intact skin are also reliable, although needle biopsies are less sensitive than larger samples.[22] Material obtained from infected wounds, fistulas or ulcers that are often contaminated may suffice when a single organism such as *Staph. aureus* is repeatedly isolated, but the results of such cultures are often misleading, leading to either undertreatment or overtreatment.[6,12,23]

For septic arthritis, joint aspiration to obtain material for Gram stain and culture should be accompanied by fluid analysis for cells, protein and glucose content to distinguish infectious from non-infectious arthritis. Imaging studies are not as important as with osteomyelitis, but may be helpful to detect joint destruction or define associated bone or soft-tissue involvement.[3–5,15,24]

ANTIMICROBIAL CHOICE

The choice of antimicrobial regimen to treat a bone or joint infection is largely dependent on identifying the pathogen(s) and determining antimicrobial susceptibilities. The bacterial species that commonly cause skeletal infections are shown in Table 55.1.[1–7,9,10,12,25–29]

Antimicrobials that have proven most effective in treating skeletal infections include the β-lactams,[5,12,27] clindamycin,[27,30–32] and the fluoroquinolones.[12,33–36] Vancomycin, teicoplanin, fusidic acid, trimethoprim–sulfamethoxazole, and metronidazole have more limited indications. Prolonged aminoglycoside administration is not very efficacious and irreversible toxicity may be unpredictable. Monitoring blood levels does not assure the absence of delayed disabling ototoxicity. Macrolides and tetracyclines should generally be avoided.

Antimicrobial selection should be based on the clinical experiences enumerated above, with only minor consideration given to achievable bone and joint concentrations. Bone concentrations are quite variable and technically difficult to measure,[37] although concentrations in synovial fluid are more predictive of therapeutic response.[4,38–40] Drug selection should generally also be independent of the site of infection, the route by which it was acquired, or the degree of chronicity: these three characteristics are more important in determining route of administration, dose, and duration of treatment.

STAPHYLOCOCCAL AND STREPTOCOCCAL INFECTIONS

β-Lactams, in high doses, are the preferred drugs for streptococcal and staphylococcal infections.[5,12,27] Intravenous penicillin G is usually used for the former and nafcillin, flucloxacillin or oxacillin for the latter because most staphylococci produce penicillinase. In penicillin-allergic patients, cephalosporins such as cefotaxime or ceftriaxone may be substituted. For oral administration, when appropriate, drugs such as penicillin V, amoxicillin, cloxacillin, dicloxacillin,

Table 55.1 Common pathogens in suppurative bone and joint infections

Hematogenous spread	Contiguous spread		
	Acute skin and soft-tissue infections	Orofacial and dental infections	Diabetic foot and pressure sores
Staphylococcus aureus	*Staphylococcus aureus*	*Streptococcus* spp.	*Staphylococcus aureus*
Streptococcus spp.	*Streptococcus agalactiae*	Anaerobic cocci	*Staphylococcus epidermidis*
Haemophilus influenzae[a]	*Streptococcus pyogenes*	*Fusobacterium* spp.	*Streptococcus* spp.
Enterobacteriaceae[b]		*Prevotella melaninogenica*	Enterobacteriaceae
Streptococcus epidermidis[c,d]		*Pasteurella multocida*[g]	*Pseudomonas aeruginosa*
Candida[d]		*Eikenella corrodens*[h]	*Enterococcus faecalis*
Neisseria gonorrhoeae[e]			Anaerobic cocci
Pseudomonas aeruginosa[f]			*Bacteroides* spp.
			Clostridium spp.

[a] Infants and unimmunized children.
[b] Elderly and neonates.
[c] Bone and joint prostheses.
[d] Intravenous devices.
[e] Young adults.
[f] Injection drug use and foot puncture wounds.
[g] Dog and cat bites.
[h] Human bites.

flucloxacillin, cefuroxime and cefpodoxime may be used. Blood levels can be increased by the coadministration of probenecid.[41] Clindamycin has been used extensively for the treatment of staphylococcal osteomyelitis (including susceptible strains of methicillin-resistant staphylococci (MRSA)) with excellent results.[27,30,31] For prolonged courses, oral clindamycin provides serum concentrations nearly comparable to those achieved intravenously.[31,42] In an animal model of *Staph. aureus* osteomyelitis, clindamycin was more effective than cefazolin, presumably due to better bone penetration and possibly due to inhibition of glycocalyx formation.[32]

Fusidic acid is not available in the USA, but is used to treat methicillin-resistant as well as methicillin-susceptible *Staph. aureus* skeletal infections in Europe, where it is combined with drugs such as penicillins, erythromycin or rifampicin (rifampin) to reduce the emergence of resistance during treatment.[43–46]

The glycopeptides vancomycin and teicoplanin are consistently active against Gram-positive cocci including methicillin-resistant staphylococci. They are not as effective, however, as β-lactams for treating serious infections caused by methicillin-susceptible *Staph. aureus*,[47,48] and should be used only to treat infections caused by multiresistant Gram-positive organisms.

Like clindamycin, trimethoprim–sulfamethoxazole can be given orally as well as intravenously for prolonged periods of time to avoid the hazards of intravenous lines when the isolates are susceptible.[49] Minocycline (combined with rifampicin) has been suggested as another oral alternative for methicillin-resistant staphylococci,[41] but published clinical experience in the treatment of osteomyelitis is limited.

Two new antimicrobials have been marketed for the treatment of multiresistant Gram-positive cocci. While they are most important as agents to treat vancomycin-resistant *Enterococcus faecium* (VRE), they may have an occasional role in the treatment of MRSA skeletal infections. Linezolid is an oxazolidinone,[50] and quinupristin–dalfopristin a combination of two semisynthetic pristinamycin derivatives (*see* Chapters 28 and 31).[51] There is little experience with either in treating skeletal infections; both are inordinately expensive and have serious problems with administration. Linezolid is available orally but causes a high incidence of thrombocytopenia. Quinupristin–dalfopristin be given intravenously and is problematic to administer.

HAEMOPHILUS INFLUENZAE INFECTIONS

Ampicillin or amoxicillin are preferred for β-lactamase-negative *H. influenzae* infections; for resistant strains, expanded-spectrum cephalosporins,[27] ampicillin–sulbactam or amoxicillin–clavulanate[52] are recommended. In adults and older children, a fluoroquinolone is probably preferred. Few of these infections have been encountered since the advent of *H. influenzae* type b vaccination in children.

ENTEROBACTERIACEAE AND *PSEUDOMONAS AERUGINOSA* INFECTIONS

A β-lactam plus an aminoglycoside has traditionally been recommended to treat serious infections caused by the Enterobacteriaceae and *Ps. aeruginosa*, but monotherapy with highly active expanded-spectrum β-lactams is satisfactory for many infections. Aminoglycoside toxicity, poor penetration and the necessity for prolonged parenteral administration can complicate their use, and aminoglycosides should be avoided when possible.[12]

There is now extensive experience using fluoroquinolones, particularly ciprofloxacin, in treating aerobic Gram-negative skeletal infections.[12,33,35,36] Ciprofloxacin is highly active, available parenterally and orally, well tolerated during prolonged administration and has established efficacy. The presence of Gram-positive cocci and/or anaerobes requires the addition of a second agent (Fass, unpublished results). Newer fluoroquinolones such as gatifloxacin and moxifloxacin, with enhanced activity against Gram-positive cocci, might be useful as monotherapy for treating mixed infections, but there is little experience with them in treating skeletal infections and the safety of long-term administration is unknown.[53,54]

GONOCOCCAL INFECTIONS

Skeletal involvement with gonococci is the result of hematogenous seeding and most commonly presents as tenosynovitis, with or without dermal lesions, rather than as osteomyelitis or overt septic arthritis. Despite a high frequency of resistance to penicillin G and ampicillin among gonococci, strains that disseminate are usually susceptible.[4] Because of the high prevalence of penicillin resistance among gonococci causing genital infections, however, expanded-spectrum cephalosporins (such as ceftriaxone parenterally or cefixime orally) are usually recommended.[5] The fluoroquinolones would probably also be effective, but there is little clinical experience with these drugs in treating gonococcal skeletal infections. Concomitant treatment of chlamydial genital infection is also indicated.

OROFACIAL AND DENTAL INFECTIONS

Orofacial and dental infections are caused by oropharyngeal streptococci and anaerobes, and are appropriately treated with a penicillin–β-lactamase inhibitor combination or clindamycin.[55] Human and animal bites may also include the Gram-positive skin flora of the victim as well as the mouth flora of the attacker.[5,25,26] Amoxicillin–clavulanate (or ampicillin–sulbactam) has an ideal spectrum against the organisms isolated from these infections; cephalosporins, macrolides, tetracyclines and fluoroquinolones are less consistently active.[5,26,28] Clindamycin is also useful to treat infected bites, but it is not active against *Eikenella corrodens*[56] (associated with human bites) or *Pasteurella multocida*[57] (associated with animal bites).

THE INFECTED DIABETIC FOOT AND PRESSURE SORES

Selecting the optimal antimicrobial regimen for treating these infections is difficult because infection may be caused by combinations of staphylococci, streptococci, enterococci, Enterobacteriaceae, *Ps. aeruginosa* and fecal anaerobes.[6,7] The antimicrobial spectra of drugs potentially useful for treating these infections are shown in Table 55.2. If acute, severe and life threatening, broad-spectrum treatment covering appropriate potential pathogens is appropriate. Many of these infections are more indolent, however, and oral monotherapy or combination therapy may be adequate and appropriate. Amoxicillin–clavulanate and clindamycin–ciprofloxacin are useful oral combinations. Metronidozole–ciprofloxacin has also been used but it leaves aerobic streptococci and enterococci virtually untreated. Trimethoprim–sulfamethoxazole covers staphylococci and Enterobacteriaceae but is poor for some streptococci and inadequate for enterococci or anaerobes.

DOSE, ROUTE AND DURATION OF TREATMENT

Skeletal infections have traditionally been treated with relatively high doses of intravenous antimicrobials, septic arthritis for 2–3 weeks and osteomyelitis for 4–6 weeks.[2,5,12,58] In children, however, shorter courses of treatment are often adequate. Acute infections caused by *H. influenzae*, *Neisseria* spp. or streptococci should be treated for at least 10–14 days and those caused by *Staph. aureus*, Enterobacteriaceae or *Ps. aeruginosa* for at least 3 weeks.[5,27,58,59]

Acute infections in adults and chronic infections at any age need to be treated for longer.[3] After initiating intravenous therapy in the hospital, it has become common practice to continue treatment after discharge using a central venous catheter (inserted either peripherally or directly into the subclavian vein) and long half-life antibiotics in an attempt to reduce the length of hospital stay and associated costs.[12] Complication rates of 20% have been reported,[60] however, and costs are still appreciable.

While prolonged intravenous treatment would be appropriate for some infections, such as those associated with acute staphylococcal bacteremia, it is probably unnecessary for many

Table 55.2 Clinically useful spectra of antimicrobials for treating mixed aerobic-anaerobic bone and joint infections such as the diabetic foot and infected pressure sores

Antimicrobial	Staphylococci[a]	Streptococci	Enterococcus faecalis	Enterobacteriaceae	Pseudomonas aeruginosa	Anaerobes (oral)	Anaerobes (fecal)
Penicillin G, ampicillin, amoxicillin	+	+++	+++	±	0	++	+
Ampicillin–sulbactam, amoxicillin–clavulanate[b]	+++	+++	+++	++	0	+++	+++
Mezlocillin, piperacillin	±	+++	+++	++	++	+++	+
Piperacillin–tazobactam[b]	+++	+++	+++	+++	++	+++	+++
Cefotaxime, ceftriaxone	+++	+++	0	+++	±	++	+
Ceftazidime	+++	±	0	+++	++	±	±
Cefoperazone	+++	+++	±	+++	++	+++	++
Imipenem	+++	+++	+++	+++	++	+++	+++
Ciprofloxacin	±	±	±	+++	++	±	±
Trimethoprim–sulfamethoxazole	+++	+	0	++	0	0	0
Aminoglycosides	±	0	0	+++	+++	0	0
Clindamycin	+++	+++	0	0	0	+++	++
Metronidazole	0	0	0	0	0	+++	+++
Vancomycin, teicoplanin	+++	+++	+++	0	0	±	±

[a] Methicillin-susceptible strains; vancomycin or teicoplanin for resistant strains.
[b] Not necessary for non-β-lactamase-producing strains.
0, Little or no clinical utility; ±, some in-vitro activity but not very useful clinically; +, good for a limited number of strains or organisms; ++, good for many strains or organisms; +++, good for most or all strains or organisms.

chronic infections. The availability of highly active, predictably absorbed oral agents has obviated the need for prolonged intravenous antimicrobials with the attendant discomfort, complications and costs. Indeed, for some patients, such as those with chronic, recalcitrant osteomyelitis, treatment with an appropriate oral agent for 3–12 months may be associated with more favorable results, better patient tolerance, fewer adverse reactions and lower costs.[2,6,30,41,59]

Oral penicillins, cephalosporins or clindamycin, after 5–10 days of initial intravenous therapy, have been effective in children.[30,31,59,61,62] Similarly, treatment with intravenous, and then oral, ampicillin-sulbactam has also been used successfully.[52]

Switching from intravenous to oral therapy has also been successful in adults: 21 adults with osteomyelitis or septic arthritis caused primarily by *Staph. aureus* and/or Enterobacteriaceae treated intravenously for a mean of 3.6 days followed by a mean of 43 days orally, had a satisfactory outcome.[63] Cloxacillin, cefalexin (6–9 g/day plus probenecid) or trimethoprim–sulfamethoxazole (160/800 mg four times daily) were prescribed for the staphylococcal infections and trimethoprim–sulfamethoxazole for those caused by the Enterobacteriaceae. Trimethoprim–sulfamethoxazole, at the same dose, was also used successfully to treat MRSA osteomyelitis, usually after initial intravenous vancomycin.[49]

Ciprofloxacin and, to a lesser extent, ofloxacin and pefloxacin, initially available only orally, have been extensively used to treat skeletal infections.[12,33–36] Because of borderline activity against streptococci and enterococci and the emergence of staphylococcal resistance during treatment,[64] monotherapy with these fluoroquinolones should be restricted to the treatment of aerobic Gram-negative skeletal infections. Our early experience with oral ciprofloxacin in treating 21 patients with osteomyelitis was uniformly successful for those caused by Enterobacteriaceae and/or *Ps. aeruginosa*, but only 2 of 11 (18%) with concomitant Gram-positive and/or anaerobic pathogens had a satisfactory response (Fass, unpublished data). The use of fluroquinolones is not approved for children in most countries of the world. Alternative antibiotics remain most acceptable.

Oral therapy requires predictable gastrointestinal absorption. Although β-lactams are often the preferred drugs for skeletal infections, oral derivatives are often much less potent and unpredictably absorbed, even at high doses with probenecid.[59,65] Serum concentrations of intravenous and oral clindamycin far exceed those necessary to inhibit most staphylococci and streptococci.[30,31,42] Serum concentrations of trimethoprim–sulfamethoxazole after intravenous and oral administration are virtually identical (data on file, Glaxo SmithKline Co.) and are inhibitory to most staphylococci and Enterobacteriaceae. Oral administration of ciprofloxacin[66] and other quinolones is equivalent to intravenous administration and results in serum concentrations higher than those needed to inhibit most Enterobacteriaceae and *Ps. aeruginosa*. Serum concentrations of metronidazole after intravenous and oral

Table 55.3 Comparison of intravenous and oral antimicrobial regimens to treat infections in adults

Drug	Intravenous			Oral		
	Dose	Approximate peak serum concentration (mg/l)	Usual MIC (mg/l) of appropriate pathogens	Drug	Dose[a]	Approximate peak serum concentration (mg/l)
β-Lactams						
Penicillin G	1–2 MU every 4–6 h	10–20 (U/ml)	≤0.12	Penicillin V	500 mg four times daily	5
Ampicillin	1–2 g every 4–6 h	20–50	≤0.12, 0.5–2[b]	Amoxicillin	500 mg three times daily	5–10
Ampicillin–sulbactam	1.5–3 g every 6 h	50–150	≤2, 2–8[c]	Amoxicillin–clavulanate	500 mg three times daily	5–10
Nafcillin	2 g every 4–6 h	40–80	≤0.5	Dicloxacillin	0.5–1 g four times daily	10–25
Cefazolin	1–2 g every 8 h	80–150	≤2	Cefalexin[d]	0.5–1 g four times daily	15–25
Ceftriaxone	1–2 g every 24 h	100–250	≤4	Cefixime[e]	400 mg once daily	4
Non-β-lactams						
Clindamycin	600 mg every 8 h	8	≤0.5	Clindamycin	300 mg four times daily	5
Trimethoprim–sulfamethoxazole[f]	160/800 mg every 8 h	6/120	≤0.5/9.5	Trimethoprim–sulfamethoxazole	160/800 mg three times daily	4/100
Ciprofloxacin	400 mg every 8–12 h	4	≤0.25, 0.12–2[g]	Ciprofloxacin	500–750 mg twice daily	3–4
Metronidazole	500 mg every 6 h	15–25	≤4	Metronidazole	500 mg four times daily	12

[a] For the β-lactams, higher doses and/or coadministration of probenecid are appropriate for skeletal infections.
[b] MIC ≤0.12 mg/l for most susceptible organisms; 0.5–2 mg/l for *E. faecalis*.
[c] MIC ≤2 mg/l for β-lactamase-positive *H. influenzae*; 2–8 mg/l for susceptible Enterobacteriaceae.
[d] Cefalexin is 4-fold less active than cefazolin against *Staph. aureus*; cefpodoxime or cefuroxime are preferred.
[e] Cefixime is for Gram-negative organisms only.
[f] Peak serum concentrations at steady state are extrapolated from multiple studies.
[g] MIC ≤0.25 mg/l for Enterobacteriaceae; 0.12–2 mg/l for susceptible *Ps. aeruginosa*.

administration are virtually identical[67] and exceed those needed to inhibit most anaerobes. Linezolid is the only oral drug available to treat skeletal infections caused by vancomycin-resistant enterococci and those methicillin-resistant staphylococcal infections that are resistant to trimethoprim–sulfamethoxazole, clindamycin and minocycline.

In Table 55.3, intravenous antimicrobials commonly used to treat skeletal infections are shown with recommended doses, observed peak serum concentrations and the usual minimum inhibitory concentrations (MICs) for pathogens appropriate for treatment. For each drug, doses of the oral preparation (or similar drug in the case of the β-lactams) with observed peak serum concentrations are provided for comparison. For the antipseudomonal β-lactams and glycopeptides, no oral equivalents are available and switching to oral therapy requires changing drug class. Direct instillation or irrigation of infected bones or joints is no longer necessary with currently available antibiotics and thus the risk of secondary infection and chemical synovitis with a treatment of uncertain efficacy are avoided. Antibiotic-impregnated cements are sometimes introduced temporarily during surgical management of osteomyelitis to fill dead space and provide high local concentrations of antibiotics in combination with systemically administered agents, but clinical efficacy data is scant.[68]

MONITORING ANTIMICROBIAL THERAPY

Clinical and microbiological follow-up are important to ensure that resolution of skeletal infections is progressing satisfactorily. This is particularly the case when the microbiological diagnosis has been equivocal or lacking. Serum bactericidal tests (SBTs) have been used to monitor the adequacy of treatment,[41] but this is usually unnecessary. The tests suffer from poor standardization and the absence of validated guidelines for interpretation of results.[59,69,70] In-vivo treatment success has been observed in situations where SBT results were unfavorable.[71] Infections due to gonococci and streptococci usually respond favorably, while staphylococcal and Gram-negative bacillary infections often do poorly,[1,3] regardless of the SBT test results.

Determining SBT titers or, more simply measuring drug levels, may be useful to confirm adequacy of drug concentrations, particularly when bioavailability is poor or unpredictable or when treating with marginally active antimicrobials. From a practical point of view, this is most helpful with the penicillins and cephalosporins but not with other recommended oral agents as indicated above.[31,52,58,59,61,63,65]

SURGERY

Surgical procedures are indicated for a variety of reasons in the diagnosis and management of bone and joint infec-

tions.[1–6,10,27,37,72] Needle aspiration or biopsy may suffice for diagnosis or drainage. Arthroscopic drainage of joints may facilitate breaking up fibrinous joint material and removal of debris. More extensive procedures may be indicated to resect fistulas, debride ulcers or necrotic devascularized bone, remove foreign bodies, including joint prostheses, as well as improving locomotor stability, restoring vascular supply and joint reconstruction.

In some patients with diabetic foot ulcers, the vascular supply may be so poor or the infection so extensive that antimicrobial administration and debridement is insufficient to ensure eradication of infection and ultimate healing.[6] In such instances, prolonged chemotherapy may be futile and unnecessarily subject a patient to adverse drug effects, expenses and disability. Amputation may be advisable for cure and a return to a more satisfactory lifestyle. An analogous situation may occur with extensive decubitus ulcers. Early excision of the ulcer, aggressive debridement of the involved bone and flap grafting to cover the wound may result in a more rapid, satisfactory outcome than protracted ineffectual antimicrobial therapy.[73] Risk factors predisposing to the initial infection should be reduced to avoid recurrence after this time-consuming and expensive procedure.

INTERNAL FIXATION AND PROSTHETIC DEVICES

It is particularly difficult to eradicate infection in the presence of foreign bodies, including prostheses.[10] Overtly infected or unstable fixation devices and prosthetic joints should be removed. When it is not clear that they are infected or are required for stability, prolonged treatment may be tried, sometimes with removal at a later date. Alternately, one can remove the prostheses, use external fixation on a temporary basis, and then insert a new device at a later date once the infection has been eradicated.[37]

Joint replacement is now a commonly performed operative procedure. Initially, deep wound infection rates were about 10% but with greater experience, prophylactic antibiotics and unidirectional airflow systems infection rates should be less than 2%. The use of gentamicin-impregnated cement and personnel isolator systems may also have contributed to reduced infection rates at some centers. The most commonly used prophylactic antimicrobial has been cefazolin or a similar cephalosporin. If infection does occur, therapeutic agents should be selected, as for the treatment of other skeletal infections, based on microbial etiology. Staphylococci are most common, but infections caused by streptococci, Gram-negative bacilli and, occasionally, anaerobes may be seen. Removal of the prosthesis, infected tissue and cement should be done with immediate (one-stage) or, preferably, delayed (two-stage) replacement of the prosthesis.[29,74]

References

1. Cooper C, Cawley MID 1986 Bacterial arthritis in an English health district: a 10 year review. *Annals of Rheumatic Disease* 45: 458–463.

2. Waldvogel FA, Medoff G, Swartz MN 1970 Osteomyelitis: a review of clinical features, therapeutic considerations and unusual aspects. *New England Journal of Medicine* 282: 198–206, 260–266, 316–322.

3. Esterhai JL Jr, Gelb I 1991 Adult septic arthritis. *Orthopedic Clinics of North America* 22: 503–514.

4. Goldenberg DL, Reed JI 1985 Bacterial arthritis. *New England Journal of Medicine* 312: 764–771.

5. Smith JW, Piercy EA 1995 Infectious arthritis. *Clinical Infectious Diseases* 20: 225–231.

6. Lipsky BA, Pecoraro RE, Wheat LJ 1990 The diabetic foot. Soft tissue and bone infection. *Infectious Disease Clinics of North America* 4: 409–432.

7. Sugarman B, Hawes S, Musher DM et al 1983 Osteomyelitis beneath pressure sores. *Archives of Internal Medicine* 143: 683–688.

8. Gillespie WJ 1990 Epidemiology in bone and joint infection. *Infectious Disease Clinics of North America* 4: 361–376.

9. Inman RD, Gallegos KV, Brause BD et al 1984 Clinical and microbial features of prosthetic joint infection. *American Journal of Medicine* 77: 47–53.

10. Gillespie WJ 1990 Infection in total joint replacement. *Infectious Disease Clinics of North America* 4: 465–484.

11. Gillespie WJ 1997 Prevention and management of infection after total joint replacement. *Clinical Infectious Diseases* 25: 1310–1317.

12. Gentry LO 1990 Antibiotic therapy for osteomyelitis. *Infectious Disease Clinics of North America* 4: 485–499.

13. Boutin RD, Brossmann J, Sartoris DJ et al 1998 Update on imaging of orthopedic infections. *Orthopedic Clinics of North America* 29: 41–66.

14. Schauwecker DS, Braunstein EM, Wheat LJ 1990 Diagnostic imaging of osteomyelitis. *Infectious Disease Clinics of North America* 4: 441–463.

15. Wegener WA, Alavi A 1991 Diagnostic imaging of musculoskeletal infection. *Orthopedic Clinics of North America* 22: 401–418.

16. Huang AB, Schweitzer ME, Hume E et al 1998 Osteomyelitis of the pelvis/hips in paralyzed patients: accuracy and clinical utility of MRI. *Journal of Computer Assisted Tomography* 22: 437–443.

17. Eckman MH, Greenfield S, Mackey WC et al 1995 Foot infections in diabetic patients Decision and cost-effectiveness analyses. *Journal of the American Medical Association* 273: 712–720.

18. Grayson ML, Gibbons GW, Balogh K et al 1995 Probing to bone in infected pedal ulcers a clinical sign of underlying osteomyelitis in diabetic patients. *Journal of the American Medical Association* 273: 721–723.

19. Palestro CJ, Mehta HH, Patel M et al 1998 Marrow versus infection in the Charcot joint: Indium-111 leukocyte and technetium-99m sulfur colloid scintigraphy. *Journal of Nuclear Medicine* 39: 346–350.

20. Palestro CJ, Torres MA 1997 Radionuclide imaging in orthopedic infections. *Seminars in Nuclear Medicine* 27: 334–345.

21. Tomas MB, Patel M, Marwin SE et al 2000 The diabetic foot. *British Journal of Radiology* 73: 443–450.

22. Perry CR, Pearson RL, Miller GA 1991 Accuracy of cultures of material from swabbing of the superficial aspect of the wound and needle biopsy in the preoperative assessment of osteomyelitis. *Journal of Bone and Joint Surgery* 73A: 745–749.

23. Mackowiak PA, Jones SR, Smith JW 1978 Diagnostic value of sinus-tract cultures in chronic osteomyelitis. *Journal of the American Medical Association* 239: 2772–2775.

24. Perry CR 1999 Septic Arthritis. *American Journal of Orthopedics* 28: 168–178.

25. Goldstein EJC, Citron DM, Finegold SM 1984 Role of anaerobic bacteria in bite-wound infections. *Reviews of Infectious Diseases* 6 (Suppl. 1): S177–S183.

26. Brook I 1987 Microbiology of human and animal bite wounds in children. *Pediatric Infectious Disease Journal* 6: 29–32.

27. Nelson JD 1990 Acute osteomyelitis in children. *Infectious Disease Clinics of North America* 4: 513–522.

28. Goldstein EJC, Citron DM 1993 Comparative susceptibilities of 173 aerobic and anaerobic bite wound isolates to sparfloxacin, temafloxacin, clarithromycin, and older agents. *Antimicrobial Agents and Chemotherapy* 37: 1150–1153.

29. Goldenberg DL 1998 Septic arthritis. *Lancet* 351: 197–202.

30. Feigin RD, Pickering LK, Anderson D et al 1975 Clindamycin treatment of osteomyelitis and septic arthritis in children. *Pediatrics* 55: 213–223.

31. Kaplan SL, Mason EO Jr, Feigin D 1982 Clindamycin versus nafcillin or methicillin in the treatment of *Staphylococcus aureus* osteomyelitis in children. *Southern Medical Journal* 75(2): 138–142.

32. Mader JT, Adams K, Morrison L 1989 Comparative evaluation of cefazolin and clindamycin in the treatment of experimental *Staphylococcus aureus* osteomyelitis in rabbits. *Antimicrobial Agents and Chemotherapy* 33: 1760–1764.

33. Norrby SR 1989 Ciprofloxacin in the treatment of acute and chronic osteomyelitis: a review. *Scandinavian Journal of Infectious Diseases* 60 (Suppl.): 74–78.

34. Waldvogel FA 1989 Use of quinolones for the treatment of osteomyelitis and septic arthritis. *Reviews of Infectious Diseases* 11 (Suppl. 5): S1259–S1263.

35. Mader JT 1990 Fluoroquinolones in bone and joint infections. In: Sanders WE, Sanders CC (eds). *Fluoroquinolones in the treatment of infectious diseases.* Glenview, IL, Physicians & Scientists Publishing Co., pp. 71–86.

36. Gentry LO 1991 Oral antimicrobial therapy for osteomyelitis. *Annals of Internal Medicine* 114: 986–987.

37. Waldvogel FA, Vasey H 1980 Osteomyelitis: the past decade. *New England Journal of Medicine* 303: 360–370.

38. Nelson JD 1971 Antibiotic concentrations in septic joint effusions. *New England Journal of Medicine* 284: 349–353.

39. Nelson JD, Howard JB, Shelton S 1978 Oral antibiotic therapy for skeletal infections of children. I. Antibiotic concentrations in suppurative synovial fluid. *Journal of Pediatrics* 92: 131–134.

40. Sattar MA, Barrett SP, Cawley MID 1983 Concentrations of some antibiotics in synovial fluid after oral administration, with special reference to antistaphylococcal activity. *Annals of Rheumatic Disease* 42: 67–74.

41. Haas DW, McAndrew MP 1996 Bacterial osteomyelitis in adults: evolving considerations in diagnosis and treatment. *American Journal of Medicine* 101: 550–561.

42. Fass RJ 1980 Lincomycin and clindamycin. In: Kagan BM (ed.) *Antimicrobial therapy*, 3rd edn. Philadelphia, WB Saunders, pp. 97–116.

43. Atkins B, Gottlieb T 1999 Fusidic acid in bone and joint infections. *International Journal of Antimicrobial Agents* 12 (Suppl. 2): S79–93.

44. Coombs RRH 1990 Fusidic acid in staphylococcal bone and joint infection. *Journal of Antimicrobial Chemotherapy* 25 (Suppl. B): 53–60.

45. Drancourt M, Stein A, Argenson JN et al 1997 Oral treatment of *Staphylococcus* spp. infected orthopaedic implants with fusidic acid or ofloxacin in combination with rifampicin. *Journal of Antimicrobial Chemotherapy* 39: 235–240.

46. Drugeon HB, Caillon J, Juvin ME 1994 In-vitro antibacterial activity of fusidic acid alone and in combination with other antibiotics against methicillin-sensitive and -resistant *Staphylococcus aureus*. *Journal of Antimicrobial Chemotherapy* 34: 899–907.

47. Fortún J, Pérez-Molina JA, Alnón MT et al 1995 Right-sided endocarditis caused by *Staphylococcus aureus* in drug abusers. *Antimicrobial Agents and Chemotherapy* 39: 525–528.

48. Small PM, Chambers HF 1990 Vancomycin for *Staphylococcus aureus* endocarditis in intravenous drug users. *Antimicrobial Agents and Chemotherapy* 34: 1227–1231.

49. Yeldandi V, Strodtman R, Lentino JR 1998 In-vitro and in-vivo studies of trimethoprim-sulphamethoxazole against multiple resistant *Staphylococcus aureus*. *Journal of Antimicrobial Chemotherapy* 22: 873–880.

50. Chien JW, Kucia ML, Salata RA 2000 Use of linezolid, an oxazolidinone, in the treatment of multidrug-resistant gram-positive bacterial infections. *Clinical Infectious Diseases* 30: 146–151.

51. Nichols RL, Graham DR, Barriere SL et al 1999 Treatment of hospitalized patients with complicated Gram-positive skin and skin structure infections: two randomized, multicentre studies of quinupristin/dalfopristin versus cefazolin, oxacillin or vancomycin. *Journal of Antimicrobial Chemotherapy* 44: 263–273.

52. Aronoff SC, Scoles PV, Makley JT et al 1986 Efficacy and safety of sequential treatment with parenteral sulbactam/ampicillin and oral sultamicillin for skeletal infections in children. *Reviews of Infectious Diseases* 8 (Suppl. 5): S639–S643.

53. Hosaka M, Yasue T, Fukuda H et al 1992 In vitro and in vivo antibacterial activities of AM-1155, a new 6-fluoro-8-methoxy quinolone. *Antimicrobial Agents and Chemotherapy* 36: 2108–2117.

54. Fass RJ 1997 In vitro activity of bay 12–8039, a new 8-methoxyquinolone. *Antimicrobial Agents and Chemotherapy* 41: 1818–1824.

55. von Konow L, Köndell PÅ, Nord CE et al 1992 Clindamycin versus phe-

noxymethylpenicillin in the treatment of acute orofacial infections. *European Journal of Clinical Microbiology and Infectious Diseases* 11: 1129–1136.

56. Robinson JVA, James AL 1974 In vitro susceptibility of *Bacteroides corrodens* and *Eikenella corrodens* to ten chemotherapeutic agents. *Antimicrobial Agents and Chemotherapy* 6: 543–546.

57. Goldstein EJC, Citron DM, Richwald GA 1988 Lack of in vitro efficacy of oral forms of certain cephalosporins, erythromycin, and oxacillin against *Pasteurella multocida*. *Antimicrobial Agents and Chemotherapy* 32: 213–215.

58. Syrogiannopoulos GA, Nelson JD 1988 Duration of antimicrobial therapy for acute suppurative osteoarticular infections. *Lancet* 1: 37–40.

59. Nelson JD 1983 A critical review of the role of oral antibiotics in the management of hematogenous osteomyelitis. In: Remington JS, Swartz MN (eds) *Current clinical topics in infectious diseases.* New York, McGraw-Hill, pp. 64–74.

60. Couch L, Cierny G, Mader JT 1987 Inpatient and outpatient use of the Hickman catheter for adults with osteomyelitis. *Clinical Orthopedics* 219: 226–235.

61. Tetzlaff TR, McCracken GH Jr, Nelson JD 1978 Oral antibiotic therapy for skeletal infections of children. II. Therapy of osteomyelitis and suppurative arthritis. *Journal of Pediatrics* 92: 485–490.

62. Newton PO, Ballock T, Bradley JS 1999 Oral antibiotic therapy of bacterial arthritis. *Pediatric Infectious Disease Journal* 18: 1102–1103.

63. Black J, Hunt TL, Godley PJ et al 1987 Oral antimicrobial therapy for adults with osteomyelitis or septic arthritis. *Journal of Infectious Diseases* 155: 968–972.

64. Fass RJ, Barnishan J, Ayers LW 1995 Emergence of bacterial resistance to imipenem and ciprofloxacin in a university hospital. *Journal of Antimicrobial Chemotherapy* 36: 343–353.

65. Prober CG, Yeager AS 1979 Use of the serum bactericidal titer to assess the adequacy of oral antibiotic therapy in the treatment of acute hematogenous osteomyelitis. *Journal of Pediatrics* 95: 131–135.

66. Heller AH 1992 Pharmacokinetic studies demonstrating equivalent doses of intravenous and oral ciprofloxacin. *Infections in Medicine 9* (Suppl. B): 32–40.

67. Houghton GW, Smith J, Thorne PS et al 1979 The pharmacokinetics of oral and intravenous metronidazole in man. *Journal of Antimicrobial Chemotherapy* 5: 621–623.

68. Wininger DA, Fass RJ 1996 Antibiotic-impregnated cement and beads for orthopedic infections. *Antimicrobial Agents and Chemotherapy* 40: 2675–2679.

69. Weinstein MP, Stratton CW, Hawley HB et al 1987 Multicenter collaborative evaluation of a standardized serum bactericidal test as a predictor of therapeutic efficacy in acute and chronic osteomyelitis. *American Journal of Medicine* 83: 218–222.

70. Wolfson JS, Swartz MN 1985 Serum bactericidal activity as a monitor of antibiotic therapy. *New England Journal of Medicine* 312: 968–975.

71. Fass RJ 1984 Laboratory tests for defining bactericidal activity as predictors of antibiotic efficacy in the treatment of endocarditis due to *Staphylococcus aureus* in rabbits. *Journal of Infectious Diseases* 149: 904–912.

72. Tetsworth K, Cierny G 1999 Osteomyelitis debridement techniques. *Clinical Orthopedics* 360: 87–96.

73. Mathes SJ 1982 The muscle flap for management of osteomyelitis. *New England Journal of Medicine* 306: 294–295.

74. Saravolatz LD 1993 Infection in implantable prosthetic devices. In: Wenzel RP (ed.) *Prevention and control of nosocomial infections*, 2nd edn. Baltimore, Williams & Wilkins, pp. 683–707.

56 Infections of the eye

D. V. Seal and A. J. Bron

This chapter outlines the therapy of ocular infections. The reader is referred to the previous edition of this book for further information and to references 1–3.

DEFENSE OF THE OCULAR SURFACE

The commensals of the ocular surface are chiefly Gram-positive organisms (*Staphylococcus aureus*, coagulase-negative staphylococci, diphtheroids and *Propionibacterium acnes*), with occasional Gram-negative organisms, especially in elderly people. They are found with greater frequency on the lid margin than in the conjunctival sac. Pathogens such as *Staph. aureus* are found in about 10% of normal eyes.

The cornea and conjunctiva are protected by a tear film with an outer lipid, a middle aqueous and an inner mucin layer. The aqueous layer is of lacrimal origin and contains several antibacterial proteins. Non-specific defense mechanisms in the tears include lysozyme, lactoferrin and the defensins, while specific mechanisms involve IgA antibodies directed against a wide range of organisms. There is co-operation between specific and non-specific mechanisms. At the ocular surface potent antimicrobials (such as lysozyme, IgA and SLPI) are entrained in the mucus film and maintain an antimicrobial presence in the surface microenvironment. With age, tear secretion and the concentration of protective lacrimal proteins falls. This situation is magnified in dry eye, including Sjögren's syndrome, where lacrimal secretion is compromised and surface defenses are lowered.

Infection at the ocular surface involves binding of organisms by bacterial ligands or adhesins to specific surface molecules, which initiate the process of invasion. For example, *Pseudomonas aeruginosa* lipopolysaccharide binds to the lectin galectin-3 present on corneal epithelial cells and experimental infection can be inhibited passively by antibodies against either molecule, or actively, by immunization against lipopolysaccharide.

PHARMACOKINETICS

The bulbar conjunctiva and corneal epithelium are relatively impermeable to water-soluble drugs, which penetrate poorly into the anterior chamber. Water-soluble, proprietary ophthalmic preparations, such as gentamicin sulfate, are available as eye drops or ointments at high concentration (e.g. 0.3%) relative to their effective antimicrobial concentration and are thus active in the treatment of surface ocular infections such as conjunctivitis. In contrast, agents with a relatively high lipid-water solubility (such as the fluoroquinolones, fusidic acid, chloramphenicol and the sulfonamides) readily penetrate the conjunctiva and cornea to enter the tissues of the anterior segment.

If the surface epithelium is breached, as by corneal ulceration, water-soluble drugs can diffuse more readily into the anterior segment in high concentration. This can be enhanced using antibiotic concentrations exceeding those of commercially available preparations (fortified drops). The topical route is unable to produce therapeutic concentrations in the posterior segment of the eye because of diffusion barriers across the lens and zonule and the vitreous. Also, drug is lost from the vitreous and aqueous to the systemic circulation across the iris and retina or by aqueous drainage.

The surface epithelial barrier can be circumvented by delivering a bolus of drug under the conjunctiva (subconjunctival injection) or close to the surface of the globe (sub-Tenon's injection). These periocular routes deliver effective antimicrobial concentrations into the anterior segment of the eye (e.g. cornea and anterior chamber) and, less, the posterior segment (e.g. the vitreous). Drugs may, however, be injected directly into the vitreous to treat infections of the vitreous and retina and controlled-release devices may be implanted in the scleral wall or suspended in the vitreous to provide long-term drug delivery.

THE BLOOD–OCULAR BARRIERS

In the uninflamed eye, barriers exist to the transfer of antibiotic from the circulation into the eye. A blood–aqueous barrier inhibits the entry of water-soluble drugs across the epithelium of the ciliary body into newly formed aqueous, and a blood–retinal barrier limits the entry of such drugs into the vitreous humor. Although drugs may reach a high concentration within the choroid via its fenestrated capillaries, diffusion across the outer retina is obstructed by tight junctions between the cells of the retinal pigment epithelium (the outer blood–retinal barrier), and across the retinal capillaries by endothelial tight junctions (the inner blood–retinal barrier).

In addition, anionic drugs (such as penicillins, cephalosporins and quinolones) present in the vitreous are actively transported out of the eye by the iris and ciliary epithelia, the retinal capillary endothelial cells and the retinal pigment epithelium (RPE), giving a half-life of about 8 h for such drugs introduced into the vitreous. There is also a *passive* route for outflow of the drugs, regardless of charge, by forward diffusion into the aqueous.

These barriers affect the potential for drugs to enter the vitreous space after systemic administration, as well as their retention after direct delivery into the vitreous. In the uninflamed eye, the highest aqueous concentrations using the systemic route are achieved by lipid-soluble drugs such as chloramphenicol or the fluoroquinolones. Negligible concentrations are achieved using water-soluble drugs, particularly those in anionic form (such as the penicillins and cephalosporins), which are actively transported out of the eye.

In the inflamed eye, breakdown of the blood–ocular barriers allows higher concentrations of antibiotic to be achieved in the ocular compartments following systemic therapy. Effective antimicrobial concentrations may be reached in the aqueous, but concentrations in the vitreous are still too low to provide adequate therapeutic levels, for instance in the treatment of endophthalmitis. Vitreous concentrations after high-dose systemic therapy in such situations will be subtherapeutic (0.5–2 mg/l) and much lower than those achievable by direct injection into the vitreous (up to 1000 mg/l). The latter route is always favored in the treatment of endophthalmitis and reliance should not be made on intravenous therapy alone.

The above barriers (Figure 56.1) do not exist for other orbital structures. Thus, infections within the orbit or ocular adnexae (the eyelids, lacrimal gland and nasolacrimal system) are readily accessible to systemic antibiotics.

MODES OF DELIVERY OF ANTIBIOTICS TO THE EYE

Some modes of delivery discussed here that are outside the specifications of the product licence and should be used at the clinician's responsibility.

TOPICAL PREPARATIONS

Drops and ointments are the standard means of administering antibiotics to the surface of the eye, either for prophylaxis or

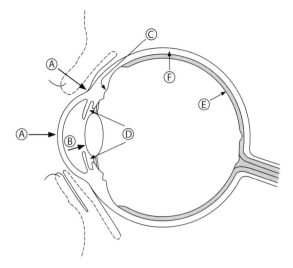

Fig. 56.1 (A) Epithelial barrier (breached by an ulcer; negotiated by topical drops or subconjunctival injection). (B) Aqueous-vitreous barrier. (C) Blood-aqueous barrier limits entry into the aqueous from the blood. (D) Iris pigment epithelial pump removes anions from the aqueous. (E) Blood-retinal barrier; external, pigment-epithelial barrier. (F) Internal, capillary-endothelial barrier. There is an outward pumping of anions across the retina.

treatment. Ointments prolong contact and permit less frequent instillation. Prior to the availability of commercial, topical quinolone drugs (0.3%), the preparation of fortified antibiotic eye drops was advocated for the treatment of suppurative keratitis. Their use still has a place. Fortified drops are prepared by combining commercially available parenteral preparations with artificial tear preparations or sterile water to widen the range and concentration of agents used.

PERIOCULAR INJECTION

Subconjunctival delivery involves the injection of 0.25–1.0 ml of antibiotic solution under the conjunctiva. There is some leakage of antibiotic back into the conjunctival sac, but the bolus chiefly acts as a depot for diffusion which will produce transient high levels of antibiotic in cornea, sclera, choroid and aqueous and, to a lesser and variable extent, the vitreous. Vitreous levels are lower because of the absorption of drug into the choroidal and retinal circulations, and because of the natural barriers to penetration into the vitreous across the retina (see above). Appropriate doses for subconjunctival injection are given in Table 55.3.

Peak aqueous levels are achieved in the first hour and effective levels are maintained for about 6 h. Inclusion of adrenaline in the subconjunctival injection prolongs antibiotic activity for 24 h or more, so that injections may be repeated less frequently. This is contraindicated in patients with cardiac disease, and caution must be exercised in the aged, or when patients are receiving general anesthesia with halothane. Where

Table 56.1 Selected topical antimicrobial drops: commercially available and fortified extemporaneous preparations

Antibacterial eye drops	Fortified[a] preparation	Commercial
Amikacin	25/50 mg/ml	
Bacitracin		10 000 U/ml (Not in UK)
Cefazolin	50 mg/ml	
Ceftazidime	50 mg/ml	
Cefuroxime	50 mg/ml	
Cephalotin	50 mg/ml	
Chloramphenicol[b]		5 mg/ml
Ciprofloxacin		3 mg/ml (0.3%)
Gentamicin	15 mg/ml	3 mg/ml
Framycetin		5 mg/ml
Fusidic acid gel		10 mg/ml
Levofloxacin	5 mg/ml	
Neomycin		5 mg/ml
Ofloxacin		3 mg/ml
Oxacillin	66 mg/ml	
Penicillin G	5000 U/ml (0.3%)	
Piperacillin	50 mg/ml	
Propamidine isethionate		1 mg/ml
Sulfacetamide		100–300 mg/ml
Tetracycline		10 mg/ml, oil vehicle
Ticarcillin	50 mg/ml	
Tobramycin	15 mg/ml	3 mg/ml
Teicoplanin	25 mg/ml	
Vancomycin	50 mg/ml	
Combinations		
Neosporin®:		
Polymyxin B		5000 U/ml
Gramicidin		25 U/ml
Neomycin		2.5 mg/ml
Polytrim®:		
Polymyxin B		10 000 U/ml
Trimethoprim		1 mg/ml
Antifungal eye drops		
Amphotericin[c]	1.5–3.0 mg/ml	
Clotrimazole	1% in arachis oil	
Econazole	1% in arachis oil	
Fluconazole	1% in arachis oil	
Flucytosine	1%	
Itraconazole	1% in arachis oil	
Miconazole	1% in arachis oil	
Natamycin[c]	50 mg/ml	
Antiprotozoal eye drops[d]		
Propamidine isethionate		0.1% (1 mg/ml)
Chlorhexidine digluconate	0.02% (200 mg/l)	

[a] Produced in hospital pharmacy.
[b] There is no evidence from new studies that topical chloramphenicol use in the eye contributes to bone marrow toxicity.[81,82]
[c] Aqueous suspension.
[d] For the treatment of *Acanthamoeba* keratitis.[38,83,84]

Box 56.1 Topical antimicrobial ointments

Antibacterial eye ointments	
Chloramphenicol[a]	1%
Chlortetracycline	1%
Erythromycin	0.5% (not commercially available)
Framycetin	0.5%
Gentamicin	0.3%
Neomycin	0.5%
Rifampicin	2.5% (not commercially available)
Sulfacetamide	2.5–10%
Tetracycline	1%
Antibacterial ointment combinations	
Graneodin®:	
Neomycin	0.25%
Gramicidin	0.025%
Polyfax®:	
Bacitracin	500 U/g
Polymyxin B	10 000 U/g
Polytrim®:	
Trimethoprim	0.5%
Polymyxin B	10 000 U/g
Antiprotozoal eye ointment	
Dibromopropamidine	0.15%

[a] There is no evidence from new studies that topical chloramphenicol use in the eye contributes to bone marrow toxicity.[81,82]

possible, the injection is delivered close to the site of infection, since tissue levels are highest near the site of the injection.

A sub-Tenon's injection is delivered in a similar volume but more deeply into the orbit, beneath Tenon's capsule and close to the sclera. Care must be taken to avoid penetration of the globe. It is said to achieve higher levels in the posterior eye than the more anterior, subconjunctival route.

Ofloxacin and ciprofloxacin have not yet been used routinely by the intravitreal route to treat endophthalmitis, although ciprofloxacin has been shown to be relatively nontoxic intravitreally in rabbits and to be removed by the active transport route similarly to cephalosporins. Recent studies by other routes[4,5] have shown that insufficient intravitreal levels are achieved to treat serious infective endophthalmitis.

Periocular injections require local anesthesia, and are not without complications. Conjunctival ischemia and necrosis may occur locally and orbital hemorrhage and penetration of the globe have been reported. Although high aqueous levels can be achieved, they are not sustained, and the use of frequent topical application of fortified antibiotic preparations is generally preferred to repeated periocular injections in the treatment of microbial keratitis.

INTRAVITREAL INJECTION

Intravitreal antibiotic injection is the standard treatment for endophthalmitis. Injected antibiotic persists in the vitreous in effective concentrations, for up to 96 h. Only a small volume is injected (up to 0.2 ml), and an equal volume of vitreous withdrawn, to minimize ocular pressure elevation and to provide a specimen for culture. The retina is sensitive to toxic damage; amounts injected are based on animal toxicity studies. Selected doses are indicated in Table 56.2.

The vitreous is entered via the pars plana to avoid retinal injury and sampling may be combined with a total vitrectomy to reduce the infective load and facilitate drug diffusion. The injection can be repeated at 48–72 h intervals according to clinical response. Subsequent vitreous samples can be used to assay the vitreous level of antibiotic.

Cationic drugs such as gentamicin have longer half-lives in the vitreous than anionic drugs such as penicillin, which are actively transported out of the vitreous space. This effect is less in the inflamed eye. Persistence of drug can be prolonged if the same drug is given systemically, since the outward diffusion gradient is decreased. In the case of certain anionic drugs, such as the penicillins, cephalosporins and ciprofloxacin, levels can be further increased by parenteral probenecid. This raises plasma levels by inhibiting renal tubular excretion, and blocks active transport out of the eye.

THE SYSTEMIC ROUTE

Systemic medication may be used to treat preseptal and orbital cellulitis, dacryoadenitis, acute dacryocystitis and the rare condition of ocular erysipelas (necrotizing fasciitis of the eyelids, which may need surgical debridement). In the management of chronic blepharitis, tetracyclines used in low dose (e.g. oxytetracycline 250 mg twice daily) may act by an effect on meibomian oil composition through inhibition of bacterial lipases.[6] In rosacea-associated blepharitis, oral tetracycline 250 mg twice daily or doxycycline 100 mg once daily will be effective in 50% of patients.[7]

Systemic medication may be combined with local therapy in the treatment of ophthalmia neonatorum due to *Neisseria gonorrhoeae*. *Chlamydia* or, rarely, *Pseudomonas* spp. It is also used in the treatment of adult chlamydial or gonococcal eye disease.

Systemic chemotherapy has no place in the management of uncomplicated bacterial keratitis. It is often employed in high dosage as adjunctive treatment of bacterial endophthalmitis but must *not* be used alone without intravitreal injection. It is mandatory in the management of metastatic endophthalmitis associated with septicemia. High-dose regimens should be closely monitored.

THE ROLE OF BIOFILMS IN OCULAR INFECTION

Many serious ocular infections are caused by virulent organisms invading a compromised eye. However, increasingly, indolent infections result from organisms harbored in biofilms, carried by a therapeutic device, including contact lenses, lens

Table 56.2 Selected intravitreal and parenteral antibiotics

Intravitreal injection[a] Agent	Dose (μg)	Effective Duration (h)	Intravenous injection, dose
Amikacin	400	24–28	15 mg/kg every 24 h[c]
Ampicillin	500	24	1 g 4-hourly
Amphotericin	5–10	–	0.1–1.0 mg/kg every 24 h[c]
Cefazolin	2000	16–24	1 g 4-hourly
Cefuroxime	2000	16–24	1.5 g 6-hourly
Ceftazidine	2000	–	1.5 g 6-hourly
Chloramphenicol[b]	–	–	0.75 g 6-hourly
Clindamycin	1000	16–24	0.75 g 8-hourly
Erythromcyin	500	50	0.5 g 6-hourly
Flucloxacillin	–	–	1 g 6-hourly
Gentamicin	100–200	48	5 mg/kg every 24 h[c]
Methicillin	2000	40	1 g 4-hourly
Penicillin	–	–	3 MU (1.8 g) 4-hourly
Vancomycin	1000	25	1 g 12-hourly

[a] Maximum intravitreal injection volume is usually 0.2 ml, i.e. 0.1 ml of each agent used in combination.
[b] Chloramphenicol given systemically penetrates to the vitreous to treat acute bacterial endophthalmitis satisfactorily providing the organism is sensitive to it; it should be reserved for therapy when intravitreal antibiotics cannot be given, but must be used within 48 h of the start of endophthalmitis if useful vision is to be saved.
[c] Administered in three divided doses.

cases, sutures and explants, keratoprostheses and intraocular lens implants.[8] Similar infections occur on heart valves, joint prostheses and indwelling catheters. The polymer becomes a physical vector, conveying the biofilm to the eye.

THE BIOFILM

Micro-organisms responsible

A biofilm is an association of replicating micro-organisms within their polysaccharide glycocalyx. Certain strains of *Staphylococcus epidermidis* or *Pseudomonas* spp. secrete a glycocalyx, which will attach to and encase the biopolymer, dividing slowly and colonizing the device. For *Staph. epidermidis* and *Staph. aureus*, attachment may be enhanced by the presence of fibronectin.

Free-swimming organisms such as *Ps. aeruginosa* are ideally suited to the formation of biofilms. Having formed a glycocalyx they divide at a slower rate than in the planktonic conditions (5–15 times slower). Bacteria within the biofilm are relatively inaccessible to antibiotics, biocides, surfactants, antibodies, bacteriophages and neutrophils, and are consequently better able to survive attack. The levels of antibiotics required to inhibit growth within the biofilm may be 20–1000 times higher than that required to inhibit planktonic growth. Antigens expressed at the biofilm surface can activate complement.

Biofilm-related infections tend to be chronic, resistant to antibiotics, polymicrobial and culture negative, since treatment may effectively free tissue fluids from planktonic forms, and shedding may be intermittent. The sensitivity to antibiotics of shed forms is usually higher than that of organisms within the biofilm.[9] To obtain positive cultures it may be necessary to sample directly from the device and to release the bacteria with ultrasound. Simple or non-nutrient agar should be used in addition to normal cultural procedures.

Antibiotic resistance within the biofilm results in part from binding of the antibiotic, with a variable effect on sensitivity. Thus ciprofloxacin is inhibited more than tobramycin. Also, antibacterial enzymes, such as β-lactamases produced by resistant staphylococci, are concentrated within the biofilm and reduce the antibiotic action of some penicillins and cephalosporins.

BIOFILMS ON OPHTHALMIC BIOMATERIALS

Silicone polymers, polymethylmethacrylate, hydrogels, nylon, polypropylene, aluminium oxide ceramics and Teflon, may be non-specifically colonized. The subject is fully reviewed by Wilson.[10] Biofilms are encountered in the following situations:

Contact lenses

The incidence of contact lens-associated keratitis increased greatly with the introduction of hydrogel lenses, particularly for extended wear lenses and to a lesser extent with daily wear lenses. Risk is associated with overnight wear and poor lens hygiene. A number of studies have demonstrated the same strains of organism in the lens case and in saline dispensers used for lens care.

The sequence of events leading to infection is as follows:

1. Organisms, such as staphylococci, are transferred to the surface of a contact lens from the commensal population of the eye or by lens handling when there is poor lens hygiene.
2. Overnight wet storage of a soft hydrogel lens provides an environment which encourages the glycocalyx formation.
3. Home-made storage solutions from a saline dispenser increase the bacterial load by adding organisms from the dispenser nozzle.
4. Organisms within an established biofilm are relatively protected from storage preservatives, although the preservatives may kill organisms shed from the biofilm. Lens storage cases tend to be washed in tap water, contaminating the case with coliforms and *Ps. aeruginosa*. The lens and its case become a reservoir for organisms and a physical vector from which organisms or their products can be transferred to the ocular surface during wear, to establish an infection.

The risk of infection is multiplied 5–10 times when there is extended, overnight wear of the lens, because of the increased exposure time and because conditions at the ocular surface are altered during prolonged eye closure. During sleep, the ocular surface is in a pro-inflammatory state and the tears are rich in polymorphonuclear neutrophils and their digestive enzymes. Tear flow is almost at a standstill and IgA makes up the major fraction of the tear proteins. The new extended-wear silicone hydrogel lenses provide greater oxygen transmission and reduce the risk of hypoxia. Cases of microbial keratitis have been reported with this new lens, although the incidence may be less than with non-silicone hydrogels. This suggests, that, while hypoxic edema may be an important element in the pathogeneticity of lens-associated infections, it is not the sole risk factor.

Contact lens – associated keratitis

Ps. aeruginosa is the most common cause of contact lens-associated keratitis, while among the Gram-positive organisms, *Staph. aureus* and coagulase-negative staphylococci are the next most common. Those coagulase-negative strains with virulence factors for contact lens-associated keratitis adhere more effectively to biomaterials and resist disinfection.

Acanthameba are of particular interest because their growth is encouraged by the presence of other organisms and they feed on bacterial products. The trophozoite and cyst stages are introduced from tap water, showers and hot tubs. In the USA and UK, about 85% of infections have been contact lens-associated; in South India, where most of the infections arise from corneal trauma to the eyes of paddy-field workers, the figure is 1%.

Mycotic keratitis in soft lens wearers occurs most frequently in relation to extended-wear therapeutic lenses, when yeasts predominate, or with aphakic lenses, when filamentous fungi are more frequent.

Prevention of biofilm-related, contact lens-associated keratitis

Preventive measures include:

1. Good hygiene and removal of proteinaceous contact lens deposits.
2. The use of cleaners and surfactants to remove adherent micro-organisms, or multipurpose solutions that clean and disinfect (polyhexamethylene biguanide or polyquat) with little toxic residual activity.
3. Avoidance of home-prepared saline, or chlorine tablet-based solutions, which are prone to microbial contamination.[10]

Hydrogen peroxide within 10 minutes is an effective microbicide against bacteria and within 60 minutes against some filamentous fungi. Hydrogen peroxide 3% is effective against the trophozoites and cysts of *Acanthamoeba* over a period of 6 hours.[11] Catalytic neutralization of hydrogen peroxide allows microbial contamination and is not recommended. The 'gold standard' for soft lenses is 3% hydrogen peroxide overnight followed by neutralization with a thiosulfate/catalase solution made up from tablets.

Sutures

Biofilms can form around unburied sutures with a sequence of events including attachment to the hydrophobic polymer, colonization and biofilm formation. Once formed, a suture biofilm may give rise to a stitch abscess, corneal abscess, or infectious crystalline keratopathy.

Infectious crystalline keratopathy is an indolent condition of intrastromal, bacterial multiplication within a biofilm, in which the close packing of micro-organisms and disturbance of stromal lamellae gives rise to a crystalline appearance on biomicroscopy.[12] Most cases occur as a complication of surgery or keratitis. The organism responsible for infectious crystalline keratopathy is usually an α-hemolytic streptococcus, although other bacteria and, rarely, fungi or amebae, have been incriminated. For streptococci, intensive treatment with topical vancomycin or bacitracin is recommended, although penetration is poor in the absence of an epithelial defect.

Punctal plugs

Punctal plugs are used to provide long-term occlusion of the lacrimal puncta, in order to conserve tears in dry eye states. Biofilms around punctal plugs occasionally give rise to canaliculitis or dacryocystitis. Infected canalicular plugs may be removed under direct vision, or flushed down the nasolacrimal duct.

Explants for retinal surgery

Both solid and sponge explants cause infection by means of a biofilm, although bacteria adhere more readily to sponge explants, presumably because of their greater surface area. Organisms include *Staph. aureus*, coagulase-negative staphylococci, *Ps. aeruginosa*, *Proteus spp.*, *Moraxella spp.*, *Branhamella catarrhalis*; coagulase-negative staphylococci predominates. The frequency of infection has been estimated to be 0.6%.

Intraocular lens implants

While 15% of aqueous samples at the end of cataract surgery contain bacteria, endophthalmitis is not an inevitable consequence. Lens implantation can none the less be associated with a chronic, saccular or capsular bag-associated endophthalmitis due to coagulase-negative staphylococci, diphtheroids and *P. acnes* from a biofilm around the implant or due to macrophage-associated bacteria within the capsule remnant.[13] The non-purulent inflammatory reaction probably reflects a loss of anterior chamber-associated immune deviation. Systemic azithromycin or clarithromycin can provide effective therapy and high intracellular concentrations.[14]

MICROBIAL INFECTIONS OF THE EYE

BLEPHARITIS

Blepharitis is an inflammation of the lid margins involving either the lash line (anterior blepharitis) or the meibomian oil glands (posterior blepharitis). Both forms are often associated with skin diseases, such as seborrheic and atopic dermatitis and acne rosacea.[3,15]

Anterior blepharitis

Staphylococcal blepharitis implies an anterior blepharitis with lash collarettes, crusting, lid ulceration and folliculitis, and a positive culture for *Staph. aureus*. This is an indication for antimicrobial treatment. However, a positive culture alone does not warrant treatment since the lid margins are colonized with *Staph. aureus* in 6–15% of normal lids, rising to 50% in atopes. Similarly, coagulase-negative staphylococci are isolated from over 80% of normal lid margins.

Chronic anterior blepharitis is common and requires regular cleansing of the lid margins with dilute bicarbonate or baby lotion to remove adherent scales. Misdirected lashes must also be removed. Culture of the lid margin requires 'scrubbing' with a swab soaked in sterile broth, and plating directly onto blood agar and a selective medium for *Staph. aureus*. A staphylococcal blepharitis is treated with topical ophthalmic fusidic acid gel 1%, 2–4 times daily, or with Oc. polytrim or Oc. tetracycline. A highly active staphylococcal blepharitis merits a course of systemic antistaphylococcal therapy, such as flucloxacillin (oxacillin) or erythromycin (500 mg four times daily for 4 days). Patients should be encouraged to wash with antiseptic soaps to suppress the carriage of *Staph. aureus* at other skin sites with a disinfectant such as chlorhexidine.[16]

Anterior blepharitis may respond to short courses of hydrocortisone lotion or ointment, 0.5%, applied sparingly to the lid margin.

Posterior blepharitis

The most common form of posterior blepharitis is obstructive meibomian gland dysfunction (MGD), which is highly symptomatic. Lid margins are thickened and red, there is plugging of the meibomian gland orifices and lid oil is poorly expressible. MGD is treated by daily heat to the lids, to increase oil fluidity and firm massage to express retained secretions.

Generally, MGD is not an infective condition but both anterior and posterior blepharitis are accompanied by an increase in commensals, which produce lipases capable of releasing fatty acids from the lipid esters of the tear oils. These contribute to the inflammation and the lipases are inhibitable by sub-antimicrobial levels of tetracycline, given intermittently as oxytetracycline (250 mg twice daily) or doxycycline (50 mg daily), for 3 months, which can be repeated after a 3-month interval. Minocycline has been proposed for recalcitrant staphylococcal blepharitis[17] and erythromycin in children, to avoid dental abnormalities.

Atopy

Atopic blepharitis should not be confused with staphylococcal blepharitis, although they may co-exist. Non-inflamed lids in patients with atopic dermatitis are colonized with *Staph. aureus*,[18] as is the conjunctiva and nasal mucosa and skin. While tear IgE levels are high, they are not directed against *Staph. aureus* antigens. Both anterior and posterior blepharitis occurring in association with atopic dermatitis is treated as in non-atopes.

Rosacea

Acne rosacea is also associated with blepharitis and the lids are often colonized by *Staph. aureus*. Although cell-mediated immunity to *Staph. aureus* is enhanced, it is not known whether this is cause or effect. In a randomized, placebo-controlled crossover trial, symptomatic improvement of blepharitis in mild rosacea occurred in 90% of patients receiving topical fusidic acid (Fucithalmic) compared with 50% in those on oral oxytetracycline. This improvement did not occur in non-rosacea blepharitis. The non-infective keratitis of rosacea is treated with topical steroid.

STYES

Styes are painful microabscesses of the lid margin, at the base of a lash follicle. Colonization of the lash base with *Staph. aureus* is well recognized. Styes may respond to the application of heat, combined with a topical antibiotic with good tissue-penetration, 4–6 times daily (e.g. ofloxacin, ciprofloxacin, chloramphenicol, or fusidic acid gel). Resistant cases may require treatment with a systemic antistaphylococcal agent.

CHALAZIA

A chalazion is a granuloma within the meibomian glands, associated with obstruction of the gland orifices. It usually forms a painless swelling, which may resolve without treatment or may require incision and curettage. Although heat and antibiotic ointment are prescribed, there is no evidence for infection, but acute chalazion is a painful, infective condition which responds to systemic antimicrobials.

CONJUNCTIVITIS

Conjunctivitis can be due to bacteria, chlamydia, viruses, fungi, protozoa and helminths (Box 56.2). Non-infective causes include allergy or toxicity. Toxicity may be due to preservatives, such as benzalkonium chloride, associated with tear substitutes or, occasionally to circulating bacterial toxins.

Clinical presentation

Bacterial conjunctivitis presents with an acute purulent discharge, which frequently becomes bilateral. Viral conjunctivitis is usually associated with a watery discharge and in both viral and chlamydial conjunctivitis there is often a follicular conjunctival response. Bacterial conjunctivitis may sometimes be confused with viral or chlamydial disease but an associated urethritis or proctitis points to chlamydial infection.

Microbial diagnosis and treatment

The patient's history will often give a clue to the organism responsible.

Presumed bacterial conjunctivitis
Swabs should be collected for smears (for Gram and acridine orange stains) and for culture on blood and chocolate agars (and a selected gonococcal agar if relevant). Culture should take place in carbon dioxide at 37°C for 48 h. Treatment is listed in Table 56.1 and Box 56.1 (p. 745).

Presumed chlamydial conjunctivitis
The diagnosis is confirmed by polymerase chain reaction or using a monoclonal antibody (e.g. the 'Syvamicrotrak' test).

Box 56.2 Microbial and other causes of conjunctivitis

Bacteria
- *Staph. aureus*, associated with blepharitis.
- *Streptococcus pneumoniae*, associated with sinus disease.
- *Str. pyogenes*, associated with throat infections.
- *Listeria monocytogenes*, associated with rural and farmyard dust (Farmer's eye).
- *Corynebacterium diphtheriae*, associated with a pseudomembrane.
- *Neisseria meningitidis/gonorrhoeae*, associated with throat/genital infection.
- *Pseudomonas aeruginosa*, associated with contact lens wear.
- *Klebsiella pneumoniae* and *other* Enterobacteriaceae, associated with contact lens wear.
- *Proteus* spp., associated with old age (more in men than women).
- *Moraxella* spp., associated with damaged ocular surface.
- *Haemophilus influenzae*, associated with intrinsic throat flora.

Chlamydia
- *Chlamydia trachomatis*, associated with overcrowding, poor hygiene and flies (encouraged by cattle dung) in the Near and Middle East and tropics.
- Trachoma/inclusion conjunctivitis, associated with genital infection in Western countries (may be transmitted in swimming pools).

Viruses
- *Herpes simplex*, associated with corneal disease.
- *Herpes zoster*, associated with affection of the fifth nerve.
- Adenovirus, associated with epidemics from shipyards, close living quarters, and eye clinics (via tonometers and staff handling of patients); early diagnosis is required to bring outbreaks to a quick halt.
- Acute hemorrhagic conjunctivitis: enterovirus 70, poliovirus and Coxsackie A24v are associated with epidemics and occasional paralysis; it is associated with foreign travel, especially Singapore, Hong Kong and Calcutta.
- Conjunctivitis occurs with systemic infection in measles, mumps and dengue, glandular fever and hepatitis A infection.

Fungi
Fungal conjunctivitis is uncommon, but may complicate fungal keratitis.

Helminths
- *Thellazia capillaris* and *Thellazia californensis*, associated with birds in the Middle East and the USA.
- *Loa loa*, subconjunctival worm occurring in tropical countries.

Protozoa
Protozoa include *Acanthamoeba* spp. associated with contact lens wear, or rural corneal trauma and keratitis.

Conjunctival cells are scraped using a spatula and placed on special slides provided in the kit.

The older and cheapest method involved Giemsa staining for intracytoplasmic (Bedson) bodies (complete chlamydial cells lacking a traditional bacterial cell wall). Under ultraviolet light, the stained chlamydiae fluoresce yellow, non-specifically, rendering the method more sensitive.

Presumed viral conjunctivitis

A conjunctival swab is placed in viral transport medium. Inoculation into tissue culture or immunofluoresce testing offer rapid and sensitive tests.

Therapy

Bacterial conjunctivitis

Therapy requires antibacterial drops or ointment for 5 days. If a primary culture is not collected, treatment with a broad spectrum antibiotic should be given, such as chloromycetin, gentamycin or Polytrim®. Fluoroquinolone drops may be kept in reserve. (e.g. ciprofloxacin, levofloxacin, lomefloxacin, or ofloxacin.). If treatment fails, then conjunctival specimens should be collected, after stopping drop therapy, including specimens for chlamydia where appropriate. (A positive culture for chlamydia is more likely in this situation after gentamycin use, since the aminoglycosides do not suppress chlamydial growth.).

Ophthalmia neonatorum

Ophthalmia neonatorum is defined as any purulent discharge from the eyes during the first 28 days of life. The presentation may be hyperacute and infection may progress rapidly to keratitis and perforation, leading to blindness. It is an important cause of blindness in low-income countries.[19] Ophthalmia neonatorum in the UK occurs in up to 12% of live births but gonococcal infection is now rare. Elsewhere, the incidence of gonococcal conjunctivitis varies from 0.04% of live births in the West to 1.0% in parts of Africa. The incidence of neonatal chlamydial ophthalmia in London has been estimated to be less than 1%.

Neonatal prophylaxis with topical oxytetracycline provides protection against both gonococcal and chlamydial ophthalmia, without the toxicity of silver nitrate drops (Créde's solution).[20]

Systemic treatment for gonococcal keratoconjunctivitis is essential, with 30 mg of benzylpenicillin/kg in two daily doses for 7 days. Isolation of penicillin-resistant strains has led to the use of β-lactamase-stable cephalosporins such as ceftriaxone 25–40 mg/kg intravenously every 12 h for 3 days, combined with topical saline lavage and antibiotic ointment (e.g. Oc. gentamicin). Single-dose intramuscular therapy may be appropriate when there is no corneal involvement. As is the case with neonatal chlamydial ophthalmia, the infection must be treated systemically.

TRACHOMA AND OTHER CHLAMYDIAL DISEASE

Ocular infection by *Chlamydia trachomatis* takes three forms: trachoma, adult chlamydial ophthalmia and neonatal chlamydial ophthalmia.

Trachoma affects 500 million people in developing countries and accounts for 5–10 million blind patients. It is caused by the chlamydial serovars A, B and C and is transmitted by 'eye-seeking' flies. In hyperendemic areas 30–50% of the population have active disease and 10% exhibit blinding sequelae. Although infection may be encountered as early as the second month of life, active inflammatory disease is most common in preschool children, when the infection leads to conjunctival scarring, ectropion and trichiasis, causing recurrent microbial keratitis from repeated corneal infection and trauma. Blinding sequelae occur after the age of 40 years. Public health intervention is required to prevent spread of the infection and reinfection during childhood. The World Health Organization program for the elimination of trachoma (GET 2020) has adopted the SAFE strategy of control measures (Surgery for ectropion and entropion, Antibiotics for infectious trachoma, Facial cleanliness to reduce transmission by the fly vector and Environmental improvements, such as control of disease-spreading flies, improved access to clean water, and provision of latrines).[21]

Adult chlamydial ophthalmia, also known as inclusion conjunctivitis, and neonatal chlamydial ophthalmia result from sexual transmission. They are caused by serotypes D–K. The adult disease has its greatest prevalence between the ages of 15 and 20 years. The neonatal form may rarely occur immediately after birth, but presents most commonly in the first week or up to 6 weeks later. Treatment of maternal genital chlamydia trachomatis infection during pregnancy, usually with erythromycin, is an important preventive measure.

Treatment

C. trachomatis is unresponsive to aminoglycosides and only partially susceptible to chloramphenicol and penicillin, which adversely affect growth in culture media. For this reason, transport media for chlamydial culture do not contain penicillin. The organism is fully sensitive to the tetracyclines, erythromycin and other macrolides including azithromycin, rifampicin and the quinolones. Some authorities regard quinolones as second-line treatment. It is also sensitive to chlorhexidine.

Topical treatment of trachoma with tetracycline or erythromycin ointment or quinolone drops can be effective given 2–3 times daily for 6 weeks. In trachoma, treatment of other family members, or whole villages, is necessary to prevent reinfection. Treatment of the early, active, inflammatory stages is effective with a single dose of azithromycin, which is now the preferred therapy, but the cost is higher.[22]

Systemic therapy is necessary for the treatment or prophylaxis of systemic manifestations such as cervicitis, uveitis, upper respiratory or ear disorders and Reiter's disease in adult chlamydial ophthalmia, and for pharyngitis, vaginitis and a potentially fatal pneumonitis in the neonatal disease.

Adult chlamydial ophthalmia treatment with oral tetracycline, erythromycin or rifampicin for 2 weeks has been recommended but long-acting tetracyclines, such as doxycycline and minocycline, offer convenience and improved compliance, as fewer doses are required and dietary constraints are not necessary. Oral azithromycin therapy is effective with a single dose. The patient and partner(s) should be checked for genital carriage and treated with erythromycin or azithromycin if positive.

A suitable treatment for neonatal chlamydial ophthalmia is oral erythromycin 50 mg/kg per 24 h in four divided doses for 2–3 weeks. Topical therapy may be used adjunctively, but is inadequate on its own (see also Ch. 59).

VIRAL CONJUNCTIVITIS

Primary herpes simplex causes a watery blepharoconjunctivitis, which responds well to aciclovir ointment 3% five times daily.

Adenovirus conjunctivitis may begin unilaterally, but commonly becomes bilateral and may cause a disabling punctate keratitis. In its acute form it lasts up to 21 days, but full recovery from visual sequelae may take several months. While no commercial agent is currently available, promising results have been obtained with cidofovir. Current management is palliative; cultures should be undertaken to confirm the diagnosis and inform in relation to potential epidemics.

Acute hemorrhagic conjunctivitis may occur in epidemics and is due to enterovirus 70; mild paralysis occasionally ensues. Diagnosis is usually clinical. Viral culture should be performed if possible for epidemiologic reasons. No specific antiviral therapy is available and treatment is symptomatic.

OTHER FORMS OF CONJUNCTIVITIS

Treatment of *Acanthamoeba* conjunctivitis and (epi)scleritis is dealt with in the section on keratitis (p. 751).

CANALICULITIS

Recurrent unilateral conjunctivitis due to an antibiotic-sensitive bacterium such as *H. influenzae*, can be the presenting symptom of a canaliculitis due to *Actinomyces* spp. (formerly *Streptothrix* or *Leptothrix*), or *Arachnia propionica*. The organism does not usually invade the canaliculus wall but forms a 'fungal' ball that obstructs the lumen. The canaliculus provides a microaerophilic environment, which supports the growth of non-fastidious anaerobic bacteria, and becomes infected with endogenous flora.

Pus, massaged along the canaliculus to the punctum, can be Gram stained to show typical, branching Gram-positive bacilli. Prolonged anaerobic culture on blood agar plates is necessary to demonstrate actinomycetes. Thioglycolate broth should also be inoculated. Sensitivity tests should be performed.

Actinomycetes and *Arachnia* spp. are usually sensitive to penicillin, tetracycline and erythromycin but resistant to aminoglycosides. Initial treatment involves irrigating the canaliculus with penicillin. If this fails the canaliculus is opened and debrided and material removed is Gram-stained and cultured. The canaliculus should be treated with 5% povidone iodine for 5 min as an effective antiseptic, syringed daily for 7 days with penicillin, and the patient reviewed at 3 months.

DACRYOCYSTITIS

Acute dacryocystitis is caused by nasolacrimal stasis, with *Staph. aureus* or streptococci as the usual causes. Infection may respond to systemic chemotherapy or require drainage of a lacrimal sac abscess and ultimately dacryocystorhinostomy.

Chronic dacryocystitis, commonly involving Gram-negative organisms, can only be treated effectively by relieving the nasolacrimal duct obstruction.

The postoperative infection rate in patients undergoing dacryocystorhinostomy is greatly reduced by a single dose of intraoperative cefuroxime intravenously (750 mg).

MICROBIAL KERATITIS

Suppurative bacterial keratitis presents clinically with acute pain, globe redness, lid swelling, watering and visual loss, accompanying a corneal stromal infiltrate or abscess with an overlying ulcer. Common causes are given in Box 56.3. It is usually central, but can be peripheral, particularly if traumatic. Because the cornea is only about 0.5 mm thick, such an ulcer may rapidly progress to perforation within 24 h of onset. In this case, in the aphakic or in the pseudophakic eye with a capsulotomy, there is access to the vitreous space and a secondary endophthalmitis may supervene. There is an urgent need to treat bacterial keratitis with high doses of effective antibiotic. Corneal transplantation may be required later, to deal with corneal scarring or perforation.

Box 56.3 Bacteria causing bacterial keratitis

Gram-positive cocci
Staphylococcus aureus
Coagulase-negative staphylococci
Streptococcus pneumoniae
Streptococcus pyogenes
Viridans streptococci
Anaerobic streptococci (rare)

Gram-negative coccobacilli
Moraxella spp.
Neisseria gonorrhoeae
Neisseria meningitidis

Gram-positive rods
Corynebacterium diphtheriae (rare)
Diphtheroids (rare)

Gram-negative rods
Pseudomonas aeruginosa
Proteus spp.
Klebsiella pneumoniae
Escherichia coli
Serratia marcescens
Acinetobacter spp.
Morganella morganii
Other enteric bacteria

Acid-fast bacteria
Mycobacterium chelonei
Nocardia asteroides

In northern climates bacteria account for over 80% of cases, with 60% in the south, where fungal keratitis is more common. In tropical regions the risk of fungal infection is even higher.[23] Mixed bacterial and fungal infections are common in the tropics.

In the past, suppurative keratitis was due chiefly to trauma, or occurred in compromised eyes with existing corneal disease. In recent years, however, there has been a rapid increase in contact lens-associated keratitis, most of which is bacterial. In general, the risk is much lower for wearers of hard lenses than soft-lens wearers and is greater with extended wear than daily wear. The risk has not been removed by the introduction of 'disposable' contact lenses or oxygen-permeable silicone hydrogels.

In three multicenter case-controlled studies, the overall risk for ulcerative keratitis with extended-wear lenses was four times greater than that for daily wear. In addition, overnight wear of contact lenses increased the risk of keratitis to 10–15 times that occurring with daily wear alone.[23] Wearing soft contact lenses in corneal graft patients also increases the risk of microbial keratitis.

The incidence of contact lens-associated microbial keratitis has been estimated to be 1 in 500 for extended-wear patients and 1 in 2500 in daily-wear patients.[23] The bacteria responsible for contact lens-associated keratitis include those usually associated with suppurative keratitis, but Gram-negative bacteria are more common than Gram-positive, with *Ps. aeruginosa* the most frequent. Contamination of contact lens care solutions is an important potential source of keratitis, with homemade solutions a major risk factor.[11]

Diagnosis

Diagnosis depends on smears and cultures from direct scrapes of the corneal ulcer.[24] The base and edge of the ulcer are most likely to yield organisms.

One drop of unpreserved amethocaine or benoxinate is instilled. The first scrape should be taken for microscopy, using a platinum spatula, large-gauge needle, or surgical blade. A fresh sterile instrument is used for each sample and the material gathered is spread onto a clean glass slide. This is air-dried and a second scrape is taken for a second slide. A third scrape should be cultured by plating out on to blood, chocolate and Sabouraud agars; then a fluid medium, preferably brain–heart infusion, should be inoculated with the same instrument. In addition, a Löwenstein–Jensen slope should be inoculated if the keratitis is chronic, although the atypical *Mycobacterium chelonae* will grow on blood agar if incubated for one week at 37°C. With chronic ulcers, blood agar should be incubated for 1 week in 4% CO_2 in order to culture *Nocardia* spp.

When *Acanthamoeba keratitis* is suspected an appropriate specimen should be taken (p. 751).

Media should be inoculated directly at the slit lamp or operating microscope. If possible, duplicate specimens should be taken, to culture at different temperatures. Transport media should not be necessary. Culture of agar plates should always take place at 37°C for one week. The fluid media should be incubated at 30°C in 4% CO_2 for at least 3 weeks. Anaerobic cultures should be considered when there is an unsatisfactory response to therapy.

Stains include Gram stain and acridine orange for common bacteria, modified Ziehl–Neelsen stain (decolorizing with 5% acetic acid only) for nocardia and mycobacteria, full Ziehl–Neelsen stain for mycobacteria and periodic acid Schiff (PAS) or methenamine silver (Grocott) stains for fungi and protozoal cysts. Selective stains include the use of labelled polyclonal or monoclonal antibodies. Acridine orange and Gram stains together will identify organisms in about 80% of cases. It is also possible to maximize the available material and decolorize and restain the same slide with a further intermediate stain and finally, an end stain.

TREATMENT OF SUPPURATIVE KERATITIS

An historical review of current therapy is provided by Baum and Barza[25]. Treatment is usually initiated with either a commercial preparation of ofloxacin 0.3%, or ciprofloxacin 0.3%, or alternatively, with combination drop therapy using fortified preparations prepared in the hospital pharmacy. A common empirical combination is gentamicin or tobramycin 1.5% (15 mg/ml) with cefazolin or 5% cefuroxime (50 mg/ml).

Trials have demonstrated that monotherapy with fluoroquinolones is as effective as combination therapy in the treatment of bacterial keratitis,[26–29] with greater toxicity in the combined group. Fortified preparations may have an advantage in the management of advanced disease, and the growing recognition of bacterial resistance to the fluoroquinolones[30] suggests that there should be caution in adopting monotherapy as a universal approach.

Drops are given every 15–30 min day and night, and then hourly, for the first 3 days, then 2-hourly by day and night, weaning according to response and cultural findings. It is unusual to modify therapy on the basis of the smear report alone, unless fungi are identified. An exception is the identification of *Str. pneumoniae*, when penicillin drops should be substituted. Successful eradication of bacterial infection is reported in about 90% of patients treated in this way. Ofloxacin treatment causes less irritation. Topical ciprofloxacin can leave microcrystalline corneal deposits. Fortified gentamicin drops cause an inferior, perilimbal conjunctival necrosis which resolves on withdrawing therapy.

Where frequent application is not possible, as in a child or a disturbed individual, subconjunctival injections of gentamicin 40 mg and cefazolin 100 mg can be delivered under general anesthetic. In the absence of cardiac disease, inclusion of epinephrine 0.3 ml (of 1:1000) in 1 ml of solution prolongs the tissue concentration of antibiotic from 6 to 24 h. Other regimens are given in Box 56.4.

Drop use varies from center to center. Where monotherapy is used, a loading dose of one drop every minute for five doses

Box 56.4 Suppurative bacterial keratitis: specific antibiotic regimens for topical or periocular therapy

---

Initial therapy

To treat unknown organism(s) (new case or no growth on presentation):

- ofloxacin 0.3% or ciprofloxacin 0.3%, or
- cefuroxime (5%) + gentamicin (1.5%).

These therapies will treat the following organisms:

- *Staph. aureus*
- Coagulase-negative staphylococci
- *Streptococcus* spp.
- *Haemophilus influenzae*
- *Klebsiella* spp.
- *Proteus* spp.
- Other Enterobacteriaceae

***Pseudomonas aeruginosa* infection (culture-proven or suspected)**

Ticarcillin or piperacillin (5%) + gentamicin (1.5%) and/or ceftazidime (5%) and/or ciprofloxacin (ofloxacin) (0.3%).

Note: Ticarcillin and piperacillin should not be used when penicillin allergy is suspected. Cephalosporins should also be avoided when there is a history of an anaphylactic reaction to penicillin.

Nocardial and mycobacterial keratitis

See text.

Fungal keratitis (hyphae or yeasts seen on smear or fungus cultured)

Hyphal infection (*Aspergillus* spp., *Fusarium* spp.): natamycin (5%) or amphotericin B (0.15–0.3%).

Yeast infection (*Candida* spp.): clotrimazole (or other imidazole) at 1% in arachis oil eye drops or flucytosine 1% drops.

---

can be initiated, and repeated hourly, to achieve high initial levels in the cornea. In the USA, a regimen of fortified drops every 15–30 min, day and night is recommended on an outpatient basis for 3 days in the first instance. In the UK it is usual to admit patients to hospital. Antibiotic ointment may be given at night once infection is under control. Systemic antibiotics have no place in the management of bacterial keratitis in the absence of limbal involvement or perforation.

Antibiotics are modified according to the results of cultures and clinical response. If there is a clear clinical response, the same regimen should be continued. Susceptibility tests may be misleading because they assume lower tissue antibiotic levels than achievable in the cornea during topical therapy: therapy is reduced by increasing the interval between drops every 3–4 days, not by reducing their concentration. The decision to terminate therapy is based on clinical response and nature of the causative organism.

If there is no response, topical therapy is stopped, the clinical condition reappraised after 24 or 48 h and the cornea rescraped. A full search must be made for fastidious organisms.

If no organism is identified, a second-line broad-spectrum empirical antibiotic regimen should be started, to include antimicrobial action against resistant streptococci, nocardia and mycobacteria. This may include drop therapy with topical vancomycin 50 mg/ml (5%) plus amikacin 50 mg/ml (5%) and trimethoprim 0.1% (given as Polytrim®), substituting erythromycin (0.5%) or rifampicin (2.5%) ointment at night). This situation is less likely since the introduction of topical quinolone therapy, since quinolones are effective against nocardia and mycobacteria, although not against resistant streptococci.

Special cases

Treatment of *M. chelonae* infection requires topical amikacin or ciprofloxacin. This mycobacterium, which causes a chronic keratitis and may follow radial keratotomy, is resistant to the common antituberculosis drugs.

Nocardia causes a refractory keratitis. Therapy usually demands surgery to debulk the infectious load, plus antibiotics. Antibiotics alone often fail, despite apparent full in-vitro sensitivity. A combination of topical amikacin (always) plus erythromycin and/or vancomycin and/or trimethoprim has been used successfully. Isolates are resistant to penicillin but may be sensitive to sulfonamides. The new generation of macrolides (azithromycin and clarithromycin) may prove useful.

Acanthamoeba infection

Acanthamebae are free-living protozoa, found in fresh-water ponds, lakes, domestic water supplies, swimming pools and soil. Subclinical exposure occurs frequently and antibodies against *Acanthamoeba* are common. *Acanthamoeba* keratitis was first recognized between 1973 and 1975 and this was followed in the 1980s by a virtual epidemic of cases, related to the expansion of contact lens use:[31] in various series, 71–85% of patients have been contact lens wearers.[32] In the UK, this infection has occurred in 1 in 6750 contact lens wearers[11,33] but the figure has reduced since multipurpose solutions were introduced for lens storage and disinfection.[34] In Asia it is associated with rural, traumatic eye disease and presentation is often late.[35] The subject is reviewed by McCulley et al.[36] and O'Day and Head.[37]

Persons who present with an unusual keratitis after exposure to hot tubs or natural springs may have *Acanthamoeba* keratitis. A high index of suspicion must be maintained for all contact lens-related keratopathies presenting with epithelial infiltrations, especially with a 'snowstorm' appearance, multiple superficial abscesses or dendritiform ulcers. A keratoneuritis (corneal nerve infiltration) is diagnostic and *Acanthamoeba* cysts may be visible in vivo by confocal microscopy. Suppurative keratitis that is 'culture-negative' and resistant to standard therapy may be due to *Acanthamoeba* infection.

Diagnosis

Early diagnosis, when the infection is confined to epithelium or anterior stroma, is important for a successful outcome. Sheets of cells should be removed for both culture and microscopy. Identification of cysts in wet mounts may establish the diagnosis within 10 min of collection. The epithelial material is placed in a conical tube containing 2 ml saline, agitated on a vibrator, centrifuged, and the deposit inspected by wet-field microscopy at × 100.

If the disease has progressed to a stromal ring abscess, epithelial scrapes may not yield viable organisms. Cysts from the midst of the abscess may fail to excyst, and results may be delayed. Corneal biopsy allows sampling of the deep infiltrate for viable trophozoites. Both culture and electron microscopy are useful to demonstrate stromal amebae.

For culture, scrapes are inoculated onto non-nutrient agar, ideally made up in Page's amebal saline. If non-nutrient agar without Page's saline is used, then the plate should be inoculated again with a suspension of heat-killed *K. pneumoniae* or other Enterobacteriaceae as a nutrient source for the amebae. The plate is incubated at 32°C for 4 weeks. Amebae are usually visible by light microscopy after 1 week; after 2 weeks the whole plate is covered by the typical double-walled, star-shaped cysts. Isolates should be sent to a reference laboratory for in-vitro drug sensitivity testing.

Treatment

Acanthamoeba exists in two forms: the free-living trophozoite is relatively responsive to therapy, whereas cysts may be highly resistant. Cysts form in response to adverse conditions and may remain viable for years. *Acanthamoeba* does not invade the epithelial cells themselves but is found between them, where host defense depends on phagocytosis by macrophages. Drugs are therefore targeted to the stroma, to amebae internalized within cysts, rather than to the epithelial cells. Thus the cationic antiseptics chlorhexidine and polyhexamethylene biguanide, which do not penetrate the epithelial cell, are none the less highly effective in the treatment of *Acanthamoeba* keratitis and other forms of amebic keratitis.

Treatment should begin with either 0.02% (200 mg/l) chlorhexidine in physiological saline[38] or with polyhexamethylene biguanide (0.02%),[39] which, however, is less available and not licensed for use as a drug. Both agents are highly effective against the trophozoite and cystic forms of the organism. Propamidine isethionate (Brolene®) 0.1% or hexamidine isethionate (Desmodine®) 0.1% are usually used in combination with the above drugs. Propamidine has been used effectively in combination with neomycin but most cysts are resistant to neomycin, and propamidine is moderately toxic with intensive use.

Drops are given hourly day and night for the first 3 days, reducing to 2-hourly by day only. This requires admission to hospital. Adjunctive therapy includes oral flurbiprofen, for both non-steroidal anti-inflammatory and analgesic effects, and topical mydriatic. Thereafter, combination therapy is given 3-hourly by day for 2 months and then 4-hourly by day for 2 months more. Treatment may be needed for 2–6 months.

If infection is diagnosed early, cure is possible, with complete recovery of vision. One week after starting therapy, however, there may be a corneal reaction to the lysis of dead amebae, with localized stromal edema and anterior chamber activity, which lasts up to 3 weeks.[38] Although this may be suppressed with steroids, their use is not encouraged. Steroid treatment, necessary in cases presenting late with considerable pain, ring abscess and episcleritis, prolongs treatment but can relieve intolerable pain. Steroids appear to have a role in controlling the late immunoinflammatory responses, when the amebae have been killed and antigens remain bound to the corneal stroma or sclera. Adjunctive immunosuppression has been advocated for *Acanthamoeba* scleritis.

Prevention

Contact-lens storage cases become contaminated with *Acanthamoeba* from the domestic water supply and airborne dust. Prevention involves use of acanthamebicidal disinfectants in storage and cleaning solutions, of which the best is hydrogen peroxide 3%; if polyhexamethylene biguanide is included as the disinfectant, the minimum concentration for an acanthamebicidal effect is 5 mg/l or parts per million (0.0001%). Chlorine is ineffective against cysts. Storage cases should never be washed in tap water, but with boiled water only, and should be stored dry. This is important because Enterobacteriaceae die quickly in dry conditions, and amebae cannot then multiply.

ENDOPHTHALMITIS

Endophthalmitis implies infection of the vitreous, retina and uveal coats of the eye. It is commonly exogenous and encountered as a complication of intraocular surgery or refractive surgery, or following suture removal after cataract or corneal graft surgery. Alternatively, it may be caused by penetrating eye injury. Organisms introduced into the anterior chamber at the time of cataract surgery may give rise to an acute endophthalmitis. Less pathogenic organisms may induce chronic infection. Some cases of endophthalmitis result from contaminated irrigation fluids, which may lead to an epidemic of infections. The formation of thin-walled drainage blebs after glaucoma operations using mitomycin C may predispose to late infections. The risk of infection is reduced by careful preoperative preparation and the use of povidone iodine immediately before or after surgery.

Less commonly, endogenous or metastatic endophthalmitis may arise in association with septicemia. This may result from bacterial endocarditis, infusion of contaminated fluids, the presence of infected intravenous lines or in drug addicts, using contaminated needles or syringes. Contaminated needles are commonly associated with *Candida albicans* infection. In East Asian populations, patients at highest risk are those with diabetes or hepatobiliary infection; *Klebsiella pneumoniae* is reported as the most common organism (60%).[40] In Caucasians, endocarditis or skin or joint infections are more frequent predisposing factors. In children, pneumonia due to *Ps. aeruginosa* may be the cause of a bilateral endophthalmitis which rapidly leads to blindness.

Following cataract surgery, patients can present with a ful-minant endophthalmitis within 5 days of surgery, often leading to permanent loss of vision. Alternatively, a subacute or chronic endophthalmitis may occur within 12 weeks of surgery, often presenting as a hypopyon uveitis. Risk factors include diabetes, duration of surgery, iris manipulation, torn posterior capsule (especially with vitreous loss), lens fragments in the vitreous, type of intraocular lens (with polypropylene haptics being more commonly associated with infection), and the experience of the surgeon.

Causes of acute endophthalmitis include *Str. pyogenes*, *Staph aureus* and Enterobacteriaceae and, with penetrating injury, *Bacillus* spp. and clostridia.[41] Acute endophthalmitis occasionally follows squint surgery, when infection is usually due to *Staph. aureus*. Surgeons should use appropriate prophylaxis against *Staph. aureus* in atopic or allergic patients. Causes of chronic endophthalmitis include coagulase-negative staphylococci, *Propionibacterium acnes* and, occasionally, viridans streptococci. Polymicrobial endophthalmitis is also reported, particularly after injury.

Fungal endophthalmitis is dealt with on p. 755.

Diagnosis and treatment

Acute endophthalmitis

Endophthalmitis is potentially blinding from irreversible retinal damage occuring within 24–48 h of onset. Early diagnosis and prompt treatment are essential. Bacterial endophthalmitis is treated with a combination of intravitreal and systemic antibiotic therapy. Subconjunctival therapy currently has no place in treatment and reliance should *not* be placed on intravenous therapy alone.

The clinical diagnosis of endophthalmitis is based on the presence of pain, visual loss, lid swelling and redness of the eye, including chemosis. A hypopyon uveitis may be present and, most importantly, loss of the red reflex. Microbiological diagnosis requires a vitreous biopsy for smears and cultures. Polymerase chain reaction-based techniques have a role to play in diagnosis and may yield a higher positive rate than direct culture[42] especially for Gram-negative organisms.[43] A simultaneous intravitreal injection of an antibiotic combination is given at the time of sampling and repeated at intervals (e.g. 48–72 h) depending on the expected intravitreal persistence of the selected drug and the clinical response (see Table 56.2, p. 743 for dosages). Dexamethasone (400 μg) is added to the intravitreal injection to reduce the vitreous inflammatory response and subsequent vitreous organization.

Additional systemic therapy, ideally with the same antibiotics as used for intravitreal therapy, will maintain effective intravitreal levels for longer by reducing the outward diffusion. High doses are required and there is a need to be aware of the risks of systemic toxicity.

Dexamethasone is added to the intravitreal injection. Antibiotic therapy is modified after 24–48 h according to the clinical response and to the antibiotic sensitivity profile of the cultured organism.

Chronic endopthalmitis

A diagnosis of chronic endophthalmitis should be considered in patients presenting late, several days or weeks after surgery, with a 'hypopyon uveitis' that has failed to respond to routine topical antibiotic and steroid therapy. Symptoms are less marked than in acute endophthalmitis. Visual loss may be more evident than pain. Chronic endophthalmitis is usually caused by indolent organisms such as coagulase-negative staphylococci or *P. acnes*, capable of forming a biofilm on the lens implant.[44]

Diagnosis may be established as late as 1 year after surgery, by an aqueous or vitreous tap, followed by Gram stain and culture, or polymerase chain reaction analysis, but microbiological diagnosis may await explantation of the implant and histological examination of the implant and capsular bag.

Initial treatment should commence with oral clarithromycin 500 mg twice daily for 1 week, followed by 250 mg twice daily for 3 weeks, as a 'trial of therapy'.[14] A good response, when it occurs, may be due to concentration of the drug within macrophages containing bacteria.[3] If this treatment fails, then further intravitreal therapy should be given, with emphasis on drugs against Gram positive organisms, such as vancomycin. Capsulectomy, vitrectomy and removal of the intraocular lens, with or without lens exchange, may be necessary to eradicate the organism.[44]

Prophylaxis against postoperative infection

Several approaches can reduce the risk of endophthalmitis following intraocular surgery.

- Meticulous preoperative preparation with occlusive drapes.
- Irrigation of the operative field with povidone-iodine (5%).
- Avoidance of contamination of the intraocular lens during insertion.
- Use of antimicrobials.

Postoperative infection is the most common form of exogenous bacterial endophthalmitis. Sources of organisms include the patients themselves, surgeon (hands, gloves, nose, technique), contaminated instruments, implants, drugs, irrigations and infusions, and environmental sources. Phako machines, vitrectomy machines and viscoelastic materials may all be sources of infection. Metastatic endophthalmitis occurs after intravenous infusions and blood transfusions.

Eyelid and conjunctival sac commensals are responsible for 80% of postcataract surgery endophthalmitis. Since eyelid cultures vary from day to day, preoperative cultures are no longer performed, and reliance is placed on preoperative antiseptic preparation with povidone-iodine and an aseptic technique.[45]

Although topical preoperative antibiotics are given by some clinicians, it is not established that they reduce postoperative infection.

Cataract surgery

The rate of endophthalmitis following modern cataract surgery is 0.1–0.7%. While this rate is low, the risk of blindness presents a challenge to reduce infection.

Some bacteria (predominantly coagulase-negative staphylococci or *P. acnes*) enter the chamber during cataract surgery. Re-entry of the anterior chamber increases this risk. DNA typing of postoperative staphylococcal cultures from lids and those causing endophthalmitis has shown similarity in 85% of cases,[46] suggesting that most patients become infected by their own bacterial flora. To combat this, some surgeons add an antibiotic, such as gentamicin 5 mg/l or vancomycin 10 mg/l, to the irrigant fluid. While this is controversial, there is anecdotal evidence that this approach reduces the incidence of postextraction endophthalmitis. Intracameral injection with 1 mg cefuroxime around the intraocular lens at the end of surgery has been associated with an incidence of endophthalmitis as low as 0.06%.[47,48] Contact between implant and conjunctiva during insertion can be avoided, using injectable, foldable lenses Careful wound closure is also important.

Subconjunctival antibiotics are routinely given, usually a subconjunctival injection of cefuroxime 125 mg, or gentamicin 20 mg, at the end of surgery. Cefuroxime provides good antibiotic prophylaxis against *Staph. aureus*, *Str. pyogenes*, coagulative-negative staphylococci and *P. acnes*. Gentamicin gives poor streptococcal and *P. acnes* coverage.

Topical antibiotics are continued four times daily for one week after cataract surgery.

Management of surgery in atopy

In the atope *Staph. aureus* colonizes the skin, including the lids and nasal mucosa, to a high degree.[18] Care is needed when planning intraocular surgery, particularly in the presence of blepharitis. The following additional regimen is suggested.

- Whole-body bathing, including shampooing with 4% chlorhexidine soap, for 72 h before surgery.
- Topical antistaphylococcal prophylaxis with fusidic acid (Fucithalmic®) for 24 h before surgery.
- Intracameral cefuroxime 1 mg around the intraocular lens if having cataract surgery).
- Fusidic acid 750 mg three times a day postoperatively (enteric coated capsules), or trimethoprim for 5 days.

Prevention of endophthalmitis due to an intraocular foreign body

An intraocular foreign body represents a medical emergency, especially metal fragments arising from hammering farmyard equipment, soil-contaminated items and machinery. Seal and Kirkness[41] found that 8% of patients with an intraocular foreign body developed endophthalmitis, and half became blind.

Bacillus spp. are the most virulent pathogens carried by an intraocular foreign body, while *Staph. aureus*, Enterobacteriaceae, streptococci (and, occasionally, *Clostridium perfringens*) are equally likely to cause sight-threatening endophthalmitis. All patients undergoing removal of a foreign body require intravitreal antibiotic prophylaxis. Any delay, or dependence on intravenous antibiotics alone, will risk blindness.[49] Intravitreal dexamethasone may reduce early inflammatory signs, but may not influence visual outcome.[50]

The regimen shown in Box 56.5 is suggested; cephalosporins are excluded because *Bacillus* spp. produce β-lactamses that inactivate them.

Box 56.5 Prophylaxis against endophthalmitis following intraocular foreign body

Essential prophylaxis

Intravitreal gentamicin 200 μg (or amikacin 400 μg) + vancomycin 1 mg (or clindamycin 1 mg)

Adjunctive prophylaxis

Subconjunctival gentamicin 40 mg + clindamycin 34 mg

Topical gentamicin (forte) 15 mg/ml + clindamycin 20 mg/ml

Intravenous therapy (with same drugs as given intravitreally) – give adequate dosage for weight but assay to avoid systemic toxicity, especially to the kidney and eighth nerve.

ORBITAL CELLULITIS

Orbital cellulitis is an extraocular infection presenting with pain, proptosis and diplopia. A few cases follow penetrating injury or panophthalmitis, but most are secondary to sinusitis. The condition commonly affects children, spreading to the orbit across the thin orbital plate of the ethmoid bone. Delayed or inadequate treatment may lead to blindness or death. Retroseptal infection requires multidisciplinary management because of the risk of extension to the eye or cranial cavity. Loculated pus must be drained.

The lid swelling of preseptal cellulitis may resemble orbital cellulitis, but ocular movements are normal and globe inflammation absent in preseptal disease. Diagnosis can be resolved by magnetic resonance imaging. It is associated with sinusitis, ocular infection and infected wounds.

Parenteral therapy is directed against common causative organisms: *H. influenzae*, *Staph. aureus*, *Str. pneumoniae* and *Str. pyogenes*. *H. influenzae* is the prominent cause of orbital cellulitis in young children and in this age group amoxicillin–clavulanic acid or cefuroxime are the drugs of choice. In view of the emergence of multiresistant strains of *H. influenzae*, consideration should be given to the use of a group 4 cephalosporin such as cefotaxime, particularly when the clinical response is poor or resistant organisms are isolated from nasal swabs. In adults, therapy is directed against streptococci and *Staph. aureus*, with high-dose intravenous benzylpenicillin and flucloxacillin (or otherisoxazolypenicillin) or clindamycin or vancomycin.

LYME DISEASE (SEE ALSO CH. 63)

Although ocular manifestations are rare in this tick-borne disease, the spirochete *Borrelia burgdorferi* invades the eye early and remains dormant, accounting for both early and late ocular manifestations. A follicular conjunctivitis occurs in approximately 10% of patients with early Lyme disease, and an interstitial keratitis within a few months of onset. Inflammatory events include orbital myositis, episcleritis, vitritis, uveitis and retinal vasculitis. When serology is negative, a vitreous tap may be required for diagnosis. Neuro-ophthalmic manifestations include bilateral mydriasis, neuroretinitis, pigmentary retinopathy, involvement of multiple cranial nerves, optic atrophy, and disc edema. Seventh nerve paresis can lead to neuroparalytic keratitis. In endemic areas, Lyme disease may be responsible for approximately 25% of presenting Bell's palsy.

Diagnosis is based on a history of exposure in an endemic area, positive serology and response to treatment. Antibodies may be measured by enzyme-linked immunosorbent assay and Western blot. The polymerase chain reaction has been used successfully for vitreous and cerebrospinal fluid. Serum reagin tests are non-reactive in Lyme borreliosis, but false-positive specific tests for syphilis (viz. fluorescent treponemal antibody) can occur. Spirochetes have been identified in the vitreous of a seronegative patients with vitritis and choroiditis and cultured from an iris biopsy in a treated patient.

Therapy with doxycycline or amoxicillin is effective in the earliest stages, but serious late complications require high doses of intravenous penicillin or ceftriaxone.

WHIPPLE'S DISEASE

Whipple's disease is a rare systemic disorder with malaise, fever, migrating arthralgias, fatigue, abdominal discomfort, diarrhea and weight loss. Ocular signs include uveitis, vitritis and retinal vasculitis. Small bowel biopsy shows diastase-resistant PAS-positive macrophages in the mucosal lamina propria. The cause is a Gram-positive actinomycete called *Tropheryma whippelii*. There may be a predisposing immunodeficiency.

Antibiotics that penetrate the blood–brain barrier minimize central nervous system (CNS) complications. Relapse is not uncommon. Combination therapy is recommended – e.g. parenteral streptomycin and benzylpenicillin for 2 weeks followed by sulfamethoxazole (800 mg) and trimethoprim (160 mg) (co-trimoxazole) orally twice daily for 1 year.

TOXOPLASMA RETINOCHOROIDITIS
(SEE ALSO CH. 65)

The intracellular protozoan *Toxoplasma gondii* can enter the fetal retina during intrauterine life to cause retinochoroiditis in the second and third decades, when it is the most common cause of posterior uveitis. However, primary toxoplasmosis, which may be subclinical or cause a glandular fever-like syndrome with lymph-node enlargement, can produce an acute primary retinochoroiditis. Evidence from Brazil, where the prevalence of ocular toxoplasmosis is high, suggests that the condition is most commonly acquired post-natally.[51–53]

Therapy is directed against the dividing organism and the inflammatory host response. Small peripheral retinal lesions may be allowed to run their course, but lesions near the macula, optic disc or maculopapular nerve fibre bundle, or those associated with severe vitritis, should be treated. Treatment is complicated because tissue cysts, multiplying within retinal cells, are impervious to drug penetration, so that recurrence can be expected. *Toxoplasma* infection is encountered in immunocompromised patients.

Treatment

Pyrimethamine and sulfadiazine act synergistically to interfere with folic acid synthesis. They should be commenced early in the course of the disease and continued for 4–6 weeks (Box 56.6). Pyrimethamine therapy should be avoided in early pregnancy and monitored to exclude bone marrow depression. Folinic acid supplements reduce this risk, but platelet and white cell counts should be performed weekly.

Clindamycin has also been shown to be effective in the treatment of ocular toxoplasmosis, but does carry the risk of pseudomembranous colitis.

Box 56.6 Treatment of *Toxoplasma* retinochoroiditis

Regimen

Pyrimethamine[a] 100 mg immediately then 25 mg/day orally for 4–6 weeks

and

Sulfadiazine 2 g immediately then 1 g orally four times daily for 4–6 weeks

and

Folinic acid 3 mg orally or i.m. twice weekly.

Alternative regimen

Clindamycin[b] 300 mg orally four times daily for 4–6 weeks

and

Sulfadiazine 2 g immediately then 1 g orally four times daily for 4–6 weeks.

[a] Pyrimethamine may cause bone marrow depression; leukocyte and platelet counts should be monitored weekly.
[b] Clindamycin may cause pseudomembranous colitis.

Recently it has been recognised that Onchocercal oocytes contain endosymbiotic organisms (*Wolbachia spp.*), which are passed on to the microfilaria and are essential to embryogenesis in the female worm. *Wolbachia spp.* are sensitive to tetracyclines, rifampicin, chloramphenicol and azithromycin. In a trial where doxycycline 200mg daily for 4–6 weeks was combined with ivermectin, embryogenesis was disrupted for 24 months, and microfilaria were absent from the skin after 18 months.[54]

Oral corticosteroid therapy is indicated in vision-threatening disease, but should not be used without concurrent, specific antiprotozoal therapy or in immunocompromised patients.

OCULAR *TOXOCARA* (LARVA MIGRANS) INFECTION

Toxocara canis is a worm whose natural host is the dog. Humans are accidental hosts, infected by ingesting the ova from contaminated soil. The larval stage causes visceral and ocular larva migrans, but adult worms are not found. These larvae migrate and are deposited in the CNS, including the retina. Here, they can present as a (usually unilateral) possible tumor, for which eyes have been enucleated in the past.

Serological tests only confirm previous exposure and may be negative when a choroidal lesion is present. Fine-needle biopsy in a reference center with cytology for tumor cells and a test system for *Toxocara* antigen is the best approach.

If the retinal lesion is close to the macula, treatment is warranted, with oral diethylcarbamazine 3 mg/kg for 3 weeks. There may be symptoms of allergic reaction to the dying larvae, for which prednisolone is given. Albendazole or a single dose of ivermectin are alternative therapies.

OCULAR ONCHOCERCIASIS (SEE ALSO CH. 66)

Ocular onchocerciasis, or 'river blindness', results from infection with the filarial parasite Onchocerca volvulus. The disease is endemic in areas of Africa and Central and South America, where it is a major cause of blindness. The ocular manifestations include keratitis, anterior uveitis, glaucoma, chorioretinitis and optic neuritis.

For several decades diethylcarbamazine and sumarin have been used systemically and have a positive effect on keratitis and uveitis; they are, however, less beneficial in posterior segment disease. The use of diethylcarbamazine may be followed by a severe systemic reaction, which is largely prevented by the use of systemic corticosteroids. An appropriate therapeutic regimen has been provided by Taylor and Dax.[55]

Ivermectin (a 12 mg single dose) represents an important advance in the mass therapy of onchocerciasis in endemic areas. It inhibits reproduction by adult female worms, so that no new microfilariae are produced for several months. It also kills microfilariae in tissues, including skin and the eye, slowly eliminating them from the anterior chamber with minimal ocular inflammation and little systemic reaction. It has to be given yearly so that the eradication program is a continuous one. Ivermectin should not be given to children under 5 years, to pregnant women or to patients with other severe infections such as trypanosomiasis.

OCULOMYCOSIS (SEE ALSO CH. 62)

Fungal infections of the eye are invariably sight-threatening and include keratomycosis, exogenous or endogenous endophthalmitis and orbital mycosis. Although oculomycosis is rare in the UK, it may account for one-third or more of infective corneal ulcers in some rural settings and in developing countries.[23] The management of keratomycosis has been summarized by O'Day and Head.[37]

The fungi responsible for keratomycosis, with the exception of *Candida* spp. (common in the UK), are mainly filamentous. Those most frequently encountered are *Aspergillus*, *Fusarium* and *Curvularia*, but prevalence varies geographically. *Candida* is an important cause of endogenous endophthalmitis in drug addicts and immunocompromised individuals. Penetration of drugs such as natamycin and amphotericin B in the treatment of a fungal ulcer is greatly enhanced by the absence of an epithelial barrier.

Because of the toxicity of the most effective antifungal agents, the relatively narrow activity spectrum of some and the difficulties of clinical diagnosis, treatment is rarely instituted in the absence of direct evidence of fungal etiology, based at least on the results of smears. Some filamentous fungi such as *Fusarium* have been detected in the cornea in vivo by confocal microscopy.

Effective therapy requires mycological identification and, preferably, information about drug sensitivity. The number of drugs available for local ocular use is limited, not only by problems of local and systemic toxicity, but also by poor solubility or ocular penetration. No commercial antifungal preparations are available in the UK for local ocular use; eye drops are usually formulated from parenteral preparations.

Amphotericin B is active against a wide range of fungal organisms causing oculomycosis, including *Aspergillus* spp., *Fusarium* spp. and *Candida* spp. It may be given topically as drops, subconjunctivally or intravitreally. Although it is toxic when used topically at high concentration, in part due to the presence of deoxycholate in the parenteral preparation, the 0.15% formulation is virtually non-toxic. Amphotericin B is given parenterally by slow intravenous infusion in the management of endophthalmitis, often in a background of more widespread systemic infection, in addition to intravitreal therapy. Renal and hematological status must be kept under surveillance and drug levels monitored (Ch. 9).

Natamycin (pimaricin) is a tetraene antifungal agent, which has been used in the topical treatment of a wide range of filamentous fungi causing keratitis such as *Fusarium* spp. (particularly *F. solani*) and to a lesser extent *Aspergillus*. A 5% suspension is available commercially in the USA. It has some topical toxicity.

Imidazoles have also been used effectively in the topical treatment of keratomycosis: clotrimazole, miconazole and econazole are effective against *Candida* spp. and *Aspergillus* spp. but not against the majority of *Fusarium* spp. Generally they have been considered to be less effective than amphotericin B in clinical use.[37] They can be locally toxic. Ketoconazole is well absorbed after oral administration and is generally well tolerated, although there is a risk of hepatotoxicity. It has been used effectively in oculomycosis caused by *Fusarium*, combined with another antifungal agent to prevent the emergence of resistance.

Topical fluconazole is effective in animal models and patients in the treatment of *Candida* keratitis[56] and shows less protein binding than the imidazoles. Itraconazole also has an enhanced therapeutic index compared to the imidazoles. *Candida* endophthalmitis can be effectively treated with oral fluconazole combined with intravitreal amphotericin B, but vitrectomy and fluconazole alone have also been reported to be successful. Aqueous levels of fluconazole over 2 h after oral treatment with 200 mg were 2.7–5.4 mg/l and vitreous levels up to 1.7 mg/l. Corneal levels were low (0.031 mg/l).

5-Fluorocytosine is only active against *Candida* spp. It is well absorbed by the oral route and achieves high blood and tissue levels. It has been used effectively in the treatment of *Candida* endophthalmitis, in combination with systemic or intravitreal amphotericin to prevent the otherwise rapid emergence of resistant strains. 5-Fluorocytosine has also been used topically (1% suspension) in the treatment of *Candida albicans* keratomycosis.

Thomas, reviewing the results of treating 318 patients with culture-proven keratitis,[57] found oral and/or topical ketoconazole and itraconazole useful in treating severe keratitis, especially that due to *Aspergillus*.

Fungal keratitis usually responds slowly to antifungal therapy over a period of weeks. Signs of toxicity (conjunctival chemosis and injection, recurrent corneal erosions) should also be looked for. Negative scrapings during treatment do not always indicate that the fungus has been eradicated, since it may become deep-seated; hence therapy should be maintained for 6 weeks or more.

Patients who respond most poorly to topical antifungal therapy are those with deep corneal infections and those who have received corticosteroids prior to diagnosis. Fungal growth is aided by corticosteroids and argues against their use alone, or in combination with antifungal agents.

Therapeutic surgery may be required for cases which respond poorly to medical therapy. However, therapy should be prolonged, to render the infecting fungus non-viable prior to surgery.

VIRAL INFECTIONS OF THE EYE

HERPES SIMPLEX EYE DISEASE

Primary ocular herpes simplex (HSV) infection is a self-limiting disease, expressed as blepharitis, conjunctivitis or punctate keratitis. Zosteriform spread along along the fifth cranial nerve axons can establish latency in the trigeminal ganglion even in asymptomatic infections. Subsequent ocular disease results from viral reactivation, with peripheral shedding, and is termed 'recurrent' disease. Recurrent eye disease includes epithelial keratitis (dendritic and geographic ulcers), stromal keratitis (disciform and necrotizing), limbitis, keratouveitis, secondary glaucoma and, rarely, acute retinal necrosis.

Ocular disease may be caused by HSV types 1 or 2. HSV-1 usually produces non-genital infections and is transmitted by direct or indirect non-sexual contact; HSV-2 is chiefly transmitted sexually. Most neonatal eye disease is caused by HSV-

2, transmitted during transit through the birth canal, and most non-infantile ocular disease is caused by HSV-1. Of HSV keratoconjunctivitis, 1% is caused by HSV-2. HSV-1 is generally more sensitive to antivirals than HSV-2 and drug resistance does not appear to be a significant problem. Trifluorothymidine may be more effective against the HSV-2, which can produce a more severe form of keratouveitis. Not all primary eye disease is followed by recurrent eye disease.

Herpetic antiviral therapy

The earliest antivirals available for the topical treatment of superficial ocular infection with HSV were idoxuridine, adenine arabinoside and trifluorothymidine. This last is available commercially in the USA but not in the UK; However, a 1.0% solution in normal saline can be prepared from the dry powder. All three agents are extremely effective in blocking herpes virus replication but, as they are incorporated into DNA of both infected and uninfected cells, they show significant toxicity with prolonged use.

The newer antivirals are activated by virus-induced enzymes (e.g. thymidine kinase) and exert their action chiefly in infected cells. These drugs are more inhibitory to herpetic DNA polymerase than cellular polymerase and preferentially inhibit viral DNA synthesis. They are less toxic than the earlier agents and include aciclovir, bromovinyldeoxyuridine and ethyldeoxyuridine. Aciclovir reaches effective aqueous levels in the intact eye after topical use. Two agents with greatly improved bioavailability after oral therapy are famciclovir, which is converted to its active form penciclovir, and valaciclovir, which is converted to aciclovir. The topical regimens advocated for some of these compounds are listed in Table 56.3. In addition to these agents, human interferon has been used clinically.

Treatment of specific herpes simplex eye infections

Epithelial keratitis

Dendritic ulcer is the most common form of keratitis, seen as a branching lesion, which may expand into a broader, geographic ulcer. Dendritic ulcer may be self-limiting, with about 26% of placebo-treated cases resolving within 2–3 weeks, but antiviral therapy will produce a clinical cure in 76–100% and shorten the median healing time to as little as 3 days. Simple debridement of the infected epithelium also promotes healing by reducing the viral load.

Aciclovir is highly effective against the dendritic ulcer, in some studies appearing to be more effective than idoxuridine and in others equally effective as adenine arabinoside. Since aciclovir is less toxic than any of the earlier antivirals, it would appear to be the treatment of choice for dendritic ulcer, with trifluorothymidine and adenosine arabinoside as alternatives. Bromovinyldeoxyuridine and ethyldeoxyurldine also appear to be highly effective agents. Ganciclovir gel (0.15%) has also been shown to be effective by Colin et al.[58] Alternative therapies for epithelial keratitis are presented in Box 56.7 and Table 56.3.

Box 56.7 Topical therapies for dendritic ulcer

Aciclovir ointment 3% five times daily for 10–14 days (not currently available in the USA) *or*

Trifluorothymidine drops 1% nine times daily for 10–14 days, *or*

Vidarabine 3% five times daily for 14–21 days.

Idoxuridine, 0.1% hourly by day and 2-hourly at night, is less efficacious and carries a greater risk of ocular toxicity.

Table 56.3 Antiviral drugs for ocular therapy (modified from Pavan-Langston and Grene 1984)[59]

Drug	Form	Concentration/Dose	Frequency	Available in UK
Idoxuridine	Ointment	0.5%	Five times daily for 14 days	Yes
	Drops	0.1%	1-hourly by day, 2-hourly by night for 14 days	Yes
Vidarabine	Ointment	3.0%	Five times daily for 14 days	Yes
	i.v.	1 mg in 2 ml 5% dextrose up to 1 mg/kg per 24 h		Yes
Trifluorothymidine	Drops	1.0%	Hourly by day, 2-hourly by night for 14 days	No[a]
Aciclovir	Ointment	3.0%	Five times daily for 14 days	Yes
	Tablets	200 mg	400–800 mg 4-hourly for 5 days	Yes
	i.v.		5 mg/kg over-1 h every 8 h	Yes
Bromovinyldeoxyuridine	Drops	0.1%	1–2-hourly by day	No
	Ointment	0.5%	5 times daily for 14 days	No
Ethyldeoxyuridine	Drops		1–2-hourly by day	No
	Gel		Nightly	No
Penciclovir	Tablet	125/250 mg	8-hourly for 5 days	Yes
Valaciclovir	Tablet	125/250 mg	8-hourly for 5 days	Yes

[a] Not commercially available; can be produced in a hospital pharmacy.

Where topical instillation is not feasible (e.g. children, patients with severe arthritis, where instillation is difficult), systemic therapy can be effective (e.g. in the adult – oral aciclovir 200 mg five times daily for 14–21 days).[60]

Steroid use converts untreated dendritic ulcer into the expanded and aggressive, geographic ulcer. Trifluorothymidine is claimed to be the most effective treatment for geographic keratitis. Where prolonged use is required, aciclovir would be preferable.

Disciform keratitis

This is a disk-shaped zone of stromal edema, associated with a variable keratouveitis. It represents an immune reaction to viral antigen in the corneal stroma. Treatment is with topical steroid, directed against the immune response, while providing prophylactic cover against dendritic ulcer, with aciclovir or a similar agent. A typical regimen would be Predsol eyedrops 0.5% five times daily, with oc. aciclovir 3% five times daily. Treatment is continued for 14 days after healing and then tapered by reducing instillation by one dose per week over the next 5 weeks.[61]

Stromal keratitis

Stromal keratitis occurs in two forms. Focal stromal infiltration may accompany a dendritic ulcer, or occur independently. Necrotizing stromal keratitis may ulcerate or perforate. They are presumed to be caused by a combination of active viral invasion and an immune reaction to viral antigen. In patients receiving topical steroid at the time of diagnosis, the condition may be greatly exacerbated by steroid withdrawal, which leads to a rebound increase in inflammation. In this situation, steroids should be weaned slowly to an adequately suppressive level.

Treatment involves topical steroid to suppress inflammation, together with a topical antiviral agent. Both agents are weaned slowly over a period of many weeks. Some patients must be maintained on low-dose steroids (prednisolone phosphate, 0.1% and 0.03%) to avoid rebound inflammation.

The regimen reported by the Herpetic Eye Disease Study Group[62] employed trifluorthymidine (Table 56.5). In the UK aciclovir would be used. No additional benefit is obtained when oral aciclovir is combined with topical therapy.

Table 56.4 Topical therapy for herpes simplex stromal keratitis

Prednisolone phosphate	Trifluorthymidine 1%	Week
1% 8 ×/day	4 ×/day	1
1% 6 ×/day	4 ×/day	2
1% 4 ×/day	4 ×/day	3
1% 2 ×/day	2 ×/day	4
1% 1 ×/day	2 ×/day	5
0.125% 4×/day	2 ×/day	6
0.125% 2 ×/day	2 ×/day	7
0.125% 1 ×/day	2 ×/day	8–10

Iritis

Herpetic iritis is heralded by an aqueous flare and cells and keratic precipitates, occurring independently or accompanying a stromal keratitis. In an eye that has suffered past herpes simplex keratitis, iritis should be regarded as herpetic in origin unless proved otherwise. Iritis may be accompanied by secondary glaucoma. Treatment involves topical steroid therapy combined with oral antiviral treatment. The Herpetic Eye Disease Study[63] reported a beneficial trend for oral aciclovir 400 mg five times daily for 10 weeks in combination with trifluorthymidine and prednisolone eyedrops indicated in Table 56.5.

Necrotizing herpetic retinopathies

These necrotizing retinopathies are accompanied by vasculitis and vitritis. Visual loss may result from retinal detachment or ischemic optic neuropathy. HSV retinitis due to HSV-2 infection is a rare but serious neonatal infection. Acute retinal necrosis may affect healthy adults of all ages and, occasionally, immunocompromised patients. Progressive outer retinal necrosis typically occurs in immunocompromised patients.

Treatment is with high-dose antiviral therapy (Box 56.8). Retinal edema and inflammation is suppressed with oral prednisolone 20 mg/day, starting on the third day of antiviral treatment. Laser photocoagulation or surgery may be required to prevent progression of or to treat retinal detachment.

Box 56.8 Systemic therapy for necrotizing herpetic retinopathy

Intravenous aciclovir 13 mg/kg/day in three divided doses for 14 day, *then*	
Oral aciclovir 800 mg × 5/day	
Oral famciclovir 500 mg × 3/day for 3 months	More effective in immunocompromised patients
Intravitreal ganciclovir 400 mg × 2/week, *combined with* Intravenous foscarnet 60 mg/kg, × 3/week	May delay progress in immunocompromised patients

Prophylactic antiviral therapy

HSV keratitis recurrence

Recurrence of herpes simplex keratitis is due to reactivation of latent virus. The risk of recurrence is increased after a first attack, with a 25% chance in the first year, increasing to 72% in 10 years.[64] The risk of recurrence (including blepharitis, conjunctivitis, iritis and epithelial and stromal keratitis) is reduced by long-term prophylactic treatment with aciclovir 400 mg twice daily.[65]

Keratoplasty

Keratoplasty for postherpetic corneal scarring carries with it the risk of reactivating latent herpes, in part because of the trigeminal damage at the time of surgery, and also because of the postoperative use of topical corticosteroids. Graft failure has been reported variously at between 66% at 2 years and 71% at 5 years. Graft failure is due to viral recurrence in about

15% of cases and to rejection in 64%. Graft survival is enhanced by prophylactic antiviral therapy,[66] and it is customary to treat patients prophylactically with aciclovir 400 mg twice daily, preoperatively and in the long-term during the postoperative period.

There is less agreement as to the benefit of long-term topical antiviral therapy. A rational approach is to reserve topical prophylaxis for episodes of increased topical steroid use, for instance during episodes of graft rejection.

Strains of virus resistant to idoxuridine, adenine arabinoside and trifluorothymidine have been identifid and have been responsible for clinical disease. Culture of HSV with aciclovir has permitted the emergence of aciclovir-resistant strains within 10 days, and has raised some concerns as to the long-term expectation of clinical resistance to aciclovir and related drugs. Adenine arabinoside may be effective in the treatment of keratitis resistant to idoxuridine and trifluorothymidine, and aciclovir in disease resistant to adenine arabinoside and idoxuridine. Bromovinyldeoxyuridine can be effective in cases resistant to idoxuridine, adenine arabinoside and trifluorothymidine.

HERPES ZOSTER VIRUS

Involvement of the first division of the fifth cranial nerve by varicella zoster virus (VZV) is associated with ocular features ranging from blepharitis, to persistent conjunctivitis, keratouveitis, glaucoma, papillitis, ocular nerve palsy and neuralgic ocular pain. This is termed herpes zoster ophthalmicus (HZO).

Oral administration of aciclovir is now standard treatment for HZO at a dose of 600–800 mg five times daily, initiated within 72 h of the onset of skin lesions.[67] It is well tolerated and reduces the incidence and severity of epithelial and stromal keratitis and uveitis. Treatment reduces pain in the acute phase, but not neurotrophic keratitis or postherpetic neuralgia. The higher bioavailability of valaciclovir and famciclovir has allowed their use in more convenient dosing schedules at 1 g three times daily and 500 mg three times daily for × 7 days respectively, with faster resolution of acute pain in herpes zoster infection. Placebo-treated patients in a trial of intravenous aciclovir therapy suffered progression until topical aciclovir was started

Intravenous aciclovir has replaced vidarabine as the treatment of choice in the management for HZO in AIDS and other immunocompromised patients, and intravenous foscarnet has been used effectively for the treatment of those patients with aciclovir-resistant HZO.[68]

Although the use of topical ocular steroids to suppress the inflammation does not have the dire consequences seen with HSV eye disease (e.g. induction of dendritic or geographic ulceration), outcome in those treated with aciclovir alone may be better than in those receiving steroids alone (aciclovir 3% ointment versus betamethasone 0.1% ointment, five times daily). No recurrence occurred in the aciclovir-treated group, whereas the recurrence rate was 63% in the steroid-only group. Such recurrences were more difficult to suppress than the initial disease features. Corneal epithelial disease healed significantly more quickly in the aciclovir patients.

ADENOVIRUS KERATOCONJUNCTIVITIS

Adenovirus (ADV) infection causes epidemic forms of clinical disease, including pharyngeal conjunctival fever (ADV-3,4 and 7), follicular conjunctivitis (ADV-1–11 and ADV-19) and epidemic keratoconjunctivitis (EKC). EKC is a self-limiting disorder characterized by a follicular conjunctivitis and a multifocal keratitis, with subepithelial features developing at 10–14 days after the onset of the disease. These infiltrates may persist for weeks or months, giving rise to disabling symptoms of glare and discomfort. Although subepithelial infiltrates may be suppressed by topical steroids, they reappear on steroid withdrawal, with a return of symptoms. Therefore in practice, steroids are used only for selected, highly symptomatic patients and are weaned slowly, over a period of months. It appears that topical cyclosporin can be used in a similar fashion. Nosocomial, hospital outbreaks of EKC may be reduced by establishing appropriate infections control policies.[69]

Although no antiviral agents are available commercially for the treatment of adenovirus infection, several, such as cidofovir, hydroxyphosphonylmethoxypropyl adenine and 2-nor cyclic guanosine monophosphate, have shown efficacy in experimental models. Phase I/II clinical trials of cidofovir 0.5% twice daily for 7 weeks have shown rapid clearing of adenovirus and suppression of infiltrate formation compared with placebo.[70]

OTHER VIRAL INFECTIONS

Most cases of measles are associated with conjunctivitis. Measles keratitis is a major cause of blindness in developing nations where secondary infection and vitamin A deficiency may be compounding factors. Although there is no specific antiviral agent available, topical antibiotics and systemic vitamin A supplements improve the prognosis.

ACQUIRED IMMUNE DEFICIENCY SYNDROME

Human immunodeficiency virus (HIV) has been identified in tear fluid, conjunctiva, corneal epithelium and retina and can give rise to a retinal microangiopathy, but the principal ophthalmic manifestations of acquired immune deficiency syndrome (AIDS) relate to florid opportunistic infections and to conjunctival and orbital involvement with Kaposi's sarcoma and other neoplasms. Therapy is directed against the relevant organism and generally is more intense and prolonged than is required in immunocompetent individuals. Highly active antiretroviral therapy (HAART) in AIDS patients leads to a striking fall in HIV load and substantial improvements in immune functions, including increases in total CD4 and CD8 cell counts, in memory and naïve T-cell subsets, and in antigen responses to certain opportunistic pathogens. HAART leads to improved survival and reduced progression of HIV disease, with complete or partial resolution of infections or malignancies (*see* Ch. 46).

CYTOMEGALOVIRUS

Cytomegalovirus (CMV) is the most common of the ocular opportunists and produces a hemorrhagic, necrotizing retinitis. Because the onset of retinitis is often asymptomatic, it is recommended that in patients with AIDS with blood CD4$^+$ counts below 50 cells/μl, ophthalmological examinations are carried out on a monthly basis.[71] The onset or reactivation of CMV retinitis is heralded by elevated or rising blood CMV DNA levels.

During the first 7 years after infection, fewer than 1% of HIV-infected persons present with CMV retinopathy as the initial manifestation of AIDS, but CMV retinitis is found in 16–19% of terminal AIDS patients, bilateral in about 17%. The delay from presentation with HIV infection is shorter in bilateral cases. HSV, Epstein-Barr virus and toxoplasma occasionally cause a clinically similar retinitis.

In a study of CMV retinitis in AIDS patients, 58% presented with unilateral disease and 15% of these developed contralateral infection, despite treatment with ganciclovir. The risk factors for progression or involvement of the fellow eye have been reviewed by Holbrook et al.[72]

The incidence of CMV disease and of CMV relapses has fallen significantly since the introduction of HAART[73] including the frequency of CMV-related retinal detachment. However, subclinical infections may be awakened at the initiation of HAART and CMV retinitis may be activated when it is necessary to interrupt HAART for reasons of toxicity. At present with use of nucleoside and non-nucleoside analogs and protease inhibitors, CMV retinitis does not frequently pose an immediate threat to vision, but it may do so with development of retinal detachment, in association with peripapillary disease or by affecting the central retina. Retinal detachment, an important cause of blindness from CMV retinitis, can be treated successfully by vitrectomy, silicone oil, and endolaser.

In patients with AIDS receiving HAART and treated additionally for CMV retinitis, it has been possible to withdraw anti-CMV therapy without major risk of reactivation of the retinitis for at least 48 weeks after ceasing antiviral therapy.[74] Reactivation, if it occurs, is more likely in those patients whose CD4$^+$ counts fall below 50 cells/μl and in whom there are signs of virological failure. At the time when the CMV retinitis has become inactive, patients receiving HAART are at risk of developing a visually symptomatic 'immune recovery' vitritis or uveitis and macular edema, thought to represent a T-cell mediated reaction to latent CMV antigens. The vitritis responds to treatment with periocular steroids without reactivation of the retinitis.

CMV retinitis occurring in AIDS patients implies a high risk for the development of CMV encephalitis. On the other hand, in patients with AIDS without CMV retinitis, CNS symptoms are unlikely to be attributable to CMV encephalitis.[75]

Systemic therapy

Progression of CMV retinitis may be delayed in the short term by intravenous ganciclovir or foscarnet.[76] Repeated, local intravitreal therapy is more effective, and particularly valuable when there are no signs of disseminated CMV disease. Ganciclovir, a virustatic drug similar in structure to aciclovir and foscarnet, improves or temporarily stabilizes the retinitis in the majority of patients receiving long-term maintenance therapy. Ganciclovir and foscarnet are equally effective in controlling CMV retinitis, but foscarnet is less well tolerated. Repeated therapy is indicated because of the high relapse rate. Ganciclovir is given by intravenous infusion over 1 h in a dose of 5 mg/kg every 12 h. Valganciclovir, the oral prodrug of ganciclovir, has excellent oral bioavailability, giving high ganciclovir blood levels without the need for prolonged intravenous access.

Intravenous administration of ganciclovir results in intravitreal concentrations which are subtherapeutic (0.93 ± 0.39 mg/ml) for many CMV isolates, which explains the difficulty of long-term complete suppression of CMV retinitis by this route.

Combined daily therapy with ganciclovir and foscarnet has recently been shown to be beneficial,[77] with prolonged intervals between progression, without increased toxicity. Such therapy may halt the progress of peripheral outer retinal necrosis in AIDS patients.

Improved results have been achieved with cidofovir treatment with 5 mg/kg once weekly for 2 weeks, then 5 mg/kg every other week, which retarded the progression of retinitis in AIDS patients compared to delayed therapy. Toxicity to cidofovir may occur in the form of proteinuria (23%), neutropenia (15%) and uveitis, and may lead to discontinuation of the drug.

Intraocular delivery

Intravitreal injection of antiviral agents is effective in the treatment of CMV retinitis, and avoids the risk of systemic toxicity. Intravitreal ganciclovir or foscarnet have been given on a weekly basis with little local ocular complication and no greater risk of retinal detachment. An intravitreal dose of ganciclovir (0.2–0.4 mg) is as effective as intravenous therapy and a dose of 2 mg in 0.05–0.1 ml probably provides adequate intravitreal levels (0.25–1.22 μg/l) for up to 7 days. Levels at 24 h have been recorded as 143.4 μg/l and at 72 h as 23.4 μg/l. This higher dose (2 mg) has been used effectively to produce prolonged remission, with a low relapse rate (5% at 44 weeks).[78] The intravitreal dose of foscarnet is 2.4 mg in 0.1 ml. A lower dose of these agents has been given in patients whose eyes contain silicone oil in relation to retinal surgery.

Intravitreal cidofovir together with oral probenecid has also been effective in halting progression of CMV retinitis. Fomivirsen is an antisense oligonucleotide newly approved for intravitreal use (see Ch. 40).

More recently, the development of intraocular controlled-release devices has provided the opportunity to deliver drugs for prolonged periods with minimum local toxicity. Rhegmatogenous detachments can occur in CMV retinitis, with or without systemic treatment or GCV implant therapy but implants do not appear to increase the risk of detachment.[79]

TOXOPLASMA

Ocular toxoplasmosis in patients with AIDS is less common than CNS involvement. It may be the cause of presention, with blurred vision and floaters, or pronounced visual loss from macular, papillomacular bundle or optic nerve head involvement

The retinochoroiditis is unassociated with a pre-existing retinochoroidal scar, suggesting that the lesions are a manifestation of acquired rather than congenital disease. Lesions may be single or multifocal, in one or both eyes, or consist of massive areas of retinal necrosis. They may resemble those of CMV retinitis and may occur concurrently in the same eye. In comparison, toxoplasmic lesions tend to be thick and opaque, with smooth borders and a relative lack of hemorrhage.

Treatment of the toxoplasmic ocular infection with pyrimethamine, clindamycin and sulfadiazine is effective in over 75% of patients. Once resolution is observed, maintenance therapy is continued, as relapses occur in the absence of treatment. Corticosteroid treatment is unnecessary and its use has been associated with the development of CMV retinitis.

PNEUMOCYSTIS CARINII

This organism can cause a choroidopathy in patients, due to systemic spread from primary lung infections. Multiple yellow placoid fundus lesions are seen.

CANDIDA ALBICANS AND CRYPTOCOCCUS NEOFORMANS

These can also produce retinal lesions or endophthalmitis, particularly in AIDS patients who are intravenous drug users. A bilateral epithelial keratopathy caused by encephalitozoon has been described in an HIV-positive patient with cryptococcal meningitis, which responded to itraconazole given for the meningitis.

HERPES ZOSTER OPHTHALMICUS

This occurs in a more severe and chronic form in AIDS and may require prolonged systemic penciclovir therapy.

MICROSPORIDIA

Microsporidial keratoconjunctivitis in a patient with AIDS have responded to treatment with dibromopropamidine isethionate ointment.

OTHER INFECTIONS

VIBRIO SPECIES

In the coastal regions of the gulf of Mexico, vibrio infections are responsible for infections including gastroenteritis, wound infections and septicemia. Penland et al.[80] reported *Vibrio* spp. as a cause of conjunctivitis, keratitis and endophthalmitis, in this part of the world, often following eye trauma by shellfish from contaminated water or exposure to brackish sea water. Responsible organisms include *V. vulnificus*, *V. albensis*, *V. fluvialis* and *V. parahaemolyticus*.

References

1. Pepose JS, Holland GN, Wilhelmus KR 1995 *Ocular Infection and Immunity*, Edition Mosby, St. Louis.
2. Leibowitz HM, Waring GO III 1998 *Corneal Disorders: Clinical Diagnosis and Management*, 2nd edn. W.B. Saunders Company, Philadelphia.
3. Seal DV, Bron AJ, Hay J 1998 *Ocular Infection – Investigation and Treatment in Practice*, edition. Martin Dunitz, London.
4. von Gunten S, Lew D, Paccolat F et al 1994 Aqueous humor penetration of ofloxacin given by various routes. American Journal of Ophthalmology 117: 87–89.
5. El Baba F, Trousdale M, Gauderman J et al 1992 Intravitreal penetration of oral ciprofloxacin in humans. *Ophthalmology* 99: 483–486.
6. Dougherty JM, McCulley JP, Silvany ME, Meyer DR 1991 The role of tetracycline in chronic blepharitis. Investigative *Ophthalmology and Vision Science* 32: 2970–2975.
7. Seal DV, Wright P, Ficker L, Hagan K, Troski M, Menday P 1995 Placebo controlled trial of fusidic acid gel and oxtetracycline for recurrent blepharitis and rosacea. British Journal of Ophthalmology 79: 42–45.
8. Elder MJ, Stapleton F, Evans E, Dart JKG 1995 Biofilm-related infections in ophthalmology. *Eye* 9: 102–109.
9. Evans DJ, Allison DG, Brown MR 1991 Susceptibility of *Pseudomonas aeruginosa* and *Escherichia coli* bioforms towards ciprofloxacin: effect of specific growth rate. *Journal of Antimicrobiology & Chemotherapy* 27: 177–184.
10. Wilson LA 1996 Biomaterials and ocular infection. In Wilhelmus K, Pepose G (eds) *Ocular Infection and Immunity*. Mosby, Chicago. pp. 215–231.
11. Seal DV, Kirkness CM, Bennett HGB, Peterson M, Group KS 1999 *Acanthamoeba keratitis* in Scotland: risk factors for contact lens wearers. *Contact Lenses and the Anterior Eye* 22: 58–68.
12. Fulcher TP, Dart JK, McLaughlin-Borlace L, Howes R, Matheson M, Cree I 2001 Demonstration of biofilm in infectious crystalline keratopathy using ruthenium red and electron microscopy. *Ophthalmology* 108: 1088–1092.
13. Abreu JA, Cordoves L, Mesa CG, Mendez R, Dorta A, De-la-Rosa MG 1997 Chronic pseudophakic endophthalmitis versus saccular endophthalmitis. *Journal of Cataract and Refractive Surgery* 23: 1122–1125.
14. Warheker PT, Gupta SR, Mansfield DC, Seal DV, Lee WR 1998 Post-operative saccular endophthalmitis caused by macrophage-associated staphylococci *Eye* 12: 1019–1021.
15. McCulley JP, Dougherty JM, Deneau DG 1982 Classification of chronic blepharitis. *Ophthalmology* 89(10): 1173–1180.
16. Ficker L, Seal DV, Wright P 1996 Staphylococcal blepharitis. In Wilhelmus K, Pepose G, G Holland, (eds). *Ocular Infection and Immunity*. Mosby, Chicago.
17. McCulley JP, Shine WE 2000 Changing concepts in the diagnosis and management of blepharitis. *Cornea* 19: 650–658.
18. Tuft SJ, Ramakrishnan M, Seal DV, Kemeney DM, Buckley RJ 1992 Role of staphylococcus aureus in chronic allergic conjunctivitis. *Ophthalmology* 99: 180–184.
19. Gilbert C, Foster A 2001 Childhood blindness in the context of VISION 2020 – the right to sight. *Bulletin of the World Health Organization* 79: 227–232.
20. van Bogaert LJ 1998 Ophthalmia neonatorum revisited. *African Journal of Reproductive Health* 2: 81–86.

21. Bailey R, Lietman T 2001 The SAFE strategy for the elimination of trachoma by 2020: will it work? *Bulletin of the World Health Organization* 79: 233–236.

22. Bowman RJ, Sillah A, Van Dehn C, et al 2000 Operational comparison of single-dose azithromycin and tropical tetracycline for trachoma. *Investigative Ophthalmology & Visual Science* 41: 4074–4079.

23. Houang E, Lam D, Fan D, Seal D 2001 Microbial keratitis in Hong Kong – relationship to climate, environment and contact lens disinfection. *Transactions of the Royal Society of Tropical Medicine and Hygiene* 95: 361–367.

24. Ficker L, Kamakrishnan M, Seal DV et al 1991 Role of cell-mediated immunity to staphyloccal blepharitis. In: Wilhelmus K, Pepose G (eds) *Ocular Infection and Immunity*. Mosby, Chicago.

25. Baum J, Barza M 2000 The evolution of antibiotic therapy of bacterial conjunctivitis and keratitis: 1970–2000. *Cornea* 19: 659–672.

26. O'Brien TP, Maguire MG, Fink NE, Alfonso E, McDonnell P 1995 Efficacy of ofloxacin vs cefazolin and tobramycin in the therapy for bacterial keratitis. Report from the Bacterial Keratitis Study Research Group. *Archives of Ophthalmology* 113: 1257–1265.

27. Hyndiuk RA, Eiferman RA, Caldwell DR et al 1996 Comparison of ciprofloxacin ophthalmic solution 0.3% to fortified tobramycin-cefazolin in treating bacterial corneal ulcers. Ciprofloxacin Bacterial Keratitis Study Group. 103: 1854–1862.

28. Ofloxacin Study Group 1997 Ofloxacin monotherapy for the primary treatment of microbial keratitis: a double-masked, randomized, controlled trial with conventional dual therapy. *Ophthalmology* 104: 1902–1909.

29. Khokhar S, Sindhu N, Mirdha BR 2000 Comparison of topical 0.3% ofloxacin to fortified tobramycin-cefazolin in the therapy of bacterial keratitis. *Infection* 28: 149–152.

30. Alexandrakis G, Alfonso EC, Miller D 2000 Shifting trends in bacterial keratitis in south Florida and emerging resistance to fluoroquinolones. *Ophthalmology* 107: 1497–1502.

31. Schaumberg DA, Snow KK, Dana MR 1998 The epidemic of *Acanthamoeba keratitis*: Where do we stand? *Cornea* 17: 3–10.

32. Alizadeh H, Niederkorn JY, McCulley JP 1996 Acanthamoebic keratitis In Pepose JS Holland GN, Wilhelmus KR, (eds) *Ocular Infection & Immunity* Mosby, St. Louis, pp. 1062–1071.

33. Seal DV, Kirkness CM, Bennett HGB, Peterson M, Group KS 1999 Population-based cohort study of microbial keratitis in Scotland: incidence and features *Contact Lenses and the Anterior Eye* 22: 49–57.

34. Rosenthal RA, McAnally CL, McNamee LS, Buck SL, Schlitzer RL, Stone RP 2000 Broad spectrum antimicrobial activity of a new multi-purpose disinfecting solution *CLAO Journal* 26: 120–126.

35. Sharma N, Vajpayee RB, Pushker N, Vajpayee M 2000 Infectious crystalline keratopathy. *CLAO Journal* 26: 40–43.

36. McCulley JP, Alizadeh H, Niederkorn JY 2000 The diagnosis and management of Acanthamoeba keratitis. *CLAO Journal* 26: 47–51.

37. O'Day DM, Head WS 2000 Advances in the management of keratomycosis and *Acanthamoeba* keratitis. *Cornea* 19: 681–687.

38. Seal DV, Hay J, Kirkness CM et al 1996 Successful medical therapy of *Acanthamoeba* keratitis with chlorhexidine and propamidine. *Eye* 10(4): 413–421.

39. Larkin DF, Kilvington S, Dart JK 1992 Treatment of *Acanthamoeba* keratitis with polyhexamethylene biguanide. *Ophthalmology* 99: 185–191.

40. Wong JS, Chan TK, Lee HM, Chee SP 2000 Endogenous bacterial endophthalmitis: an east Asian experience and a reappraisal of a severe ocular affliction. *Ophthalmology* 107: 1483–1491.

41. Seal DV, Kirkness CM 1992 Criteria for intravitreal antibiotics during surgical removal of intraocular foreign bodies. *Eye* 6: 465–468.

42. Lohmann CP, Linde HJ, Reischl U 2000 Improved detection of microorganisms by polymerase chain reaction in delayed endophthalmitis after cataract surgery. *Ophthalmology* 107: 1047–1051, 1051–1052.

43. Okhravi N, Adamson P, Carroll N et al 2000 PCR-based evidence of bacterial involvement in eyes with suspected intraocular infection. *Investigative Ophthalmology and Visual Science* 41: 3474–3479.

44. Clark WL, Kaiser PK, Flynn HWJ, Belfort A, Miller D, Meisler DM 1999 Treatment strategies and visual acuity outcomes in chronic postoperative propionibacterium acnes endophthalmitis. *Ophthalmology* 106: 1665–1670.

45. Bohigian GM 1999 A study of the incidence of culture-positive endophthalmitis after cataract surgery in an ambulatory care center. *Ophthalmic Surgery with Lasers* 30: 295–298.

46. Speaker MG, Milch FA, Shah MK, Eisner W, Kreiswirth BN 1991 Role of external bacterial flora in the pathogenesis of acute postoperative endophthalmitis. *Ophthalmology* 98: 639–649.

47. Montan PG, Wejde G, Koranyi G et al 2002 Prophylactic intracameral cefuroxime. Efficicay in preventing endophthalmitis after cataract surgery. *Journal of Cataract and Refractive Surgery* 28: 977–981.

48. Montan PG, Wejde G, Setterquist H et al 2002 Prophylactic intracameral cefuroxime. Evaluation of safety and kinetics in cataract surgery. *Journal of Cataract and Refractive Surgery* 28: 982–987.

49. Jonas JB, Knorr HL, Budde WM 2000 Prognostic factors in ocular injuries caused by intraocular or retrobulbar foreign bodies. *Ophthalmology* 107: 823–82.

50. Das T, Jalali S, Gothwal VK, Sharma S, Naduvilath TJ 1999 Intravitreal dexamethasone in exogenous bacterial endophthalmitis: results of a prospective randomised study. *British Journal of Ophthalmology* 83: 1050–1055.

51. Glasner PD, Silveira C, Kruszon-Moran D et al 1992 An unusually high prevalence of ocular toxoplsasmosis in southern Brazil. *American Journal of Ophthalmology* 114: 136–144.

52. Nussenblatt RB, Belfort R Jr. 1994 Ocular toxoplasmosis. An old disease revisited. *JAMA* 271: 304–307.

53. Silveira C, Belfort R Jr, Muccioli C et al 2001 A follow-up study of Toxoplasmas gondii infection in southern Brazil. *American Journal of Ophthalmology* 130: 351–354.

54. Hoerauf A, Büttner DW, Adjei O et al 2003 Onchocerciasis. *British Medical Journal* 326: 207–210.

55. Taylor HR, Dax EM 1986 Ocular onchocerciasis. In: Tabbara KF, Hyndiuk RA (eds) Infections of the eye. Little Brown and Co., Boston, pp. 653–664.

56. Yee RW, Sullivan LS, Lai HT et al 1997 Linkage mapping of Thiel-Behnke corneal dystrophy (CDB2) to chromosome 10q23–q24. *Genomics* 46: 152–154.

57. Thomas PA 1995 Oral azole antifungals: promising agents in treatment of mycotic keratitis. *Abstracts of International Conference on Ocular Infections, Jerusalem, 18–22 June*.

58. Colin J, Hoh HB, Easty DH et al 1997 Ganciclovir ophthalmic gel (Virgan: 0.15%) in the treatment of herpes ketatitis. *Cornea* 16: 393–399.

59. Pavan-Langston D, Grene B 1984 Herpes simplex ocular disease. *Comprehensive Therapy* 10: 30–36.

60. Simon AL, Pavan-Langston D 1996 Long-term oral acyclovir therapy. Effect on recurrent infectious herpes simplex keratitis in patients with and without grafts. *Ophthalmology* 103:1399–1404.

61. Collum LM, Power WJ, Collum A 1992 The current management of herpetic eye disease. *Document Ophthalmologica* 80: 201–205.

62. Wilhelmus KR, Gee L, Hauck WW et al 1994 Herpetic Eye Disease Study. A controlled trial of topical corticosteroids for herplex simplex stromal keratitis. *Ophthalmology* 101: 1883–1896.

63. Group H.E.D.S. 1998 Acyclovir for the prevention of recurrent herpes simplex virus eye disease. *New England Journal of Medicine* 339: 300–306.

64. Liesegang TJ 1989 Epidemiology of ocular herpes simplex. Natural history in Rochester, Minn, 1950 through 1982. *Archives of Ophthalmology* 107: 1160–1165.

65. HEDS Group 1998 Acyclovir for the prevention of recurrent herpes simplex virus eye disease. *New England Journal of Medicine* 339: 300–306.

66. Larkin DF, 1998 Corneal transplantation for herpes simplex keratitis. *British Journal of Ophthalmology* 82: 107–108.

67. Hoang-Xuan T, Buchi ER, Herbort CP 1992 Oral acyclovir for herpes zoster ophthalmicus. *Ophthalmology* 99: 1062–1071.

68. Cohen J, Brunell PA, Straus SE et al 1999 Recent advances in varicella-zoster infection. *Annals of Internal Medicine* 130: 922–932.

69. Gottsch JD, Froggatt JW, Smith DM et al 1999 Prevention and control of epidemic keratoconjunctivitis in a teaching eye institute. *Ophthalmic Epidemiology* 6: 29–39.

70. Gordon YJ 2000 The evolution of antiviral therapy for external ocular viral infections over twenty-five years. *Cornea* 19: 673–680.

71. Kitagawa M, Nagata Y, Fujino Y, Mochizuki M 2001 Usefulness of routine ophthalmologic examination for cytomegalovirus retinitis in acquired immunodeficiency syndrome patients. *Nippon Ganka Gakkai Zasshi* 105: 31–36.

72. Holbrook JT, Davis MD, Hubbard LD et al 2000 Risk factors for advancement of cytomegalovirus retinitis in patients with acquired immunodeficiency syndrome. Studies of Ocular Complications of AIDS Research Group *Archives of Ophthalmology* 118: 1196–1204.

73. Deayton JR, Wilson P, Sabin CA et al 2000 Changes in the natural history of cytomegalovirus retinitis following the introduction of highly active antiretroviral therapy. *AIDS* 14: 1163–1170.

74. Jouan M, Saves M, Tubiana R et al 2001 Discontinuation of maintenance therapy for cytomegalovirus Retinitis in HIV-infected patients receiving highly active antiretroviral therapy. *AIDS* 15: 23–31.

75. Bylsma SS, Achim CL, Wiley CA et al 1995 The predictive value of cytomegalovirus retinitis for cytomegalovirus encephalitis in acquired immunodeficiency syndrome. *Archives of Ophthalmology* 113(1): 89–95.

76. Hoffman VF, Skiest DJ 2000 Therapeutic developments in cytomegalovirus retinitis. *Expert Opinion on Investigational Drugs* 9: 207–220.

77. Weinberg DV, Murphy R, Naughton K 1994 Combined daily therapy with intravenous ganciclovir and foscarnet for patients with recurrent cytomegalovirus retinitis. *American Journal of Ophthalmology* 117: 776–782.

78. Cochereau I, Diraison MC, Mousalatti H et al 2000 Ganciclovir intravitreen a fortes doses pour le traitement de la retinite a CMV. [High-dose intravitreal ganciclovir in CMV retinitis]. *Journal Français d'Ophtalmologie* 23: 123–126.

79. Kempen JH, Jabs DA, Dunn JP, West SK, Tonascia J 2001 Retinal detachment risk in cytomegalovirus retinitis related to the acquired immunodeficiency syndrome. *Archives of Ophthalmology* 119: 33–40.

80. Penland RL, Boniuk M, Wilhelmus KR 2000 Vibrio ocular infections on the U.S. Gulf Coast. *Cornea* 19: 26–29.

81. Walker S, Diaper CJ, Bowman R, Sweeney G, Seal DV, Kirkness CM 1998 Lack of evidence for systemic toxicity following topical chloramphenicol use. *Eye* 12: 875–879.

82. Robert PY, Adenis JP 2001 Comparative review of topical ophthalmic antibacterial preparations. *Drugs* 61: 175–185.

83. Seal DV, Hay J, Kirkness CM 1995 Chlorhexidine or polyhexamethylene biguanide for *Acanthamoeba* keratitis. *Lancet* 345: 136.

84. Seal DV, Hay J, Kirkness CM et al 1996 Successful medical therapy of *Acanthamoeba* keratitis with topical chlorhexidine and propamidine. *Eye* 10: 413–421.

 Further information

Abu-el-Asrar AM, Kadry AA, Shibl AM, al-Kharashi SA, al-Mosallam AA 2000 Antibiotics in the irrigating solutions reduce *Staphylococcus epidermidis* adherence to intraocular lenses. *Eye* 14 (Pt.2): 225–230.

Caballes RL, Caballes RA Jr 1999 Primary cryptococcal prostatitis in an apparently uncompromised host. *Prostate* 39: 119–122.

Callegan MC, Booth MC, Jett BD, Gilmore MS 1999 Pathogenesis of gram-positive bacterial endophthalmitis. *Infection and Immunity* 67: 3348–3356.

Chuang LH, Song HS, Lee SC, Lai CC, Ku WC 2000 Endogenous *Klebsiella pneumoniae* endophthalmitis associated with prostate abscess: case report. *Chang. Keng. I. Hsueh. Tsa. Chih* 23: 240–245.

Ciulla TA 1999 Update on acute and chronic endophthalmitis [editorial; comment]. *Ophthalmology* 106: 2237–2238.

Culbert RB, Devenyi RG 1999 Bacterial endophthalmitis after suture removal. *Journal of Cataract and Refractive Surgery* 25: 725–727.

Ferencz JR, Assia EI, Diamantstein L, Rubinstein E 1999 Vancomycin concentration in the vitreous after intravenous and intravitreal administration for postoperative endophthalmitis. *Archives of Ophthalmology* 117: 1023–1027.

Fiscella RG, Nguyen TK, Cwik M et al 1999 Aqueous and vitreous penetration of levofloxacin after oral administration. *Ophthalmology* 106: 2286–2290.

Gangopadhyay N, Daniell M, Weih L, Taylor HR 2000 Fluoroquinolone and fortified antibiotics for treating bacterial corneal ulcers. *British Journal of Ophthalmology* 84: 378–384.

Holm SO, Jha HC, Bhatta RC et al 2001 Comparison of two azithromycin distribution strategies for controlling trachoma in Nepal. *Bulletin of the World Health Organization* 79: 194–200.

Horio N, Horiguchi M, Murakami K, Yamamoto E, Miyake Y 2000 *Stenotrophomonas maltophilia* endophthalmitis after intraocular lens implantation. *Graefes Archive for Clinical and Experimental Ophthalmology* 238: 299–301.

Jaeger EE, Carroll NM, Choudhury S et al 2000 Rapid detection and identification of *Candida*, *Aspergillus*, and *Fusarium* species in ocular samples using nested PCR. *Journal of Clinical Microbiology* 38: 2902–2908.

Jonas JB, Budde WM 1999 Early versus late removal of retained intraocular foreign bodies. *Retina* 19: 193–197.

Kunimoto DY, Sharma S, Garg P, Rao GN 1999 In vitro susceptibility of bacterial keratitis pathogens to ciprofloxacin. Emerging resistance. *Ophthalmology* 106: 80–85.

Lesser RL 1995 Ocular manifestations of Lyme disease. *American Journal of Medicine* 98(4A): 60S–62S.

Liu SM, Way T, Rodrigues M, Steidl SM 2000 Effects of intravitreal corticosteroids in the treatment of *Bacillus cereus* endophthalmitis. *Archives of Ophthalmology* 118: 803–806.

Mallari PL, McCarty DJ, Daniell M, Taylor H 2001 Increased incidence of corneal perforation after topical fluoroquinolone treatment for microbial keratitis *American Journal of Ophthalmology* 131: 131–133.

Manfredi R, Nanetti A, Ferri M, Chiodo F 2000 Clinical and microbiological survey of *Serratia marcescens* infection during HIV disease. *European Journal of Clinical Microbiology and Infectious Diseases* 19: 248–253.

Mikkila HO, Seppala IJ, Viljanen MK, Peltomaa MP, Karma A 2000 The expanding clinical spectrum of ocular lyme borreliosis. *Ophthalmology* 107: 581–187.

Mino-de-Kaspar H, Grasbon T, Kampik A 2000 Automated surgical equipment requires routine disinfection of vacuum control manifold to prevent postoperative endophthalmitis. *Ophthalmology* 107: 685–690.

Morlet N, Graham GG, Gatus B et al 2000 Pharmacokinetics of ciprofloxacin in the human eye: a clinical study and population pharmacokinetic analysis. *Antimicrobial Agents and Chemotheraphy* 44: 1674–1679.

Moyes AL, Sugar A, Musch DC, Barnes RD 1994 Antiviral therapy after penetrating keratoplasty for herpes simplex keratitis. *Archives of Ophthalmology* 112: 601–607.

Nujjuka HO, Seppal IJ, Viljanen MK, Peltomaa MP, Karma A 2000 The expanding clinical spectrum of ocular lyme borreliosis. *Ophthalmology* 107: 581–587.

O'Day DM 1985 Studies in experimental keratomycosis. *European Journal of Clinical Microbiology and Infectious Diseases* 4: 243–252.

Ozturk F, Kortunay S, Kurt E et al 1999 Effects of trauma and infection on ciprofloxacin levels in the vitreous cavity. *Retina* 19: 127–130.

Ozturk F, Kortunay S, Kurt E, Ilker SS, Basci NE, Bozkurt A 1999 Penetration of topical and oral ciprofloxacin into the aqueous and vitreous humor in inflamed eyes. *Retina* 19: 218–222.

Perez-Santonja JJ, Ruiz-Moreno JM, de-la-Hoz F, Giner-Gorriti C, Alio JL 1999 Endophathalmitis after phakic intraocular lens implantation to correct high myopia. *Journal of Cataract and Refractive Surgery* 25: 1295–1298.

Perrine D, Chenu JP, Georges P, Lancelot JC, Saturnino C, Robba M 1995 Amoebicidal efficiencies of various diamidines against two strains of *Acanthamoeba polyphaga*. *Antimicrobial Agents and Chemotherapy* 39: 339–342.

Rosenbaum AL 2000 Endophthalmitis after strabismus surgery. *Archives of Ophthalmology* 118: 982–983.

Saluski S, Clayman HM, Karsenti G et al 1999 *Pseudomonas aeruginosa* endophthalmitis coused by contamination of the internal fluid pathways of a phacoemulsifier. *Journal of Cataract and Refractive Surgery* 25: 540–545.

Seal DV, Dalton A, Doris D 1999 Disinfection of contact lenses without tap water rinsing: is it effective? *Eye* 13: 226–230.

Seal DV, Ficker LA, Wright P 1996 Staphylococcal blepharitis. In Pepose JS, Holland GN, Wjilhelmus KR (eds). *Ocular Infection & Immunity*. Mosby, St. Louis, pp. 788–798.

Spector SA, Weingeist T, Pollard RB et al 1993 A randomized, controlled study of intravenous ganciclovir therapy for cytomegalovirus peripheral retinitis in patients with AIDS. AIDS Clinical Trials Group and Cytomegalovirus Cooperative Study Group. *Journal of Infectious Diseases* 168: 557–563.

Swaddiwudhipong W, Linlawan P, Prasantong R, Kitphati R, Wongwatcharapaiboon P 2000 A report of an outbreak of postoperative endophthalmitis. *Journal of the Medical Association of Thailand* 83: 902–97.

Takourt B, de-Barbeyrac B, Khyatti M et al 2001 Direct genotyping and nucleotide sequence analysis of VS1 and VS2 of the Omp 1 gene of chlamydia trachomatis from Moroccan tracomatous specimens. *Microbes and Infection* 3: 459–466.

Teichmann KD 2000 *Propionibacterium acnes* endophthalmitis requiring intraocular lens removal after failure of medical therapy. *Journal of Cataract and Refractive Surgery* 26: 1085–1088.

Tuft SJ, Kemeny DM, Dart JKG, Buckley RJ 1991 Clinical features of atopic keratoconjunctivitis. *Ophthalmology* 98: 150–158.

Wasserman BN, Sondhi N, Carr BL 1999 Pseudomonas-induced bilaterial endophthalmitis with corneal perforation in a neonate. *Journal of the American Association for Pediatric Ophthalmology and Strabismus* 3: 183–184.

Wisniewski SR, Capone A, Kelsey SF, Groer-Fitzgerald S, Lambert HM, Doft BH 2000 Characteristics after cataract extraction or secondary lens implantation among patients screened for the Endophthalmitis Vitrectomy Study. *Ophthalmology* 107: 1274–1282.

Zell K, Engelmann K, Bialasiewicz AA, Richard G 2000 Endophthalmitis after cataract surgery: predisposing factors, infectious agents and therapy. *Ophthalmologe* 97: 257–263.

57 Urinary tract infections

S. Ragnar Norrby

This chapter deals with cystitis, pyelonephritis, prostatitis, and urethritis caused by pathogens other than sexually transmitted ones such as *Neisseria gonorrhoeae*, *Chlamydia trachomatis*, *Trichomonas vaginalis* and *Ureaplasma urealyticum*. Cystitis and pyelonephritis are characterized by significant bacteriuria, which was originally defined by Kass as 10^5 colony forming units (cfu) or more per ml in each of two voided urine samples or any bacterial count in urine obtained by catheterization or bladder puncture.[1] This concept has now been redefined (Table 57.1), based on studies showing that by lowering the bacterial counts and including pyuria, the diagnostic sensitivity can be increased without marked loss of specificity.[2–4]

Table 57.1 Definitions of bacteriuria in midstream urine samples. Note that in all patients with symptomatic infections, pyuria must also be present.[4]

Type of infection	Definition
Acute uncomplicated cystitis in women	
Infections caused by Gram-negative bacteria	$\geq 10^3$ cfu/ml
Infections caused by staphylococci	$\geq 10^2$ cfu/ml
Acute uncomplicated pyelonephritis	
Infections caused by Gram-negative bacteria	$\geq 10^4$ cfu/ml
Infections caused by staphylococci	$\geq 10^3$ cfu/ml
Complicated infections and infections in men	$\geq 10^4$ cfu/ml
Patients with asymptomatic bacteriuria	$\geq 10^5$ cfu/ml in two samples

Both cystitis and pyelonephritis can be classified as symptomatic or asymptomatic, complicated or uncomplicated, and sporadic or recurrent. This classification is meaningful because etiology, choice of antibiotics and treatment times differ considerably between the various types of infections. The approximate frequencies of the various types are outlined in Table 57.2.

Asymptomatic bacteriuria is common in girls and occurs in 1–7% of adult women, depending on age. All patients with long-term urinary catheters have significant bacteriuria, which in most is asymptomatic. Many patients with cystitis who do not respond bacteriologically to

Table 57.2 Approximate frequencies of various types of symptomatic urinary tract infections in an unselected material of outpatients with significant bacteriuria

Type of urinary tract infection	Approximate frequency (%)
Cystitis	90
Pyelonephritis	10
Uncomplicated infections	98
Complicated infections	2
Sporadic infections	75
Recurrent infections	25

antibiotic treatment but have persistent bacteriuria are also asymptomatic.

Complicated cystitis or pyelonephritis is defined as infections in patients with anatomical or functional defects which facilitate establishment of bacteriuria. Examples of such defects are congenital anomalies of the urethra, ureters or kidneys, foreign bodies (stones, catheters), residual bladder urine due to obstruction or neurological disease, tumors and obstructions of the urethra by strictures, prostate hyperplasia, prostate cancer or prostatitis. Diseases that may aggravate the course of pyelonephritis (e.g. diabetes mellitus with nephropathy and malignant hypertension) are sometimes considered complicating factors. However, these conditions do not increase the risk of establishment of bacteriuria. Significant bacteriuria in a man should always be considered a complicated urinary tract infection: the length of the male urethra prevents ascending infections and establishment of bacteriuria in a healthy man.

Cystitis and pyelonephritis are often recurrent infections, both in patients with uncomplicated and complicated infections but more commonly in the latter. Recurrent urinary tract infections can be subclassified into relapse, when the same bacterial strain that caused the previous episode is isolated, or reinfection, when the causative pathogen is a new strain. There is no internationally accepted definition of a recurrent urinary tract infection. In clinical trials it is often defined as more than one episode in 6 months or more than two episodes in 1 year. Consequently, sporadic infections occur less than twice per 6 months or less than three times per year. It should be noted that this classification does not include chronic infections; chronic pyelonephritis and chronic glomerulonephritis are inflammatory diseases, albeit often aggravated by infections.

Urethritis is an inflammation of the urethra without concomitant significant bacteriuria. In patients with sexually transmitted diseases urethritis is a well defined concept (see Ch. 59). However, when such organisms are not identified and significant bacteriuria is not present the 'urethral syndrome' becomes a microbiologically poorly defined disease usually without identified etiology.

Prostatitis is an inflammation of the prostate gland, which often also involves the seminal vesicles. When prostatitis is caused by bacterial pathogens it is subdivided into acute and chronic bacterial prostatitis, which may or may not be associated with significant bacteriuria.

EPIDEMIOLOGY AND PATHOGENESIS

Urinary tract infections occur in all ages and are most common in sexually active women. Below the age of 3 years, symptomatic cystitis or pyelonephritis is somewhat more common in boys than in girls due the higher frequency of congenital defects of the male urethra. In very old people bacteriuria is more common in men than in women due to the high frequency of prostate disease.

Cystitis and pyelonephritis are infections resulting from the aerobic fecal flora. The pathogenesis of these infections should be considered from two aspects: host factors and virulence factors of the infecting organisms.

HOST FACTORS

Host factors of importance for establishment of bacteriuria are the ones mentioned above defining a complicated cystitis or pyelonephritis. In addition, the short length of the female urethra explains the higher frequency of bacteriuria in adult women than in adult men. Also in women without urinary tract defects bacteria can ascend the urethra and reach the bladder. In postmenopausal women atrophy of the vaginal mucosa constitutes an important and usually treatable (with topical estrogen) complicating factor, which is surprisingly often overlooked.

Establishment of significant bacteriuria in a woman is facilitated by a high number of bacteria in the periurethral area. This is achieved during sexual intercourse, which often leads to bacteriuria if the bladder is not emptied post-coitus.

In men, especially those who are sexually active, the source of a bacteriuria may be prostatitis. Otherwise a prerequisite for bacteria to reach the bladder in sufficient amounts to establish bacteriuria is a turbulent urine flow, which may result from strictures or obstruction of the urethra. Irrespective of age and

gender, pyelonephritis almost invariably results from bacteria ascending the ureters. This is facilitated by defects in the ureteral bladder sphincters causing ureteric reflux during micturition. Such defects may be congenital but are also common in pregnant women during the latter half of pregnancy due to the pressure of the uterus on the bladder. Pyelonephritis is also common in patients with ureteral stones or stones in the renal pelvis. Pyelonephritis and renal abscesses resulting from hematogenous dissemination of bacteria from other infectious foci is extremely rare but may be seen in patients with endocarditis.

VIRULENCE FACTORS

Virulence factors of the organisms causing cystitis and pyelonephritis have been extensively studied. With the most common etiologic agent, *Escherichia coli*, it has been demonstrated that an important virulence factor is the ability of the bacterial cells to adhere to epithelial cells in the urinary tract mucosa.[5] This is achieved by antigens located to the fimbriae of the bacteria, which adhere to glycosphingolipid receptors on the epithelial cells. As a result of adherence, transportation of bacteria in the urethra and the ureters is facilitated. Another consequence of adherence is that cytokines (e.g. interleukins 1, 6 and 8) are released and that invasive infections are facilitated.[6–8] Adherence is important in patients without complicating factors but seems less important when such factors are present.[9] Other defined bacterial virulence factors are the antigenic structures of Enterobacteriaceae, the O, H and K antigens and the polysaccharide capsules. Virulence factors in Gram-positive organisms of importance in urinary tract infections are less extensively studied. In some situations (e.g. after treatment of bacteriuria caused by Gram-negative bacteria) the pathogenicity of Gram-positives in an asymptomatic patient should be questioned.[10]

ETIOLOGY

Bacteriuria is acquired by the fecal-genital route, often via periurethral colonization in women. With the exception of patients who have rectovesical fistulas or other abnormal communications between the bladder and the intestines or vagina, anaerobic bacteria rarely cause bacteriuria. The most common organisms causing bacteriuria are listed in Table 57.3.

In women with sporadic uncomplicated cystitis or pyelonephritis, the etiology is quite predictable; about 85% of these patients will have infections caused by *Escherichia coli*. The second most common organism is *Staphylococcus saprophyticus*, which accounts for about 10% of the infections. However, in north Europe *Staph. saprophyticus* has a seasonal pattern:[11] it is normally not found between November and March and reaches a peak in July and August, when it causes up to 40% of all uncomplicated infections. The reason for this

Table 57.3 Etiology of cystitis and pyelonephritis

Bacterial species	Dominating type of infection
Escherichia coli	All types
Staphylococcus saprophyticus	Uncomplicated cystitis and pyelonephritis in women during April to September
Klebsiella spp.	Recurrent/complicated infections
Enterobacter spp.	Recurrent/complicated infections
Enterococcus spp.	Recurrent/complicated infections
Proteus spp.	Tumors or stones
Morganella morganii	Recurrent/complicated infections
Pseudomonas spp.	Recurrent/complicated infections, bladder catheters
Other organisms	Recurrent infections

variation is unknown and it is not seen in the Southern Hemisphere.[12]

Also in recurrent and/or complicated cystitis and pyelonephritis *Esch. coli* is the most common etiology but other Gram-negatives as well as enterococci become increasingly frequent. Of importance in these patients is the antibiotic treatment given for the preceding episode, which is likely to have selected resistant organisms. Organisms such as *Enterobacter* spp., *Pseudomonas aeruginosa*, *Pseudomonas* spp., *Acinetobacter* spp. and *Citrobacter* spp. typically appear in patients who have received repeated antibiotic courses or who have acquired their bacteriuria in hospital.

Proteus spp., *Morganella morganii* and *Providencia* spp., which all grow in alkaline pH are common findings in patients with kidney or bladder stones or tumors. Since *Proteus* spp. is also common in the preputial flora, it is often a contaminant in urine samples from young boys.

Fungal growth in the urine is in most cases due to *Candida albicans* or other *Candida* spp. The clinical importance of funguria is uncertain or doubtful in patients with bladder catheters. In patients without catheters growth of *Candida* may reflect a renal infection resulting from hematological dissemination of the organisms. In rare cases candiduria is also seen as a result of the formation of a mycelial ball in the bladder.

DIAGNOSIS

CLINICAL DIAGNOSIS

Patients with cystitis are afebrile and the dominating symptoms are dysuria, frequent micturition and/or suprapubic pain. Sometimes macroscopic hematuria is present, especially in infections caused by *Staph. saprophyticus*.[11] With the exception of hematuria these symptoms are difficult or impossible to dif-

ferentiate from those of urethritis unless the patient has a urethral discharge.

Pyelonephritis is a systemic infection, the patients develop fever and may have signs of septicemia, which occurs in up to 30% of patients with this infection.[9] Other symptoms are chills and flank pain. Differential diagnoses are urinary stones, cholecystitis, appendicitis and basal pneumonia. The clinical symptoms of pyelonephritis are often masked by patients taking drugs with analgesic and/or antipyretic activity.

In children urinary tract infections often present with few clinical symptoms and fever may be the only symptom of pyelonephritis.

Acute prostatitis is characterized by symptoms similar to those of cystitis but the patient also has a distinct tenderness and enlargement of the prostate at rectal palpation. In chronic prostatitis the symptoms may be more diffuse and the prostate is often normal at rectal examination.

RADIOLOGIC DIAGNOSIS

Radiological examinations are rarely indicated in the acute phase of a urinary tract infection. An exception is when an obstruction of a ureter is suspected in a patient with signs of pyelonephritis. In children with pyelonephritis or with recurrent cystitis radiological examinations for identification of congenital anatomical defects and/or ureteral reflux should be performed after treatment of the acute infection.

In adults who have recovered from pyelonephritis it is recommended that ultrasound or a radiological examination is performed to exclude renal scars from childhood episodes of pyelonephritis.[13,14]

LABORATORY DIAGNOSIS

The keystone in the diagnosis of cystitis and pyelonephritis is the demonstration of significant bacteriuria. The reference technique is the quantitative urine culture. The sample can be obtained as a clean-catch (midstream) urine or by bladder puncture or catheterization. Bladder puncture is the preferred technique in small children, especially boys. After sampling the urine must be kept chilled (but not frozen) until analyzed. If there is likely to be a delay in transportation to a laboratory, a dip-slide culture can be used. With this technique an agar-covered slide is dipped in urine and incubated overnight at room temperature or a small incubator. It provides results in terms of quantity of bacteria and differentiation of Gram-negative and Gram-positive organisms. The slide can then be sent to a microbiological laboratory for determination of species and antibiotic susceptibility.

In patients with infections caused by Gram-negative bacteria other than *Pseudomonas* spp. bacteriuria can also be demonstrated by the nitrite test, a rapid paper-strip test. Nitrite is formed by bacterial metabolism of nitrate and is not normally present in urine. A positive nitrite test has a very high specificity. The sensitivity, however, is low because the method requires bladder incubation and because Gram-positive bacteria and *Pseudomonas* do not form nitrite.

Urine cultures should always be obtained in patients with complicated infections, recurrent infections or pyelonephritis. In patients with sporadic uncomplicated cystitis etiological diagnosis should be optional.

A marker for significant bacteriuria is pyuria. Demonstration of pyuria is best achieved by microscopy of unspun urine using a Bürker counting chamber and defining pyuria as $>10 \times 10^6$ leukocytes per liter of urine. The second-best method is to use a leukocyte esterase paper-strip test. Sediment microscopy has a low reliability because it is a technique that can not be standardized.[10] Marked pyuria in a patient with negative bacteriological cultures should lead to a suspicion of renal tuberculosis (*see* Ch. 61).

There is no specific laboratory test for the differentiation of cystitis from pyelonephritis. Patients with pyelonephritis normally have increased serum concentrations of C-reactive protein and peripheral white blood cell counts may be increased. Erythrocyte sedimentation rate is not always increased when the patient is first seen but is likely to rise during the following days. A regular finding in patients with acute pyelonephritis is that the concentration ability of the kidneys is reduced. This can be measured as urine osmolality after 12 h of no fluid intake or, more easily, by a subcutaneous (not nasal) challenge with anti-diuretic hormone. However, this test cannot be used when the patient is febrile and it is therefore a confirmatory test, which can be done once the patient's condition has improved.

Bacteria causing pyelonephritis form complexes with antibodies. Therefore, detection of antibody coated bacteria by immunofluorescence has been used as a method to differentiate cystitis and pyelonephritis. However, this test has tended to show a high frequency of false-positive results if a reasonable sensitivity is strived for, or too many false-negative results if the specificity of the test is high.

The etiologic diagnosis of prostatitis is difficult. The most ambitious technique is to culture four samples:

- the first portion of a voided urine sample;
- a midstream urine portion;
- prostate secretion obtained by rectal massage of the prostate; and
- the first portion of new voided urine sample.[15,16]

Patients with acute or chronic bacterial prostatitis should be culture positive with the same organism in all four of these samples.

ANTIBIOTIC TREATMENT

Antibiotic treatment of cystitis and pyelonephritis is normally empiric. Women with acute cystitis are rarely willing to wait 24 h for treatment and patients with acute pyelonephritis should be treated as soon as possible to avoid damage to the kidneys and reduce the risk of serious systemic manifestations of the infections.

PHARMACOKINETIC REQUIREMENTS

All antibiotics used for treatment of urinary tract infections with significant bacteriuria should be excreted via the kidneys. This makes drugs such as chloramphenicol and the tetracyclines less suitable because they are lipid soluble, with elimination mainly via liver metabolism resulting in very low urine concentrations. In patients with pyelonephritis it is also important that the antibiotic achieves serum concentrations sufficiently high to eliminate bacteremia. With renally excreted antibiotics therapeutic concentrations are normally achieved in the renal parenchyma.

In patients with prostatitis special pharmacokinetic requirements apply. The prostate tissue is a difficult-to-penetrate compartment. Moreover, the pH of the prostatic and vesicular fluid vary and is often altered by infection. Hence, the drugs used must be active at a wide range of pH values. Finally, in chronic prostatitis calculi may be present, which reduce the efficacy of antibiotic treatment.

SAFETY CONSIDERATIONS

Uncomplicated cystitis is an infection that constitutes no threat to the patient if adequately treated. When such infections are treated it is a prerequisite that the antibiotics used have the highest possible degree of safety; serious or life-threatening adverse effects cannot be accepted even if they appear in very low frequencies. On the other hand, in patients with pyelonephritis the infection per se constitutes a considerable risk to the patient, which makes adverse effects to the treatment given more acceptable if a high degree of efficacy can be expected.

CHOICE OF ANTIBIOTICS

Of paramount importance in this respect is the local antibiotic resistance pattern: it is not possible to extrapolate susceptibility data generated in one country to another. In the hospital environment there may be marked differences between hospitals in the same country in the frequency of resistance to commonly used antibiotics. The local microbiological laboratories must provide data from regular resistance surveillance studies performed on clinically relevant collections of bacterial strains. Results obtained in outpatients should be considered separately from hospital-generated data. Preferably, resistance surveillances should be prospective and denominator driven. If they are made (as is often the case) on routine samples sent to a diagnostic laboratory, they are likely to overestimate frequencies of resistance because cultures are more often taken in patients with recurrent infections or treatment failures.

DOCUMENTATION OF ANTIBIOTIC EFFICACY

Treatment of urinary tract infections with antibiotics aim at eliminating the symptoms and, most importantly in patients with cystitis or pyelonephritis, the bacteriuria. Systematic evaluation of antibiotic efficacy is made in clinical trials. Table 57.4 lists minimal requirements on clinical trials of antibiotic treatment of cystitis and pyelonephritis. Most trials initiated by pharmaceutical companies today fulfill these criteria. However, before the mid-1980s many clinical trials included too few patients to allow any conclusions to be drawn.

Table 57.4 Requirements of clinical trials of antibiotic treatment of urinary tract infections

Criterion	Requirements
Type of infection	Only one – e.g. uncomplicated cystitis in women or complicated infections in either sex
Sample size	For trials in cystitis at least 200 patients with confirmed bacteriuria per treatment group; smaller samples for complicated infections and pyelonephritis
Entry criteria	Verified pyuria and/or positive nitrite test, typical symptoms, urine for culture
Control	Well documented regimen
Design	Always prospective, controlled and randomized. Preferably double-blind
Endpoints	Bacteriological efficacy, clinical efficacy and safety. Efficacy to be analyzed 5–9 days and 4–6 weeks after treatment
Analyses	Both intention-to-treat analysis of outcome in all patients randomized and per-protocol analysis of patients fulfilling defined criteria (e.g. minimum treatment time, bacteriuria pretreatment and at least one follow-up visit)

TREATMENT OF CYSTITIS

Cystitis accounts for approximately 90% of all infections with significant bacteriuria. Typically, about 75% of women with cystitis have sporadic infections and 25% recurrent infections in an unselected sample. Complicated infections are seen in only about 2% of unselected patients. Most of the patients with cystitis are women aged 15–50 years.

In addition to antibiotic treatment, it is important to provide advice to the patient on how to prevent recurrences. Sexually active women should be told that emptying of the bladder after intercourse will reduce the risk of recurrences.

Although cystitis is a self-limiting benign infection in most patients, antibiotic treatment is recommended,[17] the most important reason being to prevent ascending infections and pyelonephritis.

A large number of antibiotics are used for treatment of uncomplicated cystitis. A general rule is that oral β-lactam antibiotics (ampicillin, amoxicillin, carbacephems, cephalosporins, amoxicillin–clavulanic acid and other β-lactam–β-lactamase inhibitor combinations and pivmecillinam) seem to be considerably less efficacious in eradicating bacteriuria than trimethoprim-sulfonamide combinations, trimethoprim or fluoroquinolones (Table 57.5).[10,18] This is not due to more frequent resistance to β-lactams than to other antibiotics in bacteria causing bacteriuria: a possible explanation is that β-lactam antibiotics are rapidly eliminated (i.e. the urine becomes free from antibacterial drug about 12 h after the last treatment dose). On the other hand, with trimethoprim, trimethoprim-sulfamethoxazole and fluoroquinolones high concentrations of drug are maintained in the urine for 24 h or more after the end of treatment. Another possibility is that the latter drugs reduce the periurethral inoculum more effectively than β-lactams, thereby reducing the risk of recurrences.

There are no major differences in clinical efficacy between antibiotics used for treatment of uncomplicated cystitis. Irrespective of whether the bacteriuria is eliminated or not, symptoms tend to disappear after 3 days. Thus, there is a poor correlation between clinical efficacy and bacteriological efficacy.

Table 57.5 Bacteriological efficacy in a study comparing a β-lactam (ritipenem acoxil) with a fluoroquinolone (norfloxacin) for 5 days treatment of uncomplicated cystitis in women[10]

Follow-up and outcome	Treatment	
	Ritipenem acoxil	Norfloxacin
5–9 Days post-treatment:		
No bacteriuria	51/122 (42%)[a]	77/114 (68%)
Superinfection	22/122 (18%)	20/114 (18%)
Persistence	41/122 (34%)[a]	12/114 (11%)
Not assessable	8/122 (7%)	5/114 (4%)
3–4 Weeks post-treatment:		
no bacteriuria	31/59 (53%)	52/82 (63%)
recurrence	17/59 (29%)	16/82 (20%)
reinfection	11/59 (19%)	8/82 (10%)
not assessable	0/59	6/82 (7%)

[a] $p < 0.001$

The treatment time in uncomplicated cystitis is a controversial issue. Recommendations range from a large single dose to 7 days or more treatment. A short treatment time offers better patient compliance, reduces costs and minimizes risks of adverse effects; however, all antibiotics tested in sufficiently large trials have been found to be less effective if used as a single-dose than in a longer treatment time (Table 57.6).[18] Differences exist between antibiotics. For trimethoprim–sulfamethoxazole and other combinations of trimethoprim and sulfonamides, high cure rates could be demonstrated after administration of a single dose. Treatment for 3 days improved the efficacy but no further benefits were achieved with longer

Table 57.6 Comparative efficacy of trimethoprim–sulfonamide combinations and β-lactam antibiotics when used for different treatment times in patients with uncomplicated cystitis[18]

Treatment time	Rate of eradication of bacteriuria and treatment	
	Trimethoprim–sulfonamide	β-lactam
Single-dose	267/300 (89%)	58/60 (66%)
3-day	139/147 (95%)	282/343 (82%)
>5-day	294/308 (96%)	370/423 (88%)

treatment times. However, with prolonged treatment the frequencies of adverse events increased markedly in patients receiving trimethoprim-sulfonamide combinations while the safety of β-lactam antibiotics was far less affected by the treatment time (Table 57.7). Fluoroquinolones seem also to be relatively effective if used for 3 days or less and probably little is gained by increasing the treatment time to 5 days or more.

Table 57.7 Frequencies of adverse events reported after treatment of uncomplicated cystitis[18]

Treatment time	No. of patients with adverse events and treatment	
	Trimethoprim – sulfonamide	β-lactam
Single-dose	30/404 (7%)	23/212 (11%)
3-day	13/195 (7%)	55/630 (9%)
>5-day	101/406 (25%)	126/934 (14%)

It is recommended that a short course (3 days or less) of trimethoprim–sulfamethoxazole, another trimethoprim–sulfonamide combination or trimethoprim alone is used as first-line treatment of sporadic uncomplicated cystitis when the local susceptibility pattern so allows. The documentation of efficacy is less comprehensive for trimethoprim because for many years trimethoprim–sulfamethoxazole was the gold standard in clinical trials. In pregnant women nitrofurantoin or a β-lactam antibiotic for 5–7 days should be used. β-Lactam antibiotics should otherwise generally be used restrictively due to their poor bacteriological efficacy.

Older, non-fluorinated quinolones should not be used for treatment of any type of urinary tract infections because they are considerably less active than the fluorinated quinolones and resistance emerges in high frequencies with these antibiotics. Moreover, resistance to older quinolones increases the risk of resistance to fluoroquinolones. Resistance to these antibiotics is chromosomal. With the non-fluorinated derivatives a single mutation of one the bacterial genes coding for the DNA-gyrase (topoisomerase I), which is the main target for quinolones, will result in resistance (see Ch. 3). Such mutations occur in a frequency of about 10^{-8} The new fluoroquinolones are 100–1000 times more active and require two consecutive mutations in species such as *Esch. coli* before the organisms become resistant, which is likely to occur at a frequency of 10^{-16}. If an old quinolone is used the first mutation is often initiated, and the risk for mutation to resistance against the fluoroquinolones (if they are used) then increases from 10^{-16} to 10^{-8}.

Patients with recurrent uncomplicated cystitis are more likely to have bacteriuria caused by organisms other than *Esch. coli* or *Staph. saprophyticus*. Pathogens that should be covered are enterococci and *Klebsiella* spp. The choice of antibiotics will depend on the treatment used for the preceding episode. Fluroquinolones, if they have not been used in the same patient recently, are very likely to be effective. To preserve the usefulness of the fluoroquinolones for treatment of these more serious infections and patients with pyelonephritis, these antibiotics are not recommended as first-line drugs for treatment of uncomplicated sporadic cystitis.

In women with frequently recurring cystitis and in whom underlying complicating factors have been excluded short-term self-treatment has been proven to be effective.[19,20]

No follow-up procedures are warranted following treatment of uncomplicated sporadic cystitis. The patient should be told to come back if she again experiences clinical symptoms. However, advice should always be given about ways to avoid recurrences – e.g. double- or triple-voiding, generous fluid intake and (as mentioned above) post-coital bladder emptying.

Antibiotics for treatment of uncomplicated sporadic cystitis can often be chosen without urine cultures, based on knowledge of the local antibiotic susceptibility pattern. In patients with complicated infections (which are typically recurrent), and in patients with uncomplicated infections that recur, urine cultures should be performed routinely.

Antibiotics used for treatment of complicated and recurrent cystitis are the same as those used in sporadic uncomplicated infections. However, β-lactams tend to perform even less well than in sporadic cases and treatment must last 5 days or longer. In these patients the urine should be cultured after treatment to identify and eliminate any complicating factors.

TREATMENT OF PYELONEPHRITIS

Pyelonephritis may be a life-threatening infection. In adults, septicemia may lead to septic shock. In children, there is a marked risk for developing renal scars, which may lead to permanent renal damage if the patient develops recurrent urinary tract infections involving the affected kidney.[13,14] Correct choice of empiric antibiotic treatment is therefore essential.[17,18] The first therapeutic decision to be taken is whether or not the patient needs parenteral treatment. If an injectable antibiotic is needed, there are several alternatives for empiric treatment. In patients with community-acquired sporadic infections, a group 3 cephalosporin (e.g. cefuroxime), an aminoglycoside or, in some countries, trimethoprim–sulfamethoxazole is likely to be effective: ampicillin, amoxicillin and groups 1 and 2 cephalosporins (cephalotin, cefazolin, cefadine and others), against which more than 10% of *Esch. coli* strains are resistant, are not recommended. In patients with hospital-acquired infections a group 4 or group 6 cephalosporin such as ceftazidime, cefotaxime or ceftriaxone, a carbapenem (imipenem or meropenem), an aminoglycoside or a fluoroquinolone (e.g. ciprofloxacin or levofloxacin), are effective in most countries.

In the acute phase of pyelonephritis the renal function is always reduced. This, together with the fact that β-lactams, aminoglycosides and quinolones all achieve high concentrations in urine, blood and renal tissues, allows the use of low doses (e.g. cefuroxime 750 mg three times daily, 3 mg/kg body weight per day of gentamicin, netilmicin or tobramycin, and 200 mg twice daily of intravenous ciprofloxacin). Some patients with pyelonephritis may be given oral antibiotics throughout the course of treatment. Antibiotics to be preferred are the fluoroquinolones, which are more efficacious than oral β-lactam antibiotics.[21] Because quinolones are not recommended for pregnant women, and since the therapeutic efficacy of oral (but not parenteral) β-lactams must be questioned, oral treatment is not recommended initially in pregnant women with signs of pyelonephritis.

An insufficiently studied problem is what to use when a patient started on parenteral treatment is to be switched to an oral regimen. Clinical trials of antibiotics have traditionally not been directed towards this problem and few studies have evaluated the normal clinical situation – i.e. that a patient is treated parenterally for 24–48 h and then continued on an oral antibiotic. At present the best choice for oral follow-up to an injectable antibiotic in a patient with pyelonephritis seems to be a fluoroquinolone.

The treatment time is traditionally 2 weeks in pyelonephritis. Longer periods seem not to increase the cure rates but are likely to result in higher frequencies of adverse reactions to the antibiotics used. One study comparing ciprofloxacin for 7 days with trimethoprim–sulfamethoxazole for 14 days showed equally good results in the two groups. Further studies are needed in this field. The efficacy of treatment for pyelonephritis should be followed up with urine cultures at least once after treatment.

ASYMPTOMATIC BACTERIURIA

Most patients with asymptomatic bacteriuria should not be treated. This is certainly true for patients with bladder catheters: in such cases treatment will only result in selection of increasingly resistant bacterial strains and, if the patient should develop a systemic infection, it may be difficult to find an active antibiotic. Early studies indicated that asymptomatic bacteriuria in elderly people was correlated to an increased mortality; however, more recent investigations have not shown that bacteriuria per se is an independent risk factor for increased mortality.[23–25] In one such study antimicrobial treatment of asymptomatic bacteriuria did not affect mortality.

Exceptions to this rule are pregnant women and patients who are to undergo urogenital tract surgery: both these categories should be screened for bacteriuria and treated if positive. Antibiotics recommended are those used for treatment of uncomplicated cystitis. In other categories of patients (e.g. elderly people and those with diabetes mellitus) screening for bacteriuria is not recommended because treatment of asymptomatic bacteriuria has not been proven to have beneficial effects.

PROPHYLAXIS AND LONG-TERM TREATMENT

Antibiotic prophylaxis of cystitis and pyelonephritis should be used very restrictively. Patients with frequent recurrences of these infections should be investigated in order to find and eradicate complicating factors leading to the recurrences. In some patients episodes of cystitis or pyelonephritis may require prolonged treatment to prevent recurrence before surgery is performed. An important group in which such prophylaxis is indicated is children with congenital anatomical defects. Several studies have indicated that reflux and pyelonephritis in young children is correlated with renal cortical damage and scarring.

In a small fraction of patients with recurrent cystitis or pyelonephritis, mainly girls and young women, no complicating factor can be identified. Such patients benefit from prophylaxis and should be given nitrofurantoin or trimethoprim once-daily at bedtime to ensure high bladder concentrations of drug during sleep. The treatment time is normally 6 months but several years of treatment may be required.

As mentioned above, cystitis in older women is often due to atrophic changes of the vaginal mucosa, increasing the periurethral bacterial inoculum. Elderly women should therefore be examined for vaginal atrophy; if present, atrophy should be treated with estrogen to prevent recurrence. Intravaginal treatment with estriol seems to give the lowest frequencies of adverse reactions.[26,27]

TREATMENT OF PROSTATITIS

Antibiotic treatment of prostatitis differs from that of cystitis and pyelonephritis, both in choice of antibiotic and in treatment time. In patients in whom gonorrhea and chlamydial infection have been excluded, identification of the etiology can be attempted using segmented urine culture (*see above*). However, in most cases this procedure is too cumbersome and treatment is started without etiological verification. Drugs frequently used and well documented are trimethoprim–sulfamethoxazole, tetracyclines (e.g. doxycycline) and fluoroquinolones. Treatment lasts 3 weeks or longer.

TREATMENT OF FUNGURIA

When *Candida* sp. is isolated in the urine and considered clinically relevant, treatment should be given. Amphotericin B is generally active against *Candida* and resistance has never been reported. However, the drug is difficult to administer and has considerable nephrotoxicity. One alternative in selected patients is local instillation of amphotericin B.[28] The azole derivatives (e.g. fluconazole and itraconazole) are liver metabolized and achieve low urine concentrations. Resistance to these drugs may occur; *Candida krusei* and *Candida glabrata* are normally fluconazole resistant. An alternative choice for treatment of candiduria, if the isolated organisms are susceptible, is 5-fluorocytosine (flucytosine) which is excreted by the kidneys and achieves high concentrations in renal tissue. However, caution should be taken not to use too high a dose of this drug, which may lead to adverse reactions. Optimally, serum concentrations of flucytosine should be kept between 25 and 75 mg/l during the entire dose period.

References

1. Kass EH 1957 Bacteriuria and diagnosis of infections of the urinary tract: with observations on the use of methenamine as a urinary antiseptic. *Archives of Internal Medicine* 100: 709–714.
2. Stamm WE, Counts GW, Running KR, Fihn S, Turck M, Holmes KK 1982 Diagnosis of coliform infection in acutely dysuric women. *New England Journal of Medicine* 307: 463–468.
3. Stamm WE 1983 Measurement of pyuria and its relation to bacteriuria. *American Journal of Medicine* 75: 53–58.
4. Rubin EH, Shapiro ED, Andriole VT, Davis RJ, Stamm WE 1992 Evaluation of new anti-infective drugs for the treatment of urinary tract infections. *Clinical Infectious Diseases* 15 (Suppl. 1): S216–227.
5. Svanborg-Edén C, HansonL, Jodal U, Sohl-Åkelund A 1976 Variable adherence to normal urinary tract epithelial cells of *Escherichia coli* strains associated with various forms of urinary tract infections. *Lancet* 1: 490–492.
6. Wullt B, Bergsten G, Samuelsson M, Gebretsadik N, Hull R, Svanborg C 2001 The role of *P fimbriae* for colonization and host response induction in the human urinary tract. *Journal of Infectious Diseases* 183 (Suppl. 1): S43–46.
7. Hedlund M, Rui-Dong D, Nilsson Å, Svensson M, Karpman D, Svanborg C 2001 Fimbriae, transmembrane signaling, and cell activation. *Journal of Infectious Diseases* 183 (Suppl. 1): S47–50.
8. Frendelis B, Godaly G, Hang L, Karpman D, Svanborg C 2001 Interleukin-8 receptor deficiency confers susceptibility to acute pyelonephritis. *Journal of Infectious Diseases* 183 (Suppl. 1): S43–46.
9. Otto G, Sandberg T, Marklund BI, Ulleryd P, Svanborg C 1993 Virulence factors and pap genotype in *Escherichia coli* isolates from women with acute pyelonephritis, with or without bacteremia. *Clinical Infectious Diseases* 17: 448–456.
10. The Swedish Urinary Tract Infection Study Group 1995 Interpretation of the bacteriological outcome of antibiotic treatment for uncomplicated cystitis: impact of the definition of significant bacteriuria in a comparison of ritipenem axetil with norfloxacin. *Clinical Infectious Diseases* 20: 507–503.
11. Hovelius B, Mårdh PA 1984 *Staphylococcus saprophyticus* as a common cause of urinary tract infections. *Reviews of Infectious Diseases* 6: 328–337.
12. Schneider PF, Riley TV 1996. *Staphylococcus saprophyticus* urinary tract infections: epidemiological data from Western Australia. *European Journal of Epidemiology* 12: 51–54.
13. Ditchfield MR, Decampo JF, Nolan TM et al 1994 Risk factors in the development of early renal cortical defects in children with urinary tract infections. *American Journal of Roentgenology* 162: 1393–1397.
14. Smellie JM, Poulton A, Prescod NP 1994 Retrospective study of children with renal scarring associated with reflux and urinary infection. *British Medical Journal* 308: 1193–1196.
15. Domingue GR Sr, Hellstrom WJ 1998 Prostatitis. *Clinical Microbiological Reviews* 11: 604–613.
16. Krieger JN, Jacobs R, Ross SO 2000 Detecting urethral and prostatic inflammation in patients with chronic prostatitis. *Urology* 55: 186–191.
17. Warren JW, Abrutyn E, Hebel JR, Johnson JR, Schaeffer AJ, Stamm WE 1999 Guidelines for antimicrobial treatment of uncomplicated acute bacterial cytitis and acute pyelonephritis in women. *Clinical Infectious Diseases* 29: 745–758.
18. Norrby SR 1990 Short-term treatment of uncomplicated urinary tract infections in women. *Reviews of Infectious Diseases* 12: 458–467.
19. Wong ES, McKevitt M, Running K, Counts GW, Turck M 1985 Management of recurrent urinary tract infections with patient-administered single-dose therapy. *Annals of Internal Medicine* 102: 301–307.
20. Schaeffer AJ, Stuppy BA 1999 Efficacy and safety of self-start therapy in women with recurrent urinary tract infections. *Urology* 161: 207–211.
21. Sandberg T, Englund K, Lincoln K, Nilsson LG 1990 Randomized double-blind study of norfloxacin and cefadroxil in the treatment of acute pyelonephritis. *European Journal of Clinical Microbiology and Infectious Diseases* 9: 317–322.
22. Talan DA, Stamm WE, Hooton TM et al 2000 Comparison of ciprofloxacin (7 days) and trimethoprim-sulfamethoxazole (14 days) for acute uncomplicated pyelonephritis in women. *Journal of the American Medical Association* 283: 1583–1590.
23. Abrutyn E, Mossey J, Berlin JA, Levison M, Pitsakis P, Kaye D 1994 Does asymptomatic acteriuria predict mortality and does antimicrobial treatment reduce mortality in elderly ambulatory women? *Annals of Internal Medicine* 120: 827–833.
24. Nicolle LE, Mayhew WJ, Bryan L 1987 Prospective randomized comparison of therapy or no therapy for asymptomatic bacteriuria in institutionalized elderly women. *American Journal of Medicine* 83: 27–33.
25. Nicolle LE, Bjornson J, Harding GK, MacDonell JA 1983 Bacteriuria in elderly institutionalized men. *New England Journal of Medicine* 309: 1420–1425.
26. Raz R, Stamm WE 1993 A controlled trial of intravaginal estriol in postmenopausal women with recurrent urinary tract infections. *New England Journal of Medicine* 329: 753–756.
27. Raz R 2001 Hormone replacement therapy or prophylaxis in postmenopausal women with recurrent urinary tract infection. *Journal of Infectious Diseases* 183 (Suppl. 1): S74–76.
28. Fisher FJ 2000 Candiduria: When and how to treat it. *Current Infectious Diseases Reports.* 2: 523–530.

58 Infections in pregnancy

Phillip Hay and Rüdiger Pittrof

On a global scale, infection during or after pregnancy is an important public health problem and a leading cause of pregnancy-related health loss. The prevention and appropriate treatment of infection in pregnancy must have a high priority in any health service. Healthcare interventions during pregnancy, the puerperium and the lactational period differ from those occurring at other times as they may affect the health of both mother and fetus/baby.

Possible outcomes of pregnancy-related infections are shown in Table 58.1. The United States Food and Drug Administration (FDA) categories for prescribing antimicrobials are shown in Table 58.2.

While treating infections in pregnancy can improve the health of mother and fetus/baby, it may result in congenital or neonatal health problems or litigation. In affluent countries approximately 1 in 400 babies is affected by a birth defect with a teratogenic etiology. If nutritional supplements are excluded, medication to treat infection constitutes the largest single group of prescribed drugs. As patients often assume that congenital malformations are secondary to a drug taken in pregnancy[1] and attorneys offer 'no-cost litigation,' litigation following antimicrobial treatment is a real risk of prescribing in pregnancy.

GENERAL PRINCIPLES OF DRUG USE IN PREGNANCY AND THE PUERPERIUM

As for any medical intervention, antimicrobial treatment in pregnancy aims to maximize expected benefits while minimizing expected harms. The frequency of harmful outcomes of treatment or its omission is uncertain for most conditions and drugs. When estimating the risks of a treatment, teratology studies in non-human primates offer the best predictors of human teratogenicity as they have a sensitivity and specificity of >90%.[2]

Table 58.1 Theoretically possible outcomes of pregnancy-related infections

Outcome	Example
Healthy mother and healthy fetus	Common cold (most infections)
Mother without apparent health problems, congenital infection with abortion, stillbirth, or long-term morbidity of the child	Untreated latent syphilis infection
Maternal infection causing minimal maternal illness but resulting in congenital infection	Cytomegalovirus infection causing mental retardation. Parvovirus infection causing non-immune hydrops fetalis, toxoplasmal congenital eye disease
Maternal infection causing (preterm) delivery of non-infected child	Urinary tract infection with high maternal fever, malaria
Maternal infection causing (preterm) delivery of an infected child	Chorioamnionitis secondary to ascending lower genital tract infection (group B streptococcus, bacterial vaginosis, toxoplasmosis, rubella)
Maternal death or long-term morbidity following inadequate treatment (this may also affect the health of the fetus/baby)	Postabortion or puerperal sepsis leading to maternal death or infertility
Treatment of maternal illness causing fetal problems	Treatment of maternal infection with aminoglycosides resulting in 8th cranial nerve damage of the fetus
Treatment of maternal illness causing neonatal problems	Neonatal gray syndrome following maternal chloramphenicol treatment. Neonatal kernicterus following maternal long-acting sulfonamides
Litigation of the prescribing physician (not uncommon)	Treatment of maternal illness and birth of a child with congenital abnormalities not related to the infection or treatment

Table 58.2 US FDA categories for prescribing antimicrobials in pregnancy

	Food and Drug Administration (FDA) pregnancy category		
	B	**C**	**D**
FDA definition	Animal reproduction studies fail to demonstrate a risk to the fetus and adequate and well controlled studies of pregnant women have not been conducted	Safety in human pregnancy has not been determined, animal studies are either positive for fetal risk or have not been conducted, and the drug should not be used unless the potential benefit outweighs the potential risk to the fetus	Positive evidence of human fetal risk based on adverse reaction data from investigational or marketing experiences, but the potential benefits from the use of the drug in pregnant women may be acceptable despite its potential risks
Antimicrobials	Amoxicillin, ampicillin, azithromycin, carbenicillin, cefazolin, cefotaxime, cefoxitin, ceftriaxone, cefuroxime, cefalexin, cefalotin, clindamycin, cloxacillin, dicloxacillin, erythromycin, metronidazole, nafcillin, nitrofurantoin, sulfonamides, vancomycin	Aciclovir, amikacin, chloramphenicol, ciprofloxacin, clarithromycin, fluconazole, gentamicin, imipenem, trimethoprim	Tetracyclines, tobramycin

Antiretroviral agents Shown in Table 58.4

Group A
FDA definition: Adequate and well-controlled studies of pregnant women fail to demonstrate a risk to the fetus during the first trimester of pregnancy (and there is no evidence of risk during later trimesters).
Antimicrobials: there are no antimicrobials in this group

Group X
FDA definition: Studies in animals or reports of adverse reactions have indicated that the risk associated with the use of the drug for pregnant women clearly outweighs any possible benefit
Antimicrobials: there are no antimicrobials in this group

When treating infection in pregnancy and the puerperium the prescriber has to decide:

1. When to initiate treatment; when the diagnosis is suspected, as in possible maternal pyelonephritis.
2. When the diagnosis is confirmed, for example maternal tuberculosis, or when the risk of congenital or neonatal problems is minimized as in maternal HIV infection after the first trimester of pregnancy.

3. Which medication to use – whether scientific data are available regarding the safety of various treatments options in pregnancy. Unfortunately, little information is available to assess the frequency of maternal side effects.
4. How the physiological changes in normal and abnormal pregnancy (Table 58.3) affect the pharmacokinetics, dose regimen and side effects of the treatment chosen.

Table 58.3 Implications of physiological changes in pregnancy

Physiological effects in pregnancy	Therapeutic implications
Increased blood volume (>40% at term) and total body water	Possibly larger loading dose
Decreased serum albumin concentration	Possible underestimation of free active drug
Increased hepatic metabolism, increased creatinine clearance	Possible increased drug clearance and need for higher doses and/or shorter dose intervals
Decreased gastrointestinal motility	Unpredictable absorption of oral medication. Possibly increased frequency of gastrointestinal side effects
Pathophysiological changes in pre-eclampsia (proteinuric hypertension in pregnancy). Compared with normal pregnancy: reduced intravascular volumes and total body water, serum albumin and creatinine clearance	Use high doses for drugs with a wide safety margin (such as penicillins) and/or monitor therapeutic levels of drugs with narrow safety margin (such as aminoglycosides) frequently

While there is little information as to how these changes affect the pharmacokinetics of antimicrobial medication, it is reasonable to assume that for a given dose and dose interval serum levels of antimicrobial agents will be 10–15% lower than in a similar non-pregnant patient.[3]

SPECIAL CONSIDERATIONS FOR ANTIMICROBIAL TREATMENT IN PREGNANCY OR DURING LACTATION

ANTIBACTERIALS

Aminogycosides

Aminoglycosides readily cross the placenta, and fetal blood concentrations reach 20–60% of maternal blood levels. Following the long-term use of streptomycin for the treatment of maternal tuberculosis eighth nerve damage has been reported in the neonate,[4] but short-term use of aminoglycosides at therapeutic dose is extremely unlikely to result in fetal ototoxicity.[3] The physiological changes in pregnancy may make it very difficult to maintain therapeutic levels of aminoglycosides in mother (or fetus) and regular monitoring of serum is indicated.

Cephalosporins

The cephalosporins are the most commonly prescribed antibiotics in pregnancy. All cephalosporins cross the placenta and no adverse fetal effects have been reported in humans. However, testicular damage has been observed in male rats following intrauterine exposure to *N*-methylthiotetrazole cephalosporins. Many group 3 and group 4 cephalosporins contain this side chain (*see* Ch. 15) and should be used with caution in pregnancy. Cefoxitin (a group 3 cephalosporin) does not contain the side chain.

Clindamycin

Cord blood levels of clindamycin are only 15–50% of those in maternal blood. Clindamycin has not been linked to congenital abnormalities.

Chloramphenicol

Chloramphenicol has not been associated with an increased risk of congenital malformation. However, when given in late pregnancy there is a theoretical risk of 'gray baby syndrome' (cyanosis vascular collapse and death in premature neonates).

Macrolides

The most commonly used macrolides are erythromycin, azithromycin and clarithromycin. Placental transfer of these antibiotics is low and no fetal problems have been reported.

While there is considerable evidence of the safety of azithromycin in pregnancy it is still labeled as a category B drug by the manufacturer.

Clarithromycin is usually used for the treatment or prophylaxis of *Mycobacterium avium* complex in HIV-positive patients. There are no large studies of this drug in pregnancy and its manufacturer rates it as category C.

Erythromycin has been extensively used in pregnancy and has not been linked to fetal adverse effects, with the exception of erythromycin estolate, which may have increased maternal adverse effects (particularly hepatotoxicity) in pregnancy.

Metronidazole

Metronidazole is the treatment of choice for trichomoniasis and anaerobic infections. It crosses the placenta readily and cord blood levels are similar to maternal blood levels. In mice and bacteria it is tumorigenic and mutagenic but no such observations have been made in humans, and administration to over 1000 women during the first trimester of pregnancy did not result in an increased rate of malformations.[5] However, metronidazole should be used during the first trimester only if the benefits outweigh the potential risks. Metronidazole concentrates in breast milk, causing it to taste bitter and may thus cause problems with breastfeeding.

Nitrofurantoin

Nitrofurantoin is commonly used for the treatment of urinary tract infections in pregnancy. As it crosses the placenta, it could cause hemolysis in a fetus with glucose-6-phosphate dehydrogenase deficiency.

Penicillins

Although all penicillins cross the placenta rapidly and result in cord blood concentrations that may be higher than those observed in maternal blood there is no evidence that they are teratogenic.

Quinolones

In a study of 549 pregnancies exposed to quinolones during the first trimester (70 ciprofloxacin, 318 norfloxacin, 93 ofloxacin and 57 pefloxacin) no increased rate of malformations was observed.[6] However, quinolones are not recommended in pregnancy as they can cause lesions of the cartilage leading to lameness and arthropathy in immature dogs.

Sulfonamides and trimethoprim

Sulfonamides inhibit folate synthesis and may thus be associated with an increased risk of congenital malformations. They cross the placenta readily and compete for fetal and neonatal bilirubin binding sites. In the neonate this could cause hyperbilirubinemia.

Tetracyclines

Tetracyclines readily cross the placenta and when given in the second half of pregnancy are deposited in the long bones (no adverse effects) and deciduous teeth (causing yellow-brown discoloration) of the fetus. The impact of pregnancy on the frequency or severity of adverse side effects of tetracyclines in the mother is unknown but gastrointestinal problems appear to be more frequent. Except for the treatment of penicillin-allergic patients for whom desensitization is not available, tetracyclines are rarely indicated in pregnancy or during lactation.

Vancomycin

There are insufficient data to comment on the safety of vancomycin in pregnancy. Vancomycin can be ototoxic and nephrotoxic and, as it crosses the placenta, similar effects could also occur in the fetus.

Aztreonam and imipenem

There are insufficient data to comment on the safety of these agents in pregnancy.

Antituberculosis drugs

There is good evidence that antituberculosis drugs do not increase the frequency of congenital malformations. Rifampicin (rifampin), ethambutol and isoniazid have no apparent adverse effects and, therefore, are considered safe throughout pregnancy. As pyridoxine requirements in pregnancy are likely to be increased, pregnant women taking isoniazid should also take 50 mg pyridoxine/day. Insufficient data are available for pyrazinamide, which may best be avoided during the first trimester. Streptomycin is not recommended in pregnancy.

ANTIFUNGALS

Nystatin, clotrimazole and miconazole are frequently used for the treatment of candidiasis. There are no reports of increases in malformations from their use and they can be regarded as safe to take in pregnancy. Butoconazole, terconazole and ketoconazole are unlikely to cause malformations but have not been adequately investigated in large studies. Congenital malformations (craniosynostosis, radial-humeral bowing and the tetralogy of Fallot) have been reported following repeated high doses of fluconazole in pregnancy

No controlled studies have evaluated the safety of amphotericin B in pregnancy but case reports do not suggest teratogenicity. Case reports suggest that griseofulvin in early pregnancy could be associated with conjoined twins. Furthermore, fetal skeletal and central nervous system abnormalities have been reported in animal experiments and thus griseofulvin is not recommended in pregnancy.

INTRODUCTION

During the nineteenth century maternal death from puerperal sepsis was a feared and common outcome of delivery. It is now rare in industrialized countries, but infections continue to present more subtle problems for pregnant women. The unique vulnerability of the developing fetus to infection and the role of subclinical infections in preterm birth (and possibly cerebral palsy) are being unraveled.

CHORIOAMNIONITIS AND INTRA-AMNIOTIC INFECTION

Premature delivery is a continuing and serious neonatal problem. Most neonatal deaths and morbidity (in the form of chronic lung disease and neurological impairment) occur in preterm births. Algorithms have been produced to enable obstetricians to estimate the risk of preterm birth for a particular pregnancy. A history of previous preterm birth is the greatest risk factor; this, and most of the other risk factors, are not easily modified during pregnancy. Few interventions have been shown to reduce the incidence of preterm birth, and the incidence has changed little in the last 40–50 years in Europe and USA.[7] Currently the incidence of birth at less than 37 weeks' gestation is 5–7% in Europe and 11% in North America. Most of the mortality and morbidity occurs in babies born before 34 weeks' gestation.

Histologic chorioamnionitis and subsequent amniotic fluid infection are associated with preterm birth; this association is strongest in very preterm birth (< 29 weeks). Animal models have demonstrated putative mechanisms through which infection leads to the release of proinflammatory cytokines such as interleukin-6 and tumor necrosis factor-α.[8] These cytokines in turn stimulate production of arachidonic acid metabolites, including prostaglandins, leading to cervical ripening, uterine contractions and preterm birth. This process is often subclinical, but in its most acute forms is associated with maternal fever, a raised C-reactive protein and an elevated erythrocyte sedimentation rate (ESR) in the mother. Recent studies have implicated elevated levels of proinflammatory cytokines with adverse sequelae in the neonate, including the pathogenesis of fetal cerebral white matter damage and bronchopulmonary dysplasia, precursors of cerebral palsy and chronic lung disease respectively. This has been reviewed in more detail elsewhere.[9]

Most chorioamnionitis is due to ascending spread of bacteria from the lower genital tract either during or before pregnancy. The organisms found most frequently in association with chorioamnionitis and amniotic fluid infection include mycoplasmas (*Ureaplasma urealyticum* and *Mycoplasma hominis*), *Bacteroides* (*Prevotella*) species, *Gardnerella vaginalis*, peptostreptococci, and group B streptococci.[10] Most of these organisms are found in high concentration in the vaginal fluid of women with bacterial vaginosis, but also make up part of the normal flora in healthy women.

Bacterial vaginosis (BV) is the most common cause of vaginal discharge in women of childbearing age. The principal symptom is an offensive fishy-smelling vaginal discharge that is often more apparent during menstruation or following unprotected intercourse. BV may resolve and occur spontaneously. In some populations its prevalence is greater than 50%, although in the UK it occurs in 10 and 15% of women. It is thought to represent a disturbance of the vaginal ecosystem in which the usually dominant lactobacilli are overwhelmed by an overgrowth of predominantly anaerobic organisms including *Gardnerella vaginalis*, *Bacteroides* spp. *Mycoplasma hominis* and *Mobiluncus* spp. There is an increase in the vaginal pH from a normal below 4.5 to up to 7.0. BV is not a sexually transmitted infection and there is no benefit from treating male partners. Many observational studies have confirmed that women with BV have an increased risk of second-trimester loss and preterm birth, with odds ratios between 1.4 and 6.9:[11] indeed, it may be the most important cause of idiopathic preterm birth.

Several studies have evaluated the use of antibiotics to treat women in pregnancy with BV to prevent preterm birth. Some studies of selected women at high risk have shown a benefit from treatment with metronidazole, or with a combination of erythromycin and metronidazole. The largest study, however, used short courses or metronidazole orally and showed no benefit in unselected asymptomatic women, or the subgroup with a previous preterm delivery.[12] Further studies are being performed, but at present no definitive conclusions can be reached on the value of such treatment. Current guidelines from the USA (Centers for Disease Control and Prevention guidelines), the UK (Medical Society for the Study of Venereal Disease Clinical effectiveness group) and a recent Cochrane review[13] do not advocate routine screening for asymptomatic infection, but allow screening and treatment of women with a history of preterm birth or second-trimester miscarriage at the discretion of the clinician.

Standard treatment in the UK for BV is metronidazole 400 mg twice a day for 5 days, resulting in resolution within a few days; however, relapse occurs in as many as 30% of women within 1 month. Alternative treatments include intravaginal 0.75% metronidazole gel, 2% clindamycin cream and oral clindamycin 300 mg twice a day for 5 days. Physicians have been wary of prescribing metronidazole during pregnancy because of reputed teratogenicity, but this has not been proven by human experience. If a woman requires treatment, it is sensible to discuss the potential risks and weigh them against the benefits. Both oral and intravaginal clindamycin have been associated with pseudomembranous colitis, a potentially fatal condition. Women who develop diarrhea following such treatment, particularly with blood, should cease treatment and seek medical advice.

PRETERM LABOR AND PRETERM PREMATURE RUPTURE OF MEMBRANES

Many of the infections that trigger preterm, premature rupture of membranes and preterm birth are subclinical, without accompanying fever, maternal tachycardia, raised white cell count or raised ESR. A large multicenter UK-based study (ORACLE) of antibiotic treatment for women presenting in preterm labour has been completed recently. There was a reduction in adverse neonatal outcome for the use of erythromycin, but not amoxicillin–clavulanic acid, compared with the placebo group. There was an increase in neonatal morbidity with amoxicillin–clavulanic acid, with 2.3% of infants whose mothers received it developing necrotizing enterocolitis (compared with 0.8% in the other groups).[14]

Symptomatic intrauterine infection should be managed by delivery and intrapartum antibiotics, as described for postpartum infection.

ANTIBIOTIC PROPHYLAXIS AND CESARIAN SECTION

Randomized trials provide conflicting evidence as to the value of antibiotic prophylaxis on the prevention of postoperative febrile illness and wound infection following cesarian section. While the most recent and largest study[15] showed no significant benefit, a Cochrane review showed that prophylactic antibiotics reduce the risk of febrile illness by two-thirds to three-quarters. This effect was independent of the timing of administration, the specific antibiotic used and the indication for cesarian section[16] In a 'litigation-friendly environment' obstetricians are currently advised to follow local or national guidelines. If antibiotic prophylaxis is used, ampicillin or a group 1 cephalosporin is a reasonable choice.[17]

URINARY TRACT INFECTION

Asymptomatic bacteriuria occurs in 5–10% of all pregnancies. If it is left untreated, 20–30% of mothers will develop acute pyelonephritis.[18] A Cochrane review compared antibiotic treatment with placebo or no treatment. It found that antibiotic treatment was effective in clearing asymptomatic bacteriuria (odds ratio 0.07, 95% confidence interval 0.05–0.10), reducing the incidence of pyelonephritis (odds ratio 0.24, 95% confidence interval 0.19–0.32) and the incidence of preterm delivery or low birthweight babies (odds ratio 0.60, 95% confidence interval 0.45–0.80).[19,20] Furthermore, screening for and treatment of asymptomatic bacteriuria in pregnancy has been shown to be cost-effective.[21]

It is uncertain whether single-dose therapy is as effective as longer conventional antibiotic treatment[22] (*see* Ch. 57).

POSTPARTUM INFECTION

Following pregnancy the genital tract offers ideal culture conditions for many bacteria. The presence of virulent bacteria (group A and B streptococci, aerobic Gram-negative rods, *Neisseria gonorrhoeae*, organisms associated with bacterial vaginosis or *Mycoplasma hominis*) increases the risk of endometritis,[23] as do prolonged rupture of membranes and multiple vaginal examinations.

A Cochrane review of antibiotic regimens for endometritis after delivery concluded: 'the combination of gentamicin and clindamycin is appropriate for the treatment of endometritis. Regimens with activity against penicillin-resistant anaerobic bacteria are better than those without. There is no evidence that any one regimen is associated with fewer side effects. Once uncomplicated endometritis has clinically improved with intravenous therapy, oral therapy is not needed.'[24]

SPECIFIC INFECTIONS

BACTERIAL INFECTIONS

Syphilis

Syphilis is a sexually transmitted infection caused by the sphirochete *Treponema pallidum*. It can also be spread nosocomially through contact with infected secretions, occasionally through blood products, and transplacentally. Syphilis is common in many developing countries, where up to 10% of pregnant women may have positive serological tests. In Western Europe and the United States the incidence fell progressively over the course of the second half of the twentieth century. An increase in incidence in the USA during the late 1980s was linked to substance abuse, particularly 'crack' cocaine, as was a small epidemic in Bristol in the UK in 1998. Such outbreaks, including the epidemic reported in Russia and Eastern Europe during the 1990s, reinforce the importance of continued vigilance and surveillance against this infection. Syphilis is described fully in Ch. 59, so only the aspects relevant to pregnancy are reviewed here.

Syphilis may infect the fetus at any time during gestation and can be transmitted during any stage of maternal disease; at least two-thirds of all babies born to untreated women with syphilis are infected.[25] The spectrum of congenital syphilis varies, from a severe fetal infection causing intrauterine death to a neonate with symptomatic disease (early congenital syphilis), late congenital syphilis presenting after more than 2 years of age, or asymptomatic infection.

Penicillin is the treatment of choice for syphilis. Current UK guidelines recommend treating early syphilis (primary, secondary or early latent) with procaine penicillin 1.2 million units (1.2 g) daily, intramuscularly, for 12 days. Later stages require 21 days of treatment. Particularly during early syphilis, a Jarisch–Herxheimer reaction may occur. This is mediated by the release of proinflammatory cytokines in response to dying organisms, and presents as a worsening of symptoms with fever for 12–24 h after starting treatment. It does not represent an allergic reaction and may be associated with uterine contractions and preterm labor.

Women who are allergic to penicillin represent a problem. Tetracycline, the second-line treatment, is relatively contraindicated in pregnancy. Erythromycin is less reliable, and resistance has been reported. If erythromycin is to be used, it is best administered intravenously. The neonate should receive treatment with penicillin. The alternative is to perform penicillin desensitization with assistance from a clinical allergist. Current and recent sexual partners of women with syphilis must be screened, as well as older children in the family, if the date of acquisition is unknown.

Treatment in pregnancy should be instituted before 20 weeks gestation to prevent the development of the stigmata of congenital syphilis.[26] In one population studied in the USA, a third of the cases of syphilis diagnosed in pregnant women were acquired during the course of the index pregnancy, suggesting that rescreening may be an appropriate policy in some populations.[27]

The ideal treatment for syphilis in pregnancy is currently uncertain. A Cochrane review found that none of the 26 studies included met the predetermined criteria.[28] Further studies are needed to evaluate the impact of HIV on the effectiveness of the currently recommended treatment regimens.

Stoll comprehensively reviewed the management of an infant born to a mother with reactive serological tests for syphilis.[29] In principle, if the mother has not received definitive treatment with penicillin, the infant *should* be treated with penicillin. The infant should be evaluated clinically, through serological tests and examination of the cerebrospinal fluid (CSF).

Gonorrhea

Neisseria gonorrhoeae is a sexually transmissible agent causing cervicitis, urethritis, endometritis, salpingitis and perihepatitis in women. In men it causes urethritis and epididymitis. In both men and women it causes proctitis and pharyngitis. Gonorrhea is common worldwide, although the incidence has decreased in developed countries since the Second World War. Infection in both sexes may be asymptomatic (*see* Ch. 59). Like chlamydia, gonorrhea is most common in young, sexually active women, with the incidence declining over the age of 25. Its importance in obstetrics is due to a neonatal eye infection that, if untreated, can progress to blindness due to corneal scarring. The introduction of silver nitrate drops as prophylaxis produced a dramatic decline in the incidence of this complication.

The diagnosis is confirmed by culture. DNA detection-based tests are available and might be used for screening, but do not currently provide information about antibiotic sensitivity. *N. gonorrhoeae* has demonstrated a great ability to acquire resistance to antibiotics. It readily exchanges plasmids with other bacterial species and plasmid-mediated resistance to penicillin and tetracycline appear rapidly under selection pressure with such antibiotics. In many developing countries the price of antibiotics is prohibitive for most individuals, so that suboptimal doses are used; this encourages the development of resistant strains, which are then exported worldwide.

Chromosomal mutation has also produced moderate levels of penicillin resistance and is responsible for resistance to quinolones. Quinolones are contraindicated in pregnancy, because of potential damage to developing cartilage and therefore in a penicillin-allergic woman or a woman with penicillin-resistant infection a cephalosporin such as cefotaxime (2 g in a single intramuscular dose) should be administered. In 1996, a Cochrane review of the treatment of gonorrhea in pregnancy concluded that amoxicillin with probenicid or spectinomycin or ceftriaxone are similarly effective.[30]

Neonates may present with ophthalmia neonatorum due to gonorrhea a few days after birth. If *N. gonorrhoeae* is cultured, topical and systemic treatment should be administered according to antibiotic sensitivities (*see* Ch. 56). In a similar way to *Chlamydia trachomatis* infection gonorrhea is associated with chorioamnionitis and preterm birth.

Chlamydia trachomatis

Chlamydia trachomatis is important in pregnancy because it causes neonatal eye infection (ophthalmia neonatorum) and infant pneumonitis. Its role in miscarriage, chorioamnionitis and preterm birth is unclear, with some studies finding associations and others none. Nevertheless, chlamydia infections need to be treated at whatever stage of pregnancy they are diagnosed.

Estimates of the prevalence of genital *C. trachomatis* infection vary between 2% and 10% of women in the UK. The organism is detected much more commonly in young sexually active women, particularly those under the age of 25. The spectrum of disease varies from chronic asymptomatic infection to cervicitis, endometritis, salpingitis (pelvic inflammatory disease) and intraperitoneal spread leading to perihepatitis (Fitz-Hugh–Curtis syndrome). In men it causes non-gonococcal urethritis, which may present with urethral discharge and dysuria.

Approximately 15–25% of babies born to women with chlamydial infection develop ophthalmia neonatorum. The treatment of choice for *C. trachomatis* in the non-pregnant woman is tetracycline, usually doxycycline. Tetracycline should be avoided in the second and third trimesters of pregnancy because it binds to developing bones and teeth in the fetus, causing brown staining of the teeth and dysplastic bones: erythromycin 500 mg twice a day for 2 weeks is therefore prescribed. This may cause nausea, and lower plasma levels are obtained than in non-pregnant women. A test of cure should therefore be performed 2 weeks after completing treatment. It is essential that male partners are screened and treated before sexual intercourse is resumed.

Amoxicillin appears as effective as erythromycin in achieving microbiological cure and is better tolerated than erythromycin.[31] Azithromycin, as a single 1-g dose, is licensed for the treatment of *C. trachomatis* and may be useful if the woman is unable to tolerate erythromycin. Caution is advised if it is used in pregnancy, although no teratogenicity has been reported. Although penicillins are not considered adequate treatment to eradicate *C. trachomatis*, amoxicillin–clavulanic acid is effective in preventing neonatal infection and may be used if macrolides are contraindicated. Definitive treatment with a tetracycline should be administered after completion of pregnancy and breast-feeding. Neonates with ophthalmia neonatorum should be treated with tetracycline eye ointment. Because there is a risk of subsequent chlamydial pneumonitis they should also be treated with a 2-week course of erythromycin syrup.

Chlamydophila abortus

This organism, formerly classified as a strain of *Chlamydia psittaci*, causes epidemic abortion in ewes. In humans it causes an atypical pneumonia. Exposure to lambing ewes, and the products of conception can lead to infection of pregnant women, resulting in intrauterine infection and abortion. It occurs most commonly in veterinarians and farm workers. All pregnant women should be advised to avoid sheep during the lambing season. Treatment is as for *C. trachomatis*.

Listeriosis

Listeria monocytogenes is commonly found in the stool samples of pregnant women; however, invasive disease in pregnancy is very rare. Most maternal disease results in influenza-like symptoms and does not usually require treatment.

Vertical transmission can occur transplacentally or, more frequently during birth from cervicovaginal secretions. Intrauterine infection often leads to premature labor, fetal distress and meconium-stained amniotic fluid. Infection with *L. monocytogenes* responds to treatment with high-dose penicillin, ampicillin or trimethoprim–sulfamethoxazole (not a first-choice drug in the first trimester or in late pregnancy). While most causes of chorioamnionitis call for the early termination of pregnancy (delivery), chorioamnionitis caused by *L. monocytogenes* can be treated medically.[32]

Group B streptococci

Colonization of the vagina with group B streptococci is very common in pregnancy.[33] While it does not usually cause morbidity in mothers, it is a common cause of neonatal infection. A Cochrane review[19,20] concluded that intrapartum antibiotic treatment reduces the rate of infant colonization and early-onset neonatal infection with group B streptococci but does not significantly reduce neonatal mortality. The five randomized trials reviewed by Smaill[19,20] used intrapartum intravenous ampicillin 1 g 6-hourly, benzylpenicillin or erythromycin.

Some guidelines recommend intrapartum treatment of women in preterm labor (<37 weeks), with intrapartum fever or prolonged rupture of membranes if culture results are not available or if the woman is known to be colonized or to have had a previously affected child or a group B streptococcal urinary tract infection.[34]

The best method of screening in pregnancy or labor has not been established. Bergeron and colleagues[35] used the polymerase chain reaction (PCR) in labor. In their hands the test had a sensitivity of 97% and a specificity of 100% and yielded results within 30–45 minutes.

VIRAL INFECTIONS

Specific therapeutic agents to treat viral infections systemically have not been available for more than a few years, with the exception of aciclovir for herpes simplex virus. Their role and safety in pregnancy is not fully established. The potential harm caused by intrauterine or congenital infections means that clinicians must consider the use of many such agents in pregnancy. Nevertheless, for many viral infections that can harm a fetus specific treatments are either not available (e.g. parvovirus and rubella) or have not been studied sufficiently in pregnancy (e.g. cytomegalovirus).

Cytomegalovirus

Cytomegalovirus (CMV) is a herpes virus with the ability to establish latency. In the UK approximately 40% of pregnant women are susceptible. The incidence of primary infection in pregnancy is unknown, but estimated to be about 1%. In healthy women reactivation of latent CMV infection is unusual but may occur in pregnancy. The exposed fetus is less likely to have severe manifestations than in primary maternal infection: the principal features are microcephaly, blindness and deafness but some affected children have sensorineural hearing loss as the only sign of congenital CMV infection. A definitive diagnosis of congenital CMV infection can be made by isolating the virus in cell culture from throat swabs, urine, blood or cerebrospinal fluid (CSF) in the first 3 weeks of life. Serological diagnosis is made by the demonstration of a rising titer of IgG antibody or specific CMV IgM antibody.

Specific antiviral agents such as ganciclovir, foscarnet and cidofovir are available for CMV; however, none should be used routinely. Only ganciclovir has an oral preparation, which produces lower plasma levels than the intravenous formulation. These agents are used in immunosuppressed individuals with AIDS or following transplantation. A trial of intravenous ganciclovir in infected infants has shown some benefit in reducing deafness, but no role for treatment in pregnancy has been established.

Herpes simplex virus

Herpes is important in pregnancy because a devastating neonatal infection can occur with involvement of skin, liver and CNS. Neonatal mortality may reach 75%, but can be reduced to 40% if aciclovir is administered rapidly to the neonate. This syndrome is more common in the USA than the UK, with rates of 1 in 5000 and 1 in 33 000 live births, respectively. The vast majority of these cases are associated with a primary herpes infection in the mother in the weeks before delivery. The baby has no protective antibody and is vulnerable to disseminated infection, or localized herpes encephalitis. The incidence of neonatal herpes is remarkably low considering the high prevalence of both symptomatic and asymptomatic genital herpes in these populations. The risk of neonatal herpes is greatest if primary infection occurs shortly before delivery, when there is no maternal IgG to cross the placenta, providing partial protection to the neonate.

In adults herpes is initially a clinical diagnosis. Typical vesicles or ulcers are seen on the genital mucosa. In primary infection lesions may be widespread, and persist for up to 3 weeks; secondary or recurrent episodes are usually localized and resolve in 3–7 days. In pregnancy recurrences may resemble primary infections, making clinical staging more difficult. Type-specific serological tests are becoming available, which may help to clarify the diagnosis. If antibody to the same type of virus as is isolated on culture or is present in the serum, then it is not a primary infection.

In the non-pregnant woman primary herpes is treated with a 5-day course of aciclovir 200 mg 5 times a day. This prevents further lesions from developing and allows current ulcers to heal. Recurrent episodes do not usually require treatment, as use of antivirals has not been shown to usefully reduce the time to healing.

There are insufficient data to confirm that aciclovir is safe during pregnancy and the manufactures (Glaxo–SmithKline) currently maintain a register. To date there is no excess of birth defects associated with its use but the potential benefits and risks must be discussed with individual mothers. The authors have used aciclovir to control symptoms in pregnant women with primary herpes following such discussions. Like any febrile illness, primary herpes may be associated with early miscarriage. Use of continuous aciclovir to suppress recurrent herpes throughout pregnancy is inadvisable.

Neonatal infection usually follows exposure to active lesions in the mother during delivery. When lesions are present the risk increases in proportion to the time between rupture of the membranes and delivery. In many units if active lesions are identified clinically, and the membranes have not been ruptured for more than 4 h, cesarean section is advocated. As the risk of neonatal herpes is so small for recurrent herpes, this policy cannot be recommended routinely. In the Netherlands cesarean section for recurrent herpes was abandoned in 1987 and there was no subsequent increase in neonatal herpes.[36]

If primary herpes presents around the time of delivery, the pediatrician should be informed. Cesarean section generally provides protection to the infant as long as the membranes have not been ruptured for more than 4 h. Genital swabs should be cultured from mother and throat swabs from the baby within 24 h of birth. Intravenous aciclovir should be administered to the neonate. The role of aciclovir administration for the last 2–4 weeks of pregnancy in women with recurrent herpes has not been evaluated fully because neonatal herpes in such cases is rare.

Human immunodeficiency virus

The acquired human immunodeficiency virus (HIV) pandemic has been spreading around the world since before the original descriptions of AIDS in 1981. Worldwide, approximately equal numbers of men and women are infected; most affected women are of childbearing age. In some cities in sub-Saharan Africa more than 30% pregnant women are HIV infected. In London some hospitals have a prevalence of greater than 0.5% of antenatal attendees. In the UK, approximately 300 children are born to HIV-infected women annually. Since the vast majority of HIV-infected children acquire the infection by perinatal transmission, the prevention of vertical transmission is of paramount importance in reducing the prevalence of pediatric HIV.

Vertical transmission

Mother to child (vertical) transmission of HIV may occur during pregnancy, during childbirth or through breastfeeding. In the absence of intervention, vertical transmission of HIV infection is reported in 15–20% of babies born to HIV-positive women in European/American populations and in 25–35% in Africa and Asia.[36–38] Transmission is more likely if the mother has advanced HIV disease, as shown by a high viral load and a low CD4 count. Other risk factors include prolonged rupture of membranes and exposure to events that brings the fetus in contact with maternal blood such as vaginal/instrumental delivery, the use of fetal scalp electrodes and episiotomy.[37] Premature birth, low birthweight and breastfeeding are also established risk factors associated with increased risk of vertical transmission.

The exact mechanisms for perinatal transmission of HIV and the gestational age of greatest risk have not yet been determined. Viral DNA has been detected in fetal tissues as early as 12 weeks of gestation.[39] At birth, the virus can be detected in 30–50% of infected children,[40] suggesting that the remaining 50–70% of the infected infants without viral markers at birth may have been infected late in pregnancy, during delivery or after birth, mainly through breast feeding. The additional risk of transmission through breastfeeding in infants of infected mothers, over and above transmission in utero or during birth, is estimated to be 16%.[41]

The duration of breast feeding is important and correlates with the risk of transmission. Nevertheless, in developing countries, the negative nutritional impact on overall infant morbidity and mortality of not breast feeding may outweigh the benefit of avoiding HIV transmission from breast milk.

PREVENTING VERTICAL TRANSMISSION

Three interventions have been shown to reduce the risk of vertical transmission: elective cesarean section; bottle feeding; and

antiretroviral treatment for the mother and neonate. In Europe and the USA the rate is currently below 2% in pregnancies in which the mother undertakes the recommended regimens to reduce the risk of transmission.

ANTIRETROVIRAL THERAPY

The aims of antiretroviral therapy in pregnancy are to prevent vertical transmission and maintain maternal health. Current UK guidelines for treatment of adults recommend starting combination antiretroviral therapy if there are clinical indications, or if the CD4 count is below 350 cells/ml (British HIV Association guidelines).

The safety of antiretrovirals in pregnancy has not been assessed adequately. The US FDA guidelines (Table 58.4) rate the nucleoside analogs as category C, with the exception of didanosine, which is category B. Three protease inhibitors are also category B: nelfinavir, saquinavir and ritonavir. All the non-nucleoside analog drugs are category C. A discussion of choice of agents in a standard triple-therapy regimen is beyond the scope of this chapter, but is discussed fully in the FDA guidelines and updated by the perinatal HIV working group at www.hivatis.org. Efavirenz is associated with congenital abnormalities in Rhesus macaque monkeys and its use is not recommended, particularly in the first trimester. To date, when used in human pregnancy, no increased rate of birth defects has been reported.

Potential hazards for the mother and fetus include the usual side effects of triple therapy, such as increased insulin resistance and diabetes mellitus, mitochondrial toxicity and lactic acidosis. Recently a case of maternal death from lactic acidosis in the third trimester was reported. A further hazard is the risk of resistant virus emerging if monotherapy is used. If monotherapy is prescribed to women with low viral loads, CD4 counts > 350 cells/ml and who are clinically well, the risk of developing zidovudine resistance mutations is low. A continuing study from London reported a single resistance mutation in only 3 of 70 women prescribed zidovudine monotherapy in the last 3 years (P.E. Hay, personal communication).

THE ROLE OF SINGLE AGENT (MONO-) THERAPY

The efficacy of zidovudine monotherapy in reducing vertical transmission was demonstrated in a landmark randomized, double-blind, placebo-controlled trial.[41] Treatment was started at between 14 and 34 weeks of gestation, administered intravenously during delivery, and the neonate received oral treatment for 6 weeks. The rate of vertical transmission was reduced by 67% in women treated with zidovudine (25.5% placebo v 8.3% zidovudine) Apart from a mild self-limiting anemia, no adverse effects were observed after a 4-year follow up.

Nevirapine is the only other single drug (other than zidovudine) that has been shown in a randomized controlled trial to significantly reduce vertical transmission. In the HIVNET 012 trial, 600 pregnant women were randomized to receive zidovudine during and at the onset of labor followed by 1 week of neonatal treatment, or a single 200 mg dose of nevirapine at

Table 58.4 FDA categories for antiretroviral agents in pregnancy

Antiretroviral drug	FDA category	Placental passage (newborn to mother ratio)	Long-term animal carcinogenicity studies	Animal teratogen studies
Nucleoside analog reverse transcriptase inhibitors				
Zidovudine (Retrovir, AZT, ZDV)	C	Yes (human) (0.85)	Positive (rodent, non-invasive vaginal epithelial tumors)	Positive (rodent near-lethal dose)
Zalcitabine (HiVID, ddC)	C	Yes (rhesus monkey) (0.30–0.50)	Positive (rodent, thymic lymphomas)	Positive (rodent hydrocephalus at high dose)
Didanosine (Videx, ddl)	B	Yes (human) (0.5)	Negative (no tumors, lifetime rodent study)	Negative
Lamivudine (Epivir, 3TC)	C	Yes (human) (c. 1.0)	Negative (no tumors, lifetime rodent study)	Negative
Abacavir (Ziagen, ABC)	C	Yes (rats)	Not completed	Positive (rodent anasarca and skeletal malformations at 1000 mg/kg (35× human exposure) during organogenesis; not seen in rabbits)
Non-nucleoside reverse transcriptase inhibitors				
Nevirapine (Viramune)	C	Yes (human) (c. 1.0)	Not completed	Negative
Delavirdine (Rescriptor)	C	Unknown	Not completed	Positive (rodent ventricular septal defect)
Efavirenz (Sustiva)	C	Yes (cynomologus monkey, rat,) (c. 1.0)	Not completed	Positive (cynomologus monkey anencephaly, anophthalmia, micro-ophthalmia)
Protease inhibitors				
Indinavir (Crixivan)	C	Yes (rats, rabbits) (substantial in rats, low in rabbits)	Not completed	Negative (but extra ribs in rodents)
Ritonavir (Norvir)	B	Yes (rats) (mid-term fetus, 1.15; late-term term fetus, 0.15–0.64)	Positive (rodent, liver adenomas and carcinomas in male mice)	Negative (but cryptorchidism in rodents)
Saquinavir (Fortovase)	B	Minimal (rats, rabbits)	Not completed	Negative
Nelfinavir (Viracept)	B	Unknown	Not completed	Negative
Amprenavir (Agenerase)	C	Unknown	Not completed	Negative (but deficient ossification and thymic elongation in rats and rabbits)
Lopinavir/ritonavir (Kaletra)	C	Unknown	Not completed	Negative (but delayed skeletal ossification and increase in skeletal variations in rats at maternally toxic doses)

the onset of labor with a single dose administered to the neonate within 3 days of delivery.[42] At 14–16 weeks of age, 13.1% of the nevirapine-treated group were HIV infected, compared with 25.1% in the zidovudine group, a 47% reduction in transmission. Nevirapine monotherapy is relatively inexpensive, easy to administer and has immense potential for use in developing countries. There are concerns about the risk of resistance developing, as it occurred in 23% of women in a small substudy.

COMBINATION THERAPY

Triple therapy is recommended for pregnant women with advanced HIV disease, high viral load or low CD4 counts because the risk of mother-to-infant transmission correlates with these parameters.[43] Nevertheless, the marked reduction in viral load produced by triple therapy, and the resultant reduction in transmission, may be outweighed by potential and unquantified risks of these interventions on the neonate. For women with advanced HIV disease who are reluctant to expose their babies to combination therapy, zidovudine monotherapy plus an elective cesarean section is recommended.[44]

For women who present too late in pregnancy to allow formal virological/immunological assessment, the consensus guidelines recommend a zidovudine regimen with possible addition of lamivudine and/or nevirapine. In women who conceive while on antiretroviral therapy treatment should be continued, although a change to (or the addition of) zidovudine should be considered while it remains the main agent of proven efficacy and safety in human pregnancy.

Hepatitis

In pregnancy the liver appears to be particularly vulnerable to infectious agents. Thus, hepatitis A, for which there is no specific antiviral agent, may cause fulminant, fatal infection in pregnancy, as may hepatitis E. Vaccination against hepatitis A and the use of human immunoglobulin may provide some protection if initiated in the incubation period. In non-pregnant adults ribavirin and interferon are used to treat hepatitis C, but their effects have not been studied in pregnancy. The risk of vertical transmission is low (< 3%), but increases if there is a high level of maternal viremia.

Hepatitis B

Hepatitis B is a more severe infection, which may be followed by chronic carriage and disease ending in cirrhosis. Infection is transmitted sexually through blood or blood products or vertically to the fetus from an infected mother. The majority of acute infections are not clinically recognized, as only 20% of individuals develop jaundice. The earlier in life the infection occurs the more likely the person is to become a carrier: 80% of infants infected perinatally become carriers. Infection is particularly common in China and South-East Asia but prevalent in most tropical countries (*see* Ch. 51).

Pregnant women are screened for hepatitis B at booking. Treatment is available with interferon under the guidance of a liver specialist, and antiviral drugs with specific activity against hepatitis B are being introduced. However, the safety of interferon in pregnancy is not adequately evaluated.[45] Vertical transmission can be prevented by vaccination of neonates born to mothers with hepatitis B. Hepatitis B immune globulin is also given at birth if the mother is antigen e positive. Many countries have a policy of universal vaccination of all infants.

PROTOZOAL AND FUNGAL INFECTIONS

Toxoplasmosis

Maternal infection with the intracellular protozoan parasite *Toxoplasma gondii* is usually asymptomatic and the risk to an immunocompetent mother is minimal. Transplacental fetal infection occurs in 20–50% of primary infections and may cause chorioretinitis, intracranial calcifications and hydro-

cephalus. Diagnosis of primary infection during pregnancy depends on serological screening for *Toxoplasma*-specific IgG in pregnant women followed by confirmatory testing and, ultimately, amniocentesis or cordocentesis. Where the incidence of primary toxoplasmosis in pregnancy is low (e.g. in the USA and UK) screening is currently not recommend. Women who seroconvert during pregnancy should be treated with spiramycin (a macrolide that does not cross the placenta) and, if fetal infection is confirmed, treatment should be changed to pyrimethamine and sulfadiazine plus folate supplements (after 18 weeks' gestation).[46]

Mothers should be informed (a) that such treatment will not always prevent transmission but will reduce the risk of severe congenital malformations developing and (b) that maternal side effects and congenital abnormalities may occur as a result of the treatment.

Trichomoniasis

Trichomonas vaginalis causes a severe vulvovaginitis in susceptible women. It is generally sexually transmitted, although infection may persist asymptomatically for many months in women and in some men. In men it causes urethritis but is frequently asymptomatic. Male partners should be screened for sexually transmitted diseases and treated with metronidazole.

Transient infection may be transmitted to newborn female infants who have stratified squamous epithelium in the vagina, similar to that of an adult, due to the influence of high levels of maternal estrogen in utero. These infants are susceptible to infection and may present with purulent vaginal discharge. As the influence of maternal estrogen wanes over the first few weeks of life, infection usually resolves spontaneously and specific treatment is rarely necessary.

The only established treatments for trichomoniasis are metronidazole and tinidazole. As discussed above, there is no evidence of teratogenicity from metronidazole use, and it should be used to treat symptomatic infection whatever the stage of pregnancy. Treatment of asymptomatic trichomoniasis with metronidazole did not prevent preterm birth in a randomized controlled trial.[47]

Malaria

Malaria is prevalent throughout the tropics and is a major cause of mortality in both children and adults. *Plasmodium falciparum* causes the most severe type of malaria, which can present with hepatic and cerebral manifestations. It is transmitted between human hosts by the female *Anopheles* mosquito. *P. falciparum* has been able to develop resistance to most antimalarials, creating a need for new agents. The other strains of malaria seldom cause fatal disease but cause considerable morbidity; they are virtually always chloroquine sensitive (*see* Ch. 64).

Pregnant and puerperal women are at increased risk of malaria infection. If they become infected with malaria complications, particularly hypoglycemia and lactic acidosis, are more frequent. Infection may also trigger a miscarriage or premature labor. In hyperendemic areas the disease may present as severe anemia, with a negative blood film. In women at risk of malaria regular chemoprophylaxis is associated with fewer episodes of fever in the mother, fewer women with severe anemia antenatally, and higher average birthweight in infants than treatment of symptomatic malaria.[48] Even non-falciparum malaria has been associated with intrauterine growth retardation. Congenital malaria has been described.

The diagnosis should be suspected in anybody who has been to the tropics and presents with a febrile illness. A history of taking prophylaxis does not exclude the diagnosis, as no prophylaxis is 100% effective. A blood film should be requested and stained for malaria parasites. Repeated blood films should be taken during episodes of fever if the initial test is negative. As well as anemia there may be thrombocytopenia and elevation of liver enzymes. Fever in the tropics or in people recently returned may be caused by many other infections including typhoid, food poisoning organisms, and viral infections such as dengue fever.

Pregnant women with malaria should be admitted to hospital and monitored closely as sudden deterioration requiring intensive care may occur. Confirmed or possible falciparum malaria is usually treated with quinine sulfate. The dose regimen and mode of administration is not affected by pregnancy. Quinine does not cause abortion or preterm labor (unless massively overdosed) but can induce hypoglycemia and lactic acidosis. Malariae, vivax and ovale malaria should be treated with standard doses of choloroquine. Vivax and ovale malaria can develop persisting forms (hypnozoites). The best method of eradication therapy in pregnancy is currently controversial and expert advice should be obtained. A treatment course of pyrimethamine–sulfadoxine may be appropriate.

Individuals living in endemic areas acquire immunity to malaria but lose it within a few months of moving away. Therefore, anyone travelling from a non-malarial country to an endemic area should take prophylaxis (*see* Ch. 64 for recommendations). A randomized controlled trial in Kenya found that intermittent sulfadoxine-pyrimethamine (Fansidar) was safe and prevented severe anemia secondary to malaria in pregnancy.[49]

The choice of prophylactic agent should be made after consulting current recommendations giving details of resistance patterns. Chloroquine is probably the least toxic prophylactic agent for pregnant women. Those travelling to areas of chloroquine resistance must balance the risk of malaria against the potential toxicity of prophylactic agents. It is safest to avoid travel to such areas when pregnant but if the mother cannot be persuaded to delay travel the potential risks and benefits of chemoprophylaxis (and/or standby treatment) must be discussed.

Vaginal candidiasis

Over three-quarters of women have at least one episode of vaginal candidiasis during their lifetime. The organism is carried in the gut, under the nails, in the vagina and on the skin. The yeast *Candida albicans* is implicated in more than 80% cases; *Candida glabrata*, *Candida krusei* and *Candida tropicalis* account for most of the rest (*see* Ch. 62). *Candida* is an opportunist, growing under favorable conditions. Symptomatic episodes are common in pregnancy; its growth is favored by the high levels of estrogen, increased availability of sugars, and subtle alterations in immunity.

In general it is better to use a topical treatment rather than systemic one. This minimizes the risk of systemic side effects and exposure of the fetus. Vaginal creams and pessaries can be prescribed at a variety of doses and duration of treatment. For uncomplicated candidosis, a single dose treatment, such as clotrimazole 500 mg, is adequate. If oral therapy has to be used, a single 150 mg tablet of fluconazole is usually effective, although the safety of fluconazole in pregnancy has not been established.

References

1. Brent LB 1998 Legal considerations of drug use in pregancy. In: Gilstrap LC, Little BB (eds). *Drugs and Pregnancy*. New York, pp. 33–42.
2. Little BB, Gilstrap LC 1998 Human teratology principles. In Gilstrap LC, Little BB (eds). *Drugs and Pregnancy*. New York, pp. 7–24.
3. Gilstrap LC, Little BB 1998 Antimicrobial agents during pregnancy. In: Gilstrap LC, Little BB (eds). *Drugs and Pregnancy*. New York, pp. 77–102.
4. Donald PR, Sellars SL 1981 Streptomycin ototoxicity in the unborn child. *South African Medical Journal* 60: 316–318.
5. Rosa FW, Baum C, Shaw M 1987 Pregnancy outcomes after first-trimester vaginitis drug therapy. *Obstetrics and Gynecology* 69: 751–755
6. Schaefer C, Amoura-Elefant E, Vial T et al 1996 Pregnancy outcome after prenatal quinolone exposure. Evaluation of a case registry of the European Network of Teratology Information Services (ENTIS). *European Journal of Obstetrics, Gynecology and Reproductive Biology* 69: 83–89.
7. Gibbs RS, Romero R, Hillier SL, Eschenbach DA, Sweet RL 1992 A review of premature birth and subclinical infection. *American Journal of Obstetrics and Gynecology* 166: 1515–1528.
8. Gravett MG, Witkin SS, Haluska GJ, Edwards JL, Cook MJ, Novy MJ 1994 An experimental model for intraamniotic infection and preterm labor in rhesus monkeys. *American Journal of Obstetrics and Gynecology* 171: 1660–1667.
9. Hay PE, Ugwumadu A, Sharland M 2001 Infections in obstetrics. In: *Turnbull's Obstetrics* Chamberlain G, Steer P (eds). London
10. Hillier SL, Martius J, Krohn M, Kiviat N, Holmes KK, Eschenbach DA 1998 A case control study of chorioamnionic infection and histologic chorioamnionitis in prematurity. *New England Journal of Medicine* 319: 972–978.
11. Hillier SL, Nugent RP, Eschenbach DA et al 1995 Association between bacterial vaginosis and preterm delivery of a low-birth-weight infant. The Vaginal Infections and Prematurity Study Group. *New England Journal of Medicine* 333: 1737–1742.
12. Carey JC, Klebanoff MA, Hauth JC et al 2000 Metronidazole to prevent preterm delivery in pregnant women with asymptomatic bacterial vaginosis. *New England Journal of Medicine* 342: 534–540.
13. Brocklehurst P, Hannah M, McDonald H 2001 Interventions for treating bacterial vaginosis in pregnancy (Cochrane Review). In: *The Cochrane Library*, Issue 3. Oxford, Update Software.
14. Kenyon SL, Taylor DJ, Tarnow-Mordi W, ORACLE Collaborative Group 2001 Broad-spectrum antibiotics for spontaneous preterm labour: the ORACLE II randomised trial. ORACLE Collaborative Group. *Lancet* 357: 989–994.
15. Bagratee JS, Moodley J, Kleinschmidt I, Zawilski W 2001 A randomised controlled trial of antibiotic prophylaxis in elective caesarian delivery. *British Journal of Obstetrics and Gynaecology* 108: 143–148.
16. Smaill F, Hofmeyr GJ 2001 Antibiotic prophylaxis for cesarean section (Cochrane Review). In: *The Cochrane Library*, Issue 3. Oxford, Update Software.

17. Hopkins L, Smaill F 2001 Antibiotic prophylaxis regimens and drugs for cesarean section (Cochrane Review). In: *The Cochrane Library*, Issue 3. Oxford, Update Software.

18. Whalley P 1967 Bacteriuria of pregnancy. *American Journal of Obstetrics and Gynecology* 97: 723–738.

19. Smaill F 2001 Intrapartum antibiotics for Group B streptococcal colonisation (Cochrane Review). In: *The Cochrane Library*, Issue 3. Oxford, Update Software.

20. Smaill F 2001 Antibiotics for asymptomatic bacteriuria in pregnancy (Cochrane Review). In: *The Cochrane Library*, Issue 3. Oxford, Update Software

21. Rouse DJ, Andrews WW, Goldenberg RL, Owen J 1995 Screening and treatment of asymptomatic bacteriuria of pregnancy to prevent pyelonephritis: a cost-effectiveness and cost-beneficial analysis. *Obstetrics and Gynecology* 86: 119–123.

22. Villar J, Lydon-Rochelle MT, Gülmezoglu AM, Roganti A 2001 Duration of treatment for asymptomatic bacteriuria during pregnancy (Cochrane Review). In: *The Cochrane Library*, Issue 3. Oxford, Update Software.

23. Newton ER, Prihoda TJ, Gibbs RS 1990 A clinical and microbiologic analysis of risk factors for puerperal endometritis. *Obstetrics and Gynecology* 75(3): 402–406.

24. French LM, Smaill FM 2001 Antibiotic regimens for endometritis after delivery (Cochrane Review). In: *The Cochrane Library*, Issue 3. Oxford, Update Software.

25. Zenker PN, Rolfs RT 1990 Treatment of syphilis, 1989. *Reviews of Infectious Diseases* 12 (Suppl. 6). S590–S609.

26. Wendel GD 1988 Gestational and congenital syphilis. *Clin Perinatol* 15(2): 287–303.

27. Goldmeier D, Hay P 1993 A review and update on adult syphilis with particular reference to its treatment. *International Journal of STD and AIDS* 4: 70–82.

28. Walker GJA 2001 Antibiotics for syphilis diagnosed during pregnancy (Cochrane Review). In: *The Cochrane Library*, Issue 3. Oxford, Update Software.

29. Stoll BJ 1994 Congenital syphilis: evaluation and management of neonates born to mothers with reactive serologic tests for syphilis *Pediatric Infectious Diseases Journal* 13: 845–853.

30. Brocklehurst P 2001 Interventions for treating gonorrhoea in pregnancy (Cochrane Review). In: *The Cochrane Library*, Issue 3. Oxford, Update Software.

31. Brocklehurst P, Rooney G 2001 Interventions for treating genital chlamydia trachomatis infection in pregnancy (Cochrane Review). In: *The Cochrane Library*, Issue 3. Oxford, Update Software.

32. Silver HM 1998 Listeriosis in pregnancy. *Obstetric and Gynecology Surveys* 53: 737–740.

33. Campbell JR, Hillier SL, Krohn MA, Ferrieri P, Zaleznik DF, Baker CJ 2000 Group B streptococcal colonization and serotype-specific immunity in pregnant women at delivery. *Obstetrics and Gynecology* 96(4): 498–503.

34. Centers for Disease Control 1996 Prevention of perinatal group B streptococcal disease: a public health perspective. *Morbidity and Mortality Weekly Report* 45 (No RR-7).

35. Bergeron MG, Ke D, Menard C et al 2000 Rapid detection of group B streptococci in pregnant women at delivery. *New England Journal of Medicine* 343(3): 175–179.

36. van Everdingen JJ, Peeters MF, ten Have P 1993 Neonatal herpes policy in the Netherlands. Five years after a consensus conference. *Journal of Perinatal Medicine* 21: 371–375.

37. Peckham C, Gibb D 1995 Mother-to-child transmission of the human immunodeficiency virus. *New England Journal of Medicine* 333: 298–302.

38. Newell ML, Gray G, Bryson YJ 1997 Prevention of mother-to-child transmission of HIV-1 infection. *AIDS* 11(Suppl. A): S165–S172.

39. Backe E, Unger M, Jimenez E, Siegel G, Schafer A, Vogel M 1993 Fetal organs infected by HIV-1. *AIDS* 7: 896–897.

40. Burgard M, Mayaux MJ, Blanche S et al 1992 The use of viral culture and p24 antigen testing to diagnose human immunodeficiency virus infection in neonates. The HIV Infection in Newborns French Collaborative Study Group. *New England Journal of Medicine* 327: 1192–1197.

41. Nduati R, John G, Mbori-Ngacha D et al 2000 Effect of breastfeeding and formula feeding on transmission of HIV-1: a randomized clinical trial. *Journal of the American Medical Association* 283: 1167–1174.

42. Connor EM, Sperling RS, Gelber R et al 1994 Reduction of maternal-infant transmission of human immunodeficiency virus type 1 with zidovudine treatment. Pediatric AIDS Clinical Trials Group Protocol 076 Study Group. *New England Journal of Medicine* 331: 1173–1180.

43. Guay LA, Musoke P, Fleming T et al 1999 Intrapartum and neonatal single-dose nevirapine compared with zidovudine for prevention of mother-to-child transmission of HIV-1 in Kampala, Uganda: HIVNET 012 randomised trial. *Lancet* 354: 795–802.

44. Taylor GP, Lyall EG, Mercey D et al 1999 British HIV Association guidelines for prescribing antiretroviral therapy in pregnancy (1998). *Sexually Transmitted Infections* 75: 90–97.

45. Watanabe M, Kohge N, Akagi S, Uchida Y, Sato S, Kinoshita Y 2001 Congenital anomalies in a child born from a mother with interferon-treated chronic hepatitis B. *American Journal of Gastroenterology* 96(5): 1668–1669.

46. Jones JL, Lopez A, Wilson M, Schulkin J, Gibbs R 2001 Congenital toxoplasmosis: a review. *Obstetric and Gynecology Surveys* 56(5): 296–305.

47. Klebanoff MA, Carey JC, Hauth JC et al 2001 Failure of metronidazole to prevent preterm delivery among pregnant women with asymptomatic *Trichomonas vaginalis* infection. *New England Journal of Medicine* 345(7): 487–493.

48. Garner P, Gülmezoglu AM 2001 Prevention versus treatment for malaria in pregnant women (Cochrane Review). In: *The Cochrane Library*, Issue 3. Oxford, Update Software.

49. Shulman CE, Dorman EK, Cutts F et al 1999 Intermittent sulphadoxine-pyrimethamine to prevent severe anaemia secondary to malaria in pregnancy: a randomised placebo-controlled trial. *Lancet* 353(9153): 632–636.

 Further information

Anonymous 1998 Guidelines for Treatment of Sexually Transmitted. 47. 23–1–1998. Centers for Disease Control and Prevention Recommendations and Reports.

Clinical Effectiveness Group (Association of Genitourinary Medicine and the Medical Society for the Study of Venereal Diseases) 1999 National guideline for the management of bacterial vaginosis. *Sexually Transmitted Infections* 75(Suppl. 1): S16–S18.

59 Sexually transmitted diseases

Vicky Johnston and Adrian Mindel

Many infections are sexually transmitted, as listed in Table 59.1. Some infections, including HIV, hepatitis B and hepatitis C, can be transmitted by blood or blood products. Others, like human papillomavirus, herpes simplex virus, and molluscum contagiosum can be transmitted by close bodily contact.

In 1995 the World Health Organization (WHO) estimated that there were 333 million cases of the four major curable sexually transmitted diseases (trichomoniasis, chlamydia, gonorrhea and syphilis) among people aged 15–49.[1] 90% of cases occur in developing countries. Viral sexually transmitted diseases (STDs), in particular HIV, have become an increasing problem over recent years: the joint United Nations programme on HIV/AIDS estimated that at the end of 2000 there were 36.1 million people living with HIV/AIDS, most in developing countries.[2]

The rate of spread of any STD within a community is dependent on a number of factors, including exposure to an infected individual, efficiency of transmission and the duration of infectiousness. The epidemiologic pattern of individual infections depends on the interplay between these factors and the social, economic and political environment. This interplay to an extent explains the different patterns of infection in developed versus developing countries. One of the more dramatic examples of the effect of social, economic and political changes on STDs is demonstrated by the epidemic growth of such diseases in the former USSR with the breakdown in communism. The growth in the sex industry, exchange of sex for drugs, economic crisis and a change in healthcare provision and disease reporting have all played a part in this epidemic.

At an individual level there are a number of risk factors. For example, early coitarche, multiple sexual partners within the last 3 months, choice of partners from high-risk groups, failure to use barrier contraception and drug use.

Both the infection itself and its complications have important health, social and economic consequences for the individual and their community. These complications include pelvic inflammatory disease leading to infertility and ectopic pregnancy, complications of pregnancy and the puerperium (congenital, perinatal and postnatal infections) and a variety of cancers (cervical, vaginal, vulval, penile, anal, Kaposi's sarcoma and lymphoma). Clearly, STDs, and in particular genital ulcer disease, affect the spread of HIV,[3] increasing the transmission of the virus. Control of STDs is becoming increas-ingly important for control of individual infections and to halt the spread of HIV.

CHLAMYDIA

Chlamydiae are obligate intracellular bacteria, which infect eukaryotic cells, depending on these cells for many of the nutrients they require for growth and replication. There are several species, two of which infect humans as their primary host (*Chlamydia trachomatis* and *Chlamydophila pneumoniae*). *C. trachomatis* can be further divided into biovars, distinct group of biological variants, each producing a different disease spectrum. Serovariants or serovars of the trachoma biovar result in trachoma (serovars A–C) or sexually transmitted diseases (serovar D–K). Lymphogranuloma venereum compromises the serovars L1, L2 and L3 and forms the second biovar in the *C. trachomatis* species.

EPIDEMIOLOGY

C. trachomatis has the highest prevalence of any sexually transmitted bacterial infection in developed countries.[4] The WHO estimated that worldwide in 1995 there were 89 million new cases of *C. trachomatis* infection in people aged 15–49. This makes it second only to trichomoniasis as the leading cause of curable STD. It is difficult to obtain accurate data with regard to prevalence and incidence, as up to 80% of women and 50% of men may be asymptomatic. In both sexes the prevalence of infection ranges from 3 to 5% in low-prevalence general medical settings to 15 to 20% in high-prevalence STD clinics.

In common with other STDs, risk factors include age below 25, new sexual partner or more than one partner in the recent past, lack of barrier contraception, use of the oral contraceptive pill, termination of pregnancy and non-White race.

The disease results in significant complications, including pelvic inflammatory disease, infertility, ectopic pregnancy,

Table 59.1 Sexually transmitted infections

Disease	Causative organism	Complications
Bacterial		
Gonorrhea	*Neisseria gonorrhoeae*	Pelvic inflammatory disease, bartholinitis and bartholin's abscess, systemic dissemination, epididymo-orchitis
Chlamydia	*Chlamydia trachomatis*	Pelvic inflammatory disease, bartholinitis and bartholin's abscess, epididymo-orchitis
Syphilis	*Treponema pallidum*	Central nervous system, cerebrovascular system and gummatous infection
Chancroid	*Haemophilus ducreyi*	Local genital destruction
Lymphogranuloma venereum	*Chlamydia trachomatis*	Local abscess, fistulas, strictures and genital destruction, rarely meningoencephalitis, hepatitis, pneumonitis
Donovanosis (granuloma inguinale)	*Calymmatobacterium granulomatis*	Local genital destruction, genital lymphedema, squamous cell carcinoma, bone and liver dissemination
Viral		
Genital warts	Human papillomaviruses	Genital tract tumor (mainly cervical cancer—with 'high risk' types)
Genital herpes	Herpes simplex virus type 1 and 2	Acute systemic viremia with primary HSV-2, local recurrence
Molluscum contagiosum	Molluscum contagiosum virus	
HIV	Human immunodeficiency virus types 1 and 2	Severe immune suppression, opportunisitic infection
Hepatitis B	Hepatitis B virus	Fulminant hepatitis, chronic infection, cirrhosis, hepatocellular carcinoma
Hepatitis A	Hepatitis A virus	Fulminant hepatitis
Hepatitis C	Hepatitis C virus	Fulminant hepatitis, chronic infection, cirrhosis, hepatocellular carcinoma
Other infections and miscellaneous conditions		
Candidiasis	*Candida albicans* *Candida glabrata*	
Bacterial vaginosis	Reduced lactobacilli, high-concentration anaerobic bacteria	Pelvic inflammatory disease, and chorioamnionitis, prematurity, premature rupture of membranes, low birthweight
Trichomoniasis	*Trichomonas vaginalis*	Premature rupture of membranes, low birthweight
Non-specific genital infection	*Ureaplasma urealyticum*, *Mycoplasma genitalium*, *Mycoplasma hominis*	

neonatal infection, epididymo-orchitis and reactive arthritis, making it a personal and public economic and social burden. In the UK the annual cost of complications is estimated to be at least £50 million and in the USA the annual cost of 4–5 million cases estimated at $2.4 billion.[5,6]

PATHOGENESIS

The infective agent of chlamydia is a metabolically inactive elementary body, which attaches to epithelial cells, induces phagocytosis and, avoiding lysosomal fusion, enters the reticulate system. Once within the phagosome the elementary body undergoes morphological change to form the reticulate body. This is the metabolically active, replicating form of chlamydia. Over the next 48–72 h the reticulate body replicates with increasing numbers reorganizing into elementary bodies: a mature inclusion body may contain thousands of elementary bodies. When cell death is imminent lysosomal fusion occurs, the cell ruptures and elementary bodies are released. The disease process is thought to result from a combination of direct tissue damage secondary to chlamydial replication, a local inflammatory response and the body's humoral and cell-mediated immune responses.

The immune responses to chlamydia control the acute infection, which is often self-limiting; however, the infection evolves into a low-grade chronic infection which, unless treated, persists. One hypothesis regarding the pathogenesis is that there is a delayed hypersensitivity reaction to chlamydia heat shock protein (hsp 60).[6] Chlamydial and human hsp 60 share extensive amino acid sequence identity. Correlations have been noted between women with late-stage disease (tubal infertility and ectopic pregnancy) and antibody titers to chlamydia hsp 60.[7] Chlamydial hsp 60 shares some antigenic sites with mycobacterium and *Escherichia coli*. Infections with these pathogens could presensitize the patient, resulting in a primed response to chlamydial infection and greater disease severity.

DIAGNOSIS

Clinical

Most women with uncomplicated chlamydial infection are asymptomatic. Those that do have symptoms present with lower abdominal pain, vaginal discharge, intermenstrual or post-coital bleeding and on examination have mucopurulent cervicitis and/or contact bleeding. Men present with a varying degree of dysuria and urethral discharge. Rectal infection results in proctitis and pharyngeal infections are asymptomatic.

Investigations

Any patient who presents with the above symptoms or signs is at high risk and should be tested. The options are culture, antigen testing or nucleic acid tests. Although culture has the highest specificity, sensitivity is low, it is an invasive investigation requiring endocervical or urethral swab, prior experience is essential and it is expensive. Antigen testing is cheap, has relatively easy specimen collection and transport conditions; however, sensitivity is variable and positive predictive value in low prevalence populations is low (<5%). Nucleic acid tests such as the polymerase chain reaction (PCR) and ligase chain reaction (LCR) are highly specific and highly sensitive but expensive. PCR and LCR have gained popularity in male diagnosis due to non-invasive specimen collection (urine instead of urethral swab) and have been shown to be comparable with other test methods.[8] Urine collected needs to be a 'first-pass' sample. Further studies are required before this can be advocated over cervical culture in women.[9] When obtaining swabs an endocervical swab (not wooden) or urethral swab, preferably taken after the patient has not passed urine for 2–4 h, is required. Serology is available but is of little diagnostic value in genital disease as it fails to differentiate between previous and current infection.

MANAGEMENT

Uncomplicated infection:

- single dose azithromycin 1 g orally
- doxycycline 100 mg twice a day, for 7 days.

  Alternative regimens:

- erythromycin 500 mg four times a day for 7–14 days
- ofloxacin 200 mg twice a day for 7 days
- tetracycline 500 mg four times a day for 7 days
- amoxicillin 500 mg three times a day for 7 days (recommended in pregnancy only).

Azithromycin and doxycycline are equally efficacious.[10] Azithromycin has a very long half-life, a large volume of distribution with excellent tissue and cellular penetration (*see* Ch. 24) and can be given as a single dose. This makes it an ideal choice in patients who are non-compliant; however, they should still abstain from sex for 7 days. Its side effect profile is better than that of doxycycline, with the major problem being mild gastrointestinal disturbance. Doxycycline can also lead to gastrointestinal disturbance, in particular esophagitis, the other common side effect being photosensitivity (*see* Ch. 33). The limiting factor in prescribing azithromycin is cost, particularly in developing countries. Cost-effective analyses, however, indicate that azithromycin is more cost effective when duration of course and compliance are taken into account.[11] This is not surprising when studies have shown that about a quarter of patients prescribed doxycycline for proven of presumed chlamydial genital infection either fail to commence or complete the treatment course.[12]

Alternative therapies all have broadly comparable cure rates but use is limited either because of side effects or cost. Erythromycin has been studied at 500 mg four times a day or 500 mg twice a day for 7–14 days. The higher dose regimens are slightly more efficacious but less effective because of gastrointestinal intolerance, with up to half of patients not being able to complete the course. Ofloxacin, one of the fluroquinolones, has been shown to be as effective as doxycycline with a better side effect profile but is considerably more expensive and does not share the advantage with azithromycin of single-dose therapy.[13] Tetracyclines are as efficacious but have a greater reporting of side effects than doxycycline and have to be taken four times a day which raises concern about compliance and therefore effectiveness of the drug when used outside a trial environment.

Pregnancy and breast feeding

Doxycycline and ofloxacin are contraindicated in pregnancy. Azithromycin is not currently recommended because of insufficient data. Initial information that the drug is effective, but further confirmatory studies are required. Azithromycin in a pregnant woman will have a larger volume of distribution, may have variable absorption and will be metabolized at a greater rate by the liver. Current recommendations in pregnant woman are either erythromycin as above or amoxicillin; this has a similar cure rate to erythromycin and a better side effect profile when compared by meta-analysis.[14] However, it is not clear whether amoxicillin eliminates the organism or temporarily suppresses replication. Due to the concerns over efficacy of therapy in this sub-group, a test of cure is advised 3 weeks after completion of treatment.

Sexual partners

All sexual contacts of the index case (within 4 weeks if symptomatic, or up to 6 months if asymptomatic) should be traced, screened and treated if necessary. To optimize partner notification, counseling may be required and the method should be documented and followed up at subsequent consultations.

Screening

Since many infections with *Chlamydia* are asymptomatic and the sequelae can be devastating, screening programs should be implemented. Screening criteria are normally age related and can include behavioral and clinical measures. Where screening programs have been implemented, prevalence has decreased.[15] Not only are these programs epidemiologicaly effective but they also appear to be cost-effective at prevalence as low as 3%.[16]

GONORRHEA

Neisseria gonorrhoeae is an aerobic Gram-negative diplococcus of the genus *Neisseria*. In common with other members of this genus its primary site of infection is mucous membranes. The gonococcus and meningococcus are the two major pathogenic species seen in humans. In the case of gonorrhea primary infection leads to urethritis, cervicitis, proctitis or pharyngitis. Co-infection with *Chlamydia* has been reported in 20–40% of people.

EPIDEMIOLOGY

In 1995, the WHO estimated that there were 62 million cases of gonorrhea worldwide in adults aged 15–49. Most of these cases were in the developing world, reflecting the global population distribution. The incidence of gonorrhea in most developed countries has declined since the 1980s; however, in recent years an increase has been reported in some countries among both homosexual men and heterosexuals.[17,18] In 1999 the annual incidence in the UK varied widely, with highest incidences in London: 141 per 100 000 (males) and 55 per 100 000 (females).[19] The number of cases diagnosed rose by 25% between 1998 and 1999. In 1999 133.2 per 100 000 cases of gonococcal infections were reported in the USA, with the highest incidence in the South (202.9 per 100 000);[20] overall an increase of 1.2% over 1998.

Risk factors for gonorrhea are the same as for most STDs and have been discussed earlier. Gonorrhea also shows a distinct ethnic minority bias, as demonstrated in a number of studies both in the USA and Europe. These differences can be partly explained by accessibility to healthcare, poverty and socioeconomic class but the differences still exist even in studies that have tried to control for these factors.[21]

Transmission between partners depends partly on the frequency of exposure and sexual practice. Men have a 20% risk of acquiring urethral infection after one episode of vaginal intercourse but 60–80% after four episodes. Women who have had contact with a known male case of gonococcal urethritis have 50–90% prevalence of infection.[22,23] Pharyngeal to urethral infection is becoming increasingly recognized with the change in sexual practice seen following the emergence of HIV. Another factor that aids transmission is the number of asymptomatic cases. Although not as commonly as in chlamydial infection, up to 35% of women and 1–3% of men will be asymptomatic.

PATHOGENESIS

N. gonorrhoeae has two main patterns of infection. Most bacteria are limited to the mucosal surface, where they cause marked tissue damage, local primary infection and local complications. Some bacteria are able to disseminate throughout the body, resist serum attack and cause disseminated infection with little or no mucosal damage. Within each infection pattern exists a spectrum of pathogenicity. The surface molecules expressed determine the severity and pattern of infection seen, including those responsible for adherence, metabolite transport, and tissue toxicity and against which various antibodies are formed. Two surface molecules, pilus and opacity proteins, are responsible for adherence to cells. Both show antigenic variation, allowing them to attach in different niches and escape the host's immune responses, and show phase variation, which alters the pathogenicity of the gonococci. Once adhered to the cell the gonococci, in order to survive, must evade neutrophil phagocytosis. Pili surface proteins increase resistance to phagocytosis and killing:[24] even following phagocytosis 2% of gonococci survive.[25] Gonococci adhere to and invade mucus-secreting, non-ciliated cells. Inside this immune privileged site they multiply, divide, then exit from the basal surface by exocytosis. The tissue damage caused by gonococci is thought to be secondary to extracellular products such as enzymes (phospholipase, peptidase), lipo-oligosaccharides and peptidoglycans.[26,27]

Gonococci have developed a number of mechanisms to avoid killing by serum antibodies and complement. For example, blocking antibodies against a surface molecule, reduction modifiable protein (RMP), appear to inhibit IgM complement-fixing antibodies from recognizing their target on lipo-oligosaccharides.[28] Blocking antibodies to RMP have not only been shown to be of importance in the development of serum resistance but also appear to play a part in mucosal immunity, and therefore bacterial transmission between partners. Women with antibodies against RMP are more likely to acquire mucosal infection from their partner because these antibodies in the genital secretions block protective antibodies.[29] Serum-resistant gonococci, however, lead to limited (if any) mucosal inflammation, which correlates with their inability to trigger a chemotactic response to neutrophils. Serum-sensitive gonococci, which are limited to the mucosal surface, are throught to be able to trigger a strong chemotactic response and marked mucosal inflammation.[30]

DIAGNOSIS

Clinical[31,32]

Symptomatic women commonly present with vaginal discharge associated with cervical infection. Dysuria but not frequency is seen with urethral infection, which is present in 70–90% of infections. Less commonly, patients will present with intermenstrual bleeding or menorrhagia. Clinical findings include a mucopurulent cervical discharge with contact bleeding and ectopy. Frequently, no signs are evident in uncomplicated infection. If the infection has ascended up the genital tract to cause pelvic inflammatory disease, a different spectrum of symptoms and signs is observed as discussed later.

In men the most common presentation is urethral discharge, occurring up to 14 days after infection. About half of these will have dysuria. Asymptomatic infections do occur but are less common. The discharge tends to be purulent and associated with erythema at the urethral meatus. Epididymitis occurs in 1% of infections. Other sites of infection include rectal infection via direct inoculation in homosexual men and perineal contamination in females. In women it is often asymptomatic, but 50% of men will have discharge or proctitis. Pharyngeal infection also occurs but in most patients is asymptomatic and spontaneously resolves in about 12 weeks.

In addition to the local complications of pelvic inflammatory disease and epididymitis, disseminated infection can occur. This is rare and presents as an arthritis–dermatitis syndrome. The arthritis takes the form of either an acute, asymmetric destructive monoarthritis or a reactive arthropathy. Classically the rash is in the form of distal, tender, necrotic pustules, however, many different presentations occur. Meningitis and endocarditis are infrequently described.

Investigations

The gold standard investigation is culture on selective culture media containing antimicrobials to reduce contamination. This has a high sensitivity (80–95%) and specificity. In male urethral swabs the sensitivity of microscopy and Gram stain alone in a symptomatic individual is 90–95%, which is comparable with culture. However, the sensitivity falls to 50–75% in asymptomatic infections and 50–70% in cervical infection.[33] Microscopy and Gram stain, therefore, has a place in rapid diagnostic testing but can not supplant culture. Nucleic acid tests are growing in popularity and do have sensitivities in the range of 87–98%, but in an organism that shows increasing antibiotic resistance, culture and antimicrobial testing will always be the gold standard. Serological testing has too low a sensitivity and specificity to be of use in screening, case finding or diagnosis.

MANAGEMENT

Anogenital infection

Single dose treatment with:

- ciprofloxacin 500 mg orally;
- ofloxacin 400 mg orally;
- cefixime 400 mg orally; or
- ceftriaxone 250 mg intramuscularly.

Alternative regimen: single dose of spectinomycin 2 g intramuscularly.

Patients with positive microscopy, positive culture or a recent partner with confirmed gonorrhea should receive treatment. The choice of antibiotics depends to a large extent on local resistance patterns. Since the 1950s antibiotic resistance has been documented to a number of different antibiotics, in particular penicillin, tetracycline and quinolones. Resistance is acquired through either multiple chromosomal mutations or single-step plasmid acquisition. The antibiotics chosen should eliminate infection in 95% of those treated.[34] The WHO and individual countries use sentinel surveillance systems to monitor susceptibility and guide treatment recommendations. In general, resistant strains are more prevalent in developing countries. Quinolone resistance has been increasingly documented worldwide, with the highest levels in South-east Asia and the Pacific area. In these areas quinolones are no longer recommended in the treatment of gonorrhea. In 1999 the Gonococcal Isolate Surveillance Project in the USA recorded 28.1% of isolates resistant to penicillin, tetracycline or both.[20] The proportion of isolates with decreased susceptibility to ciprofloxacin rose to 1.1%. In Honolulu, 14.3% were resistant to ciprofloxacin and fluoroquinolones are no longer recommended in the treatment of gonorrhea. Similar trends have been seen in the UK with a 66% increase in antimicrobial resistance between 1999 and 2000.[19] In both the USA and the UK gonococci remain sensitive to ceftriaxone. To date there have been no recorded isolates resistant to cephalosporins, and one record of an isolate from the UK in 1999 that was resistant to spectinomycin.

One systematic review has been carried out of studies published between 1980 and 1993 looking at single-dose antimicrobial therapy, excluding β-lactamase-sensitive penicillin and tetracyclines.[35] Of the 24 383 reviewed cases 96.7% were cured based on culture results. Cure rates were over 95% for all sites specified excluding the pharynx, which had a cure rate of 80%. A total of 21 antibiotics were looked at, including cephalosporins, fluroquinolones, azithromycin, rifampicin and spectinomycin. Those that appeared to offer the best balance of efficacy and safety in the treatment of uncomplicated gonococcal infection included ceftriaxone (125 mg), cefixime (400 mg), ciprofloxacin (500 mg) and ofloxacin (400 mg). In general all the single-dose regimens recommended above have few side effects and are well tolerated. The disadvantages of using ceftriaxone and spectinomycin are that both have to be given intramuscularly. The limiting factor in prescribing is antimicrobial resistance and therefore it is important to know the local prevalence of resistant organisms.

Pharyngeal infection

Ceftriaxone, ciprofloxacin or ofloxacin, in dosages as above, can all be used to treat pharyngeal infection.[35,36] Spectinomycin and ampicillin have poor efficacy in eradication.

Disseminated gonococcal infection

* intravenous ceftriaxone 1 g every 24 h.

   Alternative regimens:

* intravenous cefotaxime 1 g every 8 h;
* intravenous ciprofloxacin 500 mg every 12 h;
* intramuscular spectinomycin 2 g every 12 h.

No systematic reviews or studies on the treatment of disseminated gonoccocal infection have been carried out in recent years. The above regimens have been used in clinical practice with no reported adverse effects.

All patients should be admitted to hospital for initial treatment and examined for endocarditis and meningitis. Parenteral therapy is continued for 24–48 h after signs of improvement are seen, followed by oral therapy to complete a full week's course. If meningitis is present, ceftriaxone is continued parenterally for up to 2 weeks and, if endocarditis is present the drug should be taken for at least 4 weeks. Local expert opinion is advised when treating disseminated infection.

Pregnancy and breast feeding

* Intramuscular ceftriaxone 250 mg.
* Oral cefixime 400 mg.
* Oral amoxicillin 3 g given 30 min after oral probenecid 1 g.
* Intramuscular spectinomycin 2 g.

Two randomized controlled trials have studied the treatment of gonorrhea in pregnancy; one compared ceftriaxone with cefixime and the other evaluated ceftriaxone, amoxicillin and spectinomycin.[37] Eradication rates, as determined by microbiological cure, ranged from 89 to 97%. In these two trials all antibiotics were efficacious in treating the infection; however, in practice the prevalence of local antibiotic resistance must be taken into account. No serious side effects were reported. Fluroquinolones are not recommended in pregnancy because of reported arthropathy in animal studies.

Sexual partners

All sexual partners of the index case within the last 2–3 months should be evaluated and treated for gonococcal and chlamydial infection. As with all contact tracing, counseling may be required and the method of tracing chosen should be documented and followed up.

Further management

All patients should be screened for other STDs, in particular chlamydia infection. Dual infection can be seen in 20–40% of the population: at that level the cost of routine dual therapy is less than the cost of testing for chlamydia.

NON-SPECIFIC URETHRITIS

There are several infectious causes of urethritis other than gonorrhea and chlamydia, including *Trichomonas vaginalis*, Herpes simplex viruses, *Ureaplasma urealyticum*, *Mycoplasma genitalium* and *Mycoplasma hominis*. However, in practice, once gonorrhea and chlamydia have been excluded the other organisms are seldom sought; instead the condition is usually managed empirically. Tetracyclines, erythromycin and azithromycin are all effective.[38–42]

* Azithromycin 1 g orally (single dose).
* Doxycycline 100 mg twice a day, for 7 days.
* Erythromycin 500 mg four times a day for 7–14 days.
* Tetracycline 500 mg four times a day for 7 days.

PELVIC INFLAMMATORY DISEASE

There are many causes of pelvic inflammatory disease (PID) and it is beyond the scope of this chapter to review these in detail. However, PID is a major complication of two sexually transmitted organisms (*Neisseria gonorrhoea* and *Chlamydia trachomatis*) together with anaerobic organisms. Definitive diagnosis of PID is dependent on laparoscopy and, as this is regarded as an invasive procedure, many individuals are treated

Box 59.1 Treatment for PID as recommended by CDC[44]

Inpatient treatment
Regimen A:

Cefoxitin 2 g intravenously every 6 h or a group 4 cephalosporin plus doxycycline 100 mg intravenously or orally every 12 h.

Regimen B:

Clindamycin 900 mg intravenously every 8 h plus intravenous or intramuscular gentamicin loading dose 2 mg/kg body weight followed by 1.5 mg/kg every 8 h.

Intravenous therapy for both regimens should be continued for at least 48 h and followed by doxycycline 100 mg twice daily or clindamycin 450 mg daily for 14 days.

Outpatient treatment
Regimen A:

Cefoxitin 2 g intramuscular plus probenecid 1 g orally or group 4 cephalosporin plus doxycycline 100 mg orally twice daily for 14 days.

Regimen B:

Ofloxacin 400 mg orally twice daily for 14 days plus clindamycin 450 mg orally four times daily or metronidazole 500 mg orally twice daily for 14 days.

presumptively. This results in over-diagnosis of PID and under-diagnosis of other causes of pelvic pain.[43] As microbiological confirmation is seldom undertaken treatment is directed at the most likely organism(s).

The Centers for Disease Control and Prevention (CDC) recommend the treatments shown in Box 59.1.[44]

Cure rates (i.e. microbiological resolution and clearance of symptoms) are achieved with most regimens. A recent meta-analysis showed that regimens with two or more drugs had a better than 90% success rate.[45] However, damage to the fallopian tubes and subsequent infertility are long-term consequences of PID, particularly where this occurs more than once.

EPIDIDYMO-ORCHITIS

Epididymo-orchitis is a complication of gonorrhea and chlamydia, particularly in men under the age of 35. Treatment should be directed at these organisms and should include intramuscular ceftriaxone 250 mg as a single dose (or other group 4 cephalosporin) plus doxycycline 100 mg twice daily for 10 days. An alternative regimen is to use ofloxacin 300 mg twice daily for 10 days.[44]

In men over 35 years of age, treatment should be directed at urinary tract infections.

LYMPHOGRANULOMA VENEREUM

EPIDEMIOLOGY

Lymphogranuloma venereum (LGV) is a disease of developing countries, where it is often endemic. Sporadic cases do occur in developed countries, often secondary to sexual contact overseas. Within endemic countries, cases tend to occur in the sexually promiscuous, low socioeconomic class groups, and in urban areas. Most patients presenting with acute LGV are in their 20s and male: the male to female ratio varies but can reach as high as 5:1. This gender bias is due to a greater proportion of asymptomatic cases in women. The later complications, however, are reported more frequently in women.

PATHOGENESIS

LGV is a disease of the lymphatics, with the organism inducing a thrombolymphangitis and perilymphangitis in the drainage site of the primary infection. The endothelial cells lining the lymphatic vessels proliferate and central necrosis occurs. These areas coalesce to form abscesses from which fistula or sinuses can develop. This acute inflammatory process lasts weeks to months and is followed by fibrosis, resulting in further destruction to the lymphatics. Chronic edema devel-

ops secondary to lymphatic obstruction and the areas often become indurated with break down of the overlying skin. When the rectum is involved a picture similar to that of Crohn's disease develops with transmural inflammation, mucosal ulceration and inflammatory strictures.

DIAGNOSIS

Clinical

Like syphilis, LGV is divided into three stages.

- The first stage is the development of a painless non-scarring ulcer or papule most commonly found on the glans penis, vaginal wall or labia. It occurs 3–12 days after sexual contact and often heals unnoticed. Less commonly, lesions can be found intraurethrally, leading to a non-specific urethritis, on the cervix, leading to cervicitis, or in the rectum, leading to proctitis. Lymphangitis develops in the field of drainage.
- The second stage manifests as tender lymphadenopathy in the inguinal and/or femoral region. In two-thirds of cases this is unilateral. The area can feel matted and ulceration with sinus formation can develop. When both inguinal and femoral regions are affected the taut inguinal ligament forms a groove, which is said to be pathognomonic of LGV. This stage is often associated with a fever, and meningoencephalitis, hepatitis, pneumonitis, erythema nodosum and erythema multiforme have been described. The time period between the primary lesion and lymphadenopathy is on average 10–30 days but may be as long as 6 months.
- Not all cases progress to the tertiary stage, where spread and destruction of surrounding areas results in proctocolitis, abscess formation, fistulas and strictures. This is more common in females and homosexual men. Alternatively, a lesion (esthiomene) occurs when the primary infection has involved the lymphatics of the scrotum, penis or vulva. Lymphangitis, lymphatic obstruction and fibrosis result in induration, enlargement and ulceration of the affected parts. This is a destructive process most commonly seen in women.

Investigations

LGV is one of a number of differential diagnoses for genital ulceration and lymphadenopathy. Investigations need to exclude other diagnoses and other coexisting sexually transmitted diseases. Various techniques can be used to assess lymph node aspirates or ulcer base exudates. These include culture, immunofluoresence, enzyme immunoassay and detection of nucleic acid by PCR. Alternatively, serological testing including micro-immunofluoresence, complement fixation or enzyme-linked immunosorbent assay may be used. Culture is the most specific method but its sensitivity is poor (50–85%). Culture and immunofluorescence are labor intensive and expensive. Enzyme immunoassay is relatively easy but has poor sensitivity and needs confirmation by another method. PCR, used in non-LGV chlamydia, has not been used to any great extent in LGV; although it is of high sensitivity and specificity PCR is prohibitively expensive for many developing countries. Of the serological tests micro-immunofluorescence is one of the most sensitive and specific and can distinguish the serotype, making it the diagnostic test of choice if available.

MANAGEMENT

Studies regarding the treatment of LGV are few. Assessment of treatment outcome is difficult because spontaneous resolution can occur. CDC guidelines suggest the following:[44]

- doxycycline 100 mg orally twice a day for 21 days;
- erythromycin 500 mg orally four times a day for 21 days.

Treatment must be commenced early to limit the chronic phase. Resolution of symptoms should be seen within a few days and (in the case of uncomplicated proctocolitis) the rectal mucosa should heal within a few weeks. In the presence of further complications such as fistulas, sinuses or strictures, surgery may be required, always under antibiotic cover.

SYPHILIS

The causative organism of syphilis is *Treponema pallidum*, subspecies pallidum, a spirochetal organism belonging to the genus *Treponema*. The genus includes three other human pathogens, *T. pallidum* subspecies *pertenue* (the cause of yaws), *T. pallidum* subspecies *endemicum* (the causative organism of bejel), and *Treponema carateum*, the causative organism of pinta.

EPIDEMIOLOGY

The incidence of syphilis in the developed world has shown dramatic fluctuations during the twentieth century. The infection was extremely common throughout Europe in the early part of the century.[46] Following the First World War, social stability and improvements in living standards and healthcare resulted in a decline in incidence. However, this was short-lived, and during and immediately after the Second World War the incidence again increased.[47] The introduction of penicillin and improvements in healthcare resulted in a dramatic decline in the infection in the 15 years following the Second World War. During the 1960s and 1970s there was an increase in syphilis in many parts of the world, particularly in homosexual men.[48] However, the 1980s saw the widespread promotion of safer sex messages as a consequence of the HIV epidemic, and this led to a dramatic decline in syphilis, particularly in Europe, North America and Australia. Unfortunately, in Eastern Europe and some inner cities in North America, the incidence of syphilis has increased alarmingly in recent years as a consequence of poverty, unemployment, poor healthcare, and social breakdown. Indeed, incidence in Eastern Europe increased from approximately 5 per 100 000 cases in 1990 to 150 per 100 000 in 1994.[49]

In the developing world the situation is completely different. Syphilis has remained as a major public health problem, and in some parts of sub-Saharan Africa approximately 4% of adults between 15 and 49 years of age have serological evidence of previous syphilis.[1]

PATHOGENESIS

Treponemes enter the body via microabrasions caused by the trauma of sexual intercourse and then migrate into the dermis, where they attach to the surface of cells. They do not enter the cell, but penetrate the endothelial junctions and tissue layers. There is localized infection at the site of invasion, usually resulting in a local lesion (chancre), and then the organism disseminates throughout the body. Late complications are due to chronic inflammatory reaction that continues over many years.[50] Cardiovascular syphilis is characterized by lymphocytic and perivascular infiltrates, resulting in an obliterative endarteritis. The pathological changes of latent neurosyphilis again reflect a chronic inflammatory reaction with lymphocytes and plasma cells infiltrating the meninges and perivascular areas resulting in degeneration of neural cells.[51] *T. pallidum* has an immune evasiveness, which is its key to success as a pathogen. This may partly be due to its sequestration in immune sanctuary sites masking the organism's surface by host proteins, or the paucity of outer membrane proteins to act as antigenic targets.[52] Some of the immunogenic proteins appear to be under the cell surface and associated with the periplasmic leaflet.[53] In addition, the proteins are usually present in small numbers, further restricting their potential as immune targets.[54]

DIAGNOSIS

Clinical

The incubation for syphilis varies from 9 to 90 days, with an average of 21 days. Syphilis is divided into several stages.

- The primary infection, or chancre, is the site of local inoculation and replication. The chancre usually heals within 3–10 weeks.
- The secondary stage corresponds with dissemination of the infection and is characterized by skin and mucous membrane lesions and constitutional symptoms.[55]
- This is followed by a latent phase.
- In many individuals, latency is established without any signs or symptoms of early infection; these individuals may go on to develop the late complications of infection, including

cardiovascular, neurological or gummatous disease. Cardiovascular problems include aortitis, aortic incompetence, and aortic aneurysms. The second major late complication is neurological syphilis involving the brain and/or spinal cord. Gummatous disease represents a hypersensitivity reaction and is characterized by nodules consisting of necrotic tissue surrounded by mononuclear cells and proliferating connective tissue. They can occur in any tissue or organ, but most commonly in skin or bone.

Infection is completely curable in the primary and secondary stages; however, cardiovascular and/or neurological damage is irreversible, although progression can be prevented with treatment. The natural history of untreated syphilis is variable: around 10% develop cardiovascular disease, 10% neurological disease and 10% gummatous disease.

INVESTIGATIONS

Syphilis can be diagnosed either through direct visualization of the organism or by serological testing. Direct visualization of the organism may be possible in primary and secondary syphilis where specimens may be obtained from primary chancres or mucous membrane lesions.[56] The organism is not visible under direct light microscopy but can be viewed under dark-field microscopy of a serous exudate applied to a slide, usually moistened with a small amount of saline. The organisms can be visualized as motile spirochetes, characteristically said to display corkscrew and angular motion. The organism should have between 15 and 20 coils. Specimens may also be examined with fluorescent antibody stains, a method that can also be used on biopsy and autopsy specimens.

The mainstay of diagnosis relies on serology. There are two types of serological test for the diagnosis of syphilis: non-treponemal and treponemal tests.

Non-specific antibodies directed towards anticardiolipin, cholesterol and lecithin form the basis for the non-treponemal tests.[57] They can be detected in serum and are related to disease activity. However, these tests also become positive in response to other disorders, including acute viral and mycoplasmal infection, vaccination, pregnancy and the connective tissue disorders. The two tests commonly used are the Venereal Disease Research Laboratory test and the rapid plasma reagin test.

The treponemal tests are specific. However, once positive they tend to remain so, and consequently detection of antibodies indicates past *or present* infection. Two tests are commonly used: the fluorescent treponemal antibody absorption test,[58] and the *Treponema pallidum* hemagglutination assay.[59] Antibodies can be detected in serum and cerebrospinal fluid (CSF). In early infection no antibodies are present and the first to become positive is usually the fluorescent treponemal antibody absorption test.

MANAGEMENT

The aims of treatment are to eliminate the infection, thereby preventing onward spread, and to prevent complications. Penicillin remains the mainstay of treatment. No controlled trials have been conducted for the treatment of syphilis, but penicillin clearly revolutionized its management when it was introduced in the late 1940s and early 1950s. Despite widespread use of penicillin, *T. pallidum* remains sensitive to the drug. Treatment choices are predicated on the convenience of dosage, CSF penetration, concomitant HIV infection, and allergy. Benzathine penicillin is convenient to use and is consequently a popular choice in many parts of the world. However, it has poor CSF penetrance,[60,61] and some experts consider that procaine penicillin is a better choice, particularly when used with probenecid, which delays renal excretion and prolongs the half-life of penicillin in the blood.[62]

Primary, secondary or early latent syphilis if the CSF is negative[44,63]

Treatment is procaine penicillin 600 mg intramuscularly daily for 10 days together with probenecid 10 mg twice daily. An alternative is to use benzathine penicillin G 2.4 million units intramuscularly as a single dose.

If the patient is allergic to penicillin, doxycycline 100 mg should be administrated orally twice a day for 21 days.

Cardiovascular, gummatous or neurosyphilis[44,63]

Intramuscular procaine penicillin 1.8 g daily and probenecid 500 mg four times a day for 17 days is an effective regimen. As an alternative intramuscular benzathine penicillin G 2.4 million units may be given at weekly intervals for 3 weeks, or doxycycline 100 mg orally twice a day for 28 days.

The Jarisch–Herxheimer reaction

An influenza-like reaction with headache, myalgia and fever sometimes occurs within 24 h of starting therapy. This is believed to be due to the rapid reduction in treponemal load and can be managed with simple antipyretics.[64] Occasionally this reaction may cause severe complications in late syphilis, particularly where the cerebral vasculature or the aorta is involved. Systemic steroids are said to be useful in this circumstance, and prednisolone 30 mg daily for 3 days, commencing the day before treatment is said to be helpful. However, controlled trials have not been conducted.

Syphilis in an HIV-positive patient[44,63]

The treatment is the same as for late syphilis.

Pregnancy[44,63]

Procaine penicillin and benzathine penicillin are both suitable drugs for treatment in pregnancy; doxycycline is not recommended. However, erythromycin 500 mg orally four times a day for 21 days is a suitable alternative in patients who are allergic to penicillin. If erythromycin is used the baby should be treated with procaine penicillin (*see below*).

Congenital syphilis

Infants under 2 years should receive daily procaine penicillin 50 mg/kg intramuscularly for 14 days. For children over 2 years the adult doses, as mentioned above for late syphilis, should be used.

CHANCROID

Chancroid is one of the most common causes of genital ulceration in the developing world, often found associated with painful inguinal lymphadenopathy. The causative agent is *Haemophilus ducreyi*, a Gram-negative anaerobic coccobacillus.

EPIDEMIOLOGY

In 1995 the WHO estimated the annual incidence of chancroid to be 7 million.[65] The burden of this infection is in developing countries, where it is endemic. Genital ulcer disease (GUD) is a common presentation: in one study in Malawi over 50% of males presenting to a STD clinic had GUD;[66] 1% of patients attending a Nairobi primary healthcare clinic were diagnosed with GUD. *Haemophilus ducreyi* can be isolated from 20–60% of patients with GUD. In developed nations both incidence and prevalence are low, with occasional outbreaks described in Canada and US southern states. These outbreaks are thought to occur when infected individuals travel to nonendemic areas. They have often been associated with the exchange of sex for money or drugs and the use of crack cocaine or alcohol. In these epidemics the number of male cases exceeds females by 10:1.

H. ducreyi is transmitted through sexual contact, with occasional case reports of autoinoculation to non-genital sites. Low socioeconomic groups are at greatest risk. Infection is twice as common among uncircumcized men as in circumcized men. Female sex workers with subclinical disease form a reservoir of infection but there is no evidence for asymptomatic carriers. If not treated the infection is thought to last about 45 days. The probability of transmitting chancroid to an uninfected individual during a single act of sexual intercourse is 0.35%.[67]

The presence of GUD, in particular chancroid, is an important risk factor in the transmission of HIV.[3] The mechanism behind this is thought to be that *H. ducreyi* recruits CD4 cells and macrophages to the genital surface, providing an increased target population of cells for HIV to infect. Where there is coinfection with HIV and chancroid, the risk of transmission is thought to be greater with an increase in viral replication as CD4 cells and macrophages are activated.

PATHOGENESIS

H. ducreyi can penetrate the epidermis only through an abrasion or trauma. It incites a predominantly TH1 response, with recruitment of CD4 and CD8 lymphocytes, macrophages and granulocytes to the site of infection. The initial lesion is commonly intraepidermal and organisms can be found both within polymorphs and in the interstitium. The more virulent strains of *H. ducreyi* are able to withstand phagocytosis and killing by neutrophils. In addition to the cellular immune response a humoral immune response is elicited, with antibodies targeted particularly against lipo-oligosaccharide. The role of these immune responses in the pathogenesis of chancroid, both the ulcer and the associated lymphadenopathy, are not fully understood and require further evaluation.

DIAGNOSIS

Clinical

Chancroid has an incubation period of 3–10 days. It presents differently in men and women. Men present having noticed the ulcer or because of inguinal tenderness; women, however, have a wide range of symptoms depending on the initial site of infection. These include dysuria, dyspareunia, vaginal discharge and pain or bleeding on defecation.[68] The ulcer can be single or multiple. Women often have a number of discrete ulcers whereas over half of affected men will only have a single ulcer. The ulcer classically has ragged, undermined edges, a necrotic base with purulent exudate and bleeds easily on contact. It is non-indurated and has little surrounding inflammation. Pain is characteristic of chancroid in men but is less frequently described in women, where infection can be subclinical. The ulcers are sited where the incidence of trauma is greatest: in men they are therefore found either on the internal or external surface of the prepuce, the frenulum or in the coronal sulcus; in women, on the fourchette, labia, vestibule or clitoris. Ulcers can, however, extend into the vagina and have been described on the cervix.

Associated painful inguinal lymphadenopathy is described in up to 50% of cases, being unilateral and extensive. Buboes form, become fluctuant and rupture leading to extensive ulceration. Superinfection of both these and the primary ulcers by anaerobic organisms can lead to phagodenic ulceration and extensive tissue destruction. Another complication in men is that of phimosis, which occurs late and often requires circumcision.

Investigations

Diagnosis requires identification of the organism and exclusion of other differential diagnoses, in particular herpes simplex, syphilis and LGV. At present the 'gold standard' is culture of swabs taken from the base of the ulcer. Pus aspirated from the bubo can also be cultured but has a far lower yield as the number of organisms here are low. For optimum results a selective culture medium is required – for example gonococcal agar base, supplemented with either fetal calf serum or charcoal. With these methods, sensitivities of at least 80% are reached. Samples can also be looked at with Gram staining and appear as Gram-negative coccobacilli with occasional chains. This is only 50% sensitive when compared with culture. PCR is the most sensitive method (>95%) but is only commercially available as a combined test for *H. ducreyi*, *T. pallidum* and herpes simplex.

Serology is available in the form of an enzyme-linked immunosorbent assay, although it is unable to distinguish between new and old infection.

MANAGEMENT

- Azithromycin 1 g orally (single dose).
- Erythromycin 500 mg orally twice a day for 7 days.

Alternative regimen:

- Spectinomycin 2 g intramuscularly (single dose).

With the emergence of plasmid-mediated antimicrobial resistance tetracyclines, penicillins, streptomycin, chloramphenicol and sulfonamides are no longer reliable. Trimethoprim also shows widespread resistance, although the mechanism behind this has not been characterized. Intermittent resistance to ciprofloxacin and erythromycin has been described in several isolates worldwide although not in sufficient numbers to limit the use of these antibiotics. If *H. ducreyi* is not eradicated from the ulcer within 72 h of commencing therapy clinical failure can be anticipated.

All of the regimens recommended above have been proven effective in randomized controlled trials.[69,70] The advantages of azithromycin and ceftriaxone are that they are single-dose regimens and therefore have high compliance. Some studies have raised concern about the use of these single-dose regimens in patients coinfected with HIV: in one study looking at ceftriaxone 30% of patients failed treatment.[71] Treatment failures have also been described for azithromycin.[69] Single-dose regimens should therefore be used with caution, particularly in patients co-infected with HIV. Erythromycin has been found effective at a lower dose of 250 mg thrice-daily; however this was not in a randomized controlled trial. Since azithromycin and fluoroquinolones cannot be used in pregnancy, during breast-feeding or in children, erythromycin or ceftriaxone are the treatment of choice in these populations.

Fluctuant buboes are classically managed by repeated aspiration of pus through adjacent healthy skin. Incision and drainage have been shown to be effective and safe in a randomized study conducted during an outbreak in the USA[72] but whether the results are transferable to an under-resourced setting in developing countries is uncertain.

Patients should be re-assessed after initiation of treatment to ensure that there has been objective improvement in the ulcer. Re-epithelialization will be evident by day 7, although the time to complete healing of the ulcer depends on the ulcer's initial size. Failure to respond to therapy may be because of antibiotic resistance or the presence of a co-infection. Sensitivity testing and exclusion of syphilis and herpes simplex are warranted.

Contact tracing is necessary for any sexual contact in the 10 days before the onset of symptoms, and contacts should be examined for possible chancroid and treated if necessary. Active tracing and treating contacts, together with syndromic management at first presentation and condom promotion programs, make eradication of *H. ducreyi* achievable. This goal attains an even higher priority due to the enhanced HIV transmission seen in patients with chancroid.

DONOVANOSIS (GRANULOMA INGUINALE)

Donovanosis is a form of GUD seen predominantly in tropical countries and is caused by the Gram-negative bacillus *Calymmatobacterium granulomatis*.

EPIDEMIOLOGY

At present Donovanosis is seen in small endemic foci in only a few developing countries – in particular, Papua New Guinea, southern Africa, north-east Brazil, French Guyana and the aboriginal communities of Australia.[73] Most cases occur in the sexually active population, with men outnumbering women by up to 6:1.[74] Conjugal infection appears to be infrequent, with co-infection rates in marital partners varying from 1–2% in a Papua New Guinea case series to up to 50% in an Indian case series.[74,75] Most cases are associated with poor standards of personal hygiene. Vertical transmission has been reported, as has primary infection in children. HLA-B57 has been associated with Donovanosis and HLA-A23 with resistance to infection.

PATHOGENESIS

Trauma or an abrasion is thought to be a pre-requisite of infection. A small firm nodule forms containing Donovan bodies, which are classical for the disease. These consist of large mononuclear cells in which intracytoplasmic inclusion bodies contain the bacteria. These inclusion bodies rupture, releasing the infective organisms.

DIAGNOSIS

Clinical

At the site of primary inoculation a small, non-tender papule or subcutaneous nodule forms; this either ulcerates or becomes a hypertrophic growth. In some cases the ulcer can become necrotic and destructive and in others leads to the formation of extensive scar tissue. The primary ulcer, in contrast to chancroid, is painless, can be single or multiple and (like chancroid) bleeds easily on contact. The genitals are affected in 90% of cases, sites corresponding to areas of likely trauma as in chancroid. Extragenital ulcers are found in 6% of cases, usually associated with primary disease. Sites include the oropharynx, neck and chest. Inguinal lesions occur in 10% of cases secondary to spread of the infection from the lymph nodes to the overlying skin.

Some cases may resolve but others develop into a chronic form leading to extensive tissue destruction. Other complications include hemorrhage, genital elephantiasis secondary to lymphedema, squamous cell carcinoma and rarely dissemination to bone and liver. Disseminated disease is seen more frequently in pregnancy. Cervical and oral ulcers can be mistaken for malignant lesions.

Investigations

The aim of investigation is demonstration of a Donovan body. In endemic areas this should be achievable in 60–80% of patients suspected clinically to have the disease. Samples can be taken either as a swab or a scraping from the base of the ulcer or by tissue biopsy. These samples are stained with Giemsa or suitable alternative and studied under direct microscopy. Donovan bodies are found within histiocytes. They are Gram-negative with bipolar staining and are characteristic of infection. *C. granulomatis* has been cultured but culture is not yet used in practice; nor are PCR or serology.

MANAGEMENT

All patients with proven Donovanosis or clinically suspected Donovanosis from endemic areas should be treated. The choice of antibiotics to a large extent depends on local availability. The following regimens have all been evaluated in prospective studies.[74,78–80]

- Azithromycin orally 1 g weekly or 500 mg daily.
- Erythromycin orally 500 mg four times a day.
- Doxycycline orally 100 mg twice a day.
- Trimethoprim–sulfamethoxazole orally 160/800 mg twice a day.
- Norfloxacin orally 400 mg twice a day.
- Gentamicin (intramuscular or intravenous) 1 mg/kg three times a day.
- Ceftriaxone (intramuscular or intravenous) 1 g daily.

The Australian antibiotic guidelines recommend azithromycin, and in view of the long duration of therapy often required with these patients this may be one of the most cost-effective regimens. In general therapy should continue until the ulcer has healed, which varies with the extent of ulceration. Like chancroid, there is some evidence that patients with HIV may not respond to first-line therapy and may require longer courses of antibiotics; however, further evidence is needed before recommendations can be made.

Sexual contacts of the index case should be assessed and treated. This will reduce the transmission of not only Donovanosis but also of HIV in endemic areas. This known association, together with the fact that the disease is limited to a number of geographic areas, makes Donovanosis, like chancroid, an important target for global eradication.

BACTERIAL VAGINOSIS

Bacterial vaginosis (BV) is a syndrome characterized by an alteration in the normal bacterial flora found in the vagina from a predominance of lactobacilli to high concentrations of anaerobic bacteria (*Gardnerella vaginalis*, *Prevotella* species, *Mycoplasma hominis*, *Mobiluncus* species). The condition presents with an offensive vaginal discharge, and is believed to be associated with pelvic inflammatory disease, an increased risk of prematurity and chorionamniotitis in pregnant women.

EPIDEMIOLOGY

The infection is common in most countries. The highest reported rates are seen in women in rural parts of sub-Saharan Africa (over 50%),[81] followed by commercial sex workers and women attending STD clinics (24–37%).[82–86] Higher prevalence appears to be related to ethnicity, being sexually active and having symptoms.[87] BV is not just confined to the sexually active population: *G. vaginalis* has been isolated in culture from 10–31% of sexually inexperienced adolescent girls. However, overall this population has a lower prevalence of BV than sexually experienced adolescents.[88]

In common with other infections discussed in this chapter the presence of BV appears to increase a woman's risk of contracting HIV. Rural Ugandan women with BV in one cross-sectional study were twice as likely to be HIV-positive as women with a normal vaginal flora.[81] It is not clear whether HIV infection in turn increases the risk of BV or it's complications.

PATHOGENESIS

The pathogenesis of BV is unclear. Inoculation studies in humans and animal models, together with epidemiological data, suggest that sexual intercourse may introduce a set of bacteria that in some women set in motion a chain of events leading to alteration in the bacterial flora and subsequent BV. However, the fact that BV is also found in sexually naïve individuals indicates that this is not the full story. One factor that is thought to influence the host's susceptibility to infection is the predominant strain of lactobacillus present. Some strains of lactobacillus produce hydrogen peroxide, which may inhibit the growth of anaerobic rods, *Gardnerella*, *Mobiluncus*, and *Mycoplasma*; certainly these strains are found more frequently colonizing the vagina of normal women than those with BV. One prospective study also demonstrated that women colonized with hydrogen peroxide-producing strains were less likely to develop BV than those colonized with non-producing strains.[89] What is also of note is the lack of, or limited, inflammation present in the vaginal epithelial cells. Infection therefore appears to result in a change in the bacterial flora and composition of the vaginal fluid rather than a true infection of the vaginal epithelial cells.

DIAGNOSIS

Clinical

BV is asymptomatic in many women. The characteristic symptom is a malodorous vaginal discharge which appears as a thin, white, homogenous discharge coating the walls of the vagina.

In pregnancy BV is associated with chorioamnionitis, amnionitis, preterm labor, low birthweight and premature rupture of membranes. In addition to this post-partum pelvic inflammatory disease (following cesarean and vaginal delivery), postabortion pelvic inflammatory disease and postoperative infection following gynecological surgery are recognized associations. Spontaneous pelvic inflammatory disease in patients with no history of recent abortion or instrumentation is also recognized. It is not clear, however, if treatment of women with asymptomatic BV reduces their risk of developing pelvic inflammatory disease.

Investigations

The diagnosis of BV is based on the presence of symptoms, signs and physical examination. Cultures for specific bacteria are of limited use, as these bacteria can be found in normal vaginal flora. The diagnostic criteria consist of three of the following four signs:

1. Characteristic, white adherent vaginal discharge.
2. Vaginal pH <4.5.
3. Fishy odor (from release of amines) when vaginal fluid is mixed with 10% potassium hydroxide.
4. Presence of clue cells.[88]

Clue cells are vaginal squamous cells covered with bacteria giving them a stippled appearance. They can be visualized by placing a drop of vaginal fluid on a slide mixing with a drop of normal saline, covering, and viewing under high-power microscopy.[83,90]

A Gram stain will reveal clue cells as well as the presence of large numbers of Gram-negative or Gram-variable coccobacilli.

MANAGEMENT

- Metronidazole 400–500 mg orally twice a day for 7 days.
- Metronidazole 2 g orally (single dose).
- Metronidazole gel (0.75%) intravaginally once daily for 5 days.
- Clindamycin cream (2%) intravaginally once a day for 7 days.
- Clindamycin 300 mg orally twice a day for 7 days.

BV can remit spontaneously both in pregnant and non-pregnant women and, even with treatment, recurs in one-third of women. With this in mind treatment is indicated in all symptomatic women, women with BV undergoing a surgical procedure and some pregnant women. The aim of treatment is to reduce the anaerobic flora present.

Metronidazole and clindamycin have been evaluated in a number of randomized controlled trials both in oral and intravaginal preparations and appear to have similar efficacy. Most of these trials have demonstrated cure rates at one month of 71–89%. A systematic review of oral and intravaginal preparations for metronidazole and clindamycin in non-pregnant women revealed no significant difference in cumulative cure rates: at 4 weeks post-therapy the cumulative cure rates were 78% for oral metronidazole, 82% for intravaginal clindamycin and 71% for intravaginal metronidazole.[91] One randomized controlled trial comparing oral metronidazole and clindamycin in 143 women showed no difference in cure rates at short-term follow up (94–96% at 7–10 days).[92] Comparison of metronidazole 2 g single dose with 500 mg twice a day for 7 days suggests that a single dose may be less effective than a multi-dosage regimen.[93] Clindamycin has few side effects but has been associated with pseudomembranous colitis and vaginal candidiasis. Up to two-thirds of women treated with oral metronidazole will experience side effects, in particular gastrointestinal side effects. Intravaginal preparations have fewer side effects, but are more expensive.

A number of randomized controlled trials looking at the treatment of BV in pregnant women with a history of preterm birth indicates that this group should receive oral metronidazole or clarithromycin early in the second trimester.[94–97] Evidence does not support the use of intravaginal clindamycin to prevent preterm birth in women with BV.[98] The only patients who require test of cure are pregnant women with BV. These patients should be tested again at one month to assess whether further treatment is required. There is insufficient data to support the treatment of all asymptomatic pregnant women.

Data on the use of prophylactic treatment before gynecological procedures are limited. One study has shown a reduction in the incidence of postabortion Pelvic inflammatory disease by treating BV before the procedure.[99] There is no information at present to support the use of treatment before other gynecological procedures, in particular insertion of intrauterine devices.

Although the recurrence rate among women treated for bacterial vaginosis is high, there is no evidence from several placebo-controlled trials to support the treatment of male sexual partners with either metronidazole or clindamycin.[100,101] Various other alternative treatments have been tried, including acidifiers, yoghurt and lactobacillus preparations. These on the whole have been small studies and have shown a wide range of efficacies. Additional studies are required.

GENITAL HERPES

EPIDEMIOLOGY

Genital herpes is caused by infection with one of the two herpes simplex viruses (HSV): HSV-1 or HSV-2. Most genital infections are caused by HSV-2 as a consequence of direct genital-to-genital spread; however, in some countries, particularly in the developed world, HSV-1 accounts for a considerable proportion of genital herpes infections.[102,103] HSV-1 is spread to the genitals during orogenital sex and the proportion of genital infections caused by HSV-1 depends on the popularity of orogenital sex in the community, and the proportion of young adults reaching maturity who have not been exposed to the virus. Most individuals infected with HSV-1 or -2 do not develop symptoms,[104] although some shed the virus from the genital tract from time to time and can infect their sexual partners.[105]

Type-specific serology has been used in a large number of epidemiological studies to determine seroprevalence. However, many of these studies have been in a small number of highly selected populations. These have shown that among pregnant women HSV-2 seroprevalence ranges from 7 to 50%,[106,107,108] in STD clinics from 15 to 75%[106,109] and among commercial sex workers from 74 to 96%. Population-based studies in the USA demonstrated that HSV-2 seroprevalence increased from 16% in 1976–80 to 22% in 1988–94.[110,111] Many seroprevalence studies have shown that presence of HSV-2 antibodies is related to age at first sexual intercourse, the lifetime number of sexual partners, age, ethnic origin, socioeconomic status, gender (women are infected more commonly than men), and previous sexually transmitted infections.[109,112–114]

PATHOGENESIS

HSV enters the body via the skin or mucous membranes of the genital tract. The virus is then taken up by sensory nerve cells and retrogradely transported to sensory or autonomic ganglia.

The virus remains in the sensory neurones, where it may reactivate, and then be taken and via anterograde transport to the cutaneous surface, where viral replication occurs. This results in either asymptomatic viral excretion or a clinical recurrence of the disease.[115] The nature of the latent virus and the cause of recurrences remain to be fully elucidated.

DIAGNOSIS

Clinical

Most individuals exposed to HSV do not develop any symptoms.[116,117] In those that do, the first episode is usually more severe than recurrences, particularly individuals who have never been exposed to these viruses in the past (commonly due to the acquisition of HSV-2 in adulthood in an individual who has not been exposed to HSV-1 during childhood). Individuals may present with symptoms suggestive of a viremia with headache, fever and myalgia.[118] Local symptoms include genital pain, dysuria and sometimes a vaginal or rectal discharge. The first sign of infection is erythema followed by vesicles. These soon break down to superficial ulcers that will heal by crusting on dry skin. The lesions are excruciatingly painful and the entire illness, without treatment, may last from 2 to 4 weeks. The lesions may occur anywhere on the genitalia, are often bilateral and extensive, and may involve extensive areas. The draining lymph glands are often enlarged and painful.[118]

Recurrences are usually of shorter duration, often consisting of a single lesion or small group of lesions on the external genitalia, usually healing within 7–10 days.[118,119] Many individuals with recurrent herpes have prodromal or warning symptoms consisting of neuralgia-type pain in the dermatomal distribution of the lesions. The frequency of recurrences is variable: HSV-2 genital infections tend to recur more often than HSV-1 infections, and lesions recur more often in the first year of the infection. Some individuals may have 12 or more recurrences a year.[120]

Investigations

HSV may be grown in cell culture from appropriate specimens, such as vesicle fluid or material from the base of ulcers. The virus produces a typical cytopathic effect in infected cells. Additional methods of identification include direct immunofluorescence, cytology (where typical cytological changes can be seen) and PCR. This last has been extensively used in experimental situations,[105] but its use has not yet been widely evaluated in the clinical setting. Serological tests can be divided into group-specific and type-specific: group-specific serological tests will indicate whether the individual has been exposed to one or other of the two HSV viruses in the past; type-specific serology will differentiate between the two viruses. A number of enzyme-linked immunosorbent assay tests are currently available for type-specific serology;[121] however, the most reliable technology is Western blot.[122] IgG antibodies take approximately 6–8 weeks to develop, and consequently type-specific serology is of little use in primary infection. In addition, as many individuals are asymptomatic, type-specific serological tests should be used with caution.

MANAGEMENT

Several nucleoside analogs are available for the management of genital herpes. These include aciclovir, valaciclovir (the prodrug of aciclovir), and famciclovir (a prodrug of penciclovir, converted to the active agent in the liver). The two active drugs aciclovir and penciclovir have a similar mode of action.[123,124] (*see* Ch. 2). There are a number of pharmacokinetic differences between the agents (*see* Ch. 40).

All three drugs may be used in the management of genital herpes.

First-episode genital herpes

All three nucleoside analogs have been evaluated for the treatment of first episode genital herpes. Numerous randomized, double-blind, placebo-controlled trials of intravenous, oral and topical aciclovir have demonstrated considerable efficacy in reducing constitutional symptoms and fever within 48 h, preventing new lesion formation and reducing the duration of lesions by many days.[129,130–133] Intravenous and oral therapy appears to be better than topical treatment. Oral valaciclovir and famciclovir have similar efficacy to aciclovir. Recommended regimens are:

- aciclovir 200 mg five times a day for 5–10 days *or*
- valaciclovir 500 mg twice daily for 5–10 days *or*
- famciclovir 125 mg twice daily for 5–10 days.

Treatment should be initiated as early as possible, and results in a significant reduction in the duration of lesions, symptoms and viral shedding. None of the drugs has any effect on the likelihood of frequency of subsequent recurrences. The efficacy of all three agents appears to be similar, although the superior bioavailability of valaciclovir and famciclovir offer better dosing regimens.

Recurrent genital herpes

There are two approaches to the treatment of recurrent genital herpes: the drugs can be used intermittently to treat each episode or continuously over a period of time to prevent episodes from occurring. The latter approach is referred to as 'suppressive therapy'. Intermittent therapy will reduce the duration of each episode by a small amount, and may be particularly useful for individuals who have severe but infrequent recurrences. Intermittent treatment also may be beneficial when used during the prodrome when it may abort episodes. However, not all individuals have prodromal symptoms, and not all prodromal symptoms lead to full-blown recurrences. All three available drugs have been evaluated in placebo-controlled trials and have demonstrated similar efficacy.[134–137]

Doses for intermittent treatment

- Aciclovir 200 mg five times a day for 5 days.
- Valaciclovir 500 mg twice daily for 3–5 days.
- Famciclovir 125 mg twice daily for 5 days.

The second approach is the use of suppressive therapy. This is particularly useful for individuals who have frequent recurrences where continuous treatment is highly effective. Most individuals on suppressive therapy will have no recurrences, and the few that do occur are usually short-lived and virus culture negative. All three drugs have similar efficacy,[138–141] although the superior bioavailability of valaciclovir and famciclovir allow for less frequent and more convenient dosing schedules.[140–143] Many patients will have an improvement in psychosexual morbidity.

Doses for suppressive treatment

- Aciclovir 200 mg four times a day or 400 mg twice a day.
- Valaciclovir 500 mg once daily for individuals with 10 or fewer recurrences per year; 500 mg twice a day for individuals with more than 10 recurrences per year.
- Famciclovir 250 mg twice daily.

Treatment should be continued for approximately 1 year and then stopped to see if recurrences are still occurring with similar frequency and determine whether further therapy is necessary. Suppressive therapy does not appear to affect the natural history of recurrences. Individuals on treatment should be advised that viral shedding may still occur, and that barrier contraception is necessary. Symptomatic therapy may be helpful, including saline bathing and the use of systemic analgesics.

Pregnancy

None of the drugs have been formally evaluated during pregnancy. However, the 'Aciclovir Pregnancy Register' looking at inadvertent use of the drug during pregnancy, did not suggest any adverse events during pregnancy.[144] Information about the other two agents is limited and these drugs can not be recommended for use during pregnancy, particularly during the first trimester. However, as primary herpes may be very severe during pregnancy, treatment with aciclovir in standard doses should be considered. It has been suggested that suppressive antiviral treatment could be used in women with a history of recurrent genital herpes to reduce the likelihood of recurrences in late pregnancy and thereby the need for cesarean section and possibly spread to the neonate.[145] Unfortunately breakthrough recurrences occur on standard doses of aciclovir,[146] and neither of the other two drugs have, as yet, been assessed in this situation. Consequently this form of treatment is not recommended.

GENITAL HUMAN PAPILLOMAVIRUS INFECTIONS – GENITAL WARTS

EPIDEMIOLOGY

A large number (over 40) of human papillomavirus (HPV) infections can involve the genital tract. These may result in genital warts or subclinical infection. Some of these HPV types have been associated with the subsequent development of cervical cancer.[147] Types with low transforming potential are associated with condylomata acuminata (genital warts). All the HPV types found in the genital tract are transmitted by sexual intercourse.[148]

The true prevalence of these infections in the community is unknown as a large number of individuals are asymptomatic, and currently no reliable serological tests are available for the diagnosis of these infections. The incidence of genital warts appears to have increased in Europe, North America and Australia.[149] DNA detection techniques have detected HPV in 4–55% of sexually active women, 0–86% of heterosexual men and 0.8–78% of homosexual men.[149] However, these data are difficult to interpret as many of the studies were small, the detection techniques varied, and the population groups were different. Finally, recent studies have suggested that genital warts and HPV infection may be more common in individuals co-infected with HIV.[150,151,152]

PATHOGENESIS

HPV infects the stratified squamous epithelium of the genital tract. The infection does not result in cell lysis; rather, infected cells are shed from the surface of the skin or mucous membranes. This means that no viral proteins are released, and consequently the immune response is limited. It takes approximately 6 months after infection for natural immunity to develop.[153] T-cell function appears to be critical in modifying the effects of HPV and allowing for persistence and spontaneous regression. Individuals with depressed cellular immunity often have persistent ongoing and proliferative HPV infections.[154]

In benign lesions, HPV remains extrachromosomal. However, in cervical and other genital tract tumors viral DNA is incorporated into the host chromosome.[153]

DIAGNOSIS

Clinical

Most individuals infected with genital tract HPV's are asymptomatic. Some will develop genital warts, which can occur in women on the vulva, inside the vagina or on the cervix, in men, on the penis, the scrotal skin and occasionally within the urethra. In both sexes, perianal and anal warts can occur.

Internal warts in women tend to be asymptomatic and HPV infections associated with cervical intraepithelial neoplasia or cervical cancer are usually aysmptomatic.[155]

Investigations

There are no routine diagnostic tests available for the detection of HPV. DNA amplification tests have been widely used in research and epidemiological studies. However, their use in routine clinical management is yet to be fully evaluated.[156]

MANAGEMENT

There are no agents that specifically eradicate HPV or limit its replication.[157] Treatments are directed at obliterating genital warts or removing dysplastic lesions. A number of ablative techniques can be used to remove warts. These include cryotherapy, electrocautery, laser therapy, or surgical removal.[157] Choice depends on the site and number of warts, the availability of individual treatments, the expertise of the operator, cost and side effects.[158] The success rate for all these treatments appears to be similar, with initial removal of warts achievable in most cases. However, recurrences are common.

A number of chemical treatments are also used. These include the antimitotic drug podophyllin and its purified counterpart podophyllotoxin. The advantage of podophyllotoxin is that it does not contain any of the toxic ligands present in podophyllin, the consistency and strength of the agent can be guaranteed, and it is suitable for self-application on external warts. This drug is not recommended for use during pregnancy or for lesions on the cervix. Podophyllin should be applied once or twice weekly for three to six weeks. Podophyllotoxin is applied twice daily for 3 days, repeated in 7-day cycles. Complete clearance occurs in 50–90% of patients.[159–163] Relapses occur in up to 38% of patients.[164–166]

The use of imiquimod, an immune-modulating agent that acts by inducing α and γ interferon and recruitment of CD4+ T lymphocytes, results in 'immune-induced' regression of warts and HPV DNA.[167,168] The 5% cream should be applied three times a week for up to 16 weeks, and clearance occurs in 56–62% of cases.[167,169,179] The agent sometimes causes local irritation,[167,169,170] and recurrences do occur but there is limited evidence to suggest that recurrences may be less frequent in individuals treated with imiquimod than with other treatment modalities.[169]

MOLLUSCUM CONTAGIOSUM

Molluscum contagiosum is an infectious skin condition characterized by umblicated papules of up to 5–10 mm. The infective agent has been isolated as a pox virus but little is known about its life cycle and pathogenesis due to its inability to grow in tissue culture. The infection is mainly found in two population groups: children and young adults. Transmission of the virus is via skin contact, which is reflected in the distribution of lesions in these two groups: most lesions in children are on the trunk and upper limbs and in adults on the buttocks, thighs and perineal area. The exception to this is in HIV-infected adults where lesions are widespread, often affecting the face.[171] The lesions in this group often tend to be larger in size and more abundant. The fact that HIV-positive individuals have an exaggerated infection and that the lesions often respond to commencement of antiretrovirals suggests a role for cellular immune response in contolling the infection.

Diagnosis of molluscum contagiosum is clinical; however, the histological appearance will confirm the diagnosis. Detection of viral DNA by PCR can differentiate between types 1 and 2; IgG antibodies can be detected by enzyme-linked immunosorbent assay. Molluscum contagiosum lesions may resolve spontaneously over a period of months and treatment can leave residual scarring. The decision to treat must therefore be discussed carefully with the patient. Options include extrusion or chemical ablation of the central core of the papule, topical creams including podophyllotoxin, acidified nitrite, an imiquimod analog and physical ablation with cryotherapy.[172–174]

VIRAL HEPATITIS

Hepatitis A, B (and very occasionally C) can be acquired sexually. These infections are considered fully in Ch. 51.

TRICHOMONAS VAGINALIS

This flagellated protozoan is found in the genitourinary tract of both women and men. It is transmitted primarily by sexual intercourse and in women is often found in association with other sexually transmitted diseases. Documentation of the infection indicates the need for counseling and behavioral change to reduce the risk of acquiring other sexually transmitted diseases, in particular HIV, which is thought to have a 2–4-fold increased transmission rate in the presence of trichomonas infection.[175]

EPIDEMIOLOGY

The WHO in 1995 estimated there to be 170 million cases of trichomoniasis in adults between the ages 15 and 49[1]. Prevalence rates vary widely according to the population studied, with figures as disparate as 5% in the general population and 60% in commercial sex workers and other high-risk groups.[176] Individuals with multiple sex partners, poor personal hygiene, previous sexually transmitted disease and from low socioeconomic groups are at increased risk.

The incubation period is thought to be 5–28 days. Transmission from men to women is greater than women to men: 14–60% and 67–100%, respectively.[176]

PATHOGENESIS

Infection with *T. vaginalis* elicits a cellular and humoral immune response. One of the initial events is an influx of polymorphonuclear leukocytes, and there is evidence that molecules of the organism act as a chemoattractant for these cells.[177] Leukocytes can then kill these organisms and the fragments are phagocytosed by macrophages. A second line of attack is complement mediated: C3 binds to the organism, activating the alternative complement pathway leading to its death.[178] Multiple environmental factors are thought to influence the susceptibility of *T. vaginalis* to complement-mediated lysis. Iron has been shown to induce resistance to lysis, probably by the induction of cysteine protease, which degrades C3.[179] Antibodies (IgA, IgG, IgM) against a number of different surface molecules are found both locally and in serum. The level of protection in resolving the initial infection and protecting against future reinfection has not been defined.

DIAGNOSIS

Clinical

The main site of infection in women is the vaginal epithelium. The organism may also be isolated from the urethra in most infected individuals, although the urinary tract is seldom the sole site of infection. Paraurethral glands may also be infected but endocervical infection is rare. In men the urethra is the most common site infected, although the organism has also been isolated from external genitalia, epididymal aspirates and the prostate. The clinical presentation is often an overlap between that of trichomonal infection and other STDs.

Even with trichomoniasis alone the symptomatology is multifactorial depending on a number of organism and host factors. Between 20 and 50% of infected women are asymptomatic. Symptoms, when present, include vaginal discharge, which can be malodorous, and vulvar itch. Abdominal pain is described but is commonly thought to be secondary to co-infective agents. On examination patients will have vulvar and vaginal erythema with a small percentage having a 'strawberry' appearance to the cervix; 5–15% of women will have no signs of infection.[180,181] Men often present on contact tracing and, like women, up to half will have no symptoms of infection. Symptoms, if present, are those of a urethritis with or without urethral discharge. Frequently there are no signs of infection but balanitis has been described. Spontaneous resolution and prolonged asymptomatic infection do occur in men.[182]

Investigations

Direct microscopy of a wet preparation of vaginal discharge will diagnose 50–70% of infections.[183] The characteristic jerky movements caused by the beating of the anterior flagella can be observed, along with an increased number of polymorphonuclear cells. Culture remains the 'gold standard' and can diagnose up to 95% of cases. The diagnostic sensitivities are not as good for men: direct microscopy of urethral discharge will pick up on only 30% of cases and culture of urethral discharge or first-pass urine has a sensitivity of 60–80%.[184]

MANAGEMENT

- Metronidazole 2 g orally (single dose).
- Metronidazole 400 mg orally twice a day for 5–7 days.

Metronidazole or its related compounds remains the mainstay of treatment, with the only debate surrounding the dosage regimen used. Between 20 and 25% of cases will resolve spontaneously but metronidazole achieves a 95% cure rate if both partners are treated.[185] The concern regarding the single-dose regimen is that, unless the partner is treated, the failure rate will be high due to reinfection. Other reasons for failure include non-compliance and co-infections. Some organisms are capable of living under aerobic conditions and as yet there are no effective treatments for these organisms. Prolonged courses, higher doses and parenteral route have all been tried with some reports of success.

T. vaginalis is now recognized to be associated with an adverse effect on pregnancy, with reports of premature delivery and low birthweight. There have been no reports of metronidazole having an adverse effect in pregnancy or on the breast-fed neonate.[186]

CANDIDIASIS

As much as 85% of genital tract candidal infections are caused by *Candida albicans*. The remainder are caused by non-albicans species, the most common of which is *Candida glabrata*.[187]

EPIDEMIOLOGY

Over 70% of women will have one or more episodes of vulvovaginal candidiasis in their lifetime, and about half will have a recurrence.[188] However, frequent recurrences are uncommon. Several factors appear to predispose women to the infection including pregnancy, diabetes mellitus, the oral contraceptive pill, steroids and HIV infection.[189–191] Candidiasis is not usually a sexually transmitted condition and infection is uncommon in men who have been circumcised.

PATHOGENESIS

C. albicans is a common bowel commensal and gains access to the vagina via the perianal area. Whether it is ever a commen-

sal in the vagina is disputed.[192] How and why the organism causes inflammation is unclear, although there are a number of recognized predisposing factors. A possible mechanism relates to the production of proteases and phospholipases produced by *Candida* organisms.[193]

DIAGNOSIS

Clinical

In women candida causes a vulvovaginitis, characterized by vulval pruritus and a white curdy vaginal discharge. On examination there may be vulval and/or or vaginal erythema. The discharge is white and often adheres to the walls of the vagina.[193] However, many women present with atypical features and laboratory confirmation is important, particularly if there is a possibility of STD. Infected males usually present with an acute balanoposthitis.

Investigations

A 'wet mount' or Gram-stain microscopic examination of vaginal fluid may reveal yeast cells and mycelia.[193] On Gram stain, the cells and mycelia stain Gram-positive. *Candida* species can readily be cultured on Sabaroud's medium.

MANAGEMENT

Topical agents with activity against *Candida*, include the imidazole agents and nystatin. Topical preparations usually come in the form of cream or pessary for intravaginal and vulval use. The imidazole agents commonly used are miconazole or clotrimazole and econazole. Several dosing options are available. All appear to have similar efficacy (over 80%) and a low relapse rate.[194] Nystatin is now less often used as it is felt to be less effective and messy. The oral azole agents (ketoconazole, fluconazole and itraconazole) have efficacy similar to those of the topical agents,[195–199] and are preferred by many women.[198] In addition, single-dose oral fluconazole was has been shown in the UK to be a cost-effective treatment. However, some concerns about toxicity, particularly hepatotoxicty with ketoconazole, may limit their use.[200]

Vulvo-vaginal candidiasis

Topical agents

Numerous topical regimens are available and all appear to have similar efficacy. Some of these are listed below.

- Clotrimazole pessaries 500 mg dose single dose.
- Clotrimazole pessaries or 200 mg/day for 3 days.
- Clotrimazole pessaries 100 mg/day for 6 days.
- Clotrimazole cream 5 g/day for 3 days.
- Miconazole cream 200 mg/day for 3 days.
- Miconazole cream 100 mg/day for 7 days.

- Miconazole pessaries 100 mg/day for 7 days.
- Econazole cream 5 g twice daily for 3 days.
- Econazole pessaries 150 mg/day for 3 days.

Oral treatments

- Fluconazole 150 mg single dose.
- Itraconazole 200 mg single dose.

Candidal balanitis

Topical therapy with any of the azoles is usually successful.

References

1. Gerbase AC, Rowley JT, Heymann DHL et al, 1998 Global prevalence and incidence estimates of selected curable STDs. *Sexually Transmitted Infections* 74(Suppl. 1): S12–S16.
2. UNAIDS/WHO 2000 AIDS epidemic update: December.
3. Plummer FA, Simonsen JN, Cameron DW et al 1991 Cofactors in male-female transmission of human immunodeficiency virus type 1. *Journal of Infectious Diseases* 163: 233–239.
4. Quinn TC, Gaydos C, Shepherd M et al, 1996 Epidemiologic and microbiologic correlates of *Chlamydia trachomatis* infection in sexual partnerships. *Journal of the American Medical Association* 276: 1732–1742.
5. Taylor-Robinson D 1994 *Chlamydia trachomatis* and sexually transmitted disease. *British Medical Journal* 308: 150–151.
6. Centres for Disease Control 1995 *Chlamydia trachomatis* genital infections – United States, 1995. *Morbidity and Mortality Weekly Report* 45: 883–884.
7. Brunham RC, Peeling RW 1994 *Chlamydia trachomatis* antigens: Role in immunity and pathogenesis. *Infective Agents and Disease* 3: 218–233.
8. Chernesky MA, Lee H, Schacter J et al, 1994 Diagnosis of *Chlamydia trachomatis* urethral infections in symptomatic and asymptomatic men by testing first-void urine in a ligase chain reaction assay. *Journal of Infectious Diseases* 170: 1308–1311.
9. Lee HH, Chiang WH, Chaing SH et al 1995 Diagnosis of *Chlamydia trachomatis* genitourinary infection in woman by ligase chain reaction assay of urine. *Lancet* 345: 213–216.
10. Martin DH, Mrocskowski TF, Dalu ZA et al 1992 A controlled trial of a single dose of azithromycin for the treatment of chlamydial urethritis and cervicitis. The Azithromycin for Chlamydial Infections Study Group. *New England Journal of Medicine* 327: 921–925.
11. Magid D, Douglas JM Jr, Schwartz JS 1996 Doxycycline compared with azithromycin for treating woman with genital *Chlamydia trachomatis* infections: an incremental cost-effectiveness analysis. *Annals of Internal Medicine* 124: 389–199.
12. Augenbraun M, Bachmann L, Wallace T et al 1998 Compliance with doxycycline therapy in sexually transmitted diseases clinics. *Sexually Transmitted Diseases* 1998; 25: 1–4.
13. Hooton TM, Battieger BE, Judson FN et al 1992 Ofloxacin versus doxycycline for treatment of cervical infection with chlamydia trachomatis. *Antimicrobial Agents and Chemotherapy* 36: 1144–1146.
14. Brocklehurst P, Rooney G 1997 The treatment of genital *Chlamydia trachomatis* infection in pregnancy. In: Neilson JP et al (eds) Pregnancy and Childbirth Module of The Cochrane database of Systematic Reviews (updated 2 December 1997). The Cochrane Library.
15. Katz BP, Blythe MJ, Van der Pol B et al 1996 Declining prevalence of chlamydial infection among adolescent girls. *Sexually Transmitted Diseases* 23: 226–229.
16. Howell MR, Quinn TC, Gaydos CA et al 1998 Screening for *Chlamydia trachomatis* in asymptomatic women attending family planning clinics. A cost-effective analysis of three strategies. *Annals of Internal Medicine* 128: 277–284.
17. van Duynhoven YT 1999 The epidemiology of *Neisseria gonorrhoeae* in Europe. *Microbes and infection* 1999 May; 1: 455–464.
18. Centers for Disease Control and Prevention 1997 Gonorrhea among men who have sex with men – selected sexually transmitted diseases clinics, 1993–1996. *Morbidity and Mortality Weekly Report* 46: 889–892.
19. Public Health Laboratory Service Sexually transmitted infections quarterly report 2001 Gonorrhoea in England and Wales. *CDR Weekly* 11.
20. Centers for Disease Control and Prevention 1999 Sexually transmitted disease surveillance report.
21. Ellen JM, Kohn RP, Bolan GA et al 1995 Socioeconomic differences in sexually transmitted disease rates among black and white adolescents, San Francisco, 1990 to 1992. *American Journal of Public Health* 85: 1546–1548.
22. Holmes KK, Johnson DW, Trostle HJ et al 1970 An estimate of the risk of men acquiring gonorrhoea by sexual contact with infected females. *American Journal of Epidemiology* 91: 170–174.
23. Hooper RR, Reynolds GH, Jones OG et al 1978 Cohort study of venereal disease. 1: The risk of gonorrhoea transmission from infected women to men. *American Journal of Epidemiology* 108: 136–144.
24. Densen P, Mandell GL 1978 gonococcal interactions with polymorphonuclear neutrophils: importance of the phagosome for bactericidal activity. *Journal of Clinical Investigation* 62: 1161–1171.
25. Casey SG, Shafer WM, Spitznagel JK 1986 *Neisseria gonorrhoeae* survive intraleukocytic oxygen-independent antimicrobial capacities of anaerobic and aerobic granulocytes in the presence of pyocin lethal for extracellular gonococci. *Infection and Immunity* 52: 384–389.
26. Gregg CR, Melly MA, Hellerqvist CG et al 1981 Toxic activity of purified lipopolysaccharide of *Neisseria gonorrhoea* for human fallopian tube mucosa. *Journal of Infectious Diseases* 143: 532–439.
27. Melly MA, Gregg CR, McGee ZA 1984 Ability of mononieric peptidoglycan fragments from *Neisseria gonorrhoeae* to damage human fallopian tube mucosa. *Journal of Infectious Diseases* 149: 378–386.
28. Rice PA, Kasper DL 1982 Characterisation of serum resistance of *Neisseria gonorrhoeae* that disseminate: Roles of blocking antibodies and gonococcal outer membrane proteins. *Journal of Clinical Investigation* 70: 157–167.
29. Rice PA, McQuillen DP, Gulati S et al 1994 Serum resistance of *Neisseria gonorrhoeae*. Does it thwart the inflammatory response and facilitate the transmission of infection? *Annals of the New York Academy of Sciences* 730: 7–14.
30. Densen P, Gulati S, Rice PA 1987 Specificity of antibodies against *Neisseria gonorrhoeae* that stimulate neutrophil chemotaxis: Role of antibodies directed against lipooligosaccharides. *Journal of Clinical Investigation* 80: 78–87.
31. Sherrard J, Barlow D 1996 Gonorrhoea in men: clinical and diagnostic aspects. *Genitourinary Medicine* 72: 422–426.
32. Barlow D, Phillips I 1978 Gonorrhoea in women: diagnostic, clinical and laboratory aspects. *Lancet* 1(8067): 761–764.
33. Hook EW III, Handsfield HH 1999 Gonoccocal infections in the adult. In: Holmes KK, Sparling PF, Mardh P-E (eds). *Sexually Transmitted Diseases*, 3rd edn. New York, McGraw-Hill, pp. 451–466.
34. Fitzgerald M, Bedford C 1996 National standards for the management of gonorrhoea. *International Journal of STD and AIDS* 7: 298–300.
35. Moran JS, Levine WC 1995 Drugs of choice for the treatment of uncomplicated gonococcal infections. *Clinical Infectious Diseases* 20: S47–65.
36. Moran JS 1995 Treating uncomplicated Neisseria gonorrhoea infections: is the anatomic site of infection important? *Sexually Transmitted Diseases* 22: 39–47.
37. Brocklehurst P 2001 Interventions for treating gonorrhoea in pregnancy (Cochrane Review). The Cochrane Library, Issue 1. Oxford, Update Software.
38. Handsfield HH, Alexander ER, Pin Wang S et al 1976 Differences in the therapeutic response of chlamydia-positive and chlamydia-negative forms of nongonococcal urethritis. *Journal of the American Venereal Disease Association* 2: 5–9.
39. Bowie WR 1978 Etiology and treatment of nongonococcal urethritis. *Sexually Transmitted Diseases* 5: 27–33.
40. Stamm WE 1991 Azithromycin in the treatment of uncomplicated genital chlamydial infections. *American Journal of Medicine* 91: 19S–22S.
41. Laurharanta J, Saarinen K, Mustonen MT et al 1993 Single-dose oral azithromycin versus seven-day doxycycline in the treatment of non-gonococcal urethritis in males. *Journal of Antimicrobial Chemotherapy* 31(Suppl. E) 177–183.
42. Stamm WE, Hicks CB, Martin DH et al 1995 Azithromycin for empirical treatment of the nongonococcal urethritis syndrome in men. A randomized double-blind study. *Journal of the American Medical Association* 274: 545–549.

43. Marks C, Tideman RL, Estcourt CS et al 2000 Diagnosing PID – getting the balance right. *International Journal of STD and AIDS* 11: 545–547.

44. Centres for Disease Control and Prevention 1998 Guidelines for treatment of sexually transmitted diseases. *Morbidity and Mortality Weekly Report* 47: 1–111.

45. Walker CK, Kahn JG, Washington AE et al 1993 Pelvic inflammatory disease: metaanalysis of antimicrobial regimen efficacy. *Journal of Infectious Diseases* 168: 969–978.

46. Adler MW 1980 The terrible peril: a historical perspective on the venereal diseases. *British Medical Journal* 281: 206–211.

47. Aral SO, Holmes KK 1990 Epidemiology of sexual behavior and sexually transmitted diseases. In: Holmes KK, Mardh P-A, Sparling PE et al (eds). *Sexually Transmitted Diseases*. New York, McGraw-Hill.

48. Mindel A, Tovey SJ, Williams P 1987 Primary and secondary syphilis, 20 years' experience. 1. Epidemiology. *Genitourinary Medicine* 63: 361–364.

49. WHO 1996 Epidemic of sexually transmitted diseases in Eastern Europe. Report on a WHO Meeting, Copenhagen, Denmark, pp. 13–15.

50. Sell S, Norris SJ 1983 The biology, pathology and immunology of syphilis. *International Review of Experimental Pathology* 24: 203–276.

51. Swartz MN, 1990 Neurosyphilis. In: Holmes KK, Mardh P-A, Sparling PF et al (eds). *Sexually Transmitted Diseases*, 2nd edn. McGraw-Hill, pp. 231–250.

52. Norris SJ 1993 Polypeptides of *Treponema pallidum*: progress toward understanding their structural, functional, and immunologic roles. Treponema Pallidum Polypeptide Research Group. *Microbiology Review* 57: 750–779.

53. Cox DL, Chang P, McDowall A et al 1992 The outer membrane, not a coat of host proteins, limits antigenicity of virulent *Treponema pallidum. Infection and Immunity* 60: 1076–1083.

54. Blanco DR, Reimann K, Skare J et al 1994 Isolation of the outer membranes from *Treponema pallidum* and *Treponema vincentii. Journal of Bacteriology* 176: 6088–6099.

55. Mindel A, Tovey SJ, Timmins DJ et al 1989 Primary and secondary syphilis, 20 years' experience. 2. Clinical features. *Genitourinary Medicine* 65: 1–3.

56. Manual of Tests for Syphilis 1969 Atlanta Venereal Disease Program, US Communicable Disease Center. USPHS Publication 411.

57. Larsen SA, Steiner BM, Rudolph AH 1995 Laboratory diagnosis and interpretation of tests for syphilis. *Clinical Microbiology Reviews* 8: 1–21.

58. Scotti AT, Logan L 1968 A specific IgM antibody test in neonatal congenital syphilis. *Journal of Pediatrics* 73: 242–243.

59. Jaffe HW, Larsen SA, Jones OG et al 1978 Haemagglutination tests for syphilis antibody. *American Journal of Clinical Pathology* 70: 230–233.

60. Rein MF 1981 Treatment of neurosyphilis. *Journal of the American Medical Association* 246: 2613–2614.

61. Dunlop EM 1985 Survival of treponemes after treatment: Comments, clinical conclusions and recommendations. *Genitourinary Medicine* 61: 293–301.

62. Goh BT, Smith GW, Samarasinghe L et al 1984 Penicillin concentrations in serum and cerebrospinal fluid after intramuscular injection of aqueous procaine penicillin 0.6 MU with and without probenecid. *British Journal of Venereal Diseases* 60: 371–373.

63. Thin RN, Barlow D, Bingham JS et al 1995 Investigation and management guide for sexually transmitted disease (excluding HIV). *International Journal of STD and AIDS* 62: 130–136.

64. Catterall RD (ed) 1974 The treatment of syphilis and the treponematoses. In: *A Short Textbook of Venereology*, 2nd edn. English Universities Press Limited, London, pp. 152–153.

65. WHO 1995 Press Release. WHO/64 Sexually transmitted diseases 333 million new curable cases. Geneva, WHO.

66. Behets FMT, Liomba G, Lule G et al 1995 Sexually transmitted diseases and human immunodeficiency vius control in Malawi: A field study of genital ulcer disease. *Journal of Infectious Diseases* 171: 451–455.

67. Brunham RC et al 19XX Epidemiology of sexually transmitted diseases in developing countries. In: Research Issues in human behaviour and STD in the AIDS era.

68. Plummer FA, D'Costa LJ, Nsanze H et al 1985 Clinical and microbiologic studies of genital ulcers in Kenyan women. *Sexually Transmitted Diseases* 12: 193–197.

69. Tyndall MW, Agoki E, Plummer FA et al 1994 Single dose azithromycin for the treatment of chancroid: A randomised comparison with erythromycin. *Sexually Transmitted Diseases* 21: 231–234.

70. Martin DH, Sargent SJ, Wendel GD Jr et al 1995 Comparison of azithromycin and ceftriaxone for the treatment of chancroid. *Clinical Infectious Diseases* 21: 409–414.

71. Tyndall M, Malisa M, Plummer FA et al 1993 Ceftriaxone no longer predictably cures chancroid in Kenya. *Journal of Infectious Diseases* 167: 317–321.

72. Ernst AA, Marvez-Valls E, Martin DH et al 1995 Incision and drainage versus aspiration of fluctuant buboes in the emergency department during an epidemic of chancroid. *Sexually Transmitted Diseases* 22: 217–220.

73. O'Farrell N 1999 Donovanosis. In: Holmes KK, Sparling PF, Mardh PA et al (eds). *Sexually Transmitted Diseases*, 3rd edn. New York, McGraw-Hill, pp. 525–561.

74. Maddocks I, Anders EM, Dennis E et al 1976 Donovonosis in Papua New Guinea. *British Journal of Venereal Diseases* 52: 190–196.

75. Lal S, Nicholas C 1970 Epidemiological and clinical features in 165 cases of granuloma inguinale. *British Journal of Venereal Diseases* 46: 461–463.

76. Bowden FJ, Mein J, Plunkett C et al 1996 Pilot study of azithromycin in the treatment of genital donovanosis. *Genitourinary Medicine* 72: 17–19.

77. Robinson HM, Cohen MM 1953 Treatment of granuloma inguinale with erythromycin. *Journal of Investigative Dermatology* 20: 407–409.

78. Lal S, Garg BR 1980 Further evidence of the efficacy of co-trimoxazole in donovonosis. *British Journal of Venereal Diseases* 56: 412–413.

79. Ramanan C, Sarma PS, Ghorpade A et al 1990 Treatment of donovanosis with norfoloxacin. *International Journal of Dermatology* 29: 298–299.

80. Merianos A, Gilles M, Chuah J et al 1994 Ceftriaxone in the treatment of chronic donovanosis in central Australia. *Genitourinary Medicine* 70: 84–89.

81. Sewankambo N, Gray RH, Wawer MJ et al 1997 HIV-1 infection associated with abnormal vaginal flora morphology and bacterial vaginosis. *Lancet* 350: 546–550.

82. Hallen A, Pahlson C, Forsum U 1987 Bacterial vaginosis in women attending STD clinic: diagnostic criteria and prevalence of *Mobiluncus* spp. *Genitourinary Medicine* 63: 386–389.

83. Eschenbach DA, Hillier S, Critchlow C et al 1988 Diagnosis and clinical manifestations of bacterial vaginosis. *American Journal of Obstetrics and Gynecology* 158: 819–828.

84. Hill LH, Ruparelia H, Embil JA 1983 Nonspecific vaginitis and other genital infections in three clinic populations. *Sexually Transmitted Diseases* 10: 114–118.

85. Harms G, Matull R, Randrianasolo D et al 1994 Pattern of sexually transmitted diseases in a Malagasy population. *Sexually Transmitted Diseases* 21: 315–320.

86. Cohen CR, Duerr A, Pruithithada N et al 1995 Bacterial vaginosis and HIV seroprevalence among female commercial sex workers in Chiang Mai, Thailand. *AIDS* 9: 1093–1097.

87. Hillier S, Holmes KK 1999 Bacterial vaginosis. In: Holmes KK, Sparling PF, Mardh P-E (eds). *Sexually Transmitted Diseases*, 3rd edn. New York, McGraw-Hill, pp. 563–586.

88. Amsel R, Totten PA, Spiegel CA et al 1983 Nonspecific vaginitis. Diagnostic criteria and microbial and epidemiologic associations. *American Journal of Medicine* 74: 14–22.

89. Hawes SE, Hillier SL, Benedetti J et al 1996 Hydrogen peroxide-producing lactobacilli and acquisition of vaginal infections. *Journal of Infectious Diseases* 174: 1058–1063.

90. Thomason JL, Gelbart SM, Anderson RJ et al 1990 Statistical evaluation of diagnostic criteria for bacterial vaginosis. *American Journal of Obstetrics and Gynecology* 162: 155–160.

91. Joesoef MR, Schmid GP, Hillier SL 1999 Bacterial vaginosis: review of treatment options and potential clinical indications for therapy. *Clinical Infectious Diseases* 28 (Suppl. 1): S57–S65.

92. Greaves WL, Chungafung J, Morris B et al 1988 Clindamycin versus metronidazole for the treatment of bacterial vaginosis. *Obstetrics and Gynecology* 72: 799–802.

93. Joesoef MR, Schmid GP 1995 Bacterial vaginosis: review of treatment options and potential clinical indications for therapy. *Clinical Infectious Diseases* 20(Suppl. 1): S72–S79.

94. McDonald HM, O'Loughlin JA, Vigneswaran R et al 1997 Impact of metronidazole therapy on preterm birth in women with bacterial vaginosis flora (*Gardnerella vaginalis*): a randomised, placebo controlled trial. *British Journal of Obstetrics and Gynaecology* 104: 1391–1397.

95. Hauth JC, Goldenberg RL, Andrews WW et al 1995 Reduced incidence of preterm delivery with metronidazole and erythromycin in women with bacterial vaginosis. *New England Journal of Medicine* 333: 1732–1736.

96. Morales WJ, Schorr S, Albritton J 1994 Effect of metronidazole in patients with preterm birth in preceding pregnancy and bacterial vaginosis: a placebo-controlled, double blind study. *American Journal of Obstetrics and Gynecology* 171(2): 345–347.

97. McGregor JA, French JI, Parker R et al 1995 Prevention of premature birth by screening and treatment for common genital tract infections: results of a prospective controlled evaluation. *American Journal of Obstetrics and Gynecology* 173: 157–167.

98. Joesoef MR, Hillier SL, Wiknjosastro G et al 1995 Intravaginal treatment for bacterial vaginosis: effects on preterm delivery and low birth weight. *American Journal of Obstetrics and Gynecology* 175: 1527–1531.

99. Larsson PG, Platz-Christensen JJ, Thejls H et al 1992 Incidence of pelvic inflammatory disease after first-trimester legal abortion in women with bacterial vaginosis after treatment with metronidazole: a double blind randomised study. *American Journal of Obstetrics and Gynecology* 166(1 Pt 1): 100–103.

100. Colli E, Landoni M, Parazzini F 1997 Treatment of male partners and recurence of bacterial vaginosis: a randomised trial. *Genitourinary Medicine* 73: 267–270.

101. Vejtorp M, Bollerup AC, Vejtorp L et al 1988 Bacterial vaginosis: a double blind randomised trial of the effect of treatment of the sexual partner. *British Journal of Obstetrics and Gynaecology* 95: 920–926.

102. Corey L 1990 Genital herpes In: Holmes KK, Mardh P, Sparling PS et al (eds). *Sexually Transmitted Diseases.* New York, McGraw-Hill.

103. Tayal Sc, Pattman RS 1994 High prevalence of herpes simplex virus type 1 in female anogenital herpes simplex in Newcastle upon Tyne 1983–92. *International Journal of STD and AIDS* 5: 359–361.

104. Koutsky LA, Stevens CE, Holmes KK et al 1992 Underdiagnosis of genital herpes by current clinical and viral-isolation procedures. *New England Journal of Medicine* 326: 1533–1539.

105. Wald A, Zeh J, Selke S et al 1995 Virologic characteristics of subclinical and symptomatic genital herpes infections. *New England Journal of Medicine* 333: 770–774.

106. Nahmias AJ, Lee FK, Beckman-Nahmias S 1990 Sero-epidemiological and - sociological patterns of herpes simplex virus infection in the world. *Scandinavian Journal of Infectious Disease Supplementum* 69: 19–36.

107. Forsgren M, Sterner G, Anzen B et al 2000 Management of women at term with pregnancy complicated by herpes simplex. *Scandinavian Journal of Infectious Disease Supplementum* 77: 58–66.

108. Mindel A, Taylor J, Tideman RL et al 2000 Neonatal herpes prevention: a minor public health problem in some communities. *Sexually Transmitted Infections* 76: 287–291.

109. Cowan FM, Johnson AM, Ashley R et al 1996 Relationship between antibodies to herpes simplex virus (HSV) and symptoms of HSV infection. *Journal of Infectious Diseases* 174: 470–475.

110. Johnson RE, Nahmias AJ, Magder LS et al 1989 A seroepidemiologic survey of the prevalence of herpes simplex virus type 2 infection in the United States. *New England Journal of Medicine* 321: 7–12.

111. Fleming DTR, McQuillan GM, Johnson RE et al 1997 Herpes simplex virus type 2 in the United States, 1976 to 1994. *New England Journal of Medicine* 337: 1105–1111.

112. Breinig MK, Kingsley LA, Armstrong JA et al 1990 Epidemiology of genital herpes in Pittsburgh: serologic, sexual and racial correlates of apparent and inapparent herpes simplex infections. *Journal of Infectious Diseases* 162: 299–305.

113. Wald A, Corey L, Cone R et al 1997 Frequent genital herpes simplex virus 2 shedding in immunocompetent women. Effect of acyclovir treatment. *Journal of Clinical Investigation* 99: 1092–1097.

114. Tideman RL, Taylor J, Marck C et al 2001 Sexual and demographic risk factors for Herpes simplex type 1 and 2 in women attending an antenatal clinic. *Sexually Transmitted Infections* 77(6) 413–415.

115. Stanberry LR, Jorgensen DM, Nahmias AJ 1997 Herpes simplex viruses 1 and 2. In: Evans AS, Kaslow RA (eds). *Viral infection of humans: epidemiology and control,* 4th edn. New York, Plenum Press, pp. 419–454.

116. Langenberg A, Benedetti J, Jenkins J et al 1989 Development of clinically recognizable genital lesions among women previously identified as having 'asymptomatic' herpes simplex virus type 2 infection. *Annals of Internal Medicine* 110: 882–887.

117. Wald A, Corey L 1996 The clinical features and diagnostic evaluation of genital herpes. In: Stanberry LR (ed.). *Genital and neonatal herpes.* John Wiley, pp. 109–138.

118. Corey L, Adams HG, Brown ZA et al 1983 Genital herpes simplex virus infections: clinical manifestations, course, and complications. *Annals of Internal Medicine* 98: 958–972.

119. Guinan ME, MacCalman J, Kern ER et al 1981 The course of untreated recurrent genital herpes simplex infection in 27 women. *New England Journal of Medicine* 304: 759–763.

120. Benedetti J, Corey L, Ashley R 1994 Recurrence rates in genital herpes after symptomatic first-episode infection. *Annals of Internal Medicine* 121: 847–854.

121. Ho DW, Field PR, Sjogren-Jansson E et al 1992 Indirect ELISA for the detection of IgG and IgM antibodies with glycoprotein G (gG2). *Journal of Virological Methods* 36: 249–264.

122. Ho DW, Field PR, Irving WL et al 1993 Detection of immunoglobulin M antibodies to glycoprotein G-2 by western blot (immunodot) for diagnosis of initial herpes simplex genital infections. *Journal of Clinical Microbiology* 31(12): 3157–3164.

123. Elion GB 1993 Acyclovir: Discovery, mechanism of action, and selectivity. *Journal of Medical Virology* (Suppl. 1): 2–6.

124. Boyd MR, Safrin S, Kern ER 1993 Penciclovir: a review of its spectrum of activity, selectivity and cross-resistance pattern. *Antiviral Chem Chemother* 4(Suppl. 1): 3–11.

125. De Miranda P, Blum MR 1983 Pharmacokinetics of acyclovir after intravenous and oral administration. *Journal of Antimicrobial Chemotherapy* 2(Suppl. B): 29–37.

126. Soul-Lawton J, Seaber E, On N et al 1995 Absolute bioavailability and metabolic disposition of valaciclovir, the L-valyl ester of acyclovir, following oral administration to humans. *Antimicrobial Agents and Chemotherapy* 39: 2759–2764.

127. Pue MA, Benet LA 1993 Pharmacokinetics of famciclovir in man. *Antiviral Chemistry and Chemotherapy* 4(Suppl. 1): 47–55.

128. Weinberg AA, Bate BJ, Mastern HB 1992 In vitro activities of penciclovir and acyclovir against hepres simplex virus types 1 and 2. *Antimicrobial Agents and Chemotherapy* 36: 2037–2038.

129. Mindel A, Adler MW, Sutherland S et al 1982 Intravenous acyclovir treatment for primary genital herpes. *Lancet* 1: 697–700.

130. Corey L, Nahmias AJ, Guinan ME et al 1982 A trial of topical acyclovir in genital herpes simplex virus infections. *New England Journal of Medicine* 306: 1313–1319.

131. Mertz GJ, Critchlow CW, Benedetti J et al 1984 Double-blind placebo-controlled trial of oral acyclovir in first-episode genital herpes simplex virus infection. *Journal of the American Medical Association* 252: 1147–1151.

132. Corey L, Fife KH, Benedetti JK et al 1983 Intravenous acyclovir for the treatment of primary genital herpes. *Annals of Internal Medicine* 98: 914–921.

133. Bryson YJ, Dillon M, Lovett M et al 1983 Treatment of first episodes of genital herpes sdimplex virus infection with oral acyclovir. A randomised double-blind controlled trial in normal subjects. *New England Journal of Medicine* 308: 916–921.

134. Neilsen AE, Aasen T, Halsos AE et al 1982 Efficacy of oral acyclovir in the treatment of initial and recurrent genital herpes. *Lancet* 2: 571–573.

135. Reichman RC, Badger GJ, Mertz GJ et al 1984 Treatment of recurrent genital herpes simplex infections with oral acyclovir: a controlled trial. *Journal of the American Medical Association* 251: 2103–2107.

136. Sacks SL, Aoki FY, Diaz-Mitoma F et al 1996 Patient-initiated, twice-daily oral famciclovir for early recurrent genital herpes. A randomized, double-blind multicenter trial. *Journal of the American Medical Association* 276: 44–49.

137. Spruance SL, Tyring SK, DeGregorio B et al 1996 A large-scale, placebo-controlled, dose-ranging trial of peroral valaciclovir for episodic treatment of recurrent herpes genitalis. *Archives of Internal Medicine* 156: 1729–1735.

138. Mindel A, Weller IVD, Faherty et al 1984 Prophylactic oral acyclovir in recurrent genital herpes. *Lancet* 2: 57–62.

139. Douglas JM, Critchlow C, Benedetti J et al 1984 A double-blind study of oral acyclovir for suppression of recurrences of genital herpes simplex virus infection. *New England Journal of Medicine* 310: 2551–1556.

140. Mertz GJ, Loveless MO, Levin MJ et al 1997 Oral famciclovir for suppression of recurrent genital herpes simplex virus infection in women. A multicenter, double-blind, placebo-controlled trial. *Archives of Internal Medicine* 157: 343–349.

141. Reitano M, Tyring S, Lant W et al 1998 Valaciclovir for the suppression of recurrent genital herpes simplex virus infection: A large-scale dose range-finding study. *Journal of Infectious Diseases* 178: 603–610.

142. Mindel A, Faherty A, Carney O et al 1988 Dosage and safety of long-term suppressive acyclovir therapy for recurrent genital herpes. *Lancet* 1: 926–928.

143. Patel R, Bodsworth NJ, Woolley P et al 1997 Valaciclovir for the suppresson of recurrent genital HSV infection: a placebo controlled study of once daily therapy. *Genitourinary Medicine* 73: 83–84.

144. Andrews EB, Yankaskas BC, Cordero JF et al 1992 Acyclovir in pregnancy registry: six years' experience. The Acyclovir in Pregnancy Registry Advisory Committee. 79: 7–13.

145. Stray-Pedersen B 1990 Acyclovir in late pregnancy to prevent neonatal herpes simplex (letter). *Lancet* 336: 756.

146. Brocklehurst P, Kinghorn G, Carney O et al 1998 A randomised placebo controlled trial of suppressive acyclovir in late pregnancy in women with recurrent genital herpes infection. *British Journal of Obstetrics and Gynaecology* 105: 275–280.

147. IARC Working Group on the Evaluation of Carcinogenic Risks to Humans 1995 IARC Monographs on the evaluation of carcinogenic risks to humans. Vol. 64. Human papillomaviruses. Lyon (France), WHO.

148. Oriel JD 1971 Natural history of genital warts. *British Journal of Venereal Diseases* 47: 1–13.

149. Cunningham AL, Mindel A, Dwyer DE 2000 Global epidemiology of sexually transmitted diseased. In: Stanberry LR, Bernstein DI (eds). *Sexually Transmitted Diseases, vaccines, prevention and control.* Academic Press, London, pp. 3–42.

150. Melby M, Palefsky J, Gonzales J et al 1990 Immune status as a determinant of human papillomavirus detection and its association with anal epithelial abnormalities. *International Journal of Cancer* 46: 203–206.

151. Palefsky JM, Gonzales J, Greenblat RM et al 1990 Anal intraepithelial neoplasia and anal papillomavirus infection among homosexual males with group IV HIV disease. *Journal of the American Medical Association* 263: 2911–2916.

152. De Villiers EM 1992 Laboratory techniques in the investigation of human papillomavirus infection. *Genitourinary Medicine* 68: 50–54.

153. Severson JL, Beutner KR, Tyring SK 2000 Genital papillomavirus infection. In: Stanberry LR, Bernstein DI (eds). *Sexually Transmitted Diseases, vaccines, prevention and control.* Academic Press, London, pp. 259–272.

154. Kast W, Feltkamp M, Ressing M 1996 Cellular immunity against human papillomavirus associated cervical cancer. *Seminars in Virology* 7: 117–123.

155. Sonnex C 1995 The clinical features of genital and perigenital human papillomavirus infection. In: Mindel A (ed.) *Genital warts – Human Papillomavirus Infection.* Edward Arnold, London, pp. 82–104.

156. Manos MM 2001 HPV testing for clarifying borderline cervical smear results. Recent conflicting results highlight the dilemmas of progress. *British Medical Journal* 322: 878–879.

157. Von Krogh G, Lacey CJN, Gross G et al 2000 European course on HPV associated pathology: guidelines for primary care physicians for the diagnosis and management of anogenital warts. *Sexually Transmitted Infections* 76: 162–168.

158. Maw R, von Krogh G 2000 The management of anal warts. *British Medical Journal* 321: 910–911.

159. Von Krogh G 1991 Podophyllotoxin for condylomata acuminata eradication. Clinical and experiemental comparative studies on Podophyllum lignans, colchicine and 5-fluorouracil. Thesis. *Acta Dermatovenereologica Supplementum* 98: 1–48.

160. Von Krogh G, Szpak E, Andersson M et al 1994 Self-treatment using 0.25%–0.5% podophyllotoxin ethanol solutions against penile condylomata acuminata – a placebo-controlled comparative study. *Genitourinary Medicine* 70: 105–110.

161. Claesson U, Lassu A, Happonen H et al 1996 Topical treatment of venereal warts: a comparative open study of podophyllotoxin cream versus solution. *International Journal of STD and AIDS* 7: 429–434.

162. Strand A, Brinkeborn R-M, Siboulet A 1995 Topical treatment of genital warts in men, an open study of podophyllotoxin cream compared with solution. *Genitourinary Medicine* 7: 387–390.

163. Sand Peterson C, Agner T, Ottevanger V et al 1995 A single-blind study of podophyllotoxin cream 0.5% and podophyllotoxin solution 0.5% in male patients with genital warts. *Genitourinary Medicine* 71: 391–392.

164. Beutner KR, Conant MA, Friedman-Kien A 1989 Patient-applied podofilox for treatment of genital warts. *Lancet* 1: 831–834.

165. Greenberg MD, Rutledge LH, Reid R et al 1991 A double blind rantomized trial of 0.5% podofilox and placebo in the treatment of genital warts in women. *Obstetrics and Gynecology* 77: 735–739.

166. Kirby P, Dunne A, King DH et al 1990 Double-blind randomized clinical trial of self-administered podofilox solution versus vehicle in the treatment of genital warts. *American Journal of Medicine* 88: 465–470.

167. Tyring SK, Arany I, Stanley MA et al 1998 A randomized, controlled, molecular study of condylomata acuminata clearance drug treatment with imiquimod. *Journal of Infectious Diseases* 178: 551–555.

168. Miller RL, Gerster JF, Owens ML et al 199 X Imiquimod applied topically: a novel immune response modifer and new class of drug. *International Journal of Immunopharmacology* 21: 1–14.

169. Edwards L, Ferenczy A, Eron L et al 1998 Self-administered topical; 5% imiquimod cream for external anogenital warts. *Acta Dermatologica* 134: 25–30.

170. Gollnick H, Barasso R, Jappe U et al 2001 Safety and efficacy of imiquimod 5% cream in the treatment of penile genital warts in uncircumcised men when applied three times weekly or once per day. *International Journal of STD and AIDS* 12: 22–28.

171. Schwartz JJ, Myskowski PL 1992 Molluscum contagiosum and human immunodeficiency virus. *Archives of Dermatology* 128: 223–227.

172. Ormerod AD, White MI, Shah SA et al 1999 Molluscum contagiosum effectively treated with a topical acidified nitrite, nitric oxide liberating cream. *British Journal of Dermatology* 141: 1051–1053.

173. Syed TA, Lundin S, Ahman SA et al 1994 Topical 0.3% and 0.5% podophyllotoxin cream for self-treatment of molluscum contagiosum in males. A placebo-controlled, double-blind study. *Dermatology* 189: 65–68.

174. Syed TA, Goswami J, Ahmadpour OA et al 1998 Treatment of molluscum contagiosum in males with an analog of imiquimod 1% in cream: a placebo-controlled, double blind study. *Journal of Dermatology* 25: 309–313.

175. Wasserheit JN 1992 Epidemiological synergy: Interrelationship between human immunodeficiency virus infection and sexually transmitted diseases. *Sexually Transmitted Infections* 19: 61–77.

176. Krieger JN, Alderete JF 1999 Trichomonas vaginalis and trichomoniasis. In: Holmes KK, Sparling PF, Mardh P-E (eds). *Sexually Transmitted Diseases*, 3rd edn. McGraw-Hill, New York, 587–604.

177. Mason PR, Forman L 1982 Polymorphonuclear cell chemotaxis to secretions of pathogenic and nonpathogenic *Trichomonas vaginalis. Journal of Parasitology* 68: 457–462.

178. Gillin F, Sher H 1981 Activation of the alternative complement pathway by *Trichomonas vaginalis. Infection and Immunity* 34: 268.

179. Alderete JF, Provenzano D, Lehker MW et al 1995 Iron mediates *Trichomonas vaginalis* resistance to complement lysis. *Microbial Pathogenesis* 19: 93–103.

180. Wolner-Hanssen P, Krieger JN, Stevens CE et al 1989 Clinical manifestations of vaginal trichomoniasis. *Journal of the American Medical Association* 264: 571–576.

181. Fouts AC, Kraus SJ 1980 *Trichomonas vaginalis*: re-evaluation of its clinical presentation and laboratory diagnosis. *Journal of Infectious Diseases* 141: 137–143.

182. Krieger JN, Jenny C, Verdon M et al 1993 Clinical manifestations of trichomoniasis in men. *Annals of Internal Medicine* 118: 844–849.

183. Krieger JN, Tam MR, Stevens CE et al 1988 Diagnosis of trichomoniasis: comparison of conventional wet-mount examination with cytological studies, cultures and monoclonal antibody staining of direct specimens. *Journal of the American Medical Association* 259: 1223–1227.

184. Krieger JN, Verdon M, Siegel N et al 1992 Risk assessment and laboratory diagnosis of trichomoniasis in men. *Journal of Infectious Diseases* 166: 1362.

185. Hager WD et al 1980 Metronidazole for vaginal trichomoniasis: seven day vs. single dose regimens. *Journal of the American Medical Association* 244: 1219–1220.

186. Taddio A et al 1995 Safety of metronidazole in pregnancy: a meta-analysis. *American Journal of Obstetrics and Gynecology* 172(2 Pt 1): 525–529.

187. Goldacre MJ, Watt B, Loudon N et al 1979 Vaginal microbial flora in normal young women. *British Medical Journal* 1: 1450–1455.

188. Reed BD 1992 Risk factors for Candida vulvovaginitis. *Obstetrical and Gynecological Survey* 47: 551–560.

189. Odds FC 1982 Genital candidosis. *Clinical and Experimental Dermatology* 7: 345–354.

190. Morton RS, Rashid S 1977 Candidal vaginitis: natural history, predisposing factors and prevention. *Proceedings of the Royal Society of Medicine* 70(Suppl. 4): 3–6.

191. Rhoads JL, Wright DC, Redfield RR et al 1987 Chronic vaginal candidiasis in women with human immunodeficiency virus infection. *Journal of the American Medical Association* 257(22): 3105–3017.

192. Soll DR 1988 High-frequency switching in Candida albicans and it relations to vaginal candidiasis. *American Journal of Obstetrics and Gynecology* 158: 997–1001.

193. Sobel JD 1999 Vulvovaginal candidiasis. In: Holmes KK, Sparling PF, Mardh P-E (eds) *Sexually Transmitted Diseases*, 3rd edn. New York, McGraw-Hill, pp. 629–639.

194. Forssman L, Milsom I. Treatment of recurrent vaginal candidiasis. *American Journal of Obstetrics and Gynecology* 152(7 Pt 2): 959–961.

195. Silva-Cruz A, Andrade L, Sobral L et al 1991 Itraconazole versus placebo in the management of vaginal candidiasis. *International Journal of Gynaecology and Obstetrics* 36: 229–232.

196. Kutzer E, Oittner R, Leodolter S et al 1988 A comparison of fluconazole and ketoconazole in the oral treatment of vaginal candidiasis; report of a double-blind multicentre trial. *European Journal of Obstetrics, Gynecology and Reproductive Biology* 29: 305–313.

197. Tobin JM, Loo P, Granger SE 1992 Treatment of vaginal candidosis: a comparative study of the efficacy and acceptability of itraconazole and clotrimazole. *Genitourinary Medicine* 68: 36–38.

198. Osser S, Haglund A, Westrom L 1991 Treatment of candidal vaginitis. A prospective randomized investigator-blind multicenter study comparing topically applied econazole with oral fluconazole. *Acta Obstetrics Gynecologica Scandinavica* 70: 73–78.

199. Patel HS, Peters MD, Smith CL 1992 Is there a role for fluconazole in the treatment of vulvovaginal candidiasis? *Annals of Pharmacotherapy* 26: 350–353.

200. Lewis JH, Zimmerman HJ, Benson GD et al 1984 Hepatic injury associated with ketoconazole therapy. Analysis of 33 cases. *Gastroenterology* 86: 503–551.

60 Leprosy

Diana Lockwood and Sharon Marlowe

Leprosy is one of the oldest recorded diseases. In 1988 the World Health Organization (WHO) proposed to eliminate leprosy (i.e. < 1 case per 10 000 population) by the year 2000; however, this proved over-ambitious as over 600 000 new cases were detected in India and a further 44 000 in Brazil in 1999.

In 1873 the Norwegian Armauer Hansen showed that leprosy was caused by *Mycobacterium leprae*, which invades the skin and nerves, causing a chronic granulomatous disease with peripheral neuropathy and skin lesions.

Outside endemic areas, doctors often fail to diagnose leprosy, with unfortunate consequences for the patients: for example, in the UK 40% of new cases have severe neuropathy at diagnosis. Early recognition of leprosy is important because the infection is curable and prompt treatment can reduce nerve damage and associated stigma.

EPIDEMIOLOGY

Leprosy remains a public health problem in 24 countries, mainly in the tropics. The top six endemic countries are India, Brazil, Madagascar, Indonesia, Myanmar and Nepal: 67% of the prevalent cases and 73% of the detected cases worldwide are found in India[1] (Figure 60.1). In 1999 just under 1 million cases were registered on treatment worldwide.

M. leprae is transmitted via the nasal discharge of untreated lepromatous patients and enters another human subject through the nasal mucosa, with subsequent hematogenous spread to the skin and peripheral nerves. Leprosy is a unique-ly human disease with no animal reservoir except the nine-banded armadillo; and although this animal is frequently infected or seropositive for *M. leprae*, there have been few reports of transmission from this animal to humans.

In England and Wales, where leprosy is a notifiable disease, a total of 1358 cases have been registered since 1951.[2] There are still 128 individuals who are on treatment or under sur-veillance. Since 1993 approximately nine new cases per year have been notified. Half of the new cases in the UK are found in migrants from the Indian subcontinent and there are a few cases in Caucasians who have lived in leprosy-endemic areas

for prolonged periods (8–42 years).[3] Leprosy has a long incu-bation period (2–10 years), so patients can present long after leaving endemic areas.

PATHOGENESIS

M. leprae cannot be cultivated on artificial media, but can be grown with difficulty in nude mice and the nine-banded armadillo with a 14 day doubling time and at low temperatures (30–33 °C). Recent sequencing of the *M. leprae* genome revealed that it has lost approximately one-third of the genes possessed by *M. tuberculosis*.[4]

Leprosy manifests in a spectrum of disease forms, ranging from the tuberculoid to the lepromatous (Figure 60.2).[5] The varied clinical manifestations of leprosy are determined by the host's response to the leprosy bacillus: tuberculoid (TT) patients have a uniform clinical, histological and immuno-logical response manifesting as limited clinical disease, granuloma formation and active cell-mediated immunity; lepromatous (LL) patients have multiple clinical signs, a high bacterial load and low cell-mediated immunity. Between these two extremes there is a range of variations in host response; these comprise borderline cases (BT, BB, BL).[6] Immunologically, borderline cases are unstable and polar tuberculoid and lepromatous cases are stable.

CLINICAL FEATURES AND SPECTRUM OF DISEASE

Patients present with skin or nerve lesions, or a combination of both. Leprosy affects only the peripheral nerves – *never* the central nervous system. A patient may present with a macular hypopigmented skin lesion, weakness or pain in the hand due to nerve involvement, facial palsy, acute foot drop or blisters, burns or ulcers due to neuropathy. Patients may also present with painful eyes as a first indication of lepromatous leprosy. The diagnosis of leprosy should be considered in anyone from

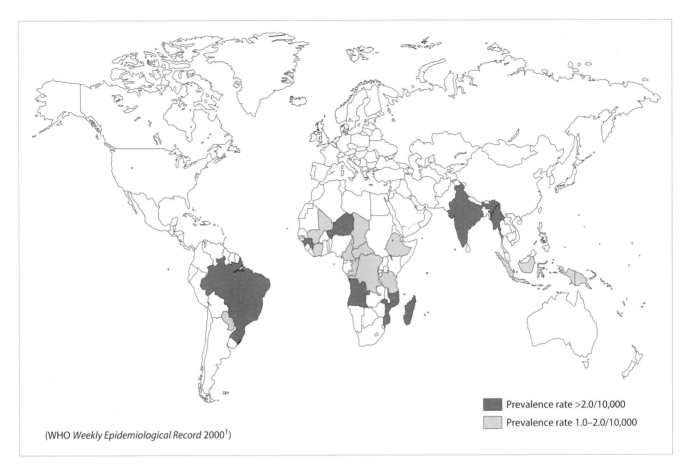

Fig. 60.1 Global leprosy prevalence 2000[1]

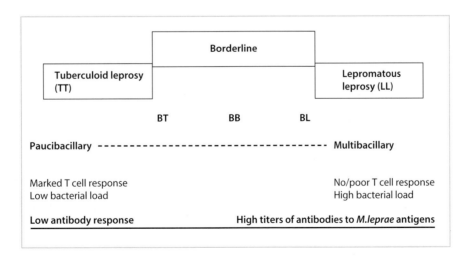

Fig. 60.2 Leprosy – a spectrum of disease

Table 60.1 Characteristic features of different types of leprosy

	TT	BT	BB	BL	LL
Skin lesions	Single, well defined, hypopigmented, erythematous macule	Few, asymmetric well demarcated macules	Few asymmetric, less well demarcated and shiny	Many symmetric shiny macules and plaques	Many symmetric erythematous, shiny, macules, papules and nodules
Sensory impairment in lesions	Marked	Marked	Moderate	Slight neuropathy	Late 'glove and stocking'
Peripheral nerve involvement	Single peripheral nerve trunk	Several and asymmetric	Multiple	Multiple and symmetric	Multiple, late, symmetric

TT, Tuberculoid; BT, borderline tuberculoid; BB, mid-borderline; BL, borderline lepromatous; LL, lepromatous.

an endemic area who presents with typical skin lesions, neuropathic ulcers or a peripheral neuropathy.

DIAGNOSIS

BACTERIOLOGICAL AND HISTOLOGICAL EXAMINATION

In a suspected case, slit skin smears are taken to look for acid-fast bacilli. *M. leprae* on the smears are counted and the bacterial index calculated on a logarithmic scale. A negative result does not exclude leprosy, as tuberculoid lesions may contain no detectable bacteria.

Histopathological evaluation is essential for accurate classification of leprosy lesions and is the best diagnostic test in a well-resourced setting, both for confirming and for excluding the diagnosis of leprosy. The presence of granulomata and lymphocytic infiltration of dermal nerves in anesthetic skin lesions confirms the diagnosis. A nerve biopsy may be required in cases with no visible skin lesions.

SEROLOGICAL TESTS AND POLYMERASE CHAIN REACTION

There is no good serological test with adequate sensitivity and specificity for leprosy.[7] Methods based on the polymerase chain reaction have proved too insensitive and non-specific for general diagnostic use.[8]

TREATMENT

The management of leprosy consists of treating the *M. leprae* infection with antibiotic chemotherapy, management of the immune mediated reactions, prevention of nerve damage and education.

CHEMOTHERAPY

Treatment of infection

Multidrug therapy (MDT) with a combination of dapsone, rifampicin and clofazimine is the current treatment for infection with *M. leprae*. Introduced by WHO in 1982, this is very successful, with a high cure rate, few side effects and low relapse rates (relapse is defined as the reappearance of signs of activity and/or appearance of new lesions and/or bacteriological positivity during or after surveillance). Relapse rates as low as 0.1% per annum have been recorded.[9] In their review of the outcome of MDT of more than 67 000 Indian patients from 1983 to 1992, Lobo et al showed that only 0.3% of all paucibacillary and multibacillary cases relapsed and that 2.7% of all patients were recorded as treatment failures.[10] They also found that 92.2% of patients completed satisfactory treatment, were declared cured and released from treatment.

The benefits of MDT include the prevention of drug resistance and better patient compliance due to a fixed duration of therapy. Another advantage is that field workers review patients and supervise the taking of their monthly medication (*see* Table 60.2). MDT is safe in pregnancy and in breastfeeding mothers.[11,12] Children should receive reduced doses of the drugs.

Dapsone

Dapsone is bacteristatic and effective against a wide range of bacteria and protozoa.[13] In 1947, Cochrane used 1.25 g of subcutaneous dapsone twice weekly to successfully treat leprosy patients.[14,15] This effectiveness was confirmed in Malaysia with a reduced subcutaneous dose of 200–400 mg. At the same time, research in Calcutta,[16] Nigeria[17,18] and the French West Indies reported good results with an oral preparation.[19] By 1951, the standard treatment for leprosy was oral dapsone, 100 mg daily, and was used widely as monotherapy in the 1950s and 1960s. However, in the late 1960s two important problems developed: primary and secondary dapsone resistance.

Table 60.2 Multidrug regimens for treatment of *M. leprae* infection

Regimen	Drug	Dosage	Frequency	Duration
Paucibacillary	Dapsone	100 mg	Daily (self-administered)	6 months
	Rifampicin	600 mg	Monthly (supervised)	
Multibacillary	Dapsone	100 mg	Daily (self-administered)	
	Clofazimine	50 mg	Daily (self-administered)	2 years
	Clofazimine	300 mg	Monthly (supervised)	
	Rifampicin	600 mg	Monthly (supervised)	

- Primary resistance refers to resistance in patients who have never been exposed to dapsone.
- Secondary resistance refers to relapse in patients who have previously been treated with dapsone.

Dapsone acts as other sulfonamides, by competing with *para*-aminobenzoic acid for the enzyme dihydropterorate synthetase and therefore inhibiting the synthesis of dihydrofolic acid (*see* Ch. 2). A dose of 100 mg of dapsone is weakly bactericidal against *M. leprae* and after a few weeks of starting dapsone therapy active lesions start to improve.

Side effects are rare with dapsone and include mild hemolysis and dapsone allergy, occurring within the first few months of treatment. Dapsone allergy usually starts 3–6 weeks after starting the drug, with fever, pruritus and a dermatitic rash. Unless dapsone is stopped immediately, the syndrome may progress to exfoliative dermatitis; hepatitis, albuminuria, pychosis and death have also been recorded.[17] Treatment is to stop dapsone and treat with corticosteroids for several weeks. The incidence of dapsone allergy is estimated at one per several hundred patients. Although dapsone-induced peripheral neuropathy has been reported in some diseases there have been few reports of it occurring in leprosy.

Clofazimine

Clofazimine was first used for the treatment of leprosy as monotherapy in the early 1960s and continued until the mid 1970s. To date there has been only one reported case of resistance.[20]

Clofazimine is bacteristatic and slowly bactericidal against *M. leprae*, similar to dapsone.[21] Clofazimine is active against other mycobacteria, this effect being more pronounced in vitro than in vivo, but the mechanism of its action against *M. leprae* is unknown. The speed of response is similar to that of dapsone but slower than that of rifampicin. At doses greater than 1 mg/kg daily clofazimine exhibits increasing anti-inflammatory activity.[22]

The main problems encountered with clofazimine are increased skin pigmentation and dryness, which occur as the drug becomes clinically effective. This icthyosis is reversible and slowly resolves on stopping the drug. Pigmentation can also be seen in the cornea and conjunctival and macular areas of the eyes. Clofazimine is lipophilic and is therefore deposited in fatty tissue and cells of the reticuloendothelial system. Autopsies carried out on patients who had been on clofazimine therapy revealed large quantities of the drug in mesenteric lymph nodes, adrenal glands, subcutaneous fat, liver, spleen, small intestine and skin but not in the central nervous system.[23]

Rifampicin

Rifampicin is used mainly for the treatment of tuberculosis and leprosy although it also inhibits the growth of other bacteria[24] (*see* Ch. 30).

Rifampicin is bactericidal and the most effective anti-leprosy drug, rendering the patient non-infectious within days of commencing therapy.[25] Resistance has been shown to be due to tightly clustered mutations in a short region of the *rpoβ* gene.[26]

Few serious side effects have been related to rifampicin, which may be due to its monthly dosing regimen, and no cases of resistance have been recorded in leprosy patients. The most common reported side effect is hepatotoxicity, which has (rarely) resulted in death. Early symptoms are anorexia, vomiting and jaundice associated with a two or threefold increase in hepatic transaminases. The elevated transaminases may be transient and return to normal despite continuing therapy.

'Flu-like' syndrome has been reported with intermittent rifampicin therapy and consists of chills, fever, headache, myalgia and arthalgia. This syndrome has a reported incidence of 0.3% in the WHO/MDT report of complications. Rifampicin also produces a red–brown discoloration of urine, feces, saliva, sputum, sweat and tears; patients should be informed that this is inconsequential and will last only 24–48 h.

Other regimens instead of MDT

Following the success of MDT there has been research into the use of other drugs that are more potent than, and as effective, as MDT, but which require a shorter duration of therapy. Other antibiotics currently available as second-line therapy to MDT are minocycline, ofloxacin and clarithromycin.

MINOCYCLINE

Minocycline has a strong bactericidal activity against *M. leprae* due to its lipophilic properties, which allow it to penetrate the outer capsule and cell wall of the organism.[27] Data from a clinical trial carried out in Mali in 1992 showed that 100 mg minocycline daily caused marked clinical improvement by 1 month. After 2 months of treatment there was a significant decrease in bacterial index, indicating that minocycline was very effective at killing *M. leprae* bacilli.[28]

The main side effect observed in minocycline-treated leprosy patients is hyperpigmentation, presenting as a patchy blue–black color at the site of skin lesions, especially on the legs and feet.[29] Dizziness is a specific side effect of minocycline and other mild adverse effects include gastrointestinal symptoms of nausea, abdominal pain or diarrhea, and headache[30] (*see* Ch. 33).

OFLOXACIN

Ofloxacin is a fluoroquinolone derivative with strong bactericidal activity against *M. leprae*.[31] A clinical trial in Côte d'Ivoire, studying the efficacy of a daily dose of 400 mg of ofloxacin[32] showed definite clinical improvement after 22 doses, 99.9% of initially viable organisms being dead at day 22.

CLARITHROMYCIN

Clarithromycin is a macrolide with potent bactericidal activity against *M. leprae*, both in mice and in lepromatous patients. A study in Mali showed that 500 mg of daily clarithromycin was as effective as 100 mg of daily minocycline. Of the 12 patients treated with clarithromycin alone, 5 (42%) showed definite clinical improvement and 6 (50%) showed marked clinical improvement after 1 month of treatment. This treatment also resulted in significant reductions in bacterial index after 3 months.[28] Mouse studies have reported additive effects of clarithromycin and minocycline, but this has not been confirmed in human trials.[33]

Single-dose therapy

A single-dose MDT is now available for single-lesion paucibacillary patients: rifampicin 600 mg, ofloxacin 400 mg and minocycline 100 mg (ROM). A large, multicentered, randomized controlled, double-blind trial carried out in India to test single-dose ROM versus 6 months of paucibacillary MDT in single-lesion cases demonstrated that 51.8% of patients treated with ROM showed marked clinical improvement, compared with 57.3% of those on WHO/MDT for patients with paucibacillary disease. Although this result showed that the WHO regimen was statistically better than single-dose ROM for single-lesion cases, ROM may still be appropriate for field situations.[34]

Other drug regimens

In the mouse model, the combination of minocycline and ofloxacin has been found to be almost as bactericidal as rifampicin, and the combination of rifapentine, moxifloxacin and minocycline significantly more bactericidal than the ROM regimen. This latest combination is currently undergoing clinical trial.[35]

Treatment of nerve damage

Nerve damage refers to peripheral sensory or motor neuropathy. Patients may present with nerve damage or develop nerve function impairment during or after MDT.

A large field study in Ethiopia looked prospectively at 650 patients treated with WHO/MDT and followed them up for 11 years (1988–1999). In this study 55% of patients had some nerve function impairment at diagnosis and 12% developed new impairment after starting MDT; 33% had no initial impairment and never developed neuropathy. Patients with no initial nerve impairment who later developed nerve damage and were treated with corticosteroids within 6 months of symptoms (defined as acute neuropathy) had full recovery in 88% of nerves. Corticosteroids were also successful in treating 51% of patients who had chronic or recurrent nerve damage. Chronic neuropathy was defined as nerve function impairment occurring within 3 months of stopping corticosteroids and recurrent neuropathy as new nerve impairment occurring at least 3 months after stopping corticosteroids.[36]

Current treatment for patients presenting with new nerve damage of less than or equal to 6 months duration is corticosteroids in addition to MDT. Oral prednisolone is started at 40 mg daily and reduced over 4–6 months depending on clinical response.

The Bangladesh Acute Nerve Damage Study (BANDS) is a prospective study of a cohort of 2664 previously untreated leprosy patients in Bangladesh. This study started in 1997 with a 12-month recruitment period and follow up of 5 and 3 years for multibacillary and paucibacillary cases respectively. The BANDS data showed that there was a delay in patients presenting for treatment, and this could be as long as 12 months after initial symptoms started. The prevalence of nerve function impairment was seven times greater in multibacillary than paucibacillary patients and twice as high in men as in women. Of the patients presenting with nerve damage almost 12% had a sensory neuropathy and just over 7% had a motor neuropathy. The nerve most commonly affected was the posterior tibial nerve (sensory neuropathy), followed by the ulnar nerve.[37]

The TRIPOD trials (Trials in the Prevention of Disability in Leprosy) followed the BANDS study, with the aim of investigating the effectiveness of prophylactic corticosteroid therapy in preventing nerve impairment and subsequent disability. Interim analysis in 1999 showed that widespread use of corticosteroids was safe if patients were selected carefully and monitored regularly. Patient recruitment was due to finish towards the end of 2001.[38]

Treatment of reactions

Leprosy is complicated by immunological phenomena called reactions: reversal reactions (type 1 reactions); ENL reactions (erythema nodosum leprosum, or Type 2, reactions). The clinical features of these reactions are listed in Table 60.4.

These sudden episodes of acute inflammation occur in approximately 30% of leprosy patients. This is due to immune reactions against antigenic components liberated from the

Table 60.3 Clinical features of leprosy reactions

	Reversal reactions	ENL reactions
Immune response	T-cell mediated	Immune complex deposition
Type of leprosy affected	BT, BB and BL	BL and LL
Clinical features	*Skin lesions:* Erythema, swelling tenderness *Peripheral nerve lesions:* pain/tenderness, increased weakness, increased sensory loss	*Skin lesions:* transient crops of small, painful red nodules, lasting 2–3 days *Other signs:* fever, malaise, lymph node enlargement, arthritis, iritis, orchitis, neuritis

ENL, erythema nodosum leprosum; LL, lepromatous; BL, borderline lepromatous; BB, mid-borderline; BT, borderline tuberculoid.

bacilli. Patients can present in reaction before MDT treatment, and a significant proportion of patients develop reactions within the first 6 months of treatment. There is also an increase in the incidence of reactions in post-partum patients. However, reactions can also occur after successful MDT treatment and are probably due to persistence of *M. leprae* antigens.

Patients may suffer from recurrent reactions or repeated reactions after treatment, resulting in increased suffering and disability.

Treatment of reversal reactions

Reversal reactions are characterized by edema, inflammation and an increase in lymphocytic infiltration in skin and/or nerves of borderline patients. Reversal reactions are due to delayed hypersensitivity at sites of localization of *M. leprae* antigens. They are characterized by CD4 cell activation and production of tissue-damaging T-cell and macrophage cytokines. Mild reactions can be treated with aspirin (600 g–1200 mg 4-hourly). Moderate and severe reactions are treated with prednisolone.

PREDNISOLONE

Oral prednisolone has proved to be an effective treatment for severe reactions. Steroid treatment should be started within the first 6 months of an episode of reaction or nerve function impairment to be effective.[39–41] Starting doses may be as high as 60 mg and tapered over several months to prevent further nerve damage; a starting dose of 40 mg is usually sufficient to suppress inflammation in the skin or nerves. The response to treatment can be seen by a decrease in skin inflammation over a few days. In a study looking at motor nerve conduction velocity, Naafs et al confirmed that there is a good response to several months of steroid therapy with remyelinization and nerve regeneration.[42]

Prednisolone has many effects on cytokines, but it down-regulates proinflammatory cytokines mainly by inhibition of NF-κB-induced transcription of cytokine mRNA. Little et al assessed the in-vivo effects of prednisolone in RR patients: they found that 1 month of prednisolone treatment reduced cellularity, cytokine production (γ-interferon, interleukin-12) and inducible nitric oxide synthetase in skin lesions of RR patients.[43]

Prednisolone is the drug of choice for severe reversal reactions, although about 30% of patients do not respond to therapy or need a protracted course of corticosteroids. Research looking into alternative treatments to prednisolone for severe reversal reactions, which are non-responsive or need chronic steroid therapy, is ongoing.

Treatment of ENL

ENL presents as a systemic illness: a patient with ENL may be very sick with high temperatures, painful subcutaneous nodules, peripheral edema and inflammation of the nerves, eyes, joints, muscles, bones and testes. In ENL, antigen–antibody complexes are deposited in the tissues with the activation of complement and migration of neutrophils into lesions.

For mild cases aspirin may be used, but many cases require treatment with prednisolone and an increased dose of clofazimine (up to 300 mg) or thalidomide. Thalidomide is the treatment of choice for severe ENL but its availability and teratogenicity limits its use.

THALIDOMIDE

Thalidomide was first synthesized in 1954 and marketed as a hypnotic in 1956. It is now being used for its anti-inflammatory properties in ENL and other diseases.[44] Thalidomide has two main actions: a potent depressant effect on the central nervous system and an immunomodulatory effect in inflammatory disease. Sampaio et al showed that it selectively inhibits transcription of the inflammatory cytokine tumor necrosis factor-alpha (TNF-α)[45] by accelerating the degradation of mRNA encoding the protein.[46] Thalidomide also enhances cell-mediated immunity by directly stimulating cytotoxic T cells and increasing the production of interleukin-10.[47]

Thalidomide has been used for treatment of ENL since the early 1960s. In 1965, Sheskin[48] reported that six patients with ENL responded well to thalidomide, and this was confirmed with other studies.[49] It has also been shown that the raised serum TNF-α levels in ENL are lowered by thalidomide.[50] Thalidomide shortens the ENL reaction. It acts rapidly, with improvement occurring after 8 h, although it may take up to 48 hours before the patient becomes afebrile. The dose used is 400 mg daily in 2–4 divided doses, with gradual reduction to 50 mg daily. Thalidomide is the most effective drug for ENL but must be used in women of childbearing age only with caution; it is absolutely contraindicated in pregnancy. All patients should be given specific advice (*see* Box 60.1) before commencing thalidomide therapy. If thalidomide is either not available or contraindicated, prednisolone is used to treat ENL.

Box 60.1 Advice for patients before commencing thalidomide therapy

- Do not share tablets with anyone else.
- Use double contraception whilst on therapy.
- Seek medical advice at the first sign of amenorrhea.
- An abortion should be considered if pregnancy is confirmed.

There have been no reports of thalidomide causing accelerated nerve damage in leprosy. However, when used in other diseases such as Behçet's disease, thalidomide is known to cause an axonal sensory neuropathy and there is evidence to suggest more widespread effects of the nervous system.[51–53] Other side effects that occur with thalidomide include a widespread rash developing 6–12 days after starting the drug, drowsiness, constipation, xerostomia, increased appetite, nausea and loss of libido.[55] It can also rarely result in menstrual abnormalities, increased urinary secretion of corticosteroids, myxedema and a euthyroid state in previous thyrotoxicosis.[56]

CHEMOPROPHYLAXIS AND IMMUNOTHERAPY

In the 1960s and 1970s chemoprophylaxis with dapsone and acedapsone was investigated. However, dapsone showed varying protection to contacts of leprosy patients and there were anxieties about dapsone resistance, so this regimen was curtailed. In the 1980s–1990s rifampicin, used either alone or in combination with other drugs, was found to have chemoprophylactic efficacy.[57] More recently a study was carried out in Micronesia of a single dose of ROM as chemoprophylaxis. Results from this study are currently being analyzed.

A meta-analysis of 14 trials showed that chemoprophylaxis gives approximately 60% protection against leprosy. Leprosy chemoprophylaxis may be an effective way of reducing incidence and is more cost-effective if it is given only to household contacts.[58] Current UK practice is for all childhood contacts of newly diagnosed patients to be given rifampicin prophylaxis (1 mg/kg). At present chemo- and immunoprophylaxis are not cost-effective measures for wide usage, because there is no means of identifying all persons who are at high risk of developing leprosy and the prophylactic measures are not close to 100% efficacy.

To date no specific vaccine has been developed to prevent infection by *M. leprae*, although there is good evidence that BCG has protective efficacy. Large field trials in Uganda, Burma, Papua New Guinea and India have all demonstrated a protective efficacy varying from 20% to 80% with BCG

vaccines. Adding *M. leprae* antigen to BCG does not increase the efficacy of the vaccine.[59]

ONGOING MANAGEMENT AND PREVENTION OF COMPLICATIONS

Education concerning factual information such as mode of transmission, treatment and complications is essential for all patients and health providers. Education is also important in equipping patients with knowledge on how to adapt their lifestyle to prevent the development of complications (e.g. comfortable footwear and cessation of smoking in order to care for the anesthetic limb).

LEPROSY AND HIV

There were concerns that an interaction between HIV and *M. leprae* infection would result in an increased incidence of leprosy cases. However, studies in Uganda, Mali, Ethiopia and South India have not shown an increased prevalence of leprosy cases associated with HIV infection.[60–62]

An association has been found between HIV infection and complications of leprosy. In a case-controlled study in Uganda, Bwire et al found that HIV seropositivity was a significant risk factor for developing reactions and neuritis; an unusual finding because reversal reactions are associated with an increase in CD4 cells. Similarly, Sampaio et al found that HIV infected patients with low CD4 counts had normal granuloma formation with numerous CD4 cells.[63]

Treatment of a leprosy patient with concurrent HIV infection does not differ from that of a seronegative leprosy patient and reactions should be managed with corticosteroids or thalidomide as appropriate.

CONCLUSION

MDT has been a success story in both the treatment of *M. leprae* infection and in the mobilization of many people involved in treatment, surveillance and leprosy control programs. In 1982 MDT was implemented in endemic areas and since then more than 90% of registered cases have received treatment, 8 million patients have been cured and global prevalence has declined.

The current treatment for leprosy reactions is still not optimal, with a significant number of patients not responding to prednisolone and some ENL patients requiring chronic thalidomide therapy. Researchers are still looking for different immunosuppressant drugs with efficacy in the treatment of reactions (e.g. azathioprine and cyclosporin A).

The stigma associated with the diagnosis of leprosy is still a very real problem and the management of someone with the disease should include discussion of their psychosocial status and education for the patient and their family.

References

1. WHO 2000 Leprosy – global situation. *Weekly Epidemiological Record* 28: 226–231.

2. Van Buynder P, Eccleston J, Leese J, Lockwood DNJ 1999 Leprosy in England and Wales. *Communicable Disease and Public Health* 2: 119–121.

3. Lockwood DNJ, Reid AJ 2001 The diagnosis of leprosy is delayed in the United Kingdom. *Quarterly Journal of Medicine* 94: 207–212.

4. Cole ST et al 2001 Massive gene decay in the leprosy bacillus. *Nature* 409 1007–1011.

5. Evans M, Lockwood D 1999 Leprosy: a clinical update. *Africa Health* 21: 14–16.

6. Hastings RC 1994 *Leprosy*, 2nd edn. Churchill Livingstone, Edinburgh.

7. Smith PG 1992 The serodiagnosis of leprosy. *Leprosy Review* 63: 97–100.

8. Wichitwechkarn J, Karnjan S, Shuntawuttisettee S, Sornprasit C, Kampirapap K, Peerpakorn 1995 Detection of *Mycobacterium leprae* by PCR. *Journal of Clinical Microbiology* 33: 45–49.

9. WHO 1994 Chemotherapy of leprosy. Report of a WO Study Group. *World Health Organization Technical Reports Series* 847: 1–24.

10. Lobo D 1992 Treatment failures with multidrug therapy. *Leprosy Review* 63: 93s–98s.

11. Maurus JN 1978 Hansen's Disease in pregnancy. *Obstetrics and Gynaecology* 52: 22–25.

12. Farb H, West DP, Pedvis-Leftick A 1982 Clofazimine in pregnancy complicated be leprosy. *Obstetrics and Gynaecology* 59: 122–123.

13. Anonymous 1999 In: Dollery C (ed) *Therapeutic Drugs* 2nd edn. Churchill Livingstone, Edinburgh, pp. D13–D18.

14. Cochrane RG 1949 A comparison of sulphone and hydnocarpus therapy of leprosy. Memoria del V Congreso Internacional de la Lepra. Editorial Cenit, Havana, Cuba, 220–224.

15. Cochrane RG, Ramanujam K, Paul H, Russell D 1949 Two and a half years' experimental work on the sulphone group of drugs. *Leprosy Review* 20: 4–64.

16. Muir E 1950 Preliminary report on 4:4'-diaminodiphenylsulphone (DDS) treatment of leprosy. *International Journal of Leprosy* 18: 299–308.

17. Lowe J, Smith M 1949 The chemotherapy of leprosy in Nigeria, with an appendix on glandular fever and exfoliative dermatitis precipitated by sulphones. *International Journal of Leprosy* 17: 181–195.

18. Lowe J 1950 Treatment of leprosy with diaminodiphenlysulphone by mouth. *Lancet* 1: 145–150.

19. Floch H, Destomes R 1949 Traitement de la lepre par la 'sulphone-mere' (diamino-diphenyl-sulphone). *International Journal of leprosy* 17: 367–377.

20. Levy L, Shepard CC, Fasal P 1972 Clofazimine therapy of lepromatous leprosy caused by dapsone-resistant *Mycobacterium leprae*. *American Journal of Tropical Medicine and Hygiene* 21: 315–321.

21. Warndorff-van Diepen T 1982 Clofazimine-resistant leprosy, a case report. *International Journal of Leprosy* 50: 139–142.

22. Browne SG, Hogerzeil L 1962 B.663 in the treatment of leprosy. Preliminary report of a pilot trial. *Leprosy Review* 33: 6–10.

23. Mansfield RE 1974 Tissue concentrations of clofazimine (B663) in man. *American Journal of Tropical Medicine and Hygiene* 50: 139–142.

24. Anonymous 1999 In: Dollery C (ed) *Therapeutic Drugs*, 2nd edn. Churchill Livingstone, Edinburgh, pp. R32–R36.

25. Levy L, Shepard CC, Fasal P 1976 The bactericidal effect of rifampicin on *M. leprae* in man: a) single doses of 600, 900, and 1200 mg; and b) daily doses of 300 mg. *International Journal of Leprosy* 44: 183–187.

26. Honoré N, Cole ST 1993 The molecular basis of rifampicin-resistance in *Mycobacterium leprae*. *Antimicrobial Agents and Chemotherapy* 37: 414–418.

27. Gelber RH 1987 Activity of minocycline in *Mycobacterium leprae*-infected mice. *Journal of Infectious Diseases* 156: 236–239.

28. Ji B, Jamet P, Perani EG, Bobin P, Grosset JH 1993 Powerful bactericidal activities of clartihromycin and minocycline against *Mycobacterium leprae* in lepromatous leprosy. *Journal of Infectious Diseases* 168: 188–190.

29. Rea TH 2000 Trials of daily, long-term minocycline and rifampicin or clarithromycin and rifampicin in the treatment of borderline lepromatous and Lepromatous leprosy. *International Journal of Leprosy* 68: 129–135.

30. Bernier C, Dreno B 2001 Minocycline. *Annals of Dermatology and Venereology* 128: 627–637.

31. Grosset JH, Geulpa-Lauras CC, Perani EG, Beoletto C 1988 Activity of ofloxacin against *Mycobacterium leprae* in the mouse. *International Journal of Leprosy* 56: 259–264.

32. Grosset JH, Ji B, Geulpa-Lauras CC, Perani EG, N'Deli LN 1990 Clinical trial of perfloxacin and ofloxacin in the treatment of lepromatous leprosy. *International Journal of Leprosy* 58: 281–295.

33. Ji B, Perani EG, Grosset JH 1991 Effectiveness of clarithromycin and an minocycline alone and in combination against experimental *Mycobacterium leprae* infection in mice. *Antimicrobial Agents and Chemotherapy* 35: 579–581.

34. Gupte MD 2000 Field trials of a single dose combination of rifampicin-ofloxacin-minocycline (ROM) for the treatment of paucibacillary leprosy. *Leprosy Review* 71: S77–S80.

35. Grosset L 2000 The new challenges for chemotherapy research. *Leprosy Review* 71(Suppl.): 100–104.

36. Saunderson P, Gebre S, Desta K, Byass P, Lockwood DNJ 2000 The pattern of leprosy-related neuropathy in the AMFES patients in Ethiopia: definitions, incidence, risk factors and outcome. *Leprosy Review* 71: 285–308.

37. Croft IRP, Richardus JH, Nicholls PG, Smith WCS 1999 Nerve function impairment in leprosy: design, methodology and intake status of a prospective cohort of 2664 new leprosy cases in Bangladesh. The Bangladesh Acute Nerve Damage Study. *Leprosy Review* 70: 140–159.

38. Smith WC 2000 Review of current research in the prevention of nerve damage in leprosy. *Leprosy Review* 71 (Suppl.): S138–144.

39. Becx-Bleumink M, Berhe D, Mannetje W 1990 The management of nerve damage in the leprosy control services. *Leprosy Review* 61: 1–11.

40. Becx-Bleumink M, Berhe D 1992 Occurrence of reaction, their diagnosis and management in leprosy patients with MDT; experience in the Leprosy Control Programme of the All Africa Leprosy and Rehabilitation Training Centre (ALERT) in Ethiopia. *International Journal of Leprosy* 60: 173–184.

41. Van Brakel WH, Kwasas IB 1996 Nerve function impairment in leprosy: an epidemiological and clinical study – Part 2: Results of steroid treatment. *Leprosy Review* 67: 104–118.

42. Naafs B, Pearson JMH, Baar AJM 1976 A follow-up study of nerve lesions in leprosy during and after reactions using motor nerve conduction velocity. *International Journal of Leprosy* 44: 188–197.

43. Little D, Khanolkar-Young S, Coulthart A, Suneetha A, Lockwood DNL 2001 Immunohistochemical analysis of cellular infiltrate and gamma-interferon, interleukin-12 and inducible nitric oxide synthetase expression in leprosy Type 1 (Reversal) Reactions before and during prednisolone treatment. *Infection and Immunity* 3413–3417.

44. Anonymous 1999 In: Dollery C (ed) *Therapeutic Drugs*, 2nd edn. Churchill Livingstone, Edinburgh, pp. T60–T74.

45. Sampaio EP, Sarno EN, Galilly R, Cohn ZA, Kaplan G 1991 Thalidomide selectively inhibits tumour necrosis factor α production by stimulated human monocytes. *Journal of Experimental Medicine* 173: 699–703.

46. Sarno EN, Grau GE, Vieira LMM, Nery JA 1991 Serum levels of tumour necrosis factor-alpha and interleukin-1 beta during leprosy reactional states. *Clinical and Experimental Immunology* 84: 103–108.

47. Singhal S et al 1999 Antitumor activity of thalidomide in refractory multiple myeloma. *New England Journal of Medicine* 341: 1565–1571.

48. Sheskin J 1965 Thalidomide in the treatment of lepra reactions. *Clinical Pharmacology and Therapeutics* 6: 303–306.

49. Leading Article 1994 Thalidomide in leprosy reaction. *Lancet* 343: 432–433.

50. Sampaio EP, Kaplan G, Miranda A et al 1993 The influence of thalidomide on the clinical and immunologic manifestations of erythema nodosum leprosum. *Journal of Infectious Diseases* 168: 408–414.

51. Fullerton PM, Kremer M 1961 Neuropathy after intake of thalidomide (Distaval). *British Medical Journal* ii: 855–858.

52. Editorial 1961 Thalidomide neuropathy. *British Medical Journal*, ii: 876.

53. Fullerton PM, O' Sullivan DJ 1968 Thalidomide neuropathy: an electrophysiological study. *Muscle and Nerve* 9: 837–844.

54. Harland CC, Steventon GB, Marsden JR 1993 Thalidomide induced neuropathy and drug metabolite polymorphism. *Clinical Research* 41: 496A.

55. Gunzler V 1992 Thalidomide in human immunodeficiency virus. A review of safety considerations. *Drug Safety* 7: 116–134.

56. Mellin GW, Katzenstein M 1962 The saga of thalidomide. *New England Journal of Medicine* 267: 1184–1193, 1238–1244.

57. Cartel JL, Chanteau S, Moulia-Pelat JP et al 1992 Chemoprophylaxis of leprosy

with a single dose of 25 mg/kg rifampicin in the Southern Marquesas: results after 4 years. *International Journal of Leprosy* 60: 416–420.

58. Smith CM, Smith WCS 2000 Chemoprophylaxis is effective in the prevention of leprosy in endemic countries: a systematic review and meta-analysis. *Journal of Infection* 41: 137–142.

59. Nordeen SK 2000 Prophylaxis – scope and limitations. *Leprosy Review* 71: S16–S20.

60. Kawuma HJS, Bwire R, Adatu-Engwau F 1994 Leprosy and infection with the human immunodeficency virus in Uganda.; a case-control study. *International Journal of Leprosy* 62: 521–526.

61. Lienhardt C, Kamate B, Jamet P et al 1996 Effect of HIV infection on leprosy: a three year survey in Bamako, Mali. *International Journal of Leprosy and Other Mycobacterial Diseases* 64: 383–391.

62. Sekar B, Jayasheela M, Chattopadhya D et al 1994 Prevalence of HIV Infection and high-risk characteristics among leprosy patients of South India; a case-control study. *International Journal of Leprosy* 62: 527–531.

63. Sampaio EP, Caneshi JRT, Nery JAC et al 1995 Cellular immune response to *Mycobacterium leprae* infection in human immunodeficiency virus infected individuals. *Infection and Immunity* 63: 18848–18854.

61

Other mycobacterial infections

L. Peter Ormerod

Tuberculosis (TB) has been increasing significantly on a worldwide basis over the last decade, to such an extent that the World Health Organization (WHO) proclaimed it a Global Emergency in 1995. The WHO estimated that in 1998 there were 7.9 million new clinical cases each year (95% confidence limit 6.3–11.1), 1.8 million (1.4–2.8) deaths each year, and 1.8 billion persons infected in the world as judged by a positive tuberculin skin test.[1] This increase has been seen both in the developing world and in developed countries, reversing the historical continuous decline seen since the Second World War. The reasons for the increase are different in the developing and developed worlds.

In developed countries, particularly in Europe, the increases seen are due to an increasing proportion of the cases of TB occurring in ethnic minority groups who have come from countries of high prevalence, and who consequently have very high TB rates. The rates in the native population continue generally to decline. In England and Wales, incidence increased nearly 40% between 1987 and 2000, but only 35% of cases are in the White ethnic population, with over 56% of cases being foreign born.[2] Rates in ethnic minority groups are 25–40 times higher than in the White ethnic group.[2] Similar trends have been seen in most European countries, with the increase being due to immigrants and refugees/asylum seekers from high-prevalence countries. In the USA the increase seen between 1985 and 1990, which was partly due to HIV-co-infection, but also due to social factors and the dismantling of TB programs[3] has been reversed but (as in Europe) an increasing proportion of cases are in the foreign born.

In developing countries the increase is largely due to the lack of funding, marked population increases and the associated economic and social deprivation. To this is now added the effect of HIV co-infection. Although first described in the USA,[4] its largest impact so far has been in sub-Saharan Africa where TB rates doubled between 1985 and 1991 in some countries (e.g. Malawi and Zambia[5]), and have continued to rise almost exponentially since. This dual epidemic, which has hit largely the younger economically active adults (and children), has further fuelled deprivation, social pressures and economic collapse. Although currently only 8–10% of TB worldwide is HIV associated,[2] this proportion is expected to rise over the next 5–10 years as dual infec-

tion increasingly occurs in South Asia, which, because of the much larger populations of these countries, will have a much greater numerical effect[2].

In this chapter the principles underlying the development of short-course treatment will be set out, together with recommendations based on those principles for individual patients and sites of disease. The complexities of treatment of HIV-infected patients with particular relation to highly active antiretroviral treatment (HAART) are also discussed. Such treatments, as well as prophylactic therapy in both HIV-negative and HIV-positive individuals, need to be within the context of a monitored TB control program. Finally, treatment of the opportunist mycobacteria that cause human disease is also considered.

SCIENTIFIC BASIS OF SHORT-COURSE CHEMOTHERAPY

Each of the main anti-tuberculosis drugs varies in its capacity to kill bacteria, to sterilize lesions and to prevent the emergence of drug resistance. Killing capacity is measured by early bactericidal activity,[6] sterilizing ability by a low relapse rate after cessation of treatment and a low culture-positive rate at 2 months of treatment.[7] The efficiency of a drug in preventing the emergence of drug resistance is more difficult to assess and is largely derived from the interpretation of clinical studies.[7]

Isoniazid (H) is the most potent bactericidal drug and kills more than 90% of bacilli within 7 days, acting on metabolically active bacilli. It is also quite effective at preventing the emergence of drug resistance. Rifampicin (R) is also a good bactericidal drug, with a potent sterilizing effect and a good ability to prevent the emergence of drug resistance. In addition to acting on rapidly dividing bacilli it kills so-called 'persisters', which remain inactive for long periods but have intermittent periods of metabolism, with only a short drug exposure. This gives it its potent sterilizing efficiency. Although bactericidal, pyrazinamide (Z) is used mainly for its sterilizing ability, it is particularly effective at killing intracellular mycobacteria sequestered inside macrophages in an acid environment.[6] Streptomycin (S) and ethambutol (E) are less potent drugs, with ethambutol probably being bactericidal only at high concentration. They are less effective at preventing the emergence of resistance to rifampicin and isoniazid.

The efficacy of regimens based on rifampicin, isoniazid and pyrazinamide has been extensively studied by many controlled trials of different durations and dosing schedules. With this type of regimen it is possible to convert over 90% of sputum smear-positive patients to culture-negative at 2 months, to cure greater than 95%, and to have a relapse rate of under 5%. The studies from which various aspects of treatment can be deduced, and from which later chemotherapy recommendations are based, are set out in Table 61.1.

A duration of 6 months seems to be the shortest period for a regimen based on isoniazid and rifampicin that will give an acceptably low relapse rate. If the duration is reduced below 6 months higher relapse rates and lower cure rates are found, which are not acceptable for developed countries. Studies in Singapore and Hong Kong comparing 2, 4 and 6 months pyrazinamide with rifampicin and isoniazid for 6 months

showed that pyrazinamide is needed only for the initial 2 months. Conversely, however, if pyrazinamide is not used or cannot be tolerated, then a 9-month duration regimen of rifampicin and isoniazid is required, supplemented by ethambutol for the initial 2 months.

The trials described in Table 61.1 covered a spectrum of dosing schedules from daily treatment throughout, a daily initial phase followed by a twice or thrice weekly continuation phase, or twice or thrice weekly dosing throughout. All of these schedules gave relapse rates of under 5% during periods of follow-up between 6 and 30 months after cessation of treatment. The dosing schedule used therefore depends on a balance of cost, side effects and tolerance, drug availability and organizational aspects.

If rifampicin is omitted from the regimen in the continuation phase because of cost constraints, a 6-month total duration gives higher relapse rates and inadequate sterilization. Before the HIV epidemic regimens with an extended continuation phase of isoniazid for 6 months with either ethambutol or thiacetazone (Th) had been tested. A regimen of 2SHRZ/6HTh had been shown to be very effective when combined with admission to hospital for the initial 2 months.[20,21]

Table 61.1 Six-month short course regimen trials for the treatment of pulmonary tuberculosis

	Regimen	No. of patients	Bacteriological relapse (%)	Reference
Daily throughout				
United Kingdom	2SHRZ/4HR	125	1	8
	2EHRZ/4HR	132	2	8
Hong Kong	2EHRZ/4EHRZ	163	1	9–11
US Trial 21	2HRZ/4HR	273	4	12
Singapore	2SHRZ/4HRZ	78	1	13–14
	2SHRZ/4HR	80	2	13–14
Daily initial phase and intermittent continuation phase				
Poland	2HRZ/4HR(3)	116	4	15
	2SHRZ/4HR(2)	56	2	15
Singapore	2SHRZ/4HR(3)	97	1	16–17
	1SHRZ/5HR(3)	94	1	16–17
	2HRZ/4HR(3)	109	1	16–17
Intermittent throughout				
Hong Kong	6SHRZE(3)	152	1	9–11
	6SHRZ(3)	151	1	9–11
	6HRZE(3)	160	2	9–11
	2SHRZ(3)/2SHR(3)/3HR(3)	149	3	18
	4SHRZ(3)/2HR(3)	133	6	18
	4SHRZ(3)/2HRZ(3)	142	1	18
	4HRZ(3)/4HRZ(3)	135	4	18
USA	0.5SHRZ/1.5SHRZ(2)/4HR(2)	125	2	19

S, streptomycin; H, isoniazid; R, rifampicin; Z, pyrazinamide; E, ethambutol. The number in front of the letters represents the duration of treatment in months. The number in brackets after the letters represents the number of doses per week.

This is no longer viable as a 'cheaper' regimen because of the rate of drug reactions to thiacetazone in HIV-positive patients (*see later*) and the costs of initial hospital care. If rifampicin is not used in the continuation phase then there is a significantly increased failure rate if the organism is found to have initial isoniazid resistance.

Regimens of various durations of between 2 and 4 months have been studied in sputum smear-negative tuberculosis. For those with positive initial cultures, relapse rates of 32% with 2 months' treatment,[22] 7–13% with 3 months' treatment,[22,23] and 4% with 4 months' treatment have been reported.[22,23] The results of the 4-month regimen varied with the initial sensitivities of those with a positive culture. For initially sensitive organisms, the relapse rate was 2%, but rose to 8% for those with initial resistance to isoniazid and/or streptomycin.[23]

RECOMMENDED REGIMENS

The recommendations made by various expert bodies are founded on the substantial body of evidence for pulmonary tuberculosis, and take into account the likelihood of drug resistance in the target population. The recommendations of the Joint Tuberculosis Committee of the British Thoracic Society are set out in Table 61.2.[24] Where there are variations between these recommendations and those of the European Respiratory Society,[25] the American Thoracic Society,[26] and the World Health Organization[27] these are also shown in Table 61.2.

In the UK, a 6-month regimen comprising isoniazid, rifampicin, pyrazinamide and ethambutol for 2 initial months followed by rifampicin and isoniazid for a further 4 months is recommended for adult respiratory tuberculosis, including isolated pleural effusion and mediastinal lymphadenopathy, irrespective of the bacteriological status of the sputum.[24] A 6-month regimen is therefore recommended for sputum smear-negative disease. Where a positive culture for *M. tuberculosis* has been obtained but susceptibility results are outstanding at 2 months, the initial four-drug phase should be continued until full susceptibility is known, but the total duration of treatment does not need to be extended. Ethambutol is included to cover the possibility of isoniazid resistance in those groups with higher prevalence of isoniazid resistance. It can be omitted only in those who are at low risk of isoniazid resistance, namely those who fulfill all of the following criteria:[2,28]

Table 61.2 Recommended regimens for treatment of tuberculosis

Type of tuberculosis	American Thoracic Society	European Respiratory Society	British Thoracic Society
Adult			
New smear positive pulmonary	2RHZ(E/S)[a]/4HR	2RHZ(E)[b]/4HR	2RHZ(E)[c]/4HR
or	*or*	*or*	*or*
New extensive smear-negative pulmonary	0.5RHZ(S/E)[a]/1.5RHZ(E)[a](2)/4HR(2) (DOT)	2RHZ(E)[b]/4HR(3)	2RHZS[c](3)/4HR(3) DOT
	or		
Extensive non-respiratory	2RHZ(E/S)[a](3)/4RHZ(E/S)[a](3) DOT		
Non-extensive smear-negative pulmonary	2RHZ/4HR	As above	As above
Adult meningitis	Presumed as extensive non-respiratory but not specified	Presumed as extensive non-respiratory but not specified	2RHZ(E/S)[c]/10HR
Children			
Pulmonary/lymph node	As adult	As adult	As adult
Central nervous system	2RHZ(S)[a]/10HR	As adult	2RHZ(E)[c]/10HR
Miliary	As above	As adult	2RHZ(E)[c]/4HR
Bone/joint	As above	As adult	2RHZ(E)[c]/4HR
Drug resistance			
Isoniazid	2RZE/4RZE or 2RE/10RE	Not specified	2RZES/7RE DOT or 2RZE/10RE
MDR-TB	Individualized	Individualized	Individualized
Other resistances	Not specified	Not specified	*See* Table 3

[a] Omit fourth drug if isoniazid resistance probability<4%.
[b] Omit fourth drug if isoniazid resistance probability<2%.
[c] Omit fourth drug on individual risk assessment
S, streptomycin; H, isoniazid; R, rifampicin; Z, pyrazinamide; E, ethambutol The number in front of the letters represents duration in months. The number in parentheses after the letters represents the number of doses per week. DOT, Directly observed therapy.

- white ethnic origin;
- previously untreated;
- known HIV-negative or thought likely to be so on risk assessment;
- not a known contact of drug-resistant disease.

Individuals who are known or suspected to be HIV-positive,[28] who are from non-White ethnic groups,[2,28] who have had previous treatment, or who are recent arrivals such as refugees or immigrants from countries of high tuberculosis prevalence, have rates of isoniazid resistance over 5% and should be commenced on a four-drug combination unless there are very strong contraindications to one of the drugs.

If a patient cannot tolerate pyrazinamide, then the treatment required to give a suitably high cure rate is 9 months rifampicin and isoniazid supplemented by 2 months initial ethambutol.[29] Routine daily pyridoxine is not required but should be given to people at higher risk of peripheral neuropathy: those with diabetes mellitus, chronic renal failure, alcohol dependency, malnourishment and the HIV-positive.

NON-PULMONARY TUBERCULOSIS

Non-respiratory tuberculosis has been subject to fewer controlled clinical trials than respiratory tuberculosis, but there are sites where evidence-based advice can be given.

Lymph-node tuberculosis

The third British Thoracic Society lymph node trial showed that a 6-month regimen was just as effective as a 9-month regimen.[30,31] From this trial,[30,31] and from earlier lymph node studies,[32,33] the course of lymph node disease is variable. In 10–15% of cases nodes may enlarge, abscesses may form, and new nodes may develop, both during or after treatment. These are usually without any bacteriological evidence of relapse or recurrence, and in the absence of a positive culture should not in themselves be taken as failure of treatment[32] or relapse.[33] The 6-month regimen recommended for respiratory tuberculosis is therefore also recommended for lymph node disease.[24]

Bone/joint tuberculosis

Approximately half of all cases are in spinal sites. This form of tuberculosis has been the subject of a number of controlled clinical trials, with 6 months of therapy being shown to give good results.[34–37] These studies also showed that chemotherapy can be fully ambulant in nearly all cases of tuberculosis of the thoracic and lumbar spine, with surgery reserved for the few patients with evidence of spinal cord compression or instability.[34–37] The 6-month regimen recommended for respiratory tuberculosis is therefore advised for bone and joint tuberculosis.[24]

Pericardium

A 6-month regimen of rifampicin and isoniazid supplemented by 3 months initial pyrazinamide and streptomycin has been shown to be highly effective.[38] The continuation of streptomycin and pyrazinamide after 2 months is not likely to confer additional benefit, so the 6-month regimen preferred for respiratory disease is recommended.[24] Trials have shown that corticosteroids confer additional benefit in this form of tuberculosis (*see later*).[39]

Central nervous system

There is lack of evidence from controlled trials but management in centers treating large numbers suggests that rifampicin and isoniazid for 12 months, supplemented by pyrazinamide and a fourth drug for at least the first 2 months, will give good results. Isoniazid, pyrazinamide and protionamide/ethionamide penetrate the cerebrospinal fluid well, but rifampicin penetrates less well.[40] Ethambutol and streptomycin penetrate the cerebrospinal fluid in adequate concentrations only when there is active meningeal inflammation early in the treatment. Although the risk of ethambutol ocular toxicity at the recommended dosage of 15 mg/kg is low,[41] ethambutol should be used with caution in unconscious patients (Stage III) as visual acuity cannot be tested. Intrathecal administration of streptomycin is unnecessary. The fourth drug in the initial phase of treatment can be ethambutol,[40] streptomycin[40] or ethionamide.[42] In the UK a 12-month regimen of rifampicin and isoniazid, supplemented by 2 months initial pyrazinamide and ethambutol, is recommended for both meningitis and tuberculoma,[24] prolonged to 18 months if pyrazinamide is not given or cannot be tolerated. Additional corticosteroids are of benefit in some cases (*see later*).

Other sites

There are few clinical trial data for other sites. In the UK, by extrapolation from respiratory disease and the more common non-respiratory data, the 6-month regimen recommended for respiratory disease is advised,[24] it is also advised for tuberculosis in multiple sites, or for miliary (classical or cryptic) disease.[43] Because of the high rates of bloodborne spread to the meninges in miliary tuberculosis, lumbar puncture is recommended in such cases so that the correct duration of therapy can be determined.[24]

Corticosteroids as an adjunct to therapy

Clinical trial data support a beneficial effect of corticosteroids in addition to the recommended antituberculosis chemotherapy for pericarditis,[38,39] for stage II and III meningitis[40,44] and for endobronchial disease in children.[45] There is clinical, but no clinical trial, data of possible benefit in pleural effusions,[46] in tuberculosis affecting the ureter,[47] in patients with extensive pulmonary disease[48] and in suppression of hypersensitivity reactions to antituberculosis drugs.[48]

TREATMENT IN PREGNANCY

Pregnancy in patients taking rifampicin is not an indication for termination. Standard treatment should be given to pregnant women, the risk to both the mother and the fetus being greater if suboptimal treatment is given.[49] None of the first-line drugs has been shown to be teratogenic in humans, but the reserve drugs (*see later*) ethionamide and protionamide may be and are best avoided. Streptomycin and other aminoglycosides are potentially ototoxic to the fetus and should be avoided in pregnancy. Women may breast-feed normally whilst taking antituberculosis drugs. Patients on rifampicin-containing regimens should be told of the reduced effectiveness of oral contraceptives and be given contraceptive advice.

TREATMENT IN CHILDREN

Recommended dosages of isoniazid vary substantially. The British Thoracic Society,[24] the International Union against Tuberculosis and Lung Diseases,[24] and the WHO[27] recommend 5 mg/kg up to a maximum dose of 300 mg daily. Other organizations such as the American Thoracic Society[26] and the American Academy of Pediatrics[51] recommend 10 mg/kg up to a maximum of 300 mg. Pharmacokinetic studies[52] show that 5 mg/kg gives serum levels 60–100 times the minimum inhibitory concentration and satisfactory clinical outcome is achieved.[53] Dosages should generally be rounded up to easily-given volumes of syrup or appropriate strengths of tablet.

The 6-month regimen advised for adults should be used for children with respiratory tuberculosis including hilar lymphadenopathy.[24] Ethambutol should also be included for the first 2 months if the criteria for its omission recommended for adults on page 823–824[24] also apply to the child. A recent literature review concluded that, use of a 15 mg/kg dosage of ethambutol, in children aged five years or older, required no more precautions to be taken than for adults.[54] The same review also concluded that ethambutol could be used in younger children without undue fear of side effects.[54]

No controlled trials examining the treatment of extrapulmonary tuberculosis in children have been reported. Recommendations are therefore made by extrapolation from adult trials. Treatment of tuberculous lymphadenopathy, pericarditis, bowel disease, bone and joint disease and other end-organ disease using the 6-month regimen advised for adults is recommended.[24] For disseminated and congenital tuberculosis treatment should also last 6 months unless there is evidence of any central nervous system involvement, when a 12-month regimen is advised[24]. Meningitis should be treated with 12 months of isoniazid and rifampicin supplemented by 2 months

initial pyrazinamide plus either ethambutol or streptomycin.[24,26,40,51]

MOLECULAR BASIS

Advances in molecular genetics over the last decade or so have demonstrated the mechanisms of resistance to specific antituberculosis drugs, and in general these come about because of mutation at a small number of sites in the chromosome (*see* p. 428). Isoniazid resistance has been linked to mutations in either the *inhA* gene which codes for an enzyme involved in mycolic acid synthesis in the cell wall[55] or the catalase peroxidase gene (*katG*) gene.[56] For streptomycin the resistance is due to changes in ribosomal S12 protein (rpsL) and 16S ribosomal RNA,[57] for fluoroquinolones the mutation is in the DNA gyrase A gene (*gyrA*);[58] rifampicin resistance is due to point mutations in the *rpoB* gene in the RNA polymerase B subunit[59] and has allowed the development of a molecular probe to detect this resistance, which is a key component of multidrug resistant TB (*see below*). Pyrazinamide resistance is due to lack of the pyrazinamidase enzyme but the exact genetics have not yet been worked out. The genetics of ethambutol resistance have yet to be fully established.

EPIDEMIOLOGY

Drug resistance is an increasing problem in developed countries, because an increasing proportion of cases come from people originally infected in underdeveloped countries. For underdeveloped countries themselves problems are increasing because of economic and population pressures on TB control services, variable drug availability, inadequate programs, and the difficulties of service delivery.[60] The incidence of drug resistance has to be differentiated into primary resistance (that found in previously untreated patients) and secondary or acquired resistance (that found in those with a history of treatment). Resistance rates to first-line antituberculosis drugs is found in all countries, with higher rates in underdeveloped countries, in parts of countries where there is economic collapse, or in certain populations (e.g. the Russian prison population[60]). Resistance rates to isoniazid of >5% are now common in most non-developed countries, and the drug resistance rates of minority ethnic groups in developed countries often follows that of their country of origin. Drug resistance data in the UK are monitored by Mycobnet, a section of the Public Health Laboratory Service Communicable Disease Surveillance Centre, which has monitored trends prospectively since 1993. The current levels of isoniazid resistance are 5–6% overall,[61] with lower rates (1–2%) in previously untreated White patients, but rates of 5–10% in ethnic minority groups.[62]

In an analysis of risk factors for drug resistance[63] independent risk factors by multivariate analysis included:

- a history of previous treatment (×3);
- HIV infection (×4);
- ethnic origin from the Indian Subcontinent (×3);
- Black–African ethnic origin (×4);
- Residence in London (×2).

In the UK, the national treatment guidelines[24] have been designed with these factors in mind.

Combined resistance to rifampicin and isoniazid, with or without additional drug resistances (so-called MDR-TB), is a particular concern, and is found worldwide. Certain countries (such as the Baltic republics, Russia, the Dominican Republic, and Côte d'Ivoire) are 'hotspots' with an incidence greater than 5%.[60] MDR-TB occurred infrequently in England and Wales between 1982 and 1991, being found in only 0.6% of isolates,[64] rose to nearly 2% in the early 1990s but fell to 1.3% in 1999,[61] representing approximately 50 cases, two-thirds of which occurred in Greater London. In England and Wales the risk factors for MDR-TB are those for drug resistance in general, but are even more pronounced:[63]

- previous treatment (×12);
- HIV infection (×9);
- birth in India (×4);
- male sex (×2);
- residence in London (×2).

Clinical suspicion of acquired resistance should also be raised by failure of clinical response to treatment or by prolonged sputum smear or culture positivity while on treatment.

Because of the rates of drug resistance, every effort should be made to obtain bacteriological confirmation of the diagnosis. In addition to proving the diagnosis, drug susceptibility information comes only from positive culture. Three sputum samples, obtained on separate mornings, should be sent for pulmonary cases. In patients unable to produce sputum, fibreoptic bronchoscopy and washings from the appropriate lung segment(s) has a good yield.[65] Pus obtained from neck glands and other sites, and fluid from serous sites, pleura, peritoneum and pericardium, should also be sent for culture. Surgeons performing biopsies on lesions in which tuberculosis is suspected should be reminded that half of the sample should be sent for TB culture *without* preservative such as formalin.

A risk assessment using the factors above should be made for the likelihood of drug resistance in all cases. If concerns are raised as to the possibility of MDR-TB, rapid molecular tests for rifampicin resistance are available on either sputum microscopy-positive or culture-positive material. These can be performed rapidly and are >95% accurate. If a test reports rifampicin resistance in a patient with *M. tuberculosis*, the patient should be managed as if he or she have MDR-TB, pending the results of full susceptibility tests, as 'isolated' rifampicin resistance accounts for under 10% of rifampicin resistance, and rifampicin resistance for more than 90% MDR-

TB. Separate isolation criteria are also advised for suspected or proven MDR-TB.[66,67]

TREATMENT OF DRUG-RESISTANT TUBERCULOSIS

Various short-course chemotherapy studies have been carried out on the efficacy of 'standard' chemotherapy in patients with prior initial drug resistance.[68] In these trials, patients with initial isoniazid and/or streptomycin resistance had a failure rate of 17% when given a 6-month regimen of rifampicin and isoniazid; the failure rate was 12% in those treated in the 2 month initial phase. As the number of drugs given in the regimen and the duration of rifampicin treatment increased, the failure rate fell, reaching only 2% of those receiving 4–5 drugs, including rifampicin throughout, in a 6-month regimen. The key exception was that of rifampicin resistance, where the outcome was much poorer.

Such a policy is appropriate in underdeveloped countries where routine drug susceptibility data is not available, but in developed countries it is thought preferable to modify treatment on the basis of the drug resistance data.[24] The recommendations are set out below and summarized in Table 61.3.

Single drug resistance

Streptomycin
Some of the drug resistance encountered, particularly in ethnic minority groups, is to streptomycin alone. Streptomycin is now seldom used, and the efficacy of the regimen recommended for both pulmonary and non-pulmonary disease in not affected.

Isoniazid
If isoniazid resistance is known about before treatment, a regimen of rifampicin, pyrazinamide, ethambutol and streptomycin for 2 months, followed by rifampicin and ethambutol for 7 months, has given good results when fully supervised.[69] For the usual scenario of isoniazid resistance being reported after treatment has started, isoniazid should be stopped and ethambutol and rifampicin given for 12 months supplemented by 2 months initial pyrazinamide[24].

Pyrazinamide
See *Mycobacterium bovis* infection later (page 824).

Ethambutol
This is uncommon; the standard regimen should be used.

Rifampicin
Isolated rifampicin resistance accounts for less than 10% of rifampicin resistance, 90% or more being due to MDR-TB. Rifampicin resistance should be managed as for MDR-TB until full first- and second-line susceptibilities are available. If true isolated rifampicin resistance is shown, a regimen of 18

Table 61.3 Management of drug resistance in tuberculosis

Resistance	Non-MDR-TB regimen	Comment
Streptomycin	2RHZ(E)/4RH	Standard treatment unaffected
Isoniazid	2RZSE/7RE if known pretreatment	Fully supervised (DOT)
Pyrazinamide	Usually *M. bovis*	
	If had 2RHZE: stop ZE then 7RH	
	If had 2RHZ: then 2RHE/7HR	
Ethambutol	2HRZ/4HR	Standard treatment unaffected
Rifampicin	Uncommon: *see text.*	
	Manage as MDR-TB until full susceptibilities known;	
	if true: 2HZE/16HE	
Streptomycin/ isoniazid	As for isoniazid resistance during treatment	Fully supervised (DOT)
Other combination	Individual regimen needed	*See text*

S, streptomycin; H, isoniazid; R, rifampicin; Z, pyrazinamide; E, ethambutol. The number in front of the letters represents the duration of treatment in months.

months ethambutol and isoniazid supplemented by 2 months initial pyrazinamide is recommended.[24]

Combined non-MDR resistance

Streptomycin and isoniazid

This is the most common dual resistance. Management should be as for isoniazid resistance found after treatment commencement but fully supervised throughout.[24]

Other combinations

These are uncommon. An individualized regimen is needed and would need to be discussed with an experienced clinician.

Multidrug-resistant TB

Where MDR-TB is suspected, using the risk criteria set out earlier, molecular methods are available for rapid detection of rifampicin resistance using genetic probes on culture material,[70] and increasingly on direct microscopy-positive samples.[71] Treatment is complex, time consuming, demanding on both the physician and the patient, must be individually planned,[72,73] and is likely to need the inclusion of reserve drugs (Table 61.4). There are also additional infection control measures required to prevent nosocomial outbreaks.[66,67] Such treatment should be carried out only in the following circumstances.

- The physician has substantial experience in managing complex resistant cases.
- Only in a hospital with appropriate isolation facilities.
- In close liaison with the appropriate mycobacteriology service.

For this to happen the patient may need to be transferred to an appropriate unit. All treatment, both as an inpatient and

Table 61.4 Reserve drugs that may be needed for multidrug-resistant tuberculosis

Injectable	Tablet
Streptomycin	Ciprofloxacin or ofloxacin
Amikacin	Ethionamide or protionamide
Kanamycin	Clarithromycin or azithromycin
Capreomycin	Cycloserine, rifabutin, thiacetazone, PAS sodium

PAS, *p*-aminosalicylic acid

as an outpatient, must be closely monitored because of increased toxicity, and must be directly observed throughout to prevent the emergence of further drug resistance. Consideration may also need to be given to resection of pulmonary lesions under drug cover.[73] Criteria for removal from isolation have been set out.[66,67]

The principles of treating such patients are to start treatment with five or more drugs to which the organism is (or is likely to be) susceptible, including one injectable if possible, and to continue these until cultures become negative. Drug treatment then should be continued with at least three drugs to which the organism is susceptible on in-vitro testing for a further minimum of 9 months. This may extend up to or beyond 24 months depending on the drug susceptibility profile, which drugs are available, and the patient's HIV status.[73]

TUBERCULOSIS IN HIV-POSITIVE PATIENTS

The incidence of tuberculosis in HIV-positive individuals is much higher than in those who are HIV-negative, and the mortality rate in such patients is also higher.[74,75] The classical type of tuberculosis with upper zone pulmonary disease tends to occur less commonly in patients with low CD4 lymphocyte counts, who are more likely to have smear-negative or non-cavitatory disease, mediastinal lymphadenopathy or disseminated disease. Although a small clinical study has suggested that standard regimens, particularly if supervised adequately, are equally effective in HIV-positive and HIV-negative patients,[76] there have been no controlled trials of adequate power in HIV-positive patients to show differences of efficacy between regimens. Because of the increased drug resistance rates in HIV-positive patients with tuberculosis, a four-drug initial phase should be used unless there are suspicions of MDR-TB (*see above*). If cultures remain positive after 3 months in HIV-positive patients, compliance and drug absorption should be assessed in detail.

Reactions to antituberculosis drugs are more common in HIV-positive individuals (in whom severe adverse effects can occur to any drug) particularly to thiacetazone, which causes Stevens–Johnson syndrome in 10% that may be fatal.[77] Important drug interactions also occur in such patients: ketoconazole can inhibit rifampicin absorption if given at the same time, which could lead to treatment failure;[78] rifampicin and isoniazid can interact with the azole antifungal drugs, reducing serum concentrations of fluconazole and itraconazole to suboptimal levels.[78–80]

The most difficult area of interaction is between antituberculosis therapy and HAART, particularly if protease inhibitors are included. Rifampicin is a potent inducer of the hepatic CYT 3A P450 enzyme through which the protease inhibitors (and other drugs) are metabolized. This causes tensions between the best antituberculosis therapy and concomitant antiviral therapy. This area has been studied in detail[81] and the relative merits of the various options for antituberculosis therapy and anti-viral therapy assessed (Table 61.5). In patients with dual infection there is no doubt that the priority is to treat the tuberculosis, especially in sputum smear-positive cases where there is also a public health element. This is also important in reversing the potentially deleterious effects of tuberculosis on the progress of the HIV infection suggested by in-vitro and in-vivo studies.[82]

Of the options set out in Table 61.5 option 1, (standard short-course chemotherapy with rifampicin throughout) is recommended in the UK whenever possible.[24] If a patient is taking protease inhibitors at the time of diagnosis these can be discontinued and an alternative regimen used during the antituberculosis therapy. Options 2 and 3 – use of rifabutin as the rifamycin either in the continuation phase (option 2), or in both the initial and continuation phases (option 3) – do not have the weight of evidence on efficacy against TB of option 1, and are only supported by small studies.[83,84] Indinavir and some of the other protease inhibitors can be used in conjunction with rifabutin. Option 5 (to use a non-rifamycin containing regimen of 18 months[85]) means prolonged antituberculosis therapy because of the lack of the main sterilizing drug group. A further option (not included in Table 61.5) of using a regimen of 9 months of streptomycin, isoniazid and pyrazi-

Table 61.5 Treatment of tuberculosis in HIV-positive persons[a]

Option	Antituberculosis regimen	Antiviral regimen
1.	2RHZE/4RH	None or triple NRTI
2.	2RHZE/4RifH	None *or*
		triple NRTI *or*
		nelfinavir, indinavir, amprenavir
		efavirenz or nevirapine
3.	2RifHZE/4RifH	Nelfinavir, indinavir, amprenavir
		efavirenz or nevirapine
4.	2RHZE/6HE	None *or* triple NRTI
		Any PI (e.g. saquinavir, ritonavir)
		Any NNRTI
5.	2HZE/16HE	Any PI
		Any NNRTI

H, isoniazid; R, rifampicin; Rif, rifabutin; Z, pyrazinamide; E, ethambutol. The number in front of the letters represents the duration of treatment in months.
NRTI, nucleoside reverse transcriptase inhibitor; PI, protease inhibitor; NNRTI, non-nucleoside reverse transcriptase inhibitor
[a] Regimens listed in preference order, with compatible antiviral regimen(s): also see text and reference 81.

namide,[86] has been heavily criticized on bacteriological and clinical grounds, and is not thought to be viable.[87]

Because of the complexities of managing such dually infected patients, detailed liaison between the TB and HIV services is needed, and drug levels of both antituberculosis and antiretroviral drugs may need monitoring. A detailed view on the complexities, with particular emphasis on drug interactions, is found in reference 81 (*see also* Ch. 6).

MYCOBACTERIUM BOVIS

Infection with *Mycobacterium bovis* can not be differentiated clinically from *M. tuberculosis* infection, and can only be diagnosed on culture. In the UK, only some 40 cases per year are diagnosed, accounting for 1.0–1.5% of bacteriologically confirmed *M. tuberculosis* complex cases.[88] Of 210 isolates reported, 200 were in patients of White ethnic origin, of whom over three-quarters were aged over 50 years, suggesting reactivation of disease acquired earlier in life.[85] Commercial molecular DNA or RNA-based tests cannot differentiate between *M. bovis* and *M. tuberculosis*, emphasizing the role of culture. Non-commercial molecular methods exist for the identification of *M. bovis*, such as identifications of mutations of the *pncA* gene.[89]

The main difference between *M. bovis* and *M. tuberculosis* is the presence of pyrazinamide resistance in the former. This influences recommended drug regimens because the inclusion of pyrazinamide is required for an effective 6-month regimen and is nullified by the presence of pyrazinamide resistance. If a four-drug initial phase has been given, then a 7-month continuation phase of rifampicin and isoniazid can be used (Table 61.3).[24] As most cases occur in White ethnic patients, only a three-drug initial phase (excluding ethambutol) will have been given. Once the diagnosis has been made, the pyrazinamide should be stopped, 9 months rifampicin and isoniazid given, supplemented by 2 months initial ethambutol (Table 61.3).[24]

Contact tracing of human contacts of human *M. bovis* disease should follow the recommendations given for human contacts of *M. tuberculosis*.[67] Where studies of human contacts of cattle with *M. bovis* disease have been undertaken, little evidence of transmission (as judged by tuberculin testing and no evidence of disease) has been found.[90] Recent advice on contact tracing of human contacts of cattle, largely based on first principles, has been published.[67]

BCG

Bacille Calmette–Guérin (BCG) is an attenuated strain of *M. bovis* and is therefore pyrazinamide resistant. There are differences between the UK[67] and the USA[26] in its use, with the USA putting a much lower emphasis on its use and efficacy. In the UK, BCG is advocated in unvaccinated children aged 10–13, and in anyone thought to be at higher risk[67] such as:

- previously unvaccinated tuberculin-negative household contacts of pulmonary disease;
- tuberculin-negative unvaccinated new immigrants from high-prevalence countries;
- neonates of African-Asian ethnic origin;
- tuberculin-negative previously unvaccinated healthcare workers.

The complications of BCG vaccination are local abscess and ulceration at the vaccination site and local lymph node disease. Complications are almost always due to faulty vaccination technique, with subcutaneous rather than intradermal administration. These may resolve spontaneously but over a prolonged period.

Antibiotic therapy with isoniazid,[91] rifampicin and isoniazid, and macrolides[92] have all been advocated. Surgical removal of regional nodes is rarely required. Disseminated BCG infection after vaccination is rare, but occurs in people with immune deficiency and has been reported in HIV infection. Prospective studies, however, have so far failed to show increased complications overall in asymptomatic neonates, and at the moment the WHO still recommends vaccination in developing countries for all neonates unless they have clinical evidence of AIDS.

Instillation of BCG into the bladder has been found to be very effective in the management of transitional cell carcinoma. Complications can occur, with mycobacterial dissemination, and focal forms of disease localized to both the urinary tract and other sites.[93] These complications require treatment as for *M. bovis* because of the pyrazinamide resistance (Table 61.3).

DELIVERY OF THERAPY

Compliance is the major determinant of outcome in treating tuberculosis,[94] both the compliance of the patient in taking medication as prescribed and the compliance of the physician in prescribing the correct regimen and monitoring it. Respiratory physicians are more likely to prescribe the standard chemotherapy than other clinicians, and drug reactions are more common with non-standard regimens.[95,96] In the UK it is advised that only physicians with full training and expertise in managing tuberculosis, and who have direct working access to TB nurses or health visitors, should manage respiratory tuberculosis.[24] It is further recommended that they also manage the drug treatment of non-respiratory tuberculosis, and manage children jointly with a general pediatrician, unless they are a specialist infectious disease pediatrician trained in tuberculosis.[24]

Tuberculosis cases should be managed by a team, as part of a district policy that covers all aspects of management including notification of disease to the proper authorities, chemotherapy, compliance and contact tracing.[97] A minimum of one full-time TB nurse or health visitor plus full clerical support is recommended for every 50 notifications per annum per district.[67]

COMPLIANCE MONITORING

Monitoring patient compliance with medication is a vital part of management, and is carried out by TB nurses or health visitors, together with checking on the accuracy and continuity of prescribing. For patients not on directly observed therapy (DOT: *see below*) tablet checks and urine tests for rifampicin should be carried out at least monthly throughout chemotherapy. If non-compliance is detected in patients being allowed self-administered therapy, they should be switched to supervised (DOT) therapy, and an assessment made of the possibility of acquired drug resistance. This may require repeat cultures and susceptibility tests, and consideration of molecular tests for rifampicin resistance.

COMBINATION TABLETS

Combination tablets are extremely useful in patients taking daily therapy and prevent the deliberate or accidental consumption of a single drug, which in active disease can very easily lead to acquired drug resistance. They have the further advantage that compliance can be checked by using the orange/pink coloration of urine of the rifampicin component, which can be inspected for either visually or in the laboratory. Rifater (Hoechst Marion Roussel), for use in the initial phase of treatment, contains rifampicin, isoniazid and pyrazinamide, and Rimactalzid (Novartis) and Rifinah (Hoechst Marion Roussel) combine rifampicin and isoniazid for use in the continuation phase. In some studies of combined preparations, the dosages of isoniazid, rifampicin and pyrazinamide[98,99] have varied slightly from those in Rifater currently available in the UK (isoniazid 50 mg, rifampicin 120 mg, pyrazinamide 300 mg). The bioavailability of the drugs in combination tablets is similar to that of the same doses given individually,[98] and gives satisfactory clinical results.[99] The slight variations in dosage are therefore not thought to be important in combined preparations of proven bioavailability. Because of the similarity in name (rifampicin, Rifinah, Rimactazid, Rifadin, Rimifon and Rifater) care must be taken in writing and dispensing prescriptions. Care is also needed with computer-generated prescribing, because if the system does not recognize the name it may default to rifampicin alone, leading to monotherapy.

For the above reasons, for patients on daily therapy in the UK, combination tablets are recommended to aid compliance and to prevent monotherapy.

PRETREATMENT SCREENING

Liver function should be checked before treatment of clinical cases: modest elevations of the hepatic transaminases (ALT/AST) are not uncommon in the pretreatment liver function tests of people with TB. Detailed advice on the monitoring of liver function and hepatotoxicity is available.[100]

Renal function should be checked before treatment with either streptomycin or ethambutol. If possible these drugs should be avoided in renal failure, but if their use is required serum concentrations should be monitored and substantial dosage reductions made unless dialysis is used.[24] Because of its rare, but possible, toxic effects on the optic nerve, visual acuity should be tested using a Snellen chart before ethambutol is given.[101] Patients should have reasonable visual acuity and ideally be able to report symptoms, although the use of ethambutol in children appears to be safe.[54] A patient should be told to stop the drug *immediately* if symptoms occur and report to the physician, and this should be documented. In those with language difficulties or in small children this advice should be given to carers and family members.

DIRECTLY OBSERVED THERAPY

Concerns about patient compliance, its effects of relapse and the development of drug resistance, has lead to the WHO advocating directly observed therapy (DOT) in the form of short-course chemotherapy or DOTS. With this method of treatment, the ingestion of every dose is monitored by a nursing or lay observer. DOT can be given daily but an intermittent regimen, with appropriate dosage adjustments, is often more convenient as doses can be scheduled to avoid weekends. A regimen of rifampicin, isoniazid, pyrazinamide and either ethambutol or streptomycin thrice weekly for 2 months, followed by thrice-weekly rifampicin and isoniazid for a further 4 months, is advised in the UK.[24]

The strategy of universal DOT, although strongly advocated by the WHO[102] and bodies such as the International Union against Tuberculosis and Lung Diseases,[103] has not been tested by randomized controlled studies. Cohort studies against historical control groups receiving self-administered therapy in different countries have shown DOT to improve outcomes (e.g. cure rates.[104–106]). Decision analyses have also suggested that both selective and universal DOT strategies are more cost-effective than conventional self-administered therapy.[107–109] However, when DOT was compared in a controlled way directly with self-administration it actually performed less well overall, although subgroups had differing results.[110] Critics of universal DOT, which they call 'supervised pill swallowing' say that the success of DOT programs is derived from the substantial financial and technical investment in tuberculosis programs that DOT represents and not the DOT element itself.[111] Even in the USA there have been dissenting analyses of DOT effectiveness.[112] Authors who admitted initial predjudice in favor of DOT conceded that treatment completion rates of over 90% could be obtained with a much lower proportion of DOT than that proposed by the advocates of universal DOT.[112] The United States Centers for Disease Control recommend that DOT treatment should be considered for all patients, but that if more than 90% of the patients in an area are completing self-administered therapy, selective DOT in unreliable patients is an alternative.[113]

In the UK, where tuberculosis is (or should be) treated by experienced physicians working with direct conjunction with tuberculosis nurses or health visitors[24] and as part of a district plan,[67,97] DOT is recommended for selective use in people thought unlikely to comply. This includes patients who are homeless, alcohol or other drug abusers, vagrants, seriously mentally ill, patients with multiple drug resistances and for those with any history of non-compliance with antituberculosis medication, either previously or shown during treatment monitoring.[67]

NOTIFICATION AND CONTACT TRACING

All cases of tuberculosis, whether respiratory or non-respiratory, should be notified to the proper authorities. The purpose of notification is two-fold.

1. It allows proper epidemiological data to be collected and outbreaks detected, so that treatment services can be planned and monitored.
2. Contact tracing procedures are activated by notification, and so it is essential that all cases, including active cases diagnosed after death, are notified.

Failure to notify could lead to failure to screen appropriate close contacts, which could result in contacts requiring treatment for active disease, or those eligible for BCG vaccination or chemoprophylaxis, being denied the appropriate intervention. Detailed guidance, recently updated, is available in the UK.[67] The emphasis on aspects of contact tracing in the UK, where BCG vaccination is more widely advised,[67] is different from that in the USA, where there is greater emphasis on chemoprophylaxis (*see below*) and less on BCG vaccination.[26]

CHEMOPROPHYLAXIS

PRINCIPLES

A proportion of people with tuberculosis infection, as judged by a positive tuberculin skin reaction, are thought to have a small number of dormant bacilli, perhaps in the order of 10^3 or 10^4. The administration of one or two drugs for a shorter period of time than for disease – chemoprophylaxis or preventive therapy – is likely to kill these organisms and hence reduce the chance of progression to disease. It is therefore important to differentiate between disease and infection.

- In tuberculosis infection, the tuberculin skin test is positive, the chest radiography is normal, and the patient is asymptomatic.
- In tuberculosis disease, the skin test is usually positive and there are clinical signs and symptoms or radiographic changes present.

This matter is further complicated in HIV-positive individuals, where anergy to tuberculin does not necessarily mean tuberculosis infection has not occurred, and it becomes difficult to differentiate between disease and infection. Most chemoprophylaxis is secondary (i.e. after infection, as judged by a positive tuberculin test, has occurred). Occasionally it may be given before evidence of infection, to prevent infection occurring (e.g. in the neonate of a sputum smear-positive mother); this is primary chemoprophylaxis.

REGIMENS

Although multiple drug regimens are required for the treatment of disease in order to prevent the emergence of drug resistance, it is not illogical to use a one- or two-drug regimen for prophylaxis. Individuals who are receiving chemoprophylaxis are thought to have a low organism burden, in the order of 10^3 to 10^4. The chance of spontaneous resistance developing to a single drug is in the order of 10^{-5} to 10^{-7}. The chance of drug resistance developing is therefore very low, particularly if a two-drug regimen is used. For instance, when mass isoniazid chemoprophylaxis was given to Inuit communities there was no increase in isoniazid-resistant disease.[114]

Many randomized placebo-controlled trials of isoniazid chemoprophylaxis have been conducted.[115] Alaskan studies showed that the maximal effect was achieved by durations up to 12 months, and that there was no additional benefit from more extended treatment.[116] Where the rate of new infection was low, protection lasted more than 15 years.[117] A multicenter

study by the International Union against Tuberculosis and Lung Disease (IUATLD)[118] showed that for small radiographic lesions (<2 cm) 6 months of treatment with isoniazid was just as effective as 12 months, and for larger lesions (>2 cm) 6 months of isoniazid provided considerable protection. As with chemotherapy for disease, compliance with therapy is important, particularly because individuals on chemoprophylaxis are clinically well and so have less incentive to complete medication: the Alaskan studies also showed that to obtain the full benefit from chemoprophylaxis more than 60% of treatment must be taken.[116] There is also concern about possible isoniazid hepatotoxicity over a longer duration of treatment. In the later US Public Health Service studies the probable isoniazid hepatitis rate was approximately 1%.[115] There was, however, a clear relationship with age: no cases under 30 years, rising to 2.3% in patients over 50 years. The hepatitis rate was lower in the IUATLD trial, at 0.5%, but was still higher than the rate of 0.1% in the placebo-treated group.[118]

These concerns have led to a search for alternative and shorter regimens. Rifampicin has been shown to have a greater sterilizing effect in animal studies,[119] either alone or with pyrazinamide, than has isoniazid. A placebo-controlled prophylaxis study from Hong Kong in patients with silicosis suggested that rifampicin alone for 3 months had similar efficacy to rifampicin and isoniazid for 3 months or isoniazid alone for 6 months.[120] In UK studies the use of rifampicin and isoniazid combined for 3 months showed a significant decrease in childhood tuberculosis.[121,122] Using these data, and others from experimental studies, the American Thoracic Society is now recommending a regimen of rifampicin and pyrazinamide for 2 months (2RZ) rather than isoniazid alone for 6 months.[123] The Joint Tuberculosis Committee of the British Thoracic Society has reviewed the same data and regards the data supporting 2RZ over rifampicin and isoniazid for 3 months (3RH) as equivocal.[67] Since 3RH is just as effective as, and better tolerated than 2RZ, together with the fact that RH combination tablets are available for this regimen, 3RH is advised as the alternative regimen to isoniazid alone for 6 months in the UK.[67] In isoniazid-resistant cases 6 months' rifampicin is recommended.[24]

In HIV-negative persons

In the UK, where there is greater emphasis on BCG, and where prior BCG vaccination modifies the tuberculin response, the following groups are recommended to receive chemoprophylaxis:[67]

1. Children under 16 years with strongly positive Heaf tests (grades 2–4 if no prior BCG, grades 3–4 if prior BCG vaccination).
2. Children under 2 years in close contact with smear positive pulmonary disease.
   (a) those without prior BCG vaccination should be given chemoprophylaxis irrespective of the initial Heaf test result. If the initial Heaf test is negative (grade 0–1)

repeat at 6 weeks and, if still negative, stop chemoprophylaxis and give BCG vaccination. If the repeat Heaf test result becomes positive (grades 2–4) give full chemoprophylaxis if chest radiography excludes disease. If the initial Heaf test is positive (grades 2–4) give full chemoprophylaxis if chest radiography excludes disease.

(b) For children who have been given BCG vaccination (confirmed by characteristic scar or vaccination record), if the initial Heaf test is strongly positive (grades 3–4) give full chemoprophylaxis if the chest radiograph excludes disease. If the Heaf test is grades 0–2, repeat the test after 6 weeks. If there is no change in the reaction, no further action is needed. If it has become positive (grades 3–4) give full chemoprophylaxis if the chest radiograph excludes disease.

3. People in whom recent tuberculin conversion has been documented (irrespective of age).

4. Babies born to mothers with infectious TB should receive chemoprophylaxis (normally isoniazid syrup 5 mg/kg) for 6 weeks and then be tuberculin tested. If negative, BCG vaccination should be given and chemoprophylaxis stopped. If the tuberculin test is positive chemoprophylaxis should be continued. Such babies may be breast-fed.

People for whom chemoprophylaxis is recommended, but who do not receive it should have radiographic follow-up at 3 and 12 months.[67]

In the USA, preventive therapy with a positive tuberculin reaction[26] (>5 mm in persons with HIV infection, close contact of infectious disease, and with fibrotic X-ray lesions; >10 mm in other at-risk persons, including infants and children younger than 4 years; and >15 mm in low-risk populations) is recommended for:

1. Close contacts of persons with newly diagnosed infectious tuberculosis.

2. Recent tuberculin skin test converters, (defined as a 10 mm or greater increase with a 2 year period for those >35 years of age, and 15 mm or greater increase for those >35 years).

3. Persons with medical conditions that have been reported to increase the risk of tuberculosis:
    (a) diabetes mellitus
    (b) prolonged therapy with adrenocorticosteroids
    (c) immunosuppressive therapy
    (d) some hematological and reticuloendothelial diseases
    (e) injecting drug users known to be HIV negative
    (f) end-stage renal disease
    (g) clinical situations associated with substantial rapid weight loss or chronic undernutrition.

4. People under 35 years with a tuberculin test >10 mm, even in the absence of the above risk categories, if:
    (a) foreign born from high-prevalence countries
    (b) from medically under-served low-income populations, including high-risk racial or ethnic minority populations
    (c) resident of a long-term care facility.

In HIV-positive persons

The identification of individuals at high risk of developing tuberculosis in HIV infection is complicated by loss of response to tuberculin, and the atypical radiological changes. Such therapy is recommended by the WHO and IUATLD.[124] When this policy has been examined in developing countries short-term benefits have been shown but there are also logistical difficulties in implementing such a policy.[125,126] A more recent study in the USA did not support isoniazid prophylaxis in high-risk patients with anergy unless they had been exposed to active tuberculosis.[127]

For the above reasons, and because of concerns about the higher rates of drug resistance in HIV-infected persons in the UK, chemoprophylaxis in HIV-positive individuals is recommended in only contacts of sputum smear-positive pulmonary disease[67] and is no longer recommended for people treated for disease after completion of chemotherapy.[67] In the USA[26] chemoprophylaxis for a tuberculin test of 5 mm is advised as it is thought that such patients have a high annual rate of disease.[128] It may also be considered for HIV-infected persons who are tuberculin negative but belong to groups in which the prevalence of tuberculosis infection is high.

For multidrug-resistant tuberculosis

There are no data on what chemoprophylaxis regimen is feasible in persons in contact with MDR-TB. Any chemoprophylaxis should include two (and ideally three) drugs to which the organism is known to be susceptible, although the resistance pattern can be so extensive that no prophylaxis regimen is available. If the drug susceptibility pattern is not known then ofloxacin or ciprofloxacin with pyrazinamide may be effective.[129] The United States Centers for Disease Control suggest this combination, or ethambutol and pyrazinamide.[130]

The view in the UK is that, since only a minority of people infected with tuberculosis develop clinical disease, and because there are no data on which to base advice, long-term regular follow-up of individual cases is currently advised.[24]

OPPORTUNIST MYCOBACTERIA

Isolates of opportunist mycobacteria (also called atypical mycobacteria, mycobacteria other than tuberculosis, non-tuberculous mycobacteria or environmental mycobacteria) are increasing. They are ubiquitous in the environment and the significance of an isolate can be established only by considering the specimen type from which the organism was isolated, the number of isolates, the degree of growth and the species of *Mycobacterium*. In general, in non-sterile sites, multiple isolates are required to establish disease, whereas one positive culture from a sterile site, particularly if supported by histopathology, is usually sufficient.

The management of opportunistic organisms has recently been reviewed by the Joint Tuberculosis Committee of the

Table 61.6 Treatment of opportunist mycobacteria[132]

Organism	Situation	Recommended management
HIV negative		
Any	Children: lymph node	Excision
M. kansasii		9RE: 15–24 RE if relapse
M. avium complex	Adult pulmonary	24R(H)E
M. malmoense	disease	
M. xenopi		Trials of 24RE plus clarithromycin or ciprofloxacin: results awaited
M. kansasii		24RE
M. avium complex	Adult non-pulmonary	
M. malmoense	disease	24R(H)E
M. xenopi		
Fast-growing organisms	Adult pulmonary	Surgery if possible. RE plus Clarithromycin:? duration. Other drugs may be indicated
M. fortuitum	Adult	Surgical debridement
M. chelonae	Non-pulmonary	Ciprofloxacin + aminoglycoside
M. marinum	Skin	Trimethoprim–sulfamethoxazole; tetracycline; RE
HIV-positive		
M. avium complex		
M. malmoense	Pulmonary	
M. kansasii	or	RE plus clarithromycin, life-long
M. xenopi	disseminated	

R, rifampicin; E, ethambutol; H, isoniozid. The number in front of the letters represents duration in months.

British Thoracic Society, and guidelines on their management produced,[131] although these are much less based on controlled trials than is the case for tuberculosis. These are summarized in Table 61.6.

In HIV-negative people, opportunistic organisms cause disease in three main settings.

- In children, usually under the age of 5 years, isolated lymphadenopathy, usually cervical, occurs and should be managed by surgical excision.[132]
- In HIV-negative patients with underlying structural lung disease, often chronic obstructive pulmonary disease, infection with M. kansasii, M. avium complex, M. malmoense, or M. xenopi can all simulate conventional tuberculosis. Unlike the management of tuberculosis where the drug susceptibility data has to be scrupulously followed, the susceptibility to individual drugs in vitro does not correspond to clinical response and should be ignored. Clinical trials on pulmonary M. kansasii have shown that 9 months of treatment with rifampicin and ethambutol is adequate for most people, but that longer treatment may be needed in some cases.[133]
- For the other mycobacteria which cause pulmonary infection treatment with rifampicin and ethambutol, sometimes with isoniazid as well, gives cure rates of approximately 80%.[134] Treatment of extrapulmonary other than M. marinum disease in adults is more complex and detailed recommendations should be followed.[131]

In HIV-positive patients restoring immune function with combinations of antiretroviral treatment is as important as, if not more so than, antimycobacterial treatment. There are important interactions between macrolides, rifamycins and protease inhibitors which may limit treatment. In those who require treatment for pulmonary or disseminated disease, rifampicin, ethambutol and clarithromycin on an indefinite basis are advised.[131] For prophylaxis against M. avium complex the first-choice recommendation is azithromycin 1200 mg weekly, with clarithromycin 500 mg twice daily as second, and azithromycin 1200 mg once weekly plus rifabutin 300 mg once daily as third choice.[132]

References

1. Dye C, Scheele S, Dolin P, Pathania V, Raviglione MC 1999 Consensus Statement: Global burden of tuberculosis: estimated incidence, prevalence and mortality by country. World Health Organization Global Surveillance and Monitoring Project. *Journal of the American Medical Association* 282: 677–686.

2. Rose AMC, Watson JM, Graham C et al 2001 Tuberculosis at the end of the 20th century in England and Wales: results of a national survey. *Thorax* 56: 173–179.

3. Brudney K, Dobkin J 1991 Resurgent tuberculosis in New York City: human immunodeficiency virus, homelessness and the decline of tuberculosis programs. *American Review of Respiratory Disease* 144: 745–749.

4. Pitchenik AE, Cole C, Russell BW, Fischl MA, Spira TJ, Snider DE 1984 Tuberculosis, atypical mycobacteriosis and the acquired immunodeficiency Syndrome among Haitian and non-Haitian patients in South Florida. *Annals of Internal Medicine* 101: 641–645.

5. Nunn P, Elliot AM, McAdam KPWJ 1994 The impact of human immunodeficiency virus on tuberculosis in developing countries. *Thorax* 49: 511–518.

6. Jindani A, Aber VR, Edwards EA, Mitchison DA 1980 The early bactericidal activity of drugs in patients with pulmonary tuberculosis. *American Review of Respiratory Disease* 121: 139–148.

7. Mitchison DA 1998 Basic concepts in the chemotherapy of tuberculosis. In: Gangadharam PRJ, Jenkins PA (eds) *Mycobacteria Vol II Chemotherapy*. Chapman and Hall, New York, pp. 15–50.

8. British Thoracic Society 1984 A controlled trial of 6-month chemotherapy in pulmonary tuberculosis. Final report: results during 36 months after the end of chemotherapy and beyond. *British Journal of Disease of the Chest* 78: 330–336.

9. Hong Kong Chest Service/British Medical Research Council 1981 First report: Controlled trial of four thrice weekly regimens and a daily regimen all given for six months for pulmonary tuberculosis. *Lancet* 1: 171–174.

10. Hong Kong Chest Service/British Medical Research Council 1982 Second Report: controlled trial of four thrice-weekly regimens and a daily regimen all given for 6 months. The results up to 24 months. *Tubercle* 63: 89–98.

11. Hong Kong Chest Service/British Medical Research Council 1987 Five year Follow-up of a controlled trial of five 6-month regimens of chemotherapy for pulmonary tuberculosis. *American Review of Respiratory Disease* 136: 1339–1342.

12. Combs DL, O'Brien R, Geiter L 1990 USPHS tuberculosis short course chemotherapy trial 21. Effectiveness, toxicity and acceptability. The report of final results. *Annals of Internal Medicine* 112: 397–406.

13. Singapore Tuberculosis Service/British Medical Research Council 1979 Clinical trial of six-month and 4 month regimens of chemotherapy in the treatment of pulmonary tuberculosis. *American Review of Respiratory Disease* 119: 579–585.

14. Singapore Tuberculosis Service/British Medical Research Council 1981 Clinical trial of 6-month and 4-month regimens of chemotherapy in the treatment of pulmonary tuberculosis. The results up to 30 months. *Tubercle* 61: 95–102.

15. Snider DE, Graczyk J, Bek E, Rogowski J 1984 Supervised six-months treatment of newly diagnosed pulmonary tuberculosis using isoniazid, rifampin and pyrazinamide with or without streptomycin. *American Review of Respiratory Disease* 130: 1091–1094.

16. Singapore Tuberculosis Service/British Medical Research Council 1985 Clinical trial of three 6-month regimens of chemotherapy given intermittently in the continuation phase in the treatment of pulmonary tuberculosis. *American Review of Respiratory Disease* 132: 374–378.

17. Singapore Tuberculosis Service/British Medical Research Council 1988 Five year follow-up of a clinical trial of three 6-month regimens of chemotherapy given intermittently in the continuation phase in the treatment of pulmonary tuberculosis. *American Review of Respiratory Disease* 137: 1147–1150.

18. Hong Kong Chest Service/British Medical Research Council 1991 Controlled Trial of 2, 4 and 6 months of pyrazinamide in 6-month, three-times-weekly regimens for smear-positive tuberculosis, including an assessment of a combined preparation of isoniazid, rifampicin and pyrazinamide. Results at 30 months. *American Review of Respiratory Disease* 143: 700–706.

19. Cohn DL, Catlin BJ, Peterson KL *et al* 1990 A 62 dose, 6 month therapy for pulmonary and extra-pulmonary tuberculosis. A twice weekly, directly observed, and cost-effective regimen. *Annals of Internal Medicine* 112: 407–415.

20. Third East African/British Medical Research Council Study 1978 First report: Controlled clinical trial of four short course regimens of chemotherapy for two durations in the treatment of pulmonary tuberculosis. *American Review of Respiratory Disease* 118: 39–48.

21. Third East African/British Medical Research Council Study 1980 Second report: controlled clinical trial of four short course regimens of chemotherapy for two durations in the treatment of pulmonary tuberculosis. *Tubercle* 61: 59–69.

22. Hong Kong Chest Service/Tuberculosis Research Centre Madras/British Medical Research Council 1981 A controlled trial of 2-month, 3-month and 12 month regimens of chemotherapy for sputum-negative pulmonary tuberculosis. The results at 30 months. *American Review of Respiratory Disease* 124: 138–142.

23. Hong Kong Chest Service/Tuberculosis Research Centre Madras/British Medical Research Council 1989 A controlled trial of 3-month, 4-month and 6-month regimens of chemotherapy for sputum smear-negative pulmonary tuberculosis. Results at 5 years. *American Review of Respiratory Disease* 139: 871–876.

24. Joint Tuberculosis Committee of the British Thoracic Society 1998 Chemotherapy and management of tuberculosis in the United Kingdom: recommendations 1998. *Thorax* 53: 536–548.

25. Migliori GB, Raviglione MC, Schaberg T *et al* 1999 Tuberculosis management in Europe. Task Force of ERS, WHO and the Europe Region of IUATLD. *European Respiratory Journal* 14: 978–992.

26. American Thoracic Society 1994 Treatment of tuberculosis and tuberculosis infection in adults and children. *American Journal of Respiratory Critical Care Medicine* 149: 1359–1378.

27. World Health Organization Tuberculosis Unit, Division of Communicable Disease 1991 Guidelines for tuberculosis treatment in adults and children in National Tuberculosis Programmes. Geneva, WHO, WHO/TB/91, pp. 1–61.

28. Hayward AC, Bennett DE, Herbert J *et al* 1996 Risk factors for drug resistance in patients with tuberculosis in England and Wales 1993–4. *Thorax* 51(Suppl. 3): S32.

29. British Thoracic and Tuberculosis Association 1976 Short-course chemotherapy in pulmonary tuberculosis. *Lancet* ii: 1102–1104.

30. British Thoracic Society Research Committee 1992 Six months versus nine months chemotherapy for tuberculosis of lymph nodes: preliminary results. *Respiratory Medicine* 86: 15–19.

31. Campbell IA, Ormerod LP, Friend JR *et al* 1993 Six months versus nine months chemotherapy for tuberculosis of lymph nodes: final results. *Respiratory Medicine* 87: 621–623.

32. Campbell IA, Dyson AJ 1977 Lymph node tuberculosis: a comparison of various methods of treatment. *Tubercle* 58: 171–179.

33. Campbell IA, Dyson AJ 1979 Lymph node tuberculosis: a comparison of treatments 18 months after completion of chemotherapy. *Tubercle* 60: 95–98.

34. Girling DJ, Darbyshire JH, Humphries MJ *et al* 1988 Extrapulmonary tuberculosis. *British Medical Bulletin* 44: 738–756.

35. Medical Research Council Working Party on Tuberculosis of the Spine 1986 A controlled trial of 6-month and 9-month regimens of chemotherapy in patients undergoing radical surgery for tuberculosis of the spine in Hong Kong. *Tubercle* 67: 243–259.

36. Medical Research Council Working Party on Tuberculosis of the Spine 1993 Controlled trial of short-course regimens of chemotherapy in ambulatory treatment of spinal tuberculosis. *Journal of Bone and Joint Surgery* 75: 240–248.

37. Indian Council of Medical Research/British Medical Research Council Working Party 1989 A controlled trial of short-course regimens of chemotherapy in patients receiving ambulatory treatment or undergoing radical surgery for tuberculosis of the spine. *Indian Journal of Tuberculosis* 36(Suppl.): 1–22.

38. Strang JIG, Kakaka HHS, Gibson DG *et al* 1987 Controlled trial of prednisolone as an adjuvant in treatment of tuberculous constrictive pericarditis in Transkei. *Lancet* ii: 1418–1422.

39. Strang JIG, Kakaka HHS, Gibson DG *et al* 1988 Controlled clinical trial of complete open surgical drainage and of prednisolone in treatment of tuberculous pericardial effusion in Transkei. *Lancet* ii: 759–763.

40. Humphries MJ 1992 The management of tuberculous meningitis. *Thorax* 47: 577–581.

41. Citron KM, Thomas GO 1986 Ocular Toxicity from ethambutol. *Thorax* 41: 737–739.

42. Donald PR, Seifart HI 1989 Cerebrospinal fluid concentrations of ethionamide in children with tuberculous meningitis. *Journal of Pediatrics* 115: 383–386.

43. Ormerod LP, Watson JM, Pozniak A *et al* 1997 Notification of tuberculosis: an updated code of practice for England and Wales. *Journal of the Royal College of Physicians of London* 31: 299–303.

44. Schoerman JF, Van Zyl LE, Laubscher JA *et al* 1997 Effects of corticosteroids on intracranial pressure, computerised tomographic findings, and clinical outcome in young children with tuberculous meningitis. *Pediatrics* 99: 226–231.

45. Toppet M, Malfroot A, Derde MP *et al* 1990 Corticosteroids in primary tuberculosis with bronchial obstruction. *Archives of Disease in Childhood* 65: 1222–1226.

46. Lee CH, Wang WJ, Lan RS *et al* 1988 Corticosteroids in the treatment of tuberculous pleurisy. A double-blind, placebo controlled, randomized study. *Chest* 94: 1256–1259.

47. Horne NW, Tulloch WS 1973 Conservative management of renal tuberculosis. *British Journal of Urology* 47: 481–487.

48. Home NW 1966 A critical evaluation of corticosteroids in tuberculosis. *Advances in Tuberculosis Research* 15: 1–54.

49. Ormerod LP 2001 Tuberculosis in pregnancy and the puerperium. *Thorax* 56: 494–499.

50. International Union against Tuberculosis and Lung Disease 1988 Antituberculosis regimens of chemotherapy. Recommendations from the committee on treatment of IUATLD. *Bulletin of the International Union against Tuberculosis and Lung Disease* 63: 60–64.

51. American Academy of Pediatrics, Committee on Infectious Diseases 1992 Chemotherapy for tuberculosis in infants and children. *Pediatrics* 89: 161–165.

52. Roy V, Tekur U, Chopra K 1996 Pharmacokinetics of isoniazid in pulmonary Tuberculosis: a comparative study at two dose levels. *Indian Pediatrics* 33: 287–291.

53. Palma Beltran OR, Pelosi F, Budani H et al 1986 The treatment of child tuberculosis with isoniazid (H), rifampicin (R) and pyrazinamide (Z). *Bulletin of the International Union against Tuberculosis and Lung Disease* 61: 17.

54. Trebucq A 1997 Should ethambutol be recommended for routine treatment of tuberculosis in children? A review of the literature. *International Journal of Tuberculosis and Lung Disease* 1: 12–15.

55. Banerjee A, Dubnau E, Quemard A et al 1994 InhA a gene encoding a target for isoniazid and ethionamide in *Mycobacterium tuberculosis*. *Science* 263: 227–230.

56. Zhang Y, Heym B, Allen B, Young D, Cole S 1992 The catalase-peroxidase gene of *Mycobacterium tuberculosis*. *Nature* 358: 591–593.

57. Finken M, Kirschner P, Meier A, Wrede A, Bottger EC 1993 Molecular basis of streptomycin resistance in *Mycobacterium tuberculosis*: alterations in the ribosomal protein S12 gene and point mutations within a functional 16S ribosomal RNA pseudoknot. *Molecular Microbiology* 9: 1239–1246.

58. Takiff HE, Salazar L, Guerrero C et al 1994 Cloning and nucleotide sequence of the *Mycobacterium tuberculosis* gyrA and gyrB genes and detection of quinolone resistance mutations. *Antimicrobial Agents and Chemotherapy* 38: 773–780.

59. Telenti A, Imboden P, Marcheu F et al 1993 Detection of rifampicin resistance mutations in *Mycobacterium tuberculosis*. *Lancet* 341: 647–650.

60. Pablos-Mendez A, Raviglione MC, Laszlo A et al 1998 Global surveillance of Antituberculosis-drug resistance 1994–97. World Health Organisation-International Union against Tuberculosis and Lung Disease Working Group on Anti Tuberculosis Drug Resistance Surveillance. *New England Journal of Medicine* 338: 1641–1649.

61. Public Health Laboratory Service 1999 Tuberculosis Update.

62. Rose AMC et al 2001 Tuberculosis at the turn of the century: A national survey of tuberculosis notifications 1998. *Thorax* 56: 173–179.

63. Hayward AC, Bennett DE, Herbert J, Watson JM 1996 Risk factors for drug resistance in patients with tuberculosis in England and Wales 1993–94. *Thorax* 51(Suppl 3): A8.

64. Warburton AR, Jenkins PA, Waight PA, Watson JM 1993 Drug resistance in Initial isolates of Mycobacterium tuberculosis in England and Wales, 1982–1991. *Communicable Diseases Review* 3: R175–179.

65. Chawla R, Pant K, Jaggi OP et al 1998 Fibreoptic bronchoscopy in smear-negative pulmonary tuberculosis. *European Respiratory Journal* 1: 804–806.

66. The Interdepartmental Working group on Tuberculosis 1998 The prevention and control of tuberculosis in the United Kingdom: UK Guidance on the prevention and control of tranmission of 1. HIV-related tuberculosis, 2. Drug-resistant, including multiple drug-resistant, tuberculosis. London, Department of Health, The Scottish Office, The Welsh Office.

67. Joint Tuberculosis Committee of the British Thoracic Society 2000 Control and prevention of tuberculosis in the United Kingdom: Code of Practice 2000. *Thorax* 55: 887–901.

68. Mitchison DA, Nunn AJ 1986 Influence of initial drug resistance on the response to short-course chemotherapy in pulmonary tuberculosis. *American Review of Respiratory Disease* 133: 423–430.

69. Babu Swai O, Alnoch JA, Githui WA et al 1988 Controlled clinical trial of a regimen of two durations for the treatment of isoniazid resistant tuberculosis. *Tubercle* 69: 5–14.

70. Drobniewski FA, Pozniak AL 1996 Molecular diagnosis, detection of drug resistance and epidemiology of tuberculosis. *British Journal of Hospital Medicine* 56: 204–208.

71. Goyal M, Shaw RJ, Banerjee DK et al 1997 Rapid detection of multi-drug resistant tuberculosis. *European Respiratory Journal* 10: 120–124.

72. Goble M, Iseman M, Madsen LA et al 1993 Treatment of 171 patients with pulmonary tuberculosis resistant to isoniazid and rifampin. *New England Journal of Medicine* 328: 527–532.

73. Iseman M 1993 Treatment of multidrug resistant tuberculosis. *New England Journal of Medicine* 328: 784–790.

74. Grosset JH 1992 Treatment of tuberculosis in HIV infection. *Tubercle and Lung Disease* 73: 378–383.

75. Ackah AN, Coulibaly D, Digbeu H et al 1995 Response to treatment, mortality and CD4 lymphocyte counts in HIV-infected persons with tuberculosis in Abidjan, Côte d'Ivoire. *Lancet* 345: 607–610.

76. Perriens JH, St Louis ME, Yiadiul B et al 1995 Pulmonary tuberculosis in HIV-infected patients in Zaire. *New England Journal of Medicine* 332: 779–784.

77. Small PM, Schecter GF, Goodman PC et al 1990 Treatment of tuberculosis in patients with advanced human immunodeficiency virus infection. *New England Journal of Medicine* 324: 289–294.

78. Englehard D, Stutman HR, Marks MI 1994 Interaction of ketoconazole with rifampicin and isoniazid. *New England Journal of Medicine* 311: 1681–1683.

79. Lazar JD, Wilner KD 1990 Drug interactions with fluconazole. *Reviews of Infectious Disease* 12(Suppl. 3): S327–333.

80. Heyden R, Miller R 1996 Adverse effects and drug interactions of medications commonly used in the treatment of adult HIV positive patients. *Genitourinary Medicine* 72: 237–246.

81. Pozniak AL, Miller R, Ormerod LP 1999 The treatment of tuberculosis in HIV-infected persons. *AIDS* 13: 435–445.

82. Goletti D, Weissman D, Jackson RW et al 1996 Effect of *Mycobacterium tuberculosis* in HIV replication: role of immune activation. *Journal of Immurology* 157: 1271–1278.

83. McGregor MM, Olliaro P, Wolramans L et al 1996 Efficacy and safety of rifabutin in the treatment of patients with newly diagnosed pulmonary tuberculosis. *American Journal of Respiratory Critical Care Medicine* 154: 1462–7.

84. Bass JB, Farer LS, Hopewell PC et al 1995 Treatment of tuberculosis and tuberculosis infection in adults and children. *Clinical Infectious Diseases* 21: 9–27.

85. Anonymous. Clinical update 1996 Impact of HIV protease inhibitors on the treatment of HIV infected tuberculosis patients with rifampicin. *Morbidity and Mortality Weekly Reports* 45: 921–925.

86. Centres for Disease Control and Prevention 1998 Prevention and treatment of tuberculosis among patients infected with human immunodeficiency virus: principles of therapy and revised recommendations. *Morbidity and Mortality Weekly Reports* 47: 1–51.

87. Pozniak AL, Ormerod LP, Miller R 1999 Reply: Treatment of tuberculosis in HIV infected persons. *AIDS* 13: 1431–1432.

88. Public Health Laboratory Service 1998 Enhanced surveillance of *Mycobacterium bovis* in humans. *Communicable Disease Weekly* 8(32): 281–284.

89. Scorpio A, Zhang Y 1996 Mutations in pncA, a gene encoding pyrazinamidase/nicotinamidase cause resistance to the antituberculosis drug pyrazinamide in the tubercle bacillus. *Nature Medicine* 2: 662–667.

90. Cawthorne D, Raashed M, Synnott M et al 1997 Contact tracing in bovine TB. *European Respiratory Journal* 11: P1388.

91. De Souza GRM, Sant'Anna CC, Silva JRL, Mano DB, Bethlem NM 1983 Intradermal BCG vaccination complications – analysis of 51 cases. *Tubercle* 64: 23–27.

92. Murphy PM, Maters DL, Brock NF, Wagner KF 1989 Cure of bacille Calmette-Guérin vaccination abscesses with erythromycin. *Reviews of Infectious Disease* 11: 335–337.

93. Lamm DL, van der Meijden PM, Morales A et al 1992 Incidence and treatment of complications of bacillus Calmette-Guérin intravesical therapy in superficial bladder cancer. *Journal of Urology* 147: 596–600.

94. Ormerod LP, Prescott RJ 1991 Interrelationships between compliance, regimen and relapse in tuberculosis. *Respiratory Medicine* 85: 339–342.

95. Ormerod LP, Bentley C for the Joint Tuberculosis Committee of the British Thoracic Society 1997 The management of of pulmonary tuberculosis in England and Wales in 1993. *Journal of the Royal College of Physicians of London* 31: 662–665.

96. Ormerod LP, Bentley C for the Joint Tuberculosis Committee of the British Thoracic Society 1997 The management of lymph node tuberculosis in England and Wales in 1993. *Journal of the Royal College of Physicians of London* 31: 666–668.

97. Interdepartmental working group on Tuberculosis 1996 Recommendations for the control and prevention of tuberculosis at a local level. London, Department of Health and Welsh Office.

98. Ellard GA, Ellard DR, Allen BW *et al* 1986 The bioavailability of isoniazid, rifampicin and pyrazinamide in two commercially available combined formulations designed for use in short course chemotherapy in tuberculosis. *American Review of Respiratory Disease* 133: 1076–1080.

99. Geiter LJ, O'Brien RJ, Coombs DL *et al* 1987 Unites States Public Health Service tuberculosis therapy trial 21. Preliminary results of an evaluation of a combination tablet of isoniazid, rifampin and pyrazinamide. *Tubercle* 68: 41–46.

100. Ormerod LP, Skinner C, Wales JM 1996 Hepatotoxicity of antituberculosis drugs. *Thorax* 51: 111–113.

101. Citron KM, Thomas GO 1986 Ocular toxicity from ethambutol. *Thorax* 41: 737–739.

102. World Health Organization, Global Tuberculosis Programme 1997 Treatment of tuberculosis. Geneva, WHO, Report WHO/TB/97.220.

103. Chaulk CP, Kazanjjian VH 1998 DOT for treatment completion of pulmonary tuberculosis: consensus statement of the Public Health Tuberculosis Guidelines Panel. *Journal of the American Medical Association* 27: 943–945.

104. Morse DI 1996 Directly observed therapy for tuberculosis. *British Medical Journal* 312: 719–720.

105. China Tuberculosis Control Collaboration 1996 Results of directly observed short-course chemotherapy in 112,842 Chinese patients with smear-positive tuberculosis. *Lancet* 347: 358–362.

106. Caminero JA, Pavon JM, Rodriguez de Castro F *et al* 1996 Evaluation of a directly observed six month fully intermittent treatment regimen for tuberculosis in patients suspected of poor compliance. *Thorax* 51: 1130–1133.

107. Moore RD, Chaulk CP, Griffiths R *et al* 1996 Cost-effectiveness of directly observed versus self administered therapy in tuberculosis. *American Journal of Respiratory Critical Care Medicine* 154: 1013–1019.

108. Sbarbaro JA 1996 The ultimate decision analysis: the confirmation of reality through theory. *American Journal of Respiratory Critical Care Medicine* 154: 835–836.

109. Miller B, Palmer CS, Halpern MT *et al* 1996 Decision model to assess the cost-effectiveness of DOT for tuberculosis. *Tubercle and Lung Disease* 77 (Suppl. 2): 74–75.

110. Zwarenstein M, Schoeman JH, Vundule C *et al* 1998 Randomised controlled trial of self-supervised and directly observed therapy for tuberculosis. *Lancet* 352: 1340–1343.

111. Garner P 1998 What makes DOT work? *Lancet* 352: 1326–1327.

112. Bayer R, Stayton C, Desvarieux M *et al* 1998 Directly observed therapy and treatment completion for tuberculosis in the United States: is universal supervised treatment necessary? *American Journal of Public Health* 88: 1052–1058.

113. Centers for Disease Control 1993 Initial therapy for tuberculosis in the era of multidrug resistance. Recommendations of the advisory council for the elimination of tuberculosis. *Morbidity and Mortality Weekly Reports* 42: RR–7.

114. Gryzbowski S, Ashley MJ, Pinkus G 1976 Chemoprophylaxis in inactive tuberculosis: long term evaluation of a Canadian trial. *Canadian Medical Association Journal* 114: 607–611.

115. Ferebee SH 1969 Controlled chemoprophylaxis trials in tuberculosis: a general review. *Advances in Tuberculosis Research* 17: 29–106.

116. Comstock GW, Ferebee SH 1970 How much isoniazid is needed for chemoprophylaxis? *American Review of Respiratory Disease* 101: 780–782.

117. Comstock GW, Baum C, Snider DE 1969 Isoniazid chemoprophylaxis amongst Alaskan Eskimos: a final report of the Bethel isoniazid studies. *American Review of Respiratory Disease* 119: 827–830.

118. Thompson NJ 1982 Efficacy of various durations of isoniazid preventive therapy in tuberculosis: 5 years of follow-up in the IUATLD Trial. *Bulletin of the World Health Organization* 60: 555–564.

119. Lecouer HF, Truffot-Pernot C, Grosset JH 1989 Experimental short-course preventive therapy of tuberculosis with rifampicin and pyrazinamide. *American Review of Respiratory Disease* 140: 1189–1193.

120. Hong Kong Chest Service/Tuberculosis Research Centre Madras/British Medical Research Council 1992 A double-blind placebo controlled clinical trial of three antituberculosis chemoprophylaxis regiemns in patients with silicosis in Hong Kong. *American Review of Respiratory Disease* 145: 36–41.

121. Ormerod LP 1987 Reduced incidence of tuberculosis by prophylactic chemotherapy in children showing strong reactions to tuberculin testing. *Archives of Disease in Childhood* 62: 1005–1008.

122. Ormerod LP 1998 Rifampicin and isoniazid prophylactic chemotherapy for tuberculosis. *Archives of Disease in Childhood* 78: 169–171.

123. American Thoracic Society and Centres for Disease Control and Prevention 2001 Targeted tuberculin testing and treatment of latent tuberculosis infection. *American Journal of Respiratory Critical Care Medicine* 161: S221–S247.

124. IUATLD, GPA(WHO) 1994 Tuberculosis preventive therapy in HIV infected individuals; a joint statement of the IUATLD and GPA(WHO). *Tubercule and Lung Disease* 75: 96–98.

125. Fitzgerald JM 1995 The downside of isoniazid chemoprophylaxis. *Lancet* 305: 404.

126. Aisu T, Raviglione MC, Van Praag E *et al* 1995 Preventive chemotherapy for HIV associated tuberculosis in Uganda: an operational assessment of a voluntary counselling and testing centre. *AIDS* 9: 267–273.

127. Gordin FM, Matts JP, Miller C *et al* 1997 A controlled trial of isoniazid in persons with anergy and human immunodeficiency virus infection who are at high risk of tuberculosis. *New England Journal of Medicine* 337: 315–320.

128. Selwyn PA, Hartel D, Lewis VA *et al* 1989 A prospective study of the risk of tuberculosis among intravenous drug users with human immunodeficiency virus infection. *New England Journal of Medicine* 320: 545–550.

129. Gallagher CT, Passannante MR, Reichman LB 1992 Preventive therapy for multidrug resistant tuberculosis (MDR-tuberculosis): a Delphi survey. *American Review of Respiratory Disease* 145: abstract.

130. Anonymous 1992 Management of persons exposed to multi-drug resistant tuberculosis. *Morbidity and Mortality Weekly Reports* 41: 61–71.

131. Joint Tuberculosis Committee of the British Thoracic Society 2000 Management of opportunist mycobacterial infections: Joint Tuberculosis Committee guidelines 1999. *Thorax* 55: 210–218.

132. MacKellar A 1976 Diagnosis and management of atypical mycobacterial lymphadenitis in children. *Journal of Paediatric Surgery* 11: 85–89.

133. British Thoracic Society 1994 *Mycobacterium kansasii* pulmonary infection: a prospective controlled study of the results of nine months treatment with rifampicin and ethambutol. *Thorax* 49: 442–445.

134. Reasearch Committee of the British Thoracic Society 2001 First randomised trial of treatments for pulmonary disease caused by *M avium intracellulare*, *M malmoense*, and *M xenopi* in HIV negative patients: rifampicin, ethambutol and isoniazid versus rifampicin and ethambutol. *Thorax* 56: 167–172.

62 Fungal infections

D. W. Denning

The treatment of most fungal infections has become considerably more complex in recent years for several reasons.

1. The increasing diversity of immunosuppression, even within the same patient population has yielded a new spectrum of fungal disease for which different therapeutic strategies have had to be devised or are being studied in clinical trials.
2. Several new antifungals have been licensed or are under investigation, giving clinicians greater choice but generating new questions such as the appropriate dose, and issues related to combination or sequential therapy.
3. A greater range of pathogens has emerged due to changes in prophylaxis, international travel and changing medical care.
4. Resistance, both intrinsic and acquired, is an increasing issue now that antifungal susceptibility testing has come of age.
5. Finally, patients are now developing multiple fungal infections concurrently or sequentially, which substantially challenge clinicians diagnostically and therapeutically.

This chapter aims to give up-to-date recommendations for the treatment of all forms of fungal disease. A classification of fungal disease, summarized in Table 62.1, will form the structure of this chapter. *Pneumocystis carinii* is now classified as a fungus taxonomically, and is also covered. Developments in antifungal therapy are occurring rapidly and new data are likely to modify some recommendations in the future.

THE ROLE OF SUSCEPTIBILITY TESTING OF FUNGI IN GUIDING TREATMENT

Susceptibility testing of antifungal agents has, until recently, had little application, but is useful when there is variability within a species to an antifungal agent. Certain fungi are intrinsically resistant to some antifungals (Table 62.2) and testing is inappropriate. In contradistinction, some fungi are apparently uniformly susceptible to certain antifungals, e.g. *Histoplasma capsulata* to itraconazole and amphotericin B. In these instances, susceptibility testing is required only if patients

Table 62.1 Classification of fungal infections

	Normal host	Compromised host
Allergic	Allergic bronchopulmonary aspergillosis Eosinophilic fungal sinusitis	
Saprophytic	Fungal sinusitis Aspergilloma	
Superficial	Tinea capitis, corporis, cruris and pedis	Tinea
	Seborrheic dermatitis	Seborrheic dermatitis
	Pityriasis versicolor	
	Paronychia	
	Onychomycosis	Onychomycosis
	Otomycosis	
Subcutaneous and submucosal	Chromoblastomycosis Subcutaneous zygomycosis Sporotrichosis Rhinosporidiosis Lobomycosis Mycetoma Mycotic keratitis	Sporotrichosis
Mucosal	Oropharyngeal candidiasis Genital candidiasis	Oropharyngeal candidiasis Esophageal candidiasis
Deep invasive	Urinary candidiasis	Candidemia Invasive candidiasis Invasive aspergillosis
	Cryptococcosis Coccidioidomycosis Histoplasmosis Blastomycosis Paracoccidioidomycosis	Cryptococcosis Coccidioidomycosis Histoplasmosis Blastomycosis Sporotrichosis Mucormycosis *Fusarium* spp. *Pseudallescheria boydii* *Trichosporon* spp. *Blastoschizomyces* spp. *Penicillium marneffei* Other rare mycoses

Table 62.2 Intrinsically resistant fungi

Species	Antifungal agents
Candida krusei	Fluconazole, ketoconazole
Candida glabrata[a]	Fluconazole, ketoconazole, itraconazole
Candida parapsilosis	Echinocandins
Candida lusitaniae[a]	Amphotericin B
Malassezia spp.	Amphotericin B
Trichosporon spp.	Amphotericin B
Aspergillus spp.	Ketoconazole, fluconazole
Mucorales	Azoles, flucytosine, echinocandins
Scedosporium apiospermum (*Pseudallescheria boydii*)	Amphotericin B
Scedosporium prolificans	Amphotericin B, azoles, flucytosine
Paecilomyces	Amphotericin B
Fusarium spp.	Azoles, flucytosine
Penicillium spp.	Ketoconazole
Madurella spp.	Amphotericin B, flucytosine

[a] A substantial proportion or majority of isolates.

fail to respond, although non-compliance, drug interactions or failure of absorption leading to low antifungal concentrations are more likely explanations.[1]

The reasons for doing susceptibility tests are given in Table 62.3. At present these tests are conducted in reference laboratories. It is not clear whether susceptibility testing to different amphotericin B preparations is clinically appropriate, and is not generally done. The utility of susceptibility testing with the echinocandins is presently unclear.

Selected antifungal combinations are useful clinically. In-vitro synergy studies are complex, but are occasionally useful clinically. In experimental murine models, combinations have shown both synergy and antagonism, which are isolate dependent. Some combinations are predictably additive or synergistic (e.g. amphotericin B and flucytosine for *Cryptococcus neoformans*), others are not. For example, in vitro the combination of amphotericin B and flucytosine is as often synergistic as antagonistic against *Aspergillus* spp. and testing can be clinically useful. In contrast, flucytosine and azoles appear to be predictably synergistic when combined.

ALLERGIC FUNGAL DISEASE

ALLERGIC BRONCHOPULMONARY ASPERGILLOSIS

Allergic bronchopulmonary aspergillosis (ABPA) was first reported in 1952. ABPA complicates asthma and cystic fibrosis.

Patients in remission require no therapy. Acute exacerbations are best treated with systemic corticosteroid therapy: usually a daily dose of 40–60 mg prednisolone for 7–10 days. Response is gauged both clinically and serologically; serum immunoglobulin E (IgE) levels should fall and radiological infiltrates should clear.

Many patients, however, require continuous corticosteroid therapy to maintain remission. For these a number of different antifungal strategies have been tried. There have been anecdotal reports of amphotericin B inhalation showing some benefit. Itraconazole in a dose of 200–400 mg/day has shown benefit in several open studies.[2] A recently completed placebo-controlled study showed clear benefit with itraconazole 200–400 mg daily in corticosteroid-dependent ABPA.[3] Reductions in steroid dose, total IgE and improvement in pulmonary function and exercise tolerance were demonstrated over 4–8 months therapy. Relapse off therapy is common. Data

Table 62.3 Indications for antifungal susceptibility testing

Fungus	Clinical setting	Antifungal
Candida spp.	Oral or esophageal candidosis in AIDS (when unresponsive to treatment)	Azoles
		Flucytosine
	Candidemia	Flucytosine, amphotericin B, azoles
	Focal deep infections	
Candida tropicalis	All infections	Fluconazole, flucytosine
Candida glabrata	Urinary tract infections	Flucytosine, fluconazole
	All other infections	Azoles
Candida lusitaniae	All infections	Amphotericin B
Rare fungi	All	Azoles, flucytosine, amphotericin B, echinocandins
All	When unresponsive to treatment or prophylaxis breakthrough	Azoles
		Amphotericin B, flucytosine
All	When in-vitro resistance documented and first-line susceptibility testing shows resistance or tolerance	Synergy tests

on the utility of itraconazole for ABPA in cystic fibrosis patients are still lacking. There is a variable ratio of sputum:serum itraconazole concentrations (<0.03–2) in cystic fibrosis patients and some patients with adequate serum concentration have very low sputum concentrations.[4] The relatively poor bioavailability of itraconazole capsules is problematic and needs addressing.

Occasionally, a syndrome similar to ABPA is not caused by *Aspergillus* spp. but by *Candida* or *Trichophyton* spp. In these circumstances, if antifungal therapy is considered appropriate, this should be guided by known activity of the agent against the fungus in question.

ALLERGIC ASPERGILLUS SINUSITIS (EOSINOPHILIC FUNGAL SINUSITIS)

This condition has recently been re-evaluated. Diagnostic criteria are in flux, but the collection of nasal mucus from sinuses onto non-absorbent material, and visualization of hyphae within the mucus is the most direct means of establishing the diagnosis.[5] It is associated with nasal polyps and the presence of eosinophils and Charcot-Leyden crystals in mucus in the context of chronic sinusitis.[6] Most cases are treated by surgical debridement. The use of corticosteroids or antifungal therapy is controversial but may be beneficial based on uncontrolled studies. Unlike ABPA, allergic aspergillus sinusitis appears to be primarily an eosinophilic disease rather than an IgE-mediated one; hence the proposed name change.

SAPROPHYTIC FUNGAL DISEASE

FUNGAL SINUSITIS

Aspergillus spp. are the most common cause of fungal sinusitis although numerous other fungi have been implicated. In the case of maxillary involvement the fungus is almost always not truly invasive and surgical aeration of the maxillary sinus and destruction of the ethmoidal air cells, usually endoscopically, is generally curative. Results of surgical therapy are dependent on the skill of the operator. Involvement of the sphenoid or frontal sinuses usually indicates that antifungal therapy is required in addition to surgery. Mucosal invasion by fungal hyphae or destruction of bone on computed tomography (CT) scan is an indication for antifungal therapy. Response to azoles (itraconazole or voriconazole) is probably inferior to amphotericin B, but worth trying if critical structures are not involved.

The next most common causes of sinusitis are the dematiaceous fungi such as *Bipolaris*, *Dreschlera* and *Exserohilum* spp. These occur in normal hosts, often young patients, and tend to be subacute in presentation. These infections tend to be highly resistant to therapy and are slowly progressive, leading to ocular palsy and cerebral invasion. Some success has been reported with very large doses of itraconazole (e.g. 800–1200 mg/day).

ASPERGILLOMA

The vast majority of fungus balls of the lungs are due to *Aspergillus* spp., with rare cases due to *Pseudallescheria boydii* or Mucorales. Distinguishing an aspergilloma from chronic necrotizing pulmonary aspergillosis can be problematic.[7] Approximately 10% of aspergillomas resolve spontaneously, making uncontrolled observations in small numbers of patients difficult to interpret.

Several therapeutic strategies have been used to treat aspergillomas. Itraconazole 200 mg/day is of marginal symptomatic and little radiological benefit:[8] a dose of 400 mg/day may be more appropriate. Adequate penetration of itraconazole into aspergillomas has been shown.[9] The chronic fibrotic changes in the surrounding lung and co-morbidity probably compound adequate evaluation. Oral ketoconazole is ineffective.

Instillation of the aspergilloma with nystatin or amphotericin B has been tried with some benefit, especially with amphotericin B. Repeated instillations are usually necessary (in one study daily for 15 days[10]). Communication between the cavity and the airways is usual, so the instilled agent usually leaks into the airways. Repeated instillations are not very effective for complex and/or bilateral aspergillomas, probably because the diagnosis is chronic necrotizing pulmonary aspergillosis, rather than aspergilloma, and systemic therapy is required. The incorporation of amphotericin B in gelatin or glycerin that solidifies at 37°C[11,12] appears to be successful (www.aspergillus.man.ac.uk/secure/treatment).

Some patients with aspergillomas are corticosteroid dependent because of other pulmonary or systemic disease. This carries a slightly greater risk of invasive aspergillosis. Whether systemic antifungal therapy prevents this is unclear, but is a reasonable course of action.

Surgery may be necessary for patients with recurrent hemoptyses, but is fraught with difficulty, particularly for complex aspergilloma, because of the adherent vascular pleura, while the remaining chest cavity may become infected with *Aspergillus*. In those patients with major hemoptysis and *simple* aspergillomas, surgery offers an 84% 5-year survival compared with a 41% survival with conservative therapy.[13] Surgical removal of pleural aspergillomas and thoracoplasty is prone to many complications and is best avoided.[14]

In most instances of hemoptysis, abnormal systemic vascular connections may arise (e.g. internal mammary or bronchial arteries). Aspergillomas may also lead to an extensive network of small vessels. In patients with recurrent hemoptyses and unfit for surgery, embolization may successfully occlude these vessels permanently. The patient must lie still for 3–4 h during the procedure, which is a major limiting factor. Approximately 50–70% of embolization procedures are successful, although 50% will relapse. Multiple procedures are possible.

SUPERFICIAL MYCOSES

Tinea capitis, cruris, corporis and pedis are common infections in the normal population. They are caused by a variety of filamentous fungi including. *Trichophyton*, *Microsporum* and *Epidermophyton* spp.

TINEA CAPITIS

Tinea capitis may manifest as alopecia with little apparent inflammation to a kerion, which is an inflammatory mass of hair, exudate, fungus and granulation tissue that can mimic a squamous cell carcinoma, and is more common in children.[15] Examination using a Wood's light and/or mycological sampling make the diagnosis. The mycological cause of tinea capitis varies geographically. Many cases are due to *Trichophyton interdigitale* and *Trichophyton verrucosum*. In the UK, *Trichophyton tonsurans* predominates over *Microsporum canis*. In Italy, *M. canis* is more common and often associated with asymptomatic infection in cats. Cats should be examined, mycologically tested and treated if infected. In other parts of the world, *Trichophyton violaceum* and *Trichophyton soudanense* are more common. *M. canis* infections are more difficult to treat and are refractory to terbinafine.[16]

Ketoconazole shampoo may be effective for *T. tonsurans* infection but has a high relapse rate.[17] There are multiple alternatives for therapy. Oral griseofulvin (500–1000 mg/day after food) for 8 weeks or longer has the disadvantage of being more protracted and having a higher relapse rate.[18] Oral terbinafine 250 mg/day for 2–4 weeks (unless *M. canis*)[19] or itraconazole 200 mg/day are appropriate but must be continued for 2–4 weeks, depending on severity[20] (Table 62.4).

Table 62.4 Treatment of tinea infections

Condition	Agent	Daily dose	Duration
Tinea capitis	Griseofulvin	10 mg/kg	2–3 months
	Itraconazole	200 mg	2–6 weeks
	Terbinafine	250 mg	2–4 weeks
Tinea cruris	Clotrimazole	Topical twice daily	2–3 weeks
	Miconazole	Topical twice daily	2–3 weeks
	Sulconazole	Topical twice daily	2–3 weeks
	Itraconazole	200 mg	1 week
	Terbinafine	250 mg	1 week
Tinea corporis	Itraconazole	200 mg	1 week
	Terbinafine	250 mg	1 week
	Terbinafine, 1% cream	Topical twice daily	1 week
Tinea pedis	Terbinafine, 1% cream	Topical twice daily	1 weeks
	Clotrimazole, 1% cream	Topical twice daily	1 week
Moccasin-type tinea pedis	Itraconazole	200 mg	3 weeks
	Terbinafine	250 mg	3 weeks

In children with tinea capitis caused by *M. canis*, a 6-week course of either itraconazole 100 mg or griseofulvin 500 mg/day exhibited equivalent efficacy of 88%, but itraconazole was better tolerated.[21] A longer course may be necessary in people with severe disease. Corticosteroids are not helpful. Higher doses of itraconazole (200 mg/day or 3 mg/kg solution) may be advantageous, especially as only 40% of patients with *T. tonsurans* infection responded to 4 weeks of itraconazole 100 mg daily.[22]

TINEA CRURIS

Tinea cruris is more common in young men than women, producing a confluent, red, scaly rash covering the groin, scrotum and thighs. It is caused by various dermatophytes but *Candida* spp. can be involved if the skin is wet and macerated (intertrigo). Topical imidazoles such as clotrimazole, miconazole or sulconazole twice daily for at least 2 weeks are usually effective (Table 62.4). Oral itraconazole (200 mg/day for 1 week)[23] or terbinafine 250 mg/day for 7 days[24] are highly effective, and may be preferred. In children, and those with limited areas affected, terbinafine 1% cream applied once daily for 1 week is effective in >90% of cases.[25] An alternative approach is once-weekly fluconazole 8 mg/kg.[26]

TINEA CORPORIS

Tinea corporis (ringworm) tends to affect exposed areas of the extremities and may be treated systemically, as for tinea cruris, or with terbinafine cream (Table 62.4).

TINEA PEDIS

Tinea pedis (athlete's foot) affects about 30% of the population, and often recurs. Terbinafine cream 1% twice daily for 1 week compares well with 1% clotrimazole cream twice daily for 4 weeks (97% versus 84% response)[27] (Table 62.4). Moccasin-type tinea pedis affecting the soles is invariably due to *T. rubrum* and is often recalcitrant to therapy: 3 weeks' therapy with either terbinafine 250 mg/day or itraconazole 200 mg/day are the best options. The combination of bifonazole cream and 10% urea ointment with occlusive dressings was curative in one study.[28]

SEBORRHEIC DERMATITIS, PITYRIASIS VERSICOLOR AND DANDRUFF

There is a range of superficial diseases related to superficial infection with *Malassezia furfur* (*Pityrosporum ovale*): namely dandruff, cradle cap, pityriasis versicolor and seborrheic dermatitis. *M. furfur* may also be associated with folliculitis.

Dandruff (or its equivalent in babies – cradle cap) is characterized by excessive scaling but minimal inflammation, and is largely a cosmetic problem. Use of medicated shampoo containing ketoconazole is effective if used frequently, but relapse is common. Alternatives include topical selenium sulfide shampoo or zinc pyrithione solutions. Cradle cap in babies requires no therapy but can be treated with olive oil, which is inoffensive and safe.

Pityriasis versicolor is a superficial skin infection of the upper trunk, usually without an inflammatory component or scaling. It can be treated with 2.5% selenium sulfide shampoo applied nightly for at least 7 days (80% response). Topical griseofulvin cream 1% and terbinafine cream are also effective. Many patients do not like topical applications; oral itraconazole 200 mg/day for 7 days is 85% effective.[29]

Seborrheic dermatitis is characterized by excess scaling of the edge of the scalp, face and anterior chest associated with an inflammatory component. The relative contribution of a cell-mediated response (or hypersensitivity) to yeast colonization of the skin versus 'simple' infection of the keratin layer of the skin is poorly understood. Seborrheic dermatitis is a common problem: some authors have stated a lifetime incidence of 10% for the normal population with an incidence of 50% in HIV-infected patients. Seborrheic dermatitis frequently accompanies symptomatic HIV infection and tends to worsen as the immune deficit progresses.

Seborrheic dermatitis is a chronic disease that relapses rapidly after treatment. It may also be difficult to effect improvement despite good antifungal therapy and anti-inflammatory agents. Topical corticosteroids have largely been supplanted by the use of topical ketoconazole with or without a steroid component. Lithium succinate 8% ointment is also effective. These treatments compare favorably with alternatives such as selenium sulfide- and zinc pyrithione-containing preparations. Patients with very inflammatory lesions benefit from combined hydrocortisone 1% and locally applied antifungals. Oral itraconazole 200 mg/day is also effective and has useful in-vitro activity against *M. furfur*.[29] Fluconazole is not very effective, especially in those with AIDS. Maintenance therapy is not recommended for seborrheic dermatitis, unless it is very severe.

FUNGAL NAIL DISEASE (PARONYCHIA AND ONYCHOMYCOSIS)

Fungi may affect the nail fold (paronychia) or the nail itself (onychomycosis). Paronychia is usually caused by *Candida albicans* and occasionally other *Candida* species. Confirmation by culture is desirable because there are more cases of paronychia due to bacteria, especially *Staphylococcus aureus*, than to *Candida* spp. Onychomycosis is caused by a variety of fungi: the most common are *T. rubrum* and *Trichophyton interdigitale* (*mentagrophytes*), which cause about 80% of cases in the UK; uncommon dermatophyte causes include *Epidermophyton floccosum*, *Trichophyton erinacea*, *T. soudanense*, *T. tonsurans*, *T. violaceum* and *M. canis*. Non-dermatophyte moulds that occasionally cause onychomycosis, usually of the toenail, include *Fusarium* spp., *Aspergillus* spp., *Acremonium* spp., *Scytalidium dimidiatum*, *Scytalidium hyalinium*, *Scopulariopsis brevicaulis* and *Onychocola*

canadensis. Some cases of onychomycosis are due to *C. albicans* and, rarely, *Candida parapsilosis*.

Candida paronychia

Candida paronychia, when mild and localized, will usually respond to imidazole or terbinafine cream or nystatin ointment applied topically for 1–3 weeks. In addition, patients should refrain from excessive washing, which is the usual primary reason for the development of paronychia. This will often mean a period off work. For patients with extensive *Candida* paronychia or an immunodeficiency state, including chronic mucocutaneous candidosis, itraconazole 200 mg/day for 3–6 weeks is usually adequate, although some patients require longer term maintenance therapy to prevent recurrence. Patients who also have onychomycosis require longer therapy. Fluconazole is also active against *Candida* spp., doses of 50–200 mg/day being effective depending on the severity of disease and how immunocompromised the patient is. Terbinafine may be an inferior choice in immunocompromised patients because it is not fungicidal against *C. albicans*, although it is against other *Candida* species.

Onychomycosis

The treatment of onychomycosis depends on the species of the infecting fungus, whether fingernails or toenails are involved, how many nails are involved, the pattern of nail involvement, the age of the patient and whether the patient is immunocompromised.[30]

Distal subungual and superficial onychomycosis

In localized distal fingernail disease in non-immunocompromised patients topical therapy is appropriate. The combination of tioconazole with undecylenic acid applied twice a day for 4–6 weeks is one option. Amorolfine nail paint applied weekly for the same duration has an equivalent efficacy rate (40%).[31] An alternative choice is bifonazole 1% combined with urea paste 40%, which has a response rate of 70% (in children),[32] or 2% butenafine with 20% urea cream.[33]

However, the cure rate of topical therapy in adults is only about 40% and many months of treatment are required. Failure is more likely if more than 30% of the nail is involved. Chemical dissolution of the nail with 40% urea paste, phenol or sodium hydroxide[34] may be the preferred option for these patients.

Proximal subungual, endonyx and total dystrophic onychomycosis

For patients with proximal nail involvement or extensive nail disease, which may also include the skin around the nails, systemic therapy is appropriate. Griseofulvin (≥500 mg/day) was the standard therapy for these infections until recently. The response rates after 4–8 months of griseofulvin therapy for fingernails is 90% and for toenails treated for 12–18 months is 40%.[35] Both itraconazole 200 mg/day or 400 mg daily for 1 week per month and terbinafine 250 mg daily yield a response in excess of 75% for fingernail involvement with dermatophytes but terbinafine is more effective than intermittent itraconazole for toenail disease.[36] Treatment is usually for 3 months for fingernails[37] and 6–12 months for toenails. Relapse may occur after discontinuation of therapy – 22% in one study.[38] Studies with itraconazole have shown slightly lower efficacy rates than terbinafine, which is also more cost effective,[39] but this depends on the infecting fungus.

In patients with non-dermatophyte onychomycosis of the toenails, itraconazole may be appropriate for those caused by *Aspergillus* spp. and possibly *Acremonium* spp. However, it will not be effective therapy for *Fusarium* onychomycosis and the data supporting its use for *Scopulariopsis* and *Scytalidium* infections are limited. Response rates in toenails are <80% and disease-free nails 1 year after therapy are seen in only 35–50% of cases.[40] Chemical dissolution may be the preferred option.

In leukemic patients with onychomycosis it is important to ascertain whether *Fusarium* is the cause. Removal of the nail may prevent disseminated *Fusarium* infection, which carries a high mortality.[41]

Onychomycosis is common in people with AIDS and includes a superficial white onychomycosis caused by *Candida* or dermatophytes or a more destructive generalized nail disease. Systemic therapy with itraconazole 200 mg/day or 200 mg twice-daily for a week, every fourth week, for 3 months for fingernails and 6–12 months for toenails, is recommended. Terbinafine 250 mg/day is another option if *Candida* is not the causative agent, although the response rate in AIDS patients is not known. Treatment is primarily for cosmetic reasons rather than to prevent dissemination, which is rare.

Onychomycosis in children is usually a dermatophyte infection. In very small children fluconazole syrup 2–3 mg/day may be preferable. In older children itraconazole 5 mg/kg is acceptable.

OTOMYCOSIS (OTITIS EXTERNA)

Otomycosis is a relatively common problem in non-immunocompromised patients. It may be caused by bacteria or fungi, the latter being more likely in humid climates and in those with poor hygiene. The causative fungi include *Aspergillus niger* and *C. albicans*. However, the diagnosis can be elusive and superficial white patches may be all that is seen in the ear canal.

The vast majority of cases of otomycosis respond to a combination of thorough cleaning of the ear canal and local antifungal therapy. Clotrimazole powder or cream, applied at least twice daily for a minimum of a week, is probably the best primary therapy. Alternatives include cresyl acetate solution, gentian violet (1%), or topical ketoconazole, econazole or amphotericin B. Care should be taken in the application of any of these compounds if the tympanic membrane is perforated, as hearing loss has been reported.

Occasionally, invasive otomycosis of the bone, in particular of the mastoid, occurs when there is perforation of the tympanic membrane. It is usually caused by *Aspergillus fumigatus*, but occasionally other organisms such as *Pseudallescheria boydii*. Many, but not all, patients are immunocompromised. These patients require systemic antifungal therapy according to the nature of the organism; surgical debridement is often necessary in addition.

SUBCUTANEOUS MYCOSES

A wide range of fungi cause subcutaneous mycoses. The clinical hallmark is chronic deep induration, usually with sinuses that extrude pus or fungal material. Management is dependent on isolation of the fungus as many different species can be involved; the clinical picture alone is not sufficiently distinct to differentiate one from another.

CHROMOBLASTOMYCOSIS (CHROMOMYCOSIS)

Chromoblastomycosis is a chronic infection of the skin and subcutaneous tissue of non-immunocompromised individuals caused by several dematiaceous fungi, including *Fonsecaea pedrosoi*, *Fonsecaea compacta*, *Phialophora verrucosa*, *Cladosporium* (or *Cladophialophora*) *carrionii*, *Rhinocladiella aquaspersa* and *Botryomyces caespitosus*. It is worldwide in distribution, but more common in tropical and subtropical areas.

Therapy is often unsatisfactory. Small lesions can be surgically excised. Reasonable results have been obtained with oral itraconazole (200 mg/day) with or without flucytosine (100 mg/kg daily).[42,43] Cost savings may be possible using pulse therapy. A small, randomized study of itraconazole (300 mg/day) and cryotherapy concluded that both were effective for *F. pedrosoi* infection.[44] Itraconazole was superior for infection in the flexures. Combined therapy may be best. Treatment with locally applied heat is sometimes efficacious, either alone or in combination with antifungal therapy.[45] Cryotherapy is also effective, especially for localized disease.[46] Response rates differ depending on the species of fungus implicated. Tiabendazole (2 g/day) is also effective with or without flucytosine.[47] Fluconazole appears to be ineffective even at doses of 400 mg/day.[48]

SUBCUTANEOUS ZYGOMYCOSIS

Subcutaneous zygomycosis is distinct from invasive zygomycosis and mucormycosis (p. 857). *Basidiobolus ranarum* causes an indolent, painless, slowly progressive disease in children and adolescents in tropical countries, particularly Uganda. It has been treated with a saturated solution of potassium iodide 1.5–2 g/day for at least 3 months.[45] Recent data suggest that conventional antifungal agents such as ketoconazole 400 mg/day, itraconazole 100–200 mg/day, trimethoprim–sulfamethoxazole, amphotericin B and fluconazole have also been effective in small numbers of patients.[49]

Conidiobolomycosis is a nasal and facial disease of adults seen primarily in central and western Africa. It causes gross nasal and facial distortion. Unfortunately, nothing has been shown to cure the disease, although it may be arrested by trimethoprim–sulfamethoxazole (960 mg three times daily for at least 6 months).[45,50] Surgery should be limited because it may spread the disease.

SPOROTRICHOSIS

Sporotrichosis is caused by *Sporothrix schenckii* and usually manifests as lymphocutaneous disease. A small proportion of non-immunocompromised patients have other sites of disease, including osteoarticular forms, pneumonia and meningitis.

Lymphocutaneous disease responds well (>90%) to potassium iodide (15–120 drops of saturated solution/day) and itraconazole 100–200 mg daily. However, potassium iodide is unpleasant to take. Treatment must continue for 3–6 months with either agent. Local application of heat or infrared treatment is also useful if applied daily for several weeks.[45] Ketoconazole and systemic amphotericin B are ineffective. Itraconazole 100–200 mg/day appears to be superior to fluconazole 200–400 mg/day. Terbinafine may also be effective.[51]

Osteoarticular and other deep forms of sporotrichosis are a major therapeutic challenge. Response rates to intravenous amphotericin B (1 mg/kg daily) and itraconazole are often poor, particularly in pulmonary disease. Depending on the severity of disease amphotericin B or itraconazole 400 mg daily is the best choice, with consideration of surgery. Itraconazole 200–400 mg/day is effective for most cases of osteoarticular disease. Probably larger doses or a new more effective antifungal agent is required. Data on the response of *Sporothrix* meningitis to antifungal therapy are lacking.

In immunocompromised patients, particularly AIDS patients, sporotrichosis may be much more aggressive, invasive and destructive and less responsive to therapy. Itraconazole 400 mg/day after a loading dose is recommended or amphotericin B (1 mg/kg daily). Repeated cultures and clinical assessment guide the response. Treatment should extend for many months, and in AIDS patients probably for life.

RHINOSPORIDIOSIS

Rhinosporidiosis is a relatively rare disease caused by *Rhinosporidium seeberi*. It occurs in India, Sri Lanka, South America and Africa. Most cases are submucosal, causing polypoid masses in the nose and conjunctiva. However, it may involve subcutaneous tissues, other parts of the respiratory or urogenital tracts or anal canal. The organism does not grow in conventional media, but is quite distinctive in histological sections. It is now classified as a member of the mesomycetozoea, an aquatic protozoan closely related to several fish parasites.[52]

The only known effective therapy is surgical excision with electrocoagulation of the base of the lesion.[45] This is highly effective for conjunctival sac disease[53] but recurrence is common in other sites. One report indicates that dapsone 100 mg/day may prevent recurrence,[54] and degenerate organisms were found in serial biopsies from some patients on dapsone.[55]

LOBOMYCOSIS

This is a rare, slowly progressive subcutaneous disease reported mostly from Latin and South America. It is caused by an uncultured fungus tentatively called *Lacazia loboi*, taxonomically close to *Paracoccidioides brasiliensis*. The disease does not disseminate. Antifungal therapy is usually unsuccessful. Surgical excision of lesions is the only effective remedy.[56]

MYCETOMA (MADUROMYCOSIS)

Mycetoma is a chronic, progressive destructive infection of the distal limbs involving all tissues. Numerous different organisms may be implicated and the appropriate treatment depends on the causative organism.[57] There are three broad groups of infecting organisms: the true fungi, the higher bacteria, such as *Actinomyces*, *Nocardia* and *Streptomyces*; and bacteria including *Staphylococcus* species. This discussion concerns only the fungi causing mycetoma, but it is essential to distinguish between the various causes for successful therapy.

The causative agent varies with the locality: *S. apiaspermum* is the most common cause in Europe and the USA, *Madurella grisea* is more common in South America and *Madurella mycetomatis* in India. Sinuses form in the affected area and spore grains are often extruded through the sinus, providing a diagnostic sample. Sometimes the color of the grain, if it is not available for culture and microscopy, can indicate a particular organism.

The agents of mycetoma are almost always resistant to amphotericin B and flucytosine. They may be sensitive to one of the azoles: for example, *S. apiaspermum* may respond to ketoconazole, itraconazole or voriconazole. Ketoconazole or itraconazole are often effective if administered for several months or years.[50,58] Doses should not be lower than 400 mg/day. Amputation is frequently required if the disease is extensive and progressive or bone pain becomes unrelenting.[57] However, many mycetomas remain relatively localized for long periods of time, with or without therapy.

FUNGAL KERATITIS

Fungal keratitis is a relatively common problem in subtropical and tropical areas. *Fusarium* and *Aspergillus* spp. are the most important causes. Mycotic keratitis may also be caused by *Candida* spp. in particular *C. albicans*, but also *Candida guilliermondii*, *Candida kefyr* and *C. parapsilosis*. Over 70 species of fungi have been reported to cause this disease, including a number of dematiaceous organisms.[59] It is more commonly associated with trauma and less with contact lens wear than bacterial keratitis.[60]

The principles involved in the management of mycotic keratitis include rapid specialist assessment to evaluate any threat of corneal perforation or malignant glaucoma, correction of predisposing factors, appropriate antifungal and judicious surgical therapy.[61]

Fusarium keratitis should be treated with 0.2% chlorhexidine gluconate.[62] It was superior to natamycin 5% in a randomized study. Topical amphotericin B deoxycholate 0.15% is the alternative treatment. Some isolates of *Fusarium* are susceptible to voriconazole and this may become an alternative. Polyhexamethylene biguanide 0.02% is also active.[63] Natamycin 5% ophthalmic solution may be superior to amphotericin B, although local bioavailability in corneal tissue is only 2% and therefore topical natamycin (and probably amphotericin B) is inappropriate for infection involving the aqueous humor or other deep sites.

Aspergillus keratitis is treated with amphotericin B, clotrimazole or econazole local solution; 1% solutions are commercially available, but the azoles can be prepared in arachis oil at the same concentration. Topical solutions should be administered hourly initially. Amphotericin B given locally has a 27% response rate. Oral itraconazole 200–400 mg/day is also effective in 75% of cases of *Aspergillus* keratitis and superior to ketoconazole and topical amphotericin B.[64] Chlorhexidine gluconate (0.2%) is another locally administered alternative.

Candida keratitis is treated with local nystatin, clotrimazole or ketoconazole 2% suspension.[65] Mycotic keratitis caused by unusual organisms should be treated with the most appropriate agent, although empirical therapy with either oral ketoconazole or oral itraconazole may be necessary.

Surgery is sometimes required for cases that fail to respond to medical therapy or where there is a threat of ocular perforation or the formation of a descemetocele. Surgical procedures include debridement or lamella keratectomy, and formation of a conjunctival flap over a severely ulcerated area of the cornea or penetrating keratoplasty if a donor cornea is available. If possible, surgery should be preceded by medical therapy for as long as possible.

MUCOSAL CANDIDOSIS

Mucosal fungal infections are extremely common. The vast majority are caused by *C. albicans* and occasionally by other yeasts, especially *C. glabrata*, and rarely by filamentous molds such as *Aspergillus* spp (*see* Table 62.2).

OROPHARYNGEAL CANDIDOSIS

Before the AIDS epidemic, oropharyngeal candidosis (OPC) was largely seen in patients at the extremes of age, those receiving inhaled steroids or antibiotic therapy, following oral cavity

radiotherapy and after cytotoxic chemotherapy. Chronic oral candidosis occurs in patients with chronic mucocutaneous candidosis (CMC). *C. albicans* is the primary pathogen and rarely *C. glabrata* and *C. krusei* (*see* Table 62.2). The most common pattern of OPC is the pseudomembranous form, but an exanthematous type is also found. Occasionally, denture related candidosis or angular cheilitis are the primary manifestations. In AIDS, the pseudomembranous form predominates.

Topical agents such as nystatin or amphotericin B oral suspension (1 ml 6-hourly for 2–3 weeks) are effective in non-immunocompromised patients. Clotrimazole troches (available in the USA) are also effective. Miconazole oral gel in a dose of 10 ml 6-hourly is particularly useful for denture-related candidosis. In patients taking inhaled steroids with oropharyngeal candidosis, the use of a large-volume spacer will minimize the problem.

In immunocompromised patients, fluconazole 100 mg/day is more effective than topical therapy and is the agent of first choice, with response rates in excess of 90%. Ketoconazole and itraconazole are also effective at doses of 200–400 mg/day but are less well absorbed in conditions of hypochlorhydria that complicate AIDS and bone marrow transplantation. Improved serum of levels of both itraconazole and ketoconazole are achieved by acid drinks such as orange juice or cola and food. Itraconazole oral solution overcomes this problem. Long-term suppressive therapy is usually required in CMC patients.

ESOPHAGEAL CANDIDOSIS

Esophageal candidosis usually co-exists with oropharyngeal disease, although in 30% of cases no oral lesions are visible. Before AIDS, most cases occurred in cancer patients, typically also on corticosteroids or neutropenic. Esophageal infection is confined to HIV-positive patients with more advanced disease, typically when the CD4 count is below $100 \times 10^6/l$, and is itself an AIDS-defining condition. There are rare reports of esophageal candidosis in immunocompetent individuals and after omeprazole therapy, suggesting that hypochlorhydria favors colonization.

The standard treatment for esophageal candidiasis is fluconazole 200 mg daily for 10–14 days. Ketoconazole 200–400 mg/day is slightly inferior but less expensive than fluconazole 100 mg/day. Itraconazole oral solution is as effective as fluconazole.[66] If the diagnosis was not proven by endoscopy and symptoms persist, endoscopy is indicated to rule out other (usually viral) causes of esophagitis. Resistance or drug interactions may account for the failure to respond; if available, serum drug concentrations can be measured. Relapse is common.

Azole resistance

The incidence of fluconazole resistance and azole cross-resistance has risen with the widespread use of azoles in the context of AIDS.[67] Estimates of the incidence of azole resistance vary from 5% to 20%, depending on the definition and the CD4 count of the cohort of patients. Baily et al[68] identified a group of patients with persistent oropharyngeal or esophageal candidosis despite a dose of ≥100 mg fluconazole for at least 10 days. Isolates from these patients were less susceptible in vitro to fluconazole (minimum inhibitory concentration (MIC) ≥ 12.5 mg/l). Several other studies have also shown a good correlation between susceptibility testing and failure in oropharyngeal candidosis in AIDS.[1,69]

The management of azole-resistant oropharyngeal or esophageal candidosis is not well studied and is somewhat empirical but can be guided by susceptibility test results (Box 62.1). Isolates with only slightly elevated MIC values to either ketoconazole or itraconazole are more likely to respond to these drugs. Itraconazole solution is moderately successful. Low doses of oral amphotericin B and nystatin are relatively ineffective, but large doses of amphotericin B solution may be helpful.

Box 62.1 Options for treatment of azole resistant oropharyngeal and esophageal candidosis in AIDS

- Itraconazole oral solution 200–600 mg/day
- Fluconazole 400–800 mg/day
- Ketoconazole 400–800 mg/day
- Amphotericin B oral solution 200 mg 4 times daily
- Combination therapy: azole + flucytosine 75 mg/kg daily
- Combination: azole + terbinafine 250–750 mg/day
- Amphotericin B 0.5–1 mg/kg i.v. daily
- Experimental antifungal therapy

When oral therapy fails, intravenous amphotericin B has been the only option. However, even this often fails. The dose should be a minimum of 0.7 mg/kg daily initially. It may be combined with flucytosine. The recent introduction of caspofungin offers another intravenous alternative. Improvement should be assessed primarily by symptomatology, not by the visual appearance of the mouth. Complete clearance of oral plaques of *Candida* is hard to achieve with any of the above regimens, although symptoms usually improve.

VULVOVAGINAL CANDIDOSIS

Vulvovaginal candidosis is common. By a mean age of 24 years, 60% of 76 women had suffered at least one episode of vulvovaginal candidosis.[70] Among these women, 36% had at least one episode a year and 3% had it 'almost all the time'. Certain conditions increase the incidence and possibly the severity of vulvovaginal candidosis. These include pregnancy, antibiotic use, diabetes mellitus and cystic fibrosis.[30,70] HIV-seropositive women are no more likely to develop vaginal candidiasis than controls[71] but in these patients there is often a worse response to initial treatment and a shorter time to relapse. Over 90% of cases are caused by *C. albicans* and about 5% by *C. glabrata*; various other species such as *C. tropicalis* comprise the remainder (*see* Table 62.3).

Treatment may be local or systemic (Table 62.5). There is a spontaneous resolution rate over 7 days of up to 50%. Local treatment regimens with azoles yield response rates of 80–90%. Many different regimens are available, which vary primarily in

Table 62.5 Examples of treatment regimens for vulvovaginal candidosis

Antifungal agent	Formulation	Dose	Duration
Local therapy			
Clotrimazole	Vaginal tablet	1–200 mg	3–7 daily doses
Clotrimazole	Vaginal tablet	500 mg	1 dose
Econazole	Vaginal tablet	150 mg	3 daily doses
Miconazole	Pessary	100–200 mg	3–7 daily doses
Miconazole	Pessary	1200 mg	1 dose
Nystatin	Vaginal tablet	100 000 U	14 daily doses
Terconazole	Pessary	300 mg	1 dose
Terconazole	Vaginal tablet	80 mg	3 days
Butoconazole	2% cream	5 g	1–3 daily doses
Clotrimazole	1% cream	5 g	7–14 daily doses
Clotrimazole	10% cream	5 g	1 dose
Econazole	1% cream		Twice daily for 3–7 days
Fenticonazole	2% cream	5 g	7 daily doses
Miconazole	2% cream	5 g	7 daily doses
Terconazole	0.4–2% cream	5 g	3 daily doses
Tioconazole	2% cream	5 g	3 daily doses
Tioconazole	6.5% cream	5 g	1 dose
Systemic therapy			
Fluconazole	Capsule	150 mg	1 dose
Itraconazole	Capsule	200 mg	2 doses, or 3 days
Ketoconazole	Tablet	400 mg	5 daily doses

cost. Women without predisposing factors such as pregnancy will usually prefer single-dose or 3-day treatments. Responses are slower in those with predisposing factors and 5–14-day treatment regimens are generally preferable, if topical therapy is preferred. Nystatin, one to two pessaries inserted high into the vaginal vault nightly for 14 nights, has a lower response rate (80%) than the azoles (and stains clothing), but is useful for azole-resistant organisms such as *C. glabrata*.

Oral therapy is preferred by many women; fluconazole as a single dose of 150 mg or itraconazole two 200 mg doses 8 h apart are effective in over 90% of patients. Itraconazole may be preferable for *C. glabrata* infections.

In pregnancy, local therapy with a clotrimazole 500 mg vaginal tablet is often effective and does not expose the fetus to an antifungal.[72] This is desirable in the first trimester, although there is no evidence that azoles are teratogenic in humans at the doses usually used.[73,74] However 4 days' therapy is more effective than single-dose therapy and 7 days' therapy even better.[75] Later in pregnancy, systemic therapy with fluconazole or itraconazole are accepted alternatives.[76] Treatment of vaginal candidiasis in pregnancy appears to reduce preterm birth.[77]

Suppressive treatment may be indicated for very frequent episodes. Continuous therapy for 3–6 months suppresses symptoms and reduces the subsequent frequency of relapse.[30] Once a month prophylaxis with itraconazole 400 mg was partially successful.[78] If symptoms recur local treatment with single-dose clotrimazole 500 mg fortnightly or intermittent single-dose oral treatment with fluconazole 150 mg may be helpful. There is no evidence to date of antifungal resistance resulting from such a regimen, although *C. glabrata* infections are more common in women who have received much azole therapy.

DEEP INVASIVE MYCOSES

SYSTEMIC *CANDIDA* INFECTION

Most cases of systemic candidiasis arise from the gastrointestinal tract. In leukemic patients mucosal involvement of the stomach, small bowel and colon are frequently demonstrable at autopsy without dissemination to other organs, indicating local invasion. Candidemia follows mucosal invasion. Candidemia may be detected by blood cultures (50–75% of autopsy-proven cases of *Candida* infection) or may be manifest subsequently by specific organ involvement, e.g. endophthalmitis and osteomyelitis.

Until recently, most candidal infections have been caused by *C. albicans* (85–90%). However, currently a higher proportion (30–60%) of non-*albicans* species cause candidemia.[79] Most *C. albicans* isolates are susceptible to fluconazole (95–98%), flucytosine (c. 90%) and amphotericin B (c. 99%). *C. glabrata* is less susceptible to all antifungal agents, but particularly fluconazole (Table 62.2; p. 834). *C. krusei* is intrinsically resistant to fluconazole, less susceptible to amphotericin B and may be resistant to itraconazole (Table 62.2). Up to

20% of *C. tropicalis* isolates are resistant to fluconazole in vitro. *C. lusitaniae* may be intrinsically resistant to amphotericin B or may develop resistance during therapy (Table 62.2). Isolates for which the MIC of amphotericin B is slightly elevated may be more commonly associated with clinical failure.[80]

Amphotericin B or, increasingly, one of the lipid-associated preparations (*see* Ch. 35) is commonly used for the treatment of systemic *Candida* infection. The appropriate doses are given in the sections below for conventional amphotericin B. If a lipid-associated preparation (e.g. AmBisome, Amphocil/Amphotec or Abelcet) is selected, then at least 3–5 times the dose of conventional amphotericin B should be used (e.g. 3–5 mg/kg daily).

Fluconazole is a useful, well-tolerated agent for susceptible systemic *Candida* infections. Combination with amphotericin B may be antagonistic.[81] Doses in adults should not be less than 400 mg/day for very ill patients, while some data support using 800 mg/day for candidemia in patients in intensive care units.[82] Details are given in the sections below. There are very few data supporting the use of ketoconazole for systemic *Candida* infection. The introduction of an intravenous preparation has allowed the study of itraconazole for life-threatening candidal infections. Oral azole therapy has a role in long-term suppressive therapy for infections in which foreign material cannot be removed. The choice of azole should be guided by susceptibility testing.

The present indications for flucytosine are shown in Box 62.2; usually it is given in combination with amphotericin B or fluconazole. If the organism is later found to be resistant to flucytosine the drug should be discontinued. Appropriate dosing depends on renal function, hemofiltration and dialysis, but in a patient with normal renal function should be 75–100 mg/kg daily in three divided doses. Serum concentrations should be monitored.[83] If the patient has any elevation of serum creatinine, the dose of flucytosine should be reduced by at least 50% and, if creatinine is more than twice normal, this dose should be reduced to 25% or less. Flucytosine is cleared by dialysis, but not hemofiltration.

Box 62.2 Indications for flucytosine in *Candida* infections

Superficial infection
Mucosal infections failing azole therapy (combined with an azole or polyene).

Urinary tract infection (without disseminated disease)
Candiduria due to fluconazole-resistant *Candida* spp.

Candidemia
Extremely ill patient[a]
C. glabrata, *C. lusitaniae* infection[a]
Neonates[a]

Focal *Candida* infection
Endophthalmitis[a]
Endocarditis or other vascular involvement[a]
Meningitis[a]

---

[a]Always in combination with amphotericin B, fluconazole or caspofungin

The echinocandins may supplant amphotericin B and/or fluconazole in the treatment of *Candida* infections, but only caspofungin is presently licensed.

Candidemia

Candidemia is the most common life-threatening form of invasive candidiasis and all patients require therapy.

Neonates

Therapy should be started if the neonate is clinically unstable or deteriorating (especially with respiratory status) with any skin breaks from which *Candida* has been grown; or exhibits positive urine microscopy or culture for yeast. A single positive blood culture is an absolute indication for treatment.

The combination of flucytosine and amphotericin B (1 mg/kg daily) remains the treatment of choice for babies with *Candida* infection.[84] The lack of an intravenous formulation of flucytosine has limited its use in the USA. Liposomal amphotericin B (3–5 mg/kg daily) has some advantages in terms of infusion time (1 h) and fluid volumes. If the platelet count allows, a lumbar puncture to exclude *Candida* meningitis should be done. It is beneficial to remove any risk factors if possible, e.g. broad-spectrum antibiotics and corticosteroids. Umbilical catheters should be changed.[85] Neonates appear to tolerate amphotericin B and flucytosine well, although the monitoring of flucytosine concentrations should be commenced with 48 h of initiating therapy and carried out 2–3 times a week. Flucytosine should be administered twice-daily initially. Complications of candidemia besides meningitis include renal outflow obstruction, osteomyelitis or arthritis, cutaneous abscesses, myocarditis and endocarditis. With combination therapy the mortality rate in neonates (10%) is substantially lower than in adults.

Fluconazole is also effective in neonates with candidemia at a minimum dose of 5 mg/kg daily.[86] As the mortality rate of neonatal candidemia is low with amphotericin B and flucytosine, and as few data have been published on the efficacy of fluconazole as primary therapy, fluconazole should be reserved for follow-on therapy, which should be continued for at least 4 weeks, or longer if significant immunocompromising factors are still present, or for isolated candiduria.

Neutropenia and bone-marrow-transplant patients

Neutropenic patients require a minimum of 1 mg/kg daily of amphotericin B, and if there is a poor or no response the dose of amphotericin B should be increased or a lipid-associated preparation used. Fluconazole is not presently recommended for patients who are profoundly neutropenic, although some data suggesting equal efficacy are now available.[87] In those who are neutropenic, granulocyte colony stimulating factor should be given.[88]

Non-neutropenic adults and children

Empirical therapy for candidemia should be started if colonization at two or more sites is documented together with dete-

riorating clinical status or signs of infection. A single positive blood culture is an absolute indication for treatment. A delay in starting therapy of more than 48 h leads to a worse outcome.[89] There is a wide spectrum of severity of illness in candidemia. Some patients are ambulant and essentially well, while others are critically ill. The intensity and duration of therapy will differ between these two groups, but all patients should receive therapy.

Randomized trials of candidemia in non-neutropenic adults[90,91] have shown that fluconazole 400 mg/day is equivalent to amphotericin B 0.5–0.6 mg/kg daily. The choice depends on the species and susceptibility of the *Candida* isolated. However, uncertainty remains about the optimal dose of fluconazole (and amphotericin B). For example, 30 surgical or intensive care unit patients with candidemia treated with 5 mg/kg had a 60% response rate, whereas the next 30 patients in the same unit treated with 10 mg/kg had an 83% response rate.[92] The dose of fluconazole should be doubled in patients undergoing hemofiltration as the drug is rapidly cleared by this route. Patients who present in septic shock due to candidemia have a poor outlook and should be treated with either amphotericin B (at least 0.6–1 mg/kg daily) and flucytosine or fluconazole and flucytosine. Doses of lipid-associated amphotericin B (*see* Ch. 35) should be: colloidal dispersion products (Amphocil or Amphotec) ≥4 mg/kg; lipid complex (Abelcet) 5 mg/kg; liposomal formulation ≥3 mg/kg. Recently presented data indicate that caspofungin is equivalent to amphotericin B (0.6 mg/kg daily) in candidaemia.

In patients with candidemia the central venous catheter should be changed without the use of a guidewire, if possible. Arterial catheters, in general, do not require changing. Controversy exists over the necessity to remove Hickman catheters in cancer patients with candidemia. Infection with *C. parapsilosis* is more commonly associated with intravenous catheters. Quantitative cultures of blood taken from the line and from a peripheral vein before treatment should indicate if the Hickman catheter is infected; colony counts ≥25 colony forming units (cfu)/culture or ≥2.5 cfu/ml are a positive indicator for an intravascular source of infection. The additional work of quantitative cultures by the microbiology laboratory is well worth the effort, given the implications of changing a Hickman catheter.

Duration of therapy

The most appropriate duration of therapy for candidemia is unclear. Short courses of amphotericin B (e.g. <500 mg) should be used only if there are immunocompromising factors such as neutropenia, no evidence of ocular, heart valve or other site of infection and a relatively stable clinical condition.[93]

Doses ranging from 0.5 to 1.5 g amphotericin B are appropriate, depending in part on the severity of the illness, the weight of the patient and the convenience of continued administration of intravenous amphotericin B. A reasonable approach now that fluconazole is available is the initial use of intravenous amphotericin B or fluconazole (with or without flucytosine) in hospital followed by continued oral fluconazole for 2–8 weeks depending on the type of patient, provided the organism is fluconazole susceptible.

Some implanted devices such as Dacron grafts, ventricular pacemakers and prosthetic joints are surgically impossible to remove. If they are infected patients are best placed on long-term fluconazole therapy if the isolate is susceptible.[94]

CANDIDA MENINGITIS

Candida meningitis is relatively uncommon and occurs in neonates (*see above*), as part of disseminated candidosis in other patients, and as a complication of ventriculoatrial or ventriculoperitoneal shunts. In the treatment of *Candida* meningitis unrelated to a shunt, amphotericin B 0.7–1 mg daily and flucytosine (75–100 mg/kg daily given 3–4 times daily) should be used because of its excellent cerebrospinal fluid (CSF) penetration. In patients with infected shunts, removal of the shunt is of critical importance. If the isolate is susceptible to fluconazole, this would be an appropriate first-line agent in combination therapy with flucytosine if the patient is not critically ill. At least 4 of weeks therapy should be given as relapse is common.[88]

CANDIDA PERITONITIS OR WOUND DRAINAGE IN SURGICAL PATIENTS

Candida peritonitis following extensive abdominal surgery can be insidious in onset and is often associated with bacterial peritonitis or mixed yeast and bacterial cultures in wound drainage. Therapy is appropriate when *Candida* is the only isolate from a deep collection or as a heavy growth from a drain with clinical features of sepsis. A combination of peritoneal lavage without further laparotomy and either fluconazole or amphotericin B with or without flucytosine is usually appropriate.

CHRONIC AMBULATORY PERITONEAL DIALYSIS

Candida peritonitis related to chronic ambulatory peritoneal dialysis (CAPD) usually responds to fluconazole or amphotericin B if the peritoneal catheter is removed. The nephrotoxicity of amphotericin B is not of concern in these patients but fluconazole is a reasonable alternative choice.

HEPATOSPLENIC CANDIDOSIS (CHRONIC DISSEMINATED CANDIDOSIS)

Hepatosplenic candidosis is a distinctive clinical entity in leukemic patients. Following recovery from neutropenia, patients complain of abdominal pain, have an enlarged liver (and sometimes spleen), have a rising plasma alkaline phosphatase, and on scanning there are small defects in the sub-

stance of the liver, spleen and kidneys. Directed biopsy or splenectomy show small or large granulomata surrounding yeasts and hyphae. Cultures are usually negative.

Management consists of prolonged high-dose antifungal therapy. The choice of initial antifungal depends on the prophylactic agent used (if any) and, if cultures are positive, the antifungal susceptibility of the organism: if the patient received fluconazole prophylaxis then amphotericin B and flucytosine would be an appropriate choice;[95] if the patient did not receive prophylaxis, but did receive empirical amphotericin B, then fluconazole 400–800 mg/day would be appropriate,[96,97] probably with flucytosine. The lipid-associated amphotericin B preparations accumulate in the liver and spleen and they may be preferable to conventional amphotericin B, but there is little data supporting their use.[98] Treatment should continue for several weeks. Delay in further cytotoxic chemotherapy is appropriate until clear improvement has been obtained. Subsequent bone-marrow transplantation is not precluded.[99]

URINARY TRACT CANDIDOSIS AND CANDIDURIA

From 1% to 9% of patients in hospital have *Candida* grown from their urine. Typically this occurs in patients who have been catheterized, have received antibiotics or who are diabetic.[100,101] For those in the intensive care unit candiduria is a good marker for candidemia, and systemic treatment is appropriate if the patient manifests features of systemic sepsis.[94] Other immunocompromised patients and those undergoing urinary tract instrumentation also require therapy. Asymptomatic patients, without structural abnormalities of the urinary tract, do not require therapy, although follow-up is desirable. Urinary tract candidiasis implies candiduria and evidence of outflow obstruction with fungal balls, a parenchymal abscess or other evidence of urinary tract disease. These patients require therapy, as 10% develop candidemia.[100] However, no criteria exist to distinguish colonization from infection[102] and a decision to treat is based on the likelihood of candidemia, local symptomatology and demonstration of obstruction or fungal balls.

Removal of stents and catheters, control of diabetes and discontinuation of antibiotics will result in 40% spontaneous clearance of funguria.[103] The penetration of amphotericin B into the urine is poor if given intravenously. However, a 10-day course of 1 mg/kg intravenously daily is effective for candiduria without obstruction.

Fluconazole 200 mg daily is an alternative first-line therapy if the species of *Candida* isolated is susceptible.[104,105] However, relapse is common and 2 weeks after treatment eradication rates were equivalent to placebo.[105] For patients with *C. glabrata* infections, susceptibility testing will help guide therapy. Obstructive nephropathy due to pelvic fungal balls usually requires surgical exploration for removal.

Patients with persistent candiduria related to long-term indwelling urinary catheters may respond (50% response) to amphotericin B bladder washouts and catheter change, but relapse is common.[103] If used, amphotericin B 5–10 mg with an intravesical dwell time of 90–120 min is appropriate once or twice daily for no longer than 2 days, although the dose of amphotericin B may not matter much.[103]

CANDIDA ENDOCARDITIS

Candida primarily causes prosthetic valve endocarditis, but occasionally causes native valve endocarditis as a complication of candidemia in non-neutropenic patients (1%). Intravenous drug abuse and total parenteral nutrition are risk factors. Amphotericin B 1 mg/kg daily or fluconazole (≥400 mg/day), both with flucytosine, is recommended, depending on the infecting species and susceptibility testing.[106] Virtually all patients, except neonates, will require valve replacement. It is not known if the timing of surgery is important in response. Relapse may occur many months after apparently successful therapy.

CANDIDA SUPPURATIVE THROMBOPHLEBITIS

Resection of the affected vein or artery in accessible sites in addition to systemic antifungal therapy is appropriate. If the great veins in the chest are involved, resection is impossible: prolonged high-dose amphotericin B and flucytosine followed by fluconazole are usually necessary to eradicate the infection.

CANDIDA OPHTHALMITIS

Candida ophthalmitis manifests as a chorioretinitis or endophthalmitis and complicates about 10% of episodes of candidemia. It rarely occurs in neutropenic patients. Most species of *Candida* have been implicated. Endophthalmitis may not be manifest until several days or weeks after treatment has commenced. Early aggressive therapy is necessary to improve the chance of retention of useful vision. Early vitrectomy is recommended.[85] Microscopy of the vitreous fluid (to distinguish bacterial and fungal endophthalmitis) while the patient is still anesthetized can guide the need for intravitreal dosing of amphotericin B (5 µg). Systemic amphotericin B and flucytosine is indicated in all cases as combination therapy, since amphotericin B penetrates into the vitreous poorly. Fluconazole is a preferred agent if the *Candida* species is susceptible, since vitreous penetration is good. Treatment for 6–12 weeks is necessary.

CANDIDA ARTHRITIS

Candida arthritis is usually a complication of candidemia (particularly in intravenous drug abusers) or follows prosthetic joint replacement. Fluconazole ≥200 mg/day may be successful, but in patients with infected non-prosthetic joints systemic ampho-

tericin B is more appropriate initially. Flucytosine should be added if there is no improvement within 5–7 days, or fluconazole substituted. In those with infected prosthetic joints, replacement of the joint together with the removal of all cement and necrotic bone should be undertaken if technically feasible. When this is difficult to achieve, long-term suppressive therapy may be necessary.

CANDIDA OSTEOMYELITIS

Candida osteomyelitis requires debridement of necrotic bone if extensive disease is present. Bone grafting may be done simultaneously if necessary in the case of vertebral osteomyelitis. Systemic amphotericin B with or without flucytosine is appropriate therapy, with fluconazole a useful alternative. Therapy should continue for several months until radiological improvement and inflammatory markers have settled.

INVASIVE ASPERGILLOSIS

Most patients with invasive aspergillosis are immunocompromised. Untreated invasive aspergillosis carries a nearly 100% mortality.[107–109] Outcome depends in part on the potential for immune recovery, extent of disease when treatment is first started and the rate of progression of disease. The rate of progression varies hugely; it is most rapid in liver and bone-marrow-transplant patients and those with profound neutropenia. In these patients death typically occurs 5–14 days from the first clinical features, which are often non-specific. A successful outcome requires at least 14 days' therapy, and therefore early empirical therapy is critically important in these highly immunocompromised patients. In contrast, in less immunocompromised patients such as AIDS patients, disease progression is often slower, allowing the diagnosis to be confirmed before treatment is given.

The standard therapeutic agent for the treatment of invasive aspergillosis has been amphotericin B deoxycholate for 40 years. The overall response rate in amphotericin B-treated patients is 35%.[109–112] This response rate is lower (25%) in severely immunocompromised patients[107,109,111] and higher (50%) in less immunocomprised patients.[107,111] A randomized double-blind study comparing a lipid-based amphotericin B (6 mg/kg/day) and conventional amphotericin B (1–1.5 mg/kg/day) showed equivalent response rates of 37% in invasive aspergillosis.[112] Even higher doses of lipid amphotericin B (7.5–15 mg/kg) do not appear to be superior.[113] If initial treatment with amphotericin B is followed by itraconazole the response rates appear to be higher (55%), (perhaps because the patients live long enough to receive oral therapy) and very similar to that of itraconazole alone (45–60%).[111,114,115] The response rate to voriconazole was 48% in a study combining primary and salvage cases.[7] This response rate appears similar to itraconazole, and is superior to amphotericin B.[116] In a salvage study, caspofungin was 40% successful.[117]

Recommended criteria for the initiation of therapy for invasive aspergillosis are shown in Box 62.3. However many patients are receiving itraconazole prophylaxis or empiric amphotericin B before the diagnosis is made. Table 62.6 contains recommendations for different circumstances.

Box 62.3 Criteria for initiation of antifungal therapy for invasive aspergillosis

---

Neutropenia (<500 × 10^6/l) including aplastic anemia
- Two positive *Aspergillus* antigen tests
- Isolation of *Aspergillus* from any site including nose swab, blood, bronchoalveolar lavage
- Positive microscopy/cytology for hyphae, etc.
- New pulmonary infiltrates on chest radiograph
- Infiltrates on CT scan of chest showing characteristic features, e.g. halo or crescent sign, pleural based sharply angulated lesion, pleural based lesion with pneumothorax
- Persistent fevers (>7 days) with any localizing clinical features, e.g. chest pain, dry cough, facial/sinus pain, epistaxis, hoarseness or new skin lesions consistent with aspergillosis
- Any sudden intracranial event including stroke or fit with or without fever

Solid organ transplantation or allogeneic stem cell transplantation
- Radiological infiltrate with isolation of *Aspergillus* from respiratory secretions, bronchoalveolar lavage or blood
- Evidence of ulcers/bronchitis on bronchoscopy with hyphae visualized in bronohoalveolar lavage
- Histological or cytological evidence of hyphae from any tissue
- Any sudden intracranial event including stroke or fit with or without fever

AIDS
- Respiratory symptoms, abnormal chest radiograph or bronchoscopy and isolation of *Aspergillus* or visualization of hyphae from respiratory source
- Cerebral lesions unresponsive to therapy for toxoplasmosis or a single enhancing lesion consistent with aspergillosis
- Histological or cytological evidence of hyphae from any sterile site (culture not obtained or pending)

Resistance in to itraconazole and amphotericin B has been described *Aspergillus* spp. but appears to be infrequent.[118] However, *Aspergillus terreus* is always resistant to amphotericin B, although testing is problematic.

Amphotericin B

If amphotericin B is used for treatment, the dose of the deoxycholate preparation should be 0.8–1.0 mg/kg daily, regardless of renal dysfunction, except in neutropenic patients in whom 1–1.25 mg/kg daily is more appropriate (Table 62.7). If renal dysfunction occurs or is likely to be a problem because of concurrent cyclosporin, then one of the lipid-associated amphotericin B preparations in dose of 4–5 mg/kg daily is appropriate (Table 62.7).[119,120] A typical regimen for amphotericin B is a minimum of 2 weeks until a therapeutic response has been obtained, followed by 2–4 weeks of amphotericin B, or longer term azole therapy. One of the lipid-associated amphotericin B preparations may be preferred, to minimize infusion-related and other side effects.

If invasive aspergillosis is progressing despite amphotericin B, alternative regimens include itraconazole, caspofungin, voriconazole, experimental therapy and occasionally surgery (*see below*).

Itraconazole

Itraconazole can be given intravenously or orally. The intravenous dose of itraconazole is 200 mg twice daily and as no loading dose can easily be given intravenously, supplemental dosing may be helpful to accelerate build up of tissue levels. The oral dose of itraconazole is 200 mg thrice-daily for 4 days, followed by 200 mg twice daily. Higher doses (e.g. 800 mg/day) may be appropriate for cerebral aspergillosis. Intravenous itraconazole should not be given to patients with moderate to severe renal dysfunction (accumulation of cyclodextrin). Drugs that induce the metabolism of cytochrome P$_{450}$ enzyme (e.g. rifampicin, phenytoin, carbamazepine, phenobarbitone), substantially reduce itraconazole

Table 62.6 Recommended antifungal choice for proven or suspected invasive aspergillosis in severely immunocompromised patients who are or are not already receiving prophylactic antifungals at time of diagnosis

Prophylaxis	Empiric therapy	Definitive therapy	Salvage therapy
None or fluconazole	None	Voriconazole or itraconazole or amphotericin B[a]	Switch class to echinocandins if not profoundly neutropenic or add echinocandin or experimental therapy
None or fluconazole	Amphotericin B	Switch to voriconazole or itraconazole	Switch to or add an echinocandin
Itraconazole	Amphotericin B	Voriconazole or echinocandin	Echinocandin or voriconazole
Any	Voriconazole	Itraconazole or Amphotericin B	Combination of echinocandin plus amphotericin B

[a] Amphotericin B 1 mg/kg or lipid-amphotericin B 4–5 mg/kg.
Few data available on combination of echinocandin plus azoles.

Table 62.7 Treatment regimens for invasive aspergillosis

Drug	Route	Daily dose	
		Neutropenia, bone-marrow transplant, cerebral aspergillosis, endocarditis	Other patient groups or sites
Voriconazole:	i.v./oral		
Loading	i.v.	6 mg/kg × 2	6 mg/kg × 2
Continuation	i.v.	8 mg/kg	8 mg/kg
Continuation	oral	400 mg	400 mg
Itraconazole:	i.v./oral		
Loading dose*	i.v./oral	600–800 mg	600 mg
Continuation*	i.v./oral	400–600 mg	400 mg
Caspofungin			
Loading dose*	i.v.	70 mg	70 mg
Continuation*	i.v.	50 mg	50 mg
Amphotericin B deoxycholate	i.v.	1–1.25 mg/kg	0.8–1.0 mg/kg
Liposomal amphotericin B	i.v.	5 mg/kg	5 mg/kg
Amphotericin B colloidal dispersion	i.v.	4 mg/kg	4 mg/kg
Amphotericin B lipid complex	i.v.	5 mg/kg	5 mg/kg

*Itraconazole i.v. dose should not exceed 200 mg twice daily.

levels. Itraconazole capsules should be taken with food or an acidic carbonated drink; itraconazole solution on an empty stomach, if possible. Serum concentrations of itraconazole should ideally be measured after 5–10 days, since reasonable response rates have been achieved if serum concentrations exceed a 1 mg/l (high-performance liquid chromatography) or 5 mg/l (bioassay).[114]

Voriconazole

Voriconazole can be given orally or intravenously. A loading dose of 6 mg/kg twice followed by 3–4 mg/kg twice daily is appropriate. Young children may need much higher doses (up to 10–12 mg/kg twice daily), guided by serum concentrations. There is no pharmacokinetic advantage in giving it intravenously, unless the patient is unable to take fluids or drugs orally. Intravenous voriconazole should not be given to patients with severe renal dysfunction (accumulation of cyclodextrin). Drug concentrations vary substantially (100-fold) between patients, but are generally consistent in individual patients. The therapeutic margin is wide. Extremely low serum concentrations (<250 µg/ml) may be associated with poorer response rates.[7] Certain patients accumulate drugs rapidly (with the potential for toxicity) and may need dose reduction. This includes those with hepatic cirrhosis and those with CYP2C19 polymorphism present in 3% of caucasians and 20% of Asians. Toxicity may be associated with high serum concentrations. It is therefore desirable to measure serum concentrations to determine optimal dosing.

Rifampicin and rifabutin accelerates the metabolism of voriconazole.

Caspofungin

Caspofungin (50 mg daily) has been licensed for the salvage treatment of invasive aspergillosis.[117] Another echinocandin (micafungin) is being evaluated in combination with amphotericin B for invasive aspergillosis. Caspofungin is fungistatic for *Aspergillus* and relatively ineffective in profoundly neutropenic patients.

Combination therapy

The place of amphotericin B and itraconazole in combination is uncertain and cannot be recommended. Theoretically, antagonism is more likely than synergy, as itraconazole inhibits the synthesis of ergosterol, to which amphotericin B binds. Limited animal data suggest that antagonism is a real phenomenon, although the magnitude of the effect may be concentration and time dependent.

The role of adjunctive therapy with either rifampicin or flucytosine is also unclear. Amphotericin B with flucytosine improves clinical response rates marginally[110] and is indicated for certain sites of disease (e.g. brain, meninges, heart valve, eye) to which amphotericin B penetrates poorly. Antagonism is well documented in vitro for amphotericin B and flucytosine in a few isolates. Azole therapy is preferable to combined amphotericin B and flucytosine.

Rifampicin and amphotericin B are often synergistic in vitro. However, rifampicin induces the metabolism of immunosuppressants, particularly corticosteroids, and thus rejection or graft-versus-host disease could develop in transplant recipients. Rifampicin is also a powerful inducer of cytochrome P_{450} enzymes, so its use for more than 3 days precludes the subsequent use of itraconazole or voriconazole. As azoles are key to the successful treatment of aspergillosis, the use of rifampicin is not advised.

Persistent profound neutropenia is often associated with a fatal outcome in invasive aspergillosis. In these patients granulocyte-colony stimulating factor or granulocyte–macrophage–colony stimulating factor may be administered, although the benefit is unproven. While there is a substantial shortening of the period of neutropenia, which reduces the period at risk, it has yet to be shown that cytokine adjunctive therapy is beneficial for an established fungal infection. In a useful series of experiments, murine granulocyte-colony stimulating factor was synergistic in a neutropenic model and antagonistic in a corticosteroid model of invasive aspergillosis.[121] Patients whose leukemia has relapsed also respond less well.

Assessment of response or failure

Assessment of response can be difficult. The faster the pace of infection, the quicker it will become apparent that therapy is failing. Many patients deteriorate in the first 3–5 days of therapy even if they subsequently improve.[122] A rising serum *Aspergillus* antigen titer is a bad prognostic sign, yet no reduction is often seen in patients who subsequently respond. Increasing volume of lesions on CT scan or chest radiograph in neutropenic patients in the first 5–7 days is not necessarily a bad feature because it is still consistent with a subsequent good response.[116] However, the appearance of new lesions is a bad feature. Fever may continue for several days after initiation of therapy, even in patients who subsequently respond. The use of corticosteroids (sometimes given with amphotericin B or as part of immunosuppression) can obscure fever and give a false impression of improvement.

Duration of therapy

Treatment of invasive aspergillosis should continue for as long as the patient is immunocompromised and until there has been either complete or near-complete resolution of disease. Aspergillosis characteristically causes vascular invasion and infarction of tissue so that drug delivery is poor, the response slow and relapse common if therapy is terminated early.[114] In the neutropenic patient treatment should continue until the neutrophil count exceeds $1.0 \times 10^9/l$ and there has been regression of disease radiologically. Eradication of the disease may require surgery (*see below*). In solid organ transplant recipients therapy should be continued until there is a complete or near-complete clinical response. Few AIDS patients and allogeneic bone marrow transplant recipients

survive with aspergillosis, but here long-term itraconazole (or voriconazole) is appropriate.[114]

Secondary prophylaxis is indicated in those with persistent *Aspergillus* disease who require further cytotoxic chemotherapy or bone marrow transplantation. Typically, amphotericin B (1 mg/kg daily) is co-administered with the cytotoxic regimen. Secondary prophylaxis is particularly indicated for patients with *Aspergillus* sinusitis, as these patients have a 50% relapse rate. Surgical resection may also be appropriate. Secondary prophylaxis is not always successful.[123]

Surgical excision

The indications for surgery in invasive aspergillosis (Box 62.4) include life-threatening hemoptysis where lesions impinge on the great vessels or major airways and early surgical resection may prevent fatal hemoptysis or tracheal perforation.[110,124,125] In patients awaiting bone-marrow transplantation, resection of a persistent *Aspergillus* lesion, despite antifungal therapy, will reduce relapse.[123]

Biopsy of the nasal mucosa is necessary for diagnosis in patients with invasive sinus aspergillosis. Surgery is also an essential part of the management of patients with *Aspergillus* endophthalmitis, endocarditis and, probably, osteomyelitis (Box 62.4).

Box 62.4 Indications for surgery in invasive aspergillosis

Absolute indication
Endocarditis
Endophthalmitis
Major hemoptysis
Epidural abscess
Possible indication
Bone aspergillosis
Invasive external otitis
Invasive sinusitis
Localized unresolved pulmonary aspergillosis

CHRONIC NECROTIZING PULMONARY ASPERGILLOSIS

Many complex aspergillomas are in fact chronic necrotizing pulmonary aspergillosis (CNPA). All patients with CPNA have radiological evidence of one or more cavitary lesions in the lung, usually in the upper lobe. Initially infiltrates are ill-defined areas of consolidation or small cavities which progress to form well defined cavities. The cavities often contain an aspergilloma. The expansion of a cavity over time and/or paracavitary infiltrates distinguishes CPNA from a simple aspergilloma. Serology is positive for *Aspergillus* and inflammatory markers are raised. CPNA patients require systemic antifungal therapy.[126, 127]

Although itraconazole (or voriconazole) have the advantage of being oral agents, neither is very effective. Many patients require admission to hospital for a 4–6 week course of amphotericin B 0.8 mg/kg daily or 4–5 mg/kg lipid-based amphotericin B. Follow-on therapy with itraconazole maintains remission as relapse is common.

Surgery is often contemplated but should be avoided if possible as multiple complications are common, including aspergillus empyema. Embolization of abnormal vascular connections is often preferable to surgery for hemoptysis.

CRYPTOCOCCAL INFECTIONS

Pulmonary cryptococcosis

Pulmonary cryptococcosis is uncommon and presents subacutely. The diagnosis is made by sputum culture, bronchoscopy, transbronchial, or open or percutaneous lung biopsy. It is essential to exclude meningeal disease in these patients. If the disease is confined to the lungs, the agents of choice are fluconazole 200–400 mg daily or itraconazole 400 mg daily, with ketoconazole or amphotericin B as alternatives, for 2–3 months. The new echinocandins are not active against *C. neoformans*.

In AIDS and other immunocompromised patients, pulmonary cryptococcosis may precede or reflect disseminated disease. Isolated pulmonary cryptococcosis requires therapy for 4–6 months initially. Maintenance therapy may be required, but should be individualized depending on resolution of disease and the immune status of the patient.

Cryptococcal meningitis

Cryptococcal meningitis may manifest few symptoms and is diagnosed by a positive cerebrospinal fluid (CSF) culture or cryptococcal antigen. Patients with altered mental status should be classified as high risk[128] as should those with low CD4 cell counts, low serum albumin or very high CSF antigen titers.[129] Untreated, the disease is uniformly fatal. Mortality can be reduced to 10% with therapy.

AIDS

All patients with cryptococcal meningitis should be treated with at least 0.7 mg/kg daily of amphotericin B and flucytosine 75–150 mg/kg daily for at least 2 weeks.[129–131] Flucytosine improves the outcome slightly in the first 2 weeks of therapy but, more importantly, has a major effect in preventing relapse over the subsequent year of therapy.

The lipid-associated preparations of amphotericin B (at 3–5 mg/kg daily) show comparable efficacy to conventional amphotericin B (40–65% response rates in AIDS without flucytosine). A small comparative study of liposomal amphotericin B 4 mg/kg versus conventional amphotericin B 0.7 mg/kg daily (but without flucytosine) showed faster CSF sterilization and reduced nephrotoxicity with the liposomal

formulation.[132] Limited clinical and model data suggests even better response rates with the triple combination of amphotericin B, flucytosine and fluconazole.

Early death and blindness in cryptococcal meningitis reflects a markedly elevated CSF pressure,[133–135] which can exceed 500 mm H_2O. CT and magnetic resonance imaging (MRI) scans can be normal when pressures are markedly elevated. Where pressures exceed 250 mm H_2O, pressure-reducing measures such as large-volume CSF drainage, repeated lumbar punctures, insertion of lumbar or ventricular drains are indicated.[135] Acetazolamide may help temporarily. Steroids are less useful.

An initial 10–14 day course of amphotericin B with flucytosine is recommended in all patients. Amphotericin B therapy should continue at high dosage if the response is suboptimal. Rarely is more than 6 weeks amphotericin B required, as long as follow-on azole therapy is given. Consolidation treatment with 400 mg of fluconazole or itraconazole for up to 12 weeks is necessary. This can then be followed by maintenance fluconazole in those with HIV infection. The prostate and meninges act as nidi of infection despite apparently successful therapy.[136] Fluconazole 200 mg/day is more effective than placebo or weekly amphotericin B[137,138] and itraconazole 200 mg/day in maintenance therapy.[128] Itraconazole 400 mg daily is effective.[139] The dose of fluconazole may need to be increased in those receiving rifampicin or other enzyme inducers, and itraconazole would be ineffective.

Non-AIDS patients

Although, in non-AIDS but immunocompromised patients, fluconazole in doses of 200 or 400 mg/day has a response rate of about 85%,[140] an initial course of amphotericin B and flucytosine is recommended. Relapse is often difficult to manage successfully and, as the diagnosis if often delayed, sequelae are common, unless control of disease is obtained rapidly. Fluconazole 400 mg daily with or without flucytosine (for 2–8 weeks) would be appropriate, after an induction period with amphotericin B and flucytosine. The duration of therapy in immunocompromised or other patients should be for many months or even years until the cryptococcal antigen titer in the CSF has fallen to zero or nearly zero. A post-treatment CSF cryptococcal reciprocal titer of >8 is predictive of relapse. It is probably more appropriate to overtreat than stop and have to treat relapse, which is often less successful. Shunting for hydrocephalus is often helpful.[141]

PNEUMOCYSTIS CARINII PNEUMONIA

Pneumonia caused by the atypical fungus *Pn. carinii* occurs in immunocompromised patients. The incidence is highest in HIV-positive patients who have not received adequate prophylaxis (*see* p. 857); over 50% of such patients will develop the infection. In other types of immunodeficiency the reported incidence varies from <2% in patients with collagen vascular disease to 22–45% in patients with acute lymphatic leukemia and bone marrow transplant recipients.

The infection leads to a pneumonitis with alveolar secretion and decreased ventilation over the alveolar wall. Prodromal symptoms are dry cough, low-grade fever and increasing dyspnea. The prodromal phase lasts 3–4 weeks in an HIV patient and less than one week in patients with other types of immunodeficiency. At admission the partial oxygen pressure is markedly decreased and the patients have metabolically compensated respiratory acidosis. Pulmonary X-ray initially shows relatively discrete perihilar interstitial infiltrates, which rapidly progress to alveolo-interstitial infiltrates and may be very extensive. The diagnosis is obtained by demonstration of *P. carinii* in induced sputum or broncho-alveolar lavage. The organisms can be found several days after start of therapy. Newer diagnostic tools, especially PCR, need to be evaluated for sensitivity and efficacy.

The recommended first-line treatment of *Pn. carinii* pneumonia is trimethoprim–sulfamethoxazole at a daily dose of 15–20 mg/kg trimethoprim and 75–100 mg/kg sulfamethoxazole divided in 2–3 doses and given orally or intravenously. Up to 50% of patients treated will develop intolerance to these high doses: skin rash (most common), nausea and vomiting, bone marrow depression and/or increased transaminases. When intolerance necessitates a change of treatment, pentamidine isethionate 4 mg/kg daily intravenously is the primary choice. Other alternatives are clindamycin 600 mg every 6 h orally or intravenously combined with primaquine 15 mg daily orally (adult doses; recommendations for children are lacking). Third-line treatments include: trimethoprim 20 mg/kg daily orally or intravenously in 2–3 doses combined with a single daily dose of 100 mg of dapsone or atovaquone suspension 750 mg twice daily; and trimetrexate 45 mg/m² once daily by intravenous infusion over 60–90 min with leucovorin, 20 mg/m² intravenously over 5–10 min, or orally every 6 h. Leucovorin must be continued for 72 h after the last dose of trimetrexate.

Antimicrobial treatment should be maintained for 3 weeks and it is recommended that it should be combined with high-dose steroids, e.g. prednisolone 40–60 mg daily for 5 days followed by tapering doses for another 14 days.

HISTOPLASMOSIS

Histoplasmosis presents in several forms, including acute pulmonary histoplasmosis shortly after exposure, chronic cavitary, nodular or mediastinal disease, localized extrapulmonary and disseminated histoplasmosis. In AIDS and other immuno-compromised conditions disseminated histoplasmosis is most common and life-threatening.

Acute pulmonary histoplasmosis

In the normal host, acute pulmonary histoplasmosis may be localized or bilateral and diffuse. Localized disease does not require therapy unless resolution has not occurred within a month, but in those with diffuse bilateral disease treatment is indicated. Severe disease with high, prolonged fever, significant hypoxemia and major systemic disturbance is best treated with intravenous amphotericin B 0.7 mg/kg daily or liposomal amphotericin B 3 mg/kg daily.[142] Corticosteroids for 2 weeks may also be beneficial. In less ill patients, itraconazole 200 mg daily for 6–12 weeks is the treatment of choice.

Patients with acute pulmonary histoplasmosis who are immunocompromised should always be treated.

Chronic pulmonary histoplasmosis

Chronic cavitary, other intrathoracic forms of histoplasmosis and localized extrapulmonary forms (e.g. oral or gastrointestinal ulcers or adrenal disease) require therapy. The response to intravenous amphotericin B 0.3–0.5 mg/kg daily for 3–4 weeks (to a total of 1.5 g) gives response rates of 59–100% and

Table 62.8 Treatment of histoplasmosis

Type of histoplasmosis	Severe manifestation	Moderately severe or mild manifestation
Acute pulmonary	Amphotericin B with corticosteroids,[a] then itraconazole for 12 weeks	Symptoms less than 4 weeks, none; persistent symptoms for more than 4 weeks, itraconazole for 6–12 weeks
Chronic pulmonary	Amphotericin B,[b] then itraconazole for 12–24 months	Itraconazole for 12–24 months
Desseminated in non-AIDS	Amphotericin B,[b] then itraconazole for 6–18 months[c]	Itraconazole for 6–18 months
Disseminated in AIDS	Amphotericin B,[b] then itraconazole for life	Itraconazole for life
Meningitis	Amphotericin B for 3 months then fluconazole for 12 months	Same as severe
Granulomatous mediastinitis	Amphotericin B, then itraconazole for 6–12 months	Itraconazole for 6–12 months
Fibrosing mediastinitis	Itraconazole for 3 months[d]	Same as non-severe

[a] Effectiveness of corticosteroids is controversial.
[b] If amphotericin B is used for the entire course of treatment, 35 mg/kg should be given over 3–4 months.
[c] Therapy should continue until *Histoplasma* antigen concentrations are <4 units in urine and serum.
[d] Therapy is controversial and probably ineffective except in cases of granulomatous mediastinitis that are misdiagnosed as fibrosing mediastinitis.

relapse rates of 9–15%.[142] Because of the inconvenience and toxicity of this regimen, certain forms of histoplasmosis were deemed inappropriate for therapy. These included those with few symptoms, thin-walled cavities and early pulmonary lesions. However, the availability and low toxicity of oral therapy with ketoconazole or itraconazole now favors treatment of all culture-positive cases.

Ketoconazole therapy (400 mg/day) has a similar response rate (84%) to amphotericin B[143] but in high dose is toxic.[144] Itraconazole 200–400 mg/day appears to be slightly more efficacious than ketoconazole (85–97% response rate).[145,146] The duration of therapy is uncertain but ranges from 6 to 12 months depending on response. Fluconazole is less active than itraconazole[48] and resistance may develop on therapy.[147] Central nervous system disease should be treated with intravenous amphotericin B initially and with itraconazole 400 mg/day as follow-on therapy.[148,149]

Medical therapy for mediastinal fibrosis due to *H. capsulata* is probably ineffective[150] but itraconazole may be tried[142] and surgical treatment carries a high complication rate. This emphasizes the importance of early effective therapy for milder forms of the disease. Other forms of histoplasmosis (pericarditis, granulomatous mediastinitis and pericarditis) are reviewed in Wheat et al[142] (Table 62.8 and Box 62.5).

Box 62.5 Alternatives for the treatment of histoplasmosis

Acute pulmonary histoplasmosis
- None
- Itraconazole

Chronic pulmonary or localized histoplasmosis
- Itraconazole
- Ketoconazole
- Amphotericin B

Disseminated histoplasmosis
- Amphotericin B
- Itraconazole

Maintenance therapy in AIDS
- Itraconazole
- Weekly amphotericin B
- Fluconazole (less effective)

Disseminated histoplasmosis

In the immunocompromised patient with disseminated histoplasmosis (usually someone with AIDS) the clinical condition of the patient determines first-line therapy. In those in whom the diagnosis is made early and do not have features of severe systemic toxicity, confusion or poor oxygenation should be treated with itraconazole initially at 400 mg/day, reducing to 200 mg/day when a response has been noted. Itraconazole levels should be measured to ensure a detectable level. In the very ill, intravenous amphotericin B 0.7–1 mg/kg daily is appropriate. Defervescence may be slightly more rapid in patients treated with amphotericin B than itraconazole, but the response to both agents exceeds 80% in patients with disseminated histoplasmosis.[151] Fluconazole 800 mg/day is slightly less effective than itraconazole 200 mg/day. Ketoconazole is not recommended (9% response rate). The echinocandins are not effective in models.[152]

Maintenance therapy of histoplasmosis is indicated as the relapse rate is extremely high. Itraconazole 200 mg/day is the preferred agent.[153] Fluconazole 400 mg/day is less effective than itraconazole or weekly amphotericin B,[147] but may be useful in those whom itraconazole and amphotericin B cannot be given. Both these regimens are preferable to long-term weekly amphotericin B.

Histoplasma capsulata var. *dubolsii* infection

A relatively rare form of histoplasmosis is caused by *H. capsulata* var. *duboisii* and occurs in central and southern Africa. It is primarily a cutaneous disease, but thin-walled pulmonary cavities are well recognized. Disseminated forms may rarely complicate AIDS. Cutaneous disease responds to itraconazole, but pulmonary disease has a high relapse rate. Amphotericin B followed by itraconazole is recommended.

COCCIDIOIDOMYCOSIS

Coccidioidomycosis is endemic to North, Central and South America and is caused by *Coccidioides immitis* acquired by inhalation.

Primary coccidioidomycosis (valley fever)

Approximately 60% of infected persons suffer a primary illness, which ranges from a mild 'flu-like' illness to severe, progressive pneumonia. Treatment is only indicated for primary coccidioidomycosis if the patient is particularly ill with persistent high fever or hypoxia, or if the patient is immunocompromised, including solid organ transplant recipients and HIV-positive patients with CD4 counts $<250 \times 10^6$/l. Indications of severity include weight loss (>10%), extensive infiltrates, high complement fixation serum titer (>32) and persistent disease.[154] Patients with severe disease and all pregnant patients should receive intravenous amphotericin B 1 mg/kg daily. Immunocompromised patients typically respond poorly. Patients with diffuse lung disease fare worse than those with focal disease. This has been well evaluated in AIDS, where the respective mortality rates are 70% and 30%.[155] Those not quite so ill should receive itraconazole 400 mg/day. Treatment should be given for 4–8 weeks only.

Chronic pulmonary coccidioidomycosis

Fewer than 10% of patients develop chronic coccidioidomycosis. This may be confined to the lung (50–70% of cases) or involve other organs. The later pulmonary manifestations include asymptomatic nodules, small thin or thick-walled cavities and progressive consolidation. The nodules are often mistaken for a malignant process and are removed surgically only to discover their nature histologically. Patients usually have serological evidence of infection or a positive skin test for *Coccidioides*. Therapy is not indicated for asymptomatic patients with nodular disease, although continued observation is appropriate.

Patients with cavitary disease and cough usually have positive sputum cultures and serological evidence of coccidioidomycosis. Therapy is indicated to control symptoms and prevent progression of disease. The results of therapy for chronic pulmonary coccidioidomycosis are summarized in Table 62.9. No agent yields better than a 60% response rate, but either itraconazole 400 mg/day or fluconazole 400 mg/day are appropriate. The initial response may take up to 9 months. Treatment should continue for 6 months beyond the last symptom or maximal improvement, which typically means 1–2 years of therapy. Even so, relapse is common, as indicated in Table 62.9. Those with a negative coccidioidin skin test during therapy and a peak complement fixation titer of ≥256 are approximately five times more likely to relapse, regardless of which therapy is used.[156]

Severely ill patients with pneumonia high fever and hypoxemia should be treated with systemic amphotericin B.

Table 62.9 Response of pulmonary coccidioidomycosis to azoles

Agent	Dose (mg)	Response rate (%)	Relapse rate (%)	Response rate 1 year post-treatment
Ketoconazole	400	23	9	21
	800	32	44	18
Itraconazole	400	57	16	49
Fluconazole	200	34	39	21
	400	61	36	39

Extrapulmonary coccidioidomycosis

Other forms of coccidioidomycosis, including lymphoreticular, cutaneous, osteoarticular and genitourinary, respond to antifungal therapy better than does pulmonary disease. Itraconazole 400 mg/day for several months or years has response rates of approximately 90%.[157] Fluconazole and ketoconazole may also be effective. In patients with osteoarticular disease, stabilization of the bone may be important to prevent pathological fractures. It may take many years for bone remodelling to occur. Surgical resection of easily accessible draining lymph nodes may be appropriate if the response to antifungal therapy is slow.

Coccidioidal meningitis

Meningitis due to *C. immitis* is a slowly progressive lymphocytic meningitis with a 100% mortality if untreated. Some patients are extremely ill and die within weeks of presentation, others have a more indolent course over a period of up to 2 years. Coccidioidal meningitis does not respond to systemic ketoconazole or amphotericin B, and for this reason intrathecal amphotericin B was the mainstay of therapy until the triazoles were introduced. Itraconazole 400 mg/day and fluconazole ≥400 mg/day are also effective in patients with coccidioidal meningitis.[158,159] Fluconazole has the theoretical advantage of better CSF penetration, but this has not been clearly translated into a better response rate. In general, the fluconazole response rate in coccidioidal meningitis is 70–90%, which contrasts with the intrathecal amphotericin B response rate of 40–100% depending on the series.

In patients who do not respond to an oral azole, intrathecal amphotericin B is currently the only alternative. It is administered daily initially, in slowly escalating doses together with narcotic premedication. Intrathecal amphotericin B is prepared in 5 ml of 5% dextrose. Cerebrospinal fluid (5 ml) is removed at lumbar puncture or cisternal puncture in patients with spinal block or in whom lumbar puncture is difficult. The 5 ml of amphotericin B in 5% dextrose is given slowly intrathecally over a period of about 3–5 min with the patient in a head-down position. The lumbar puncture needle is then removed and the patient remains head-down for 2 h. The initial dose of amphotericin B is 0.05 mg, which is increased by 0.05 mg each day until the level of tolerance is reached, up to a maximum of 1.2 mg. In general, few patients can tolerate more than 0.5 mg/day during the acute phase. During the maintenance phase higher doses can be given weekly or every other week. In patients unable to tolerate a therapeutic dose, 25 mg hydrocortisone should also be given intrathecally with some amelioration of adverse effects. The response to therapy is judged by following the CSF glucose, white cell count and antibody titers. Unfortunately, intrathecal amphotericin B often causes a rise in the CSF white cell count.

Communicating hydrocephalus and other rather complex alterations of CSF flow are common in patients with coccidioidal meningitis. CSF pressures should be measured intermittently and ventriculoperitoneal shunts inserted for those with hydrocephalus. Such shunts clearly alter CSF flow and may create additional difficulties in delivering intrathecal amphotericin B to the sites of disease. Sometimes an Ommaya reservoir is necessary. CSF flow studies are important in determining how amphotericin B is delivered in and around the brain in this context. Vasculitic and encephalitic complications are also occasional complications of coccidioidal meningitis.[160]

The treatment of coccidioidal meningitis is for life. No regimen is curative, and relapse is virtually universal in all patients.

Coccidioidomycosis in immunocompromised patients

A question that arises for patients in endemic areas of coccidioidomycosis who require a solid organ transplant is whether or not a history of coccidioidomycosis is a contraindication to transplantation. One study of six such patients showed that none treated with long-term ketoconazole reactivated.[161] In those who develop coccidioidomycosis post-transplantation, lifelong therapy is recommended. Coccidioidomycosis complicating AIDS carries a poor outlook when disseminated or of a diffuse pulmonary pattern.[155] Such patients should be treated with intravenous amphotericin B 1 mg/kg daily and followed, if successful, by an oral azole for life.

BLASTOMYCOSIS

Blastomycosis is endemic to North America and Africa.[162] It causes primary pulmonary infection. Cutaneous and osseous lesions indicate dissemination. Meningitis occurs in 3–10% of patients. The disease is usually relatively indolent. A few present with rapidly progressive pneumonia leading to the adult respiratory distress syndrome[163] and, although this is life-threatening, a successful outcome is possible. There are rare reports of blastomycosis in AIDS and other immunocompromised conditions.[164]

In patients who are acutely unwell or immunocompromised[165] amphotericin B 1 mg/kg daily is appropriate. This should be continued until the patient is improved and stable. In less acutely ill patients itraconazole 200 mg/day is the treatment of choice.[146] It is slightly superior to ketoconazole[143] and fluconazole in doses of 400–800 mg daily. Treatment should last 6–12 months in non-immunocompromised patients and longer in the immunocompromised. In patients with pulmonary and/or bone disease more prolonged treatment may be necessary.

PARACOCCIDIOIDOMYCOSIS

Paracoccidioidomycosis is caused by *Paracoccidioides brasiliensis* and is endemic to Latin America. Men are affected more frequently than women, although the frequency in prepubertal girls and post-menopausal women is similar to that in men. Chronic pulmonary or disseminated disease is common and may mimic malignancy or tuberculosis, which co-exist in 30% of patients with pulmonary involvement. Mucosal and cervical node involvement is relatively common. A few cases have been reported in AIDS patients with low CD4 counts.

Sulfadiazine 4–6 g/day (adults) or 60–100 mg/kg daily (children) in divided doses is reasonably effective for mild and moderately disseminated disease or as follow-on therapy after initial amphotericin B treatment. The dose can be reduced when clear evidence of improvement has occurred. Therapy should be continued for 2 years to avoid relapse, but the development

of resistance during treatment is relatively common. In severe or disseminated cases amphotericin B 0.5–1 mg/kg daily (to a total of 1.5–2 g) is appropriate. Whether lipid-associated amphotericin B is as effective as conventional amphotericin B is not known, but it may not be.[166] Mild cases in patients for whom sulfonamides are contraindicated may be cured by itraconazole 100–200 mg/day for 6 months.[56] The relapse rate is only 3–5%. Ketoconazole 200–400 mg/day for 12 months is an alternative, and yields a 90% response rate.[56] Fluconazole is also effective.[48]

PENICILLIUM INFECTIONS

Penicillium species are ubiquitous airborne fungi which, rarely, cause infection. Such infections are most often pulmonary (in both non-immunocompromised and immunocompromised patients) and related to surgical intervention or trauma (e.g. prosthetic valve endocarditis, CAPD peritonitis and ocular infection).[167] Responses to therapy have been poor, but amphotericin B would appear to be the optimal initial therapy.

Penicillium marneffei infections are localized to south-east China, Burma, northern Thailand, Vietnam and Indonesia.[168] *P. marneffei* is a primary pathogen and may cause focal or fatal progressive disseminated disease. It is a major problem in AIDS in northern Thailand where approximately a third of such patients develop disseminated *P. marneffei* infections with CD4 counts $<100 \times 10^6/l$.[168]

P. marneffei is highly susceptible in vitro to itraconazole, ketoconazole, terbinafine and flucytosine, but is less susceptible to amphotericin B and fluconazole.[169] The response of disseminated disease in those with AIDS parallels these in-vitro responses. Mild to moderately severe *P. marneffei* infections should be treated with itraconazole 400 mg/day or ketoconazole 400 mg/day. In patients taking rifampicin or other interacting drugs amphotericin B 0.6–1 mg/kg daily is appropriate. Seriously ill patients should be treated with amphotericin B 1 mg/kg daily for at least 2 weeks, but there is a substantial failure rate, possibly attributable (at least in part) to the seriousness of the infection. A standard regimen of 2 weeks of amphotericin B 0.6 mg/kg daily for 2 weeks followed by itraconazole 400 mg daily was succesful in 97% of patients.[170]

Relapse is common when therapy is stopped. In patients with AIDS, oral maintenance therapy with itraconazole 200 mg daily is appropriate.[171]

MUCORMYCOSIS (ZYGOMYCOSIS)

Several clinical patterns of mucormycosis are described in varying patient populations; rhinocerebral and pulmonary disease are most common. A large number of different causal genera and species are described. Subcutaneous zygomycosis affects a small subgroup (p. 838). Diagnosis is often difficult, partly because cultures are frequently negative, for reasons that are not clear. Histology is required for early diagnosis, which

Table 62.10 Treatment of zygomycosis

	Medical therapy	Surgery[a]
Subcutaneous		
Conidiobolomycosis	Yes, various, high relapse rate	No
Basidiobolomycosis	Potassium iodide 30 mg/kg	No
Wound or burn associated	Amphotericin B[b] 1.0–1.5 mg/kg ± rifampicin	Resection of affected areas (multiple if necessary)
Rhinocerebral	Amphotericin B[b] 1.0–1.5 mg/kg ± rifampicin	Resection to margins of affected tissue on CT scan
Pulmonary	Amphotericin B[b] 1.0–1.5 mg/kg ± rifampicin	Lobectomy or pneumonectomy if exclusively or predominantly unilateral
Gastrointestinal	Amphotericin B[b] 1.0–1.5 mg/kg ± rifampicin	
Cerebral	Amphotericin B[b] 1.0–1.5 mg/kg ± rifampicin	Resection of lesion
Renal	Amphotericin B[b] 1.0–1.5 mg/kg ± rifampicin	Nephrectomy
Disseminated	Amphotericin B[b] 1.0–1.5 mg/kg ± rifampicin	Not feasible

[a] Other than diagnostic biopsy.
[b] Also consider lipid-associated amphotericin B preparations in doses exceeding 4 mg/kg for life-threatening disease.

is critical for a more favorable outcome. The clinical features of zygomycosis are similar to those of invasive aspergillosis, although the histological appearances of the hyphae are distinct. Azoles are ineffective; the organism is resistant to flucytosine in vitro.

Treatment requires large doses of amphotericin B (≥1 mg/kg daily) (Table 62.10). The evidence for synergy between amphotericin B and rifampicin is anecdotal. Considerable experience with lipid-associated amphotericin B has now accrued. Liposomal, colloidal dispersion and lipid complex formulations (*see* Ch. 35) are all efficacious in mucormycosis in doses of 3–10 mg/kg daily.[172,173] Correction of any underlying immune defect such as diabetic ketoacidosis or neutropenia is highly desirable.

Surgical debridement is critically important in the management of mucormycosis, as antifungal therapy is relatively ineffective alone. In particular, the rhinocerebral form, localized pulmonary disease[174] and cutaneous varieties[175] require surgery for a successful outcome. Better control of underlying predisposing factors, early high-dose amphotericin B and possibly local amphotericin B have allowed surgery to be less radical than previously, and repeated examination under anesthesia with adequate debridement is the optimal approach. Advances in endoscopic sinus surgery may also be successful for rhinosinusitis and has the advantage of lower operative morbidity and greater operative precision.[176] Disseminated disease is usually fatal, regardless of therapy. Hyperbaric oxygen therapy, in combination with surgery and amphotericin B, has been used, often with success, but its contribution to outcome is uncertain.

FUSARIUM INFECTIONS

Most disseminated *Fusarium* infections complicate leukemia, other hematological malignancies, or bone marrow transplantation. Most are due to *Fusarium solani*, but other species have been implicated. Disseminated disease with fungemia is usual; 75% of patients have skin lesions.

Pneumonia and sinusitis also occur. Sometimes infection arises from an affected toenail.

Treatment is often ineffective. Amphotericin B in doses of at least 1 mg/kg daily together with granulocyte–macrophage colony-stimulating factor if the patient is still profoundly neutropenic is probably first-line therapy. Lipid-associated amphotericin B in doses >4 mg/kg may also be effective. Voriconazole may also be effective. No patient with persistent neutropenia has survived this infection.[41,177]

SCEDOSPORIUM INFECTIONS

Two species of *Scedosporium*, *S. apiospermum* (*Pseudallescheria boydii*) and *S. prolificans*, cause infection. The spectrum of infection is wide. *S. apiospermum* causes superficial skin disease, mycetoma, sinusitis, cerebral abscess in leukemia and rare systemic infections such as endocarditis in immunocompromised patients. Disease expression is similar to that of *Aspergillus*, but is much less common. Rarely it causes a fungal ball in the lung. *S. prolificans* may cause localized skin, soft tissue and bone disease, usually after trauma, or pulmonary disease or fungemia, usually in neutropenic patients.[178]

S. apiospermum is resistant to amphotericin B in vitro[179] and in vivo,[180] but susceptible to miconazole, ketoconazole, itraconazole and voriconazole.[181] Patients with cerebral abscess due to *S. apiospermum* require large doses of intravenous or oral itraconazole[182,183] or voriconazole.[184] Treatment should be continued for months; oral drug may be substituted for intravenous drug once the disease is stabilized. The treatment of other forms of *S. apiospermum* infection are essentially along the same lines as described for invasive aspergillosis, with itraconazole or voriconazole.

S. prolificans is a multiresistant fungus and no current antifungal drug is reliably active. Some isolates are less resistant to itraconazole than others. Syngery between itraconazole and terbinafine is marked[185] and currently offers the best therapeutic option.

TRICHOSPORON INFECTIONS

The taxonomy of the genus *Trichosporon* has been revised recently and it has become difficult to correlate the old literature with the new nomenclature. *Trichosporon capitatum* is now classified as *Blastoschizomyces capitatus* but causes a disease process in leukemia similar to that caused by *Trichosporon beigelii*.[186] Other than this, most infections are caused by *Trichosporon beigelii* or closely related species. The term *Trichosporon* spp. will be used here, although for the most part this relates to *Trichosporon beigelii*.

Trichosporon spp. cause three forms of disease:

- white piedra, a superficial infection of hair shafts found in the tropics;
- endocarditis;
- disseminated infection in neutropenic patients.[187]

Data suggest that, although isolates may be inhibited by amphotericin B, they are not killed[188] and that the preferred agents for life-threatening *Trichosporon* infections are the azoles.[189] Large doses of fluconazole (e.g. 400–800 mg/day) should be used for the control of this rapidly lethal infection, with subsequent tailoring depending on response. Most isolates are also resistant to flucytosine.

For patients with *Trichosporon* endocarditis surgery is essential, particularly in those with an infected prosthetic heart valve; large and prolonged doses of fluconazole or another azole should be given.

OTHER RARE FUNGAL DISEASES

For the management of other rare fungal infections too numerous to discuss here, the reader is referred to the recent literature.[190]

PROPHYLACTIC, EMPIRIC AND PRE-EMPTIVE THERAPY OF FUNGAL DISEASE

DEFINITIONS

Several different approaches for the prevention, early treatment or prevention of relapse of both superficial and invasive fungal infections have been described. A glossary of terms is provided here to ensure the reader is fully cognizant of the terminology and implications of different strategies (Box 62.6). Indications for prophylaxis are shown in Table 62.11.

Some populations are at such high risk of fungal disease that all such patients should receive prophylaxis; the best examples are antifungal prophylaxis for allogeneic stem cell transplant recipients and the use of pneumocystis prophylaxis in advanced HIV disease. In most other settings the benefits of prophylaxis are less clearly defined. At present, antifungal prophylaxis is not indicated for patients in intensive care units, surgical patients, most neonates, patients with burns, or those with solid tumors.

Table 62.11 Summary of current prophylaxis and the evidence base supporting it

Indication	Evidence[a]	Regimens	Duration
Stem cell transplantation	AI	Fluconazole 200–400 mg daily	75+ days
Graft-versus-host disease	CIII	Itraconazole 400 mg daily	Uncertain
		Lipid amphotericin B 3–5 mg/kg	Uncertain
Chemotherapy for leukemia	BI	Fluconazole 100–400 mg daily	Resolution of neutropenia
		Itraconazole solution 200–400 mg daily	Resolution of neutropenia
Chronic granulomatous disease	BII	Itraconazole 200 mg daily	Years
Solid organ transplantation and evidence of coccidioidal exposure or infection	BII	Itraconazole 200–400 mg daily	Years
		Fluconazole 200–400 mg daily	Years
High-risk surgical patient	BI	Fluconazole 400 mg daily	Until clinically improved
Pancreatitis	CIII	Fluconazole 400 mg daily	Until clinically improved
Liver transplantation – high risk[b]	BII	Fluconazole 200–400 mg daily	4 weeks
		Lipid amphotericin B 3–5 mg/kg daily	4 weeks
Pancreas transplantation – high risk[b]	BII	Fluconazole 200–400 mg daily	4 weeks
Neonate, <1000g	BI	Fluconazole 3 mg/kg	6 weeks

[a] Infectious Disease Society of America guidelines.
[b] High risk includes prolonged operation time, retransplantation and postoperative complications. Other factors vary from study to study.
[c] 3 mg/kg every third day for 2 weeks, then 3 mg/kg alternate days for 2 weeks, then 3 mg/kg daily for 2 weeks.

NEUTROPENIA AND STEM CELL TRANSPLANTATION

Remission induction therapy for leukemia involves multiple courses of intensive cytoreductive chemotherapy with discrete episodes of neutropenia; corticosteroids may also be used. The incidence of invasive fungal infection in these patients is as high as 25% during neutropenia and up to 15% following stem cell transplantation.[191] Patients whose leukemia does not go into remission or who relapse have a very high incidence of invasive fungal infections at autopsy. The important fungi to protect against are various species of *Candida* and *Aspergillus*, while any given choice may also protect against several other rare fungi.

Antifungal prophylaxis may be appropriate for patients who will have at least 7 days of profound neutropenia, to prevent invasive fungal infections: prophylaxis is not indicated for shorter periods. Any benefit of prophylaxis increases with the duration of profound neutropenia. Prophylaxis may also protect against mucosal candidosis, which is common in acute leukemia. Table 62.11 shows the best-studied prophylactic choices.

Clearly no topical oral regimens with amphotericin B or nystatin, or fluconazole, protect against invasive aspergillosis. Alternatives that may prevent invasive aspergillosis and other airborne fungi include aerosolized or a nasal spray of amphotericin B, but these will not protect against mucosal or invasive candidosis. Oral amphotericin B solution may protect against superficial and invasive *Candida* infections. Ketoconazole is not sufficiently effective for prophylaxis against *Candida* and has no activity against *Aspergillus*.

Fluconazole probably has some efficacy in protecting against invasive candidosis in acute leukemia, but this was not shown in a study of 257 patients.[192] One probable reason for the failure to show a difference was the high (70%) incidence of empirical amphotericin B usage, usually started on day 3 or 4 of neutropenic fever. In other studies of similar populations, lower doses of fluconazole and less frequent use of empirical amphotericin B had similar incidences of invasive fungal infection.[193,194] Thus lower doses of fluconazole (e.g. 100–200 mg/day) are probably adequate.[195] Breakthrough *C. krusei* or *C. glabrata* fungemia or invasive aspergillosis may be problematic.

Itraconazole has not yet been well evaluated for antifungal prophylaxis. It has the potential to prevent invasive aspergillosis and *C. krusei* infections, which fluconazole does not, and other more common *Candida* infections. Two large studies showed equivalence to fluconazole in preventing *Candida* infections and possibly a reduction in *Aspergillus* infection.[196,197] Optimization of the dose to produce serum concentrations above 500 mg/l, may be helpful.[198] Itraconazole may prejudice a good response to amphotericin B in invasive aspergillosis.[199]

The prophylaxis of fungal infections during and after bone-marrow transplantation has been the subject of some controlled trials. Fluconazole 400 mg/day was highly effective compared with placebo in preventing *Candida* infec-

tions, and reduced mortality due to *Candida*.[200] In one study 40% of the doses of fluconazole were given intravenously.[200] Prophylaxis extending beyond the end of neutropenia to 75 days in allogeneic bone marrow recipients reduces mortality.[201] There is some debate about whether a high daily dose of fluconazole (400 mg) is necessary for prophylaxis in the bone-marrow transplant setting. The prophylaxis of patients with graft-versus-host disease to prevent invasive aspergillosis, using itraconazole or liposomal amphotericin B, is commonly done but not convincingly shown to be beneficial by randomized studies. Criteria for the selection of these patients are unclear.

Secondary prophylaxis is indicated for patients with previous or current invasive aspergillosis, candidemia, hepatosplenic candidosis, mucormycosis and other rarer fungal infections. Management may involve surgery and will require individualization of the antifungal regimen, depending on the infecting organism and response to therapy. A typical regimen is amphotericin B 1 mg/kg or lipid amphotericin B 3–5 mg/kg, or itraconazole 400 mg daily starting on the day chemotherapy is given.[123]

SOLID ORGAN TRANSPLANTATION

Very few studies have addressed antifungal prophylaxis in the solid organ transplant patient.[202] It is generally agreed that long-term azole prophylaxis is indicated for all solid organ transplant recipients with prior markers of coccidioidal infection (serology or skin test).[161,202] The frequency of disseminated or life-threatening fungal infections is low in the renal transplant recipient unless there are major problems with rejection, and prophylaxis is not indicated for these patients. There are higher risks associated with heart transplantation, of invasive candidosis, aspergillosis and *P. carinii* pneumonia, but it is not possible to recommend routine prophylaxis in these patients.[130,202] Similarly, no data support the use of prophylaxis in the lung transplant recipient, although pre-emptive therapy for those whose airways yield *Aspergillus* is widely practised. Both itraconazole and aerosolized amphotericin B are used, the former not wholly successful, the latter with some tolerance and delivery problems.[203,204] The frequency of deep candidosis in liver transplant patients is high and therefore prophylaxis may be appropriate in the first month after transplantation for those patients at high risk (Box 62.6). An amphotericin B (e.g. the liposomal formulation 3–5 mg/kg daily) is probably most appropriate given the diversity of fungi causing disease in these patients. Low doses of lipid-based amphotericin B are associated with failure.

AIDS

Two studies have shown the benefit of fluconazole 100 mg/day for the prevention of cryptococcal disease and mucosal candidosis in patients with AIDS, although this regimen was inef-

Box 62.6 Definitions of preventive and early treatment of invasive fungal infections

Prophylaxis
- Primary – use of an antimicrobial agent in an unselected population of patients with the same condition (e.g. AIDS) or undergoing the same treatment (such as orthoptic liver transplantation), with the objective of complete or partial prevention.
- Targeted – a more focused approach to primary prophylaxis by administration of an antimicrobial agent for a subset of a patient population (e.g. patients colonized with *Candida tropicalis* or patient with grade II, III or IV graft-versus-host disease).
- Secondary – prevention of relapse of an infection that was previously fully or partially documented (e.g. intravenous amphotericin B for invasive aspergillosis in second and subsequent courses of cytotoxic chemotherapy and/or stem cell transplantation, when the infection occurred in the first episode of neutropenia).

Empiric therapy
Treatment based on early clinical features of disease, prior to confirmation (e.g. amphotericin B therapy of fever during neutropenia).

Pre-emptive therapy
Selective use of treatment in those with a laboratory marker of disease, but before disease is apparent (e.g. sputum culture growing *C. neoformans* in an AIDS patient, but without apparent disease).

fective in preventing histoplasmosis.[205,206] However, the financial cost of preventing each case of cryptococcal meningitis is high. Long-term primary fluconazole may also carry a risk of the development of fluconazole resistance. Primary prophylaxis is not warranted to prevent oral candidosis in patients with HIV infection.

Prophylaxis against *Pn. carinii* pneumonia is recommended in all patients who have had the acute infection and in HIV-positive patients with a CD4 count of $<200 \times 10^6/l$. Primary prophylaxis should also be considered in patients with other types of severe immunodeficiency. The drug of choice for prophylaxis is trimethoprim–sulfamethoxazole. Recommended adult doses at 160 mg of trimethoprim plus 800 mg of sulfamethoxazole once daily or 3 times weekly; and 80 mg of trimethoprim plus 400 mg of sulfamethoxazole once daily. The advantage of once daily high-dose prophylaxis is that it also protects against cerebral toxoplasmosis. The disadvantage is that it causes side effects more commonly than lower doses. In patients who cannot tolerate trimethoprim–sulfamethoxazole alternatives are aerosolized pentamidine, atovaquone, dapsone, and dapsone plus pyrimethamine. The latter combination is recommended for patients who have antibodies against *Toxoplasma gondii* indicating a latent infection with that organism.

In HIV-positive patients on effective antiretroviral treatment, whose CD4 counts are consistently $>200 \times 10^6/l$, prophylaxis can be discontinued.[207–209]

CHRONIC GRANULOMATOUS DISEASE

Historically controlled studies suggest a substantial reduction in invasive aspergillosis with itraconazole prophylaxis.[210,211] Antibacterial prophylaxis alone increases the incidence of fungal infections.[212] Itraconazole prophylaxis increases the incidence of bacterial infection. The dose of itraconazole can be adjusted by body weight and optimized by blood level monitoring.

INTENSIVE CARE PATIENTS

High-risk surgical candidates (perforated viscus, renal impairment or dialysis, pancreatitis) may benefit from targeted fluconazole prophylaxis with 200–400 mg daily.[213] Resistant species of *Candida* may emerge on therapy, however.

NEONATES

A recently completed placebo-controlled randomized study in extremely low birth weight babies showed a clear benefit for fluconazole (Table 62.11).[214] The clearance of fluconazole in these babies is low, hence dosing was every third day initially. More work and experience is required on this subject.

EMPIRIC THERAPY

For about 20 years, the addition of empiric amphotericin B therapy to antibacterial therapy in the neutropenic patient with fever has been standard practice. The database on which this practice is built is not substantial.[215,216] Current US guidelines recommend initiation of amphotericin B after 3 days of neutropenic fever, in all patients, regardless of antifungal prophylaxis. Resolution of fever after initiation of antibacterial therapy can take up to 7 days. In 25% of patients resolution of fever occurs between days 3 and 5 on antibiotics.[217] Most experienced physicians begin empiric amphotericin B on days 4–6 of febrile neutropenia, depending on other symptoms or signs, whether bacteremia was documented (this increases the risk of candidemia) and other perceived risk factors.

Comparisons of conventional amphotericin B and lipid-associated amphotericin have shown response rates of 50–60% and breakthrough documented fungal infection rates of 5%.[113,218] Fewer toxicities are associated with Liposomal amphotericin B than any other amphotericin B preparation apart from the lipid complex formulation.

References

1. Rex JH, Pfaller MA, Galgiani JN et al 1997 Development of interpretive breakpoints for antifungal susceptibility testing: conceptual framework and analysis of in vitro–in vivo correlation data for fluconazole, itraconazole and candida infections. *Clinical Infectious Diseases* 24: 235–247.
2. Denning DW, Van Wye J, Lewiston NJ, Stevens DA 1991 Adjunctive therapy of

allergic bronchopulmonary aspergillosis with itraconazole. *Chest* 100: 813–819.

3. Stevens DA, Kan VL, Judson MA et al 2000 Practice guidelines for diseases caused by *Aspergillus* 30: 696–709.

4. Sermet-Gaudelus, Lesne-Hulin A, Lenoir G, Singlas E, Berche P, Hennequin C 2001 Sputum itraconazole concentrations in cystic fibrosis patients. *Antimicrobial Agents and Chemotherapy* 45: 1937–1938.

5. Ponikau JU, Sherris DA, Kern EB et al 1999 The diagnosis and incidence of allergic fungal sinusitis. *Mayo Clinic Proceedings* 74: 877–884.

6. Manning SC, Schaefer SD, Close LG, Vuitch F 1991 Culture-positive allergic fungal sinusitis. *Archives of Otolaryngology and Head and Neck Surgery* 117: 174–178.

7. Denning DW, Ribaud P, Milpied N et al 2002 The efficacy and safety of voriconazole in the treatment of acute invasive aspergillosis. *Clinical Infectious Diseases* 34: 563–571.

8. Campbell JH, Winter JH, Richardson MS, Shankland GS, Banham SW 1991 Treatment of pulmonary aspergilloma with itraconazole. *Thorax* 46: 839–841.

9. Tsubura E 1997 Multicenter clinical trial of itraconazole in the treatment of pulmonary aspergilloma. Pulmonary Aspergilloma Study Group. *Kekkaku* 72: 557–564.

10. Berenguer J, Diaz-Mediavilla J, Urra D, Munoz P 1989 Central nervous system infection caused by *Pseudallescheria boydii*: case report and review. *Reviews of Infectious Diseases* 11: 890–896.

11. Giron JM, Poey CG, Fajadet PP et al 1993 Inoperable pulmonary aspergilloma: percutaneous CT-guided injection with glycerin and amphotericin B paste in 15 cases. *Radiology* 188: 825–827.

12. Munk PL, Vellet AD, Rankin RN, Müller NL, Ahmad D 1993 Intracavitary aspergilloma: transthoracic percutaneous injection of amphotericin gelatin solution. *Radiology* 188: 821–823.

13. Jewkes J, Kay PH, Paneth M, Citron KM 1983 Pulmonary aspergilloma: analysis of prognosis in relation to haemoptysis and survey of treatment. *Thorax* 38: 572–578.

14. Massard G, Roeslin N, Wihlm J-M, Dumont P, Witz J-P, Morand G 1992 Pleuropulmonary aspergilloma: clinical spectrum and results of surgical treatment. *Annals of Thoracic Surgery* 54: 1159–1164.

15. Elewski BE 2000 Tinea capitis: a current perspective. *Journal of the American Academy of Dermatology* 42: 1–20.

16. Dragos V, Lunder M 1997 Lack of efficacy of 6-week treatment with oral terbinafine for tinea capitis due to *Microsporum canis* in children. *Pediatric Dermatology* 14: 4–48.

17. Greer DL 2000 Successful treatment of tinea capitis with 2% ketoconazole shampoo. *International Journal of Dermatology* 29: 302–304.

18. Caceres-Rios H, Rueda M, Ballona R, Bustamante B 2000 Comparison of terbinafine and griseofulvin in the treatment of tinea capitis. *Journal of the American Academy of Dermatology* 42: 80–84.

19. Filho ST, Cuce LC, Foss NT, Marques SA, Santamaria JR 1998 Efficacy, safety and tolerability of terbinafine for tinea capitis in children: Brazilian multicentric study with daily oral tablets for 1, 2 and 4 weeks. *Journal of the European Academy of Dermatology and Venereology* 11: 141–146.

20. Jahangir M, Hussain I, Ul Hasan M, Haroon TS 1998 A double-blind, randomised, comparative trial of itraconazole versus terbinafine for 2 weeks in tinea capitis. *British Journal of Dermatology* 139: 672–674.

21. Lopez-Gomez S, Del Palacio A, Van Cutsem J, Soledad Cuetara M, Iglesias L, Rodriguez-Noriega A 1994 Itraconazole versus griseofulvin in the treatment of tinea capitis: a double-blind randomized study in children. *International Journal of Dermatology* 33: 743–747.

22. Abdel-Rahman SM, Powell DA, Nahata MC 1998 Efficacy of itraconazole in children with *Trichophyton tonsurans* tinea capitis. *Journal of the American Academy of Dermatology* 38: 443–446.

23. Parent D, Decroix J, Heenen M 1994 Clinical experience with short schedules of itraconazole in the treatment of tinea corporis and/or tinea cruris. *Dermatology* 189: 378–381.

24. Farag A, Taha M, Halim S 1994 One-week therapy with oral terbinafine in cases of tinea cruris/corporis. *British Journal of Dermatology* 131: 684–686.

25. Bakos L, Brito AC, Castro LC et al 1997 Open clinical study of the efficacy and safety of terbinafine cream 1% in children with tinea corporis and tinea cruris. *Pediatric Infectious Disease Journal* 16: 545–548.

26. Gupta AK, Dlova N, Taborda P et al 2000 Once weekly fluconazole is effective in children in the treatment of tinea capitis: a prospective, multicentre study. *British Journal of Dermatology* 142: 965–968.

27. Evans EGV 1994 A comparison of terbinafine (Lamisil) 1% cream given for one week with clotrimazole (Canesten) 1% cream given for four weeks, in the treatment of tinea pedis. *British Journal of Dermatology* 130 (Suppl. 43): 12–14.

28. Tanuma H, Doi M, Sato N et al 2000 Bifonazole (Mycospor cream) in the treatment of moccasin-type tinea pedis. Comparison between combination therapy of bifonazole cream and 10% urea ointment (Urepearl) and occlusive dressing therapy with the same agents. *Mycoses* 43: 129–137.

29. Delescluse J 1990 Itraconazole in tinea versicolor: a review. *Journal of the American Academy of Dermatology* 23: 551–554.

30. British Society for Medical Mycology Group on Diagnostic Mycology 1995 Management of genital candidosis. *British Medical Journal* 310: 1241–1244.

31. Zang M, Bergstraesser M 1992 Amorolfine in the treatment of onychomycosis and dermatomycoses (an overview). *Clinical and Experimental Dermatology* 17 (Suppl. 1): 61–70.

32. Bonifaz A, Ibarra G 2000 Onychomycosis in children: treatment with bifonazole-urea. *Pediatric Dermatology* 17: 310–314.

33. Syed TA, Ahmadpour OA, Ahmad SA, Shamsi S 1998. Management of toenail onychomycosis with 2% butenafine and 20% urea cream: a placebo-controlled, double-blind study. *Journal of Dermatology* 25: 648–652.

34. McInnes BD, Dockery BL 1997 Surgical treatment of mycotic toenails. *Journal of the American Podiatric Medical Association* 87: 557–564.

35. Roberts MM 1991 Developments in the management of superficial fungal infections. *Journal of Antimicrobial Chemotherapy* 28 (Suppl. A): 47–58.

36. Evans EGV, Sigurgeirsson B 1999 Double blind, randomised study of continuous terbinafine compared with intermittent itraconazole in treatment of toenail onychomycosis. The LION study group. *British Medical Journal* 318: 1031–1035.

37. Tausch I, Brautigam M, Weidinger G, Jones TC 1997 Evaluation of 6 weeks treatment of terbinafine in tinea unguim in a double-blind trial comparing 6 and 12 weeks therapy. The Lagos V Study Group. *British Journal of Dermatology* 136: 737–742.

38. Tosti A, Piraccini BM, Stinchi C Colombo MD 1998 Relapses of onychomycosis after successful treatment with systemic antifungals: a three-year follow-up. *Dermatology* 197: 162–166.

39. Arikian SR, Einarson TR, Kobelt-Nguyen G, Schubert F 1994 A multinational pharmacoeconomic analysis of oral therapies for onychomycosis. The Onychomycosis Study Group. *British Journal of Dermatology* 130: 35–44.

40. Epstein E 1998 How often does oral treatment of toenail onychomycosis produce a disease-free nail? *Archives of Dermatology* 134: 1551–1554.

41. Nelson PE, Dignani MC, Anaissie EJ 1994 Taxonomy, biology and clinical aspects of *Fusarium* species. *Clinical Microbiology Reviews* 7: 479–504.

42. Bayles MAH 1989 Chromoblastomycosis. *Baillières Clinical Tropical Medicine and Communicable Diseases* 4: 45–69.

43. Queiroz-Telles F, Purim KS, Fillus JN et al 1992 Itraconazole in the treatment of chromoblastomycosis due to *Fonsecaea pedrosoi*. *International Journal of Dermatology* 31: 805–812.

44. Bonifaz A, Martinez-Soto E, Carrasco-Gerard E, Peniche J 1997 Treatment of chromoblastomycosis with itraconazole, cryosurgery and a combination of both. *International Journal of Dermatology* 36: 542–547.

45. Randhawa HS, Budimulja U, Bazaz-Malik G et al 1994 Recent developments in the diagnosis and treatment of subcutaneous mycoses. *Journal of Medical and Veterinary Mycology* 32 (Suppl. 1): 299–307.

46. Pimentel ERA, Castro LGM, Cuce LC, Sampaio SAP 1989 Treatment of chromomycosis by cryosurgery with liquid nitrogen: a report on eleven cases. *Journal of Dermatology, Surgery and Oncology* 15: 72–77.

47. Bayles MAH 1989 Chromomycosis. *Baillières Clin Med Commun Dis* 4: 45–7.

48. Diaz M, Negroni R, Montero-Gei F et al 1992 A Pan-American 5-year study of fluconazole therapy for deep mycoses in the immunocompetent host. *Clinical Infectious Diseases* 14 (Suppl. 1): S68–S76.

49. Gugnani HC 1999 A review of zygomycosis due to *Basidiobolus ranarum*. *European Journal of Epidemiology* 15: 923–929.

50. Restrepo A 1994 Treatment of tropical mycoses. *Journal of the American Academy of Dermatology* 31: S91–S102.

51. Kauffman CA, Hajjeh R, Chapman SW 2000 Practice guidelines for the management of patients with sporotrichosis. For the Mycoses Study Group. Infectious Diseases Society of America. *Clinical Infectious Diseases* 30: 684–687.

52. Herr RA, Ajello L, Taylor JW, Arseculeratne SN, Mendoza L 1999 Phylogenetic analysis of rhinosporidium seeberi's 18s small-subunit ribosomal DNA groups this pathogen among members of the protoctistan mesomycetozoa clade. *Journal of Clinical Microbiology* 37(9): 2750–2754.

53. Shrestha SP, Hennig A, Parija SC 1998 Prevalence of rhinosporidiosis of the eye and its adnexa in Nepal. *American Journal of Tropical Medicine and Hygiene* 59: 231–234.

54. Nair KK 1979 Clinical trial of diaminodiphenylsulfone (DDS) in nasal and nasopharyngeal rhinosporidiosis. *Laryngoscope* 89: 291–295.

55. Venkateswaran S, Date A, Job A, Mathan M 1997 Light and electron microscopic findings in rhinosporidiosis after dapsone therapy. *Tropical Medicine and International Health* 12: 1128–1132.

56. Rios-Fabra A, Restrepo Moreno A, Isturiz RE 1994 Fungal infection in Latin American countries. *Infectious Disease Clinics of North America* 8: 129–154.

57. Welsh O 1993 Mycetoma. *Seminars in Dermatology* 12: 290–295.

58. Venugopal PV, Venugopal TV 1993 Treatment of eumycetoma with ketoconazole. *Australasian Journal of Dermatology* 34: 27–29.

59. Ishibashi Y, Hommura S, Matsumoto Y 1987 Direct examination vs culture of biopsy specimens for the diagnosis of keratomycosis. *American Journal of Ophthalmology* 103: 636–640.

60. Wong TY, Ng TP, Fong KS, Tan DT 1997 Risk factors and clinical outcomes between fungal and bacterial keratitis: a comparative study. *CLAO Journal* 23: 275–281.

61. Thomas PA 1994 Mycotic keratitis – an underestimated mycosis. *Journal of Medical and Veterinary Mycology* 32: 235–256.

62. Rahman MR, Minassian DC, Srinivasan M, Martin MJ, Johnson GJ 1997 Trial of chlorhexidine gluconate for fungal corneal ulcers. *Ophthalmic Epidemiology* 4: 141–149.

63. Fiscella RG, Moshifar M, Messick CR, Pendland SL, Chandler JW, Viana M 1997 Polyhexamethylene biguanide (PHMB) in the treatment of experimental *Fusarium* keratomycosis. *Cornea* 16: 447–449.

64. Thomas PA, Abraham DJ, Kalavathy CM, Rajasekaran J 1988 Oral itraconazole therapy for mycotic keratitis. *Mycoses* 31: 271–279.

65. Torres MA, Mohamed J, Cavazos-Adame H, Martinez LA 1985 Topical ketoconazole for fungal keratitis. *American Journal of Ophthalmology* 100: 293–298.

66. Wilcox CM, Darouchiche RO, Laine L, Moxkovitz BL, Mallegol I, Wu J 1997 A randomized, double-blind comparison of itraconazole oral solution and fluconazole tablets in the treatment of esophageal candidiasis. *Journal of Infectious Diseases* 176: 227–232.

67. Law D, Moore CB, Wardle HM et al 1994 High prevalence of antifungal resistance in *Candida* spp. from patients with AIDS. *Journal of Antimicrobial Chemotherapy* 34: 659–668.

68. Baily GG, Perry FM, Denning DW, Mandal BK 1994 Management of candidiasis after failure of fluconazole in an HIV cohort. *AIDS* 8: 787–792.

69. Ghannoum MA, Rex JH, Galgiani JN 1996 Susceptibility testing of fungi: current status of correlation of in vitro data with clinical outcome. *Journal of Clinical Microbiology* 34: 489–495.

70. Sawyer SM, Bowes G, Phelan PD 1994 Vulvovaginal candidiasis in young women with cystic fibrosis. *British Medical Journal* 308: 1609.

71. Sobel JD 1998 Vaginitis *New England Journal of Medicine* 337: 1896–1903.

72. Lindeque BG, Van Niekerk WG 1984 Treatment of vaginal candidiasis in pregnancy with a single clotrimazole 500 mg vaginal pessary. *South African Medical Journal* 65: 123–124.

73. Sobel JD 2000. Use of antifungal drugs in pregnancy: a focus on safety. *Drug Safety* 23: 77–85.

74. Czeizel AE, Toth M, Rochenbauer M 1999 No teratogenic effect after clotimazole therapy during pregnancy. *Epidemiology* 10: 437–440.

75. Young GL, Jewell D 2000 Topical treatment for vaginal candidiasis in pregnancy. *Cochrane Database System Review* CD000225.

76. Inman W, Pearce G, Wilton L 1994 Safety of fluconazole in the treatment of vaginal candidiasis. A prescription-event monitoring study, with special reference to the outcome of pregnancy. *European Journal of Clinical Pharmacology* 46: 115–118.

77. Czeizel AE, Rockenbauer M 1999 A lower rate of preterm birth after clotimazole therapy during pregnancy. *Pediatric and Perinatal Epidemiology* 13: 58–64.

78. Spinillo A, Colonna L, Piazzi G, Baltaro F, Monaco A, Ferrari A 1997 Managing recurrent vulvovaginal candidiasis. Intermittent prevention with itraconazole. *Journal of Reproductive Medicine* 42: 83–87.

79. Pfaller MA, Jones RN, Doern GV et al 2000 Bloodstream infections due to Candida species: SENTRY antimicrobial surveillance program in North America and Latin America. *Antimicrobial Agents and Chemotherapy* 44: 747–751.

80. Clancy CJ, Nguyen MH 1999 Correlation between in vitro susceptibility deter-

mined by E test and response to therapy with amphotericin B: results from a multicenter prospective study of candidemia. *Antimicrobial Agents and Chemotherapy* 43: 1289–1290.

81. Louie A, Liu W, Miller DA, Sucke AC, Liu QF, Drusano GL, Mayers M, Miller MH 1999. Efficacies of high-dose fluconazole plus amphotericin B and high-dose fluconazole plus 5-flurocytosine versus amphotericin B, fluconazole, and 5-fluorocytosine monotherapies in treatment of experimental endocarditis, endophthalmitis, and pyelonephritis due to Candida albicans. *Antimicrobial Agents and Chemotherapy* 43: 2831–2840.

82. Graninger W, Presterl E, Schneeweiss B, Teleky B, Georgopoulos A 1993 Treatment of *Candida albicans* fungaemia with fluconazole. *Journal of Infection* 26: 133–146.

83. British Society for Antimicrobial Chemotherapy Working Party on Fungal Infection 1991 Laboratory monitoring of antifungal chemotherapy. *Lancet* 357: 1577–1580.

84. Leibovitz E, Luster-Reicher A, Amitai M, Mogilner B 1992 Systemic candidal infections associated with use of peripheral venous catheters in neonates: a 9-year experience. *Clinical Infectious Diseases* 14: 485–491.

85. Dato VM, Dajani AS 1990 Candidemia in children with central venous catheters: role of catheter removal and amphotericin B therapy. *Pediatric Infectious Disease Journal* 9: 309–314.

86. Fasano C, O'Keefe J, Gibbs D 1994 Fluconazole treatment of neonates and infants with severe fungal infections not treatable with conventional agents. *European Journal of Clinical Microbiology and Infectious Diseases* 13: 35–41.

87. de Pauw BE, Raemaekers JMM, Donnelly JP, Kullberg B-J, Meis JFGM 1995 An open study on the safety and efficacy of fluconazole in the treatment of disseminated *Candida* infections in patients treated for hematological malignancy. *Annals of Hematology* 70: 83–87.

88. Rex JH, Walsh TJ, Sobel JD 2000 Practice guidelines for the treatment of candidiasis. *Clinical Infectious Diseases* 30: 662–678.

89. Nolla-Salas J, Sitges-Serra A, Leon-Gil C et al 1997 Candidaemia in non-neutropenic critically ill patients: analysis of prognostic factors and assessment of systemic antifungal therapy. Study Group of Fungal Infection in the ICU. *Intensive Care Medicine* 23: 23–30.

90. Rex JH, Bennett JE, Sugar AM et al 1994 A randomized trial comparing fluconazole with amphotericin B for the treatment of candidemia in patients without neutropenia. *New England Journal of Medicine* 331: 1325–1330.

91. Phillips P, Shafran S, Garber G et al 1997 Multicenter randomized trial of fluconazole versus amphotericin B for treatment of candidemia in non-neutropenic patients. Canadian Candidemia Study Group. *European Journal of Clinical Microbiology and Infectious Diseases* 16: 337–345.

92. Graninger W, Presterl E, Schneeweiss B, Teleky B, Georgopoulos A 1993 Treatment of *Candida albicans* fungaemia with fluconazole. *Journal of Infection* 26: 133–146.

93. Fichtenbaum CJ, German M, Dunagan WC et al 1999 A pilot study of the management of uncomplicated candidemia with a standardised protocol of amphotericin B. *Clinical Infectious Diseases* 29: 1551–1556.

94. British Society for Antimicrobial Chemotherapy Working Party on Fungal Infection 1994 Management of deep *Candida* infection in the surgical and intensive care unit patient. *Intensive Care Medicine* 20: 522–528.

95. Blade J, Lopez-Guillermo A, Rozman C et al 1992 Chronic systemic candidiasis in acute leukemia. *Annals of Hematology* 64: 240–244.

96. Anaissie E, Bodey GP, Kantarjian H et al 1991 Fluconazole therapy for chronic disseminated candidiasis in patients with leukaemia and prior amphotericin B therapy. *American Journal of Medicine* 91: 142–150.

97. Kauffman CA, Bradley SF, Ross SC, Weber DR 1991 Hepatosplenic candidiasis: successful treatment with fluconazole. *American Journal of Medicine* 91: 137–141.

98. Walsh TJ, Whitcomb P, Piscitelli S et al 1997 Safety, tolerance and pharmacokinetics of amphotericin B lipid complex in children with hepatosplenic candidiasis. *Antimicrobial Agents and Chemotherapy* 41: 1944–1948.

99. Bjerke JW, Meyers JD, Bowden RA 1994 Hepatosplenic candidiasis – a contraindication to marrow transplanation? *Blood* 84: 2811–2814.

100. Storfer SP, Medoff G, Fraser VJ, Powderly WG, Dunagan WC 1994 Candiduria: retrospective review in hospitalized patients. *Infectious Diseases in Clinical Practice* 3: 23–29.

101. Occhipinti DJ, Gubbins PO, Schreckenberger P, Danziger LH 1994 Frequency, pathogenicity and microbiologic outcome of non-*Candida albicans* candiduria. *European Journal of Clinical Microbiology and Infectious Diseases* 13: 459–467.

102. Wong-Beringer A, Jacobs RA, Guglielmo BJ 1992 Treatment of funguria. *Journal of the American Medical Association* 267: 2780–2785.

103. Leu H-S, Huang C-T 1995 Clearance of funguria with short-course antifungal regimens: a prospective, randomized, controlled study. *Clinical Infectious Diseases* 20: 1152–1157.

104. Voss A, Meis JFGM, Hoogkamp-Korstanje JAA 1994 Fluconazole in the management of fungal urinary tract infections. *Infection* 22: 247–251.

105. Sobel JD, Kauffman CA, McKinsey D et al and NIAID Mycoses Study Group 2000 Candiduria: a randomized, double-blind study of treatment with fluconazole and placebo. *Clinical Infectious Diseases* 30: 19–24.

106. Ellis ME, Al-Abdely H, Sandridge A, Greer W, Ventura W 2000 Fungal endocarditis: evidence in the world literature. *Clinical Infectious Diseases* 32: 50–62.

107. Denning DW 1996 Therapeutic response in invasive aspergillosis. *Clinical Infectious Diseases* 23: 608–615.

108. Holding KJ, Dworkin MS, Wan P-CT et al 2000 Aspergillosis among people infected with human immunodeficiency virus: incidence and survival. *Clinical Infectious Diseases* 31: 1253–1257.

109. Lin S-J, Schranz J, Teutsch M 2001 Aspergillosis case-fatality rate: systematic review of literature. *Clinical Infectious Diseases* 32: 358–366.

110. Denning DW, Stevens DA 1990 Antifungal and surgical treatment of invasive aspergillosis: review of 2121 published cases. *Reviews of Infectious Diseases* 12: 1147–1201.

111. Patterson TE, Kirkpatrick WR, White M et al 2000 Invasive aspergillosis – disease spectrum, treatment practices and outcomes. *Medicine* 79: 250–260.

112. Bowden R, Chandrasekar P, White M et al 1998 A double blind randomised controlled trial of Amphocil (ABCD) versus amphotericin B (AmB) for treatment of invasive aspergillosis in immunocompromised patients. *Abstracts of the 1901 International Immunocompromised Host Society Meeting, Davos, Switzerland June 21–24.*

113. Walsh TJ, Finberg RW, Arndt C et al 1999 Liposomal amphotericin B for empirical therapy in patients with persistent fever and neutropenia. *New England Journal of Medicine* 340: 764–771.

114. Denning DW, Lee JY, Hostetler JS et al 1994 NIAID Mycoses Study Group multicenter trial of oral itraconazole therapy of invasive aspergillosis. *American Journal of Medicine* 97: 135–144.

115. Stevens DA, Schwartz HJ, Lee JY et al 2000 A randomized trial of itraconazole in allergic bronchopulmonary aspergillosis. *New England Journal of Medicine* 342: 756–762.

116. Herbrecht R, Denning DW, Patterson TF et al 2002 Voriconazole versus amphotericin B for primary therapy of invasive aspergillosis. *New England Journal of Medicine* 347: 408–415.

117. Maertens J, Raad I, Sable CA et al 2000 Multicenter, non-comparative study to evaluate safety and efficacy of caspofungin (CAS) in adults with invasive aspergillosis (IA) refractory (R) or intolerant (I) to amphotericin B (AMB), AMB lipid formulations (lipid AMB) or azoles. *Program and Abstracts of the 40th Interscience Conference on Antimicrobial Agents and Chemotherapy, Toronto, September 16–20, 2000.*

118. Moore CB, Sayers N, Mosquero et al 2000 Antifungal drug resistance in Aspergillus. *Journal of Infection* 41: 203–220.

119. Mills W, Chopra R, Linch DC, Goldstone AH 1994 Liposomal amphotericin B in the treatment of fungal infections in neutropenic patients: a single-centre experience of 133 episodes in 116 patients. *British Journal of Haematology* 86: 754–760.

120. White MH, Anaissie EJ, Kusne S et al 1997 Amphotericin B colloidal dispersion vs. amphotericin B as therapy for invasive aspergillosis. *Clinical Infectious Diseases* 24: 635–642.

121. Graybill JR, Bocanegra R, Najvar LK, Loebenberg D, Luther MF 1998 Granulocyte colony-stimulating factor and azole antifungal therapy in murine aspergillosis: role of immune suppression. *Antimicrobial Agents and Chemotherapy* 10: 2467–2473.

122. Caillot D, Couaillier J-F, Bernard A et al 2001 Increasing volume and changing characteristics of IPA on sequential thoracic CT scans in neutropenic patients. *Journal of Clinical Oncology* 19: 253–259.

123. Offner F, Cordonnier C, Ljungman P et al 1998 Impact of previous aspergillosis on the outcome of bone marrow transplantation. *Clinical Infectious Diseases* 26: 1093–1098.

124. Caillot D, Casasnovas O, Bernard A et al 1997 Improved management of invasive pulmonary aspergillosis in neutropenic patients using early thoracic computer tomographic scan and surgery. *Journal of Clinical Oncology* 15: 139–147.

125. Yeghen T, Kibbler CC, Prentice HG et al 2000 Management of invasive pulmonary aspergillosis in hematology patients: a review of 87 consecutive cases at a single institution. *Clinical Infectious Diseases* 31: 859–868.

126. Saraceno JL, Phelps DT, Ferro TJ, Futerfas R, Schwartz DB 1997 Chronic necrotizing pulmonary aspergillosis. *Chest* 112: 541–548.

127. Denning DW 2001 Chronic forms of pulmonary aspergillosis. *Clinical Microbiology and Infection* (Suppl. 2): 25–31.

128. Saag MS, Cloud GC, Graybill JR et al 1999 A comparison of itraconazole versus fluconazole as maintenance therapy for AIDS-associated cryptococcal meningitis. *Clinical Infectious Diseases* 28: 291–296.

129. Bennett JE, Dismukes WE, Dumar RJ et al 1979 A comparison of amphotericin B alone and combined with flucytosine in the treatment of cryptococcal meningitis. *New England Journal of Medicine* 301: 126–131.

130. British Society for Antimicrobial Chemotherapy Working Party on Fungal Infection 1992 Treatment of fungal infections in AIDS. *Lancet* 340: 648–651.

131. Van der Horst CM, Saag MS, Cloud GA et al and the NIAID Mycoses Study Group and AIDS Clinical Trials Group 1997. Treatment of cryptococcal meningitis associated with the acquired immunodeficiency syndrome. *New England Journal of Medicine* 337: 15–21.

132. Leenders ACA, Daenen S, Jansen RLH et al 1998 Liposomal amphotericin B compared with amphotericin B deoxycholate in the treatment of documented and suspected neutropenia-associated invasive fungal infections. *British Journal of Haematology* 103: 205–212.

133. Denning DW, Armstrong RW, Lewis BH, Stevens DA 1991 Elevated cerebrospinal fluid pressure in patients with cryptococcal meningitis and acquired immunodeficiency syndrome. *American Journal of Medicine* 91: 267–272.

134. Rex JH, Larsen RA, Dismukes WE, Cloud GA, Bennett JE 1993 Catastrophic visual loss due to *Cryptococcus neoformans* meningitis. *Medicine (Baltimore)* 72: 207–224.

135. Graybill JR, Sobel J, Saag M et al and the NIAID Mycoses Study Group and AIDS Cooperative Treatment Groups 2000 Diagnosis and management of increased intracranial pressure in patients with AIDS and cryptococcal meningitis. *Clinical Infectious Diseases* 30: 47–54.

136. Larsen RA, Bozette S, McCutchan A et al 1989 Persistent *Cryptococcus neoformans* infection of the prostate after successful treatment of meningitis. *Annals of Internal Medicine* 11: 125–128.

137. Bozzette SA, Larsen RA, Chiu J et al 1991 A placebo-controlled trial of maintenance therapy with fluconazole after treatment of cryptococcal meningitis in the acquired immunodeficiency syndrome. *New England Journal of Medicine* 324: 580–584.

138. Powderly WG, Saag MS, Cloud GA et al 1992 A controlled trial of fluconazole or amphotericin B to prevent relapse of cryptococcal meningitis in patients with the acquired immunodeficiency syndrome. *New England Journal of Medicine* 326: 793–798.

139. Chotmongkol V, Sukeepaisarncharoen W 1997 Maintenance therapy with itraconazole after treatment of cryptococcal meningitis in the acquired immunodeficiency syndrome. *Journal of the Medical Association of Thailand* 80: 767–770.

140. Dromer F, Mathoulin S, Dupont B et al 1996 Comparison of the efficacy of amphotericin B and fluconazole in the treatment of cryptococcosis in human immunodeficiency virus-negative patients; retrospective analysis of 83 cases. *Clinical Infectious Diseases* 22: S154–160.

141. Park MK, Hospenthal DR, Bennett JE 1999 Treatment of hydrocephalus secondary to cryptococcal meningitis by use of shunting. *Clinical Infectious Diseases* 28: 629–633.

142. Wheat J, Sarosi G, McKinsey D et al 2000 IDSA practice guidelines for the management of patients with histoplasmosis. *Clinical Infectious Diseases* 30: 688–695.

143. Dismukes WE, Cloud G, Bowles C et al 1985 Treatment of blastomycosis and histoplasmosis with ketoconazole: results of a prospective randomized clinical trial. *Annals of Internal Medicine* 103: 861–872.

144. Sugar AM, Alsip S, Galgiani JN et al 1987 Pharmacology and toxicity of high dose ketoconazole. *Antimicrobial Agents and Chemotherapy* 31: 1874–1878.

145. Negroni R, Palmieri O, Koren F, Tiraboschi IN, Galimberti RL 1987 Oral treatment of paracoccidioidomycosis and histoplasmosis with itraconazole in humans. *Reviews in Infectious Diseases* 9 (Suppl. 1): S47–S50.

146. Dismukes WE, Bradsher RW, Cloud GC et al 1992 Itraconazole therapy for blastomycosis and histoplasmosis. *American Journal of Medicine* 93: 489–497.

147. Wheat J, MaWhinney S, Hafner R et al and the NIAID, AIDS Clinical Trials

Group and Mycoses Study Group 1997 Treatment of histoplasmosis with fluconazole in patients with acquired immunodeficiency syndrome. *American Journal of Medicine* 103: 223–232.

148. Wheat LJ, Batteiger BE, Sathapatayavongs B 1990 *Histoplasma capsulatum* infections of the central nervous system. A clinical review. *Medicine* 69: 244–260.

149. Wheat LJ, Connolly-Stringfield PA, Baker RL et al 1990 Disseminated histoplasmosis in the acquired immune deficiency syndrome: clinical findings, diagnosis and treatment and review of the literature. *Medicine* 69: 361–364.

150. Loyd JE, Tillman BF, Atkinson JB, Des Prez RM 1988 Mediastinal fibrosis complicating histoplasmosis. *Medicine* 67: 295–310.

151. Wheat LJ, Hafner R, Korzun AH et al 1995 Itraconazole treatment of disseminated histoplasmosis in patients with the acquired immunodeficiency syndrome. *American Journal of Medicine* 98: 336–342.

152. Kohler S, Wheat LJ, Connolly P et al 2000 Comparison of the echinocandin caspofungin with amphotericin B for treatment of histoplasmosis following pulmonary challenge in a murine model. *Antimicrobial Agents and Chemotherapy* 44: 1850–1854.

153. Hecht FM, Wheat J, Korzun AH et al 1997 Itraconazole maintenance treatment for histoplasmosis in AIDS: a prospective, multicenter trial. *Journal of Acquired Immune Deficiency Syndrome and Human Retrovirology* 16: 100–107.

154. Galgiani JM, Ampel NM, Catanzaro A, Johnson RH, Stevens DA, Williams PL 2000 Practice guidelines for the treatment of coccidioidomycosis. *Clinical Infectious Diseases* 30: 658–661.

155. Fish DG, Ampel NM, Galgiani JN et al 1990 Coccidioidomycosis during human immunodeficiency virus infection. A review of 77 patients. *Medicine* 69: 384–391.

156. Oldfield EC, Bone WD, Martin CR, Gray GC, Olson P, Schillaci RF 1997 Prediction of relapse after treatment of coccidioidomycosis. *Clinical Infectious Diseases* 25: 1205–1210.

157. Tucker RM, Denning DW, Arathoon EG, Rinaldi MG, Stevens DA 1990 Itraconazole therapy of non-meningeal coccidioidomycosis: clinical and laboratory observations. *Journal of the American Academy of Dermatology* 23: 593–601.

158. Tucker RM, Denning DW, Dupont B, Stevens DA 1990 Itraconazole therapy for chronic coccidioidal meningitis. *Annals of Internal Medicine* 112: 108–112.

159. Tucker RM, Galgiani JN, Denning DW et al 1990 Treatment of coccidioidal meningitis with fluconazole. *Reviews of Infectious Diseases* 12 (Suppl. 3): S380–S389.

160. Williams PL, Johnson R, Pappagianis D et al 1992 Vasculitic and encephalitic complications associated with *Coccidioides immitis* infection of the central nervous system in humans: report of 10 cases and review. *Clinical Infectious Diseases* 14: 673–682.

161. Hall KA, Sethi GK, Rosado LJ, Martinez JD, Huston CL, Copeland JG 1993 Coccidioidomycosis and heart transplantation. *Journal of Heart and Lung Transplantation* 12: 525–526.

162. Baily GG, Robertson VJ, Neill P, Garrido P, Levy LF 1991 Blastomycosis in Africa: clinical features, diagnosis, and treatment. *Reviews of Infectious Diseases* 13: 1005–1008.

163. Meyer KC, McManus EJ, Maki DG 1993 Overwhelming pulmonary blastomycosis associated with the adult respiratory distress syndrome. *New England Journal of Medicine* 329: 1231–1236.

164. Pappas PG 1997 Blastomycosis in the immunocompromised patient. *Seminars in Respiratory Infection* 12: 243–251.

165. Chapman SW, Bradsher RW, Campbell GD Jr, Pappas PG, Kauffman CA 2000 IDSA practice guidelines for the management of patients with blastomycosis. Infectious diseases society of America. *Clinical Infectious Diseases* 30: 679–683.

166. Dietze R, Fowler VG Jr, Steiner TS, Pecanha PM, Corey GR 1999 Failure of amphotericin B colliodal dispersion in the treatment of paracoccidioidomycosis. *American Journal of Tropical Medicine and Hygiene* 60: 837–839.

167. Liratsopulos G, Ellis M, Nerringer R, Denning DW. 2002 Invasive infection due to *Penicillium* species other than *P. marneffei Journal of Infection* 45: 184–195.

168. Supparatpinyo K, Khamwan C, Baosoung V, Nelson KE, Sirisanthana T 1994 Disseminated *Penicillium marneffei* infection in southeast Asia. *Lancet* 344: 110–113.

169. McGinnis MR, Nordoff NG, Ryder NS, Nunn GB 2000 In vitro comparison of terbinafine and itraconazole against *Penicillium marneffei*. *Antimicrobial Agents and Chemotherapy* 44: 1407–1408.

170. Sirisanthana T, Supparatpinyo K, Perriens J, Nelson KE 1998. Amphotericin B

171. Supparatpinyo K, Perriens J, Nelson KE, Sirisanthana T 1998. A controlled trial of itraconazole to prevent relapse of *Penicillium marneffei* infection in patients infected with the human immunodeficiency virus. *New England Journal of Medicine* 24: 1739–1743.

172. Oppenheimer BA, Herbrecht R, Kusne S 1995 The safety and efficacy of amphotericin B colloidal dispersion in the treatment of invasive mycoses. *Clinical Infectious Diseases* 21: 1145–1153.

173. Walsh TJ, Hiemenz JW, Seibel NL et al 1998 Amphotericin B lipid complex for invasive fungal infections: analysis of safety and efficacy in 556 cases. *Clinical Infectious Diseases* 26: 1383–1396.

174. Tedder M, Spratt JA, Anstadt MP, Hedge SS, Tedder SD, Lowe JE 1994 Pulmonary mucormycosis: results of medical and surgical therapy. *Annals of Thoracic Surgery* 57: 1044–1050.

175. Vainrub B, Macareno A, Mandel S, Musher DM 1988 Wound zygomycosis (mucormycosis) in otherwise healthy adults. *American Journal of Medicine* 84: 546–548.

176. Jiang RS, Hsu CY 1999 Endoscopic sinus surgery for rhinocerebral mucormycosis. *American Journal of Rhinology* 2: 105–109.

177. Martino P, Gastaldi R, Raccah R, Girmenia C 1994 Clinical patterns of *Fusarium* infections in immunocompromised patients. *Journal of Infection* 28 (Suppl. 1): 7–15.

178. Idigoras P, Perez-Trallero E, Pineiro L et al 2001 Disseminated infection and colonization by *Scedosporium prolificans*: A review of 18 cases, 1990–1999. *Clinical Infectious Diseases* 32: E158–165.

179. Walsh TJ, Peter J, McGough DA, Fothergill AW, Rinaldi MG, Pizzo PA 1995 Activities of amphotericin B and antifungal azoles alone and in combination against *Pseudallescheria boydii*. *Antimicrobial Agents and Chemotherapy* 39: 1361–1364.

180. Walsh M, White L, Atkinson K, Enno A 1992 Fungal *Pseudallescheria boydii* lung infiltrates unresponsive to amphotericin B in leukaemic patients. *Australian and New Zealand Journal of Medicine* 22: 265–268.

181. Espinel-Ingroff A 2001 In vitro fungicidal activities of voriconazole, itraconazole, and amphotericin B against opportunistic moniliaceous and dematiaceous fungi. *Journal of Clinical Microbiology* 29: 954–958.

182. Berenguer J, Diaz Mediavilla J, Urra D, Munoz P 1989 Central nervous system infection caused by *Pseudalleschria boydii*: case report and reivew. *Reviews of Infectious Diseases* 11: 890–896.

183. Goldberg SL, Geha DJ, Marshall WF, Inwards DJ, Hoagland HC 1993 Successful treatment of simultaneous pulmonary *Pseudallescheria boydii* and *Aspergillus terreus* infection with oral itraconazole. *Clinical Infectious Diseases* 16: 803–806.

184. Nesky MA, McDougal EC, Peacock Jr JE 2000 *Pseudallescheria boydii* brain abscess successfully treated with voriconazole and surgical drainage: case report and literature review of central nervous system pseudallescheriasis. *Clinical Infectious Diseases* 31: 673–677.

185. Meletiadis J, Mouton JW, Meis JF, Verweij PE 2000 Combination chemotherapy for the treatment of invasive infections by *Scedosporium prolificans*. *Clinical Microbiology and Infection* 6: 336–337.

186. Martino P, Venditti M, Micozzi A et al 1990 *Blastoschizomyces capitatus*: an emerging cause of invasive fungal disease in leukemia patients. *Reviews of Infectious Diseases* 12: 570–582.

187. Tashiro T, Nagai H, Kamberi P et al 1994 Disseminated *Trichosporon beigelii* infection in patients with malignant diseases: immunohistochemical study and review. *European Journal of Clinical Microbiology and Infectious Diseases* 13: 218–224.

188. Walsh TJ, Melcher GP, Rinaldi MG et al 1990 *Trichosporon beigelli*, and emerging pathogen resistant to amphotericin B. *Journal of Clinical Microbiology* 28: 1616–1622.

189. Anaissie E, Gokaslan A, Hachem R et al 1992 Azole therapy for trichosporonosis: clinical evaluation of eight patients, experimental therapy for murine infection, and review. *Clinical Infectious Diseases* 15: 781–787.

190. Groll AH, Walsh JJ 2000 Uncommon opportunistic fungi: new nosocomial threats. *Clin Microbiol Infect* 2001; 7 Suppl 2: 8–24. Review.

191. Walsh TJ, Lee JW 1993 Prevention of invasive fungal infections in patients with neoplastic diseases. *Clinical Infectious Diseases* 17 (Suppl. 2): S480–S486.

192. Winston DJ, Chandrasekar PH, Lazarus HM et al 1993 Fluconazole prophylaxis of fungal infections in patients with acute leukemia. *Annals of Internal Medicine* 118: 495–503.

and itraconazole for treatment of disseminated *Penicillium marneffei* infection in human immunodeficiency virus-infected patients. *Clinical Infectious Diseases* 26: 1107–1110.

193. Philpott-Howard JN, Wade JJ, Mutfi GJ, Brammer KW, Ehninger G, Multicentre Study Group 1993 Randomized comparison of oral fluconazole versus oral polyenes for the prevention of fungal infection in patients at risk of neutropenia. *Journal of Antimicrobial Chemotherapy* 31: 973–984.

194. Menichetti F, Del Favero A, Martino P et al 1994 Preventing fungal infection in neutropenic patients with acute leukemia: Fluconazole compared with oral amphotericin B. *Annals of Internal Medicine* 120: 913–918.

195. British Society for Antimicrobial Chemotherapy Working Party on Fungal Infection 1993 Chemoprophylaxis for candidiasis and aspergillosis in neutropenia and transplantation: a review and recommendations. *Journal of Antimicrobial Chemotherapy* 32: 5–21.

196. Menichetti F, Del Favero A, Martino P et al 1999 Itraconazole oral solution as prophylaxis for fungal infections in neutropenic patients with hematologic malignancies: a randomized, placebo-controlled, double-blind, multicenter trial. *Clinical Infectious Diseases* 28: 250–255.

197. Morgenstern GR, Prentice AG, Prentice HG, Ropner JE, Schey SA, Warnock DW. A randomized controlled trial of itraconazole versus fluconazole for the prevention of fungal infections in patients with haematological malignancies UK Multicentre Antifungal Prophylaxis Study Group. *British Journal of Haematology* 1999; 105: 901–911.

198. Glasmacher A, Molitor E, Mezger J et al 1996 Antifungal prophlaxis with itraconazole in neutropenic patients; pharmacological, microbiological and clinical aspects. *Mycoses* 39: 249–58.

199. Denning DW, Marinus A, Cohen J et al and the EORTC Invasive Fungal Infections Cooperative Group 1998 An EORTC multicentre prospective survey of invasive aspergillosis in cancer patients: diagnosis and therapeutic outcome. *Journal of Infection* 37: 173–180.

200. Goodman JL, Winston DJ, Greenfield RA et al 1992 A controlled trial of fluconazole to prevent fungal infections in patients undergoing bone marrow transplantation. *New England Journal of Medicine* 326: 845–851.

201. Marr KA, Seidal K, Slavin MA 2000 Prolonged fluconazole prophylaxis is associated with persistent protection against candidiasis-related death in allogeneic marrow transplant recipients: long-term follow-up of a randomized, placebo-controlled trial. *Blood* 96: 2055–2061.

202. Singh N 2000 Antifungal prophylaxis for solid organ transplant recipients: seeking clarity amidst controversy. *Clinical Infectious Diseases* 31: 545–553.

203. Nadeem I, Yeldandi V, Sheridan P et al 1997 Efficacy of itraconazole prophylaxis for aspergillosis in lung transplant recipients. In: Program and Abstracts of the 32nd Annual Meeting of the Infectious Diseases Society of America (New Orleans), abstract 58A.

204. Monforte V, Roman A, Gavald J, Bravo C, Tenorio L, Ferrer A, Maestre J, Morell F. Nebulized amphotericin B prophylaxis for Aspergillus infection in lung transplantation: study of risk factors. *Journal of Heart and Lung Transplantation* 2001; 20: 1274–1281.

205. Nightingale SD, Cal SX, Peterson DM et al 1992 Primary prophylaxis with fluconazole against systemic fungal infections in HIV-positive patients. *AIDS* 6: 191–194.

206. Powderley WG, Finkelstein D, Feinberg J et al 1995 A randomised trial comparing fluconazole with clotrimazole troches for the prevention of fungal infections in patients with advanced human immunodeficiency virus infection. *New England Journal of Medicine* 332: 700–705.

207. Bernaldo de Quiros JCL, Miro JM, Pena JM et al. 2001 A randomized trial of the discontinuation of primary and secondary prophylaxis against *Pneumocystis carinii* pneumonia after highly active antiretroviral therapy in patients with HIV infection. *New England Journal of Medicine* 344: 159–167.

208. Ledergerber B, Mocroft A, Reiss P et al. 2001 Discontinuation of secondary prophylaxis against *Pneumocystis carinii* pneumonia in patients with HIV infection who have a response to antiretroviral therapy. *New England Journal of Medicine* 344: 168–174.

209. Trikinalos TA, Ioannidis JPA 2001 Discontinuation of *Pneumocystis carinii* prophylaxis in patients infected with human immunodeficiency virus. A meta-analysis and decision analysis. *Clinical Infectious Diseases* 33: 1901–1909.

210. Mouy R, Veber F, Blanche S 1994 Long-term itraconazole prophylaxis against *Aspergillus* infections in thirty-two patients with chronic granulomatous disease. *Journal of Pediatrics* 125: 998–1003.

211. Cale CM, Jones AM, Goldblatt D 2000 Follow up of patients with chronic granulomatous disease diagnosed since 1990. *Clinical and Experimental Immunology* 120: 351–355.

212. Liese J, Kloos S, Jendrossek V et al 2000 Long-term follow-up and outcome of 39 patients with chronic granulomatous disease. *Journal of Pediatrics* 137: 687–693.

213. Eggimann P, Francioli P, Bille J et al 1999 Fluconazole prophylaxis prevents intra-abdominal candidiasis in high-risk surgical patients. *Critical Care Medicine* 27: 1033–1034.

214. Kaufman D, Boyle R, Hazen KC et al 2001 Fluconazole prophylaxis against fungal colonization and infection in preterm infants. *New England Journal of Medicine* 345: 1660–1666.

215. Pizzo PA, Robichaud KJ, Gill FA, Witebsky FG 1982 Empiric antibiotic and antifungal therapy for cancer patients with prolonged fever and granulocytopenia *American Journal of Medicine* 72: 101–111.

216. Empiric antifungal therapy in febrile granulocytopenic patients. EORTC International Antimicrobial Therapy Cooperative Group 1989 *American Journal of Medicine* 86: 668–672.

217. Cometta A, Calandra T, Gaya H et al 1996. Monotherapy with meropenem versus combination therapy with ceftazidime plus amikacin as empiric therapy for fever in granulocytopenic patients with cancer. *Antimicrobial Agents and Chemotherapy* 40: 1108–1115.

218. White MH, Bowden RA, Sandler ES et al 1998 Randomized, double-blind clinical trial of amphotericin B colloidal dispersion vs. amphotericin B in the empirical treatment of fever and neutropenia. *Clinical Infectious Diseases* 27: 296–302.

 Further information

Sepkowitz KA 2002 Opportunistic infections in patients with and patients without acquired immunodeficiency syndrome. *Clinical Infectious Diseases* 34: 1098–1107.

United States Public Health Service/Infectious Diseases Society of America Prevention of Opportunistic Infections Working Group 2000 1999 USPHS/IDSA guidelines for the prevention of opportunistic infections in persons infected with human immunodeficiency virus. *Clinical Infectious Diseases* 30 (Suppl. 1): S29–65.

Weller IVD, Williams IG 2001 ABC of AIDS. Treatment of infections. *British Medical Journal* 322: 1350–1354.

63 Zoonoses

R. N. Davidson and A. Bjöersdorff

BRUCELLOSIS

Worldwide about 500 000 human cases of brucellosis occur annually.[1] The responsible species are, in order of importance: *Brucella melitensis* (the animal hosts are goat, sheep and camels), *Brucella abortus* (cattle, buffalo, camels), *Brucella suis* (pig and reindeer), *Brucella ovis* (sheep) and *Brucella canis* (dogs). Brucellae are shed in large numbers in milk, urine and products of conception of infected animals, and humans are infected by direct contact with infected animals or, more commonly, by ingestion of unpasteurized milk or milk products. In humans the disease may be acute or chronic, though it is no longer a fashionable etiology of chronic fatigue syndromes. About 50% of cases are subclinical, and seropositive patients with no clinical disease generally need to be observed but do not need treatment. Central nervous system (CNS) brucellosis and brucella endocarditis are rare, but particularly difficult to treat.[2]

ANTIBIOTIC THERAPY – DRUG COMBINATIONS

Three principles have emerged from clinical and animal studies in relation to treatment.

1. Although *Brucella* species are extremely sensitive to many antimicrobial agents in conventional assays, such tests often do not predict clinical efficacy – for example, ceftriaxone has good in-vitro activity against *Brucella*; a dose of 2 g/day produced an initial clinical response in only 2 of 8 patients, and one of these relapsed.[3]
2. Prolonged treatment with a combination of agents is required – single-agent therapy has high relapse rates. It is unclear whether drug combinations provide synergy, prevent resistance, or act against different subpopulations of brucellae; none the less, combinations are far more effective than single agents.
3. Therapy of brucellosis is complicated by the location of the

organism within an acid compartment in reticuloendothelial cells, where optimal concentrations and effects of antibiotics are difficult to achieve. Regimens should thus include at least one agent with good intracellular penetration.[4]

For all regimens initial response rates are higher than long-term cure rates because relapses occur with all regimens. Relapses should be confirmed bacteriologically, as *Brucella* serology will remain positive in successfully treated patients as well as relapses. Relapses usually occur within the first 6 months, but can be as long as 2 years after apparently successful treatment. Nearly all relapses will respond to a repeated course of treatment.

Doxycycline remains central to combination treatments for brucellosis minimum inhibitory concentrations (MICs) of tetracycline for *Brucella* are generally <1 mg/l. Aminoglycosides are synergistic with doxycycline, and the combination of intramuscular streptomycin 1 g/day for the initial 14 days of treatment, followed by doxycycline 200 mg/day for 6 weeks has been thoroughly evaluated in at least nine clinical trials. Initial response rates are *c.* 98%, and relapse rates of 0–8% are found.[4] Combinations of doxycycline with gentamicin 5 mg/kg/day[4] or netilmicin are also effective, and if therapeutic drug levels can be monitored more easily with these, they should be chosen in preference to streptomycin. While the duration of aminoglycoside treatment can be reduced to below 14 days, the overall duration of treatment should not be less than 45 days.

MICs of rifampicin are ≤1 mg/l, yet rifampicin monotherapy is unsatisfactory. The regimen of choice recommended by the World Health Organization (WHO) Expert Committee on Brucellosis is doxycycline 200 mg/day plus rifampicin 600–900 mg/day for ≥6 weeks.[5] However, a meta-analysis of eight trials (total enrolled = 1059 patients) that compared rifampicin–doxycycline with streptomycin–doxycycline found the rifampicin-containing regimen to have a higher relapse rate (17% vs. 5%).[4] It is not clear whether longer courses of rifampicin–doxycycline would be more effective, or if the relapse rate could be reduced if a third agent were added.

Trimethoprim–sulfamethoxazole used as monotherapy for 6 weeks has a very high relapse rate.[6] This can be reduced by extending treatment for 3–6 months, or by combining it with doxycycline, rifampicin, or an aminoglycoside.[7] The quinolones, especially ofloxacin, have excellent bactericidal activity against *Brucella* spp. and penetrate neutrophils and macrophages. Ofloxacin alone has a very high failure rate, but in a small study rifampicin plus ofloxacin was better tolerated than rifampicin plus doxycycline, and the relapse rate of 3% was identical.[8] The combination of rifampicin and ciprofloxacin has also been studied in a small group of patients, with an 85% cure rate.[9] Because of the scarcity of data on rifampicin–ofloxacin, this combination cannot yet be recommended.

CHILDREN WITH BRUCELLOSIS

As tetracyclines are contraindicated in children under 8 years old a combination of trimethoprim–sulfamethoxazole and rifampicin is preferred. The recommended regimen is 45 days of trimethoprim–sulfamethoxazole 60–72 mg/kg daily plus rifampicin 15–20 mg/kg daily, both given as divided doses. This regimen has been highly effective: only 4 of 113 children relapsed, and all the relapsed patients responded to repeat therapy with the same agents.[10] An alternative regimen for children is 45 days of rifampicin plus gentamicin 5–6 mg/kg daily for the first 5 days.[7]

TREATMENT OF BRUCELLOSIS DURING PREGNANCY AND LACTATION

Early diagnosis and adequate treatment of brucellosis in pregnancy is necessary to reduce the risk of miscarriage, premature birth and stillbirth. Tetracyclines should be avoided in pregnancy and breast-feeding, and streptomycin has been associated with fetal eighth nerve damage.[11] A suitable regimen for pregnant and lactating women is trimethoprim–sulfamethoxazole plus rifampicin.

BRUCELLA SPONDYLITIS

Suppurating lesions of the vertebral column occur in brucellosis, and patients with *Brucella* spondylitis have a higher relapse rate.[6] The duration of antimicrobial therapy may need to be up to 18 months, according to clinical response and the presence of epidural and paravertebral masses.[1] As with other bacterial infections, abscesses due to *Brucella* should be surgically drained whenever possible.

NEUROBRUCELLOSIS

Involvement of the CNS is best treated with a combination of three or more drugs. Of note, doxycycline crosses the blood–brain barrier better than generic tetracycline.

Neurobrucellosis has been treated with combinations of streptomycin, doxycycline, rifampicin and trimethoprim–sulfamethoxazole, but, despite this, the clinical sequelae may be severe.[2] The duration of treatment should be at least 8–12 weeks.[12] Steroids may prevent early clinical deterioration following the commencement of antibiotics.[13]

BRUCELLA ENDOCARDITIS

In cases of *Brucella* endocarditis, surgical removal of the valve may be necessary for hemodynamic reasons. The best prospect of cure without surgery seems to be with a combination of three or more effective agents, chosen from among streptomycin (or another aminoglycoside), doxycycline, rifampicin, ofloxacin or ciprofloxacin. Treatment should be continued for a year or more.[14–16]

BRUCELLOSIS IN PATIENTS INFECTED WITH HIV

Twelve patients with brucellosis and HIV coinfection have been reported from Spain; all were cured by the combination of doxycycline and streptomycin.[17]

ANTHRAX

Bacillus anthracis is a large, Gram-positive, non-motile, spore-forming rod. The three virulence factors of *B. anthracis* are edema toxin, lethal toxin and a capsular antigen. Anthrax is considered as likely for use in acts of biological terrorism.[18] *B. anthracis* causes acute infection in wild and domestic herbivores, and 4000–8000 human cases worldwide annually,[19] with occasional epidemics.

Human anthrax has three major clinical forms: cutaneous, inhalation, and gastrointestinal. Cutaneous anthrax is a result of introduction of the spore through the skin; inhalation anthrax, through the respiratory tract; and gastrointestinal anthrax by ingestion. Human cutaneous infections follow contact with anthrax spores on animal hair or hides, either in an industrial or agricultural setting. More rarely, spores may be inhaled or ingested, causing respiratory and gastrointestinal anthrax.

If untreated, anthrax in all forms can lead to septicemia and death. Early treatment of cutaneous anthrax is usually curative, and early treatment of all forms is important for recovery. Patients with gastrointestinal anthrax have reported case fatality rates ranging from 25% to 75%.[20]

PROPHYLAXIS

An anthrax vaccine has been licensed for use in humans (BioPort, Corporation, Lansing, Michigan), and guidelines for its use are available on-line (www.cdc.gov/mmwr/preview/mmwrhtml/rr4915a1.htm). The vaccine is reported to be 93% effective in protecting against anthrax. Because anthrax is considered to be a potential agent for use in biological warfare, the vaccine is offered in some countries to military personnel who might be involved in conflict. On the basis of studies in animal models, the US Food and Drug Administration has approved the use of ciprofloxacin following aerosol exposure to *B. anthracis* spores to prevent development or progression of inhalation anthrax.

TREATMENT OF ANTHRAX

In vitro, 44 isolates of *B. anthracis* from wild game were highly susceptible to ampicillin, streptomycin, chloramphenicol, erythromycin, tetracycline, methicillin and netilmicin. More than 90% of the isolates were sensitive to clindamycin, gentamicin and cefoxitin. Only 84.1% of the isolates were highly sensitive to penicillin G, the remainder being moderately sensitive. There was complete resistance to trimethoprim–sulfamethoxazole.[21] Naturally occurring *B. anthracis* resistance to penicillin is rare, but has been reported; no naturally occurring resistance to tetracyclines or ciprofloxacin has been seen.

Cutaneous anthrax is rarely fatal if treated with intravenous penicillin G 12 g/day for 10–12 days. Patients who are allergic to penicillin should be treated with erythromycin, tetracycline or chloramphenicol.[22,23] Surgical debridement of the black, necrotic eschar is contraindicated. Systemic steroids have been used for the extensive edema, but their efficacy is unproven.

Pulmonary anthrax is frequently fatal, but survival is possible with early antibiotic treatment and intensive pulmonary and circulatory support. Corticosteroids may be useful but have not been adequately evaluated. If treatment is delayed (usually because the diagnosis is missed), death, caused by the anthrax toxin, is likely. Antibiotic resistance to beta lactams and tetracyclines should be assumed following a terrorist attack until laboratory testing demonstrates otherwise. The recommended empiric treatment for adults with suspected or proven pulmonary anthrax is intravenous ciprofloxacin 400 mg 12 hourly; for children the regimen is intravenous ciprofloxacin 10–15 mg/kg 12 hourly. If the organism is shown to be sensitive, treatment can later be changed to high dose IV penicillin or doxycycline. Risk for recurrence remains for at least 60 days because of the possibility of delayed germination of spores. Therefore, antibiotics should be continued for 60 days, with oral therapy replacing intravenous therapy when conditions improve.

ANIMAL BITES

About 85% of dog, cat and other animal bites become infected with either animal oral flora or human skin flora. Infected bites are usually polymicrobial, even if a single species is cultured – in a recent study, a median of 5 (range 0–16) species were isolated from infected dog and cat bites. Aerobes are present in most wounds, and anaerobes often accompany these. *Pasteurella* species are the most common isolates from both dog bites (50%) and cat bites (75%) – *Pasteurella canis* predominates from dog bites, and *Pasteurella multocida* from cat bites. Other common aerobes include streptococci, *Staphylococcus aureus*, *Staphylococcus intermedius*, *Moraxella* spp., *Neisseria* spp., *Capnocytophaga canimorsus* (formerly called 'dysgonic fermenter 2' (DF2)), and *Eikenella corrodens*. Common anaerobes include *Fusobacterium*, *Bacteroides*, *Porphyromonas*, and *Prevotella* spp.[24]

TREATMENT AND PROPHYLAXIS OF INFECTED ANIMAL BITES

The wound should be cleansed and debrided, and tetanus, rabies and antimicrobial prophylaxis should be considered.[25] The following bite wounds warrant antimicrobial prophylaxis:

- moderate or severe injuries <8 h old (most infections present clinically >8 h after the bite);
- possible bone or joint penetration;
- face, genital and hand wounds;
- bites suffered by patients with underlying illness such as liver disease or local conditions such as limb edema or prosthetic joints.

Amoxicillin–clavulanic acid has good activity against these organisms, and is the best choice both for prophylaxis of infection-prone bites and for empirical treatment of infected bites before the results of cultures become available. Trimethoprim–sulfamethoxazole may substitute for amoxicillin–clavulanic acid if the patient is allergic to amoxicillin, although clinical efficacy data are lacking. Prophylaxis for 3–5 days should suffice; treatment of established infections should be more prolonged, and punctures over or near a joint observed carefully for osteomyelitis or septic arthritis. Prophylaxis with amoxicillin–clavulanic acid will, incidentally, prevent rat-bite fever, though trimethoprim–sulfamethoxazole will not. Patients who have had a splenectomy or who have functional asplenia should always receive antibiotic prophylaxis because of the risk of overwhelming postsplenctomy sepsis with *Capnocytophaga canimorsus* and other organisms.

RAT-BITE FEVER

The term 'rat-bite fever' refers to two similar diseases caused by different Gram-negative facultative anaerobes: streptobacillary rat-bite fever, caused by infection with *Streptobacillus moniliformis* (a pleomorphic Gram-negative bacillus), and spirochetal rat-bite fever, caused by *Spirillum minus* (a short, thick Gram-negative spirochete with darting motility). Both organisms are common inhabitants of the pharynx of wild, pet, and laboratory rats in all parts of the world. Humans usually acquire the disease through the bite of a rat, though a history of a bite is sometimes absent in *S. moniliformis* infections, which may be acquired by oral ingestion.[26] Cases of *S. moniliformis* rat-bite fever have been associated with the bites of mice, squirrels, gerbils, and exposure to animals that prey on these rodents (e.g. cats and dogs). Sporadic cases have been reported in children who lived in rat-infested dwellings. Ingestion of food or water potentially contaminated with rat feces can also result in *S. moniliformis* bacteremia (i.e. Haverhill fever). Sometimes Haverhill fever is seen in food- or milk-borne outbreaks.[27] Both organisms are susceptible to penicillin.

Prophylaxis against rat-bite fever

Infections due to *Sp. minus* or *S. moniliformis* should, in theory, be adequately prevented by a 3-day course of penicillin 500 mg 6-hourly or doxycycline 100 mg/day; however, the efficacy of prophylaxis has not been assessed in clinical practice.

Streptobacillus moniliformis infection

The onset of rat-bite fever caused by *S. moniliformis* is usually 2–10 (range 1–22) days after the bite of a rat. The clinical syndrome is characterized by irregularly relapsing fever and asymmetric polyarthritis followed within 2–4 days by a maculopapular rash of the extremities, palms, and soles. The wound from the bite heals spontaneously. Headache, nausea, vomiting, myalgia, minimal regional lymphadenopathy, anemia, endocarditis, myocarditis, meningitis, pneumonia, and focal abscesses have been reported. Most cases resolve spontaneously within 2 weeks, but 13% of untreated cases are fatal. Uncomplicated *S. moniliformis* infection may be treated with intramuscular or intravenous benzylpenicillin for 5–7 days, followed by oral penicillin for 7 days. Mild cases can be treated with oral penicillin alone. Other appropriate therapies include tetracycline and streptomycin. Although other antibiotics (erythromycin, chloramphenicol, clindamycin, and cephalosporins) have been used with some success, the effectiveness of these agents has not been assessed rigorously[28] and erythromycin may fail.[29]

Complications such as septic arthritis, meningitis and pneumonia require more intensive treatment with intravenous penicillin. Endocarditis due to *S. moniliformis* is rare, and generally occurs on previously damaged valves. It will probably respond to standard regimens used to treat endocarditis caused by other penicillin-sensitive organisms.[30,31]

Spirillum minus infection

Sp. minus rat-bite fever occurs worldwide, but is most common in Asia where it is known as sodoku. The incubation period is longer (1–3 weeks), arthralgia is rare, and the bite wound which may reappear at the onset of symptoms or persist with edema and ulceration. *Sp. minus* is highly sensitive to penicillin, may be given intravenously, intramuscularly, or orally according to the clinical situation. Initiation of treatment may be followed by the Jarisch–Herxheimer reaction.

TULAREMIA

Tularemia is a plague-like zoonosis occurring occasionally in Europe (excluding the UK), North America and the former USSR, where it is enzootic in a large number of animal species.[19] The causative organism, *Francisella tularensis*, an extremely virulent Gram-negative coccobacillus, infects humans either by direct animal contact or by bites from ticks or biting flies that have fed on infected animals. Infection may also occur through aerosol inhalation, contamination of mucus membranes or ingestion of bacteria. Six clinical syndromes of tularemia are recognized: ulceroglandular, glandular, oculoglandular, oropharyngeal, typhoidal and pulmonary. Rare complications of tularemia include meningitis, pericarditis, and endocarditis.[32]

TREATMENT OF TULAREMIA

Streptomycin is the antibiotic of choice,[33] at a dose of 7.5–15 mg/kg intramuscularly 12-hourly for 7–14 days, the higher doses being used for more severe illness. A case of tularemic meningitis has been treated successfully with the combination of streptomycin and tetracycline given for 1 week, followed by tetracycline alone for an additional 2 weeks.[34] Gentamicin is an acceptable alternative to streptomycin; the recommended dose is 3–5 mg/kg daily in divided doses.[35,36] Cases of tularemia have also been treated with chloramphenicol and imipenem.[37,38]

Ciprofloxacin and, to a lesser extent, ofloxacin, and pefloxacin, have good in-vitro activity against *F. tularensis*. Many patients have been successfully treated with quinolones: ciprofloxacin 750 mg 12-hourly, and levofloxacin 500 mg daily.[38,39]

Tetracycline treatment for *F. tularensis* has an unacceptable relapse rate.[40] Although ceftriaxone has excellent in-vitro activity against *F. tularensis*, it fails in clinical practice.[41]

PLAGUE

Plague is caused by a bipolar staining Gram-negative bacillus, *Yersinia pestis*. A disease of worldwide distribution, plague is epizootic and enzootic in many urban and rural areas. In the bubonic form, humans are infected by the bite of an infected flea. From the infected lymph nodes the infection may spread, and death is caused by overwhelming septicemia. Patients with pulmonary involvement may transmit the disease as pneumonic plague; rare forms such as plague meningitis or pharyngitis may also occur.[42]

The true frequency of human plague is uncertain, because underreporting is likely, as well as wrong attribution of outbreaks of pneumonic or septicemic illness to plague without confirmation by culture.[43] Official estimates are of about 1000 human cases worldwide annually.[19]

PROPHYLAXIS OF PLAGUE

Household contacts of patients with bubonic plague, and casual or close contacts of a patient with pneumonic plague, should receive chemoprophylaxis for 7 days after their last exposure with tetracycline 250 mg 6-hourly, doxycycline 100 mg/day or trimethoprim–sulfamethoxazole 480 mg 12-hourly. Babies and pregnant women in the first trimester should take amoxicillin. While older children should take doxycycline, those under 8 years of age should take trimethoprim–sulfamethoxazole. Standby or prophylactic 7-day courses of the same drugs are recommended for travelers visiting areas where a plague outbreak is confirmed or suspected.

Plague vaccine is available, but is only partially protective.

TREATMENT OF PLAGUE

Untreated bubonic plague has a case fatality rate of >50%, whilst pneumonic and septicemic forms are invariably fatal without treatment.[43] Treatment reduces this dramatically, the critical factor being early initiation of antibiotic treatment. When 28 patients were treated in a well-equipped hospital, 6 deaths occurred: 3 of 8 cases of pneumonic plague and 3 of 19 cases of bubonic plague. All the fatalities were attributed to a failure to treat initially with an antibiotic appropriate for plague.[44]

Plague has an incubation period of 2–8 days, and has been reported in travelers who have returned recently from a plague-endemic area (including both tropical and temperate zones).[45]

Nearly all strains of Y. pestis are susceptible to streptomycin, tetracycline, chloramphenicol, ampicillin, cephalotin and trimethoprim–sulfamethoxazole. Drug resistance seems to be rare; Marshall et al[46] found only 2 of 156 strains resistant to streptomycin, and none was resistant to tetracycline or chloramphenicol. There is thus no rationale for the use of multiple antibiotics to treat plague. The drug of choice (except for plague meningitis) is streptomycin, at a dose of 30 mg/kg daily in two divided doses, intramuscularly for 10 days.[42,47] Treatment has reduced mortality from 40–90% to 5–18%.[47] Although combined treatment with streptomycin and tetracycline is often recommended, there is little evidence that these two drugs are more effective than streptomycin alone. Alternative regimens are tetracycline 2–4 g/day in four doses for 10 days, or chloramphenicol 4 g/day (60 mg/kg daily) in divided doses for 10 days, following an initial loading dose of 25 mg/kg.[42] Plague meningitis should be treated with chloramphenicol. It is probable that other antibiotics might be effective in plague: the most active injectable drugs in vitro against Y. pestis are cefotaxime and ceftriaxone; among oral agents, ciprofloxacin, levofloxacin and ofloxacin are highly active, MICs typically being <0.03 mg/l.[48,49]

In addition to antibiotics, patients with plague will often require intensive care for septicemic shock. There is no evidence that corticosteroids are beneficial. Patients with any form of plague should be maintained in strict isolation for the first 48 h after initiation of treatment. Relapses after treatment are very uncommon.

BARTONELLA–ASSOCIATED INFECTIONS

At least six *Bartonella* species cause human disease. Most are transmitted by ectoparasites.

- *Bartonella bacilliformis* (transmitted by sandflies) causes bartonellosis (Carrion's disease).
- *Bartonella henselae* causes cat-scratch disease, peliosis hepatis, and bacillary angiomatosis.
- *Bartonella quintana* (transmitted by the body louse) causes trench fever, endocarditis, bacillary angiomatosis and chronic or recurrent bacteremia.
- *Bartonella vinsonii*, isolated from blood of small rodents.
- *Bartonella elizabethae* (*Rattus* rats have been shown to be a reservoir), causes endocarditis.
- *Bartonella clarridgeiae* (isolated from blood of 5% of pet cats and 17% of stray cats) may be responsible for some cases of cat-scratch disease.

Available data on treatment of *Bartonella*-associated infections remain relatively sparse but would suggest that erythromycin or doxycycline provide the best responses for all the species.[50] Culture of *Bartonella* is difficult, as the bacteria are extremely fastidious. Though apparently sensitive to many antibiotics in vitro, treatment failures with β-lactams, trimethoprim–sulfamethoxazole and quinolones have occurred in immunocompromised patients.

BARTONELLOSIS (CARRION'S DISEASE)

B. bacilliformis, a Gram-negative obligate aerobic organism, is limited to the Andean river valleys of Peru and Ecuador. In these foci the *Lutzomyia* sandfly vector exists, and 5–10% of the population may be asymptomatic blood carriers, or have chronic hemangiomatous lesions (verruga peruana). The disease also occurs as an acute malaria-like illness with severe hemolytic anemia (Oroya fever). In more than 50% of acute cases, blood films show bartonellae adherent to erythrocytes or within macrophages.[51] Oroya fever may be fatal, particularly if complicated by salmonellosis, tuberculosis or other infections, or it may gradually resolve spontaneously, with the development of a chronic cutaneous phase (verruga peruana) over weeks to months. Oroya fever responds well to penicillin, streptomycin or chloramphenicol.[51,52] Antibiotics are less effective in treating verruga peruana or chronic asymptomatic carriers. It is possible that wild rodents are reservoirs of B. bacilliformis and chickens the amplification hosts.[51]

BARTONELLA HENSELAE – CAT-SCRATCH DISEASE, BACILLARY ANGIOMATOSIS, PELIOSIS HEPATIS, LYMPHADENITIS

B. henselae (formerly *Rochalimaea henselae*) is a small Gram-negative rod, which causes several syndromes that sometimes overlap. *B. henselae* causes cat-scratch disease but, like *B. quintana* (*see below*) also causes a wide range of clinical diseases including bacillary angiomatosis, peliosis hepatis, lymphadenitis, bacteremia, and aseptic meningitis. The immune status of the host determines the disease expression. In immunocompetent hosts the pathologic response is granulomatous, suppurative, extracellular and intracellular, generally self-limited and usually not altered by antibiotic treatment. In contrast, in immunocompromised hosts the organisms induce vasculoproliferation, and organisms may be seen intracellularly or in abundance in extracellular clumps. In immunocompromised hosts infection is usually severe, and response to suitable antibiotics dramatic.

B. henselae causes asymptomatic bacteremia in 20–40% of asymptomatic domestic cats.[53,54] Infection is linked to ownership of cats, particularly kittens less than a year old. Though the mode of transmission is unproven, cat scratches and bites, as well as flea or tick bites, are implicated. In cat-scratch disease, the benign lymphadenitis will resolve spontaneously during about 3 months.

Antimicrobials are generally unnecessary, but a 5-day course of azithromycin has been shown to hasten resolution of lymphadenitis.[55] In immunocompetent patients with systemic symptoms a 2–4 week course of erythromycin or doxycycline is recommended,[56] but occasional cases of unresponsiveness and relapse, requiring several combinations of antimicrobials, have been documented.[57] The Etest (*see* Ch. 9) shows that *B. henselae* has high in-vitro susceptibility to erythromycin, azithromycin, doxycycline and rifampicin.[58]

Complicated *B. henselae* infections

Occasional patients may have complicated cat-scratch disease, with the infection spreading beyond regional lymph nodes to involve the vertebral column. These patients respond to prolonged combinations of gentamicin, rifampicin and trimethoprim–sulfamethoxazole.[59] *B. henselae* may cause encephalitis with fits in children.[54] There is also evidence that *B. henselae* infections, and cat ownership, are linked to some cases of HIV-associated dementia.[60]

BARTONELLA QUINTANA – TRENCH FEVER, BACILLARY ANGIOMATOSIS, PELIOSIS HEPATIS

B. quintana (formerly *Rochalimaea quintana*) causes trench fever, a disease extensively reported during the World Wars. The organism is now also known to cause fever and bacteremia, endocarditis, bacillary angiomatosis, and chronic lymphadenopathy. HIV-infected patients and homeless people are vulnerable to infection. The body louse is the vector.[61]

In immunocompromised patients, untreated bacillary angiomatosis with or without dissemination will be progressive and potentially fatal. Doxycycline 100 mg 12-hourly or erythromycin 500 mg 6-hourly are the drugs of choice. Cutaneous lesions should begin to resolve in 4–7 days, and should have completely resolved after 4 weeks of treatment. Treatment should continue for 3 months or for as long as the underlying immunosuppressive condition lasts.[56]

LEPTOSPIROSIS

Pathogenic leptospires all belong to the species *Leptospira interrogans*; serovar *canicola* is most frequent in the USA and Europe, and *icterohaemorrhagiae* most commonly causes the severe form (Weil's disease). Leptospirosis is primarily a disease of wild and domestic animals, which may asymptomatically pass large numbers of leptospires in their urine. Humans are infected mainly due to occupational or recreational contact with contaminated surface water, commonly during the summer. In endemic areas seroprevalence is 5–10%,[19] and travel-associated leptospirosis can often be diagnosed in febrile travelers when serology is performed.[62] Rats are the most common source of human infection in developing countries, and dogs and livestock in industrialized countries. *Leptospira* may enter the body through cut or abraded skin, mucus membranes, and conjunctivae. The acute generalized illness may mimic other tropical diseases (e.g. dengue fever, malaria, and typhus) and common symptoms include fever, chills, myalgia, nausea, diarrhea, and conjunctivitis. Manifestations of severe disease may include jaundice, renal failure, hemorrhage, and shock.

PROPHYLAXIS OF LEPTOSPIROSIS

Doxycycline 200 mg once weekly was tested against placebo in 940 American soldiers undergoing 3 weeks of jungle training in Panama.[63] One of 469 men (0.2%) receiving doxycycline and 20 of 471 (4.2%) receiving placebo developed leptospirosis, a prophylactic efficacy of 95%. Leptospirosis developed after a prolonged incubation period of 40 days in a laboratory technician, who received a single dose of a triple penicillin formulation (benzathine penicillin, procaine penicillin and benzylpenicillin) within 1 h after exposure in a laboratory accident,[64] suggesting that amoxicillin or ampicillin might be ineffective as prophylaxis.

Physicians may be asked to advise on prophylaxis for cave explorers, canoeists, etc., who have ingested potentially infected water, as many clubs issue their members with cards warning about leptospirosis. Only 29–48 cases were reported annually in England and Wales during the period 1990–1992.[65] Physicians may yet feel obliged to prescribe a prophylactic drug, such as doxycycline 200 mg/day for 3 days, bearing in mind that this schedule has not been assessed for efficacy.

TREATMENT OF LEPTOSPIROSIS

Doxycycline 100 mg 12-hourly for 7 days, started within 3 days of the onset of symptoms, was more effective than placebo in 29 American soldiers.[66] The illness was shortened by 2 days, and leptospiruria did not develop. In moderately or severely ill patients, intravenous benzylpenicillin 1.2 g for 5–7 days should be used, even if the patient has been ill for several days. Watt et al[67] evaluated the effect of a 7-day course of intravenous penicillin on severe advanced leptospirosis in a randomized placebo-controlled double-blind trial involving 42 patients, all but one of whom had been ill for at least 5 days. Duration of fever, duration of renal impairment, hospital stay and duration of leptospiruria were all decreased by treatment with penicillin. Thus, treatment with penicillin is effective in leptospirosis, even when therapy begins late in the course of the disease. Intravenous ampicillin 1 g 6-hourly or cefotaxime are alternatives to penicillin, though clinical data are lacking. Chloramphenicol is ineffective in both experimental and human infections.

The Jarisch–Herxheimer reaction may occur 4–6 h after initiation of penicillin therapy in some patients.[68]

LYME BORRELIOSIS

Lyme borreliosis is a multisystem disorder caused by spirochetes of the *Borrelia burgdorferi* complex. The vectors are ticks of the genus *Ixodes*: *Ixodes ricinus* in Europe, *Ixodes dammini* (also called *I. scapularis*) and *Ixodes pacificus* in the USA. Lyme borreliosis is considered endemic in the USA, Canada, large areas of Europe and northern Asia: about 15 000 cases of are reported every year in the USA.[69] The transmission season is summer.

Lyme borreliosis is characterized in one third of cases by erythema migrans, spreading from the site of a tick bite 3–22 days earlier. As *B. burgdorferi* disseminates throughout the body a variety of systemic symptoms can occur, including secondary skin lesions, fever, headache and myalgia. Late complications, including arthritis, neurologic abnormalities and myocardial conduction defects, occur fairly frequently. The diagnosis is based on tick exposure, clinical features, and either serological tests or culture of *B. burgdorferi* from biopsies. In the first few weeks of infection, only 20–30% of patients are seropositive by enzyme-linked immunosorbent assay or Western blot; after a month the majority are seropositive.[70]

Following effective antibiotic treatment, IgM or IgG antibodies may remain detectable for years, but their persistence does not imply active infection.[71] In endemic areas, up to 25% of people may be seropositive, mostly without a history of symptomatic Lyme borreliosis.[72]

PROPHYLAXIS OF LYME BORRELIOSIS

The relative cost-effectiveness of postexposure treatment of tick bites to avoid Lyme borreliosis in endemic areas is dependent on the probability of *B. burgdorferi* infection after a tick bite. In most circumstances, treating persons for tick bite alone is not recommended.[73,74] People who are bitten by a tick should remove it promptly and seek medical attention if any signs and symptoms of early Lyme disease, ehrlichiosis, or babesiosis develop during the ensuring days or weeks. A physician may, none the less, prescribe prophylaxis for patients with a history of tick bite if follow-up of the patient cannot be assured, or to satisfy patients' expectations, as many patients are aware that chronic joint and neurological involvement does not respond consistently to antimicrobials. In highly endemic areas, >3% of tick bites are followed by Lyme disease,[75] and prophylaxis is recommended.

A single dose of doxycycline 200 mg is highly effective,[75] although longer courses of amoxicillin, erythromycin, or cefuroxime axetil are also effective. *B. burgdorferi* is resistant in vitro to rifampicin, ciprofloxacin and aminoglycosides.

A Lyme vaccine available in the USA is not expected to be effective in Europe because of variations within the *B. burgdorferi* strains.[70] European vaccine development is under way.

TREATMENT OF LYME BORRELIOSIS

The treatment of Lyme borreliosis has been extensively studied and comprehensive guidelines are available.[76,77] These are also available on-line (www.journals.uchicago.edu/CID/journal/issues/v31nS1/000342/000342.html). Treatment of pregnant women is identical to that of non-pregnant patients with the same disease manifestation, except that tetracyclines should be avoided. Children under 8 years old should not be treated with doxycycline because of the risk of discoloration of the teeth.

Treatment of early Lyme borreliosis

Doxycycline (100 mg twice daily) or amoxicillin (500 mg 3 times daily) for 14–21 days is recommended for treatment of early localized or early disseminated Lyme borreliosis associated with erythema migrans (in the absence of neurological involvement or third-degree atrioventricular heart block).[78] Doxycycline has the advantage of being effective against human granulocytic ehrlichiosis, which is transmitted by the same ticks. An effective alternative is cefuroxime axetil (500 mg orally twice daily). Children under 8 should receive amoxicillin 50 mg/kg/day divided into three doses (maximum 500 mg/dose); over 8 years old they should receive doxycycline 112 mg/kg twice per day (maximum, 100 mg/dose) or cefuroxime axetil, 30 mg/kg daily, divided into two doses (maximum 500 mg/dose).[79]

Treatment of acute Lyme borreliosis with neurologic or cardiac involvement

Acute neurological disease (meningitis or radiculopathy) or third-degree atrioventricular block is best treated with ceftriaxone (intravenous; 2 g once daily for 14–28 days), alternatives being intravenous benzylpenicillin at a dosage of 18–24 million units (10.8–14.4 g) daily (in six divided doses) or intravenous cefotaxime (2 g every 8 h). Characteristics of ceftriaxone, which may contribute to its effectiveness, are its long half-life, greater activity against *B. burgdorferi* in vitro and the high microbicidal concentrations achieved in the brain and cerebrospinal fluid.[80] For patients with isolated facial palsy, and for adults who are intolerant of both penicillin and cephalosporins, doxycycline (200–400 mg/day) in two divided doses given orally (or intravenously if the patient is unable to take oral medications) for 14–28 days may be adequate.[81] For children, the best recommendation is ceftriaxone (75–100 mg/kg daily) in a single daily intravenous dose (maximum 2 g) or cefotaxime (150–200 mg/kg daily) divided into three or four intravenous doses (maximum 6 g/day) or penicillin G (200 000–400 000 units/kg–[120–240 mg/kg] daily; maximum 18–24 million units/day [10.8–14.4 g/day]), intravenously in six divided doses.

Treatment of Lyme arthritis

Lyme arthritis without neurologic involvement can usually be treated successfully with doxycycline (100 mg twice daily orally) or amoxicillin (500 mg three times daily) for 28 days. Patients who have persistent or recurrent joint swelling after recommended courses of antibiotic therapy should be re-treated with another 4-week course of oral antibiotics or with a 2–4-week course of intravenous ceftriaxone.

Treatment of late neuroborreliosis

For patients with late Lyme borreliosis affecting the central or peripheral nervous system treatment is with ceftriaxone, cefotaxime, or benzylpenicillin, in the same regimen as for acute Lyme borreliosis with neurologic involvement. Response to treatment is usually slow and may be incomplete. However, unless relapse is shown by reliable objective measures, repeat treatment is not recommended.

Treatment of 'chronic Lyme disease' or 'post Lyme disease syndrome'

After an episode of Lyme borreliosis that has been treated appropriately some people have a variety of subjective complaints (such as myalgia, arthralgia, or fatigue). Some of these patients have been classified as having 'chronic Lyme disease' or 'post Lyme disease syndrome'. Two randomized placebo controlled trials showed no benefit of re-treating such patients with 4 weeks of intravenous ceftriaxone followed by 8 weeks of oral doxycycline.[82] The consensus of the Infectious Diseases Society of America expert panel is that there is insufficient evidence to regard 'chronic Lyme disease' as a separate diagnostic entity. Patients with chronic fatigue do not generally improve with antimicrobial treatment, even when given repeat-

ed courses. A standard recommendation is not to treat chronic fatigue with antimicrobials, even if serology for *B. burgdorferi* is positive; yet some physicians do so, being aware of the subtlety of abnormalities that neuroborreliosis can produce.[83]

Although patients occasionally relapse or become reinfected after treatment for Lyme borreliosis, the main cause of failure to respond to antimicrobials is misdiagnosis, due to false-positive Lyme serology or for other reasons.[70]

RELAPSING FEVER

Louse-borne relapsing fever, transmitted by the human body louse, is caused by *Borrelia recurrentis*; epidemics and pandemics affected approximately 50 million people during the twentieth century, with millions of deaths.[84] Relapsing fever is characterized by recurrent episodes of fever and spirochetemia, separated by afebrile intervals during which spirochetes are rarely found in the blood. Tick-borne relapsing fever, transmitted by ticks, is caused by many different species of *Borrelia*, and is milder.

TREATMENT OF RELAPSING FEVER

Tetracyclines, erythromycin, penicillin and chloramphenicol have been used successfully. Treatment with any effective antibiotic typically induces the Jarisch–Herxheimer reaction within 2 h of initiating therapy, and coincides with the clearing of spirochetemia. It is not prevented by prior treatment with prednisolone, but may be diminished with meptazinol.[83] Louse-borne relapsing fever responds to a single oral dose of tetracycline 500 mg, doxycycline 100 mg or erythromycin 500 mg.[85,86] Fever lasts longer in patients treated with penicillin, and there are more frequent failures and relapses.

Patients who cannot be treated with an oral agent may be given a single dose of tetracycline 250 mg intravenously. Tick-borne relapsing fever has a higher rate of treatment failures or relapses. Treatment should therefore be with 5–10 days of tetracycline 500 mg 6-hourly, doxycycline 100 mg 12-hourly, or erythromycin 500 mg 6-hourly.[87]

RICKETTSIOSES

These are due to *Rickettsia rickettsii*, *Rickettsia conorii*, *Rickettsia australis*, *Rickettsia sibirica*, *Rickettsia akari*, *Rickettsia prowazekii*, *Rickettsia typhi*, *Orientia tsutsugamushi* and *Coxiella burnetii*.

Rickettsiae are small, fastidious, obligate intracellular coccobacilli. With the exception of *R. prowazekii* (epidemic typhus), all are zoonoses, and with the exception of *Coxiella burnetii* (Q fever), all are unable to survive outside a mammalian host or vector.[88]

The spotted fever rickettsiae mainly circulate in hard ticks, rodents and domestic animals in rural and peridomestic habitats. They infect endothelia of small blood vessels and produce fever, malaise and, often, a vasculitic rash. The most familiar is *R. rickettsii* (Rocky Mountain spotted fever). This occurs only in the Western hemisphere and is the most severe, with a case-fatality rate of 20% if untreated. Only 3–18% of patients present with rash, fever, and a history of tick exposure on their first visit: physicians should consider Rocky Mountain spotted fever in American infants and children even when some features are lacking. Delayed diagnosis and late initiation of specific anti-rickettsial therapy (e.g. on or after day 5 of the illness) is associated with substantially greater risk for a fatal outcome.

R. africae, the cause of African tick-bite fever, has been distinguishable since 1994 from *R. conorii*, the agent of fièvre boutonneuse or Mediterranean spotted fever.[89] *R. africae* may cause particularly mild illness in some regions, as almost all adults in parts of Zimbabwe have antibodies that react to *R. conorii*, despite few clinical cases.[90] In Israel, by contrast, *R. conorii* was isolated from the blood of three previously healthy children with fatal infections.[91] *R. australis* and *R. sibirica* are similar clinically, but occur in Australia and Siberia.

R. akari (rickettsial pox) differs: it occurs in cities, has a mouse host and mite vector, and causes a papulovesicular rash.

The typhus group comprises *R. prowazekii*, responsible for epidemics among refugees (hosts, human; vectors, lice); *R. typhi* (also called *R. mooseri*) responsible for sporadic cases in slums and on farms (hosts, rodents; vectors, fleas). *Orientia tsutsugamushi* is responsible for scrub typhus in Asia (hosts, wild rodents; vectors, mites).

PROPHYLAXIS OF RICKETTSIOSES

In a large placebo-controlled study involving more than 1000 military personnel on the Pescadores Islands, a weekly dose of 200 mg doxycycline, continued throughout the period of residence in the endemic area, reduced the incidence of scrub typhus by approximately 80%.[92]

TREATMENT OF RICKETTSIOSES

For all the rickettsioses, tetracycline 0.5–1 g 6-hourly orally or 0.5 g 6-hourly intravenously, or doxycycline 100 mg 12-hourly, is highly effective. The duration of treatment is 5–7 days, or 2–3 days after the temperature returns to normal.

In a small series of cases of louse-borne relapsing fever and typhus in Ethiopia, a single 100 mg dose of doxycycline by mouth cured all patients, and there were no relapses.[85] In patients with scrub typhus a single dose of doxycycline 200 mg orally was as effective as a 7-day course of tetracycline, and no relapses occurred among the patients given single-dose doxycycline.[93] In a retrospective series of Thai patients with murine typhus, a single dose of doxycycline 200 mg (52 patients) was as effective as 5–10 day course of chloramphenicol (9 patients) and significantly shortened the duration of fever compared to placebo.[94]

Many antibiotics, including penicillins, cephalosporins, and sulfonamides, are ineffective. In almost all clinical situations, including disease in children under 8 years of age, the antibiotic of choice is doxycycline.[95] The use of tetracyclines in young children has been discouraged because of the potential for tooth discoloration and should be reserved for patients in whom a rickettsial illness is strongly suspected; however, tetracycline staining of teeth is dose related and available data suggest that one course of doxycycline for presumed rickettsiosis does not cause clinically significant staining of permanent teeth.[96] Alternatively, chloramphenicol may be used for children. Chloramphenicol appears to be highly effective against rickettsioses. The adult dose is 2–4 g/day orally or intravenously in divided doses for 7 days.

The fluoroquinolones are highly active against *Rickettsia* spp. in vitro, and limited clinical experience suggests that they are effective in the treatment of all rickettsial syndromes.[97,98] Ruiz and Herrero[99] compared ciprofloxacin 750 mg with doxycycline 100 mg, each 12-hourly for 7 days, in 70 Spanish patients with Mediterranean spotted fever (*R. conorii*), and found the two drugs to be equally effective. Brill–Zinsser disease is a recrudescence of illness in an individual previously affected by epidemic typhus, for example among immigrants from Eastern Europe whose initial infection occurred during the Second World War. It responds to treatment with tetracycline.[100]

Q FEVER

Q fever is a worldwide zoonosis caused by *Coxiella burnetii*, which differs from other rickettsiae in its high resistance to desiccation and its ability to survive for long periods in the environment. Human infection is usually acquired by inhalation of small numbers of airborne organisms when in proximity to infected domestic animals, hides, manure, dust, milk and, especially, placentas.[101] In endemic areas, over 10% of individuals may have antibodies to *C. burnetii*, and most recall no characteristic illness. The incubation period for Q fever is 14–39 days. Acute Q fever is characterized by fever and chills, severe headache and myalgia. The syndrome may be that of atypical pneumonia, and hepatitis is commonly present. Although the acute disease is usually self-limited, Q fever endocarditis occasionally develops, typically 3–20 years following the acute infection, and is often fatal.[102,103] Patients with previously damaged heart valves are at risk.

Treatment of Q fever

Untreated, acute Q fever lasts from a few days to 2 weeks. Treatment with either tetracycline 500 mg four times daily or doxycycline 100 mg twice daily usually results in defervescence within 48 h.[104] Treatment should be continued for 2 weeks. Since acute Q fever is usually a mild self-limiting disease, it is difficult to ascertain with certainty whether or not antimicrobial therapy substantially alters the course of the illness: in one large series, the duration of fever was 2 days in patients receiving tetracycline, 1.7 days in those receiving doxycycline, and 3.3 days in those who received no treatment.[104] Q fever pneumonia is usually an undiagnosed 'atypical pneumonia', and thus erythromycin is often the antimicrobial chosen. In a double-blind comparison, doxycycline 100 mg 12-hourly or erythromycin 500 mg 6-hourly, both for 10 days, were administered to 48 patients with acute Q fever pneumonia. Doxycycline produced a more rapid reduction in fever and fewer side effects than erythromycin. There were no differences in any other clinical or radiological measures, and by day 40 the chest radiograph was normal in 47 of the patients.[105] In a small series, patients with Q fever pneumonia did not respond to erythromycin at doses as high as 4 g/day, whereas the addition of rifampicin 600 mg/day resulted in cure.[106]

Prophylactic administration of tetracycline was found ineffective when given soon after infection of human volunteers.[107]

Therapy for Q fever endocarditis is controversial because combinations of antimicrobials are necessary, and relapse may follow discontinuation of therapy, even after prolonged courses.[108,109] A logical choice is doxycycline plus trimethoprim–sulfamethoxazole, or doxycycline plus rifampicin, continued for 2 years.[106]

EHRLICHIOSIS

During the period 1980–1990 two new human pathogens were found: *Ehrlichia chaffeensis* causing human monocytic ehrlichiosis, and *Anaplasma* (formerly *Ehrlichia*) *phagocytophila*, causing human granulocytic ehrlichiosis. Both ehrlichioses are transmitted to humans by a tick bite. About a week later there is an onset of fever, rigors, headache and myalgia; rash and edema may occur (particularly in children), and leukopenia, thrombocytopenia and elevated liver enzyme levels are common.[110,111] The organisms may rarely be seen in vacuoles within circulating leukocytes. The diagnosis is usually made serologically by a four-fold rise or fall in antibodies to *E. chaffeensis* and/or *A. phagocytophila* respectively. The polymerase chain reaction or cell culture are other diagnostic tools.

Many cases are asymptomatic, and serological surveys of febrile patients have shown ehrlichiosis to be as common as rickettsial infections in parts of the USA[112] and a common coinfection with Lyme borreliosis in parts of Scandinavia.[113] Clinical cases or serological evidence of both diseases have been found in many European countries. Fatal cases of both have been reported.

TREATMENT OF EHRLICHIOSIS

In vitro, *A. phagocytophila* and *E. chaffeensis* are both susceptible to doxycycline and rifampicin, and both are resistant to erythromycin and gentamicin. *A. phagocytophila* is susceptible to rifabutin but resistant to ampicillin, ceftriaxone, imipenem–cilastatin, azithromycin, clindamycin, and trimethoprim–sulfamethoxazole, while *E. chaffeensis* is resistant to chloramphenicol, trimethoprim–sulfamethoxazole, ciprofloxacin and penicillin.[114]

Doxycycline 200 mg/day for 7–14 days is highly effective.[111,115] In children, doxycycline at 2 mg/kg twice daily (maximum 200 mg per day) for 7–10 days have been used.[116] Fever resolved within 2 days in 33 of 34 doxycycline-treated adult patients with human granulocytic ehrlichiosis; while headache and myalgia usually disappeared in 3 days, weakness and fatigue were more persistent. Rifampicin has been used in 2 pregnant patients with good results.[117] When a tetracycline was given to human monocytic ehrlichiosis outpatients with non-specific febrile symptoms, only 3 of 49 were subsequently admitted to hospital, whereas 35 of 38 patients who received antimicrobials other than tetracyclines needed inpatient treatment. Among patients in hospital, those not receiving tetracyclines or chloramphenicol had a more protracted course, and severe illness was seen more commonly among patients who were over 60 years old, or who did not receive a tetracycline or chloramphenicol within the first week of symptoms.[110]

VIRAL ZOONOSES

No specific treatment is established for most viral zoonoses. The exceptions are hantavirus (hemorrhagic fever with renal syndrome, hantavirus pulmonary syndrome) and Lassa fever.

LASSA FEVER

Ribavirin (tribavirin), a guanosine analog, has broad-spectrum antiviral activity. The only important adverse effect of ribavirin in humans is mild, usually reversible, anemia. It is contraindicated in pregnant women.

Prophylaxis of Lassa fever

For needlestick or other high-risk contact, oral ribavirin 5 mg/kg 8-hourly for 2–3 weeks would be a logical step, although it is of unproven efficacy.

Treatment of Lassa fever

Ribavirin should be given intravenously in a loading dose of 30 mg/kg, followed by 15 mg/kg 6-hourly for 4 days, then 7.5 mg/kg 8-hourly for 6 days. In a study in Sierra Leone, ribavirin reduced mortality from 55% to 5%, if treatment began within 6 days of the onset of symptoms.[118]

Ribavirin has proved beneficial in Argentine hemorrhagic fever[119] and, although this is unproven, may be useful in Bolivian, Venezuelan and Brazilian hemorrhagic fevers, all of which are caused by arenaviruses.

Ribavirin is of established benefit in hantavirus infections,[120,121] and has also been used in hantavirus pulmonary syndrome.

References

1. Solera J, Martinez-Alfaro E, Espinosa A 1997 Recognition and optimal treatment of brucellosis. *Drugs* 53: 245–256.

2. McLean DR, Russell N, Khan MY 1992 Neurobrucellosis: clinical and therapeutic features. *Clinical Infectious Diseases* 15: 582–590.

3. Lang R, Dagan R, Potasman I, Einhorn M, Raz R 1992 Failure of ceftriaxone in the treatment of acute brucellosis. *Clinical Infectious Diseases* 14: 506–509.

4. Solera J, Espinosa A, Martinez-Alfaro E et al 1997 Fernandez JA Treatment of human brucellosis with doxycycline and gentamicin. *Antimicrobial Agents and Chemotherapy* 41: 80–84.

5. WHO 1986 Joint FAO/WHO Expert Committee on Brucellosis (6th report). WHO technical report series 740. Geneva, World Health Organization.

6. Ariza J, Gudiol F, Pallares R et al 1992 Treatment of human brucellosis with doxycycline plus rifampin or doxycycline plus streptomycin. A randomized, double blind study. *Annals of Internal Medicine* 117: 25–30.

7. Lubani MM, Dubin KI, Sharda DC et al 1989 A multicenter therapeutic study of 1100 children with brucellosis. *Pediatric Infectious Disease Journal* 8: 75–78.

8. Akova M, Uzun O, Akalin HE, Hayran M, Unal S, Gur D 1993 Quinolones in treatment of human brucellosis: comparative trial of ofloxacin–rifampin versus doxycycline–rifampin. *Antimicrobial Agents and Chemotherapy* 37: 1831–1834.

9. Agalar C, Usubutun S, Turkyilmaz R 1999 Ciprofloxacin and rifampicin versus doxycycline and rifampicin in the treatment of brucellosis. *European Journal of Clinical Microbiology and Infectious Diseases* 18: 535–538.

10. Khuri Bulos NA, Daoud AH, Azab SM 1993 Treatment of childhood brucellosis: results of a prospective trial on 113 children. *Pediatric Infectious Disease Journal* 12: 377–381.

11. Korzeniowski OM 1995 Antibacterial agents in pregnancy. *Infectious Disease Clinics of North America.* 9: 639–651.

12. Omar FZ, Zuberi S, Minns RA 1997 Neurobrucellosis in childhood: six new cases and a review of the literature. *Developmental Medicine and Child Neurology* 39: 762–765.

13. Habeeb YK, Al Najdi AK, Sadek SA, Al Onaizi E 1998 Paediatric neurobrucellosis: case report and literature review. *Journal of Infection* 37: 59–62.

14. Pratt DS, Tenney JH, Bjork CM, Reller LB 1978 Successful treatment of *Brucella melitensis* endocarditis. *American Journal of Medicine* 64: 897–900.

15. Jacobs F, Abramowicz D, Vereerstraeten P et al 1990 *Brucella* endocarditis: the role of combined medical and surgical treatment. *Reviews of Infectious Diseases* 12: 740–744.

16. Cakalagaoglu C, Keser N, Alhan C 1999 Brucella-mediated prosthetic valve endocarditis with brachial artery mycotic aneurysm. *Journal of Heart Valve Diseases* 8: 586–590.

17. Moreno S, Ariza J, Espinosa FJ et al 1998 Brucellosis in patients infected with the human immunodeficiency virus. *European Journal of Clinical Microbiology and Infectious Diseases* 17: 319–326.

18. Inglesby TV, Henderson DA, Bartlett JG et al 1999 Anthrax as a biological weapon: medical and public health management. Working Group on Civilian Biodefense. *Journal of the American Medical Association* 281: 1735–1745.

19. Sturchler D 1988 *Endemic areas of tropical infections*, 2nd edn. Hans Huber, Stuttgart

20. Dixon TC, Meselson M, Guillemin J, Hanna PC 1999 Anthrax. *New England Journal of Medicine* 341: 815–826.

21. Odendaal MW, Pieterson PM, de Vos V, Botha AD 1991 The antibiotic sensitivity patterns of *Bacillus anthracis* isolated from the Kruger National Park, Onderstepoort. *Journal of Veterinary Research* 58: 17–19.

22. Knudson GB 1986 Treatment of anthrax in man: history and current concepts. *Military Medicine* 151: 71–77.

23. Singh RS, Sridhar MS, Sekhar PC, Bhaskar CJ 1992 Cutaneous anthrax: a report of ten cases. *Journal of the Association of Physicians of India* 40: 46–49.

24. Talan DA, Citron DM, Abrahamian FM, Moran GJ, Goldstein EJ 1999 Bacteriologic analysis of infected dog and cat bites. Emergency Medicine Animal Bite Infection Study Group. *New England Journal of Medicine* 340: 85–92.

25. Weber DJ, Hansen AR 1991 Infections resulting from animal bites. *Infectious Diseases Clinics of North America* 5: 663–680.

26. Rygg M, Bruun CF 1992 Rat bite fever (*Streptobacillus moniliformis*) with septicemia in a child. *Scandinavian Journal of Infectious Diseases* 24: 535–540.

27. McEvoy MB, Noah ND, Pilsworth R 1987 Outbreak of fever caused by *Strep. moniliformis*. *Lancet* ii: 1361–1363.

28. Centers for Disease Control 1984 *Streptobacillus moniliformis*. In: Clark WA, Hollis DG, Weaver RE, Riley P (eds). *Identification of unusual pathogenic gram-negative aerobic and facultatively anaerobic bacteria*. Atlanta, Georgia: US Department of Health and Human Services, CDC, pp. 288–289.

29. Hagelskjaer L, Sorensen I, Randers E 1998 *Streptobacillus moniliformis* infection: 2 cases and a literature review. *Scandinavian Journal of Infectious Diseases* 30: 309–311.

30. McCormack RC, Kaye D, Hook EW 1967 Endocarditis due to *Streptobacillus moniliformis*. A report of two cases and review of the literature. *Journal of American Medical Association* 200: 77–79.

31. Rupp ME 1992 *Streptobacillus moniliformis* endocarditis: case report and review. *Clinical Infectious Diseases* 14: 769–772.

32. Alfes JC, Ayers LW 1990 Acute bacterial meningitis caused by Francisella tularensis. *Pediatric Infectious Disease Journal* 9: 300–301.

33. Penn RL, Kinasewicz GT 1987 Factors associated with a poor clinical outcome in tularemia. *Archives of Internal Medicine* 147: 265–268.

34. Hutton JP, Everett ED 1985 Response of tularemic meningitis to antimicrobial therapy. *Southern Medical Journal* 78: 189–190.

35. Mason WL, Eigelsbach HT, Little SF, Bates JH 1980 Treatment of tularemia, including pulmonary tularemia, with gentamicin. *American Review of Respiratory Disease* 121: 39–45.

36. Tancik CA, Dillaha JA 2000 *Francisella tularensis* endocarditis. *Clinical Infectious Diseases* 30: 399–400.

37. Lee HC, Horowitz E, Linder W 1991 Treatment of tularemia with imipenem–cilastatin sodium. *Southern Medical Journal* 84: 1277–1278.

38. Limaye AP, Hooper CJ 1999 Treatment of tularemia with fluoroquinolones: two cases and review. *Clinical Infectious Diseases* 29: 922–924.

39. Syrjala H, Schildt R, Raisainen S 1991 In vitro susceptibility of *Francisella tularensis* to fluoroquinolones and treatment of tularemia with norfloxacin and ciprofloxacin. *European Journal of Clinical Microbiology and Infectious Diseases* 10: 68–70.

40. Enderlin G, Morales L, Jacobs RF, Cross JT 1994 Streptomycin and alternative agents for the treatment of tularemia: review of the literature. *Clinical Infectious Diseases* 19: 42–47.

41. Cross JT, Jacobs RF 1993 Tularemia: treatment failures with outpatient use of ceftriaxone. *Clinical Infectious Diseases* 17: 976–980.

42. Butler T, Mahmoud AAF, Warren KS 1977 Algorithms in the diagnosis and management of exotic diseases. XXV. Plague. *Journal of Infectious Diseases* 136: 317–320.

43. John TJ 1994 India: is it plague? *Lancet* 344: 1359–1360.

44. Crook LD, Tempest B 1992 Plague. A clinical review of 27 cases. *Archives of Internal Medicine* 152: 1253–1256.

45. Mann JM 1982 Peripatetic plague. *Journal of American Medical Association* 247: 47–48.

46. Marshall JD, Joy RJT, Ai NV, Gibson FL 1967 Plague in Vietnam 1965–1966. *American Journal of Epidemiology* 86: 603–616.

47. Cleri DJ, Vernaleo JR, Lombardi LJ et al 1997 Plague pneumonia disease caused by *Yersinia pestis*. *Seminars in Respiratory Infection* 12: 12–23.

48. Frean JA, Arntzen L, Capper T, Bryskier A, Klugman KP 1996 In vitro activities of 14 antibiotics against 100 human isolates of *Yersinia pestis* from a southern African plague focus. *Antimicrobial Agents and Chemotherapy* 40: 2646–2647.

49. Smith MD, Vinh DX, Nguyen TT, Wain J, Thung D, White NJ 1995 In vitro antimicrobial susceptibilities of strains of *Yersinia pestis*. *Antimicrobial Agents and Chemotherapy* 39: 2153–2154.

50. Spach DH, Koehler JE 1998 Bartonella associated infections. *Infectious Disease Clinics of North America* 21: 137–155.

51. Cooper P, Guderian R, Orellana P et al 1997 An outbreak of bartonellosis in Zamora Chinchipe Province in Ecuador. *Transactions of the Royal Society of Tropical Medicine and Hygiene* 91: 544–546.

52. Schultz MG 1968 A history of bartonellosis (Carrion's disease). *American Journal of Tropical Medicine and Hygiene* 17: 503–515.

53. Koehler JE, Glaser CA, Tappero JW 1994 *Rochalimea henselae* infection: new zoonosis with the domestic cat as reservoir. *Journal of the American Medical Association* 271: 531–535.

54. Noah DL, Bresee JS, Gorensek MJ et al 1995 Cluster of five children with acute encephalopathy associated with cat-scratch disease in south Florida. *Pediatric Infectious Disease Journal* 14: 866–869.

55. Bass JW, Freitas BC, Freitas AD 1998 Prospective randomized double blind placebo-controlled evaluation of azithromycin for treatment of cat-scratch disease. *Pediatric Infectious Disease Journal* 17: 447–452.

56. Adal KA, Cockerel CJ, Petri WA 1994 Cat scratch disease, bacillary angiomatosis, and other infections due to Rochalimea. *New England Journal of Medicine* 330: 1509–1515.

57. Lucey D, Dolan MJ, Moss CW et al 1992 Relapsing illness due to *Rochalimaea henselae* in immunocompetent hosts: implication for therapy and new epidemiological associations. *Clinical Infectious Diseases* 14: 683–688.

58. Wolfson C, Branley J, Gottlieb T 1996 The E test for antimicrobial susceptibility testing of *Bartonella henselae*. *Journal of Antimicrobial Chemotherapy* 38: 963–938.

59. Robson JM, Harte GJ, Osborne DR, McCormack JG 1999 Cat-scratch disease with paravertebral mass and osteomyelitis. *Clinical Infectious Diseases* 28: 274–278.

60. Schwartzman WA, Patnaik M, Angulo FJ, Visscher BR, Miller EN, Peter JB 1995 Bartonella (Rochalimaea) antibodies, dementia, and cat ownership among men infected with human immunodeficiency virus. *Clinical Infectious Diseases* 21: 954–959.

61. Brouqui P, Lascola B, Roux V, Raoult D 1999 Chronic *Bartonella quintana* bacteremia in homeless patients. *New England Journal of Medicine* 340: 184–189.

62. Berman SJ, Tsai CC, Holmes K, Fresh JW, Watten RH 1973 Sporadic anicteric leptospirosis in South Vietman: a study in 150 patients. *Annals of Internal Medicine* 79: 167–173.

63. Takafuji ET, Kirkpatrick JW, Miller RN et al 1984 An efficacy trial of doxycycline chemoprophylaxis against leptospirosis. *New England Journal of Medicine* 310: 497–500.

64. Gilks CF, Lambert HP, Broughton ES, Baker CC 1988 Failure of penicillin prophylaxis in laboratory acquired leptospirosis. *Postgraduate Medical Journal* 64: 236–238.

65. Ferguson IR 1993 Leptospirosis surveillance: 1990–1992. *Communicable Diseases Report CDR Review* 3: R47–R48.

66. McClain JBL, Ballou WR, Harrison SM, Steinweg DL 1984 Doxycycline therapy for leptospirosis. *Annals of Internal Medicine* 100: 696–698.

67. Watt G, Padre LP, Tuazon ML et al 1988 Placebo controlled trial of intravenous penicillin for severe and late leptospirosis. *Lancet* i: 433–435.

68. Vaughan C, Cronin CC, Walsh EK, Whelton M 1994 The Jarisch–Herxheimer reaction in leptospirosis. *Postgraduate Medical Journal* 70: 118–121.

69. Centers for Disease Control and Prevention 1997 Lyme Disease – the United States, 1996: *Morbidity and Mortality Weekly Report* 46: 531–535.

70. Steere AC 2001 Lyme disease. *New England Journal of Medicine* 345: 115–125.

71. Kalish RA, McHugh G, Granquist J, Shea B, Ruthazer R, Steere AC 2001 Persistence of Immunoglobulin M or Immunoglobulin G Antibody Responses to *Borrelia burgdorferi* 10–20 Years after Active Lyme Disease. *Clinical Infectious Diseases* 33: 780–785.

72. Gustafson R, Svenungsson B, Gardulf A, Stiernstedt G, Forsgren M 1990 Prevalence of tick-borne encephalitis and Lyme borreliosis in a defined Swedish population. *Scandinavian Journal of Infectious Diseases* 22: 297–306.

73. Magid DM, Schwartz B, Craft J, Schwartz JS 1992 Prevention of Lyme disease after tick bites. *New England Journal of Medicine* 327: 534–541.

74. Dennis DT, Meltzer MI 1997 Antibiotic prophylaxis after tick bites. *Lancet* 350: 1191–1192.

75. Nadelman RB, Nowakowski J, Fish D et al 2001 Prophylaxis with single-dose doxycycline for the prevention of Lyme disease after an *Ixodes scapularis* tick bite. *New England Journal of Medicine* 345: 79–84.

76. Wormer GP, Nadelman RB, Dattwyler RJ et al 2000 Practice guidelines for the treatment of Lyme disease. The Infectious Diseases Society of America. *Clinical Infectious Diseases* 31 Suppl 1: 1–14.

77. Wormser GP, Nadelman RB, Dattwyler RJ et al 2000 Practice Guidelines for the Treatment of Lyme Disease. *Clinical Infectious Diseases* 31: 1–14.

78. Dattwyler RJ, Luft BJ, Kunkel MJ et al 1997 Ceftriaxone compared with doxycycline for the treatment of acute disseminated Lyme disease. *New England Journal of Medicine* 337(5): 289–294.

79. Luger SW, Paparone P, Wormser GP et al 1995 Comparison of cefuroxime axetil and doxycycline in treatment of patients with early Lyme disease associated with erythema migrans. *Antimicrobial Agents and Chemotherapy* 39: 661–667.

80. Dattwyler RJ, Halperin JJ, Volkman DJ, Luft BJ 1988 Treatment of late Lyme borreliosis randomized comparison of ceftriaxone and penicillin. *Lancet* i: 1191–1194.

81. Dotevall L, Hagberg L 1999 Successful oral doxycycline treatment of Lyme disease-associated facial palsy and meningitis. *Clinical Infectious Diseases* 28: 569–574.

82. Klempner MS, Hu LT, Evans J et al 2001 Two controlled trials of antibiotic treatment in patients with persistent symptoms and a history of Lyme disease. *New England Journal of Medicine* 345: 85–92.

83. Kaplan RF, Meadows ME, Vincent LC et al 1992 Memory impairment and depression in patients with Lyme encephalopathy: comparison with fibromyalgia and nonpsychotically depressed patients. *Neurology* 42: 1263–1267.

84. Teklu B, Habte Michael A, Warrell DA, White NJ, Wright DJM 1983 Meptazinoal diminishes the Jarisch–Herxheimer reaction of relapsing fever. *Lancet* i: 835–839.

85. Perine PL, Awoke S, Krause DW, McDade JE 1974 Single dose doxycycline treatment of louse borne relapsing fever and epidemic typhus. *Lancet* ii: 742–744.

86. Perine PL, Teklu B 1983 Antibiotic treatment of louse borne relapsing fever in Ethiopia: a report of 377 cases. *American Journal of Tropical Medicine and Hygiene* 32: 1096–1100.

87. Horton JM, Blaser MJ 1985 The spectrum of relapsing fever in the Rocky Mountains. *Archives of Internal Medicine* 145: 871–875.

88. Walker DH and Raoult D 2000 *Ricettsia rickettsii and other spotted fever group rickettsiae (Rocky Mountain spotted fever and other spotted fevers)* in: Mandell, Douglas and Bennett's Principles and Practice of Infectious Diseases 5th edn; Churchill Livingstone, Philadelphia, USA

89. Kelly PJ, Beati L, Matthewman LA, Mason PR, Dasch GA, Raoult D 1994 A new pathogenic spotted fever group rickettsia from Africa. *Journal of Tropical Medicine and Hygiene* 97: 129–137.

90. Kelly PJ, Mason PR 1991 Tick bite fever in Zimbabwe. Survey of antibodies to *Rickettsia conorii* in man and dogs, and of rickettsia like organisms in dog ticks. *South African Medical Journal* 80: 233–236.

91. Yagupsky P, Wolach B 1993 Fatal Israeli spotted fever in children. *Clinical Infectious Diseases* 17: 850–853.

92. Olson JG, Bourgeois AL, Fang RCY, Coolbaugh JC, Dennis DT 1980 Prevention of scrub typhus: prophylactic administration of doxycycline in a randomized double blind trial. *American Journal of Tropical Medicine and Hygiene* 29: 989–997.

93. Brown GW, Saunders JP, Singh S, Huxsoll DL, Shirai A 1978 Single dose doxycycline therapy for scrub typhus. *Transactions of the Royal Society of Tropical Medicine and Hygiene* 72: 412–416.

94. Silpapojakul K, Chayakul P, Krisanapan S, Silpapojakul K 1993 Murine typhus in Thailand: clinical features, diagnosis and treatment. *Quarterly Journal of Medicine* 86: 43–47.

95. Purvis JJ, Edwards MS 2000 Doxycycline use for rickettsial disease in pediatric patients. *Pediatric Infectious Disease Journal* 19: 871–874.

96. Lochary ME, Lockhart PB, Williams WT 1998 Doxycycline and staining of permanent teeth. *Pediatric Infectious Disease Journal* 17: 429–431.

97. Eaton M, Cohen MT, Shlim DR, Ennis B 1989 Ciprofloxacin treatment of typhus. *Journal of the American Medical Association* 262: 772–773.

98. Gudiol F, Pallares R, Carratala J et al 1989 Randomized double blind evaluation of ciprofloxacin and doxycycline for Mediterranean spotted fever. *Antimicrobial Agents and Chemotherapy* 33: 987–988.

99. Ruiz BR, Herrero JI 1992 Evaluation of ciprofloxacin and doxycycline in the treatment of Mediterranean spotted fever. *European Journal of Clinical Microbiology and Infectious Diseases* 11: 427–431.

100. Green CR, Fishbein D, Gleiberman I 1990 Brill Zinsser: still with us. *Journal of the American Medical Association* 264: 1811–1812.

101. Langley JM, Marrie TJ, Covert A et al 1988 Poker players pneumonia. An urban outbreak following exposure to a parturient cat. *New England Journal of Medicine* 319: 354–356.

102. Turck WPG, Howitt G, Turnberg LA et al 1976 Chronic Q fever. *Quarterly Journal of Medicine* 45: 193–217.

103. Wilson HG, Neilson GH, Galea EG et al 1976 Q fever endocarditis in Queensland. *Circulation* 53: 680–684.

104. Spelman DW 1982 Q fever: a study of III consecutive cases. *Medical Journal of Australia* 1: 547–553.

105. Sobradillo V, Zalacain R, Capelastegui A, Uresandi F, Corral J 1992 Antibiotic treatment in pneumonia due to Q fever. *Thorax* 47: 276–278.

106. Marrie TJ 1995 *Coxiella burnetii* (Q fever). In: Mandell GL, Bennett JE, Dolin R (eds) *Mandell, Douglas and Bennett's principles and practice of infectious diseases*, 4th edn. Churchill Livingstone, New York, pp. 1727–1735.

107. Tigertt WD, Benenson AS, Shope RE 1956 Studies on Q fever in man. *Transactions of the Association of American Physicians* 69: 98–104.

108. Levy PY, Drancourt M, Etienne J et al 1991 Comparison of different antibiotic regimens for therapy of 32 cases of Q fever endocarditis. *Antimicrobial Agents and Chemotherapy* 35: 533–537.

109. Fernandez Guerrero ML 1993 Zoonotic endocarditis. *Infectious Disease Clinics of North America* 7: 135–152.

110. Fishbein DB, Dawson JE, Robinson LE 1994 Human ehrlichiosis in the United States, 1985 to 1990. *Annals of Internal Medicine* 120: 736–743.

111. Bakken JS, Krueth J, Wilson-Nordskog C, Tilden RL, Asanovich K, Dumler JS 1996 Clinical and laboratory characteristics of human granulocytic ehrlichiosis. *Journal of the American Medical Association* 275: 199–205.

112. Dumler JS, Sutker WL, Walker DH 1993 Persistent infection with *Ehrlichia chaffeensis*. *Clinical Infectious Diseases* 17: 903–905.

113. Bjöersdorff A, Brouqui P, Eliasson I, Massung RF, Wittesjö B, Berglund J 1999 Serological evidence of Ehrlichia infection in Swedish Lyme borreliosis patients. *Scandinavian Journal of Infectious Diseases* 31: 51–55.

114. Klein MB, Nelson CM, Goodman JL 1997 Antibiotic susceptibility of the newly cultivated agent of human granulocytic Ehrlichiosis: Promising activity of quinolones and rifamycins. *Antimicrobial Agents and Chemotherapy* 41: 76–79.

115. Everett ED, Evans KA, Henry RB, McDonald G 1994 Human ehrlichiosis in adults after tick exposure. *Annals of Internal Medicine* 120: 730–735.

116. Jacobs RF, Schutze GE 1997 Ehrlichiosis in children. *Journal of Pediatrics* 131: 184–192.

117. Buitrago MI, Ijdo JW, Rinaudo P et al 1998 Human granulocytic ehrlichiosis during pregnancy treated successfully with rifampin. *Clinical Infectious Diseases* 27:213–215.

118. McCormick JB, King IJ, Webb PA et al 1986 Lassa fever: effective therapy with ribavirin. *New England Journal of Medicine* 314: 20–26.

119. Enria DA, Maiztegui JI 1994 Antiviral treatment of Argentine hemorrhagic fever. *Antiviral Research* 23: 23–31.

120. Huggins JW, Hsiang CM, Cosgriff TM et al 1991 Prospective, double blind, concurrent, placebo controlled trial of intravenous ribavirin therapy of hemorrhagic fever with renal syndrome. *Journal of Infectious Diseases* 164: 1119–1127.

121. Chapman LE, Mertz GJ, Peters CJ et al 1999 Intravenous ribavirin for hantavirus pulmonary syndrome: safety and tolerance during 1 year of open-label experience. Ribavirin Study Group. *Antiviral Therapy* 4: 211–219.

64 Malaria

N. J. White

Malaria is the most important parasitic disease of humans. It is estimated to affect approximately 200 million people, and the annual death toll from *Plasmodium falciparum* infections is between 1 and 2.5 million. Pregnant women, infants and those over 60 years old are at greatest risk. Most of the deaths are in African children, and most occur away from facilities where optimum antimalarial treatment can be given. Unlike many other infections, the mortality rate due to malaria is rising, and this is attributed directly to increasing antimalarial drug resistance.[1] Much antimalarial treatment is still administered for the empirical self-treatment of febrile illnesses in the tropics. The amounts of drug used are enormous. Despite resistance throughout most of the tropics, chloroquine is probably the second most widely used drug in the world. As malaria is one of the most common causes of fever in tropical countries it must be excluded in any febrile patient living in, or returning from, the tropics. Ideally, antimalarial drugs should be given only for the treatment of microscopically confirmed malaria infections or for the prevention of malaria in pregnant women or travelers. The rapid development of resistance to most of the available antimalarial drugs by the potentially lethal parasite *P. falciparum* has compromised considerably recommendations for both prevention and treatment.[2] The most important recent development in antimalarial chemotherapy has been the introduction of the artemisinin derivatives, and the use of combinations containing these compounds. It is now accepted that, in order to delay the emergence of resistance, just as in the treatment of tuberculosis, leprosy and HIV/AIDS, combinations of drugs with different modes of action should be used. It is likely that fixed artemisinin derivative combinations will become the treatment of choice for uncomplicated falciparum malaria everywhere.[3] The major determinant of antimalarial use in endemic areas, as with many other anti-infective drugs, is the cost of the medications. Ineffective drugs are used because most countries cannot afford more effective alternatives. Treatment recommendations must be under constant review.

ANTIMALARIAL DRUG RESISTANCE AND THE CHOICE OF DRUGS

Although it had been suspected for three centuries, the first cases of quinine resistance were documented only 85 years ago.

Fortunately, resistance has progressed very slowly and quinine still remains useful today.

Within a few years of the introduction of the dihydrofolate reductase inhibitors pyrimethamine and proguanil as antimalarial treatments in the late 1940s and early 1950s, high-level resistance was noted in both *P. falciparum* and *Plasmodium vivax*.[4] Resistance could also be selected readily in the laboratory. Nevertheless, these drugs remained useful in prophylaxis, but for treatment use of proguanil was discontinued, and pyrimethamine was later prescribed in a fixed combination with long-acting sulfonamides – most commonly sulfadoxine.

Chloroquine took over rapidly as the treatment of choice for all malaria, and was also used widely in prophylaxis. Chloroquine resistance in *P. falciparum* was first recorded in the late 1950s, and by the early 1970s had become a significant problem in South America and South-East Asia. During the 1980s, chloroquine resistance spread remorselessly across southern Asia and in the 1990s marched across the entire length and breadth of the African continent. Few tropical countries are now unaffected. High-level chloroquine resistance in *P. vivax* was reported first on the island of New Guinea, and more recently in other parts of Oceania and south-east Asia.[5,6]

Amodiaquine shares cross-resistance patterns with chloroquine, but it is significantly more effective than chloroquine against resistant parasites and has replaced chloroquine in some areas.

Resistance to combinations of pyrimethamine and long-acting sulfonamides (SP) developed rapidly after their introduction for routine treatment in south-east Asia and South America, and they are now beginning to fail in Eastern and Southern Africa, where they replaced chloroquine as first-line treatment.

The combination of chlorproguanil (or proguanil) and dapsone is more effective than SP against antifol-resistant parasites, and provides less selection pressure to the emergence of resistance.[7] A fixed-dose formulation is under development.

Mefloquine is generally effective against multiresistant strains of *P. falciparum* but, with increasing use, resistance was an increasing problem in countries in south-east Asia during the 1990s, and now there are some areas (such as the eastern and western borders of Thailand) where mefloquine alone is no longer effective.[8,9]

Although halofantrine is intrinsically more active than mefloquine, susceptibility to the two drugs is linked, and concerns over cardiotoxicity and its high cost have limited its use.[10] Fortunately, resistance to quinine has remained low grade in South America and south-east Asia (although susceptibility is declining slowly) and has not been a problem in Africa. However, because of consistent minor adverse effects compliance is very poor with the 5–7 day courses of quinine necessary for cure, and in areas with resistance failure rates up to 50% have been reported. Quinine is usually combined with either tetracycline (or doxycycline) or in some areas sulfadoxine–pyrimethamine or clindamycin to prevent recrudescences of falciparum malaria. Even in areas with a high prevalence of resistance the quinine–tetracycline combination, given for 7 days, still retains cure rates over 85%.[11]

Atovaquone–proguanil has been introduced recently. It is highly effective against all malaria parasites. High-level resistance to atovaquone was reported in early clinical trials, and remains a concern if this drug is deployed widely. But the very high cost of manufacture and consequent high price are likely to limit use. Atovaquone–proguanil is being used increasingly as a prophylactic.

The most important new additions to the antimalarial armamentarium are the antimalarial peroxides derived from qinghao or *Artemisia annua* (sweet wormwood). The artemisinin compounds were discovered in China and are the most rapidly effective, potent, and have the broadest stage-specificity of action of all antimalarial drugs.[12] They have been used extensively in south-east Asia since 1992, as they retain excellent efficacy against multiresistant parasites, and they are rapidly effective in severe malaria. They prevent gametocyte development and therefore reduce transmission. This can reduce the incidence of malaria in low transmission settings. Use in the Indian subcontinent, Africa and South America is increasing. To date, there have been no well-documented cases of resistance to artemisinin or its derivatives.[13] In uncomplicated malaria these drugs are used in combination with other antimalarial drugs. Combined with existing drugs they accelerate the initial therapeutic response, improve efficacy, reduce gametocyte carriage and in the case of mefloquine, tolerance. Artesunate–mefloquine has proved highly effective in south-east Asia, despite pre-existing mefloquine resistance.[14] The fixed combination of artemether and lumefantrine is a highly effective and well tolerated alternative to artesunate–mefloquine. Dihydroartemisinin–piperaquine is another fixed combination from China with excellent activity against multidrug-resistant parasites.

RESISTANCE

MECHANISMS

Resistance to antimalarial drugs arises through the selection of rare naturally arising mutants with reduced drug susceptibility. Unlike some bacteria, plasmodia do not have transferable resistance mechanisms, but they are eukaryotes, and they can acquire or lose polygenic resistance mechanisms during meiosis. Resistance arises readily to drugs such as the antifols or atovaquone because single-point mutations confer resistance (as opposed to a requirement for several unlinked mutations – i.e. epistasis) and per-parasite mutation frequencies for these viable mutations are relatively high (>1 in 10^{13} mitotic divisions).[15] Pyrimethamine and the active metabolites of the antimalarial biguanides (cycloguanil from proguanil, and chlorcycloguanil from chlorproguanil) interfere with folic acid synthesis in the parasite by inhibiting the bifunctional enzyme dihydrofolate reductase–thymidylate synthase (DHFR). Sulfonamides act at the previous step in the synthetic pathway by inhibiting dihydropteroate synthase (DHPS), and there is marked synergy between the two classes of compounds (*see* Ch. 2). Resistance in *P. falciparum* and *P. vivax* is associated with point mutations in the DHFR gene that lead to reduced affinity (100–1000 times less) of the enzyme complex for the drug. For *P. falciparum* the first mutation is usually at position 108 of *PfDHFR* (serine to asparagine). For *P. falciparum* this has little clinical effect initially, but mutations then arise at positions 51 and 59, which confer increasing resistance to pyrimethamine.[16] Infections with 'triple' mutants are relatively resistant but some therapeutic response is usually seen, particularly if there is background immunity. The acquisition of a fourth mutation at position 164 (isoleucine to leucine) renders the available antifols completely ineffective. This mutation is prevalent in parts of south-east Asia and South America, and has just been reported in East Africa. Mutations conferring moderate levels of pyrimethamine resistance do not necessarily confer cycloguanil resistance, and vice versa. For example mutations at position 16 (alanine to valine) plus serine to threonine at 108 confer high-level resistance to cycloguanil but not pyrimethamine. In general the biguanides (cycloguanil, chlorcycloguanil) are more active than pyrimethamine against the resistant mutants (and they are more effective clinically too), but they are ineffective against parasites with the DHFR 164 mutation. *P. vivax* shares similar antifol resistance mechanisms through serial acquisition of mutations in *PvDHFR*.

The marked synergy with sulfonamides and sulfones is very important for the antimalarial activity of sulfa-pyrimethamine or sulfone-biguanide combinations. Sulfonamide and sulfone resistance also develops by progressive acquisition of mutations in the gene encoding the target enzyme DHPS (which is a bifunctional protein with the enzyme dihydropteridine pyrophosphokinase. Specifically altered amino acid residues have been found at positions 436, 437, 540, 581, and 613 in the DHPS domain. The 581 and 631 mutations do not occur in isolation, but always on top of an initial mutation (usually alanine to glycine at 437).[17]

The mode of action and mechanisms of resistance of the quinoline antimalarials remains controversial. These drugs are weak bases, and they concentrate in the acid food vacuole of the parasite, but this in itself does not explain their antimalarial activity. Chloroquine binds to ferriprotoporphyrin IX, a product of hemoglobin degradation, and thereby chemically inhibits heme dimerization (*see* Ch. 2). Chloroquine also inhibits competitively glutathione-mediated heme degradation, another parasite detoxification pathway. Chloroquine resistance is associated with reduced concentrations of drug in the acid food vacuole. Both reduced influx and increased efflux have been implicated. Resistant parasites pump chloroquine out 40–50 times faster than drug-sensitive parasites. This efflux mechanism is similar to that found in multidrug resistant (MDR) mammalian tumor cells. One of the efflux mechanisms is through an ATP-requiring transmembrane pump, P-glycoprotein. These MDR genes (*pfmdr1*) are found in increased numbers in most quinine and mefloquine-resistant *P falciparum* parasites, and point mutations (notably asparagine to tyrosine at position 86) are associated with chloroquine resistance. Recently point mutations in CRT (a food vacuolar membrane protein thought to have a transporter function), have been shown to mediate chloroquine resistance.[18] The principal correlate of low level resistance is a *PfCRT* mutation, resulting in a change in coding from lysine to threonine at position 76. From an epidemiological standpoint multiple unlinked mutations are probably required for the development of chloroquine resistance, and it is likely that other contributors to quinoline resistance remain to be discovered. The role of these mechanisms in resistance to the other aryl aminoalcohol antimalarials (amodiaquine, halofantrine, lumefantrine, piperaquine and pyronaridine) remains to be elucidated.

The chloroquine efflux mechanism in resistant parasites can be inhibited by a number of structurally unrelated drugs such as calcium-channel blockers, tricyclic antidepressants, phenothiazines, cyproheptadine and antihistamines whereas mefloquine resistance is reversed by penfluridol, which does not reduce chloroquine efflux. Clinical trials of reversers have yielded conflicting results. Whether general use of resistance reversers will be a safe and feasible therapeutic option remains to be seen. In general, antimalarial drug resistance to mefloquine, quinine, lumefantrine, and halofantrine is linked but, as suggested by their different susceptibility to reversing agents, chloroquine resistance and mefloquine resistance are not linked closely. Indeed, within a particular geographic area there is a reciprocal relationship; mefloquine resistance is correlated inversely with chloroquine resistance.

Atovaquone interferes with parasite mitochondrial electron transport and depolarizes the parasite mitochondria, thereby blocking cellular respiration. High levels of resistance result from single point mutations in the gene encoding cytochrome

b. This gene is encoded on a small extrachromosomal plastid-like DNA-containing organelle that may have an intrinsically high mutation rate. Resistance mutations arise frequently (about 1 in 10^{12} asexual divisions).

The artemisinin drugs kill malaria parasites by generating carbon-centered free radicals, which alkylate critical proteins. Parasiticidal activity is dependent on the integrity of the peroxide bridge. Although in general multiresistant parasites are more artemisinin-resistant, and reduced susceptibility can be induced experimentally, the degree of resistance is slight and very unlikely to be of clinical relevance.

Several factors encourage the development of resistance.

- The intrinsic frequency with which the genetic changes occur.
- The degree of resistance conferred by the genetic change (pharmacodynamics).
- The proportion of all transmissible infections that are exposed to the drug.
- The drug concentration profile (pharmacokinetics).
- The pattern of drug use.
- The immunity profile of the community.[15]

Resistant parasites will be selected when parasites are exposed to subtherapeutic drug concentrations. Thus nonimmune patients infected with large numbers of parasites who receive inadequate treatment (because of poor drug quality, reduced adherence, vomiting of an oral treatment, etc.) are a potent source of resistance. This emphasizes the importance of correct prescribing and good adherence to prescribed drug regimens in slowing the emergence of resistance. Resistance develops more slowly in high-transmission areas, because the patients' background immunity may eliminate the resistant mutants and stop them being transmitted. The spread of resistant mutant parasites is facilitated by the use of drugs with long elimination phases, which provide a 'selective filter', allowing infection by the resistant parasites while the residual antimalarial activity prevents infection by sensitive parasites. Slowly eliminated drugs such as mefloquine (terminal half-life 3 weeks) or chloroquine (terminal half-life 2 months) persist in blood for months after drug administration and provide such a selective filter.

PREVENTION OF RESISTANCE USING COMBINATIONS OF ANTIMALARIAL DRUGS

The emergence of resistance can be prevented by the use of combinations of drugs with different mechanisms of action, and therefore different drug targets and unlinked resistance mechanisms.[15,19] The same rationale underlies the current treatment of tuberculosis, leprosy, HIV infections and many cancers. If two drugs with different mechanisms of action are used then the per-parasite probability of developing resistance to both drugs is the product of their individual per-parasite probabilities. For example, if the per-parasite probability of developing resistance to drug A and drug B are both 1 in 10^{12} then a simultaneously resistant mutant will arise spontaneously every 1 in 10^{24} parasites. As there are approximately 10^{17} malaria parasites in the entire world, and a cumulative total of less than 10^{20} in one year, such a simultaneously resistant parasite would arise spontaneously roughly once every 10 000 years – if the drugs always confronted the parasites in combination. Thus the lower the de-novo per-parasite probability of developing resistance, the greater the delay in the emergence of resistance. This powerful approach has several limitations. If not everyone receives the combination, and some patients only receive one of the components, or there is already high-level resistance to one of the components, then resistance can arise (emphasizing the importance of achieving high coverage when these drugs are deployed). Combinations are also more expensive. But the increased cost is outweighed by the longer term benefits. The most promising approach is the systematic deployment everywhere of artemisinin combinations, but which combinations has yet to be decided.

CLINICAL ASSESSMENT OF RESISTANCE

Low-grade resistance (R1 resistance) is usually manifest by recrudescences, which tend to occur several weeks after primary treatment. Most recrudescences occur within 6 weeks of initial treatment. For quinine and other rapidly eliminated drugs the median time to recrudescence as resistance begins is approximately 3 weeks, but for drugs that have long terminal half-lives, such as mefloquine, the recrudescences can occur up to 10 weeks, and possibly longer, after the primary treatment. Although the treatment is unable to eradicate the parasites in such cases, the multiplication rate is suppressed whilst therapeutic blood concentrations are still present in the blood. The more susceptible the parasites, the lower the blood concentrations required to suppress parasite multiplication. As resistance worsens, the median time to recrudescence becomes shorter and an increasing number of patients are seen in whom parasitemia fails to clear by 7 days following treatment (R2 resistance). Eventually the situation deteriorates further and some patients do not respond at all to antimalarial treatment (R3 resistance). Obviously, alternative treatment should be employed before this stage. In the individual patient long parasite clearance times (>4 days) are a common predictor of subsequent recrudescence.

UNCOMPLICATED MALARIA

MANAGEMENT

Infections with *P. vivax*, *Plasmodium malariae*, or *Plasmodium ovale* are very rarely fatal, but *P. falciparum* malaria may progress rapidly to severe disease and death, particularly in the non-immune patient or young children in endemic areas. If the clinician is in any doubt about the severity of the infection, the patient should remain in hospital under observation. Otherwise, uncomplicated malaria can be treated on an outpatient basis. If there is any uncertainty over speciation of the parasites they should be considered as *P. falciparum*, and if there is any doubt over drug susceptibility the infection should be considered as resistant. A thorough history and examination should pay particular attention to likely origin of the infection, and any previous antimalarial treatment. Except in areas without facilities for diagnosis, antimalarial treatment should be given only for slide- or dipstick-confirmed malaria. In general, administration of the first dose should be observed. Symptomatic measures are important. The incidence of vomiting, particularly in children, is proportional to fever. Young children with high fevers should be cooled, given paracetamol (acetaminophen) (15 mg/kg), and allowed to settle before receiving the first oral dose of antimalarial treatment. The patient should be observed for 1 h after drug administration, and if vomiting occurs within this period the drugs should be readministered (*see below*). Ideally, patients should be seen daily for a clinical examination and a blood smear until they are asymptomatic and parasite negative. They should be advised to return to the same hospital or clinic if fever recurs within 6 weeks.

SPECIFIC ANTIMALARIAL TREATMENT

P. VIVAX, P. OVALE AND *P. MALARIAE*

P. vivax is the most common cause of malaria in the Indian subcontinent, Central America, North Africa, and the Middle East. There is unequivocal evidence of chloroquine resistance in *P. vivax* from parts of south-east Asia and Oceania, but elsewhere infections with this parasite, and the other two that cause the benign human malarias, remain sensitive to chloroquine. Treatment is rapidly effective and usually well tolerated. The main adverse effect is troublesome pruritus in dark-skinned patients, which occurs in approximately 50% of cases. The quinoline antimalarials may all exacerbate the orthostatic hypotension that commonly complicates malaria, and symptomatic postural hypotension is common.[20] Rarely (less than 1 in 1000), chloroquine treatment is associated with transient neuropsychiatric abnormalities.

The total dose of chloroquine is 25 mg base/kg divided classically as 10, 10 and 5 mg/kg given on days 0, 1, and 2, respectively (adult dose 600 mg base followed by three doses of 300 mg). This schedule may be compressed into a 36 h treatment regimen, giving 10, 5, 5, and 5 mg/kg at 12-hour intervals[21] (Table 64.1). Both *P. vivax* and *P. ovale* infections produce persistent dormant hepatic forms of the parasite (hypnozoites), which are resistant to chloroquine. These become activated between 3 weeks and 1 year after the primary infection, and cause the relapses so characteristic of these infections. (A *relapse* is a recurrent infection caused by the development of persistent hypnozoites: the primary blood-stage

Table 64.1 Antimalarial drugs: recommended doses for treatment

	Uncomplicated malaria: dose	Usual adult dose	Severe malaria[a]
Chloroquine	10 mg base/kg followed by 10 mg/kg at 24 h and 5 mg/kg at 48 h or 5 mg/kg at 12, 24 and 36 h. Total dose 25 mg base/kg For *P. vivax* or *P. ovale* add primaquine 0.25 mg/kg daily for 14 days[b] for radical cure	4 × 150 mg tablets followed by 4 then 2 or 2, 2, 2	10 mg base/kg by constant-rate infusion over 8 h followed by 15 mg/kg over 24 h or 3.5 mg base/kg by intramuscular or subcutaneous injection every 6 h. Total dose 25 mg base/kg[a]
Sulfadoxine–pyrimethamine	25/1.25 mg/kg single oral dose	3 tablets	Efficacy of the parenteral formulation in severe malaria unproven
Mefloquine	25 mg/kg: give 15 mg base/kg followed by 10 mg/kg dose 8–24 h later. Alternatively, give 8.3 mg/kg daily for 3 days	3 × 250 mg tablets + 2 × 250 mg tablets	
Artesunate	In combination with a slowly eliminated drug 4 mg/kg daily for 3 days[c]. If used alone or with a tetracycline or clindamycin, 4 mg/kg followed by 2 mg/kg daily: total 7 days	4 × 50 mg daily for 3 days in combination 4 × 50 mg followed by 2 × 50 mg daily for 6 days	2.4 mg/kg i.v. or i.m. immediately followed by 1.2 mg/kg at (12), 24 h and then daily[a]
Artemether	Same oral dose regimens as for artesunate	5 × 40 mg daily for 3 days in combination	3.2 mg/kg i.m. immediately followed by 1.6 mg/kg daily[a]
Dihydroartemisinin	Same oral dose regimens as for artesunate	5 × 40 mg followed by 3 × 40 mg daily for 6 days	
Artemether-lumefantrine	80/480 mg twice daily for 3 days with food	4 tablets twice daily for 3 days.	
Halofantrine	8 mg base/kg 3 times in one day[d]	2 × 250 mg three times	
Quinine	10 mg salt/kg 8-hourly for 7 days. Often combined with tetracycline[e] (4 mg/kg) four times daily for 7 days.	2 × 300 mg three times daily	20 mg salt/kg by intravenous infusion over 4 h[f] followed by 10 mg/kg infused over 2–8 h every 8 h[a]
Quinidine	Recommended *only* if alternatives unavailable. Dose as for quinine	Do not use oral quinidine	10 mg base/kg infused at constant rate over 1 h followed by 0.02 mg/kg per minute, with electrocardiographic monitoring[a]
Atovaquone–proguanil	1000/400 mg once daily for 3 days with food.	4 tablets twice daily for 3 days	

[a] Oral treatment should be substituted as soon as the patient can take tablets by mouth.
[b] In Oceania and south-east Asia the dose should be higher: 0.33–0.5 mg base/kg. In patients with mild glucose-6-phosphate dehydrogenase deficiency give 0.7 mg/kg once weekly for 6 weeks.
[c] For hyperparasitemic patients (>4% parasitemia in a non-immune) give artesunate for 5 days; 4 mg/kg then 2 mg/kg daily for 4 days with a second drug.
[d] In 'non-immunes' it is recommended that a repeat 3-dose treatment be given on day 7.
[e] Doxycycline 3 mg/kg daily is an alternative to tetracycline. Tetracycline or doxycycline should not be given to pregnant women or children <8 years old.
[f] Alternatively for the initial loading dose, 7 mg salt/kg can be infused over 30 min followed by 10 mg salt/kg over 4 h.

infection has cleared. A *recrudescence* is a blood-stage infection that is not eradicated, but may decline below the level of microscopic detection, and then increases later causing patent parasitemia and clinical illness). The hypnozoites are sensitive only to the 8-aminoquinoloine antimalarials. The eradication of both the blood stage and the persistent liver stages of malaria is called a 'radical cure'. For this, primaquine is usually given in an adult daily dose of 15 mg base (0.25 mg/kg) for 14 days. Strains of *P. vivax* from Oceania and some parts of south-east Asia appear to be more resistant to the hypnozoitocidal effects of primaquine, and a daily dose of 22.5–30 mg base (0.375–0.5 mg/kg) should be given for 14 days for infections originating in these areas. Primaquine has weak asexual-stage activity against *P. vivax* and this may mask low-level chloroquine resistance if the two drugs are given together.

Primaquine is an oxidant drug and causes hemolysis in patients with hereditary defects in the pentose-phosphate shunt, most commonly glucose-6-phosphate dehydrogenase (G6PD) deficiency. In patients with severe variants of G6PD deficiency primaquine is contraindicated, but for patients with mild variants primaquine should be given in a weekly dose of 45 mg base (0.75 mg/kg) for 6 weeks. Although chloroquine is considered safe, primaquine should not be used in pregnancy or given to newborns. Pyrimethamine and the pyrimethamine–sulfonamide combinations are relatively ineffective against *P. vivax* in many areas because of acquired resistance. All the other antimalarial drugs are active, and so for mixed infections requiring treatment for *P. falciparum* it is not necessary to add chloroquine. However, primaquine should be given as well to prevent relapses.

UNCOMPLICATED *P. FALCIPARUM* MALARIA

Antimalarial treatments are increasingly using combinations of antimalarial drugs. Several of the artemisinin combinations (artesunate–mefloquine, artemether–lumefantrine, artesunate–atovaquone–proguanil) can be relied upon everywhere in the world. In those areas such as Central America or North Africa where *P. falciparum* remains sensitive, chloroquine can still be used in a total treatment dose of 25 mg base/kg (adult dose 1500 mg). There is no significant difference between the phosphate, sulfate or hydrochloride salts. If there is any doubt about antimalarial sensitivity in the area where malaria was acquired, *P. falciparum* infections should be considered resistant.

UNCOMPLICATED CHLOROQUINE-RESISTANT FALCIPARUM MALARIA

Amodiaquine is more effective than chloroquine against resistant strains of *P. falciparum*. It is also well tolerated. When used in prophylaxis amodiaquine was associated with a 1 in 2000 incidence of agranulocytosis. The true incidence of this in therapeutic use is not known but is certainly much lower. In some countries amodiaquine in a total dose of 25–35 mg base/kg (adult dose 1.5–2.5 g), divided over 3 days, is given where there is low-level chloroquine resistance.

A single dose of sulfadoxine–pyrimethamine (20/1 mg/kg; corresponding to three tablets in an adult) is a well tolerated and effective treatment of sensitive strains. This is now a first-line treatment for *P. falciparum* malaria in some countries in East Africa. The principal adverse effects result from sulfonamide allergy. When used in prophylaxis the incidence of serious adverse effects is approximately 1 in 7000, and fatal adverse effects occurs in 1 in 18 000.[22] In single-dose treatment the incidence of serious adverse effects appears to be significantly lower. Pyrimethamine-induced blood dyscrasias, seen usually in patients with underlying folate deficiency, are most unusual. As an alternative, combinations of chlorproguanil and dapsone are currently under evaluation. There is an increasing tendency to combine all these drugs with artesunate (4 mg/kg daily for 3 days) both to increase efficacy and to protect from resistance.[19] Alternatively, where sensitivity is retained chloroquine or amodiaquine may be combined safely with sulfadoxine–pyrimethamine. There are no significant interactions among these drugs.

MULTIDRUG-RESISTANT *P. FALCIPARUM* MALARIA

Mefloquine

Mefloquine (hydrochloride) has the advantage of a long terminal elimination half-life of 2–3 weeks and in the past it has been given in a single dose of 15 mg base/kg (adult dose

three tablets of 250 mg)[23] to semi-immune patients. A higher dose 25 mg base/kg (five tablets for an adult) is generally more effective and less likely to lead to resistance. Peak whole blood concentrations above 1000 ng/ml are effective. Recent studies suggest that absorption is augmented, but adverse effects are not increased, if the treatment dose is split (i.e. a 25 mg base/kg dose is given as 15 mg/kg initially, followed by 10 mg/kg 8–24 h later, or as 8.3 mg/kg for 3 days daily.

Mefloquine–artesunate

Combining mefloquine with artesunate (4 mg/kg daily for 3 days) further improves efficacy and reduces immediate adverse effects.[9] As with many antimalarial drugs, children tolerate mefloquine better than adults.[24] The principal adverse effect of mefloquine is immediate vomiting. This is less likely if the dosage is split, and started on the second day of the 3-day combined regimen with artesunate. Patients must be observed for 1 h after the drug has been given. If vomiting occurs within 30 min the full dose of mefloquine should be repeated. For vomiting 30–60 min later, half the dose should be given. Vomiting after 1 h does not require retreatment. Later adverse effects are all more common in adults and comprise nausea, dysphoria, dizziness or 'muzziness', poor concentration, sleeplessness, nightmares and postural hypotension. Mefloquine does not have significant cardiac effects. Adverse effects following mefloquine treatment are reported more frequently in women than in men. Serious, but reversible neuropsychiatric reactions occur in approximately 1 in 1300 Asians patients receiving high-dose mefloquine treatment, but as many as 1 in 200 European and African patients. This rises to 1 in 20 if mefloquine is given following acute treatment of severe malaria, and it should not be used in this context.[25]

Artemether–lumefantrine

The new combination of artemether and lumefantrine is as effective as artesunate–mefloquine and has several advantages.[3]

1. It is a fixed combination and lumefantrine is not available as a single drug (which improves compliance and reduces resistance selection in endemic areas).
2. It is better tolerated (indeed it does not appear to have any significant adverse effects) and, in particular, produces less vomiting and has no central nervous toxicity.
3. The lumefantrine component is more rapidly eliminated than mefloquine (half-life *c*. 4 days compared with 14 days for mefloquine in malaria), which would be expected to reduce the selection of resistant parasites. On the other hand, it needs to be given twice daily for 3 days instead of once daily, and absorption of lumefantrine is very variable (like atovaquone and halofantrine, it is highly fat dependent).

There are no pediatric formulations available yet for either combination.

Dihydroartemisinin–piperaquine

Dihydroartemisinin–piperaquine is another fixed-dose artemisinin combination from China. Although it is registered in China, Vietnam and Cambodia, and it has proved highly effective against multiresistant falciparum malaria there are outstanding questions over the optimum dose and adverse effect profile of this interesting and inexpensive compound.

Atovaquone–proguanil

Atovaquone–proguanil is very well tolerated and highly effective against all the human malaria parasites. Fortunately, resistance has not yet proved to be a problem with limited use, although many consider that this drug should be used only in combination with an artemisinin derivative in treatment. Interestingly, the synergistic activity of proguanil with atovaquone is derived from the parent compound through an uncharacterized mechanism, and not dihydrofolate reductase inhibition by the triazine metabolite cycloguanil. This is important because atovaquone–proguanil retains excellent activity against highly antifol-resistant parasites; and also in East Asia where 20% of the population have a genetic polymorphism resulting in reduced CYP_{450} 2C19 activity – the enzyme responsible for conversion of proguanil to cycloguanil. The main drawback to atovaquone–proguanil is its cost. It is given in a 3-day course. There is no pediatric formulation.

Halofantrine

Halofantrine is intrinsically more active than mefloquine, and is better tolerated.[24] It suffers the disadvantages of requiring multiple dose administration as it has very erratic oral bioavailability. The current recommendation is to give 24 mg base/kg divided into three doses 8 h apart (adult dose 500 mg × 3), and to repeat this 1 week later in non-immune subjects. In mefloquine-resistant areas, the single-day regimen has a failure rate of approximately 40%. Use of halofantrine has been associated with sudden death. Halofantrine, like quinidine, induces a predictable prolongation of the electrocardiograph QT interval (delayed ventricular repolarization).[10] This can be pro-arrhythmic. Atrioventricular conduction abnormalities (first- and, rarely, second-degree block) have also been seen. These cardiac effects are augmented by previous treatment with mefloquine. Halofantrine should not be given to patients who have received mefloquine in the previous month, or to patients either with known prolongation of the QT interval or who are receiving other drugs known to prolong the QT interval. This potentially lethal toxicity has markedly limited its use. Halofantrine absorption is augmented considerably by coadministration with fats or fatty food. The other adverse effect reported with high-dose treatment is diarrhea. Halofantrine does not have significant adverse central nervous system effects.

Quinine

Quinine sulfate, the time-honored remedy, at a dose of 10 mg/kg (adult dose 600 mg) three times daily is effective in a 7-day course. Shorter courses (3–5 days) are much less effective. Quinine is usually combined with tetracycline, doxycycline or, particularly in children or pregnant women, with clindamycin to improve cure rates. In areas where full sensitivity to all drugs is retained, a single dose of sulfadoxine–pyrimethamine (adult dose three tablets) may be added instead. Quinine is not well tolerated. The characteristic syndrome of 'cinchonism', comprising nausea, vomiting, dizziness, dysphoria and high-tone deafness is a predictable accompaniment of quinine treatment. In addition, the drug is extremely bitter and many children find it unacceptable. However, serious adverse effects, principally blindness, deafness or cardiac dysrhythmias, are unusual. Hypoglycemia is more common in severe malaria, although it may also develop in uncomplicated malaria treated by quinine, particularly in young children or pregnant women. Hypoglycemia results from stimulation of the pancreatic β-cells and consequent hyperinsulinemia.

Artemisinin derivatives

The artemisinin derivatives comprise the parent compound artemisinin, dihydroartemisinin (which is 5–10 times more potent), artemether, and artesunate. In vivo artesunate and artemether are converted back to dihydroartemisinin. The most widely used of the drugs is artesunate. These drugs are all well absorbed by mouth, and rapidly eliminated (dihydroartemisinin half-life 1 h). They are all very well tolerated with no consistent adverse effects.[26] Serious allergic reactions, (usually preceded by urticaria) have been reported in approximately 1 in 1300 patients. The parasiticidal and clinical responses are more rapid than with other antimalarials. They also reduce gametocyte carriage, and therefore the transmission potential of the infection.[27] The artemisinin derivatives are usually combined with a more slowly eliminated drug, in which case they are given over 3 days. In patients who have uncomplicated hyperparasitemia (i.e. a non-immune with more than 4% parasitemia but no vital organ dysfunction) the dose should be spread over 5 days (4 mg/kg immediately then 2 mg/kg daily for 4 days with the accompanying drug). When given alone they should be given for 7 days in a dose of 4 mg/kg initially then 2 mg/kg daily, and preferably in combination with doxycycline or clindamycin.

These drugs are currently not available in the USA or Australasia. Travelers returning to these countries with multiresistant *P. falciparum* malaria should be treated with quinine plus tetracycline or doxycycline.

Monitoring the response to treatment

If possible patients should be seen at least daily until parasite and fever clearance; this is not possible in most endemic areas.

If there is clinical deterioration, or repeated vomiting then parenteral treatment should be substituted. If there is an early failure of treatment suggesting drug resistance then a different treatment must be substituted. If there is a return of parasitemia after one week, then it may not be possible to distinguish recrudescence from reinfection in an endemic area (this requires a comparison of parasite genotypes). The choice of subsequent retreatment will then depend on the prevailing level of resistance. Most drugs can be repeated within one month, but for mefloquine this should be avoided as there is an increased risk of neuropsychiatric reactions with retreatment. Either a 7-day course of artesunate (or quinine) and doxycycline (clindamycin in children), or a 3-day, six dose course of artemether–lumefantrine should be prescribed.

SEVERE *P. FALCIPARUM* MALARIA

Management

Severe malaria is a multisystem disease requiring intensive care management. Unfortunately, optimum treatment is usually not available in most of the areas of the world where severe malaria occurs. Severe malaria has been defined as the presence of one or more of the following: unrousable coma (cerebral malaria), severe anemia (hematocrit <15% plus parasitemia >100 000/µl), renal failure (serum creatinine >265 µmol/l), pulmonary edema, hypoglycemia (glucose <2.2 mmol/l), shock, bleeding, repeated seizures, metabolic acidosis or hemoglobinuria. The clinician should not feel restricted by this definition:[28] a simpler bedside assessment based on any impairment of consciousness or inability to sit unaided (prostration), acidotic breathing (respiratory distress), anuria, hypoglycemia, severe anemia, shock or a high parasitemia (>4% in a non-immune, >20% in any patient) identifies those patients in need of intensive care. Any patient in whom there is doubt as to the severity of the infection should be managed as described below.

A rapid clinical appraisal should be made. This includes assessment of the level of consciousness or central nervous system dysfunction, exclusion of covert seizure activity (clinical evidence of seizures can be subtle), measurement of vital signs (particularly respiratory pattern and rate), questioning of the patient or relatives concerning earlier antimalarial treatment, duration of impaired consciousness, convulsions and urine output. A malaria parasite count (thick and thin blood films), blood glucose, plasma bicarbonate or blood lactate, and hematocrit should be measured immediately. The patient should be rehydrated with saline and, if there is any doubt about the jugular venous pressure, a central venous line should be inserted and central pressure monitored. If hypoglycemia is suspected or confirmed, 0.3 g/kg (25 g) of glucose should be given by slow intravenous injection. The role of prophylactic intramuscular phenobarbitone in childhood cerebral malaria is uncertain after a recent large study from Kenya showed significant protection against convulsions following 20 mg/kg of intramuscular phenobarbitone, but an *increased* mortality.[29] This was associated with repeated diazepam administration (for uncontrolled seizures) and was attributable to respiratory arrest. Some authorities still give a lower dose (7 mg/kg) of phenoloarbitone. Patients with respiratory abnormalities should be ventilated early, with care to avoid even temporary hypercapnea. Prompt anticonvulsant therapy (intravenous lorazepam, midazolam or diazepam) should be given if there are seizures. A lumbar puncture should be performed to exclude coincident meningitis. Hemofiltration should be started early in patients with acute renal failure, and blood (preferably fresh) should be transfused if the hematocrit falls below 20%. Antimalarial drugs should be given on a milligram-per-kilogram basis. The patient should be weighed and parenteral treatment given intravenously if possible. Artesunate can be given by slow intravenous injection but quinine or quinidine must be given by slow intravenous infusion. Rises in parasitemia in the first 12 h after antimalarial treatment has started should *not* be attributed to drug resistance. Conversely, a rapid decline in parasitemia shortly after drug administration does not indicate a very sensitive infection. These changes result from natural fluctuations in parasitemia related to synchronous schizogony and sequestration respectively. If, by 48 h after starting treatment, parasitemia has not fallen by more than 75% (R3 resistance), then the treatment should be changed, but this is extremely unusual. Therapeutic responses are assessed in terms of clinical measures: times to recovery of consciousness, and in adults the times to reach Glasgow coma scores of 8, 11 and 15; the time until fever falls below 37.5 °C and remains below this for 24 h; and laboratory measures, which include the rate of fall in plasma lactate and the times to reduce parasitemia by 50%, 90% and 100%. If the parasitemia has not cleared by 7 days, treatment should be continued, provided of course the counts are not rising. Adult patients receiving quinine, artesunate or artemether should receive a 7-day course of doxycycline, and children clindamycin, which starts when the patient can take oral medicine.

SPECIFIC ANTIMALARIAL THERAPY

CHLOROQUINE

In those few fully chloroquine-sensitive areas, intravenous chloroquine is still the treatment of choice. However, if there is any doubt then quinine, quinidine or, if available, one of the artemisinin derivatives should be given as described below. Intravenous artesunate is probably the best treatment of all, but it is not available in many countries. Chloroquine has unusual pharmacokinetic properties, characterized by an enormous total apparent volume of distribution and a very slow terminal elimination phase (half-life 1–2 months). As a consequence, blood concentrations in the treatment of acute malaria are determined by distribution rather than elimination processes. Provided chloroquine enters the circulation slowly, immediate toxicity (principally hypotension or cardiac dysfunction) will not occur. Intravenous chloroquine in normal saline or 5% dextrose should be given by carefully rate-controlled infusion in a dose of 10 mg base/kg over 8 h followed by 15 mg base/kg infused over 24 h. Intramuscular and subcutaneous chloroquine are absorbed rapidly, even in the most severely ill patients. Doses higher than 3.5 mg/kg risk producing transiently toxic blood concentrations. Intramuscular or subcutaneous chloroquine should be given in a dose of 3.5 mg base/kg 6-hourly, or 2.5 mg base/kg 4-hourly, until the patient recovers sufficiently to complete the total dose (25 mg/kg) of treatment by mouth.[28] The principal adverse effect of parenteral chloroquine is hypotension, but the risks may be reduced considerably by careful attention to dose and rate of administration. Although a parenteral (intramuscular) formulation of sulfadoxine–pyrimethamine is available, it has not been assessed sufficiently in the treatment of severe malaria and should not be used. There are no generally available parenteral formulations of halofantrine or mefloquine.

SEVERE CHLOROQUINE-RESISTANT MALARIA

Quinine

Parenteral quinine should be given by slow rate-controlled intravenous infusion. Where this is not possible, intramuscular administration is an effective alternative. In order to achieve therapeutic concentrations as early as possible in the course of treatment, which may be life-saving, an initial loading dose is recommended. A variety of approaches have been described. The simplest is to give a loading dose of 20 mg quinine dihydrochloride salt/kg by constant rate infusion over 4 h, dissolved in 5% or 10% dextrose, or normal (0.9%) saline.[30] Alternatively, 7 mg salt/kg may be infused over 30 min, followed immediately by 10 mg/kg over 4 h[31]. It has been suggested that in East Africa, where *P. falciparum* is considerably more susceptible to quinine than in south east Asia or South America, a loading dose of 15 mg/kg would suffice,[32] but this is unproven and could lead to undertreatment in some patients. After the initial loading dose, maintenance doses of 10 mg salt/kg should be given every 8 h. For the treatment of children in sensitive areas 12-hourly administration suffices. Maintenance dose intravenous infusions can be given over 2–12 h. Quinine should *never* by given by intravenous injection. Intramuscular bioavailability is good even in severe malaria, although there is still uncertainty as to the optimum dilution. Quinine dihydrochloride should be diluted between 2 and 5:1 with sterile water for intramuscular injection and given into the anterior thigh. The initial loading dose should be divided (10 mg/kg to each thigh). Undiluted quinine dihydrochloride (300 mg/ml) is acidic (pH 2) and painful, and may occasionally result in sterile abscesses or tetanus. The therapeutic range for quinine has not been defined previously, but total plasma concentrations between 8 and 15 mg/l are safe and effective.[33] There is an increased potential risk of toxicity with free (unbound) quinine levels over 2 mg/l (corresponding to total plasma concentrations of approximately 20 mg/l). To prevent accumulation to toxic levels the dose of quinine should be reduced by one-third on the third day of treatment if there is no clinical improvement or the patient is in acute renal failure.

The principal adverse effect of quinine in the treatment of severe malaria is hypoglycemia.[34] This is a particular problem in children and pregnant women (occurring in 50% of the latter group) and tends to occur after 24 h of treatment in those patients who remain severely ill. Management is difficult as hypoglycemia is often recurrent. A maintenance infusion of 10% glucose should be given after correction with a bolus of 0.3 g/kg (25 g) of glucose given by slow intravenous injection. Cinchonism is common in recovering patients, but does not limit dosage. Adverse cardiovascular or central nervous system effects (particularly retinal blindness or deafness) are very unusual and, in general, parenteral quinine is well tolerated in the treatment of severe malaria.[35] Electrocardiographic monitoring is not necessary except in patients with previous heart disease. In the tropics there have been concerns over the use of a loading dose in areas where patients are commonly pretreated before admission to hospital and therefore may already have therapeutic blood concentrations of quinine on admission, but these concerns have not been substantiated in large trials.[36] Undertreatment is more dangerous than overtreatment. Our practice is to give a loading dose of quinine unless the patient has definitely received 25 mg/kg of quinine or more in the preceding 48 h. We have not seen any serious complications using these guidelines.

Quinidine

In some countries, notably the USA, parenteral quinine is not available.[37] In this case quinidine (the dextrorotatory diastereoisomer) may be used as an alternative. This is usually available as the gluconate salt. Quinidine is intrinsically more active than quinine as an antimalarial, but it also has an approximately fourfold greater effect on the heart, and electrocardiographic monitoring is necessary.[38] The dose has been controversial (as there are few studies on which to base it). An infusion of 10 mg base/kg given by constant rate intravenous infusion over 1 h as a loading dose, followed by 0.02 mg/kg per minute (1.2 mg/kg per hour) thereafter until the patient can be safely switched to oral treatment will achieve therapeutic concentrations. If the QT interval is prolonged by more than 25% of the baseline value, or exceeds an absolute value of 0.6 s, the infusion should be stopped. Hypotension should be treated with intravenous saline. Quinidine has the same propensity as quinine to induce hypoglycemia. As with quinine, the therapeutic range has not been determined precisely, but total plasma concentrations of 5–8 mg/l should be achieved. Plasma concentration monitoring is advisable. If it is not available then the dose of quinidine should be reduced by one-third on the third day of treatment if there is no clinical improvement, or the patient is in renal failure.

Artemisinin, artemether, arteether and artesunate

Artemisinin and its derivatives have proved remarkably effective alternatives to quinine for the treatment of severe chloroquine-resistant *P. falciparum* malaria. In both uncomplicated and severe infections they have given consistently faster parasite and fever clearance times, and have proved rapidly effective in cerebral malaria.[12] Large randomized trials have compared artemether and quinine in severe malaria.[36,39] Intramuscular artemether was associated with 14% mortality versus 17% with quinine (odds ratio 0.8, 95% confidence interval 0.62–1.02, $P = 0.08$).[40] In the prospectively determined subgroup of adults, artemether was associated with a significantly lower mortality. Artemether was not associated with any serious adverse effects, notably there was no hypoglycemia, and no neurological abnormalities. But artemether (and the similar compound arteether) are oil-based intramuscular injections, and they are absorbed slowly and erratically in severely ill patients.[41] Thus the benefits obtained by greater intrinsic activity and broader stage specificity of action are offset partially by variable absorption. Artesunate is a water-soluble compound which can be given intravenously, and is absorbed rapidly after intramuscular injection. Although it is very widely used, it has not been subject to large comparative trials. The evident pharmacokinetic advantages over artemether and arteether suggest that this is the best drug for severe falciparum malaria. Unfortunately at the time of writing there is only one, non-'good manufacturing practice', source for this compound (Guilin No. 2 Factory, People's Republic of China).

Artesunate

This is provided for parenteral use as artesunic acid powder, which is dispensed together with an ampoule of 5% sodium bicarbonate. The two are mixed immediately before injection. The resulting sodium artesunate is hydrolyzed rapidly in vivo to the biologically active metabolite dihydroartemisinin. Artesunate is usually diluted in 5–10 ml of 5% dextrose before intravenous or intramuscular injection. The currently recommended dose is an initial dose of 2.4 mg/kg followed daily by single doses of 1.2 mg/kg. Some authorities add a 1.2 mg/kg dose at 12 h.

Artemether and arteether

These compounds are very similar. They are dissolved in groundnut or sesame oil and given by intramuscular injection to the anterior thigh in an initial dose of 3.2 mg/kg (for arteether some recommend an initial dose of 4.8 mg/kg), followed by daily injections of 1.6 mg/kg. Oral treatment is substituted as soon as possible. Mefloquine should not be used because the incidence of neurotoxicity is increased following severe malaria.

Rectal formulations

These compounds are absorbed adequately after rectal administration,[42] and this offers the prospect of treating severe malaria in the rural tropics away from health facilities, where most fatalities occur.

Use of the artemisinin derivatives has not been associated with any reported toxicity in the treatment of severe malaria. They do not have cardiovascular or metabolic adverse effects, do not need dose adjustment in renal failure, and they are equally well tolerated by adults and young children. Blackwater (massive hemolysis) seems to occur with the same frequency as with quinine use. In animal models the oil-soluble ethers, artemether and arteether, have both produced selective toxicity to brainstem nuclei. Similar neurotoxicity also followed administration of dihydroartemisinin, the common metabolite. The water-soluble artesunate, and oral administration of any of the drugs is much less neurotoxic. There is no evidence that similar effects occur in humans.

ANTIMALARIAL TREATMENT OF CHILDREN

Apart from early vomiting, children generally tolerate the antimalarial drugs better than adults. For oral treatment, particularly in younger children, care should be taken to cool and calm the patient before oral treatment is given. If the temperature is >38.5 °C, tepid sponging, and oral or rectal paracetamol (15 mg/kg) should be administered and the antimalarials given after the temperature has been lowered (usually 30–60 min). Tablets should be crushed and mixed with water or sweet drink or disguised in jam. The suspension may be drawn up into a syringe so that an accurate dose (on a milligram per kilogram basis) can be instilled into the mouth. Although the pharmacokinetic properties of some antimalarials differ in children, these differences are not great. Dose regimens on a milligram per kilogram basis are the same as in adults, except that primaquine should not be given to neonates, tetracycline should not be given to children <8 years old, and (in resistant areas) the dose of quinine should be increased to 15 mg/kg three times daily after the fourth day.

Children with severe malaria are more likely than adults to have convulsions, or become severely anemic or hypoglycemic. They are less likely to develop renal failure, pulmonary edema or jaundice. In general, children deteriorate more rapidly than adults, but they also recover more quickly.

ANTIMALARIAL TREATMENT IN PREGNANCY

Pregnant women should be treated in the same way as nonpregnant adults, except that for symptomatic women there should be a much lower threshold for admission to hospital. Tetracyclines (or doxycycline), long-acting sulfonamides at term and primaquine should not be used. Mefloquine has been associated with an increased risk of stillbirth in one study.[43] It is now generally considered that artemisinin derivatives should be used if the woman is in the second or third trimesters of pregnancy.[44] In the first trimester oral artemisinin derivatives for uncomplicated malaria should probably be avoided unless there is no alternative, as there are insufficient data to support their use. There are little or no data on the use of halofantrine, atovaquone–proguanil, artemether–lumefantrine or dihydroartemisinin–piperaquine in pregnancy.

Chloroquine, pyrimethamine, proguanil and quinine are all considered safe, although quinine–stimulated hyperinsulinemia is more problematic in late pregnancy. For severe malaria artesunate or artemether are safer and easier to administer than quinine. The risks to the mother in severe malaria dictate that they can be used at any stage of pregnancy.

Breast-feeding

Primaquine should be avoided, but the other drugs can be used as the doses received by the suckling infant are very small.

MALARIA PROPHYLAXIS

It is difficult to make generalized recommendations for antimalarial prophylaxis, as the risks of acquiring malaria and antimalarial drug sensitivity vary considerably over short geographic distances. Antimalarial prophylaxis is indicated in two circumstances:

- in non-immune travelers visiting areas where they may acquire malaria;
- in pregnant women who live in endemic areas.

Antimalarial prophylaxis is not generally recommended otherwise for the indigeneous population in malaria-endemic areas. In practice in endemic areas for prophylaxis in pregnancy this means chloroquine, where it is effective, or intermittent sulfadoxine–pyrimethamine (given twice during pregnancy). In areas in which multiresistance is prevalent there are no safe effective prophylactics for pregnant women.

Drugs are only one component of personal protection against malaria. The risks of acquiring malaria can be reduced considerably by avoiding contact with malaria vectors, by use of appropriate protective clothing, window netting, insect repellents and sleeping under insecticide-impregnated bed nets. Travelers should seek medical advice urgently if they develop a febrile illness. Standby treatment sufficient for one complete antimalarial course may be given to those who will be unable to reach medical services for extended periods. As the geographic distribution of drug resistance changes rapidly, the following general recommendations should be under constant scrutiny.

In areas where *P. falciparum* malaria remains chloroquine sensitive (such as North Africa, the Middle East and Central America north of the Panama Canal) chloroquine alone can be given. In areas where antifol sensitivity is retained and/or *P. vivax* is prevalent then the combination of chloroquine (5 mg base/kg weekly) and proguanil (3 mg/kg daily) is still effective in many areas. Chloroquine is generally well tolerated, although pruritus is common in dark-skinned patients and it may cause occasional skin eruptions or worsening of psoriasis. As chloroquine accumulates in the body, and may cause retinal damage, ophthalmologic examinations are advisable for people who take continuous chloroquine for 5 years or more (total dose >100 g). Retinal toxicity is more common when chloroquine is taken daily for rheumatic diseases, and is probably very unusual with antimalarial prophylaxis. Proguanil is given in a daily dose of 3 mg/kg (adult 200 mg). It is very safe and well tolerated. The main adverse effects are mouth ulcers and, less commonly, alopecia. In renal failure proguanil and its principal metabolite cycloguanil accumulate, and blood dyscrasias have been reported. The fixed-dose combination of pyrimethamine (12.5 mg) and dapsone (100 mg) once weekly has generally been superseded by other drugs, but it remains a second-line prophylaxis for Oceania and other areas where alternative drugs are not usable. The principal adverse effects are related to the sulfone component (methemoglobinemia and occasional blood dyscrasias).

For most endemic areas the choice is between four drugs; mefloquine, doxycycline, primaquine or atovaquone–proguanil. Weekly mefloquine (3.5 mg base/kg equivalent to an adult dose of 250 mg) is often the antimalarial prophylactic of choice. Mefloquine should be started at least 1 week, and preferably 2 weeks, before entering the malarious area, so that therapeutic levels are achieved before exposure and any adverse effects have declared themselves. Mefloquine is generally well tolerated, with an incidence of serious adverse (neuropsychiatric) effects similar to that with chloroquine prophylaxis (about 1 in 10 000 recipients). In 70% of cases these arise within the first 3 weeks of prophylaxis. Less serious central nervous system effects such as dizziness, muzziness, feelings of dissociation, difficulty concentrating, sleeplessness and nightmares are much more common, but these are usually not sufficiently troublesome to limit prophylaxis. Because of inadequate data, rather than evidence of toxicity, mefloquine is considered 'not indicated' in the first trimester of pregnancy or in children under 2 years old. Serious neuropsychiatric reactions (seizures, encephalopathy and psychosis) are more common if there is a previous history of seizures or psychiatric abnormalities, if quinine has been taken, and when mefloquine is used for treatment rather than prophylaxis. These reactions usually resolve spontaneously. Mefloquine should be continued for 1 month after leaving the endemic area. A maximum of 12 months continuous use is currently recommended.

In those few areas where multiresistant *P. falciparum* is also resistant to mefloquine (on the eastern and western borders of Thailand and adjacent Cambodia and Burma), daily doxycycline is generally recommended. As with the other prophylactic drugs this should be continued for 4 weeks after leaving the transmission area. The main adverse effects are nausea, diarrhea, photosensitivity and, in women, *Candida* vaginitis. Doxycycline should be taken after meals with copious fluids to avoid

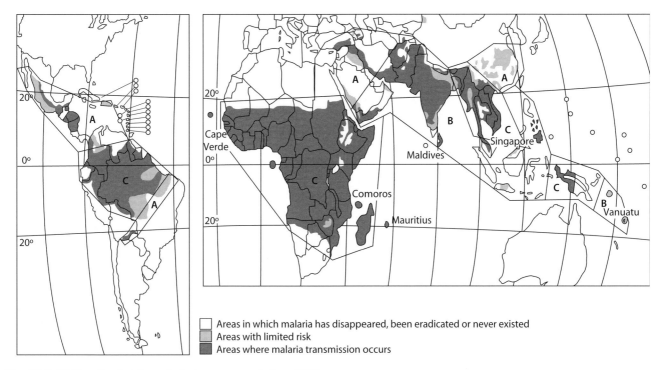

Areas in which malaria has disappeared, been eradicated or never existed
Areas with limited risk
Areas where malaria transmission occurs

Fig. 64.1 WHO antimalarial prophylaxis recommendations 2000

A Risk generally low and seasonal; no risk in many areas (for example urban areas). *P. falciparum* absent or sensitive to chloroquine prophylaxis: chloroquine or (in case of very low risk) no prophylaxis.

B Low risk in most of the areas. Chloroquine alone will protect against *P. vivax*. Chloroquine with proguanil will give some protection against *P. falciparum* and may alleviate the disease if it occurs despite prophylaxis. Prophylaxis: chloroquine + proguanil; second choice mefloquine or (in case of very low risk) no prophylaxis.

C Risk high in most areas of this zone in Africa, except in some high-altitude areas. Risk low in most areas of this zone in Asia and America, but high in parts of the Amazon basin. Resistance to sulfadoxine–pyrimethamine common in zone C in Asia, variable in zone C in Africa and America. Prophylaxis: first choice mefloquine (except areas Cambodia/Burma/Thailand border); second choice doxycycline; third choice chloroquine + proguanil or (in case of very low risk) no prophylaxis.

Note: Protection from mosquito bites should be the rule in all situations, even when prophylaxis is taken.

esophagitis. It should not be given to children under 8 years of age (in the UK a 12-year age limit is recommended as there are very limited data on prophylactic use in older children)[45] (Table 64.1; p. 880), to pregnant women or for more than 3 months in duration. Atovaquone–proguanil (250/100 mg daily) has proved effective and very well tolerated everywhere it has been tested.[46] It is a more expensive, but better tolerated alternative to mefloquine or doxycycline. Primaquine (30 mg daily) has proved remarkably well tolerated in prophylactic use, provided it is not taken on an empty stomach.[47] It has been effective even against multiresistant falciparum malaria. Side effects include abdominal pain (particularly if taken on an empty stomach) and oxidant hemolysis. Primaquine should not be given to people with G6PD deficiency. Both primaquine and atovaquone–proguanil have pre-erythrocytic activity and can be stopped immediately the transmission area is left, making them suitable for short-term visitors.

Chloroquine is certainly safe in all age groups and in preg-

nancy but, although no adverse effects have been reported with mefloquine prophylaxis in pregnancy, experience is still limited and this should remain under review. Atovaquone–proguanil is considered safe in children but there are no data in pregnancy. Primaquine and doxycycline are contraindicated in pregnancy. The artemisinin derivatives should not be used for prophylaxis. Neither the sulfadoxine–pyrimethamine combination nor amodiaquine are now recommended for prophylactic use because of toxicity. However, intermittent sulfadoxine–pyrimethamine (twice during pregnancy, four times in HIV-infected mothers) has proved very effective in reducing the impact of falciparum malaria in pregnancy in endemic areas.

Travelers should obtain detailed information on the risks of malaria, the value of vector avoidance and personal protection, and the efficacy of antimalarial drugs in the area that they will visit. Most travelers visiting South-East Asia do not enter areas of risk and do not need to take antimalarial drugs. For India and for South America the risks depend very much on the area to be visited, and for sub-Saharan Africa (north of South Africa) and Oceania malaria risks are very high and prophylaxis is required (Figure 64.1).

References

1. Trape JF, Pison G, Preziosi MP et al 1998 Impact of chloroquine resistance on malaria mortality. *Comptes Rendus de l'Académie des Sciences, Series III.* 321: 689–697.

2. White NJ 1999 Antimalarial drug resistance and mortality in falciparum malaria. *Tropical Medicine and International Health* 4: 469–470.

3. White NJ, van Vugt M, Ezzet F 1999 Clinical pharmacokinetics and pharmacodynamics of artemether-lumefantrine. *Clinical Pharmacokinetics* 37: 105–125.

4. Covell G, Coatney GR, Field JW, Singh J 1955 Chemotherapy of malaria (WHO monograph series 27). WHO, Geneva.

5. Baird JK, Basri H, Purnomo et al 1991 Resistance to chloroquine by *Plasmodium vivax* in Irian Jaya, Indonesia. *American Journal of Tropical Medicine and Hygiene* 44: 547–552.

6. Baird JK, Sustriayu Nalim MF, Basri H et al 1996 Survey of resistance to chloroquine by *Plasmodium vivax* in Indonesia. *Transactions of the Royal Society of Tropical Medicine and Hygiene* 90: 409–411.

7. Nzila AM, Nduati E, Mberu EK et al 2000 Molecular evidence of greater selective pressure for drug resistance exerted by the long-acting antifolate pyrimethamine/sulfadoxine compared with the shorter-acting chlorproguanil/dapsone on Kenyan *Plasmodium falciparum. Journal of Infectious Diseases* 181: 2023–2028.

8. Fontanet AL, Johnston BD, Walker AM, Bergqvist Y, Hellgren U, Rooney W 1994 Falciparum malaria in eastern Thailand: a randomised trial of the efficacy of a single dose of mefloquine. *Bulletin of the World Health Organization* 72: 73–81.

9. Nosten F, Luxemburger C, ter Kuile FO et al 1994 Treatment of multi-drug resistant *Plasmodium falciparum* malaria with 3-day artesunate-mefloquine combination. *Journal of Infectious Diseases* 170: 971–977.

10. Nosten F, ter Kuile FO, Luxemburger C et al 1993 Cardiac effects of antimalarial treatment with halofantrine. *Lancet* 341: 1054–1056.

11. Watt G, Loesuttivibool L, Shanks GD et al 1992 Quinine with tetracycline for the treatment of drug-resistant falciparum malaria in Thailand. *American Journal of Tropical Medicine and Hygiene* 47: 108–111.

12. Hien TT, White NJ 1993 Qinghaosu. *Lancet* 341: 603–608.

13. Brockman A, Price RN, van Vugt M et al 2000 *Plasmodium falciparum* antimalarial drug susceptibility on the northwestern border of Thailand during five years of extensive use of artesunate-mefloquine. *Transactions of the Royal Society of Tropical Medicine and Hygiene* 94: 537–544.

14. Nosten F, van Vugt M, Price R et al 2000 Effects of artesunate-mefloquine combination on incidence of *Plasmodium falciparum* malaria and mefloquine resistance in western Thailand; a prospective study. *Lancet* 356: 297–302.

15. White NJ 1999 Antimalarial drug resistance and combination chemotherapy. *Philosophical Transactions of the Royal Society of London, Series B* 354: 739–749.

16. Mberu EK, Mosobo MK, Nzila AM, Kokwaro GO, Sibley CH, Watkins WM 2000 The changing in vitro susceptibility pattern to pyrimethamine/sulfadoxine in *Plasmodium falciparum* field isolates from Kilifi, Kenya. *American Journal of Tropical Medicine and Hygiene* 62: 396–401.

17. Wang P, Lee CS, Bayoumi R et al 1997 Resistance to antifolates in *Plasmodium falciparum* monitored by sequence analysis of dihydropteroate synthetase and dihydrofolate reductase alleles in a large number of field samples of diverse origins. *Molecular and Biochemical Parasitology* 89: 161–177.

18. Fidock DA, Nomura T, Talley AK et al 2000 Mutations in the *P. falciparum* digestive vacuole transmembrane protein PfCRT and evidence for their role in chloroquine resistance. *Molecular Cell* 6: 861–871.

19. White NJ, Nosten F, Looareesuwan S et al 1999 Averting a malaria disaster. *Lancet* 353: 1965–1967.

20. Supanaranond W, Davis TME, Pukrittayakamee S, Nagachinta B, White NJ 1993 Abnormal circulatory control in falciparum malaria; the effects of antimalarial drugs. *European Journal of Clinical Pharmacology* 44: 325–330.

21. Pussard E, Lepers JP, Clavier F et al 1991 Efficacy of a loading dose of oral chloroquine in a 36-hour treatment schedule for uncomplicated *Plasmodium falciparum* malaria. *Antimicrobial Agents and Chemotherapy* 35: 406–409.

22. Miller KD, Lobel HO, Satriale RF, Kuritsky JN, Stern R, Campbell CC 1986 Severe cutaneous reactions among American travelers using pyrimethamine-sulfadoxine (Fansidar®) for malaria prophylasix. *American Journal of Tropical Medicine and Hygiene* 35: 451–458.

23. Karbwang J, White NJ 1990 Clinical pharmacokinetics of mefloquine. *Clinical Pharmacokinetics* 19: 264–279.

24. ter Kuile FO, Dolan G, Nosten F et al 1993 Halofantrine versus mefloquine in the treatment of multidrug resistant falciparum malaria. *Lancet* 341: 1044–1049.

25. Mai NTH, Day NPJ, Chuong LV et al 1996 Post-malaria neurological syndrome. *Lancet* 348: 917–921.

26. Price RN, van Vugt M, Phaipun L et al 1999 Adverse effects in patients with acute falciparum malaria treated with artemisinin derivatives. *American Journal of Tropical Medicine and Hygiene* 60: 547–555.

27. Price RN, Nosten F, Luxemburger C et al 1996 The effects of artemisinin derivatives on malaria transmissability. *Lancet* 347: 1654–1658.

28. World Health Organization 1990 Control of Tropical Diseases. Severe and complicated malaria. *Transactions of the Royal Society of Tropical Medicine and Hygiene* 84 (Suppl. 2): 1–65.

29. Crawley J, Waruiru C, Mithwani S et al 2000 Effect of phenobarbital on seizure frequency and mortality in childhood cerebral malaria: a randomised, controlled intervention study. *Lancet* 355: 701–706.

30. White NJ, Looareesuwan S, Warrell DA et al 1983 Quinine loading dose in cerebral malaria. *American Journal of Tropical Medicine and Hygiene* 32: 1–5.

31. Davis TME, Supanaranond W, Pukrittayakamee S et al 1990 A safe and effective consecutive-infusion regimen for rapid quinine loading in severe falciparum malaria. *Journal of Infectious Diseases* 161: 1305–1308.

32. Winstanley P, Mberu EK, Watkins WM, Murphy SA, Lowe B, Marsh K 1994 Towards optimal regimens of parenteral quinine for young children with cerebral malaria: unbound quinine concentrations following a simple loading dose regimen. *Transactions of the Royal Society of Tropical Medicine and Hygiene* 87: 201–206.

33. White NJ 1992 Antimalarial pharmacokinetics and treatment regimens. *British Journal of Clinical Pharmacology* 34: 1–10.

34. White NJ, Warrell DA, Chanthavanich P et al 1983 Severe hypoglycemia and hyperinsulinemia in falciparum malaria. *New England Journal of Medicine* 309: 61–66.

35. Krishna S, White NJ 1996 Pharmacokinetics of quinine, chloroquine and amodiaquine. Clinical implications. *Clinical Pharmacokinetics* 30: 263–299.

36. Hien TT, Day NPJ, Phu NH et al 1996 A controlled trial of artemether or quinine in Vietnamese adults with severe falciparum malaria. *New England Journal of Medicine* 335: 76–83.

37. Miller KD, Greenberg AE, Campbell CC 1989 Treatment of severe malaria in the United States with a continuous infusion of quinidine gluconate and exchange transfusion. *New England Journal of Medicine* 321: 65–70.

38. Karbwang J, Davis TME, Looareesuwan S, Molunto P, Bunnag D, White NJ 1993 A comparison of the pharmacokinetic and pharmacodynamic properties of quinine and quinidine in healthy Thai males. *British Journal of Clinical Pharmacology* 35: 265–271.

39. van Hensbroek MB, Onyiorah E, Jaffar S et al 1996 A comparison of the effect of artemether and quinine on survival from childhood cerebral malaria. *New England Journal of Medicine* 335: 69–75.

40. The Artemether-Quinine Meta-analysis Study Group 2001 A meta-analysis of trials comparing artemether with quinine in the treatment of severe falciparum malaria using individual patient data. *Transactions of the Royal Society of Tropical Medicine and Hygiene* 95; 637–650.

41. Murphy SA, Mberu E, Muhia D et al 1997 The disposition of intramuscular artemether in children with cerebral malaria; a preliminary study. *Transactions of the Royal Society of Tropical Medicine and Hygiene* 91: 331–334.

42. Krishna S, Planche T, Agbenyega T et al 2001 Bioavailability and preliminary clinical efficacy of intrarectal artesunate in Ghanaian children with moderate malaria. *Antimicrobial Agents and Chemotherapy* 45: 509–516.

43. Nosten F, Vincenti M, Simpson JA et al 1999 The effects of mefloquine treatment in pregnancy. *Clinical Infectious Diseases* 28: 808–815.

44. McGready R, Cho T, Keo NK et al 2001 Artemisinin antimalarials in pregnancy: a prospective treatment study of 539 episodes of multidrug resistant *P. falciparum. Clinical Infectious Diseases* 33: 2009–2016.

45. Bradley DJ, Warhurst DC 1995 Malaria prophylaxis: guidelines for travellers from Britain. *British Medical Journal* 310: 709–714.

46. Hogh B, Clarke PD, Camus D et al 2000 Atovaquone-proguanil versus chloroquine-proguanil for malaria prophylaxis in non-immune travellers: a randomised, double-blind study. Malarone International Study Team. *Lancet* 356: 1888–1894.

47. Fryauff DJ, Baird JK, Basri H et al 1995 Randomised placebo-controlled trial of primaquine for prophylaxis of falciparum and vivax malaria. *Lancet* 346: 1190–1193.

CHAPTER

65 Other protozoal infections

P. L. Chiodini and H. Schuster

TOXOPLASMOSIS

The regimen of choice is pyrimethamine plus sulfadiazine. The combination is synergistic against toxoplasma tachyzoites. Pyrimethamine is given at a dose of 25–50 mg/day, preceded by a loading dose of 100 mg twice daily for 1 day. Sulfadiazine is given as 2–8 g/day (in four divided doses). Some authors recommend a loading dose of 75 mg/kg up to 4 g. Alternatives to sulfadiazine are sulfatriad or sulfadimidine.

Therapy with pyrimethamine–sulfadiazine (or an alternative) should be accompanied by folinic acid 15 mg/day orally. Duration and dose of combination therapy is influenced by the variant of toxoplasmosis being treated and clinical progress on therapy. Where sulfonamides are contraindicated or cannot be tolerated, clindamycin 2.4–4.8 g/day in four divided doses can be substituted and given in combination with pyrimethamine.

Spiramycin 2–3 g/day in three or four divided doses is less active than pyrimethamine–sulfadiazine.[1] Its main application lies in the management of toxoplasmosis in pregnancy (Ch. 58).

Non-pregnant immunologically intact individuals

Many infections in the normal population are asymptomatic and thus not recognized. Most symptomatic cases resolve without treatment so do not require drug therapy, but severely ill patients should be treated. The regimen consists of pyrimethamine 25 mg/day plus sulfadiazine 2 g/day plus folinic acid, for 2–4 weeks. Cerebral, pulmonary, hepatic or cardiac involvement also constitute indications for giving antitoxoplasma drugs.[2]

OCULAR TOXOPLASMOSIS (SEE ALSO CH. 56)

Rothova et al[3] examined the action of pyrimethamine 100 mg on the first day followed by 25 mg twice daily, plus sulfadiazine 1 g four times daily, plus folinic acid, plus corticosteroids, with the action of clindamycin 300 mg four times daily plus sulfadiazine (as above) with an untreated control group. Pyrimethamine–sulfadiazine with corticosteroids significantly reduced the size of the retinal lesion in 52% of patients (compared with 25% of controls). Improvement on clindamycin–sulfadiazine with corticosteroids was borderline (retinal lesion reduced in size in 32% of patients). In contrast, Dutton[4] preferred clindamycin–sulfadiazine to pyrimethamine–sulfadiazine.

Pearson et al[5] conducted an open, phase I (safety and efficacy) trial of atovaquone therapy for ocular toxoplasmosis in immunocompetent patients: 17 individuals were treated with atovaquone tablets 750 mg four times daily for 3 months. Prednisolone 40 mg per day was begun on day 3 and tapered as ocular inflammation resolved. One patient stopped treatment at 6 weeks due to persistent epigastric discomfort. All patients showed improvement on treatment within 1–3 weeks and visual acuity stabilized or improved in all cases, median initial visual acuity being 20/200 and median final visual acuity 20/25. Because recurrent ocular toxoplasmosis is due to reactivation of the bradyzoite (tissue cyst) of *Toxoplasma*, atovaquone's activity against this stage in the parasite's life cycle (an attribute not possessed by conventional antitoxoplasma drugs) may limit the ultimate visual loss caused by this condition. This hypothesis should be tested by randomized clinical trials.

Antitoxoplasma drugs are indicated for ocular toxoplasmosis where there is a threat to vision, either from local posterior pole lesions or from more general inflammation. Systemic corticosteroids are indicated in the presence of posterior pole lesions if there is a possibility of large vessel involvement, or if the lesions are in the patient's only eye. Steroid therapy must be accompanied by antitoxoplasma drugs and is reserved for sight-threatening lesions.

Indications for surgical intervention include cataract, uncontrolled rise in intraocular pressure, vitreous membranes, epiretinal membranes and retinal detachment. Systemic steroid cover is administered if surgery is undertaken for ocular toxoplasmosis. Peripheral retinal lesions that are no threat to vision can be observed and do not usually require specific anti-toxoplasma drugs.[6]

TOXOPLASMOSIS IN THE IMMUNOCOMPROMISED PATIENT

Cardiac transplantation

Cardiac transplantation is the organ donation most likely to lead to toxoplasmosis in the recipient. Most instances occur when the donor heart comes from a seropositive patient and the recipient is seronegative. The other possibility is reactivation of latent toxoplasmosis secondary to immunosuppression, in an already seropositive recipient. Luft et al[7] reported a series of 50 heart or heart–lung transplant patients: of four patients who were seronegative before receiving a heart from a seropositive donor, three developed life-threatening toxoplasmosis. None of 19 patients who were seropositive before transplantation developed illness attributable to toxoplasmosis, although 10 showed significant increases in toxoplasma antibody titers. Another series studied 21 seronegative recipients of seropositive heart or heart–lung transplants.[8] Four patients (two of whom died) from the first seven suffered clinical toxoplasmosis within 17–32 days of the transplant. The next 14 transplant patients deemed at risk of toxoplasmosis received pyrimethamine prophylaxis 25 mg/day plus folinic acid 15 mg three times daily for 6 weeks postoperatively; two cases developed.

Soave[9] recommends prophylaxis with pyrimethamine 25 mg daily, plus folinic acid 15 mg three times daily, for 6 months after heart transplantation in seronegative recipients of seropositive organs. Prophylaxis should be continued beyond 6 months in patients with ongoing risk factors for reactivation of toxoplasmosis or with persistent allograft dysfunction.

Trimethoprim–sulfamethoxazole prophylaxis for *Pneumocystis carinii* pneumonia may also be effective in preventing toxoplasmosis, although a controlled trial versus pyrimethamine has not been undertaken. Treatment of acute toxoplasmosis after heart or heart–lung transplantation is with pyrimethamine–sulfadiazine with folinic acid, continuing until 4–6 weeks after all symptoms and signs have resolved.

Renal transplantation

The risk of the recipient developing toxoplasmosis after renal transplantation appears to be small,[10] but is recorded as the result of reactivation of latent infection or, more commonly, due to recently infected donor to host transmission.[11] In a review, these authors found 22 cases of disseminated toxoplasmosis following renal transplantation. Ten of 11 recipients whose serology was known were seronegative before transplantation. In the six cases for whom the corresponding donor serology was known, it was positive in five.

Hepatic transplantation

Toxoplasmosis following liver transplantation appears to be rare[12,13] and there is little published data on the efficacy of post-transplantation prophylaxis against *Toxoplasma*. However, trimethoprim–sulfamethoxazole is often used after liver transplantation as prophylaxis against *Pneumocystis carinii* so, based on its efficacy in preventing *Toxoplasma* encephalitis in AIDS, this regimen might be expected to confer protection against *Toxoplasma* in liver transplant patients.[12,13] Knowledge of the *Toxoplasma* serological status pretransplantation for both donor and recipient will help alert the clinical team to toxoplasmosis as one of the possible diagnoses to be considered in the investigation of fever after liver transplantation.

Bone marrow transplantation

In contrast to solid organ transplants, toxoplasmosis in bone-marrow-graft recipients appears to be due largely to reactivation of latent infection in the recipient, rather than infection coming from the transplanted organ.[14] There are likely to be more problems in countries with a higher toxoplasma seroprevalence rate.[15] Slavin et al reported 12 cases of toxoplasmosis in 3803 bone marrow allograft patients:[16] 2% of seropositive patients developed toxoplasmosis, which appeared to occur by reactivation within the first 6 months after marrow transplantation, in patients who were *Toxoplasma*-seropositive pretransplant, had received allogeneic marrow and had severe graft-versus-host disease. Recipients seropositive before bone-marrow transplantation should receive chemoprophylaxis from months 2 to 6 after grafting.[17] Foot et al studied the efficacy of weekly pyrimethamine–sulfadoxine prophylaxis in bone-marrow transplant recipients.[18] In 69 evaluable seropositive patients, the combination was given from the time of established engraftment (median day 40; range 13–100 days) and was scheduled to be given until 6 months, or longer in instances of continued immunosuppression (median 10 months, range 72 days to 22 months). No cases of toxoplasmosis occurred in patients receiving prophylaxis over a 21-month period.

CEREBRAL TOXOPLASMOSIS

Toxoplasma gondii may cause diffuse encephalitis, but this is an extremely rare infection and cerebral toxoplasmosis is normally manifested as solitary or multiple brain abscesses. The condition is typically seen in HIV-positive patients who have $<100 \times 10^6$ CD4 lymphocytes/l and who have positive toxoplasma serology. More rarely transplant patients and other patients with severe deficiencies of cellular immunity may get cerebral toxoplasmosis. Clinically the patients develop symptoms of intracerebral expansion; seizures, headache, and confusion are the most common manifestations. The most common differential diagnoses are cryptococcal meningitis, AIDS dementia complex, and progressive multifocal leucoencephalopathy. Diagnosis is obtained by computed tomography (CT) scan of the brain showing typical ring-enhanced lesions combined with demonstrations of *Toxoplasma* antibodies.

If diagnosed reasonably early, treatment of cerebral toxoplasmosis is normally successful. First line treatment is sulfadiazine 4–6 g per day combined with pyrimethamine 50–100 mg per day and folinic acid 15 mg per day. In patients who cannot take sulfonamides, clindamycin 600 mg 4 times daily has been recommended as replacement of sulfadiazine. Another alternative to sulfadiazine is clarithromycin 2 g per day or atovaquone 750 mg 4 times daily orally; both to be combined with pyrimethamine and folinic acid.

Both primary and secondary prevention of cerebral toxoplasmosis should be considered in HIV-positive patients. Those who lack antibodies should be advised to avoid raw and undercooked meat, which are the most common modes of transmission of the infection. Antibody tests should be repeated if the CD4 count falls below 100×10^6/l. At or below that CD4 count primary prophylaxis with a daily dose of trimethoprim 160 mg and sulfamethoxazole 800 mg (which also prevents *Pneumocystis carinii* pneumonia) is recommended for antibody-positive patients. Alternatives to trimethoprim-sulfamethoxazole are dapsone plus pyrimethamine or atovaquone with or without pyrimethamine. However, these regimens are incompletely documented. Several studies indicate that primary prophylaxis can be discontinued if the CD4 count rises to above 200×10^6/l as a result of antiretroviral treatment.

The regimens recommended for primary prophylaxis should also be administered as secondary prophylaxis to patients who have had an episode of cerebral toxoplasmosis. In these patients the evidence does not allow a recommendation to discontinue prophylaxis if the CD4 count increases.

TOXOPLASMOSIS IN PREGNANCY

This is discussed in Ch. 58

LEISHMANIASIS

CUTANEOUS LEISHMANIASIS

Old world cutaneous leishmaniasis

Most lesions heal spontaneously. Treatment may produce more rapid healing and less severe scarring and is indicated for multiple sores, those at risk of causing disfigurement or disability, or lesions sited where healing is expected to be slow. Options for local drug treatment are topical paromomycin (aminosidine) ointment[19] or infiltration of sodium stibogluconate into the edge and base of the sore.[20] Systemic treatment may be required for multiple or potentially disfiguring lesions.

New World cutaneous leishmaniasis

If infection with *Leishmania (Viannia) braziliensis* complex is suspected, the cutaneous lesion should be treated systemically to prevent the development of mucocutaneous leishmaniasis. Systemic therapy of cutaneous leishmaniasis (CL) is undertaken with pentavalent antimonials (sodium stibogluconate or meglumine antimonate; *see below*). On the basis that a course of pentamidine isethionate is cheaper and shorter than antimonial therapy, some clinicians use pentamidine in the treatment of CL. Nacher et al[21] examined the efficacy of short-course pentamidine in treating CL due to *Leishmania braziliensis guyanensis* in French Guiana. Two intramuscular injections of pentamidine 4 mg/kg each, separated by 48 hours cured 165 of 189 (87%) evaluable patients. Of the 24 patients who were not cured by one course 80% were cured by a repeat course of pentamidine. The five individuals in whom active lesions persisted after two courses of pentamidine all responded to antimonial therapy.

Diffuse cutaneous leishmaniasis

This condition requires expert assessment and follow-up. In principle, *Leishmania aethiopica* is treated with paromomycin plus sodium stibogluconate daily[22] until the parasite is thought to be eliminated, which may take a few months. Weekly pentamidine is an alternative.[23]

MUCOSAL LEISHMANIASIS

South American mucosal leishmaniasis, due to *Leishmania (Viannia) braziliensis*, is treated with antimonials at 20 mg antimony/kg daily for 6–8 weeks, provided the patient is previously untreated and does not have laryngeal involvement. For those previously treated, or in whom the larynx is involved, amphotericin B 1 mg/kg is given by intravenous infusion on alternate days for 6–8 weeks.[24]

Adjunctive therapy

Lessa et al studied 10 Brazilian patients with mucosal leishmaniasis who had failed to respond to at least two courses of conventional pentavalent antimonial therapy.[25] Based on observations that suggested a possible role of tumor necrosis factor-alpha (TNF-α) in the pathology of mucosal leishmaniasis, a TNF-α inhibitor (pentoxifylline) was assessed in combination with a pentavalent antimonial drug. Each patient received parenteral pentavalent antimony (20 mg/kg/day) plus oral pentoxifylline (400 mg three times daily) for 30 days. The criteria for cure were complete re-epithelialization of the mucosal tissue 90 days post-treatment and no evidence of relapse after 1 year of follow-up. Complete healing was found by day 60 in eight patients and by day 90 in one person: one patient was not cured, although some improvement in the lesion was reported. Mean TNF-α levels fell from 776 before treatment to 94 within 60 days after the end of treatment ($P < 0.05$). Further results from a randomized study should help to define the potential role of this combination therapy for mucosal leishmaniasis.

Oral therapy

Amato et al conducted a small open study of the efficacy of itraconazole in the treatment of mucocutaneous leishmaniasis in Brazil.[26] Ten patients received 6 weeks' therapy with itraconazole 4 mg/kg daily to a maximum of 400 mg/day in two divided doses with food; 6 of the 10 showed healing of the lesions at 3 months and none of these showed reactivation of disease after follow-up for 12–18 months. One of the six had previously failed to improve on pentavalent antimonial treatment and another had relapsed after initial healing on pentamidine therapy.

Sudanese mucosal leishmaniasis is due mainly to *Leishmania donovani* and is usually a primary mucosal disease, though it may appear during or after an attack of visceral leishmaniasis. Therapy is with sodium stibogluconate 10 mg/kg daily for 30 days.[27]

VISCERAL LEISHMANIASIS

Until recently, pentavalent antimonials were the first choice for therapy of visceral leishmaniasis (VL). Sodium stibogluconate solution contains 100 mg antimony/ml, while meglumine antimonate solution contains 85 mg antimony/ml. Antimonial resistance develops easily following inadequate treatment[28] and has now become a significant problem, notably in recent epidemics in India and the Sudan. Traditional dosage regimens recommended by the World Health Organization[29] advocated 20 mg/kg of antimony daily, subject to a maximum daily dose of 850 mg, for a minimum of 20 days, until no parasites are found in consecutive splenic aspirates taken at 14-day intervals, but this would result in suboptimal dosage of patients weighing more than 42 kg.[30] Herwaldt and Berman advocated lifting of the 850 mg ceiling for antimony dosage, with close monitoring of the patient for drug-related reactions.[31] Current regimens advocate 28–30 days of treatment.[30] In children, who tolerate pentavalent antimony better than do adults, dosage is calculated by body surface area.[32]

A successful immune response to VL is T cell-dependent, mainly Th1 type,[30] thus, Th1-derived γ-interferon was assessed to see if it would augment the response to anti-leishmanial chemotherapy. A controlled trial comparing combination therapy of Kenyan VL with alternate-day γ-interferon plus daily sodium stibogluconate and daily sodium stibogluconate alone, suggested that combination therapy accelerated the early clearance of parasites.[33] Sundar et al[34] used sodium stibogluconate, 20 mg/kg daily intravenously for 30 days, plus γ-interferon 25 μg/m² subcutaneously on day 1, 50 μg/m² on day 2 and 100 μg/m² daily for 28 days, to treat 15 Indian patients,

all of whom had failed an initial course of 30 or more days of antimony treatment at 20 mg/kg daily. Eight of the patients had received two courses and seven had received three or four treatment courses. Combination therapy was discontinued in two patients, both of whom died. After 30 days of therapy, 9 of 13 (69%) of the patients were apparently cured. All nine had negative bone-marrow smears at 6 months and none relapsed after a mean follow-up of 15.9 (± 1.7) months. Combination therapy with antimonials plus γ-interferon may have a role in selected refractory cases, but its cost renders it unsuitable for widespread use in the tropics. Furthermore, it would be unwise to use it in areas where there is significant antimony-resistant VL.

Secondary infection is an important cause of morbidity and mortality in VL. Granulocyte–macrophage colony-stimulating factor (GM-CSF) was compared to placebo as adjunctive therapy in Brazilian patients with VL and leukopenia due to *Leishmania chagasi*. Patients received antimony 10–20 mg/kg daily for 20 days plus GM-CSF 5 μg/kg daily or placebo, for 10 days. Neutrophil counts were significantly higher in the GM-CSF group at 5 and 10 days. Eosinophil and monocyte counts were significantly higher at 10 days in the patients who received GM-CSF. Significantly fewer secondary infections occurred in the GM-CSF group.[35]

Paromomycin (aminosidine) is active against antimony-resistant strains causing VL.[36] Scott et al[37] treated seven patients with Mediterranean VL with daily intravenous infusions of paromomycin 14–16 mg/kg for 21 days or for 1 week after demonstration of parasitological cure, whichever was the longer: four of the seven (treated for between 22 and 54 days) were cured; one relapsed 4 months after an apparent cure, but was successfully re-treated with a second course lasting 63 days, the remaining two showed a partial parasitological response. Jha et al compared paromomycin with sodium stibugloconate for the treatment of VL in Northern Bihar.[38] While the cure rate for pentavalent antimony was only 63%, paromomycin at 16 mg/kg daily for 30 days gave a cure rate of 93% and a cure rate of 97% at 20 mg/kg daily for 30 days.

Indian VL has become significantly less responsive to pentavalent antimonials. By the early 1990s the regimen for VL treatment in Bihar was sodium stibogluconate 20 mg/kg daily for 40 or more days, a dosage regimen associated with increased toxicity and higher costs of hospital care. A decade later, Sundar et al[39] reported a long-term cure rate of 35% for VL treated with pentavalent antimonials in Bihar, versus 86% of VL cases in Uttar Pradesh given identical treatment. They concluded that traditional pentavalent antimony therapy should be abandoned in Bihar. Following reports of a study from Kenya, where paromomycin 12 mg/kg daily in combination with sodium stibogluconate 20 mg/kg daily for 20 days appeared more effective than sodium stibogluconate alone, Thakur et al undertook a pilot study of the activity of the combination on VL in Bihar, India.[40] Twenty-four patients were assigned to receive paromomycin 12 mg/kg daily plus sodium stibogluconate, for 20 days. Two patients died before completing the course, one from hemorrhage following splenic puncture and one as a result of severe gastroenteritis. Of 22 patients who completed therapy, 18 (82%) were cured and did not relapse within a 6-month follow-up period. The remaining four patients improved clinically and parasitologically. Seaman et al[41] confirmed the efficacy of combined paromomycin plus sodium stibogluconate in a study on VL in Southern Sudan. Mishra et al[42] compared conventional amphotericin B with sodium stibogluconate in the treatment of Indian visceral leishmaniasis: eighty patients, none of whom had been previously treated with antileishmanial agents, were randomized to receive either sodium stibogluconate 20 mg/kg in two divided doses intramuscularly daily for 40 days or amphotericin B 0.5 mg/kg infused in 5% dextrose on alternate days for 14 doses. All 40 patients who received amphotericin B showed initial cure (no fever and no amastigotes in a bone-marrow smear after 6 weeks) and definitive cure (well at the end of 12 months). In the stibogluconate-treated group 28 of 40 (70%) showed initial cure and 25 of 40 (62.5%) showed definitive cure. Patients who failed to respond to stibogluconate, or who relapsed after an initial cure, were treated with, and cured by, amphotericin B. Davidson[28] regards the optimal regimen for amphotericin B deoxycholate as 20 mg/kg given as 0.5 mg/kg daily or 1 mg/kg on alternate days.

The amastigotes of *Leishmania* are found in macrophages, which also clear liposomes from the circulation. Thus, the sites of infection can be targeted by amphotericin B, itself a more active antileishmanial drug than sodium stibogluconate. Davidson et al reported a multicenter trial of liposomal amphotericin B in Mediterranean VL.[43] Ten immunocompetent patients (six of them children) received 1–1.38 mg/kg daily for 21 days and a further ten (nine of them children) received 3 mg/kg daily for 10 days. All were clinically cured after a follow-up period of at least 12 months.

Lipid-associated amphotericin B preparations all reach very high levels in liver and spleen and are less toxic than conventional amphotericin B. All three are more expensive. Liposomal amphotericin B (AmBisome) is given as a total dose of 20–30 mg/kg, split to more than five daily doses of 3–4 mg/kg over 10–21 days.[43] Liposomal amphotericin B was the first drug approved for the treatment of VL by the United States Food and Drug Administration, in a regimen of 21 mg/kg given on 7 days over a 21-day period.[44] Cost is a major issue affecting the use of liposomal amphotericin B, so short-course, low-dose regimens have been investigated as a way of reducing treatment costs. Sundar et al[45] compared single-dose infusion of liposomal amphotericin B at 5 mg/kg with once-daily infusions of 1 mg/kg for 5 days in the therapy of Indian VL. Cure rates at 6 months were 92% (84 of 91 patients) for the whole study, 91% (42 of 46) for the single-dose group and 93% (42 of 45) in the five-dose group, with no significant difference in response rates between the two groups. Further work is required to support the use of the regimens described and to see whether or not their deployment will encourage the development of amphotericin resistant strains of *Leishmania*.

Amphotericin B cholesterol dispersion (Amphocil) consists of a 1:1 molar ratio of cholesterol sulfate and amphotericin B in disk-shaped particles, 115 nm in diameter and 4 nm thick. Dietze et al treated Brazilian patients with VL using two different regimens: 10 patients received amphotericin B cholesterol dispersion 2 mg/kg daily intravenously for 10 days, and another 10 patients received a 7-day course.[46] The authors reported treatment success in all patients. One patient who received the 7-day course had scanty parasites in the bone-marrow smear 15 days after treatment, but the remainder (95%) had negative bone-marrow smears. All patients were well after 6 months of follow-up. Side-effects consisting of fever, chills and respiratory distress were noted in children under 3 years of age.

Amphotericin B lipid complex (Abelcet) at a dosage of 3 mg/kg daily for 5 consecutive days proved effective in the treatment of Indian VL unresponsive to more than 30 days' treatment with pentavalent antimony.[47]

Oral therapy

Effective, oral therapy for VL would constitute a major therapeutic advance. Miltefosine (hexadecylphosphocholine), an orally administered agent initially developed as a potential anti-cancer drug (*see* Ch. 38), was found to have antileishmanial activity in vitro and in animal models.[48] Studies in Indian VL showed very encouraging activity and have been summarized by Murray.[30] A total of 249 patients aged 12 years or more were included: 96% (224 of 234) patients treated with 50–200 mg daily for 14–42 days were regarded as long-term cures; 97% (68 of 70) of those who received 100 mg per day (in two divided doses) for 28 days were cured, but only 89% were cured by 100 mg per day for 14 days. Gastrointestinal side effects were frequent on miltefosine (up to two-thirds of cases) but were judged mild to moderate in severity.[48] Miltefosine is teratogenic in animals and should not be given in pregnancy.[30] The potential impact of miltefosine in the treatment of VL, should its efficacy and safety be confirmed in larger studies, is substantial. It should also be assessed in AIDS-related VL, both for initial treatment and for maintenance therapy, and in post-kala-azar dermal leishmaniasis.[30]

VISCERAL LEISHMANIASIS AND HIV CO-INFECTION

Before the development of highly active antiretroviral therapy (HAART), 20–70% of patients with VL in the Mediterranean area were co-infected with HIV[28] but there has been a significant decrease in the incidence of VL in HIV-infected patients since HAART was introduced.[49] Davidson[28] reports that clinical remission can be produced at first presentation of VL in approximately 65% of patients co-infected with HIV and *Leishmania* with a regimen of sodium stibogluconate or meglumine antimonate 20 mg antimony/kg daily or amphotericin B 0.7 mg/kg daily, for 28 days. Berenguer et al report the use of meglumine antimonate (as above) or liposomal amphotericin B, at doses of 4 mg/kg daily on days 1 to 5, 10, 17, 24,

31 and 38.[50] Their regimen for secondary prophylaxis in HIV/*Leishmania* co-infection was one dose of either agent per month. They studied the relapse rate in 15 patients with HIV and VL established on HAART. Although larger studies are still required, they were able to conclude that secondary prophylaxis against *Leishmania* should not be discontinued in patients who were co-infected with HIV and VL and were unable to achieve and maintain a CD4 cell count above 200 µl on HAART; however it may be safe in patients whose CD4 cell count is above 350 µl.[50] Despite recent advances, there remains significant cause for concern regarding co-infection with HIV and VL. Although most reported cases have been from the Mediterranean region, Rosenthal et al have pointed out the potential for an explosion of co-infection with HIV and *Leishmania* in Eastern Africa and the Indian subcontinent due to the simultaneous spread and geographical overlap of both infections,[49] migration of refugees and seasonal workers and periodical epidemics of VL; yet HAART is not available to the population of those areas.

TRYPANOSOMIASIS

TRYPANOSOMA BRUCEI GAMBIENSE INFECTION

Hemolymphatic disease can be treated with eflornithine or suramin or pentamidine. Eflornithine (α-difluoromethylornithine, DFMO) has been evaluated for the treatment of established gambiense sleeping sickness (i.e. with central nervous system involvement)[51–53] but can also be used to treat hemolymphatic disease due to *T. brucei gambiense*.

Suramin is used to attempt radical cure of the hemolymphatic stage of the disease or to clear trypanosomes from the blood and lymph before melarsoprol therapy. All doses are given by slow intravenous infusion of a 10% aqueous solution. A test dose of 200 mg is given first, then 20 mg/kg (maximum dose 1 g) on days 1, 3, 7, 14 and 21.

Pentamidine 4 mg/kg by intramuscular injection daily or on alternate days for 10 doses is an alternative for the hemolymphatic stage, for *T. brucei gambiense* only. Doua et al[54] evaluated pentamidine as an alternative to the expensive eflornithine and the toxic melarsoprol in early–late stage *T. brucei gambiense* trypanosomiasis (patients with cerebrospinal fluid (CSF) white cell count <20/mm^3 and/or the presence of trypanosomes by microscopy or culture). Fifty-eight patients received pentamidine 4 mg/kg on alternate days by deep intramuscular injection to a total of 10 injections per patient: three patients relapsed with trypanosomes present in the CSF, one at 15 months and two at 18 months after the end of treatment, giving a 94% cure rate at 24 months.

In the absence of treatment, late-stage infection with meningoencephalitis is uniformly fatal. Until recently the mainstay of therapy was melarsoprol, an arsenical compound with significant toxicity. The development of eflornithine has proven to be a major advance.[51] Pepin et al[52] treated 26 patients with *T. brucei gambiense* sleeping sickness resistant to arsenicals (melarsoprol or trimelarsan) with eflornithine, 100 mg/kg every 6 h (total daily dose 400 mg/kg) by intravenous infusion over 1 h for 14 days, followed by oral eflornithine 75 mg/kg every 6 h (300 mg/kg daily) for a further 30 or 21 days. Five patients died. Follow-up of the surviving 21 patients for a mean of 16 (range 6–30) months showed no relapses. Trypanosomes disappeared rapidly from the CSF, the CSF lymphocyte count gradually fell and there was improvement in symptoms after the first 2 weeks of treatment, such that most patients were asymptomatic by the time of hospital discharge. Giving 2 weeks intravenous eflornithine before commencing oral treatment appeared to give a lower relapse rate than did oral therapy reported from other studies. The authors felt that reducing the oral phase of therapy from 30 to 21 days reduced the frequency of side effects.

Milord et al examined the effect of three different eflornithine treatment regimens on a group of 207 patients with late-stage *T. brucei gambiense* sleeping sickness.[53] In some cases eflornithine was the first antitrypanosomal drug administered, while other patients had relapsed after melarsoprol or nifurtimox or pentamidine plus suramin. Of 152 patients followed for at least 1 year only 13 (9%) relapsed. Relapse after eflornithine was more frequent in children under 12 years of age and in previously untreated than in relapsing cases. Patients with a CSF leukocytosis of ≥100/µl were slightly, though not significantly, more likely to relapse than those with lower CSF white cell counts. Relapse rates in patients with trypanosomes seen in the CSF were not significantly different from those in patients in whom none were seen. Therapy with eflornithine 100 mg/kg intravenously every 6 h for 14 days, followed by 75 mg/kg orally every 6 h for 21 days showed no relapses in 28 patients followed for at least 1 year after treatment. In patients treated by the intravenous route only (200 mg/kg 12-hourly for 14 days) the relapse rate was 10 of 108 (9%), compared with 19% (3 of 16) in those treated by the oral route (75 mg/kg 6-hourly for 35 days).

Where affordable, melarsoprol has been superseded by eflornithine for the therapy of late-stage *T. brucei gambiense* sleeping sickness. Where melarsoprol has to be used, consideration should be given to the use of a new accelerated 10-day schedule recently described from Angola.[55] This consisted of 10 daily injections of melarsoprol 2.2 mg/kg. Prednisolone was given at 1 mg/kg daily for days 1–7; 0.75 mg/kg on day 8; 0.5 mg/kg on day 9 and 0.25 mg/kg on day 10. The schedule was compared with the 26-day standard Angolan schedule of three series of four daily injections of melarsoprol, increasing from 1.2 to 3.6 mg/kg within each series, with 7 days between series. A total of 250 patients on each regimen were studied. Adverse events resulting in withdrawal were 40 on standard treatment and 47 on the concise schedule. Fifty patients on the standard regimen, but only two on the new regimen, deviated or withdrew from treatment. All patients were deemed parasitologically cured 24 h after treatment. Six patients in each group died as a result of encephalopathy. Skin reactions were more common on the new regimen.[55] It should be noted that this

Table 65.1 *Treatment schedules (adults and children) for African trypanosomiasis with meningoencephalitic involvement*[a]

Day	Drug[b]	Dose (mg/kg)
For *T. brucei rhodesiense* infection, as used in Kenya and Zambia		
1	Suramin	5.00
3	Suramin	10.00
5	Suramin	20.00
7	Melarsoprol	0.36
8	Melarsoprol	0.72
9	Melarsoprol	1.10
16	Melarsoprol	1.40
17	Melarsoprol	1.80
18	Melarsoprol	1.80
25	Melarsoprol	2.20
26	Melarsoprol	2.90
27	Melarsoprol	3.60
34	Melarsoprol	3.60
35	Melarsoprol	3.60
36	Melarsoprol	3.60
For *T. brucei rhodesiense* infection, as used in Uganda and the United Republic of Tanzania		
1	Suramin	5.00
3	Suramin	10.00
5	Melarsoprol	1.80
6	Melarsoprol	2.20
7	Melarsoprol	2.56
14	Melarsoprol	2.56
15	Melarsoprol	2.90
16	Melarsoprol	3.26
23	Melarsoprol	3.60
24	Melarsoprol	3.60
25	Melarsoprol	3.60
For *T. brucei gambiense* infection, as used in Côte d'Ivoire		
1	Pentamidine i.m.	4.00
2	Pentamidine i.m.	4.00
4	Melarsoprol	1.20
5	Melarsoprol	2.40
6	Melarsoprol	3.60
17	Melarsoprol	1.20
18	Melarsoprol	2.40
19	Melarsoprol	3.60
20	Melarsoprol	3.60
30	Melarsoprol	1.20
31	Melarsoprol	2.40
32	Melarsoprol	3.60
33	Melarsoprol	3.60

[a] Reproduced with permission from WHO (1990).[28]
[b] All given intravenously unless otherwise stated.

concise regimen for melarsoprol has not been validated for the treatment of *T. brucei rhodesiense*.

Nifurtimox (Ch. 26) is too toxic to be preferred to eflornithine. Pepin et al treated 30 patients suffering from arseno-resistant *T. brucei gambiense* sleeping sickness, with high-dose nifurtimox (30 mg/kg daily for 30 days).[56] Trypanosomes disappeared from the CSF of the nine patients in whom they were shown before therapy, and the CSF white cell count fell in all but one patient. Nine of 25 (36%) patients relapsed after follow-up, seven with trypanosomes in either CSF or blood. The relapse rate was lower than in the authors' previous study of nifurtimox 15 mg/kg daily for 60 days, when only 31% (6 of 19) were cured. However, high-dose nifurtimox produced serious toxicity; one patient died and another eight developed neurological problems, the most common being a cerebellar syndrome. Pepin et al[56] advise restricting use of high-dose nifurtimox to patients who have relapsed after both melarsoprol and eflornithine, or for the treatment of arseno-resistant trypanosomiasis if eflornithine is not available.

Smith et al suggest trying a combination of eflornithine and melarsoprol in patients who relapse after melarsoprol and eflornithine given as separate treatments.[57]

TRYPANOSOMA BRUCEI RHODESIENSE INFECTION

Hemolymphatic disease is treated with suramin (see *T. brucei gambiense*). Pentamidine is ineffective against *T. brucei rhodesiense*.

For late-stage disease with CNS involvement, eflornithine is not effective against *T. brucei rhodesiense*, even when used at a dose of 800 mg/kg daily for 14 days[58] and the treatment of choice for late-stage *T. brucei rhodesiense* infection remains melarsoprol. Several different treatment regimens are currently advocated, though there is no clear evidence that one is superior.[28] The regimens usually consist of three or four daily injections, separated by 7- to 10-day periods off treatment (Table 65.1).[28]

Therapy with melarsoprol can be followed by a Jarisch–Herxheimer reaction, which may be very severe. Thus, melarsoprol therapy is usually preceded by suramin treatment in the case of *T. brucei rhodesiense* (Table 65.1). As many as 1–5% of patients die during melarsoprol therapy, so it must be used only where there is clear evidence for CNS involvement in *T. brucei rhodesiense* infection. Especially dangerous is reactive encephalopathy, with headache, tremor, slurred speech, convulsions and coma. The syndrome appears 3–10 days after the first dose of melarsoprol.[29] Pepin et al examined the effect of prednisolone on the incidence of melarsoprol-induced encephalopathy in *T. brucei gambiense* (rather than *T. brucei rhodesiense*) sleeping sickness;[59] 308 control patients received melarsoprol, preceded by a single dose of suramin to decrease peripheral parasitemia, while 290 patients received the same drugs plus prednisolone 1 mg/kg (maximum 40 mg) daily by mouth. The prednisolone group showed a significant ($P = 0.002$) reduction in the incidence of encephalopathy compared to controls. However, there was no significant difference in case-fatality rate for encephalopathy between the two groups (66.7% in the prednisolone group, 54.3% in the control group). The presence of fever during an episode of encephalopathy was associated with an adverse outcome: none of 10 patients with fever and 20 of 37 without fever survived.

Thus, reduction in encephalopathy-associated death was due to a lower incidence of encephalopathy rather than a lower case-fatality rate. Reduction of the encephalopathy rate by prednisolone supports an autoimmune etiology for this complication, since steroids seem unlikely to decrease direct toxicity of arsenicals. In contrast, the incidence of polyneuropathy, thought to be due to a direct toxic effect of arsenic, was not reduced by prednisolone.[59] The authors rightly advise exclusion of strongyloidiasis and amebiasis before giving prednisolone, in view of the propensity of these infections to fulminate in steroid-treated individuals. Although the study was undertaken in *T. brucei gambiense* sleeping sickness, the authors thought that prednisolone should be given to patients with *T. brucei rhodesiense* sleeping sickness receiving melarsoprol.

Pepin et al enlarged upon their work on melarsoprol-induced encephalopathy,[60] reporting on 1083 patients with *T. brucei gambiense*, which included data from their earlier study of 598 patients.[59] Of 1083 patients 64 (5.9%) developed drug-induced encephalopathy; 62 of these died, 43 from reactive encephalopathy, 19 from other causes, including trypanosomiasis. Prednisolone (1 mg/kg up to 40 mg daily) significantly reduced the incidence of encephalopathy and mortality on treatment, especially in patients with trypanosomes seen in the CSF and/or whose CSF white cell count was more than or equal to 100/mm³. In patients with CSF white cell counts of ≥ 100/mm³ changing the melarsoprol regimen to three series of three injections, instead of three series of four injections, halved the mortality rate.

Addition of dimercaprol to intravenous steroids and anticonvulsants for the treatment of melarsoprol-induced encephalopathy was possibly harmful and the authors gave a clear recommendation not to use dimercaprol in the treatment of this condition. They also recommended that for patients with late-stage Gambian trypanosomiasis with white cell counts ≥100/mm³ in the CSF the maximum melarsoprol dosage should be three series of three injections of 0.1 ml/kg each (maximum 5.6 ml/day).

Foulkes reported a patient with arsenical-refractory *T. brucei rhodesiense* infection with CNS involvement who responded to combined intravenous suramin and high-dose oral metronidazole.[61] The patient's CSF was normal, with no trypanosomes evident, at 1 year follow up.

TRYPANOSOMA CRUZI INFECTION

There have been few advances in the chemotherapy of this infection for many years. Both of the standard drugs (nifurtimox and benznidazole), are toxic, with adverse reaction rates of 30–55%).[62] Despite the toxicity, patients in the acute stage of the disease should receive drug therapy. Tanowitz et al,[63] reviewing Chagas' diseasae, drew attention to studies in which 42% of rabbits receiving benznidazole and 33% of rabbits receiving nifurtimox developed widely invasive lymphomas, yet none of the control animals did so. They also point out that both agents have been widely used in Latin America for several decades, without reports of an increased frequency of lymphomas in treated patients.

Nifurtimox acts against trypomastigotes and amastigotes. The treatment regimen is 10 mg/kg, divided into three equal doses, daily by mouth, for 60–90 days. The pediatric dose is 15 mg/kg daily.[64]

Patients in whom Chagas' disease is complicated by acute meningoencephalitis can be given up to 25 mg/kg of nifurtimox daily. Side effects of nifurtimox are common and dose related. Recognized side effects include headache, vertigo, excitability, myalgia, arthralgia, convulsions and peripheral polyneuritis.[29]

Benznidazole is also active against trypomastigotes and amastigotes. The dosage regimen is 5–10 mg/kg daily orally in two divided doses for 60 days; children receive 10 mg/kg daily. Side effects commonly occur, including rashes, fever, purpura, peripheral polyneuritis, leukopenia and agranulocytosis.[28,64] Response to therapy is variable; for example some central Brazilian strains are less sensitive. Andrade et al isolated 11 strains of *T. cruzi* from patients with Chagas' disease in central Brazil and characterized them biologically and by isoenzyme analysis.[65] Patients received benznidazole or benznidazole plus nifurtimox. Mice infected with the corresponding strain were treated with the drug or drugs corresponding to the regimen received by the patient. Mice underwent a test of cure 3–6 months after the end of treatment. Patients were tested by xenodiagnosis monthly on at least 25 occasions. Mice infected with type II (zymodeme 2) strains showed 66–100% cure rates, but those infected with type III (zymodeme 1) strains showed 0–9% cure rates. In humans, five of six patients with type II strains but only two of five patients with type III strains were cured. There was correlation between treatment outcome in patients and mice in nine of eleven (81.8%) cases.

Allopurinol 600 mg daily for 30–60 days has trypanosomicidal action.[64] Gallerano et al,[62] working in Argentina, compared allopurinol 600 or 900 mg/day for 60 days with benznidazole or nifurtimox therapy and with an untreated group, in a study on patients with chronic Chagas' disease. Follow-up was based on objective laboratory criteria: serology and xenodiagnosis. Significantly more patients from the four treatment groups, whether analyzed separately or together, were rendered seronegative, than in the untreated patients. There was no significant difference between the treatment regimens in seronegativity rates after therapy. The parasitemia cleared in 63–88% of treated patients, but in only 10% of those untreated (P < 0.01%). There was no difference in efficacy between treatment regimens. Adverse reaction rates were significantly higher in the nifurtimox or benznidazole groups than in the allopurinol groups; toxic hepatitis and CNS disturbances occurred with benznidazole and with nifurtimox; skin reactions were as frequent as with allopurinol. Further work is needed to define the role of allopurinol in chronic Chagas' disease. It is unclear whether or not it will have a role in treating acute cases.

Congenital Chagas' disease can be treated with nifurtimox 8–25 mg/kg daily for 30 days or more, or with benznidazole 5–10 mg/kg daily for 30–60 days.[64]

Solari et al[66] reported a patient with hemophilia and AIDS complicated by multifocal necrotic encephalitis due to *T. cruzi*: 2 weeks' therapy with benznidazole 400 mg per day failed to improve the condition, but itraconazole 200 mg/day, later changed to fluconazole 400 mg/day in an attempt to achieve better CNS penetration, was associated with resolution of fever and stabilization of the neurological symptoms. Further evaluation of triazole antifungal agents against *T. cruzi* infections should be undertaken.

While specific treatment of *T. cruzi* was originally limited to the acute phase, recent evidence has suggested that drug therapy may be indicated in chronically infected individuals. Solari et al used the polymerase chain reaction (PCR) to follow up children treated with nifurtimox in the chronic phase of *T. cruzi* infection:[67] 66 children were treated with nifurtimox 7–10 mg/kg for 60 days and followed up by repeated serology, xenodiagnosis and PCR for 36 months after therapy. Although all but two patients remained seropositive, xenodiagnosis rapidly became negative after 3 months. PCR became negative in most cases by 24 months and in all cases by 36 months post-treatment.

Estani and Segura advocate the following guidelines for the treatment of *T. cruzi* infection, which have been adopted in Argentina.[68] They recommend treatment for all patients in the acute phase, for young people in the indeterminate phase, for adult patients in the indeterminate phase or with heart lesions, for laboratory accidents and during surgery, for organ transplant recipients or donors.

Neto, based in Brazil, advocates the following treatment regimen.[69]

- For prevention of infection by *T. cruzi* following a laboratory accident and possibly after a blood transfusion from a *T. cruzi*-infected donor: benznidazole 7–10 mg/kg for 10 days.
- For treatment of adults: benznidazole 5 mg/kg daily for 60 days and for children 5–10 mg/kg daily for 60 days.
- Nifurtimox is given as 8–10 mg/kg daily for 60–90 days for adults; 15 mg/kg daily for 60–90 days for children.

Reviewing the results from a variety of sources, Neto quotes the following percentages of cure (based upon negative xenodiagnosis and serology) for persons treated at various stages of infection:[69]

- acute phase 70%;
- recent chronic phase 60%;
- long-term chronic phase 20%.

However, not all are convinced that therapy of chronically infected individuals is appropriate. In Brazil, Braga et al used nested PCR to follow up 17 treated (at least 30 days of antitrypanosomal nitrofuran or nitroimidazole treatment) and 17 untreated chronic Chagas' disease patients.[70] There was no statistically significant difference in the mean number of *T. cruzi* per ml in untreated (25.83) and treated (6.45) individuals. These authors support the view that treatment of chronic Chagas' disease remains controversial and argue that further evaluation of the benefits of treatment with nitro derivatives is

required. They reinforce the need for a precise definition of the role of treatment with nitrofuran and nitroimidazole compounds in chronic *T. cruzi* infection.

A further note of caution is sounded by Silveira et al,[71] who studied 12 children aged between 7 and 12 in the indeterminate phase of *T. cruzi* infection, with both positive serology and xenodiagnosis. Two patients had received nifurtimox 7 mg/kg for 60 and 90 days and 10 had received benznidazole 5–7 mg/kg for 60 days. The patients were residents of an area where transmission had been interrupted for more than 10 years. Eight individuals were followed up for 8 years and four for 20 years. Clinical evaluation consisted of physical examination, electrocardiogram and esophageal radiography with contrast. Only one child was negative in all examinations performed; seven (58.4%) remained in the indeterminate stage and four (33.3%) progressed to second-degree cardiopathy and/or mega-esophagus. However, the author's data showed only one of the 12 patients to be PCR and xenodiagnosis positive, the other patients being negative by both tests. As the authors pointed out, further studies, with larger numbers of patients, are required to establish the role of specific antitrypanosomal treatment in the indeterminate phase of Chagas' disease.

Iatrogenically immunosuppressed individuals in the chronic phase of *T. cruzi* infection are at risk of reactivation of the infection, with increased parasitemia. Rassi et al treated 18 adult patients in the chronic phase of Chagas' disease, who were taking corticosteroids for concomitant diseases, with benznidazole (at the start of corticosteroid treatment in 12 patients or 15 days afterwards in six patients).[72] Benznidazole therapy (10 mg/kg daily for 60 days in all but one patient) was reported to prevent the increase, and thus might potentially be useful in immunosuppressed patients with chronic Chagas' disease.

The Pan American Health Organization recommends treatment of *T. cruzi* infection as follows:[73]

- Acute phase (with trypanosomes visualized in the peripheral blood).
- Recent chronic phase (children up to 12 years old with antibodies to *T. cruzi*).
- Congenital infection (with or without clinical manifestations).
- Treatment is with nifurtimox or benznidazole. For nifurtimox, patients up to 40 kg in weight should receive 10–12 mg/kg daily. Those whose weight exceeds 40 kg should receive 8 mg/kg daily. The total daily dose is split into two or three equal doses per day and given for 30–60 days. For benznidazole, patients weighing up to 40 kg should receive 7.5 mg/kg daily. Those who weigh more than 40 kg should receive 5 mg/kg daily. The drug is administered in two or three doses per day for 30–60 days.
- Congenital infection is treated with nifurtimox 10–15 mg/kg daily or benznidazole 10 mg/kg daily.
- In preterm or low birthweight infants, treatment should be started with half the dose. If there is no evidence of leukopenia or thrombocytopenia at 72 hours, it is possible to give the definitive dose for the next 60 days.

- It should be noted that whereas acute-phase or congenital *T. cruzi* infection can be treated with either nifurtimox or benznidazole, in the case of recent chronic infection evidence of successful treatment exists only for benznidazole.
- For late chronic infection, the objectives of treatment are to eradicate the parasite, to prevent the appearance or progression of visceral lesions, and interrupt the cycle of transmission. There is no age limit to eligibility for treatment. Specific therapy is *not* recommended during pregnancy or breastfeeding, in hepatic or renal insufficiency, when there are serious coexisting lesions. Nifurtimox is given at a dose of 8–10 mg/kg daily (split to 8-hourly doses, preferably after food) for 60–90 days. Benznidazole is given at a dose of 5 mg/kg daily (split to 8 or 12-hourly doses, preferably after food) for 60 days.
- Long-term follow up with clinical assessment, electrocardiography, serology and PCR is required.

As Neto points out,[69] the decision on treatment requires consideration of each case individually, balancing the chance of a cure and the stage of the disease against the known side effects of the drugs.

For the future, new triazole derivatives (e.g. SCH56592; Schering-Plough) and biphosphonates (e.g. pamidronate) have shown encouraging activity against *T. cruzi* in murine models.[74]

ENTAMOEBA HISTOLYTICA

Choice of treatment regimen depends upon the particular clinical presentation of amebic infection.

AMEBIC DYSENTERY

The treatment of choice is metronidazole followed by diloxanide furoate. Metronidazole 800 mg three times daily for 5 days produced a cure rate in excess of 90%.[75] Other nitroimidazoles such as tinidazole (adult dose 2 g/day for 3–5 days or a single dose of the long-acting nitroimidazole secnidazole 2 g are alternative agents. The use of a single dose of secnidazole showed microscopic clearance in 81% at day 21.[76]

With the above regimens, neither nitroimidazole achieves adequate clearance of amebic cysts from the intestinal lumen; thus, a luminal amebicide is required to complete therapy. Diloxanide furoate 500 mg by mouth three times daily for 10 days is first choice, alternatives being paromomycin (aminosidine), 500 mg by mouth three times daily for 10 days, or iodoquinol (diiodohydroxyquin) 650 mg three times daily for 20 days.[77] However, diiodohydroxyquin therapy, albeit in longer courses, has been associated with the development of blindness[78] and, since there are good alternate agents available, the use of this drug is not recommended. Nitazoxanide, a nitrothiazolyl-salicylamide derivative, at a dose of 500 mg twice daily for 3 days showed cyst passage clearance rates of 81% in treated patients within 7–10 days of therapy compared with 40% in the placebo group.[79,80] This compares well with similar clearance rates after the longer treatment regimen of diloxanide furoate.

AMEBIC LIVER ABSCESS

The dose of metronidazole required in amebic liver abscess is lower than in amebic dysentery. Amebic liver abscess is treated with metronidazole 400 mg by mouth three times daily for 5 days[75] followed by diloxanide furoate (as above). Tinidazole is an alternative to metronidazole. Initial work used a dosage regimen of 800 mg three times daily for 5 days,[81] but 2 g/day by mouth for 3–5 days is currently used. Scragg and Proctor achieved a 92% cure rate in children with amebic liver abscess, with tinidazole in a mean dose of 55 mg/kg daily for 3–5 days, in combination with therapeutic aspiration.[82] Secnidazole 500 mg three times daily for 5 days is another nitroimidazole that can be used in the treatment of amebic liver abscesses.[83]

Rarely, when nitroimidazoles do not seem to be effective despite therapeutic aspiration of the abscess (see below), dehydroemetine or emetine can be considered. However, both have serious side effects, notably cardiotoxicity. Where it is essential to use one of them, dehydroemetine is preferred as it is less toxic than emetine. The dosage regimen is dehydroemetine 1.25 mg/kg (maximum daily dose 90 mg) intramuscularly or deep subcutaneously for 10 days. Emetine dosage is 1 mg/kg (maximum daily dose 60 mg) intramuscularly or deep subcutaneously for 10 days.[84,85]

Chloroquine is another alternative where nitroimidazoles fail or cannot be used. However, it is only moderately effective in amebic liver abscess and ineffective in amebic dysentery.[75] The regimen is chloroquine 150 mg base four times daily for 2 days, then 150 mg base twice daily for 19 days.[85]

Aspiration of an amebic liver abscess is occasionally necessary. Reed gives the following indications:[77]

1. To rule out a pyogenic abscess, particularly with multiple lesions. Aspiration for diagnostic purposes should only rarely be required, provided good-quality amebic serology is available and if appropriate antibacterial and antiamebic therapy can be given from the outset pending the outcome of blood cultures and amebic serology. Scragg thought there was no place for diagnostic aspiration and that aspiration should be considered as part of treatment.[86]
2. As an adjunct to medical treatment, if a patient does not respond to therapy within 3–5 days and if rupture is believed to be imminent.
3. To decrease the risk of rupture of an abscess of the left lobe of the liver into the pericardium.

ASYMPTOMATIC CYST PASSAGE

The decision whether or not to treat asymptomatic cyst passage depends on several factors. If the patient is ordinarily resident in an area highly endemic for *Entamoeba histolytica* and thus likely to become reinfected fairly quickly, the benefit of eradicating cyst carriage has to be weighed against the cost of treatment and likely benefit to the individual, bearing in mind the fact that most strains of '*E. histolytica*' are non-pathogenic. *Entamoeba histolytica* has now been split into *E. histolytica*, which is always regarded as pathogenic, and *Entamoeba dispar* (formerly non-pathogenic *E. histolytica*), which had originally been proposed by Brumpt in 1925 and was confirmed by Sargeaunt.[88] However, where asymptomatic cyst passage persists following therapy of amebic dysentery or amebic liver abscess, further treatment with a luminal amebicide is mandatory, otherwise relapse is frequent.[84]

In areas where indigenous amebiasis is very uncommon, most *E. histolytica*/*E. dispar* infections are imported, and good luminal amebicides are readily available, so the decision is more in favor of treatment. Ideally, treatment strategy should be based on the results of isoenzyme or monoclonal antibody typing (after initial culture of trophozoites from the amebic cysts) to separate *E. histolytica* from *E. dispar* (since they are morphologically identical), but the technique is time-consuming and available in only a few centers. Some population groups appear to harbor only non-pathogenic strains. For example, Allason-Jones et al studied '*E. histolytica*' cysts from male homosexuals in London and all strains had a non-pathogenic zymodeme pattern.[88] They concluded that asymptomatic '*E. histolytica*' cyst passage in homosexual men did not require treatment.

GIARDIASIS

The treatment of choice is tinidazole 2 g as a single dose, a regimen effective in approximately 90% of cases. Metronidazole 2 g/day for 3 days gives a similar cure rate. Low dose, longer duration metronidazole regimens (200 mg three times daily for 7–10 days) give cure rates of 60–87%.[89] Failure of therapy with nitroimidazole therapy may be due to a variety of possible factors: reinfection, underlying immunodeficiency, or drug resistance. Where nitroimidazole resistance is thought to be the explanation, there are few alternative agents.

Mepacrine (quinacrine, atebrin) is active against *Giardia*[90] and is given as 100 mg three times daily for 5–7 days, with reported cure rates of 90–95%.[91,92] It should be used with caution in view of its known side effects: Wolfe reported toxic psychosis in 1.5% of adult patients treated with this agent[93] and other side effects include CNS stimulation and (on prolonged therapy) yellow discoloration of the skin.

Furazolidone provides another option[94] and is given at 100 mg four times daily for 7 days, with reported cure rates of 75–90%.[91] Side effects, though usually mild, occur in approximately 20% of patients[89] and patients with glucose-6-phosphate dehydrogenase (G-6-PD) deficiency may develop hemolysis on furazolidone.

Hall and Nahar compared the efficacy of albendazole with that of metronidazole against *Giardia* infection of children in Bangladesh.[95] Albendazole, 400 mg/day for 5 days, produced a 94.8% cure rate, not statistically different from the 97.4% cure rate produced in children receiving metronidazole 375 mg/day for 5 days.

Paromomycin (aminosidine) (25–30 mg/kg daily in three divided doses for 5–10 days) is effective in 60–70% of cases.[92] As it is excreted nearly 100% unchanged in the feces, it is used by some practitioners when nitroimidazoles cannot be used in pregnancy.

Nitazoxanide 500 mg twice daily as a 3-day course showed *Giardia* cyst clearance in 91% of patients, compared with 36% clearance in the placebo group at days 7–10.[79] This clearance rate compared well with similar rates achieved with metronidazole.

TRICHOMONAS VAGINALIS

Metronidazole 2 g as a single oral dose has produced cure rates as high as 97%.[96] An alternative regimen is 400 mg twice daily for 7 days. Tidwell et al compared a single 2 g oral dose of metronidazole with a single 2 g intravaginal dose:[97] 88% of the oral group but only 50% of the intravaginal group were microbiologically cured ($P = 0.0037$).

Tinidazole 2 g as a single dose, repeated if the first dose fails to produce clinical benefit, is an alternative to metronidazole.

Secnidazole, another nitroimidazole, is also effective against *Trichomonas* when given as a single 2 g dose.[98]

The most common causes of treatment failure are reinfection or non-compliance with therapy, but metronidazole-resistant strains of *T. vaginalis* are well documented:[99] approximately 5% of all *T. vaginalis* isolates from patients had some level of resistance to metronidazole.[100] Treatment of resistant isolates requires higher doses (usually double the recommended treatment dose for an extended period of time) and, in high level resistance, intravenous metronidazole. There is likely to be cross-resistance to other nitroimidazoles and therapy with another drug class might be necessary.[101] There are few alternative agents,[102] highlighting the need for new antitrichomonal drugs.

For *T. vaginalis* infections during the first trimester of pregnancy treatment with nitroimidazole derivatives is contraindicated; 100 mg clotrimazole suppositories intravaginally at bedtime for 14 days have been tried, with a cure rate of 50%.[101] The cure rates in a multicenter study for a single oral 2 g metronidazole dose were 80% compared with 11.1% for vaginal clotrimazole (two 100 mg tablets daily) and 18.6% for vaginal suppositories (containing 1.05 g sulfanilamide, 14 mg aminacrine hydrochloride and 140 mg allantoin) intravaginally twice daily for 7 days.[103] Treatment should be reserved for those with severe symptoms. Nitroimidazoles can be used during the second trimester of pregnancy.

Breast-feeding mothers can be treated with a single dose of 2 g secnidazole with a 24-h interruption of breast-feeding after therapy.

Neonatal trichomoniasis is dependent on maternal estrogen

levels, which begin to wane in the neonate after 3–6 weeks of life; therapy for symptomatic neonates can only be considered at 2 months of age.[101]

In general, drugs delivered intravaginally are of significantly lower efficacy than systemically administered nitroimidazoles, which still remain the drugs of choice.

CRYPTOSPORIDIUM PARVUM

Diarrhea due to this organism is usually self-limiting in those with normal immunity, but can be devastating in immuno-compromised people, notably in patients with AIDS. Highly effective treatment remains elusive, but several drugs have been found to be effective in some studies. Paromomycin has been reported effective in a double-blind placebo-controlled trial.[104] Vargas et al reported successful use of azithromycin in two cases in immunocompromised children.[105] In a randomized, double-blind, placebo-controlled study nitazoxanide 500 mg twice daily for 3 days (100 mg twice daily for 1–3 year olds, 200 mg twice daily for 4–11 year olds) showed an 80% clinical resolution and 67% oocyst clearance at day 7 (values were 41% and 22% respectively in the control group).[79,80]

Therapy of the immunocompromised patient with cryptosporidiosis is difficult and the mainstay of treatment is modulation of the immune defect. HIV-infected patients or HAART showed persistent parasitological clearance after 1 month of paromomycin 2 g four times a day. Groups on triple and double therapy showed no relapses, except for two patients who stopped HAART. The groups on no antiretroviral therapy or monotherapy showed only 20% resolution after paromomycin.[106]

Hyperimmune bovine colostrum has also been used for the treatment of cryptosporidiosis in HIV-positive patients.[107,108]

ISOSPORA BELLI

The treatment of choice is trimethoprim–sulfamethoxazole.[109] A combination of pyrimethamine and sulfadiazine given for 8 weeks was successful in an HIV-positive patient in whom trimethoprim–sulfamethoxazole daily for 2 weeks had failed. Diiodohydroxyquin, paromomycin and spiramycin have also been unsuccessful.[110]

For two AIDS patients with hypersensitivity to trimethoprim–sulfamethoxazole, a combination of albendazole and ornidazole showed parasitological clearance in one patient.[111]

Furazolidone is an alternative agent for the treatment of isosporiasis.

CYCLOSPORA CAYETANENSIS

Cyclospora infection may be self-limiting, so antimicrobial therapy is not required in every case. Where specific treatment is deemed necessary, the agent of choice is trimethoprim–sulfamethoxazole 960 mg twice daily for 7 days.[112] In a cohort study of Haitian HIV-positive patients the relapse rate after initial therapy with 960 mg trimethoprim–sulfamethoxazole four times a day for 10 days was 43% and secondary prophylaxis of single dose 960 mg trimethoprim–sulfamethoxazole three times a week was required. No patient had received antiretroviral therapy.[113] For patients with hypersensitivity to sulfa drugs monotherapy with trimethoprim showed no effect[114] but ciprofloxacin 500 mg twice daily for 7 days showed a 70% parasitological clearance on day 7 (clearance was 95% in the trimethoprim–sulfamethoxazole group).[115] Ciprofloxacin could be used in patients with hypersensitivity to sulfonamides.

MICROSPORIDIOSIS

Intestinal microsporidiosis in AIDS patients is caused by *Enterocytozoon bieneusi* or *Encephalitozoon (Septata) intestinalis*. Albendazole 400 mg twice daily for 3 weeks showed excellent efficacy for the treatment and prophylaxis of *E. intestinalis* infection in patients with AIDS.[116] Albendazole lacks efficacy against *E. bieneusi* and there are no definitive treatment options so far.[117,118] Thalidomide 100 mg at night for one month showed 38% complete remission and 17% partial remission.[119] Nitazoxanide 1 g twice daily for 60 days achieved parasitological clearance in an AIDS patient who had not been on antiretroviral therapy at the time nitazoxanide was administered.[120] Immune modulation of HIV-infected patients achieved with HAART remains an important therapeutic intervention in the treatment of microsporidial infections.[106]

BABESIOSIS

BABESIA BOVIS AND BABESIA DIVERGENS

These infections are usually encountered in splenectomized humans, leading to fulminant illness and death. There are no controlled trials of treatment. Diminazene (Berenil) is active against animal babesiosis and has been used in a case of human infection with *B. divergens*, but the patient did not survive.[121] The same authors reported successful treatment of a splenectomized patient infected with this parasite using pentamidine plus trimethoprim–sulfamethoxazole. Successful treatment of three cases with massive exchange blood transfusion (2–3 blood volumes) followed by intravenous clindamycin and oral quinine was reported by Brasseur and Gorenflot.[122, 123]

Atovaquone is effective against *B. divergens* in vitro.[124] In the absence of data from randomised controlled trials, treatment for human infection with *B. divergens* should consist of exchange blood transfusion plus intravenous clindamycin and intravenous or oral quinine, depending upon the patient's condition.

BABESIA MICROTI

In most cases patients suffer a mild illness and recover spontaneously. Where illness is severe enough to merit treatment, quinine plus clindamycin is the treatment of choice.[124] Whole blood or red cell exchange transfusion has produced a rapid and substantial fall in parasitemia.[125] Krause et al compared atovaquone 750 mg every 12 h plus azithromycin 500 mg on day 1 and 250 mg daily thereafter for 7 days with clindamycin 600 mg every 8 h and quinine 650 mg every 8 h for 7 days, all drugs being given orally.[126] Atovaquone plus azithromycin proved to be as effective as clindamycin plus quinine and had fewer adverse reactions. The authors recommended the use of atovaquone plus azithromycin for the treatment of non-life threatening babesiosis in immunocompetent adult patients and in others who cannot tolerate clindamycin and quinine. Ranque has suggested that a trial of atovaquone plus clindamycin should be performed.[127]

References

1. Nguyen BT, Stadtsbaeder S 1983 Comparative effects of cotrimoxazole (trimethoprim-sulphamethoxazole), pyrimethamine–sulphadiazine and spiramycin during avirulent infection with *Toxoplasma gondii* (Beverley strain) in mice. *British Journal of Pharmacology* 79: 923–928.

2. Joss AWL 1992 Treatment. In: Ho-Yen DO, Joss AWL (eds) *Human toxoplasmosis.* Oxford University Press, Oxford, pp. 119–143.

3. Rothova A, Buitenhuis HJ, Meenken C et al 1989 Therapy of ocular toxoplasmosis. *International Ophthalmology* 13: 415–419.

4. Dutton GN 1989 Toxoplasmic retinochoroiditis – a historical review and current concepts. *Annals of the Academy of Medicine Singapore* 18: 214–221.

5. Pearson PA, Piracha AR, Sen HA, Jaffe GJ 1999 Atovaquone for the treatment of toxoplasma retinochoroiditis in immunocompetent patients. *Ophthalmology* 106: 148–153.

6. Dutton GN 1989 Recent developments in the prevention and treatment of congenital toxoplasmosis. *International Ophthalmology* 13: 407–413.

7. Luft BJ, Noat Y, Araujo FG, Stinson EB, Remington JS 1983 Primary and reactivated toxoplasma infection in patients with cardiac transplants. Clinical spectrum and problems in diagnosis in a defined population. *Annals of Internal Medicine* 99: 27–31.

8. Wreghitt TG, Hakim M, Gray JJ et al 1989 Toxoplasmosis in heart and heart and lung transplant recipients. *Journal of Clinical Pathology* 42: 194–199.

9. Soave R 2001 Prophylaxis strategies for solid-organ transplantation. *Clinical Infectious Diseases* 33: S26–31.

10. Derouin F, Debure A, Godeaut E, Lariviere M, Kreis H 1987 *Toxoplasma* antibody titres in renal transplant recipients. *Transplantation* 44: 515–518.

11. Renoult E, Biava MF, Hulin C, Frimat L, Hestin D, Kessler M 1996 transmission of toxoplasmosis by renal transplant: a report of four cases. *Transplantation Proceedings* 28: 181–183.

12. Patel R 1999 Disseminated toxoplasmosis after liver transplantation. *Clinical Infectious Diseases* 29: 705–706.

13. Lappalainen M, Jokiranta TS, Halme L et al 1999 Disseminated toxoplasmosis after liver transplant. *Clinical Infectious Diseases* 29: 706.

14. Derouin F, Devergie A, Auber P et al 1992 Toxoplasmosis in bone marrow transplant recipients: report of seven cases and review. *Clinical Infectious Diseases* 15: 267–270.

15. Ho-Yen DO 1992 Immunocompromised patients. In: Ho-Yen DO, Joss AWL (eds) *Human toxoplasmosis.* Oxford University Press, Oxford, pp. 184–203.

16. Slavin MA, Meyers JD, Remington JS, Hackman RC 1994 *Toxoplasma gondii* infection in marrow transplant recipients: a 20 year experience. *Bone Marrow Transplant* 13: 549–557.

17. McCabe R, Chirurgi V 1993 Issues in toxoplasmosis. *Infectious Disease Clinics of North America* 7: 587–604.

18. Foot AB, Garin YJ, Ribaud P, Devergie A, Derouin F, Gluckman E 1994 Prophylaxis of toxoplasmosis infection with pyrimethamine/sulfadoxine (Fansidar) in bone marrow transplant recipients. *Bone Marrow Transplant* 14: 241–245.

19. Bryceson ADM, Murphy A, Moody A 1994 treatment of 'Old World' cutaneous leishmaniasis with aminosidine ointment: results of an open study in London. *Transactions of the Royal Society of Tropical Medicine and Hygiene* 88: 226–228.

20. Harms G, Chehade AK, Douba M et al 1991 A randomized trial comparing a pentavalent antimonial drug and recombinant interferon-gamma in the local treatment of cutaneous leishmaniasis. *Transactions of the Royal Society of Tropical Medicine and Hygiene* 85: 214–216.

21. Nacher M, Carme B, Sainte Marie D 2001 Influence of clinical presentation on the efficacy of a short course of pentamidine in the treatment of cutaneous leishmaniasis in French Guiana. *Annals of Tropical Medicine and Parasitology* 95: 331–336.

22. Teklemariam S, Hiwot AG, Frommel D, Miko TL, Ganlov G, Bryceson A 1994 Aminosidine and its combination with sodium stibogluconate in the treatment of diffuse cutaneous leishmaniasis caused by *Leishmania aethiopica*. *Transactions of the Royal Society of Medicine and Hygiene* 88: 334–339.

23. Bryceson ADM 1970 Diffuse cutaneous leishmaniasis in Ethiopia: II treatment. *Transactions of the Royal Society of Tropical Medicine and Hygiene* 64: 369–379.

24. Bryceson ADM 1987 Therapy in man. In: Peters W, Killick-Kendrick RE (eds) *The leishmaniases in biology and medicine.* Academic Press, London, vol 2, pp. 848–907.

25. Lessa HA, Machado P, Lima F et al 2001 successful treatment of refractory mucosal leishmaniasis with pentoxifylline plus antimony. *American Journal of Tropical Medicine and Hygiene* 65: 87–89.

26. Amato VS, Padilha ARS, Nicodemo AC et al 2000 Use of itraconazole in the treatment of mococutaneous leishmaniasis: a pliot study. *International Journal of Infectious Diseases* 4: 153–157.

27. El-Hassan, Zijlstra EE 2001 Leishmaniasis in Sudan. *Transactions of the Royal Society of Tropical Medicine and Hygiene* 95(Suppl. 1): S1/19–S1/26.

28. Davidson RN 1999 Visceral leishmaniasis in clinical practice. *Journal of Infection* 39: 112–116.

29. WHO 1990 Drugs used in parasitic diseases. WHO, Geneva.

30. Murray HW 2000 Treatment of visceral leishmaniasis (Kala-Azar): a decade of progress and future approaches. *International Journal of Infectious Diseases* 4: 158–177.

31. Herwaldt BL, Berman JD 1992 Recommendations for treating leishmaniasis with sodium stibogluconate (pentostam) and review of pertinent clinical studies. *American Journal of Tropical Medicine and Hygiene* 46: 296–306.

32. Anabwani GM, Bryceson ADM 1982 Visceral leishmaniasis in Kenyan children. *Indian Paediatrics* 19: 819–822.

33. Squires KE, Rosenkaimer F, Sherwood JA, Forni AL, Were JBO, Murray HW 1993 Immunochemotherapy for visceral leishmaniasis: a controlled pilot trial of antimony versus antimony plus interferon-gamma. *American Journal of Tropical Medicine and Hygiene* 48: 666–669.

34. Sundar S, Rosenkaimer F, Murray HW 1994 Successful treatment of refractory visceral leishmaniasis in India using antimony plus interferon-gamma. *Journal of Infectious Diseases* 170: 659–662.

35. Badaro R, Nascimento C, Carvalho JS et al 1994 Recombinant human granulocyte-macrophage colony-stimulating factor reverses neutropenia and reduces secondary infections in visceral leishmaniasis. *Journal of Infectious Diseases* 170: 413–418.

36. Olliaro PL, Bryceson ADM 1993 Practical progress and new drugs for changing patterns of leishmanias. *Parasitology Today* 9: 323–328.

37. Scott JAG, Davidson RN, Moody AH et al 1992 Aminosidine (paromomycin) in the treatment of leishmaniasis imported into the United Kingdom. *Transactions of the Royal Society of Tropical Medicine and Hygiene* 86: 617–619.

38. Jha TK, Olliaro P, Thakur CP et al 1998 Randomised controlled trial of aminosidine (paromomycin) v sodium stibugloconate for treating visceral leishmaniasis in North Bihar, India. *British Medical Journal* 316: 1200–1205.

39. Sundar S, More DK, Singh MK et al 2000 Failure of pentavalent antimony in visceral leishmaniasis in India: report from the center of the Indian epidemic. *Clinical Infectious Diseases* 31: 1104–1107.

40. Thakur CP, Olliaro P, Gothoskar S et al 1992 Treatment of visceral leishmaniasis (kala-azar) with aminosidine (=paromomycin)-antimonial combinations, a pilot study in Bihar, India. *Transactions of the Royal Society of Tropical Medicine and Hygiene* 86: 615–616.

41. Seaman J, Pryce D, Sondorp HE, Moody A, Bryceson AD, Davidson RN 1993 Epidemic visceral leishmaniasis in Sudan: a randomized trial of aminosidine plus sodium stibogluconate versus sodium stibogluconate alone. *Journal of Infectious Diseases* 168: 715–720.

42. Mishra M, Biswas UK, Jha AM, Khan AB 1994 Amphotericin versus sodium stibogluconate in first-line treatment of Indian kala-azar. *Lancet* 344: 1599–1600.

43. Davidson RN, DiMartino L, Gradoni L et al 1994 Liposomal amphotericin B (AmBisome) in Mediterranean visceral leishmaniasis: a multi-centre trial. *Quarterly Journal of Medicine* 87: 75–81.

44. Meyerhoff A 1999 US Food and Drug Administration approval of AmBisome (Liposomal Amphotericin B) for treatment of visceral leishmaniasis. *Clinical Infectious Diseases* 28: 42–48.

45. Sundar S, Agrawal G, Rai M, Makharia MK, Murray HW 2001 Treatment of Indian visceral leishmaniasis with single or daily infusions of low dose liposomal amphotericin B: randomized trial. *British Medical Journal* 323: 419–422.

46. Dietze R, Milan EP, Berman JD et al 1993 Treatment of Brazilian Kala-Azar with a short course of Amphocil (amphotericin B cholesterol dispersion). *Clinical Infectious Diseases* 17: 981–986.

47. Sundar S, Agrawal NK, Sinha PR, Horwith GS, Murray HW 1997 Short-course, low-dose amphotericin B lipid complex therapy for visceral leishmaniasis unresponsive to antimony. *Annals of Internal Medicine* 127: 133–137.

48. Jha TK, Sundar S, Thakur CP et al 1999 Miltefosine, an oral agent, for the treatment of Indian visceral leishmaniasis. *New England Journal of Medicine* 341: 1795–1800.

49. Rosenthal E, Tempesta S, Del Giudice P et al 2001 Declining incidence of visceral leishmaniasis in HIV-infected individuals in the era of highly active antiretroviral therapy. *AIDS* 15: 1184–1185.

50. Berenguer J, Cosin J, Miralles P, Lopez JC, Padilla B 2000 Discontinuation of secondary anti-*Leishmania* prophylaxis in HIV-infected patients who have responded to highly active antiretroviral therapy. *AIDS* 14: 2946–2948.

51. McCann PP, Bacchi CJ, Clarkson AB et al 1986 Inhibition of polyamine biosynthesis by α-difluoromethylornithine in African trypanosomes and *Pneumocystis carinii* as a basis of chemotherapy: biochemical and clinical aspects. *American Journal of Tropical Medicine and Hygiene* 35: 1153–1156.

52. Pepin J, Milord F, Guern C, Schechter PJ 1987 Difluoro-methylornithine for arseno-resistant *Trypanosoma brucei gambiense* sleeping sickness. *Lancet* ii: 1431–1433.

53. Milord F, Pepin J, Loko L, Ethier L, Mpia B 1992 Efficacy and toxicity of eflornithine for treatment of *Trypanosoma brucei gambiense* sleeping sickness. *Lancet* 340: 652–655.

54. Doua F, Miezan TW, Singaro JRS, Yapo FB, Baltz T 1996 The efficacy of pentamidine in the treatment of early-late stage *Trypanosoma brucei gambiense* trypanosomiasis. *American Journal of Tropical Medicine and Hygiene* 55: 586–588.

55. Burri C, Nkunku S, Merolle A, Smith T, Blum J, Brun R 2000 Efficacy of new, concise schedule for melarsoprol in treatment of sleeping sickness caused by *Trypanosoma brucei gambiense*: a randomized trial. *Lancet* 355: 1419–1425.

56. Pepin J, Milord F, Meurice F, Ethier L, Loko L, Mpia B 1992 High dose nifurtimox for arseno-resistant *Trypanosoma brucei gambiense* sleeping sickness: an open trial in Central Zaire. *Transactions of the Royal Society of Tropical Medicine and Hygiene* 86: 254–256.

57. Smith DH, Pepin J, Stich AHR 1998 Human African trypanosomiasis: an emerging public health crisis. *British Medical Bulletin* 54: 341–355.

58. Clerinx J, Taelman H, Bogaerts J, Vervoort T 1998 Treatment of late stage rhodesian trypanosomiasis using suramin and eflornithine: report of six cases. *Transactions of the Royal Society of Tropical Medicine and Hygiene* 92: 449–450.

59. Pepin J, Milord F, Guern C, Mpia B, Ethier L, Mansinsa D 1989 Trial of prednisolone for prevention of melarsoprol-induced encephalopathy in gambiense sleeping sickness. *Lancet* i: 1246–1250.

60. Pepin J, Milord F, Khonde AN et al 1995 Risk factors for encephalopathy and mortality during melarsoprol treatment of *Trypanosoma brucei gambiense* sleeping sickness. *Transactions of the Royal Society of Tropical Medicine and Hygiene* 89: 92–97.

61. Foulkes JR 1996 Metronidazole and suramin combination in the treatment of arsenical refractory rhodesian sleeping sickness – a case study. *Transactions of the Royal Society of Tropical Medicine and Hygiene* 90: 422.

62. Gallerano RH, Marr JJ, Sosa RR 1990 Therapeutic efficacy of allopurinol in patients with chronic Chagas' disease. *American Journal of Tropical Medicine and Hygiene* 43: 159–166.

63. Tanowitz HB, Kirchhoff LV, Simon D, Morris SA, Weiss LM, Wittner M 1992 Chagas' disease. *Clinical Microbiology Reviews* 5: 400–419.

64. WHO 1991 Control of Chagas' disease. WHO technical report series 811. WHO, Geneva

65. Andrade SG, Rassi A, Magalhaes JB, Ferriolli-Filho F, Luquetti AO 1992 Specific chemotherapy of Chagas' disease: a comparison between the response in patients and experimental animals inoculated with the same strains. *Transactions of the Royal Society of Tropical Medicine and Hygiene* 86: 624–626.

66. Solari A, Saavedra H, Sepulveda C et al 1993 Successful treatment of *Trypanosoma cruzi* encephalitis in a patient with hemophilia and AIDS. *Clinical Infectious Diseases* 16: 255–259.

67. Solari A, Ortiz S, Soto A et al 2001 Treatment of *Trypanosoma cruzi*-infected children with nifurtimox: a 3 year follow-up by PCR. *Journal of Antimicrobial Chemotherapy* 48: 515–519.

68. Estani SS, Segura EL 1999 Treatment of *Trypanosoma cruzi* infection in the undetermined phase. Experience and current guidelines of treatment in Argentina. *Memorias do Instituto Oswaldo Cruz Rio de Janeiro* 94: 363–365.

69. Neto VA 1999 Etiological treatment for infection by *Trypanosoma cruzi*. *Memorias do Instituto Oswaldo Cruz, Rio de Janeiro* 94(Suppl. 1): 337–339.

70. Braga MS, Lauria-Pires L, Arganaraz ER, Nascimento RJ, Texeira ARL 2000 Persistent infections in chronic Chagas' disease patients treated with anti-*Trypanosoma cruzi* nitroderivatives. *Revista di Instituto de Medicina Tropical de São Paolo* 42: 157–161.

71. Silveira CAN, Castillo E, Castro C 2000 Avaliacao do tratamento especifico para o *Trypanosoma cruzi* em criancas, na evolucao da fase indeterminada. *Revista da Sociedade Brasiliera da Medicina Tropical* 33: 191–196.

72. Rassi A, Neto VA, Ferraz de Siqueira A, Filho FF, Amato VS, Junior AR 1999 Efeito protetor do benznidazol contra a reativacao parasitaria em pacientes cronicamente infectados pelo *Trypanosoma cruzi* e tratados com corticoide em virtude de afeccoes associadas. *Revista da Sociedade Brasiliera de Medicina Tropical* 32: 475–482.

73. Organizacion Panamericana de la Salud/Organizacion Mundial de la Salud 1999 Tratamiento Etiologico de la Enfermedad de Chagas. OPS/HCP/HCT/140/99.

74. Urbina JA 1999 Parasitological cure of Chagas disease: is it possible? Is it relevant? *Memorias do Instituto Oswaldo Cruz, Rio de Janeiro* 94 (Suppl. 1): 349–355.

75. Powell SJ, Wilmott AJ, Elsdon-Dew R 1967 Further trials of metronidazole in amoebic dysentery and amoebic liver abscess. *Annals of Tropical Medicine and Parasitology* 61: 511–514.

76. Qureshi H, Baqai R, Mehdi I, Ahmed W 1999 Secnidazole response in amoebiasis and giardiasis. *Eastern Mediterranean Health Journal* 5: 389–390.

77. Reed SL 1992 Amoebiasis: an update. *Clinical Infectious Diseases* 14: 385–393.

78. Fleisher DI, Hepler RS, Landau JW 1974 Blindness during diiodohydroxyquin (Diodoquin®) therapy: a case report. *Pediatrics* 54: 106–108.

79. Rossignol J-FA, Ayoub A, Ayers MS 2001 Treatment of diarrhea caused by *Cryptosporidium parvum*: A prospective randomized, double-blind, placebo-controlled study of nitazoxanide. *Journal of Infectious Diseases* 184: 103–106.

80. Rossignol J-FA, Ayoub A, Ayers MS 2001 Treatment of diarrhea caused by *Giardia intestinalis* and *Entamoeba histolytica* or *E. dispar*. A randomized, double-blind, placebo-controlled study of nitazoxanide. *Journal of Infectious Diseases* 184: 381–384.

81. Hatchuel W 1975 Tinidazole for the treatment of amoebic liver abscess. *South African Medical Journal* 49: 1879–1881.

82. Scragg JN, Proctor EM 1977 Tinidazole in treatment of amoebic liver abscess in children. *Archives of Diseases of Childhood* 52: 408–410.

83. Hughes MA, Petri WA 2000 Amebic liver abscess. *Infectious Disease Clinics of North America* 14: 565–582.

84. Knight R 1980 The chemotherapy of amoebiasis. *Journal of Antimicrobial Chemotherapy* 6: 577–593.

85. Du Pont HL 1994 Prevention and treatment strategies in giardiasis and amoebiasis. *Drugs under Investigation* 8 (Suppl. 1): 19–25.

86. Scragg JN 1975 Hepatic amoebiasis in childhood. *Tropical Doctor* 5: 132–134.

87. Sargeaunt PG 1993 *Entamoeba histolytica*: a question answered. *Tropical Disease Bulletin* 90: R1–R2.

88. Allason-Jones E, Mindel A, Sargeaunt P, Katz D 1988 Outcome of untreated infection with *Entamoeba histolytica* in homosexual men with and without HIV antibody. *British Medical Journal* 297: 654–657.

89. Mendelson RM 1980 The treatment of giardiasis. *Transactions of the Royal Society of Tropical Medicine and Hygiene* 74: 438–439.

90. Thomas MEM 1952 Observations upon the effects of mepacrine and other substances on *Giardia intestinalis. Parasitology* 42: 262–268.

91. Wolfe MS 1992 Giardiasis. *Clinical Microbiology Reviews* 5: 93–100.

92. Hill DR 1993 Giardiasis. *Infectious Disease Clinics of North America* 7: 503–526.

93. Wolfe MS 1978 Giardiasis. *New England Journal of Medicine* 298: 319–321.

94. Farthing MJG 1992 *Giardia* comes of age: progress in epidemiology, immunology and chemotherapy. *Journal of Antimicrobial Chemotherapy* 30: 563–566.

95. Hall A, Nahar Q 1993 Albendazole as a treatment for infections with *Giardia duodenalis* in children in Bangladesh. *Transactions of the Royal Society of Tropical Medicine and Hygiene* 87: 84–86.

96. Lossick JG 1980 Single-dose metronidazole treatment for vaginal trichomonas. *Obstetrics and Gynaecology* 56: 508–510.

97. Tidwell BH, Lushbaugh WB, Laughlin MD, Cleary JD, Finley RW 1994 A double-blind placebo-controlled trial of single-dose intravaginal versus single-dose oral metronidazole in the treatment of trichomonal vaginitis. *Journal of Infectious Diseases* 170: 242–246.

98. Bagnoli VR 1994 An overview of the clinical experience with secnidazole in bacterial vaginosis and trichomoniasis. *Drugs under Investigation* 8 (Suppl. 1): 53–60.

99. Lossick JG, Muller M, Gorrell TE 1986 *In vitro* drug susceptibility and doses of metronidazole required for cure in cases of refractory vaginal trichomoniasis. *Journal of Infectious Diseases* 153: 948–955.

100. Narcisi EM, Secor WE 1996 In vitro effect of tinidazole and furazolidone on metronidazole-resistant *Trichomonas vaginalis. Antimicrobial Agents and Chemotherapy* 40: 1121–1125.

101. Petrin D, Delgaty K, Bhatt R, Garber G 1998 Clinical and microbiological aspects of *Trichomonas vaginalis. Clinical Microbiology Reviews* 11: 300–317.

102. Upcroft JA, Campbell RW, Benakli K, Upcroft P, Vanelle P 1999 Efficacy of New 5-nitroimidazoles against metronidazole-susceptible and -resistant *Giardia, Trichomonas,* and *Entamoeba* spp. *Antimicrobial Agents and Chemotherapy* 43: 73–76.

103. DuBochet L, Spence MR, Rein MF, Danzig MR, McCormack WM 1997 Multicenter comparison of cotrimazole vaginal tablets, oral metronidazole, and vaginal suppositories containing sulfanilamide, aminacrine hydrochloride, and allantion in the treatment of symptomatic trichomoniasis. *Sexually Transmitted Diseases* 24: 156–160.

104. White AC Jr, Chappel CL, Hayat CS, Kimball KT, Flanigan TP, Goodgame RW 1994 Paromomycin for cryptosporidiosis in AIDS: a prospective, double-blind trial. *Journal of Infectious Diseases* 170: 419–424.

105. Vargas SL, Shenep JL, Flynn PM, Pui C-H, Santana VM, Hughes WT 1993 Azithromycin for treatment of severe *Cryptosporidium* diarrhoea in two children with cancer. *Journal of Pediatrics* 123: 154–156.

106. Maggi P, Larocca AMV, Quarto G et al 2000 Effect of antiretroviral therapy on cryptosporidiosis and microsporidiosis in patients infected with Human Immunodeficiency Virus type 1. *European Journal of Clinical Microbiology and Infectious Diseases* 19: 213–217.

107. Plettenberg A, Stoehr A, Stellbrink H-J, Albrecht H, Meigel W 1993 A preparation from bovine colostrum in the treatment of HIV-positive patients with chronic diarrhoea. *Clinical Investigator* 71: 42–45.

108. Shield J, Melville C, Novelli V et al 1993 Bovine colostrum immunoglobulin concentrate for cryptosporidiosis in AIDS. *Archives of Diseases of Childhood* 69: 451–453.

109. De Hovitz JA, Pape JW, Boncy M, Johnson WD 1986 Clinical manifestations and therapy of *Isospora belli* infection in patients with the acquired immunodeficiency syndrome. *New England Journal of Medicine* 315: 87–90.

110. Ebrahimzadeh A, Bottone EJ 1996 Persistent diarrhoea caused by *Isospora belli*: Therapeutic response to pyrimethamine and sulfadiazine *Diagnostic Microbiology and Infectious Diseases* 26: 87–89.

111. Dionisio G, Sterrantino M, Meli M, Leoncini F, Orsi A, Nicoletti P 1996 Treatment of isosporiasis with combined albendazole and ornidazole in patients with AIDS *AIDS* 10: 1301–1302.

112. Hoge CW, Shlim DR, Ghimire M et al 1995 Placebo-controlled trial of co-trimoxazole for cyclospora infections among travellers and foreign residents in Nepal. *Lancet* 345: 691–693.

113. Pape JW, Verdier RI, Boncy M, Bincy J, Johnson WD Jr 1994 *Cyclospora* infection in adults infected with HIV. Clinical manifestations, treatment, and prophylaxis. *Annals of Internal Medicine* 121: 654–657.

114. Shlim DR, Pandey P, Rabold JG, Walch A, Rajah R 1997 An open trial of trimethoprim alone against Cyclospora infections. *Journal of Travel Medicine* 4: 44–45.

115. Verdier R-I, Fitzgerald DW, Johnson WD, Pape JW 2000 Trimethoprim-sufamethoxazole compared with ciprofloxacin for treatment and prophylaxis of *Isospora belli* and *Cyclospora cayetanensis* infection in HIV-infected patients. *Annals of Internal Medicine* 132: 885–888.

116. Molina J-F, Chastang C, Goguel J et al 1998 Albendazole for treatment and prophylaxis of microsporidiosis due to *Encephalitozoon interstinalis* in patients with AIDS: A randomized double-blind controlled trial. *Journal of Infectious Diseases* 177: 1373–1378.

117. Weber R, Bryan RT 1994 Microsporidial infections in immunodeficient and immunocompetent patients. *Clinical Infectious Diseases* 19: 517–521.

118. Molina J-M, Oksenhendler E, Beauvais B et al 1995 Disseminated microsporidiosis due to *Septata intestinalis* in patients with AIDS: clinical features and response to albendazole therapy. *Journal of Infectious Diseases* 171: 245–249.

119. Sharpstone D, Rowbottom A, Francis N et al 1997 Thalidomide: A novel therapy for microsporidiosis. *Gastroenterology* 112: 1823–1829.

120. Bicart-See A, Massip P, Linas M-D, Datry A 2000 Successful treatment with nitazoxanide of *Enterocytozoon bieneusi* microsporidiosis in a patient with AIDS. *Antimicrobial Agents and Chemotherapy* 44: 167–168.

121. Raoult D, Soulayrol L, Toga B, Dumon H, Casanovna P 1987 Babesiosis, pentamidine and cotrimoxazole. *Annals of Internal Medicine* 107: 944.

122. Brasseur P, Gorenflot A 1992 Human babesiosis in Europe. *Memorias do Instituto Oswaldo Cruz* 87: 131–132.

123. Pudney M, Gray JS 1997 Therapeutic efficacy of atovaquone against the bovine intraerythrocytic parasite, *Babesia divergens. Journal of Parasitology* 83: 307–310.

124. Telford SR III, Gorenflot A, Brasseur P, Spielman A 1993 Babesial infections in humans and wildlife. In: Krier JP, Baker JR (eds) *Parasitic protozoa*, 2nd edn. Academic Press, San Diego, vol 5, pp. 1–47.

125. Jacoby GA, Hunt JV, Kosinski KS et al 1980 Treatment of transfusion-transmitted babesiosis by exchange transfusion. *New England Journal of Medicine* 303: 1098–1100.

126. Krause PJ, Lepore T, Sikand VK et al 2000 Atovaquone and azithromycin for the treatment of babesiosis. *New England Journal of Medicine* 343: 1454–1458.

127. Ranque S 2001 The treatment of babesiosis. *New England Journal of Medicine* 344: 773–774.

 ## Further information

Dombrowski MP, Sokol RJ, Brown WJ, Bronsteen RA 1987 Intravenous therapy of metronidazole-resistant *Trichomonas vaginalis. Obstetrics and Gynecology* 69: 524–525.

Hughes WT, Oz HS 1995 Successful prevention and treatment of babesiosis with atovaquone. *Journal of Infectious Diseases* 172: 1042–1046.

Keiser J, Stich A, Burri C 2001 New drugs for the treatment of human African trypanosomiasis: research and development. *Trends in Parasitology* 17: 42–49.

Pepin J, Khonde N, Maiso F et al 2000 Short-course eflornithine in Gambian trypanosomiasis: a randomized controlled trial. *Bulletin of the World Health Organization* 78: 1284–1295.

Roemer E, Blau W, Basara N et al 2001 Toxoplasmosis, a severe complication in allogeneic haematopoietic stem cell transplantation: successful treatment strategies during a 5-year single-center experience. *Clinical Infectious Diseases* 32: E1–8.

United States Public Health Service/Infectious Disease Society of America Prevention of Opportunistic Infections Working Group 2000 1999 USPHS/IDSA guidelines for the prevention of opportunistic infections in persons infected with human immunodeficiency virus. *Clinical Infectious Diseases* 30 (Suppl. 1): S29–65.

Weiss LM, Wittner M, Wasserman S, Oz HS, Retsema J, Tanowitz HB 1993 Efficacy of azithromycin for treating *Babesia microti* infection in the hamster model. *Journal of Infectious Diseases* 168: 1289–1292.

Weller IVD, Williams IG 2001 ABC of AIDS. Treatment of infections. *British Medical Journal* 322: 1350–1354.

CHAPTER

66 Helminthic infections

Tim O'Dempsey

Helminths are complex, multicellular, parasitic worms occupying a wide variety of geographical, ecological and anatomical niches. They are classified into three groups: nematodes (roundworms), platy-helminths (flatworms, including trematodes and cestodes) and annelids (segmented worms, including leeches) (Table 66.1). Their life cycles vary in complexity. Some, for example *Enterobius vermicularis*, are principally dependent upon their human host, while others, such as the hepatic and intestinal flukes, require two intermediate hosts to complete their life cycle. Pathological effects in humans may be caused by the adult worms, egg deposition in tissues, or migration

Table 66.1 Clinically important helminths and their principal modes of infection

Helminth (common name)	Principal mode of infection
Intestinal helminths	
Nematodes:	
Ascaris lumbricoides (roundworm)	Ingestion of egg
Enterobius vermicularis (pinworm/threadworm)	Ingestion of egg
Trichuris trichiura (whipworm)	Ingestion of egg
Ancylostoma duodenale (hookworm)	Larval penetration of skin
Necator americanus (hookworm)	Larval penetration of skin
Strongyloides spp.	Larval penetration of skin
Cestodes:	
Taenia saginata. Taenia solium (beef/pork tapeworm)	Ingestion of cyst
Diphyllobothrium latum (fish tapeworm)	Ingestion of cyst
Larval helminths	
Nematodes:	
Trichinella spp. (trichinosis)	Ingestion of cyst
Toxocara spp. (toxocariasis)	Ingestion of egg
Cestodes:	
Taenia solium (cysticercosis)	Ingestion of egg
Echinococcus granulosus (hydatid cyst)	Ingestion of egg
Echinococcus multilocularis (alveolar hydatid)	Ingestion of egg
Trematodes (Flukes)	
Schistosoma spp. (Bilharzia)	Cercarial penetration of skin
Paragonimus spp. (lung fluke)	Ingestion of metacercariae
Fasciolopsis buski (intestinal fluke)	Ingestion of metacercariae
Fasciola hepatica, Fasciola gigantica (liver flukes)	Ingestion of metacercariae
Opisthorchis sinensis, O. viverrini (oriental liver flukes)	Ingestion of metacercariae
Filarial nematodes	
	Infective larvae from:
Onchocerca volvulus (river blindness)	Bite of *Simulium* (black fly)
Loa loa (loiasis, eye worm)	Bite of *Chrysops* (red fly)
Dracunculus medinensis (Guinea worm)	Ingestion of *Cyclops*
Wuchereria bancrofti, Brugia malayi, Brugia timori (lymphatic filariasis)	Bite of various mosquitoes

and death of larvae or microfilariae. Most infections are asymptomatic. Clinical disease is more likely in those who are immunologically naïve following substantial initial exposure, in heavy infections and in people who are immunosuppressed or malnourished.

Helminths are a major cause of morbidity and mortality worldwide. Unprecedented efforts are now being made to control or eradicate these infections by means of health education, improved hygiene and sanitation, provision of safe water, vector control, and selective and mass chemotherapy using a limited but growing repertoire of safe and effective antihelminthic agents (Table 66.2). Recently, nitazoxanide, a thiazolide compound, has been shown to be well tolerated and effective in the treatment of a wide range of helminthic and other intestinal infections, including *Ascaris lumbricoides*, *Strongyloides stercoralis*, *Trichuris trichiura*, *Enterobius vermicularis*, *Taenia saginata*, *Hymenolepis nana* and *Fasciola hepatica*. However, full prescribing information is not yet available.[1]

INTESTINAL HELMINTHS (GEOHELMINTHS)

INTESTINAL NEMATODE INFECTIONS

Ascariasis

Ascaris lumbricoides, the most common roundworm infection in humans, affects over 1 billion people worldwide. The peak prevalence and intensity of infection are among children aged 3–8 years. Infection follows ingestion of eggs contaminating vegetables, soil or dust. Larvae, liberated as the eggs pass through the stomach and small intestine, penetrate the intestinal mucosa and enter blood and lymphatic vessels. A proportion reach the lungs 4–16 days after infection. After penetrating the alveoli and molting, they migrate via the respiratory tract to the esophagus and are carried to the small intestine. Here they develop into adults, mate and start producing eggs 6–8 weeks after infection. Adults grow to a length of 15–35 cm and may survive for 1–2 years. Females are capable of producing 200 000 eggs per day. The eggs are excreted in feces and their ova mature into infective embryos within one to four weeks. Eggs may remain viable in soil for years.

Migration of larvae through the lungs may cause fever, cough, dyspnea, wheeze and urticaria. Chest pain and cyanosis occur in more severe cases and sputum may be slightly bloodstained. Chest radiographic abnormalities range from discrete densities to diffuse interstitial, or more confluent, infiltrates. *Ascaris* pneumonitis, when accompanied by eosinophilia, is known as Löffler's syndrome. The episode usually subsides spontaneously within 10 days.

Adult intestinal worms are rarely noticed unless passed in the stool. In heavy infections the worms may intertwine to form a bolus, causing intestinal obstruction, volvulus or perforation. Migrating worms may obstruct ducts or diverticuli causing biliary colic, cholangitis, liver abscess, pancreatitis or appendicitis. A well-known hazard of anesthesia is endotracheal tube

Table 66.2 Side effects of selected anthelmintic agents

Anthelmintic agent	Frequent side effects	Occasional side effects	Rare side effects
Albendazole		Abdominal pain, reversible alopecia, increased transaminases, headache	Leukopenia, rash, renal toxicity, fever
Diethylcarbamazine citrate	Mazzotti reaction with onchocerciasis	Gastrointestinal disturbances, hypersensitivity reactions	Encephalopathy, renal failure (especially in patients with loiasis and high microfilaria counts)
Ivermectin		Gastrointestinal disturbances	Mazzotti reaction in onchocerciasis, encephalopathy in loiasis, transient postural hypotension
Mebendazole		Gastrointestinal disturbances, headache	Hypersensitivity reactions, hypospermia, leukopenia, agranulocytosis
Niclosamide		Gastrointestinal disturbances, dizziness, pruritus	
Piperazine		Gastrointestinal disturbances, hypersensitivity reactions	Stevens–Johnson syndrome, angioedema, ataxia ('worm wobble'), drowsiness, confusion, convulsions in patients with neurological/renal abnormalities.
Praziquantel		Gastrointestinal disturbances, headache, dizziness, sedation, fever	Pruritus, rash, edema, hiccups
Pyrantel pamoate		Gastrointestinal disturbances, dizziness, rash, fever	
Thiabendazole	Gastrointestinal disturbances, vertigo, headache, drowsiness, pruritus	Leukopenia, crystalluria, rash, neuropsychiatric disturbances, erythema multiforme	Shock, tinnitus, intrahepatic cholestasis, convulsions, angioneurotic edema, Stevens–Johnson syndrome

obstruction by a wandering ascaris. Cases of pneumothorax and pericarditis have also been reported.[2]

Diagnosis and treatment

Ascaris pneumonitis is diagnosed on clinical grounds; the presence or absence of eggs in the stools is irrelevant. Larvae may be found in the sputum. Stool examination for eggs is the standard method for diagnosing established infection, although stools may be negative if infection is entirely due to male worms. Worms may also be identified on barium studies, ultrasonography and endoscopy.

Albendazole 400 mg in a single oral dose eliminates most infections. In heavy infections this may need to be repeated for 2–3 days. Mebendazole 100 mg orally twice daily for 3 days is also effective, although use in children under 2 years is not recommended by the manufacturer. There are also reports of ectopic migration of *Ascaris* following the use of mebendazole.

Piperazine 75 mg/kg (to a maximum of 3.5 g for adults and children over 12 years and a maximum of 2.5 g for children aged 2–12 years) is also effective. Side effects are relatively common and may be serious: therefore, piperazine should be used only if safer alternatives are unavailable. Pyrantel pamoate (10 mg/kg up to a maximum of 1 g) can be given as a single dose. Pyrantel and piperazine have antagonistic effects and should never be prescribed concurrently.

Ascaris pneumonitis is generally managed symptomatically using bronchodilators and steroids if indicated. The use of anthelmintics is questionable as symptoms may be exacerbated by larval death. Intestinal ascariasis should be treated with an anthelmintic agent. Intestinal obstruction may respond to conservative management with nasogastric aspiration, intravenous fluids and antispasmodics, followed by an anthelmintic when the obstruction has subsided. Laparotomy is required if this fails or if the patient is seriously ill. Manipulation of the worms through the ileocecal valve may be possible without having to open the bowel. Surgical or endoscopic removal of single worms blocking ducts should be reserved for patients who fail to respond to anthelmintic treatment and those with persisting pain or raised serum amylase.[3]

Enterobiasis

Enterobius vermicularis, the pinworm or threadworm, occurs worldwide and is the most common helminthic infection in Western Europe and the USA. Infection follows ingestion of the egg on contaminated food or fomites. Autoinfection occurs when perianal irritation caused by migration of gravid female worms results in scratching and transmission of eggs from anus to mouth on fingertips. Secondary bacterial infection may occur at the site of excoriation. Vulvovaginitis, enuresis, urinary tract infection and appendicitis may also be associated with *E. vermicularis*. Infection may be accompanied by mild eosinophilia.

Diagnosis and treatment

Diagnosis is usually made by collecting eggs from the perianal region using adhesive tape or a moist cotton swab. Eggs may appear in urine samples from girls.

Mebendazole, albendazole and piperazine all achieve cure rates above 90%. Mebendazole 100 mg is given as a single oral dose, repeated 2–4 weeks later. Albendazole 400 mg as a single oral dose is repeated after 7 days for adults and children over 2 years. A dose of 100 mg should be used in children aged less than 2 years. Piperazine is effective but must be given daily for 7 days and repeated after 2–4 weeks. It has been superseded by mebendazole and albendazole.

Family members and other close contacts are likely to be infected and it is usual to recommend their treatment simultaneously, except for pregnant women during the first trimester.

Trichuriasis

Trichuris trichiura, the whipworm, infects about 900 million people worldwide. Following ingestion of eggs in contaminated soil, food or fomites, larvae emerge in the cecum, penetrate the crypts of Lieberkühn and migrate within the mucosal epithelium. The adult matures and remains partly embedded in the mucosa of the cecum and ascending colon, or throughout the colon in heavy infections.

Most infections go unnoticed; however, heavy infections may cause severe gastrointestinal symptoms. The friable mucosa bleeds easily, resulting in iron deficiency anemia in children on marginal diets. Chronic trichuris colitis is associated with growth retardation. Severe trichuris dysentery syndrome frequently leads to rectal prolapse.

Diagnosis and treatment

Diagnosis may be obvious on identifying adult worms attached to the mucosa of prolapsed bowel. In less dramatic circumstances, the characteristic eggs may be identified in the stool, by concentration techniques if necessary for light infections. Trichuriasis may cause a significant eosinophilia.

A single oral dose of mebendazole 500 mg appears to be more effective than albendazole 400 mg.[4] Severe infections require either mebendazole 100 mg twice daily for 3 days or albendazole 400 mg daily for 3 days. Single-dose combination treatment using albendazole 400 mg plus ivermectin 200 μg/kg is also highly effective.[5]

Hookworm

Ancylostoma duodenale and *Necator americanus* are the principal hookworms infecting humans, affecting 900 million people worldwide. Both species are widely distributed in tropical Africa and Asia. *N. americanus* is the most common species in the Americas; *A. duodenale* also occurs in the Middle East, North Africa, southern Europe, the Caribbean, Central and South America. Lower incidence, prevalence and intensity of infection have been noted among children who have received BCG.[6]

Hookworm eggs passed in the feces hatch in soil in warm, moist conditions, liberating rhabditiform larvae. These subsequently develop into filariform larvae, which inhabit the surface layer of soil. When these larvae come into contact with the skin of the human host, they penetrate via fissures or hair follicles and are carried in the venous circulation to the lungs. Here they penetrate the alveoli and migrate to the pharynx. They are then carried into the small intestine where they mature into adults. Rarely, infection with *A. duodenale* may occur following ingestion of larvae on contaminated vegetables. Infantile hookworm disease has been described in China and attributed to transmammary transmission, laying infants on contaminated soil, or using nappies made of cloth bags stuffed with infected soil.

Adult hookworms attach themselves to the upper half of the small intestine and feed on blood. An adult *A. duodenale* may consume between 0.15 and 0.26 ml/day; *N. americanus* consumes a relatively modest 0.03 ml/day. Blood loss also occurs at the site of attachment. Loss of plasma proteins may result in hypoproteinemia.

Initial infection is usually asymptomatic. Ground itch at the site of larval penetration when severe may be associated with the development of vesicles or pustules. Cutaneous larva migrans is sometimes seen. Larval migration through the lungs may give rise to a pneumonitis similar to that in ascariasis.

Occasionally, 4–6 weeks after infection, abdominal symptoms occur including discomfort, flatulence, anorexia, nausea, vomiting and diarrhea, which may contain blood and mucus in heavy infections. Rarely, life-threatening gastrointestinal hemorrhage occurs in young children with severe primary infections.

Most chronic infections are asymptomatic. Problems arise when iron intake is low or demands are high. A gradually worsening iron deficiency anemia develops, often associated with hypoalbuminemia and edema, and eventually progresses to cardiac failure.

Diagnosis and treatment

Diagnosis is made by identification of the characteristic eggs in the stool. Concentration techniques may be necessary for lighter infections. Culture techniques similar to those used for strongyloides may also be helpful. If stool samples are left for a few days before examination, eggs may hatch liberating larvae that may be mistaken for strongyloides, although they are morphologically distinct. Mixed infections may also occur.

Albendazole 400 mg as a single dose is more effective than mebendazole 100 mg twice daily for 3 days.[7] Pyrantal pamoate 11 mg/kg (maximum 1 g) as a single dose is also effective. Treatment for iron-deficiency anemia may be indicated. Transfusion is rarely essential.

Other hookworm infections

Cutaneous larva migrans

Humans are accidental hosts in this infection caused by the larvae of the dog or cat hookworm, most commonly *Ancylostoma braziliense*. Larvae penetrate the skin and migrate in the dermis, their progress mapped by an itchy, erythematous, serpiginous rash. Blistering sometimes occurs. Unable to complete their life cycle, they wander about in the dermis for several weeks or months until they eventually die. Rarely, infection may trigger hypereosinophilia and pneumonitis.

Topical thiabendazole may suffice for infections involving a limited area. A paste made by grinding one 0.5 g thiabendazole tablet in 5 g of petroleum jelly is applied two or three times daily over the track, extending 1–2 cm beyond the leading edge. An occlusive dressing containing thiabendazole paste enhances the effect. Oral thiabendazole was previously recommended for more severe infections; however, this has been superseded by albendazole 400 mg daily for three days. More recently, ivermectin 200 µg/kg as a single dose has been shown to be more effective and less toxic than albendazole. Repeated doses are sometimes required.[8]

Eosinophilic enteritis

This has been described in Australia following infection with the immature adult dog hookworm, *Ancylostoma caninum*, which provokes an allergic reaction resulting in edema of the gut wall, ascites and regional lymphadenopathy. Ulceration may occur at the site of the hookworm bite. Enterobiasis and anisakiasis may also cause eosinophillic enteritis.

Strongyloidiasis

Strongyloidiasis affects 50–100 million people worldwide, occurring in warm, wet, tropical and subtropical regions and in suitable niches in temperate regions, where conditions are moist and sanitation poor. *Strongyloides stercoralis* is the predominant species affecting humans, although *Strongyloides fülleborni*, principally a parasite of primates, has also been found in humans in Africa and Papua New Guinea. Human infection follows cutaneous penetration by filariform larvae contaminating soil, in a similar manner to hookworm. Indeed, both parasites may be present in the same habitat. Filariform larvae are carried in the venous circulation to the lungs where they penetrate the alveoli, migrate to the pharynx and then travel to the small intestine. There they develop into adults that penetrate the duodenal and jejunal mucosa. Fertilized females produce embryonated eggs resembling those of hookworm, but these are rarely seen as they hatch in the intestinal mucosa, releasing the first-stage rhabditiform larvae characteristically found in the stool. In favorable soil conditions, the excreted rhabditiform larvae transform into infectious filariform larvae within 24–48 h, remaining viable in soil for a few weeks.

Autoinfection may occur if rhabditiform larvae rapidly transform into infectious dwarf filariform larvae in the lumen of the bowel. These penetrate the gut mucosa (internal autoinfection) or the perianal skin (external autoinfection). Infection may thus persist for decades without further external exposure. Person-to-person transmission has also been described.[9]

Larval penetration of the skin may result in ground itch, and an urticarial, serpiginous rash is sometimes observed.

Pneumonitis may be associated with larval migration. Initial invasion of the small-bowel mucosa by adult worms may cause abdominal pain and, in heavy infections, vomiting, malabsorption and paralytic ileus. Chronic infection may be asymptomatic or cause intermittent episodes of abdominal discomfort, sometimes associated with diarrhea and urticaria. Some patients develop malabsorption. Larva currens may appear transiently, usually on the trunk or buttocks. There may be episodes of pneumonitis and, rarely, a reactive arthritis.

Strongyloides hyperinfection syndrome occurs as a result of massive autoinfection. Risk factors include immunosuppression associated with organ transplants, cytotoxic drug therapy, corticosteroid therapy,[10] ribavirin therapy for hepatitis C,[11] malignancies (particularly leukemia and lymphoma), severe malnutrition and severe infections. HIV infection does not appear to predispose to strongyloides hyperinfection syndrome, although hyperinfection may occur in debilitated patients with advanced AIDS. Rarely, this syndrome occurs in an immunocompetent individual. A severe protein-losing enteropathy may develop in debilitated patients. More commonly, in patients who are abruptly immunosuppressed, hyperinfection syndrome presents with paralytic ileus accompanied by Gram-negative septicemia caused by enteric organisms. The condition is usually fatal if effective chemotherapy is delayed. Complications include meningitis, often caused by *Escherichia coli* and/or larvae of *S. stercoralis*; both organisms are often detected in cerebrospinal fluid (CSF). Larvae may be widely disseminated in the central nervous system (CNS) and elsewhere, causing microinfarcts. Additional complications include peritonitis, endocarditis and pneumonitis. All patients with a history of possible exposure should be screened for strongyloides before immunosuppression. Patients at high risk should be treated empirically even if investigations are negative.[12]

DIAGNOSIS AND TREATMENT

Rhabditiform larvae may be difficult to identify in feces. Various concentration techniques have been advocated and fecal culture on damp charcoal or Harada–Mori culture on vertical strips of damp filter paper may be helpful, although culture on nutrient agar plates is now emerging as the preferred technique.[13] Larvae may be identified in duodenal aspirates or using the string capsule technique (Enterotest).

Serological tests (indirect fluorescent antibody test or enzyme-linked immunosorbent assay (ELISA)) are useful for patients who are not normally resident in an endemic area; however, cross-reactions with filarial antigens remain a problem. Strongyloidiasis in immunocompetent individuals is usually accompanied by an eosinophilia. Diagnosis in patients who are immunocompromised is more difficult. Eosinophilia is less likely and its absence is associated with a poorer prognosis. Serological tests are likely to be negative. It is essential to search carefully for larvae in feces or bowel aspirates. Larvae may also be found in sputum, CSF and urine.

Ivermectin has emerged as the drug of choice for strongyloidiasis. An oral dose of 200 µg/kg daily for 2 days gives excellent cure rates with few side effects.[14] Thiabendazole 25 mg/kg (maximum 1.5 g) orally twice daily for 3 days is also effective, although it is advisable to repeat this after 1 week because of the difficulty in confirming eradication of infection. Side effects are common and may be serious. Albendazole has fewer side effects than thiabendazole. A course of 400 mg twice daily for 7 days has been used with encouraging results.

Hyperinfection syndrome poses therapeutic difficulties. In patients who are able to absorb oral treatment, ivermectin given in a multidose schedule offers the greatest promise of success. Patients who are unable to absorb oral therapy present a difficult challenge as no parenteral preparations of thiabendazole, albendazole or ivermectin are licensed for use in humans. However, parenteral ivermectin, available as a veterinary preparation, has been administered subcutaneously in the successful treatment of two patients with strongyloides hyperinfection.[15] Patients with hyperinfection syndrome may also require treatment for Gram-negative septicemia.

INTESTINAL CESTODE INFECTIONS (TAPEWORMS)

Tapeworms are flattened, segmented, hermaphroditic worms ranging in length from 10 mm to 20 m. The head (scolex) attaches to the intestinal mucosa by means of suckers or hooklets. All, with the exception of *Hymenolepis nana*, require a secondary intermediate host in which the larvae develop into cysts, usually in muscle. Human infection follows consumption of undercooked meat or fish. Larval cestode infections may also occur in humans following the ingestion of the egg, the most important being cysticercosis.

Taeniasis

Taenia saginata, the beef tapeworm, and *Taenia solium*, the pork tapeworm, are the most common tapeworms affecting humans. Infection follows consumption of undercooked beef or pork containing cysts. *T. saginata* cysts may occur in other domestic bovines and a closely related Asian species has been shown to infect pigs, ungulates and monkeys. *T. solium* cysts also occur in dogs and cats. Most infections are asymptomatic, the host only becoming aware when a proglottid segment is noticed in feces or felt as it passes through the anus. Gastrointestinal symptoms may include loss of appetite, nausea or vague abdominal pain. A patient who is vomiting profusely for whatever reason, may be further distressed when several metres of tapeworm appear in the vomit. Rarely, complications arise following migration of proglottids to unusual sites, such as the appendix or pancreatic and bile ducts.

Diphyllobothriasis

The most common of the 13 or more species of fish tapeworm affecting humans is *Diphyllobothrium latum*. Human infection follows ingestion of undercooked or raw fish or roe. Most infections involve a single worm and are asymptomatic or associated with vague, non-specific abdominal symptoms. Megaloblastic anemia may occur, resembling pernicious anemia in severe cases.

Hymenolepiasis and dipylidiasis

Hymenolepis nana, the dwarf tapeworm, occurs worldwide, principally among children. Most infections are asymptomatic, but heavy infections may cause abdominal pain, nausea, vomiting, pruritis ani and diarrhea, sometimes containing blood. Headache, dizziness, sleep and behavior disturbances are frequent. Convulsions have also been reported. Autoinfection is common.

Hymenolepis diminuta, the rat tapeworm, may affect humans who ingest the intermediate host, usually a weevil, flea or cockroach. Most infections are asymptomatic and of short duration.

Dipylidium caninum infection may occur in humans, usually young infants, following accidental ingestion of a flea, the intermediate host of this cestode whose usual host is a dog or other carnivore. Most infections are asymptomatic. Some children experience abdominal pain, diarrhea, pruritis ani and urticaria.

Diagnosis and treatment

Diagnosis is usually made by identification of characteristic eggs or proglottids in feces. There may be a variable eosinophilia, minimal in cases of *T. saginata* and often reaching 5–10% in hymenolepiasis.

Praziquantel is the drug of choice for all of the above intestinal cestode infections. A single oral dose of 10 mg/kg is usually effective. *H. nana* requires 25 mg/kg as a single dose. Praziquantel should be used with caution in populations in which cysticercosis is common, as there is a possibility of precipitating or aggravating symptoms. Niclosamide, given as a single oral dose of 2 g for adults, is also effective. Doses for children are 500 mg if <11 kg; 1 g if 11–34 kg and 1.5 g if > 34 kg. Tablets should be chewed well and swallowed with water. There is no clinical evidence to justify the routine use of purgatives and antiemetics in patients with *T. solium* before cestocidal treatment, in order to prevent retrograde peristalsis of eggs and possible risk of cysticercosis.

LARVAL HELMINTHIC INFECTIONS

CYSTICERCOSIS

Neurocysticercosis is the most common parasitic infection of the CNS and the main cause of adult-onset epilepsy worldwide. Cysticercosis occurs following ingestion of eggs of *T. solium* and can occur in strict vegetarians or those who avoid eating pork for religious reasons. The onchosphere liberated in the upper intestinal tract, penetrates the mucosa and enters the mesenteric vessels and lymphatics. Dissemination then occurs throughout the body and cysts develop in the tissues.

Living cysts usually provoke little or no immunological reaction. Clinical symptoms are more likely to arise as a result of the inflammatory response to dying cysticerci. Calcification eventually occurs at the site of dead cysticerci. Two forms of cysticerci, parenchymal and racemose, are found in the CNS. Racemose cysticerci are uncommon in children and are associated with a poorer prognosis.

Most infections are asymptomatic. The most common clinical presentations occur with neurocysticercosis and include epilepsy, symptoms of raised intracranial pressure, psychiatric disturbances, dementia, encephalitis, chronic meningitis, cranial nerve palsies and symptoms due to spinal cord lesions. Learning difficulties, behavior changes and psychomotor involution may be additional presenting symptoms in children.[16] Cysticerci may develop in the eye, most commonly in the retina, but sometimes are free floating in the anterior or posterior chamber. Subcutaneous cysticerci are present in about 50% of cases of neurocysticercosis. Cysticerci in muscles may result in increased muscle bulk and weakness. Cardiac involvement may also occur.

Diagnosis and treatment

Serological diagnosis is possible using an enzyme-linked immunoelectrotransfer blot (EITB) or ELISA.[17,18] CSF may be normal or white cells (lymphocytes or eosinophils) raised to a variable extent. Glucose may be reduced. Total protein and IgG may be elevated and the EITB may be positive. Single ring-enhancing intracranial lesions are often negative using currently available immunodiagnostic techniques. Subcutaneous nodules can be biopsied. Ophthalmoscopy may reveal ocular cysts. Calcified cysts may be evident on X-ray films in muscle and other tissue. Magnetic resonance imaging (MRI) is superior to computed tomography (CT) in diagnosing neurocysticercosis if cysts are still viable. CT is better for demonstration of calcified cysts.

Both praziquantel (50–75 mg/kg daily in three divided doses for 15 days) and albendazole (400 mg twice daily for adults or 15 mg/kg daily for children for 8–30 days) are effective in killing live cysticerci. However, the inflammatory response to dying cysticerci may precipitate or exacerbate symptoms. Simultaneous administration of steroids is usually advised to mitigate the inflammatory response.[19] A recent review of four trials, in which patients with intraparenchymatous neurocysticercosis were treated with either albendazole or praziquantel and compared with placebo or no treatment, concluded that there is insufficient evidence to determine whether cysticidal therapy is of any clinical benefit to patients with neurocysticercosis. The review did not exclude the possibility that more patients remain seizure-free when treated with cysticidal drugs.[20] The bioavailability of albendazole and praziquantel are increased with cimetidine.[21,22]

Anticysticercal therapy is usually unnecessary in asymptomatic cases of neurocysticercosis. Single-dose praziquantel treatment has been recommended for patients who have single brain-enhancing lesions and positive serology.[23] Anticysticercal therapy should also be considered for patients with viable cysticerci who present with epilepsy or with symptoms of a mass effect. In some cases, neurosurgical intervention may be indicated. Ophthalmic cysticercosis is usually treated surgically. Muscular and subcutaneous cysticercosis generally do not require treatment. If anticysticercal drugs are used, steroids or non-steroidal anti-inflammatory drugs may also be required.

HYDATIDOSIS

The larval stage of the canine tapeworm, *Echinococcus granulosus*, causes cystic hydatid diseases in humans. The disease is prevalent in sheep rearing areas throughout the world. Dogs and other carnivores are the definitive host for the adult tapeworm. Sheep and other domestic livestock become infected after ingesting ova shed in dog feces, following which hydatid cysts develop in the viscera of the infected animal. The cycle is completed when dogs ingest cysts in offal and other infected tissues. Human infection follows the accidental ingestion of eggs in dog feces. The ingested egg releases an onchosphere which penetrates the intestinal wall and is carried in the circulation to a variety of tissues, most commonly the liver and lungs.

Symptoms are usually either due to a mass effect produced by the growing cyst or occur as a result of leakage of fluid from a cyst. Hepatic cysts are more frequent in the right lobe and are usually asymptomatic until they become large. A nontender mass may be evident on examination. Secondary bacterial infection of a cyst may mimic a liver abscess. Rupture may be spontaneous, traumatic or occur during surgery, precipitating a hypersensitivity reaction ranging from urticaria, pruritus and fever to fatal anaphylaxis. Rupture into the peritoneal cavity may lead to seeding and the development of secondary cysts. Rupture into the biliary tree may cause colic, urticaria and obstructive jaundice, sometimes complicated by secondary bacterial infection.

Most lung cysts are asymptomatic, often being found incidentally on a chest radiograph. Patients may experience fever, dyspnea, chest pain and cough, sometimes with hemoptysis or productive of clear salty-tasting liquid. Collapsed cysts have a characteristic 'water lily' appearance on chest radiographs. Patients may cough up the soft, white outer membrane of the cyst. Rupture into the lung may cause a hypersensitivity reaction, or result in pneumothorax and empyema. A lung abscess may develop at the site of a cyst. Seeding of pulmonary cysts is uncommon.

Hydatid cysts occur at a variety of other sites including spleen, bone (causing pain and pathological fracture), brain (causing convulsions or a mass effect) and eye (causing proptosis and chemosis).

Diagnosis and treatment

Abdominal ultrasound is useful for detecting abdominal cysts: Radiography, CT or MRI may be useful for detecting cysts elsewhere. Of the serological tests available, the specific IgG ELISA AgB (antigen-B-rich fraction) appears to be the most sensitive.[24] Others include an EITB assay and the double diffusion test for arc 5 (DD5). All lack sensitivity for extrahepatic cysts and DD5 may give false-positive results in patients with cysticercosis. Urine antigen detection tests are promising.[25] Eosinophilia may follow leakage or rupture of a cyst.

Albendazole is useful for patients with inoperable, widespread or numerous cysts and in patients who are unfit for surgery. The recommended regimen is a 28-day course of 400 mg twice daily for adults, or 5–7.5 mg/kg twice daily for children, followed by 14 days rest, repeated for 3–12 cycles depending on response. Absorption of albendazole is enhanced when taken with fatty meals.

A combination of albendazole and praziquantel has been shown to have greater protoscolicidal activity in animal studies and in vitro than either drug alone.[26,27] Combination therapy has been used with success in treating inoperable spinal, pelvic, abdominal, thoracic and hepatic hydatidosis and as an adjunct to surgery.[28]

Surgical removal of hydatid cysts requires great care to avoid spillage. Before removal, large cysts are carefully aspirated and the aspirate replaced with an equivalent volume of hypertonic saline, a scolicide. This is aspirated after 5–10 minutes, and the procedure repeated. Following reaspiration, the membranes are removed and the cavity closed. Percutaneous aspiration of cysts under ultrasound control is being used increasingly as an alternative to surgery. Following initial aspiration of the cyst, hypertonic saline is injected into the cyst and reaspirated after 20 min. Patients undergoing surgery or percutaneous aspiration should receive concomitant albendazole, either alone or in combination with praziquantel. Percutaneous aspiration combined with an 8-week course of albendazole is more effective than either treatment alone. Laparoscopic treatment of hydatid cysts of the liver and spleen is also effective.[29] Anthelmintic treatment may reduce the need for surgery in patients with uncomplicated pulmonary cysts.[30]

ALVEOLAR HYDATID DISEASE

Echinococcus multilocularis is a tapeworm of foxes, wild canines, dogs and cats. Rodents are the usual intermediate hosts. The disease is endemic in North America, Europe, Siberia and China. Human infection follows ingestion of the egg in a similar manner to infection with *E. granulosus*. Unlike cystic hydatid disease, lesions caused by *E. multilocularis* are ill defined and more solid than cystic, developing in the manner of a slowly growing, invasive malignant tumor: it may be 30 years before a patient becomes symptomatic. The primary site of tissue invasion is usually the liver although metastatic lesions may occur in other tissues.

Clinical presentation is usually with right upper quadrant pain, hepatomegaly and a palpable mass. Complications as a result of local invasion or due to metastatic lesions involving brain, lung or mediastinum, occur in around 2% of patients. Untreated, 90% of patients die within 10 years of presentation. However, a 90% 10-year survival rate is possible with early diagnosis and appropriate treatment.

Diagnosis and treatment

Ultrasonography, CT and serology are useful in establishing the diagnosis. Histology provides confirmation.

Surgical excision is the treatment of choice for the primary lesion. Pre- and postoperative treatment with albendazole is recommended. Cyclical treatment with albendazole 10 mg/kg for 28 days followed by 14 days rest is recommended postoperatively and for inoperable patients. The optimal duration of treatment remains uncertain; patients often remain on treatment for more than 12 months. Mebendazole 40–50 mg/kg daily has also be used extensively, sometimes for up to 10 years. Serology may remain positive for several years following successful treatment.

TRICHINOSIS

Several species of *Trichinella* cause disease in humans, affecting about 50 million worldwide. The best known, *Trichinella spiralis*, occurs widely; most of the others are limited to particular geographical niches. Human infection follows consumption of larval cysts in raw or undercooked meat, especially pork. Larvae liberated in the stomach pass into the duodenum, where they burrow into the mucosa and develop into adults. Female worms produce larvae which seed throughout the body, particularly in skeletal and cardiac muscle, and form cysts invoking an inflammatory response. Cysts begin to calcify within 6–12 months, resulting in death of the encysted larvae.

Clinical symptoms may occur at the time of initial larval invasion and development in the intestinal mucosa. Early symptoms are more likely with heavy infection and include abdominal pain, anorexia, nausea, vomiting and diarrhea, sometimes accompanied by fever, headache and malaise. Systemic symptoms tend to occur a week or more after infection, when seeding of larvae in the tissues is associated with fever, headache, myalgia and malaise. Urticaria, conjunctivitis, periorbital and facial edema may be evident. Muscles become swollen and tender. Patients may experience cough, hoarseness, dyspnea and dysphagia. Splinter hemorrhages may be present. Myocarditis may develop 4–8 weeks after infection. Pericardial effusions are the most common manifestation of cardiac involvement.[31] Congestive cardiac failure and arrhythmias also occur. Larvae migrating through the CNS may cause a wide range of focal or generalized neurological symptoms including meningoencephalitis and psychosis. Convalescence may be prolonged with persisting myalgia, fatigue and headaches.

Diagnosis and treatment

There is usually a marked eosinophilia and raised creatinine phosphokinase, lactic dehydrogenase, aldolase and aminotransferase levels, reflecting muscle damage. Myocarditis should not be assumed on the basis of elevated creatinine phosphokinase isoenzyme-MB as this has been found in patients without clinical or other evidence of cardiac involvement. The most useful serological test for clinical purposes is the ELISA-IgG. Tissue diagnosis can be made from skeletal muscle biopsy using compression and histological techniques.

Either mebendazole 100 mg twice daily for 5 days or albendazole 400 mg daily for 3 days are effective in the early intestinal stage of infection. Patients with severe symptoms associated with larval seeding should be treated with prednisolone 40–60 mg daily plus either mebendazole 5 mg/kg daily or albendazole 400–800 mg daily until fever and allergic signs subside.

TOXOCARIASIS

Toxocara canis and *Toxocara cati* are parasitic roundworms of dogs and cats. Infection in humans is most common in young children, who ingest eggs in sand or soil contaminated by dog or cat feces. Clinical disease is relatively uncommon and depends on the intensity of infection and the organs involved.

Visceral larva migrans is caused by migrating larvae and includes symptoms of pneumonitis, fever, abdominal pain, myalgia, sleep and behavior disturbances and focal or generalized convulsions. Lymphadenopathy and hepatosplenomegaly may be evident. Eosinophilia, anemia, hypergammaglobulinemia and elevated titers of blood group isohemagglutinins are common. Serological diagnosis may be established by ELISA. The drug of choice is albendazole 10 mg/kg daily for 5 days. Alternatives include mebendazole 100 mg twice daily for 5 days, thiabendazole 50 mg/kg daily in three divided doses for a minimum of 5 days, or diethylcarbamazine 3 mg/kg three times daily for 21 days. Symptomatic treatment with bronchodilators, steroids or antihistamines may also be indicated.

Ocular larva migrans is more likely to occur in light infections. A single larva invades the eye, provoking a granulomatous reaction, usually in the retina. This may result in visual disturbance or blindness in the affected eye, which may go unnoticed or present as strabismus. The diagnosis is sometimes made by chance on routine ophthalmoscopy. The usual appearance is of chorioidoretinitis with a mass lesion, sometimes mistaken for a retinoblastoma. Serology is usually positive. Antibody detection in vitreous fluid is more sensitive and specific. Management of acute ocular larva migrans is directed at suppressing the inflammatory response with topical or systemic steroids. Anthelmintics are often used concurrently although there is no consistent evidence of additional benefit. Destruction of the larva is possible using laser photocoagulation. Steroids may be useful in exacerbations of chronic ocular larva migrans. Surgery is often required for adhesions.

MISCELLANEOUS TISSUE HELMINTHS

GNATHOSTOMIASIS

Gnathostoma spinigerum and related species occur principally in south-east Asia. Human infection follows ingestion of raw or undercooked flesh from certain fish, frogs and snakes. Acute gnathostomiasis is associated with fever, abdominal pain, tender hepatomegaly, pneumonitis, rashes (including a serpiginous rash resembling cutaneous larva migrans) and painless or pruritic subcutaneous swellings caused by migrating immature adult worms. Eosinophilia is usually marked. Invasion of the eye may result in subconjunctival hemorrhage and edema. Eosinophillic myeloencephalitis is an important and characteristic complication arising when the worm migrates along a large nerve trunk and invades the CNS, causing a radiculomyelitis, radiculomyeloencephalitis or subarachnoid hemorrhage. Migratory CNS lesions can be detected using MRI.[32] CSF may be bloody or xanthochromic with a raised white cell count, of which >20% are usually eosinophils. Highly sensitive and specific immunodiagnostic tests are available for use with serum or CSF. Definitive diagnosis requires identification of the worm.

Albendazole 400 mg twice daily for 21 days may be useful. Anti-inflammatory analgesics are helpful for symptomatic relief. Steroids may be required for patients with neurological complications. Cerebral gnathostomiasis is associated with a high case-fatality rate.

ANGIOSTRONGYLIASIS

Angiostrongylus meningitis

Infection with *Angiostrongylus cantonensis* occurs most commonly in south-east Asia following consumption of larvae in salads contaminated with slug or snail slime, or in undercooked snails, crabs or prawns. Clinical disease is usually mild and self-limiting. However, the parasite may cause eosinophillic meningitis, cranial nerve palsies and cerebral abscesses. Treatment with anthelmintics is contraindicated as death of the parasites may lead to worsening of symptoms.

Abdominal angiostrongyliasis

Infection with *Angiostrongylus costaricensis* follows consumption of food contaminated with slug slime. Cases have been reported in the Americas, the Caribbean and Central Africa. Children commonly present with an eosinophillic enteritis resembling acute appendicitis or with an ileocecal mass in chronic cases. Testicular infection may mimic torsion. Eggs and larvae are absent from the stool. An ELISA is available for serological diagnosis. Thiabendazole and diethylcarbamazine have been used in treatment; however, the role of anthelmintics remains uncertain. Surgery is sometimes required.

TREMATODES

Trematodes include the intestinal, liver and lung flukes and the schistosomes (blood flukes). About 750 million people are at risk worldwide. Common to all of their life cycles is the involvement of various species of fresh-water snail, which act as intermediate, amplifying hosts, liberating millions of cercaria. Schistosomiasis occurs as a result of cercarial penetration, usually via the skin. The other flukes require a second intermediate host (animal or vegetable) for the development of the metacercarial stage infectious to humans. The adult parasites develop in their human host, mate and produce eggs, which are shed in feces, urine or sputum. On contact with water, the egg releases the miracidium, which infects the preferred snail, thus completing the cycle.

Most infections could be prevented by public health measures promoting sanitation and safe preparation of food. Praziquantel is the anthelmintic of choice for all fluke infections, with the exception of *Fasciola hepatica* and *Fasciola gigantica*, where the drug of choice is now triclabendazole.

SCHISTOSOMIASIS

The three most common species of schistosome affecting humans are *Schistosoma haematobium* (endemic in most of Africa and parts of the Middle East), *Schistosoma mansoni* (endemic in most of Africa, part of the Middle East, and in some areas of the Caribbean and South America) and *Schistosoma japonicum* (endemic in East and South Asia and parts of Indonesia and the Philippines). *Schistosoma mekongi* and *Schistosoma intercalatum* are of lesser importance and are confined to parts of south-east Asia and Africa respectively.

In endemic regions, most of the population become infected at some time, peak prevalence usually occurring in older children and teenagers. Most infections are mild or asymptomatic. As immunity develops, egg production diminishes and eventually ceases in most of those infected. Susceptibility to long-term complications may be genetically mediated.

Cercarial dermatitis ('swimmer's itch') occurs within 24 h at the site of cercarial penetration, more commonly in individuals who are newly exposed. The papular, pruritic rash usually resolves spontaneously within a few days. Cercarial dermatitis may also occur following exposure to avian schistosomes. Cercariae develop into schistosomula, which migrate via the heart and lungs. Heavy initial infections may be associated with a transient pneumonitis at this stage.

The schistosomula pass through the liver, where they mature into adults without causing pathology. They then migrate to the vesical venous plexus in the case of *S. haematobium*, or to the mesenteric plexus in the case of *S. mansoni* and *S. japonicum*. Adult worms do not provoke any reaction and may survive for up to 7 years. Egg production and deposition in the tissues does, however, result in an immunopathologic response giving rise to the major clinical consequences of schistosomiasis.

Acute schistosomiasis, or Katayama fever, may occur 4–8 weeks following exposure. It is more likely in non-immunes following heavy infection and is more common with *S. japonicum* and *S. mansoni*, coinciding with the onset of egg deposition in the tissues. Symptoms include fever, cough, wheeze, urticaria, headache and malaise. Generalized lymphadenopathy and hepatosplenomegaly may be present. Investigations usually reveal an eosinophilia; however, parasitological diagnosis may be difficult as eggs are unlikely to be found in stool or urine unless sought by special techniques and serology is usually negative during the initial stages.

The intestine and liver are the principal sites of pathology in all types of human schistosomiasis apart from *S. haematobium*. Egg deposition in the intestinal mucosa may lead to abdominal pain, diarrhea, dysentery and malaise. Colonoscopy may reveal hyperemia, erosions, ulceration or polyps, evident on barium studies as filling defects. Egg deposition in the liver occurs in the perisinusoidal radicles of the portal vein, provoking a granulomatous reaction and, eventually, periportal fibrosis and portal hypertension. Hepatomegaly is followed by splenomegaly and hypersplenism as portal hypertension increases. Bleeding may occur from esophageal varices and ascites is common in advanced disease. Increase in portal pressure may open collaterals into the pulmonary circulation with egg deposition, granuloma formation and periarteritis leading to pulmonary hypertension and cor pulmonale. Rarely, pulmonary hypertension may also occur with *S. haematobium*. Liver function tests are usually normal until fibrosis is advanced. Abnormal liver function tests should raise the possibility of co-infection with hepatitis B or C, in which case the prognosis is likely to be worse.

Chronic *S. haematobium* infection principally affects the urogenital system. The most common symptoms are dysuria, frequency, terminal hematuria and hematospermia. Bladder outlet and vesicoureteric obstruction may lead to hydroureter and hydronephrosis. Secondary bacterial infections may occur, including pyelonephritis. In due course, chronic renal failure may develop. Cystoscopy may reveal 'sandy patches' on the mucosal surface, mucosal hypertrophy or polyps. Squamous carcinoma of the bladder is a well documented long-term complication. Involvement of the female genital tract may cause cervicitis, salpingitis and infertility. These may also occur with *S. japonicum* and *S. intercalatum*. Rarely, patients with *S. haematobium* complain of rectal passage of blood and mucus.

Neurological complications occur if schistosome eggs lodge in the brain or spine, leading to symptoms such as focal or generalized convulsions, and transverse myelitis. Subcutaneous egg deposition, often in the perineal region, may result in the development of painful papules.

A number of clinical conditions have been described arising from co-infection of schistosomes and salmonellae, including recurrent *Salmonella* bacteremia, nephrotic syndrome associated with co-infection with *S. mansoni* and *Salmonella enterica* serotype Typhi, and chronic urinary carriage of *Salmonella* Typhi associated with *S. haematobium* infection.

Diagnosis and treatment

Characteristic eggs may be identified in urine, semen or feces, by use of concentration techniques if necessary. Eggs of all species may be identified on rectal biopsy. Serological diagnosis is problematic as it takes 6–12 weeks for titers to become positive, positive titers persist for years following cure, and false-positive results may be caused by exposure to other helminths. Serology may be useful in returning travelers but not for residents in endemic areas. *S. mansoni* antibody detection in oral fluids appears to be as sensitive as serology.[33] Antigen from viable eggs can now be detected in serum and urine, offering new possibilities for diagnosis and monitoring of response to treatment.[34–36] Ultrasonography is useful for assessing patients with hepatic and urinary tract disease.

Praziquantel is the drug of choice for all species: 40 mg/kg as a single dose is usually sufficient for *S. haematobium*, *S. mansoni* and *S. intercalatum*. *S. japonicum* and *S. mekongi* require a larger dose: either 50 mg/kg as a single dose or three doses of 20 mg/kg 8 h apart. Side effects are uncommon. Resistance to praziquantel has been observed,[37] but this is not a significant clinical problem at present. Concomitant use of steroids is recommended in the management of patients with neurological disease to reduce inflammation around granulomata.

Katayama fever is managed with non-steroidal anti-inflammatory drugs or steroids depending on the severity, together with praziquantel.

No prophylactic drug is currently recommended for schistosomiasis. Artesunate and artemether are potential prophylactic agents,[38,39] but a major concern is the risk of promoting resistance in *Plasmodium falciparum*.

INTESTINAL FLUKES

The most important intestinal fluke in humans is *Fasciolopsis buski*, which is widely distributed from India to south-east Asia, particularly among pig-rearing communities. Human infection follows ingestion of metacercariae attached to an edible water plant, such as the water caltrop. The metacercariae excyst and attach to the mucosa of the duodenum and jejunum, where they develop into adults, causing inflammation and ulceration. Most infections are asymptomatic. Heavy infections result in epigastric pain and diarrhea, initially alternating with constipation, but later becoming persistent. Wasting and ascites may develop in severe cases. Characteristic eggs, and sometimes adult flukes, can be identified in feces.

Echinostome species, principally found in Asia, may also infect humans, causing symptoms similar to *F. buski*.

Heterophyds, the smallest of the intestinal flukes affecting humans, cause milder gastrointestinal symptoms than *F. buski*. However, ectopic eggs may be carried to other organs, particularly the CNS, causing a mass effect, and to the heart resulting in myocarditis or valve damage.

LIVER FLUKES

Fasciola hepatica and *Fasciola gigantica* are widely distributed, occurring in sheep- and cattle-rearing areas throughout the world. Human infection follows ingestion of metacercariae on water vegetables, for example watercress. Acute clinical symptoms may develop after 6–12 weeks, including abdominal pain, intermittent fever, weight loss, malaise, urticaria and respiratory symptoms. The liver may be enlarged and tender and liver enzymes are sometimes mildly elevated. Ectopic flukes may lead to granuloma or abscess formation in various organs. Migrating erythematous cutaneous nodules, another form of cutaneous larva migrans, may also occur. Mature flukes tend to migrate to the bile ducts, initially causing fever, anorexia and abdominal pain. This usually subsides spontaneously. A minority of patients develop chronic symptoms associated with recurrent cholangitis or intermittent biliary obstruction.

Diagnosis and treatment

Eosinophilia is common and pleural effusions, if present, may contain eosinophils. Ultrasound is usually normal, although CT scans of the liver may reveal numerous hypodense lesions. Peripheral, branched hypodense hepatic lesions, best seen on CT with use of contrast, are relatively specific for fascioliasis.

Serological tests are helpful in diagnosing *F. hepatica* infections in the acute phase when eggs are unlikely to be present in feces. Serology is less reliable for *F. gigantica*. In chronic disease, eggs may be present in feces or in bile aspirate. Concentration techniques may be helpful.

Praziquantel is unreliable in the treatment of fascioliasis. Bithional 30–50 mg/kg daily in three divided doses on alternate days for 10–15 days has been recommended in the past. Side effects include mild gastrointestinal upset and pruritus. A benzimidazole, triclabendazole, is simpler to use, has few side effects and is likely to become the drug of choice. A single dose of 10 mg/kg taken with food is usually effective. Severe infections require a second dose after 12 h.[40]

ORIENTAL LIVER FLUKES

Clonorchis sinensis (also known as *Opisthorchis sinensis*) and *Opisthorchis viverrini*, affect about 20 million people in China and South East Asia. A related species, *Opisthorchis felineus*, occurs in Eastern Europe and Russia. Human infection follows consumption of metacercariae in raw or undercooked freshwater fish. Metacercariae excyst in the small bowel and migrate along the common bile duct to colonize the biliary tree. Most infections are asymptomatic. Patients with heavy initial infections may present with an illness similar to Katayama fever. In established infections patients may present with vague right upper quadrant abdominal pain and hepatomegaly. Recurrent episodes of ascending cholangitis, jaundice and pancreatitis may occur. Chronic infection may lead to biliary cirrhosis and, rarely, cholangiocarcinoma.

Diagnosis and treatment

Ultrasound may reveal abnormalities of the biliary tree and gallstones. Other imaging techniques, such as endoscopic retrograde cholangiopancreatography, are useful. Diagnosis is established by identifying characteristic eggs in feces with the aid of concentration techniques, or in biliary aspirate. Immunological tests are not widely available and generally lack specificity. Stool antigen tests are being developed and show more promise.

Treatment is with praziquantel 40 mg/kg as a single dose, or 25 mg/kg three times in 24 h after meals. A 3-day course is advisable for heavy infections.

LUNG FLUKES

Eight species of *Paragonimus* cause disease in humans, the most important being *Paragonimus westermani*. Paragonimiasis is widespread in Asia and also occurs in regions of Africa, Central and South America. Human infection follows ingestion of metacercariae attached to undercooked or raw crab, crayfish, and shrimp, or, rarely, following consumption of larvae in undercooked wild boar. Most infections are initially asymptomatic. An acute illness may occur as the parasite excysts, penetrates the gut wall and migrates through the diaphragm into the pleural cavity and then to the lungs. Symptoms of abdominal pain and diarrhea 2–15 days after infection may be followed by cough, dyspnea, fatigue, fever and urticaria a few days later. This episode sometimes lasts several weeks. Pleuritic chest pain may occur, sometimes associated with an effusion. Adult flukes form cysts in the lung tissue and produce eggs, provoking an inflammatory response. Cavitatory or nodular, sometimes calcified, lesions develop which may be noticed incidentally on a chest radiograph as the first indication of infection in asymptomatic patients. Early symptoms of pulmonary paragonimiasis include cough, initially non-productive, later productive of gelatinous, rusty or bloodstained sputum. Pulmonary paragonimiasis may be mistaken for tuberculosis and both infections may coincide.

Cerebral paragonimiasis is the most important form of extrapulmonary paragonimiasis. Most patients are children. About one-third present with a clinical picture resembling acute meningoencephalitis, but more commonly presentation is insidious with a wide variety of neurological symptoms and signs depending on the area of the brain or spinal cord affected.

Wandering flukes may cause painless, migratory subcutaneous swellings, subcutaneous nodules or a variety of other symptoms depending on the site involved.

Diagnosis and treatment

Diagnosis can be confirmed by identifying characteristic eggs in sputum, feces or, rarely, pleural effusion. Eosinophilia is usual and should alert one to the possibility of paragonimiasis in patients presenting with a clinical picture mimicking tuberculosis. Serological tests are available, including ELISA and a complement fixation test. Paragonimus-specific IgM is useful for diagnosing patients with extrapulmonary disease and pleurisy.[41]

Praziquantel 25 mg/kg three times daily for 2 days is highly effective. A higher dose may be required for treatment of cerebral paragonimiasis and steroid cover is advisable.

FILARIAL INFECTIONS

Insect vectors play a role in the transmission of all of the medically important parasitic filarial nematodes, with the exception of *Dracunculus medinensis*. Both the parasite and the insect vector depend on favorable climatic and environmental conditions naturally occurring in certain regions of the tropics. Human infections occur when the insect vector feeds, introducing infective larvae. These mature into adult worms, which produce microfilariae, which in turn infect the insect vector. Clinical disease is caused by the adult worms, the microfilariae, or both.

Progress is being made in community control of these infections. One of the obstacles facing these programs is the longevity of the adult worms and their relative lack of response to anthelmintic agents. The development, motility and fertility of adult filarial worms depend on *Wolbachia*, intracellular, endosymbiotic bacteria. These organisms are susceptible to tetracyclines and several other antibiotics, offering fascinating new possibilities in the management and control of filarial infections.[42]

LYMPHATIC FILARIASIS

Wuchereria bancrofti, *Brugia malayi* and *Brugia timori* are transmitted by various species of mosquito. *W. bancrofti* is distributed widely in the tropics, affecting about 90 million people. *B. malayi* and *B. timori* are endemic in south-east Asia and Indonesia. The adult worms develop in the lymphatics and range in length from 20 to 100 mm. Their microfilariae enter the general circulation via the thoracic duct. Lymphatic damage is the result of inflammatory responses to living and dead adult worms, and due to the inflammatory response provoked by dead microfilariae sequestered in the lymphatics.

Most infections are asymptomatic. Acute adenolymphangitis is often the first manifestation of disease. An abrupt onset of fever is accompanied by lymphadenitis affecting one or more group of nodes. Lymphangitis proceeds away from the affected node. In severe cases, an abscess may develop at the site of an affected node and secondary bacterial infection may follow. Episodes often recur several times a year. Acute filarial fever without lymphadenitis may be mistaken for malaria.

Chronic lymphatic filariasis may develop months or years after the acute symptoms, or without a history of acute disease. Lymphatic obstruction leads to lymphedema of the affected extremity and, eventually, to elephantiasis. The sites most

commonly affected are the legs, scrotum, arms and breast. Recurrent secondary bacterial skin infections, often streptococcal, may cause acute episodes of pain and fever and lead to glomerulonephritis.

Other presentations of chronic lymphatic filariasis include hydrocele, lymph scrotum, acute epidydimitis and funiculitis. Chyluria, chylous diarrhea and chylous ascites may also occur with considerable loss of fat-soluble vitamins and protein, resulting in malnutrition and vitamin deficiencies.

Diagnosis and treatment

Eosinophilia is common during the acute stages. Parasitological diagnosis may be made by examination of a Giemsa-stained thick blood film taken at the peak of microfilarial periodicity according to the species (usually 22.00 h–02.00 h for *W. bancrofti*). However, this is relatively insensitive other than for high microfilaremias (>100 microfilariae/ml). Concentration techniques greatly improve sensitivity. Tests for circulating *W. bancrofti* antigen are now available, including an ELISA and a rapid immunochromatographic card test, and these may replace microscopy.[43] PCR assays have also been developed for *W. bancrofti* and *B. malayi*.[44,45] Ultrasound may also be useful.

For decades the recommended treatment of lymphatic filariasis has been diethylcarbamazine (DEC). The usual dose is 6 mg/kg daily in two or three divided doses for 10–14 days, up to a maximum total dose of 72 mg/kg. Side effects are less likely with lower doses (1 mg/kg three times daily on days 1 and 2). The microfilaria count falls within a month and remains low for 6–12 months. If necessary, the course of DEC may be repeated one month after completion of the initial course. DEC has limited effect in killing the adult worms. DEC is best avoided in areas endemic for onchocerciasis or *Loa loa* because of the risk of provoking a Mazzotti reaction or encephalopathy.

Recent community-based studies have shown that DEC in a single dose of 6 mg/kg given annually together with a single dose of either ivermectin 400 μg/kg or albendazole 400 mg is as effective in reducing microfilaremia and longevity of adult worms. In areas endemic for onchocerciasis or *Loa loa*, ivermectin 150 μg/kg is given with albendazole 400 mg as single doses. These strategies are now being implemented on an annual basis for community control of lymphatic filariasis.

TROPICAL PULMONARY EOSINOPHILIA

Tropical pulmonary eosinophilia occurs in areas endemic for lymphatic filariasis, particularly Sri Lanka and Southern India. Microfilarial death triggers a high eosinophilia associated with gradually worsening, non-productive cough and wheeze, and sometimes fever and malaise. Symptoms are worse at night. Chest radiography shows diffuse infiltrates. Pulmonary function tests may reveal restrictive, obstructive or mixed defects. IgE is elevated and filarial serology positive. The diagnosis is supported by a prompt response to treatment with DEC.

LOIASIS

Loa loa is transmitted by flies of the genus *Chrysops* that breed in tropical forests of Africa. Larval parasites migrate in the subcutaneous tissues, where they mature into adults over the course of a year. Clinical symptoms include urticaria, pruritus, arthralgia and malaise. Transient, migratory angiedema (Calabar swelling) occurs most commonly on the extremities where trauma to a migrating adult worm provokes a localized inflammatory reaction. Subconjunctival migration causes pain and inflammation. If instruments are readily to hand, the worm can be removed from the eye after applying local anesthetic. Other complications include proteinuria in up to 30% of patients, hematuria, and, less commonly, neurological complications (particularly meningoencephalitis). Rare presentations include pulmonary infiltrates, pleural effusions, arthritis, lymphangitis and hydrocele. Hypereosinophilia is common and *Loa loa* has been implicated in the etiology of endomyocardial fibrosis, although this condition is well described in association with numerous other causes of hypereosinophilia.

Diagnosis and treatment

Diagnosis of loiasis is often indicated by the history, particularly if an 'eye worm' has made an appearance. Dead, calcified worms are sometimes seen on radiography.

Microfilaremia peaks between 10.00 h and 15.00 h. Parasites can be identified in thick blood films with Giemsa or Wright stains, or by concentration techniques. Assessing the microfilarial load is useful in determining the likelihood of an adverse reaction to treatment. Serological tests are available and may be helpful for diagnosis in travelers from endemic areas, but other filarial parasites cross-react.

DEC 2 mg/kg orally three times daily for 7–10 days is commonly used in the treatment of loiasis. The course is repeated at intervals of 2 or 3 months if the patient remains symptomatic. Ivermectin 150 µg/kg as a single dose before treatment with DEC will reduce the likelihood of a Mazzotti reaction in patients who also have onchocerciasis. Caution is needed in managing patients with loiasis who have high microfilarial loads (>2500 microfilariae/ml) as treatment with DEC or ivermectin may precipitate meningoencephalitis or renal failure due to massive release of antigens from dying microfilariae.[46] Plasmapheresis has been used successfully to reduce microfilarial load in heavy infections before treatment with DEC under steroid cover; however, albendazole 200 mg twice daily for 3 weeks causes a gradual reduction in microfilaremia, usually without serious adverse effects.[47] This may well become the preferred strategy for managing patients with high microfilaremia.

ONCHOCERCIASIS

Onchocerciasis is one of the most important causes of blindness in the tropics. The disease is endemic in tropical Africa, the Arabian peninsular and parts of Latin America. Over 17 million people are infected, of whom almost one million are blind or visually impaired. The parasite is transmitted by blackflies of the genus *Simulium* that breed along fast flowing rivers: hence the common name 'river blindness'. Humans are the only definitive host for *Onchocerca volvulus*. Larvae injected when an infected blackfly feeds migrate in the subcutaneous tissues and mature into adults. Adult worms, measuring up to 80 cm in length, intertwine and become encapsulated in the subcutaneous tissues, forming painless nodules measuring up to 3 cm in diameter. These may be palpable over bony prominences but otherwise cause few clinical symptoms. Microfilariae produced by the adult worms are responsible for the most serious clinical effects of onchocerciasis, principally affecting the skin and eye.

Onchodermatitis initially presents as an intensely itchy papular rash. A chronic popular dermatitis ensues with gradual loss of elasticity in the skin and subcutaneous tissues, resulting in a prematurely aged appearance. Depigmentation, sparing sweat glands and hair follicles, leads to the 'leopard skin' appearance, most commonly seen on the shins. Enlarged inguinal and femoral lymph nodes may hang in apron-like folds of inelastic skin, the so-called 'hanging groin' appearance. Rarely, elephantiasis may occur. 'Sowda', a lichenified dermatitis, presents as intensely pruritic, hyperpigmented papules and plaques, usually affecting one limb and accompanied by edema and enlargement of the regional nodes.

Ocular onchocerciasis results from microfilarial invasion of the eye. Live microfilariae may be visible in the anterior chamber or aqueous humor on slit-lamp examination. They provoke a reversible inflammatory reaction, resulting in punctate keratitis or 'snowflake' corneal opacities. Microfilarial death in longstanding cases results in more severe and irreversible damage, including sclerosing keratitis, iridocyclitis, uveitis, choroidoretinitis and optic atrophy. Glaucoma and cataract may also occur. Eye complications are more likely to occur in patients who have onchocercal nodules on the head or upper body.

Diagnosis and treatment

The most common method for diagnosis is examination for the emergence of microfilariae from a skin snip placed in a drop of saline. Nodules may be excised and examined for adult worms. In the past, for diagnosis of patients with negative skin snips, DEC was used in a dose of 25–50 mg to provoke a Mazzotti reaction with considerable worsening of the rash and pruritus in the ensuing 24 h. Application of topical DEC under an occlusive dressing produces a similar, localized effect and is less distressing and safer for the patient.

Recent diagnostic advances include the development of a rapid-format antibody card test,[49] an ELISA, and DNA probes.[48] Antibody detection may be useful for screening populations, whereas PCR and antigen detection in serum and urine are potentially more useful for diagnosing active infection in individuals and for monitoring the success of therapy.

Both the treatment and the community control of onchocerciasis have been greatly improved following the introduction of ivermectin. A single oral dose of 150 µg/kg clears microfilariae for several months and suppresses microfilaria production, but does not kill adult worms. Therefore, the dose should be repeated at 6–12-monthly intervals for up to 12 or more years, until the adult worms eventually die. Other than in very heavy infections, ivermectin causes little or no Mazzotti reaction.

Ivermectin should be used with caution in *Loa loa*-endemic areas as it may precipitate meningoencephalitis in patients with high *Loa loa* microfilarial loads. In these circumstances, it is advisable to prescribe a course of albendazole before treatment with ivermectin. Nodulectomy is advised for head nodules, possibly reducing the likelihood of eye infection, but is not indicated for nodules elsewhere. Suramin, previously used in selected cases for killing adult worms, and DEC are no longer recommended in the management of onchocerciasis because of toxicity.

The onchocerciasis control program in West and Central Africa has been successful in eliminating new infections by a combination of chemotherapy, education and vector control.

GUINEA WORM

Dracunculus medinensis is acquired by swallowing a tiny copepod, *Cyclops*, harboring the larval stage of the parasite. Following digestion of *Cyclops*, the liberated larva penetrates the intestinal mucosa, migrates to loose connective tissue and develops into an adult worm. After mating, the female worm continues to mature with an enlarging gravid uterus and migrates in search of a site suitable for discharge of her larvae. Clinical symptoms occur as the worm prepares to emerge. Patients often complain of prodromal symptoms including rashes, gastrointestinal symptoms, weakness and fever. The emergence of the worm is heralded by the development of a large, indurated erythematous papule with a vesicular center. Over the next few days this develops into a painful, pruritic blister, which the patient seeks to immerse in water for relief. The larvae are thus discharged and, in suitable conditions, complete the cycle by infecting another *Cyclops*. The site of the blister tends to ulcerate and secondary bacterial infection may occur, including tetanus.

Migrating adult worms may penetrate and perish in other tissues, including the spinal cord, peritoneal cavity, pancreas, pericardium and lung, causing symptoms due to focal inflammation.

Management of guinea worm infection has changed little since ancient times. Emerging worms are encouraged to discharge their uterine contents by immersion of the affected part in water. At this stage, the tip of the worm begins to emerge and can be gently and gradually wound onto a match stick, a few centimetres each day, until the entire worm has been removed. The process can take several days as female worms may exceed 1 m in length. Administration of oral metronidazole or mebendazole may facilitate extraction. Surgical intervention is often required in the management of disease caused by ectopic worms. A highly successful program for the global eradication of guinea worm, based on the provision of safe drinking water or the use of fine filters to trap *Cyclops*, has resulted in a dramatic fall in the incidence of infection in recent years.

CONCLUSION

Most helminth infections occur in tropical developing countries. As with most infectious diseases in such countries, they are primarily diseases of poverty. Paradoxically, in affluent countries these infections occur most commonly among people who can afford to travel to or from the tropics. Presumptive use of albendazole has been recommended as a cost-effective strategy for the treatment of geohelminth infections in newly arrived immigrants in the USA.[50]

The integration of geohelminth, schistosomiasis, onchocerciasis and filariasis control programs offers a cost-effective strategy for controlling these infections.[51,52] Regular anthelmintic treatment of schoolchildren in developing countries is being promoted by the World Health Organization as a means of improving anemia, nutritional status and cognitive development in anticipation of long-term benefits to health and economic development.[53–55] Many of the most useful anthelmintic agents available to us today were originally developed for veterinary use and some of these drugs have been generously donated for use in developing countries. Unfortunately, economic imperatives dictate that there is greater profit in developing anthelmintic drugs for the treatment of animals than there is in addressing the needs of impoverished human beings. 'The poor must be grateful for a mouthful of crumbs, fallen from the table where the rich feed their dogs.'

References

1. Gilles HM, Hoffman PS 2002 Treatment of intestinal parasitic infections: a review of nitazoxanide. *Trends in Parasitology* 18: 95–97.
2. Papadopoulos GS, Eleftherakis NG, Thanopoulos BD 2000 Cardiac tamponade in a child with ascariasis. *Cardiology in the Young* 10: 539–541.
3. Gonzalez AH, Regaldo VC, Van den Ende J 2001 Non-invasive management of *Ascaris lumbricoides* biliary tact migration: a prospective study in 69 patients from Ecuador. *Tropical Medicine and International Health* 6: 146–150.
4. Jackson TF, Epstein SR, Gouws E et al 1998 A comparison of mebendazole and albendazole in treating children with *Trichuris trichiura* infection in Durban, South Africa. *South African Medical Journal* 88: 880–883.
5. Ismail MM, Javakody RL 1999 Efficacy of albendazole and its combinations with ivermectin or diethylcarbamazine (DEC) in the treatment of *Trichuris trichiura* infections in Sri Lanka. *Annals of Tropical Medicine and Parasitology* 93: 501–504.
6. Barrteo ML, Rodrigues LC, Silva RC et al 2000 Lower hookworm incidence, prevalence and intensity of infection in children with a Bacillus Calmette-Guérin scar. *Journal of Infectious Diseases* 182: 1800–1803.
7. Sacko M, De Clerq D, Behnke JM et al 1999 Comparison of the efficacy of mebendazole, albendazole and pyrantel in treatment of human hookworm infections in the southern region of Mali, West Africa. *Transactions of the Royal Society of Tropical Medicine and Hygiene* 93: 195–203.

8. Bouchard O, Houze S, Schiemann R et al 2000 Cutaneous larva migrans in travelers: A prospective study, with assessment of therapy with ivermectin. *Clinical Infectious Diseases* 31: 434–498.

9. Czachor JS, Jonas AP 2000 Transmission of *Strongyloides stercoralis* person to person. *Journal of Travel Medicine* 7: 211–212.

10. Thomas MC, Costello SA 1998 Disseminated strongyloidiasis arising from a single dose of dexamethasone before stereotactic radiosurgery. *International Journal of Clinical Practice* 52: 520–521.

11. Parana R, Portugal M, Vitvitski L et al 2000 Severe strongyloidiasis during interferon plus ribavirin therapy for chronic HCV infection. *European Journal of Gastroenterology and Hepatology* 12: 245–246.

12. Avery RK, Ljungman P 2000 Prophylactic measures in the solid-organ recipient before transplantation. *Clinical Infectious Diseases* 33(Suppl. 1): S15–S21

13. Jongwutiwes S, Charoenkorn M, Sitthichareonchai P et al 1999 Increased sensitivity of routine laboratory detection of *Strongyloides stercoralis* and hookworm by agar-plate culture. *Transactions of the Royal Society of Tropical Medicine and Hygiene* 93: 398–400.

14. Zaha O, Hirata T, Kinjo F et al 2000 Strongyloidiasis – progress in diagnosis and treatment. *Internal Medicine* 39: 695–700.

15. Chiodini PL, Reid AJ, Wiselka MJ et al 2000 Parenteral ivermectin in *Strongyloides* hyperinfection. *Lancet* 355: 43–44.

16. Morales NM, Agapejev S, Morales RR et al 2000 Clinical aspects of neurocysticercosis in children. *Pediatric Neurology* 22: 287–291.

17. Garcia HH, Parkhouse RM, Gilman RH et al 1998 A specific antigen-detection ELISA for the diagnosis of human neurocysticercosis. *Transactions of the Royal Society of Tropical Medicine and Hygiene* 92: 411–414.

18. Garcia HH, Parkhouse RM, Gilman RH et al 2000 Serum antigen detection in the diagnosis, treatment, and follow-up of neurocysticercosis patients. *Transactions of the Royal Society of Tropical Medicine and Hygiene* 94: 673–676.

19. Sotelo J, Jung H 1998 Pharmacokinetic optimisation of the treatment of neurocysticercosis. *Clinical Pharmacokinetics* 34: 503–515.

20. Salinas R, Prasad K 2001 Drugs for treating neurocysticercosis (tapeworm infection of the brain) (Cochrane Review) In: The Cochrane Library, Oxford 2.

21. Jung H, Medina R, Castro N et al 1997 Pharmacokinetic study of praziquantel administered alone and in combination with cimetidine in a single-day therapeutic regimen. *Antimicrobial Agents and Chemotherapy* 41: 1256–1259.

22. Yee T, Barakos JA, Knight RT 1999 High-dose praziquantel with cimetidine for refractory neurocysticercosis: a case report with clinical and MRI follow-up. *Western Journal of Medicine* 170: 112–115.

23. Pretell EJ, Garcia HH, Custodio N et al 2000 Short regimen of praziquantel in the treatment of single brain enhancing lesions. *Clinical Neurology and Neurosurgery* 102: 215–218.

24. Sbihi Y, Rmiqui A, Rodriguez-Cabezas MN et al 2001 Comparative sensitivity of six serological tests and diagnostic value of ELISA using purified antigen in hydatidosis. *Journal of Clinical Laboratory Analysis* 15: 14–18.

25. Ravinder PT, Parija SC, Rao KS 2000 Urinary hydatid antigen detection by coagglutination, a cost-effective and rapid test for diagnosis of cystic echinococcosis in a rural or field setting. *Journal of Clinical Microbiology* 38: 2972–2974.

26. Urrea-Paris MA, Moreno MJ, Casado N et al 2000 In vitro effect of praziquantel and albendazole combination therapy on the larval stage of *Echinococcus granulosus*. *Parasitology Research* 86: 957–964.

27. Mohamed AE, Yasawy MI, Al Karawi MA 1998 Combined albendazole and praziquantel versus albendazole alone in the treatment of hydatid disease. *Hepato-Gastroenterology* 45: 1690–1694.

28. Cobo F, Yarnoz C, Sesma B et al 1998 Albendazole plus praziquantel versus albendazole alone as a pre-operative treatment in intra-abdominal hydatidosis caused by Echinococcus granulosus. *Tropical Medicine and International Health* 3: 462–466.

29. Khoury G, Abaid F, Geagea T et al 2000 Laparoscopic treatment of hydatid cysts of the liver and spleen. *Surgical Endoscopy* 14: 243 245.

30. Keshmiri M, Baharvahdat H, Fattahi SH et al 1999 A placebo controlled study of albendazole in the treatment of pulmonary echinococcosis. *European Respiratory Journal* 14: 503–507.

31. Lazarevic AM, Neskovic AN, Goronja M et al 1999 Low incidence of cardiac abnormalities in treated trichinosis: a prospective study of 62 patients from a single-source outbreak. *American Journal of Medicine* 107: 18–23.

32. Chandenier J, Husson S, Canaple C et al 2001 Medullary gnathostomiasis in a white patient: Use of immunodiagnosis and Magnetic Resonance Imaging. *Clinical Infectious Diseases* 32: 154–157.

33. Santos MM, Garcia TD, Orsini M et al 2000 Oral fluids for the immunodiagnosis of *Schistosoma mansoni* infection. *Transactions of the Royal Society of Tropical Medicine and Hygiene* 94: 289–292.

34. Nibbeling HA, Van Lieshout L, Deelder AM 1998 Levels of circulating soluble egg antigen in urine of individuals infected with *Schistosoma mansoni* before and after treatment with praziquantel. *Transactions of the Royal Society of Tropical Medicine and Hygiene* 92: 675–677.

35. Kahama AI, Kremsner PG, Van Dam GJ et al 1998 The dynamics of a soluble egg antigen of *Schistosoma haematobium* in relation to egg counts, circulating anodic and cathodic antigens and pathology markers before and after chemotherapy. *Transactions of the Royal Society of Tropical Medicine and Hygiene* 92: 629–633.

36. Van Lieshout L, Polderman AM, Deedler AM 2000 Immunodiagnosis of schistosomiasis by determination of the circulating antigens CAA and CCA, in particular in individuals with recent or light infections. *Acta Tropica* 77: 69–80.

37. Ismail M, Botros S, Metwally A et al 1999 Resistance to praziquantel: direct evidence from *Schistosoma mansoni* isolated from Egyptian villagers. *American Journal of Tropical Medicine and Hygiene* 60: 932–935.

38. Li S, Wu L, Liu Z et al 1996 Studies on prophylactic effect of artesunate on schistosomiasis japonica. *Chinese Medical Journal* 109: 848–853.

39. Utzinger J, N'Goran EK, N'Dri A et al 2000 Oral artemether for prevention of *Schistosoma mansoni* infection: randomised controlled trial. *Lancet* 355: 1320–1325.

40. Graham CS, Brodie SB, Weller PF 2001 Imported *Fasciola hepatica* infection in the United States and treatment with triclabendazole. *Clinical Infectious Diseases* 32: 1–6.

41. Nakamura-Uchyama F, Onah D, Nawa Y 2001 Clinical features of paragonimiasis cases recently found in Japan: parasite-specific immunoglobulin M and G antibody classes. *Clinical Infectious Diseases* 32: 171–175.

42. Taylor MJ, Hoerauf A 1999 *Wolbachia* bacteria of filarial nematodes. *Parasitology Today* 15: 437–442.

43. Schuetz A, Addiss DG, Eherhard ML et al 2000 Evaluation of the whole blood filariasis ICT test for short-term monitoring after antifilarial treatment. *American Journal of Tropical Medicine and Hygiene* 62: 502–503.

44. Dissanayaka S, Rocha A, Noroes J et al 2000 Evaluation of PCR-based methods for the diagnosis of infection in bancroftian filariasis. *Transactions of the Royal Society of Tropical Medicine and Hygiene* 94: 526–530.

45. Thanomsub BW, Chansiri K, Sarataphan N et al 2000 Differential diagnosis of human lymphatic filariasis using PCR-RELP. *Molecular and Cellular Probes* 14: 41–46.

46. Gardon J, Gardon-Wendel N, Demanga-Ngangue et al 1997 Serious reactions after mass treatment of onchocerciasis with ivermectin in an area endemic for *Loa loa* infection. *Lancet* 350: 18–22.

47. Klion AD, Massougboudji A, Saddler B-C et al 1991 Albendazole in human loiasis: Results of a double-blind, placebo-controlled trial. *Journal of Infectious Diseases* 168: 202.

48. Vincent JA, Lustigman S, Zhang S et al 2000 A comparison of newer tests for the diagnosis of onchocerciasis. *Annals of Tropical Medicine and Parasitology* 94: 253–258.

49. Weil GJ, Steel C, Liftis F et al 2000 A rapid-format antibody card test for diagnosis of onchocerciasis. *Journal of Infectious Diseases* 182: 1796–1769.

50. Muenning P, Pallin D, Sell RL et al 1999 The cost effectiveness of strategies for the treatment of intestinal parasites in immigrants. *New England Journal of Medicine* 340: 773–779.

51. Beach MJ, Streit TG, Addiss DG et al 1999 Assessment of combined ivermectin and albendazole for treatment of intestinal helminth and *Wuchereria bancrofti* infections in Haitian schoolchildren. *American Journal of Tropical Medicine and Hygiene* 60: 479–486.

52. Olds GR, King C, Hewlett R et al 1999 Double-blind placebo-controlled study of concurrent administration of albendazole and praziquantel in schoolchildren with schistosomiasis and geohelminths. *Journal of Infectious Diseases* 179: 996–1003.

53. World Health Organization 1998 Guidelines for the evaluation of soil-transmitted helminths and schistosomiasis at community level. WHO/CTD/SIP 98.1.

54. World Health Organization 1999 Monitoring helminth control programmes. WHO/CDS/CPC/SIP/99.3.

55. Dickson R, Awasthi S, Williamson P et al 2000 Effects of treatment for intestinal helminth infection on growth and cognitive performance in children: systematic review of randomised trials. *British Medical Journal* 320: 1697–1701.

Index